di Fiore's

Atlas *of* Histology

WITH FUNCTIONAL CORRELATIONS

NINTH EDITION

P9-DYO-539

di Fiore's
Atlas *of* Histology

WITH FUNCTIONAL CORRELATIONS

NINTH EDITION

■

Victor P. Eroschenko, Ph.D.

Professor of Anatomy
Department of Biological Sciences
WWAMI Medical Program
University of Idaho
Moscow, Idaho

◆ LIPPINCOTT WILLIAMS & WILKINS
A **Wolters Kluwer** Company
Philadelphia · Baltimore · New York · London
Buenos Aires · Hong Kong · Sydney · Tokyo

Property of Library
Cape Fear Comm College
Wilmington, N. C.

Publisher: Susan Katz
Managing Editor: Ulita Lushnycky
Marketing Manager: Aimee Sirmon
Production Editor: Lisa JC Franko

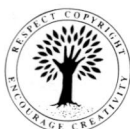

Copyright © 2000 Lippincott Williams & Wilkins

351 West Camden Street
Baltimore, Maryland 21201-2436
530 Walnut Street
Philadelphia, Pennsylvania 19106-3621

All rights reserved. This book is protected by copyright. No part of this book may be reproduced in any form or by any means, including photocopying, or utilized by any information storage and retrieval system without written permission from the copyright owner.
The publisher is not responsible (as a matter of product liability, negligence, or otherwise) for any injury resulting from any material contained herein. This publication contains information relating to general principles of medical care, which should not be construed as specific instructions for individual patients. Manufacturers' product information and package inserts should be reviewed for current information, including contraindications, dosages, and precautions.

Printed in Canada

FIRST EDITION 1957 Reprinted 1958, 1959, 1960, 1961, 1962
SECOND EDITION 1963 Reprinted 1964, 1965
THIRD EDITION 1967 Reprinted 1968, 1969, 1970, 1971, 1972, 1973
FOURTH EDITION 1974 Reprinted 1975, 1976, 1977, 1978, 1979, 1980, 1981
FIFTH EDITION 1981 Reprinted 1981, 1982, 1983, 1985, 1987
SIXTH EDITION 1989 Reprinted 1989, 1992
SEVENTH EDITION 1993 Reprinted 1994
EIGHTH EDITION 1996 Reprinted 1997, 1999

Library of Congress Cataloging-in-Publication Data

Eroschenko, Victor P.
  Di Fiore's atlas of histology with functional correlations / Victor P. Eroschenko.—9th ed.
    p. ; cm.
  Includes index.
  ISBN 0-683-30749-5 (spiral bound) —ISBN 0-7817-2676-X (perfect bound)
   1. Histology—Atlases. I. Title: Atlas of histology with functional correlations. II.
  Fiore, Mariano S. H. di. III. Title
   [DNLM: 1. Histology—Atlases. QS 517 E71d 2000]
  QM557 .F5513 2000
  611'.018—dc21   00-020713

The publishers have made every effort to trace the copyright holders for borrowed material. If they have inadvertently overlooked any, they will be pleased to make the necessary arrangements at the first opportunity.

To purchase additional copies of this book call our customer service department at **(800) 638-3030** or fax orders to **(301) 824-7390**. International customers should call **(301) 714-2324**.

Visit Lippincott Williams & Wilkins on the Internet: http://www.lww.com <http://www.lww.com>. Lippincott Williams & Wilkins customer service representatives are available from 8:30 am to 6:00 pm, EST, Monday through Friday, for telephone access.

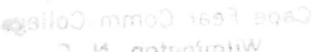

To the those that matter so much

McKenzie
Sarah
Shannon

       and
       Diane
       Kathryn
       Tatiana
       Sharon

              and
              Todd
              Shaun

                    and most especially
                      Elke

Preface to the Ninth Edition

The rapid advances in all fields of scientific research has strengthened the author's belief that histology will remain an enduring and fundamental science in the new millennium for understanding the intricate morphologies of our organs, in both normal and abnormal conditions. In revising the ninth edition of the *Atlas of Histology With Functional Correlations* for publication, the needs of the students and instructors of histology were of paramount importance. Thus, this revised, updated, and improved *Atlas of Histology* has been especially prepared to serve the needs of histology students and their instructors in the new century, as it has served them for so many years in the past century. Furthermore, the information and illustrations in this atlas will assume even greater importance as teaching of histology begins to shift from formal classroom presentations and laboratories to a more independent form of self-learning. The publication of the new edition of this atlas should meet the future needs of students preparing for different biological, medical, and/or health-related professions.

THE CHANGES

The Art

One of the most noticeable changes in the ninth edition of the atlas is the appearance of new art. Most of the illustrations in the atlas are composite drawings, prepared from viewing numerous areas of a given tissue or organ. These beautiful illustrations have served the atlas well for many years. However, numerous requests from students and instructors of histology indicated the need for photomicrographs of the same tissues and organs for comparison. These requests have been fulfilled with the publication of the ninth edition of the atlas. Each chapter now contains approximately two to three high-quality photomicrographs of selected tissues or organs to supplement some of the art illustrations. The photomicrographs, however, represent only a small fraction of the total number of images that are found in the atlas. Supplemental three-dimensional, computer-generated illustrations were prepared in addition as lead-in art for each chapter of the atlas. The addition of photomicrographs and three-dimensional art to the atlas should give the student a better idea of the complexities of structures that are viewed with a microscope.

The publication of the ninth edition of the *Atlas of Histology* marks the first appearance of the three-dimensional lead-in art and photomicrographs. Also, six old illustrations were deleted from the atlas and replaced with similar number of new images, texts, and labels.

The Update

Updating the specific functions of different cells, tissues, and organs illustrated in this atlas with new information was also of primary importance. As a result, each chapter has been rewritten and updated with new information, when it was available and where it was necessary. Also, in the previous edition, the Functional Correlations were presented in the introductory portion of each chapter. In the present edition, Functional Correlations were moved to the interior of the chapter and placed below a particular illustration of a tissue or an organ. As a result, the functional correlations are now directly related to an illustration of a specific structure. This arrangement improves the dynamics between the structure and function.

FOR THE STUDENT

One of the first difficulties that histology students encounter is the recognition of three-dimensional structures on a flat histology slide. To assist the students in properly identifying different microscopic structures, an introductory chapter has been prepared to show how solid and hollow structures change shape when they are sectioned in different planes. In addition, a low power photomicrograph of the testis tubules has been added to the drawings. The testis consists of numerous, highly convoluted or twisted tubules. When this organ is cut, the tubular morphology becomes highly variable with every plane of section. Thus, understanding how the shape of a sectioned material is altered with the plane of section will enhance the identification of histologic material.

In addition, further aid for identifying histologic structures is provided by the addition of lead-in art for each chapter. This art form allows the student to first visualize the three-dimensional details prior to examining the same structures with a microscope. Additional aid to the student is provided by the incorporating high quality photomicrographs into each chapter. Comparing the art images with photomicrographs should strengthen the students' confidence in the illustrations of this atlas and in understanding the microscopic anatomy of different structures.

ACKNOWLEDGMENTS

The completion and publication of this atlas would not have been possible without the contribution of highly professional individuals. The artwork of two talented artists is gratefully acknowledged. The talents of E. Roland Brown of Salt Lake City, Utah, who has prepared approximately 47 new illustrations for the last edition of the atlas, were again used to replace 5 older images with new images. Also, the computer expertise of Sonja Oei-Gerard of Oei Graphics, Bellevue, Washington, is visible in the striking and beautiful three-dimensional, lead-in art for each chapter of the atlas.

The editorial, production, marketing, and managerial personnel at Lippincott Williams & Wilkins have been most helpful in this endeavor. A special recognition is extended to Ulita Lushnycky, Associate Managing Editor. Her efforts in collecting, organizing, and preparing all of the finished material for publication of the atlas are greatly appreciated.

Victor P. Eroschenko, Ph.D.   Moscow, Idaho

Contents

CHAPTER SIX · Nervous Tissue   87

PART TWO

Organs

CHAPTER SEVEN · Circulatory System   111

CHAPTER ELEVEN	Digestive System: Esophagus and Stomach 177	

CHAPTER TWELVE	Digestive System: Small and Large Intestines 199	

CHAPTER THIRTEEN	Digestive System: Liver, Gallbladder, and Pancreas 219	

CHAPTER EIGHTEEN   Female Reproductive System   301

CHAPTER NINETEEN   Organs of Special Senses   337

PART ONE

Tissues

Interpretation of Histologic Sections

Histologic sections are thin, flat slices of fixed and stained tissues and/or organs mounted on glass slides. Such sections are normally composed of cellular, fibrous, and tubular structures. The cells exhibit a variety of shapes, sizes, and layers. The fibrous structures are solid and are found in the connective, nervous, and muscle tissues. The tubular structures are hollow and represent various types of blood vessels, ducts, and glands of the body.

In the tissue or organ, the cells, fibers, and tubes have a random orientation in space and are a part of a three-dimensional structure. During the preparation of histology slides, the thin sections do not have depth. In addition, the plane of section does not always cut these structures exactly in the transverse or cross section. This produces a variation in the appearance of cells, fibers, and tubes, depending on the angle of the plane of section. As a result of these factors, it is difficult to perceive correctly the three-dimensional structure from which the sections were prepared on a flat slide. Therefore, correct visualization and interpretation of these sections in their proper three-dimensional perspective on the slide becomes important criteria for mastering histology.

For a better orientation and interpretation of the three-dimensional composition of tissues and organs on the histology slide, the first two figures of the atlas have been especially prepared to illustrate how the appearance of cells and tubes changes with the plane of section.

Figure I-1   Planes of Section of a Round Object

To illustrate how a shape of a three-dimensional cell can be altered in a histologic section, a hard-boiled egg has been sectioned in longitudinal and transverse (cross) planes. The composition of a hard-boiled egg serves as a good example of a cell, with the yellow yolk representing the nucleus and the surrounding egg white representing the cytoplasm. Enclosing these structures are the soft egg shell membrane and a hard egg shell (yellow). At the rounded end of the egg is the air space (blue).

The **midline** sections of the egg in the **longitudinal (a)** and **transverse plane (d)** disclose its correct shape and size, as they appear in these planes of section. In addition, these two planes of section reveal the correct appearance, size, and distribution of the internal contents within the egg.

Similar but more **peripheral** sections of the egg in the **longitudinal (b)** and **transverse plane (e)** still show the external shape of the egg; however, because the sections were cut peripheral to the midline, the internal contents of the egg are not seen in their correct size or distribution within the egg white. In addition, the size of the egg appears smaller.

The **tangential planes (c, f)** of section graze or only pass through the outermost periphery of the egg. These sections reveal that the egg is oval (c) or a small round (f) object. The egg yolk is not seen in either section because it was not located in the plane of section. As a result, such tangential sections do not reveal sufficient detail for correct interpretation of the egg size, its contents, or their distribution within the internal membrane.

Figure I-2   Planes of Section of a Tube

Tubular structures are often seen in histologic sections. Tubes are most easily recognized when they are cut in transverse (cross) sections. However, if the tubes are sectioned in other planes, they must first be visualized as three-dimensional structures in order to be recognized as tubes. To illustrate how a blood vessel, duct, or glandular structure may appear in a histologic section, a curved tube with a simple (single) epithelial cell layer is sectioned in longitudinal, transverse, and oblique planes.

A **longitudinal (a)** plane of section that cuts the tube in the midline produces a U-shaped structure. The sides of the tube are lined by a single row of cuboidal (round) cells around an empty lumen except at the bottom, where the tube begins to curve; in this region the cells appear multilayered.

Transverse (d, e) planes of section of the same tube produce round structures lined by a single layer of cells. The variations that are seen in the cytoplasm of different cells are due to the planes of section through the individual cells, as explained above. A transverse section of a straight tube can produce a single image (e). The double image (d) of the same structure can represent either two tubes running parallel to each other or a single tube that has curved in space of the tissue or organ that is sectioned.

A **tangential (b)** plane of section through the tube produces a solid, multicellular, oval structure that does not resemble a tube. The reason for this is that the plane of section grazed the outermost periphery of tube as it made a turn in space; the lumen was not present in the plane of section. An **oblique (c)** plane of section through the tube and its cells produces an oval structure that includes an oval lumen in the center and multiple cell layers at the periphery.

A **transverse (f)** section in the region of a sharp curve in the tube grazes the innermost cell layer and produces two oval structures connected by a multiple, solid layer of cells (f). These sections of the tube also contain an oval lumen, indicating that the plane of section passed at an angle to the structure.

Thus, in a histologic section, individual structure shape and size may vary, depending on the plane of section. Some cells may exhibit full cross-sections of their nuclei and they appear prominent in the cells. Other cells may exhibit only a fraction of the nucleus and the cytoplasm appears large. Still other cells may appear only as clear cytoplasm, without any nuclei. All these variations are due to different planes of section through the nuclei. Understanding these variations in cell and tube morphology will result in a better interpretation of the histologic sections.

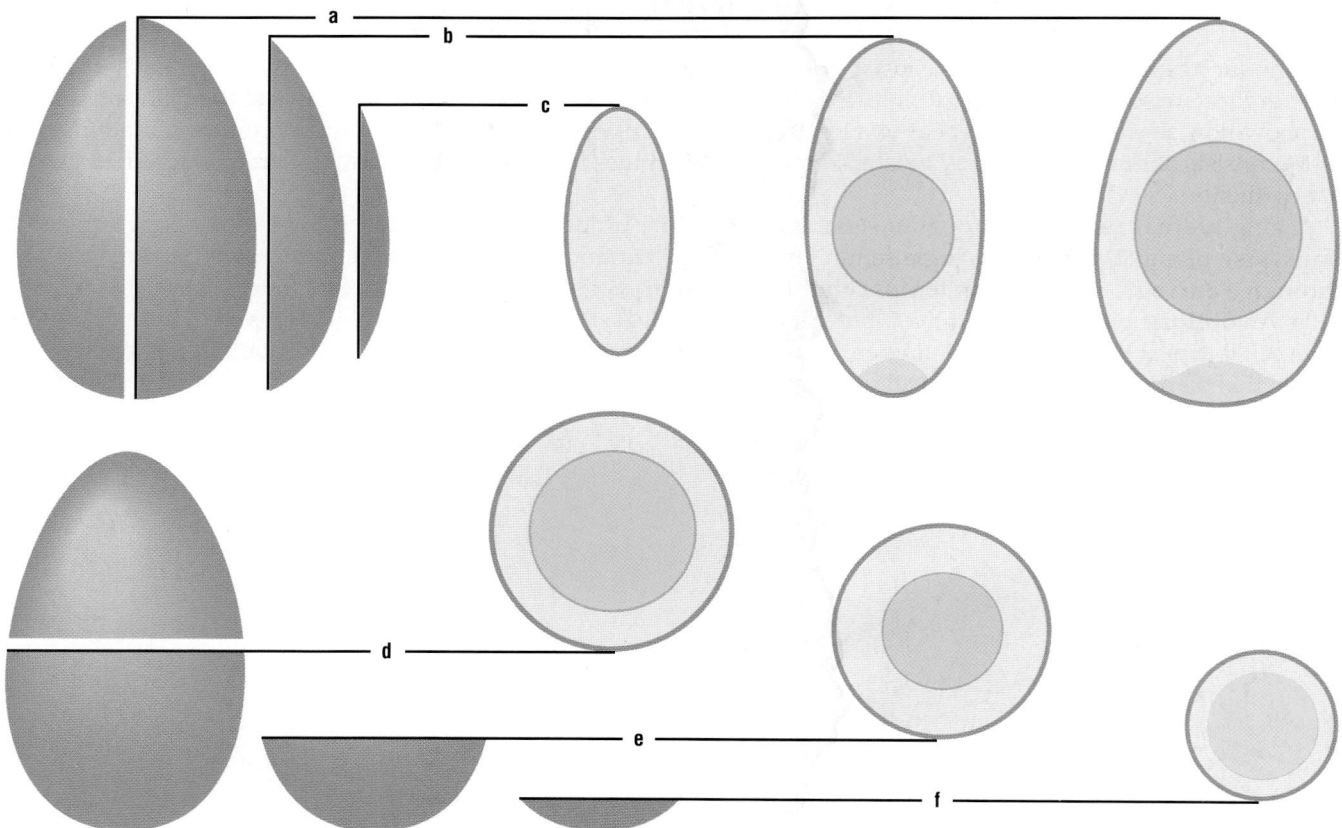

Fig. I-1   Planes of Section of a Round Object.

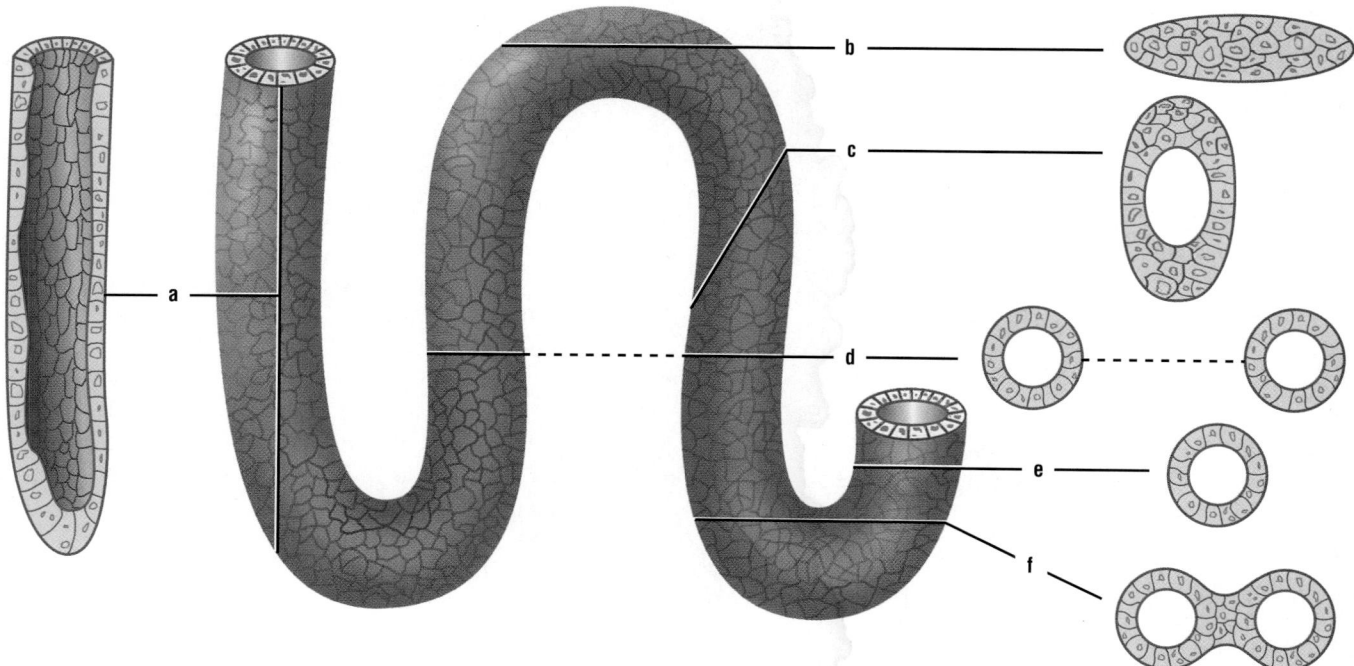

Fig. I-2   Planes of Section of a Tube.

Figure I-3   Tubules of the Testis in Different Planes of Section

Organs such as testes and kidneys consist primarily of highly twisted or convoluted tubules. When flat sections of such organs are seen on a histology slide, the cut tubules exhibit a variety of shapes because of the plane of section. To show how twisted tubules appear in a histologic slide, a portion of a testis was prepared for examination. Each testis consists of numerous, highly twisted seminiferous tubules that are lined by multi-layered or stratified germinal epithelium.

A **longitudinal plane (1)** through a seminiferous tubule produces an elongated tubule with a long lumen. A **transverse plane (2)** through a single seminiferous tubule produces a round tubule. Similarly, a **transverse plane through a curve (3, 5)** of a seminiferous tubule produces two oval structures that are connected by solid layers of cells. An **oblique plane (4)** through a tubule produces an oval structure with an oval lumen in the center and multiple cell layers at the periphery. A **tangential plane (6)** of a seminiferous tubule passes through its periphery. As a result, this plane produces a solid, multicellular, oval structure that does not resemble a tube because the lumen is not seen.

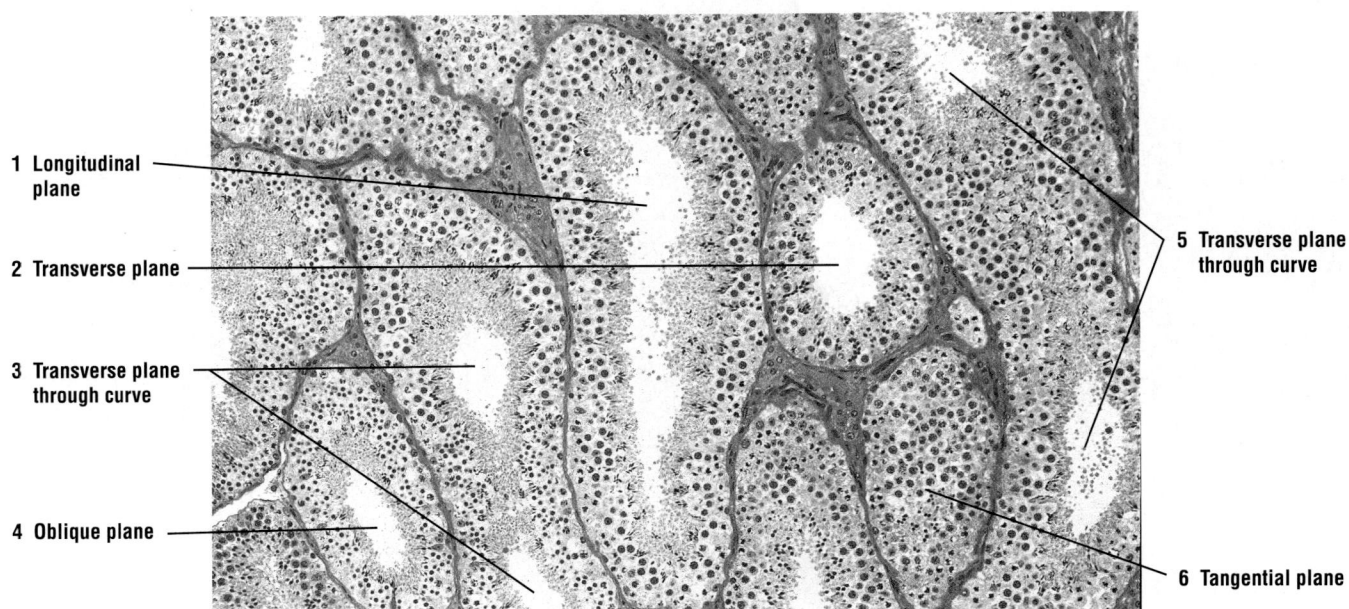

1 Longitudinal plane

2 Transverse plane

3 Transverse plane through curve

4 Oblique plane

5 Transverse plane through curve

6 Tangential plane

Fig. I-3   Tubules of the Testis in Different Planes of Section. Stain: hematoxylin-eosin (plastic section). 30×

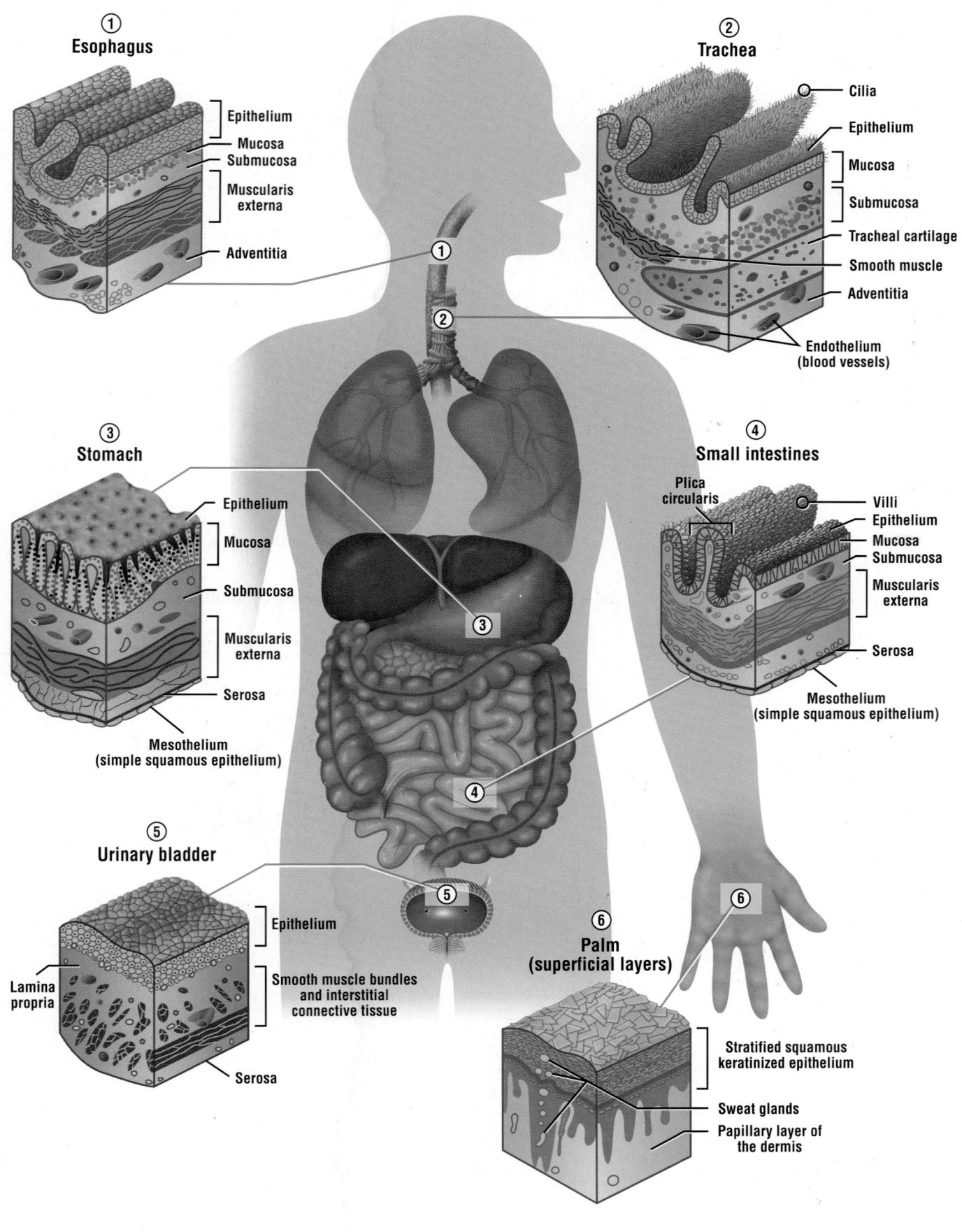

① **Esophagus**

Epithelium
— Mucosa
— Submucosa
Muscularis externa
— Adventitia

② **Trachea**

Cilia
Epithelium
Mucosa
Submucosa
Tracheal cartilage
Smooth muscle
Adventitia
Endothelium (blood vessels)

③ **Stomach**

Epithelium
Mucosa
Submucosa
Muscularis externa
Serosa
Mesothelium (simple squamous epithelium)

④ **Small intestines**

Plica circularis
Villi
Epithelium
Mucosa
Submucosa
Muscularis externa
Serosa
Mesothelium (simple squamous epithelium)

⑤ **Urinary bladder**

Epithelium
Lamina propria
Smooth muscle bundles and interstitial connective tissue
Serosa

⑥ **Palm (superficial layers)**

Stratified squamous keratinized epithelium
Sweat glands
Papillary layer of the dermis

Epithelial Tissue

SECTION 1
Classification of Epithelial Tissue

LOCATION OF EPITHELIUM

The four basic tissue types in the body are the epithelial, connective, muscular, and nervous tissue; these tissues exist and function in close association with one another.

The **epithelial tissue,** or epithelium, consists of sheets of cells that cover the **external surfaces** of the body, line the **internal cavities,** form various **organs** and **glands,** and line their **ducts.** The histology of the lining epithelium, however, differs from organ to organ, depending on its location and its function.

CLASSIFICATION OF EPITHELIUM

The epithelium is classified based on the number of **cell layers** and the **morphology** of the **surface cells.** An epithelium with a single layer of cells is called **simple,** and that with numerous cell layers is called **stratified.** A **pseudostratified** epithelium consists of a single layer of cells in which all cells attach to the **basement membrane,** but not all cells reach the surface. An epithelium with flat surface cells is called **squamous.** When the surface cells are round or they are as tall as they are wide, the epithelium is **cuboidal.** When the cells are taller than they are wide, the epithelium is called **columnar.**

The epithelium is normally separated from the underlying **connective tissue** by a **basement membrane.** Also, the epithelium is **nonvascular;** that is, it does not have blood vessels. As a result, oxygen, nutrients, and metabolites **diffuse** from the blood vessels in the underlying connective tissue to the epithelium.

SPECIAL SURFACE MODIFICATIONS ON EPITHELIAL CELLS

Epithelial cells in different organs exhibit special cell membrane modifications on their **apical surfaces.** These are either cilia, stereocilia, or microvilli. The **cilia** are motile structures that are found on certain cells in the **uterine tubes, uterus,** and conducting tubes of the **respiratory system.** The **microvilli** are small, nonmotile projections that line all absorptive cells in the small intestine and proximal convoluted tubules in the kidney. The **stereocilia** are long, nonmotile, branched microvilli that line the cells in the **epididymis** and **vas deferens.**

TYPES OF EPITHELIA
Simple Epithelium

Simple squamous epithelium that lines the external surfaces of the digestive organs, lungs, and heart is called **mesothelium.** Similarly, a simple squamous epithelium that lines the lumina of heart, blood vessels, and lymphatic vessels is called **endothelium (Figs. 1-1–1-3)**

Simple cuboidal epithelium lines small excretory **ducts** in different organs. In proximal convoluted tubules of the kidney, the apical surfaces of the simple cuboidal epithelium are lined with a **brush border (microvilli) (Fig. 1-3).**

Simple columnar epithelium is found lining the surfaces in the **digestive organs (Fig. 1-4)** (stomach, small and large intestines, and gallbladder). In the small intestine, the surfaces of absorptive cells that line the **villi** exhibit a **striated border (microvilli) (Fig 1-5).**

Pseudostratified Columnar Epithelium

Pseudostratified columnar epithelium lines the **respiratory passages,** and lumina of the **epididymis** and **vas deferens.** In trachea, bronchi, and larger brochioles, the surface cells are lined by motile **cilia (Fig. 1-6);** in the epididymis and vas deferens, the surface cells are lined by nonmotile **stereocilia (Fig. 17-16).**

Stratified Epithelium

Transitional epithelium changes shape and can resemble either the stratified squamous or stratified cuboidal epithelia, depending on whether it is stretched or contracted. When **contracted,** the surface cells appear **dome-shaped;** when **stretched,** the epithelium appears **squamous.** Transitional epithelium lines the minor and major calyxes, pelvis, ureter, and bladder of the **urinary system (Fig. 1-7).**

Stratified squamous epithelium contains multiple cell layers. The basal cells are cuboidal to columnar; these give rise to cells that migrate toward the surface and become squamous. There are two types of stratified squamous epithelia. The **nonkeratinized epithelium** exhibits live surface cells with nuclei and lines such moist cavities such as the mouth, pharynx, esophagus **(Fig. 1-8),** vagina, and anal canal. The **keratinized epithelium** covers the skin and the surface layers contain nonliving, keratinized cells that are filled with **keratin.** The epithelium that covers the palms and soles exhibits especially thick layers of dead or keratinized cells **(Fig. 1-9).**

Stratified cuboidal epithelium and **stratified columnar epithelium** have a limited distribution. Both types line the **excretory ducts** of pancreas, salivary glands, and sweat glands **(Fig. 1-10).**

Figure 1-1   Simple Squamous Epithelium: Surface View of Peritoneal Mesothelium

To visualize the surface of the simple squamous epithelium, a small piece of mesentery was fixed and treated with silver nitrate and counterstained with hematoxylin. The cells of the simple squamous epithelium (mesothelium) appear flat, adhere tightly to each other, and form a sheet with the thickness of a single cell layer. The irregular **cell boundaries (1)** are highly visible because of silver deposition and form a characteristic mosaic pattern. The blue-gray **cell nuclei (2)** exhibit a central location in the yellow- to brown-stained **cytoplasm (3).**

The simple squamous epithelium is common in the body. It lines the surfaces that allow passive transport of gases or fluids, and it lines the pleural, pericardial, and peritoneal cavities.

Figure 1-2   Simple Squamous Epithelium: Peritoneal Mesothelium (transverse section)

Examination of the simple squamous epithelium, the **mesothelium (1)** of jejunum, in transverse section, illustrates that the cells are spindle-shaped with prominent, oval nuclei. Cell boundaries are not seen distinctly but are indicated at **cell junctions (2).** A thin **basement membrane (3)** is observed under the mesothelium (1). In surface view, these cells appear similar to those illustrated in Figure 1-1.

Mesothelium and the underlying **connective tissue (4)** form the serosa of the peritoneal cavity, which is the outermost layer of the jejunal wall. Serosa is attached to the muscularis externa, which consists of **smooth muscle fibers (6).** In the connective tissue are small blood vessels, lined by a simple squamous epithelium called the **endothelium (5).**

■ Functional Correlations–Simple Squamous Epithelium

In the peritoneal cavity, simple squamous epithelium aids in smooth **movement** of the viscera, **reduces friction** between organs, and allows for **fluid transport.** In the cadiovascular system, this epithelium or endothelium allows for passive **transport** of fluids, nutrients, or metabolites across capillary walls. In the lungs, simple squamous epithelium provides for efficient **gaseous exchange** across the thin-walled capillaries and alveoli.

Figure 1-3   Different Epithelial Types: Kidney Cortex

This high power photomicrograph of the kidney illustrates the different types of epithelia that are present in its cortex. **Simple squamous epithelium (1)** lines the interior of the **Bowman's capsule (4).** This capsule surrounds the **glomerulus (6)** of the kidney, which filters blood through its numerous capillaries. A special type of simple squamous epithelium called **endothelium (3, 9)** lines the **capillaries (2)** and all other blood vessels (8). **Simple cuboidal epithelium (5)** lines the lumina of the surrounding **convoluted tubules (7).** The blue-stained fibers surrounding the capsule (4), convoluted tubules (7), and the blood vessels (8) in the kidney cortex are the collagen fibers of the **connective tissue (10).**

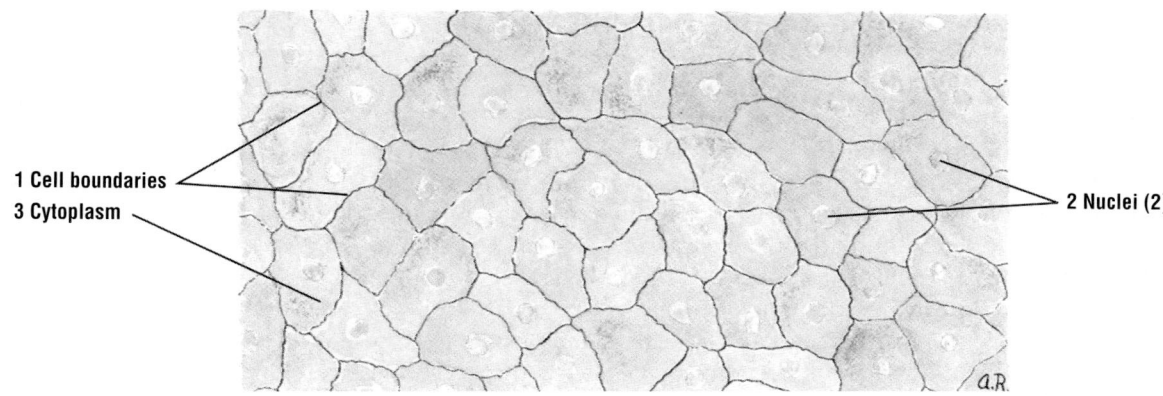

Fig. 1-1 Simple Squamous Epithelium: Surface View of Peritoneal Mesothelium. Stain: silver nitrate with hematoxylin. High magnification.

1 Cell boundaries
3 Cytoplasm
2 Nuclei (2)

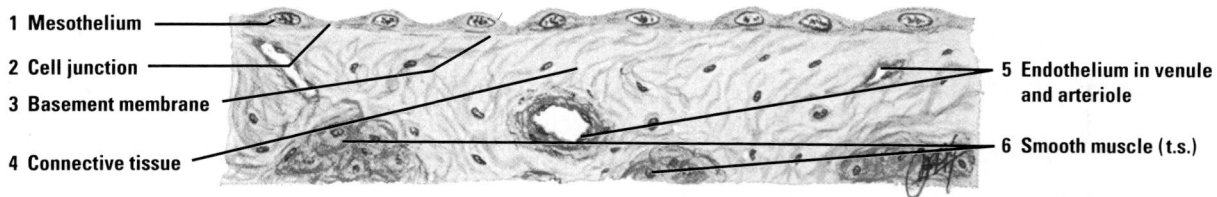

1 Mesothelium
2 Cell junction
3 Basement membrane
4 Connective tissue
5 Endothelium in venule and arteriole
6 Smooth muscle (t.s.)

Fig. 1-2 Simple Squamous Epithelium: Peritoneal Mesothelium (transverse section). Stain: hematoxylin-eosin. High magnification.

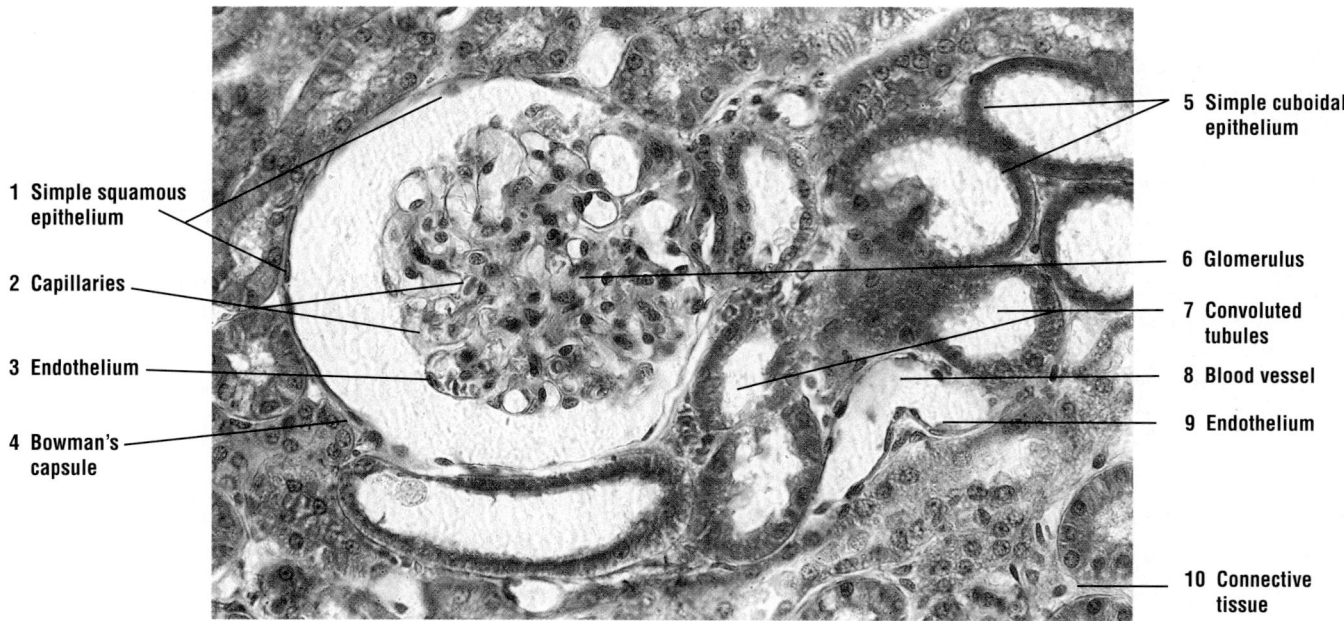

1 Simple squamous epithelium
2 Capillaries
3 Endothelium
4 Bowman's capsule
5 Simple cuboidal epithelium
6 Glomerulus
7 Convoluted tubules
8 Blood vessel
9 Endothelium
10 Connective tissue

Fig. 1-3 Different Epithelial Types: Kidney Cortex. Stain: Masson's trichrome. 100×

Figure 1-4   Simple Columnar Epithelium: Stomach

In a **simple columnar epithelium (2),** as seen on the stomach's surface, the cells are arranged in a single row. Their ovoid **nuclei (7)** are located in the basal region and exhibit a perpendicular orientation. A thin **basement membrane (3)** separates the epithelium from the underlying **connective tissue (4, 10),** the lamina propria of the gastric mucosa. Small **blood vessels (5)** lined with endothelium are seen in the connective tissue.

In some areas, the epithelium has been sectioned transversely or obliquely. When a plane of section passes close to the free surface of the epithelium, the sectioned **apical regions (1)** of these cells resemble a mosaic of enucleated polygonal cells. When a plane of section passes through **basal regions (6)** of the epithelial cells, the nuclei are cut transversely and resemble a stratified epithelium.

The surface cells of the stomach secrete mucus. The pale appearance of the cell cytoplasm in these cells is owing to the routine preparation of the tissues. The mucigen droplets that filled these **cell apices (9)** were lost during section preparation. The more granular cytoplasm is located basally **(8)** and stains more acidophilic.

Examples of other columnar epithelia may be seen in the lining of the gallbladder (Fig. 13-9:14); in salivary gland ducts (Fig. 10-12:4, IV; Fig. 10-13:17, IV); in bile ducts of the liver (Fig. 13-3:7, 14).

A simple cuboidal epithelium is illustrated in the smallest ducts of the pancreas (Fig. 10-14) and in the follicles of the thyroid gland (Figs. 16-5:3 and 16-6:5).

■ Functional Correlations–Simple Columnar Epithelium of the Stomach

Simple columnar epithelium lines the surface of the stomach. These cells are **secretory** and produce a product called **mucus.** The mucus covers the stomach surface and protects its lining from the very corrosive secretions that are normally found in this organ.

Figure 1-5   Simple Columnar Epithelium: Cells With Striated Borders and Goblet Cells (Small Intestine)

The intestinal **villi (1)** are lined by simple columnar epithelium, which consists of two types of cells: columnar cells with **striated borders (2, 13)** and **goblet cells (8, 12).** The striated border **(13)** is seen as a reddish outer membrane with faint vertical striations; these are the microvilli on the apices of the columnar cells. In an area of contiguous cells, the striated border appears continuous. The cytoplasm of these cells is finely granular and the oval nuclei are in the basal portions of the cells.

The goblet cells **(8, 12)** are interspersed among the columnar cells. During routine histologic preparation, the mucus is lost; hence, the goblet cell cytoplasm appears clear or only lightly stained **(12).** Normally, the mucigen droplets occupy the cell apices and the nucleus remains in the basal region of the **cytoplasm (8).**

The epithelium at the tip of the villus in the lower center of the figure has been sectioned in an oblique plane. As a result, the apices of the columnar cells appear as a mosaic **(7)** of enucleated cells while the basal regions, where the plane of section passed through the nuclei, appear stratified **(7).**

The **basement membrane (5)** is more visible in this illustration than in Figure 1-3. Visible in the connective tissue **(lamina propria) (10)** are a lymphatic vessel, the **central lacteal (3),** a **capillary (9)** lined with endothelium, and **smooth muscle fibers (4, 11),** seen as either single fibers or a small group of fibers.

■ Functional Correlations–Epithelium With Striated Borders (Small Intestine) and Brush Borders (Kidney)

The main function of the epithelium in the small intestine is **absorption.** This function is enhanced by the presence of finger-like **villi,** which are covered by simple columnar epithelium with **striated borders** or **microvilli.** These microvilli absorb nutrients and fluids from the intestinal contents. The intestinal epithelium also contains numerous goblet cells. These cells secrete mucus, which protects the surface lining from corrosive secretions that enter the small intestine during digestion.

Production of urine by the kidney involves filtration, absorption, and excretion. The simple cuboidal epithelium in the proximal convoluted tubules of the kidney is also lined with **brush borders** or **microvilli.** The function of these microvilli is to **absorb** the nutrient material and fluid from the filtrate that passes through these tubules.

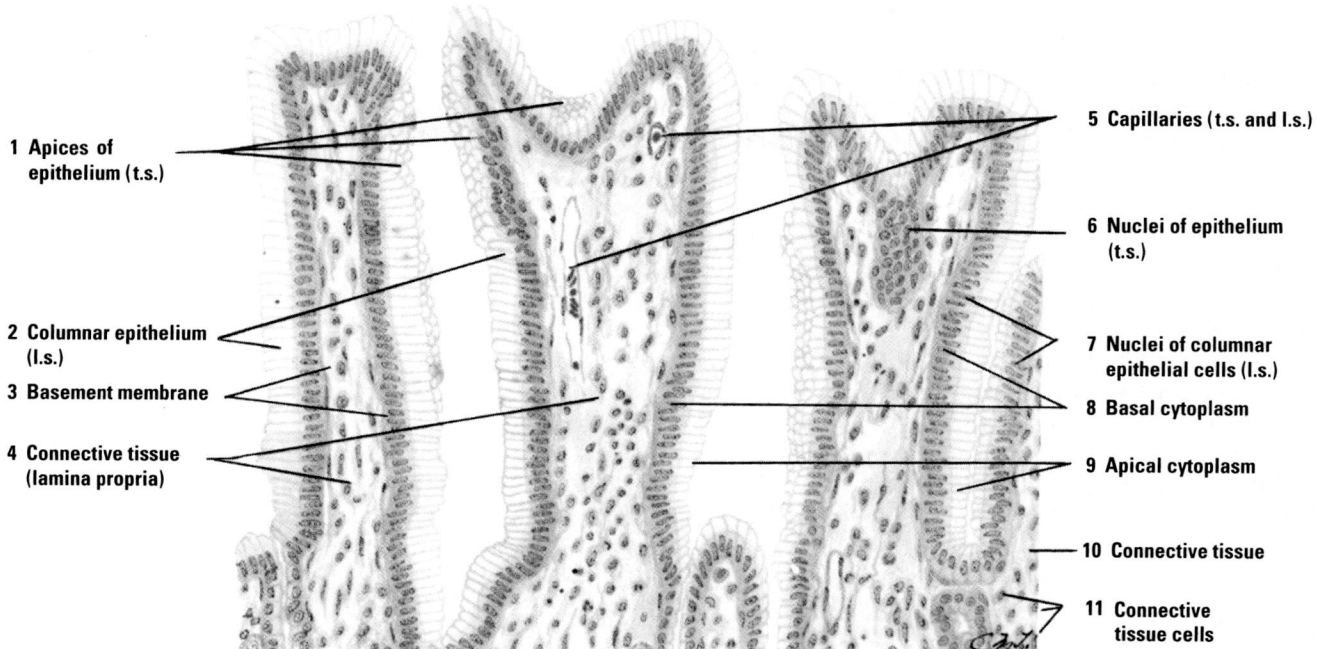

1 Apices of epithelium (t.s.)

2 Columnar epithelium (l.s.)

3 Basement membrane

4 Connective tissue (lamina propria)

5 Capillaries (t.s. and l.s.)

6 Nuclei of epithelium (t.s.)

7 Nuclei of columnar epithelial cells (l.s.)

8 Basal cytoplasm

9 Apical cytoplasm

10 Connective tissue

11 Connective tissue cells

Fig. 1-4   Simple Columnar Epithelium: Stomach. Stain: hematoxylin-eosin. Medium magnification.

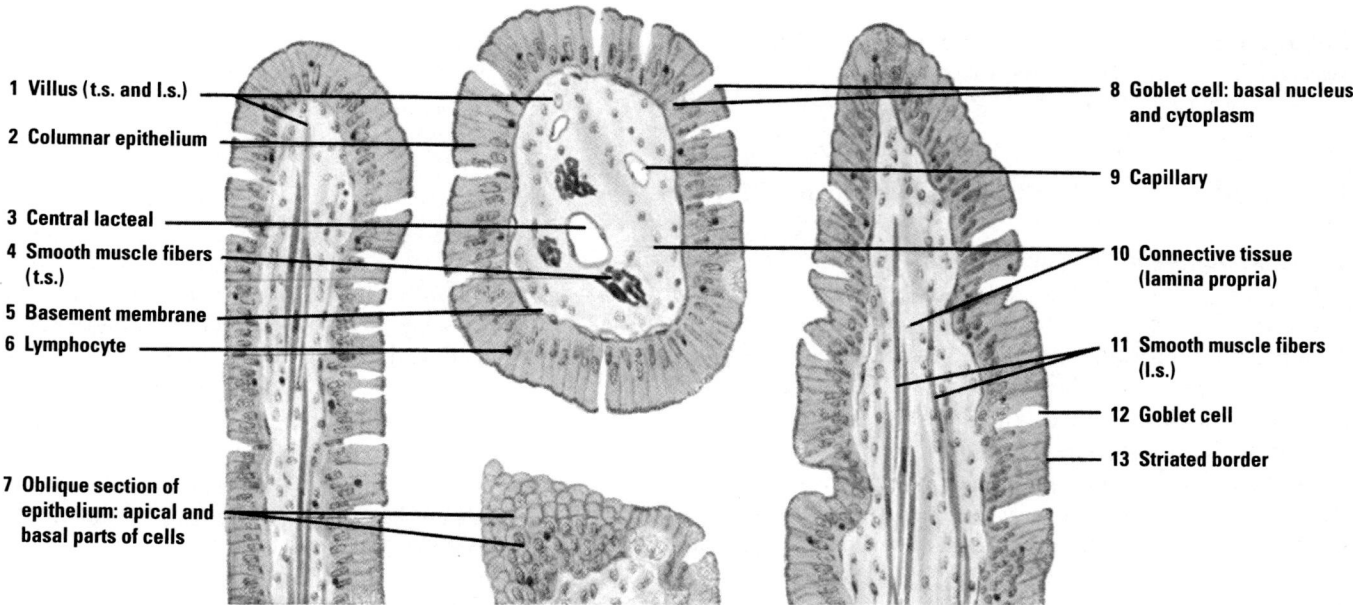

1 Villus (t.s. and l.s.)

2 Columnar epithelium

3 Central lacteal

4 Smooth muscle fibers (t.s.)

5 Basement membrane

6 Lymphocyte

7 Oblique section of epithelium: apical and basal parts of cells

8 Goblet cell: basal nucleus and cytoplasm

9 Capillary

10 Connective tissue (lamina propria)

11 Smooth muscle fibers (l.s.)

12 Goblet cell

13 Striated border

Fig. 1-5   Simple Columnar Epithelium: Cells With Striated Borders and Goblet Cells (Small Intestine). Stain: hematoxylin-eosin. Medium magnification.

Figure 1-6   Pseudostratified Columnar Ciliated Epithelium: Respiratory Passages

The **pseudostratified columnar ciliated epithelium (1)** is characteristic of the upper respiratory passages such as the trachea and variously sized bronchi. In this epithelium, the cells appear in several layers because their nuclei are at different levels. Serial sections show that all cells reach the **basement membrane (8)**; however, because the cells are of different shapes and heights, not all reach the surface. For this reason, this type of epithelium is called pseudostratified rather than stratified.

The deeper nuclei belong to the intermediate and short **basal cells (7)**. The more superficial, oval nuclei belong to the **columnar ciliated cells (5)**. Interspersed among these cells are **goblet cells (6)**. The small, round, heavily stained nuclei without any visible surrounding cytoplasm are those of **lymphocytes (9)**, which migrate from the connective tissue through the epithelium.

The short, motile **cilia (3)** are numerous and closely spaced at the cell apices. Each cilium arises from a **basal body (4)**, which is identical to the centriole. The basal bodies are located beneath the cell membrane and adjacent to each other; they often give the appearance of a continuous membrane (4).

The clearly visible **basement membrane (8)** separates the surface epithelium (1) from the underlying connective tissue of the **lamina propria (2, 11)**.

Visible in the **connective tissue (11)** are collagen fibers, cells (fibroblasts), scattered lymphocytes, and small **blood vessels (10)**. Deeper in the connective tissue are found glands with **serous acini (12)** and **mucous acini (13)**.

Other examples of pseudostratified columnar ciliated epithelium are seen in Figures 14-2, 14-3, and 14-6.

■ Functional Correlations–Epithelium With Cilia or Stereocilia

In the **respiratory passages,** the **psedostratified epithelium** contains both **goblet cells** and **ciliated cells**. The ciliated cells cleanse the inspired air and conduct **mucus** and **particulate material** across the cell surfaces to the exterior of the body. The **epididymis** and **vas deferens** are lined by pseudostratified epithelium with **stereocilia**. The functions of stereocilia in these organs is to absorb fluids produced by the testes. The simple columnar ciliated cells in the **uterine tubes** conduct the ovulated oocyte and sperm across their surfaces. In the **efferent ductules** of the **testes,** the ciliated cells **transport** sperm out of the testis and into the epididymis.

Figure 1-7   Transitional Epithelium: Bladder (contracted)

The **transitional epithelium (2)** is found exclusively in the excretory passages of the urinary system. It lines the renal calyces, pelvis, ureters, and bladder. This stratified epithelium is composed of several cell layers of similar cells, and changes its shape in response to stretching or contraction during the passage of urine. In relaxed, unstretched condition, the **surface cells (8)** are usually cuboidal and bulge out. Frequently, **binucleate (two nuclei) cells (1, 7)** are visible in the superficial or **surface cells (8)** in the bladder. When the transitional epithelium (2) is distended or stretched, the number of cell layers is reduced. The cells in the outer layers are then more elongated or flattened, but not to the degree seen in squamous epithelium. In the stretched condition, the transitional epithelium may resemble stratified squamous epithelium found in other regions of the body. (Compare transitional epithelium with stratified squamous epithelium of the cornea, Fig. 19-3.) However, the similarity in cell morphology differentiates this epithelium from stratified squamous epithelium, in which cells of various layers have different shapes.

Transitional epithelium (2) rests on a **connective tissue (4, 10)** layer, composed primarily of cells, the **fibroblasts (10a)** and **collagen fibers (10b)**. Between the connective tissue (4, 10) and the transitional epithelium (2), a thin **basement membrane (3, 9)** is visible. The base of the epithelium is not indented by connective tissue papillae, and it exhibits an even contour. Small **blood vessels (venules) (5)** and **arterioles (11)** of various sizes are present in the connective tissue (4, 10). Visible deeper in the connective tissue are strands of **smooth muscle fibers (6, 12),** sectioned in different planes from muscle layers that are located below the connective tissue (4, 10).

Other examples of transitional epithelium are illustrated in Chapter 15, Figures 15-6 to 15-9.

■ Functional Correlations–Transitional Epithelium

The major function of **transitional epithelium** is to allow **distention** in the urinary organs during urine accumulation and **contraction** during the emptying of the urinary passages without breaking the cell contacts in the epithelium. In addition, transitional epithelium forms an important **osmotic barrier** between urine and the underlying tissue fluids.

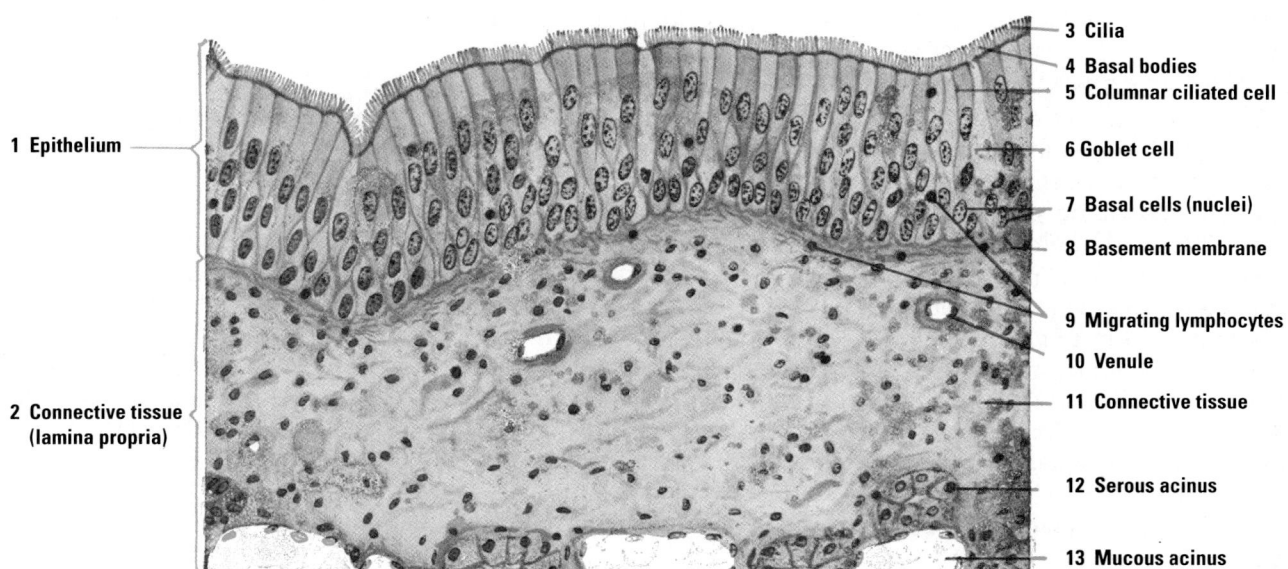

1 Epithelium

2 Connective tissue
   (lamina propria)

3 Cilia
4 Basal bodies
5 Columnar ciliated cell

6 Goblet cell

7 Basal cells (nuclei)

8 Basement membrane

9 Migrating lymphocytes

10 Venule

11 Connective tissue

12 Serous acinus

13 Mucous acinus

Fig. 1-6   Pseudostratified Columnar Ciliated Epithelium: Respiratory Passages. Stain: hematoxylin-eosin. High magnification.

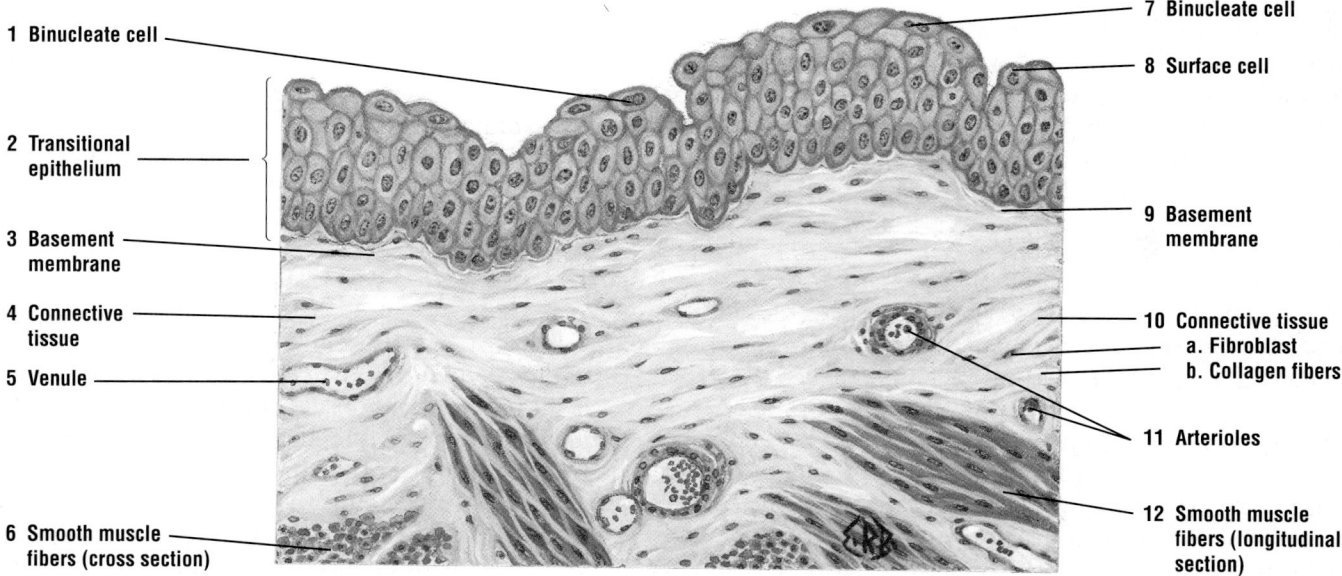

1 Binucleate cell

2 Transitional
   epithelium

3 Basement
   membrane

4 Connective
   tissue

5 Venule

6 Smooth muscle
   fibers (cross section)

7 Binucleate cell

8 Surface cell

9 Basement
   membrane

10 Connective tissue
    a. Fibroblast
    b. Collagen fibers

11 Arterioles

12 Smooth muscle
    fibers (longitudinal
    section)

Fig. 1-7   Transitional Epithelium: Bladder (contracted). Stain: hematoxylin-eosin. High magnification.

Figure 1-8   Stratified Squamous Nonkeratinized Epithelium: Esophagus (transverse section)

The stratified squamous epithelium is composed of numerous cell layers. Its thickness varies among the regions of the body and, as a result, the cell arrangement is altered.

Illustrated in this figure is an example of a moist, nonkeratinized **epithelium (1),** which lines the oral cavity, esophagus, vagina, and anal canal. The **basal cells (5)** are cuboidal or low columnar. The cytoplasm is finely granular and the oval, chromatin-rich nucleus occupies most of the cell. Cells in the intermediate layers are **polyhedral (4),** with round or oval nuclei and more visible cell membranes. **Mitoses (7)** are frequently observed in cells of the deeper layers and in the basal cells. Above the polyhedral cells are several rows of **squamous cells (3).** Cells and nuclei become progressively flatter as the cells migrate toward the free surface.

A fine **basement membrane (8)** separates the epithelium (1) from the underlying **connective tissue,** the **lamina propria (2). Papillae (12)** of connective tissue indent the lower surface of the epithelium (1), giving it a characteristic wavy appearance. The connective tissue contains **collagen fibers (11), fibroblasts (10), capillaries (6, 9, 14)** and **arterioles (13).** Other examples of moist stratified squamous epithelium may be seen in Figures 10-3, 11-1, 11-2, 18-16, and 18-17.

When stratified squamous epithelium is exposed to increased wear and tear, the outermost layer, the stratum corneum, becomes thick and keratinized, as illustrated in the epidermis of the palm in Fig. 8-2.

An example of thin, stratified squamous epithelium without connective tissue papillae indentation is illustrated in the cornea of the eye, Figure 19-3; the surface underlying the epithelium is smooth. This type of epithelium is only a few cell layers thick but shows the characteristic arrangement of basal columnar, polyhedral, and squamous cells, the most superficial cells on the cornea.

■ Functional Correlations–Stratified Epithelium

The stratified squamous epithelium is well adapted to withstand wear and tear in the moist cavities of the body. Its multilayered cellular composition serves an important protective function in these regions. Formation of keratin layers on the skin surface provides additional protection from abrasion, dessication, or bacterial invasion of the body. In large excretory ducts, stratified cuboidal or columnar epithelium serves similar protective functions.

Figure 1-9   Stratified Squamous Keratinized Epithelium: Palm of Hand

The skin of the body is covered with a layer of **stratified squamous keratinized epithelium (1).** The outermost layer of the skin is composed of dead cells and is called the **stratum corneum (5).** In the palms and soles, stratum corneum (5) is especially thick, whereas in the rest of the body, this layer is thinner. Under the stratum corneum (5) are different cell layers that give rise to this layer. This photomicrograph illustrates the different cell layers that compose the stratified squamous keratinized epithelium (1). These cell layers are **stratum granulosum (6), stratum spinosum (7),** and the basal cell layer, **stratum basale (8).** The epithelium is attached to the **connective tissue (3)** layer, which is composed of dense collagen fibers and fibroblasts. **Papillae (2)** of the connective tissue indent the lower surface of the epithelium, forming a characteristic wavy appearance. Passing through the connective tissue layer (3) and the epithelium (1) are **excretory ducts of the sweat glands (4),** which are located deep to the epithelium.

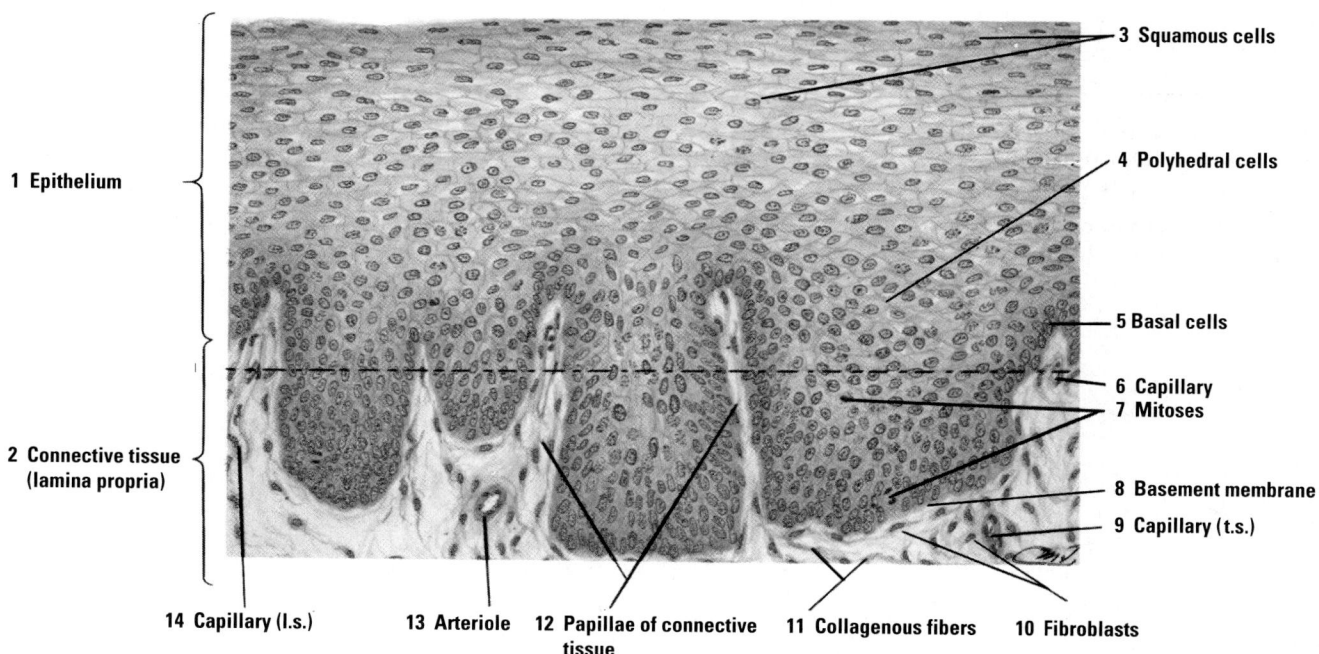

Fig. 1-8   Stratified Squamous Nonkeratinized Epithelium: Esophagus (transverse section). Stain: hematoxylin-eosin. Medium magnification.

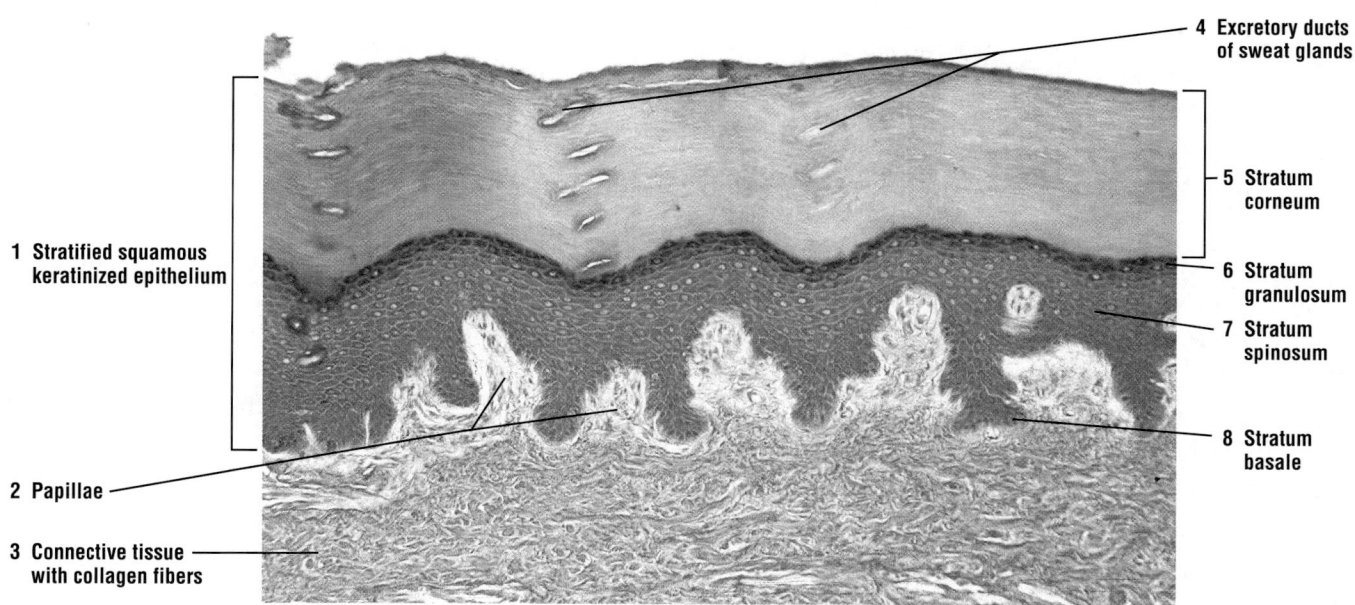

Fig. 1-9   Stratified Squamous Keratizined Epithelium: Palm of Hand. Stain: hematoxylin-eosin. 40×

Figure 1-10   Stratified Cuboidal Epithelium: Excretory Duct in Salivary Gland

Stratified cuboidal epithelium has a limited distribution in the body and is seen only in certain organs. The larger excretory ducts of the salivary glands and pancreas are lined by such stratified cuboidal epithelium. Illustrated in this figure is a high power photomicrograph of a large excretory duct of a salivary gland. Its lining consists of two layers of cuboidal cells, forming the **stratified cuboidal epithelium (1).** Surrounding the excretory duct are collagen fibers of the **connective tissue (2, 7)** and **blood vessels (3, 5),** which are lined by simple squamous epithelium called **endothelium (4, 6).**

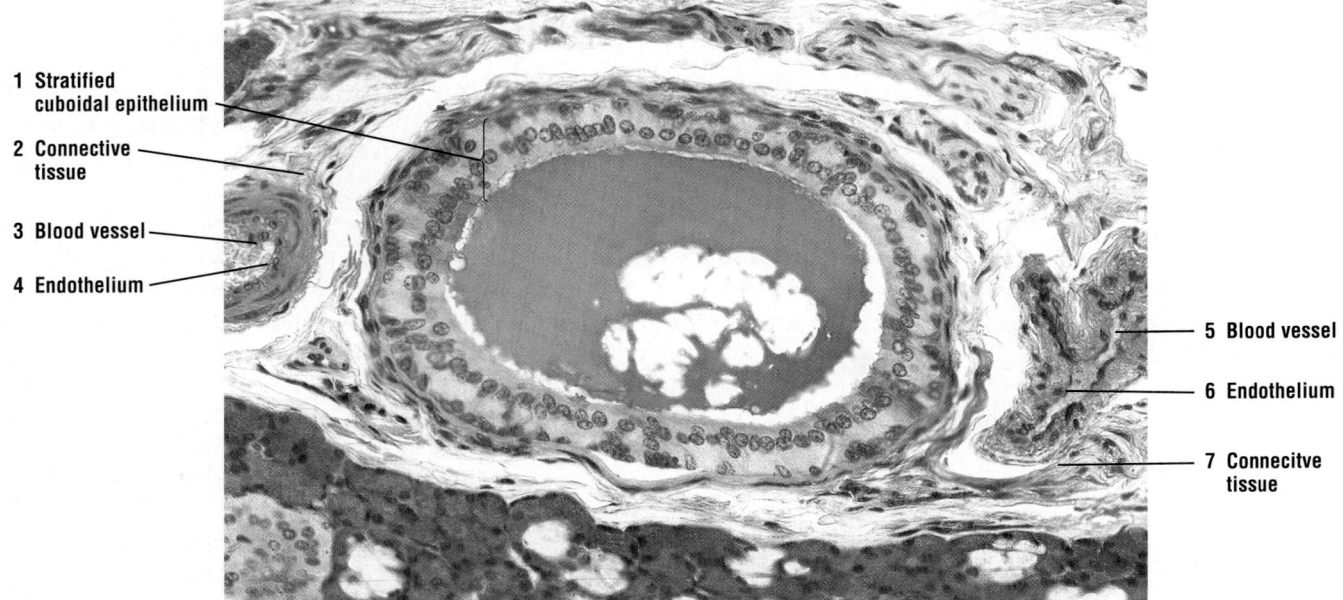

1 Stratified cuboidal epithelium

2 Connective tissue

3 Blood vessel

4 Endothelium

5 Blood vessel

6 Endothelium

7 Connecitve tissue

Fig. 1-10   Stratified Cuboidal Epithelium: Excretory Duct in Salivary Gland. Stain: hematoxylin-eosin. 100×

SECTION 2
Glandular Tissue

The body contains a variety of glands. They are classified as either **exocrine glands** or **endocrine glands.** The cells or parenchyma of these glands develop from epithelial tissue. Exocrine glands secrete their products into **ducts,** whereas endocrine glands deliver their secretory products into the **circulatory system.**

The figures on the pages that follow illustrate the morphology of various glands. The figures on the left are diagrams of the glands and those on the right illustrate examples of their histology.

SIMPLE TUBULAR EXOCRINE GLANDS

There are **unicellular** and **multicellular** exocrine glands. The unicellular glands consist of single cells. The mucus-secreting **goblet cells** found in the epithelia of the small or large intestines or in the respiratory passages are the best examples of unicellular glands.

The multicellular glands are characterized by a **secretory portion,** an endpiece where the epithelial cells secrete a product, and an epithelium-lined **ductal portion,** through which the secretion from the secretory regions is delivered to the exterior of the gland. The larger ducts are usually lined by stratified epithelium.

Multicellular exocrine glands are divided into two major categories, depending on the structure of their ductal portion. A **simple exocrine gland** exhibits an unbranched duct, which may be straight or coiled. Also, if the terminal secretory portion of the gland is shaped in the form of a tube, the gland is called a **tubular gland (Figs. 1-11–1-13).**

COMPOUND EXOCRINE GLANDS

An exocrine gland that shows a repeated branching pattern of the ducts that drain the secretory portions is called a **compound exocrine gland.** Furthermore, if the secretory portions of the gland are shaped in a form of a flask or a tube, the glands are called **acinar (alveolar) glands** or **tubular glands,** respectively. Certain exocrine glands exhibit a mixture of both tubular and acinar secretory portions. Such glands are called **tubuloacinar glands (Figs. 1-14, 1-15).**

Exocrine glands may also be classified based on the secretory products of their cells. Glands that contain cells which produce a viscous secretion that lubricates and/or protects inner lining of organs are **mucous glands.** Glands with cells that produce watery secretions that are often rich in enzymes are **serous glands.** Certain glands in the body contain a mixture of both mucous and serous secretory cells; these are the **mixed glands (Figs. 1-15A, 1-15B, 1-16).**

The exocrine glands may also be classified according to the method of discharging their secretory product. The **merocrine glands** release their secretion by exocytosis without any loss of cellular components. Most exocrine glands in the body secrete their product in this manner. In **holocrine glands,** the cells become the secretory product. These gland cells accumulate lipid, die, and degenerate to become sebum in the sebaceous glands of the skin. In the intermediate type, apocrine, parts of the cell were believed to be discharged as the secretory product. Almost all glands that were once classified apocrine are now regarded as merocrine glands.

ENDOCRINE GLANDS

The endocrine glands differ from the exocrine glands in that they do not have ducts for their secretory products. Instead, endocrine glands are characterized by being **ductless** and highly vascularized, with their secretory cells surrounded by rich **capillary networks.** The close proximity of the secretory cells to the capillaries allows efficient release of the secretory products into the **blood stream** and their distribution to different organs via the systemic circulation **(Figs. 1-17A, 1-17B, 1-18).**

The **endocrine glands** can be either **individual cells** (unicellular glands), **endocrine tissue** in mixed glands (both endocrine and exocrine), or separate and distinct **endocrine organs.** Individual endocrine cells are found in the digestive organs as the enteroendocrine cells. Endocrine tissues are seen in such mixed glands as the pancreas and the reproductive organs of both sexes.

Figure 1-11   Unbranched Simple Tubular Exocrine Glands: Intestinal Glands

Unbranched simple tubular glands without excretory ducts are best represented by the **intestinal glands** (crypts of Lieberkühn) in the **large intestine (Figs. 1-11A, 1-11B)** and rectum. The **surface epithelium** and the **secretory cells** of the glands in the intestines are lined with numerous goblet cells; these are unicellular exocrine glands. Similar but shorter intestinal glands with goblet cells are also found in the small intestine (Fig. 12-1).

Figure 1-12   Simple Branched Tubular Exocrine Glands: Gastric Glands

The simple or slightly branched tubular glands without excretory ducts are found in the stomach. These are the **gastric glands (Figs. 1-12A, 1-12B).** In the fundus and body of the stomach, they are lined with modified columnar cells that are highly specialized for secreting hydrochloric acid and the precursor for the proteolytic enzyme pepsin (Figs. 11-6 and 11-7).

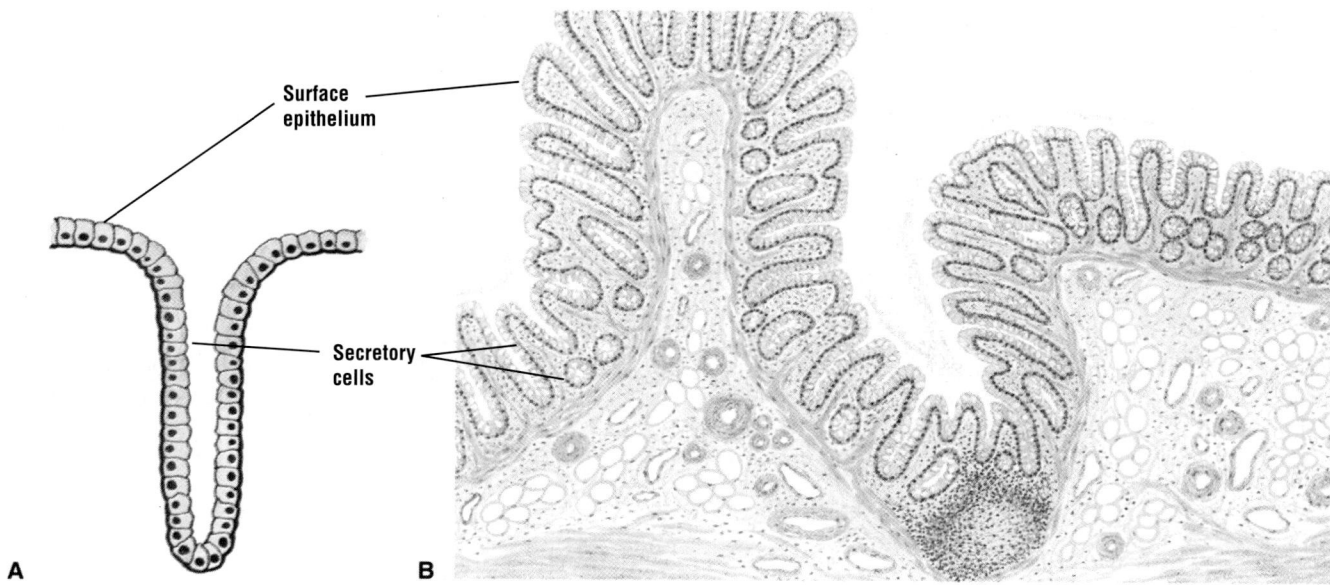

Fig. 1-11   Unbranched Simple Tubular Exocrine Glands: Intestinal Glands. (A) Diagram of gland. (B) Transverse section. Stain: hematoxylin-eosin. Medium magnification.

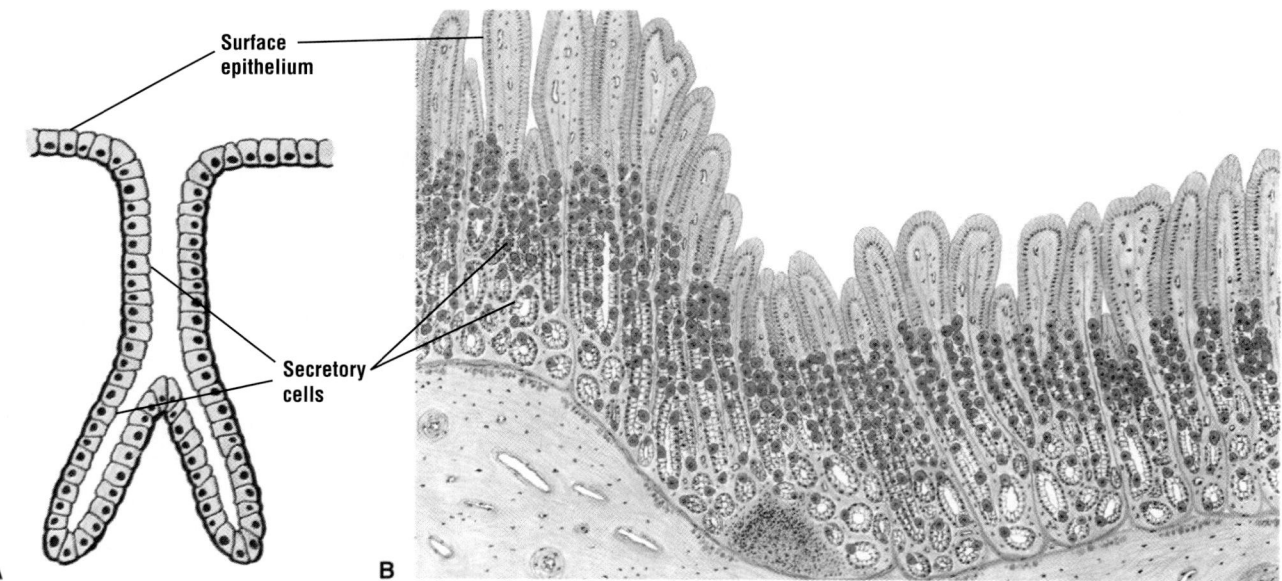

Fig. 1-12   Simple Branched Tubular Exocrine Glands: Gastric Glands. (A) Diagram of gland. (B) Transverse section. Stain: hematoxylin-eosin. Low magnification.

Figure 1-13   Coiled Tubular Exocrine Glands: Sweat Glands

Coiled tubular glands with long, unbranched ducts are found in the skin (Figs. 9-3 and 9-4); these are the **sweat glands (Figs. 1-13A, 1-13B).** Note the **secretory cells** of the gland and the **excretory duct,** lined by stratified cuboidal epithelium, that delivers the secretory product to the surface.

Figure 1-14   Compound Acinar (Exocrine) Gland: Mammary Gland

The mammary gland is an example of **compound acinar (alveolar) gland (Figs. 1-14A, 1-14B, 18-22, 18-23).** The lactating mammary gland contains enlarged **secretory acini (alveoli)** with large lumina that are filled with milk. Draining these acini (alveoli) are **excretory ducts,** some of which contain secretory material and are lined by stratified epithelium.

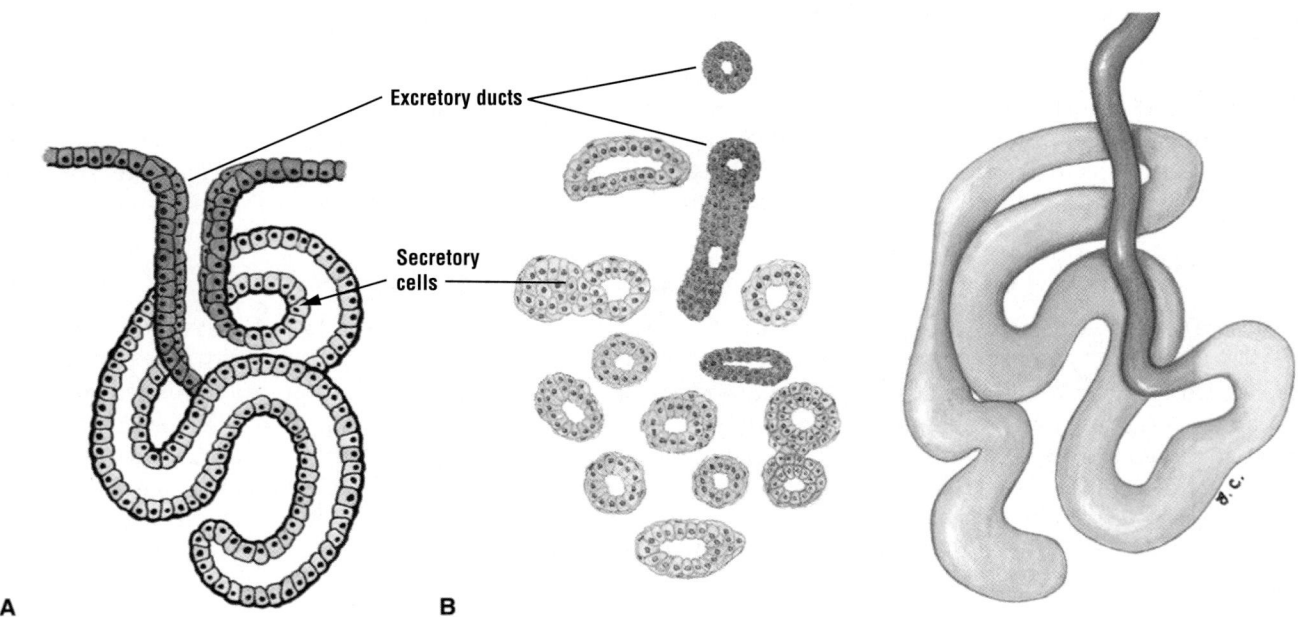

Fig. 1-13   Coiled Tubular Exocrine Glands: Sweat Glands. (A) Diagram of gland. (B) Cross section. Stain: hematoxylin-eosin. Medium magnification.

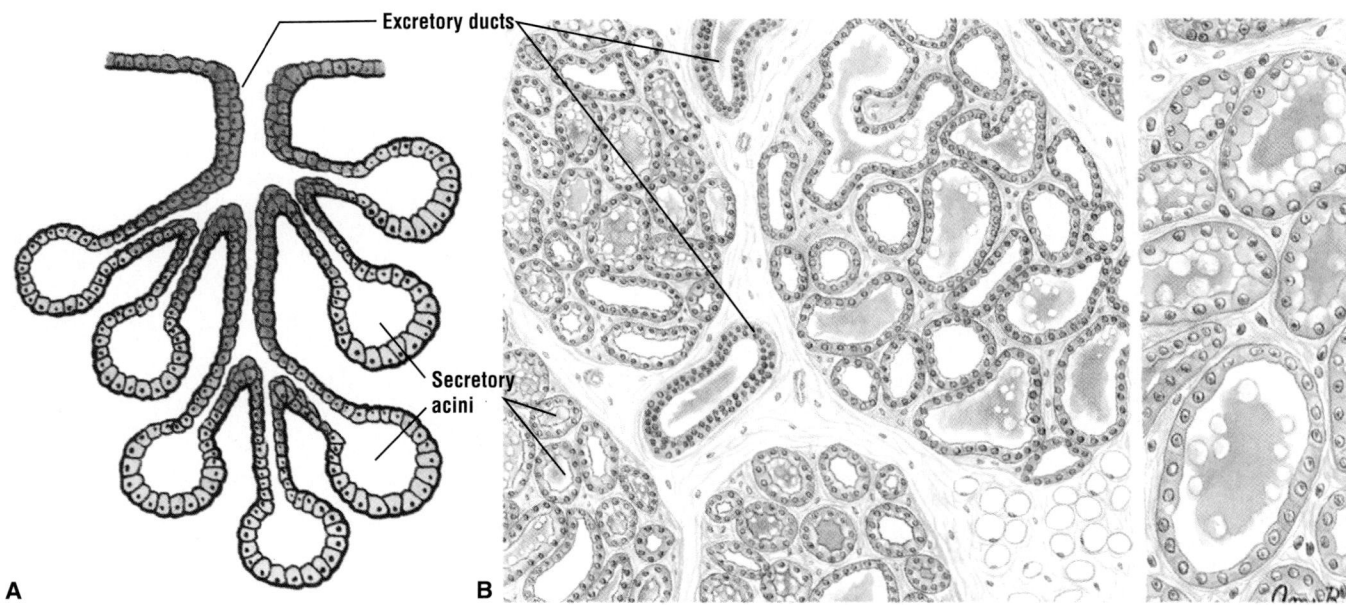

Fig. 1-14   Compound Acinar (Exocrine) Gland: Mammary Gland. (A) Diagram of gland. (B) During lactation. Stain: hematoxylin-eosin. (A) Low magnification. (B) Medium magnification.

Figure 1-15   Compound Tubuloacinar (Exocrine) Gland: Salivary Gland

The salivary glands (parotid, submandibular, and sublingual) best illustrate the **compound tubuloacinar glands (Figs. 1-15A, 1-15B, 10-16).** The glands contain **secretory acinar elements** and **secretory tubular elements.** In addition, the submandibular and sublingual salivary glands contain both serous and mucous acini. Details and comparisons of these acini are described on pages 155–163 and illustrated in Figures 10-12 to 10-17. The **excretory ducts** are lined with cuboidal, columnar, or stratified epithelium, and are named according to their location in the gland.

Figure 1-16   Compound Tubuloacinar (Exocrine) Gland: Submaxillary Salivary Gland

A photomicrograph of a submaxillary salivary gland shows the secretory units of a compound tubuloacinar gland. The grape-like **secretory acinar elements (1)** are circular in section and are distinguished from the longer **secretory tubular elements (7)** of the gland. Empty lumina can be seen in some sections of both types of secretory elements. This salivary gland is a mixed gland and contains both the **mucous cells (4),** which stain light, and **serous cells (5),** which stain dark. Draining the secretory elements of the gland are **excretory ducts (3, 6, 8).** The small excretory ducts are lined by simple cuboidal epithelium and surrounded by **connective tissue (2),** which also surrounds all of the secretory elements.

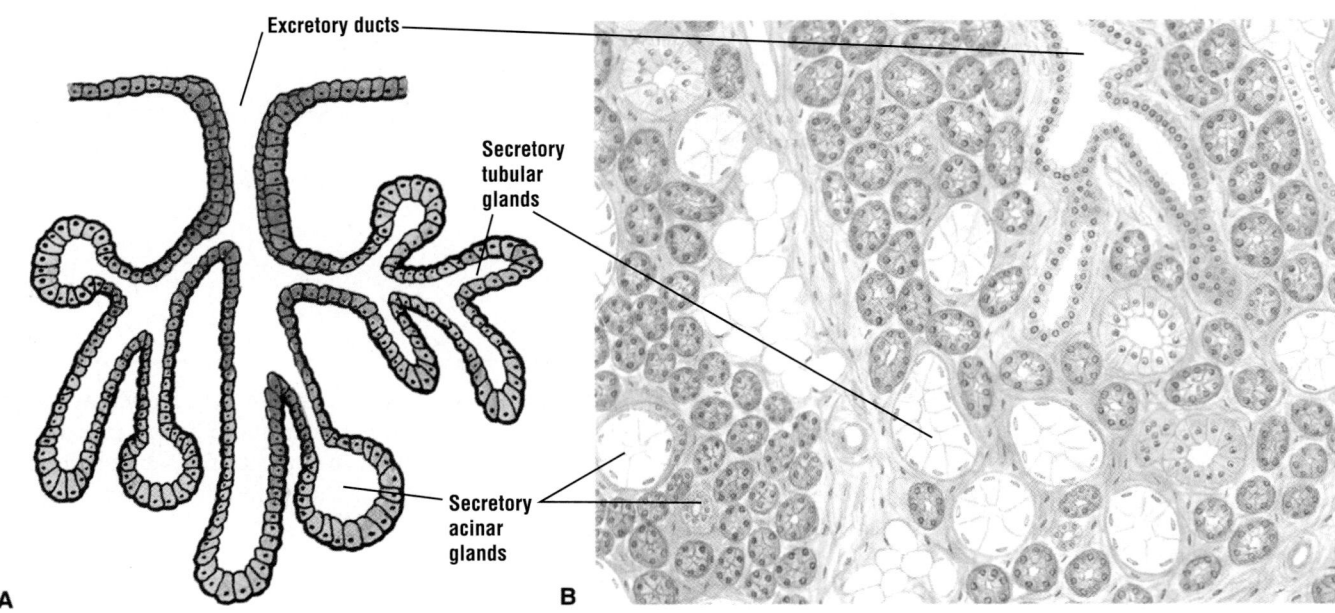

Fig. 1-15   Compound Tubuloacinar (Exocrine) Gland: Salivary Gland. (A) Diagram of gland. (B) Submandibular salivary gland. Stain: hematoxylin-eosin. Low magnification.

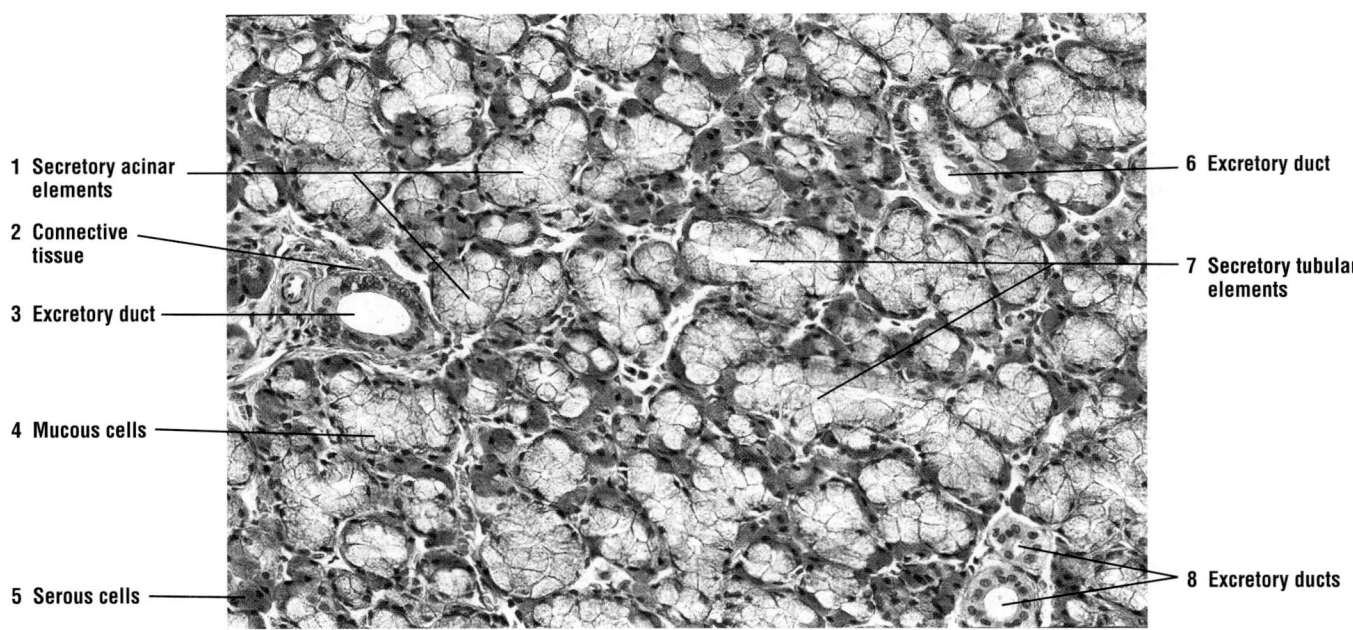

1 Secretory acinar elements

2 Connective tissue

3 Excretory duct

4 Mucous cells

5 Serous cells

6 Excretory duct

7 Secretory tubular elements

8 Excretory ducts

Fig. 1-16   Compound Tubuloacinar (Exocrine) Gland: Submaxillary Salivary Gland. Stain: hematoxylin-eosin. 64×

Figure 1-17   Endocrine Gland: Pancreatic Islet

An example of an endocrine gland is illustrated as a pancreatic islet from the pancreas. This organ is a mixed gland, containing both **exocrine portion** and **endocrine portion.** In the pancreas, the exocrine acini surround the endocrine pancreatic islets **(Figs. 1-17A, 1-17B).**

The structure and function of other endocrine organs (glands) are presented in greater detail and illustrated in Chapter 16.

Figure 1-18   Pancreas

A photomicrograph of a pancreas shows a mixed gland. The endocrine portion of the pancreas, the **pancreatic islet (4),** is separated from the secretory acini of the **exocrine pancreas (1)** by a thin connective tissue. The pancreatic islet (4) does not contain excretory ducts. Instead, it is highly vascularized and all of its secretory products leave the islet via numerous **blood vessels (capillaries) (3).** In contrast, the secretory elements of the exocrine pancreas deliver their secretory product directly into an **excretory duct (2).**

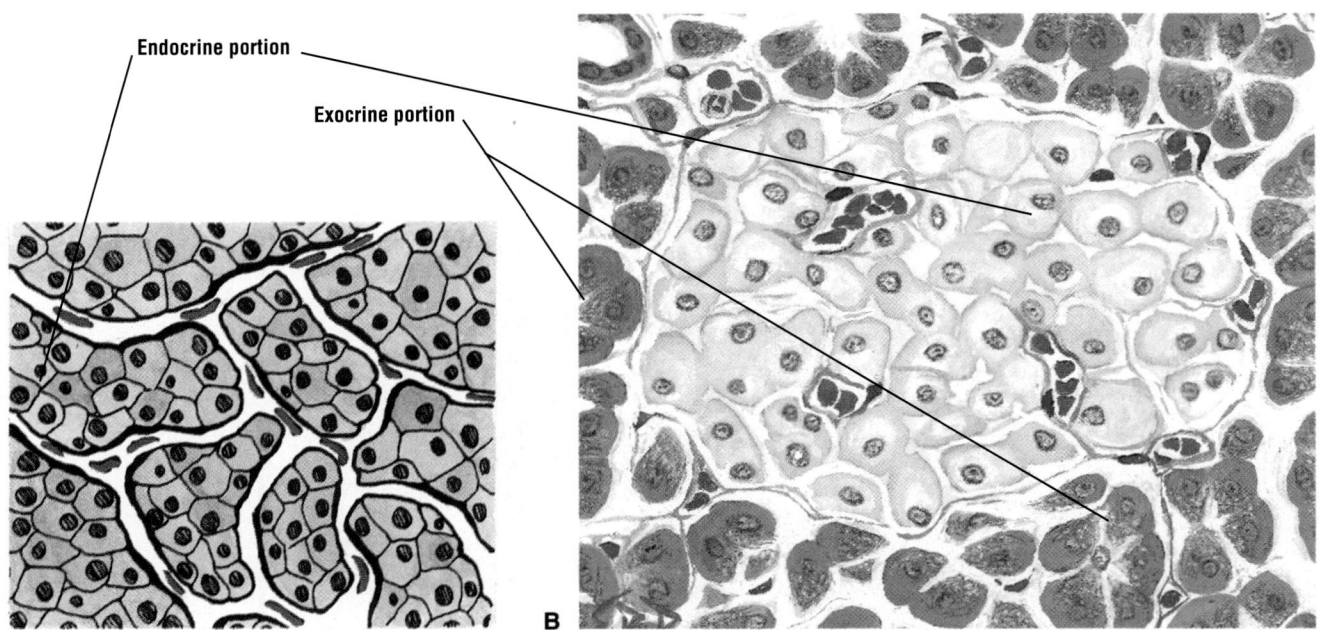

Fig. 1-17   Endocrine Gland: Pancreatic Islet. (A) Diagram of gland. (B) High magnification. Stain: hematoxylin-eosin.

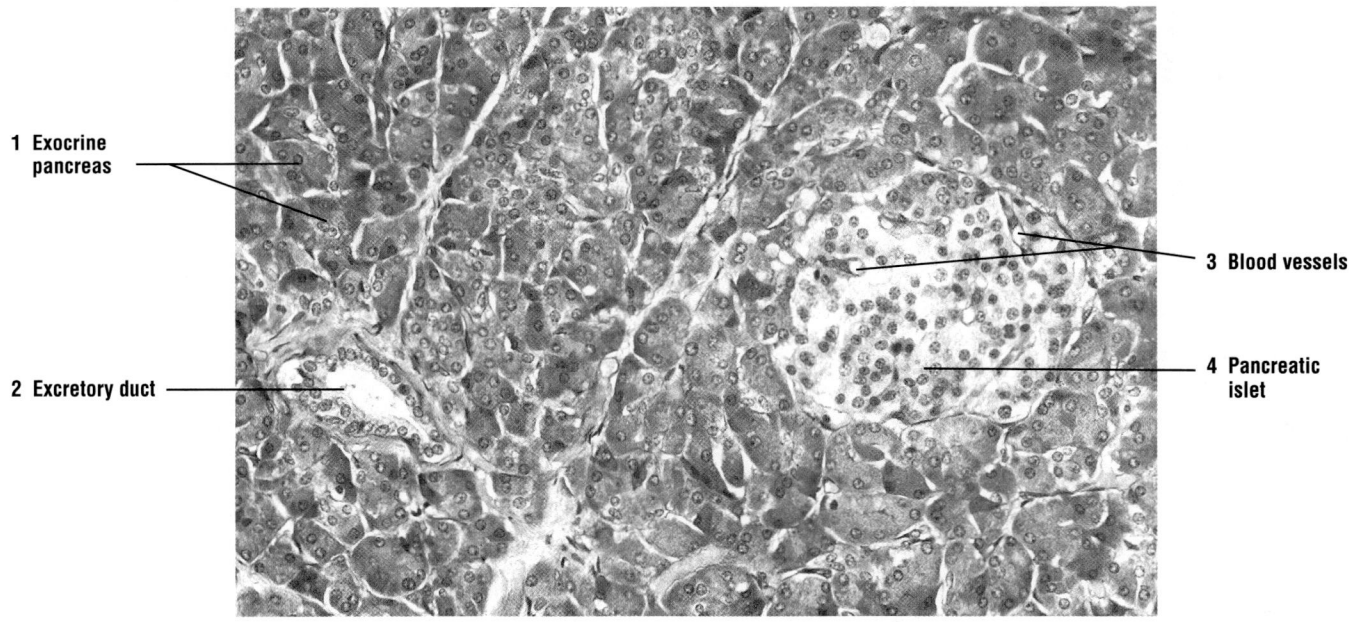

Fig. 1-18   Pancreas. Stain: hematoxylin-eosin. 80×

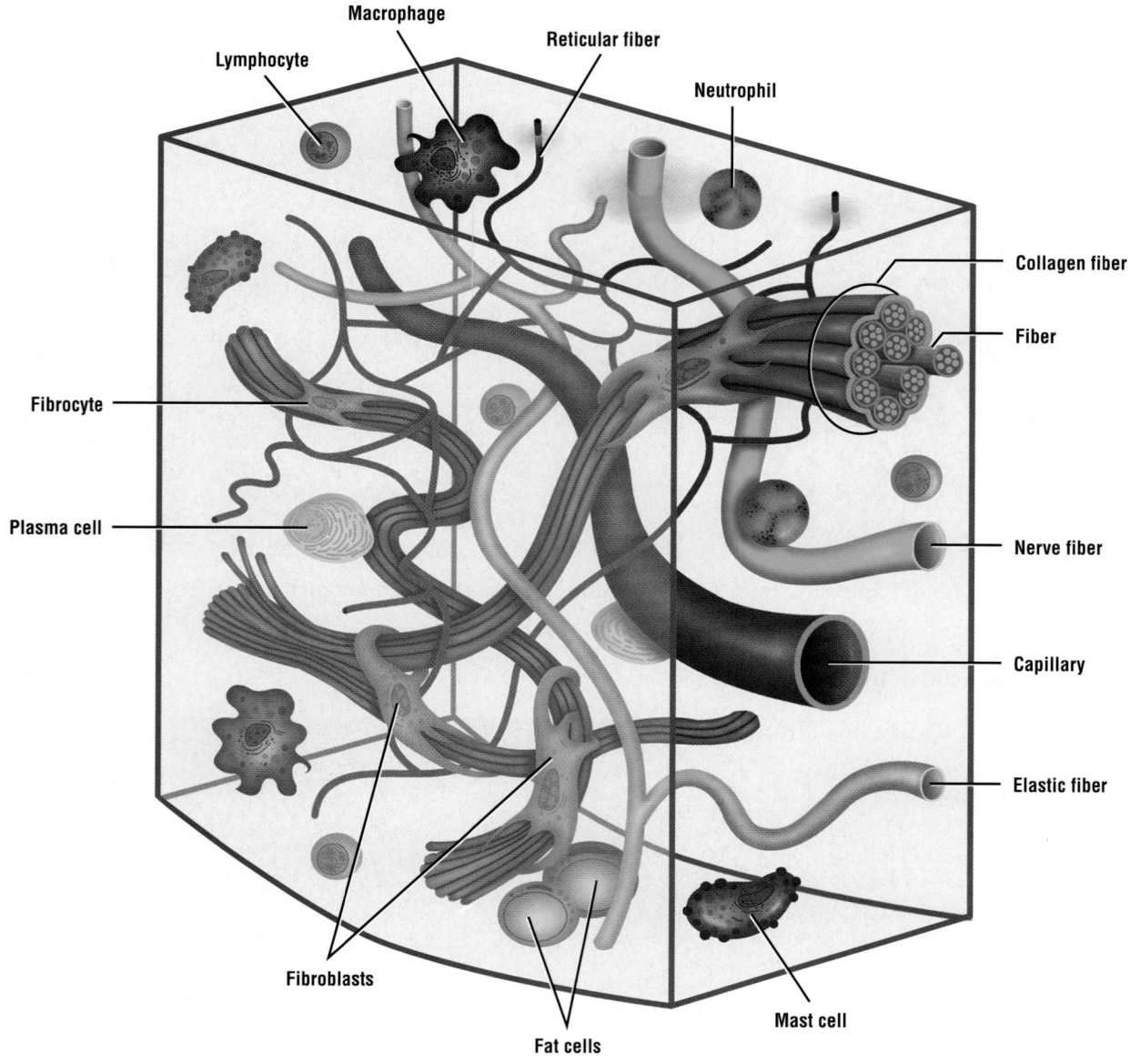

Lymphocyte

Macrophage

Reticular fiber

Neutrophil

Collagen fiber

Fiber

Fibrocyte

Plasma cell

Nerve fiber

Capillary

Elastic fiber

Fibroblasts

Fat cells

Mast cell

Connective Tissue

CLASSIFICATION OF CONNECTIVE TISSUE

With the exceptions of blood and lymph, the **connective tissue** consists of **cells** and **extracellular material**, called **matrix.** The matrix consists of connective tissue **fibers, ground substance,** and **tissue fluid.** Connective tissue binds, anchor, and supports various tissues, organs, and body parts.

The connective tissue is normally divided into **loose connective tissue** and **dense connective tissue,** depending on the amount, type, arrangement, and abundance of cells, fibers, and ground substance.

The **loose connective tissue** is more prevalent. It is characterized by a loose, irregular arrangement of its connective tissue fibers and abundant ground substance. As a result, there are numerous connective tissue cells in its matrix. **Collagen fibers, fibroblasts,** and **macrophages** predominate in the loose connective tissue **(Figs. 2-1–2-5).**

In contrast, the **dense connective tissue** contains more thick and densely packed collagen fibers. As a result, there are fewer cell-types and less ground substance. **Dense irregular connective tissue** exhibits a random and irregular orientation of its collagen fibers. It is present in the dermis of skin, in capsules of different organs, and in areas for strong support. **Dense regular connective tissue** exhibits densely packed collagen fibers with regular and parallel arrangement. This type of tissue is found in the tendons and ligaments **(Figs. 2-5–2-8).**

CELLS OF THE CONNECTIVE TISSUE (FIGS. 2-1, 2-2, 2-4, 2-6)

The connective tissue contains a variety of cell types. The fusiform-shaped **fibroblasts** are the most common connective tissue cells; these young cells synthesize connective tissue fibers and the surrounding ground substance. The **adipose (fat) cells** in the connective tissue store fat and may occur singly or in groups. When adipose cells predominate, it is called **adipose tissue.**

In addition to fibroblasts, the **macrophages** or **histiocytes** are phagocytic and are most numerous in the loose connective tissue regions. They are different to distinguish from the fibroblasts unless they exhibit phagocytic activity.

The **mast cells,** usually closely associated with blood vessels, are widely distributed in the connective tissue of the skin, and in digestive and respiratory organs. Mast cells are spherical cells filled with fine, dark-staining granules.

The **plasma cells** arise from the lymphocytes that migrate into the connective tissue. These cells are found in great abundance in the loose connective tissue and lymphatic tissue of the respiratory and digestive tracts, respectvely.

The white blood cells, or **leukocytes,** migrate into the connective tissue from the blood vessels. Their main function is to defend the organism against bacterial invasion or foreign matter.

The **fibroblasts** and the **adipose cells** are permanent connective tissue cells. Leukocytes, plasma cells, mast cells, and macrophages migrate from the blood into in the connective tissue of different regions of the body.

FIBERS OF THE CONNECTIVE TISSUE

There are three types of connective tissue fibers: **collagen, elastic,** and **reticular.** The amount, arrangement, and concentration of these fibers depends on the function of the tissues or organs in which they are found.

The **collagen fibers** are tough, fibrous protein that are thick and that do not branch. They are the most abundant fibers and found in almost all connective tissue of all organs.

The **elastic fibers** are thin and small that branch; they have less tensile strength than collagen fibers. When stretched, these fibers return to their original size (recoil) without deformation. The elastic fibers are found in large numbers in the lungs, bladder, and skin. In the wall of aorta, elastic fibers allows for stretching of the vessel without breakage or distortion, which is essential for its function.

The **reticular fibers** are thin and form a delicate net-like framework in the liver, lymph nodes, spleen, hemopoietic organs, and others where they filter blood and lymph. Reticular fibers also support capillaries, nerves, and muscle cells. These fibers are visible when stained with silver.

THE GROUND SUBSTANCE

The **ground substance** in the connective tissue is an amorphous, transparent, colorless material with the properties of a semi-fluid gel and high water content. It supports the connective tissue and surrounds its cells and fibers. The ground substance mainly consists of **glycosaminoglycans** and **glycoproteins,** with **hyaluronic acid** its principal glycosaminoglycan. The density of ground substance depends on its content of tissue fluid or water. Mineralization of ground substance changes its density, rigidity, and permeability to diffusion, as seen in cartilage and developing bone.

Figure 2-1   Loose Connective Tissue (spread)

The plate illustrates subcutaneous connective tissue from a rat, stained by injection of a dilute solution of neutral red in saline. With this preparation, fibers and cells are separated and readily identified.

The unstained **collagen fibers (2, 9)** are thickest, largest, and the most numerous. They course in all directions, are thick and somewhat wavy, and exhibit faint longitudinal striations (parts of their component fibrils).

The **elastic fibers (1, 10)** are thin, fine, single fibers that are usually straight; however, after sectioning, the fibers may become wavy because of release of tension. Elastic fibers form branching and anastomosing networks. Although unstained, the fibers are highly refringent, in contrast to the dull collagenous fibers. Fine reticular fibers are also present in loose connective tissue but are not included in this illustration.

The fixed permanent cells of this and other connective tissues are the **fibroblasts (8, I).** Here, the fibroblasts (8) are illustrated as flattened, branching cells with an oval nucleus, sparse chromatin, and one or two **nucleoli (14, 15).** Fixed **macrophages,** or **histiocytes (4, 11, II),** are always present. When inactive, they appear similar to fibroblasts, although their processes may be more irregular and their nuclei smaller. Phagocytic inclusions, however, alter the cytoplasm of the macrophages. In the illustration, the phagocytic vacuoles in the cytoplasm are filled with neutral red (small vacuoles in 4, larger vacuoles in 11 and II:17).

Mast cells (7, III) are also present in loose connective tissue and are seen as single or grouped cells along small blood vessels (7). They are usually ovoid, with a small, pale, centrally placed **nucleus (18)** and cytoplasm filled with fine, closely packed **granules (7, 19, III)** that stain deep red with neutral red stain.

The **adipose (fat) cells (3)** are seen as spherical, colorless globules without visible nucleus.

Blood and other connective tissue cells are not stained with neutral red. The **eosinophils (5)** have lobulated nuclei and coarse, cytoplasmic granules. In the small round **lymphocytes (6),** the nucleus occupies most of the cell. The faint background stain is the ground substance.

Figure 2-2   Individual Cells of Connective Tissue

This figure illustrates some cells of loose connective tissue as they appear in histologic sections after fixation and hematoxylin-eosin staining.

The free **macrophages (1)** usually appear round with slightly irregular cell outlines. Macrophages are variable in appearance: in the illustration, the macrophage exhibits a small nucleus rich in chromatin and slightly acidophilic cytoplasm. The **fibroblast (2)** is elongated with cytoplasmic projections, an ovoid nucleus with sparse chromatin, and one or two nucleoli. The **fibrocyte (3)** is a more mature, smaller cell without cytoplasmic projections; the nucleus is similar but smaller than that in the fibroblast.

The **large (4)** and **small (5) lymphocytes** are spherical cells that differ principally in the greater amount of cytoplasm in the former. The dark-staining nuclei of the lymphocytes have condensed chromatin clumps but no nucleoli.

The **plasma cells (6)** are distinguished from large lymphocytes (4) by a smaller, eccentrically placed nucleus with condensed, coarse chromatin clumps distributed in a characteristic radial pattern and one central mass. A prominent, clear area in the cytoplasm is seen adjacent to the nucleus.

Eosinophils (7) of the circulating blood are readily distinguished by their large size, a bilobate nucleus, and large, cytoplasmic granules that stain intensely with eosin.

Occasional **pigment cells (8)** may be seen. The **adipose cells (9)** are large cells with a narrow rim of cytoplasm and eccentric nuclei. In histologic sections, the large fat globule in the living cell has been dissolved by reagents used in section preparation, leaving a large, empty space.

■ Functional Correlations–Individual Cells in Connective Tissue

Macrophages or *histiocytes* are **phagocytes** whose main function is to ingest bacteria, dead cells, cell debris, and other foreign matter of connective tissue.

Fibroblasts are the dominant cells of the connective tissue. They are highly active and their main function is to synthesize **collagen fibers, reticular fibers,** and **elastic fibers,** in addition to the **extracellular matrix.**

Fibrocytes are smaller than the fibroblasts and are the more inactive or mature cells of the fibroblast line.

Lymphocytes are most numerous in the connective tissue of respiratory and gastrointestinal tracts. The lymphocytes respond to **pathogens** and foreign material. They mediate immune responses to antigens by producing antibodies.

Plasma cells synthesize and secrete **antibodies** (immunoglobulins) into circulation, aiding the body in its defense against bacterial infections.

Adipose cells **store fat** (lipid) and provide protective packing material in and around numerous organs.

The Leukocytes and other Connective Tissue Cells. The **neutrophils** are active phagocytes. They engulf and destroy bacteria, and are found in great numbers at sites of infections. The **eosinophils** increase in number following parasitic infections or allergic reactions. They phagocytize antigen-antibody complexes formed during allergic reactions. The **basophils** contain basophilic granules, which contain heparin and histamine. Their function is similar to that of the mast cells.

Mast cells synthesize and release **heparin** and **histamine.** Heparin from human mast cells is a weak anticoagulant of the blood. Histamine is a potent mediator of inflammation; it dilates blood vessels, increases their permeability to fluid, and produces edema.

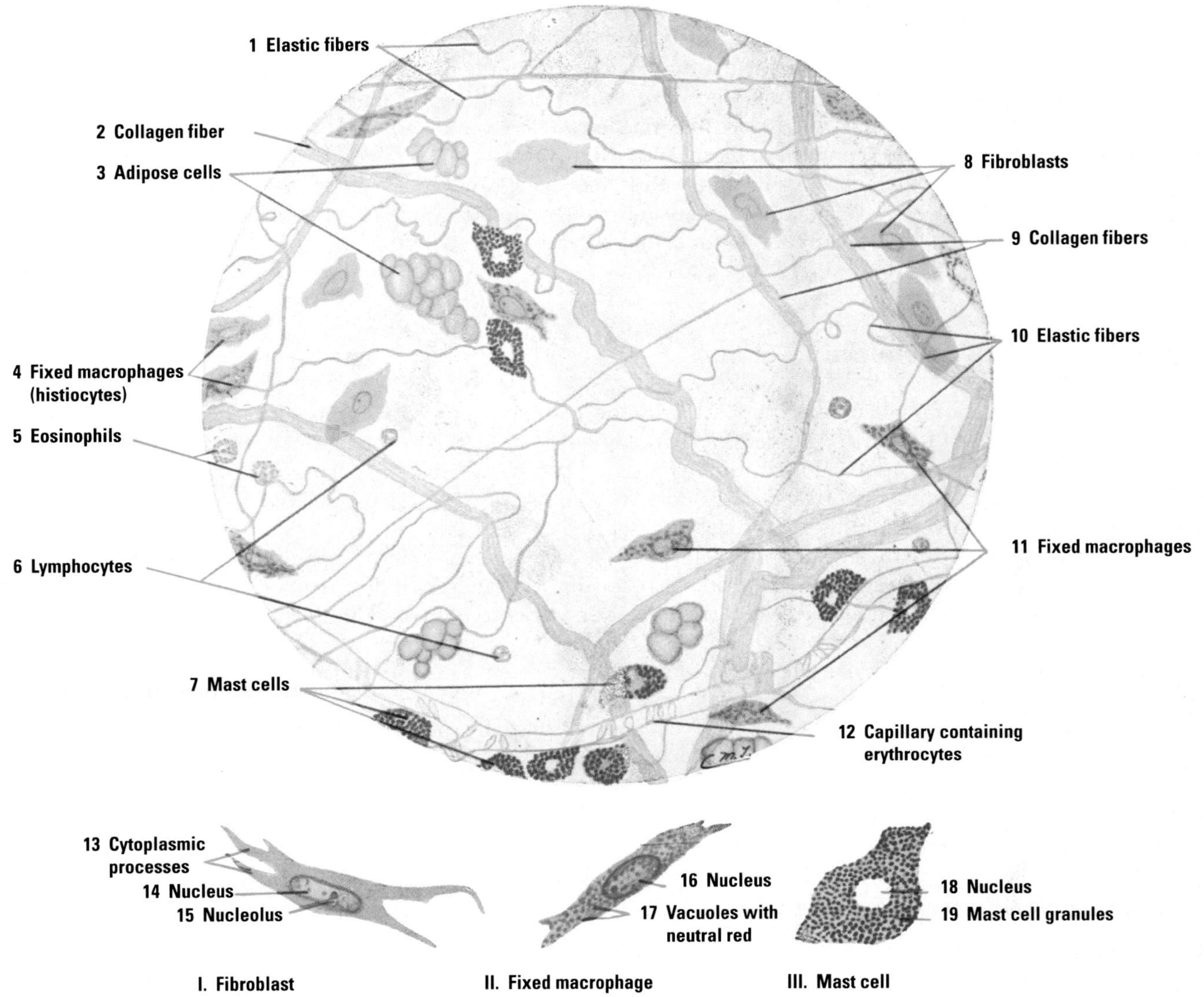

1 Elastic fibers

2 Collagen fiber

3 Adipose cells

8 Fibroblasts

9 Collagen fibers

10 Elastic fibers

4 Fixed macrophages (histiocytes)

5 Eosinophils

6 Lymphocytes

11 Fixed macrophages

7 Mast cells

12 Capillary containing erythrocytes

13 Cytoplasmic processes
14 Nucleus
15 Nucleolus

16 Nucleus
17 Vacuoles with neutral red

18 Nucleus
19 Mast cell granules

I. Fibroblast

II. Fixed macrophage

III. Mast cell

Fig. 2-1   Loose Connective Tissue (spread). Supravital staining with neutral red. Upper: high magnification. Lower: oil immersion.

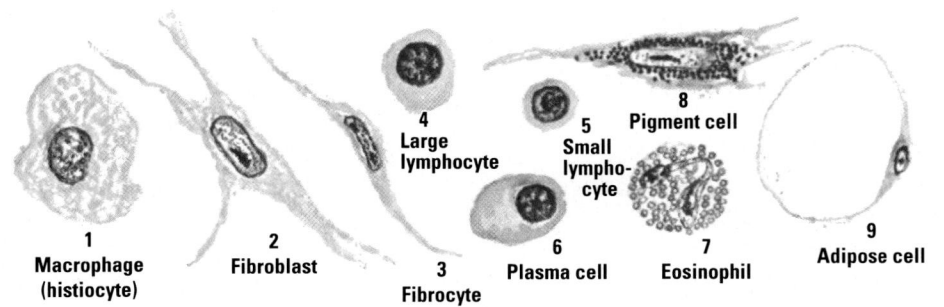

4 Large lymphocyte

5 Small lymphocyte

8 Pigment cell

1 Macrophage (histiocyte)

2 Fibroblast

3 Fibrocyte

6 Plasma cell

7 Eosinophil

9 Adipose cell

Fig. 2-2   Individual Cells of Connective Tissue. Stain: hematoxylin-eosin. Oil immersion.

Figure 2-3   Embryonic Connective Tissue

The embryonic connective tissue resembles the mesenchyme or mucous connective tissue, which is loose and irregular. The difference in ground substance (semi-fluid versus jelly-like) is not apparent in these sections.

The **fibroblasts (2)** are numerous, and fine **collagen fibers (3)** are found between them, some coming in close contact with fibroblasts. Embryonic connective tissue is vascular **(1, 4).**

At higher magnification, a primitive **fibroblast (5)** is seen as a large, branching cell with abundant cytoplasm, prominent cytoplasmic processes, an ovoid nucleus with fine chromatin, and one or more nucleoli. The widely separated **collagen fibers (6)** are more apparent at this magnification.

Figure 2-4   Loose Connective Tissue

Collagen fibers (6) predominate in loose connective tissue, course in many directions, and form a loose meshwork. In the illustration, these fibers are sectioned in various planes, and transverse ends may be seen. Collagen fibers have various diameters and appear longitudinally striated because of their fibrillar structure. The fibers are acidophilic and stain pink with eosin. Thin elastic fibers are also present in loose connective tissue but are difficult to distinguish with this stain and at this magnification.

The **fibroblasts (1)** are the most numerous cells in the loose connective tissue and may be sectioned in various planes, so that only parts of the cells may be seen. Also, during section preparation, the cytoplasm of these cells may shrink. A typical fibroblast (1) shows an oval nucleus with sparse chromatin and lightly acidophilic cytoplasm, with few short processes.

Also present in loose connective tissue are various blood cells such as the **neutrophils (3),** with lobulated nuclei, and small **lymphocytes (2),** with dense nuclei and sparse cytoplasm. The **fat** or **adipose cells (11, 12)** appear characteristically empty with a thin rim of cytoplasm (11) and peripherally displaced flat **nuclei (12).**

The connective tissue is highly vascular. **Capillaries (7, 13),** which are visible, are sectioned in several planes and lined with endothelium. Larger blood vessels, such as the **arterioles (4, 9, 10)** and **venules (5, 8)** sectioned in several planes, are also seen in the loose connective tissue.

Other examples of loose connective tissue are illustrated in Figure 16-7.

■ Functional Correlations–Loose Connective Tissue and Ground Substance

Loose connective tissue is characterized by increased amounts of **ground substance,** in which are found numerous cell types. The ground substance facilitates **diffusion** of oxygen, electrolytes, nutrients, fluids, metabolites, and other products between the cells and the blood vessels. Waste products from the cells diffuse through the ground substance back into the blood vessels. The ground substance also serves as a barrier: it prevents the spread of pathogens from the connective tissue into the bloodstream. However, certain bacteria produce hyaluronidase, an enzyme that hydrolyzes hyaluronic acid and reduces the viscosity of the ground substance, allowing pathogens to invade the surrounding tissues.

Figure 2-5   Dense Irregular and Loose Connective Tissue (elastin stain)

This figure illustrates an area with dense irregular connective tissue on the left side, a transition zone in the middle, and loose connective tissue on the right.

The **elastic fibers (1, 4)** are selectively stained a deep blue using Verhoeff's method. Using Van Gieson's as a counterstain, acid fuchsin stains **collagen fibers** red **(2, 5).** Cellular details of fibroblasts are not revealed but the **fibroblast nuclei (3, 6)** stain deep blue.

The characteristic features of dense irregular and loose connective tissues become apparent with this staining technique. In dense irregular connective tissue the collagen fibers (2) are larger, more numerous, and more concentrated. Elastic fibers are also larger and more numerous (1). In contrast, in the loose connective tissue, both fiber types are smaller (4, 5) and more loosely arranged. Fine elastic networks are seen in both types of connective tissue.

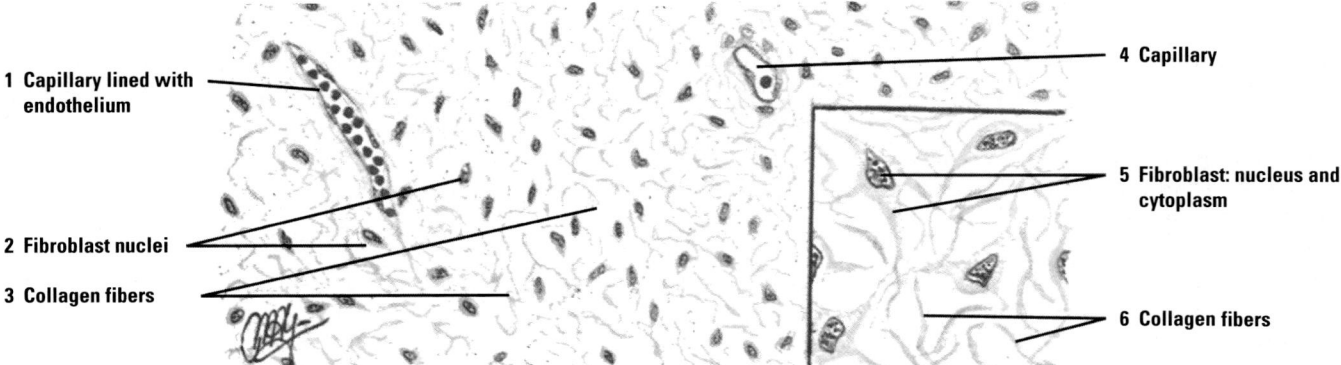

1 Capillary lined with endothelium

2 Fibroblast nuclei

3 Collagen fibers

4 Capillary

5 Fibroblast: nucleus and cytoplasm

6 Collagen fibers

Fig. 2-3   Embryonic Connective Tissue. Stain: hematoxylin-eosin. Medium magnification (inset: oil immersion).

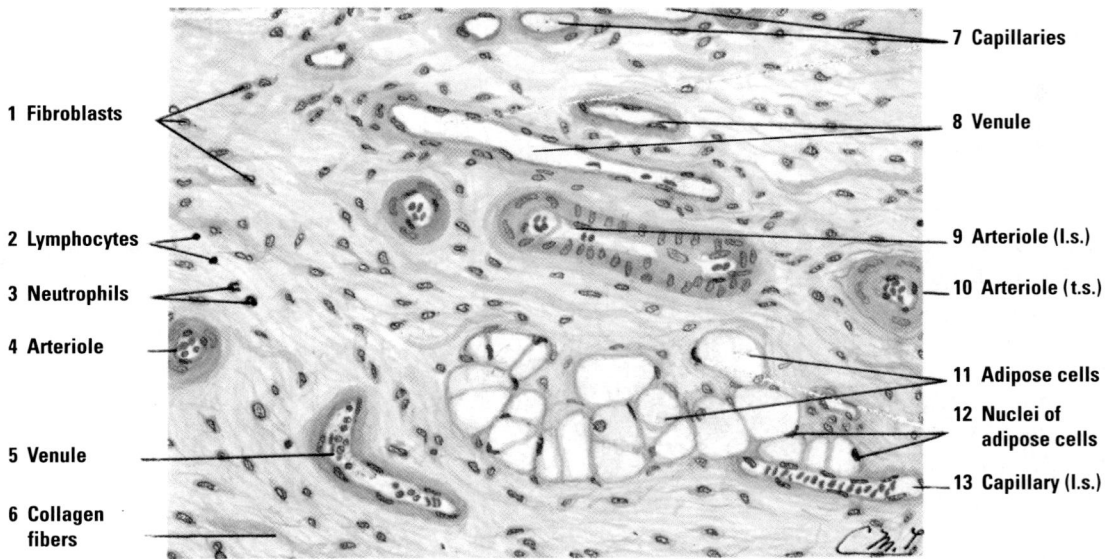

1 Fibroblasts

2 Lymphocytes

3 Neutrophils

4 Arteriole

5 Venule

6 Collagen fibers

7 Capillaries

8 Venule

9 Arteriole (l.s.)

10 Arteriole (t.s.)

11 Adipose cells

12 Nuclei of adipose cells

13 Capillary (l.s.)

Fig. 2-4   Loose Connective Tissue. Stain: hematoxylin-eosin. High magnification.

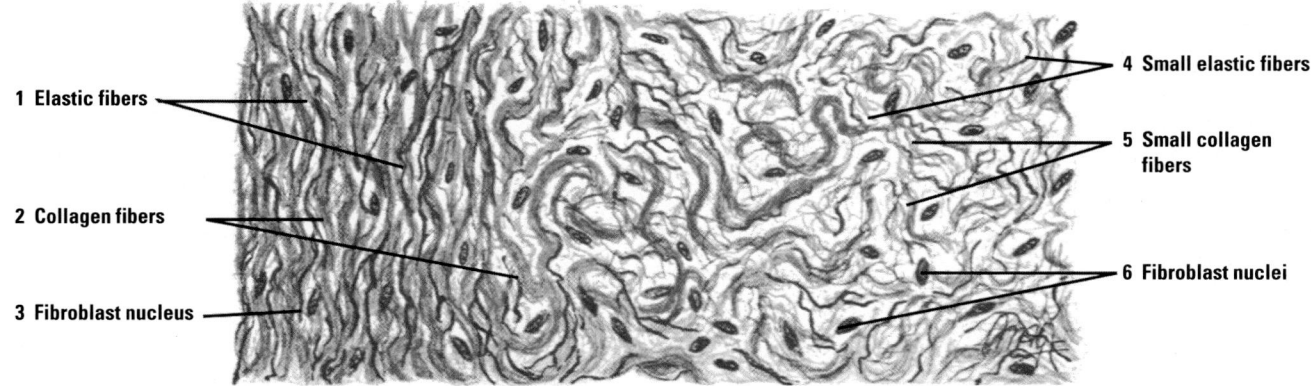

1 Elastic fibers

2 Collagen fibers

3 Fibroblast nucleus

4 Small elastic fibers

5 Small collagen fibers

6 Fibroblast nuclei

Fig. 2-5   Dense Irregular and Loose Connective Tissue (elastin stain). Stain: Verhoeff's elastin stain and Van Gieson's. Medium magnification.

Figure 2-6   Dense Irregular Connective Tissue

This figure illustrates dense irregular connective tissue from the dermis of the skin. The arrangement of fibers and cells is similar to that in loose connective tissue; however, this is modified for areas in the body where more firm support and strength are required.

The **collagen fibers (1, 2)** are large, typically found in thick bundles, and sectioned in several planes because they course in various directions. This type of fiber arrangement is compact. Also present here are thin, wavy **elastic fibers (10),** which form fine networks.

The **fibroblasts (5, 11)** are often found compressed among the collagen fibers. Also illustrated are a **perivascular cell (6)** along a small blood vessel and a few blood cells, **neutrophils (3)** with lobulated nuclei, and **lymphocytes (9)** with large round nuclei without visible cytoplasm. **Small blood vessels (4, 8)** are also illustrated.

Additional illustration of dense irregular connective tissue in the dermis of the skin is found in Figure 9-1:3.

■ Functional Correlations–Dense Irregular Collagen Fibers

The collagen fibers exhibit great tensile strength and their main function is support. They are most highly concentrated in those areas of the organs or body where such strong support is needed to resist forces pulling from different directions.

Figure 2-7   Dense Irregular Connective Tissue and Adipose Tissue

Illustrated in this photomicrograph is a deep section of the skin called the dermis. This region contains **dense irregular connective tissue (1)** and the collagen-producing cells known as **fibroblasts (3).** In this type of connective tissue, the **collagen fibers (2)** show a very random and irregular orientation. Adjacent to the dense irregular connective tissue (1) is a region of **adipose tissue (4)** with its numerous **adipose cells (5).** Owing to the tissue preparation with different chemicals, the individual adipose cells appear empty, and only their flattened, dense-staining nuclei are visible. Deep in the skin are also found numerous sweat glands. The light-staining regions are the **secretory cells of the sweat gland (7).** The dark-staining cells form a **stratified cuboidal epithelium of the excretory duct of the sweat gland (6, 8).** The excretory duct (6, 8) continues through the connective tissue and the statified squamous epithelium of the skin, and exits on the surface of the skin (See Figure 1-9).

1 Collagen fibers (t.s.)

2 Collagen fibers (l.s.)

3 Neutrophils

4 Venules

5 Fibroblasts

6 Perivascular cell

7 Endothelial cell

8 Venule

9 Lymphocytes

10 Elastic fibers

11 Fibroblasts

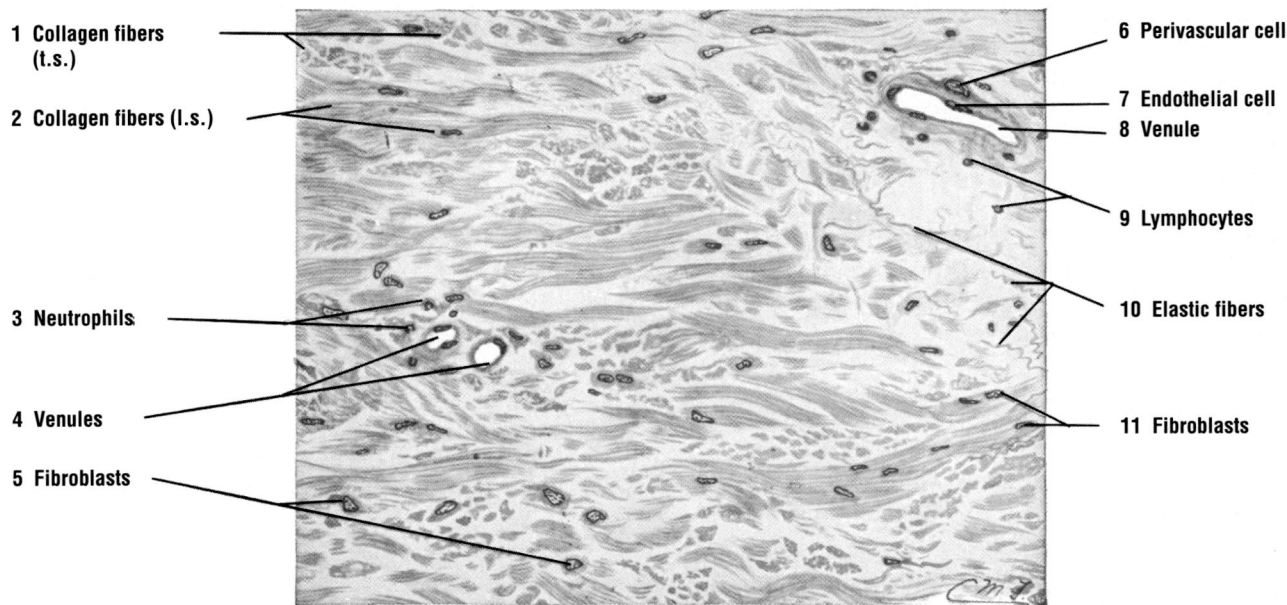

Fig. 2-6   Dense Irregular Connective Tissue. Stain: hematoxylin-eosin. High magnification.

1 Dense irregular connective tissue

2 Collagen fibers

3 Fibroblasts

4 Adipose tissue

5 Adipose cells

6 Stratified cuboidal epithelium of excretory duct of sweat gland

7 Secretory cells of a sweat gland

8 Stratified cuboidal epithelium of excretory duct of sweat gland

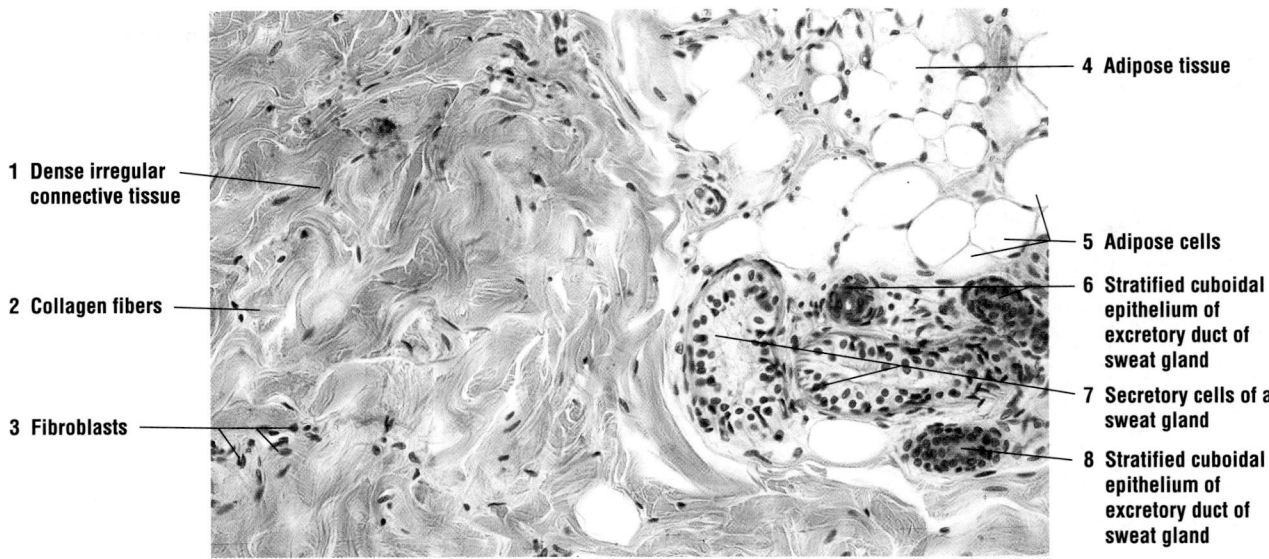

Fig. 2-7   Dense Irregular Connective Tissue and Adipose Tissue. Stain: hematoxylin-eosin. 64×

Figure 2-8   Dense Regular Connective Tissue: Tendon (longitudinal section)

Dense regular connective tissue is present in ligaments and tendons. A section of a tendon in logitudinal plane is illustrated.

The **collagen fibers (2, 3)** are arranged in compact, parallel bundles. Between these bundles are thin partitions of looser connective tissue that contain parallel rows of **fibroblasts (1, 4, 5).** These cells have short processes (not visible here) and nuclei ovoid that appear when seen in surface view (4) or rod-like in lateral view (5).

Dense regular connective tissue with less regular fiber arrangement than in the tendon also forms fibrous membranes or capsules around various organs in the body. Examples of such connective tissue are perichondrium around the tracheal cartilage (Fig. 14-5:2), the dura mater around the spinal cord (Fig. 6-19:2), and the tunica albuginea surrounding the testis (Fig. 17-1:1).

■ Functional Correlations–Dense Regular Collagen Fibers

Dense regular connective tissue is present where great tensile strength is required, such as in ligaments and tendons. The regular and dense arrangement of collagen fibers offer strong resistance to forces pulling along a single axis. Tendons and ligaments are constantly subject to such forces.

Figure 2-9   Dense Regular Connective Tissue: Tendon (longitudinal section)

A photomicrgraph of dense regular connective tissue of a tendon shows that it has a compact, regular, and parallel arrangement of **collagen fibers (1).** Between the densely packed collagen fibers are seen flattened nuclei of the **fibroblasts (2).** A small **blood vessel (3)** with blood cells courses between the dense bundles of collagen fibers to supply the connective tissue cells of the tendon.

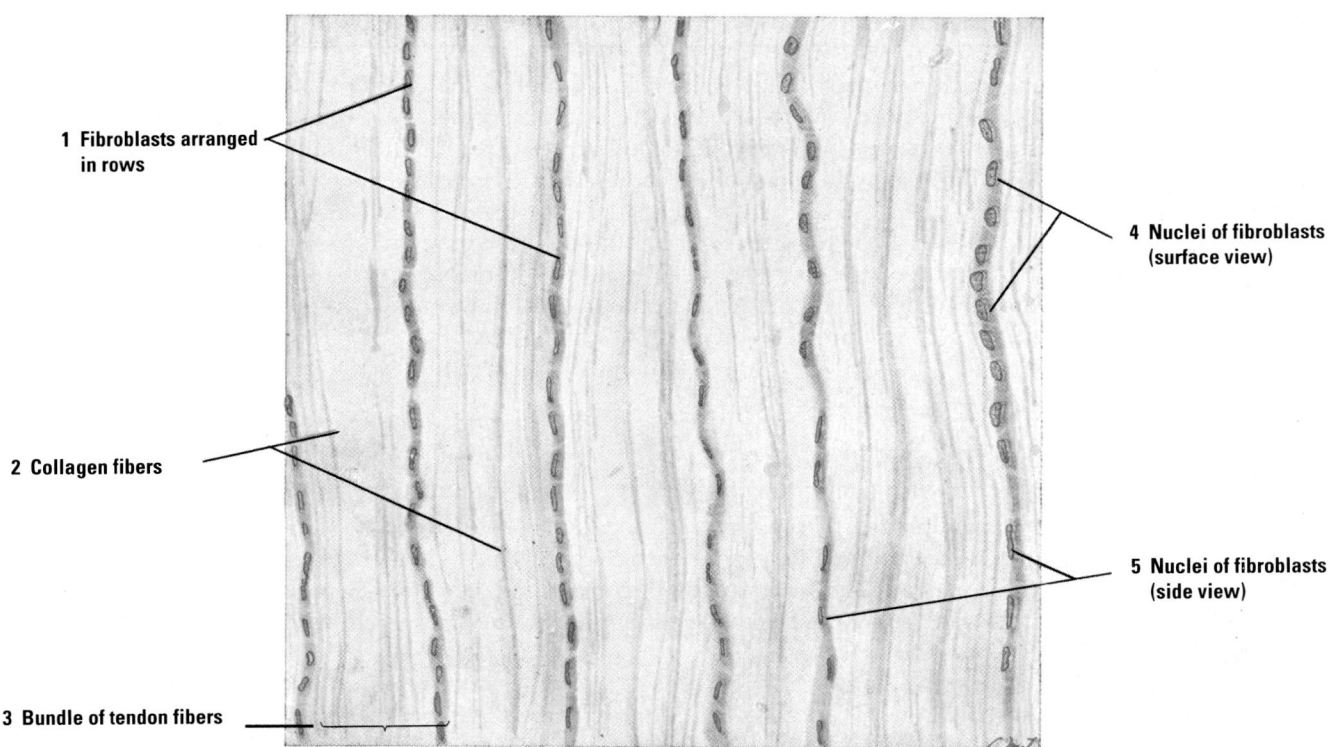

1 Fibroblasts arranged
  in rows

2 Collagen fibers

3 Bundle of tendon fibers

4 Nuclei of fibroblasts
  (surface view)

5 Nuclei of fibroblasts
  (side view)

Fig. 2-8   Dense Regular Connective Tissue: Tendon (longitudinal section). Stain: hematoxylin-eosin. Medium magnification.

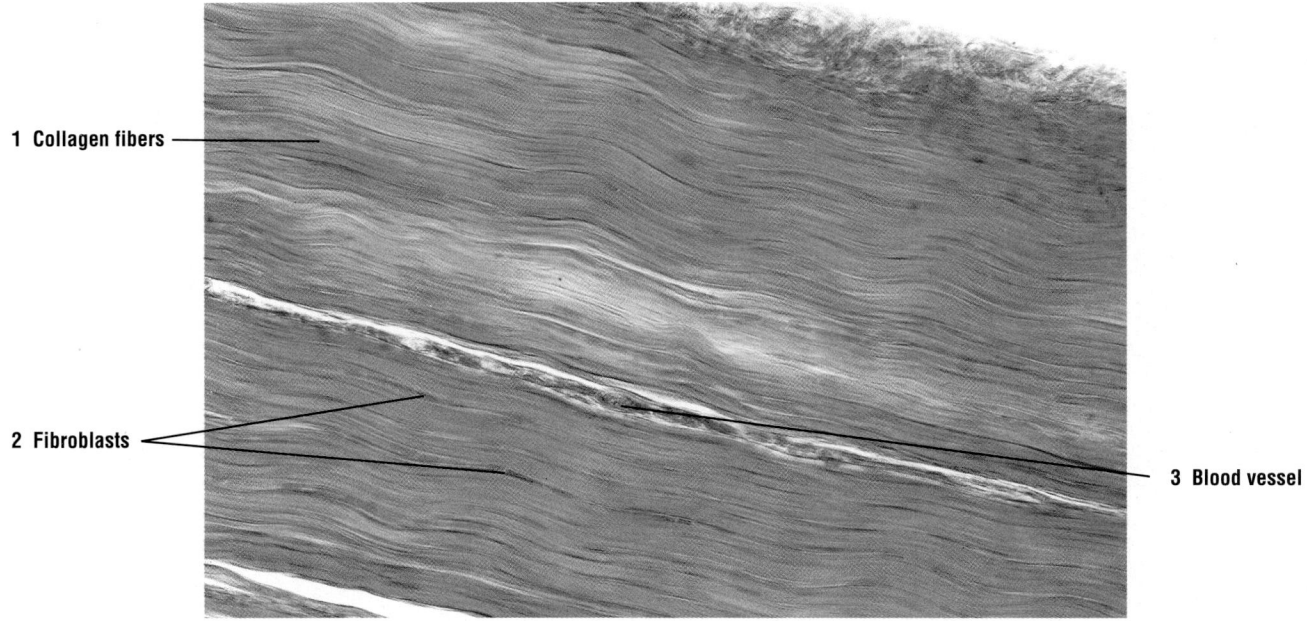

1 Collagen fibers

2 Fibroblasts

3 Blood vessel

Fig. 2-9   Dense Regular Connective Tissue: Tendon (longitudinal section). Stain: hematoxylin-eosin. 64×

Figure 2-10   Dense Regular Connective Tissue: Tendon (transverse section)

A tendon in transverse section is illustrated at a lower magnification than that in Figure 2-1. Within each large bundle of collagen fibers (1, 10) are **fibroblasts (nuclei) (2, 9)** sectioned transversely. The fibroblasts are located between small bundles of collagen fibers. These are better distinguished at the higher magnification in the inset, which shows bundles of collagen fibers (10) and the branched shape of fibroblasts (9) in transverse section.

Between the large collagen bundles are thin partitions of **connective tissue (3).** Collagen bundles are grouped into fascicles, with larger partitions (septa or trabeculae) of interfascicular **connective tissue (4, 8)** coursing between them. These partitions contain **blood vessels (5),** nerves, and, occasionally, lamellated **Pacinian corpuscles (6),** which are sensitive pressure receptors. Also illustrated in the figure is a transverse section of **skeletal muscle (7),** which is adjacent to the tendon but separated from it by connective tissue.

Figure 2-11   Adipose Tissue

A small section of a mesentery is illustrated in which large accumulations of **adipose (fat) cells (2, 8)** are organized into adipose tissue. The connective tissue of the **peritoneum (6)** serves as a capsule around the adipose tissue.

Adipose cells (2) are closely packed and separated by thin strips of connective tissue, which contains the compressed **fibroblasts (7).** Lobules of adipose tissue are separated by **connective tissue septa (3),** in which are found **blood vessels (1, 4),** nerves, and **capillaries (5).**

Individual adipose cells appear as empty cells (2) because the fat was dissolved by chemicals used during routine histologic preparation of the tissue. Their nuclei (8) are compressed in the peripheral rim of the cytoplasm, and in certain sections, it is difficult to distinguish between fibroblast nuclei (7) and adipose cell nuclei (8).

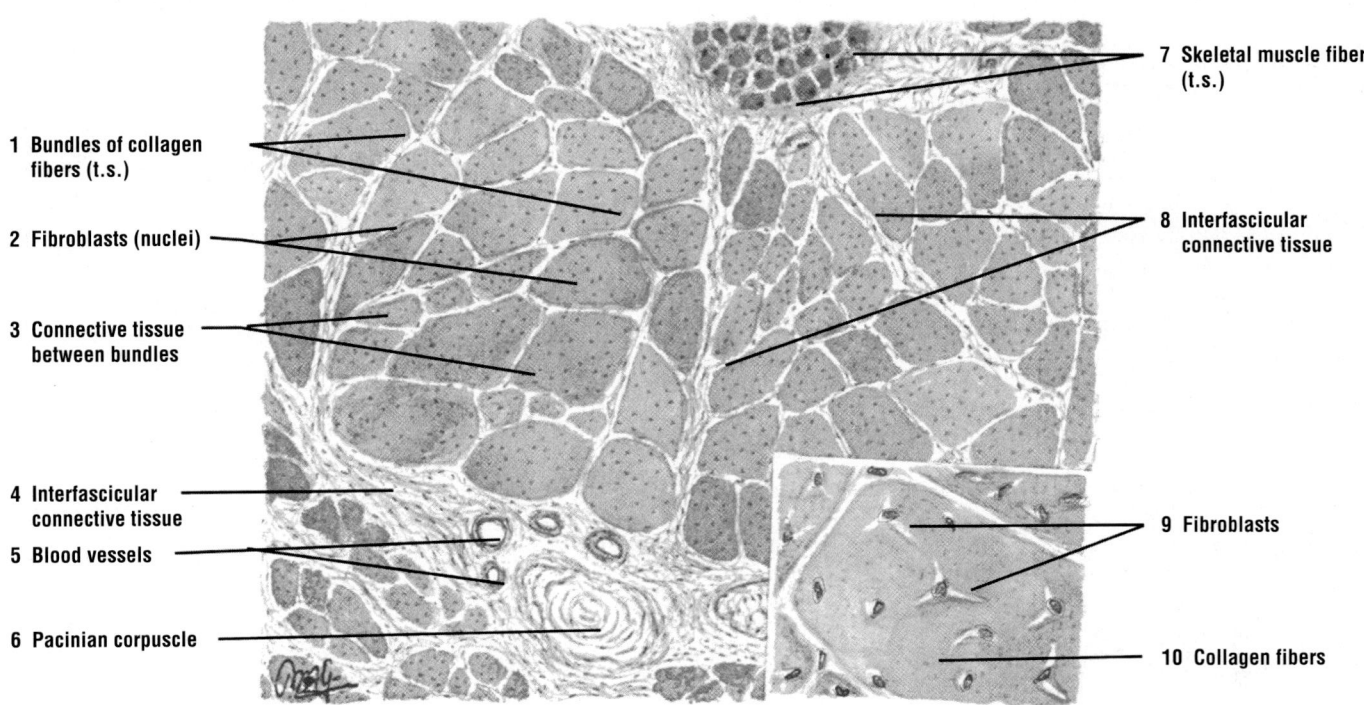

1 Bundles of collagen fibers (t.s.)

2 Fibroblasts (nuclei)

3 Connective tissue between bundles

4 Interfascicular connective tissue

5 Blood vessels

6 Pacinian corpuscle

7 Skeletal muscle fibers (t.s.)

8 Interfascicular connective tissue

9 Fibroblasts

10 Collagen fibers

Fig. 2-10 Dense Regular Connective Tissue: Tendon (transverse section). Stain: hematoxylin-eosin. Low magnification (inset: high magnification).

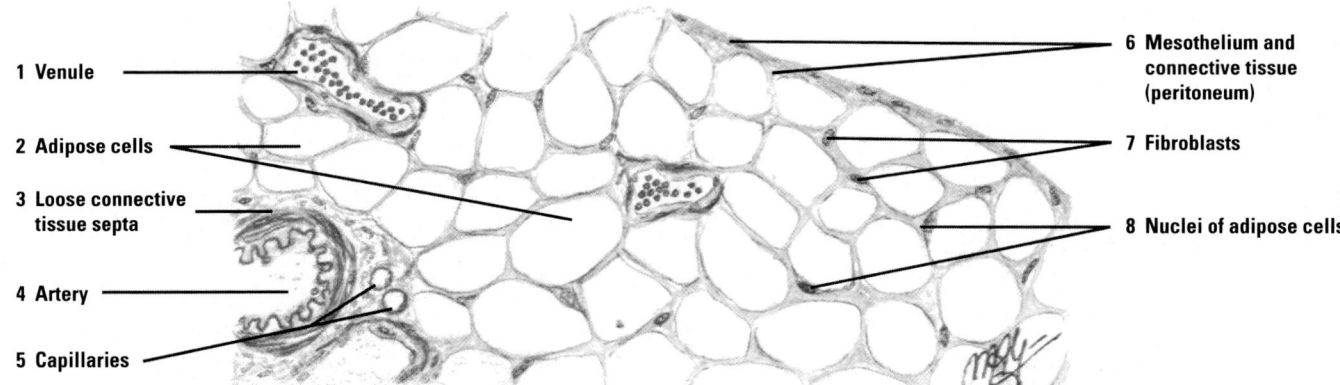

1 Venule

2 Adipose cells

3 Loose connective tissue septa

4 Artery

5 Capillaries

6 Mesothelium and connective tissue (peritoneum)

7 Fibroblasts

8 Nuclei of adipose cells

Fig. 2-11 Adipose Tissue. Stain: hematoxylin-eosin. Medium magnification.

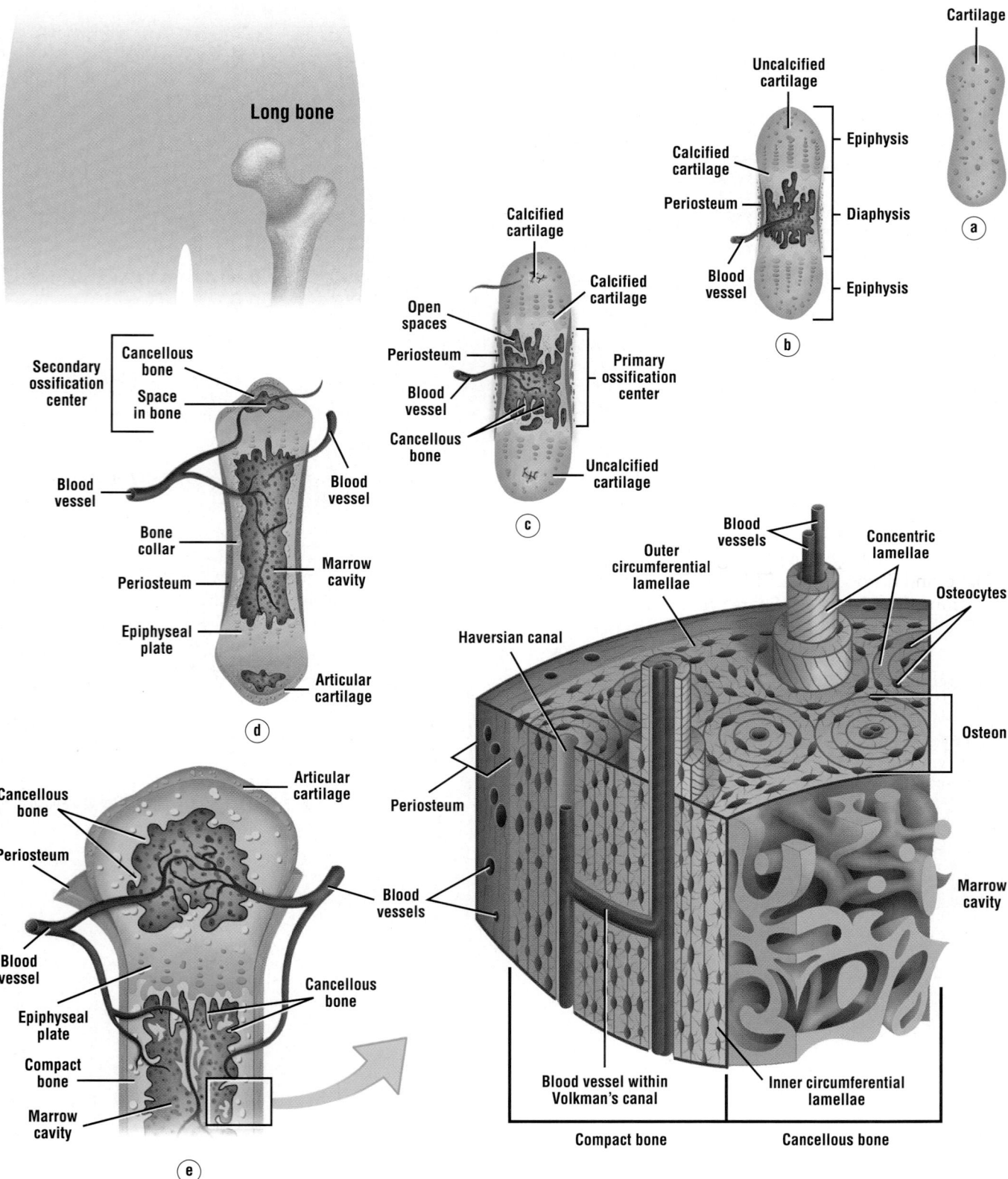

Long bone

Cartilage

Uncalcified cartilage

Calcified cartilage

Periosteum

Blood vessel

Epiphysis

Diaphysis

Epiphysis

(a)

(b)

Calcified cartilage

Calcified cartilage

Open spaces

Periosteum

Blood vessel

Cancellous bone

Primary ossification center

Uncalcified cartilage

(c)

Secondary ossification center

Cancellous bone

Space in bone

Blood vessel

Blood vessel

Bone collar

Periosteum

Marrow cavity

Epiphyseal plate

Articular cartilage

(d)

Articular cartilage

Cancellous bone

Periosteum

Blood vessel

Epiphyseal plate

Compact bone

Marrow cavity

Cancellous bone

(e)

Blood vessels

Concentric lamellae

Outer circumferential lamellae

Osteocytes

Haversian canal

Osteon

Periosteum

Blood vessels

Marrow cavity

Blood vessel within Volkman's canal

Inner circumferential lamellae

Compact bone

Cancellous bone

Cartilage and Bone

SECTION 1
Cartilage

Cartilage is a special form of connective tissue that has the main function of supporting soft tissues. It consists of **cells** (chondrocytes and chondroblasts) and the **matrix** (fibers and ground substance). The matrix contains **collagen** or **elastic fibers,** which give the cartilage its firmness and resilience. As a result, cartilage exhibits tensile strength, provides structural support, and allows flexibility without distortion.

TYPES OF CARTILAGE: HYALINE, ELASTIC, AND FIBROCARTILAGE

There are three types of cartilage in the body: hyaline, elastic, and fibrocartilage. This classification is based on the amount and types of fibers present in the matrix.

The **hyaline cartilage** is the most common type in the body. In the embryo, hyaline cartilage serves as a **skeletal model** for most bones, which form by the process of **endochondral ossification.** In adults, most of the hyaline cartilage has been replaced by bone, except on the articular surfaces of bones, ends of ribs (costal cartilage), nose, larynx, and the trachea, as well as in the bronchi.

Elastic cartilage is similar to hyaline cartilage, except that numerous elastic fibers are present in its matrix. Elastic cartilage is found in the external ear, in the walls of the auditory tube, in the epiglottis, and in the larynx.

Fibrocartilage is characterized by the presence of irregular, dense bundles of collagen fibers. In contrast to other cartilage types, fibrocartilage consists of alternating layers of cartilage matrix and thick dense layers of collagen fibers. The collagen fibers exhibit an orientation in the direction of functional stresses. Fibrocartilage is found in the intervertebral disks, the symphysis pubis, and certain joints.

Most of the cartilage in the body is surrounded by a layer of connective tissue called the **perichondrium.** An exception to this is the hyaline cartilage on the articulating surfaces of the bones. Also, because it is always associated with dense connective tissue, the fibrocartilage does not exhibit an identifiable perichondrium.

Figure 3-1   Fetal Hyaline Cartilage

This figure illustrates a cartilage model of a bone in an early stage of development. Most of the model consists of young **chondroblasts (1)** that still resemble mesenchymal cells, having spherical nuclei and cytoplasmic processes. Lacunae have not developed at this stage. The chondroblasts are numerous, crowded into a specific area, and randomly distributed in the cartilage without forming isogenous groups. At this stage of development, cartilage **matrix (3)** is secreted.

On the periphery of the cartilage model (left side), mesenchymal cells are concentrated and exhibit a parallel arrangement **(2)**. The nuclei of these cells are elongated and flattened, and the cell membranes are not distinct. This peripheral area of the cartilage develops into perichondrium, a sheath of dense connective tissue that surrounds hyaline and elastic cartilage. The inner portion of perichondrium is the chondrogenic layer from which chondroblasts (2) develop; there is some indication of such transition in the illustration.

Figure 3-2   Mature Hyaline Cartilage

This section illustrates an interior or central region of the hyaline cartilage. Distributed throughout the homogeneous ground substance, the **matrix (5, 6)**, are ovoid spaces called **lacunae (2)** with mature cartilage cells, the **chondrocytes (1)**. In intact cartilage, chondrocytes fill the lacunae. Each cell has a granular cytoplasm and a **nucleus (3)**. During histologic preparations, however, the chondrocytes (1) shrink and the lacunae (2) appear as clear spaces. Cartilage cells in the matrix are observed either singly or in isogenous groups.

The **matrix (6)** appears homogeneous and is usually basophilic; however, this condition can vary. The matrix between cells or groups of cells is called **interterritorial matrix (6)**. The more basophilic matrix around the cartilage cells is the **territorial matrix (5)**. Around each of the lacunae, the matrix forms a thin **cartilage capsule (4)**.

Figure 3-3   Hyaline Cartilage of the Trachea

This illustration depicts lacunae with **chondrocytes** appearing either singly **(12)** or in **isogenous groups (13)**. Because the chondrocytes fill their lacunae, only margins of lacunae, the **cartilage capsules (16)**, are visible. Lacunae and chondrocytes in the middle of the cartilage are large and spherical (12, 13), but become progressively flatter in the periphery; these flat cells are young chondrocytes **(11)**.

The **interterritorial** (intercellular) **matrix (14)** stains lighter, whereas the **territorial matrix (15)** stains deeper.

A **perichondrium (4, 9, 18)** of dense connective tissue surrounds the entire cartilage plate. Its inner layer is **chondrogenic (10)** where the chondrocytes are formed by proliferation and differentiation of mesenchymal cells **(17)**.

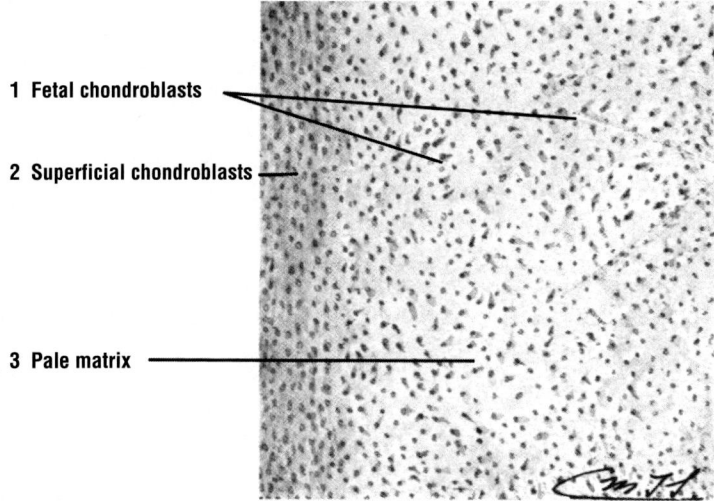

1 Fetal chondroblasts

2 Superficial chondroblasts

3 Pale matrix

Fig. 3-1   Fetal Hyaline Cartilage. Stain: hematoxylin-eosin. Low magnification.

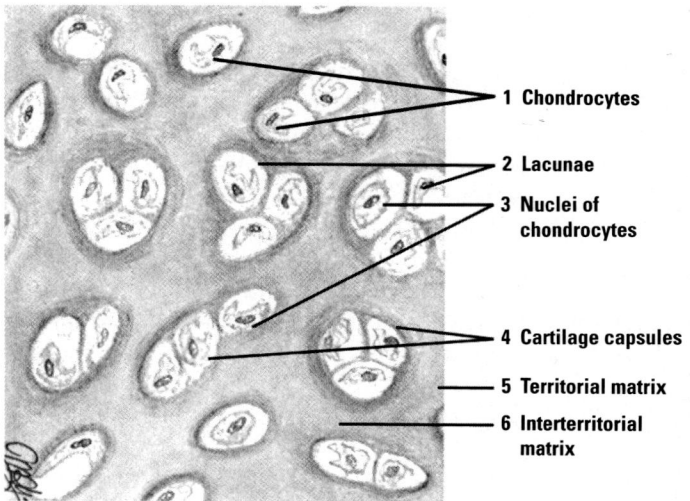

1 Chondrocytes

2 Lacunae

3 Nuclei of chondrocytes

4 Cartilage capsules

5 Territorial matrix

6 Interterritorial matrix

Fig. 3-2   Mature Hyaline Cartilage. Stain: hematoxylin-eosin. High magnification.

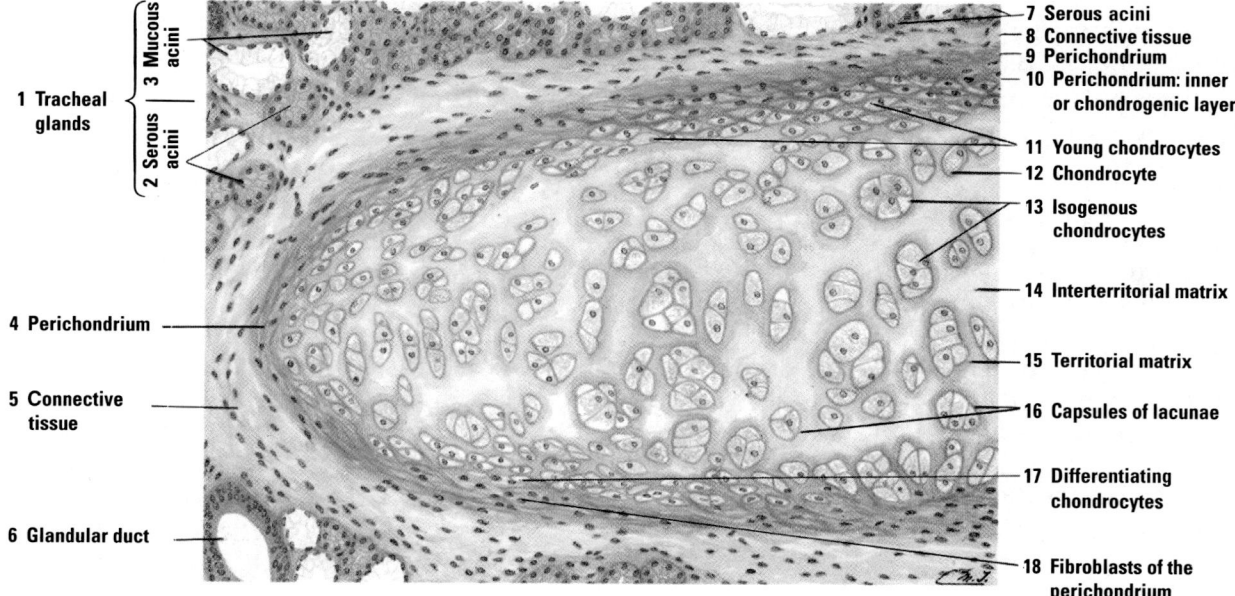

1 Tracheal glands

3 Mucous acini

2 Serous acini

4 Perichondrium

5 Connective tissue

6 Glandular duct

7 Serous acini
8 Connective tissue
9 Perichondrium
10 Perichondrium: inner or chondrogenic layer

11 Young chondrocytes
12 Chondrocyte

13 Isogenous chondrocytes

14 Interterritorial matrix

15 Territorial matrix

16 Capsules of lacunae

17 Differentiating chondrocytes

18 Fibroblasts of the perichondrium

Fig. 3-3   Hyaline Cartilage of the Trachea. Stain: hematoxylin-eosin. Medium magnification.

Figure 3-4   Fibrous Cartilage: Intervertebral Disk

In fibrous cartilage, the matrix (6) is permeated with **collagen fibers (5),** which frequently exhibit parallel fiber arrangement, as seen in tendons. Small **chondrocytes (2, 4)** in **lacunae (1)** are usually distributed in **rows (3)** within the fibrous matrix rather than at random or in isogenous groups, as is normally seen in hyaline or elastic cartilage. All chondrocytes and lacunae are of similar size; there is no gradation from larger central chondrocytes to smaller and flatter peripheral cells.

A perichondrium, normally present around hyaline and elastic cartilage, is absent because fibrous cartilage usually forms a transitional area between hyaline cartilage and tendon or ligament.

The proportion of collagen fibers to matrix, the number of chondrocytes, and their arrangement may vary. The collagen fibers may be so dense that matrix becomes invisible; in such cases, chondrocytes and lacunae appear flattened. Fibers within a bundle may be parallel, but bundles may course in many directions.

Figure 3-5   Elastic Cartilage: Epiglottis

Elastic cartilage differs from hyaline cartilage principally by the presence of **elastic fibers (1, 3)** in its matrix. After staining the cartilage with orcein (3), these are visible as deep purple fibers. The fibers enter the cartilagenous matrix from the **perichondrium (4),** usually as small fibers, and are distributed in the interior as branching and anastomosing fibers of varying size (3). Some of the fibers exhibit considerable thickness (3, middle leader). The density of fibers in the matrix varies among elastic cartilages as well as among different areas of the same cartilage.

As in hyaline cartilage, larger **chondrocytes (2, 5)** in lacunae are seen in the interior of the plate. The smaller ones are more peripheral; the latter finally become fibroblasts in the perichondrium (4).

■ Functional Correlations–Cartilage

Cartilage develops from **mesenchyme cells** that differentiate into **chondroblasts.** These cells divide mitotically, grow, and synthesize the cartilage **matrix** and the **extracellular material.** Gradually, individual chondroblasts become surrounded by the extracellular matrix and trapped in compartments called **lacunae** (singular, *lacuna*). These are the mature cartilage cells called **chondrocytes,** whose function is to maintain the cartilage matrix. Some lacunae may contain more than one chondrocyte; these groups of chondrocytes are called **isogenous groups.** Mesenchyme cells can also differentiate into **fibroblasts,** which form the **perichondrium,** a connective tissue that invests the cartilage. The inner layer of perichondrium contains **chondrogenic cells,** which can differentiate into chondroblasts.

Cartilage is **non-vascular,** but it is surrounded by vascular connective tissue. All nutrients enter and metabolites leave the cartilage by **diffusion** through the matrix. Also, because its matrix is soft and pliable, and not as hard as bone, cartilage grows by two different means simultaneously: interstitially and appositionally. **Interstitial growth** involves mitosis of the chondrocytes within the matrix and the deposition of new matrix between the cells. This process increases the cartilage size from within. **Appositional growth** occurs peripherally: chondroblasts differentiate from the inner connective tissue perichondrium and deposit a layer of cartilage that is apposed to the existing cartilage layer.

In those organs where hyaline cartilage is found, it provides important structural and flexible support. Elastic cartilage, due to the presence of elastic fibers, allows increased flexibility and support to the organs. The presence of fibrocartilage is important in the areas where durability, tensile strength, weight bearing, and resistance to stretch or compression are essential.

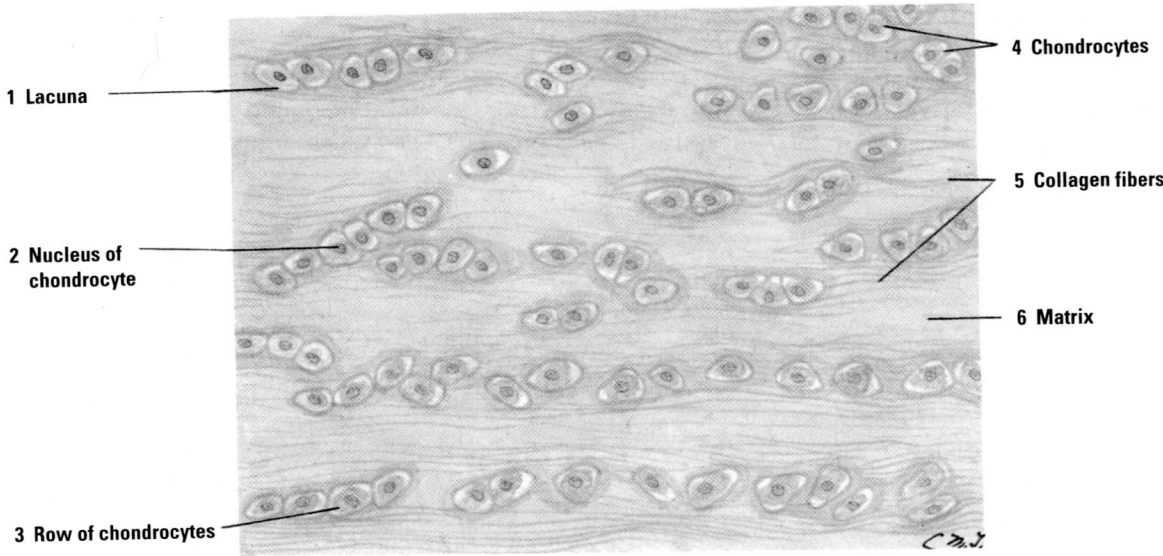

1 Lacuna

2 Nucleus of chondrocyte

3 Row of chondrocytes

4 Chondrocytes

5 Collagen fibers

6 Matrix

Fig. 3-4   Fibrous Cartilage: Intervertebral Disk. Stain: hematoxylin-eosin. High magnification.

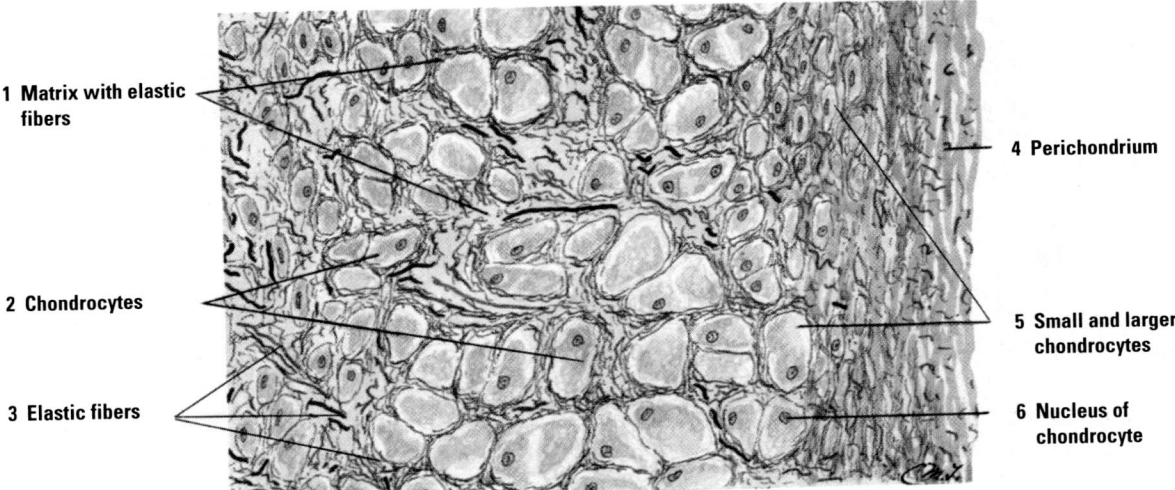

1 Matrix with elastic fibers

2 Chondrocytes

3 Elastic fibers

4 Perichondrium

5 Small and larger chondrocytes

6 Nucleus of chondrocyte

Fig. 3-5   Elastic Cartilage: Epiglottis. Stain: hematoxylin-eosin. High magnification.

Figure 3-6   Hyaline Cartilage: Developing Bone

A photomicrograph of a section through a developing bone shows a portion of the hyaline cartilage and its characteristic homogenous **matrix (1).** Located within the matrix (1) are the mature hyaline cartilage cells **chondrocytes (3)** in their **lacunae (2).** Surrounding the hyaline cartilage is the dense, irregular connective tissue **perichondrium (5).** On inner surface of the perichondrium (5) is the **chondrogenic layer (4).**

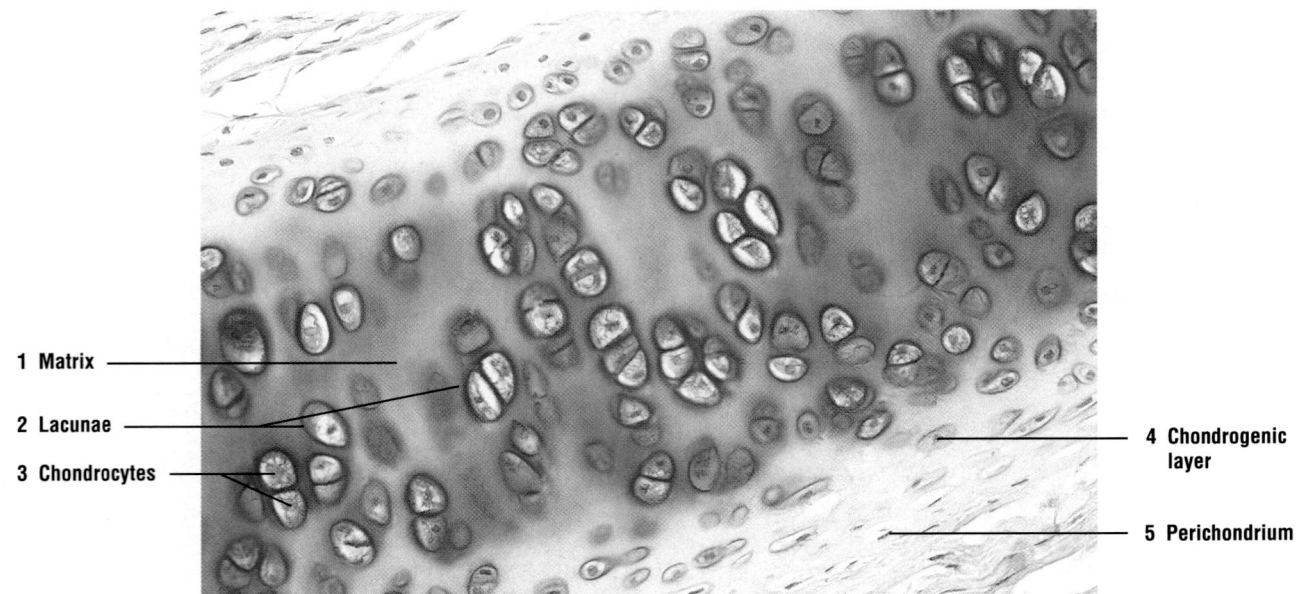

1 Matrix

2 Lacunae

3 Chondrocytes

4 Chondrogenic layer

5 Perichondrium

Fig. 3-6   Hyaline Cartilage: Developing Bone. Stain: hematoxylin-eosin. 80×

Figure 3-7   Elastic Cartilage: Epiglottis

A photomicrograph of a section of an epiglottis shows that this type of structure is characterized by the presence of a cartilage with fine, branching **elastic fibers (2)** in its **matrix (5),** in addition to distinct **chondrocytes (3)** and **lacunae (4).** Presence of elastic fibers (2) gives this cartilage flexibility in addition to support. Surrounding the elastic cartilage is a layer of dense, irregular connective tissue **perichondrium (1).**

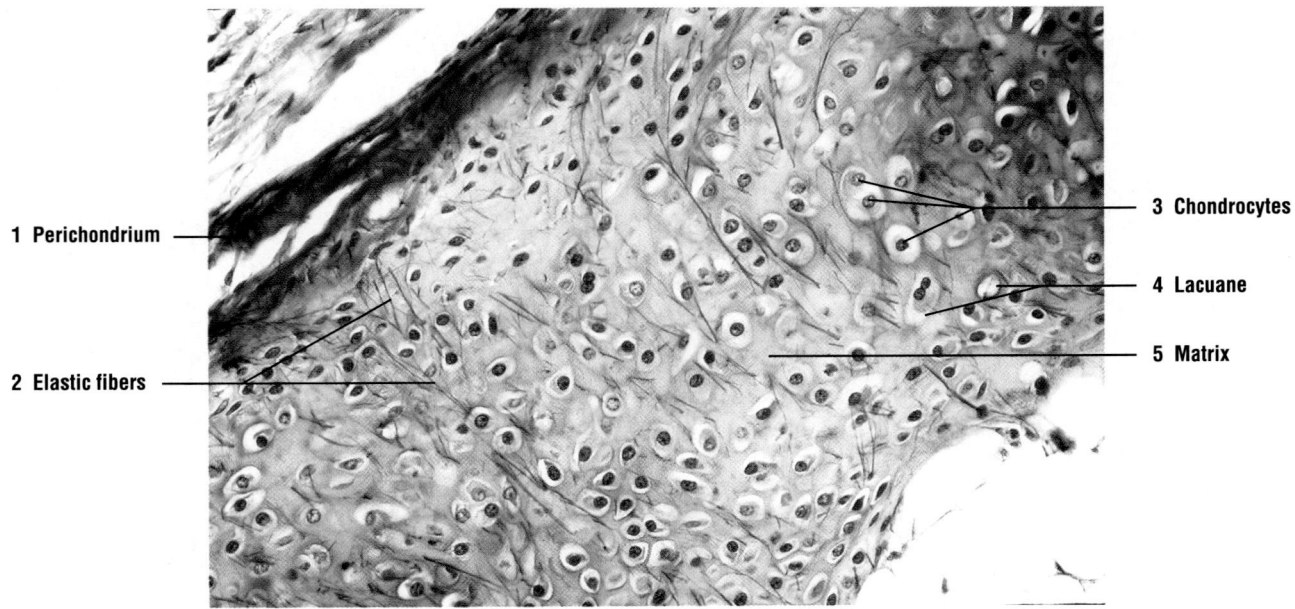

1 Perichondrium

2 Elastic fibers

3 Chondrocytes

4 Lacuane

5 Matrix

Fig. 3-7   Elastic Cartilage: Epiglottis. Stain: silver. 80×

SECTION 2
Bone

Bone is also a special form of connective tissue. Like other connective tissues, bones consist of **cells, fibers,** and **matrix.** Because of mineral deposition in their matrix, bones can bear weight, serve as a rigid skeleton for the body, and provide sites of attachment for muscles and organs. Bones also provide protection for the brain in the skull, heart and lungs in the thorax, and the urinary and reproductive organs between the pelvic bones. In addition, the bones function in **hemopoiesis** (blood cell formation) and serve as **reservoirs** for calcium, phosphate, and other minerals. Almost all (99%) of the calcium in the body is stored in bones, and the body receives some of its daily calcium needs from this source.

THE PROCESS OF BONE FORMATION (OSSIFICATION)

Bone development begins in the embryo by two distinct processes: intramembranous ossification and endochondral ossification. Bones produced by the two different methods, however, have the same histologic structures.

Endochondral Ossification (Figures 3-8–3-12)

Endochondral ossification forms most of the bones of the skeleton. Each bone is first preceded by a temporary **hyaline cartilage model.** This model first continues to grow; then the chondrocytes hypertrophy and mature, and the growing cartilage model **calcifies.** As the cartilage calcifies, **diffusion** of nutrients and gases through the calcified matrix decreases. As a result, the chondrocytes die and the fragmented calcified matrix then begins to serve as a structural framework for the deposition of the bony material. The calcified cartilage is then replaced by bone.

Osteoprogenitor cells** and blood vessels from the surrounding connective tissue **periosteum** invade the calcified and degenerating cartilage model. Osteoprogenitor cells proliferate and give rise to **osteoblasts.** Mesenchyme tissue, osteoblasts, and blood vessels form an **ossification center** in the developing bone. In developing long bones, there is first an appearance of **primary ossification center** in the **diaphysis,** which is followed by a **secondary ossification center** in the epi-

physis. Osteoid matrix** is then produced and mineralized into bone. In long bones, the cartilage in the diaphysis and epiphysis is replaced by bone, except in the epiphyseal plate region. Growth in this region is responsible for continued growth of bone until maturity is reached and bone growth stops. Expansion of the ossification centers eventually replaces all cartilage model with bone tissue, except over the free ends of the long bones. Here, a layer of permanent hyaline cartilage covers the bone as the **articular cartilage.**

Intramembranous Ossification (Figures 3-13, 3-14)

In **intramembranous ossification,** bone develops not from a cartilage model, but from the connective tissue **mesenchyme.** Some of the mesenchyme cells differentiate directly into **osteoblasts** and produce the bony matrix. The **mandible, maxilla, clavicles,** and most of the flat bones of the **skull** are formed by the intramembranous method. In the developing skull, the centers of bone development grow radially, replace the connective tissue, and then fuse. In newborns, the **fontanelles** in the skull are the soft membranous regions where intramembranous ossification of skull bones has not been completed.

Bone Matrix (Figures 3-15–3-19)

Because the mineralized bone matrix is much harder than cartilage, nutrients and metabolites cannot freely diffuse through it to the bone cells. Consequently, bones become highly vascular and exhibit a unique system of channels or canals called **canaliculi.** Cytoplasmic processes from osteocytes that are now located in their individual lacunae extend into the canaliculi, which radiate in all directions from each lacuna. The canaliculi contain extracellular fluid, and the cytoplasmic extensions allow individual osteocytes to communicate with adjacent osteocytes and with materials present in the blood vessels that supply the bone matrix. In this manner, the canaliculi allow for a very efficient exchange mechanism: nutrients are brought to the osteocytes, gaseous exchange takes place between the blood and cells, and metabolic wastes are removed from the osteocytes.

Figure 3-8   Endochondral Ossification: Developing Long Bone (panoramic view, longitudinal section)

In the process of endochondral ossification, the future bone is first formed as a model composed of embryonic hyaline cartilage. As development progresses, the cartilage model is gradually replaced by bone. In the center of the illustration, this process has already begun. In addition, most of the original spongy bone that was formed has been replaced and resorbed to form the central marrow cavity, leaving only scattered, thin spicules of **bone of endochondral origin (11, 30)**. **Red marrow (13)** now fills the cavity of newly formed bone with hemopoietic (blood-forming) cells. The fine reticular connective tissue fibers are obscured by masses of developing erythrocytes, granulocytes, **megakaryocytes (14)**, numerous **sinusoids (12)**, capillaries, and blood vessels.

The process of endochondral ossification can be followed from the upper part of the illustration downward to the central marrow cavity. In the uppermost region is seen the zone of **reserve hyaline cartilage (17)**, in which the **chondrocytes in lacunae (2)** are distributed singly or in small groups. Chondrocytes then proliferate rapidly and become arranged in **columns (3, 18)**; cells and lacunae increase in size toward the lower area of this **zone of proliferating cartilage (18)**. The chondrocytes then **hypertrophy (19)** because of the swelling of nucleus and cytoplasm. The **lacunae** enlarge **(4)**, the cells degenerate, and the thin partitions of intervening cartilage matrix calcify **(20)**. The calcified cartilage stains a deep purple.

Tufts of **vascular marrow (5)** invade the **zone of calcifying cartilage (20)**, erode the lacunar walls and the calcified cartilage **(20)**, and form new, small marrow cavities. Osteoprogenitor cells from the **inner periosteum (9)** differentiate into osteoblasts and deposit **osteoid** and **bone (6)** around the remaining spicules of calcified cartilage **(6)**. This region in the developing bone is now the **zone of ossification (21)**.

The lower, lateral two-thirds of the illustration shows the development of periosteal bone. Osteoblasts differentiate from osteoprogenitor cells in the inner layer of the periosteum (9) and form a **bone collar (10)**. Formation of new **periosteal bone (22)** keeps pace with formation of new endochondral bone. The bone collar (10) increases in thickness and compactness as development of bone proceeds. The thickest portion of the bone collar (10) is seen in the central part of the diaphysis at the initial site of **periosteal bone (29)** formation around the primary ossification center.

Surrounding the shaft of the developing bone are soft tissues: **muscle (7), subcutaneous connective tissue,** and **dermis of skin (15, 25)**. The skin, lined on the external surface by the **epidermis (24)**, contains a few **hair follicles (26), sebaceous glands (28),** and **sweat glands (16)**.

1 **Perichondrium**

2 **Chondrocytes in lacunae**

3 **Column of chondrocytes**

4 **Hypertrophied chondrocytes and calcified matrix**

5 **Vascular tufts of osteogenic marrow**

6 **Osteoid and bone around calcified cartilage**

7 **Muscle**

8 **Periosteum (outer layer)**

9 **Periosteum (inner layer with osteoblasts)**

10 **Periosteal bone (bone collar)**

11 **Spicules of bone**

12 **Sinusoid**

13 **Red bone marrow**

14 **Megakaryocytes**

15 **Subcutaneous connective tissue and dermis**

16 **Sweat gland**

17 **Zone of reserve cartilage**

18 **Zone of proliferating hyaline cartilage**

19 **Zone of hypertrophying cells and lacunae**

20 **Zone of calcifying cartilage**

21 **Zone of erosion and ossification**

22 **New periosteal bone**

23 **Younger and older bony spicules**

24 **Epidermis**

25 **Dermis and subcutaneous layer**

26 **Hair follicles**

27 **Primitive marrow cavities in periosteal bone**

28 **Sebaceous gland**

29 **Periosteal bone**

30 **Spicules of bone**

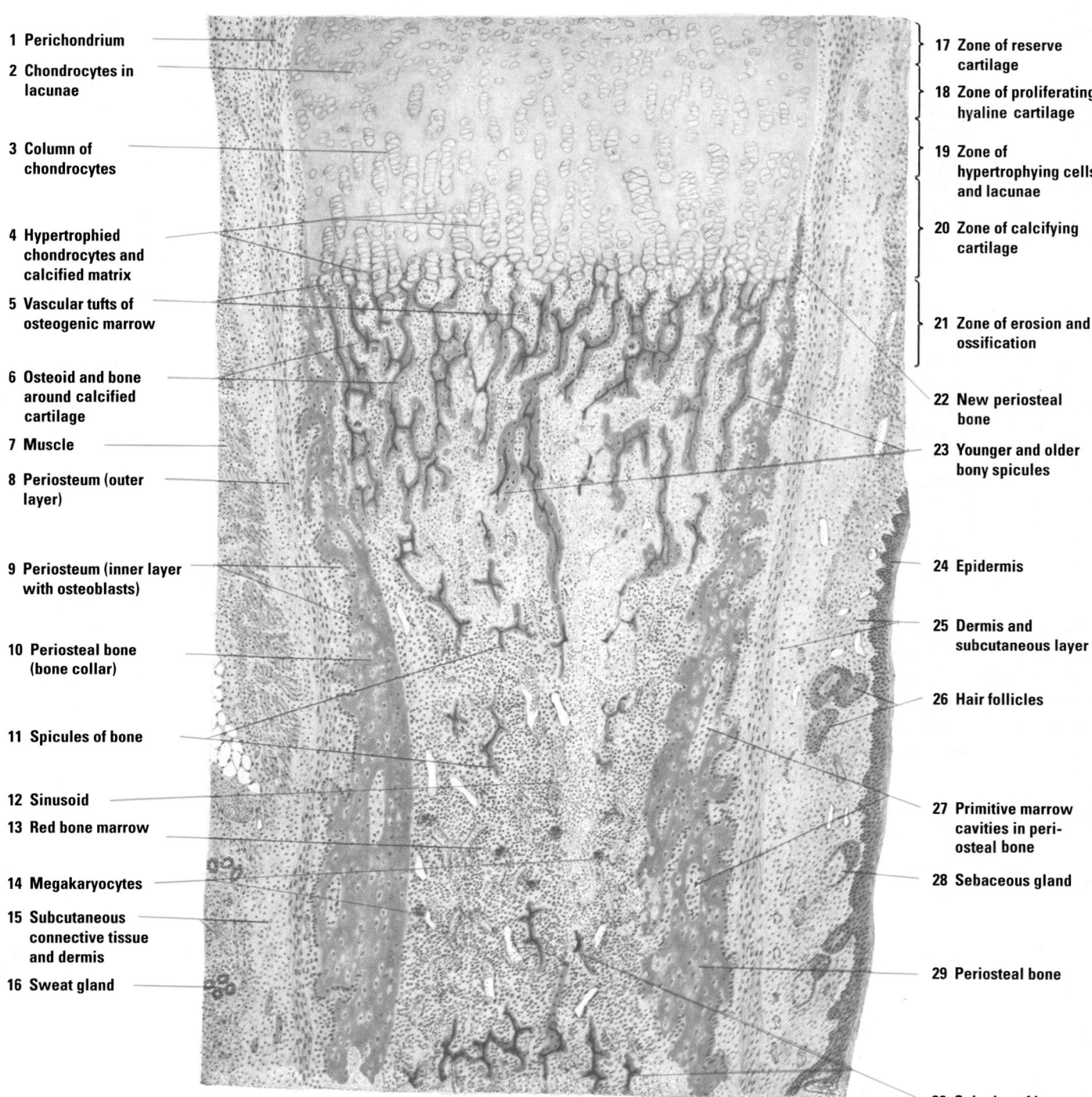

Fig. 3-8   Endochondral Ossification: Developing Long Bone (panoramic view, longitudinal section). Stain: hematoxylin-eosin. Low magnification.

Figure 3-9   Endochondral Ossification: Zone of Ossification

A higher magnification of endochondral ossification illustrates the process in greater detail. The region shown in this figure corresponds to the zone of ossification and adjacent areas (labelled 3 through 6 in Fig. 3-13).

Proliferating **chondrocytes (1, 14)** are arranged in distinct columns. Below the proliferating chondrocytes is the zone of **hypertrophied chondrocytes (2, 15).** Hypertrophy of chondrocytes occurs because of increased glycogen and lipid accumulations in the cytoplasm and nuclear swelling; lacunae also hypertrophy simultaneously. The cytoplasm of hypertrophied chondrocytes then becomes **vacuolized (16),** the nuclei become pyknotic, and the thin cartilage partitions become surrounded by **calcified matrix (5, 17).**

Tufts of **capillaries (8, 18)** from the **marrow cavity (10)** invade this area and form the zone of erosion. **Osteoblasts (6, 20)** are formed and line up along remaining spicules of calcified cartilage (5, 17), and lay down **osteoid (19)** and bone. Osteoblasts trapped in the osteoid or bone become **osteocytes (9, 21).**

The marrow cavity (10) contains pluripotential stem cells which give rise to **blood cells (23)** belonging to the erythrocytic and granulocytic series as well as **megakaryocytes (13, 24).** Multinucleated **osteoclasts (11, 22),** which lie in shallow depressions called the **Howship's lacunae (11, 22),** are situated adjacent to bone that is being resorbed.

On the left side of the illustration is an area of **periosteal bone (7)** with osteocytes (9) in the lacunae. The new bone is added peripherally by osteoblasts (6), which develop from osteoprogenitor cells of the **inner periosteum (12).** The outer layer of periosteum continues as the connective tissue **perichondrium (3),** passing superiorly over the cartilage that has not changed into bone.

Figure 3-10   Endochondral Ossification: Zone of Ossification

This photomicrograph illustrates the transformation of hyaline cartilage into bone through endochondral ossification. In the **hyaline cartilage matrix (6)** are seen the **proliferating chondrocytes (7)** and the **hypertrophied chondrocytes (1)** with **vacuolated cytoplasm (2).** Below these cells are the **spicules of calcified cartilage (3)** that are surrounded by bone-producing cells, **osteoblasts (4).** As the cartilage calcifies, a **marrow cavity (5)** is formed, in which are seen blood vessels, **hematopoietic tissue (10),** osteogenic cells, and osteoblasts (4). The hyaline cartilage is surrounded by the connective tissue **perichondrium (8).** The marrow cavity with the forming bony tissue is surrounded by the connective tissue **periosteum (9).**

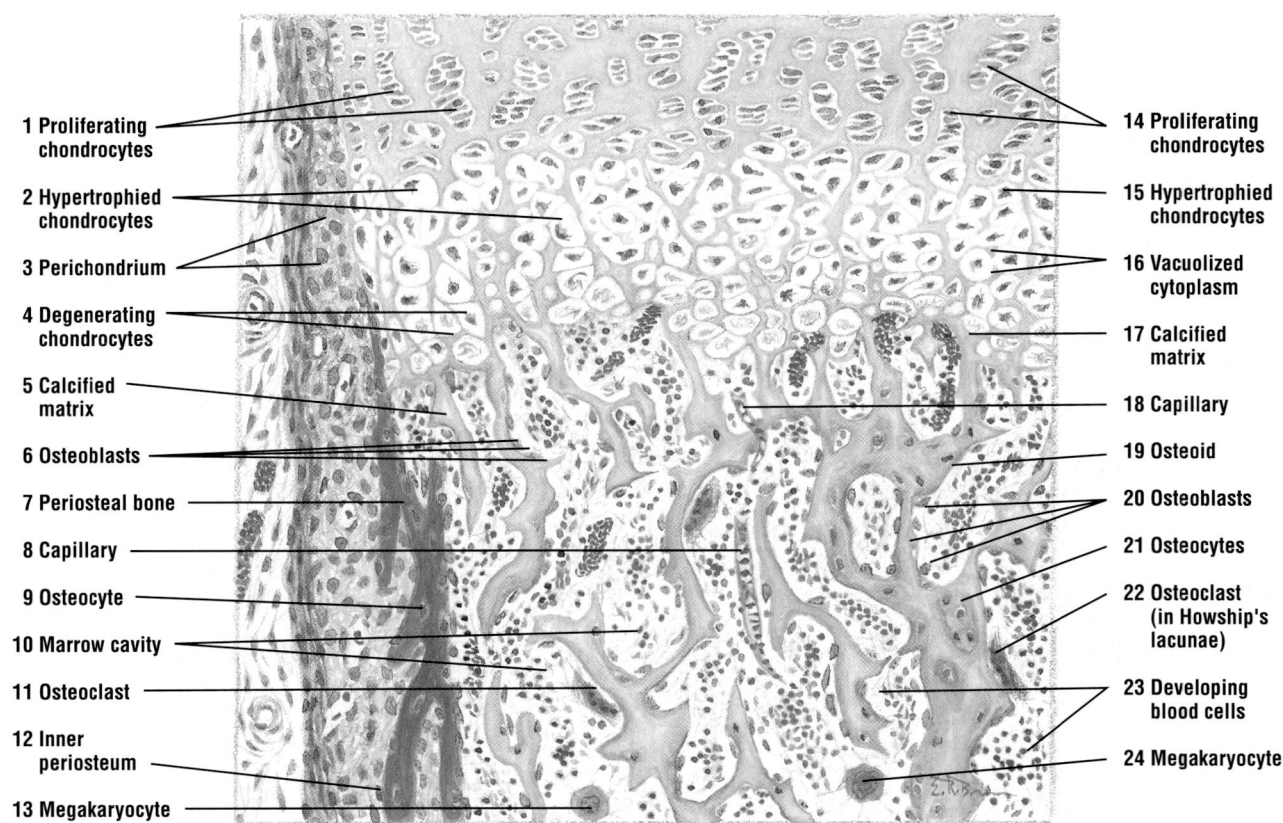

1 Proliferating chondrocytes
2 Hypertrophied chondrocytes
3 Perichondrium
4 Degenerating chondrocytes
5 Calcified matrix
6 Osteoblasts
7 Periosteal bone
8 Capillary
9 Osteocyte
10 Marrow cavity
11 Osteoclast
12 Inner periosteum
13 Megakaryocyte

14 Proliferating chondrocytes
15 Hypertrophied chondrocytes
16 Vacuolized cytoplasm
17 Calcified matrix
18 Capillary
19 Osteoid
20 Osteoblasts
21 Osteocytes
22 Osteoclast (in Howship's lacunae)
23 Developing blood cells
24 Megakaryocyte

Fig. 3-9   Endochondral Ossification: Zone of Ossification. Stain: hematoxylin-eosin. Medium magnification.

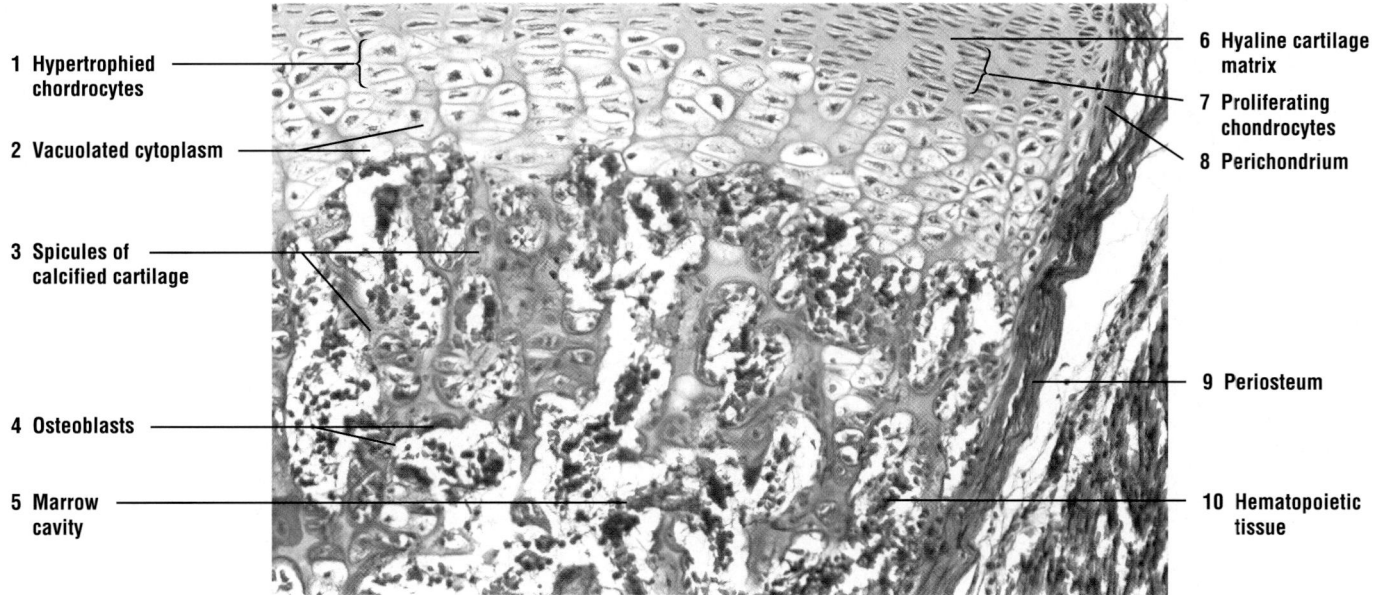

1 Hypertrophied chondrocytes
2 Vacuolated cytoplasm
3 Spicules of calcified cartilage
4 Osteoblasts
5 Marrow cavity

6 Hyaline cartilage matrix
7 Proliferating chondrocytes
8 Perichondrium
9 Periosteum
10 Hematopoietic tissue

Fig. 3-10   Endochondral Ossification: Zone of Ossification. Stain: hematoxylin-eosin. 50×

Figure 3-11   Formation of Bone: Secondary (Epiphyseal) Ossification Centers (longitudinal section, decalcified)

The cartilage in the epiphyseal ends (articular cartilages) of two developing bones is illustrated. Both bones contain a **secondary center of ossification (2, 6).** The ossification center (2) in the upper bone is in an earlier stage of development than that in the lower bone (6). The **synovial** or **joint cavity (5, 11)** is located between the two developing cartilage models.

In the upper epiphysis, the peripheral or superficial **articular cartilage (3)** with flattened chondrocytes and lacunae is visible. Toward the center of the cartilage, the chondrocytes and lacunae are rounder. At the margins of the calcification center, the chondrocytes show **hypertrophy (10)** in preparation for ossification. Small spicules of red-stained bone and primitive marrow cavities are seen in the center of ossification (2).

Similar structural components and changes are visible in the secondary center of ossification **(6, 13–15)** in the lower bone. **Bony spicules (13)** are larger and more numerous because the secondary center of ossification (6) is in a more advanced stage of development than that in the upper bone. A small area of ossification is apparent in the **metaphysis (9),** a transitional zone where cartilage is being replaced by bone. This area illustrates the typical features of the **zone of ossification (8, 9, 16, 17).** The connective tissue **periosteum** surrounds the developed bone on the right side **(18)** and on the left side (8, 9).

The synovial or joint cavity (5, 11) is covered by a joint capsule (a diarthritic joint). A portion of the outer fibrous layer of the **articular capsule (7)** is illustrated. The inner synovial membrane of squamous cells lines the cavity, except over the articular cartilages (3). The synovial membrane, together with the connective tissue of the capsule, may extend into the joint cavity as a simple **synovial projection (12)** or as more complex **synovial folds (4).**

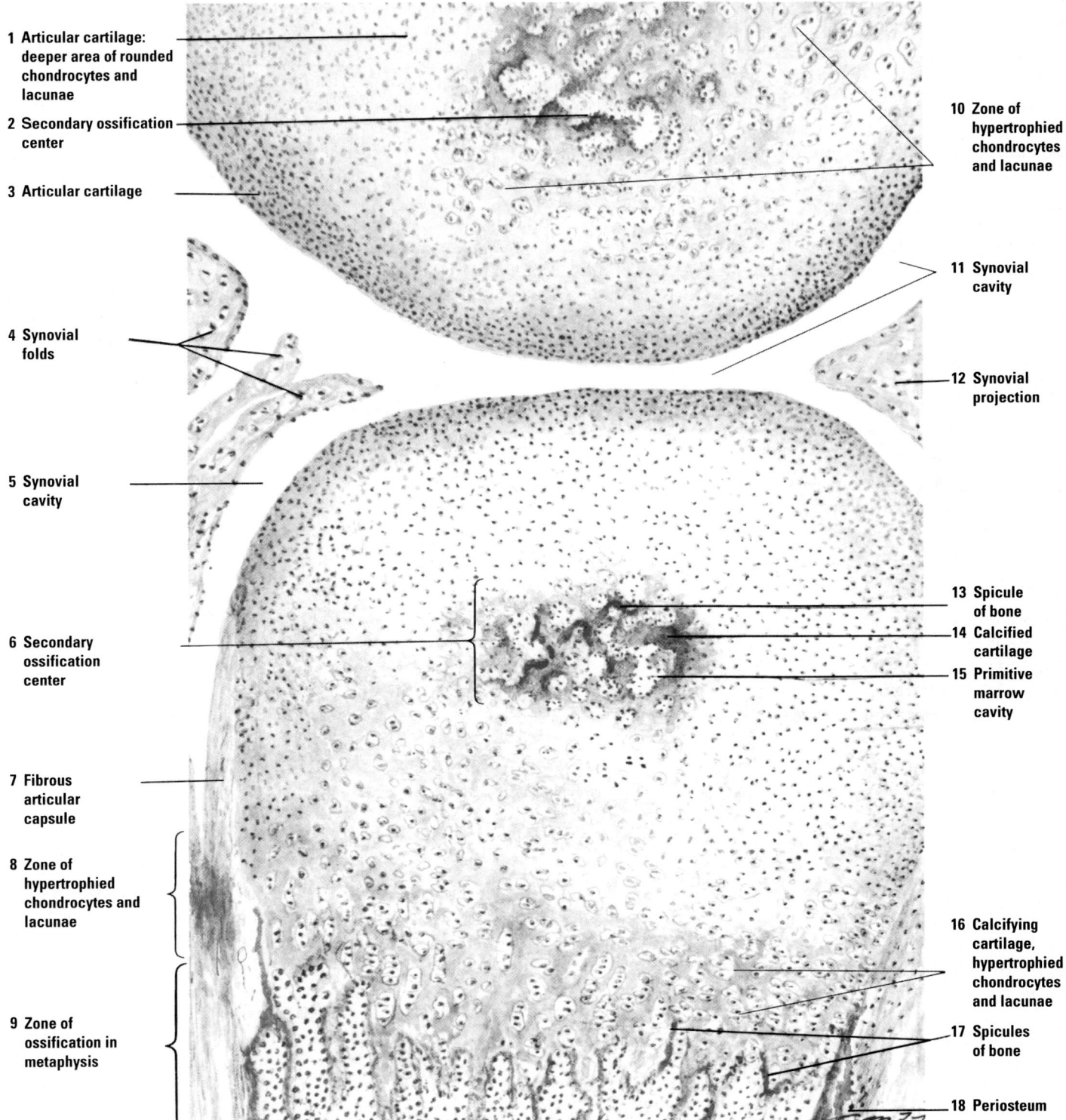

1 Articular cartilage: deeper area of rounded chondrocytes and lacunae

2 Secondary ossification center

3 Articular cartilage

4 Synovial folds

5 Synovial cavity

6 Secondary ossification center

7 Fibrous articular capsule

8 Zone of hypertrophied chondrocytes and lacunae

9 Zone of ossification in metaphysis

10 Zone of hypertrophied chondrocytes and lacunae

11 Synovial cavity

12 Synovial projection

13 Spicule of bone

14 Calcified cartilage

15 Primitive marrow cavity

16 Calcifying cartilage, hypertrophied chondrocytes and lacunae

17 Spicules of bone

18 Periosteum

Fig. 3-11   Formation of Bone: Secondary (Epiphyseal) Ossification Centers (longitudinal section, decalcified). Stain: hematoxylin-eosin. Low magnification.

Figure 3-12   Formation of Bone: Development of Osteons (Haversian Systems) (transverse section, decalcified)

This illustration represents a late stage in the development of compact bone. Primitive osteons (Haversian systems) have already formed, and others are in the process of development. In a long bone, such as in Figure 3-13, the initial compact bone is formed by deposition in the subperiosteal region (Fig. 3-13:29). Vascular tufts of connective tissue from periosteum or endosteum then invade and erode this bone and form primitive osteons, visible in this illustration. Bone reconstruction will continue as these initial osteons, and then later ones, are broken down, followed by the formation of new osteons.

This figure illustrates a section of immature compact bone whose **matrix (11)** is stained deep with eosin. Primitive osteons are visible in transverse section, with large **central (Haversian) canals (8)** surrounded by a few concentric **lamellae (3)** of bone and **osteocytes (1)**. The central (Haversian) canals contain primitive connective tissue and **blood vessels (6, 8)**. Bone deposition is continuing in some of these primitive osteons (8), as indicated by the presence of **osteoblasts (9)** along the central (Haversian) canal (8) periphery and the margin of the innermost bone lamella. In some of the primitive osteons, the **osteoclasts (2)** have already formed and are resorbing and remodeling the bone.

A longitudinal channel of **osteogenic connective tissue (10)** passes through the bone. From it arise tufts of vascular connective tissue, which give rise to new central (Haversian) canals (4). Osteoblasts (9) are already found along the periphery of the canal.

In the lower part of the figure is a large **bone marrow cavity (14)**, in which hemopoiesis (blood cell formation) is in progress; this is the red marrow. Also present in the bone marrow cavity (14) are developing erythrocytes and granulocytes, **megakaryocytes (16)**, **blood vessels (7)**, **bone spicules (15)**, and **osteoclasts (13)** in **Howship's lacunae (12)** along the wall of the bone.

■ Functional Correlations–Bone

Bones are **dynamic** structures; they are continually being renewed, remodeled, or both in response to the body's mineral needs, mechanical stresses, bone thinning caused by aging or disease, or fracture healing. Essential minerals are either stored in the bones or released into body fluids when needed for homeostasis. **Calcium** is essential for muscle contraction, blood coagulation, cell membrane permeability, transmission of nerve impulses, and other vital functions. Calcium releases into the blood stream from the bones, or its deposition in the bones depends on the **hormones** released from either the **parathyroid glands** or the **thyroid gland**, respectively. These hormones and their important functions are discussed in more detail in Chapter 16, "Endocrine System."

BONE CELLS

Developing and adult bones contain four different cell types: osteogenic (osteoprogenitor) cells, osteoblasts, osteocytes, and osteoclasts.

Osteogenic cells are undifferentiated, pleuropotential stem cells derived from the connective tissue mesenchyme. During bone development, osteogenic cells proliferate by mitosis and differentiate into osteoblasts. In mature bones, the osteogenic cells are found externally in the connective tissue **periosteum** and in the single layer of the internal **endosteum**. The periosteum and endosteum provide new osteoblasts for growth, remodeling, and repair of the bones.

Osteoblasts are present on the surfaces of bone tissue. They synthesize, secrete, and deposit the organic components of new bone matrix called **osteoid**. Osteoid is uncalcified, newly formed bone matrix that does not contain any minerals; however, shortly after its deposition, it undergoes rapid mineralization and becomes bone.

Osteocytes are the principal cells of the bone. Like the chondrocytes in cartilage, osteocytes are trapped by the surrounding bone matrix and lie within **lacunae**. In contrast to cartilage, however, only one osteocyte is found in each lacuna. The main function of the osteocytes is the maintenance of bone matrix.

Osteoclasts are large, multinucleated cells that are found along the bone surfaces where resorption, remodeling, and repair of bone take place. Their main function is to resorb bone during remodeling. Osteoclasts are often located on the resorbed or enzymatically etched shallow depressions in the bone, which are called Howship's lacunae. Osteoclasts originate in the bone from precursors that resemble monocytes.

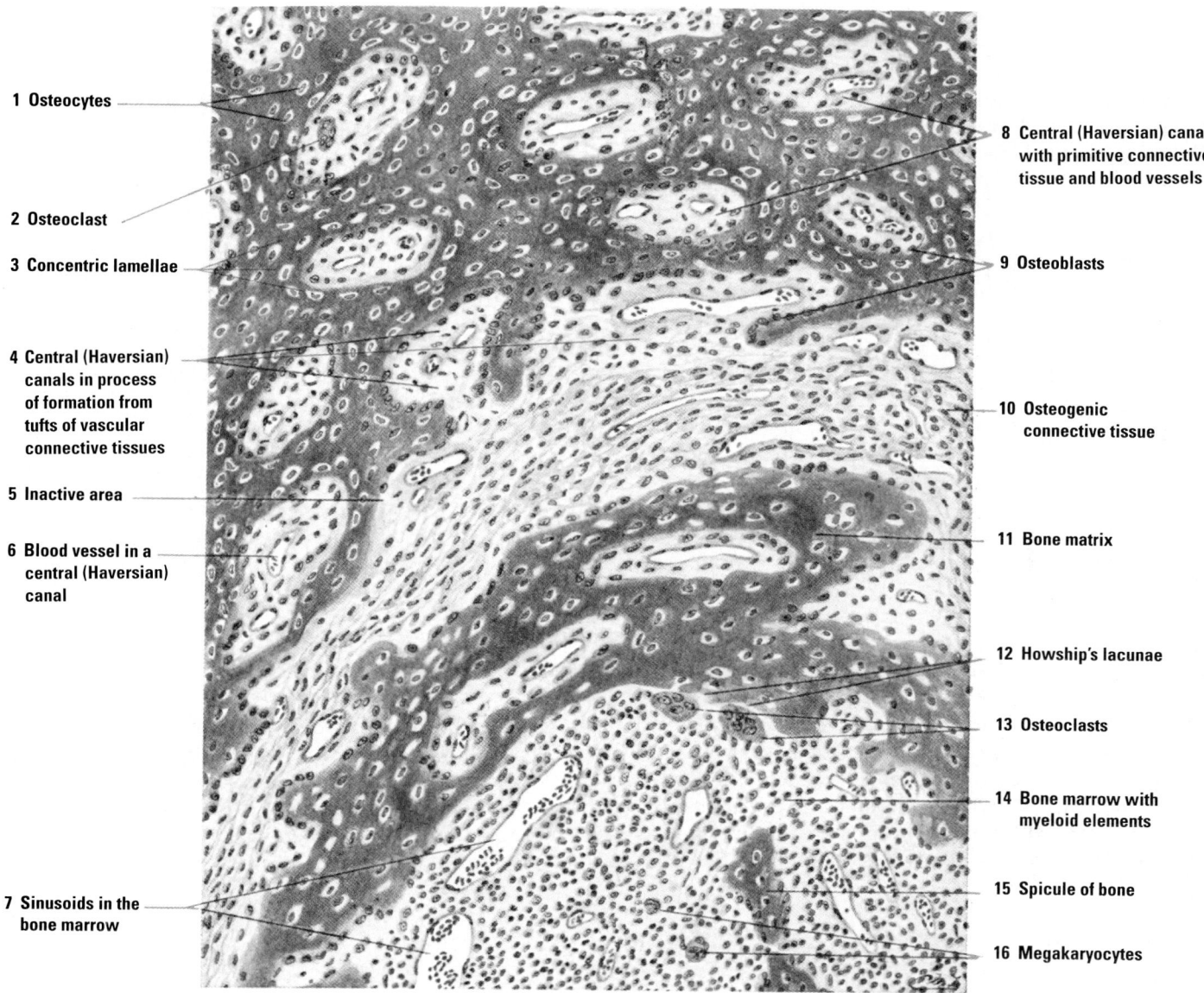

1 Osteocytes

2 Osteoclast

3 Concentric lamellae

4 Central (Haversian) canals in process of formation from tufts of vascular connective tissues

5 Inactive area

6 Blood vessel in a central (Haversian) canal

7 Sinusoids in the bone marrow

8 Central (Haversian) canals with primitive connective tissue and blood vessels

9 Osteoblasts

10 Osteogenic connective tissue

11 Bone matrix

12 Howship's lacunae

13 Osteoclasts

14 Bone marrow with myeloid elements

15 Spicule of bone

16 Megakaryocytes

Fig. 3-12   Formation of Bone: Development of Osteons (Haversian Systems) (transverse section, decalcified). Stain: hematoxylin-eosin. Medium magnification.

Figure 3-13   Intramembranous Ossification: Developing Mandible (transverse section, decalcified)

The upper left part of this illustration depicts the gum that covers the developing mandible. The mucosa of the gum consists of **stratified squamous epithelium (1)** situated above the **lamina propria (2),** a wide connective tissue with blood vessels and nerves.

Below the lamina propria (2) is the developing bone. The cells in the **periosteum (3)** have differentiated into **osteoblasts (12)** and formed the numerous anastomosing **trabeculae of bone (18)**. These trabeculae surround the primitive **marrow cavities (14)** of various sizes. Located within the marrow cavities are embryonic connective tissue, blood vessels, and nerves (16). Peripherally, collagen fibers of the periosteum (3) are in continuity with the fibers of the embryonic connective tissue of adjacent **marrow cavities (6)** and with collagen fibers within the **bone trabeculae (10).**

Osteoblasts (7, 15) actively deposit in the bony matrix and are seen in linear arrangement along the developing bone trabeculae (18). **Osteoclasts (5, 8)** are multinucleated giant cells associated with bone resorption and remodeling. The **osteocytes (4, 9)** are bone cells located in lacunae of the bone trabeculae (18).

Although collagen fibers embedded in the bony matrix are obscured, the continuity with embryonic connective tissue fibers in the marrow cavities may be seen at the margins of numerous trabeculae (13).

Formation of new bone is not a continuous process. Inactive areas appear where ossification has temporarily ceased; osteoid (newly synthesized bony matrix) and osteoblasts are not present in these areas. In some primitive marrow cavities, fibroblasts enlarge and differentiate into **osteoblasts (12)**. In other areas, **osteoid (11, 17)** is seen on the margins of bone trabeculae; osteoblasts may (11) or may not (17) be present.

Figure 3-14   Intramembranous Ossification: Developing Skull Bone

A higher power photomicrograph illustrates the developing skull bone, formed by the process of intramembranous ossification. The connective tissue **periosteum (5)** surrounds the developing bone, from which arise the **osteoblasts (6)** that form the **bone (7).** Osteoblasts (6) are located along the developing **bony trabeculae (3).** Trapped within the formed bone (7) and the bony trabeculae (3) are the **osteocytes (2)** in their lacunae. Also associated with the bony trabeculae (3) are multinuclear cells **osteoclasts (8)** that remodel the developing bone. A primitive **marrow cavity (4)** with **blood vessels (9), blood cells (9),** and hematopoietic tissue is located between the formed bony trabeculae (3).

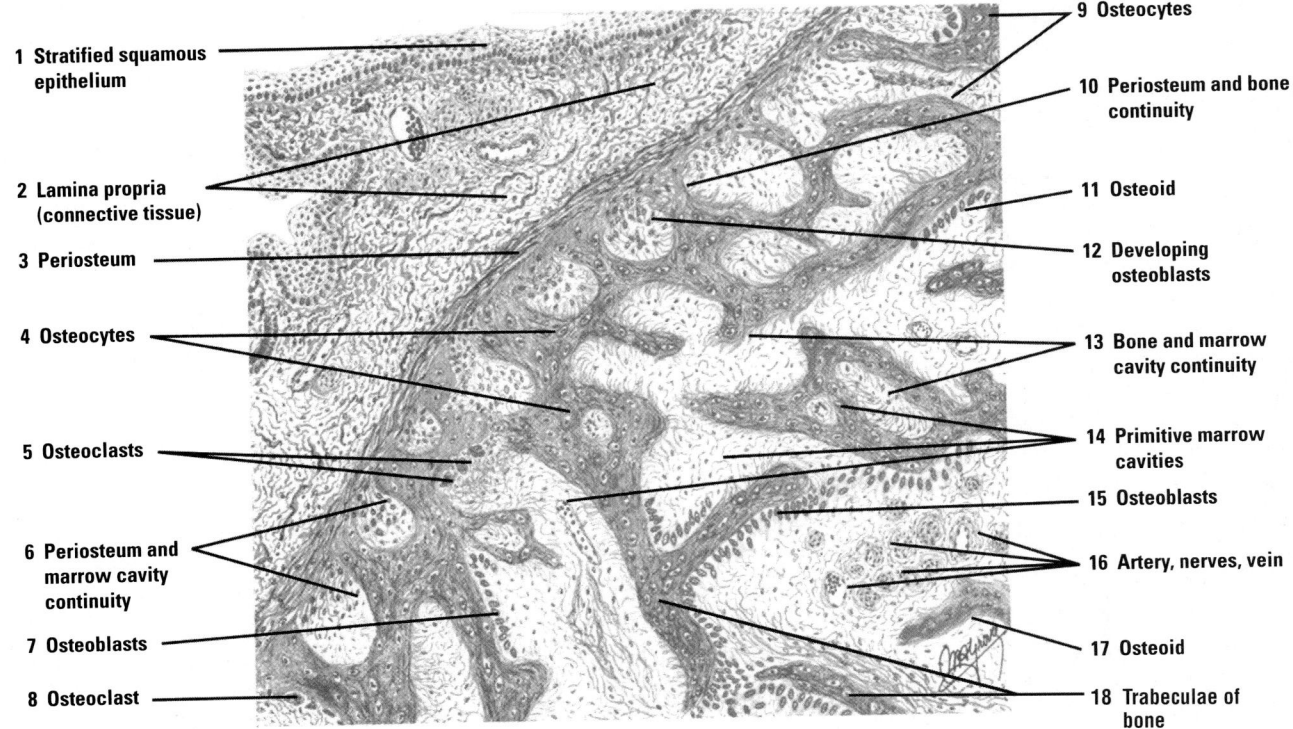

1 Stratified squamous epithelium

2 Lamina propria (connective tissue)

3 Periosteum

4 Osteocytes

5 Osteoclasts

6 Periosteum and marrow cavity continuity

7 Osteoblasts

8 Osteoclast

9 Osteocytes

10 Periosteum and bone continuity

11 Osteoid

12 Developing osteoblasts

13 Bone and marrow cavity continuity

14 Primitive marrow cavities

15 Osteoblasts

16 Artery, nerves, vein

17 Osteoid

18 Trabeculae of bone

Fig. 3-13   Intramembranous Ossification: Developing Mandible (transverse section, decalcified). Stain: Mallory-azan. Low magnification.

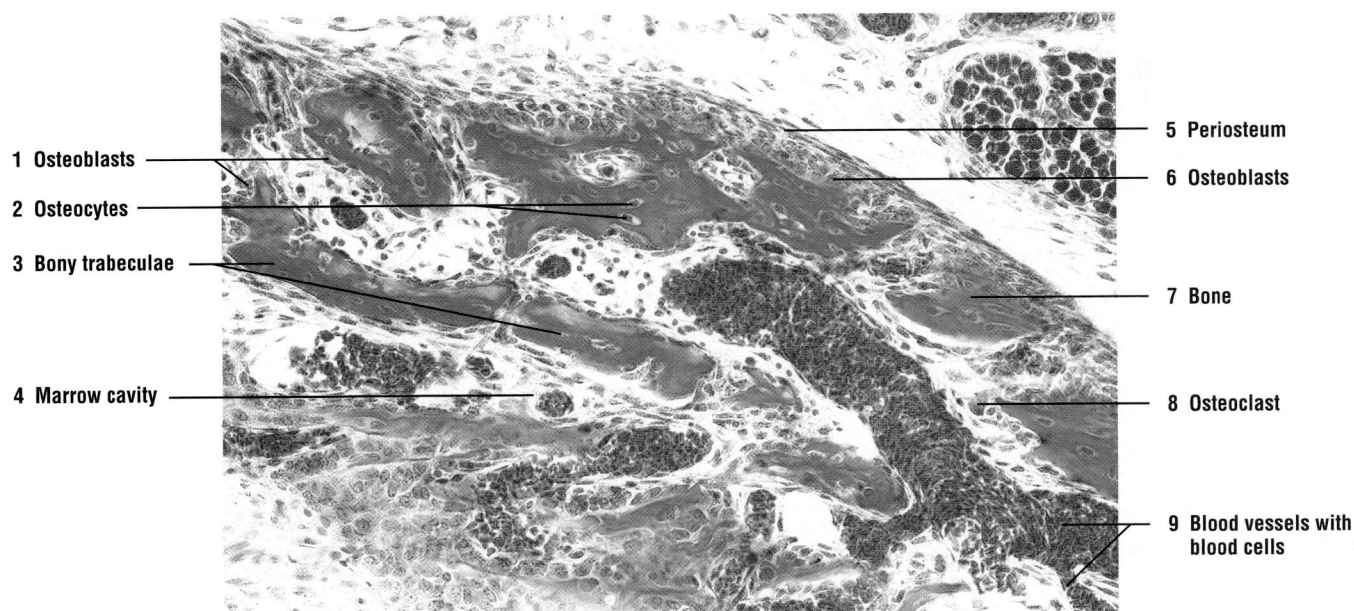

1 Osteoblasts

2 Osteocytes

3 Bony trabeculae

4 Marrow cavity

5 Periosteum

6 Osteoblasts

7 Bone

8 Osteoclast

9 Blood vessels with blood cells

Fig. 3-14   Intramembranous Ossification: Developing Skull Bone. Stain: Mallory-azan. 64×

Figure 3-15   **Cancellous Bone: Sternum (transverse section, decalcified)**

Cancellous bone consists primarily of slender, bony **trabeculae (6),** which ramify, anastomose, and enclose irregular **marrow cavities (5).** Peripherally, these trabeculae merge with a thin layer of **compact bone (3),** which contains scattered **osteons (Haversian systems) (4, 7).** The surrounding **periosteum (2)** may descend into the bone at intervals or merge with adjacent **connective tissue (1).**

Except for concentric lamellae in the osteons (4, 7), the **peripheral bone (3)** and the **trabeculae of bone (6)** exhibit **parallel lamellae (8).** In this illustration, the lamellae (8) are more apparent on the margins of bony areas. Lacunae with **osteocytes (9)** are visible in all regions of the bone.

The reticular connective tissue in the marrow cavities is obscured by **adipose cells (10)** and **hemopoietic (blood-forming) tissue (11).** Arteries are clearly visible in this illustration but sinusoids are too small to distinguish. Marrow (5) fills the cavities; however, a thin, inner layer of cells, the **endosteum (12),** becomes visible when marrow separates from the bone.

Figure 3-16   **Cancellous Bone: Sternum (transverse section, decalcified)**

This photomicrograph shows the cancellous bone of the sternum. This bone is composed of numerous **bony trabeculae (1)** that are separated by the **marrow cavity (5),** in which are found **blood vessels (7)** and different types of formed **blood cells (8).** The bony trabeculae (1) are lined by a thin inner layer of cells called the **endosteum (4, 6),** which contain the osteoprogenitor cells that give rise to osteoblasts. The formed bone contains numerous **osteocytes in their lacunae (2).** Eroding or remodeling the formed bone are the large, multinuclear cells **osteoclasts (3).** The osteoclasts erode part of the bone and are housed in these depressions, which are called the Howship's lacunae.

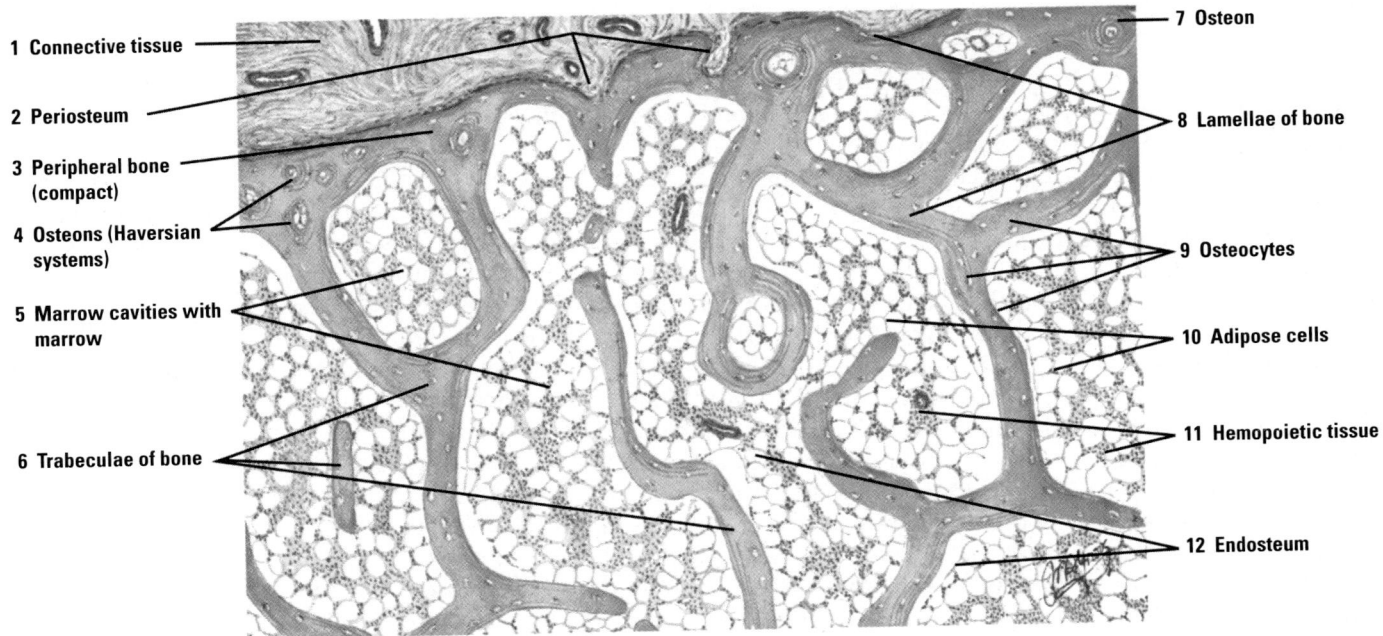

1 Connective tissue
2 Periosteum
3 Peripheral bone (compact)
4 Osteons (Haversian systems)
5 Marrow cavities with marrow
6 Trabeculae of bone
7 Osteon
8 Lamellae of bone
9 Osteocytes
10 Adipose cells
11 Hemopoietic tissue
12 Endosteum

Fig. 3-15   Cancellous Bone: Sternum (transverse section, decalcified). Stain: hematoxylin-eosin. Low magnification.

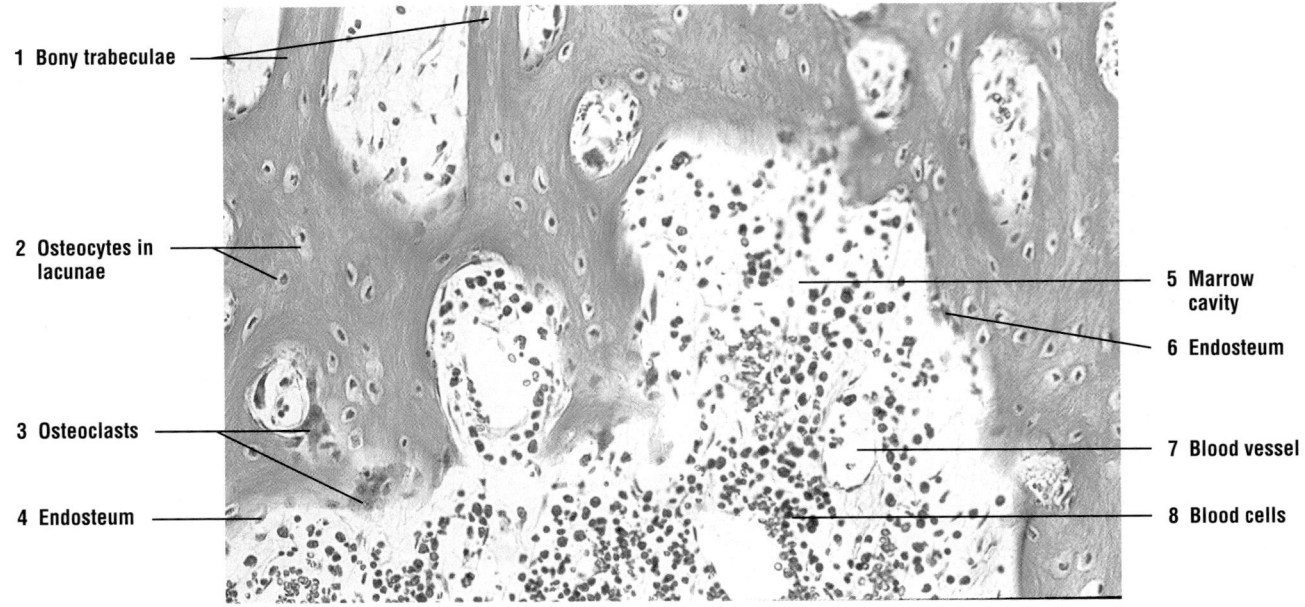

1 Bony trabeculae
2 Osteocytes in lacunae
3 Osteoclasts
4 Endosteum
5 Marrow cavity
6 Endosteum
7 Blood vessel
8 Blood cells

Fig. 3-16   Cancellous Bone: Sternum (transverse section, decalcified). Stain: hematoxylin-eosin. 64×

Figure 3-17   Compact Bone, Dried (transverse section)

Dried bone is prepared by grinding a small piece of bone to a thin section. This method removes the bone cells and only empty spaces become visible—the canals for blood vessels, lacunae where osteocytes or bone cells reside, and canaliculi that connect the adjacent lacunae.

Compact bone is characterized by the arrangement of the bone matrix into layers called lamellae (3b, 8). These are thin plates of bony tissue that contain osteocytes or bone cells in almond-shaped spaces called **lacunae (3c, 9).** Radiating from the lacunae in all directions are tiny canals, the **canaliculi (2).** These penetrate the lamellae (3b, 8), anastomose with canaliculi (2) from other lacunae (3c, 9), and provide communication links with other osteocytes. Some of the canaliculi (2) open into **central (Haversian) canals (3a)** of the osteon (3) and marrow cavities of the bone.

The external wall of the compact bone (beneath the connective tissue periosteum) is formed by the **external circumferential lamellae (7);** these run parallel to each other and to the long axis of the bone. The internal wall (the endosteum along the marrow cavity) is composed of **internal circumferential lamellae (1).** Between the internal and external circumferential lamellae (1, 7) are the **osteons (Haversian systems) (3, 10),** the structural units of the bone. Each osteon (10) consists of a number of **concentric lamellae (3b)** that surround a **central (Haversian) canal (3a).** These are shown in both transverse (3a) and oblique planes of section (10, middle leader) in this illustration. The small irregular areas of bone between osteons (3, 10) are **interstitial lamellae (5, 12).**

In living bone, the lacunae (3c, 9) contain the osteocytes, and the central canals (3a) of the osteons (3, 10) contain reticular connective tissue, blood vessels, and nerves. The boundary between each osteon (3, 10) is outlined by a refractile line called the **cement line (11),** which consists of modified matrix. Anastomoses between **central canals (3a)** are frequently seen in the cross section of the bone and are called **perforating (Volkmann's) canals (6).**

Figure 3-18   Compact Bone, Dried (longitudinal section)

This figure represents a small area of compact bone, prepared in a longitudinal section. Because the central canals (1, 9) course in the longitudinal direction in the bone, each central canal is seen as a tube, often branched, and sectioned parallel to the long axis of the bone. The central canal is surrounded by numerous **lamellae (2),** within or between which are the **lacunae (4),** and from which radiate numerous **canaliculi (5).** The lamellae (2), lacunae (4), and the osteon boundaries (the **cement lines) (8)** are typically parallel to the corresponding central canals (1, 9). The cement lines (8) indicate the extent of an osteon, as seen in longitudinal section.

Other canals in the longitudinal section of the bone extend in either a transverse or oblique direction. These are the **perforating (Volkmann's) canals (7).** They join the central canal (1, 9) of one osteon with the central canal of the adjacent osteon or with the marrow cavity. The perforating canals (7) do not have concentric lamellae; instead, they penetrate directly through the lamellae (2).

Figure 3-19   Compact Bone, Dried: An Osteon (transverse section)

A higher magnification of a compact bone in transverse section illustrates the characteristic features of one osteon and portions of adjacent osteons. Located centrally in the osteon is the prominent, dark-staining **central (Haversian) canal (3),** around which are seen the concentric arrangements of **lamellae (4).** Situated between adjacent osteons are the interstitial **lamellae (5).** The dark, fusiform-shaped structures between the lamellae (4) are the **lacunae (1, 7).** In living bone, bone cells or osteocytes reside in these spaces.

Numerous tiny **canaliculi (2)** radiate from individual lacunae (1, 7) to contact the adjacent lacunae. In this manner, a system of complex communicating canaliculi (2) is formed throughout the bony matrix, with connections to the central canals (3). Each of the canaliculi (2) contain tiny cell processes of the osteocytes. In this manner, the osteocytes around the osteon come in contact with each other and the central canals, which contain the blood vessels. Located on the outer boundary of the osteon is a layer formed by amorphous material, the **cement line (6).**

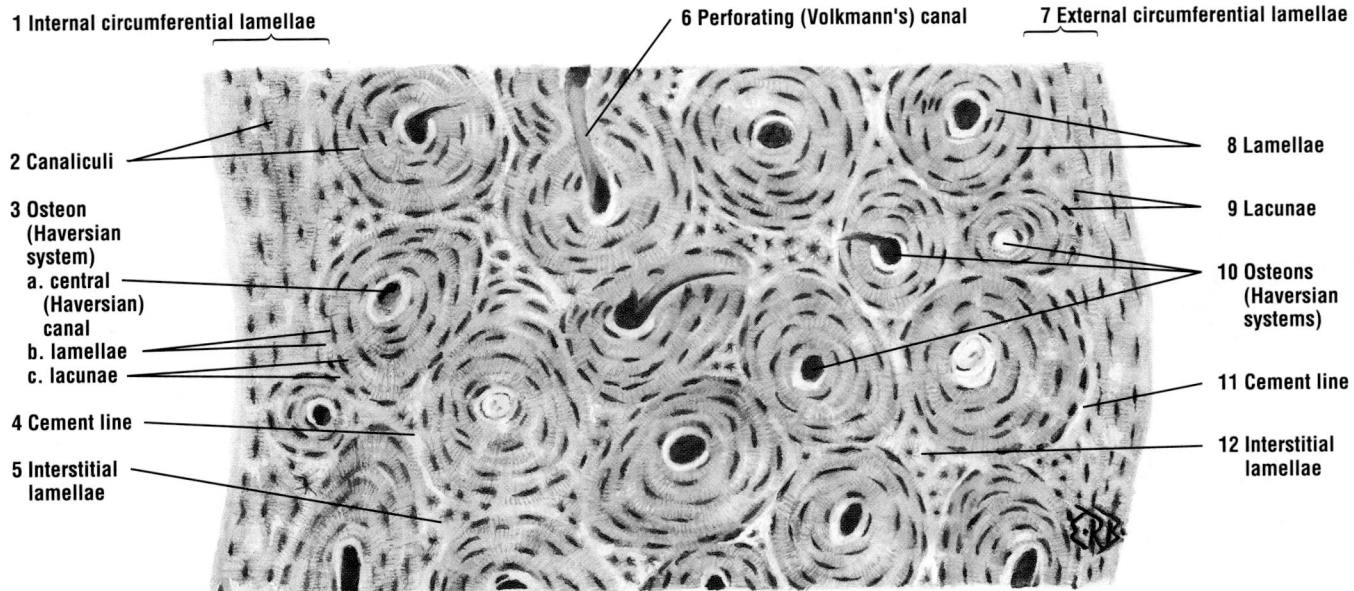

1 Internal circumferential lamellae

6 Perforating (Volkmann's) canal

7 External circumferential lamellae

2 Canaliculi

3 Osteon (Haversian system)
  a. central (Haversian) canal
  b. lamellae
  c. lacunae

4 Cement line

5 Interstitial lamellae

8 Lamellae

9 Lacunae

10 Osteons (Haversian systems)

11 Cement line

12 Interstitial lamellae

Fig. 3-17   **Compact Bone, Dried (transverse section).** Low magnification.

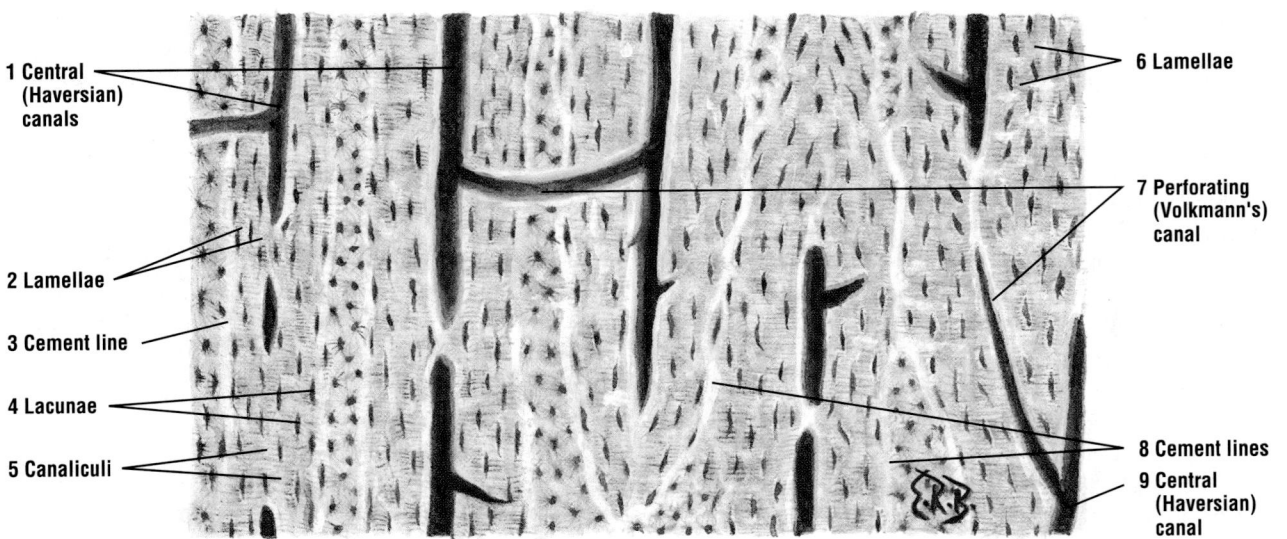

1 Central (Haversian) canals

2 Lamellae

3 Cement line

4 Lacunae

5 Canaliculi

6 Lamellae

7 Perforating (Volkmann's) canal

8 Cement lines

9 Central (Haversian) canal

Fig. 3-18   **Compact Bone, Dried (longitudinal section).** Low magnification.

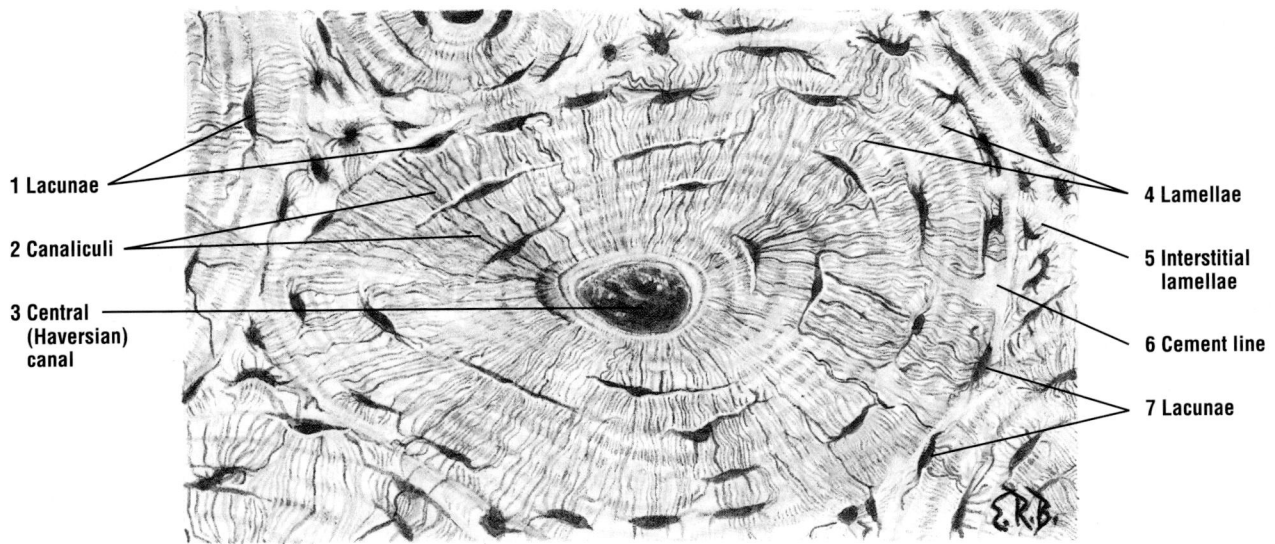

1 Lacunae

2 Canaliculi

3 Central (Haversian) canal

4 Lamellae

5 Interstitial lamellae

6 Cement line

7 Lacunae

Fig. 3-19   **Compact Bone, Dried: An Osteon (transverse section).** High magnification.

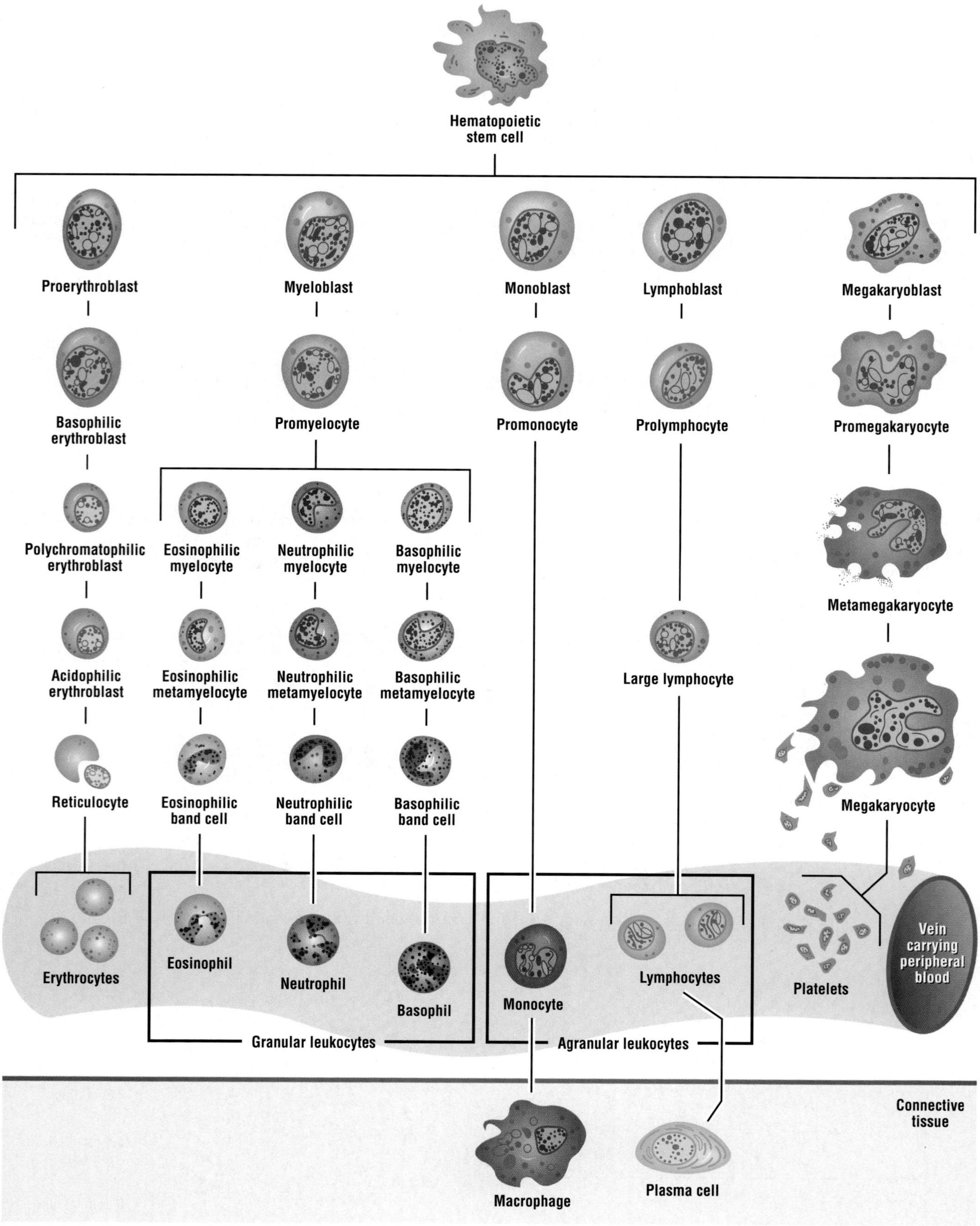

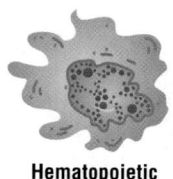

Hematopoietic stem cell

Proerythroblast **Myeloblast** **Monoblast** **Lymphoblast** **Megakaryoblast**

Basophilic erythroblast **Promyelocyte** **Promonocyte** **Prolymphocyte** **Promegakaryocyte**

Polychromatophilic erythroblast **Eosinophilic myelocyte** **Neutrophilic myelocyte** **Basophilic myelocyte**

Acidophilic erythroblast **Eosinophilic metamyelocyte** **Neutrophilic metamyelocyte** **Basophilic metamyelocyte** **Metamegakaryocyte**

Reticulocyte **Eosinophilic band cell** **Neutrophilic band cell** **Basophilic band cell** **Large lymphocyte** **Megakaryocyte**

Erythrocytes **Eosinophil** **Neutrophil** **Basophil** **Monocyte** **Lymphocytes** **Platelets** **Vein carrying peripheral blood**

Granular leukocytes **Agranular leukocytes**

Macrophage **Plasma cell**

Connective tissue

Blood

Blood is a unique form of **connective tissue** that primarily consists of three major types of cells: erythrocytes (red blood cells), leukocytes (white blood cells), and platelets (thrombocytes). These cells or the formed elements are suspended in a liquid medium called **plasma.** The blood cells **transport** gases, nutrients, waste products, hormones, antibodies, cells, various chemicals, ions, and other substances in the plasma to cells in different parts of the body.

BLOOD CELLS
(Figures 4-1–4-7, 4-11–4-13)

Blood cells are formed by a process called **hemopoiesis.** In this process, all blood cell types are derived from **pluripotential hemopoietic stem cells.** These stem cells multiply, differentiate, and develop into the various forms of specialized mature blood cells in the bone marrow and lymphoid organs. Hemopoiesis occurs in different sites of the body, depending on the stage of development of the individual. In the **embryo,** hemopoiesis occurs in the **yolk sac,** and later in the development, it takes place in the **liver, spleen,** and the **lymph nodes.** After birth, hemopoiesis continues almost exclusively in the **red marrow** of different bones. (In the newborn, all bone marrow is red). In adults, red marrow is found primarily in the **flat bones** of the skull, sternum and ribs, vertebrae, and pelvic bones. The remaining bones gradually accumulate fat, their marrow becomes yellow, and they lose the hemopoietic functions.

Microscopic examination of a stained blood smear reveals the major cell types. The **erythrocytes** or red blood cells are nonnucleated, and the **platelets** are cytoplasmic remnants of larger bone marrow cells called **megakaryocytes.** Erythrocytes and platelets perform their major functions within the blood vessels. The **leukocytes,** or white blood cells, on the other hand, perform their major functions outside of the blood vessels. The leukocytes migrate out of the blood vessels through the capillary walls and enter connective tissue, lymphatic tissue, and bone marrow. Leukocytes are **nucleated cells** and are subdivided into **granulocytes** or **agranulocytes,** depending on the presence or absence of granules in their cytoplasm. The leukocytes function primarily as a **defense system** against bacterial invasion or the presence of foreign material in the body. Consequently, most of the leukocytes are concentrated in the **connective tissue.**

PLATELETS (Figures 4-11–4-13)

Platelets or thrombocytes are the **smallest** formed elements that are found in the blood. They are nonnucleated **cytoplasmic fragments** of **megakaryocytes,** which are the largest, multilobed cells in the **bone marrow.** Platelets are produced when small, uneven portions of the cytoplasm separate or **fragment** from the peripheries of the megakaryocytes **(Fig. 4-10).** The main function of platelets is to promote blood clotting.

Figure 4-1   Human Blood Smear

A smear of human blood examined under lower magnification illustrates various formed elements of the blood. The most abundant elements of the blood are the **red blood cells** or **erythrocytes (1).** These cells are enucleated (without nucleus) and stain pink with eosin. They are uniform in size, approximately 7.5 μm in diameter, and can be used as a size reference for other cell types. The erythrocytes (1) are the most prevalent elements in the blood smear and are the easiest to identify.

In addition to numerous erythrocytes (1), several white blood cells or leukocytes are visible in the blood smear. Leukocytes are subdivided into different categories according to the shape of their nuclei, the absence or presence of cytoplasmic granules, and the staining affinities of their granules. Two **neutrophils (2, 4),** one **eosinophil (7),** and one small **lymphocyte (5)** are shown in this illustration. Scattered around these cells are small, blue-staining fragments of a blood cell, the **platelets (3, 6).** All of these formed blood elements are illustrated in greater detail and higher magnification.

Figure 4-2   Erythrocytes and Platelets

This illustration shows numerous **erythrocytes (1)** and the tiny **platelets (2)** that usually are seen in a blood smear. Blood platelets (2) are the smallest of the formed elements; they are cytoplasmic remnants of a large-cell megakaryocyte, which is found in red bone marrow. Platelets (2) appear as irregular masses of basophilic (blue) cytoplasm, and they tend to form clumps in blood smears.

■ Functional Correlations–Erythrocytes and Platelets

Mature erythrocytes are highly specialized to transport **oxygen** and **carbon dioxide.** The ability to transport respiratory gases depends on the presence of protein **hemoglobin** in the erythrocytes. Iron molecules in hemoglobin bind with oxygen molecules, and most of the oxygen in the blood is carried to tissues in the form of **oxyhemoglobin.** Carbon dioxide from the cells and tissues is carried to the lungs, partly dissolved in the blood and partly in combination with hemoglobin, as **carbaminohemoglobin.**

During differentiation and maturation processes, erythrocytes synthesize large amounts of hemoglobin. Before erythrocytes are released into the systemic circulation, the nucleus is extruded from cytoplasm, and the mature erythrocytes assume a biconcave shape. This shape provides more surface area for carrying respiratory gases. Thus, mature mammalian erythrocytes in the circulation are **nonnucleated** biconcave discs that are surrounded by a membrane and contain hemoglobin and some enzymes.

The main function of platelets is to promote **blood clotting.** When the wall of the blood vessel is broken or damaged, the platelets **adhere** to the damaged region of the wall, become activated, and release chemicals that initiate the very complex process of blood clotting. After a blood clot is formed and the bleeding ceases, the aggregated platelets contribute to the **clot retraction.**

Figure 4-3   Neutrophils

The leukocytes that contain granules and a lobulated nucleus are the polymorphonuclear granulocytes, of which the neutrophils (1) are the most abundant. The cytoplasm of neutrophils (1) contains fine violet or pink granules; these are difficult to see with a normal light microscope. As a result, the cytoplasm of neutrophils (1) appears clear. The nucleus of neutrophils (1) consists of several lobes that are connected by narrow chromatin strands; a fewer number of nuclear lobes in these cells indicates that the neutrophils (1) are immature. The neutrophils (1) constitute approximately 60 to 70% of the leukocyte population in the blood and are easy to locate in a blood smear.

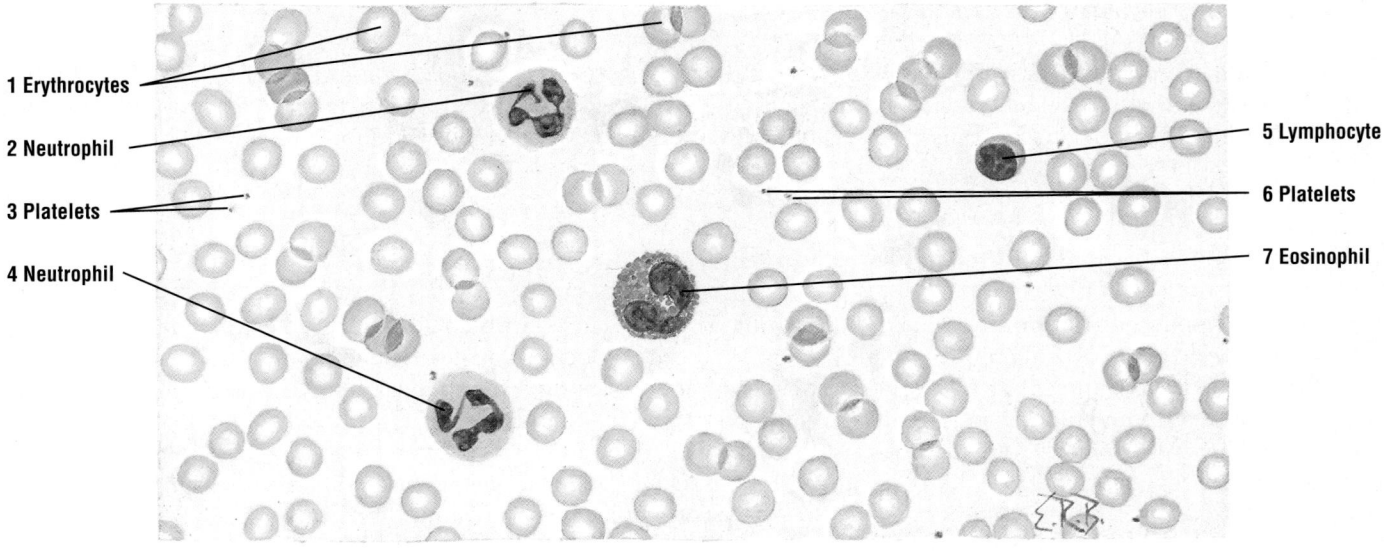

1 Erythrocytes

2 Neutrophil

3 Platelets

4 Neutrophil

5 Lymphocyte

6 Platelets

7 Eosinophil

Fig. 4-1   Human Blood Smear. Wright's stain. High magnification.

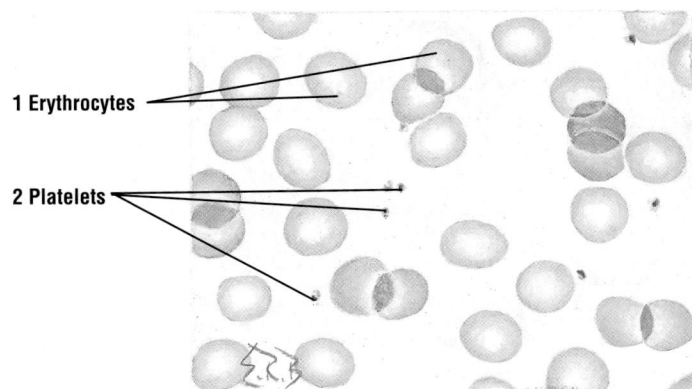

1 Erythrocytes

2 Platelets

Fig. 4-2   Erythrocytes and Platelets. Wright's stain. Oil immersion.

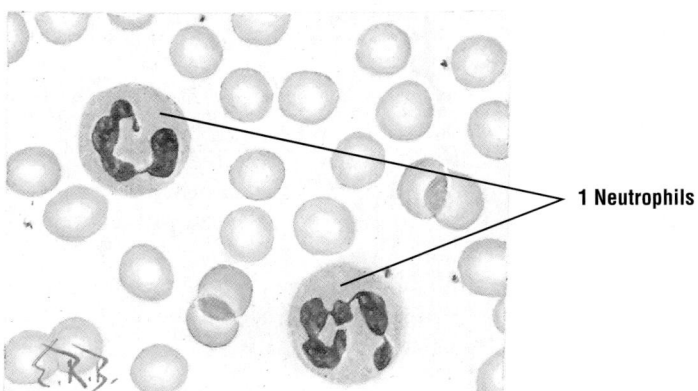

1 Neutrophils

Fig. 4-3   Neutrophils. Wright's stain. Oil immersion.

Figure 4-4   Eosinophils

Eosinophils (1) constitute approximately 2 to 4% of the leukocytes in the blood. These cells usually can be identified without difficulty in a blood smear because their cytoplasm is filled with distinct, large, eosinophilic (bright pink) granules. The nucleus in eosinophils (1) typically is bilobed, but a small third lobe may be present.

Figure 4-5   Lymphocytes

Agranular leukocytes have few or no cytoplasmic granules and exhibit round to horseshoe-shaped nuclei. **Lymphocytes (1, 2)** constitute approximately 20 to 30% of the blood leukocytes. They vary from cells smaller than erythrocytes to those almost twice as large. For size comparison among different lymphocytes and erythrocytes, this illustration of a human blood smear depicts a **large lymphocyte (1)** and a **small lymphocyte (2),** both surrounded by the erythrocytes. In small lymphocytes (2), the densely stained nucleus occupies most of the cytoplasm, and the cytoplasm is seen as a thin basophilic rim around the nucleus. The cytoplasm is agranular but may contain a few azurophilic granules. In large lymphocytes (1), basophilic cytoplasm is more abundant around the nucleus, and the larger and paler nucleus may contain one or two nucleoli.

Figure 4-6   Monocytes

Monocytes (1) are the largest leukocytes. The nucleus varies from round or oval to indented or horseshoe-shaped and stains lighter than in lymphocytes. Chromatin is more finely dispersed; abundant cytoplasm is lightly basophilic and often contains a few fine azurophilic granules. Monocytes (1) constitute approximately 3 to 8% of the blood leukocytes.

Figure 4-7   Basophils

The granules in the **basophils (1)** are not as numerous as in eosinophils (Fig. 4-4); however, they are more variable in size, less densely packed, and stain dark blue or brown. Although the nucleus is not markedly lobulated and stains pale basophilic, it is usually obscured by the density of the granules. The basophils constitute less than 1% of the blood leukocytes and are, therefore, the most difficult cells to find and identify in a blood smear.

■ Functional Correlations–Leukocytes

Neutrophils are **phagocytic** cells. They are attracted by **chemotactic factors** to sites of microorganisms, especially bacteria, which they ingest and destroy.

Eosinophils are also **phagocytic** cells with a particular affinity for **antigen-antibody complexes.** The cells increase in number during parasitic infestation and may have an important role in their destruction.

Lymphocytes have a central role in **immulogical** defense mechanism of the body. When stimulated by specific antigen, some of the lymphocytes (B cells) differentiate into **plasma cells,** which then produce **antibodies.**

Monocytes are powerful **phagocytes** that at the site of infection differentiate into **tissue macrophages,** which then destroy bacteria, foreign matter, and cellular debris.

Basophils have functional similarity with mast cells. Release of their granules liberates histamine and heparin in allergic reactions, leading to increased inflammatory response.

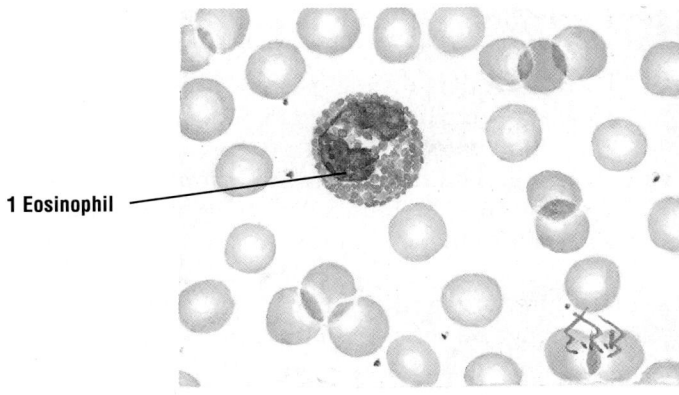

1 Eosinophil

Fig. 4-4   Eosinophils. Wright's stain. Oil immersion.

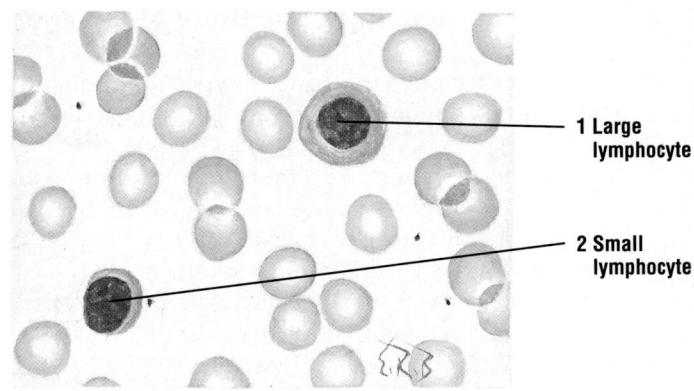

1 Large lymphocyte

2 Small lymphocyte

Fig. 4-5   Lymphocytes. Wright's stain. Oil immersion.

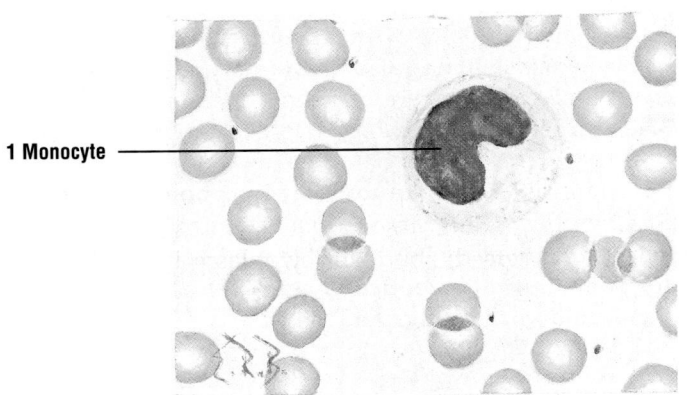

1 Monocyte

Fig. 4-6   Monocytes. Wright's stain. Oil immersion.

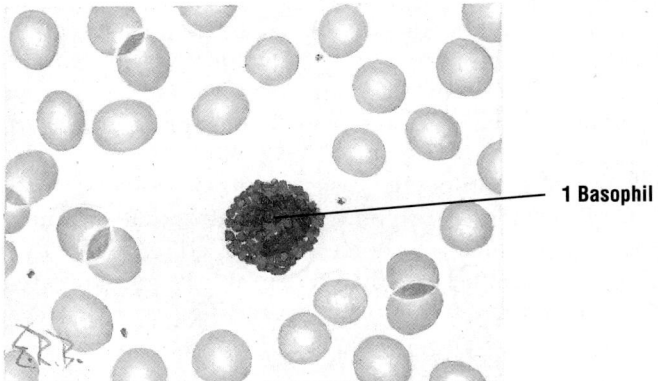

1 Basophil

Fig. 4-7   Basophils. Wright's stain. Oil immersion.

Figure 4-8   Hemopoietic Bone Marrow of a Rabbit (section)

In a section of red bone marrow, all types of developing blood cells are difficult to distinguish. The cells are packed densely, and different cell types are intermixed although some of the erythrocytic forms often occur in groups or "nests" (6, 18).

This section is stained with hematoxylin-eosin. At low magnification, little differentiation of cytoplasm is visible—except for bright-staining **eosinophilic granules (4)** in the precursor eosinophilic cells. Different individual blood cells from a bone marrow smear are illustrated below the figure at a higher magnification to show more details of the cytoplasm, its contents, and its nucleus.

The stroma of the reticular connective tissue in the marrow is obscured primarily by hemopoietic cells. In less dense areas, the reticular **connective tissue (8)** can be seen, and the elongated **reticular cells (22)** often are recognized. Different types of **blood vessels (9, 10, 17, 23)** that contain erythrocytes and leukocytes in their lumina also are seen in the bone marrow. Also conspicuous in the bone marrow are large **adipose cells (2, 13)**, each exhibiting a large vacuole (because of fat removal during routine section preparation) and small, peripheral cytoplasm that surrounds the **nucleus (2).** Other cells that are identified easily in the bone marrow are large **megakaryocytes (5, 21)** with varied nuclear lobulation.

Erythrocytes (12) are abundant in the bone marrow. The most easily recognizable of the earlier erythrocytic cells are the **normoblasts (16),** which are characterized by small, dark-staining nuclei (as in 28); numerous normoblast cells also exhibit **mitotic activity (16). Polychromatophilic erythroblasts (20)** may also occur in groups or "nests." These cells are larger than normoblasts (16), with a larger nucleus that exhibits a more evident "checkerboard" distribution of chromatin (as in 27). **Basophilic erythroblasts (3)** are larger cells that exhibit a large, less-dense nuclei and basophilic cytoplasm (as in 26).

In the granulocytic series of blood cells, the most easily recognizable cells are the **polymorphonuclear heterophils (15)** (corresponding to neutrophils in humans) and eosinophils. Their earlier forms, the **metamyelocytes (19),** have a bean- or horseshoe-shaped nuclei (as in 25). **Heterophilic myelocytes (1, 4, 24)** have larger, round, or ovoid nuclei. Less easily recognizable in a section are the pale-staining primitive **reticular cells (11).**

An alternate terminology for the developing erythrocytic forms, in use clinically, is as follows:

Proerythroblast = rubriblast
Basophilic erythroblast = prorubricyte
Polychromatophilic erythroblast = rubricyte
Normoblast (orthochromatophilic erythroblast) = metarubricyte

Figure 4-9   Bone Marrow of a Rabbit, India Ink Preparation (section)

A section of a hemopoietic bone marrow from a rabbit, injected with India ink, is illustrated. Carbon particles have been ingested by the **stromal macrophages (1, 7)** and by **fixed macrophages (3)** that are adjacent to the endothelium of the **sinusoids (3, 5).** Ingestion and accumulation of dense carbon particles in some phagocytic cells can obscure their nuclei (1, 7).

Reticular cells (10) of the connective tissue may be seen occasionally, but are obscured frequently by developing blood cells. Various cells of the **erythrocytic** and **granulocytic series (4, 6, 11)** as well as **megakaryocytes (9)** can be identified.

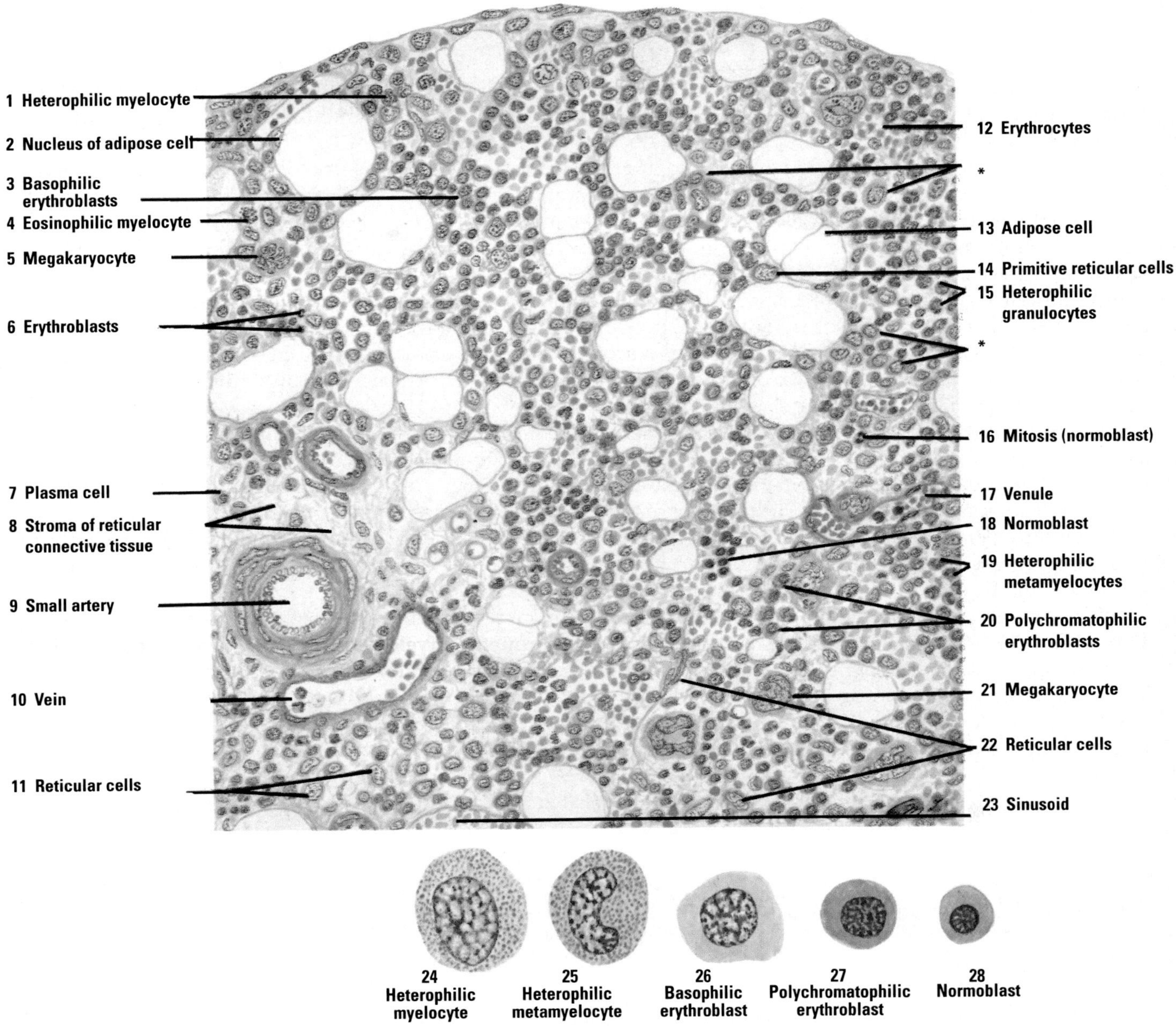

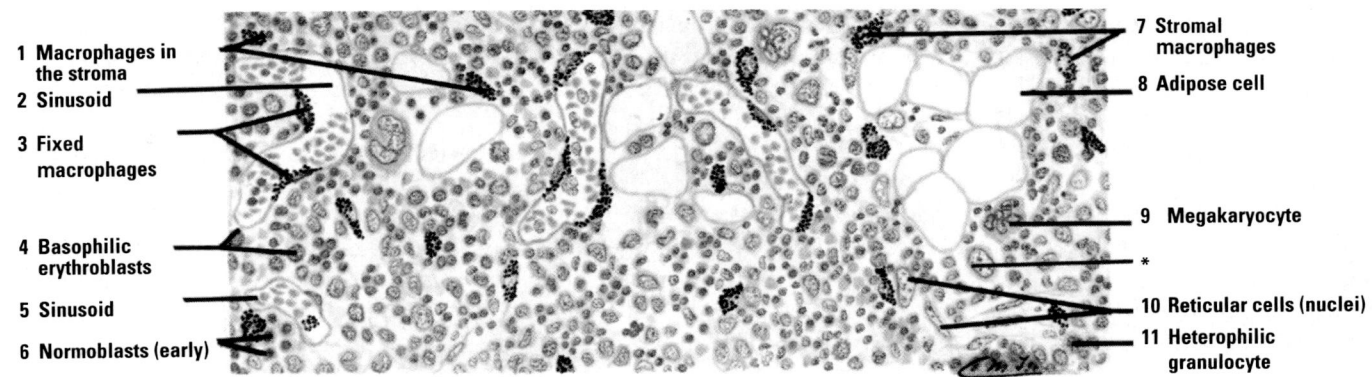

1 Heterophilic myelocyte

2 Nucleus of adipose cell

3 Basophilic erythroblasts

4 Eosinophilic myelocyte

5 Megakaryocyte

6 Erythroblasts

7 Plasma cell

8 Stroma of reticular connective tissue

9 Small artery

10 Vein

11 Reticular cells

12 Erythrocytes

*

13 Adipose cell

14 Primitive reticular cells

15 Heterophilic granulocytes

*

16 Mitosis (normoblast)

17 Venule

18 Normoblast

19 Heterophilic metamyelocytes

20 Polychromatophilic erythroblasts

21 Megakaryocyte

22 Reticular cells

23 Sinusoid

24 Heterophilic myelocyte

25 Heterophilic metamyelocyte

26 Basophilic erythroblast

27 Polychromatophilic erythroblast

28 Normoblast

Fig. 4-8   Hemopoietic Bone Marrow of a Rabbit (section). Stain: hematoxylin-eosin. Upper: high magnification. Lower: oil immersion.

1 Macrophages in the stroma

2 Sinusoid

3 Fixed macrophages

4 Basophilic erythroblasts

5 Sinusoid

6 Normoblasts (early)

7 Stromal macrophages

8 Adipose cell

9 Megakaryocyte

*

10 Reticular cells (nuclei)

11 Heterophilic granulocyte

Fig. 4-9   Bone Marrow of a Rabbit, India Ink Preparation (section). Stain: hematoxylin-eosin. Medium magnification.

Figure 4-10   Bone Marrow: Smear

A microscopic field of human bone marrow smear that was obtained by sternal puncture is represented in the center of the illustration. Around the periphery, the typical bone marrow cells are illustrated in greater detail. The formed elements that are normally found in the blood easily are recognized: **erythrocytes (18, 31)**, granulocytes **(eosinophil, 32; neutrophils, 33)**, and **platelets (24)**.

A common stem cell is believed to give rise to different hemopoietic cell lines from which arise such functional blood cells as the erythrocytes, granulocytes, lymphocytes, and megakaryocytes. Because of its ability to differentiate into all blood cells, this cell is called **pluripotential hemopoietic stem cell (1)**. Although this cell cannot be recognized microscopically, it resembles a large lymphocyte. In adults, the greatest concentration of pluripotential stem cells is found in the bone marrow.

In the erythrocytic series, the precursor cell is the **proerythroblast (3, 8)** (for alternate terminology, see page text accompanying Fig. 4-8); it measures 20 to 30 μm in diameter and contains a thin rim of basophilic cytoplasm and a large, oval nucleus that occupies most of the cell. Azurophilic granules are absent in all cells of this series. The chromatin is dispersed uniformly, and two or more nuclei may be present. Early proerythroblasts divide to form smaller basophilic erythroblasts approximately 15 to 17 μm in size.

Basophilic erythroblasts (4, 7) exhibit less intensely basophilic cytoplasm; however, sufficient basophilia is present in the cytoplasm to obscure the small amount of hemoglobin that is being synthesized by these cells. The nucleus has decreased in size; the chromatin is coarse and exhibits the characteristic "checkerboard" pattern. Nucleoli are either inconspicuous or absent. The progeny of mitotic divisions of basophilic erythroblasts (4, 7) are the **polychromatophilic erythroblasts (5, 13, 14)**. These cells are similar in size (12 to 15 μm in diameter). Their cytoplasm becomes progressively less basophilic and more acidophilic as a result of increased hemoglobin accumulation. The nuclei are smaller and exhibit the coarse "checkerboard" pattern.

When the cells acquire an acidophilic cytoplasm because of an increased amount of hemoglobin, they are called **normoblasts (6, 11);** their size is approximately 8 to 10 μm in diameter. Initially, the nucleus exhibits a concentrated "checkerboard" chromatin pattern (6, 11), and the cell division continues. The nucleus then decreases in size, becomes pyknotic, and is extruded from the cytoplasm. The resulting flattened cell is the **reticulocyte (9, 16, 17)** or a young erythrocyte, exhibiting a bluish-pink cytoplasm. With special supravital staining, a delicate reticulum is demonstrated in their cytoplasm. Mature **erythrocytes (18, 31)** are smaller and have a homogenous acidophilic cytoplasm.

The granulocytes also originate from the pluripotential stem cell, and the **myeloblast (2, 25)** is the first recognizable precursor in the granulocytic series. The myeloblasts (2, 25) are small cells (10 to 13 μm in diameter) with a large nucleus that contain two or three nucleoli and a distinctly basophilic cytoplasm that lacks specific granules. During its development, the cell enlarges, acquires azurophilic granules, and is now called a **promyelocyte (early, 19; later, 23)**. The cell measures approximately 15 to 20 μm in diameter. The chromatin in the oval nucleus is dispersed, and multiple nucleoli are evident. In more advanced promyelocytes **(neutrophilic, 23)**, the cells are smaller, nucleoli become inconspicuous, azurophilic granules increase, and specific granules appear with different staining properties in the perinuclear region.

Myelocytes are smaller than promyelocytes. The nucleus is eccentric, and the chromatin is more condensed. The cytoplasm is less basophilic, with few azurophilic granules evident, and specific granules increase **(neutrophilic early myelocyte, 26; basophilic early myelocyte, 20)**. More **mature myelocytes (12, 21, 22, 27, 29, 34, 35)** have an abundance of specific granules, slightly acidophilic cytoplasm, and a smaller nucleus. The myelocyte is the last cell of granulocytic series capable of mitosis; myelocytes then mature into metamyelocytes.

In the **metamyelocytes,** the shape of the nucleus changes from oval to that with deep indentation, which is seen in mature cells. The greatest change takes place in the **neutrophilic** forms (in succession, **30** and **36, 28, 33**). Similar structural alterations can be seen in **eosinophils** and **basophils (12, 20; lower leader, 27; upper leader, 32)**.

Megakaryoblasts (37) are large cells that measure approximately 40 to 60 μm in diameter. The cytoplasm is basophilic and largely free of specific granules. The voluminous nucleus is ovoid or indented and exhibits a loose chromatin pattern and poorly defined nucleoli. The mature cells, **megakaryocytes (15, 38)**, are giant cells approximately 80 to 100 μm in diameter and have a large, slightly acidophilic cytoplasm that is filled with fine azurophilic granules. The nucleus of these cells is large and convoluted, with multiple irregular lobes interconnected by constricted regions. The chromatin is condensed and coarse, and nucleoli are not visible. In mature megakaryocytes (38), plasma membrane invaginates the cytoplasm and forms demarcation membranes. This delimits the areas of the megakaryocyte cytoplasm that is shed into the blood as small cell fragments in the form of **platelets (39).** The platelets measure approximately 2 to 4 μm in diameter.

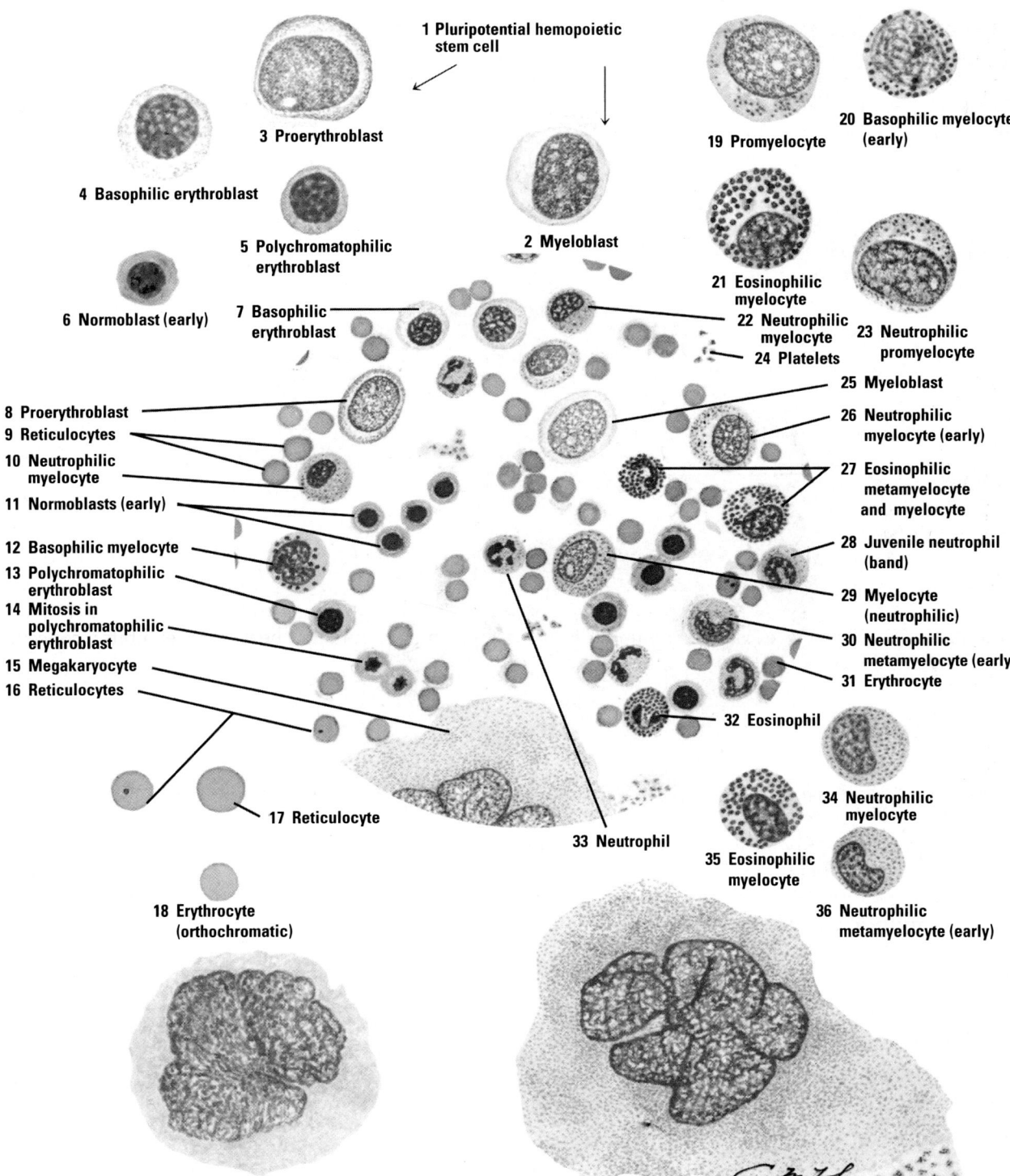

1 Pluripotential hemopoietic stem cell

3 Proerythroblast

4 Basophilic erythroblast

5 Polychromatophilic erythroblast

6 Normoblast (early)

7 Basophilic erythroblast

2 Myeloblast

19 Promyelocyte

20 Basophilic myelocyte (early)

21 Eosinophilic myelocyte

22 Neutrophilic myelocyte

23 Neutrophilic promyelocyte

24 Platelets

8 Proerythroblast

9 Reticulocytes

10 Neutrophilic myelocyte

11 Normoblasts (early)

12 Basophilic myelocyte

13 Polychromatophilic erythroblast

14 Mitosis in polychromatophilic erythroblast

15 Megakaryocyte

16 Reticulocytes

17 Reticulocyte

18 Erythrocyte (orthochromatic)

25 Myeloblast

26 Neutrophilic myelocyte (early)

27 Eosinophilic metamyelocyte and myelocyte

28 Juvenile neutrophil (band)

29 Myelocyte (neutrophilic)

30 Neutrophilic metamyelocyte (early)

31 Erythrocyte

32 Eosinophil

33 Neutrophil

34 Neutrophilic myelocyte

35 Eosinophilic myelocyte

36 Neutrophilic metamyelocyte (early)

37 Megakaryoblast

38 Megakaryocyte

39 Platelets

Fig. 4-10   Bone Marrow: Smear. Stain: May-Grunwald-Giemsa. Oil immersion.

Figure 4-11   Human Blood Smear: Red Blood Cells, Neutrophils, Large Lymphocyte, and Platelets

A photomicrograph of human blood shows different types of blood cells that are normally seen in a smear. The most numerous blood cell types are the **erythrocytes (red blood cells) (1)**. Also visible are two **neutrophils (2, 4)**, a **large lymphocyte (5)**, and numerous examples of **platelets (3)**.

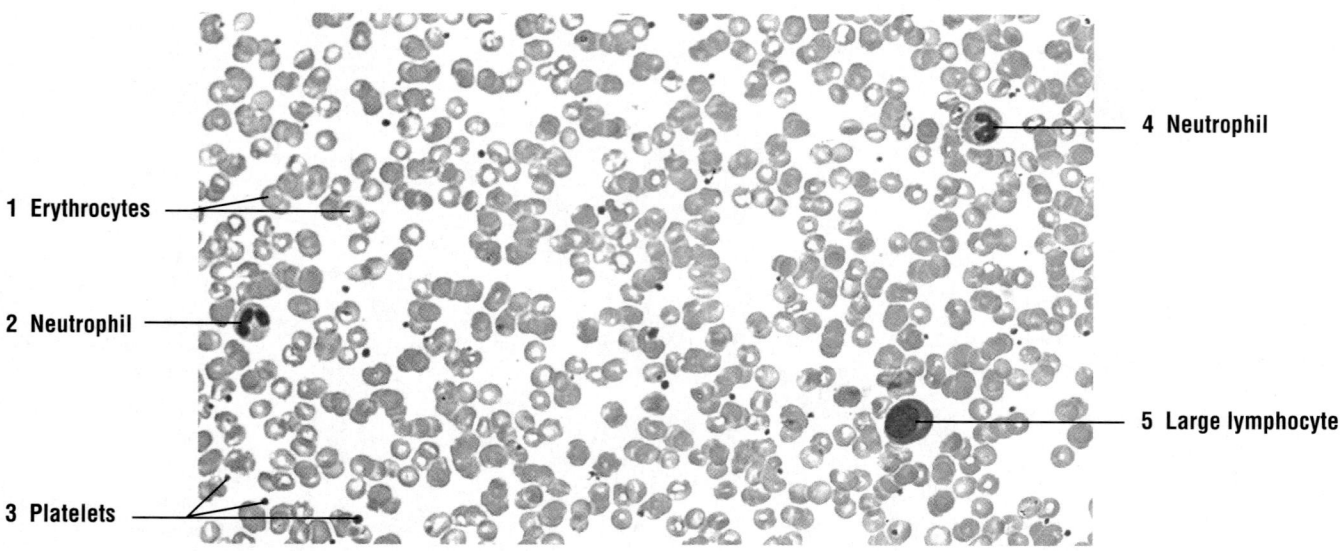

Fig. 4-11   Human Blood Smear: Red Blood Cells, Neutrophils, Large Lymphocyte, and Platelets. Stain: Wright's stain. 205×

Figure 4-12   Human Blood Smear: Basophil, Neutrophil, Red Blood Cells, and Platelets

A higher magnification photomicrograph of human blood shows **erythrocytes (3)**, a **basophil (1)**, a **neutrophil (5)**, and numerous **platelets (4)**. The basophil (1) cytoplasm is typically filled with dense **basophilic granules (2)** that normally obscure the nucleus. In contrast, the neutrophil (5) cytoplasm under light microscopy does not show granules and its **multilobed nucleus (6)** is clearly visible.

Figure 4-13   Human Blood Smear: Monocyte, Red Blood Cells, and Platelets

A photomicrograph prepared with oil immersion objective illustrates numerous **erythrocytes (1)**, **platelets (2)**, and a large **monocyte (3)** with the characteristic kidney-shaped nucleus and a nongranular cytoplasm.

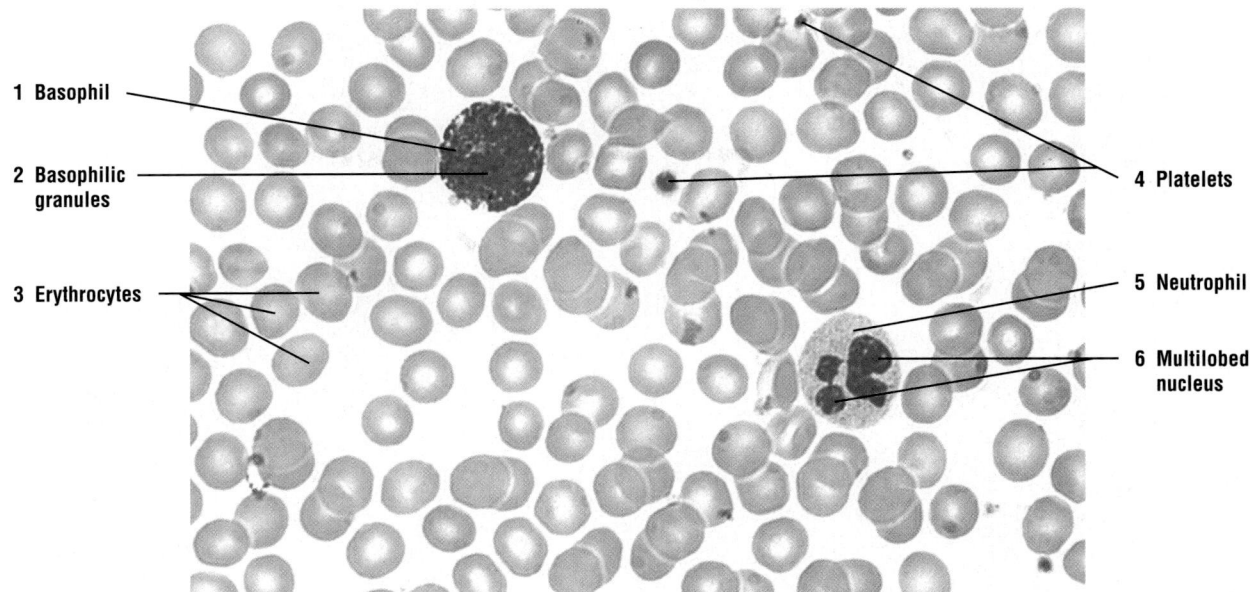

1 Basophil

2 Basophilic granules

3 Erythrocytes

4 Platelets

5 Neutrophil

6 Multilobed nucleus

Fig. 4-12   Human Blood Smear: Basophil, Neutrophil, Red Blood Cells, and Platelets. Stain: Wright's stain. 320×

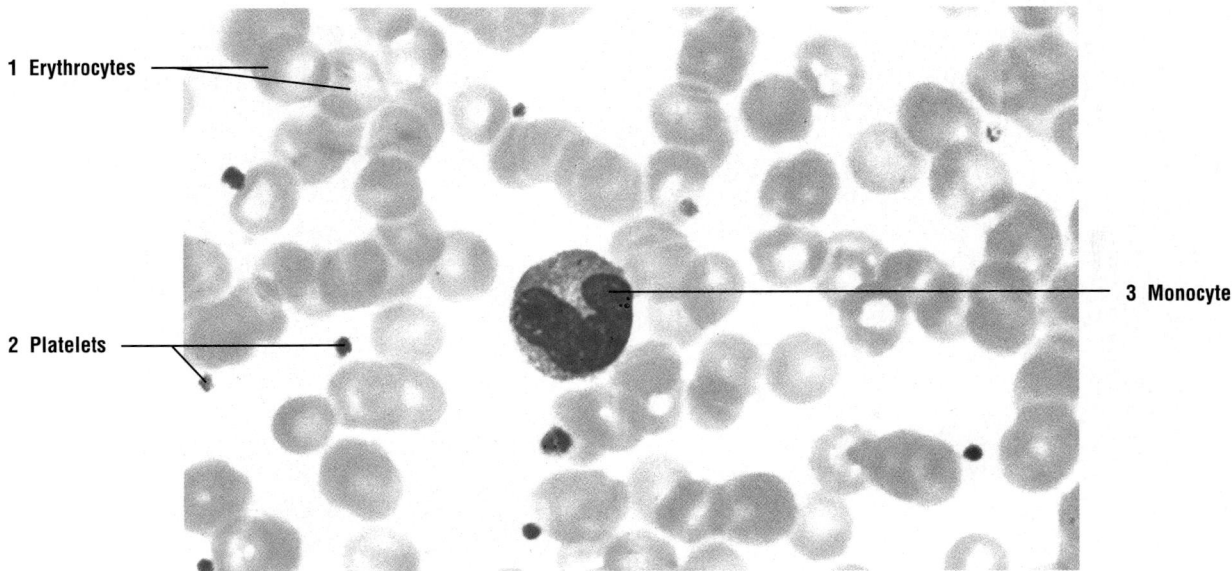

1 Erythrocytes

2 Platelets

3 Monocyte

Fig. 4-13   Human Blood Smear: Monocyte, Red Blood Cells, and Platelets. Stain: Wright's stain. 320×

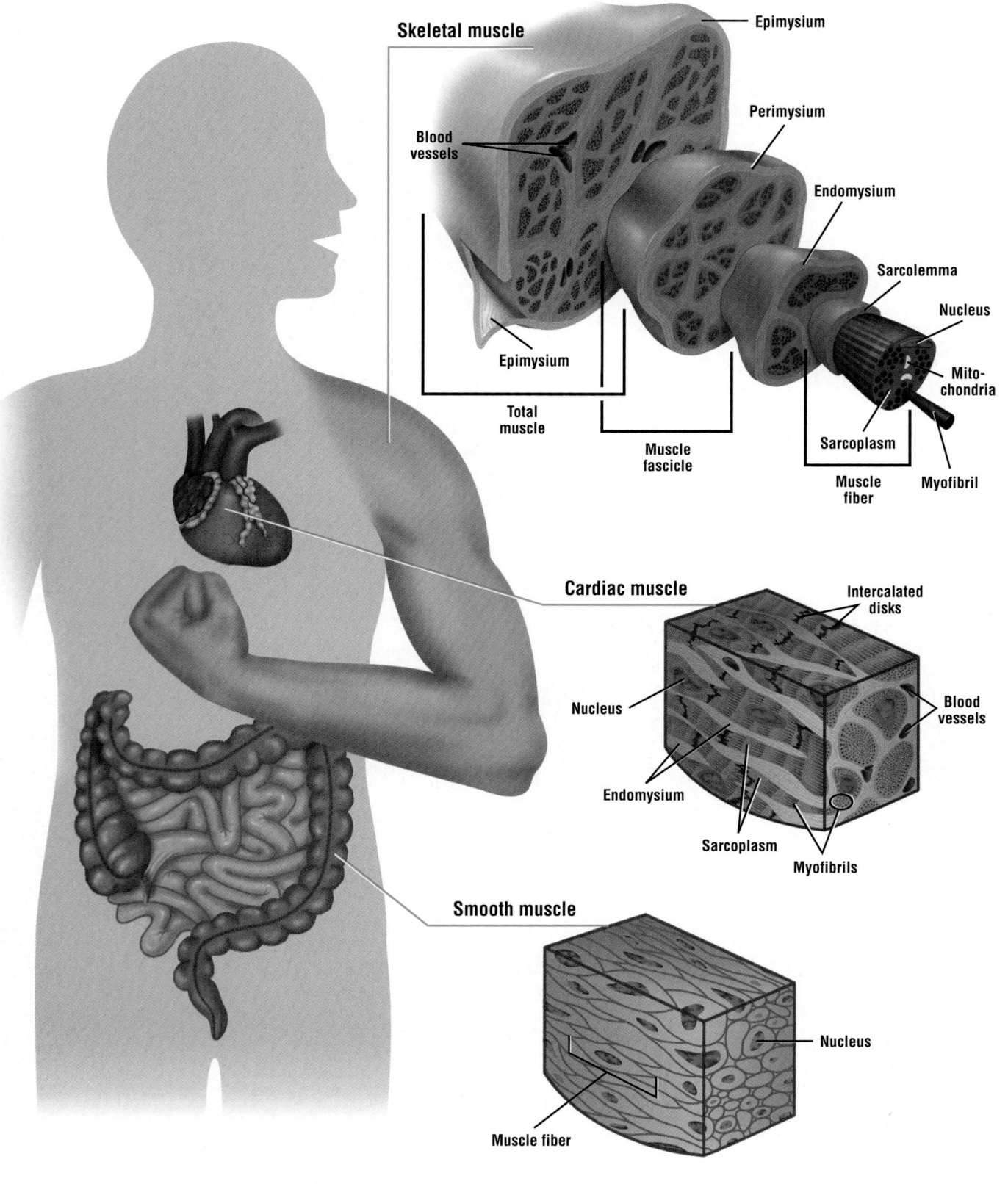

Skeletal muscle

Epimysium

Perimysium

Endomysium

Sarcolemma

Nucleus

Mito-chondria

Myofibril

Muscle fiber

Sarcoplasm

Muscle fascicle

Total muscle

Epimysium

Blood vessels

Cardiac muscle

Intercalated disks

Nucleus

Blood vessels

Endomysium

Sarcoplasm

Myofibrils

Smooth muscle

Nucleus

Muscle fiber

Muscle Tissue

There are three types of muscle tissue in the body: **skeletal muscle, cardiac muscle,** and **smooth muscle.** Each muscle type has certain structural and functional similarities with as well as differences from the others. All muscle tissues consist of elongated cells called **fibers.** Each muscle fiber cytoplasm contains numerous **myofibrils,** which contain two tpes of contractile protein filaments, **actin** and **myosin.**

SMOOTH MUSCLE

Smooth muscle fibers contain actin and myosin filaments; however, they are not arranged in striated patterns as seen in skeletal or cardiac muscles. As a result, these muscles appear **smooth** or **nonstriated.** Smooth muscle fibers are **involuntary muscles;** they are small, spindle-shaped or fusiform in shape, and contain a **single central nucleus (Figs. 5-1–5-2).** Smooth muscles are often seen as individual fibers or slender bundles or fascicles; however, they are predominantly found lining the **visceral organs** and **blood vessels.** In hollow visceral organs, such digestive tract, uterus, ureters, and others, smooth muscles occur in large **sheets.** In the blood vessels, these muscle fibers are arranged in a circular pattern; they control blood pressure by altering the vessel diameter.

SKELETAL MUSCLE

Skeletal muscles are **voluntary** because their contraction and relaxation are due to conscious control. In the cytoplasm of a skeletal muscle, the arrangement of actin and myosin filaments is very regular. As a result, these contractile filaments form distinct **cross-striations,** which are seen under a microscope as light **I bands** and the dark **A bands** across each muscle fiber. Because of these cross-striations, the skeletal muscles are also called **striated muscles.**

Skeletal muscles are long, multinucleated fibers, with the nuclei located **peripherally.** Skeletal muscles are surrounded by connective tissue. The entire skeletal muscle is invested by a dense, irregular connective tissue layer called **epimysium.** A less dense, irregular connective tissue layer, called **perimysium,** surrounds bundles or **fascicles** of skeletal muscle fibers; perimysium is an inward extension of the epimysium. A thin layer of connective tissue fibers, called **endomysium,** invests individual muscle fibers. Located in the connective tissue are blood vessels, nerves, and lymphatics of the skeletal muscle.

Skeletal muscles are richly innervated by large motor nerves or **axons.** Near the skeleton muscle, the motor nerve branches, and then a smaller axon branch innervates a single muscle fiber. Because of this **direct innervation,** each skeletal muscle fiber contracts only when stimulated by that **nerve (Figs. 5-3–5-4).**

Each skeletal muscle fiber exhibits a specialized site where the axon terminates. This is called the **neuromuscular junction** or **motor endplate,** a site where the impulse from the axon is transmitted to the skeletal muscle fiber. Between the axon terminal and the muscle fiber is a shallow trough called the **synaptic cleft.** Also, sensitive **stretch receptors** called **neuromuscular spindles** are located within all skeletal muscles. These spindles consist of special muscle fibers called **intrafusal fibers** and **nerve endings,** which are surrounded by a connective tissue **capsule (Figs. 5-5–5-6).**

CARDIAC MUSCLE

The cardiac muscle is located primarily in the walls and septa of the **heart** and in the walls of the large vessels attached to the heart. Just as the skeletal muscles, the cardiac muscles exhibit distinct **cross-striations** because **actin** and **myosin** filaments have similar and regular arrangement. In contrast, however, the cardiac muscle is **involuntary** and contracts **rhythmically** and **automatically.** This rhythmicity is influenced by nerve fibers from the **autonomic nervous system** and different **hormones.**

Cardiac muscle fibers usually exhibit one or two **central nuclei,** are also shorter than skeletal muscle fibers, and are branched. The terminal ends of adjacent cardiac muscle fibers form unique and distinct end-to-end junctional complexes called **intercalated disks.** In these regions, the opposing cell membranes contact each other and form small **gap junctions (Figs. 5-7–5-10).**

The **impulse-generating** and **impulse-conducting** system in the cardiac muscles is located within the heart wall itself. This system consists of specialized or modified cardiac muscle fibers found in the **sinoatrial (SA) node** and **atrioventricular (AV) node, bundle of His,** and **Purkinje fibers** (Chapter 7). The cardiac cells in the SA node exhibit a rapid rhythm of stimulating the heart contraction and set the pace for the heart rate. The SA node is therefore considered as the pacemaker of the heart.

Purkinje fibers are thicker and larger than cardiac muscle fibers and contain an increased amount of **glycogen.** Also, they contain fewer contractile filaments. Purkinje fibers deliver stimulation from the nodes to the rest of the heart musculature, resulting in ventricular contraction and blood ejection.

Figure 5-1   Smooth Muscle Layers of the Small Intestine

In the muscular region of the small intestine, smooth muscles are arranged in two concentric layers, an inner circulation and an outer longitudinal. In these layers, muscle fibers are packed tightly, with the cells of one layer arranged at right angles to those of the adjacent layer.

The upper region of the illustration shows the smooth muscle fibers in the inner circular layer cut in the longitudinal section. **Smooth muscle fibers (1, 7)** are spindle-shaped cells with tapered ends. The cytoplasm (sarcoplasm) of each muscle is stained deeply with an elongated or ovoid **nucleus (7)** present in the center.

The lower region of the figure shows the muscles of the adjacent longitudinal layer cut in a transverse section. Because the spindle-shaped cells are sectioned at different places along their length, the cells exhibit different shapes and sizes. The large **nuclei (5, 9)** are seen only in those sections in which the **smooth muscle fibers (3, 5, 9)** have been sectioned in the middle. The muscle fibers that were not sectioned in the center appear only as deeply stained areas of clear **cytoplasm (sarcoplasm) (3, lower leader; 9, lower leader).**

In the wall of the small intestine, the smooth muscle layers are applied closely to each other with only a minimum amount of **connective tissue fibers** and **fibroblasts (2, 4, 8, 10)** visible between the two layers. The smooth muscles also have a rich blood supply, as seen by the presence of numerous **capillaries (6, 11)** between individual fibers and between the layers.

■ Functional Correlations–Smooth Muscles

Smooth muscles usually exhibit **spontaneous activity** in a wavelike manner that passes in slow, sustained contraction throughout the entire muscle, producing a continuous contraction of low force. Smooth muscles make close contacts with each other by specialized connections called the **gap junctions.** These allow the passage of **stimuli** between the smooth muscle fibers. Smooth muscles are also **innervated** by nerves from the **sympathetic** and **parasympathetic divisions** of the **autonomic nervous system;** these innervations influence their contractility.

Figure 5-2   Smooth Muscle: Wall of the Small Intestine (transverse section and longitudinal section)

A photomicrograph through a wall of a small intestine illustrates its muscular outer wall. The smooth muscle fibers in the small intestine are arranged in two layers, an **inner circular layer (7)** and an **outer longitudinal layer (8).** In the inner circular layer (7), a single **nucleus (1)** of each smooth muscle fiber is visible in the center of the **cytoplasm (2).** In the longitudinal layer (8), which in this image is cut in transverse section, the **cytoplasm (5)** appears empty, and the single **nucleus (6)** of individual muscle fibers is only visible if the plane of section passes through it. Located between the two smooth muscle layers in the small intestine is a group of autonomic **neurons** of the **myenteric nerve plexus (3).** Small **blood vessels (4)** are seen between individual muscle fibers.

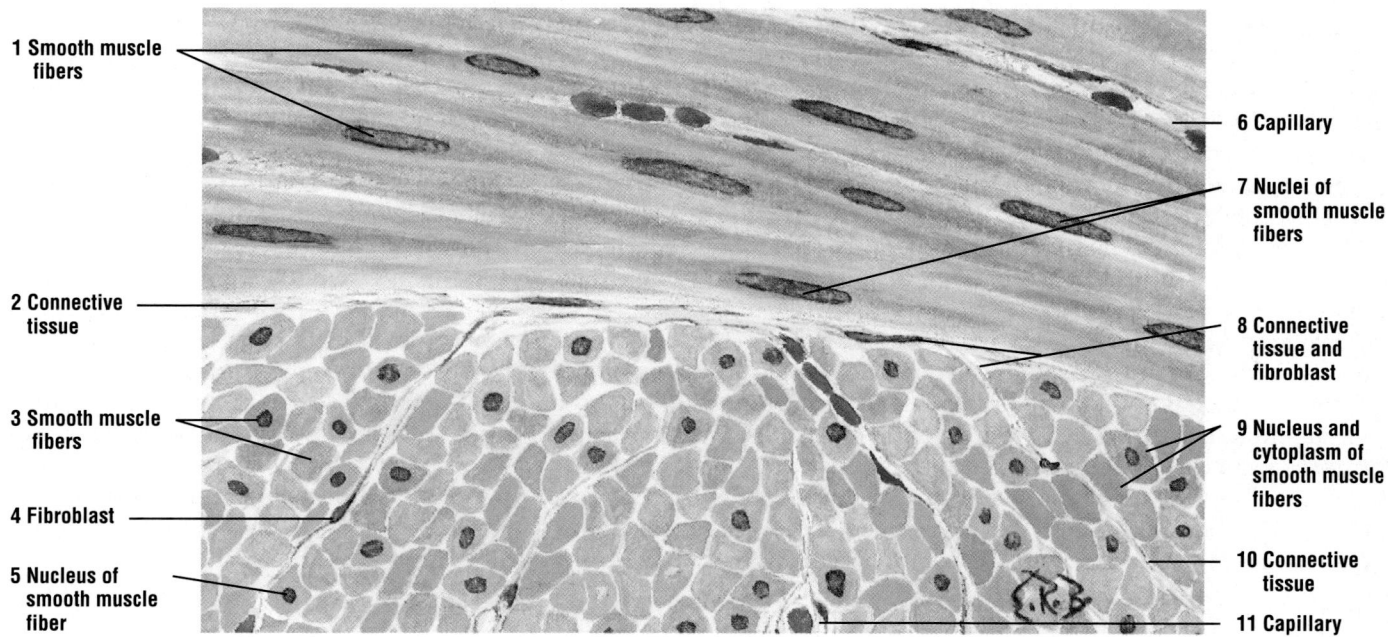

1 Smooth muscle
fibers

2 Connective
tissue

3 Smooth muscle
fibers

4 Fibroblast

5 Nucleus of
smooth muscle
fiber

6 Capillary

7 Nuclei of
smooth muscle
fibers

8 Connective
tissue and
fibroblast

9 Nucleus and
cytoplasm of
smooth muscle
fibers

10 Connective
tissue

11 Capillary

Fig. 5-1   Smooth Muscle Layers of the Small Intestine. Stain: hematoxylin-eosin. High magnification.

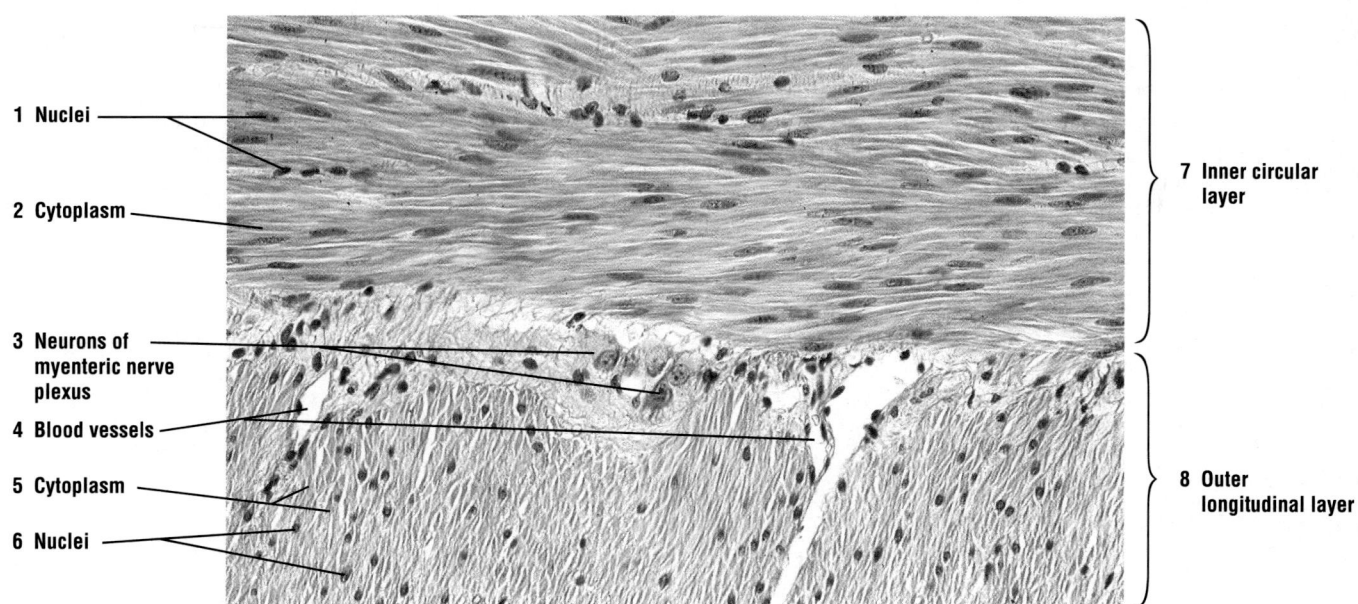

1 Nuclei

2 Cytoplasm

3 Neurons of
myenteric nerve
plexus

4 Blood vessels

5 Cytoplasm

6 Nuclei

7 Inner circular
layer

8 Outer
longitudinal layer

Fig. 5-2   Smooth Muscle: Wall of the Small Intestine (transverse section and longitudinal section). Stain: hematoxylin-eosin. 80×

Figure 5-3   Skeletal (Striated) Muscles of the Tongue

Skeletal muscle fibers are much longer and larger in diameter than smooth muscle fibers. In the tongue, these muscle fibers course in different directions. This figure illustrates the tongue muscle fibers in both the longitudinal (upper region) and transverse (lower region) sections.

Skeletal **muscles fibers (9, in transverse section; 11, in longitudinal section)** are multinucleated, with the **nuclei (1, 6)** situated peripherally and immediately below the sarcolemma. (Sarcolemma is not illustrated in the figure.) Each skeletal muscle fiber shows distinct **cross-striations (3),** which are visible as alternating dark or **A bands (3a)** and light or **I bands (3b).** With higher magnification, additional details of the cross-striations are visible in Figure 5-4.

Skeletal muscle fibers are aggregated into **fascicles (15)** and surrounded by **connective tissue fibers (5).** The connective tissue (5) sheath around each muscle fascicle is the **perimysium (12).** From the perimysium (12), thin partitions of connective tissue (5), called the **endomysium (4, 7),** extend into each muscle fascicle (15) and invest individual muscle fibers (9, 11). Small **blood vessels (8)** and **capillaries (2, 14)** are present throughout the connective tissue sheaths (5) that surround each muscle fiber.

Skeletal muscle fibers that have been sectioned longitudinally (11) show light and dark cross-striations, the A bands and I bands (3a, 3b). The muscle fibers that were sectioned transversely (9) exhibit cross sections of **myofibril bundles (13)** and peripheral nuclei (6).

Figure 5-4   Skeletal (Striated) Muscles of the Tongue (longitudinal section)

A higher magnification photomicrograph of the tongue illustrates individual **skeletal muscle fibers (1)** and their characteristic **cross striations (2).** The skeletal muscle fibers (1) are multinucleated and their **nuclei (3)** are located on the periphery of each fiber. Within each skeletal muscle fiber are seen tiny **myofibrils (6).** Surrounding each skeletal muscle fiber (1) is a thin layer of connective tissue **endomysium (5).** Aggregate of muscle fibers or a fascicle is invested by a thicker connective tissue layer **perimysium (4).** Associated with the connective tissue layers around the muscle fibers are the empty-appearing **adipose cells (7).**

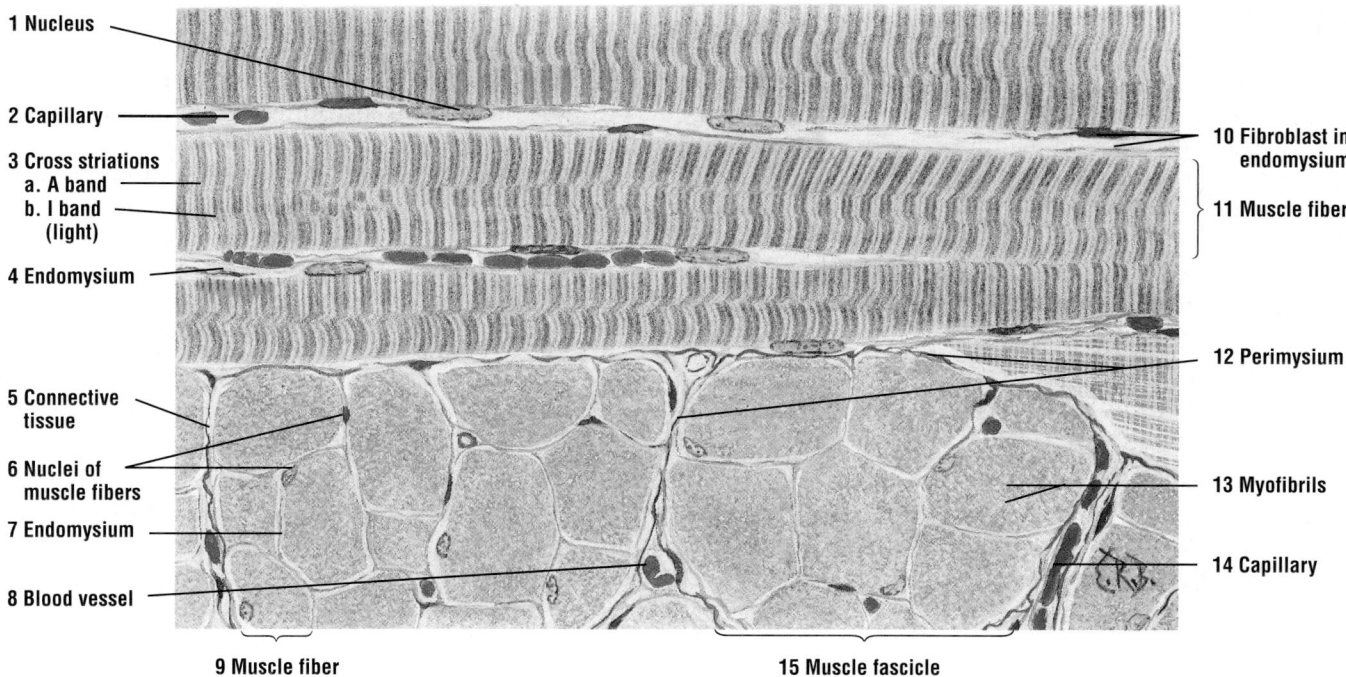

1 Nucleus

2 Capillary

3 Cross striations
   a. A band
   b. I band
      (light)

4 Endomysium

5 Connective
   tissue

6 Nuclei of
   muscle fibers

7 Endomysium

8 Blood vessel

10 Fibroblast in
   endomysium

11 Muscle fiber

12 Perimysium

13 Myofibrils

14 Capillary

9 Muscle fiber

15 Muscle fascicle

Fig. 5-3   Skeletal (Striated) Muscles of the Tongue. Stain: hematoxylin-eosin. High magnification.

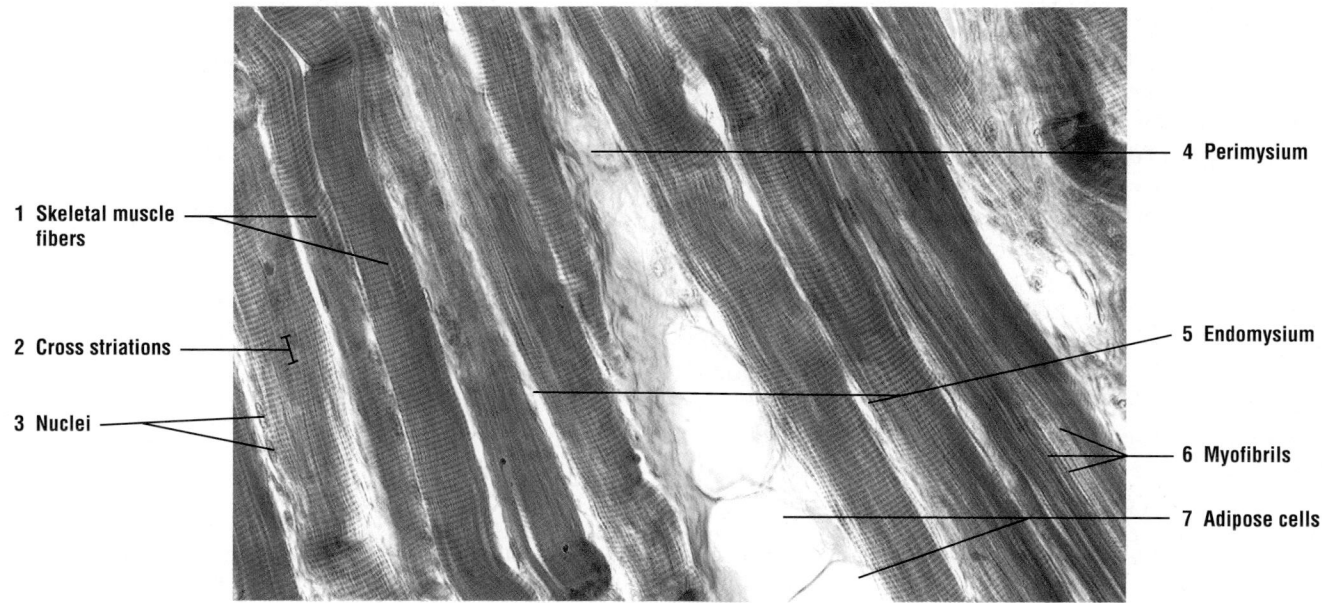

1 Skeletal muscle
   fibers

2 Cross striations

3 Nuclei

4 Perimysium

5 Endomysium

6 Myofibrils

7 Adipose cells

Fig. 5-4   Skeletal (Striated) Muscles of the Tongue (longitudinal section). Stain: Masson's trichrome. 130×

Figure 5-5   Skeletal Muscle and Motor Endplates

A group of skeletal muscle fibers (6, 7) have been teased apart and stained to illustrate the nerve terminations or myoneural junctions on the muscle fibers. In this illustration, the characteristic **cross-striations (2, 8)** of the skeletal muscle fibers (7) are seen readily. The dark-stained, string-like structures between the separated muscle fibers (7) are the myelinated motor **nerve (3)** and its terminal branches, the **axons (1, 5, 10).** The motor nerve (3) courses to the muscle, branches, and distributes its axons (1, 5, 10) to the individual muscle fibers (7). As the axons (1, 5, 10) reach the muscle fibers, they terminate on individual muscle fibers as specialized junctional regions called **motor endplates (4, 9).** The small, round structures seen in the motor endplates (4, 9) represent the terminal expansion of the axons (1, 5, 10). **Axon terminals (1),** whose motor endplates are not present in this section, are seen also in this figure.

■ Functional Correlations–Skeletal Muscle and Motor Endplates

The terminal end of each axon that innervates the muscle fiber exhibits numerous **vesicles** that contain the **neurotransmitter acetylcholine.** Arrival of a nerve impulse or the **action potential** at the axon terminal causes the synaptic vesicles to fuse with the plasma membrane and release the acetylcholine into the **synaptic cleft,** a small gap between the axon and the muscle fiber. The released neurotransmitter then diffuses across the synaptic cleft, combines with **acetylcholine receptors** on the muscle fiber membrane, and **stimulates** the muscle fiber. This action produces **contraction** of the skeletal muscle fiber. An enzyme called **acetylcholinesterase,** located on the muscle fiber membrane, **inactivates** the released acetylcholine. Inactivation of acetylcholine prevents further muscle stimulation and muscle contraction until the arrival of the next impulse at the axon terminal.

Figure 5-6   Skeletal Muscle and Muscle Spindle (transverse section)

A transverse section of an extraocular skeletal muscle shows individual **muscle fibers (2)** surrounded by a thin connective tissue fibers **endomysium (6).** The muscle fibers (2), in turn, are grouped into numerous **fascicles (1)** and surrounded by interfascicular connective tissue septa, the **perimysium (4).** Located within the numerous muscle fascicles (1) is a cross-section of an encapsulated **muscle spindle (3).** Surrounding the muscle fibers (2) and the muscle spindle (3) are numerous **arterioles (5)** in the connective tissue septa (4).

The muscle spindle (3) is an encapsulated sensory end organ. The ovoid connective tissue **capsule (8)** around the muscle spindle (3), derived from the adjacent **perimysium (11),** encloses several components of the spindle. Specialized muscle fibers that are located in the spindle and surrounded by the capsule (8) are called the **intrafusal fibers (10).** This is in contrast to the ordinary skeletal muscle fibers, the **extrafusal fibers (7)** that are located outside of the spindle capsule (8). Small nerves fibers associated with the muscle spindles (3) represent the incoming myelinated and terminal unmyelinated **nerve fibers (axons) (9)** that are surrounded by the Schwann cells. Small blood vessels are present in the capsule of the muscle spindle (3), as well as an adjacent **arteriole (12).** These vessels come from blood vessels that are located in the **perimysium (11)** of the muscle proper.

■ Functional Correlations–Muscle Spindle

Muscle spindles are sensitive **stretch receptors** located in all skeletal muscles. Their main function in the muscle is to detect changes in the **length** or stretch of the muscle fibers. An increase in the length or stretch of muscle fibers stimulates the muscle spindle and sends **impulses** via the afferent axons into the spinal cord. These impulses produce a **muscle stretch reflex** that immediately causes **contraction** and **shortening** of the stretched muscle. A decrease in muscle length ceases the stimulation of the fibers in the muscle spindle and the conduction of impulses to the spinal cord.

1 Axon terminals

2 Cross-striations

3 Myelinated nerve

4 Motor end plates

5 Axons

6 Skeletal muscle fibers

7 Skeletal muscle fibers

8 Cross-striations

9 Motor endplates

10 Axons

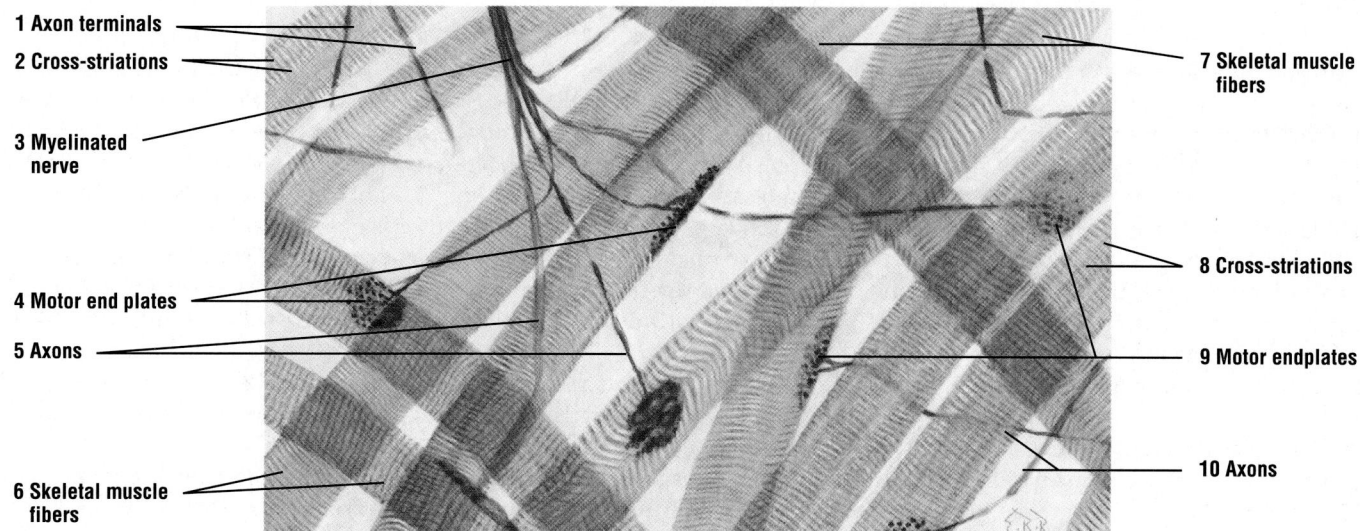

Fig. 5-5   Skeletal Muscle and Motor Endplates. Stain: silver. High magnification.

1 Fascicles

2 Skeletal muscle fibers

3 Muscle spindle

4 Perimysium

5 Arterioles

6 Endomysium

7 Extrafusal fibers

8 Capsule of muscle spindle

9 Nerve fibers with Schawann cells

10 Intrafusal fibers

11 Perimysium

12 Arteriole

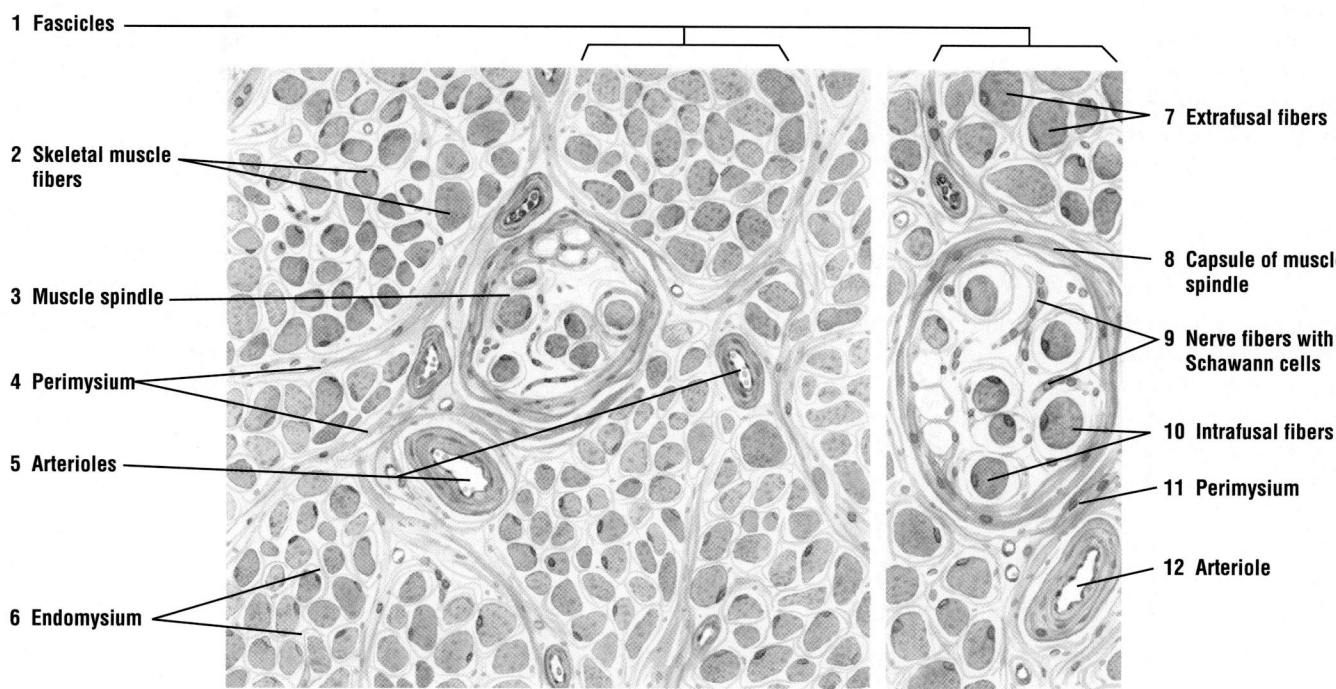

Fig. 5-6   Skeletal Muscle and Muscle Spindle (transverse section). Frozen section stained with modified Van Giesen method (hematoxylin, picric acid-ponceau S). Left, medium magnification; right, high magnification. (Tissue samples courtesy of Dr. Mark DeSantis, WWAMI Medical Program, University of Idaho, Moscow, Idaho).

Figure 5-7   Cardiac Muscle

Cardiac muscle fibers exhibit some of the features seen in the skeletal muscles. This figure illustrates a section of a cardiac muscle cut in both the longitudinal (upper portion) and transverse (lower portion) section. The **cross-striations (2)** in cardiac muscle fibers closely resemble those seen in skeletal muscles; however, cardiac muscles **branch (5, 10)** without their diameters changing much. Also, unlike the multinucleated, elongated skeletal muscles, each cardiac muscle fiber is shorter and contains a single, centrally located **nucleus (3, 7). Binucleate (two nuclei) muscle fibers (8)** also are seen occasionally. The location of the nuclei (7) in the center is clearly visible when the muscle fibers are cut in a transverse section. Around these nuclei (3, 7, 8) are the clear zones of nonfibrillar **perinuclear sarcoplasm (1, 13).** In transverse sections of the cardiac fibers, the perinuclear sarcoplasm (13) appears as a clear space if the cut is not through the nucleus. Also visible in transverse sections are the **myofibrils (14)** of individual cardiac muscle cells.

A distinguishing and characteristic feature of the cardiac muscles are the **intercalated disks (4, 9).** These disks (4,9) are dark-staining structures that are found at irregular intervals in the cardiac muscle; they represent the specialized junctional complexes between adjacent cardiac muscle fibers.

The cardiac muscle has a vast blood supply. Numerous small blood vessels are found in the **connective tissue (11)** that surrounds the muscle fibers. **Capillaries (6)** are abundant in the delicate **endomysium (12)** between individual muscle fibers.

Other examples of cardiac muscles are seen in Chapter 7 (Figs. 7-5–7-8).

■ Functional Correlations–Cardiac Muscle

Intercalated disks bind and functionally couple all cardiac muscle fibers to allow a rapid spread of stimuli for contraction of the entire heart musculature. The diffusion of ions through the pores in the **gap junctions** of cardiac muscle fibers allows for the **functional coupling** and coordination of the activities in the entire heart. As a result, the cardiac muscle acts in unison as a **functional syncytium.**

Both the **parasympathetic** and **sympathetic divisions** of the autonomic nervous system innervate the heart in the vicinity of the nodes. Nerves fibers from the parasympathetic division, by way of vagus nerves, **slow** the heart and **decrease** blood pressure. Nerve fibers of the sympathetic division produce the opposite effect; they **increase** the **rhythmicity** of the pacemaker cells and, consequently, heart rate and blood pressure.

Figure 5-8   Cardiac Muscle (longitudinal section)

A higher magnification photomicrograph illustrates a section of the cardiac muscle cut in a longitudinal plane. The **cardiac muscle fibers (2)** exhibit **cross striations (4), branching (3),** and a single central **nucleus (5).** The characteristic dark-staining **intercalated disks (1)** connect individual cardiac muscle fibers (2). Small **myofibrils (6)** are visible within each cardiac muscle fiber. Delicate **connective tissue fibers (7)** surround the individual cardiac muscle fibers.

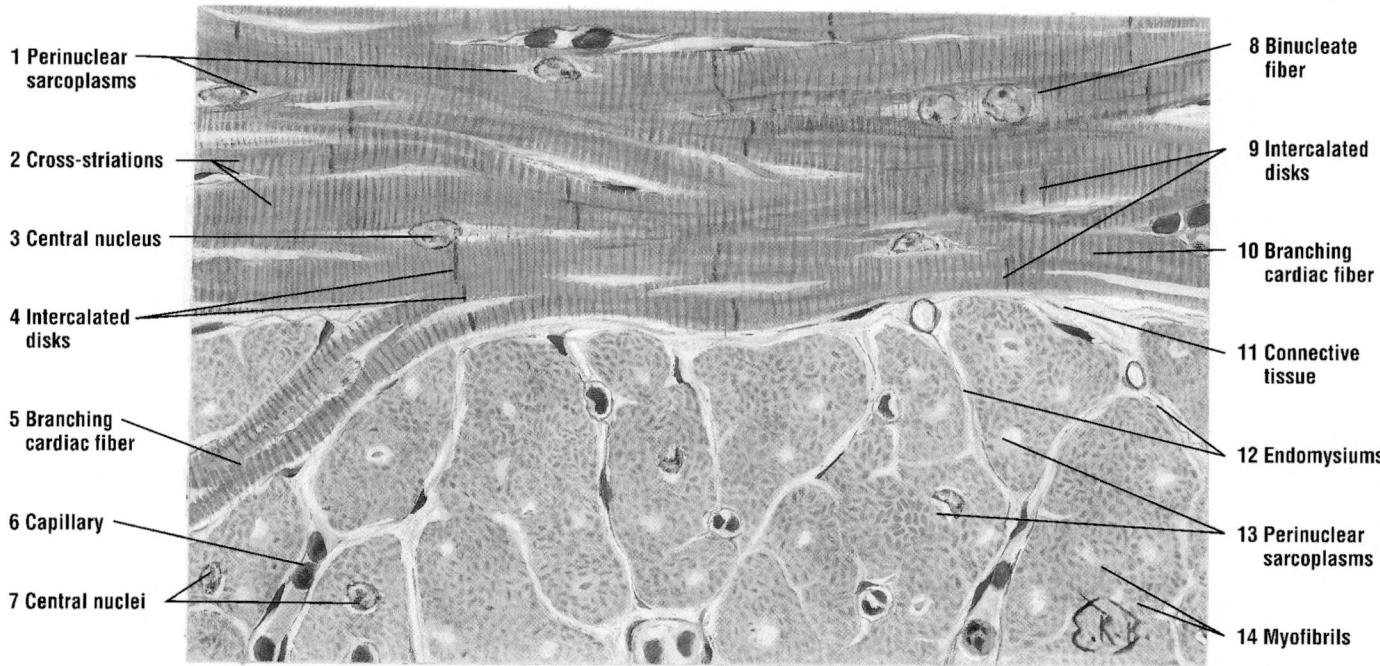

1 Perinuclear sarcoplasms

2 Cross-striations

3 Central nucleus

4 Intercalated disks

5 Branching cardiac fiber

6 Capillary

7 Central nuclei

8 Binucleate fiber

9 Intercalated disks

10 Branching cardiac fiber

11 Connective tissue

12 Endomysiums

13 Perinuclear sarcoplasms

14 Myofibrils

Fig. 5-7   Cardiac Muscle. Stain: hematoxylin-eosin. High magnification.

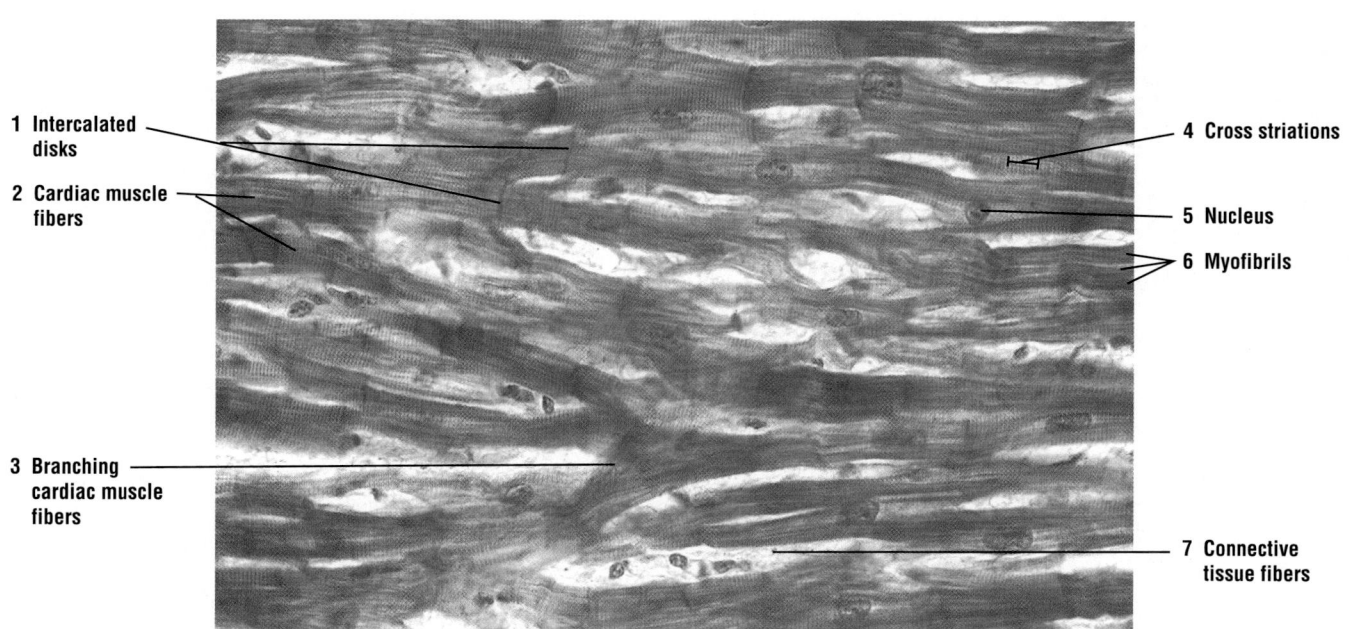

1 Intercalated disks

2 Cardiac muscle fibers

3 Branching cardiac muscle fibers

4 Cross striations

5 Nucleus

6 Myofibrils

7 Connective tissue fibers

Fig. 5-8   Cardiac Muscle (longitudinal section). Stain: Masson's trichrome. 130×

Figure 5-9   Skeletal Muscle (longitudinal section)

High magnification of muscle fibers demonstrates the cross-striations. The anisotropic or **A bands (2)** are the prominent, dark-staining bands; a lighter middle region, the H band, is not visible. The isotropic bands, or I bands, are equally prominent and are lightly stained acidophilic bands. Crossing each central portion of the I bands are distinct, narrow lines, the **Z lines (3).**

The closely arranged parallel myofibrils give a longitudinally striated appearance to the muscle fibers. Where the **myofibrils (6)** are separated because of rupture of the sarcolemma, the A, I, and Z lines are visible on the myofibrils and are aligned next to each other on adjacent myofibrils.

Slender ovoid or **elongated nuclei (4)** of muscle fibers are seen peripherally. In the **endomysium (1)** between muscle fibers, **fibroblasts (5)** and a **capillary (7)** are seen.

Figure 5-10   Cardiac Muscle (longitudinal section)

Comparison of cardiac muscle with skeletal muscle at the same magnification and the same stain illustrates the similarities and differences between the two muscle types.

Branching **cardiac fibers (3)** are in distinct contrast to individual skeletal fibers. **Cross-striations (2, 5)** are similar to both but less prominent in cardiac muscle fibers. The prominence of the **intercalated disks (7)** and their irregular structure are seen more clearly at higher magnification. The area between two intercalated disks represents one cardiac muscle cell.

Large, oval **nuclei (1),** usually one per cell, occupy the central position and much of the width of the cardiac fibers, in contrast to the many elongated peripheral nuclei of the skeletal fibers. The **perinuclear sarcoplasm (6)** region is distinct. **Endomysium (4)** fills the spaces between fibers.

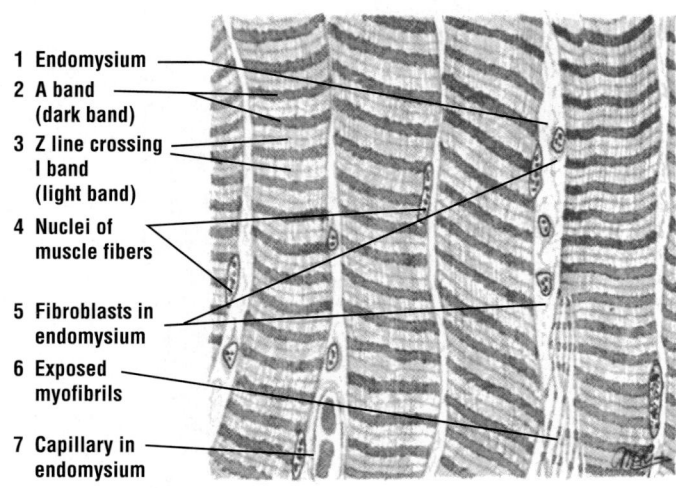

1 Endomysium
2 A band (dark band)
3 Z line crossing I band (light band)
4 Nuclei of muscle fibers
5 Fibroblasts in endomysium
6 Exposed myofibrils
7 Capillary in endomysium

Fig. 5-9   Skeletal Muscle (longitudinal section). Stain: Iron hematoxylin-eosin. Oil immersion.

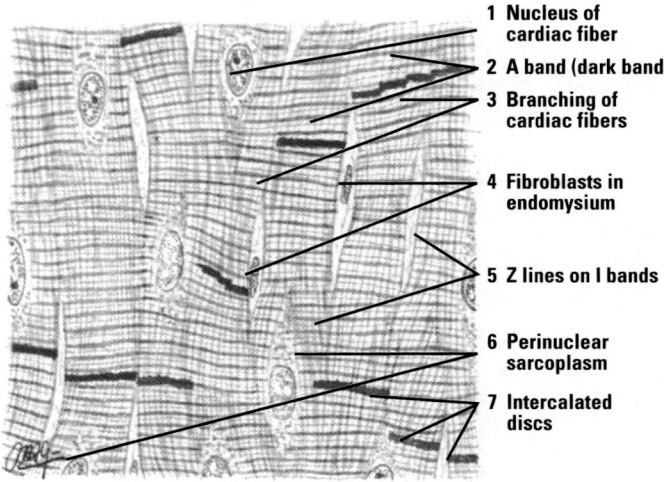

1 Nucleus of cardiac fiber
2 A band (dark band)
3 Branching of cardiac fibers
4 Fibroblasts in endomysium
5 Z lines on I bands
6 Perinuclear sarcoplasm
7 Intercalated discs

Fig. 5-10   Cardiac Muscle (longitudinal section). Stain: Iron hematoxylin-eosin. Oil immersion.

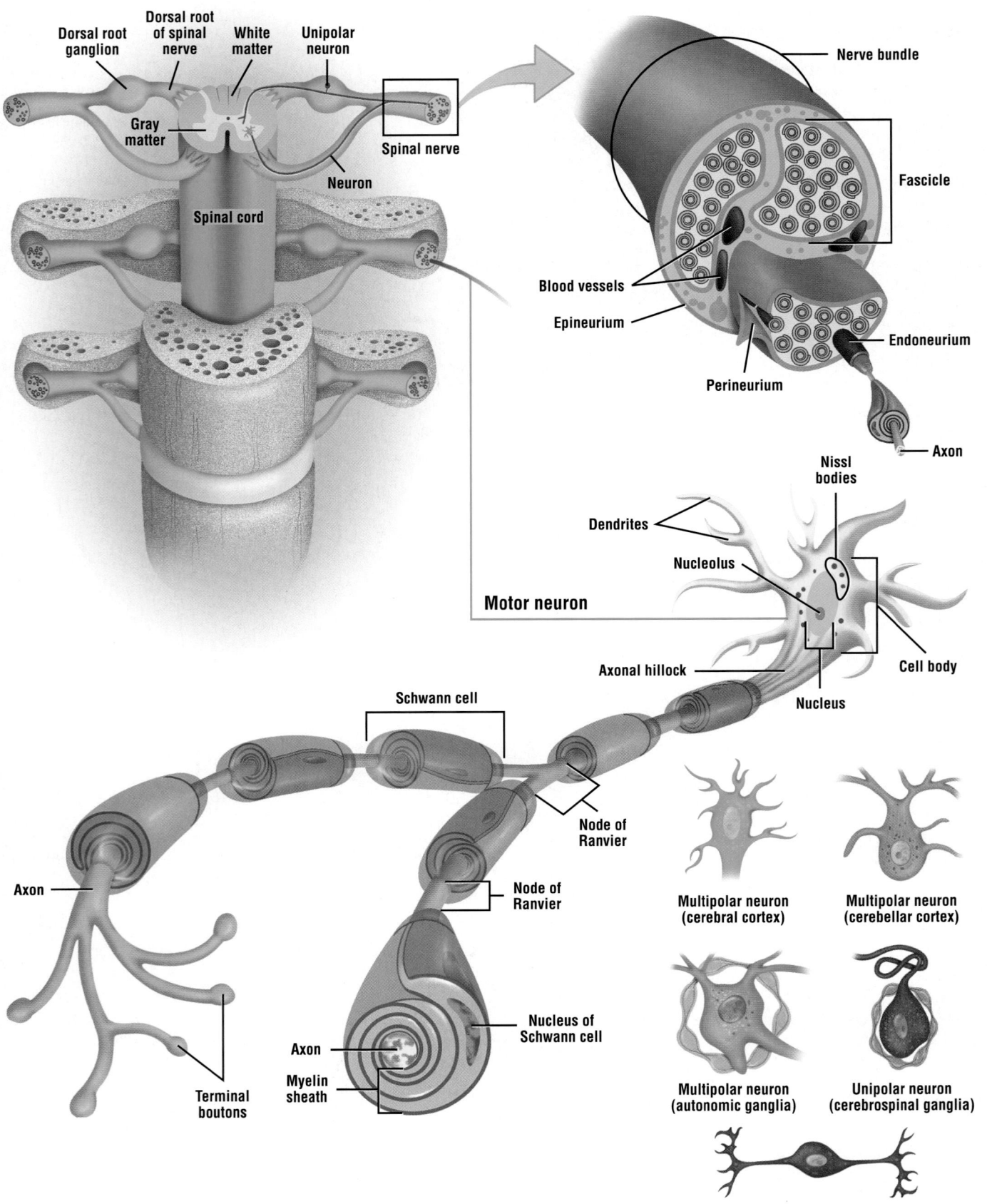

Dorsal root ganglion

Dorsal root of spinal nerve

White matter

Unipolar neuron

Gray matter

Spinal cord

Neuron

Spinal nerve

Nerve bundle

Fascicle

Blood vessels

Epineurium

Perineurium

Endoneurium

Axon

Nissl bodies

Dendrites

Nucleolus

Nucleus

Motor neuron

Axonal hillock

Cell body

Schwann cell

Node of Ranvier

Node of Ranvier

Axon

Nucleus of Schwann cell

Axon

Myelin sheath

Terminal boutons

Multipolar neuron (cerebral cortex)

Multipolar neuron (cerebellar cortex)

Multipolar neuron (autonomic ganglia)

Unipolar neuron (cerebrospinal ganglia)

Bipolar neuron (retina)

Nervous Tissue

The nervous system is divided into two major parts, the **central nervous system (CNS)** and the **peripheral nervous system (PNS).** The CNS consists of **neurons** and **axons** located in the **brain** and the **spinal cord;** it is the integrating and communicating center of the body. The PNS consists of neurons and axons located outside the CNS. These include cranial nerves from the brain, the spinal nerves from the spinal cord, and both of their associated ganglia. The brain and the spinal cord consist of **white matter** and **gray matter.** White matter consists primarily of **myelinated axons,** some unmyelinated axons, and the supporting cells. Presence of **myelin sheaths** around the axons imparts a white color to this region. Gray matter is composed of neurons, dentrites, and neuroglial cells. Lack of myelin sheaths imparts a gray color to this area of the central nervous system.

NEURONS

The nervous tissue consists of two principal cell types: **neurons** (nerve cells) and **neuroglia** (supporting cells). The structural and functional cells of the nervous tissue are the neurons. Neurons form the highly complex **intercommunicating network** of nerve cells that receive and conduct **impulses** along their neural pathways or **axons** to the CNS for analysis, integration, interpretation, and response. The appropriate response to a given stimulus from the CNS is the activation of muscles and/or glands.

The three major groups of neurons are multipolar, bipolar, and unipolar. Their anatomic classification is based on the number of dendrites and axons that originate from the cell body. **Multipolar neurons** are the most common type in the CNS and include **motor neurons** and **interneurons** of the brain and spinal cord. Projecting from the cell body of the multipolar neuron are numerous branched **dendrites.** On the opposite side of the neuron is a single process, the **axon. Bipolar neurons,** which are less common, are purely **sensory neurons.** In these neurons, a single dendrite and a single axon leave the cell body. Bipolar neurons are the sensory **receptor cells** found in the retina of the eye, in the organ of hearing in the inner ear, and in the olfactory epithelium in the upper region of the nose. Most neurons in the adult organism that exhibit only one process leaving the cell body were initially bipolar. These are the **unipolar neurons;** they are also **sensory.** Unipolar neurons are found in numerous craniosacral ganglia of the body **(Figs. 6-1–6-2, 6-14–6-16, 6-18, 6-20, 6-25–6-26).**

SUPPORTING CELLS IN THE CNS: NEUROGLIA

Neuroglia are the highly branched, supportive, nonneuronal cells in the CNS that are located between the neurons. These cells do not conduct impulses and are morphologically and functionally different from the neurons. They can be distinguished by their much smaller size and their dark-staining nuclei. There are about 10 times more neuroglial cells than neurons in the nervous system. The three types of neuroglia cells are: **astrocytes, oligodendrocytes,** and **microglia (Figs. 6-3—6-5).**

SUPPORTING CELLS IN THE PNS

There are also supportive cells found in the PNS; these are the **Schwann cells (**neurolemmocytes**)** and the **satellite cells.** The Schwann cells surround and lie along the length of the axons. The satellite cells are small cuboidal cells found in paravertebral and peripheral ganglia. Here, the satellite cells surround the neuronal cells in the ganglia **(Figs. 6-9–6-13).**

NERVE FIBERS: MYELINATED AND UNMYELINATED AXONS

Nerves are composed of **axons** of various size and their surrounding sheaths. In the **PNS,** all axons are surrounded by **Schwann cells** (neurilemma). These cells extend along the length of peripheral axon, from its origin to its termination in the muscle or gland. The Schwann cells form the lipid-rich **myelin sheath** around the larger axons. In the CNS, myelin sheath formation and myelination of axons is accomplished by **oligodendrocytes.**

Smaller axons, such as those of the autonomic nervous system (ANS), are surrounded only by the Schwann cell cytoplasm. Such axons do not have a myelin sheath and are **unmyelinated.** Larger axons are wrapped by successive layers of the **plasma membrane** of the Schwann cell, which produces the insulating myelin sheath; axons surrounded by a myelin sheath are **myelinated.** Along the entire length of a myelinated axon are small gaps in the myelin sheath between individual Schwann cells called the **nodes of Ranvier.** These nodal gaps represent the discontinuity between the Schwann cells and exposure of the axon to the **extracellular environment (Figs. 6-8, 6-11, 6-27).**

Figure 6-1   Motor Neurons: Anterior Horn of the Spinal Cord

The large, multipolar **motor neurons (7)** of the CNS have a large central **nucleus (11)**, a prominent **nucleolus (12)**, and several radiating cell processes, the **dendrites (10, 16)**. A single, thin **axon (5, 14)** arises from a cone-shaped, clear area of the neuron; this is the **axon hillock (6, 13)**. The axons (5, 14) that leave the motor neurons (7) are thinner and much longer than the thicker but shorter dendrites (10, 16).

The cytoplasm or perikaryon of the neuron is characterized by numerous clumps of coarse granules (basophilic masses). These are the **Nissl bodies (4, 8),** and they represent the granular endoplasmic reticulum of the neuron. When the plane of section misses the nucleus (4), only the dark-staining Nissl bodies (4) are seen in the perikaryon of the neuron. The Nissl bodies (4, 8) extend into the dendrites (10, 16) but not into the axon hillock (6, 13) or into the axon (5, 14). This feature distinguishes the axons (5, 14) from the dendrites (10, 16). The nucleus of the neuron (11) is outlined distinctly and stains light because of the uniform dispersion of the chromatin. The nucleolus (12), on the other hand, is prominent, dense, and stains dark. The **nuclei (2, 9)** of the surrounding **neuroglia (2, 9),** are stained prominently, whereas their small cytoplasm remains unstained. The neuroglia (2, 9) are nonneural cells of the central nervous system; they provide the structural and metabolic support for the neurons (7).

Surrounding the neurons (7) and the neuroglia (2, 9) are numerous blood vessels **(1, 3, 15)** of various sizes.

Figure 6-2   Gray Matter: Anterior Horn of the Spinal Cord

This section of the anterior horn of the spinal cord was prepared by silver impregnation (Cajal's method) to demonstrate neurofibrils. Typical **neurofibril (2, 13)** arrangements are seen in the **perikaryon (cytoplasm)** of the **motor neurons (3, 6, 11)** and in their **dendrites (7, 12)**. Axons are not illustrated in this figure, but neurofibrils would be seen in similar parallel arrangement.

Other details of the motor neurons are not revealed with silver impregnation technique. As a result, the nuclei of these **neurons (3, 11, 14)** appear as lightly stained or almost clear spaces. The **nucleolus (15)** may stain light (11) or dark (15). In the intercellular areas, many fibrillar processes, some of which arise from the anterior horn neurons or the associated adjacent neuroglia, are seen.

The **nuclei (1, 4, 5, 8, 9, 10)** of neuroglial cells are stained and show same characteristics as described in Figure 6-1.

■ Functional Correlations–Neurons

Functionally, neurons are classified as **afferent** (sensory), **efferent** (motor), or **interneurons.** Sensory neurons conduct impulses from internal or external receptors to the CNS. Motor neurons convey impulses from the CNS to the effector muscles or glands. Interneurons serve as intermediary cells and are located between sensory and motor neurons in the CNS.

Neurons are highly specialized for **irritability, conductivity,** and the **synthesis** of such neuroactive substances as the **neurotransmitters** and **neurohormones.** During a mechanical or chemical stimulus, these specializations allow the neurons to react (irritability) to the stimulus and to transmit (conductivity) the information to other neurons in different regions of the nervous system. Strong stimuli create a wave of excitation or nervous impulses (action potential) from the neurons that are then **self-propagated** along the entire length of the axon (nerve fiber) over a long distance.

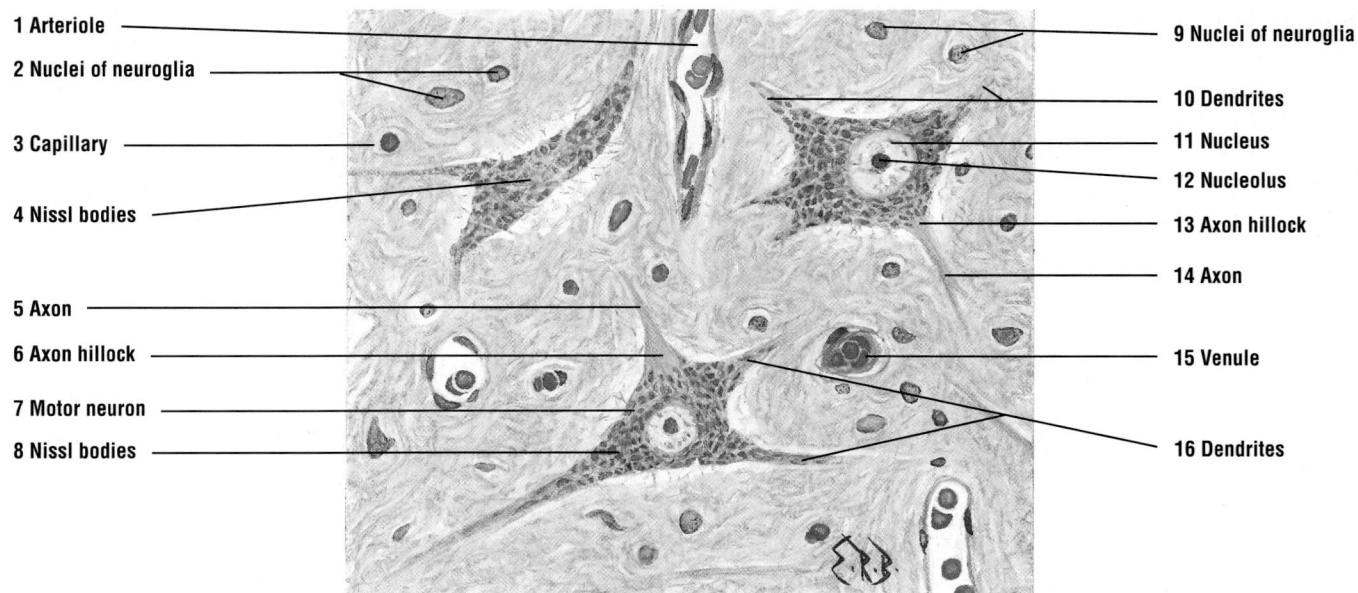

1 Arteriole

2 Nuclei of neuroglia

3 Capillary

4 Nissl bodies

5 Axon

6 Axon hillock

7 Motor neuron

8 Nissl bodies

9 Nuclei of neuroglia

10 Dendrites

11 Nucleus

12 Nucleolus

13 Axon hillock

14 Axon

15 Venule

16 Dendrites

Fig. 6-1   Motor Neurons: Anterior Horn of the Spinal Cord. Stain: hematoxylin-eosin. High magnification.

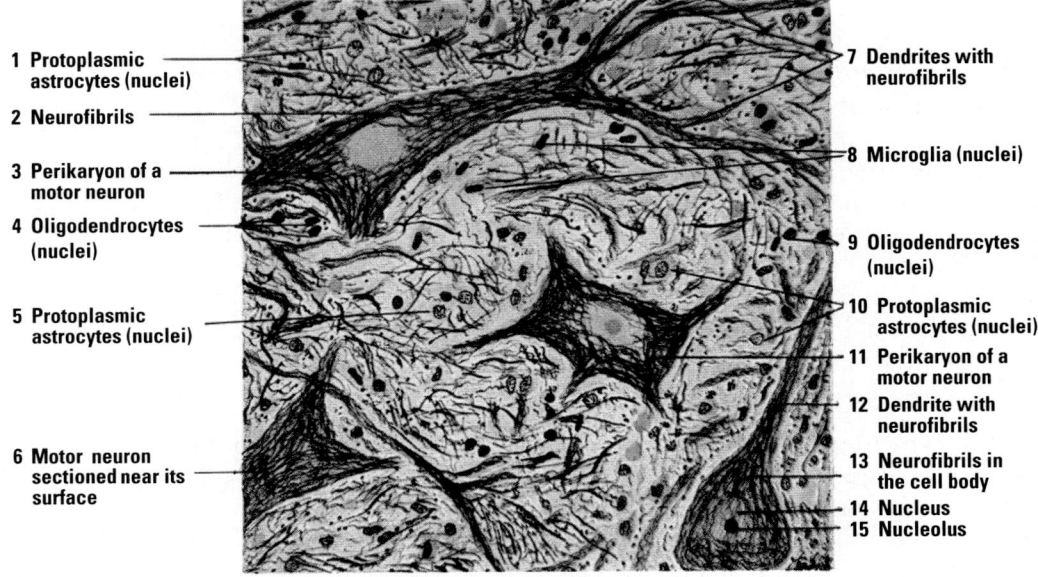

1 Protoplasmic astrocytes (nuclei)

2 Neurofibrils

3 Perikaryon of a motor neuron

4 Oligodendrocytes (nuclei)

5 Protoplasmic astrocytes (nuclei)

6 Motor neuron sectioned near its surface

7 Dendrites with neurofibrils

8 Microglia (nuclei)

9 Oligodendrocytes (nuclei)

10 Protoplasmic astrocytes (nuclei)

11 Perikaryon of a motor neuron

12 Dendrite with neurofibrils

13 Neurofibrils in the cell body

14 Nucleus

15 Nucleolus

Fig. 6-2   Gray Matter: Anterior Horn of the Spinal Cord. Stain: Cajal's method for neurofibrils. High magnification.

Figure 6-3   Fibrous Astrocytes of the Brain

A section of the brain was stained by Del Rio Hortega's method to demonstrate the cell outlines, processes, and fibers of astrocytes and oligodendrocytes.

In the center of the figure is a **fibrous astrocyte (5)**. It exhibits a small cell body, a large nucleus, and numerous long, smooth, slightly branched **processes (2)** extending in all directions. A number of these processes (2) from different astrocytes, seen in the upper left of the figure, terminate on a blood vessel as **vascular pedicles (4)** or foot plates.

Figure 6-4   Oligodendrocytes of the Brain

In the upper right corner of the figure is a **protoplasmic astrocyte (4)**. It exhibits a small cell body, large nucleus, and numerous, thick-branched processes.

In comparison, the **oligodendrocytes (2, 5)** have smaller oval cell bodies and nuclei than the astrocytes and exhibit few, thin, short processes without excessive branching. The processes may be extremely thin (5) or somewhat thicker (2).

The oligodendrocytes (2, 5) are found in both the gray and white matter of the CNS. In the white matter, the oligodendrocytes (2, 5) form myelin sheaths around numerous **axons (6)** and are analogous to the Schwann cells that myelinate the axons in the nerves of the PNS.

A portion of the **neuron (1)** in the upper left of the figure provides a size contrast with the astrocytes (4) and oligodendrocytes (2, 5).

Figure 6-5   Microglia of the Brain

In this section of the brain are the **microglia (1, 4)**. Their cell bodies are extremely small, vary in shape, and often exhibit irregular contours. The small, deeply stained nucleus almost fills the entire cell. The cell processes are few, short, slender, tortuous, and covered with small **"spines" (5)**. The **neuron (3),** located superiorly in the figure, provides a size contrast with the microglia (1, 4).

Microglia are usually not numerous, but are found in both the white and gray matter of the CNS. Microglia are the main phagocytes of the CNS.

■ Functional Correlations–Neuroglia

Astrocytes are the largest neuroglia cells and consist of two types: fibrous astrocytes and protoplasmic astrocytes. In the CNS, both types of astrocytes are attached to the walls of the **capillaries** and to **neurons.** They support **metabolic exchanges** between neurons and the capillaries of the CNS. In addition, the astrocytes control the **chemical environment** around neurons. They regulate or clear intercellular spaces of **potassium ions** and released **neurotransmitters** during neuronal activities in order to maintains a proper ionic environment for their function.

Oligodendrocytes are smaller than the astrocytes and exhibit fewer cytoplasmic processes. Oligodendrocytes form **myelin sheaths** around the **axons** in the **CNS.** Because oligodendrocytes have several processes, a single oligodendrocyte can surround and myelinate numerous axons. This same function of myelination of axons in the PNS is carried out by a different type of supporting cells called **schwann cells.**

Microglia are the smallest, dark-staining neuroglial cells. The microglia are believed to be part of the **mononuclear phagocyte system** of the CNS. Their main function is that of the **macrophages** and the microglia are found throughout the CNS. When nervous tissue is injured or damaged, microglia migrate to the region, proliferate, become phagocytic, and remove dead or foreign tissue from the CNS.

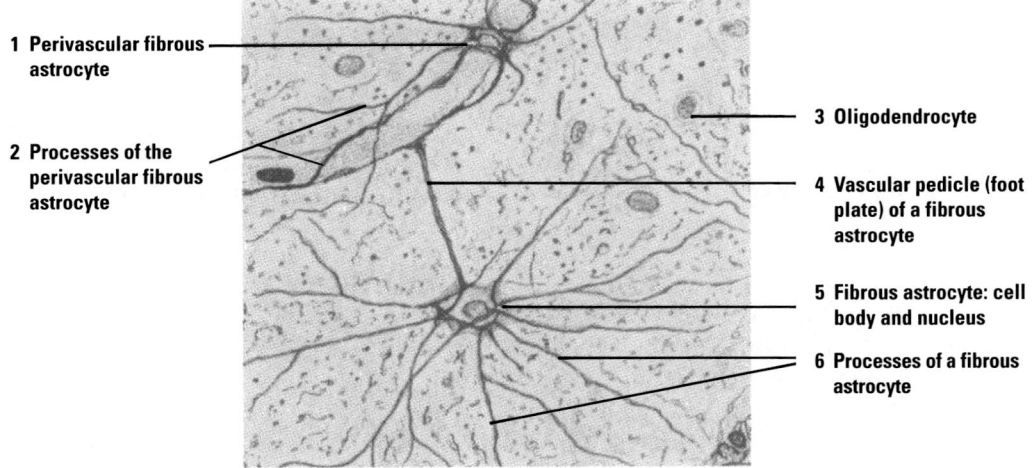

1 Perivascular fibrous astrocyte

2 Processes of the perivascular fibrous astrocyte

3 Oligodendrocyte

4 Vascular pedicle (foot plate) of a fibrous astrocyte

5 Fibrous astrocyte: cell body and nucleus

6 Processes of a fibrous astrocyte

Fig. 6-3 **Fibrous Astrocytes of the Brain.** Stain: Del Rio Hortega's method. Medium magnification.

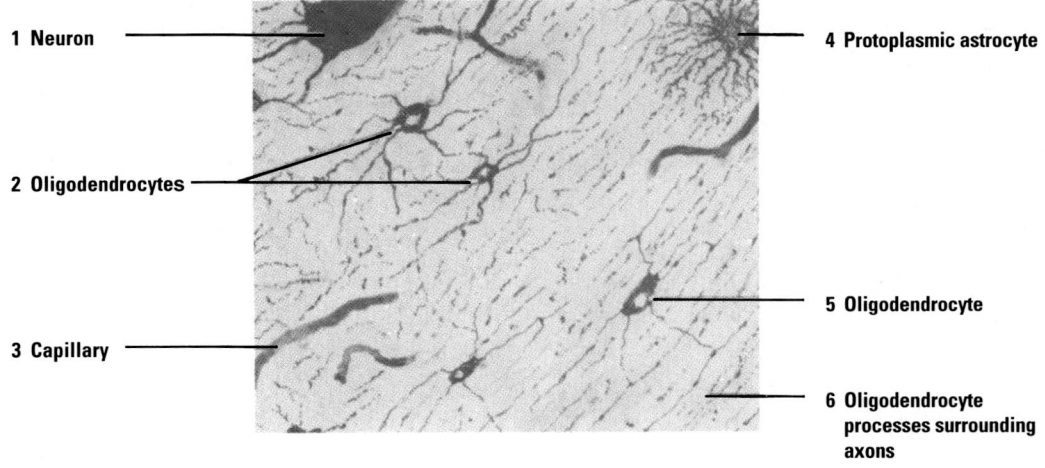

1 Neuron

2 Oligodendrocytes

3 Capillary

4 Protoplasmic astrocyte

5 Oligodendrocyte

6 Oligodendrocyte processes surrounding axons

Fig. 6-4 **Oligodendrocytes of the Brain.** Stain: Modified Del Rio Hortega's method. Medium magnification.

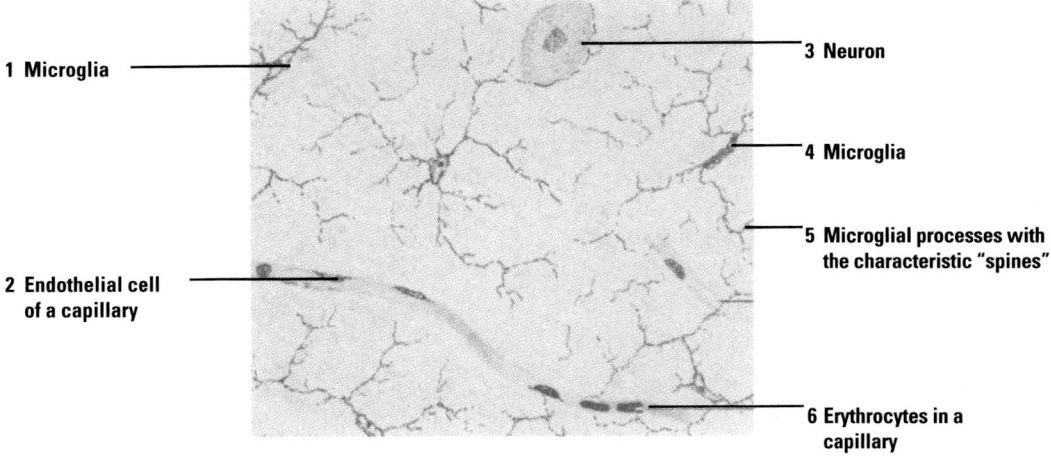

1 Microglia

2 Endothelial cell of a capillary

3 Neuron

4 Microglia

5 Microglial processes with the characteristic "spines"

6 Erythrocytes in a capillary

Fig. 6-5 **Microglia of the Brain.** Stain: Del Rio Hortega's method. Medium magnification.

Figure 6-6   Myelinated Nerve Fibers

Schwann cells surround the axons of the peripheral nerves and form a myelin sheath. To illustrate the myelin sheath, nerve fibers are fixed with an osmic acid; this preparation stains the lipid in the myelin sheath black. In this illustration, a portion of the peripheral nerve has been prepared in a longitudinal section (upper figure) and in a cross section (lower figure).

In the longitudinal section, the **myelin sheath (1)** appears as a thick, black band surrounding a lighter, central **axon (2)**. At intervals of a few microns, the myelin sheath exhibits discontinuity between adjacent Schwann cells. This region represents the **node of Ranvier (4)**.

A group of nerve fibers or fascicle is also illustrated. The fascicle is surrounded by a light-appearing connective tissue layer called the **perineurium (3, 5, 8)**. Each individual nerve fiber or axon, in turn, is surrounded by a thin layer of connective tissue called the **endoneurium (7, 11)**.

In the cross section, different sizes of myelinated axons are seen. The **myelin sheath (9)** appears as a thick, black ring around the light, unstained **axon (13)**, which in most fibers is seen in the center.

The connective tissue surrounding individual nerve fibers or the fascicle exhibits a rich supply of **blood vessels (6, 12)** of different sizes.

Figure 6-7   Peripheral Nerve (transverse section)

Several **bundles (fascicles) (1)** of nerve fibers have been sectioned in transverse **(1)** or oblique **(8)** planes. Each nerve fascicle is surrounded by a connective tissue sheath, the **perineurium (2)**, which merges with surrounding **interfascicular connective tissue (17)**. Perineurial septa may separate larger nerve fascicles. From these or directly from the perineurium, delicate connective tissue strands surround individual nerve fibers in a fascicle and form the **endoneurium (5)**.

Numerous nuclei are seen between individual nerve fibers. Most of these are **Schwann cell nuclei (3)**; others are **fibroblast nuclei of the endoneurium (5)**. (See Fig. 6-9).

Numerous **blood vessels (9–12, 16)** that course in the interfascicular connective tissue send branches into each fascicle that ultimately divide into capillaries in the endoneurium (5).

■ Functional Correlations–Axon Myelination

The function of the **Schwann cells** in the **PNS** is to wrap themselves around larger axons and form the insulating lipid-rich **myelin sheaths**. Thus, the function of Schwann cells is similar to that of the **oligodendrocytes** of the **CNS**.

Myelinated axons exhibit the **nodes of Ranvier**. The nodes accelerate the conduction of the **nerve impulses** (actions potentials) along the axons. Small unmyelinated axons conduct nerve impulses at a slower rate than the larger myelinated axons. In larger myelinated axons, the nerve impulse jumps from node to node, resulting in a much more efficient and faster conduction of the impulse. This type of impulse conduction in myelinated axons is called **saltatory conduction**. In unmyelinated axons, the impulse travels along the entire length of the axon and, as a result, conduction efficiency of the impulse and velocity is reduced. Thus, the larger, heavy-myelinated axons have the highest velocity of impulse conduction. This rate of conduction depends directly on the axon size and the myelin sheath.

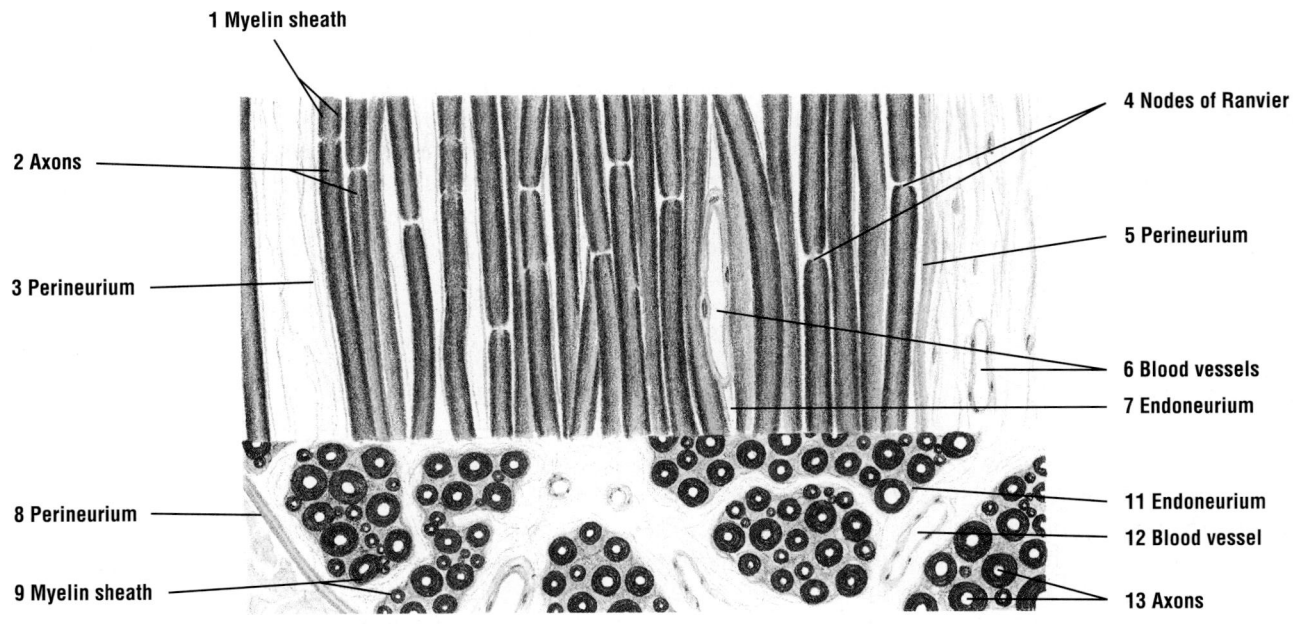

1 Myelin sheath

2 Axons

3 Perineurium

8 Perineurium

9 Myelin sheath

4 Nodes of Ranvier

5 Perineurium

6 Blood vessels

7 Endoneurium

11 Endoneurium

12 Blood vessel

13 Axons

Fig. 6-6   Myelinated Nerve Fibers. Stain: osmic acid. High magnification.

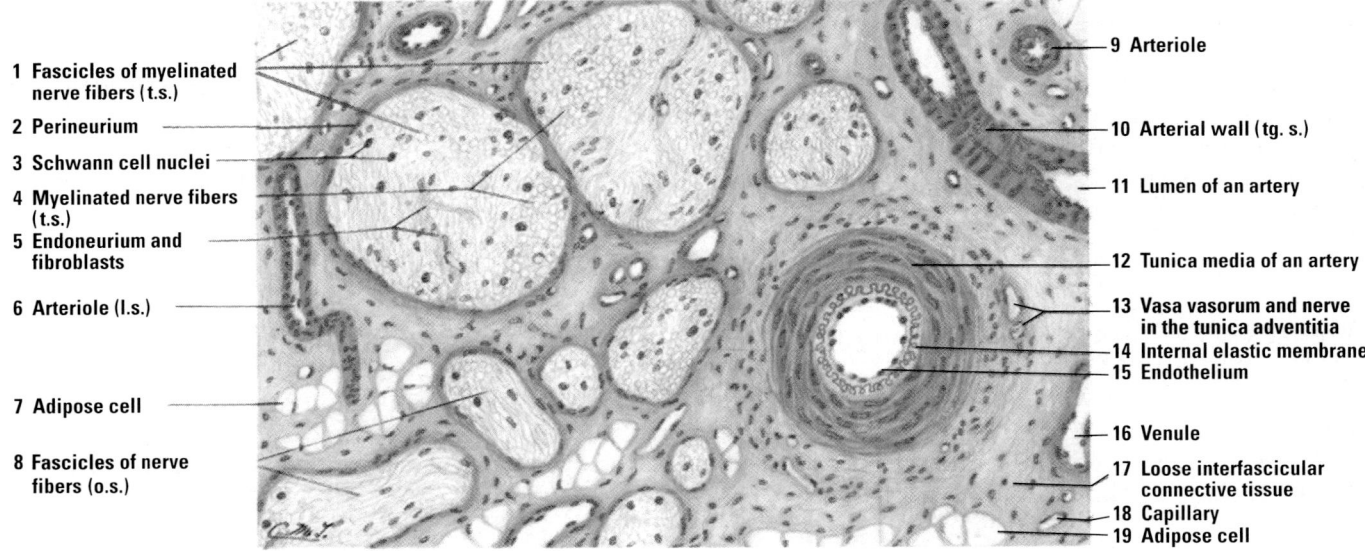

1 Fascicles of myelinated nerve fibers (t.s.)

2 Perineurium

3 Schwann cell nuclei

4 Myelinated nerve fibers (t.s.)

5 Endoneurium and fibroblasts

6 Arteriole (l.s.)

7 Adipose cell

8 Fascicles of nerve fibers (o.s.)

9 Arteriole

10 Arterial wall (tg. s.)

11 Lumen of an artery

12 Tunica media of an artery

13 Vasa vasorum and nerve in the tunica adventitia

14 Internal elastic membrane

15 Endothelium

16 Venule

17 Loose interfascicular connective tissue

18 Capillary

19 Adipose cell

Fig. 6-7   Peripheral Nerve (transverse section). Stain: hematoxylin-eosin. Medium magnification.

Figure 6-8   Nerve: Sciatic (panoramic view, longitudinal section)

A portion of sciatic nerve is illustrated at a low magnification, as it appears in a routine histologic preparation stained with hematoxylin-eosin. The complete outer layer of dense connective tissue, the epineurium, is not shown in the illustration. The deeper part of the epineurium contains **adipose tissue (2)** and **blood vessels (1). Extensions of the epineurium (3)** surround large **nerve fascicles (5). Perineurium (4)** is the connective tissue sheath that surrounds individual nerve fascicles. The numerous nuclei that are arranged along nerve fibers are the Schwann cell nuclei (neurolemma nuclei) or fibroblast nuclei of the endoneurium connective tissue. Schwann cells and fibroblasts cannot be differentiated at this magnification

Figure 6-9   Nerve: Sciatic (longitudinal section)

A small portion of the nerve illustrated in Figure 6-8 is shown at a higher magnification. The **axons (1)** appear as slender threads stained lightly with hematoxylin. The surrounding myelin sheath has been dissolved as a result of routine histologic preparation, leaving a distinct **neurokeratin network (3)** of protein. The **sheath (4)** of Schwann cells is not always distinguishable from the surrounding connective tissue; however, in certain areas it is seen as a thin, peripheral boundary and at the **node of Ranvier (2)** as it descends toward the axon. Two **Schwann cell nuclei (5)** and the connective tissue **endoneurium (7)** are seen in the illustration. The **fibroblasts (6)** in the endoneurium are distinguished from Schwann cell nuclei (5).

Figure 6-10   Nerve: Sciatic (transverse section)

The transverse section of sciatic nerve, as seen in Figure 6-9 illustrates the central **axons (2)**, the **neurokeratin network (3)** of protein as peripheral radial lines, and the peripheral **Schwann cell sheath (4). Schwann cell nucleus (1)** appears to encircle the axon (2).

Collagen fibers of the endoneurium are faintly distinguishable; however, the **fibroblasts (5)** are seen clearly. **Perineurium (6)** surrounds a fascicle of nerve fibers and contains a small **venule (7)**.

Figure 6-11   Nerve: Sciatic (longitudinal section)

This section is stained with Protargol and aniline blue. The axons (1), stained black, are prominent because of silver impregnation of the neurofibrils. The scattered black droplets probably represent remnants of neurofibrils remaining after axon shrinkage. The neurokeratin network is not stained. Other visible structures are the **nodes of Ranvier (4, 8), Schwann cell nuclei (7)**, and **fibroblast nuclei (5)** in the **endoneurium (6)**.

Figure 6-12   Nerve: Sciatic (transverse section)

As described in Figure 6-11, Protargol stains the **axons (1)** black, as seen in the cross section. The surrounding gray area and small, black droplets probably indicate the original axon diameter. The **endoneurium (4, 6)** is well demonstrated by aniline blue–staining of the collagen fibers. Other visible structures are **Schwann cell sheath (3)** and **fibroblasts (5)**.

Figure 6-13   Nerve: Branch of the Vagus (transverse section)

This figure illustrates still another staining method for nerve fibers and shows myelinated axons of varying size in a branch of the vagus nerve. The **fibroblast (1)** and **Schwann cell (6)** nuclei, **axons (3)**, and **neurokeratin network (4)** stain red with azocarmine. **The endoneurium (7)** is demonstrated clearly, especially in areas where axons are close together and within groups of **small nerve fibers (8)**.

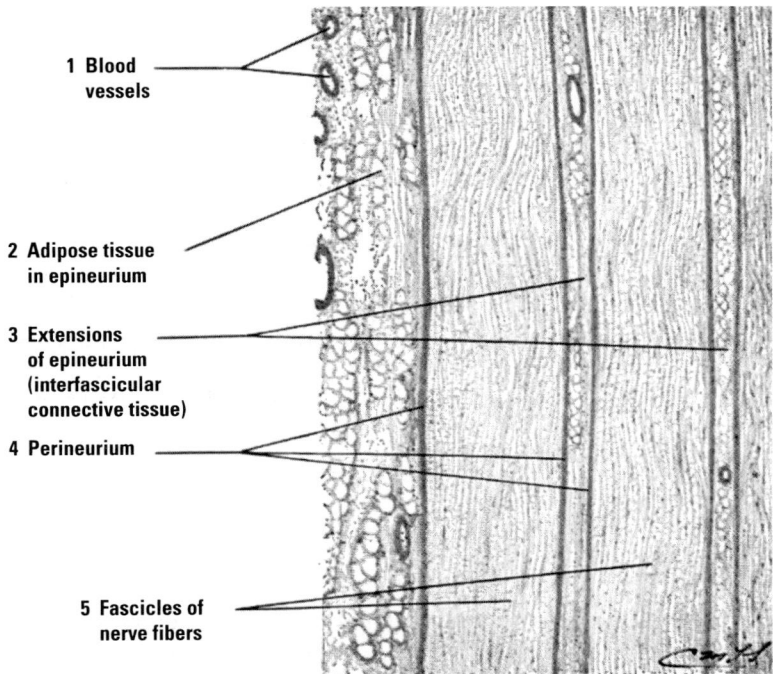

1 Blood vessels

2 Adipose tissue in epineurium

3 Extensions of epineurium (interfascicular connective tissue)

4 Perineurium

5 Fascicles of nerve fibers

Fig. 6-8   Nerve: Sciatic (panoramic view, longitudinal section). Stain: hematoxylin-eosin. Low magnification.

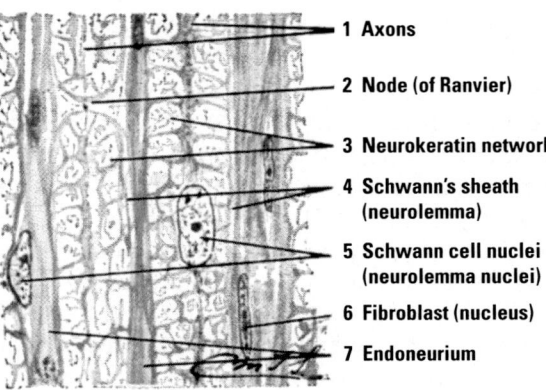

1 Axons

2 Node (of Ranvier)

3 Neurokeratin network

4 Schwann's sheath (neurolemma)

5 Schwann cell nuclei (neurolemma nuclei)

6 Fibroblast (nucleus)

7 Endoneurium

Fig. 6-9   Nerve: Sciatic (longitudinal section).

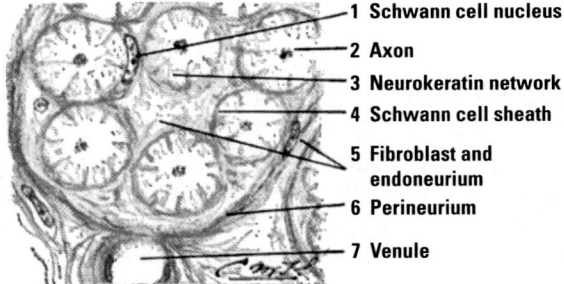

1 Schwann cell nucleus

2 Axon

3 Neurokeratin network

4 Schwann cell sheath

5 Fibroblast and endoneurium

6 Perineurium

7 Venule

Fig. 6-10   Nerve: Sciatic (transverse section). Stain: hematoxylin-eosin. Oil immersion.

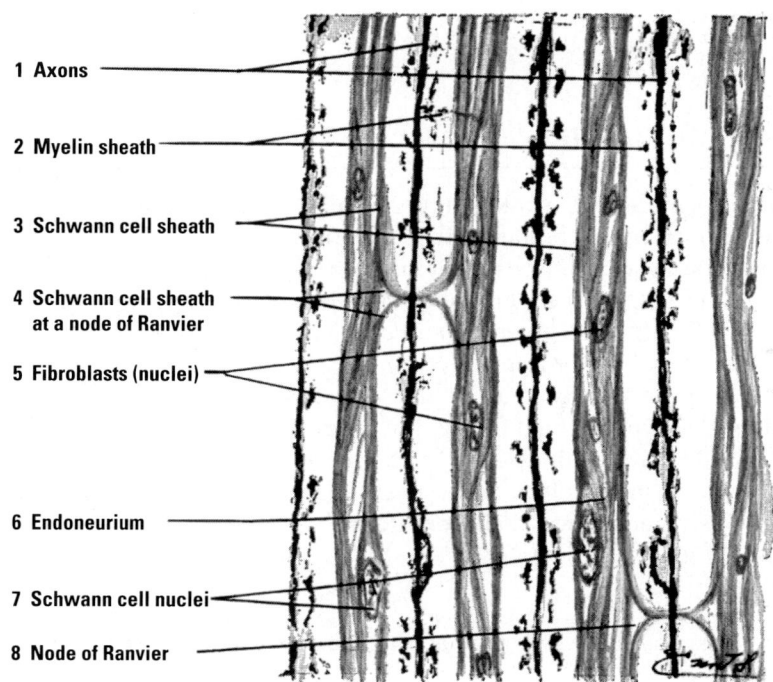

1 Axons

2 Myelin sheath

3 Schwann cell sheath

4 Schwann cell sheath at a node of Ranvier

5 Fibroblasts (nuclei)

6 Endoneurium

7 Schwann cell nuclei

8 Node of Ranvier

Fig. 6-11   Nerve: Sciatic (longitudinal section) Stain: Protargol and aniline blue. Oil immersion.

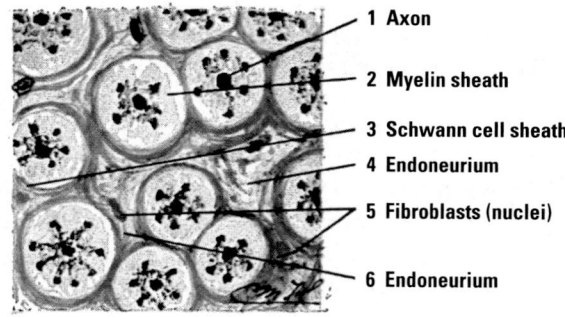

1 Axon

2 Myelin sheath

3 Schwann cell sheath

4 Endoneurium

5 Fibroblasts (nuclei)

6 Endoneurium

Fig. 6-12   Nerve: Sciatic (transverse section).

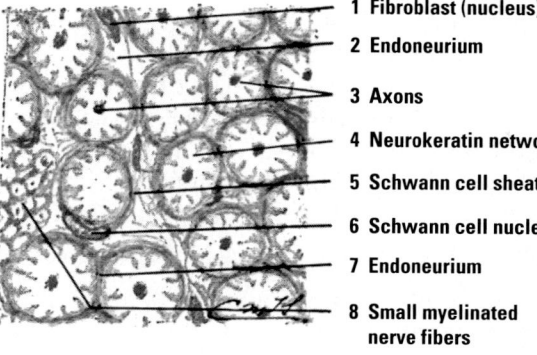

1 Fibroblast (nucleus)

2 Endoneurium

3 Axons

4 Neurokeratin network

5 Schwann cell sheath

6 Schwann cell nucleus

7 Endoneurium

8 Small myelinated nerve fibers

Fig. 6-13   Nerve: Branch of the Vagus (transverse section). Stain: Mallory-azan. Oil immersion.

Figure 6-14   Dorsal Root Ganglion (panoramic view, longitudinal section)

A connective tissue layer (1, 13), rich in adipose cells, nerves, and blood vessels (13), surrounds the nervous tissue of a **dorsal root ganglion (8)**. This layer merges with the external connective tissue capsule of the ganglion, the **epineurium (2)**, which is continuous with the **epineurium of the dorsal root (3)** and **epineurium of the spinal nerve (10, 11)**. The perineurium and the endoneurium of the spinal nerve are not distinguishable at this magnification.

The round **(pseudo)unipolar neurons (8)** of varying size constitute the majority of the ganglion (8); these neurons or ganglion cells are conspicuous because of their large size and staining. Numerous fascicles of **nerve fibers (9)** are located between the ganglion cells and course either in the **dorsal root (4)** or the **spinal nerve (11)**. These nerve fibers represent, respectively, the central processes and peripheral processes formed by bifurcation of a single axon process, which emerges from each ganglion cell.

The nerve fibers of the **ventral root (7)**, surrounded by its **epineurium (6)**, join the nerve fibers that emerge from the **ganglion (8, 12)** and form the **spinal nerve (11)**.

Figure 6-15   Section of a Dorsal Root Ganglion

At higher magnification, ganglion cells or unipolar neurons (2, 3) appear variable in size. The characteristic vesicular **nucleus (2)** with its prominent, dark-staining **nucleolus (2)** is conspicuous. The cytoplasm of these cells is filled with **Nissl bodies (3)**. Each ganglion cell contains an axon hillock; however, it is not visible in this illustration. Some of the ganglion cells contain small clumps of **lipofuscin pigment (5)** in their cytoplasm.

Within the perineuronal space and in close association with the ganglion cells (2, 3) are the much smaller **satellite cells (6)**. These cells have spherical nuclei, are of neuroectodermal origin, and form a loose inner layer of the capsule around the ganglion cells (2, 3). An outer **capsule (7)** of more flattened **fibroblasts (8)** and connective tissue fibers is continuous with the endoneurium. In different plane of sections, these two layers are not always clearly distinguishable; often the two cell types appear intermingled, as seen around the cell with the lipofuscin pigment (5).

Between ganglion cells (2, 3) are numerous **fibroblasts (4)**, randomly arranged in the connective tissue, or in rows in the endoneurium between **nerve fibers (1)**. With hematoxylin-eosin stain, small axons and connective tissue fibers are not defined clearly. Large **myelinated fibers (1)** are recognizable when sectioned longitudinally.

Figure 6-16   Section of a Sympathetic Trunk Ganglion

Similar to the dorsal root ganglion cells, the cells of the sympathetic trunk ganglion exhibit a characteristic nucleus, a dark-staining nucleolus (sometimes multiple nucleoli), and Nissl bodies in their cytoplasm.

In contrast to cells in the dorsal root ganglion, however, the cells in the sympathetic trunk are multipolar neurons and are smaller and more uniform in size. As a result, the ganglion cell outlines and their processes appear often irregular in the sections. The nuclei of the **ganglion cells (6)** are often eccentric and binucleated cells are not uncommon. Most of these cells (6) contain lipofuscin pigment in their cytoplasm.

Satellite cells (2, 5) are usually less numerous than around the cells in the dorsal root ganglion. Also, the connective tissue capsule with its **capsule cells (3)** may not be well defined. Present in the **intercellular area (4)** are fibroblasts, supportive connective tissue, blood vessels, and unmyelinated and myelinated axons. Nerve fibers aggregate into **bundles (1, 7)** and course through the sympathetic trunk. These nerve fibers represent the preganglionic fibers, postganglionic visceral efferent fibers, and visceral afferent fibers.

■ Functional Correlations–Satellite Cells

The **satellite cells** surround the neurons in different ganglia. These cells play an important role in providing **structural** and **metabolic support** to the neurons that they surround.

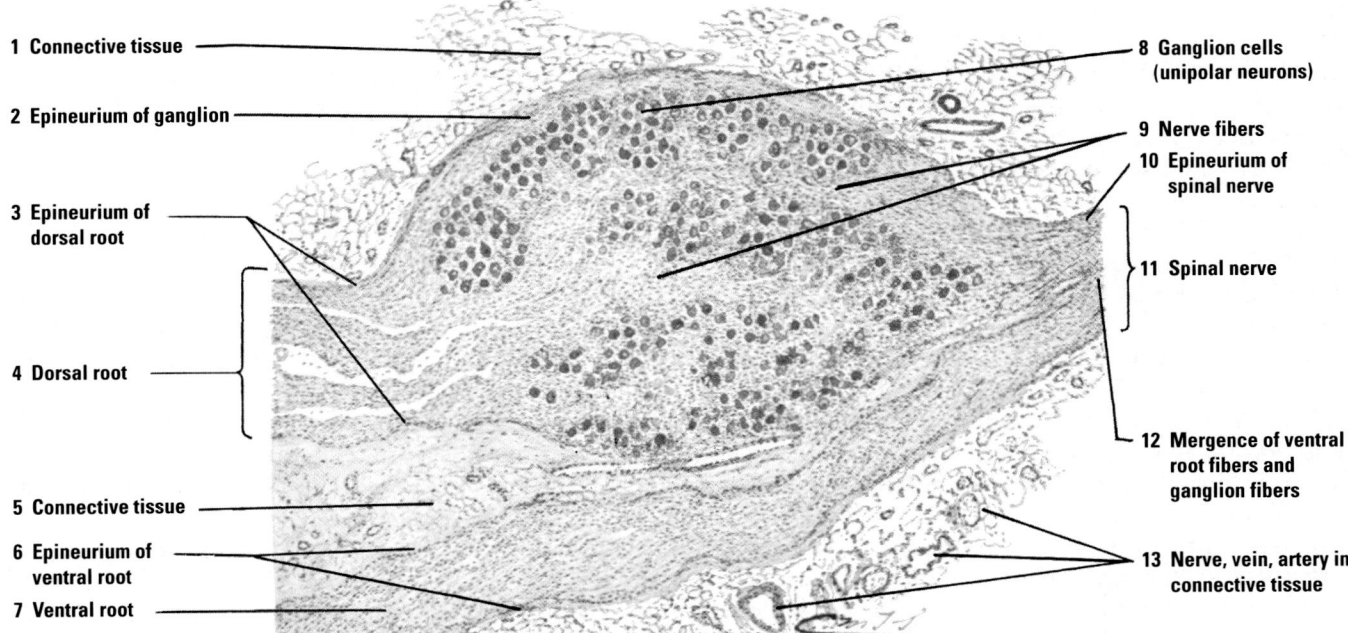

1 Connective tissue

2 Epineurium of ganglion

3 Epineurium of dorsal root

4 Dorsal root

5 Connective tissue

6 Epineurium of ventral root

7 Ventral root

8 Ganglion cells (unipolar neurons)

9 Nerve fibers

10 Epineurium of spinal nerve

11 Spinal nerve

12 Mergence of ventral root fibers and ganglion fibers

13 Nerve, vein, artery in connective tissue

Fig. 6-14   Dorsal Root Ganglion (panoramic view, longitudinal section). Stain: hematoxylin-eosin. Low magnification.

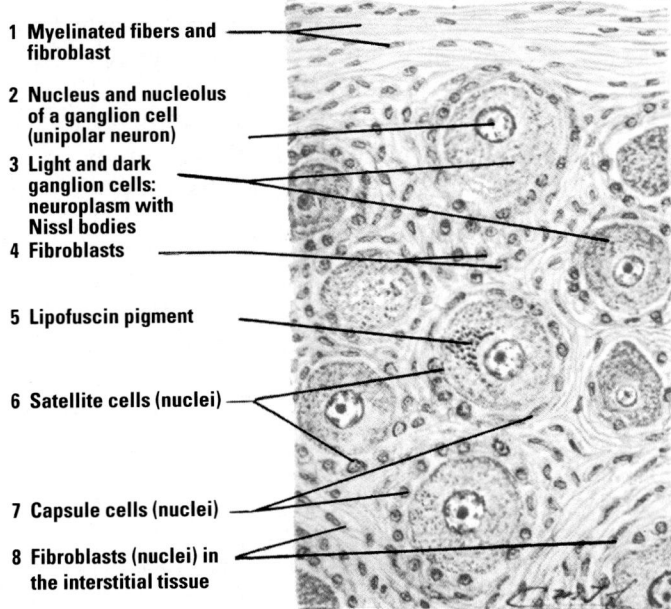

1 Myelinated fibers and fibroblast

2 Nucleus and nucleolus of a ganglion cell (unipolar neuron)

3 Light and dark ganglion cells: neuroplasm with Nissl bodies

4 Fibroblasts

5 Lipofuscin pigment

6 Satellite cells (nuclei)

7 Capsule cells (nuclei)

8 Fibroblasts (nuclei) in the interstitial tissue

Fig. 6-15   Section of a Dorsal Root Ganglion. Stain: hematoxylin-eosin. High magnification.

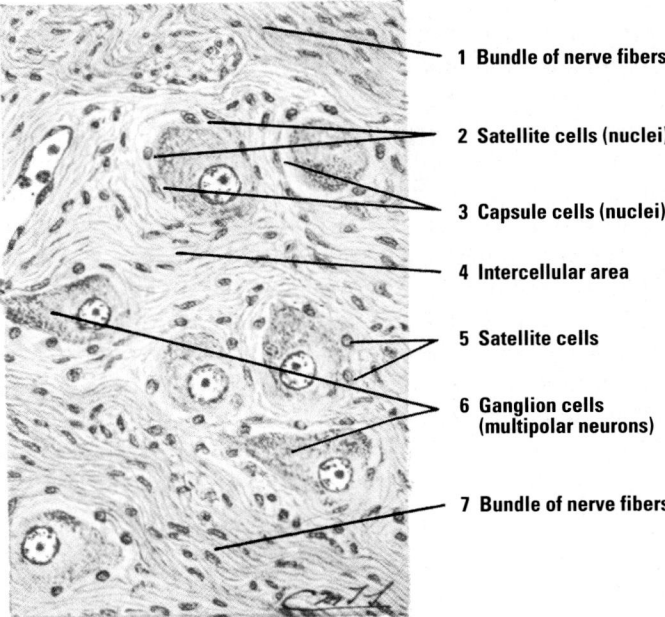

1 Bundle of nerve fibers

2 Satellite cells (nuclei)

3 Capsule cells (nuclei)

4 Intercellular area

5 Satellite cells

6 Ganglion cells (multipolar neurons)

7 Bundle of nerve fibers

Fig. 6-16   Section of a Sympathetic Trunk Ganglion. Stain: hematoxylin-eosin. High magnification.

Figure 6-17   Spinal Cord: Cervical Region (transverse section)

To illustrate the white matter and the gray matter of the spinal cord, a cross section of the cord was prepared with silver impregnation technique. After staining, the dark brown, outer white matter (3) and the light-staining, inner **gray matter (4, 14)** are clearly visible. The white matter (3) consists primarily of ascending and descending myelinated nerve fibers or axons. By contrast, the gray matter contains the cell bodies of neurons, interneurons, and their axons. The gray matter also exhibits a symmetrical H-shape, whose two sides are connected across the midline of the spinal cord by the **gray commissure (15)** in whose center is located the **central canal (16)** of the spinal cord.

The **anterior horns (6)** of the gray matter extend toward the front of the cord and are more prominent than the **posterior horns (2, 13).** The anterior horns contain the cell bodies of the large **motor neurons (7, 17).** Some **axons (8)** from the motor neurons of the anterior horns cross the white matter and exit from the spinal cord as components of the **anterior roots (9, 21)** of the peripheral nerves. The posterior horns (2, 13) are the sensory areas and contain cell bodies of smaller neurons.

The spinal cord is surrounded by connective tissue meninges, consisting of an outer dura mater, a middle **arachnoid (5),** and an inner **pia mater (18).** The spinal cord is also partially divided into right and left halves by a narrow, posterior (dorsal) groove, the **posterior median sulcus (10),** and a deep, anterior (ventral) cleft, the **anterior median fissure (19).** In this illustration, pia mater (18) is best seen in the **anterior median fissure (19).**

Between the posterior median sulcus (10) and the posterior horns (2, 13) of the gray matter are the prominent dorsal columns of the white matter. In the cervical region of the spinal cord, each dorsal column is subdivided into two fascicles, the posteromedial column, the **fasciculus gracilis (11)** and the posterolateral column, the **fasciculus cuneatus (1, 12).**

Figure 6-18   Spinal Cord: Anterior Gray Horn, Motor Neurons, and Adjacent Anterior White Matter

A small section of the white matter and the gray matter of the anterior horn of the spinal cord are illustrated at a higher magnification. The gray matter of the anterior horn contains large, **multipolar motor neurons (2, 3).** These are characterized by numerous **dendrites (5, 6)** that extend in different directions from the parikaryon (cell bodies). In some sections of the neurons, the **nucleus (8)** is visible with its prominent **nucleolus (8).** In other neurons, the plane of section has missed the nucleus and the parikaryon appears empty **(2).** Located in the vicinity of the motor neurons are the small, lightstaining, supportive cells, the **neuroglia (7).**

The white matter contains closely packed groups of myelinated axons. In cross sections, the **axons (1)** appear dark-stained and surrounded by clear spaces, which are the remnants of the myelin sheaths. The axons of the white matter represent the ascending and descending tracts of the spinal cord. On the other hand, the **axons (4)** of the anterior horn motor neurons aggregate into groups, pass through the white matter, and exit from the spinal cord as the anterior (ventral) root fibers (Fig. 6-17).

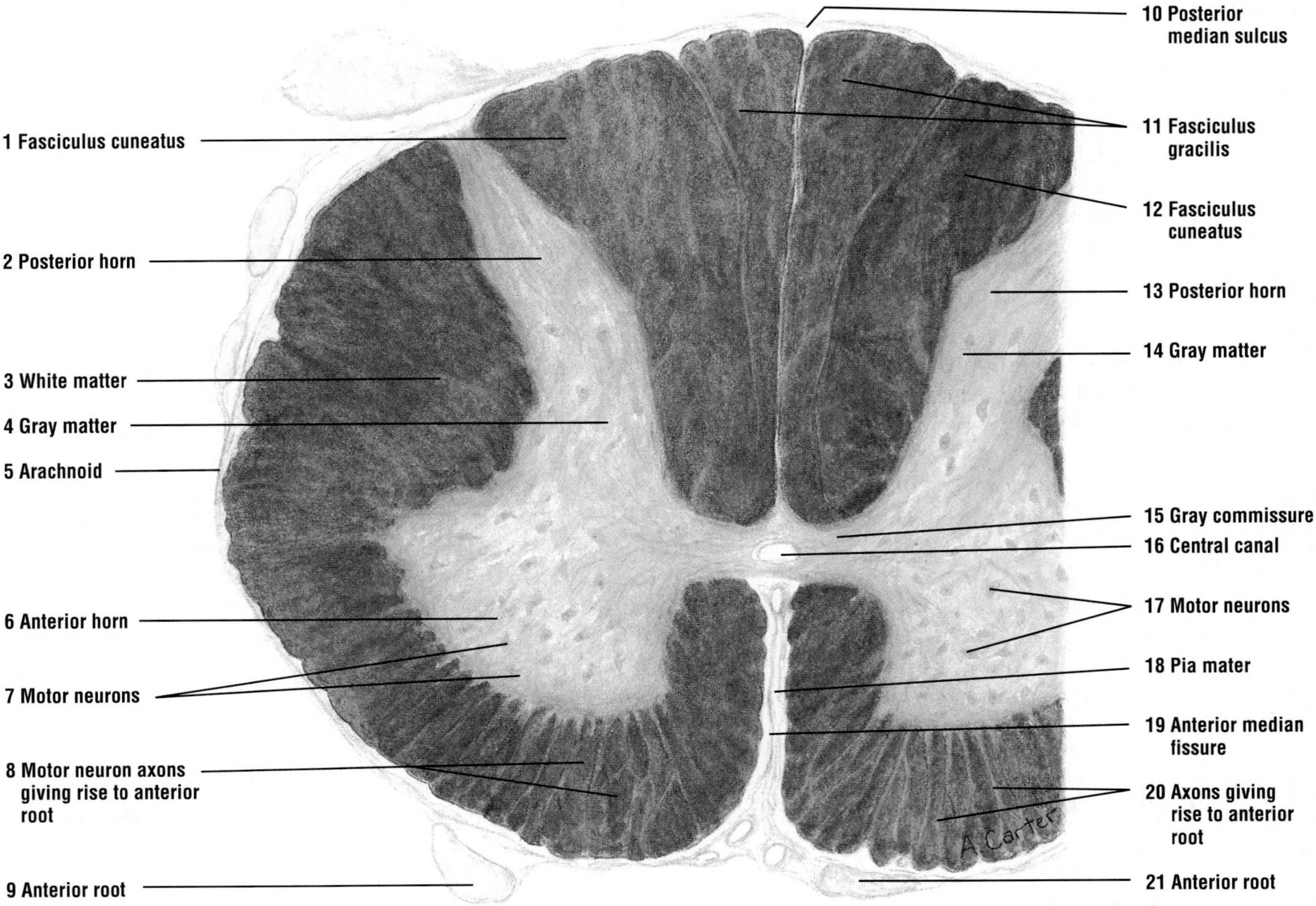

1 Fasciculus cuneatus

2 Posterior horn

3 White matter

4 Gray matter

5 Arachnoid

6 Anterior horn

7 Motor neurons

8 Motor neuron axons giving rise to anterior root

9 Anterior root

10 Posterior median sulcus

11 Fasciculus gracilis

12 Fasciculus cuneatus

13 Posterior horn

14 Gray matter

15 Gray commissure

16 Central canal

17 Motor neurons

18 Pia mater

19 Anterior median fissure

20 Axons giving rise to anterior root

21 Anterior root

Fig. 6-17   Spinal Cord: Cervical Region (transverse section). Stain: silver impregnation (Cajal's method). Low magnification.

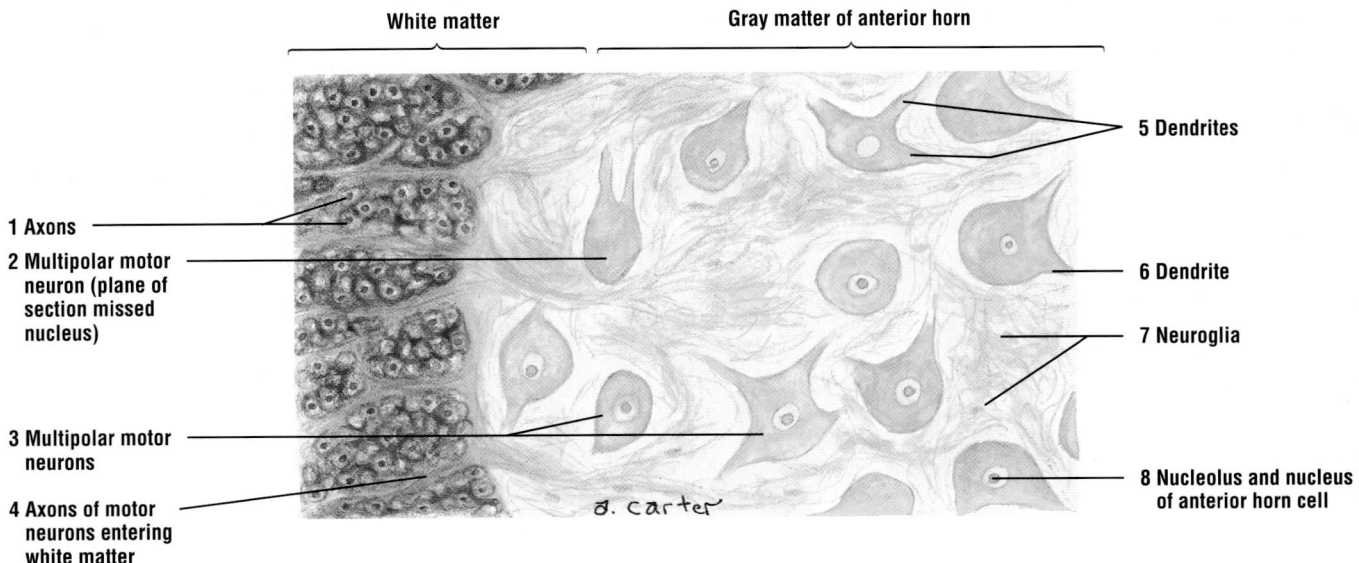

White matter

Gray matter of anterior horn

1 Axons

2 Multipolar motor neuron (plane of section missed nucleus)

3 Multipolar motor neurons

4 Axons of motor neurons entering white matter

5 Dendrites

6 Dendrite

7 Neuroglia

8 Nucleolus and nucleus of anterior horn cell

Fig. 6-18   Spinal Cord: Anterior Gray Horn, Motor Neurons, and Adjacent Anterior White Matter. Stain: silver impregnation (Cajal's method). Medium magnification.

Figure 6-19   Spinal Cord: Midthoracic Region (transverse section)

A transverse section of a spinal cord cut in the midthoracic region and stained with hematoxylin-eosin is illustrated. Although a basic structural pattern is seen throughout the spinal cord, shape and structure of the cord vary at different levels (cervical, thoracic, lumbar, and sacral).

The thoracic region of the spinal cord differs from the cervical region illustrated on the previous page in Figure 6-17. The thoracic spinal cord exhibits slender **posterior gray horns (6)** and smaller **anterior gray horns (10, 20)** with fewer **motor neurons (10, 20)**. The **lateral gray horns (8, 19)**, on the other hand, are well developed in the thoracic region of the spinal cord. These contain the **motor neurons (8, 19)** of the sympathetic division of the autonomic nervous system.

The remaining structures in the midthoracic region of the spinal cord closely correspond to the structures illustrated in the cervical cord region in Figure 6-17. These are the **posterior median sulcus (15), anterior median fissure (22), fasciculus gracilis (16)** and **fasciculus cuneatus (17)** (seen in the mid to upper thoracic region of the spinal cord) of the **posterior white column (16, 17), lateral white column (7), central canal (9)**, and the **gray commissure (18)**. Associated with the posterior gray horns (6) are axons of the **posterior roots (5)** and leaving the anterior gray horns (10, 20) are the **axons (11, 21)** of the **anterior roots (11)**.

Surrounding the spinal cord are the connective tissue layers of the meninges. These are the thick and fibrous outer **dura mater (2)**, the thinner and middle **arachnoid (3)**, and the delicate inner **pia mater (4)**, which closely adheres to the surface of the spinal cord. Located in the pia mater (4) are numerous anterior and posterior **spinal blood vessels (1, 12)** of various sizes. Between the arachnoid (3) and the pia mater (4) is the **subarachnoid space (14)**. Fine trabeculae located in the subarachnoid space (14) connect the pia mater (4) with the arachnoid (3). In life, the subarachnoid space (14) is filled with circulating cerebrospinal fluid. Between the arachnoid (3) and the dura mater (2) is the **subdural space (13)**. In this preparation, the subdural space (13) appears unusually large because of the artifactual retraction of the arachnoid during the specimen preparation.

Figure 6-20   Spinal Cord: Anterior Gray Horn, Motor Neurons, and Adjacent Anterior White Matter

A higher magnification of a small section of the spinal cord illustrates the appearance of gray matter, white matter, neurons, neuroglia, and axons stained with hematoxylin-eosin. The cells in the anterior gray horn of the thoracic region of the spinal cord are **multipolar motor neurons (2, 6)**. Their cytoplasm is characterized by a prominent vesicular **nucleus (7)**, a distinct **nucleolus (7)**, and course clumps of basophilic material called the **Nissl substance (3)**. The Nissl substance extends into the **dendrites (5)** but not the axons. One such neuron exhibits the root of an axon from the **axon hillock (4)**, which is devoid of the Nissl substance.

The nonneural **neuroglia (8)** cells, seen only as basophilic nuclei, are small in comparison to the prominent multipolar neurons (2, 4). The neuroglia (8) occupy the spaces between the neurons. The anterior white matter of the spinal cord contains myelinated axons of various sizes. Because of the histologic preparation of this section, the myelin sheaths appear as clear spaces around the dark-staining **axons (1)**.

In certain neurons (2), the plane of section did not include the nucleus, and the cytoplasm appears enucleated (without nucleus).

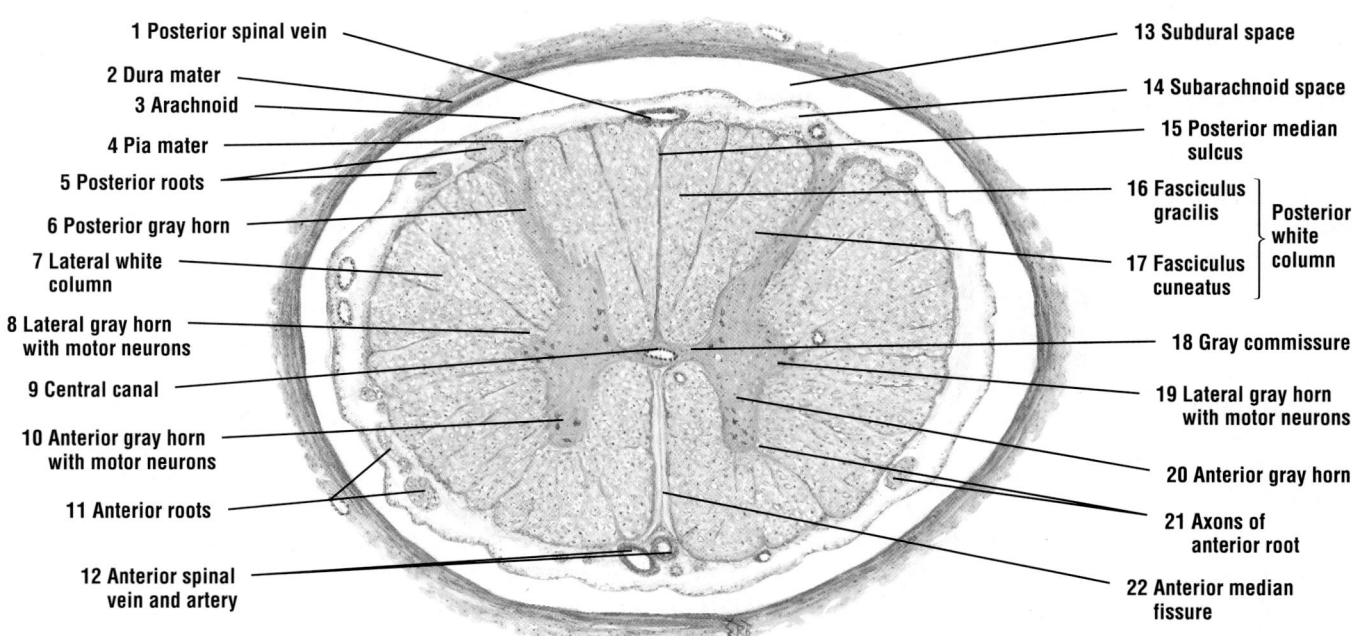

1 Posterior spinal vein
2 Dura mater
3 Arachnoid
4 Pia mater
5 Posterior roots
6 Posterior gray horn
7 Lateral white column
8 Lateral gray horn with motor neurons
9 Central canal
10 Anterior gray horn with motor neurons
11 Anterior roots
12 Anterior spinal vein and artery

13 Subdural space
14 Subarachnoid space
15 Posterior median sulcus
16 Fasciculus gracilis
17 Fasciculus cuneatus
Posterior white column
18 Gray commissure
19 Lateral gray horn with motor neurons
20 Anterior gray horn
21 Axons of anterior root
22 Anterior median fissure

Fig. 6-19 Spinal Cord: Midthoracic Region (transverse section). Stain: hematoxylin-eosin. Low magnification.

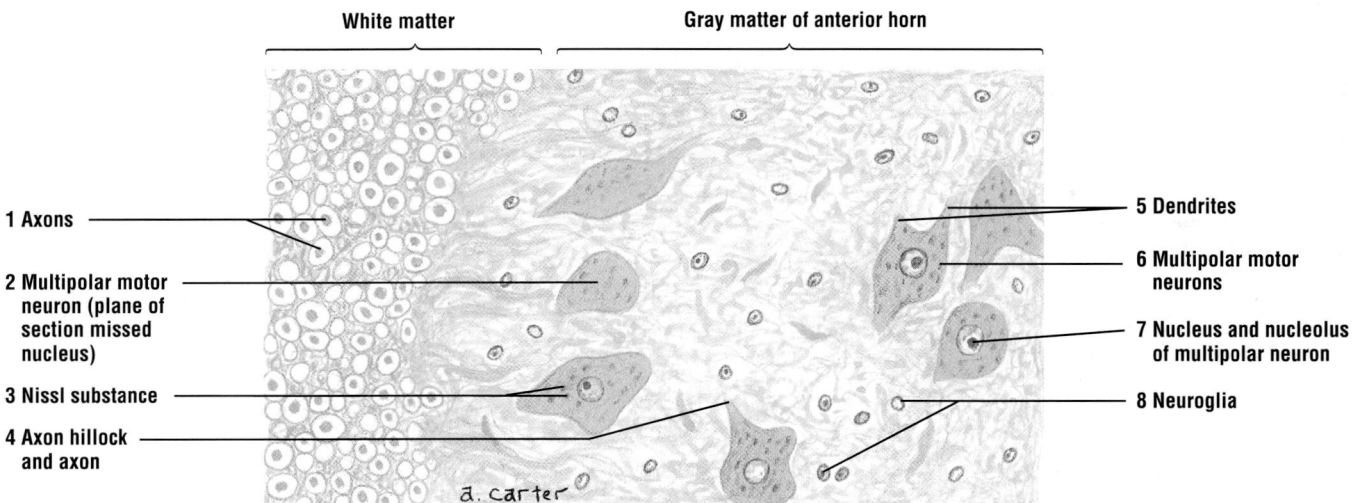

White matter
Gray matter of anterior horn

1 Axons
2 Multipolar motor neuron (plane of section missed nucleus)
3 Nissl substance
4 Axon hillock and axon

5 Dendrites
6 Multipolar motor neurons
7 Nucleus and nucleolus of multipolar neuron
8 Neuroglia

a. carter

Fig. 6-20 Spinal Cord: Anterior Gray Horn, Motor Neurons, and Adjacent Anterior White Matter. Stain: hematoxylin-eosin. Medium magnification.

Figure 6-21   Cerebellum (sectional view, transverse section)

The cerebellum consists of an outer cortex of **gray matter (3)** and an inner **white matter (4, 10).** The white matter (4, 10) consists of myelinated nerve fibers or axons. These fibers are the afferent and efferent fibers of the cerebellar cortex. Their ramification (10) forms the core of the numerous cerebellar folds.

The gray matter constitutes the cortex, and three distinct cell layers can be distinguished in the cortex: an **outer molecular layer (6)** with few cells and horizontally directed fibers, an **inner granular layer (7)** with numerous small cells with intensely stained nuclei, and a central layer of **Purkinje cells (8).** The Purkinje cells are pyriform in shape with ramified dendrites that extend into the molecular layer.

Figure 6-22   Cerebellum: Cortex

Purkinje cells (9) typically are arranged in a single row at the junction of the **molecular (8)** and **granular cell (10)** layers. Their large "flask-shaped" bodies give off one or more thick **dendrites (3),** which extend through the molecular layer to the surface, giving off complex branchings along their course. The thin **axon (5)** leaves the base of the Purkinje cell, passes through the granular layer, and becomes myelinated as it enters the **white matter (12).**

The molecular layer contains scattered outer **stellate cells (8)** whose unmyelinated axons normally course in a horizontal direction. Descending collaterals of more deeply placed **basket cells (4)** arborize around the Purkinje cells **(9)** in a "basketlike" arrangement. Axons of the **granule cells (6)** in the granular layer extend into the molecular layer and also course horizontally **(2)** as unmyelinated fibers.

In the granular layer, numerous small granule cells (6, 10) with dark-staining nuclei (an exception to the usual vesicular nucleus of nerve cells) and little cytoplasm are found. In the granular layer scattered larger **stellate cells** or **Golgi type II cells (7)** with typical vesicular nuclei and more cytoplasm are present. Throughout the granular layer are small, irregularly dispersed, clear spaces called the **"glomeruli" (11).** In these regions, the cells are absent and synaptic complexes occur.

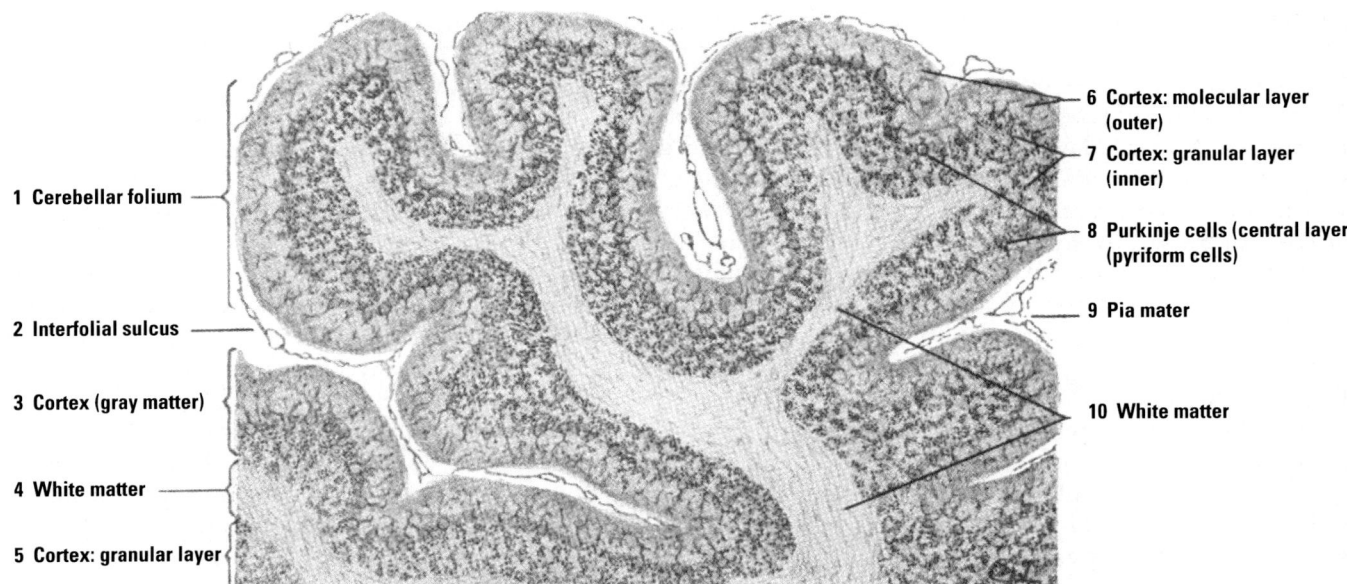

1 Cerebellar folium

2 Interfolial sulcus

3 Cortex (gray matter)

4 White matter

5 Cortex: granular layer

6 Cortex: molecular layer (outer)

7 Cortex: granular layer (inner)

8 Purkinje cells (central layer) (pyriform cells)

9 Pia mater

10 White matter

Fig. 6-21   Cerebellum (sectional view, transverse section). Stain: silver impregnation (Cajal's method). Low magnification.

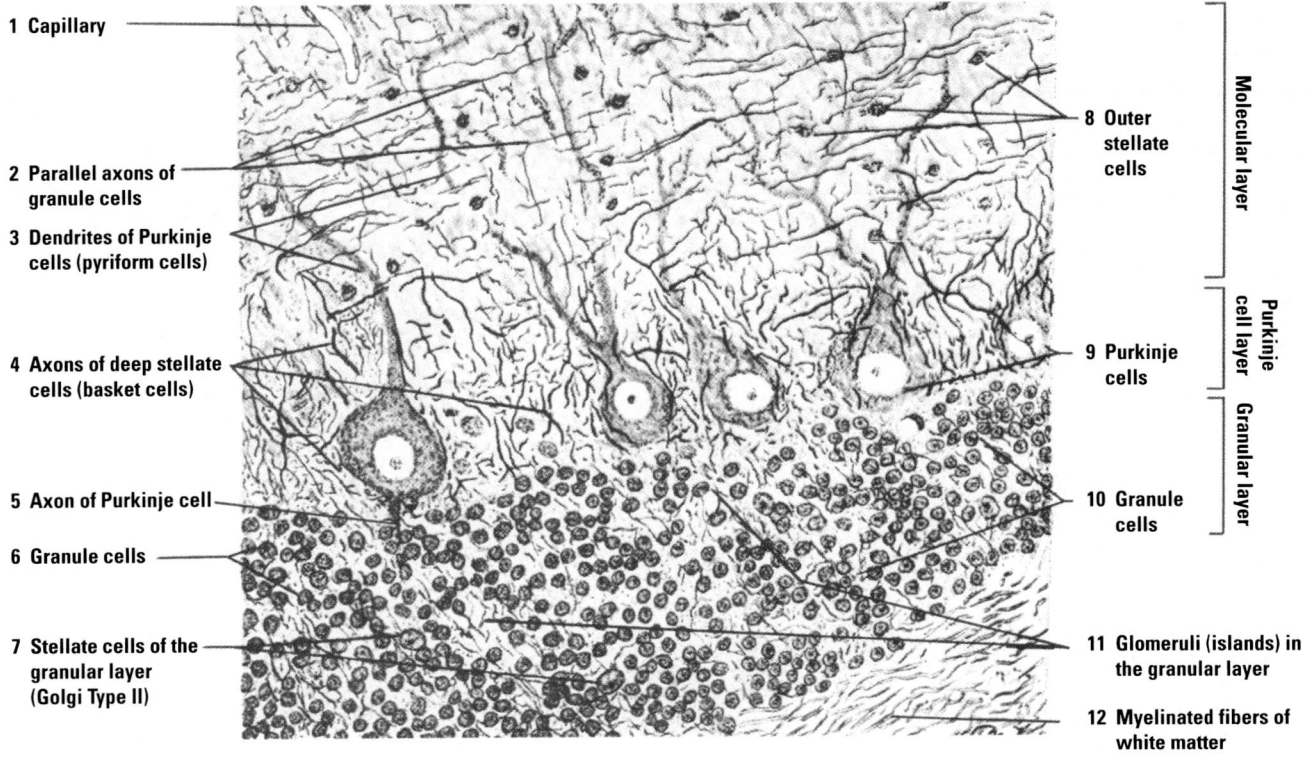

1 Capillary

2 Parallel axons of granule cells

3 Dendrites of Purkinje cells (pyriform cells)

4 Axons of deep stellate cells (basket cells)

5 Axon of Purkinje cell

6 Granule cells

7 Stellate cells of the granular layer (Golgi Type II)

8 Outer stellate cells

9 Purkinje cells

10 Granule cells

11 Glomeruli (islands) in the granular layer

12 Myelinated fibers of white matter

Molecular layer

Purkinje cell layer

Granular layer

Fig. 6-22   Cerebellum: Cortex. Stain: silver impregnation (Cajal's method). High magnification.

Figure 6-23   Cerebral Cortex: Section Perpendicular to the Cortical Surface

The silver nitrate stain used for this section of cerebral cortex demonstrates the neurofibrils.

The different cell types that constitute the cerebral cortex are distributed in layers, with one or more cell types predominant in each layer. Horizontal fibers associated with each layer give the cortex a laminated appearance. Fibers exhibiting a **radial arrangement (14)** are also present.

Although there are variations in arrangement of cells in different parts of the cerebral cortex, six distinct layers are recognized. These layers are labeled on the left side of the figure.

Starting in the periphery of the cortex, the outermost layer is the **molecular layer (1).** Its peripheral portion is composed predominantly of horizontally directed neuronal processes, both dendrites and axons. Deep in the molecular layer lie the infrequent, stellate or spindle-shaped **horizontal cells of Cajal (10);** their axons contribute to the horizontal fibers. Overlying and covering the molecular cell layer is the delicate connective tissue of the brain, the **pia mater (8).**

In the next four layers, the predominant cells are the characteristic pyramidal cells of the cerebral cortex; these cells exhibit variable sizes. The figure illustrates that the **pyramidal cells (11, 13)** get progressively larger in layers 2, 3, 4, and 5. Their **dendrites (13)** are directed toward the periphery of the cortex and their axon extends from the cell base. In the **internal granular layer (4),** numerous smaller and larger **stellate cells (12)** form numerous complex connections with the pyramidal cells.

The **multiform layer (6)** lacks the pyramidal cells; however, the fusiform cells predominate and the granule cells, stellate cells, and cells of Martinotti are intermixed. All of these cells vary in size. Axons of the cells of Martinotti are directed peripherally, whereas the axons from other cells enter the **white matter (16).**

Figure 6-24   Central Area of the Cerebral Cortex

Higher magnification of the cerebral cortex illustrates the large pyramidal cells (1, 8). Neurofibrils (1, 8) in the cell bodies have a characteristic network arrangement, whereas neurofibrils in the **dendrites (6)** and the **axons (7)** exhibit a more parallel arrangement. The typical large vesicular **nucleus (3)** with its prominent **nucleolus (3,** lower leader) is outlined. The most prominent cell process is the apical **dendrite (6),** which is directed toward the surface of the cortex. Several **collaterals (5)** are given off along its course through the cortex. Smaller dendrites (6, middle leader) arise from other parts of the cell body. The **axon (7)** arises from the base of the cell body and passes into the white matter.

The intercellular area is occupied by **nerve fibers (2)** of various cells in the cortex, small **astrocytes (4),** and blood vessels.

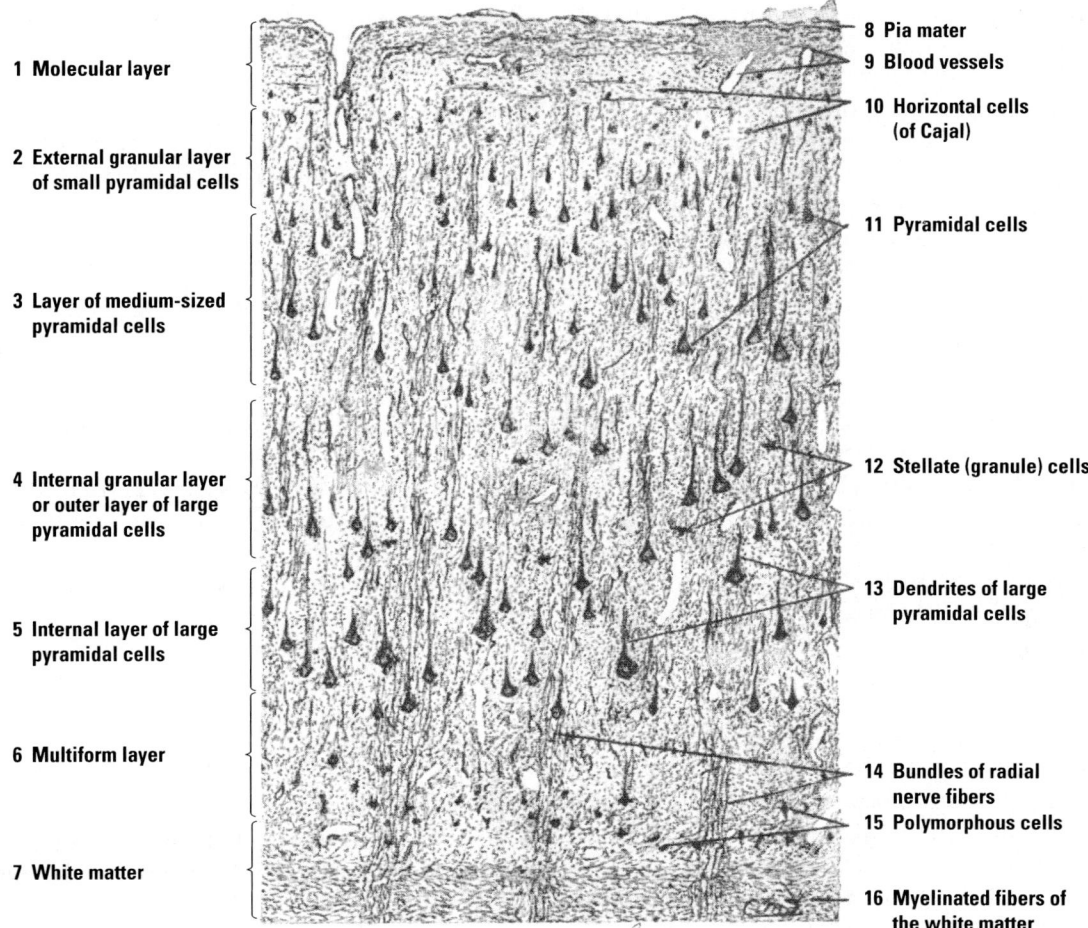

1 Molecular layer

2 External granular layer of small pyramidal cells

3 Layer of medium-sized pyramidal cells

4 Internal granular layer or outer layer of large pyramidal cells

5 Internal layer of large pyramidal cells

6 Multiform layer

7 White matter

8 Pia mater

9 Blood vessels

10 Horizontal cells (of Cajal)

11 Pyramidal cells

12 Stellate (granule) cells

13 Dendrites of large pyramidal cells

14 Bundles of radial nerve fibers

15 Polymorphous cells

16 Myelinated fibers of the white matter

Fig. 6-23   Cerebral Cortex: Section Perpendicular to the Cortical Surface. Stain: reduced silver nitrate method of Cajal. Medium magnification.

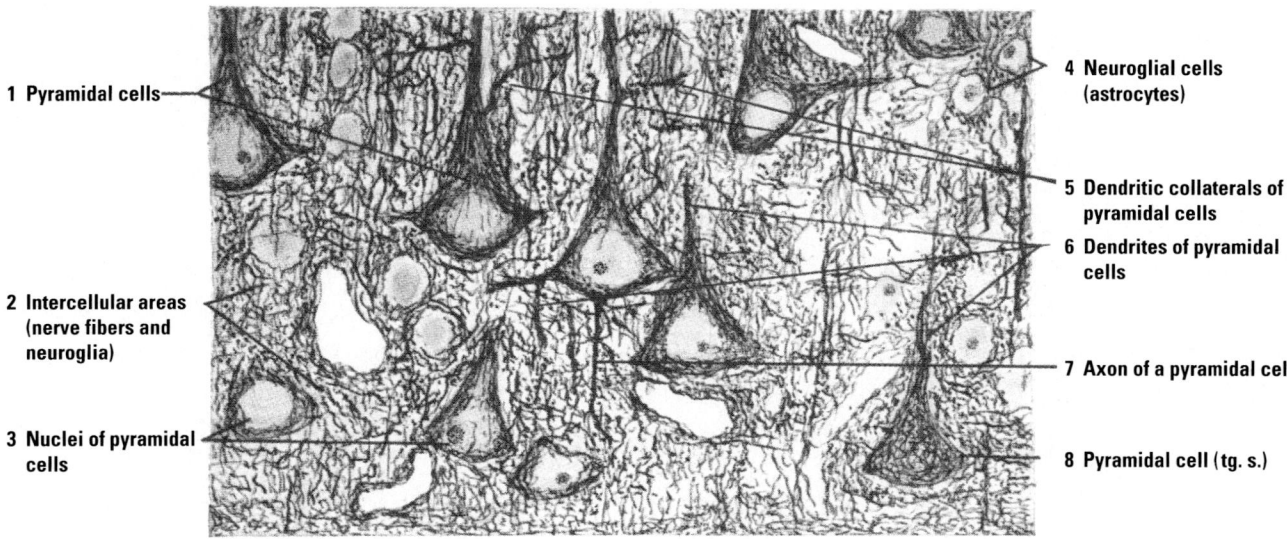

1 Pyramidal cells

2 Intercellular areas (nerve fibers and neuroglia)

3 Nuclei of pyramidal cells

4 Neuroglial cells (astrocytes)

5 Dendritic collaterals of pyramidal cells

6 Dendrites of pyramidal cells

7 Axon of a pyramidal cell

8 Pyramidal cell (tg. s.)

Fig. 6-24   Central Area of the Cerebral Cortex. Stain: reduced silver nitrate method of Cajal. High magnification.

Figure 6-25   Anterior Gray Horn of Spinal Cord: Multipolar Motor Neurons, Axons, and Neuroglial Cells

This medium magnification photomicrograph of anterior horn of the spinal cord was prepared with silver stain to show the morphology of neurons and axons of the central nervous system. The large multipolar **motorneurons (1)** of the gray horn exhibit numerous **dendrites (4).** Each motor neuron (1) contains a distinct **nucleus (5)** and a prominent **nucleolus (6).** Within the cytoplasm of the motorneurons (1) is the cytoskeleton, which consists of numerous **neurofibrils** (3) that course through the cell body and extend into the dendrites (4) and **axons (8).** Coursing past the motorneurons (1) are numerous axons of different size (8) from other nerve cells in the spinal cord. Surrounding the motorneurons (1) are numerous **nuclei** of **neuroglial cells (2)** and a **blood vessel (7)** with blood cells.

Figure 6-26   Dorsal Root Ganglion: Unipolar Neurons and Surrounding Cells

A medium magnification photomicrograph of the dorsal root ganglion illustrates the spherical shape of the sensory **unipolar neurons (2).** The cytoplasm of these neurons contains a central **nucleus (6)** and a prominent **nucleolus (5).** Surrounding the unipolar neurons (2) are the much smaller **satellite cells (1).** Other cells outside of the satellite cells are the connective tissue **fibroblasts (3).** Coursing through the dorsal root ganglion between the unipolar neurons (2) are numerous **bundles of sensory axons (4)** from the periphery.

Figure 6-27   Peripheral Nerve: Nodes of Ranvier and Axons

A medium magnification photomicrograph of a peripheral nerve sectioned in a longitudinal plane. The myelin sheaths that normally surround the axons have been washed out in this preparation and only **myelin spaces (7)** are seen. A centrally located **axon (2, 8)** can be seen in some of the nerve fibers that exhibited myelin sheaths. At regular intervals along the axon are seen indentations in the myelin sheaths. These represent the **nodes of Ranvier , (1, 9),** which indicate the edges of two different myelin sheath that enclose the axon. A possible **Schwann cell nucleus (3)** is seen associated with one of the axons (2, 8) and a thin, blue connective tissue layer **endoneurium (6)** that surrounds some of the axons (2, 8). Outside of the axons (2, 8) are seen a **capillary (4)** with blood cells and **fibroblasts (5)** of the surrounding connective tissue layers.

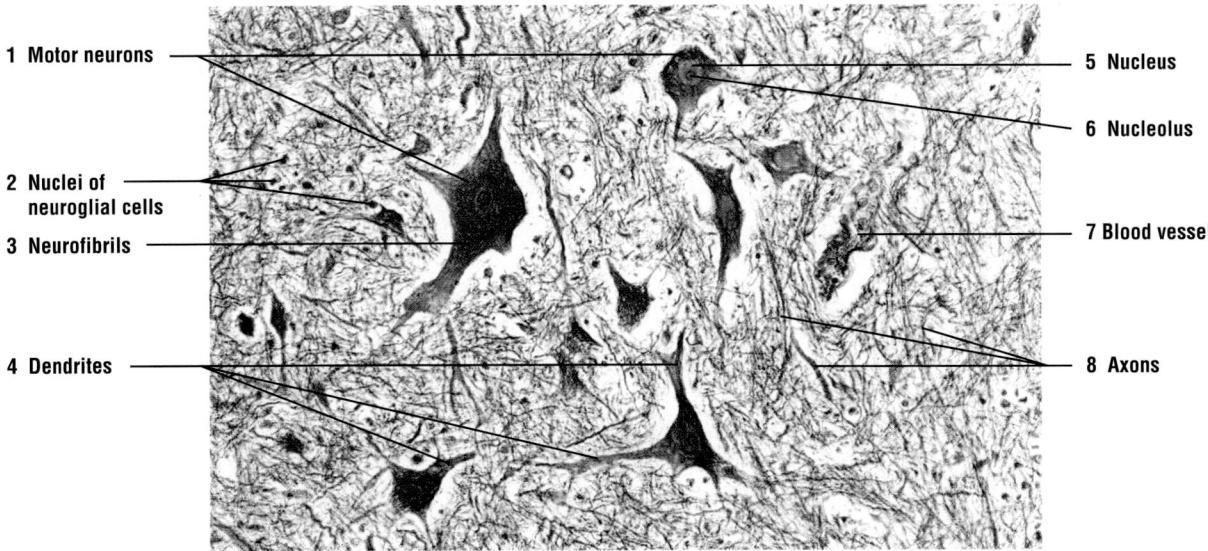

1 Motor neurons

2 Nuclei of neuroglial cells

3 Neurofibrils

4 Dendrites

5 Nucleus

6 Nucleolus

7 Blood vessel

8 Axons

Fig. 6-25   Anterior Gray Horn of Spinal Cord: Multipolar Motor Neurons, Axons, and Neuroglial Cells. Stain: silver. 80×

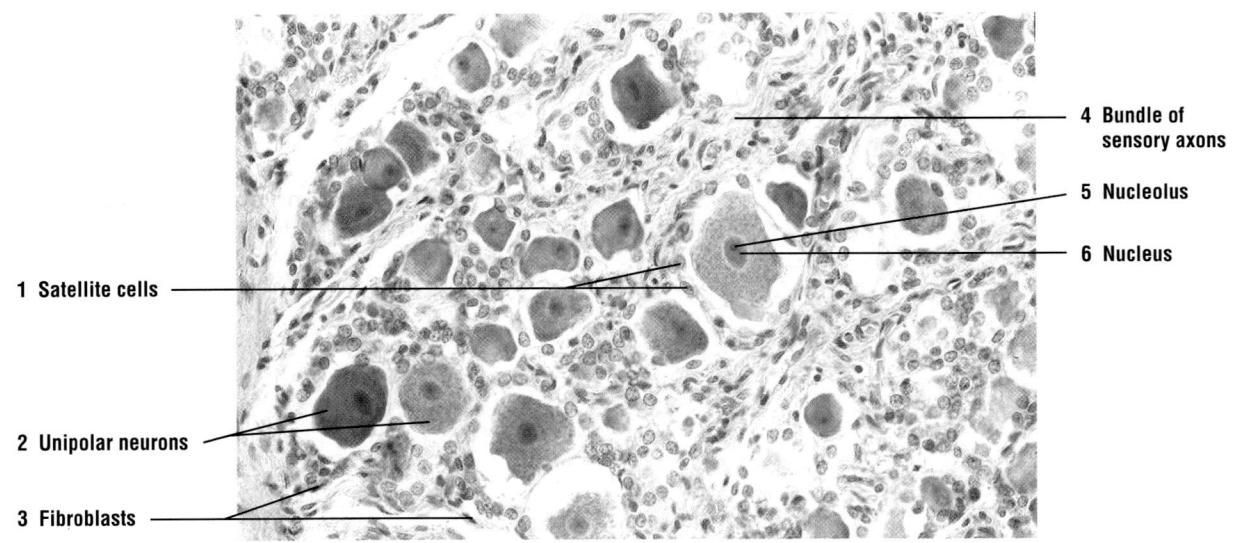

1 Satellite cells

2 Unipolar neurons

3 Fibroblasts

4 Bundle of sensory axons

5 Nucleolus

6 Nucleus

Fig. 6-26   Dorsal Root Ganglion: Unipolar Neurons and Surrounding Cells. Stain: hematoxylin-eosin. 100×

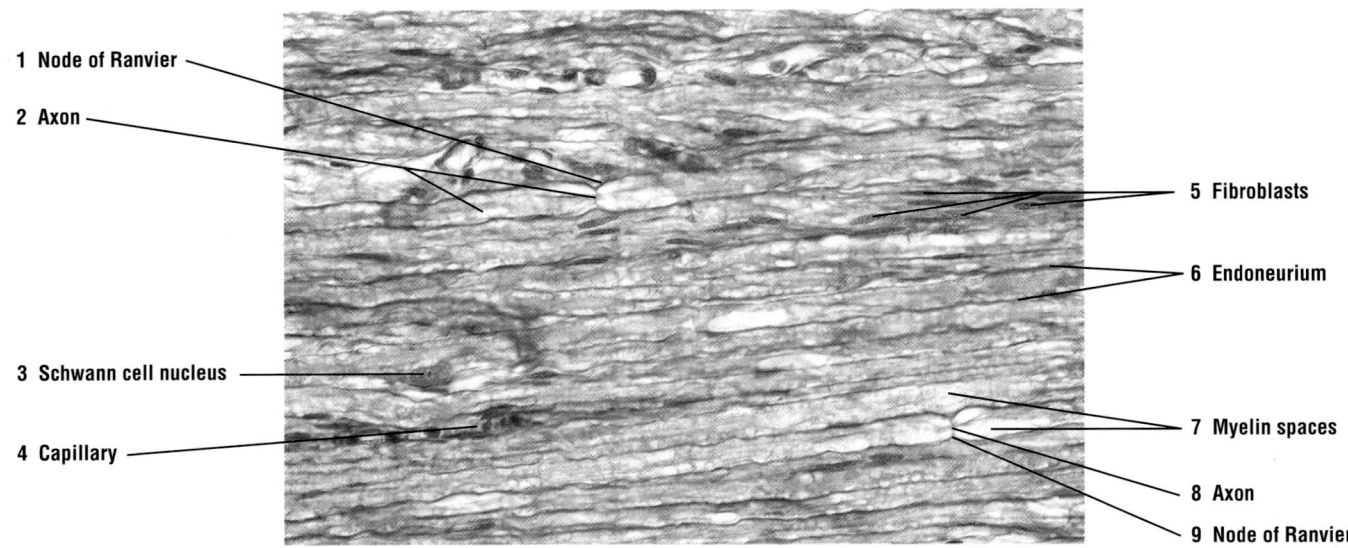

1 Node of Ranvier

2 Axon

3 Schwann cell nucleus

4 Capillary

5 Fibroblasts

6 Endoneurium

7 Myelin spaces

8 Axon

9 Node of Ranvier

Fig. 6-27   Peripheral Nerve: Nodes of Ranvier and Axons. Stain: Masson's trichrome. 100×

PART TWO

Organs

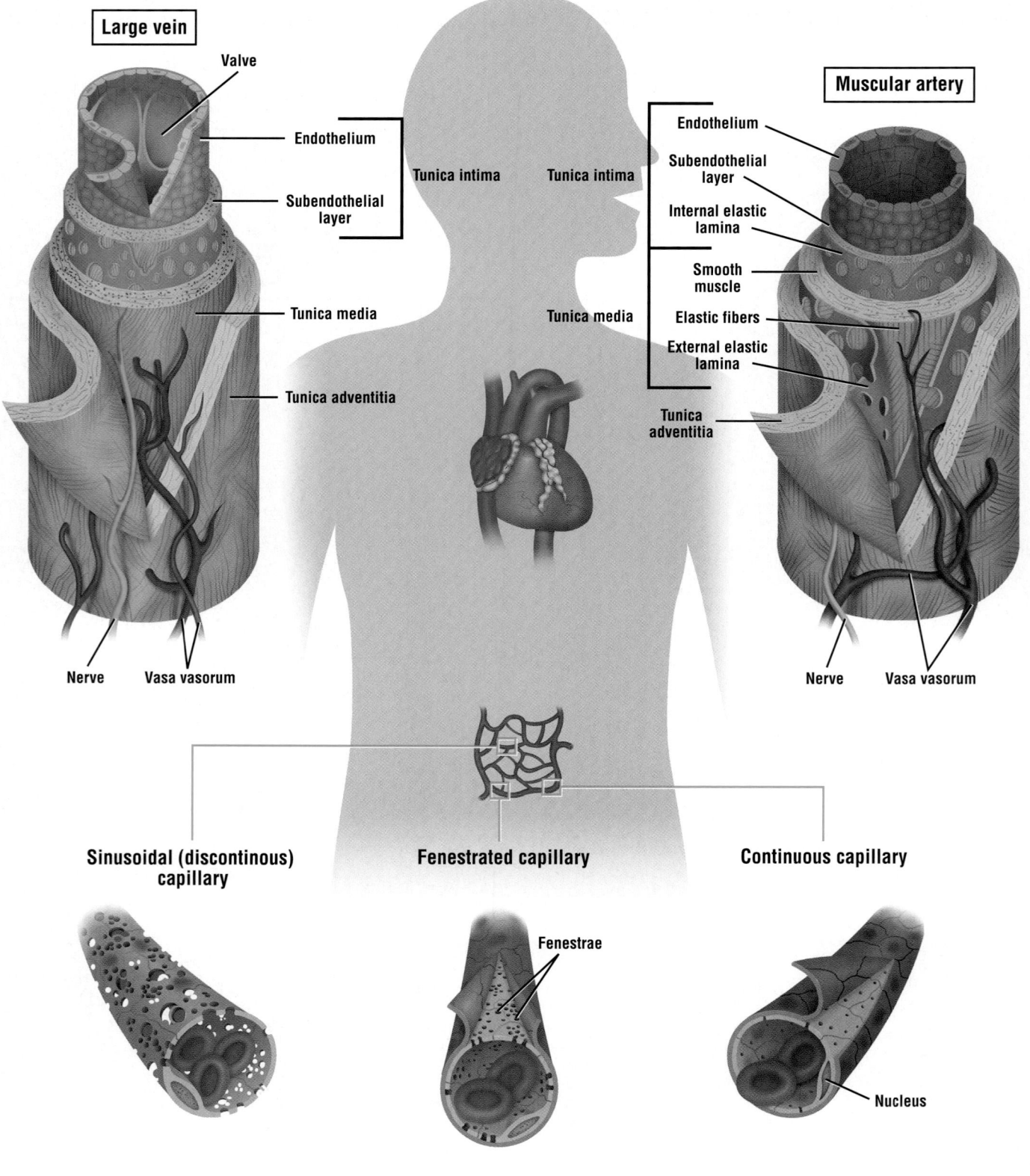

Large vein

Valve

Endothelium

Subendothelial layer

Tunica intima

Tunica media

Tunica adventitia

Nerve   Vasa vasorum

Muscular artery

Endothelium

Subendothelial layer

Internal elastic lamina

Smooth muscle

Elastic fibers

External elastic lamina

Tunica intima

Tunica media

Tunica adventitia

Nerve   Vasa vasorum

Sinusoidal (discontinous) capillary

Fenestrated capillary

Fenestrae

Continuous capillary

Nucleus

Circulatory System

THE BLOOD VASCULAR SYSTEM

The **blood vascular system** consists of the heart, the major arteries, arterioles, capillaries, venules, and veins. The histology of the heart muscle has been described in detail in Chapter 5 as one of the four main tissues **(Figs. 5-2, 5-8–5-10).** In this chapter, the heart histology is only illustrated as part of the cardiovascular system.

ARTERIES: ELASTIC AND MUSCULAR

The three major categories of arteries are the elastic arteries, the muscular arteries, and the smaller arterioles. The diameters of the arteries gradually decrease with each branching, until the smallest vessel, the capillary, is formed.

The **elastic arteries** are the largest blood vessels in the body. These include the **pulmonary trunk** and **aorta** and its major branches. The walls of these vessels are primarily composed of elastic fibers, which provide great resilience and flexibility during blood flow. The elastic arteries branch to become the medium-sized, **muscular arteries,** which are the most numerous vessels in the body. The muscular arteries contain increased amounts of smooth muscle fibers in their walls. The **arterioles** are the smallest branches of the arterial system. Their walls consist of one to five layers of **smooth muscle fibers (Figs. 7-1, 7-3, 7-9).**

The wall of a typical artery contains three concentric layers of **tunics.** The innermost layer is the **tunica intima;** it consists of **endothelium** and the underlying **subendothelial connective tissue.** The middle layer is the **tunica media;** it is composed primarily of smooth muscle fibers that surround the lumen of the vessel. The outermost layer is the **tunica adventitia;** it is composed primarily of connective tissue fibers. The medium-sized muscular arteries also exhibit a thin, wavy band of elastic fibers called an **internal elastic lamina,** located adjacent to tunica intima. Another band of wavy elastic fibers is seen on the periphery of the tunica media. This is the **external elastic lamina.**

VEINS

Capillaries gradually form larger **venules;** venules usually accompany arterioles. The returning blood initially flows into **postcapillary venules** and then into veins of increasing size. The veins are arbitrarily classified as small, medium, and large. Compared to arteries, veins typically are more numerous and have **thinner walls, larger diameters,** and greater structural **variation (Figs. 7-1, 7-2, 7-9).**

Small-sized and medium-sized veins, particularly in the extremities, have **valves.** When the blood flows toward the heart, the valves are opened. As the blood flows backward, the valve flaps close the lumen, and

prevent backflow of blood. Venous blood between the valves in the extremities flows toward the heart due to **muscular contractions.** Valves are absent in veins of the central nervous system, in inferior or superior vena cava, and in veins of the viscera.

The walls of the veins also exhibit three layers. However, the muscular layer is much less prominent. **Tunica intima** in large veins exhibits endothelium and subendothelial connective tissue. **Tunica media** is thin and **tunica adventitia** is the thicker layer in the wall.

VASA VASORUM

The **walls** of larger **arteries** and **veins** are too thick to receive nourishment by direct diffusion from their lumina. As a result, these walls are supplied by their own small blood vessels called the **vasa vasorum** (vessels of the vessel).

CAPILLARIES

Capillaries are the smallest blood vessels, with an average diameter of about **8 μm,** nearly equaling the diameter of an **erythrocyte.** There are three types of capillaries: continuous capillaries, fenestrated capillaries, and sinusoids.

The **continuous capillaries** are the most common and are found in most tissues and organs. In these capillaries, the **endothelial cells** are joined and form an uninterrupted endothelial lining **(Fig. 7-1).**

In contrast, the **fenestrated capillaries** exhibit circular openings or **fenestrations** (pores) in the cytoplasm of endothelial cells. Fenestrated capillaries are found in the **endocrine organs,** the **small intestine,** and the kidney **glomeruli.**

The **sinusoids** are blood vessels that follow irregular, tortuous paths and have much wider diameters than the other two types of capillaries. Sinusoids are found in the **liver, spleen,** and **bone marrow.** Endothelial cell junctions are rare in sinusoids, and wide **gaps** exist between individual endothelial cells. Also, the **basement membrane** is incomplete or absent in the sinusoids.

THE LYMPH VASCULAR SYSTEM

The **lymphatic system** consists of lymph capillaries and lymph vessels. This system starts as blind-ending tubules or lymphatic capillaries in the connective tissue. These vessels collect the excess **interstitial fluid (lymph),** filter it through **lymph nodes,** and return it to the blood vascular system via the larger **lymph vessels.** The **endothelium** in lymph capillaries and vessels is extremely thin for greater permeability. The structure of larger lymph vessels is similar to that of veins except that their walls are thinner. Lymph movement in the vessels is similar to blood movement; however, the lymph vessels contain more **valves.** Lymph vessels are found in all tissues except the central nervous system, cartilage, bone and bone marrow, thymus, placenta, and teeth.

Figure 7-1   Blood and Lymphatic Vessels

This plate illustrates various types of blood and lymphatic vessels, surrounded by loose connective and **adipose tissue (13, 28)**. Most vessels have been cut in a transverse or oblique plane of section.

A **small artery (4)**, with its basic wall structure, is shown at the top center of the plate. In contrast to a vein (22), an artery has a relatively thick wall and a small lumen. In cross section, the wall of an artery exhibits the following layers:

a. **tunica intima,** composed of an inner layer of **endothelium (16)**, a **subendothelial (17)** layer of connective tissue, and an **internal elastic lamina (membrane) (19),** which marks the boundary between the tunica intima and tunica media.

b. **tunica media (4),** composed predominantly of circular smooth muscle fibers. A loose network of fine elastic fibers is interspersed among the smooth muscle cells.

c. **tunica adventitia (6),** composed of connective tissue containing **small nerves (14)** and blood vessels (15). The blood vessels in the adventitia are collectively called **vasa vasorum (15),** or "blood vessels of blood vessel."

When arteries acquire about 25 or more layers of smooth muscle in tunica media, they are called muscular or distributing arteries. Elastic fibers become more numerous, but are still present as thin fibers and networks.

A **medium-sized vein (22)** is illustrated at the lower center of the plate. It has a relatively thin wall and a large lumen. In cross section, the wall of the vein exhibits the following layers:

a. **Tunica intima,** composed of **endothelium (24)** and an extremely thin layer of fine collagen and elastic fibers, which blend with the connective tissue of the tunica media.

b. **Tunica media (25),** consisting of a thin layer of circularly arranged smooth muscle loosely embedded in connective tissue. This layer is much thinner in veins than in arteries.

c. **Tunica adventitia (26),** consisting of a wide layer of connective tissue. In veins, this layer is much thicker than the tunica media.

Arterioles (1, 5, 8) are also illustrated. The smallest arteriole (1) has a thin internal elastic lamina and one layer of smooth muscle cells in the tunica media. One **arteriole (8)** with a branching **capillary (9)** is sectioned longitudinally. Also illustrated are smaller **veins (18, 27), venules (3, 10), capillaries (9, 11, 20),** and small **nerves (2, 23).**

A **lymphatic vessel (12)** can be recognized by the thinnest of its walls and the flaps of a valve in the lumen. Many veins in the extremities have similar valves.

Figure 7-2   Large Vein: Portal Vein (transverse section)

In large veins, the outstanding feature is the thick, muscular adventitia, in which the smooth muscle fibers exhibit a longitudinal orientation. In the illustrated transverse section of the portal vein, the typical arrangement in its wall is visible: the **smooth muscle fibers (1)** are segregated into bundles and seen mainly in cross section, with varying amounts of connective tissue of the tunica **adventitia (2)** dispersed among them. **Vasa vasorum (3, 7)** are present in the intervening connective tissue.

In contrast to the thick tunica adventitia, the **tunica media (6)** is a thinner layer of circularly arranged smooth muscle fibers and a more loosely arranged connective tissue. In other large veins, the tunica media may be extremely thin and compact. As seen in other vessels, the tunica intima is part of the **endothelium (4)** and is supported by a small amount of connective tissue. In addition, large veins usually exhibit an **internal elastic lamina (5),** which is not as well developed as in the arteries.

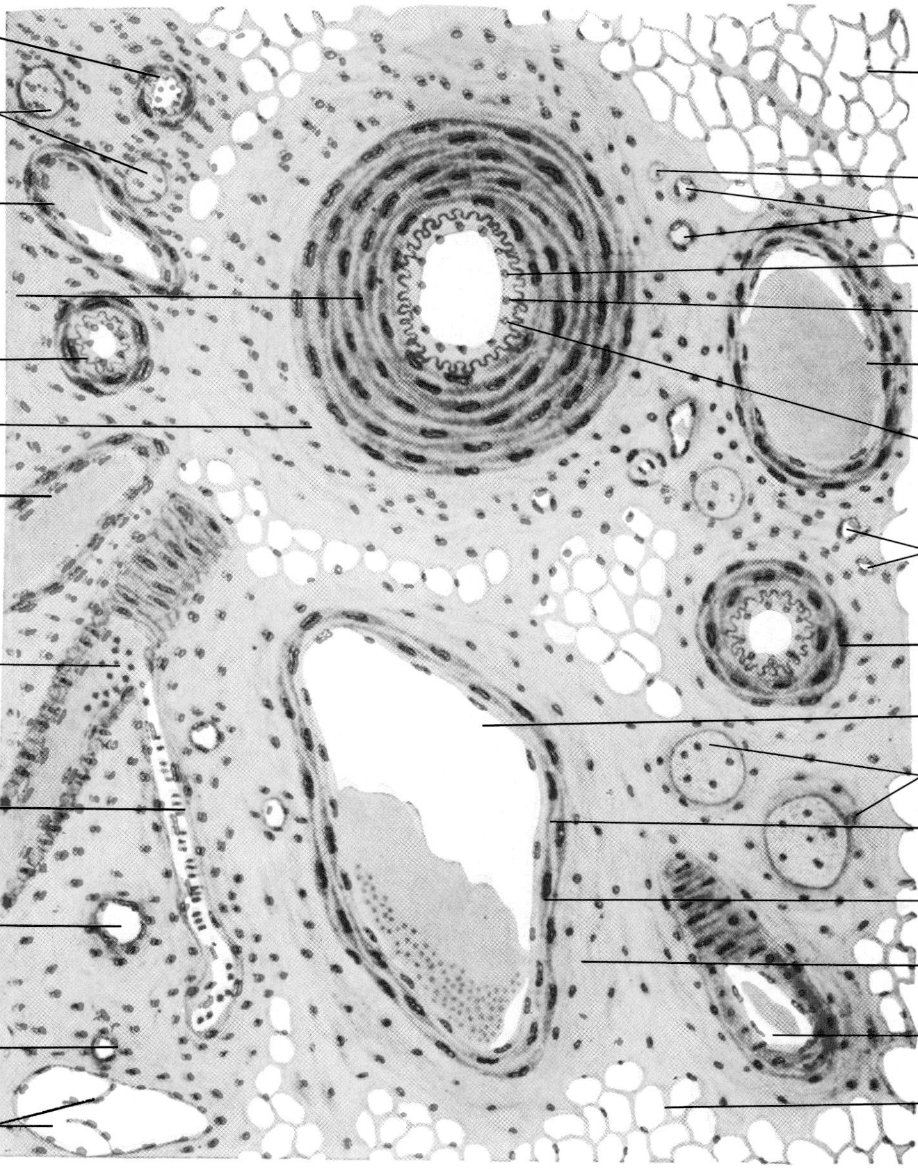

1 Arteriole

2 Nerves (t.s.)

3 Venule (o.s.)

4 Small artery: tunica media

5 Arteriole

6 Tunica adventitia of small artery

7 Vein (o.s.)

8 Arteriole with a clot (l.s.)

9 Capillary (l.s.)

10 Venule

11 Capillary

12 Lymphatic vessel with a valve

13 Adipose tissue

14 Nerve

15 Vasa vasorum

16 Endothelium

17 Subendothelial layer

18 Vein with blood clot

19 Internal elastic lamina (membrane)

20 Capillaries

21 Small artery

22 Medium-sized vein

23 Nerves (t.s.)

24 Endothelium

25 Tunica media

26 Tunica adventitia

27 Vein (o.s.)

28 Adipose tissue

Fig. 7-1   Blood and Lymphatic Vessels. Stain: hematoxylin. Medium magnification.

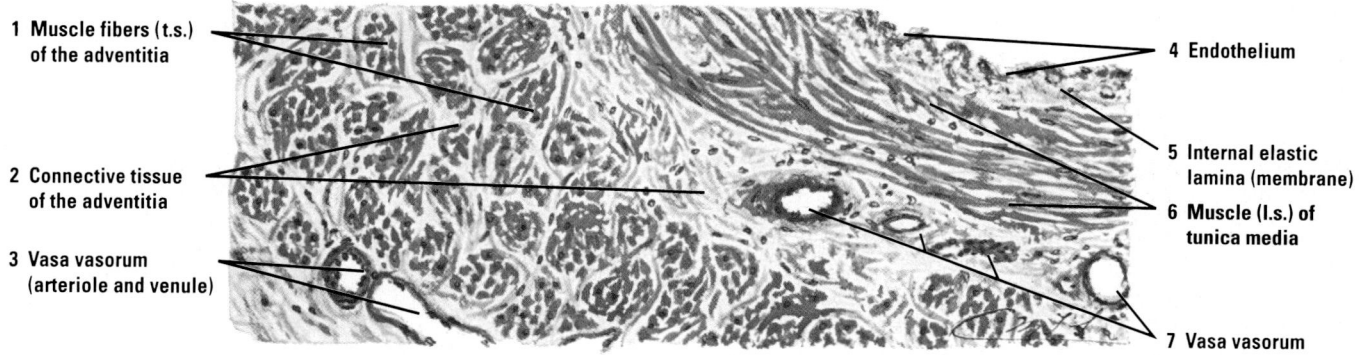

1 Muscle fibers (t.s.) of the adventitia

2 Connective tissue of the adventitia

3 Vasa vasorum (arteriole and venule)

4 Endothelium

5 Internal elastic lamina (membrane)

6 Muscle (l.s.) of tunica media

7 Vasa vasorum

Fig. 7-2   Large Vein: Portal Vein (transverse section). Stain: hematoxylin-eosin. Medium magnification.

Figure 7-3   Muscular Artery and Vein (transverse section)

The walls of blood vessels contain certain amount of elastic tissue in order to expand and contract. In this illustration, a muscular **artery (1)** and **vein (4)** have been cut in transverse plane and the section prepared with an elastic stain to illustrate the distribution of elastic fibers. In this preparation, the elastic fibers stain black and the collagen fibers light yellow. This illustration shows that the wall of artery (1) is much thicker and contains more smooth muscle fibers than the wall of the vein (4). The innermost layer tunica intima of the artery (1) is stained dark because of the thick **internal elastic lamina (1a).** The thick middle layer of the muscular artery, the **tunica media (1b),** consists of several layers of smooth muscle fibers, arranged in a circular pattern around the lumen, and thin dark strands of **elastic fibers (1b).** On the periphery of the tunica media (1b) is seen the less conspicuous **external elastic lamina (1c).** Surrounding the artery is the connective tissue **adventitia (1d).** In the adventitia (1d) are seen both the light staining **collagen fibers (2)** and the dark staining **elastic fibers (3).** In the wall of the vein (4) are also visible the layers **tunica intima (4a), tunica media (4b),** and **tunica adventitia (4c)** in cross section. However, these three layers in the vein are much more reduced in thickness in comparison to the wall of the artery. Surrounding both vessels are **capillary (5), arteriole (7), venule (6),** and cells of the **adipose tissue (8).** Present in the lumina of both vessels are numerous erythrocytes and leukocytes.

Figure 7-4   Large Artery: Wall of the Aorta (transverse section)

The structure of the wall of the aorta is similar to that of the artery wall illustrated in Figure 7-3. However, the dark brown **elastic fibers (2)** constitute the bulk of the tunica media, with **smooth muscle cells (3)** in lesser abundance than in some of the muscular arteries. Other tissues in the wall of the aorta remain colorless or are only lightly stained. The size and arrangement of elastic lamina in the tunica media are clearly demonstrated with the elastic stain. However, smooth muscle cells (3) and fine elastic fibers between the laminae remain unstained.

The extent of **tunica intima (4)** is indicated but remains unstained. The first elastic membrane is the **internal elastic lamina (membrane) (5).** At times, smaller laminae appear in the subendothelial connective tissue, and a gradual transition is made to larger laminae of the tunica media.

The **tunica adventitia (1),** also unstained, is a narrow zone of collagen fibers. In the aorta and pulmonary arteries, tunica media occupies most of the wall of the vessel, whereas tunica adventitia is reduced to a proportionately small area, as illustrated in the figure.

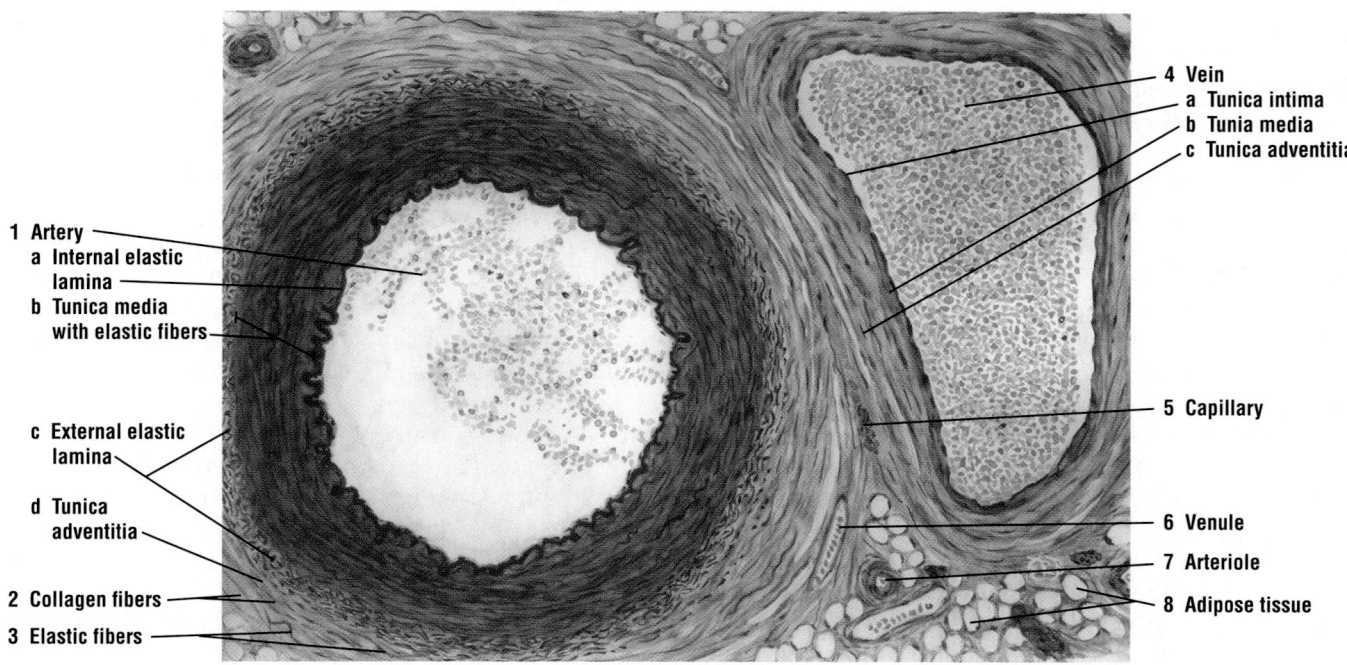

1 **Artery**
  a **Internal elastic lamina**
  b **Tunica media with elastic fibers**

  c **External elastic lamina**

  d **Tunica adventitia**

2 **Collagen fibers**

3 **Elastic fibers**

4 **Vein**
  a **Tunica intima**
  b **Tunia media**
  c **Tunica adventitia**

5 **Capillary**

6 **Venule**

7 **Arteriole**

8 **Adipose tissue**

Fig. 7-3   Muscular Artery and Vein (transverse section). Stain: Elastic stain. Low magnification.

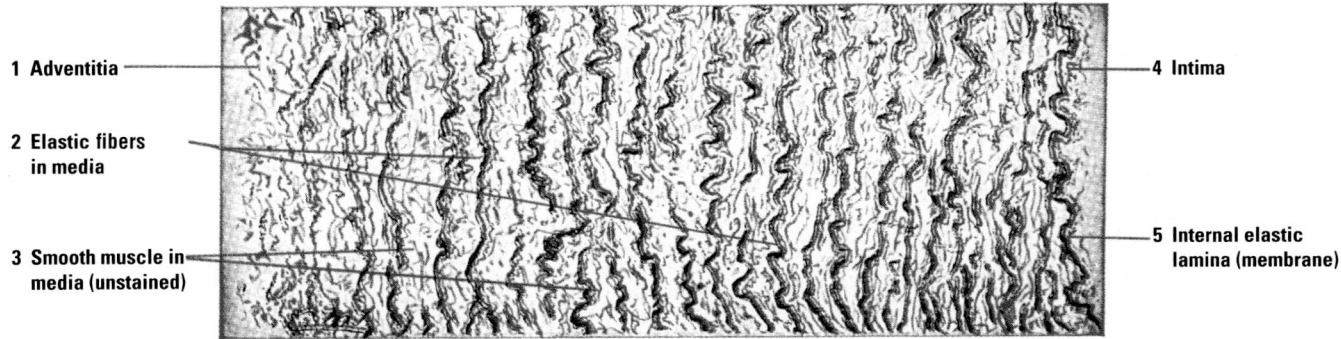

1 **Adventitia**

2 **Elastic fibers in media**

3 **Smooth muscle in media (unstained)**

4 **Intima**

5 **Internal elastic lamina (membrane)**

Fig. 7-4   Large Artery: Wall of the Aorta (transverse section). Orcein stain: aorta. Elastic fibers selectively stained dark brown. High magnification.

Figure 7-5   Heart: Left Atrium and Ventricle (panoramic view, longitudinal section)

This figure illustrates a longitudinal section of the left side of the heart, showing a portion of the **atrium (1)**, the **atrioventricular (mitral) valve (4)**, and the **ventricle (6)**. In this plane of section, the cardiac musculature is seen in various planes.

In the atrial wall, the **endocardium (1)** consists of endothelium, a thick subendothelial layer of connective tissue, and a thick **myocardium (2)** of loosely arranged musculature. The **epicardium (13)** covers the heart and is lined externally by a single layer of mesothelium. A **subepicardial layer (14)** contains connective tissue and fat, which vary in amount in different regions of the heart. This layer also extends into the coronary (atrioventricular) and interventricular sulcus of the heart.

In the ventricle, the **endocardium (6)** is thin in comparison with that in the atrium (1), whereas the **myocardium (7)** is thick and more compact. The **epicardium** and **subepicardial (16)** connective tissue are continuous with those in the atrium.

Between the atrium and ventricle is seen the **annulus fibrosus (3),** which consists of dense fibrous connective tissue. The leaflet of the **atrioventricular (mitral) valve (4)** is formed by a double membrane of the **endocardium (4a)** and a core of dense **connective tissue (4b),** which is continuous with the annulus fibrosus (3). On the ventral surface of the valve is seen the insertion of a section of **chorda tendinae (5)** into the valve.

The inner surface of the ventricular wall exhibits the characteristic prominence of myocardium and endocardium: the **apex of papillary muscle (18)** and **trabeculae carnaea (17).**

The **Purkinje fibers (8),** or impulse-conducting fibers, located in the loose subendocardial tissue, distinguished by their larger size and lighter-staining properties. The small area within the rectangle **(9)** is illustrated in greater detail and higher magnification in Figure 7-7.

The larger blood vessels, such as the **coronary artery (10),** course in the **subepicardial connective tissue (14).** Below the coronary artery is a section through the **coronary sinus (11).** Entering the coronary sinus is a **coronary vein (12)** with its valve. Smaller coronary **vessels (15)** are seen in the subepicardial connective tissue (14) and in the **perimyseal septa (15)** that extend into the myocardium (7).

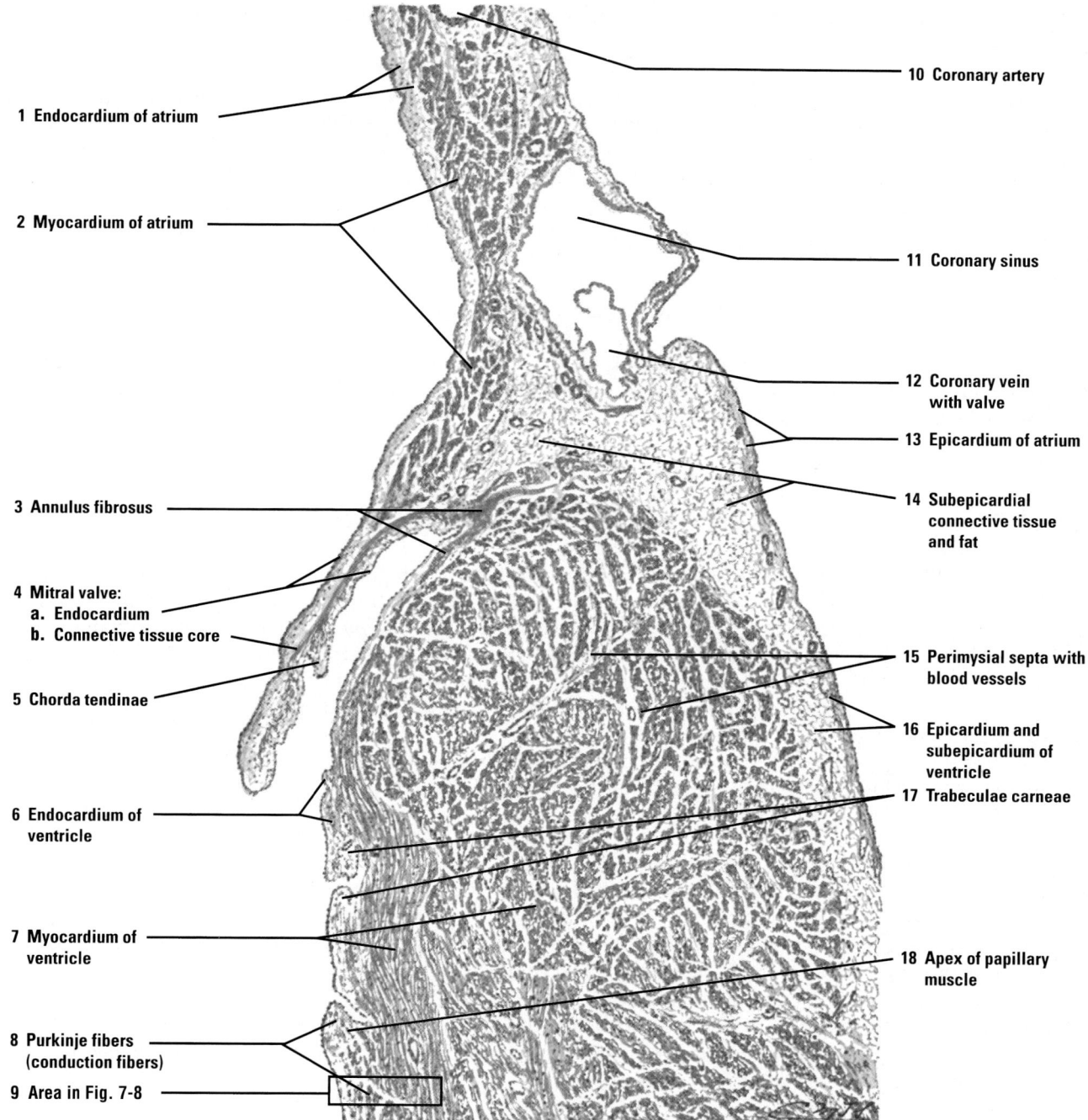

1 Endocardium of atrium

2 Myocardium of atrium

3 Annulus fibrosus

4 Mitral valve:
   a. Endocardium
   b. Connective tissue core

5 Chorda tendinae

6 Endocardium of ventricle

7 Myocardium of ventricle

8 Purkinje fibers (conduction fibers)

9 Area in Fig. 7-8

10 Coronary artery

11 Coronary sinus

12 Coronary vein with valve

13 Epicardium of atrium

14 Subepicardial connective tissue and fat

15 Perimysial septa with blood vessels

16 Epicardium and subepicardium of ventricle

17 Trabeculae carneae

18 Apex of papillary muscle

Fig. 7-5   Heart: Left Atrium and Ventricle (panoramic view, longitudinal section). Stain: hematoxylin-eosin. Low magnification.

Figure 7-6   Heart: Pulmonary Trunk, Pulmonary Valve, Right Ventricle (panoramic view, longitudinal section)

A portion of the right ventricle and a section of the **pulmonary trunk (6)** are illustrated. The endothelium of the tunica intima is visible on the surface to the right. Tunica media constitutes the thickest portion of the wall of the pulmonary trunk; however, its thick, elastic laminae are not apparent at this magnification. A thin adventitia merges into the surrounding **subepicardial connective tissue (2),** which is filled with fat in this specimen.

The **pulmonary trunk (8)** arises from the **annulus fibrosus (9).** One cusp of its **semilunar (pulmonary) valve (7)** is illustrated. Like the mitral valve (illustrated in Fig. 7-5), it is covered with endocardium. The connective tissue from the annulus fibrosus extends into the base of the **pulmonary valve (10)** and forms its central core.

The thick **myocardium (4)** of the right ventricle is lined internally by **endocardium (11).** The endocardium extends over the pulmonary valve (7) and the annulus fibrosus (9) and blends in with tunica intima of the pulmonary trunk (8).

The external surface of the **pulmonary trunk (6)** is lined by the **subepicardial connective tissue** and **fat (2),** which, in turn, is covered by **epicardium (1).** Both of these layers cover the external surface of the ventricle. **Coronary vessels (3, 5)** are seen in the subepicardium (2).

Figure 7-7   Heart: Purkinje Fibers (Impulse-conducting Fibers)

The area outlined by a rectangle **(9)** in Figure 7-5 is illustrated here at higher magnification to show the impulse-conducting fibers. Located under the **endocardium (1)** are groups of **Purkinje fibers (2, 4).** These fibers are different from typical **cardiac (myocardial) muscle fibers (5)** because of their larger size and less intense staining. Some Purkinje fibers are sectioned transversely (2) and others longitudinally (4). In transverse section, Purkinje fibers exhibit fewer myofibrils, distributed peripherally, leaving a perinuclear zone of comparatively clear sarcoplasm. A nucleus is seen in some transverse sections; in others, a central area of clear sarcoplasm is seen, with the plane of section bypassing the nucleus.

Purkinje fibers merge with cardiac fibers at a **transitional fiber (3);** the upper part of the fiber corresponds to a Purkinje fiber and the lower part to an ordinary cardiac muscle fiber.

Figure 7-8   Heart: Purkinje Fibers (Impulse-conducting Fibers)

This figure illustrates a cardiac region with Purkinje fibers that are stained with Mallory-azan; for this preparation, the same magnification as in Figure 7-7 was used. The characteristic features of **Purkinje fibers (2)** are demonstrated in both longitudinal and transverse sections.

With a hematoxylin-eosin preparation, the connective tissue does not stain well. In this preparation, the blue-stained collagen fibers accentuate the **subendocardial connective tissue (3)** around the Purkinje fibers (2). A **capillary (1)** with red blood cells is seen near these fibers.

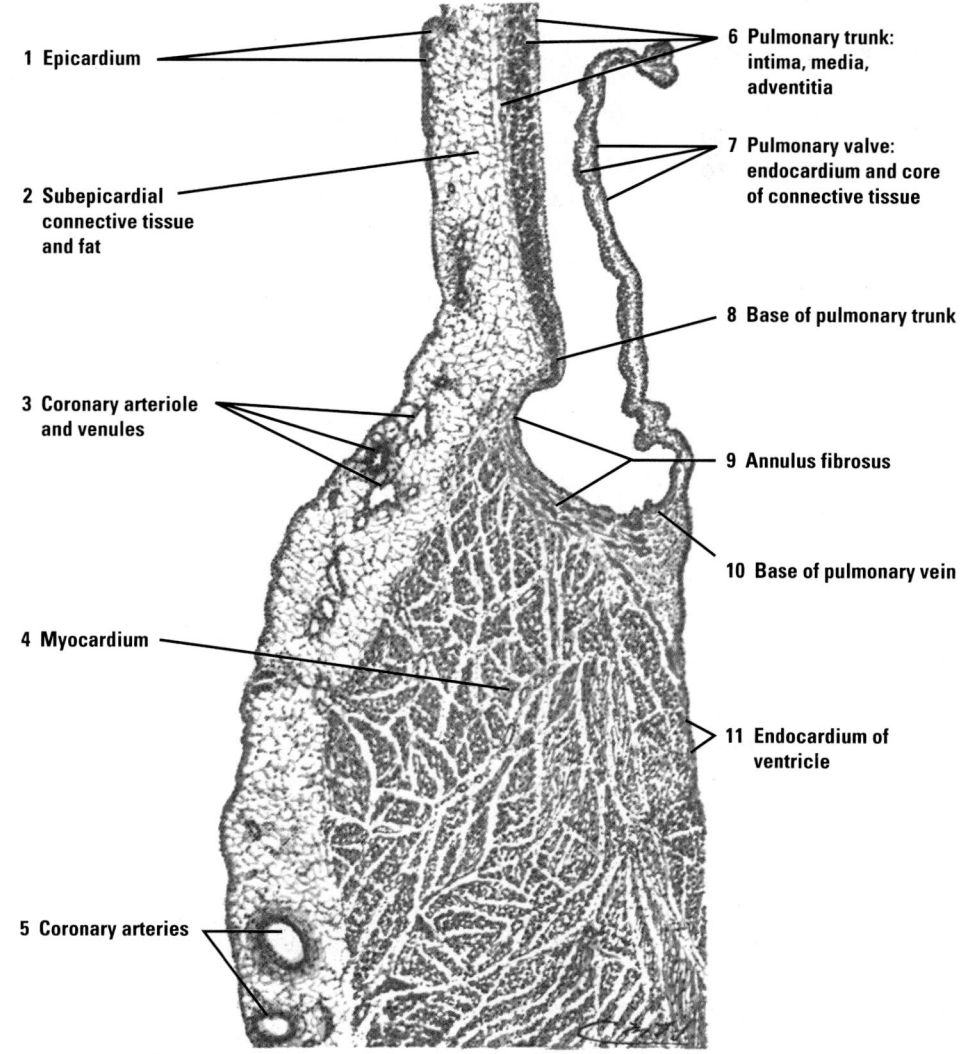

1 Epicardium

2 Subepicardial connective tissue and fat

3 Coronary arteriole and venules

4 Myocardium

5 Coronary arteries

6 Pulmonary trunk: intima, media, adventitia

7 Pulmonary valve: endocardium and core of connective tissue

8 Base of pulmonary trunk

9 Annulus fibrosus

10 Base of pulmonary vein

11 Endocardium of ventricle

Fig. 7-6   Heart: Pulmonary Trunk, Pulmonary Valve, Right Ventricle (panoramic view, longitudinal section). Stain: hematoxylin-eosin. Low magnification.

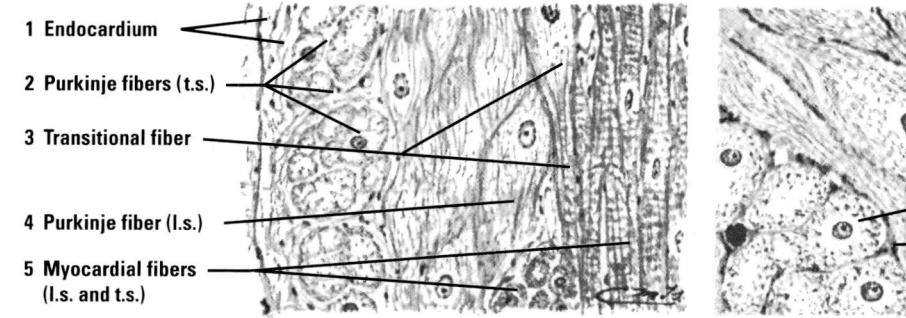

1 Endocardium

2 Purkinje fibers (t.s.)

3 Transitional fiber

4 Purkinje fiber (l.s.)

5 Myocardial fibers (l.s. and t.s.)

Fig. 7-7   Heart: Purkinje Fibers (Impulse-conducting Fibers). Stain: hematoxylin-eosin. High magnification.

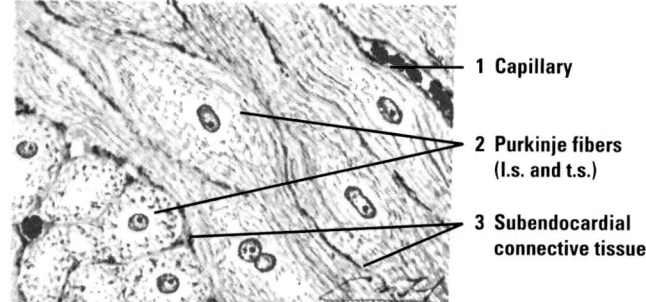

1 Capillary

2 Purkinje fibers (l.s. and t.s.)

3 Subendocardial connective tissue

Fig. 7-8   Heart: Purkinje Fibers (Impulse-conducting Fibers). Stain: Mallory-azan. High magnification.

Figure 7-9   Artery and Vein in Connective Tissue of Vas Deferens

A phtomicrograph illustrates and compares the differences between a **small artery (1)** and a small **vein (6)** surrounded by dense irregular **connective tissue (5).** The small artery (1) has a relatively thick wall and a small lumen. The arterial wall consists of the **tunica intima (2),** composed of an inner layer of **endothelium (2a),** a **subendothelial (2b)** layer of connective tissue, and an **internal elastic lamina (membrane) (2c).** This membrane (2c) separates the tunica intima (2) from **tunica media (3),** which consists predominantly of circular smooth muscle fibers. Surrounding the tunica media (3) is the connective tissue layer **tunica adventitia (4).**

Adjacent to the small artery (1) is a small vein (6) with a much larger lumen that is filled with blood cells. The wall of the vein is thinner in comparison to that of the artery (1) and consists of **tunica intima (7),** which is composed of **endothelium (7a),** a thin layer of circular smooth muscle that forms the **tunica media (8),** and the layer of connective tissue **tunica adventitia (9).**

Figure 7-10   Heart Wall: Purkinje Fibers

A photomicrograph of the ventricular heart wall illustrates the **endothelium (3)** of the heart chamber, **subendothelial connective tissue (4),** and the underlying **Purkinje fibers (5)** of the endocardium. In comparison to the adjacent, red-staining **cardiac (myocardial) muscle fibers (1),** the Purkinje fibers (5) are larger in size and exhibit less intense staining. In addition, these fibers exhibit fewer myofibrils, which are distributed peripherally and which leave a perinuclear zone of clear sarcoplasm. Purkinje fibers (5) gradually merge with the cardiac fibers (1), as shown in the illustration. Surrounding both the Purkinje fibers (5) and the cardiac muscle fibers (1) are bundles of **connective tissue fibers (2).**

■ Functional Correlations–Blood Vessels

The **elastic arteries** transport the blood from the heart and move it along the systemic vascular path. The presence of a high proportion of **elastic fibers** in their walls allows the elastic arteries to greatly expand in diameter during **systole** (heart contraction) when a large volume of blood is ejected from the ventricles into their lumina. During **diastole** (heart relaxation), the expanded elastic walls recoil on the volume of blood in their lumina and force the blood to move forward through the vascular channels. In this manner, necessary arterial pressure is maintained. Also, because of these elastic fibers in their walls, the elastic arteries provide for a less variable systemic blood pressure and a more even blood flow through the body during the heart cycles.

In contrast to elastic arteries, the **muscular arteries** control blood flow and blood pressure through **vasoconstriction** or **vasodilation** of their lumina. This is caused by the high proportion of **smooth muscle fiber**s in their walls. These effects are produced primarily by the innervation of the smooth muscles fibers by the **unmyelinated axons** of the **sympathetic division** of the **autonomic nervous system.**

Similarly, by autonomic **constriction** or **dilation** of their lumen, the smooth muscle fibers in the smaller arteries or **arterioles** regulate the flow of blood into the capillary beds. The terminal arterioles give rise to the smalles blood vessels, the capillaries. Capillaries are normally described as continuous, fenestrated (porous), and sinusoidal (discontinuous).

Because of their very thin walls, capillaries allow for a very efficient exchange of gases, metabolites, nutrients, and waste products between blood and tissues. Most capillaries in the body are **continuous type;** that is, the **endothelium** forms a continuous lining of the blood vessel. The **fenestrated (porous) capillaries** allow a more rapid exchange of molecular substances between blood and the tissues than would normally occur in continuous capillaries. In **sinusoids,** the endothelium is fenestrated, discontinuous, and there is partial or total absence of **basement membrane** underlying the endothelium. As a result, plasma, as well as formed elements, can pass through the sinusoids and make direct contact with the surrounding cells. This allows for an enhanced exchange between the contents of the blood and the surrounding tissue.

In **veins,** blood pressure is lower than in the arteries. As a result, venous blood flow is **passive.** Venous blood flow in the head and trunk is primarily owing to negative pressure in the thorax and abdominal cavities resulting from respiratory movements. Venous blood return from the extremities is aided by **muscle contractions.**

■ Functional Correlations–Lymphatic Vessels

The main function of the **lymph vascular system** is to passively collect excess tissue fluid and proteins, called **lymph,** from the intercellular spaces of the connective tissue and return it into the blood vascular system. Lymph is a clear fluid and an **ultrafiltrate** of the blood plasma. The lymph vessels also bring to the systemic blood stream **lymphocytes, fatty acids** absorbed through the capillary lymph vessels called **lacteals** in the small intestine, and **immunoglobulins** (antibodies) produced in the lymph nodes.

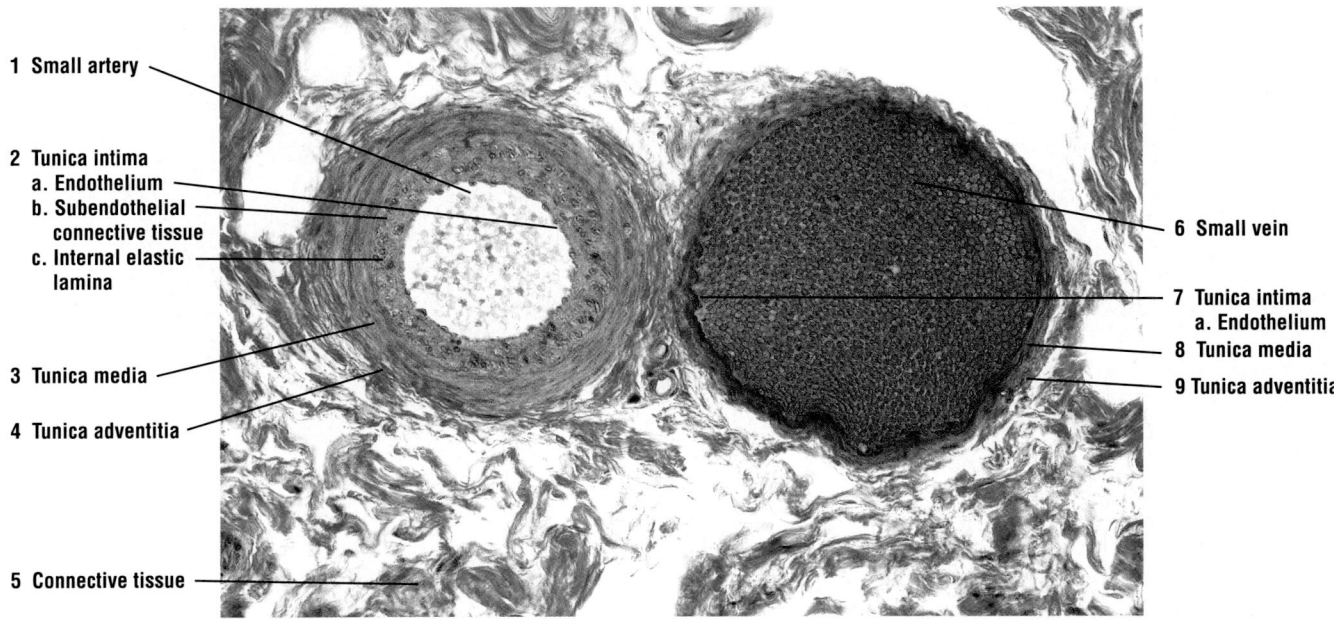

1 Small artery

2 Tunica intima
  a. Endothelium
  b. Subendothelial
    connective tissue
  c. Internal elastic
    lamina

3 Tunica media

4 Tunica adventitia

5 Connective tissue

6 Small vein

7 Tunica intima
  a. Endothelium
8 Tunica media
9 Tunica adventitia

Fig. 7-9 Artery and Vein in Connective Tissue of Vas Deferens. Stain: iron hematoxylin and alcian blue. 64×

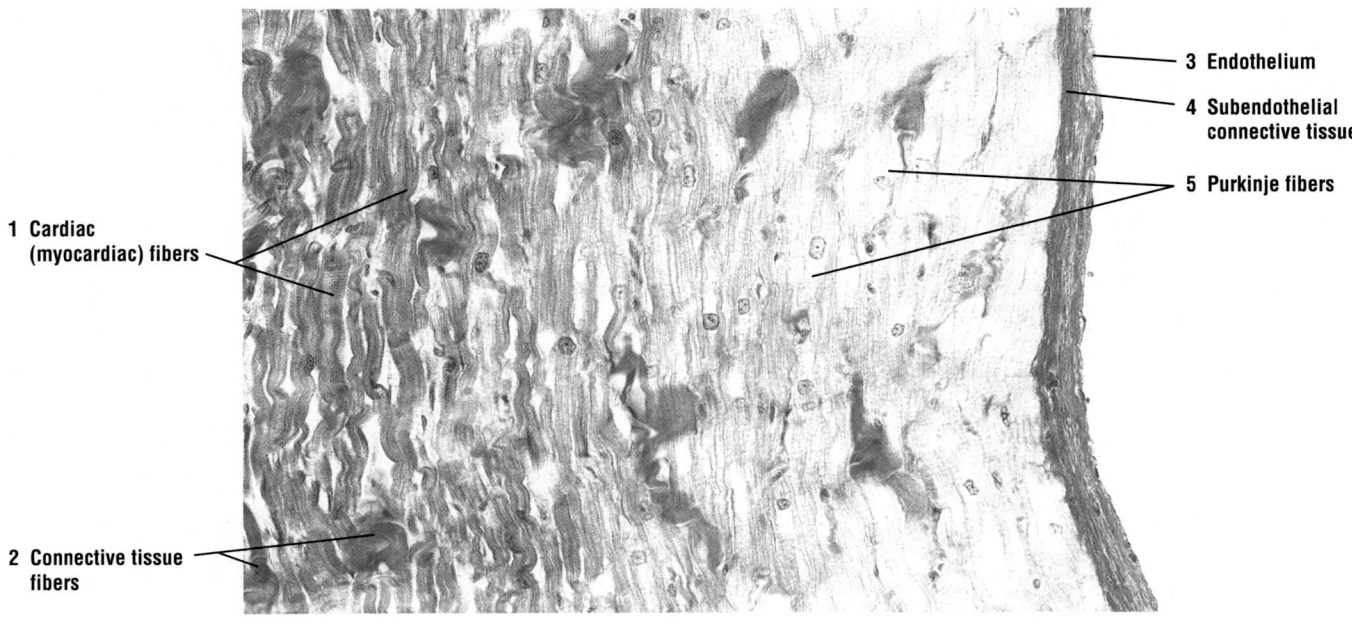

3 Endothelium

4 Subendothelial
  connective tissue

5 Purkinje fibers

1 Cardiac
  (myocardiac) fibers

2 Connective tissue
  fibers

Fig. 7-10 Heart Wall: Purkinje Fibers. Stain: Mallory-azan. 64×

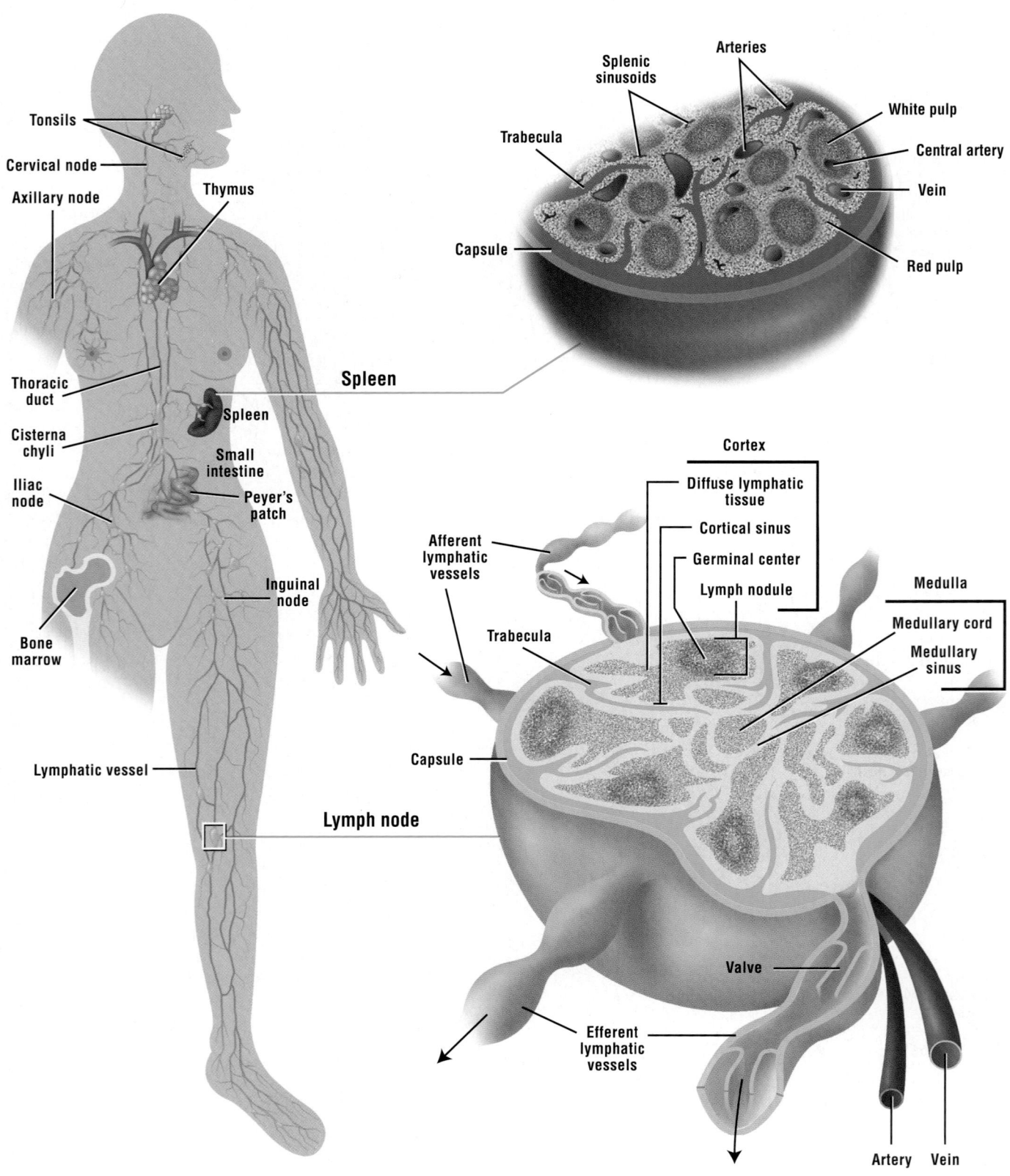

Tonsils

Cervical node

Axillary node

Thymus

Thoracic duct

Cisterna chyli

Iliac node

Bone marrow

Lymphatic vessel

Spleen

Small intestine

Peyer's patch

Inguinal node

Spleen

Splenic sinusoids

Arteries

Trabecula

White pulp

Central artery

Vein

Capsule

Red pulp

Lymph node

Afferent lymphatic vessels

Trabecula

Capsule

Cortex

Diffuse lymphatic tissue

Cortical sinus

Germinal center

Lymph nodule

Medulla

Medullary cord

Medullary sinus

Valve

Efferent lymphatic vessels

Artery

Vein

Lymphoid System

The **lymphoid system** includes all cells, tissues, and organs that contain aggregates of **lymphocytes.** The lymphocytes are distributed throughout the body either as isolated aggregates of cells, as distinct non-encapsulated lymphatic nodules in the loose connective tissue, or as encapsulated individual lymphoid organs. Because the bone marrow produces lymphocytes, it can also be considered a lymphoid organ and part of the lymphoid system. The major lymphoid organs of the body that are filled with lymphocyte aggregation are the **lymph nodes (Figs. 8-1–8-4, 8-10), tonsils (Fig. 8-5), thymus (Figs. 8-6, 8-7, 8-11),** and **spleen (Figs. 8-8, 8-9, 8-12).**

The lymphoid cells, tissue, and organs are important components of the **immune system.** They protect the internal environment of the body against foreign substances or **antigens.** This crucial protective function is performed by **lymphocytes** because they recognize antigens and react specifically against them by producing **antibodies.** An antigen is any foreign macromolecule that provokes an immune response. Antibodies are circulating plasma glycoproteins, which are also called immunoglobulins. They react with the antigens and initiate a complex immune response that protects the body from damage by eventually destroying the foreign substance.

A large variety of lymphocytes are present in the body's various organs. Morphologically, these lymphocytes are similar, but functionally they are different. Lymphoid tissue consists mainly of **T lymphocytes** and **B lymphocytes.** These two functionally distinct types of lymphocytes have important roles in the immune system and are found in the **blood, lymph,** and **lymphoid tissues.** Just as all blood cells, both types of lymphocytes originate from precursor **hemopoietic stem cells** in the **bone marrow** and enter the bloodstream. Whether the developing lymphocytes become B lym-

phocytes or T lymphocytes depends on where they mature and become **immunocompetent.**

B lymphocytes mature and become immunocompetent in the **bone marrow.** After maturation, B lymphocytes are carried by the blood to the nonthymic lymphoid tissue such as the **lymph nodes, spleen,** and **connective tissue.** When the immunocompetent B lymphocytes encounter a specific antigen, they become activated, proliferate, and differentiate into **plasma cells. T lymphocytes** arise from lymphocytes that are carried from the bone marrow to the **thymus gland.** Here, they mature and acquire **immunocompetence** before migrating to other peripheral lymphoid tissues and organs.

Thymus gland produces mature T lymphocytes early in life. After their stay in the thymus gland, T lymphocytes are distributed throughout the body in the blood and populate the lymph nodes, spleen, and different lymphoid aggregates in the connective tissue. In these regions, the T lymphocytes can carry out immune responses when stimulated.

There are two types of closely related immune responses. In the **cell-mediated immune response,** the **T lymphocytes** proliferate, come in close contact, attack, and destroy foreign microorganisms, viral infections, or antigens. T lymphocytes may also attack indirectly by activating B lymphocytes or **macrophages** of the immune system. T lymphocytes provide specific immune protection without secreting antibodies. In the **humoral immune response,** exposure of **B lymphocytes** to antigen transforms some cells into **plasma cells** that secrete specific **antibodies** into blood and lymph. These antibodies then bind to, inactivate, and/or destroy the specific foreign substance or antigen. The activation and proliferation of B lymphocytes to most antigens require the cooperation (help) of T lymphocytes that respond to the same antigen.

Figure 8-1   Lymph Node (panoramic view)

The lymph node consists of lymphocyte aggregations intermeshed with lymphatic sinuses, supported by a reticular fiber framework and surrounded by a **connective tissue capsule (2).** The lymph node has a **cortex (5)** and a **medulla (6).**

The cortex (5) of the lymph node contains lymphocytes that are aggregated into **lymphatic nodules (5, 16).** In many of the **cortical nodules (16)** the centers are lightly stained. These lighter-stained areas represent the **germinal centers (18),** which are the active sites of lymphocyte proliferation.

In the medulla (6) of the lymph node, the lymphocytes are arranged as irregular cords of lymphatic tissue, the **medullary cords (14),** in which are found macrophages, plasma cells, and small lymphocytes. The **medullary sinuses (13)** course between these cords.

The capsule (2) of the node is surrounded by **connective tissue and pericapsular fat (1).** From the capsule, **connective tissue trabeculae (7)** extend into the node, initially between the cortical nodules (7, upper leader) and then ramifying throughout the **medulla (15)** between medullary cords and sinuses. The trabeculae contain the major **blood vessels (15)** of the lymph node.

Afferent lymphatic vessels (4) course in the connective tissue of the lymph node and, at intervals, pierce the capsule to enter the **subcapsular sinus (9, 17).** From here, the trabecular sinuses (cortical sinuses) extend along the trabeculae to pass into medullary sinuses (13).

At the upper right section are the **hilus (12)** of the lymph node and the **efferent lymphatic vessels (11),** which drain lymph from the node. Also found here are nerves, small arteries, and veins, which supply and drain the node.

1 Pericapsular fat and connective tissue

2 Capsule

3 Lymphatic tissue

4 Capsule and afferent lymphatic vessels

5 Cortex

6 Medulla

7 Trabeculae

8 Blood vessels in trabeculae

9 Subcapsular sinus (marginal)

10 Arterioles

11 Efferent lymphatic vessels

12 Hilus

13 Medullary sinuses

14 Medullary cords

15 Trabeculae (t.s.) in the medulla with blood vessels

16 Lymphatic nodules

17 Subcapsular sinus (marginal)

18 Germinal centers

19 Veins

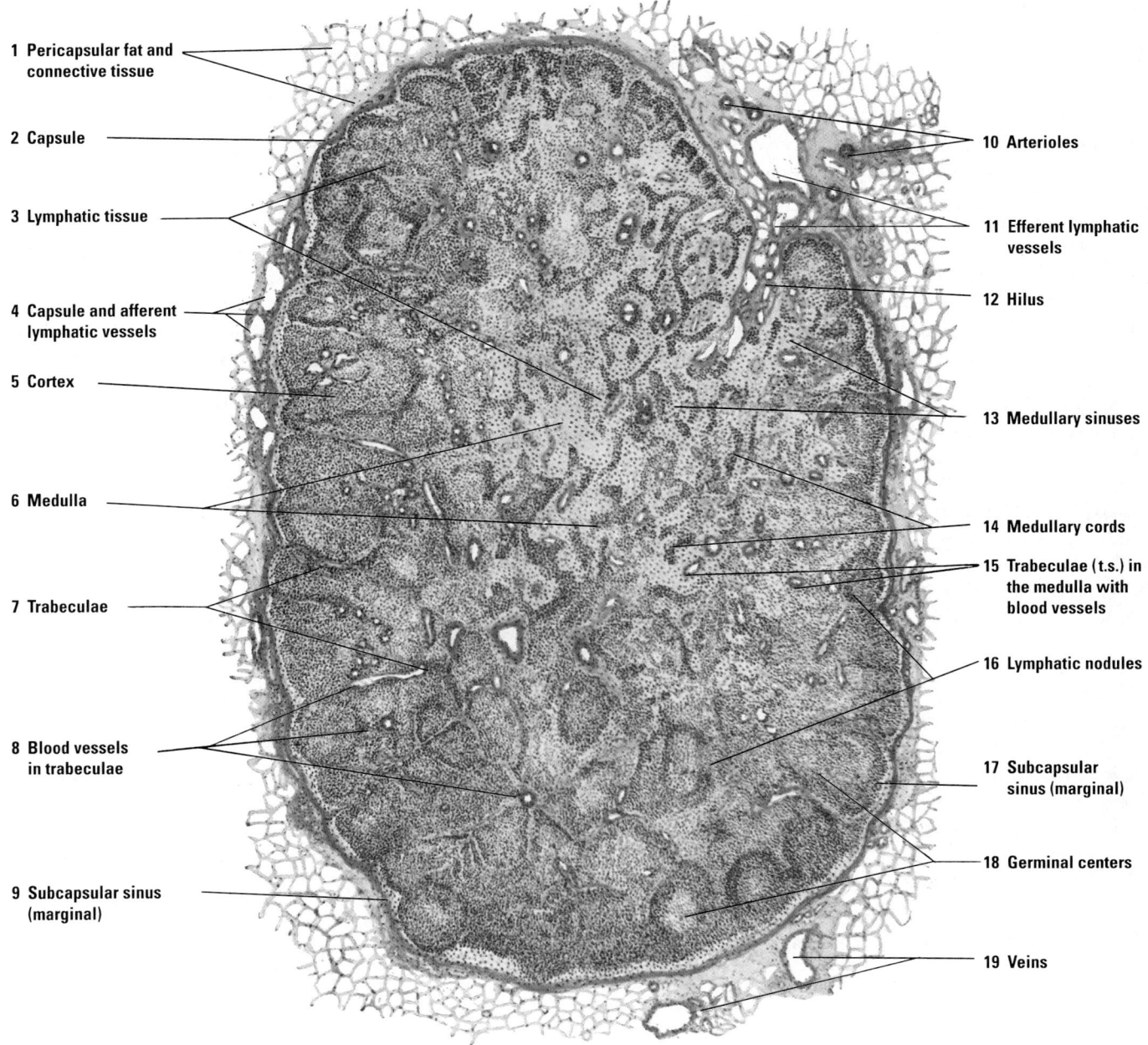

Fig. 8-1   Lymph Node (panoramic view). Stain: hematoxylin-eosin. Low magnification.

Figure 8-2   Lymph Node (sectional view)

A small section of a cortical region of the lymph node is illustrated at a higher magnification.

The lymph node **capsule (5)** is surrounded by loose **connective tissue (1)** containing **blood vessels (2, 3, 4)** and afferent **lymphatic vessels (13)**; the latter are lined with endothelium and contain **valves (14)**. Arising from the inner surface of the capsule (5), connective tissue **trabeculae (15)** extend through the cortex and medulla. Associated with these connective tissue partitions are **trabecular blood vessels (18)**.

The **cortex (7)** of the lymph node is separated from the connective tissue capsule (5) by the **subcapsular (marginal) sinus (6)**. The cortex consists of lymphatic nodules situated adjacent to each other but incompletely separated by inter-nodular trabeculae (15) and **trabecular (cortical) sinuses (16)**. In this figure, one complete **lymphatic nodule** (7, lower leader; 8; 17, lower leader) and portions of two other nodules (7, upper leader; 17, upper leader) are illustrated. The deeper portion of the cortex, the **paracortical region (19)**, is the thymus-dependent zone and is occupied by T lymphocytes. This is a transition area from the nodules to the medullary cords. The medulla consists of anastomosing cords of lymphatic tissue, the **medullary cords (12, 20)**, interspersed with **medullary sinuses (11, 21)**, which drain into the efferent lymphatic vessels located at the hilus.

Reticular connective tissue forms the stroma of the cortical nodules, the medullary cords, and all sinuses. Relatively few lymphocytes are seen in the sinuses (6, 11, 16, 21); thus, it is possible to distinguish the reticular framework (21) of the node. In the lymphatic nodules (7) and the medullary cords (12, 20) lymphocytes are so abundant that the reticulum is obscured unless it is specially stained, as shown in Figure 8-3. Most of the lymphocytes are small and contain large, deep-staining nuclei with condensed chromatin. The cells exhibit either a small amount of cytoplasm or none at all.

Lymphatic nodules often exhibit **germinal centers (8)**, which stain less intensely than the surrounding peripheral portion of the nodule (7). In the germinal center (8), the cells are more loosely aggregated and the developing lymphocytes have larger, lighter nuclei with more cytoplasm than the small lymphocytes (see Fig. 8-4).

Figure 8-3   Lymph Node: Reticular Fibers of the Stroma

A section of a lymph node has been stained with the Bielschowsky-Foot silver method to illustrate the intricate arrangement of the **reticular fibers (4, 7)**.

The various zones illustrated in Figure 8-2 are readily recognizable: the **cortex (1)**, **subcapsular (marginal) sinus (2)**, **medullary cords (5)**, and **medullary sinuses (6)**. All of these regions contain a stroma of delicate reticular fibers (4, 7), which form the fine meshwork of the lymph node.

■ Functional Correlations–Lymph Nodes

The **lymph nodes** are an important part of the **defense mechanism**. They are distributed throughout the body along the paths of **lymphatic vessels**. The lymph nodes are most prominent in the **inguinal** and **axillary regions**. Their major functions are **lymph filtration** and **phagocytosis** of bacteria or foreign substances from the lymph. Trapped within the reticular fiber network of each node are fixed or free **macrophages**. Thus, as lymph is filtered, the nodes participate in localizing and preventing the spread of infection into the general circulation.

Lymph nodes also produce, store, and recirculate **B lymphocytes** and **T lymphocytes**. B lymphocytes congregate in the **lymphoid nodules** of the lymph node while the T lymphocytes concentrate below the nodules in the deep **cortical** or **paracortical regions**. The lymph nodes are also the sites of **antigenic recognition** and **antigenic activation** of B lymphocytes, which give rise to **plasma cells**. Plasma cells then synthesize and secrete specific **antibodies** against the particular antigens into the **blood** and **lymph**.

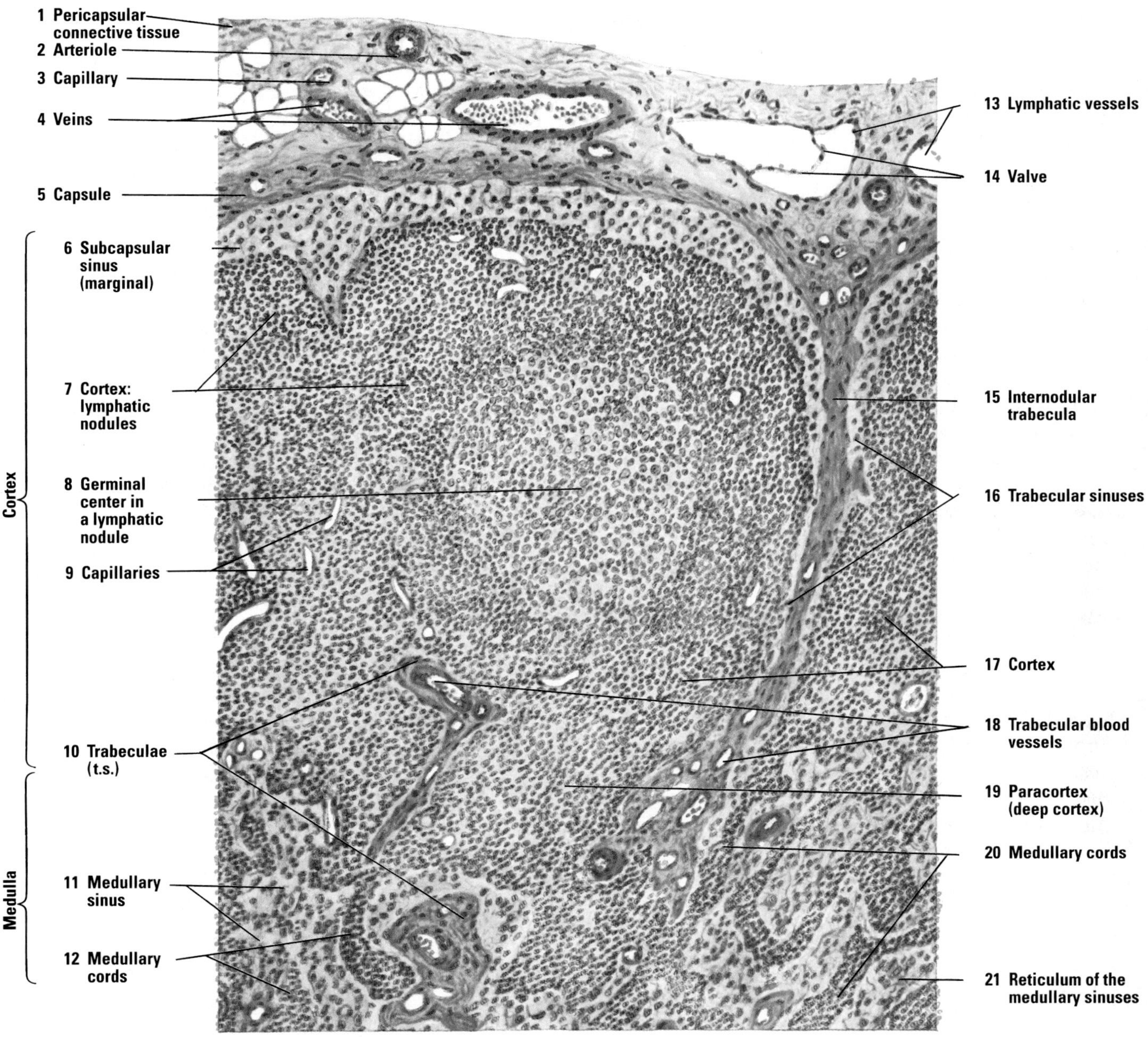

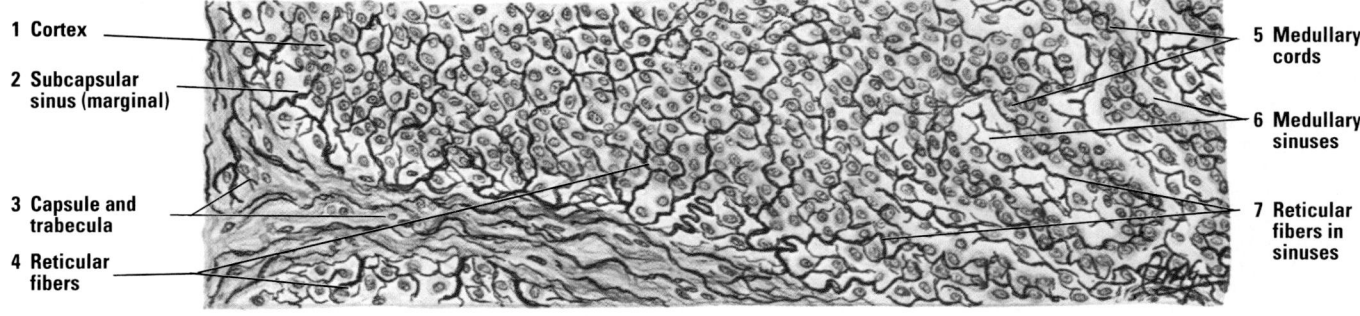

1 Pericapsular connective tissue
2 Arteriole
3 Capillary
4 Veins
5 Capsule

Cortex

6 Subcapsular sinus (marginal)
7 Cortex: lymphatic nodules
8 Germinal center in a lymphatic nodule
9 Capillaries
10 Trabeculae (t.s.)

Medulla

11 Medullary sinus
12 Medullary cords

13 Lymphatic vessels
14 Valve

15 Internodular trabecula
16 Trabecular sinuses

17 Cortex

18 Trabecular blood vessels
19 Paracortex (deep cortex)
20 Medullary cords
21 Reticulum of the medullary sinuses

Fig. 8-2 Lymph Node (sectional view). Stain: hematoxylin-eosin. Medium magnification.

1 Cortex
2 Subcapsular sinus (marginal)
3 Capsule and trabecula
4 Reticular fibers

5 Medullary cords
6 Medullary sinuses
7 Reticular fibers in sinuses

Fig. 8-3 Lymph Node: Reticular Fibers of the Stroma. Stain: Bielschowsky-Foot silver method. Medium magnification.

Figure 8-4   Lymph Node: Proliferation of Lymphocytes

This figure illustrates, at a higher magnification than that in Figure 8-2, a portion of the lymph node **capsule (1)**, the **subcapsular (marginal) sinus (2)**, a lymphatic nodule with its **peripheral zone (5)**, and a **germinal center (6)** containing developing lymphocytes.

The reticular connective tissue of the node is seen in the subcapsular sinus (2), where **reticular cells (9)** and their processes and associated delicate fibers are distinguishable. **Small lymphocytes (11, upper leader)** and free **macrophages (3, 10)** are also visible in the subcapsular sinus. **Endothelial cells (limiting cells) (4)** form an incomplete cover over the surface of the node. Occasional **reticular cells (15)** and free macrophages (3, 7, 10) may be seen in different regions of the node.

The peripheral zone (5) of the lymphatic nodule is dense because of the accumulations of **small lymphocytes (11, lower leader),** which are characterized by dark-staining nuclei, condensed chromatin, and little or no cytoplasm.

The **germinal center (6)** contains a majority of cells that are **medium-sized lymphocytes (12).** These are characterized by larger, lighter nuclei and more cytoplasm than seen in the small lymphocytes; the nuclei exhibit variations in size and density of chromatin. The largest lymphocytes, with less condensed chromatin, are derived from **lymphoblasts (14).** With successive **mitosis (8),** chromatin condenses and cell size decreases, resulting in the formation of small lymphocytes.

The lymphoblasts (14) are visible in small numbers in the germinal center (6). These are large, round cells with a broad band of cytoplasm and a large vesicular nucleus with one or more nucleoli. **Mitotic divisions of lymphoblasts (13)** produce other lymphoblasts and medium-sized lymphocytes.

Figure 8-5   Palatine Tonsil

The surface of the palatine tonsil is covered with **stratified squamous epithelium (1),** which also lines the deep invaginations or **tonsillar crypts (3, 10).** In the underlying connective tissue are numerous **lymphatic nodules (2)** distributed along the crypts. The lymphatic nodules are embedded in reticular connective tissue stroma and diffuse lymphatic tissue. The nodules frequently merge with each other **(8)** and usually exhibit a **germinal center (7).**

The fibroelastic connective tissue underlies the tonsil and forms its **capsule (11).** The **septa (trabeculae) (5, 9)** arise from the capsule (11) and pass upward as a core of connective tissue between the lymphatic nodules that form the walls of the crypts. **Skeletal muscle fibers (6, 12)** form an underlying layer of the tonsil.

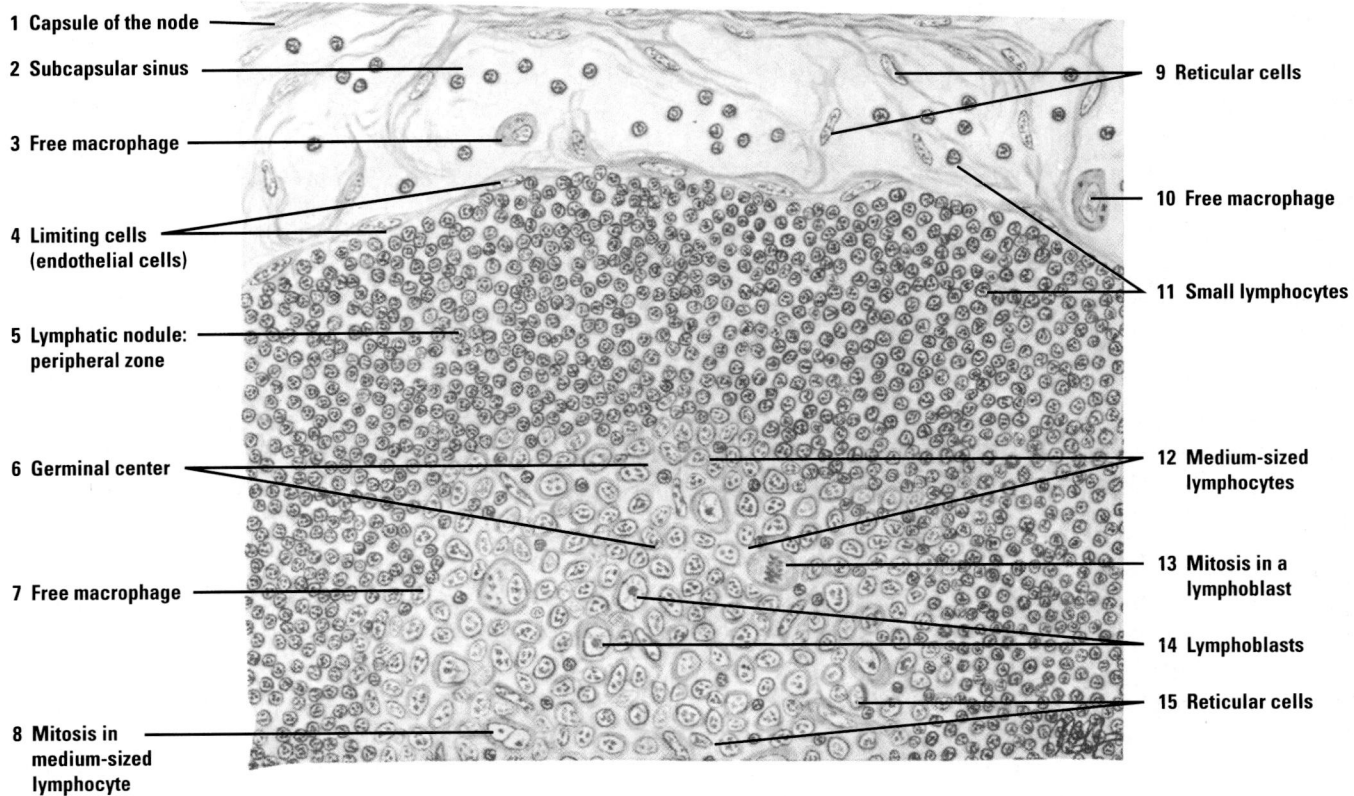

1 Capsule of the node

2 Subcapsular sinus

3 Free macrophage

4 Limiting cells (endothelial cells)

5 Lymphatic nodule: peripheral zone

6 Germinal center

7 Free macrophage

8 Mitosis in medium-sized lymphocyte

9 Reticular cells

10 Free macrophage

11 Small lymphocytes

12 Medium-sized lymphocytes

13 Mitosis in a lymphoblast

14 Lymphoblasts

15 Reticular cells

Fig. 8-4 Lymph Node: Proliferation of Lymphocytes. Stain: hematoxylin-eosin. High magnification.

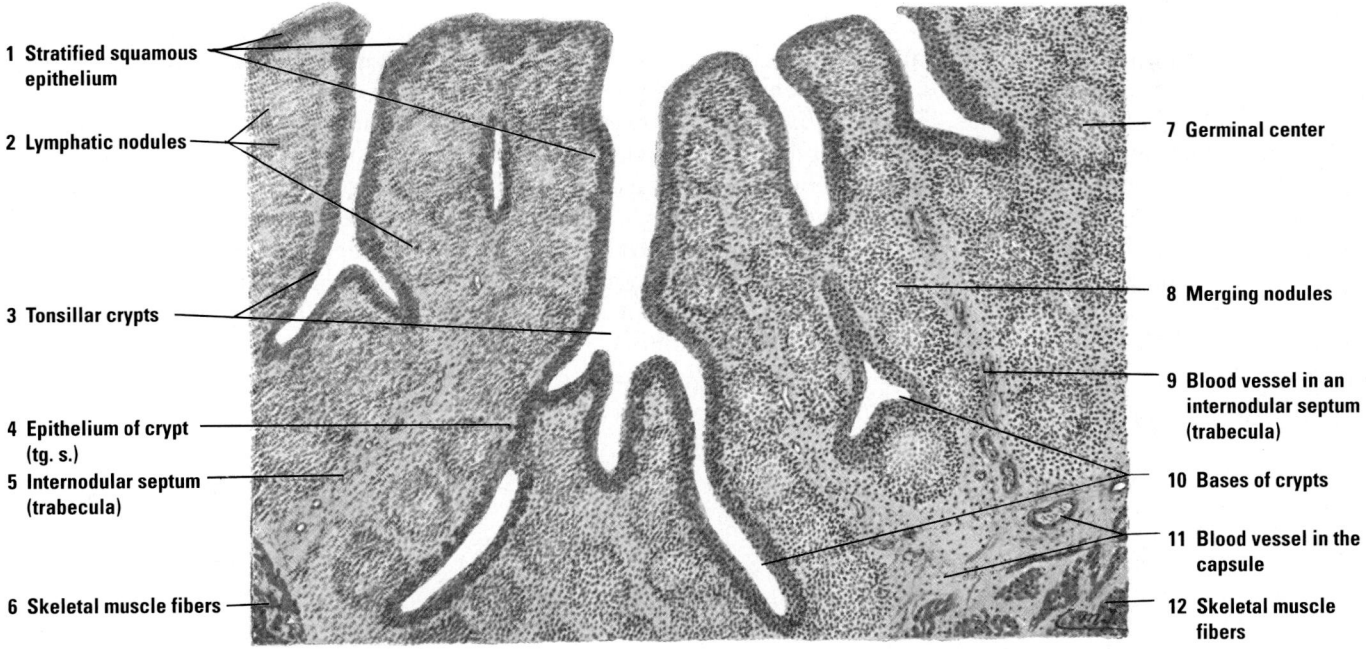

1 Stratified squamous epithelium

2 Lymphatic nodules

3 Tonsillar crypts

4 Epithelium of crypt (tg. s.)

5 Internodular septum (trabecula)

6 Skeletal muscle fibers

7 Germinal center

8 Merging nodules

9 Blood vessel in an internodular septum (trabecula)

10 Bases of crypts

11 Blood vessel in the capsule

12 Skeletal muscle fibers

Fig. 8-5 Palatine Tonsil. Stain: hematoxylin-eosin. Low magnification.

Figure 8-6   Thymus Gland (panoramic view)

The thymus gland is a lobulated lymphoid organ. It is enclosed by a connective tissue **capsule (1)** from which arise numerous **trabeculae (2, 10).** The trabeculae extend into and subdivide the thymus gland into incomplete **lobules (8).** Each lobule consists of a dark-staining outer **cortex (3, 13)** and a light-staining inner **medulla (4, 12).** Because the lobules are incomplete, the medulla exhibits continuity between neighboring lobules (4, 12). Numerous **blood vessels (5, 14)** pass into the thymus gland by way of the connective tissue of the capsule (1) and the trabeculae (2, 10).

The cortex (3, 13) of each lobule contains numerous densely packed lymphocytes without forming lymphatic nodules. In contrast, the medulla (4, 12) contains fewer lymphocytes but more epithelial reticular cells. The medulla also contains numerous **thymic (Hassall's) corpuscles (6, 9),** which are highly characteristic features of the thymus gland.

The histology of the thymus gland varies with the age of the individual. The gland attains its greatest development shortly after birth; however, by puberty, it begins to involute. Lymphocyte production declines, and the thymic (Hassall's) corpuscles (6, 9) become larger. In addition, the parenchyma of the gland is gradually replaced by loose **connective tissue (10)** and **adipose cells (7, 11).** The thymus gland depicted in this illustration exhibits involution changes associated with age.

Figure 8-7   Thymus Gland (sectional view)

A small section of the cortex and medulla of a thymus gland lobule is illustrated at a higher magnification. The thymic lymphocytes in the **cortex (1, 5)** exhibit dense aggregations. In the **medulla (3),** there are fewer lymphocytes but more **epithelial reticular cells (7, 10).**

The **thymic (Hassall's) corpuscles (8)** are oval structures consisting of round or spherical aggregations of flattened epithelial cells. The corpuscles also exhibit calcification or **degeneration centers (9),** which stain as highly eosinophilic. The functional significance of these corpuscles is unknown.

Blood vessels (6) and **adipose cells (4)** are seen in both the lobules and the connective tissue **trabecula (2).**

■ Functional Correlations–Thymus Gland

The **thymus gland** is also an important component of the **immune system.** It performs an important role early in the childhood in developing the **immune system** of the organism. Undifferentiated **lymphocytes** are carried by blood to the thymus gland. Here, the lymphocytes **proliferate** and differentiate into **immunocompetent T lymphocytes.** The T lymphocytes then leave the thymus gland via the blood and populate **lymph nodes, spleen,** and other thymus-dependent **lymphatic tissues.** Found also in the thymus gland are the **epithelial reticular** cells, which secrete **hormones** necessary for proliferation, differentiation, maturation of T lymphocytes, and expression of their surface markers. These hormones are **thymulin, thymopoietin, thymosin,** and **thymic humoral factor.**

Under experimental conditions, if the thymus gland is removed in a newborn, the lymphoid organs will not receive the immunocompetent T lymphocytes, and the organism does not develop immunological competence to fight pathogens. Death may occur early in life from the complications of an infection.

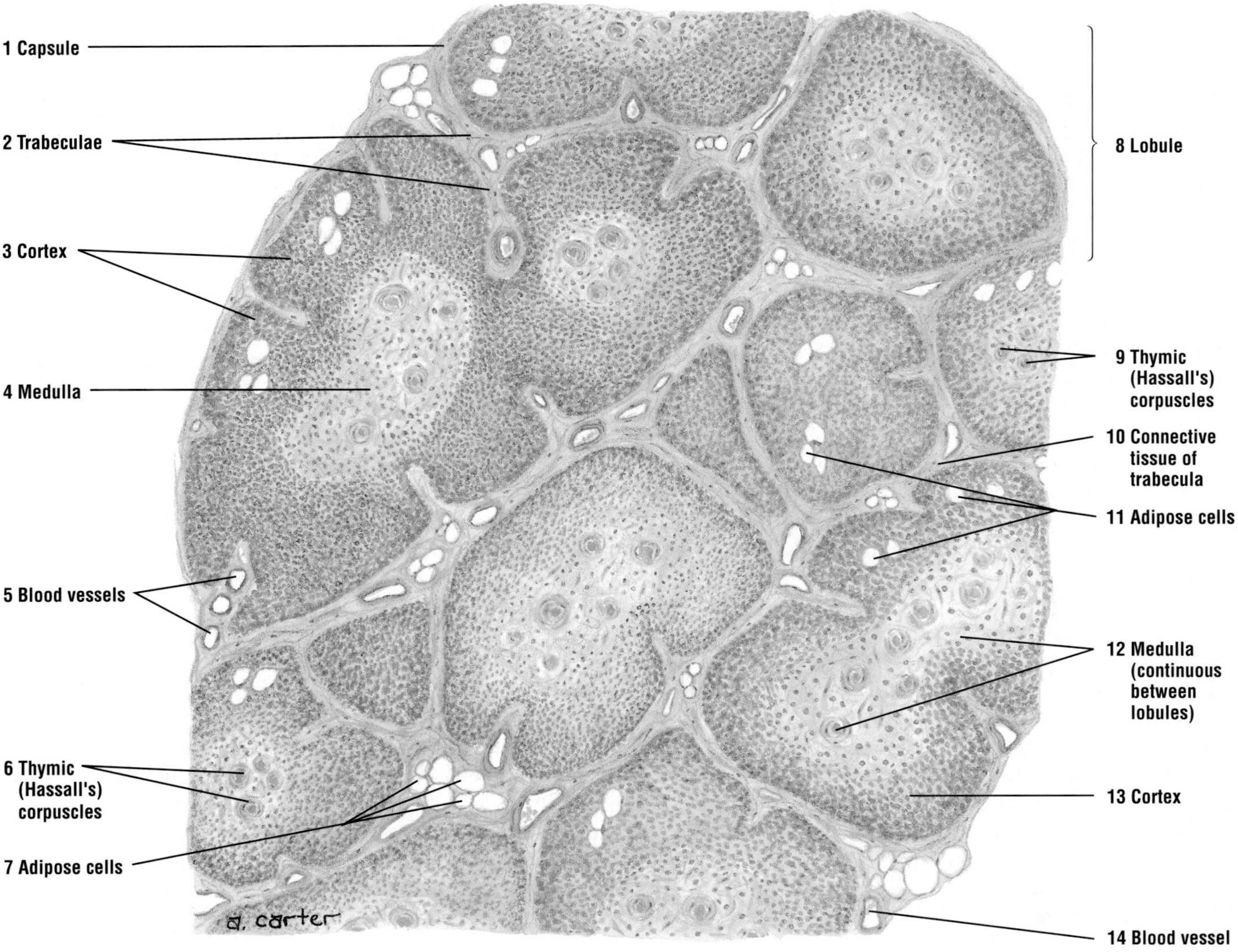

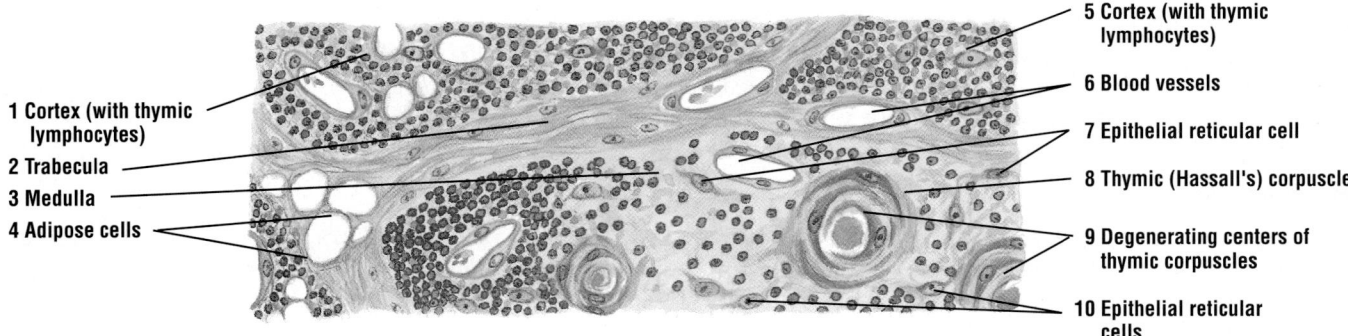

1 Capsule

2 Trabeculae

3 Cortex

4 Medulla

5 Blood vessels

6 Thymic (Hassall's) corpuscles

7 Adipose cells

d. carter

8 Lobule

9 Thymic (Hassall's) corpuscles

10 Connective tissue of trabecula

11 Adipose cells

12 Medulla (continuous between lobules)

13 Cortex

14 Blood vessel

Fig. 8-6 Thymus Gland (panoramic view). Stain: hematoxylin-eosin. Low magnification.

1 Cortex (with thymic lymphocytes)

2 Trabecula

3 Medulla

4 Adipose cells

5 Cortex (with thymic lymphocytes)

6 Blood vessels

7 Epithelial reticular cell

8 Thymic (Hassall's) corpuscle

9 Degenerating centers of thymic corpuscles

10 Epithelial reticular cells

Fig. 8-7 Thymus Gland (sectional view). Stain: hematoxylin-eosin. High magnification.

Figure 8-8   Spleen (panoramic view)

The spleen is enclosed by a dense connective tissue **capsule (1),** from which connective tissue **trabeculae (3)** extend deep into the spleen's interior. The main trabeculae enter the spleen at the hilus and branch throughout the organ. Located in the trabeculae (3) are the **trabecular arteries (5b)** and **trabecular veins (5a).** Trabeculae that are cut in transverse section (11) appear round or nodular.

The spleen is characterized by the presence of numerous aggregations of **lymphatic nodules (4, 6);** these nodules constitute the **white pulp** of the organ. The lymphatic nodules contain **germinal centers (8, 9);** these progressively decrease in number as the individual ages. Passing through each lymphatic nodule (4, 6) is a **central artery (2, 7, 10);** however, these arteries are usually displaced to one side, thus losing the central position. Central arteries are branches of trabecular arteries (5b) that become sheathed with lymphatic tissue as they leave the trabeculae. This sheath also forms the lymphatic nodules (4, 6), which then constitute the spleen's white pulp.

Surrounding the lymphatic nodules (4, 6) and intermeshed with the trabeculae (3) is a diffuse cellular meshwork that makes up the bulk of the organ and collectively forms the **red** or **splenic pulp (12, 13).** In fresh preparations, red pulp exhibits a red color because of its vascular tissue. The red pulp also contains **pulp arteries (14), venous sinuses (13)** and **splenic cords (Billroth's) (12);** these appear as diffuse strands of lymphatic tissue between the venous sinuses (13). The splenic cords (12) form a spongy meshwork of reticular connective tissue, which is usually obscured by the density of other tissue.

The spleen does not exhibit a cortex and a medulla, as seen in lymph nodes; however, lymphatic nodules (4, 6) are found throughout the spleen. In addition, the spleen contains venous sinuses, in contrast to lymphatic sinuses found in the lymph nodes. However, the spleen does not exhibit subcapsular or trabecular sinuses. The capsule (1) and trabeculae (3) in the spleen are thicker than those around the lymph nodes and contain some smooth muscle cells.

Figure 8-9   Spleen: Red and White Pulp

A higher magnification of a section of the spleen illustrates a small area of red and white pulp along with such associated structures as the connective tissue trabeculae, various blood vessels, venous sinuses, and the splenic cords.

The large **lymphatic nodule (3)** represents the white pulp of the spleen. Each nodule normally exhibits a peripheral zone, the periarterial lymphatic sheath, densely packed small lymphocytes, a **germinal center (5),** which may not always be present, and an eccentric **central artery (4).** The cells found in the periarterial lymphatic sheath are mainly T lymphocytes. In the more lightly stained germinal center (5) are found the B lymphocytes, mainly medium-sized lymphocytes, some small lymphocytes, and lymphoblasts.

The red pulp contains the **splenic cords (1, 8)** (Billroth's) and **venous sinuses (2, 9)** that course between the cords. The splenic cords (1, 8) are thin aggregations of lymphatic tissue containing small lymphocytes, associated cells, and various blood cells. Venous sinuses (2, 9) are dilated vessels lined with modified endothelium; their elongated cells appear cuboidal in transverse sections.

Also present in the red pulp are **pulp arteries (10);** these are the branches of the central artery (4) as it leaves the lymphatic nodule (3). Capillaries and pulp veins (venules) are also present.

Trabeculae containing **trabecular artery (6)** and **trabecular vein (7)** are also clearly illustrated. These vessels have the endothelial tunica intima and the muscular tunica media but no apparent connective tissue adventitia; connective tissue of the trabeculae surrounds the tunica media.

■ Functional Correlations–Spleen

The **spleen** is the largest lymphoid organ. One of its main functions is to **filter blood.** Because of its dense **reticular network,** the spleen functions as an effective filter for antigens, microorganisms, platelets, and aged or abnormal red blood cells. The trapped material in the reticular meshwork is then removed from the blood by numerous resident **macrophages** and **phagocytic reticular cells.**

The spleen also recycles **iron.** Macrophages breakdown **hemoglobin** of worn-out red blood cells. Iron is then returned to the **bone marrow,** where it is reused during the synthesis of new hemoglobin by the developing red blood cells. The **heme** from the hemoglobin is degraded and excreted in **bile** by the liver cells.

In fetal life, the spleen is a **hemopoietic organ,** producing **granulocytes** and **erythrocytes.** This hemopoietic capability, however, ceases after birth. The spleen also serves as an important **reservoir** for blood. Because it has a sponge-like structure, much blood can be stored in its interior. When needed, the stored blood is returned from the spleen to the general circulation.

The spleen also has a major role in producing **antibodies** to fight **antigens** in the blood. This is due to the presence in the spleen of numerous **B lymphocytes** and **T lymphocytes,** as well as **macrophages.** Antigens stimulate the proliferation of B lymphocytes, which give rise to plasma cells. These, in turn, produce large quantities of antibodies. Although the spleen performs various important functions in the body, it is not essential to life.

1 Capsule

2 Central artery

3 Trabeculae

4 Lymphatic nodule
(white pulp)

9 Germinal center

10 Central artery

5 Trabecular
a. vein
b. artery

11 Trabeculae

12 Splenic cords
(in red pulp)

13 Venous sinuses
(in red pulp)

6 Lymphatic nodule
(white pulp)

7 Central artery

8 Germinal center

14 Pulp arteries

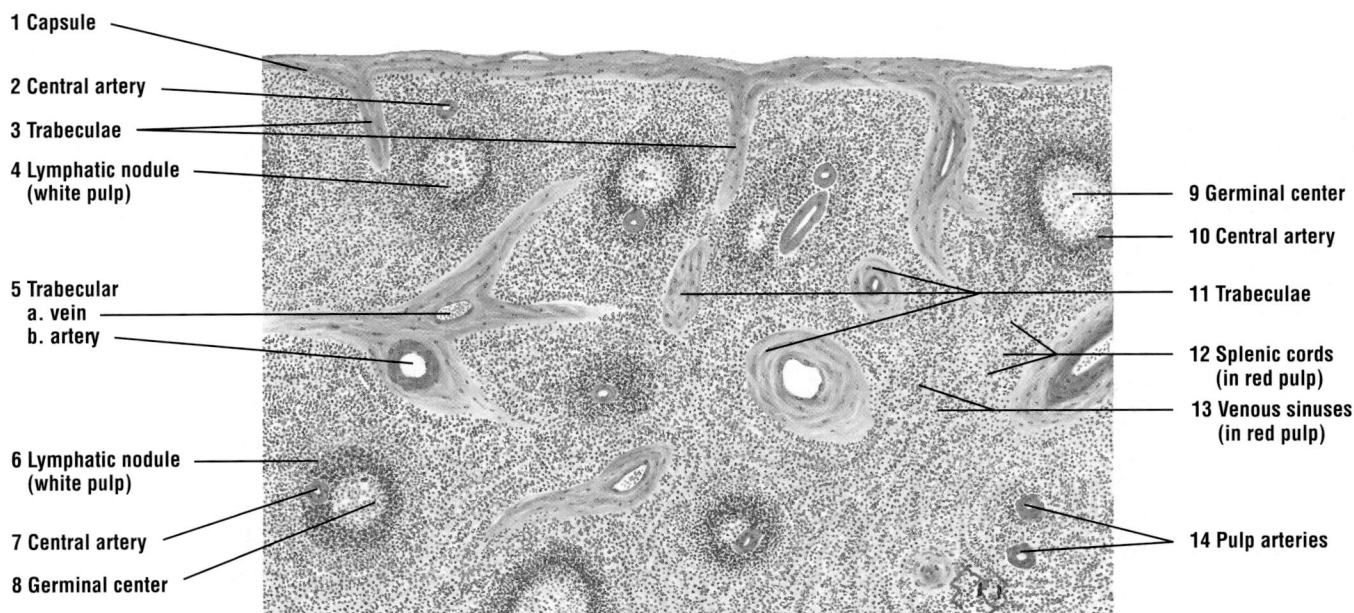

Fig. 8-8   Spleen (panoramic view). Stain: hematoxylin-eosin. Low magnification.

1 Splenic cords

2 Venous sinuses

3 Lymphatic nodule

4 Central artery

5 Germinal center

6 Trabecular artery

7 Trabecular vein

8 Splenic cords

9 Venous sinuses

10 Pulp arteries

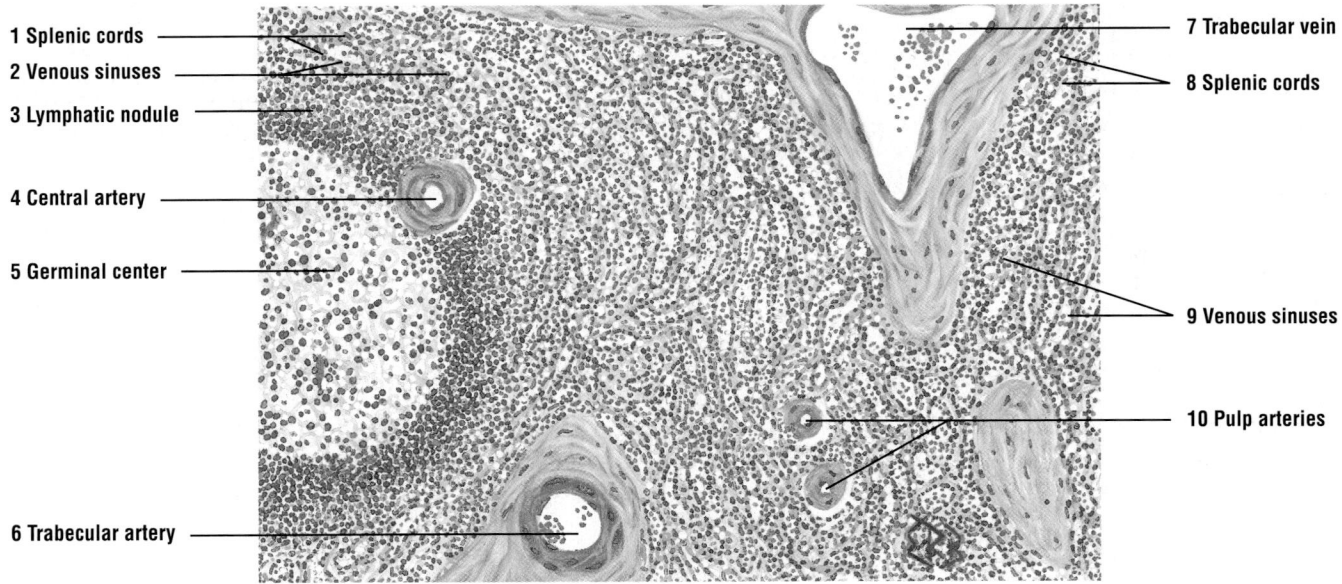

Fig. 8-9   Spleen: Red and White Pulp. Stain: hematoxylin-eosin. Medium magnification.

Figure 8-10   Cortex and Medulla of a Lymph Node

This low-power photomicrograph illustrates a section of the lymph node. A loose connective tissue **capsule (4)** with blood vessels and **adipose cells (7)** covers the lymph node. Inferior to the capsule (4) is the **subcapsular (marginal) sinus** (5), which overlies the darker staining and peripheral lymph node **cortex (3)**. In the cortex (3) are found numerous lymphatic **nodules (1, 6),** some of which contain a lighter staining **germinal center (2)**.

The central region of the lymph node is the lighter-staining **medulla (9).** Here are found the light-staining **medullary sinuses (11),** and the dark-staining **medullary cords (12).** The medullary sinuses (11) drain the lymph and converge toward the hilum of the node. In the hilum are found numerous blood **arteries (8)** and veins, and **efferent lymphatic vessels** with **valves (10)** that drain lymph from the hilum of the lymph node.

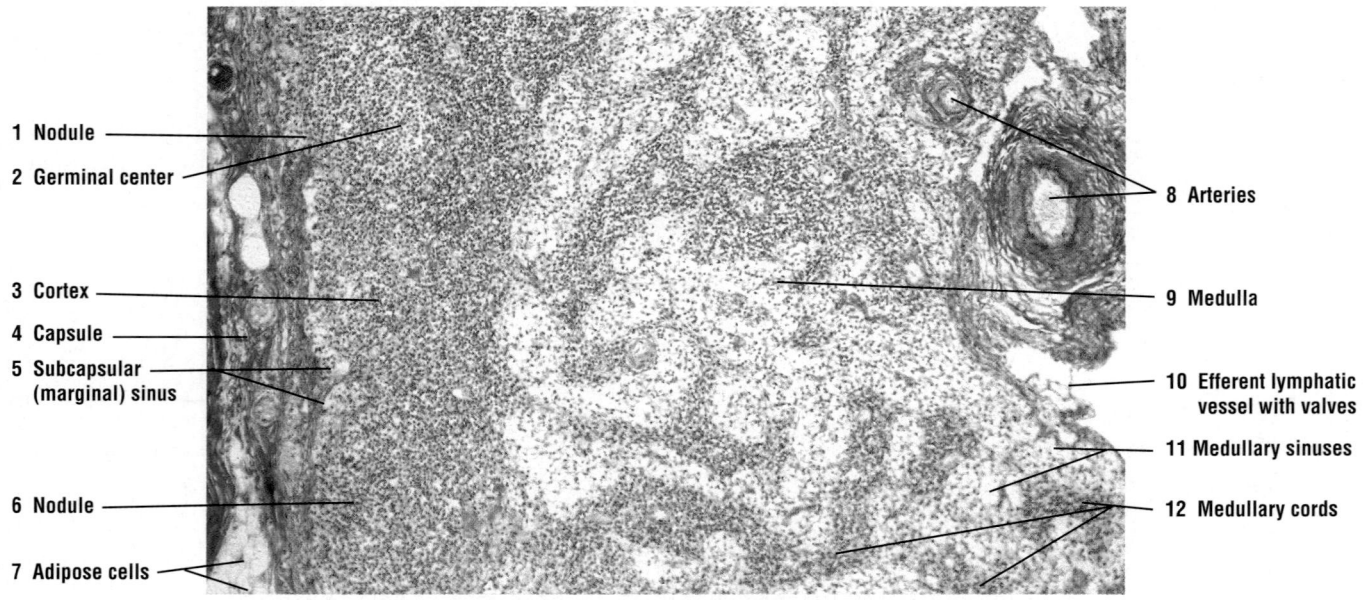

1 Nodule
2 Germinal center
3 Cortex
4 Capsule
5 Subcapsular (marginal) sinus
6 Nodule
7 Adipose cells
8 Arteries
9 Medulla
10 Efferent lymphatic vessel with valves
11 Medullary sinuses
12 Medullary cords

Fig. 8-10   Cortex and Medulla of a Lymph Node. Stain: Mallory-azan. 25×

Figure 8-11   Cortex and Medulla of a Thymus Gland

A low-magnification photomicrograph shows a portion of the lobule of the thymus gland. A **connective tissue trabecula (1)** subdivides the gland into incomplete lobules. The lobules consist of the darker staining **cortex (2)** and the lighter-staining **medulla (3).** A characteristic **thymic (Hassall's) corpuscle (4)** is seen in the medulla of one of the lobules.

Figure 8-12   Red and White Pulp of the Spleen

A low-magnification photomicrograph illustrates a section of the spleen. A dense, irregular **connective tissue capsule (1)** covers the spleen. From the capsule (1), **connective tissue trabeculae (3)** with blood vessels extend into the interior of the organ. The spleen is composed of white pulp and red pulp. **White pulp (2)** consists of lymphocytes and aggregations of **lymphatic nodules (2a).** Within the lymphatic nodule (2a) are found the **germinal center (2b)** and a **central artery (2c)** that has an off-center location in the nodule (2a). Surrounding the white pulp lymphatic nodules (2) is the **red pulp (4)**; it is primarily composed of **venous sinuses (4a)** and **splenic cords (4b).**

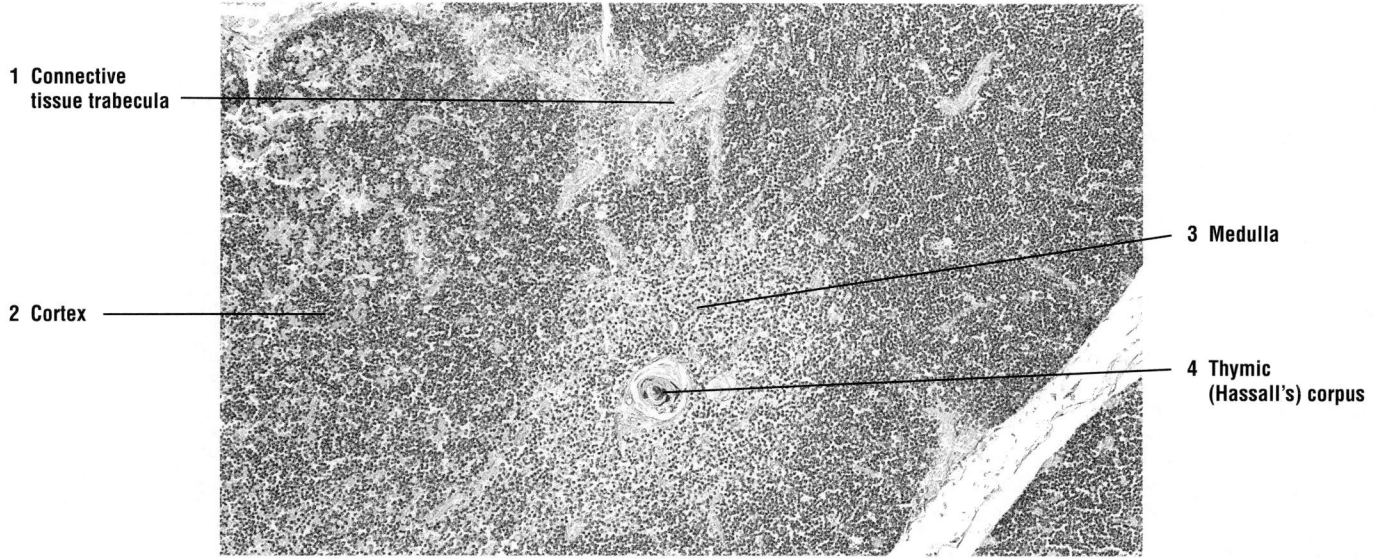

1 Connective tissue trabecula

2 Cortex

3 Medulla

4 Thymic (Hassall's) corpus

Fig. 8-11 Cortex and Medulla of a Thymus Gland. Stain: hematoxylin-eosin. 30×

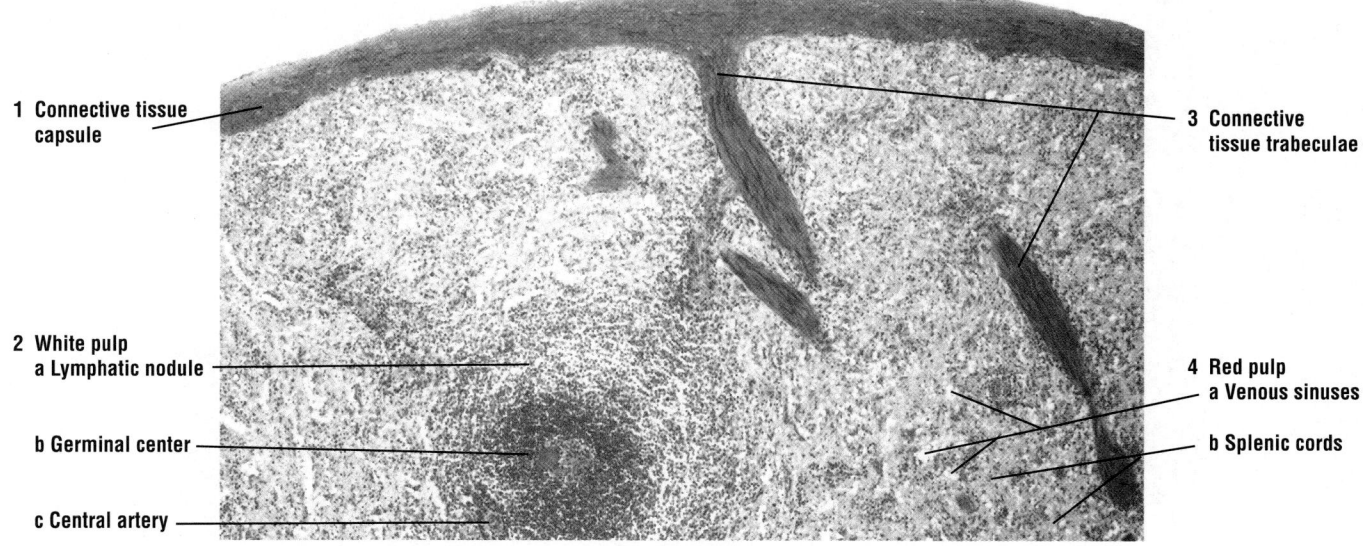

1 Connective tissue capsule

2 White pulp
a Lymphatic nodule

b Germinal center

c Central artery

3 Connective tissue trabeculae

4 Red pulp
a Venous sinuses

b Splenic cords

Fig. 8-12 Red and White Pulp of the Spleen. Mallory-azan. 21×

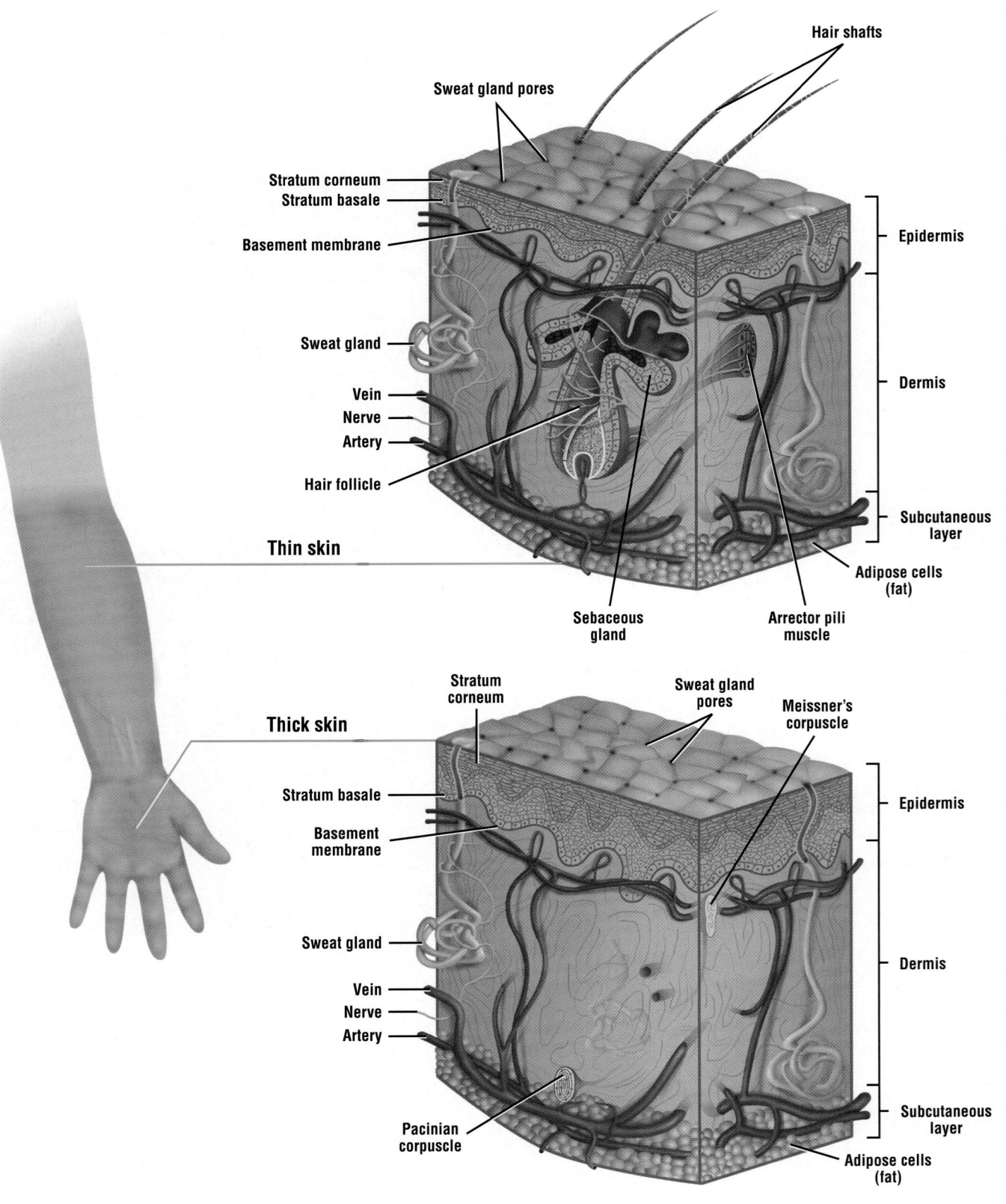

Hair shafts

Sweat gland pores

Stratum corneum

Stratum basale

Basement membrane

Epidermis

Sweat gland

Dermis

Vein

Nerve

Artery

Hair follicle

Thin skin

Subcutaneous layer

Adipose cells (fat)

Sebaceous gland

Arrector pili muscle

Stratum corneum

Sweat gland pores

Meissner's corpuscle

Thick skin

Stratum basale

Basement membrane

Epidermis

Sweat gland

Dermis

Vein

Nerve

Artery

Pacinian corpuscle

Subcutaneous layer

Adipose cells (fat)

Integument

Skin and its derivatives or appendages form the **integumentary system.** In humans, skin derivatives include the nails, hair, and several types of sweat and sebaceous glands. Skin, or integument, consists of two distinct regions, the epidermis and dermis. The **epidermis** is the superficial, nonvascular layer that contains **keratinized, stratified squamous epithelium.** This epithelium consists of numerous cell layers and different cell types. The outermost cell layer in the epidermis consists of stratified keratinized dead cells. The **dermis** is situated directly inferior to the epidermis. This skin layer is deeper, thicker, and vascular. The superficial layer of the dermis interdigitates with the epidermis and forms indentations called **dermal papillae.** This is the **papillary layer** of the dermis, and it contains loose, irregular connective tissue. The deeper layer of the dermis with dense connective tissue is the **reticular layer (Figs 9-1, 9-2, 9-4).** Dermis blends inferiorly with the **hypodermis,** or **subcutaneous layer,** which consists of superficial fascia and adipose tissue. The connective tissue of the dermis is highly vascular and contains numerous blood vessels and nerves. Such fine sensory receptors as **Meissner's corpuscles** are located closer to the surface of the skin in the dermal papillae, but the **Pacinian corpuscles** are found deeper in the connective tissue of the dermis **(Figs. 9-2, 9-4, 9-9).**

The skin's histology is basically similar in different regions of the body; however, the thickness of the epidermis varies. **Palms** and **soles** are constantly exposed to increased wear, tear, and abrasion. As a result, the epidermis in these regions of the body is thick, especially the outermost stratified keratinized layer **(Figs. 9-2, 9-9, 9-10).** These regions of the body have the **thick skin.** The thick skin contains numerous sweat glands but lacks hair follicles, sebaceous glands, or the smooth muscle fibers called arrector pilli muscles. The remainder of the body surfaces are covered by **thin skin.** In these regions, the epidermis is thinner, and its cellular composition simpler than in the thick skin. Associated with the thin skin are **hair follicles, sebaceous glands,** and **sweat glands.** Attached to the connective tissue sheath of the hair follicle and the papillary layer of the dermis are the **arrector pili muscles (Figs. 9-1, 9-4, 9-11).**

Figure 9-1   Thin Skin

Skin is composed of two principal layers: **epidermis (1)** and **dermis (2, 3)**. The epidermis (1) is the most superficial and cellular layer. The dermis (2, 3) is located directly below the epidermis (1) and consists of **connective tissue (2, 3)** components. This illustration depicts a section of skin from the general body surface, where wear and tear is minimal. In this type of skin, the epidermis (1) consists of stratified squamous epithelium and a thin layer of keratinized cells. This type of skin is thin and is in contrast to thick skin found on the palms and soles, which are covered with a thick layer of keratinized cells.

The single layer of low columnar cells at the base of the epidermis (1) is the **stratum basale,** or **germinativum (7).** Located directly above this layer are a few rows of polygonal-shaped cells that form the **stratum spinosum (6).** Above these cells are usually found one or two layers of granular cells; these blend with the elongated, cornified cells of the **stratum corneum (5).**

The narrow zone of dense, irregular connective tissue below the epidermis (1) is the **papillary layer (2)** of the dermis. This papillary layer (2) indents into the base of the epidermis and forms the **dermal papillae (8).** The deeper **reticular layer (3)** of the dermis consists of dense, irregular connective tissue; this layer comprises the bulk of the dermis. A small portion of **hypodermis (4),** the superficial region of the underlying subcutaneous tissue, is also illustrated.

Most of the skin appendages are located in the dermis. Illustrated in this figure are parts of hair follicles and a sweat gland, which is illustrated in greater detail on the next page in Figure 9-3. The lower portion of the hair follicle is in longitudinal section and exhibits the **hair bulb** and **papilla (13)** at its base; these structures are located deep in the dermis. The section of the upper portion of another **hair follicle (9)** exhibits the smooth muscle, **arrector pili muscle (10),** and a **sebaceous gland (11).** An **oblique section** of the **hair follicle (14)** is illustrated deep in the subcutaneous tissue.

The **dermis (2, 3)** contains numerous examples of the cross sections of a coiled portion of the **sweat gland (12).** The sections with light-staining epithelium are from the **secretory (12a)** portion of the gland, whereas the darker-staining sections are from the **duct (12b)** portion.

Figure 9-2   Thick Skin, Palm: Superficial Layers

A section of palm skin is illustrated here at higher magnification. The epidermis is much thicker and more complex than in the thin skin illustrated in Figure 9-1 and exhibits five distinct cell layers. The outermost layer, the **stratum corneum (1),** is a wide layer of flattened, dead cells that are constantly desquamated or shed **(10)** from the surface. Beneath the stratum corneum is a narrow, lightly stained **stratum lucidum (2).** At higher magnification, outlines of flattened cells and eleidin droplets in this layer are occasionally seen. Located under the stratum lucidum is the **stratum granulosum (3),** whose cells contain dark-staining **keratohyalin granules (7),** better seen at a higher magnification in the insert (bottom left). Below this layer is the thick **stratum spinosum (4),** composed of several layers of polyhedral-shaped cells. The deepest cell layer is the basal layer, the **stratum basale (5),** consisting of columnar cells that rest on the basement membrane.

Cells of **stratum spinosum (4, 8)** are connected by spinous processes or **intercellular bridges (9,** in the insert), which represent the desmosomes (macula adherens). **Mitotic activity (12)** is normally seen in the deeper layers of stratum spinosum (4) and stratum basale (5).

Ducts of **sweat glands (11)** penetrate the epidermis between two dermal papillae, lose their epithelial wall, and spiral through the cell layers of the **epidermis (1–5)** to the skin surface as small channels with a thin cuticular lining.

Dermal papillae (6) are prominent in thick skin. Some of the dermal papillae contain **tactile corpuscles (13)** (Meissner's corpuscles); other papillae have capillary loops.

■ Functional Correlations–Skin Cells

There are four different cell types in the epidermis of the skin. **Keratinocytes,** the dominant epithelial cells in the epidermis, divide, grow, move up, undergo **keratinization,** and form a protective surface covering for the body. **Melanocytes,** located in the basal layer of the epidermis, synthesize the pigment **melanin,** which is then incorporated into keratinocytes. Melanin imparts a dark color to the skin and exposure of the skin to sunlight promotes increased synthesis of melanin. **Langerhans' cells** are epidermal cells that participate in the body's immune responses. These cells may be involved in foreign **antigen recognition** and may be **antigen-presenting cells.** A small number of **Merkel cells** are also found in the epidermis. These cells are closely associated with **unmyelinated axons** and are believed to function as **mechanoreceptors.**

Unless the skin section is prepared with special stains, melanocytes, Langerhans' cells, and Merkel cells are not easily seen with routine histologic preparations.

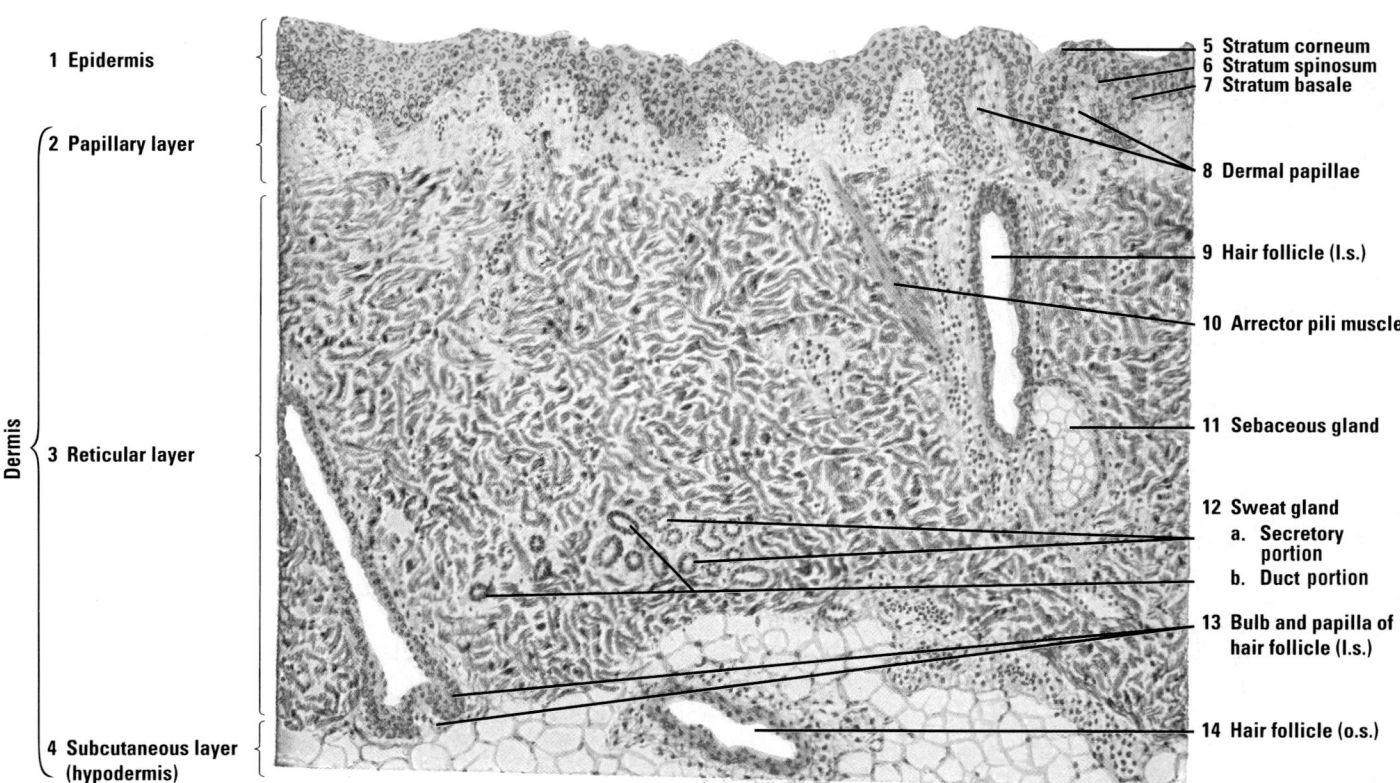

1 Epidermis

2 Papillary layer

Dermis

3 Reticular layer

4 Subcutaneous layer (hypodermis)

5 Stratum corneum
6 Stratum spinosum
7 Stratum basale

8 Dermal papillae

9 Hair follicle (l.s.)

10 Arrector pili muscle

11 Sebaceous gland

12 Sweat gland
   a. Secretory portion
   b. Duct portion

13 Bulb and papilla of hair follicle (l.s.)

14 Hair follicle (o.s.)

Fig. 9-1 Thin Skin. Stain: Cajal's trichrome. Cytoplasm: orange; nuclei: bright red; collagen fibers: deep blue. Low magnification.

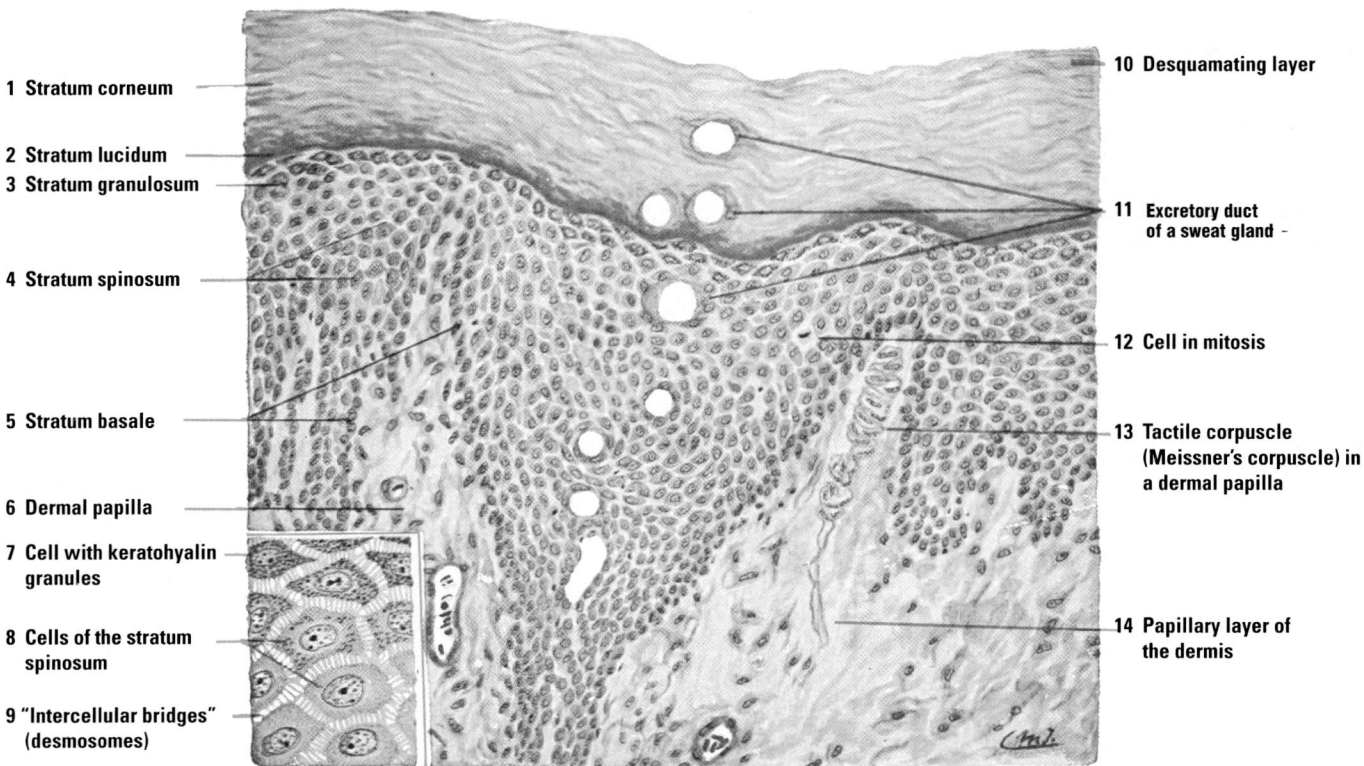

1 Stratum corneum

2 Stratum lucidum
3 Stratum granulosum

4 Stratum spinosum

5 Stratum basale

6 Dermal papilla

7 Cell with keratohyalin granules

8 Cells of the stratum spinosum

9 "Intercellular bridges" (desmosomes)

10 Desquamating layer

11 Excretory duct of a sweat gland -

12 Cell in mitosis

13 Tactile corpuscle (Meissner's corpuscle) in a dermal papilla

14 Papillary layer of the dermis

Fig. 9-2 Thick Skin, Palm: Superficial Layers. Stain: hematoxylin-eosin. Medium magnification.

Figure 9-3   Sweat Glands

The sweat gland is a simple, highly coiled tubular gland that extends deep into the dermis or the upper portion of the hypodermis. To illustrate this, the sweat gland is shown in both cross-sectional (left side) and diagrammatic views (right side).

The coiled portion of the sweat gland located deep in the dermis represents its **secretory (8)** region. The **secretory cells (3, 4)** in this region are large, columnar, and stain light eosinophilic. Surrounding the secretory cells are thin, spindle-shaped **myoepithelial cells (5);** these are located between the base of the secretory cells (3, 4) and the basement membrane (not illustrated).

Leaving the secretory region of the sweat gland is a thinner, darker-staining **excretory duct (2, 7).** The cells of excretory duct are smaller than the cells of the secretory acini. Also, the duct is smaller in diameter and is lined by two layers of deep-staining cuboidal cells. There are no myoepithelial cells around the excretory duct. As the excretory duct ascends through the dermis, it straightens out and penetrates the cell layers of the **epidermis (1, 6),** where it loses its epithelial wall. In the epidermis (1, 6), the duct follows a spiral course through the cells to the surface of the skin.

■ Functional Correlations–Skin

The skin is the outer covering of the body and comes in direct contact with the external environment. As a result, the skin performs numerous important functions.

Protection. The **keratinized stratified epithelium** of the skin epidermis protects the body surfaces from mechanical abrasion and forms a physical barrier to pathogenic microorganisms that may otherwise enter the body. Because of the presence of **glycolipid** between cells, the epidermis is also **impermeable** to water and prevents the loss of body fluids through dehydration.

Temperature Regulation. The skin plays an important role in regulating the temperature of the body. Physical exercise or a warm environment increases **sweating.** This mechanism allows for some heat loss from the body following **evaporation** of sweat from the skin surfaces. In addition to sweating, thermoregulation also occurs owing to increased **dilation** of blood vessels for maximum blood flow to the skin; this function increases the dissipation of heat from the body core to the exterior. Conversely, in cold climates, sweating does not occur, and the core body heat is conserved by **constriction** of blood vessels and decreased blood flow to the skin.

Sensory Perception. The skin is a large **sense organ** and the main source for general sensations of the body's **external environment.** Numerous encapsulated and free **sensory nerve endings** within the skin respond to stimuli for temperature (heat and cold), touch, pain, and pressure.

Excretory Organ. Through production of sweat by the **sweat glands,** water, sodium salts, and nitrogenous wastes can be excreted to the surface of the skin.

Formation of Vitamin D. When the skin is exposed to the **ultraviolet** rays from the sun, **vitamin D** is formed from precursors synthesized in the epidermis. Vitamin D is essential for **calcium absorption** from the intestinal mucosa and proper mineral metabolism.

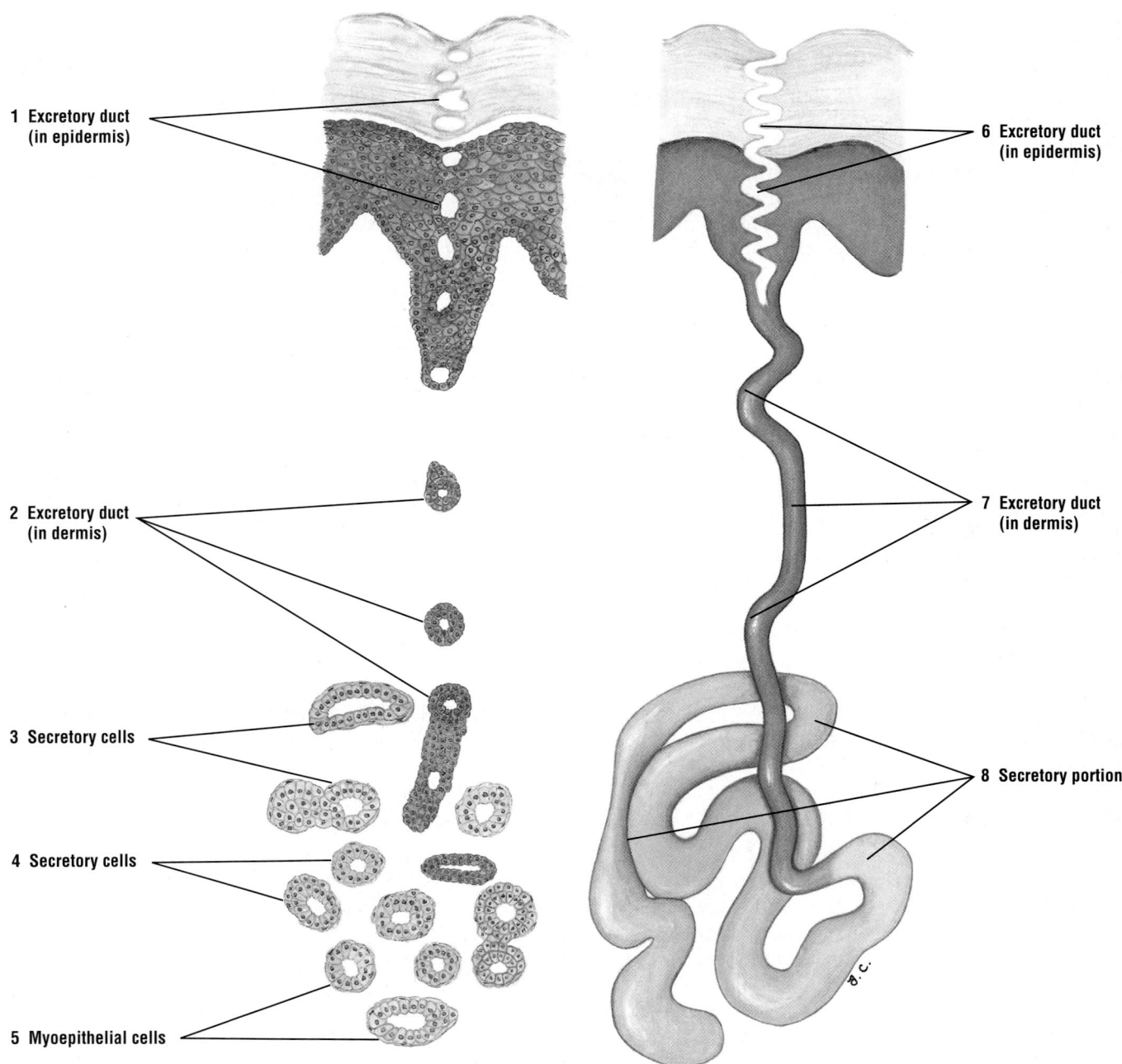

1 Excretory duct (in epidermis)

2 Excretory duct (in dermis)

3 Secretory cells

4 Secretory cells

5 Myoepithelial cells

6 Excretory duct (in epidermis)

7 Excretory duct (in dermis)

8 Secretory portion

Fig. 9-3   Sweat Glands. Stain: hematoxylin-eosin. Low magnification.

Figure 9-4   Skin: Scalp

This low magnification section of the thin skin of the scalp illustrates cell layers in the epidermis and some skin derivatives in the underlying connective tissue. In the epidermis are visible cell layers **stratum corneum (1)** with cornified superficial cells, **stratum spinosum (2),** and the basal cell layer, the **stratum basale (3)** with brown **melanin (pigment) granules (3).**

The connective tissue **dermal papillae (4)** form typical indentations on the underside of the epidermis. The thin connective tissue papillary layer of the dermis, located immediately under the epidermis, is not visible at this magnification. The thicker connective tissue **reticular layer (12)** of the dermis extends from just below the epidermis to the **subcutaneous layer (8),** which contains increased amounts of **adipose tissue (8).** Located beneath the subcutaneous layer (8) are **skeletal muscle fibers (9),** which are sectioned in different planes.

Hair follicles (13) in the skin of the scalp are very numerous, closely packed, and placed at an angle to the surface of the skin. A complete hair follicle in longitudinal section is illustrated in the figure. Parts of other hair follicles, sectioned in different planes, are also visible (13). Each hair follicle (13) consists of the following structures: cuticle, **internal root sheath (13a), external root sheath (13b), connective tissue sheath (13c), hair bulb (13d),** and connective tissue **papilla (13d).** The hair passes upward through the follicle (13) and to the surface of the skin. Numerous **sebaceous glands (11)** surround each hair follicle (13). These follicles are aggregated clusters of clear cells, which are connected to a duct that opens into the hair follicle (see Fig. 9-5).

The **arrector pili muscles (5, 10)** are smooth muscles that are aligned at an oblique angle to the hair follicles (13). These muscles bind to the papillary layer of the dermis and to the **connective tissue sheath (13c)** of the hair follicle. The contraction of arrector pili muscles (5, 10) causes the hair shaft to move into a more vertical position.

Deep in the dermis or in the subcutaneous layer (8) are found the basal portions of the highly coiled **sweat glands (6).** Sections of the sweat gland (6) that exhibit lightly stained columnar epithelium are the **secretory portions (6b)** of the gland. These are distinct from the **excretory ducts (6a)** of the sweat glands (6), which exhibit two layers of smaller, darker-stained cells. The excretory ducts (6a) are lined by stratified cuboidal epithelium. Each sweat gland duct (6a) is coiled and located deep in the dermis; then it straightens out in the upper dermis and follows a spiral course through the epidermis to the surface of the skin (See Figure 9-3).

The skin is highly **vascular (14)** and has a rich sensory innervation. Some of these sensory endings, the **Pacinian corpuscles (7),** are located in the subcutaneous tissue (8). These corpuscles are important sensory receptors for pressure and vibration. The Pacinian corpuscles (7) are illustrated in greater detail and higher magnification in Figure 9-8.

■ Functional Correlations–Skin Derivatives or Appendages

The **nails, hairs,** and **sweat glands** are derivatives of the skin that develop directly from the surface epithelium of the epidermis. During development, the appendages grow into and reside deep within the connective tissue of the **dermis.** Often the sweat glands extend deeper into the **subcutaneous layer** or **hypodermis,** a connective tissue layer situated below the dermis that exhibits increased amounts of **adipose tissue.**

Hairs are the hard, cornified, cylindrical structures that arise from the **hair follicles** of the skin. One portion of the hair projects through the epithelium of the skin to the exterior surface; the other portion remains embedded in the dermis. Hair grows in the expanded portion at the base of the hair follicle called the **hair bulb.** The base of the hair bulb is indented by a **connective tissue papilla.** This papilla is highly vascularized and brings essential nutrients to the cells of the hair follicle. Here, the hair cells divide, grow, cornify, and form the hair.

Associated with each hair follicle are one or more **sebaceous glands** that produce an oily secretion called **sebum.** Also, extending from the connective tissue around the hair follicle to the **papillary layer** of the **dermis** is a bundle of smooth muscle called the **arrector pili.** The sebaceous glands are located between the arrector pili muscle and the hair follicle. Arrector pili muscles are controlled by the **autonomic nervous system** and contract during strong emotions, fear, and/or cold. This contraction erects the hair shaft, depresses the skin at the point of insertion, and produces a small bump on the surface of the skin often called a "goose bump." In addition, contraction of the arrector pili muscle forces the sebum from the sebaceous glands onto the hair follicle and the skin. Sebum oils and keeps the skin smooth, prevents it from drying, as well as providing it with some antibacterial protection.

The **sweat glands,** widely distributed in the skin, are of two types: eccrine and apocrine. **Eccrine** sweat glands are simple, coiled tubular glands. Their **secretory portion** is found deep in the dermis, from which a coiled **excretory duct** leads to the skin surface. The eccrine sweat glands contain two types of cells: **clear cells** without secretory granules and **dark cells** containing secretory granules. Surrounding the secretory cells of the sweat gland are **myoepithelial cells,** whose contraction expels the secretion (sweat) from the sweat glands. The eccrine sweat glands are most numerous in the skin of the palms and soles. The sweat consists primarily of water and some sodium salts, ammonia, uric acid, and urea.

The **apocrine sweat** glands are limited primarily to the axillary, anal, and areolar regions of the breast. These sweat glands are larger than eccrine sweat glands and their ducts open into the hair follicle. The apocrine sweat glands produce a viscous secretion, which acquires a distinct odor following bacterial decomposition.

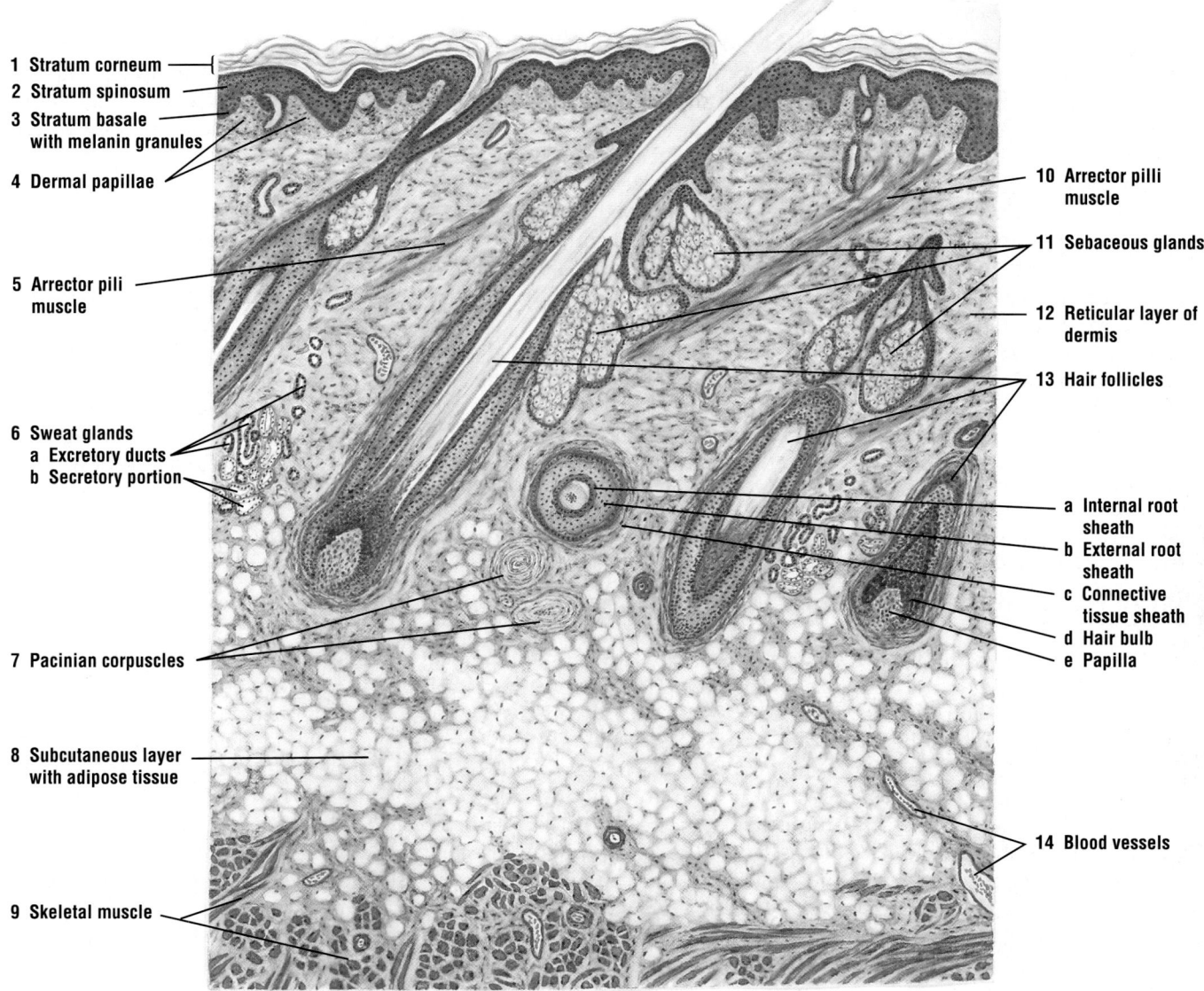

1 Stratum corneum
2 Stratum spinosum
3 Stratum basale
   with melanin granules
4 Dermal papillae

5 Arrector pili
   muscle

6 Sweat glands
   a Excretory ducts
   b Secretory portion

7 Pacinian corpuscles

8 Subcutaneous layer
   with adipose tissue

9 Skeletal muscle

10 Arrector pilli
    muscle
11 Sebaceous glands

12 Reticular layer of
    dermis

13 Hair follicles

a Internal root
   sheath
b External root
   sheath
c Connective
   tissue sheath
d Hair bulb
e Papilla

14 Blood vessels

Fig. 9-4   Skin: Scalp. Stain: hematoxylin-eosin. Low magnification.

Figure 9-5   Sebaceous Gland and Adjacent Hair Follicle

This figure illustrates a **sebaceous gland (2–6)** sectioned through the middle. The potential lumen is filled with secretory cells undergoing **cytolysis (3)** (holocrine secretion), a process in which the cells degenerate to become the oily secretory product of the gland, called sebum. The sebaceous gland (2–6) is lined with a stratified epithelium that has continuity with the **external root sheath (1)** of the hair follicle. The gland's epithelium is modified, and along its base is a single row of columnar or cuboidal cells, the **basal cells (5)**, whose nuclei may be flattened. These cells rest on a basement membrane, which is surrounded by the connective tissue of the dermis. The basal cells (5) exhibit mitotic activity and fill the acinus of the gland with larger, polyhedral cells, which enlarge, accumulate secretory material, and become round (4, 6). The cells in the interior of the acinus undergo cytolysis (3) and, together with the secretory product sebum, pass through the short **duct (2)** of the gland into the lumen of the hair follicle. The sebaceous glands (2–6) lie in the connective tissue of the dermis and in the angle between the hair follicles and the **arrector pili muscles (11)**.

The various layers of the hair follicle at the level of the sebaceous gland (2–6) may be identified. The follicle is surrounded by a **connective tissue sheath (7)** of the dermis. The **external root sheath (8)** is composed of several cell layers; these layers are continuous with the epithelial layer stratum spinosum of the epidermis. The **internal root sheath (9)** is composed of a thin, pale epithelial stratum (Henle's layer) (9) and a thin, granular epithelial stratum (Huxley's layer) (9). The latter is in direct contact with the cortex of the **hair (10)**, illustrated as a pale yellow layer with cells.

Figure 9-6   Bulb of Hair Follicle and Adjacent Sweat Gland

This figure illustrates the bulb of a hair follicle and its surrounding cell layers. A sheath of fibrous **connective tissue (7)** surrounds the bulb. The **external root sheath (1)** at this level of the bulb is a single layer of cells. The cells are columnar above the bulb and flat at the base of the bulb, where they cannot be distinguished from the matrix cells of the hair follicle. Above the bulb is the **internal root sheath (2, 3)** composed of a thin, pale **epithelium stratum (Henle's layer) (2)**, and a thin, **granular stratum (Huxley's layer) (3)**. These two cell layers become indistinguishable as their cells merge with the cells of the bulb. Internal to these cell layers are the **cuticles (4)**, **cortex (5)**, and **medulla (6)** of the hair. In the bulb, these layers merge into undifferentiated cells of the **hair matrix (12)**, which caps the **connective tissue papilla (11)** of the hair follicle. Cell **mitosis (10)** can be seen in the matrix cells.

In the dermal connective tissue and adjacent to the hair follicle are sections through the basal portion of a coiled **sweat gland (8, 9)**. The **secretory cells (9)** of the sweat gland are tall, columnar, and stain light. Along their bases may be seen the flattened nuclei of the contractile **myoepithelial cells (14)**. The **excretory ducts (8)** of the sweat gland are smaller in diameter, are lined with a stratified cuboidal epithelium, and stain characteristically darker than the secretory cells.

Figure 9-7   Glomus in the Dermis of Thick Skin

Arteriovenous anastomoses are numerous in the thick skin of fingers and toes. Some anastomoses form direct connections; in others, the arterial portion of the anastomosis forms a specialized thick-walled structure called the **glomus (2)**. The vessel is coiled and, as a result, more than one lumen may be seen in a transverse section. The smooth muscle cells in the tunica media have hypertrophied and the specialized muscle cells with the epithelioid appearance are now called the **epithelioid cells (5)**. The tunica media wall, however, becomes thin again before the arteriole empties into a venule. The small artery (3, middle leader) may represent the terminal part of the glomus.

Small nerves and capillaries are present in the glomus and a **connective tissue sheath (6)** encloses the entire structure.

The dermis that surrounds the glomus contains **blood vessels (3)**, **nerves (4)**, and **ducts (1, 7)** of sweat glands. The PAS and hematoxylin (PASH) stains demonstrate the basement membrane of these ducts.

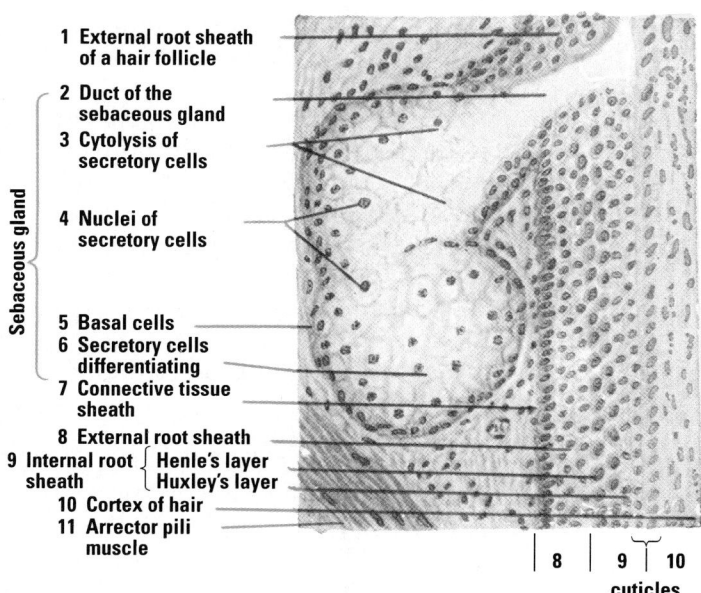

1 External root sheath of a hair follicle
2 Duct of the sebaceous gland
3 Cytolysis of secretory cells
4 Nuclei of secretory cells
5 Basal cells
6 Secretory cells differentiating
7 Connective tissue sheath
8 External root sheath
9 Internal root sheath { Henle's layer, Huxley's layer
10 Cortex of hair
11 Arrector pili muscle

Sebaceous gland

8 | 9 | 10
cuticles

Fig. 9-5 Sebaceous Gland and Adjacent Hair Follicle. Stain: hematoxylin-eosin. Medium magnification.

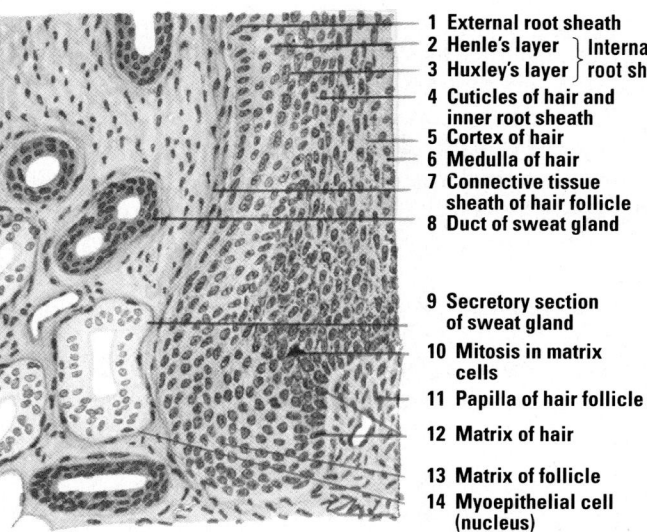

1 External root sheath
2 Henle's layer ⎱ Internal
3 Huxley's layer ⎰ root sheath
4 Cuticles of hair and inner root sheath
5 Cortex of hair
6 Medulla of hair
7 Connective tissue sheath of hair follicle
8 Duct of sweat gland
9 Secretory section of sweat gland
10 Mitosis in matrix cells
11 Papilla of hair follicle
12 Matrix of hair
13 Matrix of follicle
14 Myoepithelial cell (nucleus)

Fig. 9-6 Bulb of Hair Follicle and Adjacent Sweat Gland. Stain: hematoxylin-eosin. Medium magnification.

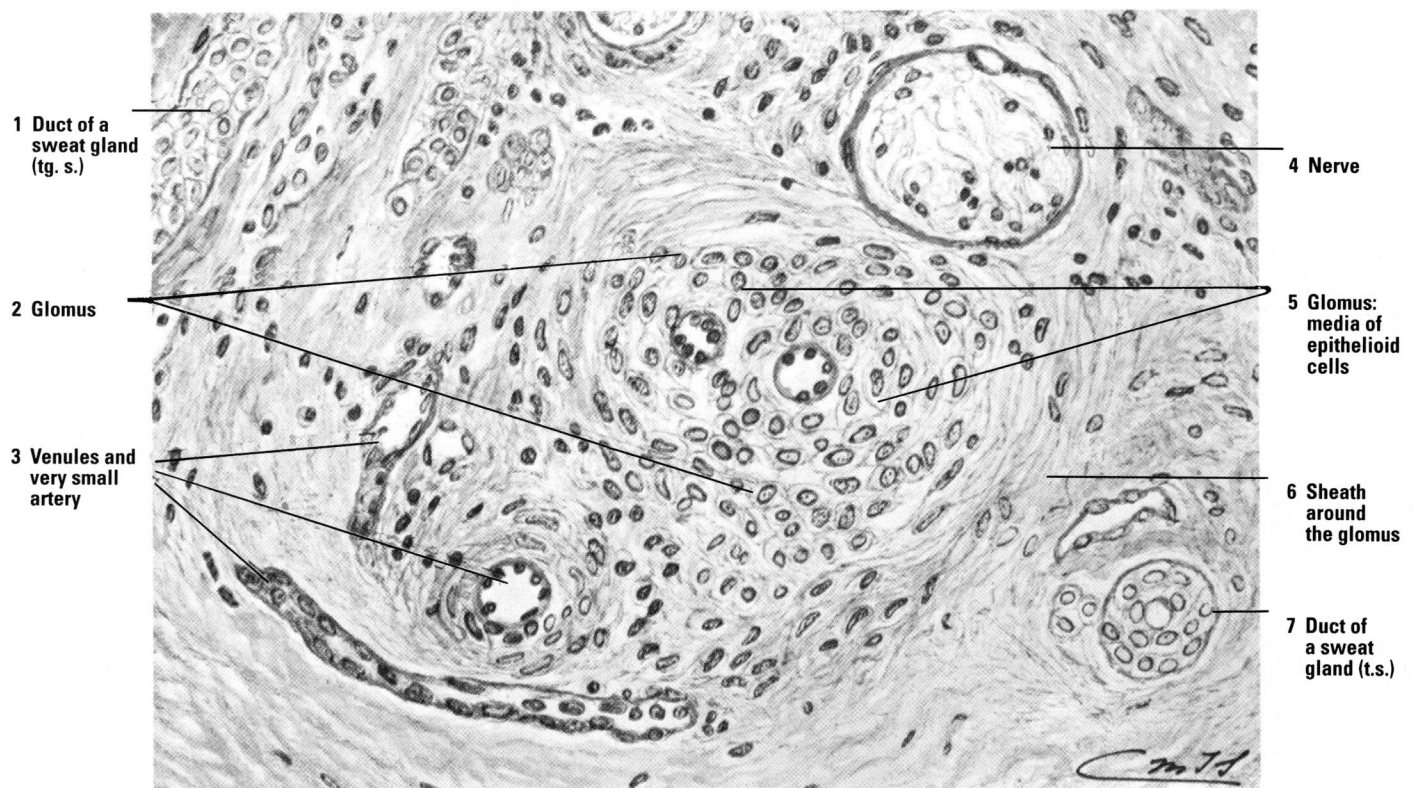

1 Duct of a sweat gland (tg. s.)
2 Glomus
3 Venules and very small artery
4 Nerve
5 Glomus: media of epithelioid cells
6 Sheath around the glomus
7 Duct of a sweat gland (t.s.)

Fig. 9-7 Glomus in the Dermis of Thick Skin. Stain: PASH. High magnification.

Figure 9-8   Pacinian Corpuscles in the Deep Dermis of Thick Skin

Pacinian corpuscles (1, 6) in the thick skin are located deep in the dermis and subcutaneous tissue. The corpuscles are important sensory receptors for pressure and possibly vibration. One corpuscle is illustrated in a transverse section (1) and another in an oblique section (6).

The Pacinian corpuscles are ovoid structures when seen in longitudinal or oblique sections (6) and contain an elongated central core, the **inner bulb (8).** This area usually appears empty in sections, but in life, the corpuscle contains a terminal myelinated nerve fiber. The inner bulb (8) is surrounded by **concentric lamellae (10)** of compact collagenous fibers, which become denser peripherally (inner and outer lamellae). Between the lamellae is a small amount of loose connective tissue with flat **fibroblasts (6).** A thin, dense connective tissue **sheath (9)** encloses the Pacinian corpuscle.

In a transverse section of the corpuscle (1), the layers of lamellae surrounding the inner bulb resemble a sliced onion.

In the dense irregular connective tissue of the **dermis (3), adipose cells (5), blood vessels (7), nerves (2, 11),** and a **sweat gland (4)** surround the Pacinian corpuscle.

Figure 9-9   Thick Skin: Epidermis, Dermis, and Hypodermis of the Palm

A low power photomicrograph illustrates the appearance of the superficial and deep structures in the thick skin of the palm. In the **epidermis (6)** of the thick skin are seen the following cell layers: **stratum corneum (7), stratum granulosum (8),** and **stratum basale (9).** Inferior to the epidermis (6) is the dense irregular connective tissue of the **dermis (5). Dermal papillae (11)** extend from the dermis (5) and indent the base of the epidermis (6). Deep in the dermis and extending into the hypodermis are cross sections of the **sweat glands (3)** and the darker-staining **excretory ducts of the sweat glands (10).** A layer of **adipose tissue (1)** with the connective tissue deep to the dermis (5) is the **hypodermis (4)** or the superficial fascia. This layer is not part of the integument. Two sensory receptors called the **Pacinian corpuscles (2)** are seen deep in the skin.

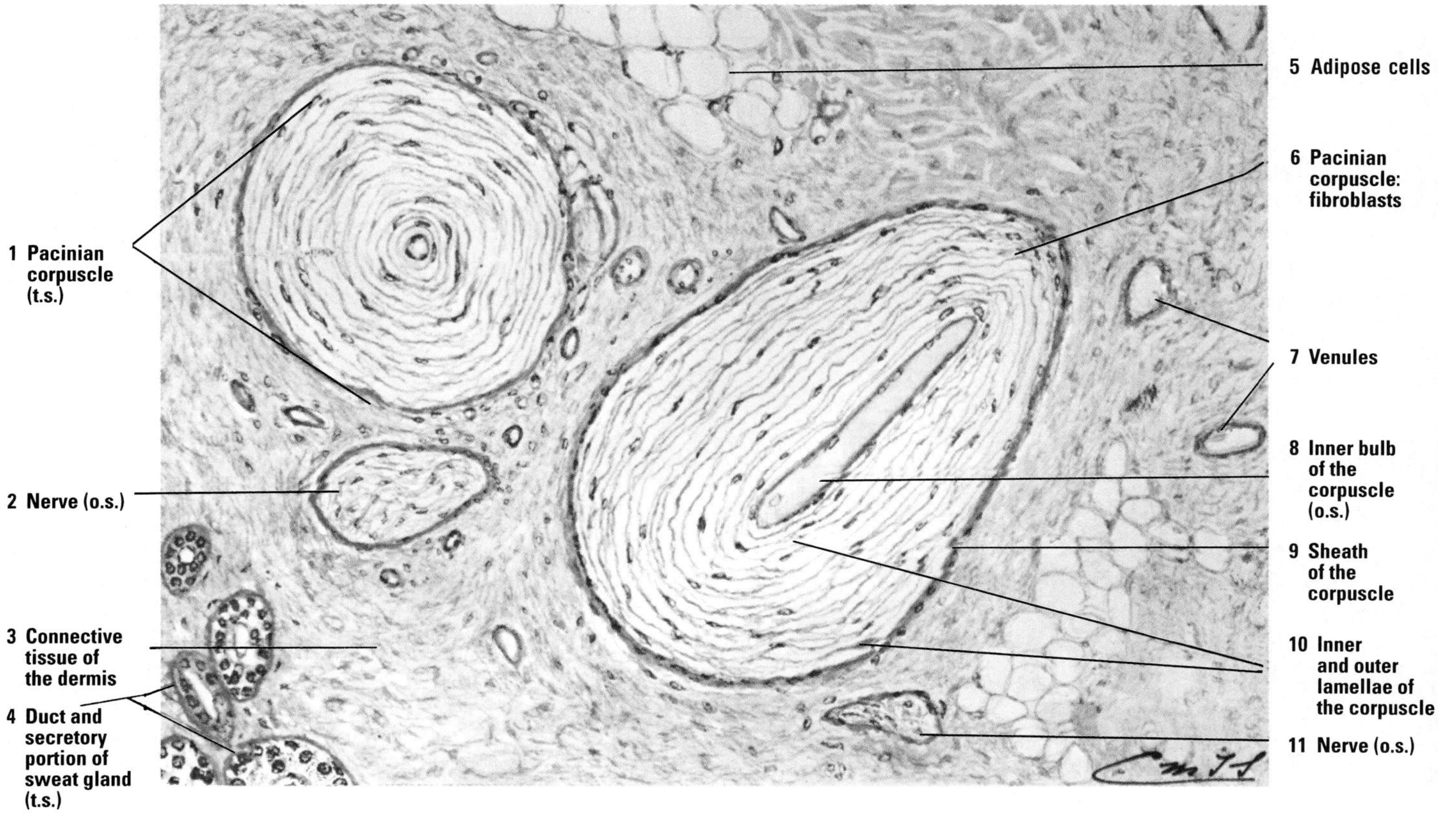

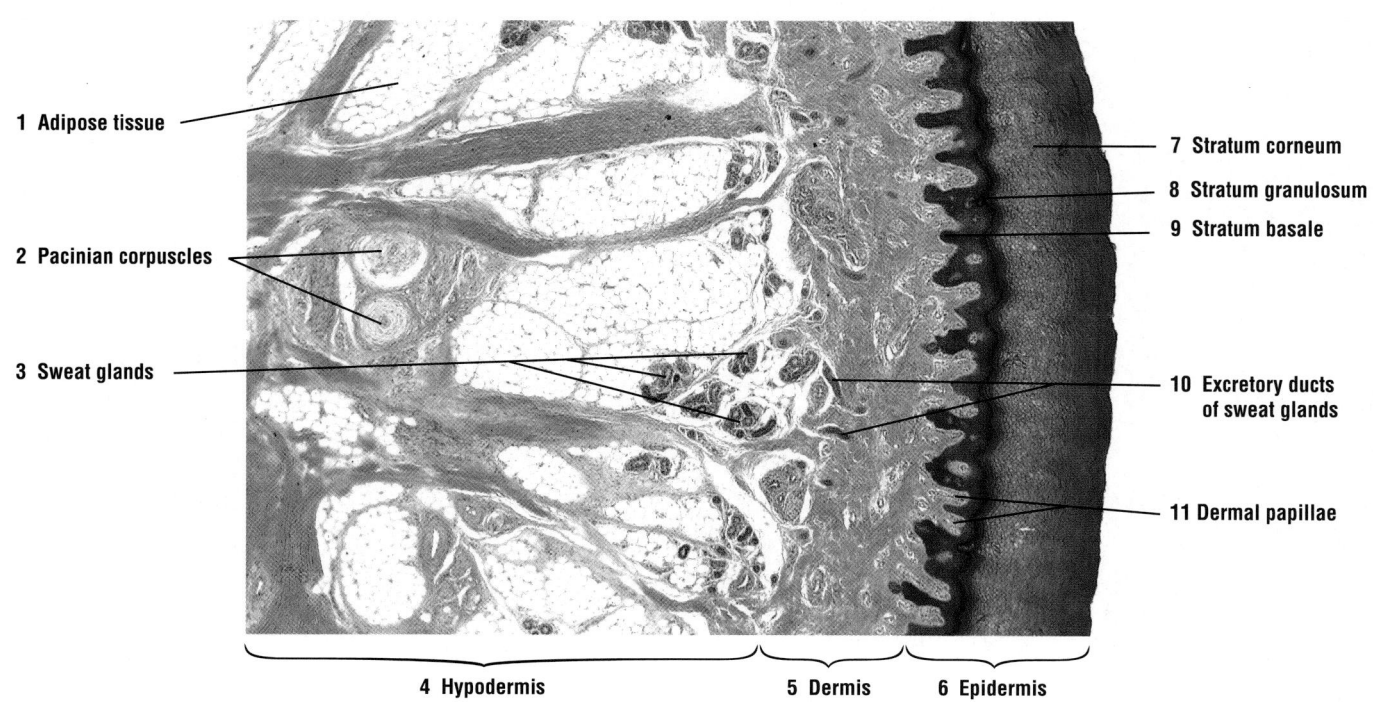

1 Pacinian corpuscle (t.s.)

2 Nerve (o.s.)

3 Connective tissue of the dermis

4 Duct and secretory portion of sweat gland (t.s.)

5 Adipose cells

6 Pacinian corpuscle: fibroblasts

7 Venules

8 Inner bulb of the corpuscle (o.s.)

9 Sheath of the corpuscle

10 Inner and outer lamellae of the corpuscle

11 Nerve (o.s.)

Fig. 9-8   Pacinian Corpuscles in the Deep Dermis of Thick Skin. Stain: PASH. High magnification.

1 Adipose tissue

2 Pacinian corpuscles

3 Sweat glands

7 Stratum corneum

8 Stratum granulosum

9 Stratum basale

10 Excretory ducts of sweat glands

11 Dermal papillae

4 Hypodermis   **5 Dermis**   **6 Epidermis**

Fig. 9-9   Thick Skin: Epidermis, Dermis, and Hypodermis of the Palm. Stain: hematoxylin-eosin. 17×

Figure 9-10   Thick Skin: Epidermis and Superficial Cell Layers

With increased magnification, this photomicrograph shows a clear distinction between the different cell layers in the **epidermis (1)** of the thick skin of the palm. The outermost and the thickest layer is the **stratum corneum (1a).** The dark layer with two to three cell layers with granules inferior to the stratum corneum (1a) is the **stratum granulosum (1b).** Below this layer is the **stratum spinosum (1c),** a thicker layer of polyhedral cells. The deepest cell layer in the epidermis (1) is the **stratum basale (1d).** In this cell layer are seen numerous brown **melanin granules (6).** Stratum basale (1d) is attached to a thin **basement membrane (4)** that separates the epidermis (1) from the underlying dense irregular connective tissue of the **dermis (2),** which indents the epidermis (1) with its numerous **dermal papillae (5).** Passing through the dermis (2) and the cell layers of the epidermis (1) is the **excretory duct (3)** of a sweat gland that is located somewhere deep in the dermis.

Figure 9-11   Hairy Thin Skin of the Scalp: Hair Follicles and Surrounding Structures

This photomicrograph illustrates a section of the hairy, thin skin of the scalp. In the **epidermis (1)** of the thin skin, **stratum corneum (1a), stratum granulosum (1b),** and **stratum spinosum (1c)** layers are thinner than the same layers seen in the thick skin. The hairy skin of the scalp also contains numerous **hair follicles (3)** and their associated **sebaceous glands (2, 5),** surrounded by the dense irregular connective tissue of the **dermis (4).** A strip of smooth muscle, the **arrector pili muscle (6),** extends from the connective tissue of the hair follicle (3) into the connective tissue of the dermis (1).

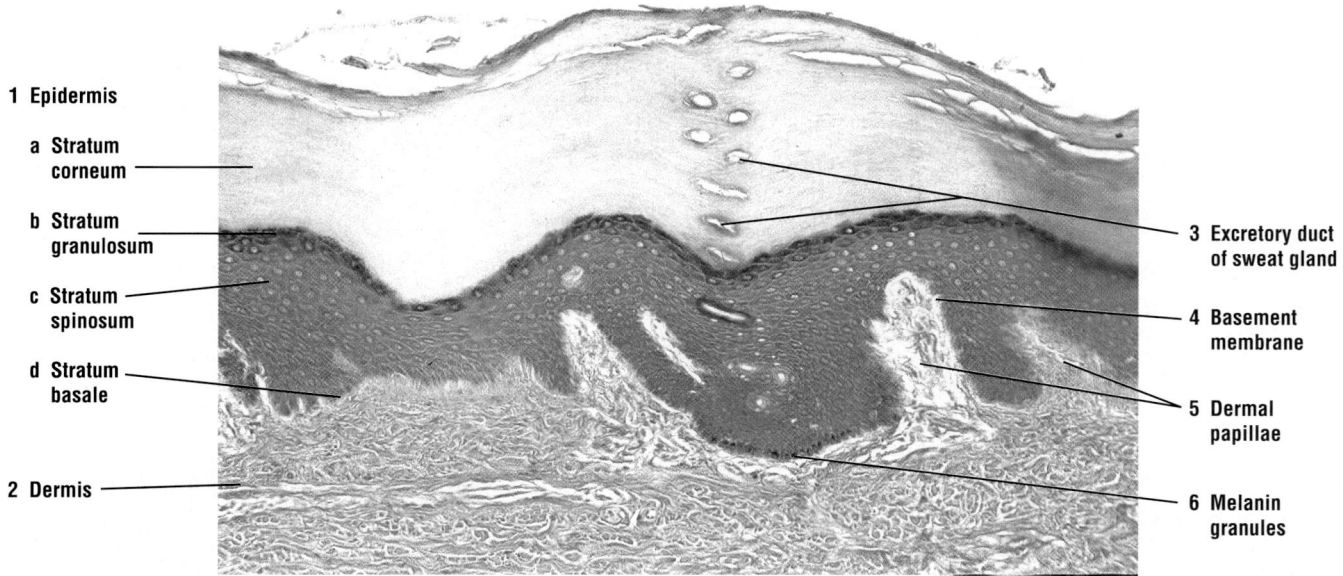

1 **Epidermis**

  a **Stratum corneum**

  b **Stratum granulosum**

  c **Stratum spinosum**

  d **Stratum basale**

2 **Dermis**

3 **Excretory duct of sweat gland**

4 **Basement membrane**

5 **Dermal papillae**

6 **Melanin granules**

Fig. 9-10   Thick Skin: Epidermis and Superficial Cell Layers. Stain: hematoxylin-eosin. 40×

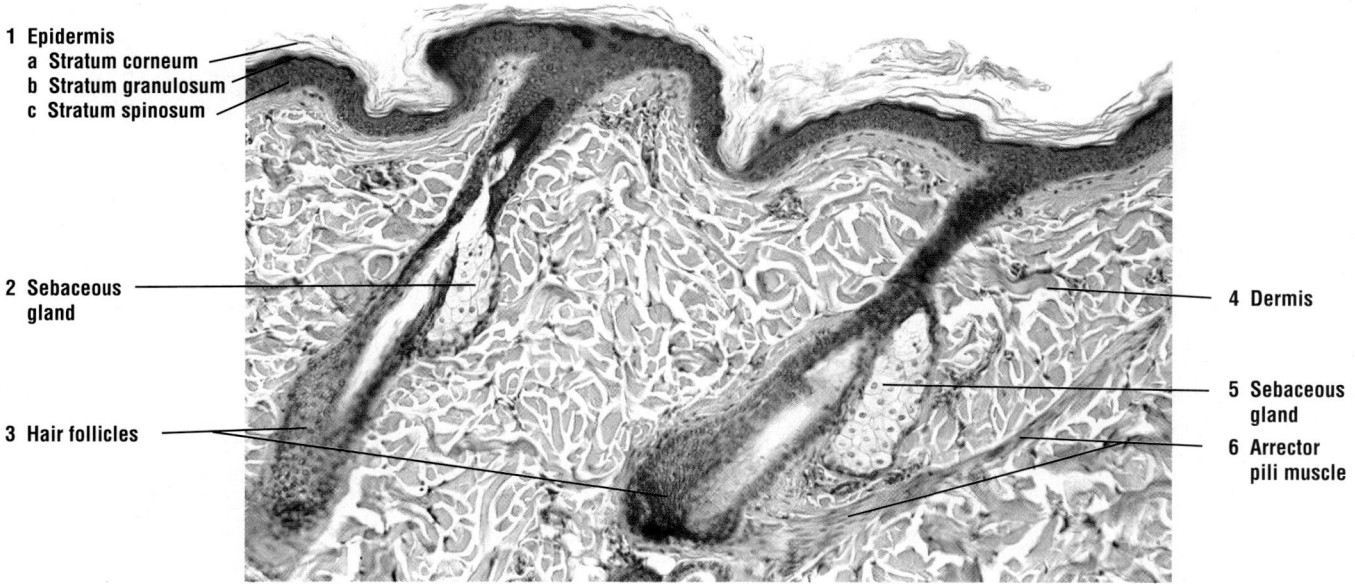

1 **Epidermis**
  a **Stratum corneum**
  b **Stratum granulosum**
  c **Stratum spinosum**

2 **Sebaceous gland**

3 **Hair follicles**

4 **Dermis**

5 **Sebaceous gland**

6 **Arrector pili muscle**

Fig. 9-11   Hairy Thin Skin of the Scalp: Hair Follicles and Surrounding Structures. Stain: hematoxylin-eosin. 40×

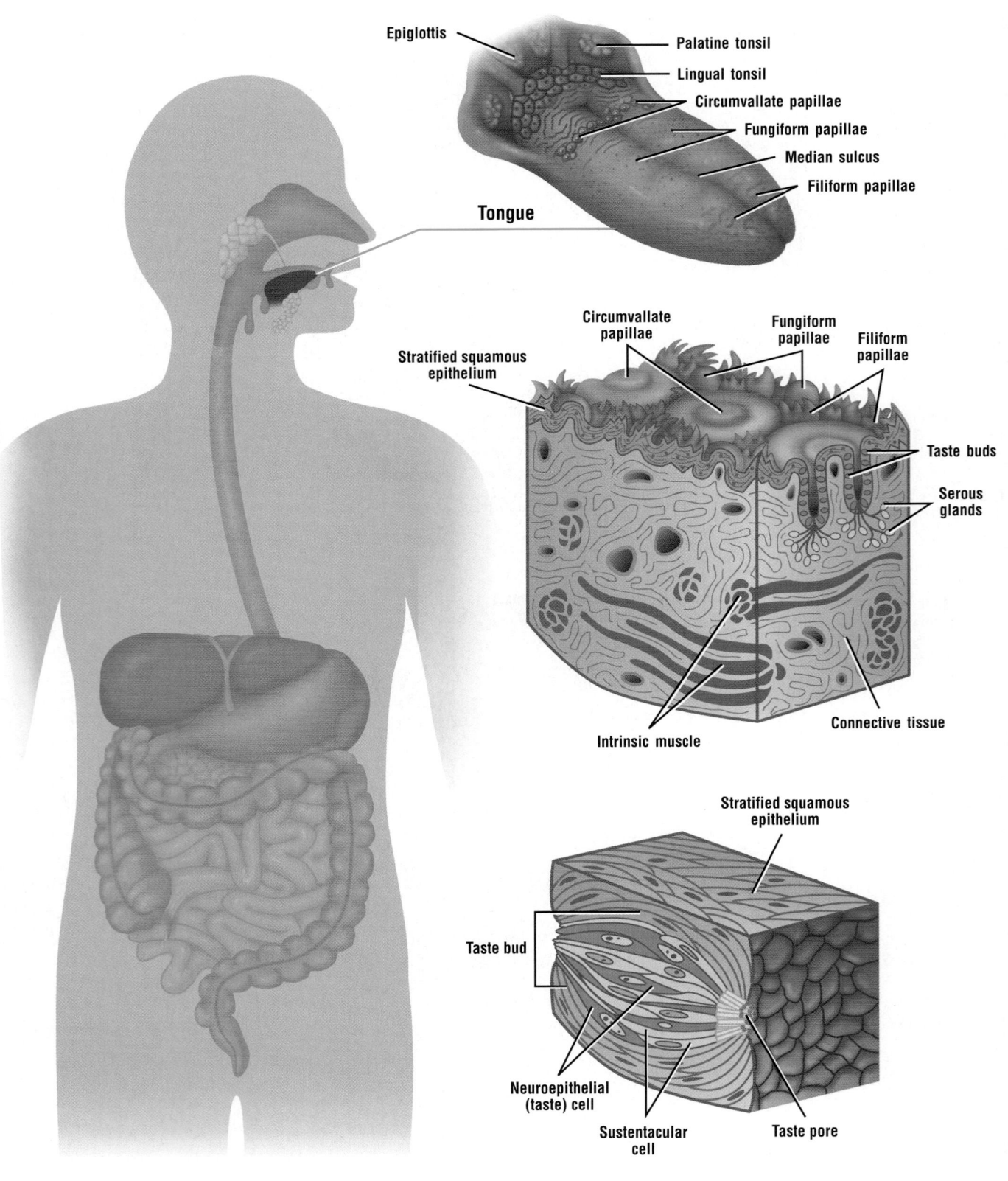

Epiglottis

Palatine tonsil

Lingual tonsil

Circumvallate papillae

Fungiform papillae

Median sulcus

Filiform papillae

Tongue

Circumvallate
papillae

Fungiform
papillae

Filiform
papillae

Stratified squamous
epithelium

Taste buds

Serous
glands

Intrinsic muscle

Connective tissue

Stratified squamous
epithelium

Taste bud

Neuroepithelial
(taste) cell

Sustentacular
cell

Taste pore

Digestive System: Tongue and Salivary Glands

THE DIGESTIVE SYSTEM

The digestive system consists of a long hollow tube or tract that starts at oral cavity and terminates at the anus. The systems consists of the **oral cavity, esophagus, stomach, small intestine, large intestine, rectum,** and **anal canal.** Associated with the digestive tract are the accessory organs **salivary glands, liver,** and **pancreas.** These organs produce numerous secretions that enter the digestive tract through the excretory ducts. These secretions aid in the digestion of the ingested material and its eventual absorption.

THE ORAL CAVITY

In the oral cavity, food is ingested, masticated (chewed), and lubricated by saliva for swallowing. Because food is physically broken down in the oral cavity, this region is lined by a protective, nonkeratinized, **stratified squamous epithelium,** which also lines the inner or labial surface of the lips **(Fig. 10-1).**

THE TONGUE

The **epithelium** on the dorsal surface of the tongue is very irregular and covered with numerous elevations or projections called **papillae** that are indented by a connective tissue **lamina propria (Figs. 10-2–10-4, 10-5).** There are four types of papillae on tongue. These are the filiform, fungiform, circumvallate, and foliate. The most numerous papillae on the tongue are the narrow, conical-shaped **filiform papillae.** They cover the entire dorsal surface of the tongue. Less numerous but larger

and broader are the **fungiform papillae (Fig. 10-2,10-15).** These papillae exhbit a mushroom-like shape and are more prevalent in the anterior region of the tongue. The **circumvallate papillae** are much larger than the fungiform or filiform papillae and consist of large 8 to 12 papillae that are located in the posterior region of the tongue. These papillae are surrounded by deep moats or **furrows.** Numerous excretory ducts of the underlying **serous** (von Ebner's) **glands,** which are located in the connective tissue of the tongue, empty into the base of the furrows **(Figs. 10-3, 10-4).** Foliate papillae are well developed in some animals, but are rudimentary in humans.

The papillae of the tongue are covered by **stratified squamous epithelium** that shows partial keratinization. Also, located in the epithelium of the fungiform and on the lateral sides of the circumvallate papillae are barrel-shaped structures called the **taste buds (Figs. 10-3, 10-4, 10-15).** The free surface of each taste bud contains an opening called the **taste pore.** Located within each taste bud are the receptor **taste cells** and the supporting **sustentacular cells.** In contrast to the dorsal surface, the epithelium on the ventral surface of the tongue is smooth and does not exhibit any papillae.

The **tongue** is a muscular structure. Its interior consists of a core of **connective tissue** and interlacing bundles of **skeletal muscle fibers (Figs. 10-2, 10-3).** The distribution and random orientation of the individual skeletal muscle fibers in the tongue allows the tongue high mobility during chewing and swallowing of the food, and speaking.

Figure 10-1   Lip (longitudinal section)

The core of the lip contains fibers of the striated muscle, **orbicularis oris (8).** Special stains would reveal the presence of intermixed dense fibroelastic connective tissue in the core. The right side illustrates the skin of the lip and the left side the mucosal lining of the mouth.

The skin of the lip is lined with **epidermis (9)** composed of stratified squamous, keratinized epithelium. Beneath the epidermis (9) is the **dermis (10)** with **sebaceous glands (11), hair follicles (12),** and **sweat glands (14);** all of these are epidermal derivatives. The dermis also contains the **arrector pili muscles (13, 15)** and a **neurovascular bundle (7)** on the lip periphery.

The labial mucosa is lined with a stratified squamous, nonkeratinized **epithelium (1).** The surface cells, without becoming cornified, slough off in the fluids of the mouth. Underlying the mucosal epithelium is the connective tissue **lamina propria (2),** the counterpart of the dermis as related to the epidermis. In the submucosa are found tubuloacinar **labial glands (4),** which are predominantly mucous with occasional serous demilunes. Their secretion moistens the oral mucosa and their **small ducts (4,** lower leader**)** open into the oral cavity.

Transition of the skin epidermis to epithelium of oral mucosa illustrates a mucocutaneous junction. The "red line" or vermilion **border of the lip (6)** is illustrated. Epithelium (1) of the lip and oral mucosa is relatively smoother than that of the epidermis (9). The underlying papillae of the lip and oral mucosa are high, numerous, and abundantly supplied with capillaries. The color of the blood shows through the overlying cells, giving the lips a characteristic red color. The epithelium of the labial mucosa (1) is also thicker than the epidermis of the skin (9).

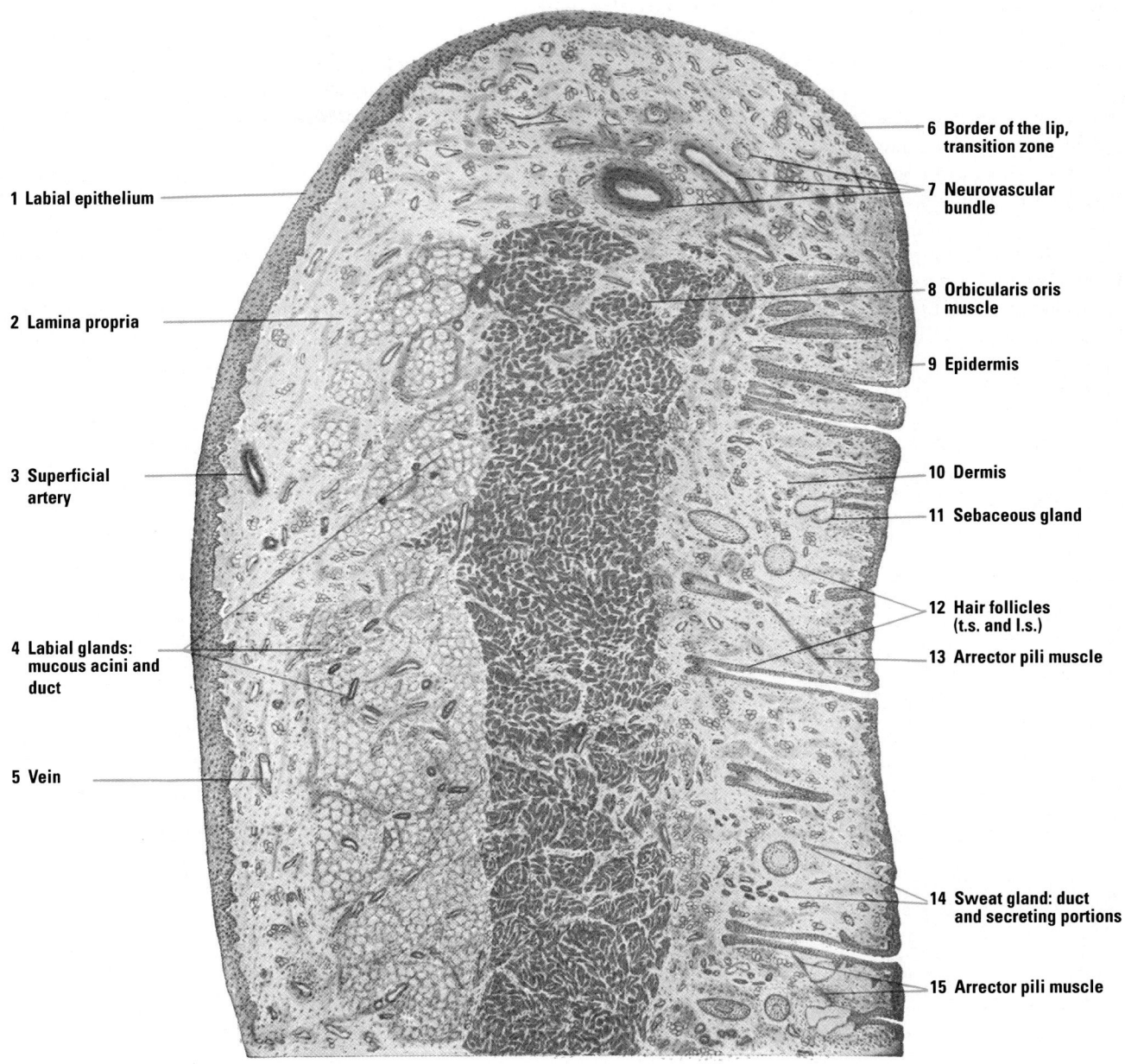

1 Labial epithelium

2 Lamina propria

3 Superficial artery

4 Labial glands: mucous acini and duct

5 Vein

6 Border of the lip, transition zone

7 Neurovascular bundle

8 Orbicularis oris muscle

9 Epidermis

10 Dermis

11 Sebaceous gland

12 Hair follicles (t.s. and l.s.)

13 Arrector pili muscle

14 Sweat gland: duct and secreting portions

15 Arrector pili muscle

Fig. 10-1   Lip (longitudinal section). Stain: hematoxylin-eosin. Low magnification.

Figure 10-2   Tongue: Apex (longitudinal section, panoramic view)

The mucosa of the tongue consists of a **stratified squamous epithelium (1)** and a thin papillated **lamina propria (1)**, which may contain diffuse lymphatic tissue. The dorsal surface of the tongue is characterized by mucosal projections called **papillae (4, 6, 7)**. Most numerous are the slender **filiform papillae (6)** with cornified tips. Less numerous are the **fungiform papillae (4, 7)**, which exhibit a broad, round surface of noncornified epithelium and a prominent core of **lamina propria (4)**. All papillae are located on the dorsal surface of the tongue but are absent on the entire ventral (lower) surface **(18)**, where the mucosa is smooth.

The core of the tongue consists of crisscrossing bundles of **skeletal muscle (3, 5)**. As a result, the tongue muscle is typically seen in longitudinal, transverse, or oblique planes of section. In the connective tissue around the muscle bundles may be seen numerous **blood vessels (9, 10, 15, 16)** and **nerves (8, 17)**.

In the lower half of the tongue near the apex and embedded in the muscle (3, 5) a portion of the anterior lingual gland is illustrated. This gland is of a mixed type and contains **serous (11)**, **mucous (13)**, and mixed acini with serous demilunes (not illustrated). The **interlobular ducts (12)** pass into the larger **excretory ducts (14)**, which then open into the oral cavity on the ventral surface of the tongue.

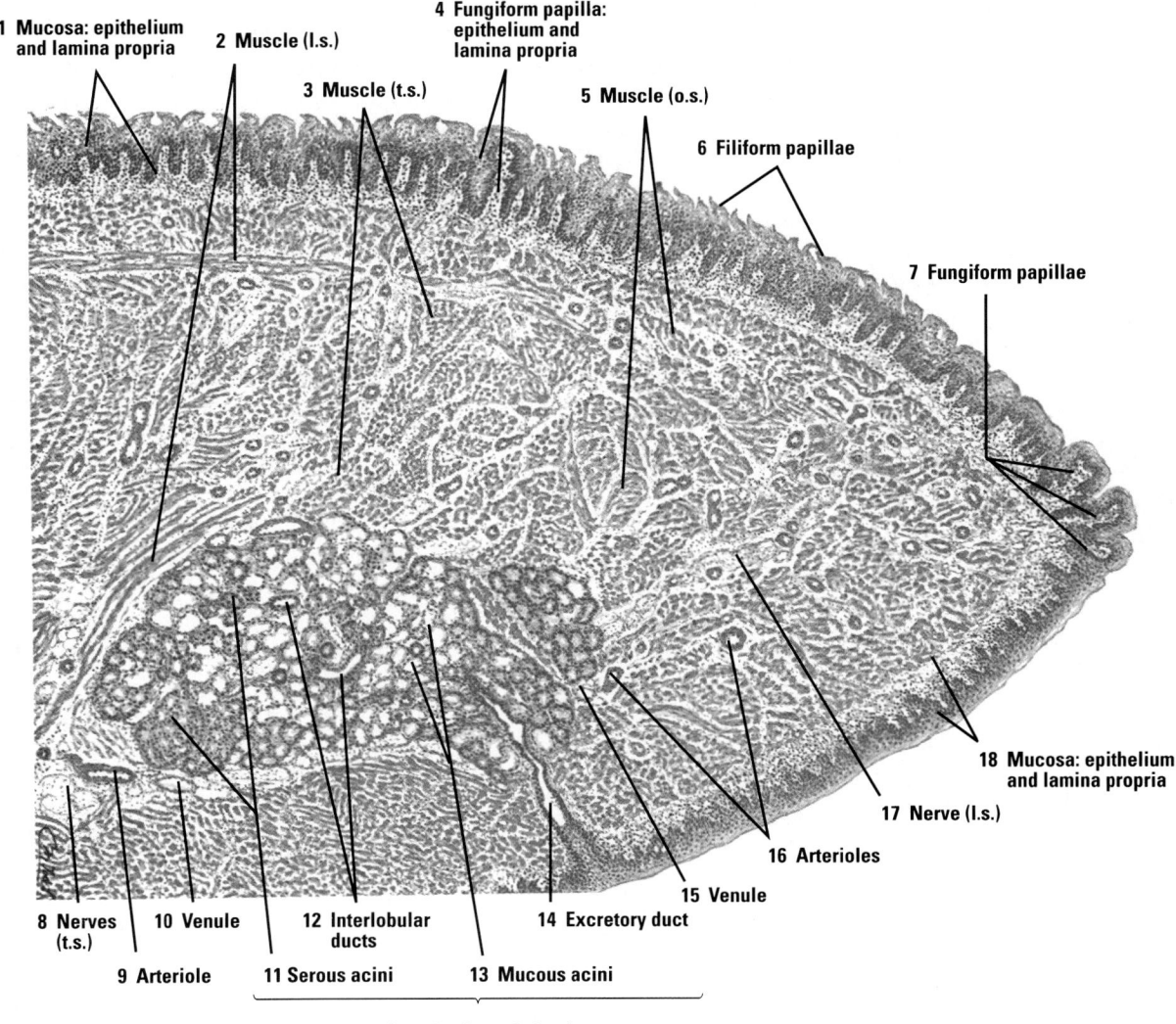

1 Mucosa: epithelium
and lamina propria

2 Muscle (l.s.)

3 Muscle (t.s.)

4 Fungiform papilla:
epithelium and
lamina propria

5 Muscle (o.s.)

6 Filiform papillae

7 Fungiform papillae

18 Mucosa: epithelium
and lamina propria

17 Nerve (l.s.)

16 Arterioles

15 Venule

14 Excretory duct

13 Mucous acini

12 Interlobular
ducts

11 Serous acini

10 Venule

9 Arteriole

8 Nerves
(t.s.)

Anterior lingual gland

Fig. 10-2   Tongue: Apex (longitudinal section, panoramic view). Stain: hematoxylin-eosin. Low magnification.

Figure 10-3   Tongue: Circumvallate Papilla (cross section)

A cross section of a circumvallate papilla of the tongue is illustrated in this figure. The epithelium of the tongue, **lingual epithelium (2),** and that covering the circumvallate papilla is **stratified squamous (1).** The underlying connective tissue, the **lamina propria (3),** exhibits numerous, **secondary papillae (7)** that project into the overlying stratified squamous epithelium (1, 2) of the papilla. A deep trench or **furrow (5, 10)** surrounds the base of each circumvallate papilla.

Numerous oval **taste buds (4, 9)** are found in the epithelium of the lateral surfaces of the circumvallate papilla and on the outer wall of the furrow (5, 10). Higher magnification and greater details of the taste buds (4, 9) are illustrated in Figure 10-4. Located deep in the lamina propria (3) and core of the tongue are numerous, tubuloacinar **serous (von Ebner's) glands (6, 11),** whose **excretory ducts (6a, 11a)** open at the base of the circular furrows (5, 10) in the circumvallate papilla. The secretory product from these glands acts as a solvent for taste-inducing substances.

Most of the core of the tongue consists of interlacing bundles of **skeletal (striated) muscles (12)** running in different directions. Examples of skeletal muscle fibers sectioned in longitudinal (12a) and transverse planes (12b) are abundant. This arrangement of muscles allows the tongue great mobility, which is necessary for phonating, chewing, and swallowing of food. The lamina propria (3) surrounding the serous glands (6, 11) and muscles also contains an abundance of **blood vessels (8).**

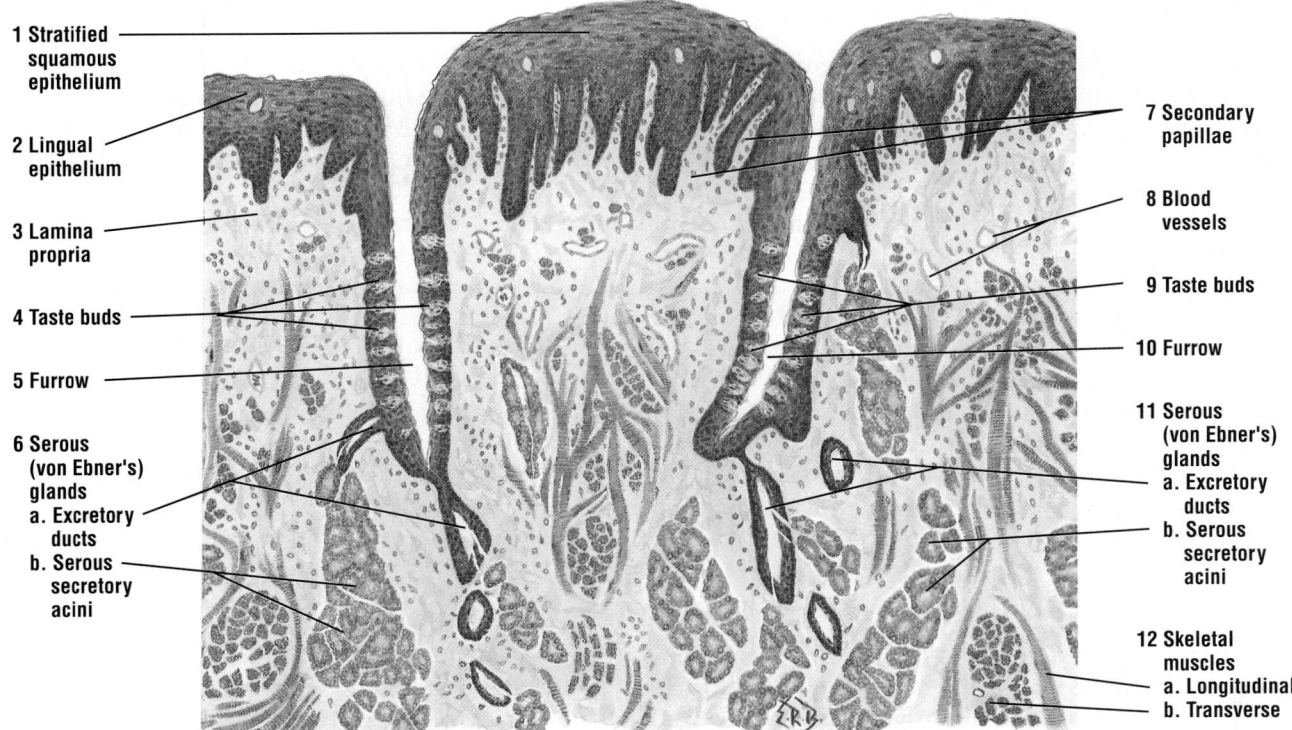

1 Stratified squamous epithelium

2 Lingual epithelium

3 Lamina propria

4 Taste buds

5 Furrow

6 Serous (von Ebner's) glands
  a. Excretory ducts
  b. Serous secretory acini

7 Secondary papillae

8 Blood vessels

9 Taste buds

10 Furrow

11 Serous (von Ebner's) glands
  a. Excretory ducts
  b. Serous secretory acini

12 Skeletal muscles
  a. Longitudinal
  b. Transverse

Fig. 10-3   Tongue: Circumvallate Papilla (cross section). Stain: hematoxylin-eosin. Medium magnification.

Figure 10-4   Tongue: Taste Buds

The **taste buds (5, 12)** at the bottom of a **furrow (14)** (Fig. 10-3) are illustrated at a higher magnification and in greater detail. The taste buds (5, 12) are actually embedded within and extend the full thickness of the stratified **lingual epithelium (1)** of the circumvallate papilla. The taste buds (5, 12) are distinguished from the surrounding stratified epithelium (1) by their oval shape and elongated cells (modified columnar) arranged perpendicularly to the surface of the epithelium (1).

There are several types of cells in taste buds (5, 12). Three different types of cells can be identified in this illustration. The dark supporting or **sustentacular cells (3, 8)** are elongated with a darker cytoplasm and slender, dark nucleus. The light **taste** or **gustatory cells (7, 11)** exhibit a lighter cytoplasm and a more oval, lighter nucleus. A third type of cell, the **basal cells (13)** are located at the periphery of the taste bud (5, 12) near the basement membrane.

At this present time, no consensus exists that defines the specific gustatory role to a certain cell type. However, because unmyelinated nerve fibers are associated with both sustentacular cells (3, 8) and gustatory cells (7, 11), both types may serve some taste receptor functions. Basal cells (13) give rise to both the sustentacular cells (3, 8) and gustatory cells (7, 11).

The apical surfaces of both the sustentacular cells (3, 8) and gustatory cells (7, 11) have long **microvilli (taste hairs) (4)** that extend into and protrude through the **taste pore (9)** into the furrow (14) that surrounds the circumvallate papilla. The surrounding **lamina propria (2)** consists of loose connective tissue and numerous **blood vessels (6, 10).**

■ Functional Correlations–Tongue and Taste Buds

The main functions of the tongue during food processing are to perceive **taste** and to assist in mastication (chewing) and swallowing of bolus (food). In the oral cavity, taste sensations are detected by specialized receptor taste cells located in **taste buds** of the **fungiform** and **circumvallate papillae** of the tongue.

Substances that are to be tasted must first be dissolved in **saliva** that is normally present in the oral cavity and which is increased during food intake. In addition to the saliva, taste buds located in the epithelium of the circumvallate papillae are continuously washed by watery secretions produced by **serous** (von Ebner's) **glands** located in the **connective tissue** of the tongue. This secretion enters the **furrow** at the base of the papillae, dissolves different substances, and allows them to enter the **taste pores** in the **taste buds** to stimulate the taste or **gustatory cells** for taste perception. In addition to the tongue, where the taste buds are most numerous, taste buds are also found in the mucous membrane of the **soft palate, pharynx,** and **epiglottis.**

There are four primary taste sensations to which the taste buds respond: **sour, salt, bitter,** and **sweet.** All remaining taste sensations are combinations of these four. The tip of the tongue is most sensitive to sweet and salt, the posterior portion of the tongue to bitter, and the lateral edges to sour taste sensations.

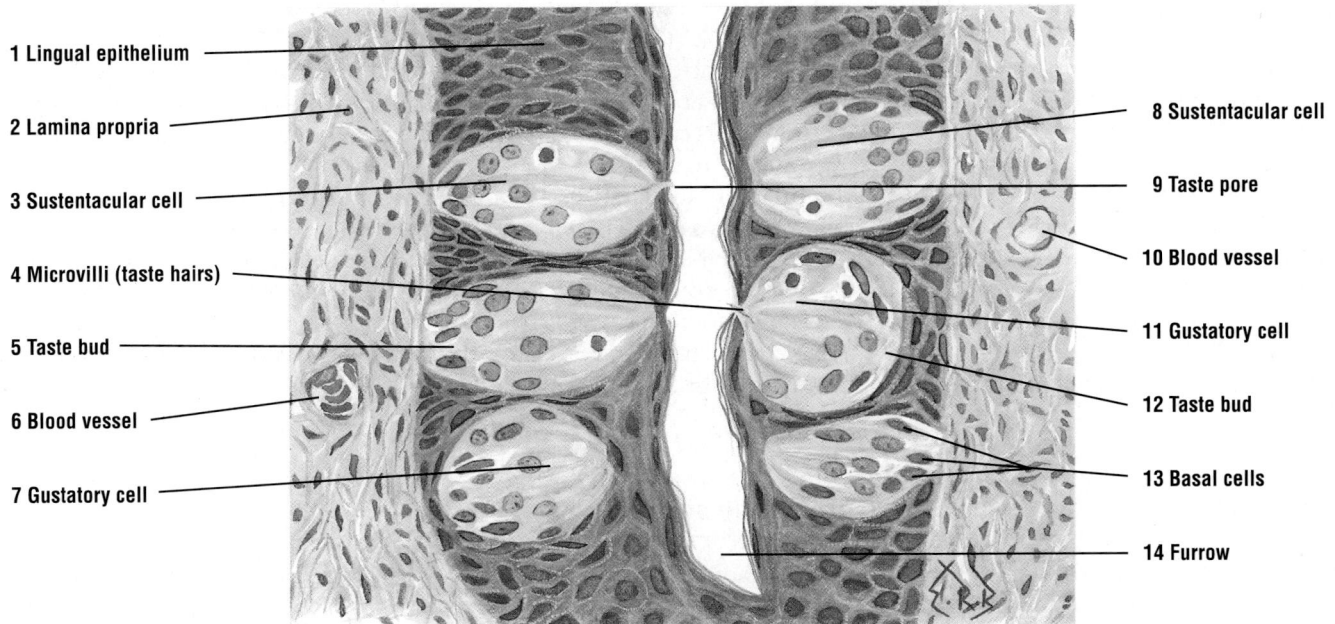

1 Lingual epithelium

2 Lamina propria

3 Sustentacular cell

4 Microvilli (taste hairs)

5 Taste bud

6 Blood vessel

7 Gustatory cell

8 Sustentacular cell

9 Taste pore

10 Blood vessel

11 Gustatory cell

12 Taste bud

13 Basal cells

14 Furrow

Fig. 10-4   Tongue: Taste Buds. Stain: hematoxylin-eosin. High magnification.

Figure 10-5   Posterior Tongue Near Circumvallate Papilla (longitudinal section)

The posterior region of the tongue is located behind the circumvallate papillae and near the lingual tonsils. Its dorsal surface typically exhibits large **mucosal ridges (1)** and round **elevations** or **folds (6)** that resemble large fungiform papillae. Lymphatic nodules of the lingual tonsils can be seen in such elevations; however, the typical filiform and fungiform papillae normally seen in the anterior region of the tongue are absent.

The lamina propria of the mucosa is wider but similar to that in the anterior two thirds of the tongue. Under the epithelium are seen diffuse **lymphatic tissue (2), adipose cells (3)**, blood vessels, and **nerves (9)**.

Numerous mucous **acini (4)** of the posterior lingual mucosal glands lie deep in the lamina propria and connective tissue between the **skeletal muscles (5, 10)**. The **excretory ducts (7)** of the lingual glands open onto the dorsal surface of the tongue, usually between bases of the mucosal ridges and folds (1, 6); however, in this figure, the duct opens at the apex of a ridge. Anteriorly, these glands come in contact with the serous glands (von Ebner's) of the circumvallate papilla; posteriorly, the glands extend through the root of the tongue.

Figure 10-6   Lingual Tonsils (transverse section)

The **lingual tonsils** are several aggregations of small, individual tonsils, each with its own **tonsillar crypt (2, 8)**. These tonsils are situated on the dorsal surface of the posterior region of the tongue. A non-keratinized **stratified squamous epithelium (1)** lines the tonsils and their crypts (2, 8), which form deep invaginations of the surface and may extend deep into the **lamina propria (5)**. Numerous **lymphatic nodules (3, 9)**, some with **germinal centers**, are located in the lamina propria (5) below the stratified squamous surface epithelium (1). **Lymphatic infiltration (4, 10)** surrounds the individual lymphatic nodules (3, 9).

Deep in the lamina propria are the fat cells of the **adipose tissue (7)** and the secretory **mucous acini** of the **posterior lingual glands (11)**. Small excretory ducts from the lingual glands (11) unite to form larger **excretory ducts (6)**, most of which open into the tonsillar crypts (2, 8), although some may open on the lingual surface. Interspersed among the connective tissue of the lamina propria (5), adipose tissue (7), and the secretory mucous acini of the posterior ingual glands (11) are fibers of the **skeletal muscles (12)** of the tongue.

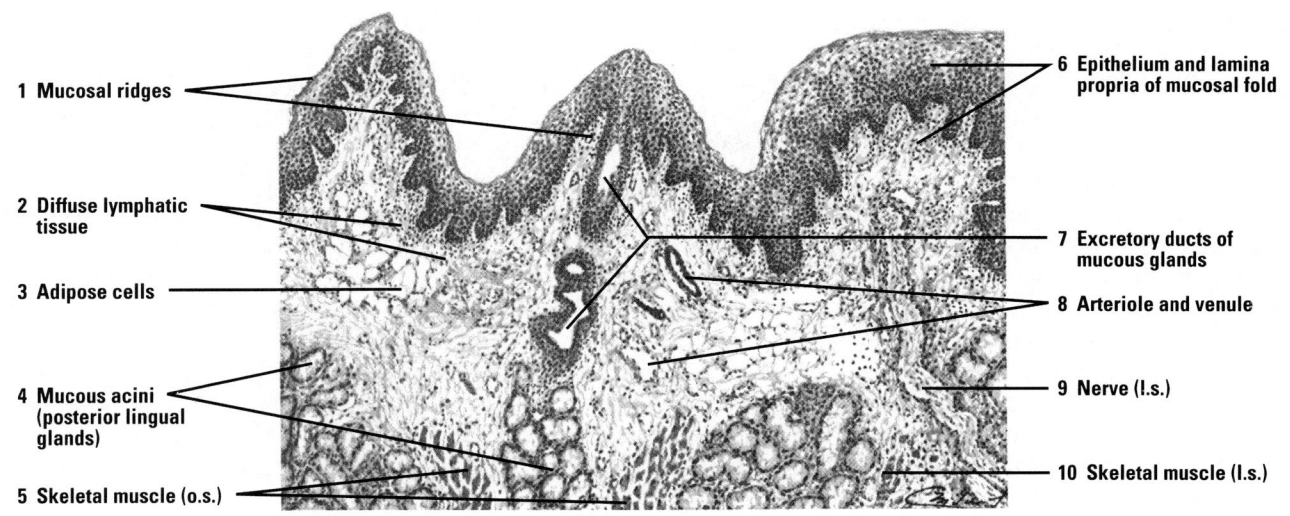

1 Mucosal ridges

2 Diffuse lymphatic tissue

3 Adipose cells

4 Mucous acini (posterior lingual glands)

5 Skeletal muscle (o.s.)

6 Epithelium and lamina propria of mucosal fold

7 Excretory ducts of mucous glands

8 Arteriole and venule

9 Nerve (l.s.)

10 Skeletal muscle (l.s.)

Fig. 10-5   Posterior Tongue Near Circumvallate Papilla (longitudinal section). Stain: hematoxylin-eosin. Low magnification.

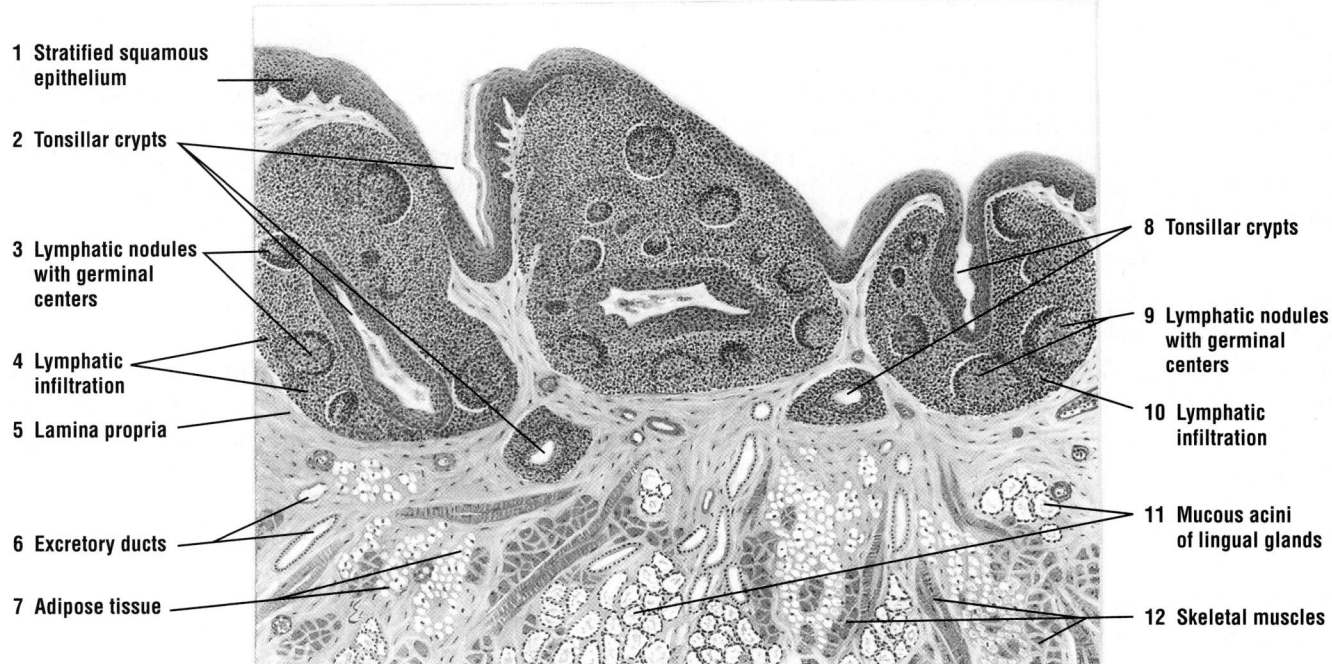

1 Stratified squamous epithelium

2 Tonsillar crypts

3 Lymphatic nodules with germinal centers

4 Lymphatic infiltration

5 Lamina propria

6 Excretory ducts

7 Adipose tissue

8 Tonsillar crypts

9 Lymphatic nodules with germinal centers

10 Lymphatic infiltration

11 Mucous acini of lingual glands

12 Skeletal muscles

Fig. 10-6   Lingual Tonsils (transverse section). Stain: hematoxylin-eosin. Low magnification.

Figure 10-7   Dried Tooth (panoramic view, longitudinal section)

Dentin (3, 5) surrounds the **pulp cavity (4)** and its extension, the **root canal (6).** In life, the pulp cavity and root canal are filled with fine connective tissue, which contains fibroblasts, histiocytes, odontoblasts, blood vessels, and nerves. Dentin (3) exhibits wavy, parallel dentinal tubules. The earlier or primary dentin (3) is located at the periphery of the tooth; the later or secondary dentin (5) lies along the pulp cavity, where it is formed throughout life by odontoblasts. In the crown of a dried tooth and at the junction of dentin with **enamel (1)** are numerous irregular, air-filled spaces that appear black in the section. These are the **interglobular spaces (12)** which, in life, are filled with incompletely calcified dentin (interglobular dentin). Similar areas, but smaller and spaced closer together, are present in the root, close to the dentinal-cementum junction, where they form the **granular layer (of Tomes) (13).**

The dentin in the crown of the tooth is covered with a thicker layer of enamel (1), composed of enamel rods or prisms held together by an interprismatic cementing substance. The incremental **growth lines (of Retzius) (8)** represent the variations in the rate of enamel deposition. Light rays passing through a dried section of the tooth are refracted by twists that occur in the enamel rods as they course toward the surface of the tooth. These are the light **bands of Schreger (9).** At the dentinoenamel junction may be seen **enamel spindles (10)** and **enamel tufts (11);** these are illustrated at a higher magnification in Figure 10-8.

Cementum (7) covers the dentin of the root. In life, cementum contains **lacunae (14)** with cementocytes and canaliculi.

Figure 10-8   Dried Tooth: Layers of the Crown

A section of **enamel (1)** and **dentin (6)** are illustrated at a high magnification. The enamel consists of elongated **enamel rods** or **prisms (1).** In the enamel region, near the junction with dentin **(4),** are the **enamel spindles (2).** These are pointed or spindle-shaped processes of dentin that penetrate the enamel. The **enamel tufts (3),** which are the poorly calcified, twisted enamel rods, extend from the **dentinoenamel junction (4)** into the enamel. Dentin (6) is clearly visible with its dentinal tubules (6) and black, air-filled **interglobular spaces (5).**

Figure 10-9   Dried Tooth: Layers of the Root

Dentin (1) and **cementum (4)** are illustrated at a high magnification. Near the dentinoenamel junction is the **granular layer (of Tomes) (2).** Internal to this layer are the large, irregular **interglobular spaces (3)** which are commonly seen in the crown of the tooth but may also be present in the root. **Cementum (4)** contains **lacunae (5)** with their canaliculi.

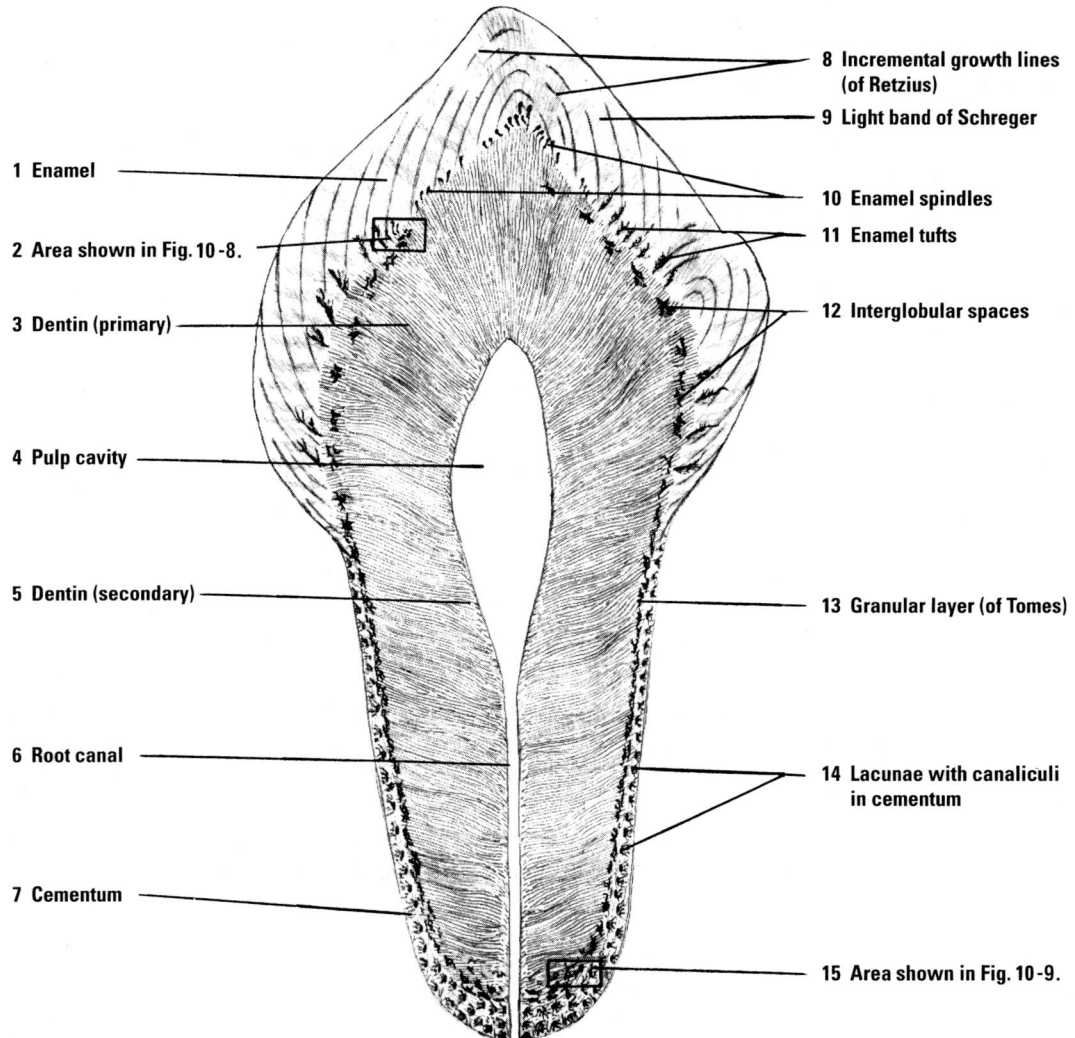

1 Enamel

2 Area shown in Fig. 10-8.

3 Dentin (primary)

4 Pulp cavity

5 Dentin (secondary)

6 Root canal

7 Cementum

8 Incremental growth lines (of Retzius)

9 Light band of Schreger

10 Enamel spindles

11 Enamel tufts

12 Interglobular spaces

13 Granular layer (of Tomes)

14 Lacunae with canaliculi in cementum

15 Area shown in Fig. 10-9.

Fig. 10-7   Dried Tooth (panoramic view, longitudinal section).

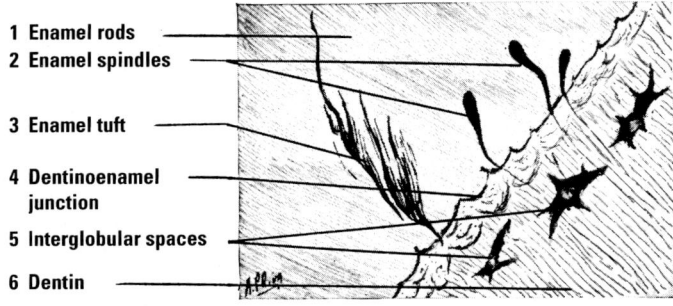

1 Enamel rods
2 Enamel spindles
3 Enamel tuft
4 Dentinoenamel junction
5 Interglobular spaces
6 Dentin

Fig. 10-8   Dried Tooth: Layers of the Crown. Area corresponding to (2) in Fig 10-7. Medium magnification.

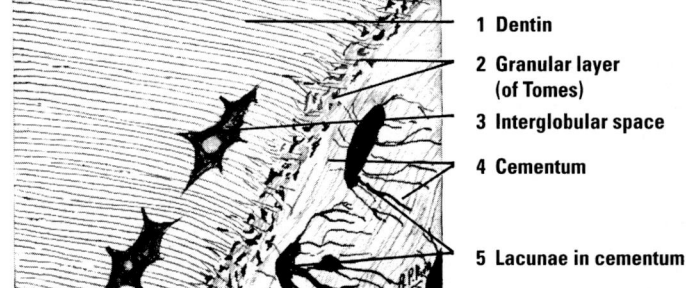

1 Dentin
2 Granular layer (of Tomes)
3 Interglobular space
4 Cementum
5 Lacunae in cementum

Fig. 10-9   Dried Tooth: Layers of the Root. Area corresponding to (15) in Fig 10-7. Medium magnification.

Figure 10-10   Developing Tooth (panoramic view)

A developing deciduous tooth is shown embedded in a socket, the **dental alveolus (22),** in the **bone (4)** of the jaw. A layer of **connective tissue (3)** surrounds the developing tooth and forms a compact layer around the tooth, the **dental sac (5).** Enclosed within the sac is the enamel organ. It is composed of the **external enamel epithelium (18),** the **stellate reticulum** of **enamel pulp (6, 19),** the **intermediate stratum (20),** and the **ameloblasts** or **inner enamel epithelium (7).** All of these structures differentiate from the downgrowth of the **gum epithelium (1).** The ameloblasts secrete enamel around the **dentin (9, 16).** The **enamel (8, 15)** appears as a narrow band of deep-staining pink material.

The **dental pulp (21)** originates from the primitive connective tissue and forms the core of the developing tooth. Blood vessels and nerves extend into and innervate the dental pulp from below. The mesenchymal cells in the dental papilla differentiate into **odontoblasts (11)** and form the outer margin of the dental pulp (21). The odontoblasts (11) secrete **predentin (10, 17),** which is an uncalcified dentin. As predentin calcifies (10, 17), it forms a layer of dentin (9, 16) adjacent to enamel (8, 15).

The **oral mucosa (1, 13)** covers the developing tooth. An epithelial downgrowth from the oral epithelium indicates the **germ of a permanent tooth (2).** At the base of the tooth, the outer and inner enamel epithelium form the **epithelial root sheath (of Hertwig) (12).**

Figure 10-11   Developing Tooth (sectional view)

The left side of the figure shows a small area of dental pulp, fibroblasts (1), and fine fibers, illustrated at a higher magnification. The **odontoblasts (2)** are located at the margin of the pulp and secrete the **uncalcified predentin (3),** which later calcifies as **dentin (4).** The odontoblasts (2) remain in the predentin and dentin as the **odontoblast processes (of Tomes) (3).**

On the right side of the figure is a small area of **stellate reticulum (7)** of enamel. Seen here are the processes of its modified epithelial cells, the **intermediate stratum (8),** a transition region, and the tall columnar **ameloblasts (6)** that secrete the **enamel (5, 10)** in the form of enamel rods or prisms. During enamel (5, 10) formation, the apical ends of ameloblast become transformed into a terminal processes of Tomes. In advanced enamel formation, these processes appear as a separate layer of **enamel processes (of Tomes) (9).**

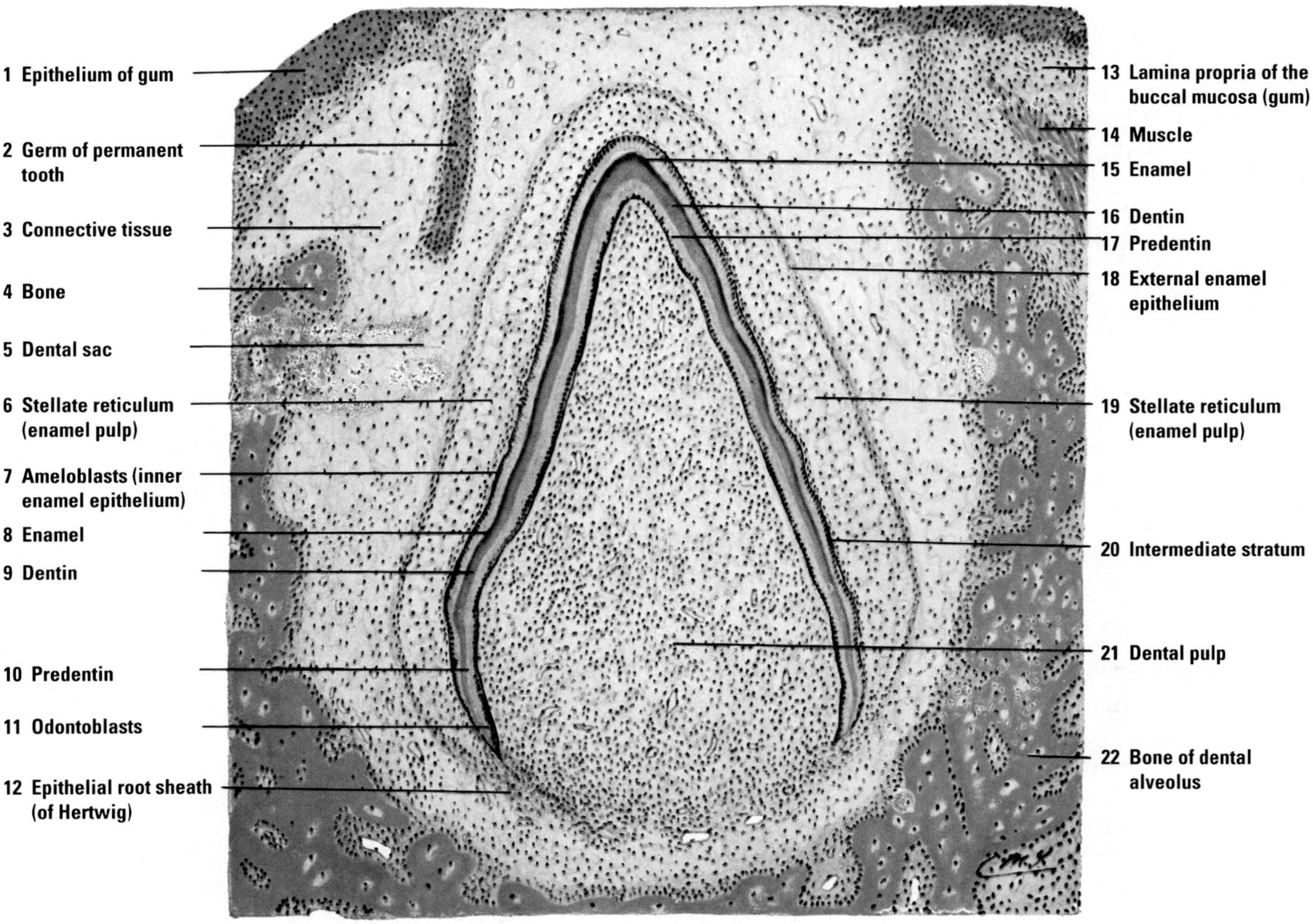

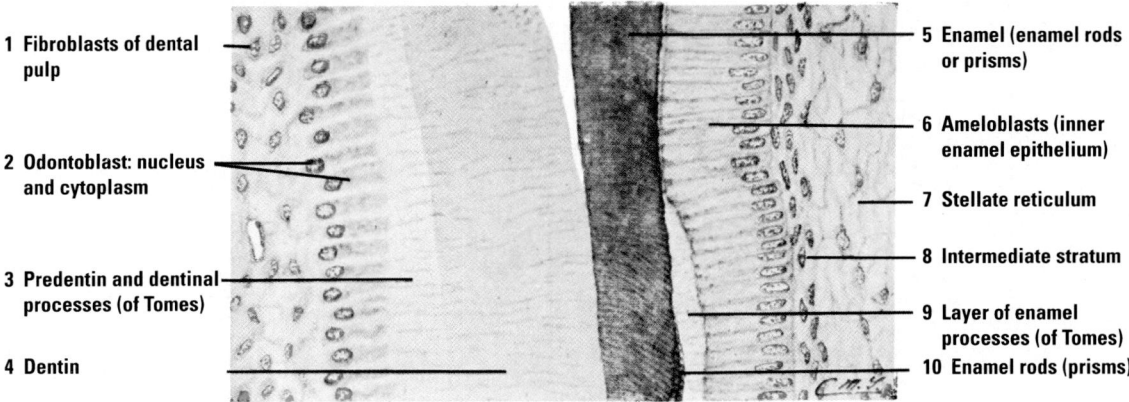

1 Epithelium of gum

2 Germ of permanent tooth

3 Connective tissue

4 Bone

5 Dental sac

6 Stellate reticulum (enamel pulp)

7 Ameloblasts (inner enamel epithelium)

8 Enamel

9 Dentin

10 Predentin

11 Odontoblasts

12 Epithelial root sheath (of Hertwig)

13 Lamina propria of the buccal mucosa (gum)

14 Muscle

15 Enamel

16 Dentin

17 Predentin

18 External enamel epithelium

19 Stellate reticulum (enamel pulp)

20 Intermediate stratum

21 Dental pulp

22 Bone of dental alveolus

Fig. 10-10   Developing Tooth (panoramic view). Stain: hematoxylin-eosin. Low magnification.

1 Fibroblasts of dental pulp

2 Odontoblast: nucleus and cytoplasm

3 Predentin and dentinal processes (of Tomes)

4 Dentin

5 Enamel (enamel rods or prisms)

6 Ameloblasts (inner enamel epithelium)

7 Stellate reticulum

8 Intermediate stratum

9 Layer of enamel processes (of Tomes)

10 Enamel rods (prisms)

Fig. 10-11   Developing Tooth (sectional view). Stain: hematoxylin-eosin. High magnification.

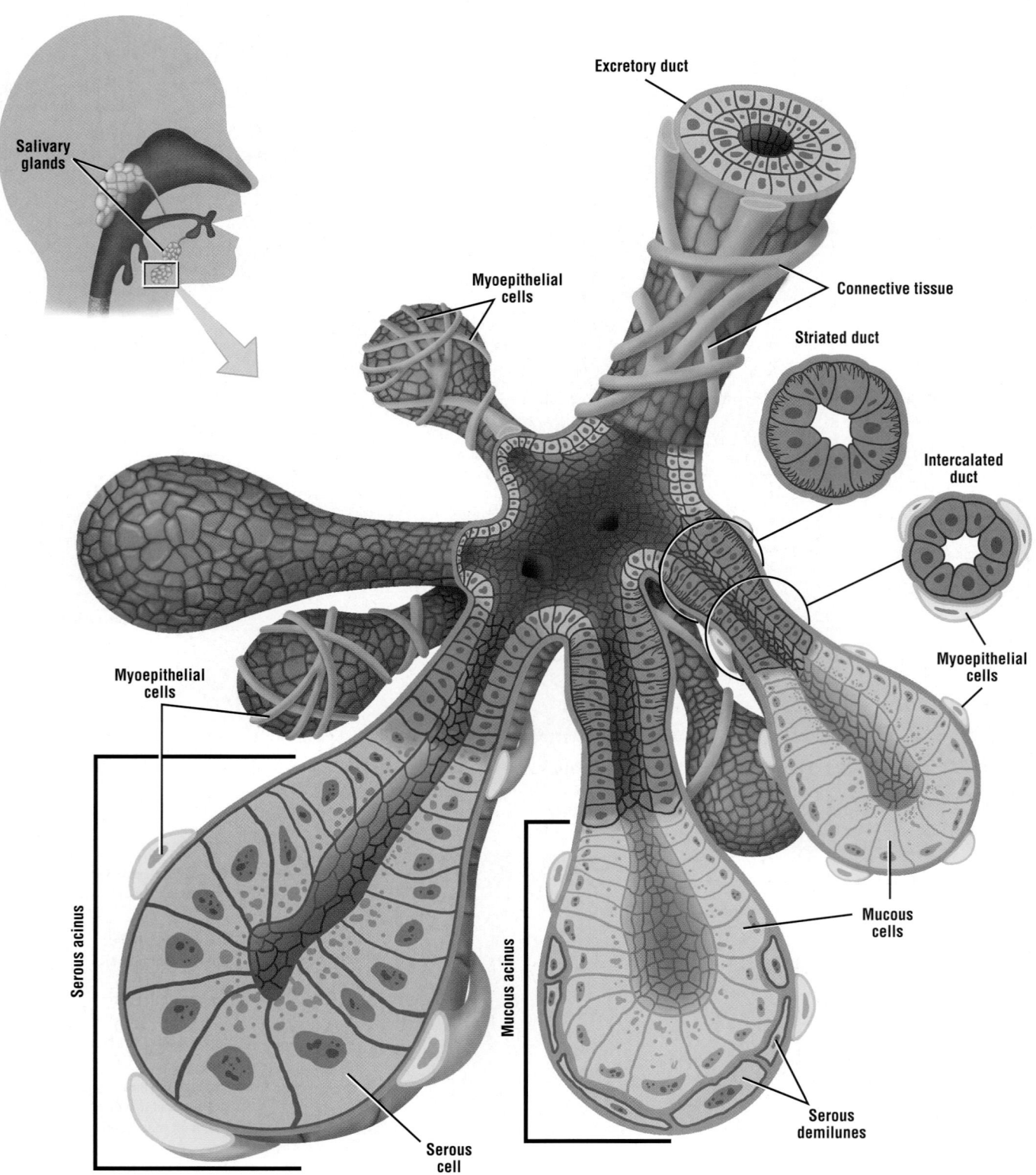

Salivary glands

Excretory duct

Connective tissue

Myoepithelial cells

Striated duct

Intercalated duct

Myoepithelial cells

Myoepithelial cells

Mucous cells

Serous acinus

Mucous acinus

Serous cell

Serous demilunes

THE MAJOR SALIVARY GLANDS (FIGS. 10-12–10-14, 10-16, 10-17)

There are three major **salivary glands,** the parotid, submandibular, and sublingual. The salivary glands are located outside of the oral cavity and convey their secretions into the mouth via large **excretory ducts.** The paired **parotid glands** are the largest of the salivary glands. These glands are located in front and below the external ear. The smaller, paired **submandibular (submaxillary) glands** are located inferior to the mandible in the floor of the mouth. The smallest of the salivary glands are the **sublingual glands,** which are aggregates of smaller glands that are located inferior to the tongue.

The salivary glands are composed of common cellular **secretory units** called **acini** (singular-acinus) and numerous **excretory ducts.** The secretory units are small, sac-like dilations located at the end of the first segment of the duct system, the **intercalated ducts.** The cells that comprise the secretory acini are of two types, **serous** and **mucous.** The serous cells exhibit round nuclei and secretory granules in their cytoplasm. The mucous cells are light staining and filled with the secretory product mucus. As a result, their nuclei are flattened and located at base of the cytoplasm.

Both the secretory cells and their intercalated ducts are surrounded by a **basal lamina** and by the finger-like processes of the contractile **myoepithelial (basket) cells,** respectively. Fibers of the connective tissue subdivide the salivary glands into numerous **lobules,** which contain the secretory units and their excretory ducts. Several intercalated ducts merge to form the larger **striated ducts,** which in turn join to form **excretory intralobular ducts** of gradually increasing size. These are surrounded by increased layers of connective tissue fibers. Intralobular ducts join to form **interlobular ducts, interlobar duct,** and the terminal portion of these large ducts conveys saliva from the salivary glands to the oral cavity.

Figure 10-12   Salivary Gland: Parotid

The parotid salivary gland is a large serous gland, classified as a compound tubuloacinar gland (Fig. 1-14). In this illustration, a section of the parotid gland is depicted at lower magnification, while the specific features of the gland are presented at a higher magnification in separate boxes below.

The parotid gland is surrounded by a connective tissue capsule from which arise numerous **septa (2, 8)** that subdivide the gland into several lobes and lobules. Located in the connective tissue septa (2, 8) between the lobules are small **arterioles (12), venules (13), interlobular excretory ducts (1, 4, 9, IV)** and numerous **adipose cells (3).**

Each lobule consists of closely packed masses of secretory cells, the **serous acini (5, 10, 16, I).** These acini (I) consist of pyramid-shaped cells arranged around a small lumen. The spherical nuclei of these cells are located at the base of the slightly basophilic cytoplasm. In certain sections, the lumen is not always visible in all acini. At a higher magnification, small **secretory granules (15, I)** are visible in the cell apices. The number of secretory granules in these cells varies with the functional activity of the gland. The serous acini (5, 10, 16, I) are also surrounded by thin, contractile **myoepithelial cells (14, I),** located between the basement membrane and the serous cells; usually, only their nuclei are visible.

The secretory acini empty their product into narrow channels, the **intercalated ducts (6, 11, II).** These ducts have small lumina, are lined by a simple squamous or low cuboidal epithelium, and are often surrounded by myoepithelial cells (see Fig. 10-13:23, III). The secretory product from the intercalated ducts drains into larger **striated ducts (7, III).** These ducts have larger lumina and are lined by simple columnar cells that exhibit **basal striations (17, III);** the striations are formed by deep infolding of the basal cell membrane.

The striated ducts empty their product into the **interlobular excretory ducts (1, 4, 9, IV)** that are located in the connective tissue septa (2, 8). Their lumina become progressively wider and the epithelium taller as the ducts increase in size. The ductal epithelium (IV) varies from columnar to pseudostratified or stratified columnar in large excretory (lobar) ducts that drain the lobes of the parotid gland.

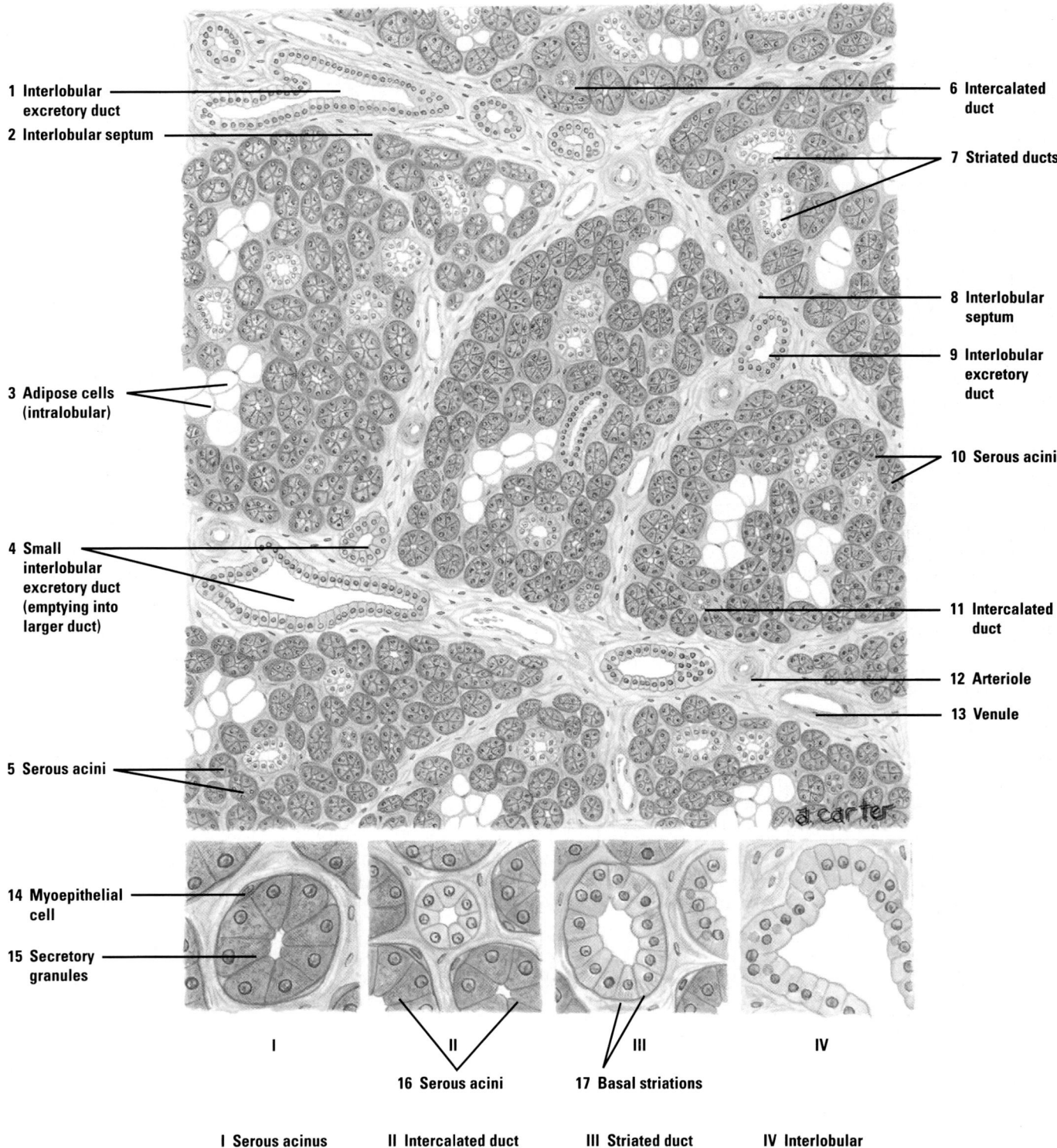

1 Interlobular excretory duct
2 Interlobular septum
3 Adipose cells (intralobular)
4 Small interlobular excretory duct (emptying into larger duct)
5 Serous acini

6 Intercalated duct
7 Striated ducts
8 Interlobular septum
9 Interlobular excretory duct
10 Serous acini
11 Intercalated duct
12 Arteriole
13 Venule

14 Myoepithelial cell
15 Secretory granules

16 Serous acini
17 Basal striations

I   Serous acinus   II   Intercalated duct   III   Striated duct   IV   Interlobular excretory duct

Fig. 10-12   Salivary Gland: Parotid. Stain: hematoxylin-eosin. Upper: medium magnification. Lower: high magnification.

Figure 10-13   Salivary Gland: Submandibular

Like the parotid salivary gland, the submandibular is also a compound tubuloacinar gland. The submandibular gland, however, is a mixed type, being composed predominantly of serous acini. The presence of serous and mucous acini distinguishes the submandibular gland from the parotid gland, which is a purely serous gland. This low-power illustration depicts portions of several lobules of the submandibular gland in which a few **mucous acini (6, 11, 14)** are intermixed with **serous acini (7, 18).** The more detailed features of the gland are illustrated at higher magnification in separate boxes below.

The **serous acini (7, 18, I)** are similar to those observed in the parotid gland (Fig. 10-12). These acini are characterized by smaller size, darker-stained pyramidal cells, spherical nucleus located basally, and **secretory granules (20)** in the cell apices, visible at higher magnification (I). The **mucous acini (6, 11, 14, II)** are larger than the serous acini (7, 18, I) and are more variable in their size and shape. The mucous cells are more columnar and exhibit pale or almost colorless cytoplasm after routine histologic staining. Their **nuclei (II)** are flattened and pressed against the base of the cell membrane. The mucous acini also have a somewhat larger and more apparent lumina.

The mixed acini (serous and mucous) are normally mucous acini surrounded or capped by one or more groups of serous cells, forming a crescent-shaped **serous demilune (8, 12).** The thin, contractile **myoepithelial cells (21, 22, 23)** surround the serous (I), mucous (II), and intercalated duct cells (III).

The duct system of the submandibular gland is similar to that of the parotid gland. The intralobular **intercalated ducts (9, 13, 15, 19, III)** have small lumina and are shorter while the **striated ducts (5, 16, IV)** are longer than in the parotid gland. Illustrated is a **mucous acinus (14)** that opens into an **intercalated duct (15),** which then opens into a larger **striated duct (16).** Numerous **interlobular excretory ducts (3, 17)** of different sizes are located in the interlobular connective tissue **septa (4).** These septa (4) penetrate and divide the gland into lobes and lobules. Also located in the connective tissue septa (4) are nerves and numerous, different-sized **arterioles (1)** and **venules (2).** Numerous **adipose cells (10)** are seen scattered among the various acini and in the connective tissue septa.

■ Functional Correlations–Salivary Glands and Saliva

The salivary glands produce a watery secretion called **saliva,** which enters the oral cavity via different excretory ducts. The **myoepithelial cells,** which surround the secretory acini and the intercalated ducts, contract and assist in expelling the secretory products from these structures. Saliva is a mixture of secretions produced by all of the different salivary glands. Although the major composition of saliva is **water,** it also contains ions, mucus, enzymes, and immunoglobulins. The sight, smell, thought, taste, or the actual presence of food in the mouth cause an **autonomic** increase of saliva secretion from the salivary glands and its release into the oral cavity.

Saliva performs numerous important functions in the oral cavity. It moistens the chewed food and lubricates the bolus to facilitate swallowing and passage of the food through the esophagus toward the stomach. Saliva also contains numerous **electrolytes** (calcium, potassium, sodium, chloride, bicarbonate ions, and others). The digestive enzyme **amylase** is produced mainly by the **serous acini** of the salivary glands and is found in the saliva. This salivary enzyme initiates the breakdown of starch into smaller carbohydrates during the short time that the food is present in the oral cavity.

Saliva also controls **bacterial flora** in the mouth and protects the oral cavity against pathogens. The salivary enzyme **lysozyme,** secreted also by the serous cells, hydrolyzes the cell walls of bacteria and inhibits their growth in the oral cavity. Also, the **immunoglobulins** in saliva, primarily the IgA produced by the **plasma cells** in the connective tissue of the glands, assist in immunological defense against bacteria found in the mouth.

As the saliva flows through the duct systems of the salivary glands, the **striated ducts** modify the ionic content by selective transport of material to and from the saliva. Sodium and chloride ions are actively reabsorbed from the fluid in the lumen while potassium and bicarbonate ions are added to the salivary secretions.

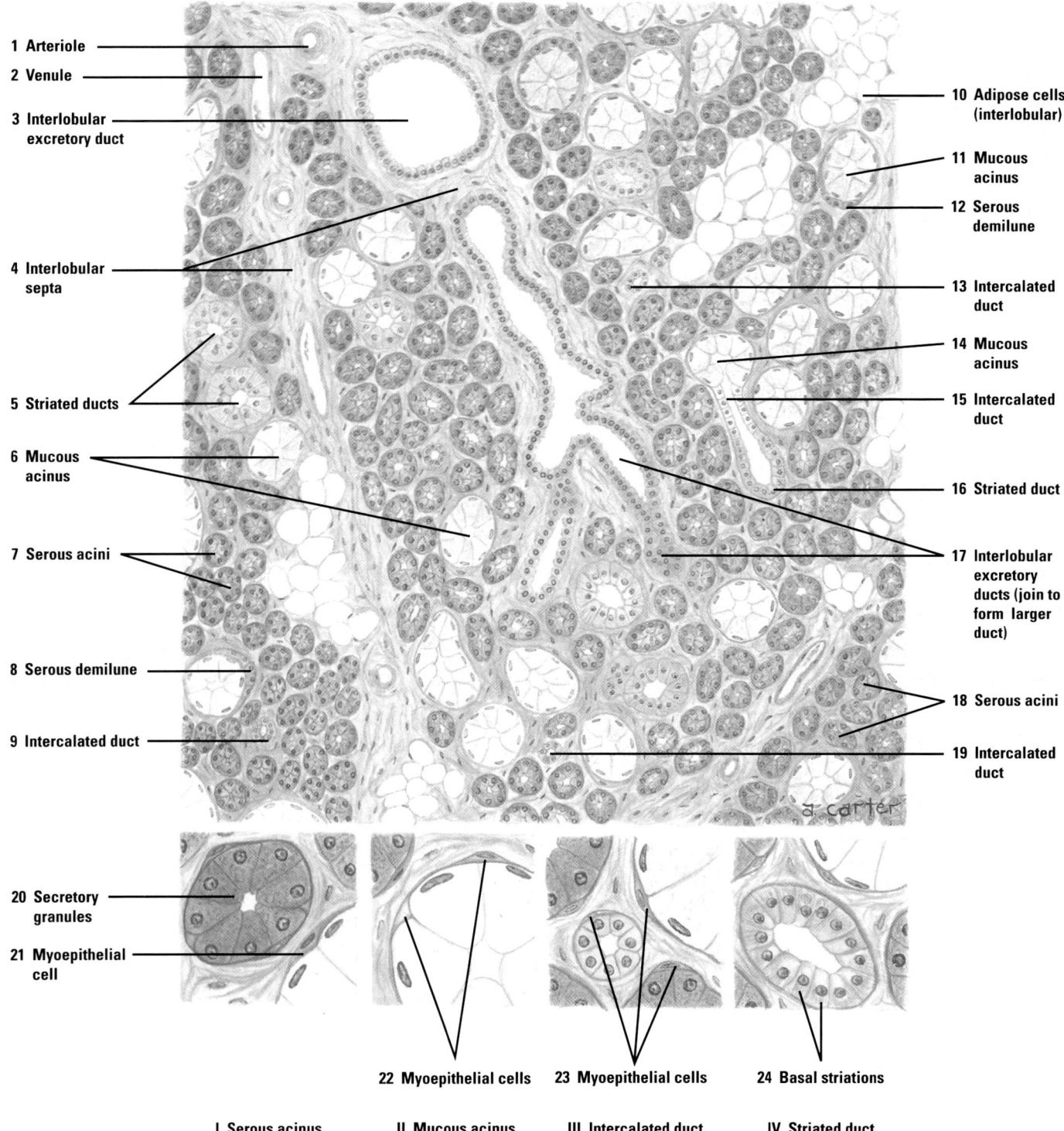

1 Arteriole

2 Venule

3 Interlobular excretory duct

4 Interlobular septa

5 Striated ducts

6 Mucous acinus

7 Serous acini

8 Serous demilune

9 Intercalated duct

10 Adipose cells (interlobular)

11 Mucous acinus

12 Serous demilune

13 Intercalated duct

14 Mucous acinus

15 Intercalated duct

16 Striated duct

17 Interlobular excretory ducts (join to form larger duct)

18 Serous acini

19 Intercalated duct

20 Secretory granules

21 Myoepithelial cell

22 Myoepithelial cells

23 Myoepithelial cells

24 Basal striations

I Serous acinus   II Mucous acinus   III Intercalated duct   IV Striated duct

Fig. 10-13   Salivary Gland: Submandibular. Stain: hematoxylin-eosin. Upper: medium magnification. Lower: high magnification.

Figure 10-14   Salivary Gland: Sublingual

The sublingual gland is a compound mixed tubuloacinar gland. This gland resembles the submandibular gland because it is composed of both serous and mucous acini. Most of the secretory acini, however, are **mucous (5, 15, I, II)** and mucous acini capped with **serous demilunes (9, 14, 18, 19, II, III).** The light-stained mucous acini (5, 15, I, II) are conspicuous in this section. Purely serous acini are scarce; however, the composition of the gland is variable. In this low-magnification illustration, **serous acini (3, 16)** appear frequently, whereas in other sections of the sublingual gland such serous acini may be absent. At higher magnification, the **myoepithelial cells (17, I)** are seen around individual acini.

In comparison to other salivary glands, the duct system is somewhat different. Typical **intercalated ducts (2, 10, III)** are infrequent or are absent. In the sublingual gland, the intercalated ducts (2, 10, III) are short and are not readily observed in a given section. The nonstriated **intralobular excretory ducts (4, 6, IV)** are more prevalent in the sublingual glands. These ducts are equivalent to the striated ducts of the submandibular and parotid glands, but lack the extensive basal striations.

The interlobular connective tissue **septa (13)** are more abundant in the sublingual than in the parotid and submandibular glands. Numerous **arterioles (12), venules (8),** nerve fibers, and **interlobular excretory ducts (1, 11)** are seen in the septa. The epithelial lining of the interlobular excretory ducts (1, 11) varies from low columnar in the smaller ducts to pseudostratified or stratified columnar in the larger ducts.

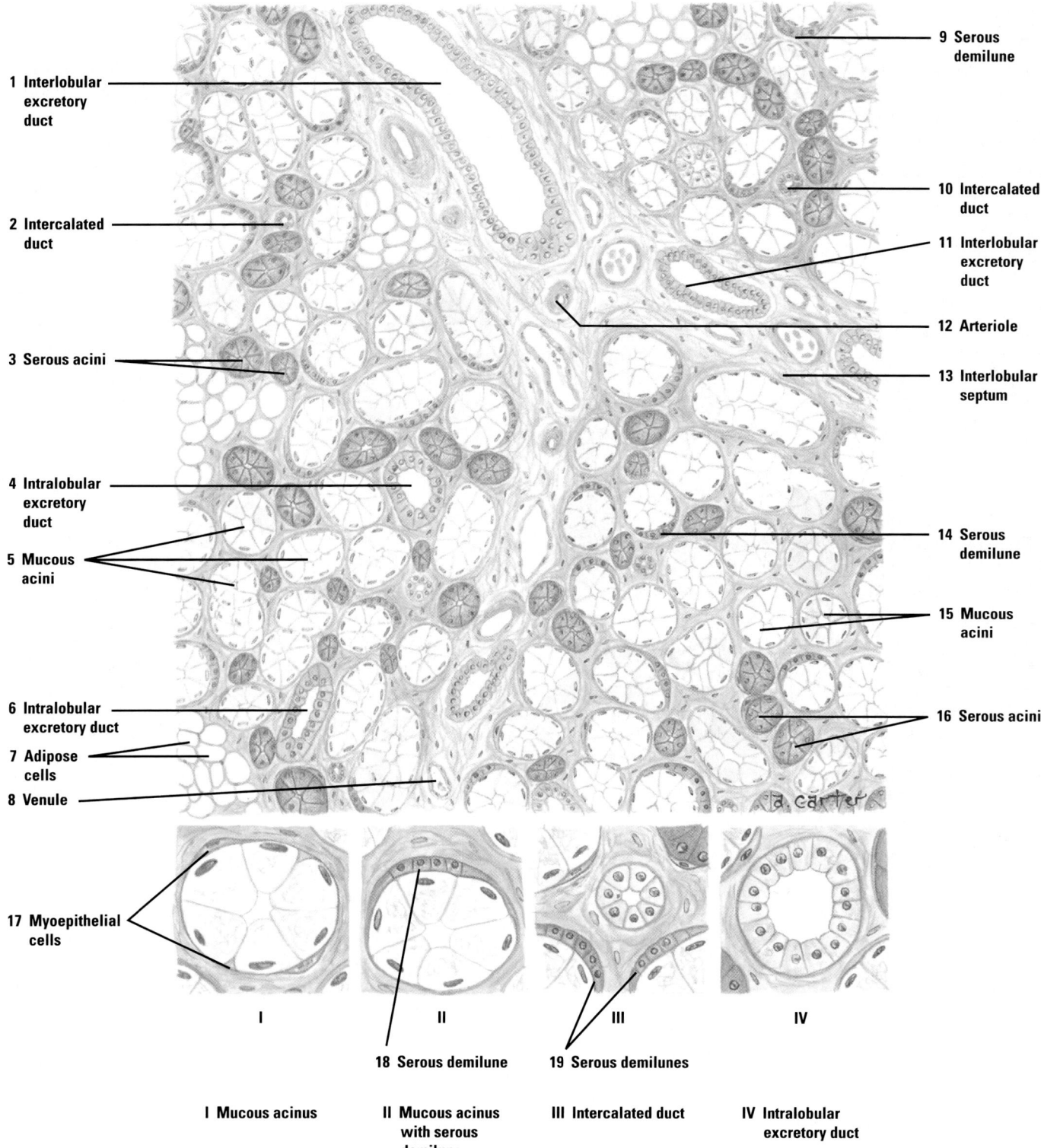

1 Interlobular excretory duct

2 Intercalated duct

3 Serous acini

4 Intralobular excretory duct

5 Mucous acini

6 Intralobular excretory duct

7 Adipose cells

8 Venule

9 Serous demilune

10 Intercalated duct

11 Interlobular excretory duct

12 Arteriole

13 Interlobular septum

14 Serous demilune

15 Mucous acini

16 Serous acini

17 Myoepithelial cells

I

II

III

IV

18 Serous demilune

19 Serous demilunes

I Mucous acinus

II Mucous acinus with serous demilune

III Intercalated duct

IV Intralobular excretory duct

Fig. 10-14   Salivary Gland: Sublingual. Stain: hematoxylin-eosin. Upper: medium magnification. Lower: high magnification.

Figure 10-15   Tongue: Filiform and Fungiform Papillae

A low power photomicrograph shows a dorsal section of the tongue. In the center of the photograph is a large **fungiform papilla (2).** Its surface epithelium is covered by **stratified squamous epithelium (3)** that is not cornfield or keratinized. The fungiform papilla (2) also exhibits numerous **taste buds (4)** that are located in the epithelium on the dorsal surface. An underlying connective tissue core, the **lamina propria (5),** projects into the surface epithelium of the fungiform papilla (2) to form numerous indentations. Surrounding the fungiform papilla (2) are the slender **filiform papillae (1),** whose conical tips are covered by stratified squamous epithelium that exhibits partial keratinization.

Figure 10-16   Serous Salivary Gland: Parotid Gland

This photomicrograph illustrates a section of the parotid salivary gland. In humans, this salivary gland is entirely composed of **serous acini (1)** and the excretory ducts. In this illustration, the cytoplasm of the serous cells is filled with tiny secretory granules. A small **intercalated duct (2)** with its cuboidal epithelium is surrounded by the serous acini (1). Also visible on the right side of the illustration is a larger, lighter stained excretory duct, the **striated duct (3).**

Figure 10-17   Mixed Salivary Gland: Sublingual Gland

The sublingual salivary gland is a mixed gland and exhibits both the **mucous acini (2)** and **serous acini (3).** The mucous acini (2) are larger and lighter staining than the serous acini (3), and their cytoplasm is filled with the secretory product **mucus (1).** The serous acini (3) are darker staining with tiny secretory granules in their cytoplasm. The serous acini (3) that surround the mucous acini (2) form crescent-shaped structures called **serous demilunes (4).** Between the secretory acini are visible a tiny excretory **intercalated duct (5)** lined by cuboidal epithelium and the larger **striated duct (6),** whose lining epithelium appears columnar.

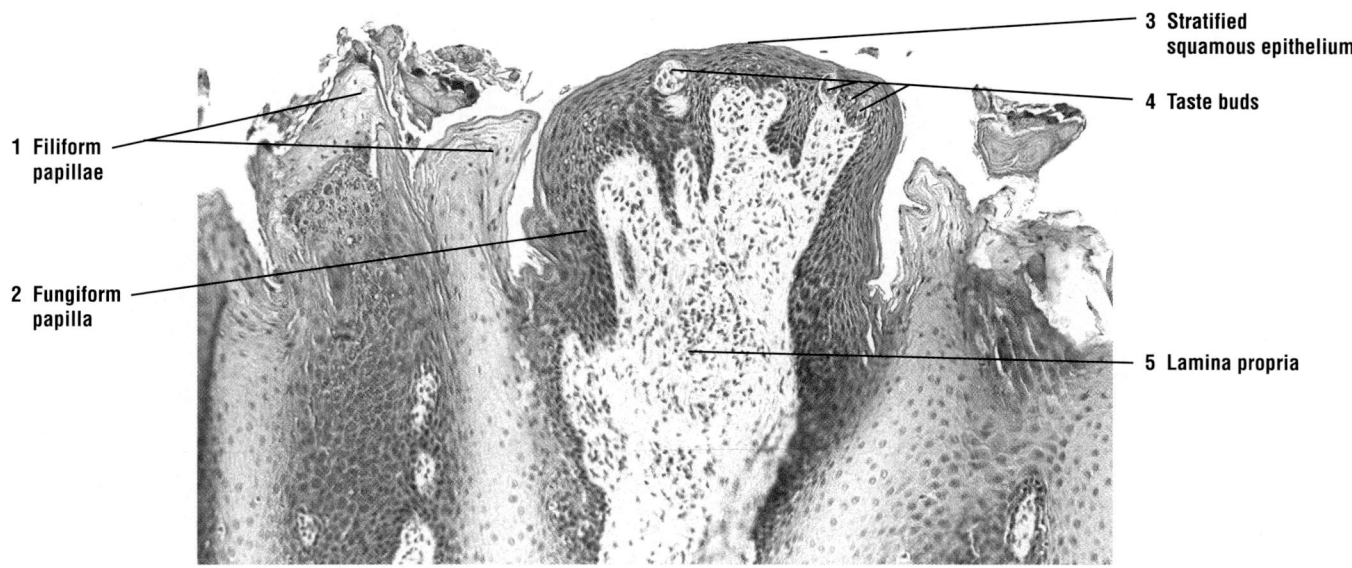

Fig. 10-15   Tongue: Filiform and Fungiform Papillae. Stain: hematoxylin-eosin. 25×

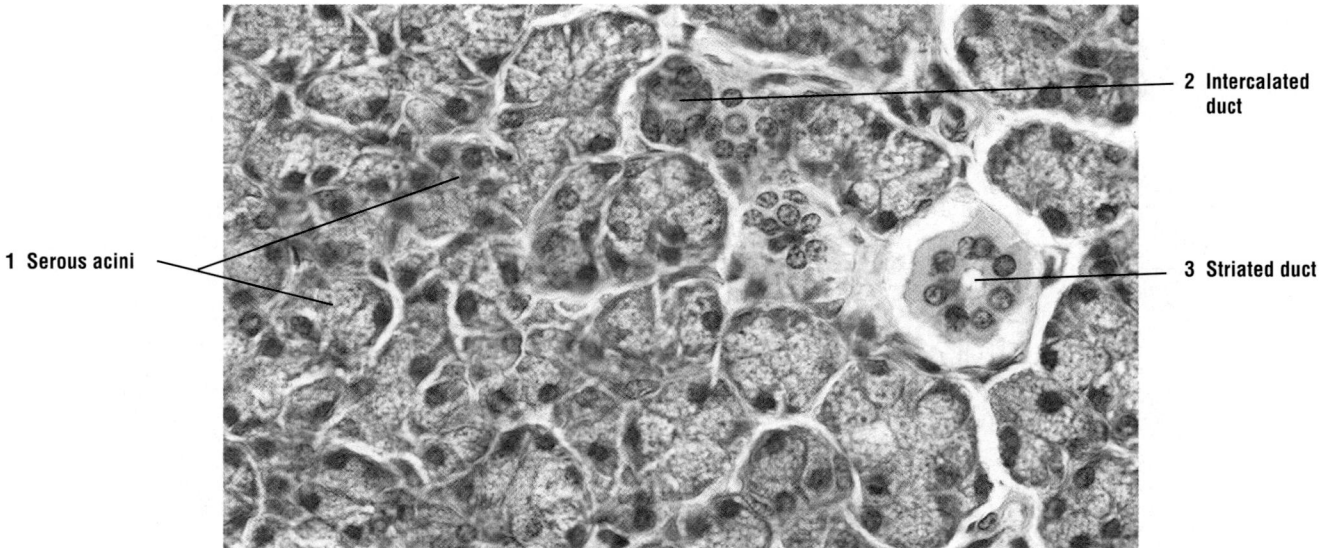

Fig. 10-16   Serous Salivary Gland: Parotid Gland. Stain: hematoxylin-eosin. 165×

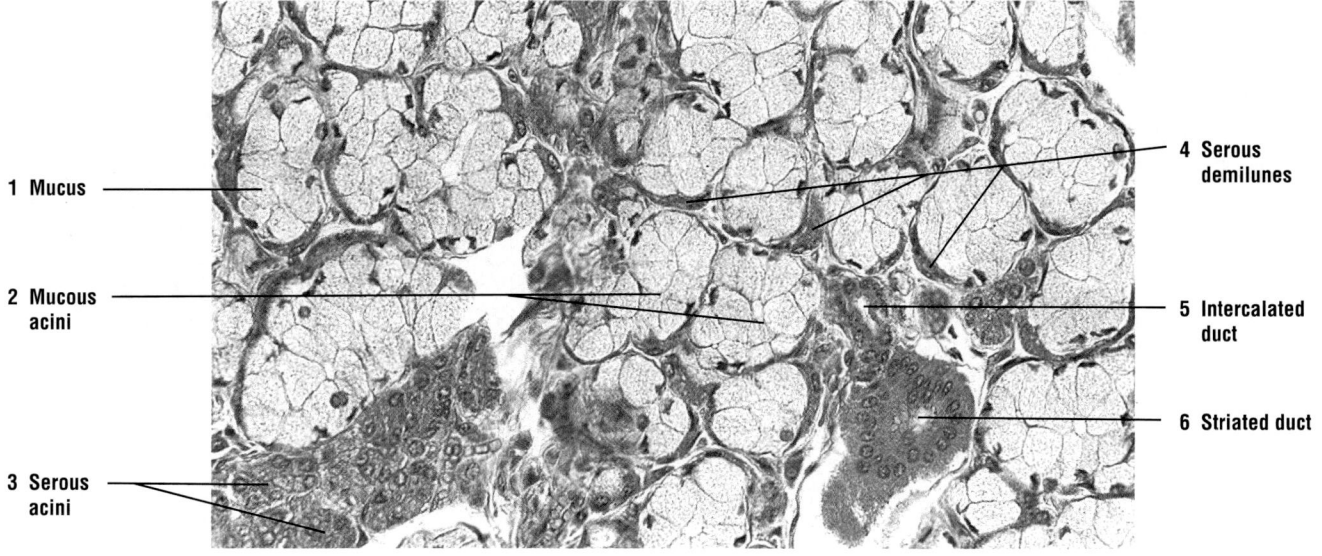

Fig. 10-17   Mixed Salivary Gland: Sublingual Gland. Stain: hematoxylin-eosin. 165×

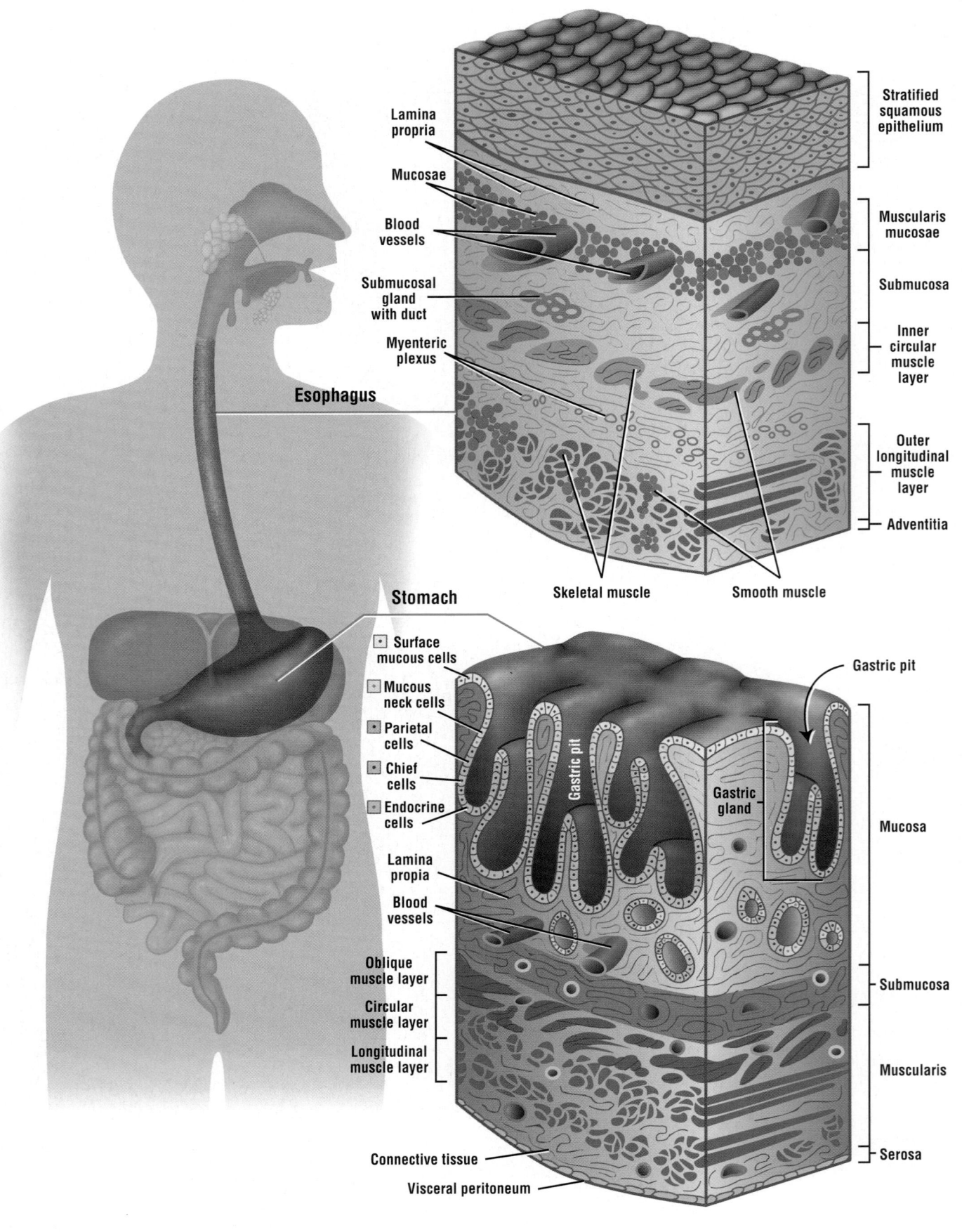

Esophagus

Lamina propria

Mucosae

Blood vessels

Submucosal gland with duct

Myenteric plexus

Stratified squamous epithelium

Muscularis mucosae

Submucosa

Inner circular muscle layer

Outer longitudinal muscle layer

Adventitia

Skeletal muscle

Smooth muscle

Stomach

Surface mucous cells

Mucous neck cells

Parietal cells

Chief cells

Endocrine cells

Lamina propria

Blood vessels

Oblique muscle layer

Circular muscle layer

Longitudinal muscle layer

Connective tissue

Visceral peritoneum

Gastric pit

Gastric pit

Gastric gland

Mucosa

Submucosa

Muscularis

Serosa

Digestive System: Esophagus and Stomach

GENERAL PLAN

The digestive tube or tract is a long hollow structure that extends from the esophagus to the rectum. The wall of the tube exhibits four common layers: **mucosa, submucosa, muscularis externa,** and **serosa.** Where the digestive tube is retroperitoneal, the outermost layer consists of connective tissue called the **adventitia.** The four layers of the digestive tube, however, show obvious histologic variations. This variation depends on the location of the digestive tube and the specific function that it performs during digestive process. The characteristic features of each layer in the digestive tube and its function are discussed with each illustration of the different digestive organ.

THE ESOPHAGUS

The **esophagus** is a long, soft tube approximately 10 inches long that extends from the **pharynx** to the **stomach.** It is located posterior to the trachea and most of it found in the mediastinum of the **thoracic cavity.** The esophagus penetrates the muscular **diaphragm,** and a short section of the organ enters the abdominal cavity before it terminates at the **stomach.** In the thoracic cavity, the esophagus is surrounded by the connective tissue **adventitia.** In the abdominal cavity, a simple squamous epithelium, the **mesothelium,** surrounds the esophagus to form the **serosa.** The esophageal lumen is lined with **nonkeratinized stratified squamous epithelium.** When empty, the lumen exhibits numerous but temporary **longitudinal folds** of the mucosa. Also, the outer wall of the esophagus contains either **skeletal muscles** (upper third of esophagus), mixed **skeletal** and **smooth muscles** (middle region of esophagus), or **smooth muscles** (lower third of esophagus) **(Figs. 11-1–11-4, 11-12, 11-13).**

STOMACH

The **stomach** is an expanded hollow organ situated between the **esophagus** and **small intestine.** At the esophageal–stomach junction, an abrupt transition occurs from the stratified squamous epithelia of the esophagus to **simple columnar** of the stomach **(Figs. 11-5, 11-13).** Also, the luminal surface of the stomach is pitted with numerous tiny openings called **gastric pits.** These are formed by the the luminal epithelium that invaginates the underlying connective tissue **lamina propria** of the **mucosa.** The tubular **gastric glands** are located below and open directly into the gastric pits to deliver their contents into the stomach lumen. The gastric pits extend through the lamina propria to the **muscularis mucosae (Figs. 11-5–11-8, 11-14).**

Below the mucosa of the stomach is the dense connective tissue **submucosa,** in which are found large blood vessels and nerves of the stomach. The thick muscular wall of the stomach, the **muscularis externa,** consists of three muscle layers, instead of the two layers that are normally seen in the esophagus and the small intestine. The outer layer of the stomach is covered by **serosa** or visceral peritoneum **(Fig. 11-6).**

Anatomically, the stomach is divided into small **cardia,** where the esophagus terminates, an upper dome-shaped **fundus,** a lower **body** or **corpus,** and a **pylorus.** The fundus and the body comprise about two-thirds of the stomach and have identical histology. As a result, the stomach has only three distinct histologic regions. The fundus and body form the major portions of the stomach. Their mucosa consists of deep **gastric glands** that produce most of the **gastric secretions** or juices for digestion. Also, all stomach regions exhibit **rugae,** the longitudinal folds of the mucosa and submucosa. These folds are temporary and disappear when the stomach is distended with fluid or solid material.

GASTRIC GLANDS AND THEIR CELL TYPES

The **cardia** and **pylorus** are located at the opposite ends of the stomach. The cardia surrounds the entrance of the esophagus into the stomach. The pylorus is the most inferior region in the stomach and it terminates at the border of the duodenum of the small intestine. In the cardia, the gastric pits are shallow, whereas in the pylorus, the gastric pits are deep. However, the gastric glands in these two regions have similar histology and their cells are predominantly **mucus-secreting (Figs. 11-5, 11-10, 11-13).** In contrast, the gastric glands in the fundus and body of the stomach are composed of three major cell types. Located in the upper region of the gastric glands near the gastric pits are the **mucous neck cells (Figs. 11-7, 11-8, 11-14).** Also, the large polygonal cells with distinctive eosinophilic cytoplasm that are located primarily in the upper half of the gastric glands and squeezed between other cells are the **parietal cells.** Located predominantly in the lower region of these gastric glands are basophilic cuboidal cells, the **chief (zymogenic) cells (Figs. 11-6–11-9, 11-14)**

ENTEROENDOCRINE (APUD) CELLS OF THE DIGESTIVE TRACT

In addition to the cells in the different gastric glands described above, the mucosa of the digestive tract also contains a wide distribution of **enteroendocrine (endocrine)** or **APUD (amine precursor uptake and decarboxylation) cells.** Unless the sections are prepared with special staining techniques, these cells are poorly seen in histologic sections.

Figure 11-1   Upper Esophagus: Wall (transverse section)

The esophagus is a long, hollow tube whose wall is composed of the mucosa, submucosa, muscularis externa, and adventitia.

The **mucosa (1, 2, 3)** consists of an inner lining of nonkeratinized **stratified squamous epithelium (1);** an underlying thin layer of fine connective tissue, the **lamina propria (2);** and a layer of longitudinal smooth muscle fibers, the **muscularis mucosae (3),** illustrated in either cross sections or oblique sections. The connective tissue papillae in the lamina propria indent the epithelium. The lamina propria (2) contains small blood vessels, diffuse lymphatic tissue, and a small **lymphatic nodule (9).**

The **submucosa (4)** is a wide layer of moderately dense, irregular connective tissue that often contains **adipose cells (14).** The **esophageal glands proper (11)** are present in the submucosa at intervals throughout the length of the esophagus. These are the tubuloacinar mucous glands, and their excretory **ducts (12)** pass through the **muscularis mucosae (3, 10)** and the lamina propria (2) and then open into the esophageal lumen. The ductal epithelium merges with stratified squamous surface epithelium of the esophagus (see Fig. 11-2). Large **blood vessels (13)** are present in the connective tissue of the submucosa (4).

Located beneath the submucosa (4) is the **muscularis externa (5, 6, 7),** composed of two well-defined muscle layers. The inner muscle layer is **circular (5)** and, in this transverse section of the esophagus, sectioned longitudinally. The outer muscle layer is **longitudinal (7),** and the muscle fibers are seen mainly in transverse sections. A thin layer of **connective tissue (6)** lies between the two muscle layers.

The muscularis externa of the esophagus is highly variable in different species. In humans, the muscularis externa in the upper third of the esophagus consists primarily of striated skeletal muscles. In the middle third, both layers exhibit a mixture of smooth muscle; in the lower third of the esophagus, only smooth muscle is found.

The **adventitia (8)** of the esophagus consists of a loose connective tissue layer that blends with the adventitia of the trachea and the surrounding structures. **Adipose tissue (16),** large **blood vessels (17, 18),** and **nerves (19)** forming the neurovascular bundles are present in the adventitia.

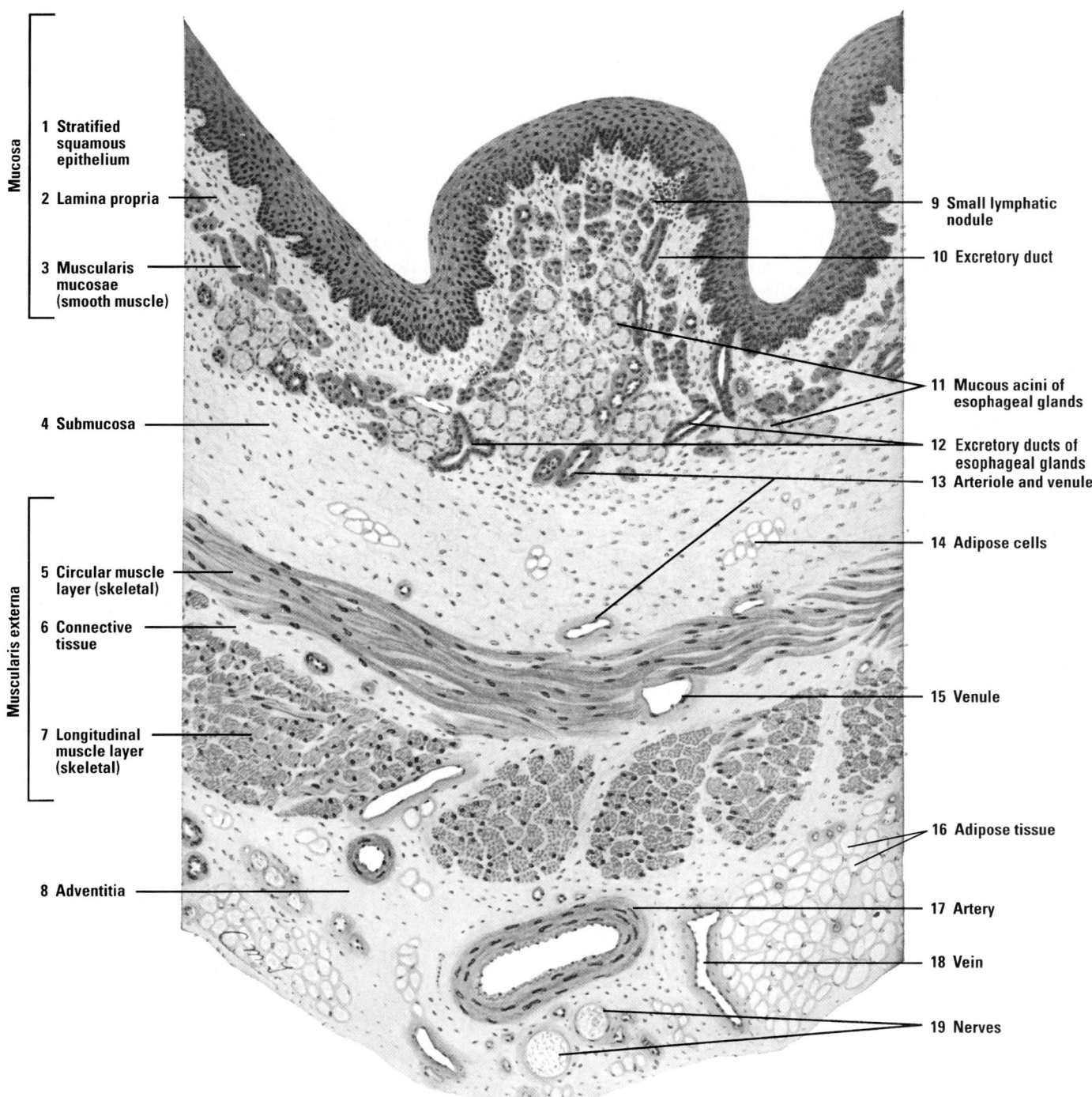

Mucosa

1 **Stratified squamous epithelium**

2 **Lamina propria**

3 **Muscularis mucosae (smooth muscle)**

4 **Submucosa**

Muscularis externa

5 **Circular muscle layer (skeletal)**

6 **Connective tissue**

7 **Longitudinal muscle layer (skeletal)**

8 **Adventitia**

9 **Small lymphatic nodule**

10 **Excretory duct**

11 **Mucous acini of esophageal glands**

12 **Excretory ducts of esophageal glands**

13 **Arteriole and venule**

14 **Adipose cells**

15 **Venule**

16 **Adipose tissue**

17 **Artery**

18 **Vein**

19 **Nerves**

Fig. 11-1   Upper Esophagus: Wall (transverse section). Stain: hematoxylin-eosin. Low magnification.

Figure 11-2   Upper Esophagus: Mucosa and Submucosa (transverse section)

Higher magnification of the upper esophageal wall illustrates the **mucosa (1, 2, 3)** with the **stratified squamous epithelium (1)** and the **submucosa (4).** In the luminal epithelium, the **squamous cells (6)** form the outer layers, the numerous **polyhedral cells (7)** form the intermediate layers, and **low columnar cells (9)** form the basal layer. **Mitotic activity (8)** is seen in the deeper layers of the epithelium.

The **lamina propria (2, 10)** contains **blood vessels (11)** and aggregates of **lymphocytes (12).** The smooth muscle of **muscularis mucosae (13)** is illustrated as bundles of muscle fibers sectioned in a transverse plane.

The submucosa (4) contains **mucous acini (15)** of the esophageal glands proper. Small **excretory ducts (16,** lower leaders) from these glands, lined with simple epithelium, join the larger excretory ducts (16, upper leader) that are lined with stratified epithelium. A large **duct,** sectioned tangentially **(14),** reveals that its epithelium is continuous with the stratified squamous epithelium of the esophageal lumen.

In the submucosa (4) are also seen **blood vessels (17, 18), nerves (19),** and **adipose cells (20).** A section of skeletal muscle fibers from the inner circular layer of the **muscularis externa (5)** is illustrated in the lower left corner of the figure.

■ Functional Correlations–Esophagus

The major function of the esophagus is to convey liquids and/or chewed food or **bolus** from the oral cavity to the stomach. For this function, the lumen of the esophagus is lined by a protective, **nonkeratinized stratified squamous epithelium.** Aiding in this conduction function are the **esophageal glands** that are located in the connective tissue of the wall. These glands produce the secretory product **mucus,** which is conducted in **excretory ducts** through the epithelium to lubricate the esophageal lumen. The swallowed material is forced from one end of the esophagus to other by strong muscular contractions called **peristalsis.** At the lower end of the esophagus, a muscular **gastroesophageal sphincter** constricts the lumen and prevents regurgitation of swallowed material into the esophagus.

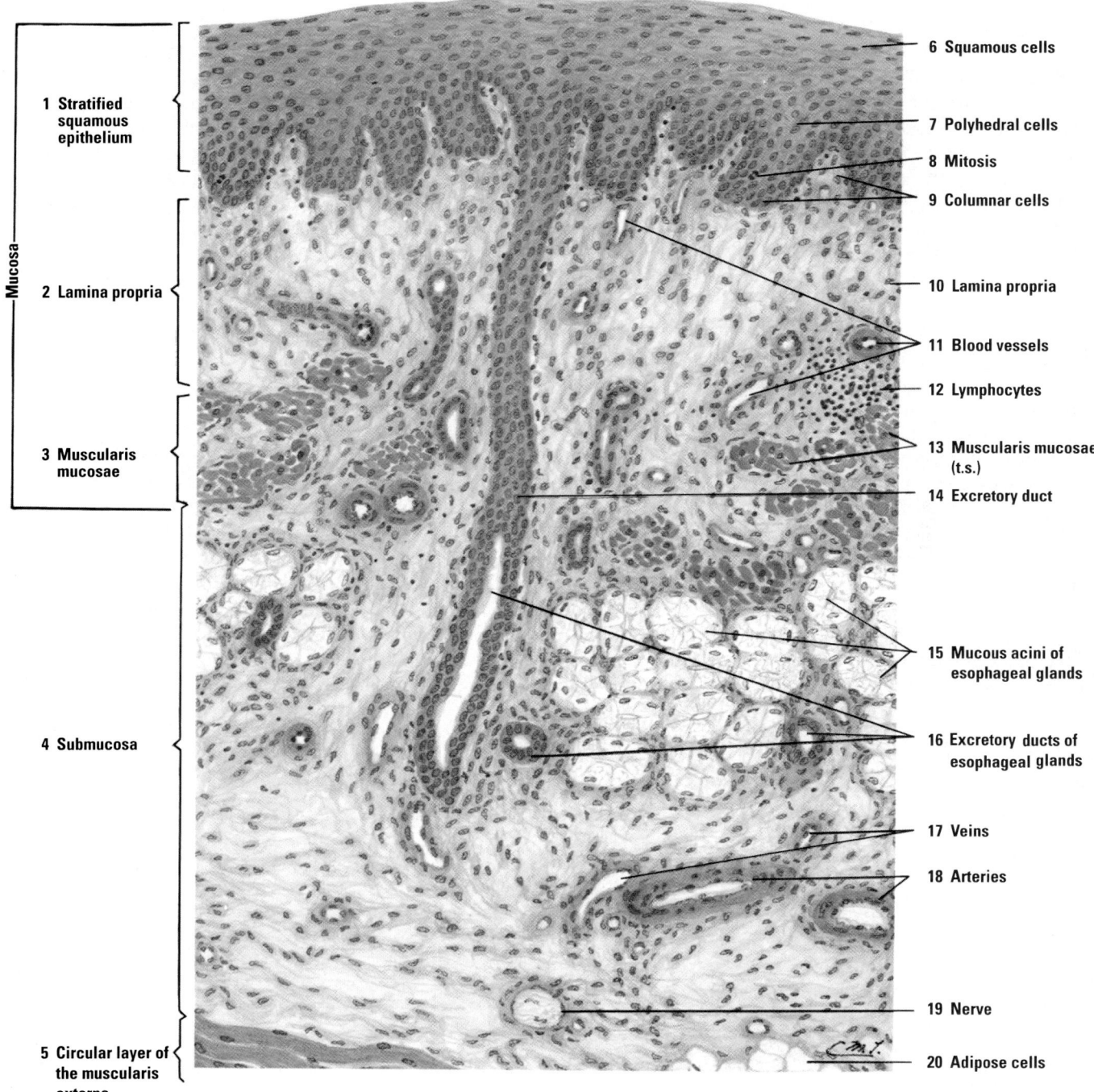

Mucosa

1 Stratified squamous epithelium

2 Lamina propria

3 Muscularis mucosae

4 Submucosa

5 Circular layer of the muscularis externa

6 Squamous cells

7 Polyhedral cells

8 Mitosis

9 Columnar cells

10 Lamina propria

11 Blood vessels

12 Lymphocytes

13 Muscularis mucosae (t.s.)

14 Excretory duct

15 Mucous acini of esophageal glands

16 Excretory ducts of esophageal glands

17 Veins

18 Arteries

19 Nerve

20 Adipose cells

Fig. 11-2   Upper Esophagus: Mucosa and Submucosa (transverse section). Stain: hematoxylin-eosin. Medium magnification.

Figure 11-3   Upper Esophagus (transverse section)

This section of the upper esophagus is similar to the illustration in Figure 11-1 except that it is stained with Heidenhain's modification of Mallory's trichrome (Mallory-azan). Azocarmine stains the nuclei an intense red. A mixture of aniline blue and orange G selectively stains other tissues. The collagen fibers of the **connective tissue (1, 4, 5, 7, 9)** stain bright blue, whereas the cytoplasm of **epithelium (6)** and **muscle cells (2, 3, 8)** stains orange to red.

The different layers of the esophagus are easily distinguishable. In the upper esophagus (as in Fig.11-2), the outermost layer is the **adventitia (1)**, and the **muscularis externa (2, 3)** is skeletal muscle. Aniline blue stains the large amounts of connective tissue in the **submucosa (9)** and adventitia (1) and the smaller amounts between (4) and within muscle layers (5). The connective tissue of the **lamina propria (7)** appears distinct from the smooth muscle of the **muscularis mucosae (8).**

Figure 11-4   Lower Esophagus (transverse section)

This section of the terminal portion of the esophagus (in the peritoneal cavity near the stomach) is stained with Van Gieson's trichrome, which uses iron hematoxylin (Wiegert's or Heidenhain's) as a nuclear stain and picrofuchsin to stain other components. As a result, cellular details are not well defined, but the connective tissue (3, 5, 7) and **smooth muscle (2, 4, 8)** are nicely differentiated. Nuclei are stained dark brown. Collagen fibers (3, 5, 7) are stained red with acid fuchsin, whereas muscle (and other tissues) (2, 4, 6, 8, 9) are stained yellow with picric acid.

The layers in the wall of the lower esophagus are similar to those in the upper region, except for regional modifications. The outermost layer is the **serosa (1)** (visceral peritoneum). This is in contrast to the adventitia, which lines the esophagus in the thoracic region. The **muscularis externa (2, 4)** layers in lower esophagus are entirely smooth muscle although this is not apparent with this stain and this magnification. Distribution of the **mucous glands (9)** in the submucosa is variable, and in some regions, they may be absent; however, some are illustrated in this section.

The collagen fibers in the **submucosa (5)** are abundant. The distribution of finer **connective tissue fibers (3, 8)** in lesser amounts is seen between and around **smooth muscle fibers (2, 3)**, in **serosa (1)**, and in the **lamina propria (7).**

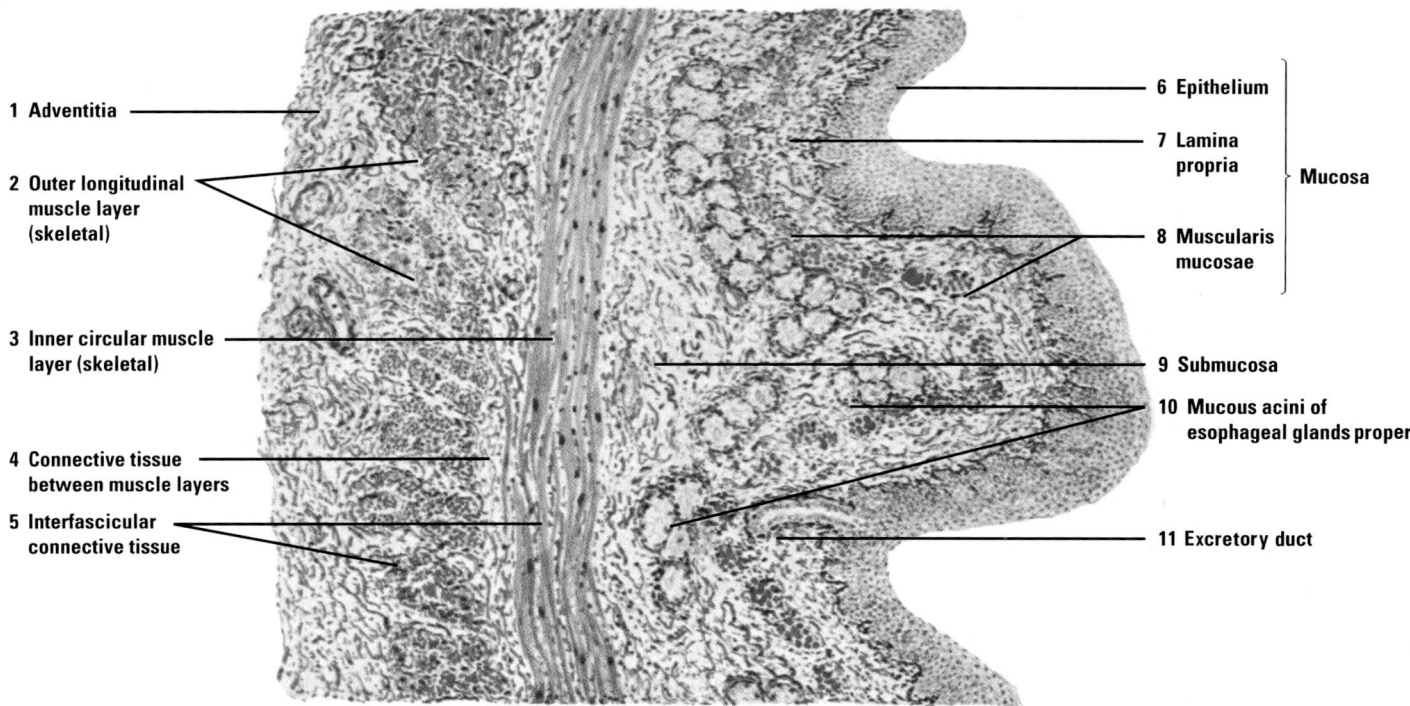

1 Adventitia

2 Outer longitudinal
  muscle layer
  (skeletal)

3 Inner circular muscle
  layer (skeletal)

4 Connective tissue
  between muscle layers

5 Interfascicular
  connective tissue

6 Epithelium

7 Lamina
  propria   } Mucosa

8 Muscularis
  mucosae

9 Submucosa

10 Mucous acini of
   esophageal glands proper

11 Excretory duct

Fig. 11-3   Upper Esophagus (transverse section). Stain: Mallory's trichrome. Nuclei: red; connective tissueL blue; epithelium and muscle: orange and red. Low magnification.

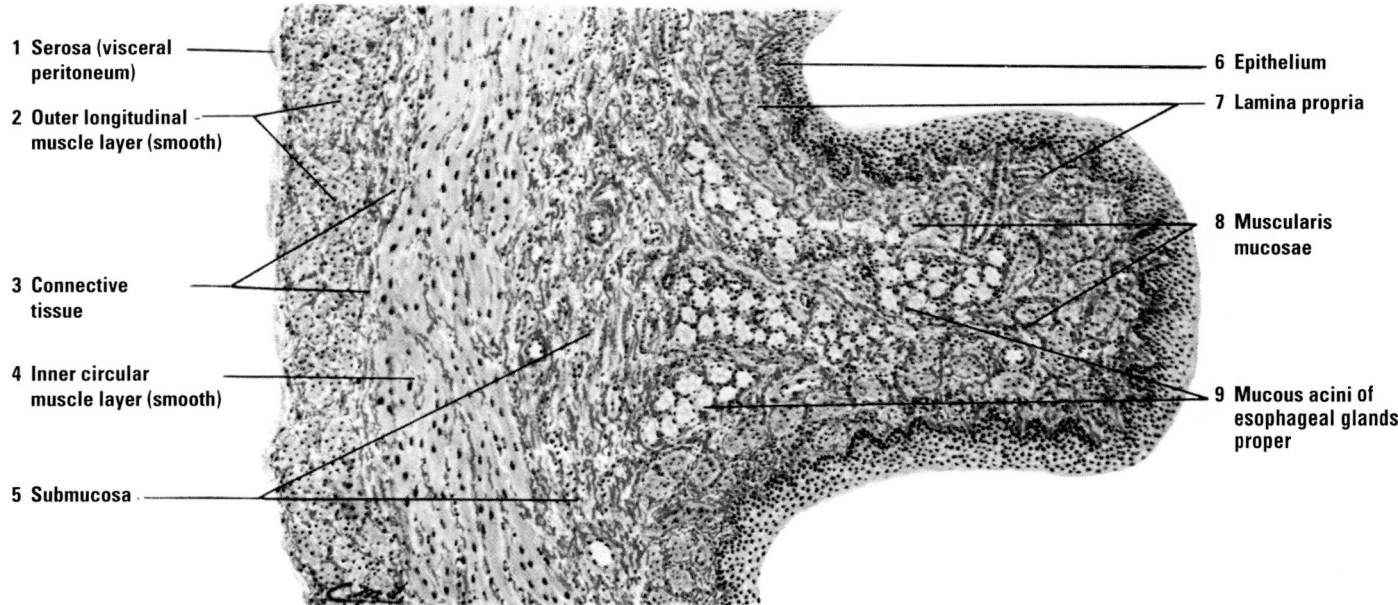

1 Serosa (visceral
  peritoneum)

2 Outer longitudinal
  muscle layer (smooth)

3 Connective
  tissue

4 Inner circular
  muscle layer (smooth)

5 Submucosa

6 Epithelium

7 Lamina propria

8 Muscularis
  mucosae

9 Mucous acini of
  esophageal glands
  proper

Fig. 11-4   Lower Esophagus (transverse section). Stain: Van Gieson's trichrome. Nuclei: dark brown; connective tissue: red; epithelium and muscle: yellow. Low magnification.

Figure 11-5   Esophageal–Stomach Junction

At its terminal end, the esophagus joins the stomach, forming the esophageal–stomach junction. The nonkeratinized **stratified squamous epithelium (1)** of the **esophagus** abruptly changes to simple columnar, mucus-secreting **gastric epithelium (10)** of the cardia of the **stomach.** Consequently, this junction between stomach and esophagus exhibits a distinct histologic mark.

At the esophageal–stomach junction, the **esophageal glands proper (7)** of the esophagus may be seen in the **submucosa (8). Excretory ducts (4, 6)** from these glands course through the **muscularis mucosae (5)** and the **lamina propria (2)** of the esophagus into its lumen. In the lamina propria (2) of the esophagus near the stomach region are also seen a group of glands called the **esophageal cardiac glands (3).** Both the esophageal glands proper (7) and the cardiac glands (3) are mucus-secreting.

The **lamina propria of the esophagus (2)** is continuous with the **lamina propria of the stomach (12),** where it becomes a wide layer filled with **glands (16, 17)** and diffuse lymphatic tissue. The lamina propria of the stomach (12) is penetrated by numerous shallow **gastric pits (11)** into which empty the numerous gastric glands (16, 17) of the mucosa.

In the upper region of the stomach are found two types of glands. The simple tubular **cardiac glands (17)** are primarily limited to the transition region, the cardia of the stomach. These glands are lined with a single type of cell, the pale-staining, mucus-secreting columnar cell. Below the cardiac region of the stomach are the simple tubular **gastric glands (16),** some of which exhibit basal branching.

In contrast to the cardiac glands (17), the gastric glands (16) contain four different cell types: the pale-staining **mucous neck cells (13),** large, eosinophilic **parietal cells (14),** basophilic **chief** or **zymogenic cells (15),** and several different types of endocrine cells (not illustrated), collectively called the enteroendocrine cells. These cells are illustrated in greater detail in Figure 12-3.

The **muscularis mucosae of the stomach (18)** is also continuous with the **muscularis mucosae of the esophagus (5).** In the esophagus, the muscularis mucosae (5) is usually a single layer of longitudinal smooth muscle fibers, whereas in the stomach, a second layer of smooth muscle is added, called the inner circular layer.

The connective tissue of the **submucosa (8, 19)** and the smooth muscles of **muscularis externa (9, 21)** of the esophagus are continuous with those of the stomach. Numerous **blood vessels (20)** are found in the submucosa (8, 19). From here, smaller blood vessels are distributed to other regions of the organ.

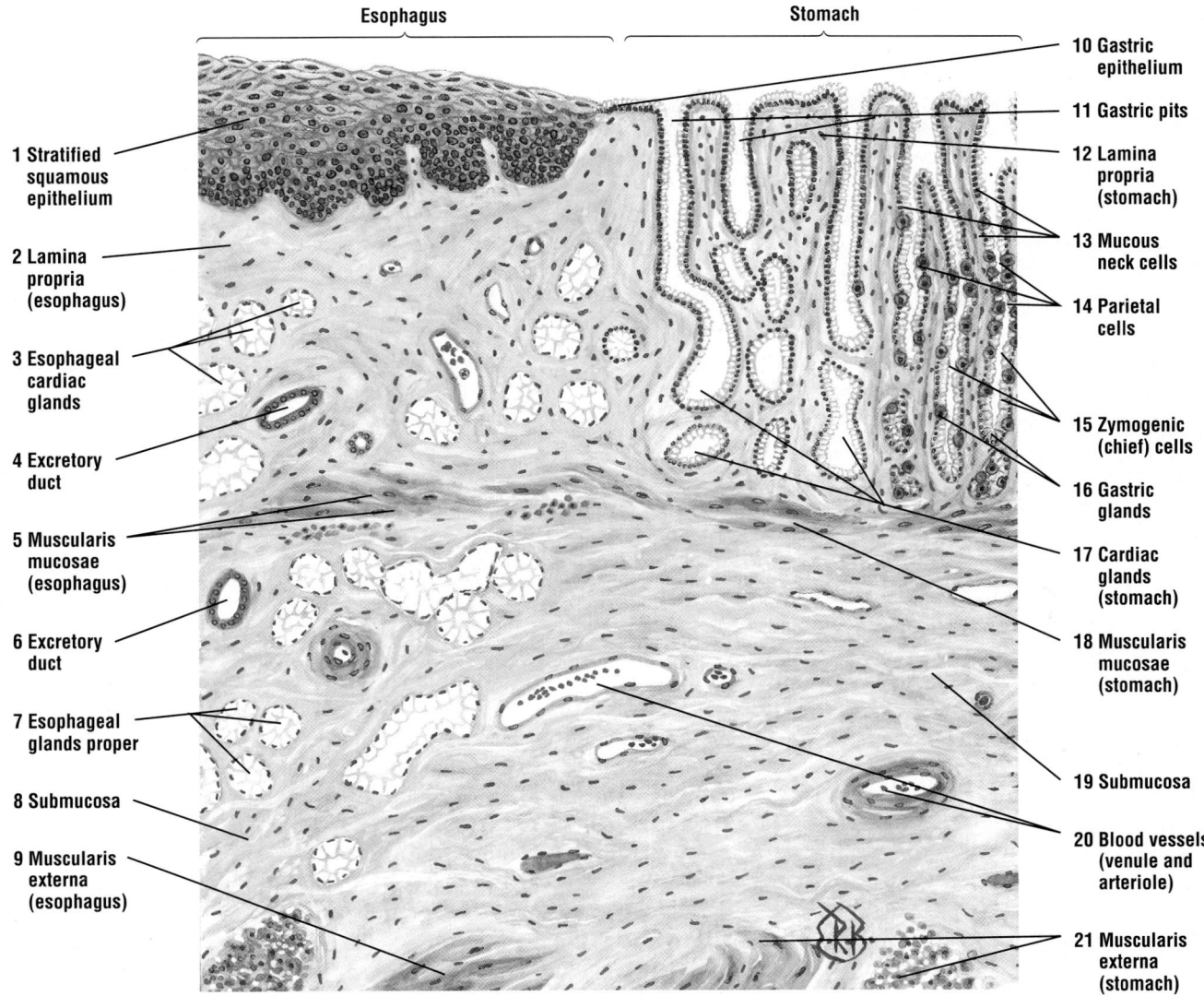

Esophagus

Stomach

1 Stratified squamous epithelium

2 Lamina propria (esophagus)

3 Esophageal cardiac glands

4 Excretory duct

5 Muscularis mucosae (esophagus)

6 Excretory duct

7 Esophageal glands proper

8 Submucosa

9 Muscularis externa (esophagus)

10 Gastric epithelium

11 Gastric pits

12 Lamina propria (stomach)

13 Mucous neck cells

14 Parietal cells

15 Zymogenic (chief) cells

16 Gastric glands

17 Cardiac glands (stomach)

18 Muscularis mucosae (stomach)

19 Submucosa

20 Blood vessels (venule and arteriole)

21 Muscularis externa (stomach)

Fig. 11-5   Esophageal–Stomach Junction. Stain: hematoxylin-eosin. Low magnification.

Figure 11-6   Stomach: Fundus and Body Regions (transverse section)

The human stomach is divided into three distinct histologic areas: the cardia, the fundus and body, and pylorus. The fundus and body is the most extensive region in the stomach.

This low magnification figure illustrates a transverse section of the fundic stomach. The stomach wall exhibits four general regions that are characteristic of the entire digestive tract: the **mucosa (1, 2, 3), submucosa (4), muscularis externa (5, 6, 7),** and **serosa (8).**

Mucosa (1, 2, 3): The mucosa of the stomach consists of three layers: the epithelium, lamina propria, and muscularis mucosae. The luminal surface of the mucosa is lined by a layer of **simple columnar epithelium (1, 11).** This epithelium also extends into and lines the **gastric pits (10),** which are tubular infoldings of the surface epithelium **(11).** In the fundic region of the stomach, the gastric pits (10) are not deep and extend into the mucosa approximately one-fourth of its thickness. Beneath the surface epithelium is a layer of loose connective tissue, the **lamina propria (2, 12),** which fills the narrow spaces between the gastric glands. The outer layer of mucosa is lined by a thin band of smooth muscle, the **muscularis mucosae (3, 15),** consisting of an inner circular and an outer longitudinal layer. Thin slips of muscle from the muscularis mucosae (3, 15) extend into lamina propria (2, 12) between the **gastric glands (13, 14)** toward the surface epithelium (1, 11) (See Fig. 11-7:8).

The gastric glands (13, 14) are packed tightly in the lamina propria and occupy the entire thickness of the mucosa (1, 2, 3). These glands open in small groups into the bottom of the gastric pits (10). The surface epithelium of the entire gastric mucosa contains the same cell type, from the cardiac to the pyloric region; however, there are distinct regional differences in the type of cells that comprise the gastric glands. At lower magnification, two distinct cell types can be identified in the gastric glands of the fundic stomach. The acidophilic **parietal cells (13)** are seen in the upper portions of the glands; the more basophilic **chief (zymogenic) (14)** cells occupy the lower regions. The subglandular regions of the lamina propria may contain small accumulations of lymphatic tissue or **nodules (16).**

The mucosa of an empty stomach exhibits numerous folds called the **rugae (9).** These folds are temporary and are formed from the contractions of the smooth muscle layer, the muscularis mucosae (3, 15). As the stomach fills with solid or liquid material, the rugae disappear and the mucosa appears smooth.

Submucosa (4): The prominent layer directly beneath the muscularis mucosae (3, 15) is the submucosa (4). In an empty stomach, this layer can extend into the folds or the rugae (9). The submucosa (4) contains denser irregular connective tissue and more **collagen fibers (17)** than does the lamina propria (2, 12). In addition to the normal complement of connective tissue cells, the submucosa (4) contains numerous lymph vessels, **capillaries (22),** large **arterioles (18),** and **venules (19).** Isolated or small clusters of the parasympathetic ganglia of the **submucosal (Meissner's) nerve plexus (21)** are also seen in the deeper regions of the submucosa.

Muscularis externa (5, 6, 7): In the stomach, the muscularis externa (5, 6, 7) consists of three layers of smooth muscle, each oriented in a different plane: an inner **oblique (5),** a middle **circular (6),** and an outer **longitudinal (7)** layer. The oblique layer is not complete and, as a result, this layer is not always seen in sections of stomach wall. In this illustration, the circular layer has been sectioned longitudinally and the longitudinal layer transversely. Located between the circular and longitudinal smooth muscle layers is a prominent **myenteric (Auerbach's) nerve plexus (23)** of parasympathetic ganglia and nerve fibers.

Serosa (8): The outermost layer of the stomach wall is the serosa (8). This is a thin layer of connective tissue that overlies the muscularis externa (5, 6, 7). Externally, this layer is covered by a simple squamous mesothelium of the **visceral peritoneum (8).** The connective tissue covered by the visceral peritoneum can contain numerous **adipose cells (24).**

■ Functional Correlations–Stomach

The main functions of the stomach are to **receive, store, mix,** and **digest** the ingested food products. Some of these stomach functions are performed by **mechanical** and **chemical** actions, which reduce the ingested food material **bolus** to a semi-liquid mass called **chyme.** The mechanical reduction of bolus in the stomach is produced by strong, muscular **peristaltic contractions** of its thick wall, when the food enters and distends the stomach wall. With the pylorus closed, the muscular contractions churn and mix the food with **gastric juices** that are produced by the **gastric glands. Neurons** and **axons** that are located in the **submucosal nerve plexus** and **myenteric nerve plexus** of the stomach wall regulate its peristaltic activity. The stomach also has some absorptive functions; however, these are primarily limited to the absorption of water, alcohol, salts, and certain drugs.

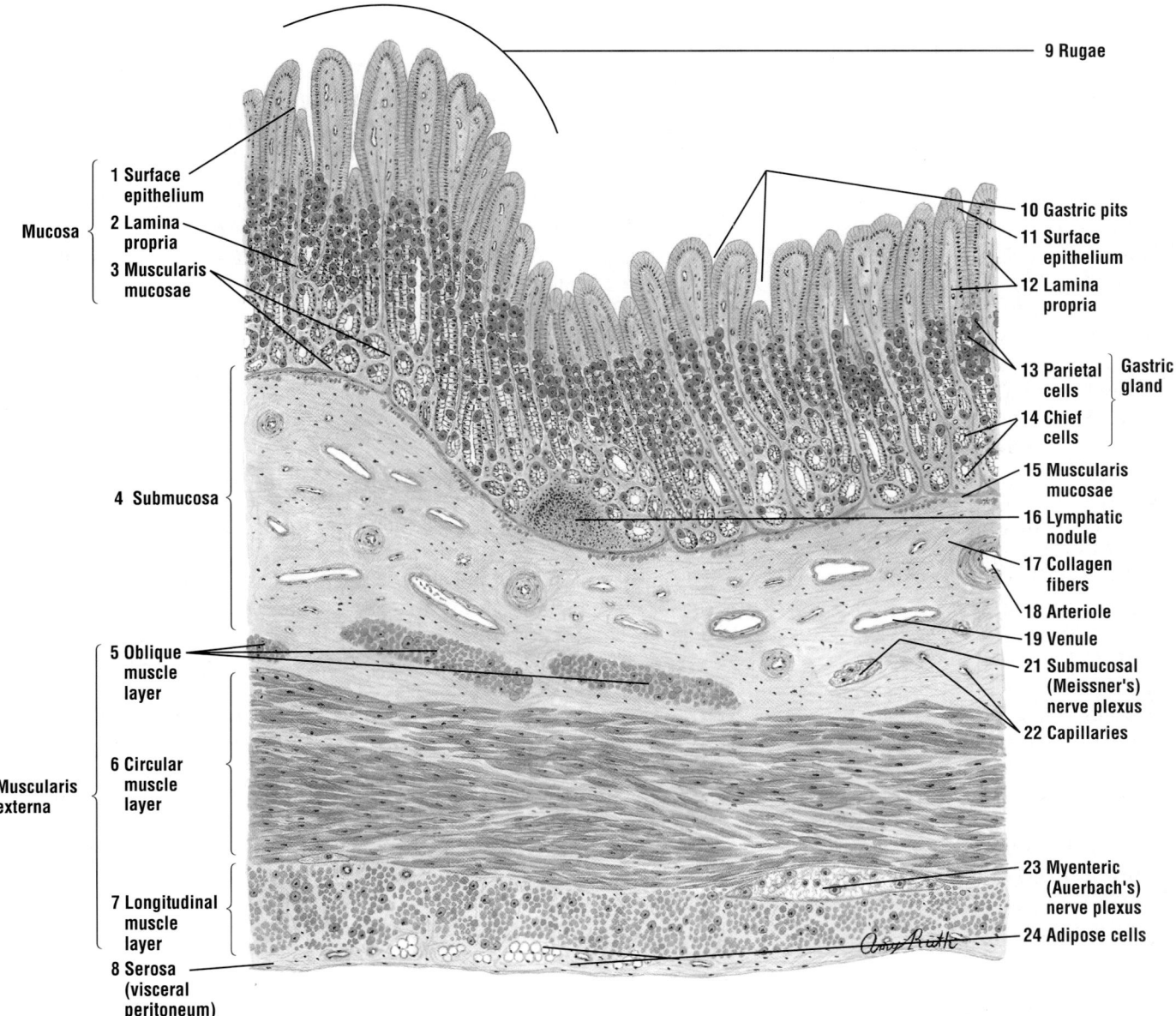

Fig. 11-6   Stomach: Fundus and Body Regions (transverse section). Stain: hematoxylin-eosin. Low magnification.

Figure 11-7   Stomach: Mucosa of the Fundus and Body (transverse section)

The mucosa and submucosa of the fundic region of the stomach are illustrated at a higher magnification. The extension of the simple columnar **surface epithelium (1, 13)** into the **gastric pits (11)** and the opening of the tubular **gastric glands (5)** into these pits are clearly seen. The loose irregular connective tissue of the **lamina propria (6)** fills the narrow spaces between the tightly packed gastric glands (5) and extends from the surface epithelium (1) to the **muscularis mucosae (9).**

The lamina propria (6) is better seen in the **mucosal ridges (2);** it consists primarily of fine reticular and collagen fibers. Scattered throughout this connective tissue are the oval nuclei of the fibroblasts. Also seen in the lamina propria (6) are accumulations of lymphoid tissue in the form of **lymphatic nodules (17),** in addition to individual lymphocytes and other cell types normally encountered in the loose connective tissue.

The gastric glands (5) extend the entire length of the mucosa. In the deeper regions of the mucosa, the gastric glands may branch, as seen by the numerous transverse and oblique sections. Each gastric gland typically consists of three regions. At the junction of the gastric pit with the gastric gland is the **isthmus (14),** containing the surface epithelial cells (1, 13) and **parietal cells (4).** Lower in the gland is the **neck (15),** composed primarily of **mucous neck cells (3)** and also parietal cells (4). The base or **fundus (16)** is the deep portion of the gland, composed predominantly of **chief (zymogenic) cells (7)** with a few scattered parietal cells (4). In addition to these cells, the fundic glands contain undifferentiated cells and a variety of enteroendocrine cells (not illustrated) that belong to the APUD group. (The characteristics of the APUD cells are discussed and illustrated in greater detail in Figure 12-3.)

In the hematoxylin-eosin preparations, three types of cells can be easily identified in the fundic gastric glands. In this illustration, the parietal cells stain intensely and uniformly acidophilic (4). This staining characteristic distinguishes clearly the parietal cells from other cells in the fundic glands. In contrast, the chief cells (zymogenic) (7) are distinctly basophilic and are readily distinguishable from the surrounding acidophilic parietal cells. The mucous neck cells (3) are located just below the gastric pits (11) and are interspersed between the parietal cells in the neck region of the glands.

The muscularis mucosae (9) is well illustrated in this stomach section. It is composed of two thin strips of smooth muscle, the **inner circular layer (9a)** and **outer longitudinal layer (9b).** In this illustration, the circular layer is sectioned longitudinally and the outer layer is sectioned transversely. Extending into the lamina propria (6) from the muscularis mucosae (9) toward the surface epithelium (1, 13) are strands of **smooth muscle (8, 12).**

Directly below the muscularis mucosae is a prominent layer of denser connective tissue, the **submucosa (10).** In this section, abundant **collagen fibers (18)** and the nuclei of numerous **fibroblasts (19)** are readily seen. The submucosa layer also contains numerous vessels, including **arterioles (20), venules (21),** lymphatics, and capillaries. Some adipose cells may also be seen in this layer.

■ Functional Correlations–Cells in Gastric Glands

The chemical reduction of food in the stomach is the function of the watery gastric secretions produced by different cells in the gastric glands, especially those located in the fundus and body regions of the stomach. The main components of the gastric secretions are **pepsin, hydrochloric acid, mucus, intrinsic factor, water, lysozyme,** and different **electrolytes.**

The **luminal cells** of the stomach secrete thick layers of **mucus,** whose main function is to cover, lubricate, and protect the stomach surface from the corrosive action of the strong gastric juices. The **parietal cells** of the gastric glands secrete **hydrochloric acid,** which is a major component of the gastric juice. In humans, the parietal cells also produce **gastric intrinsic factor,** a glycoprotein that is necessary for absorption of **vitamin B$_{12}$** from the small intestine. Vitamin B$_{12}$ is necessary for **erythrocyte** (red blood cell) production in the red bone marrow; deficiency of this vitamin leads to anemia.

The cytoplasm of **chief** or **zymogenic cells** contain numerous secretory granules. These granules contain **pepsinogen,** a precursor of the inactive **pepsin.** Release of pepsinogen during gastric secretion into the acidic environment of the stomach converts the inactive pepsinogen into the highly active, proteolytic enzyme pepsin.

The **enteroendocrine cells** secrete a variety of **polypeptides** and **proteins** with hormonal activity that influence various functions of the digestive tract. These cells are not confined to the gastrointestinal tract but are also found in the respiratory organs and other organs of the body. Additional details, description, and illustration of the enteroendocrine (APUD) cells are found in Chapter 12, Figure 12-3.

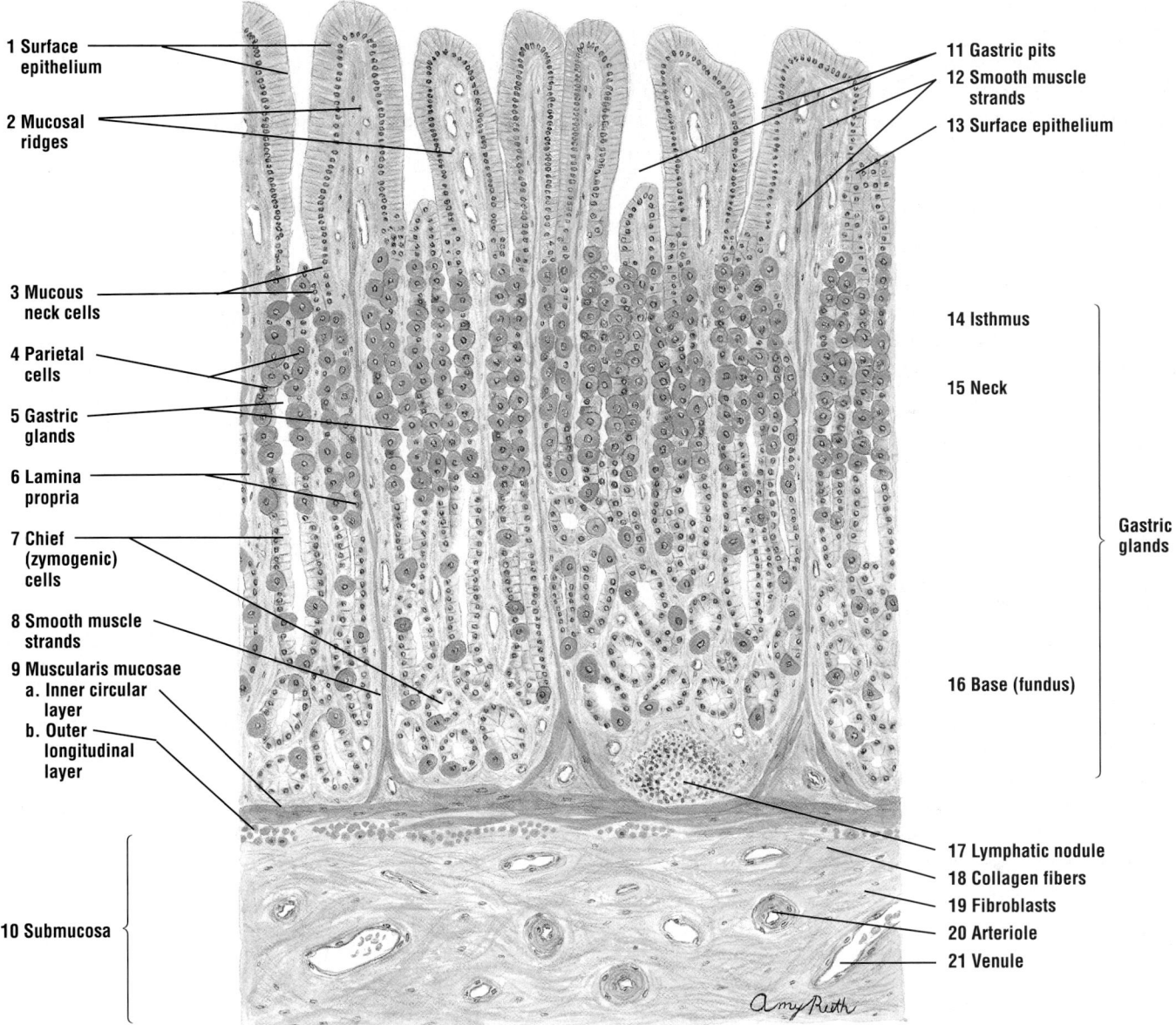

Fig. 11-7   Stomach: Mucosa of the Fundus and Body (transverse section). Stain: hematoxylin-eosin. Medium magnification.

1 Surface epithelium
2 Mucosal ridges
3 Mucous neck cells
4 Parietal cells
5 Gastric glands
6 Lamina propria
7 Chief (zymogenic) cells
8 Smooth muscle strands
9 Muscularis mucosae
  a. Inner circular layer
  b. Outer longitudinal layer
10 Submucosa

11 Gastric pits
12 Smooth muscle strands
13 Surface epithelium
14 Isthmus
15 Neck
16 Base (fundus)
Gastric glands
17 Lymphatic nodule
18 Collagen fibers
19 Fibroblasts
20 Arteriole
21 Venule

Figure 11-8   Stomach: Superficial Region of Gastric Mucosa

Higher magnification of the stomach illustrates the characteristic features of different cells that compose the superficial region of the gastric mucosa of the fundus and body.

The tall columnar **surface epithelium (1)** exhibits basal oval nuclei and is lightly stained because of the presence of mucigen droplets in the cytoplasm. It is delimited from the adjacent fibroelastic connective tissue **lamina propria (3)** by a thin but distinct **basement membrane (2).** The surface epithelium extends downward into the **gastric pits (4, 8).**

The **gastric glands (5, 12)** lie in the **lamina propria (11)** below the **gastric pits (4, 9).** The **necks (5, 10)** of the gastric glands are also lined with low columnar **mucous neck cells (6)** that have round, basal nuclei. The constricted necks of the gastric glands (10) open by a short transition region into the bottom of the gastric pit (8).

The prominent **parietal cells (7)** are interspersed among the mucous neck cells (6); their free surfaces are on the border of the **glandular lumen (12).** The parietal cells (7) are most conspicuous in the gastric mucosa and are predominantly found in the upper half of the gastric glands. These cells are large and pyramidal in shape with round nucleus and highly acidophilic cytoplasm; some pyramidal cells may be binucleate.

Deeper in the gastric glands (5, 12), toward the lower half or third of the gland, the mucous cells are replaced by basophilic **chief** or **zymogenic cells (13),** which border on the lumen of the gland. Parietal cells (7) are also seen here; however, they are displaced peripherally and lie against the basement membrane without reaching the lumen.

Figure 11-9   Stomach: Deep Region of the Mucosa

The **gastric glands (1, 10)** are branched tubular glands; the branching is normally seen at the base of the glands. A section through the deep region of the mucosa illustrates basal portions of the gastric glands (1, 10) sectioned in various planes.

As in the higher region of the gland, the **chief** or **zymogenic cells (4, 9, 12)** border the glandular lumen. The **parietal cells (3, 8, 11)** are wedged against the basement membrane and are not in direct contact with the lumen. This is well demonstrated in several transverse sections of the glands (3, lower leader).

Also illustrated in this figure are the **lamina propria (2)** between the gastric glands (1, 10) and a narrow zone of **subglandular lamina propria (5),** which is not always distinguishable.

The two layers, inner circular and outer longitudinal, of **muscularis mucosae (13, 14),** are also illustrated.

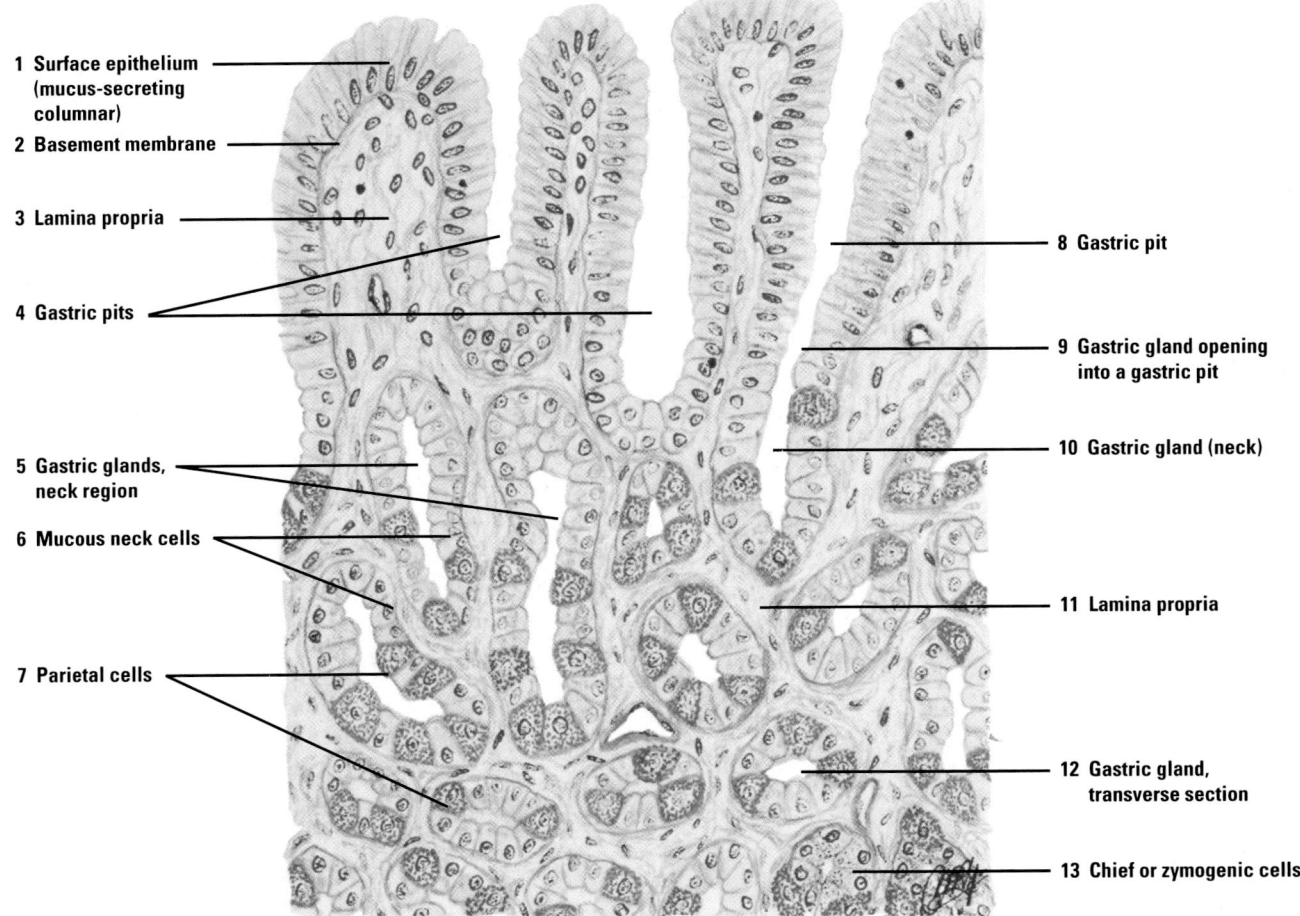

1 Surface epithelium
(mucus-secreting
columnar)

2 Basement membrane

3 Lamina propria

4 Gastric pits

5 Gastric glands,
neck region

6 Mucous neck cells

7 Parietal cells

8 Gastric pit

9 Gastric gland opening
into a gastric pit

10 Gastric gland (neck)

11 Lamina propria

12 Gastric gland,
transverse section

13 Chief or zymogenic cells

Fig. 11-8   Stomach: Superficial Region of Gastric Mucosa. Stain: hematoxylin-eosin. High magnification.

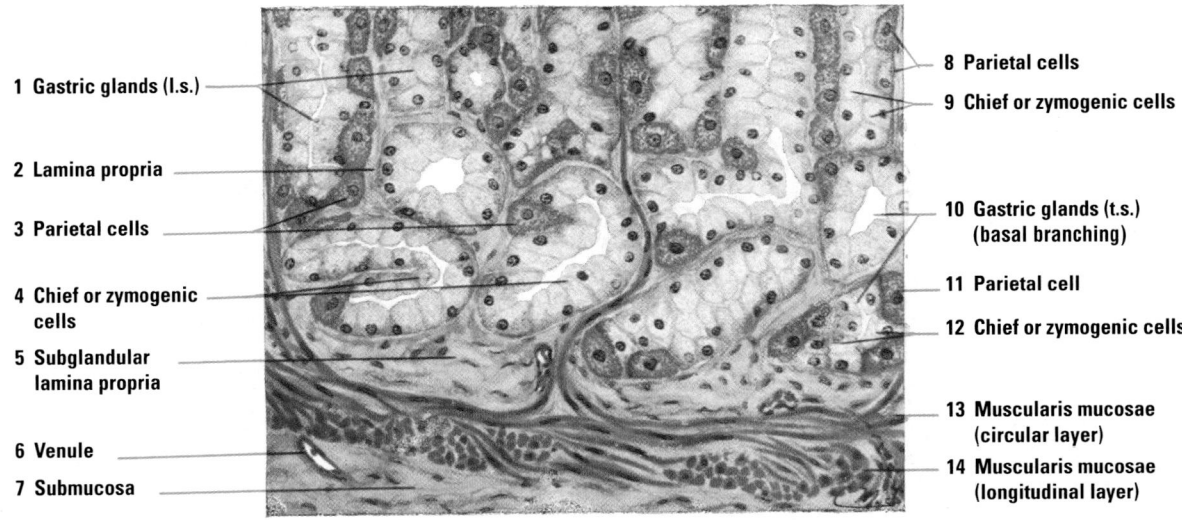

1 Gastric glands (l.s.)

2 Lamina propria

3 Parietal cells

4 Chief or zymogenic
cells

5 Subglandular
lamina propria

6 Venule

7 Submucosa

8 Parietal cells

9 Chief or zymogenic cells

10 Gastric glands (t.s.)
(basal branching)

11 Parietal cell

12 Chief or zymogenic cells

13 Muscularis mucosae
(circular layer)

14 Muscularis mucosae
(longitudinal layer)

Fig. 11-9   Stomach: Deep Region of the Mucosa. Stain: hematoxylin-eosin. High magnification.

Figure 11-10   Stomach: Mucosa of the Pyloric Region

In the pyloric region of the stomach, the **gastric pits (4, 12)** are deeper than those in the body or fundus regions of the stomach. The gastric pits (4, 12) extend into the mucosa to about one half or more of its thickness. The simple columnar mucous **epithelium (10)** that lines the surface of the stomach extends into and lines the gastric pits (4, 12).

The **pyloric gastric glands (5, 6, 14)** are either branched or coiled tubular mucous glands. As in the cardia region of the stomach, only one type of cell is normally found in these glands. This is a tall columnar cell, with slightly granular cytoplasm, lightly stained because of mucigen content, and a flattened or oval nucleus at the base. The pyloric glands (5, 6, 14) open into the bottom of the gastric pits (4, lower leader). Enteroendocrine or APUD cells are also present in this region of the stomach and can be demonstrated usually with special training techniques.

The remaining structures in this region are similar to those in the upper stomach. The **lamina propria (13)** contains diffuse lymphatic tissue, an occasional **lymphatic nodule (16)** may be seen in its deepest part. The lymphatic nodules may increase in size and penetrate through the **muscularis mucosae (18)** into the **submucosa (20)**. **Smooth muscle fibers (7, 15)** from the circular layer of the **muscularis mucosae (18)** pass upward into the lamina propria (13) between the pyloric glands (6) and into **mucosal ridges (2, 3)**.

■ Functional Correlations–Cells in Pyloric Gastric Glands

The pyloric glands contain the same cell types as those present in the cardiac glands. In addition to producing **mucus,** these cells also secrete an enzyme called **lysozyme,** which destroys bacteria in the stomach.

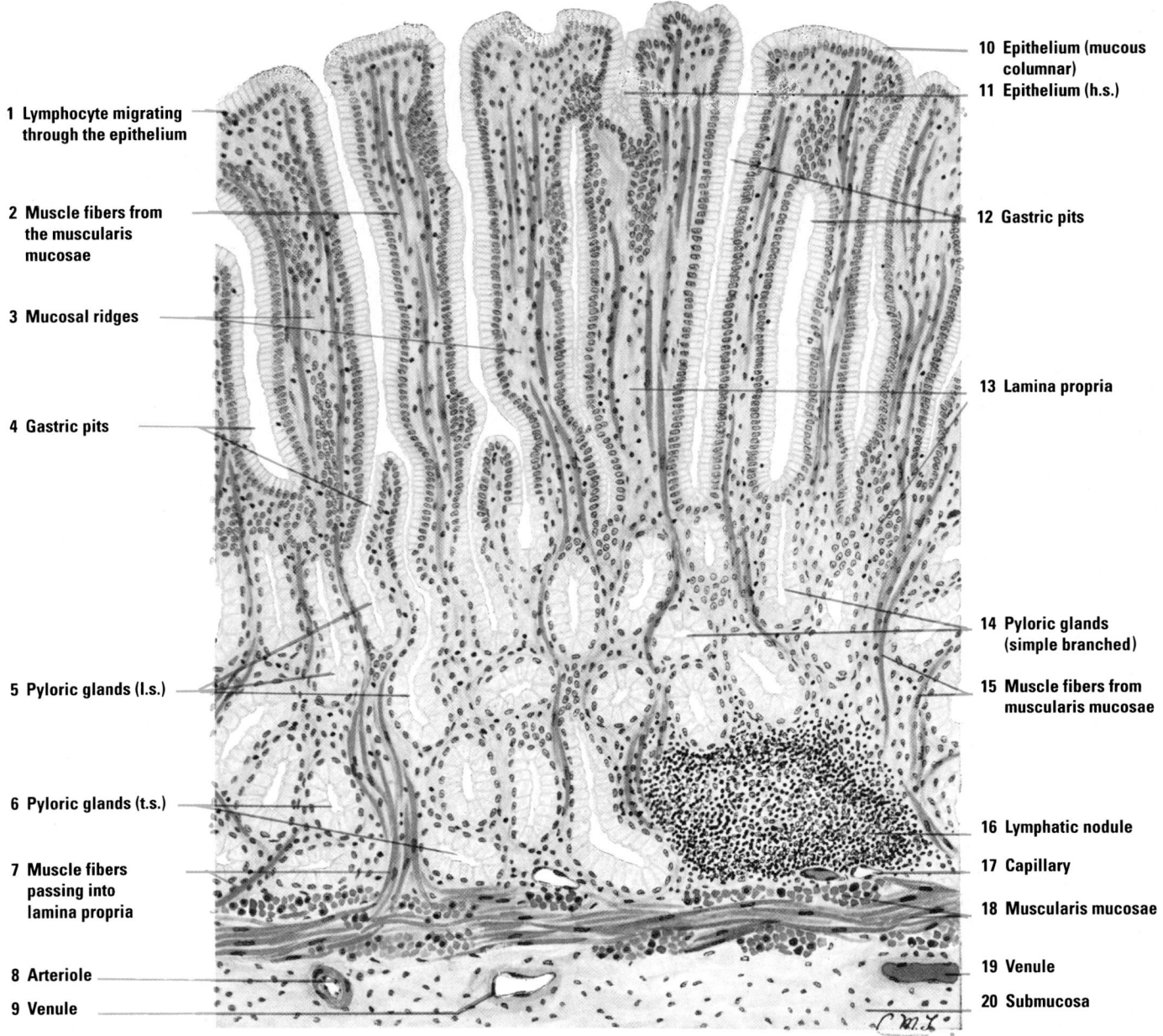

1 Lymphocyte migrating through the epithelium

2 Muscle fibers from the muscularis mucosae

3 Mucosal ridges

4 Gastric pits

5 Pyloric glands (l.s.)

6 Pyloric glands (t.s.)

7 Muscle fibers passing into lamina propria

8 Arteriole

9 Venule

10 Epithelium (mucous columnar)

11 Epithelium (h.s.)

12 Gastric pits

13 Lamina propria

14 Pyloric glands (simple branched)

15 Muscle fibers from muscularis mucosae

16 Lymphatic nodule

17 Capillary

18 Muscularis mucosae

19 Venule

20 Submucosa

Fig. 11-10   Stomach: Mucosa of the Pyloric Region. Stain: hematoxylin-eosin. Medium magnification.

Figure 11-11   Pyloric–Duodenal Junction (longitudinal section)

The **pylorus (1)** of the stomach is separated from the **duodenum (11)** of the small intestine by a thick smooth muscle layer called the **pyloric sphincter (8).** This prominent sphincter is formed by the thickened circular layer of the **muscularis externa of the stomach (9).**

As the pylorus joins the duodenum, the **mucosal ridges (4)** around **gastric pits (3),** become broader and more irregular, and their shape more variable. Coiled tubular **pyloric (mucous) glands (6),** located in the **lamina propria (5),** open at the bottom of the gastric pits (3). **Lymphatic nodules (16)** are frequently seen in the transition region between the stomach (1) and the small intestine (11).

The mucus-secreting **stomach epithelium (2)** changes abruptly to **intestinal epithelium (12)** in the duodenum. This epithelium consists of goblet cells and columnar cells with striated borders (microvilli), which are present throughout the length of the small intestine.The duodenum (11) exhibits specialized surface modification in the form of **villi (13).** Each villus (singular) (13) is a leaf-shaped surface projection with a pointed end. Between individual villi are **intervillous spaces (14)** that represent the continuation of the intestinal lumen.

Short, simple tubular **intestinal glands (crypts of Lieberkühn) (15)** are now seen in the lamina propria of the duodenum. These glands consist primarily of goblet cells and cells with striated borders (microvilli) from the surface epithelium.

Duodenal glands (Brunner's) **(18)** occupy most of the **submucosa (19)** in the upper duodenum (11) and are a characteristic features of this region of the small intestine. Here, the ducts of the duodenal glands (18) penetrate the **muscularis mucosae (7)** of the **duodenum (17)** and enter the base of the instestinal glands (15). As a result, muscularis mucosae (17) is disrupted in this region. Except for the esophageal (submucosal) glands proper, the duodenal glands (18) are the only submucosal glands in the digestive tract. In the **muscularis externa of the stomach (9)** and the **muscularis externa of the duodenum (20)** are seen neurons of the **myenteric nerve plexus (10, 21).**

1 Pylorus   **11 Duodenum**

2 Stomach
  epithelium

3 Gastric pits

4 Mucosal ridges

5 Lamina propria
  (stomach)

6 Pyloric glands

7 Muscularis mucosae

8 Pyloric sphincter

9 Muscularis externa
  (stomach)

10 Myenteric
   nerve plexus
   (stomach)

12 Intestinal epithelium

13 Villi

14 Intervillous spaces

15 Intestinal glands

16 Lymphatic nodule

17 Muscularis mucosae

18 Duodenal glands

19 Submucosa

20 Muscularis externae
   (duodenum)

21 Myenteric nerve
   plexus (duodenum)

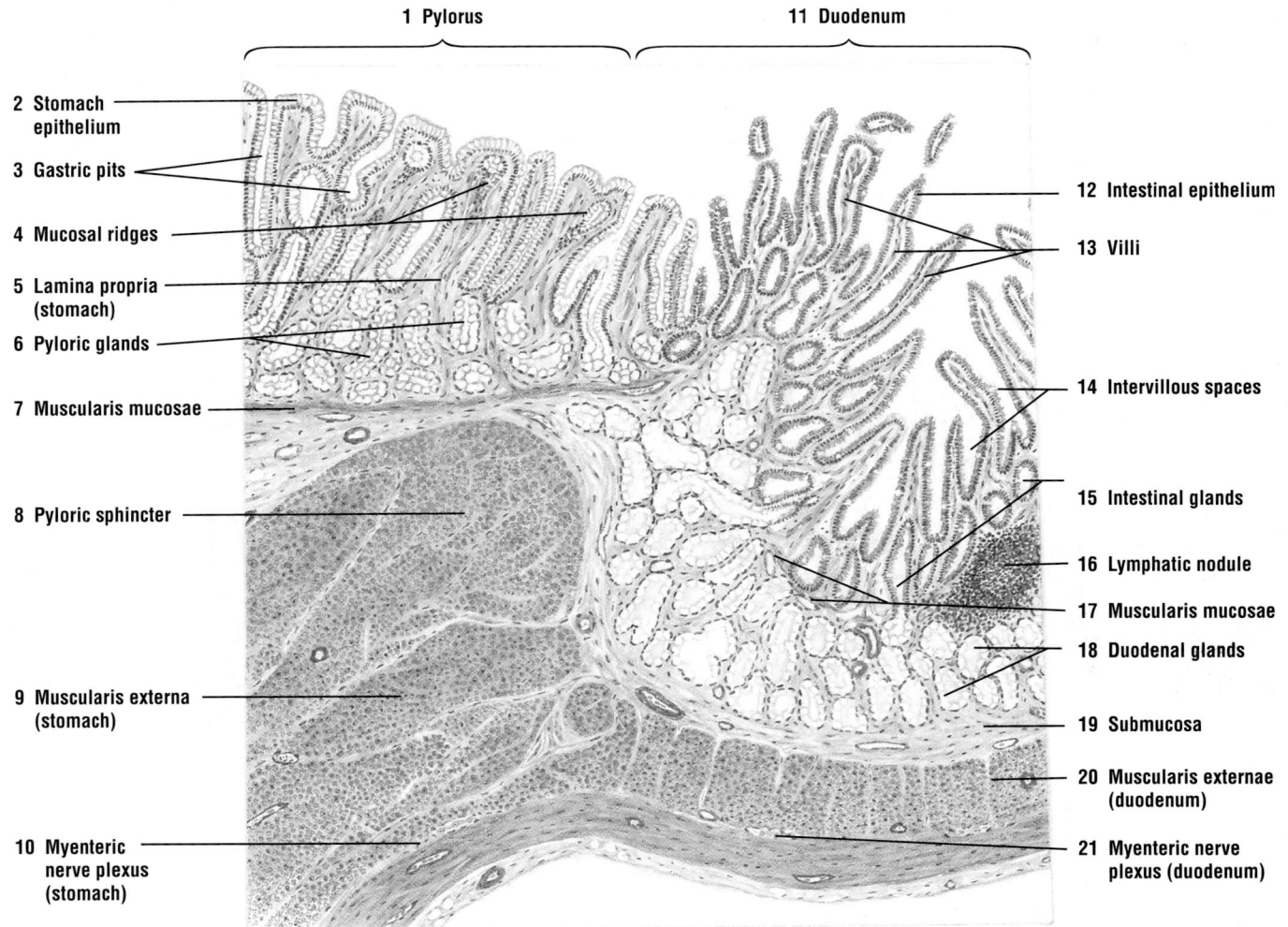

Fig. 11-11   Pyloric–Duodenal Junction (longitudinal section). Stain: hematoxylin-eosin. Low magnification.

Figure 11-12   Lower Esophagus Wall (transverse section)

A low magnification photomicrograph illustrates the lower portion of an esophagus and all of the layers of the mucosa. In the esophagus, the mucosa consists of a thick but nonkeratinized **stratified squamous epithelium (1),** a connective tissue **lamina propria (2),** and a thin strip of a muscle **muscularis mucosae (3).** In the lower regions of the esophagus, muscularis mucosae (3) is composed primarily of smooth muscle.

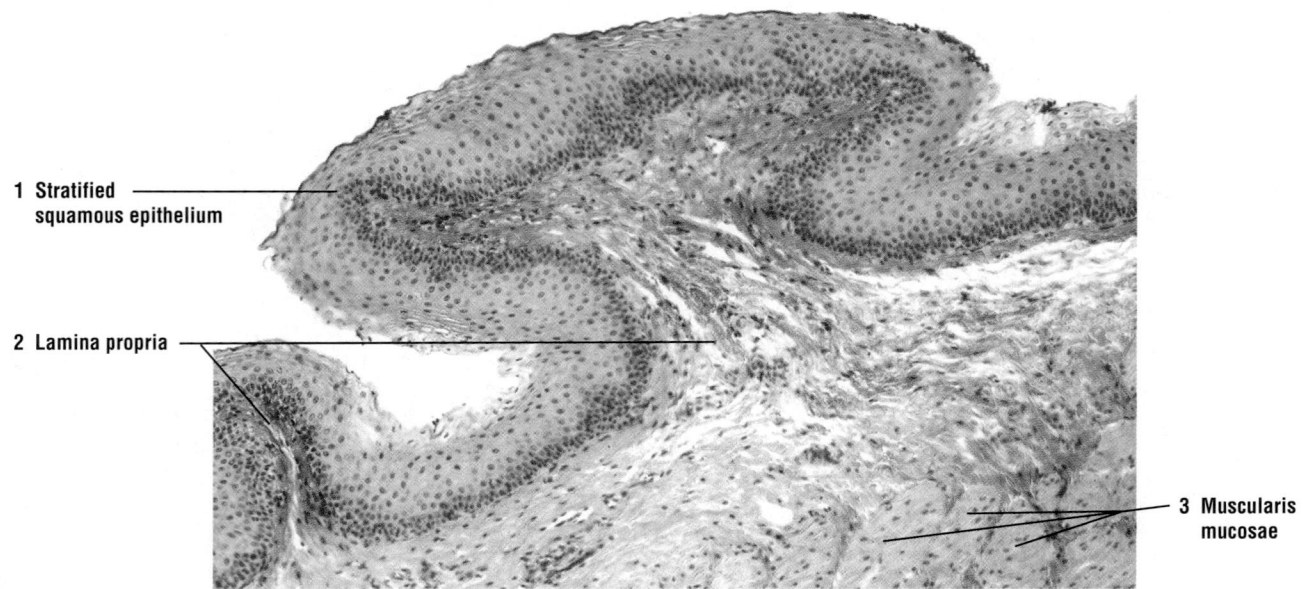

1 Stratified
squamous epithelium

2 Lamina propria

3 Muscularis
mucosae

Fig. 11-12   Lower Esophagus Wall (transverse section). Stain: Mallory-azan. 30×

Figure 11-13   Esophageal–Stomach Junction

A low magnification photomicrograph illustrates the junction of the **esophagus** and the **stomach.** The esophagus is characterized by a thick, protective, nonkeratinized **stratified squamous epithelium (1).** Inferior to the epithelium is the connective tissue **lamina propria (2),** below which are seen small strips of the smooth muscle **muscularis mucosae (3).** The lamina propria (2) indents the undersurface of the esophageal epithelium and forms numerous connective tissue papillae. The junction between the esophagus and stomach is characterized by abrupt transition. The stratified squamous epithelium (1) of the esophagus is replaced by **simple columnar epithelium (4)** of the stomach. In addition, the surface of the stomach exhibits numerous **gastric pits (5)** into which open the **gastric glands (6).** The **lamina propria (7)** of the stomach, in contrast to the esophagus, is seen as thin strips of connective tissue between the tightly packed gastric glands (6).

Figure 11-14   Stomach: Fundus and Body Regions (plastic section)

This low magnification photomicrograph illustrates the entire mucosa of a stomach wall. In terms of histology, the fundus and body regions of the stomach are identical. The stomach surface is lined by mucus-secreting, **simple columnar epithelium (1)** that extends downward into the **gastric pits (2),** which are shallow in these regions of the stomach. Draining into the gastric pits (2) are the long **gastric glands (5),** which contain different cell types. The cells of the gastric glands (5) are tightly packed and their lumina are not clearly visible. The large, pale-staining cells in the gastric glands (5) are the acid-secreting **parietal cells (3).** These cells are more numerous in the upper regions of the gastric glands (5). The darker-staining cells are the **chief (zymogenic) cells (6)** and they are mostly located in the basal regions of the gastric glands (5). Between the numerous gastric glands (5) are thin strips of the connective tissue **lamina propria (7).** A thin strip of the smooth muscle **muscularis mucosae (8)** separates the mucosa from the **submucosa (4)** of the stomach.

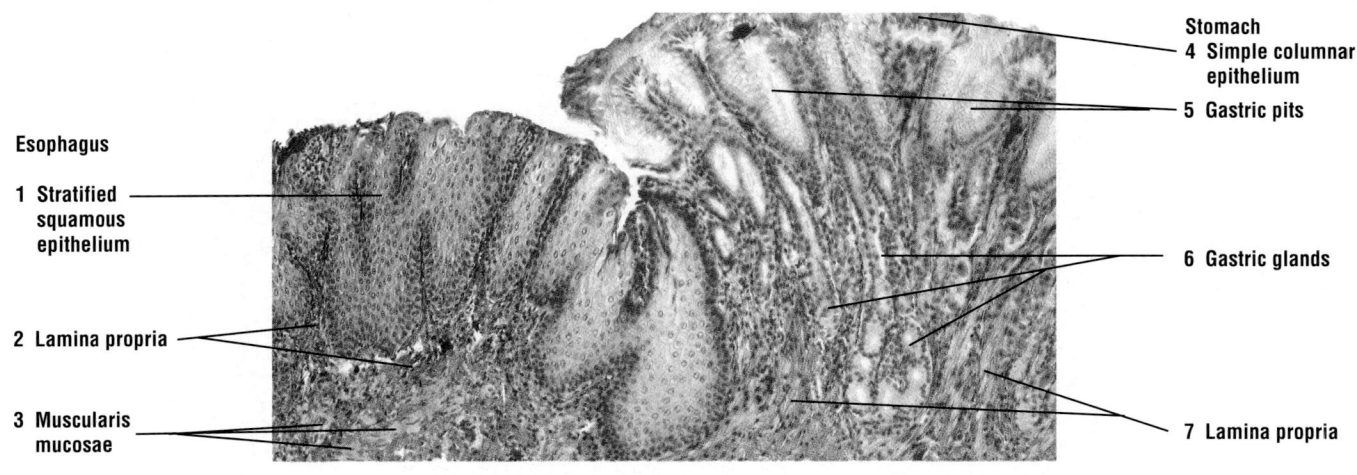

Esophagus

1 Stratified squamous epithelium

2 Lamina propria

3 Muscularis mucosae

Stomach
4 Simple columnar epithelium

5 Gastric pits

6 Gastric glands

7 Lamina propria

Fig. 11-13   Esophageal–Stomach Junction. Stain: Mallory-azan. 30×

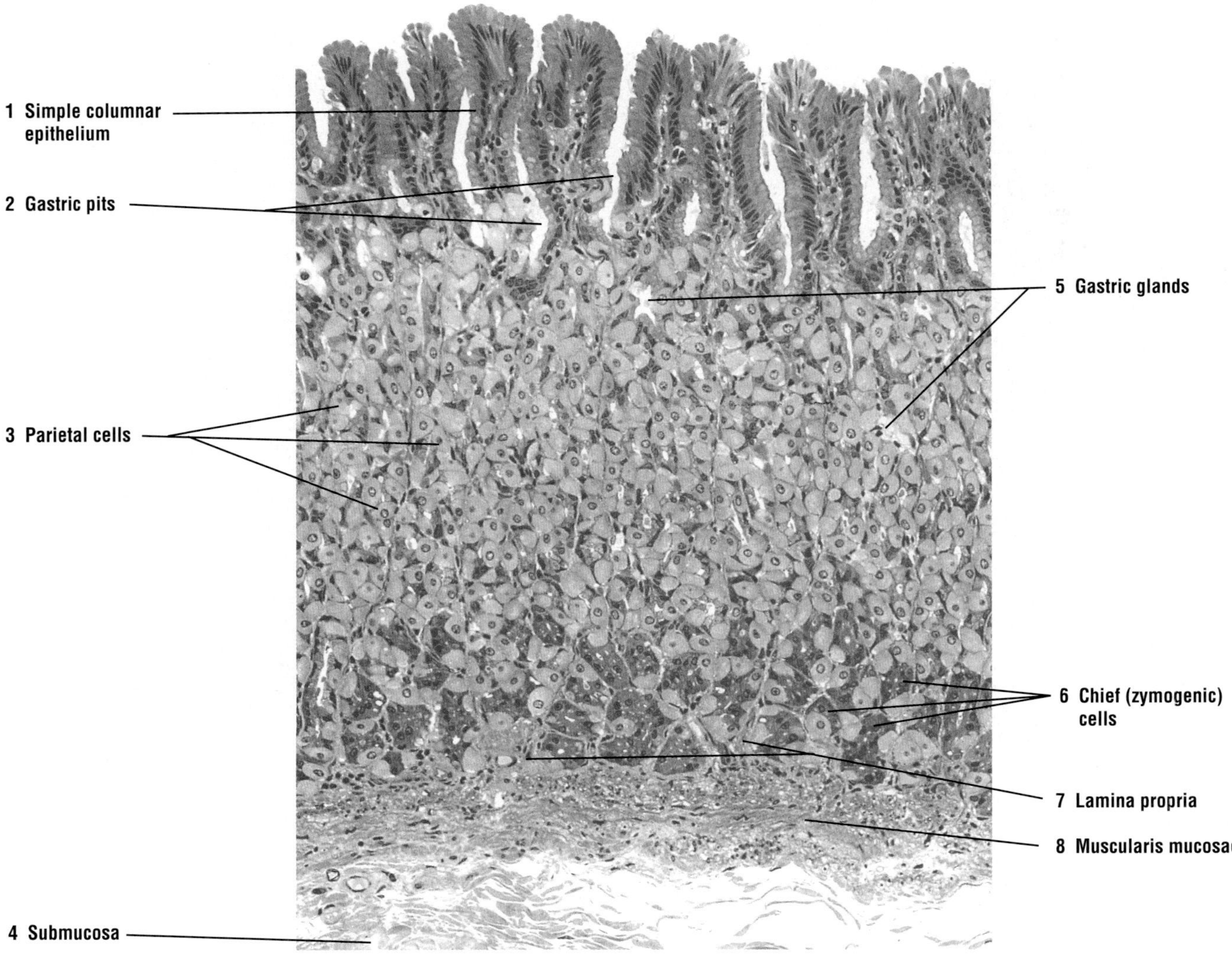

1 Simple columnar epithelium

2 Gastric pits

3 Parietal cells

4 Submucosa

5 Gastric glands

6 Chief (zymogenic) cells

7 Lamina propria

8 Muscularis mucosae

Fig. 11-14   Stomach: Fundus and Body Regions (plastic section). Stain: hematoxylin-eosin. 50×

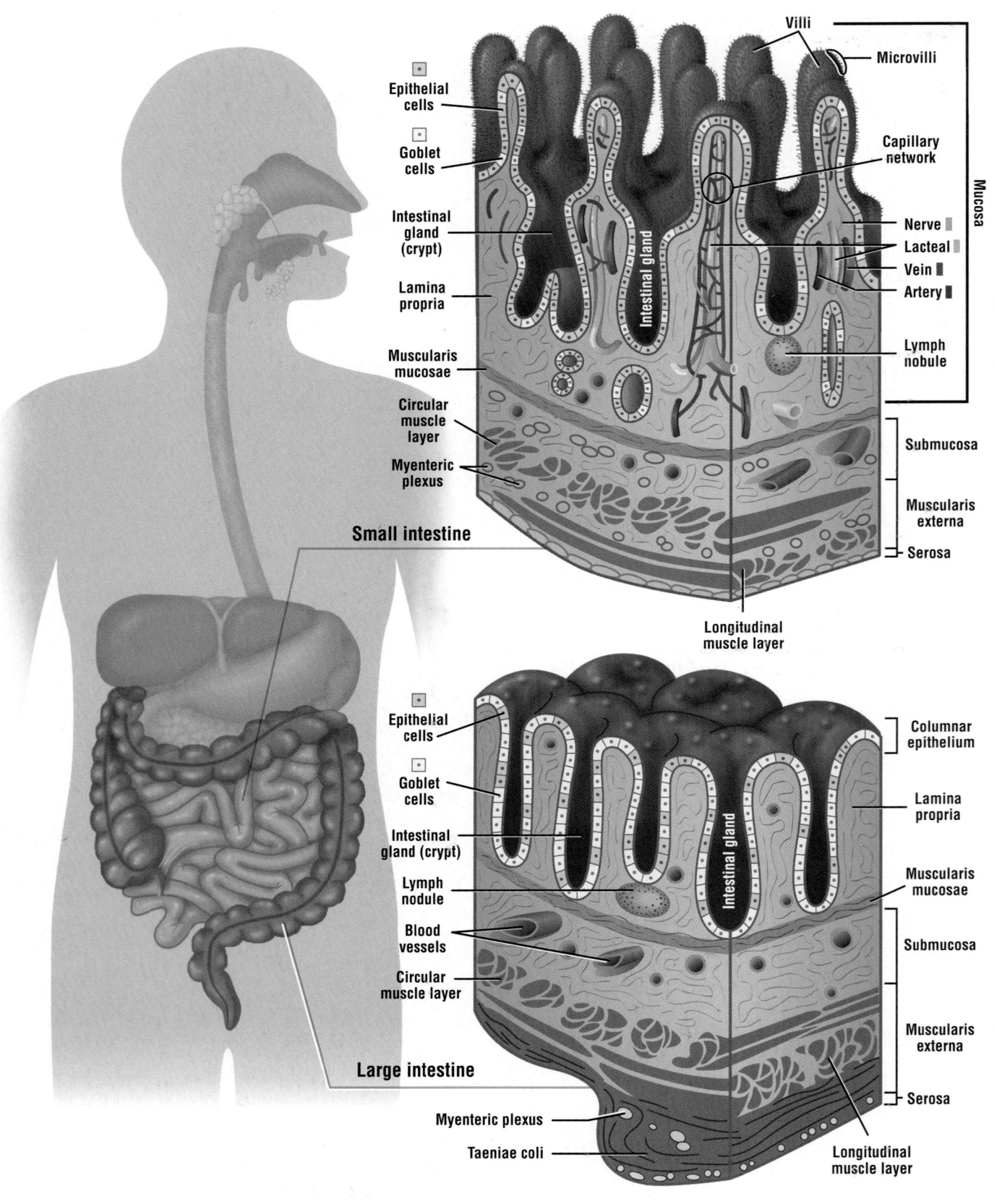

Villi

Microvilli

Epithelial cells

Goblet cells

Capillary network

Mucosa

Intestinal gland (crypt)

Intestinal gland

Nerve

Lacteal

Vein

Artery

Lamina propria

Lymph nobule

Muscularis mucosae

Circular muscle layer

Myenteric plexus

Submucosa

Muscularis externa

Serosa

Small intestine

Longitudinal muscle layer

Epithelial cells

Columnar epithelium

Goblet cells

Lamina propria

Intestinal gland (crypt)

Intestinal gland

Muscularis mucosae

Lymph nodule

Submucosa

Blood vessels

Circular muscle layer

Muscularis externa

Large intestine

Serosa

Myenteric plexus

Taeniae coli

Longitudinal muscle layer

Digestive System: Small and Large Intestines

SMALL INTESTINE

The **small intestine** is a long, convoluted tube approximately 5 meters long. It extends from the junction with the stomach to the junction with the **large intestine** or **colon**. For descriptive purposes, the small intestine is divided into three parts: the **duodenum, jejunum,** and **ileum.** The transition and microscopic differences among these three segments are minor.

The mucosa of the small intestine exhibits specialized structures that increase its surface area for absorption. These include the plicae circulares, the villi, and the microvilli. The **plicae circulares** are permanent, spiral folds or elevations of the mucosa (with submucosal core) that extend into the intestinal lumen; they are most prominent in the proximal portion of the small intestine, where most of the absorption takes place, and decrease in prominence closer to the ileum **(Fig. 12-2).** The **villi** are permanent fingerlike projections of the **lamina propria** of the mucosa that also extend into the lumen. They are covered by **simple columnar epithelium** and are more prominent in the proximal portion of the small intestine. The connective tissue core of each villus contains a lymphatic capillary called **lacteal,** blood capillaries, and strands of smooth muscles **(Figs. 12-1, 12-2, 12-4, 12-5, 12-11).** The **microvilli** are cytoplasmic extensions that cover the apices of the intestinal absorptive cells. They are visible under a light microscope as a **striated (brush) border (Fig. 12-5).**

The epithelium that lines the stomach surface is made up of only one cell type (mucus-secreting). In contrast, the surface of the mucosa of the small intestine contains numerous cell types. Most cells in the intestinal epithelium are tall, **columnar absorptive cells** with a prominent striated (brush) border (microvilli) covered by a thick **glycocalyx** coat. Interspersed among the columnar absorptive cells are the **goblet cells,** which increase in number toward the distal region of the small intestine (ileum).

The small intestine also contains numerous **intestinal glands** (crypts of Lieberkühn). These glands are located in the intestinal mucosa and open into the intestinal lumen at the base of the villi. The surface epithelium of the villi also extends into and lines the intestinal glands. **Undifferentiated cells** in the intestinal glands exhibit mitotic activity and produce the columnar absorptive cells and the goblet cells of the intestinal epithelium. Located at the base of the intestinal glands are the **Paneth cells,** characterized by the presence of deep-staining eosinophilic granules in their cytoplasm **(Figs. 12-3, 12-12).** Numerous **enteroendocrine** or APUD (amine precursor uptake and decarboxylation) cells are also found in the epithelium of the villi and intestinal glands. In the wall of the terminal end of the small intestine, the ileum, are found numerous aggregations of closely packed lymphoid nodules called **Peyer's patches.** These nodules are very prominent and occupy a large portion of the submucosa of the ileum **(Fig. 12-4).**

LARGE INTESTINE (COLON)

The large intestine is situated between the anus and the terminal end of the ileum. It is composed of an initial segment **cecum,** and the **ascending, transverse, descending,** and **sigmoid colon,** as well as **rectum** and **anus.** Unabsorbed and undigested food residues in the small intestine are forced into the large intestine by strong peristaltic action of the muscles in muscularis externa of the small intestine. The residues that enter the large intestine are in a semifluid state; by the time they have reached the terminal portion of the large intestine, however, these residues have acquired the semisolid consistency of **feces.** Although present in the small intestine, the **goblet cells** in the epithelium appear more numerous in the large intestine than in the small intestine. Also, the number of goblet cells increases from the cecum to the sigmoid colon. The large intestine does not contain **plicae circulares** or **villi,** and the **intestinal glands** are deeper than in the small intestine. The intestinal glands of the large intestine also lack the **Paneth cells** but contain different enteroendocrine (APUD) cells. **(Figs. 12-6, 12-7, 12-13).**

Figure 12-1   Small Intestine: Duodenum (longitudinal section)

The wall of the duodenum (first part) consists of four layers: the mucosa with its **lining epithelium (7a), lamina propria (7b),** and the **muscularis mucosae (9, 12);** the underlying connective tissue **submucosa** with the mucous **duodenal (Brunner's) glands (3, 13);** the two smooth muscle layers of the **muscularis externa (14);** and the visceral peritoneum **serosa (15).** These layers are continuous with those in the stomach and in the small and large intestine.

The small intestine is characterized by numerous finger-like extensions called **villi (7)** (singular: villus); a lining epithelium (7a) of columnar cells lined with microvilli, which form the striated borders; light-staining **goblet cells (2);** and short, tubular **intestinal glands (crypts of Lieberkühn) (4, 8)** in the lamina propria (7b). The presence of duodenal glands **(3, 13)** in the submucosa (13) characterizes the upper duodenum. These glands are absent in the rest of the small and large intestine.

The villi (7) are mucosal surface modifications. **Intervillous spaces (1)** are visible between the villi (7). The lining epithelium (7a) covers each villus and continues into the intestinal glands (4, 8). Each villus (7) has core of lamina propria (7b), strands of **smooth muscle fibers (10)** that extend upward into the villi from the **muscularis mucosae (9, 12),** and a central lymphatic vessel, called the **lacteal (11).** (See Fig. 12-5 for a detailed structure of a villus, the central lacteal, and the contents of the lamina propria.)

The lamina propria (7b) contains the intestinal glands (4, 8); these open into the intervillous spaces (1). In certain sections of the duodenum, the submucosal duodenal glands (13) can be seen extending into the lamina propria (3). The lamina propria (7b) also contains fine connective tissue fibers with reticular cells, diffuse lymphatic tissue, and/or **lymphatic nodules (5).**

In the duodenum, the submucosa (13) is almost completely filled with highly branched, tubular duodenal glands (13). The muscularis mucosae (9, 12) may be interrupted if the duodenal glands penetrate into the mucosal lamina propria (3). The duodenal glands (3) deliver their secretory product to the bottom of the intestinal glands (3, 4, 8).

In a normal cross section of the duodenum, the muscularis externa (14) consists of an **inner circular layer (14a)** and **outer longitudinal layer (14b)** of smooth muscle. However, because in this figure the duodenum has been cut in a longitudinal plane, the direction of fibers in these two smooth muscle layers is reversed. Nests of parasympathetic ganglion cells of the **myenteric (Auerbach's) nerve plexus (6)** are also visible in the connective tissue between the two muscle layers of the muscularis externa (14). This nerve plexus is found between these muscle layers throughout the small and large intestine. Similar but smaller nests of ganglion cells are likewise found in the submucosa (not illustrated) throughout the small and large intestine.

The **serosa (visceral peritoneum) (15)** contains the connective tissue cells, blood vessels, and adipose cells; the serosa forms the outermost layer of the duodenum (first part).

■ Functional Correlations–Duodenum

A characteristic feature of the first portion of the small intestine, the duodenum, is the presence in the submucosa of branched tubuloalveolar **duodenal (Brunner's) glands.** The excretory ducts of these glands penetrate the muscularis mucosae and deliver their secretion into the lumen of the duodenum at the base of the intestinal glands. The main function of the duodenal glands is to protect the duodenal mucosa from the highly corrosive action of gastric contents. This function is performed by secreting alkaline **mucus** and **bicarbonate ions,** which then buffer or neutralize the acidic chyme that enters the duodenum from the stomach. Duodenal glands secrete their products into the lumen in response to the entrance of acidic chyme and to the parasympathetic stimulation by the vagus nerve. These alkaline secretions also provide a more favorable environment for the continued action of the digestive enzymes. The duodenal glands also produce a polypeptide hormone called **urogastrone.** This hormone inhibits hydrochloric acid secretion by the parietal cells in the stomach and increases epithelial proliferation in the small intestine.

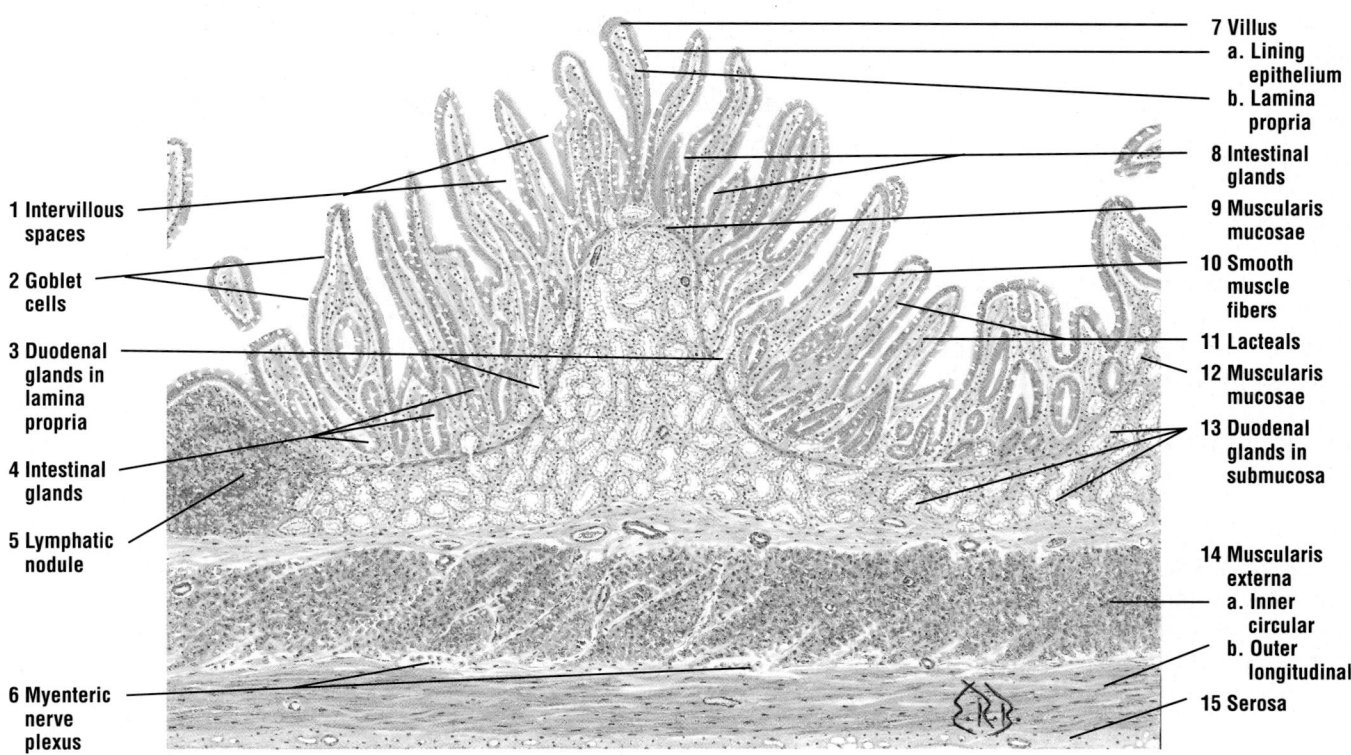

1 Intervillous
  spaces

2 Goblet
  cells

3 Duodenal
  glands in
  lamina
  propria

4 Intestinal
  glands

5 Lymphatic
  nodule

6 Myenteric
  nerve
  plexus

7 Villus
  a. Lining
     epithelium
  b. Lamina
     propria

8 Intestinal
  glands

9 Muscularis
  mucosae

10 Smooth
   muscle
   fibers

11 Lacteals

12 Muscularis
   mucosae

13 Duodenal
   glands in
   submucosa

14 Muscularis
   externa
   a. Inner
      circular
   b. Outer
      longitudinal

15 Serosa

Fig. 12-1   Small Intestine: Duodenum (longitudinal section). Stain: hematoxylin-eosin. Low magnification.

Figure 12-2   Small Intestine: Jejunum-Ileum (transverse section)

The histology of the lower duodenum, jejunum, and ileum is similar to that of the upper duodenum illustrated in Figure 12-1. The only exception are the duodenal glands (Brunner's); these are usually limited to submucosa in the upper part of the duodenum. The villi exhibit variable shapes and lengths in different regions of the small intestine; however, this is not usually apparent in histologic sections. Also, in the lower regions of the ileum, large aggregates of lymphatic nodules (Peyer's patches) are visible at intervals (See Fig. 12-4).

This figure illustrates numerous **villi (2)** sectioned in different planes and a prominent, permanent fold of the small intestine, the **plica circulares (10)**. Both the mucosa and **submucosa (4, 16)** constitute the plica circulares (10). In the lumen, each villus (2) exhibits a typical structure: a columnar **lining epithelium (1)** with striated border and goblet cells, a core of **lamina propria (3)** with diffuse lymphatic tissue, and strips of smooth muscle fibers from the **muscularis mucosae (6)**. Within the villi are also seen a central lacteal and small blood vessels; these are illustrated in Figure 12-5. The **intestinal glands** (crypts of Lieberkühn) **(5, 12)** extend into the lamina propria (3). These glands are closely packed, and in the figure are seen in both the longitudinal and cross sections. The intestinal glands (5, 12) open into the **intervillous spaces (11)**. A **lymphatic nodule (14)** is visible extending from the lamina propria (3) of the mucosa into the submucosa (16), disrupting the surrounding **muscularis mucosae (15)**.

The appearance and distribution of the muscularis mucosae (6, 15), submucosa (4, 16), **muscularis externa (7, 8)**, and **serosa (18)** are typical of the small intestine. Parasympathetic ganglion cells of the **myenteric plexus (17)** are seen in the connective tissue between the inner circular smooth muscle layer (7) and the outer longitudinal muscle layer (8) of the muscularis externa. Ganglion cells of the submucosal plexuses are also present in the small intestine but are not illustrated in this figure.

Figure 12-3   Intestinal Glands With Paneth Cells and Enteroendocrine Cells

Adjacent to the smooth muscle of the **muscularis mucosae (5, 10)** several **intestinal glands (7)** are visible. The characteristic **goblet cells (2)** and cells with striated borders are seen in the glands. Visible at the base of these glands are pyramid-shaped cells with large, acidophilic granules, which fill most of the cytoplasma and displace the nucleus toward the base of the cell. These cells are the **Paneth cells (4, 9)** and are found throughout the small intestine.

Enteroendocrine cells (3, 8) are interspersed among the intestinal gland cells, **mitotic gland cells (1, 6)**, goblet cells (2), and Paneth cells (4, 9). Enteroendocrine cells are characterized by fine granules located in the basal portions of the cytoplasm, with the nucleus situated above the granules. Most enteroendocrine cells take up and decarboxylate precursors of biogenic monoamines and are therefore considered part of a larger group of cells designated as the amine precursor uptake and decarboxylation (APUD) cell series. The APUD cell types are found in the epithelia of the gastrointestinal tract (stomach, small and large intestines), respiratory tract, pancreas, and thyroid glands.

■ Functional Correlations–Paneth Cells and Enteroendocrine Cells

Paneth cells produce **lysozyme**, an antibacterial enzyme whose function is to digest the cell walls of some bacteria and to control the microbial flora of the small intestine. **Enteroendocrine cells** secrete numerous **regulatory hormones** of the intestine, including **gastric inhibitory peptide, secretin,** and **cholecystokinin (pancreozymin)**. These intestinal hormones control the release of gastric and pancreatic secretions, intestinal motility, and contractions of the gall bladder.

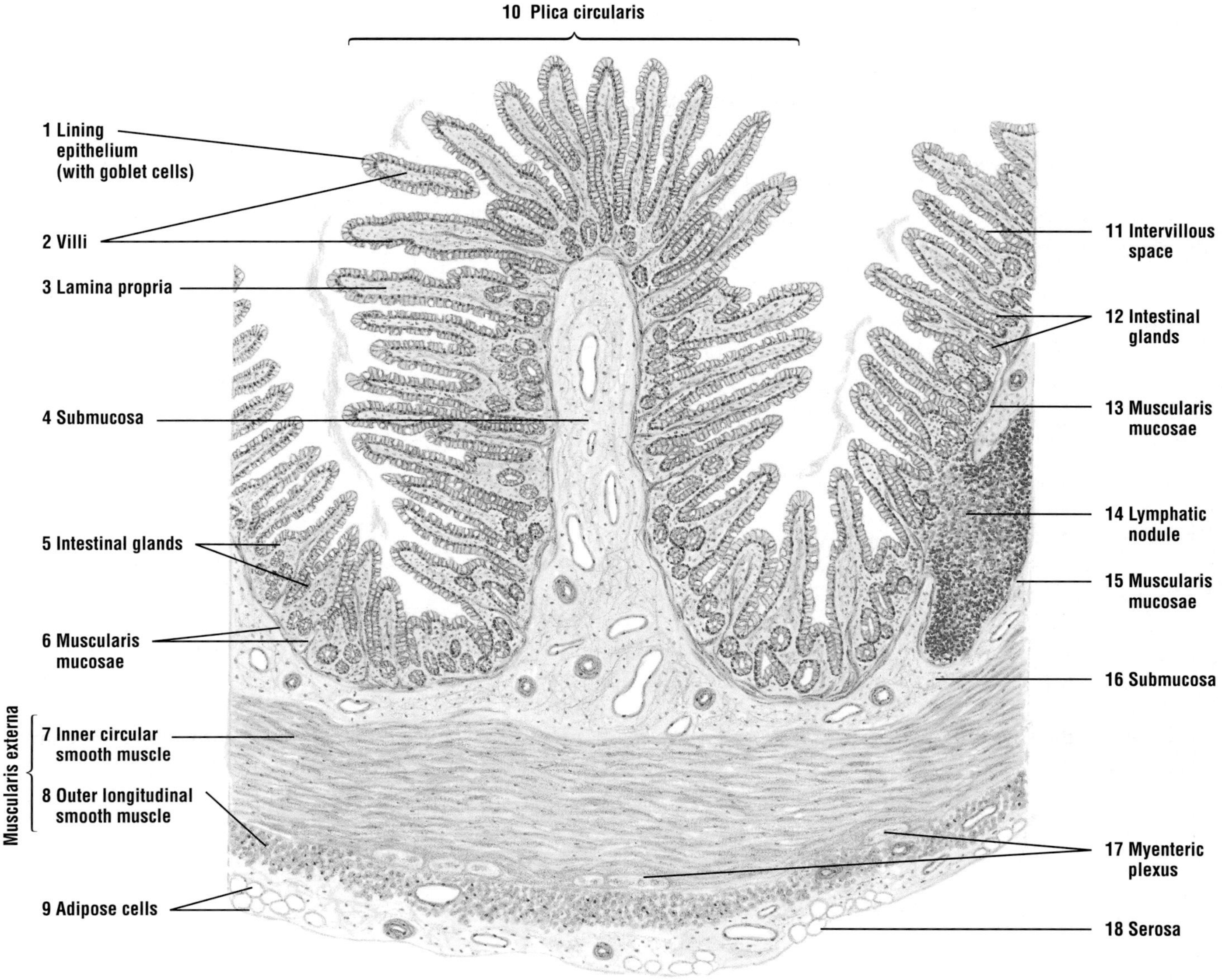

10 Plica circularis

1 Lining epithelium (with goblet cells)

2 Villi

3 Lamina propria

4 Submucosa

5 Intestinal glands

6 Muscularis mucosae

Muscularis externa

7 Inner circular smooth muscle

8 Outer longitudinal smooth muscle

9 Adipose cells

11 Intervillous space

12 Intestinal glands

13 Muscularis mucosae

14 Lymphatic nodule

15 Muscularis mucosae

16 Submucosa

17 Myenteric plexus

18 Serosa

Fig. 12-2   Small Intestine: Jejunum–Ileum (transverse section). Stain: hematoxylin-eosin. Low magnification.

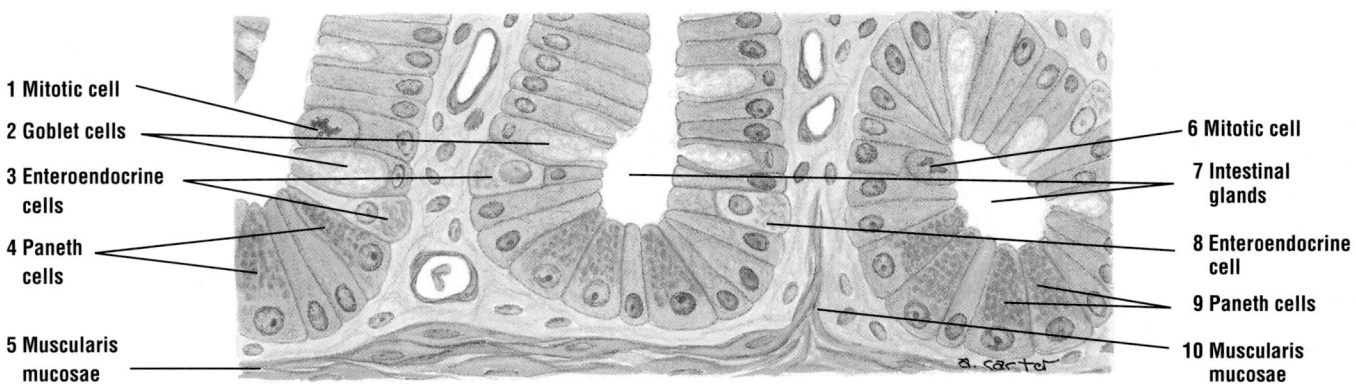

1 Mitotic cell

2 Goblet cells

3 Enteroendocrine cells

4 Paneth cells

5 Muscularis mucosae

6 Mitotic cell

7 Intestinal glands

8 Enteroendocrine cell

9 Paneth cells

10 Muscularis mucosae

Fig. 12-3   Intestinal Glands With Paneth Cells and Enteroendocrine Cells. Stain: hematoxylin-eosin, plastic section. High magnification.

Figure 12-4   Small Intestine: Ileum With Lymphatic Nodules (Peyer's Patch) (transverse section)

This cross section of the ileum illustrates the four layers of the intestinal wall **(9–16)**. The **villi (1, 2, 9)** have been sectioned in various planes and thus appear irregular. The **intestinal glands (crypts of Lieberkühn) (3, 10)** are located in the lamina propria; two of these glands are illustrated opening into an intervillous space (upper leader 3, upper leader 10).

A characteristic feature of the ileum are the aggregations of lymphatic nodules called **Peyer's patches (5)**. Each Peyer's patch is an aggregation of ten or more lymphatic nodules, which are located in the wall of the ileum opposite the attachment of the mesentery. The portion of the Peyer's patch illustrated in this figure shows nine lymphatic nodules (4, 5, and others), most of which exhibit **germinal centers (5)**. The lymphatic nodules coalesce and the boundaries between them are usually not discernible.

The nodules originate in the diffuse lymphatic tissue of the **lamina propria (11)**. Villi are absent in the area of the intestinal lumen where the nodules reach the surface of the **mucosa (4)**. Typically, the lymphatic nodules extend into the **submucosa (7, 13)**, disrupt the **muscularis mucosae (6)**, and spread out in the loose connective tissue of the submucosa (7, 13).

Figure 12-5   Small Intestine: Villi

The distal parts of several **villi (1)** are sectioned in several planes and illustrated at a higher magnification. The two villi on the left are sectioned longitudinally and the villi the right side sectioned transversely. All villi contain numerous **goblet cells (7)** that secrete mucus. In order to show this secretion in the goblet cells, the sections were stained for carbohydrates. As a result, the goblet cells (7) are stained magenta red.

The **surface epithelium (2)** of the villi contains numerous goblet cells (7) and columnar absorptive cells with **striated borders (microvilli) (3)**. A thin **basement membrane (8)** is visible between the surface epithelium (2) and the **lamina propria (4)**. In the core of the lamina propria (4) are found connective tissue cells and fibers, different types of blood cells, and **smooth muscle fibers (5)**. Also present in each villus (but not always seen in sections) is a **central lacteal (6)**—a dilated lymphatic vessel lined with endothelium. Arterioles, one or more venules, and **capillaries (9)** are also visible in the villi.

■ **Functional Correlations**–Small Intestine

The small intestine performs many important digestive functions, including (1) completing **digestion** (initiated in the stomach) of food products (chyme) by chemicals and enzymes produced in the liver and pancreas, and by cells in its own mucosa; (2) selective **absorption** of nutrients into the blood and lymph capillaries; (3) **transportation** of chyme and digestive waste material to the large intestine; and (4) release of **hormones** that regulate the digestive processes. On the surface epithelium, **goblet cells** secrete **mucus** that lubricates, coats, and protects the intestinal surface from the corrosive action of digestive chemicals and enzymes. The outer **glycocalyx** coat on the principal absorptive cells not only protects the intestinal surface from digestion, but also contains the enzymes required for the terminal digestion of various food products. These are the pancreatic enzymes that are present in the lumen and are absorbed into the glycocalyx of the absorptive cells. Transport proteins then bring the products of digestion into the cell interior. Intestinal cells absorb **amino acids, glucose,** and **fatty acids**—the end products of protein, carbohydrates, and fat digestion, respectively. Amino acids and glucose are transported through intestinal cells to the **blood capillaries.** Most of the fatty acids, however, do not enter the blood capillaries but instead enter the lymphatic vessels **lacteals** located in the lamina propria of the villi.

■ **Functional Correlations**–Peyer's Patches in the Ileum

The lymphatic nodules of the Peyer's patches contain **B lymphocytes,** some **T lymphocytes, macrophages,** and **plasma cells.** Overlying these lymphoid nodules of the Peyer's patches are the **M (membranous epithelial) cells,** which replace the columnar epithelial cells of the small intestine. M cells continually sample the **antigens** of the intestinal lumen, ingest the antigens, and present them to the underlying lymphocytes and macrophages in the lamina propria, where specific **antibodies** and proper immune response to foreign antigens are developed.

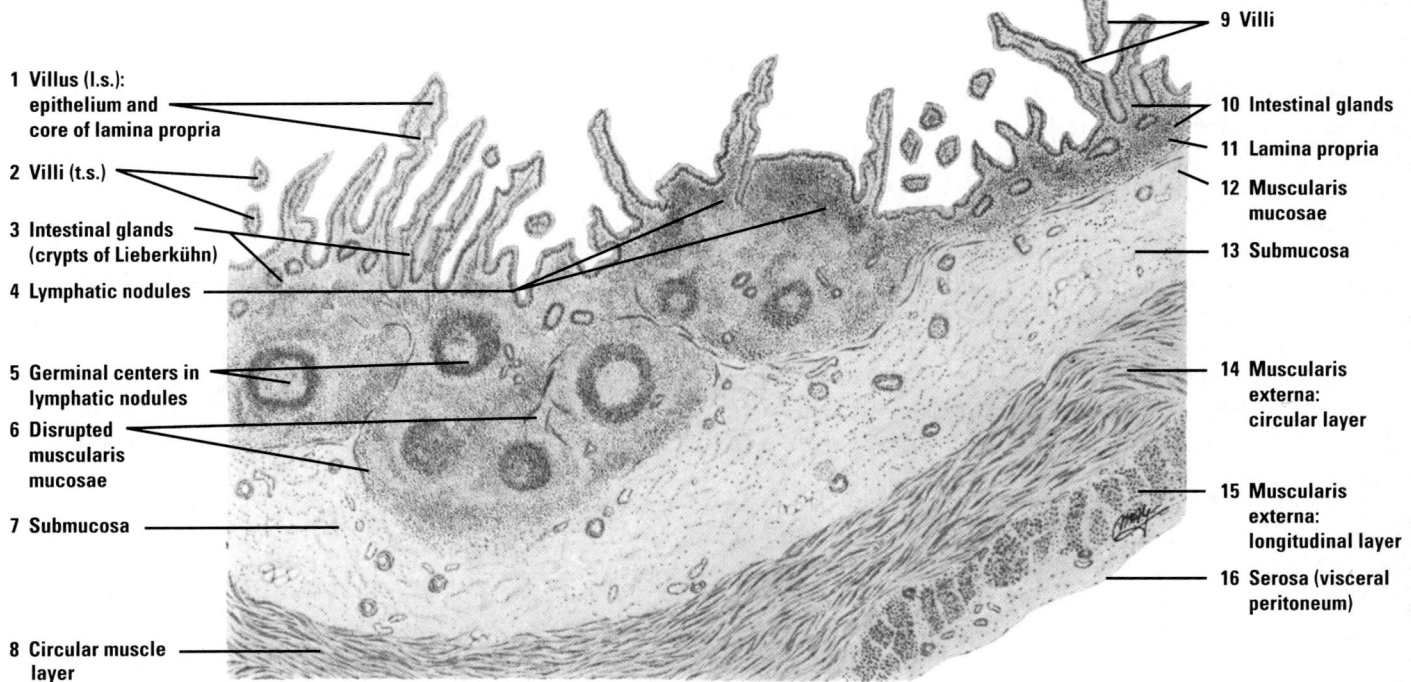

1 Villus (l.s.):
    epithelium and
    core of lamina propria

2 Villi (t.s.)

3 Intestinal glands
    (crypts of Lieberkühn)

4 Lymphatic nodules

5 Germinal centers in
    lymphatic nodules

6 Disrupted
    muscularis
    mucosae

7 Submucosa

8 Circular muscle
    layer

9 Villi

10 Intestinal glands

11 Lamina propria

12 Muscularis
    mucosae

13 Submucosa

14 Muscularis
    externa:
    circular layer

15 Muscularis
    externa:
    longitudinal layer

16 Serosa (visceral
    peritoneum)

Fig. 12-4   Small Intestine: Ileum With Lymphatic Nodules (Peyer's Patch) (transverse section). Stain: hematoxylin-eosin. Low magnification.

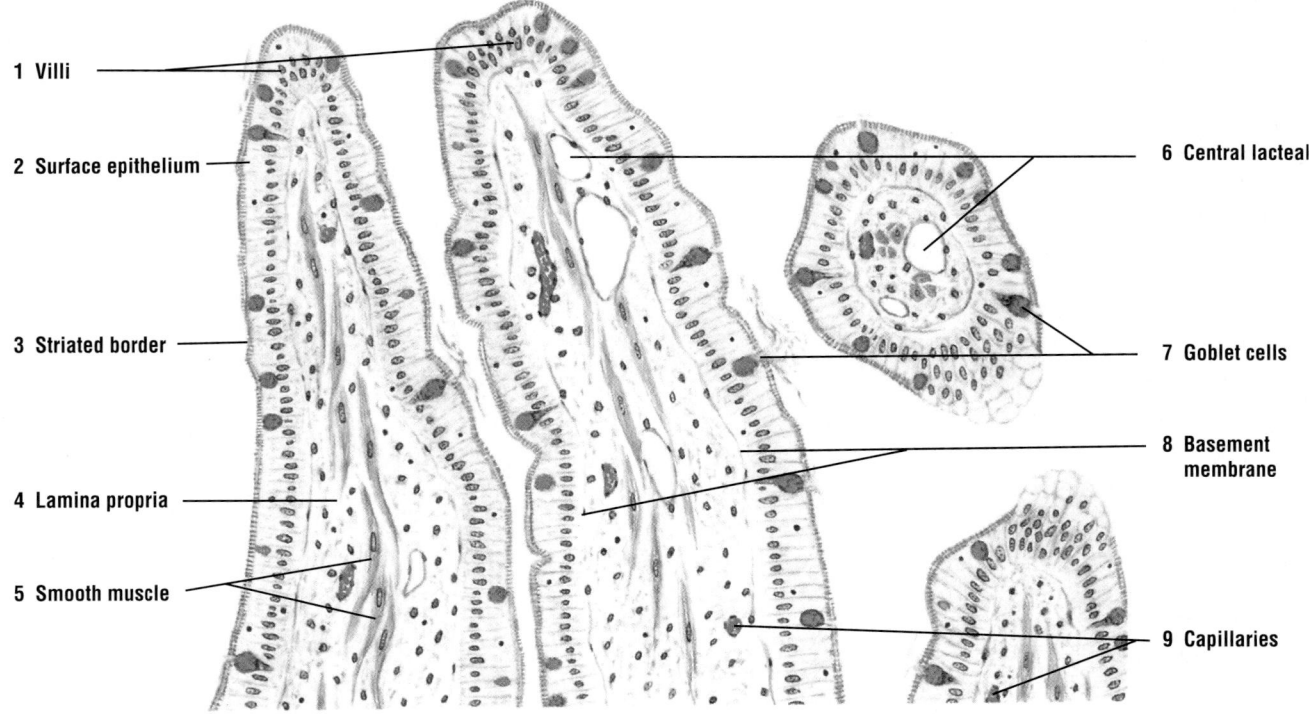

1 Villi

2 Surface epithelium

3 Striated border

4 Lamina propria

5 Smooth muscle

6 Central lacteal

7 Goblet cells

8 Basement
    membrane

9 Capillaries

Fig. 12-5   Small Intestine: Villi. Stain: PAS. Medium magnification.

Figure 12-6   Large Intestine: Colon and Mesentery (panoramic view, transverse section)

The colon has the same basic layers of epithelium, connective tissue, and smooth muscle in its wall as the small intestine. The **mucosa (4, 5, 6, 7)** consists of columnar surface **epithelium (4), intestinal glands (5), lamina propria (6),** and **muscularis mucosae (7).** The underlying **submucosa (8)** contains connective tissue cells and fibers, various blood vessels, and nerves. Two smooth muscle layers are visible in the **muscularis externa (13).** The **serosa (visceral peritoneum** and **mesentery) (3, 17)** covers the transverse colon and sigmoid colon regions. Several distinct modifications in the wall of the colon, however, clearly distinguish it from other regions of the digestive tract (tube).

In contrast to the small intestine, the colon does not have villi or plicae circulares. As a result, the luminal surface of the mucosa in the colon is smooth. When the colon is undistended, however, the mucosa (4, 5, 6, 7) and submucosa (8) exhibit numerous **temporary folds (12).** In the lamina propria (6) and the submucosa (8) of the colon wall various-sized **lymphatic nodules (9, 11)** may be found.

The smooth muscle layers in the muscularis externa (13) of the colon are also modified. The **inner circular muscle layer (16)** is continuous in the colon wall, whereas the outer smooth muscle layer is condensed into three broad, longitudinal bands called **taeniae coli (1, 10).** In the rest of the colon wall, a very thin **outer longitudinal muscle layer (15)** can be found between the taeniae coli (1, 10); this outer longitudinal muscle layer, however, is often discontinuous. The parasympathetic ganglion cells of the **myenteric (Auerbach's) nerve plexus (2, 14)** are found between the two smooth muscle layers of the muscularis externa (13).

Both the transverse and sigmoid portions of the colon are attached to the body wall by a **mesentery (18).** As a result, the serosa (3, 17) becomes the outermost layer in these two regions of the colon. Within the mesentery loose connective tissue, adipose cells, blood vessels, and nerves are found.

A more detailed description and illustration of each layer in the colon wall are presented at a higher magnification in Figure 12-7.

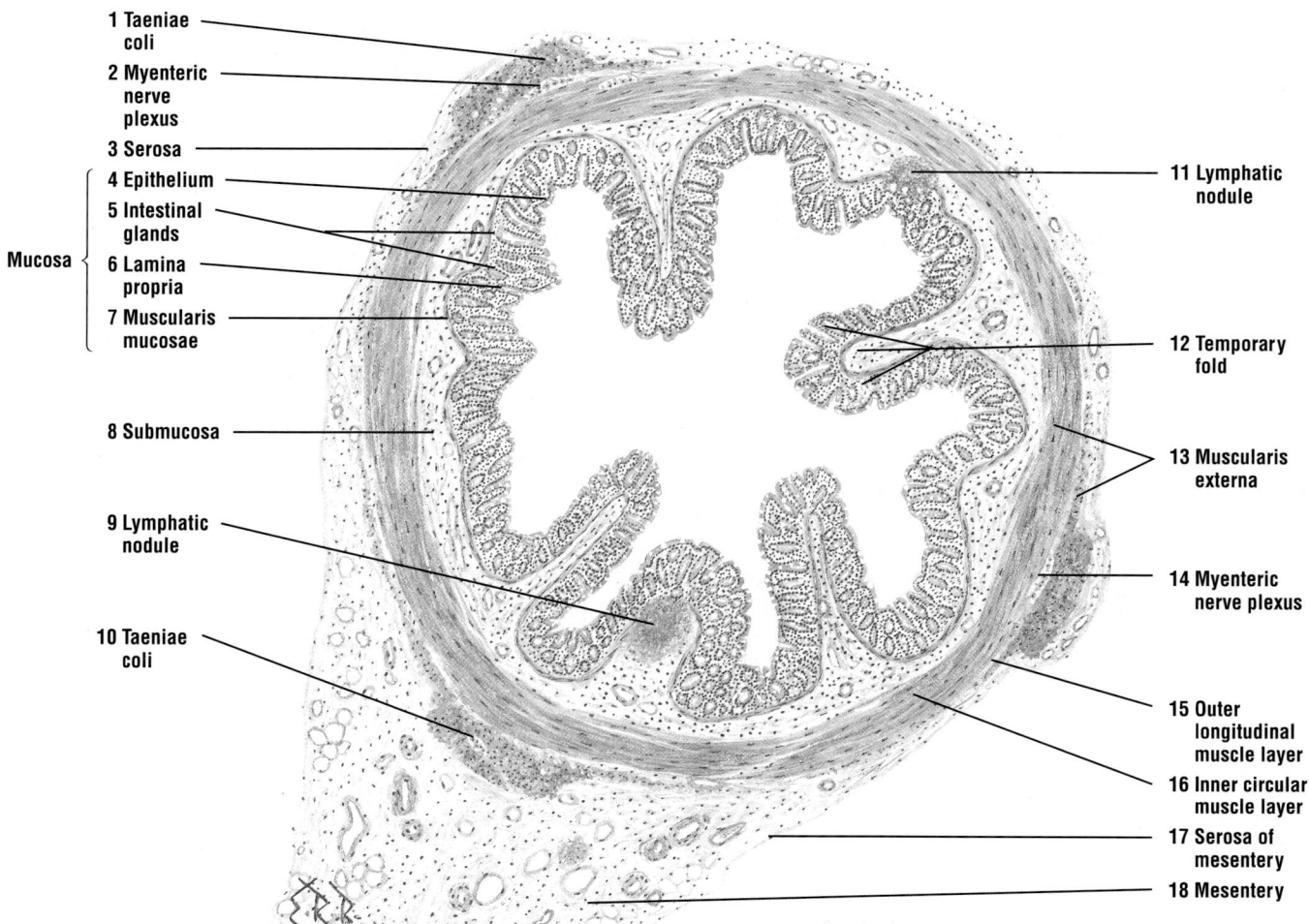

1 Taeniae coli
2 Myenteric nerve plexus
3 Serosa
Mucosa {
4 Epithelium
5 Intestinal glands
6 Lamina propria
7 Muscularis mucosae
8 Submucosa
9 Lymphatic nodule
10 Taeniae coli

11 Lymphatic nodule
12 Temporary fold
13 Muscularis externa
14 Myenteric nerve plexus
15 Outer longitudinal muscle layer
16 Inner circular muscle layer
17 Serosa of mesentery
18 Mesentery

Fig. 12-6   Large Intestine: Colon and Mesentery (panoramic view, transverse section). Stain: hematoxylin-eosin. Low magnification.

Figure 12-7   Large Intestine: Colon Wall (transverse section)

A small section of undistended colon wall is illustrated in greater detail. The four layers of the wall are the **mucosa (2, 3, 4)**, **submucosa (5)**, **muscularis externa (6)**, and **serosa (7).** These layers are continuous with those of the small intestine. This section of the colon wall shows the **temporary fold (9)** of the mucosa (2, 3, 4) and submucosa (5).

Villi are absent in the colon. The mucosa, however, is indented by long tubular **intestinal glands** (crypts of Lieberkühn) **(1, 10),** which extend through the **lamina propria (3)** to the **muscularis mucosae (4, 11).**

The **lining epithelium (2)** in the colon is primarily columnar, with thin striated borders and numerous goblet cells. This epithelium continues into the intestinal glands (1, 10), where goblet cells are abundant. Some of the intestinal glands (1, 10) are visible sectioned in longitudinal, transverse, or oblique planes.

The lamina propria (2), similar to that in the small intestine, contains abundant diffuse lymphatic tissue. A distinct **lymphatic nodule (13)** is visible deep in the lamina propria (2). Some of the larger lymphatic nodules may extend through the muscularis mucosae (4, 11) into the submucosa (5).

The appearance and distribution of the muscularis mucosae (4, 11), submucosa (5), and serosa (7) are typical for the digestive tract. The muscularis externa (6), however, appears atypical. In this section, the longitudinal layer of the muscularis externa (6) is arranged into strips or bands of smooth muscle called the **taeniae coli (15).** The parasympathetic ganglia of the **myenteric plexus (8, 14)** are visible between the muscle layers in the muscularis externa (6).

The serosa (7) covers the transverse and sigmoid colon; however, the ascending and descending colon are retroperitoneal and the outer layer on their posterior surface is the adventitia.

■ Functional Correlations–Large Intestine

The principal functions of the large intestine are to absorb **water** and **minerals (electrolytes)** from the residual contents and to form feces. Consistent with these functions, the epithelium of the large intestine contains **columnar absorptive cells** (similar to those in the epithelium of the small intestine) and mucus-secreting **goblet cells,** which produce mucus for lubricating the lumen of the larger intestine to facilitate passage of the hardened feces. No digestive enzymes are produced by the cells of the large intestine.

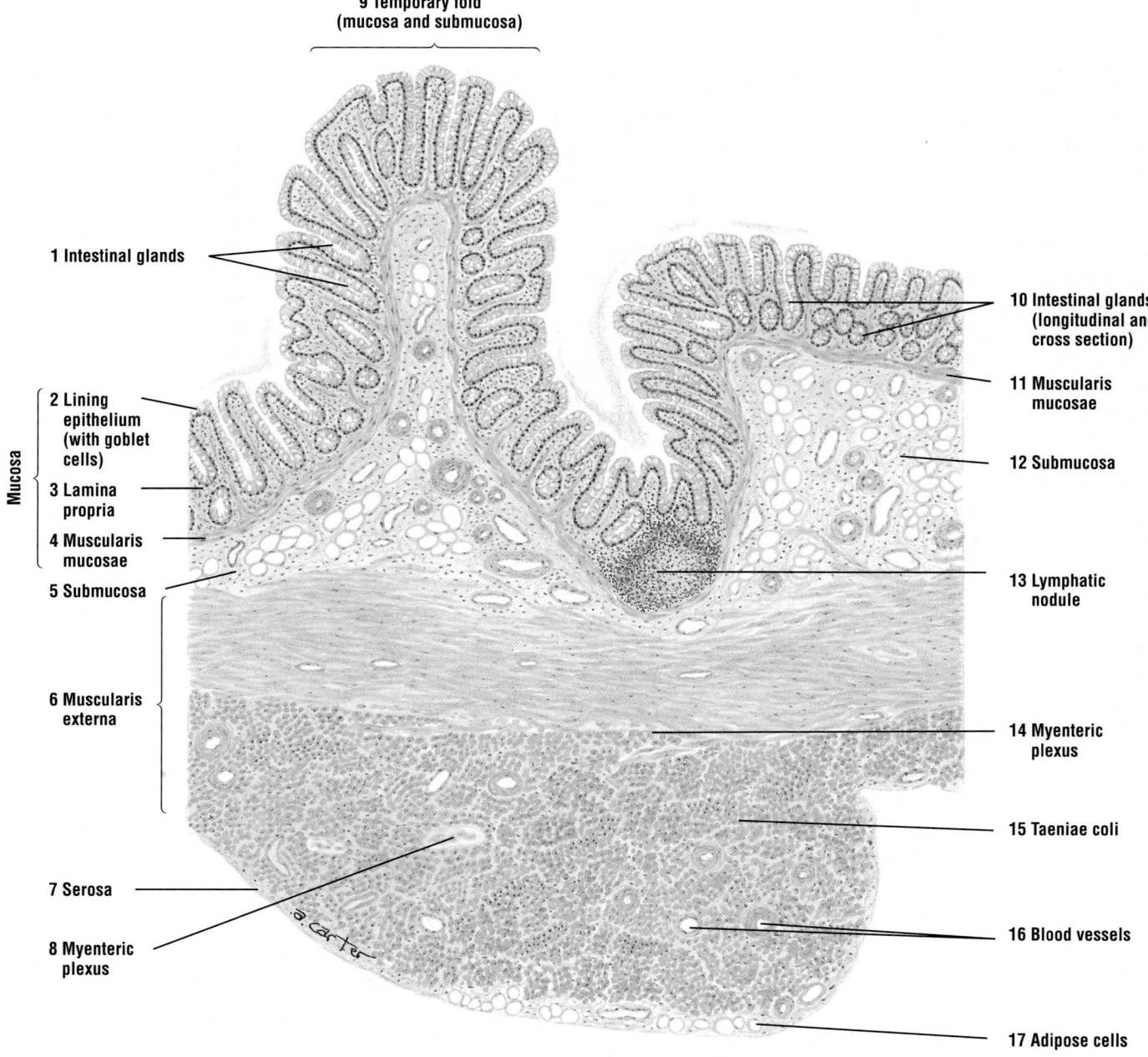

9 Temporary fold (mucosa and submucosa)

1 Intestinal glands

Mucosa

2 Lining epithelium (with goblet cells)

3 Lamina propria

4 Muscularis mucosae

5 Submucosa

6 Muscularis externa

7 Serosa

8 Myenteric plexus

10 Intestinal glands (longitudinal and cross section)

11 Muscularis mucosae

12 Submucosa

13 Lymphatic nodule

14 Myenteric plexus

15 Taeniae coli

16 Blood vessels

17 Adipose cells

Fig. 12-7   Large Intestine: Colon Wall (transverse section). Stain: hematoxylin-eosin. Medium magnification.

Figure 12-8   Appendix (panoramic view, transverse section)

This figure illustrates a cross section of the vermiform appendix at low magnification. It is structurally similar to the colon except for certain modifications characteristic of the appendix.

In comparing the mucosa of the appendix with that of the colon, several similar features are apparent: a **lining epithelium (1)** with numerous goblet cells; the underlying **lamina propria (3)** containing the **intestinal glands (5)** (crypts of Lieberkühn); and the **muscularis mucosae (2).** The intestinal glands (5) in the appendix are less well developed, shorter, and often spaced farther apart than those in the colon. **Diffuse lymphatic tissue (6)** in the lamina propria (3) is abundant and is often observed in the adjacent **submucosa (8).**

Lymphatic nodules (4, 9) with germinal centers are very numerous and highly characteristic of the appendix. These nodules originate in the lamina propria (3); however, because of their large size, the nodules may extend from the surface epithelium (1) to the submucosa (8).

The submucosa (8) is highly vascular and has numerous **blood vessels (11).** The **muscularis externa (7)** consists of the characteristic **inner circular layer (7a)** and **outer longitudinal layer (7b)** of smooth muscle; these muscle layers may vary in thickness. The **parasympathetic ganglia (12)** of the **myenteric plexus (12)** are seen between the inner (7a) and outer (7b) smooth muscle layers. The outermost layer of the appendix is the **serosa (10).**

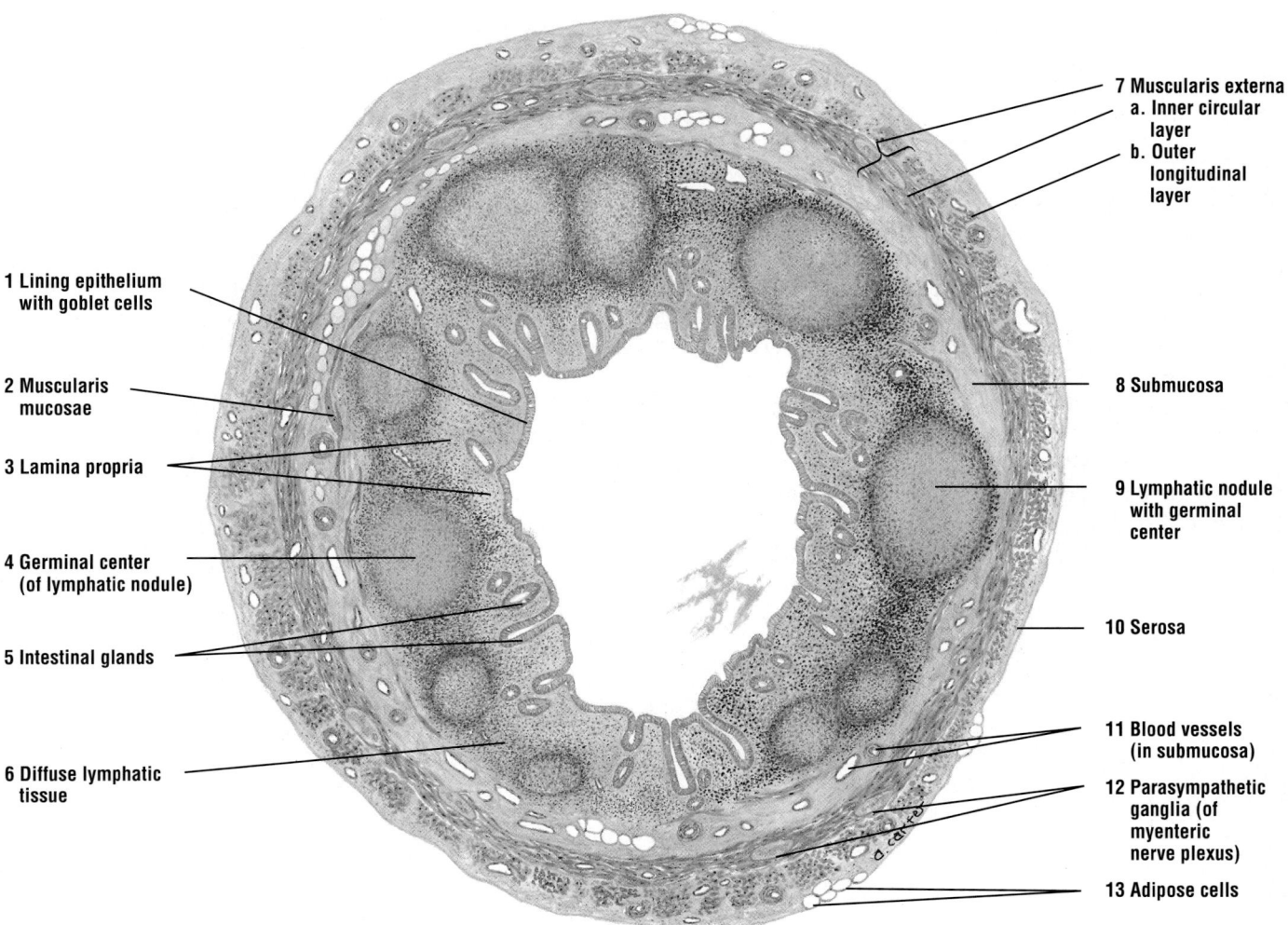

1 Lining epithelium with goblet cells

2 Muscularis mucosae

3 Lamina propria

4 Germinal center (of lymphatic nodule)

5 Intestinal glands

6 Diffuse lymphatic tissue

7 Muscularis externa
a. Inner circular layer
b. Outer longitudinal layer

8 Submucosa

9 Lymphatic nodule with germinal center

10 Serosa

11 Blood vessels (in submucosa)

12 Parasympathetic ganglia (of myenteric nerve plexus)

13 Adipose cells

Fig. 12-8   Appendix (panoramic view, transverse section). Stain: hematoxylin-eosin. Low magnification.

Figure 12-9   Rectum (panoramic view, transverse section)

The histology of the transverse section through the upper rectum appears similar to that of the colon; the same layers are present in the wall of the organ and the same components are found in each layer. Except for the longitudinal muscle layer surrounding the lumen, this figure could be a section of the colon.

The surface epithelium (1) facing the **lumen (5)** is lined by columnar cells with striated borders and goblet cells. The **intestinal glands (4), adipose cells (12),** and scattered **lymphatic nodules (10)** in the **lamina propria (2)** are similar to those in the colon; however, the glands are longer, closer together, and are mainly filled with goblet cells. Beneath the lamina propria (2) are the thin smooth muscle layers of **muscularis mucosae (11).**

The **longitudinal folds (3)** seen in the upper rectum and colon are temporary. These folds (3) have a core of **submucosa** (8) that is covered by the mucosa. Permanent transversal folds of the rectum, if present in a section, contain smooth muscle fibers from the circular layers of the muscularis externa. Permanent longitudinal folds (rectal columns) are found in the lower rectum, the anal canal.

Taeniae coli of the colon, illustrated in Figures 12-6 and 12-7, continue into the rectum. Here, however, the muscles of the **muscularis externa (13a, b)** again acquire the typical **inner circular (13a)** and **outer longitudinal (13b)** smooth muscle layers that are found in the rest of the digestive tract. Visible between these two smooth muscle layers are the **parasympathetic ganglia** of the **myenteric (Auerbach's) plexus (14).**

Adventitia (9) covers a portion of the rectum and serosa covers the remainder. Numerous **blood vessels (6, 7, 15)** are visible in both the submucosa (8) and adventitia (9).

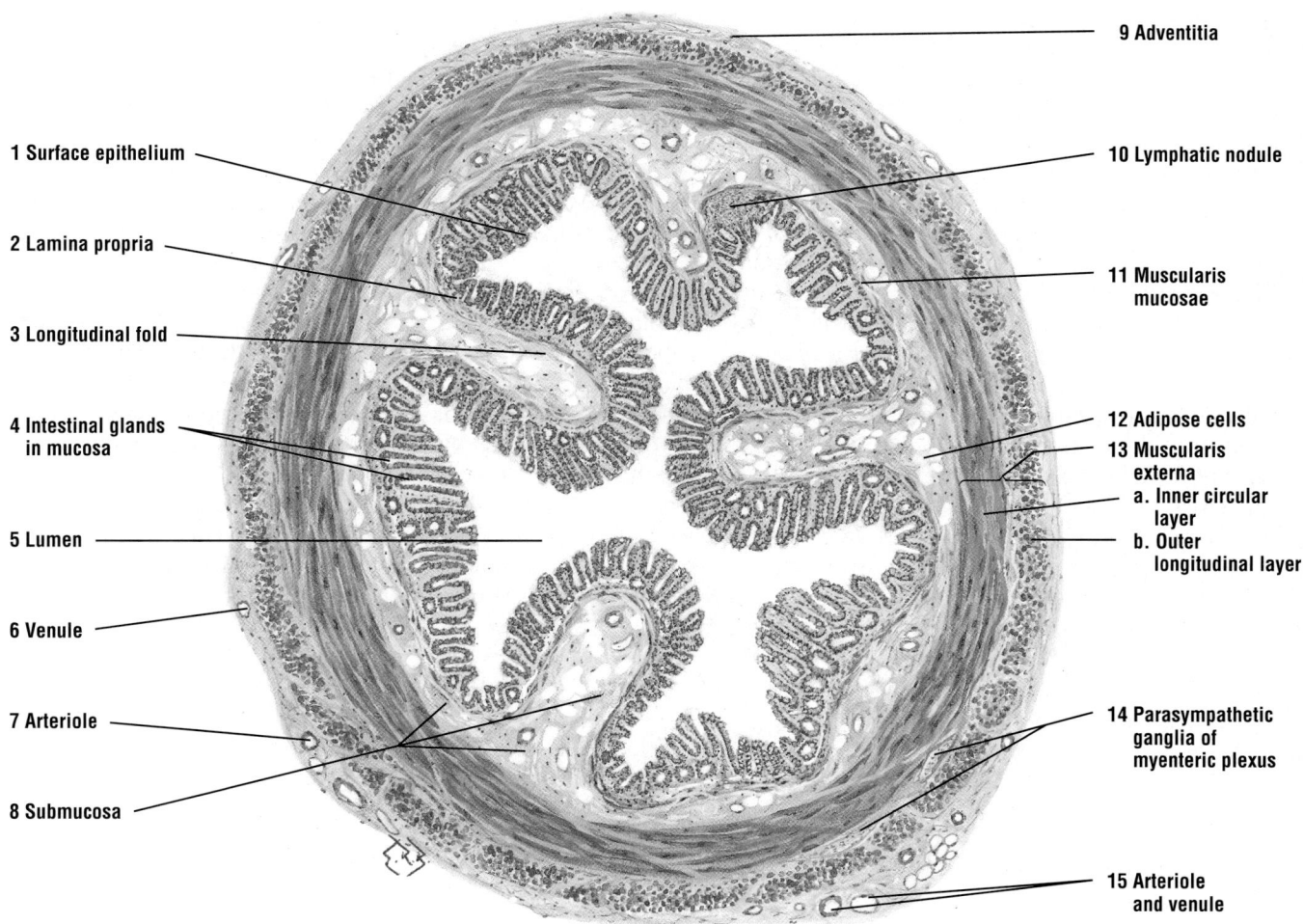

1 Surface epithelium

2 Lamina propria

3 Longitudinal fold

4 Intestinal glands in mucosa

5 Lumen

6 Venule

7 Arteriole

8 Submucosa

9 Adventitia

10 Lymphatic nodule

11 Muscularis mucosae

12 Adipose cells

13 Muscularis externa
  a. Inner circular layer
  b. Outer longitudinal layer

14 Parasympathetic ganglia of myenteric plexus

15 Arteriole and venule

Fig. 12-9   Rectum (panoramic view, transverse section). Stain: hematoxylin-eosin. Low magnification.

Figure 12-10   Anal Canal (longitudinal section)

The **upper portion of the anal canal (A),** above the **anal valves (11),** represents the lowermost part of the rectum. The **lower part of the anal canal (B),** below the anal valves (11), shows the transition from the simple columnar epithelium to the stratified squamous epithelium of the skin. The change from the rectal mucosa to the anal mucosa occurs at the apex of the anal valves (10, 11). This region is the **anorectal junction (10).**

The **rectal mucosa (4–8)** is similar to the mucosa of the colon; however, the **intestinal glands (7)** are shorter and farther apart. As a result, the **lamina propria (8)** is more prominent, diffuse lymphatic tissue is more abundant, and solitary **lymphatic nodules (6)** are more numerous.

The **muscularis mucosae (5, 12)** and the intestinal glands (7) of the digestive tract terminate in the vicinity of the anal valve (11). The lamina propria (8) of the rectum is replaced by the dense irregular connective tissue of the **lamina propria of the anal canal (13,** lower leader**).** The **submucosa (9)** of the rectum merges with the connective tissue in the lamina propria of the anal canal, a region that is highly vascular; the **internal hemorrhoidal plexus of veins (15)** lies in the mucosa of the anal canal. Blood vessels from this region continue into the submucosa (9) of the rectum. Internal hemorrhoids develop from chronic dilation of these vessels. External hemorrhoids develop from vessels of the external venous plexus of the anus (not illustrated in this figure).

The circular smooth muscle layer of the **muscularis externa (1)** increases in thickness in the upper region of the anal canal (A) and forms the **internal anal sphincter (1, 14).** Lower in the anal canal, this sphincter is replaced by skeletal muscles, the **external anal sphincter (16).** External to this sphincter is the skeletal **levator ani muscle (3).** The longitudinal muscle layer of the **muscularis externa (2)** becomes thin and disappears in the connective tissue of the external anal sphincter (16).

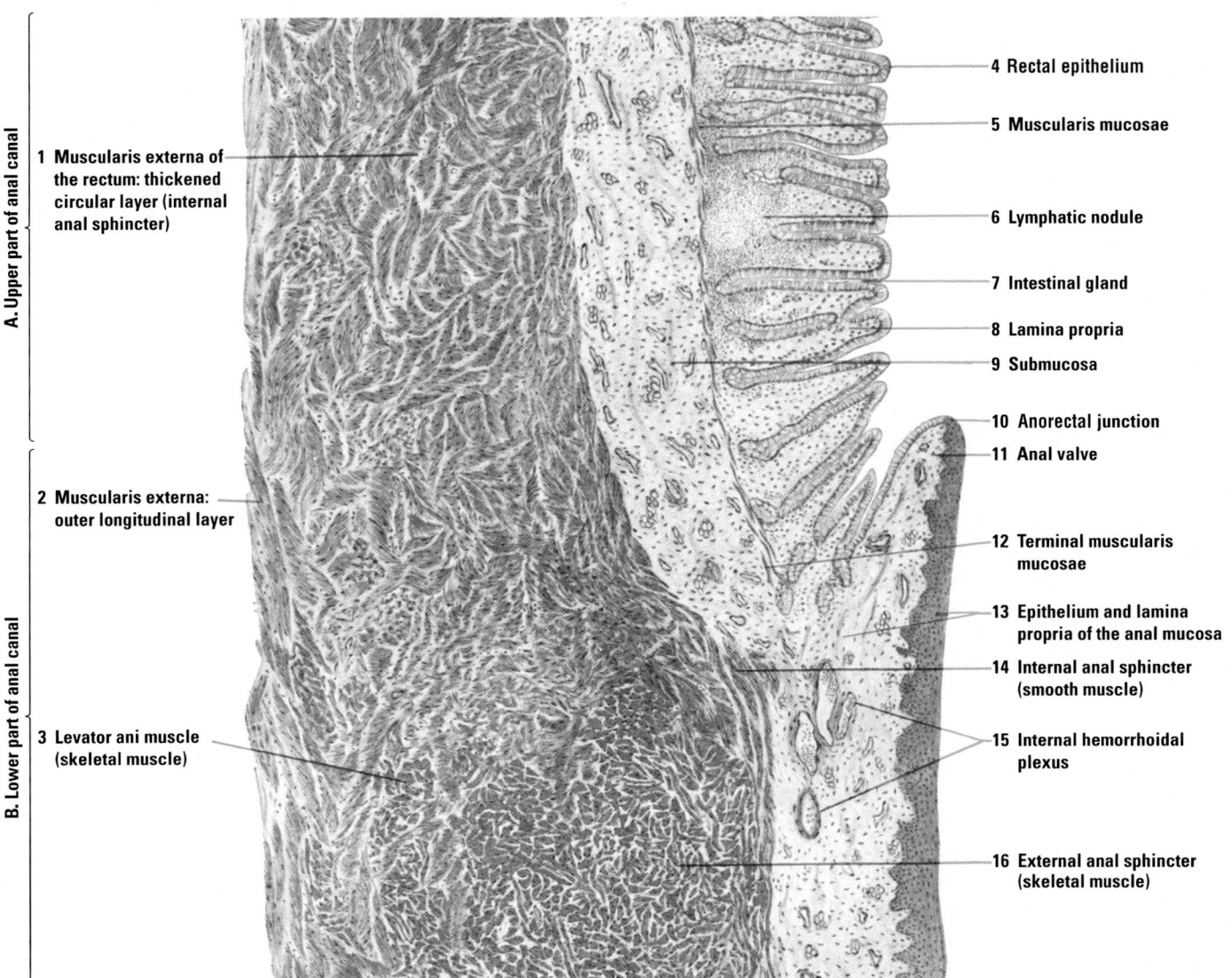

A. Upper part of anal canal

B. Lower part of anal canal

1 **Muscularis externa of the rectum: thickened circular layer (internal anal sphincter)**

2 **Muscularis externa: outer longitudinal layer**

3 **Levator ani muscle (skeletal muscle)**

4 **Rectal epithelium**

5 **Muscularis mucosae**

6 **Lymphatic nodule**

7 **Intestinal gland**

8 **Lamina propria**

9 **Submucosa**

10 **Anorectal junction**

11 **Anal valve**

12 **Terminal muscularis mucosae**

13 **Epithelium and lamina propria of the anal mucosa**

14 **Internal anal sphincter (smooth muscle)**

15 **Internal hemorrhoidal plexus**

16 **External anal sphincter (skeletal muscle)**

Fig. 12-10   Anal Canal (longitudinal section). Stain: hematoxylin-eosin. Low magnification.

Figure 12-11   Small Intestine: Duodenum (transverse section)

A low magnification photomicrograph illustrates a transverse section of the duodenum. The luminal surface of the duodenum exhibits finger-like extensions called **villi (2)**, which are covered by **simple columnar epithelium (1)** with a brush border. The core of each villus exhibits a dark stained **lamina propria (4, 6)** that contains an abundance of connective tissue cells, lymphoid cells, macrophages, smooth muscle cells, and other cells. Lamina propria (4, 6) also contains numerous blood vessels and the dilated, blind ending lymphatic channels called **lacteals (3)**. Between the villi (2) are the **intestinal glands (7)**; these extend down to the smooth muscle layer of the **muscularis mucosae (8)**. Inferior to muscularis mucosae (8) is the dense irregular connective tissue of **submucosa (9)**. In duodenum, the submucosa (9) is filled with the light-staining, mucus-secreting **duodenal glands (5)**, whose ducts pierce the muscularis mucosae (8) and deliver their secretory product into the bases of the intestinal glands (7). Surrounding the submucosa (9) and the duodenal glands (5) is the smooth muscle layer of **muscularis externa (10)**.

Figure 12-12   Small Intestine: Jejunum With Paneth Cells

A low magnification photomicrograph illustrates the mucosa of the jejunum of the small intestine. The **villi (1)** of the jejunum are lined by **simple columnar epithelium (2)** with brush border. Interspersed between the columnar cells are the round, mucus-filled **goblet cells (3)**. Located in the **lamina propria (6)** of each villus are numerous lymphoid cells, macrophages, smooth muscle cells, **blood vessels (7)**, and the lymphatic channels lacteals, which in this illustration appear collapsed and are not visible. Between the villi are the **intestinal glands (8)**, whose bases exhibit cells filled with large, red-staining or eosinophilic secretory granules. These are the **Paneth cells (9)**. The intestinal glands (8) terminate near the **muscularis mucosae (4)**, inferior to which is found the connective tissue of **submucosa (5)**.

Figure 12-13   Large Intestine: Colon Wall (transverse section)

A low magnification photomicrograph illustrates a portion of the colon wall in transverse section. The epithelium of the colon surface is lined by both the **absorptive columnar cells (1)** and the mucus-filled **goblet cells (2, 6)**, which increase in number toward the terminal end of the organ. The straight tubular **intestinal glands (4)** in the colon are deep and extend through the **lamina propria (3)** to the **muscularis mucosae (8)**. The lamina propria (3) and **submucosa (9)** of the colon are filled with individual lymphoid cells and large aggregations of lymphoid tissue or **lymphatic nodules (5, 7)**.

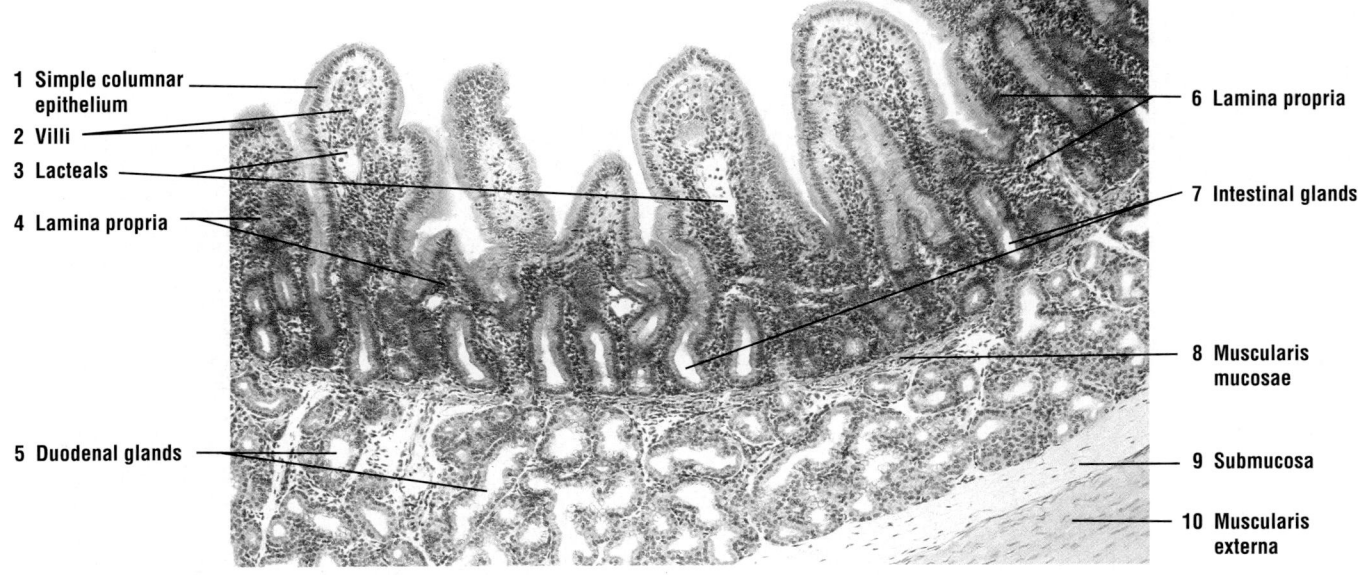

1 Simple columnar epithelium
2 Villi
3 Lacteals
4 Lamina propria
5 Duodenal glands
6 Lamina propria
7 Intestinal glands
8 Muscularis mucosae
9 Submucosa
10 Muscularis externa

Fig. 12-11   Small Intestine: Duodenum (transverse section). Stain: hematoxylin-eosin. 25×

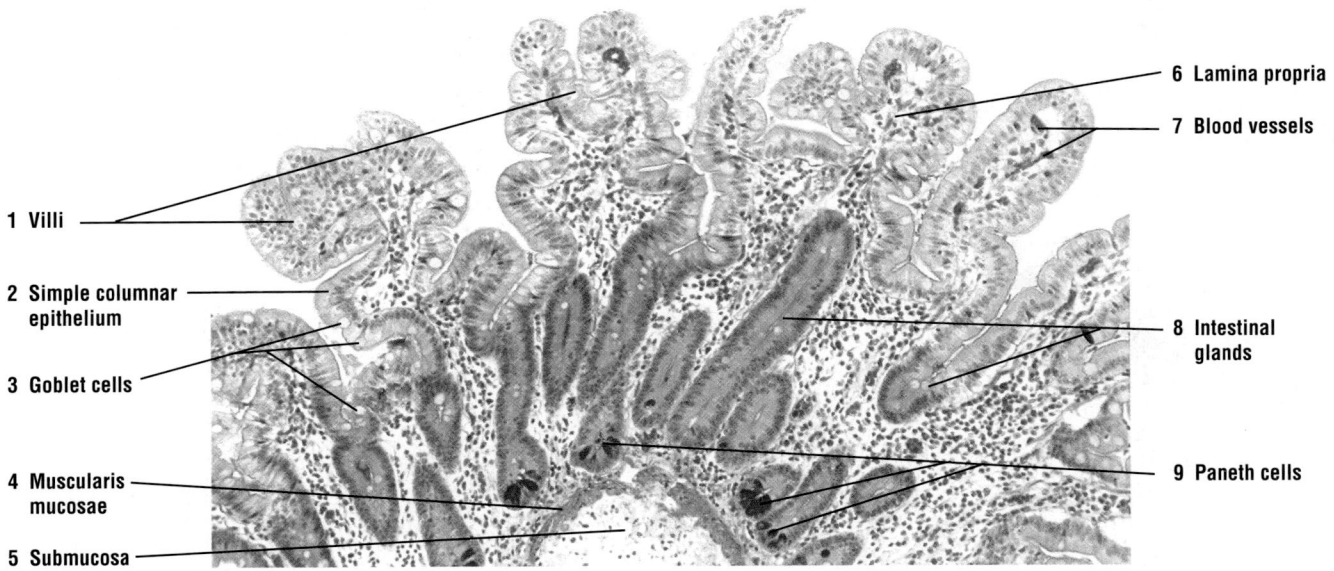

1 Villi
2 Simple columnar epithelium
3 Goblet cells
4 Muscularis mucosae
5 Submucosa
6 Lamina propria
7 Blood vessels
8 Intestinal glands
9 Paneth cells

Fig. 12-12   Small Intestine: Jejunum With Paneth Cells. Stain: Mallory-azan. 40×

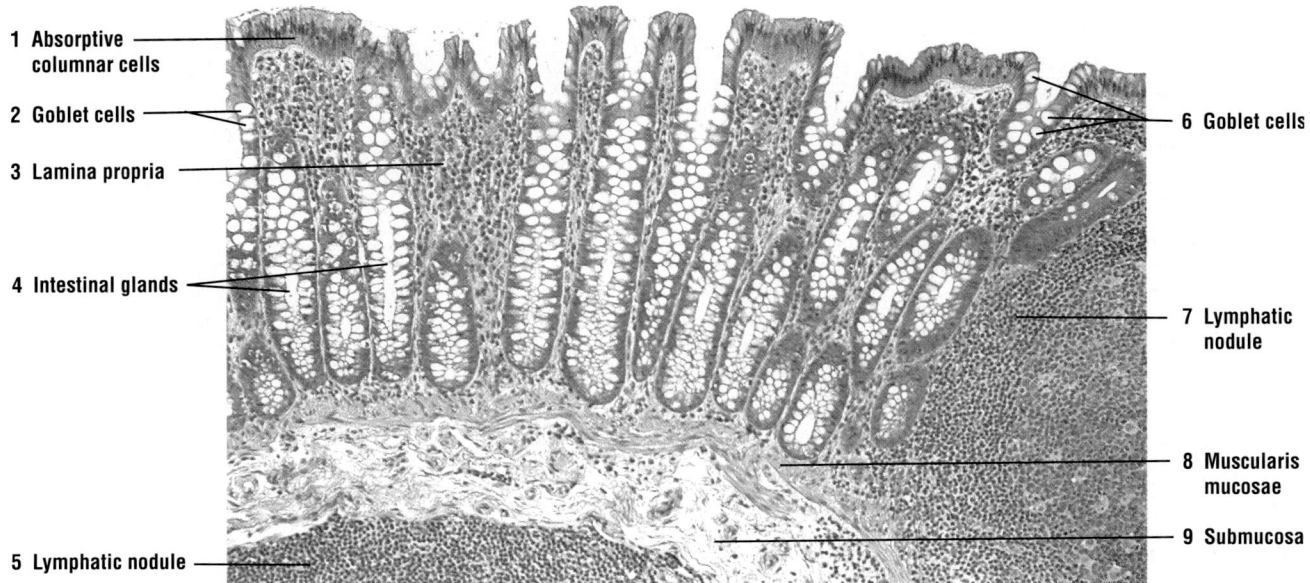

1 Absorptive columnar cells
2 Goblet cells
3 Lamina propria
4 Intestinal glands
5 Lymphatic nodule
6 Goblet cells
7 Lymphatic nodule
8 Muscularis mucosae
9 Submucosa

Fig. 12-13   Large Intestine: Colon Wall (transverse section). Stain: hematoxylin-eosin. 30×

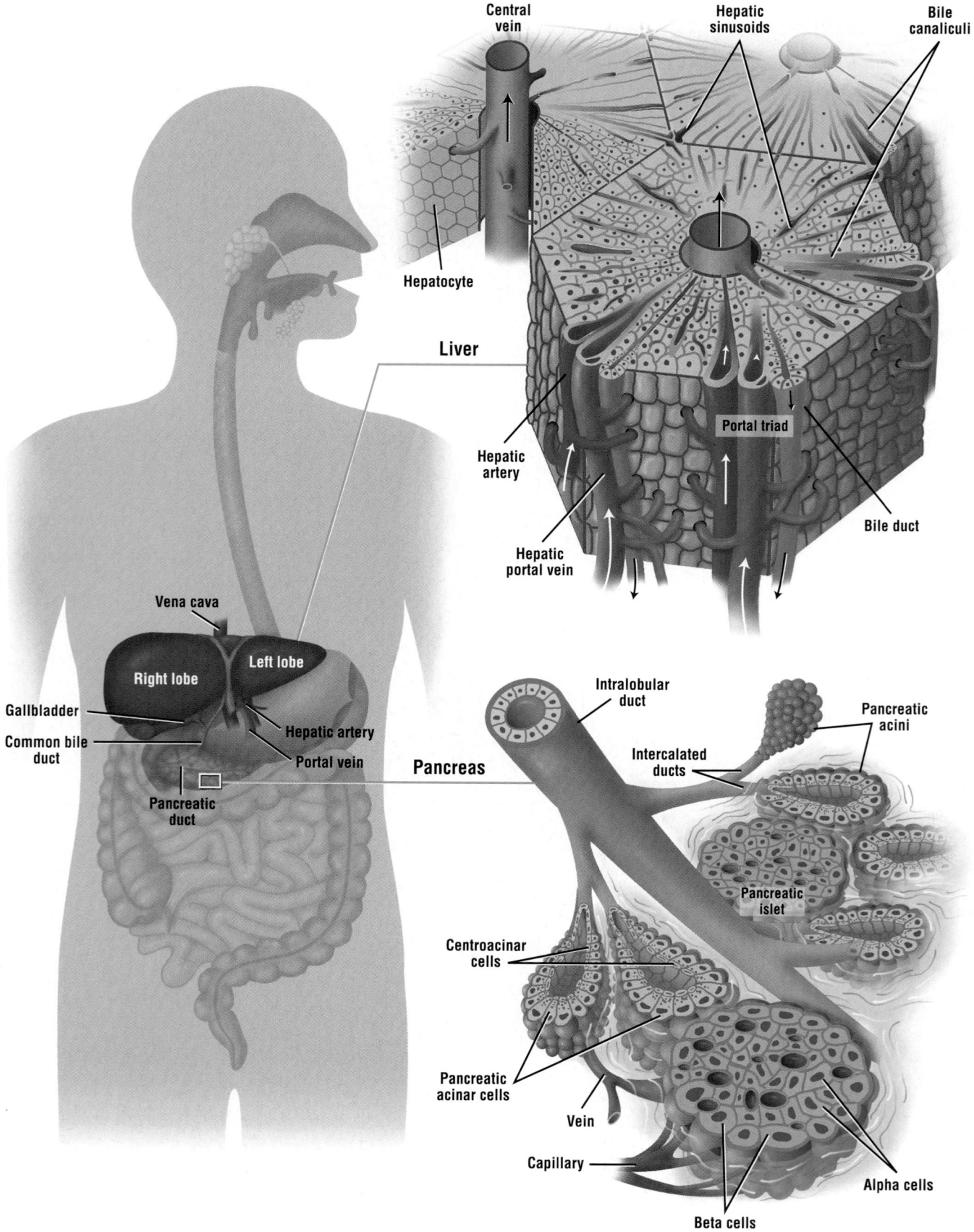

Central vein

Hepatic sinusoids

Bile canaliculi

Hepatocyte

Liver

Hepatic artery

Portal triad

Hepatic portal vein

Bile duct

Vena cava

Right lobe

Left lobe

Gallbladder

Common bile duct

Hepatic artery

Portal vein

Pancreatic duct

Pancreas

Intralobular duct

Pancreatic acini

Intercalated ducts

Pancreatic islet

Centroacinar cells

Pancreatic acinar cells

Vein

Capillary

Beta cells

Alpha cells

Digestive System: Liver, Gallbladder, and Pancreas

ACCESSORY DIGESTIVE ORGANS

The **liver, gallbladder,** and **pancreas** also constitute the **accessory organs** of the digestive tract. These organs are located outside of the digestive tract, but are connected to the small intestine by an excretory duct. The **common bile duct** from the liver and the **main pancreatic duct** from the pancreas join in the duodenal loop to form a single duct common to both organs. The duct then penetrates the duodenal wall and enters the lumen of the small intestine. The gallbladder joins the common bile duct via the cystic duct. **Bile** enters the small intestine from the gallbladder and the **digestive enzymes** from the pancreas via a common duct.

LIVER

The liver has an important strategic location. Absorbed products of digestion first percolate through the liver capillaries, called **sinusoids,** via the **hepatic portal vein** before entering the general circulation. Because venous blood is poor in oxygen, the liver is also supplied by the **hepatic artery** from the aorta, forming a dual blood supply **(Figs. 13-1–13-3).**

The liver exhibits repeating hexagonal units called **liver lobules.** In the middle of each lobule is a **central vein,** from which radiate plates of liver cells, called **hepatocytes,** and sinusoids toward the periphery. Here the connective tissue forms **portal triads** or **portal areas,** where branches of hepatic artery, hepatic portal vein, and **bile duct** can be seen. Venous and arterial blood first mix in the liver sinusoids as it flows toward the central vein. From here, the blood enters the general circulation through the hepatic veins **(Figs. 13-1–13-3, 13-13).**

The hepatic sinusoids are tortuous, dilated blood channels lined by a discontinuous layer of **fenestrated endothelial cells,** which are separated from the underlying liver cells, the **hepatocytes,** by a **perisinusoidal space** (of Disse). As a result, ingested material carried in the sinusoids percolates through the discontinuous endothelial wall and comes in direct contact with the hepatocytes. This allows for a more efficient exchange of materials in the blood with those in the hepatocytes and vice versa **(Figs. 13-1–13-3, 13-13).**

Hepatocytes secrete bile into tiny channels called **bile canaliculi** that are located between the hepatocytes. These canaliculi converge at the periphery of each lobule in the portal areas as **bile ducts (Figs. 13-1–13-3, 13-5).** The bile ducts then drain into larger hepatic ducts that carry bile out of the liver. In the liver lobules, bile flows bili canaliculi toward the bile duct in the portal area and blood in the sinusoids toward the central vein. As a result, bile and blood do not mix.

GALLBLADDER

The gallbladder is a small, hollow organ attached to the inferior surface of the liver. Bile from the liver is stored in the gallbladder. Bile leaves the gallbladder by the **cystic duct** and enters the duodenum via the **common bile duct.** The gallbladder is not a gland because it only stores and concentrates bile, which is then released into the digestive tract following hormonal stimulation. When the gallbladder is empty, the mucosa exhibits deep **folds (Fig. 13-9)**

EXOCRINE PANCREAS

Pancreas is a soft, elongated organ located posterior to the stomach. The head of the pancreas lies in the duodunal loop and the tail extends to the spleen. Pancreas contains both exocrine cells and endocrine cells. Most of the pancreas is an **exocrine, compound tubuloacinar gland.** The exocrine secretory units are the pyramidal-shaped **acinar cells** filled with secretory granules, which are precursors of the pancreatic **digestive enzymes** that are secreted into the excretory ducts in an inactive form. The secretory acinin are subdivided into **lobules** and bound together by loose connective tissue. The **excretory ducts** in the exocrine pancreas start from within the center of individual acinus as pale-staining **centroacinar cells,** which continue into the short **intercalated ducts.** These short ducts merge to form **intralobular ducts** in the connective tissue, which, in turn, join to form **larger interlobular ducts,** and these empty into the **main pancreatic duct (Fig. 13-10, 13-14).**

ENDOCRINE PANCREAS

The endocrine portion of the pancreas are scattered among the exocrine acini as pale-staining, vascularized units called **pancreatic islets** (of Langerhans). Each islet is surrounded by a reticular connective tissue fibers. With special immunocytochemical processes, four cell types can be identified in the islets: **alpha, beta, delta, and F (PP) cells.** The alpha cells comprise about 20% of the islets and are located primarily in the peripheries. The beta cells are most numerous, comprising about 70% of the islet cells. These cells are concentrated in the center of the islet. The remaining islet cells are few in number and exhibit variable location **(Figs. 13-11–13-12, 13-14).**

Figure 13-1   Pig's Liver (panoramic view, transverse section)

The connective tissue from the liver hilus extends between the liver lobes as interlobular septa. In the pig's liver, the individual **hepatic (liver) lobules (7)** are well defined. To illustrate the boundaries of the hepatic lobules, a section of pig's liver was stained with Mallory-azan stain, which stains the connective tissue septa dark blue.

This figure illustrates, in transverse section, a complete hepatic lobule (on the left) and parts of several adjacent **hepatic lobules (7)**. The blue-staining **interlobular septa (5, 9)** contain interlobular branches of the **portal vein, bile duct,** and **hepatic artery (2, 3, 4, 11, 12, 13)**. These regions around the hepatic lobule are collectively considered **portal canals** or **areas.** Around the periphery of each lobule can be seen several portal canals within the interlobular septa (5, 9). The interlobular septa (5, 9) also contain small lymphatic vessels and nerves; however, these structures are small, inconspicuous, and seen only occasionally.

In the center of each hepatic lobule (7) is a **central vein (1, 8).** Radiating from the central vein (1, 8) toward the periphery of the lobule are **plates of hepatic cells (6).** Located between the hepatic plates (6) are the **hepatic sinusoids (10).** On entering the liver, arterial and venous blood mixes in these sinusoids and then flows toward the central veins (1, 8) of the lobule (7). Bile is formed in the liver cells and flows through the minute bile canaliculi in the opposite direction into the interlobular **bile ducts (2, 12)** (See Fig. 13-5).

The interlobular vessels and bile ducts (2, 3, 4, 11, 12, 13) exhibit numerous branches in the liver parenchyma. Thus, in a cross section of the liver lobule, it is possible to see more than one section of each of these structures within a portal area.

Figure 13-2   Primate Liver (panoramic view, transverse section)

In the primate or human liver, the connective tissue septa between individual **hepatic lobules (8)** are not as conspicuous as in the pig's liver. As a result, the liver sinusoids are continuous from one lobule to the next. Despite these differences, portal areas containing the interlobular branches of the **portal veins, hepatic arteries,** and **bile ducts (1, 2, 3, 11, 12, 13)** are visible around the peripheries of different lobules.

This figure illustrates numerous hepatic lobules (8). In the center of each hepatic lobule (8) is the **central vein (6, 9).** The **hepatic sinusoids (5)** are seen between the **plates of hepatic cells (7)** that radiate from the central veins (6, 9) toward the periphery of the hepatic lobule (8). As illustrated in Fig. 13-1, numerous branches of the interlobular vessels and bile ducts are seen within the portal areas of a given hepatic lobule (8).

■ Functional Correlations–Liver

It is believed that liver performs hundred of functions, with the hepatocytes performing a wider variety of functions than any other cells in the body. As **exocrine cells,** hepatocytes synthesize and release **bile** into a system of excretory ducts, the **bile canaliculi.** The bile salts that are present in the bile are essential for **emulsification of fats** that enter the small intestine (duodenum) from the stomach. Emulsification of fat promotes more efficient digestion of the fats by the fat-digesting enzymes, the **pancreatic lipase** produced by the pancreas. The digested fats are subsequently absorbed by cells in the small intestine and enter the lymphatic **lacteal** channels that are located in the individual villi. From the villi, the fats are carried into the larger lymphatic ducts, eventually reaching the major veins in their return to the heart.

The hepatocytes are also **endocrine cells.** They release many products directly into the bloodstream, as the blood flows through the sinusoids and comes in direct contact with individual hepatocytes. Thus, the liver cells perform both endocrine and exocrine functions. The endocrine functions of the liver involve synthesis of numerous **plasma proteins,** including albumin and the blood-clotting factors prothrombin and fibrinogen. Liver also **stores** glucose (as glycogen), fats, and various vitamins. When the cells of the body need glucose, **glycogen** stored in the liver is converted back into glucose and released into the blood stream. Liver cells also **detoxify** various drugs and harmful chemicals. **Kupffer cells** are specialized liver **phagocytes** that are derived from blood monocytes and located in the sinusoids. These large, branching cells phagocytize particulate material and cellular debris that flow through the sinusoids. In the fetus, the liver cells perform **hemopoiesis**—an important function in blood cell production. Thus, the liver is an essential organ for life.

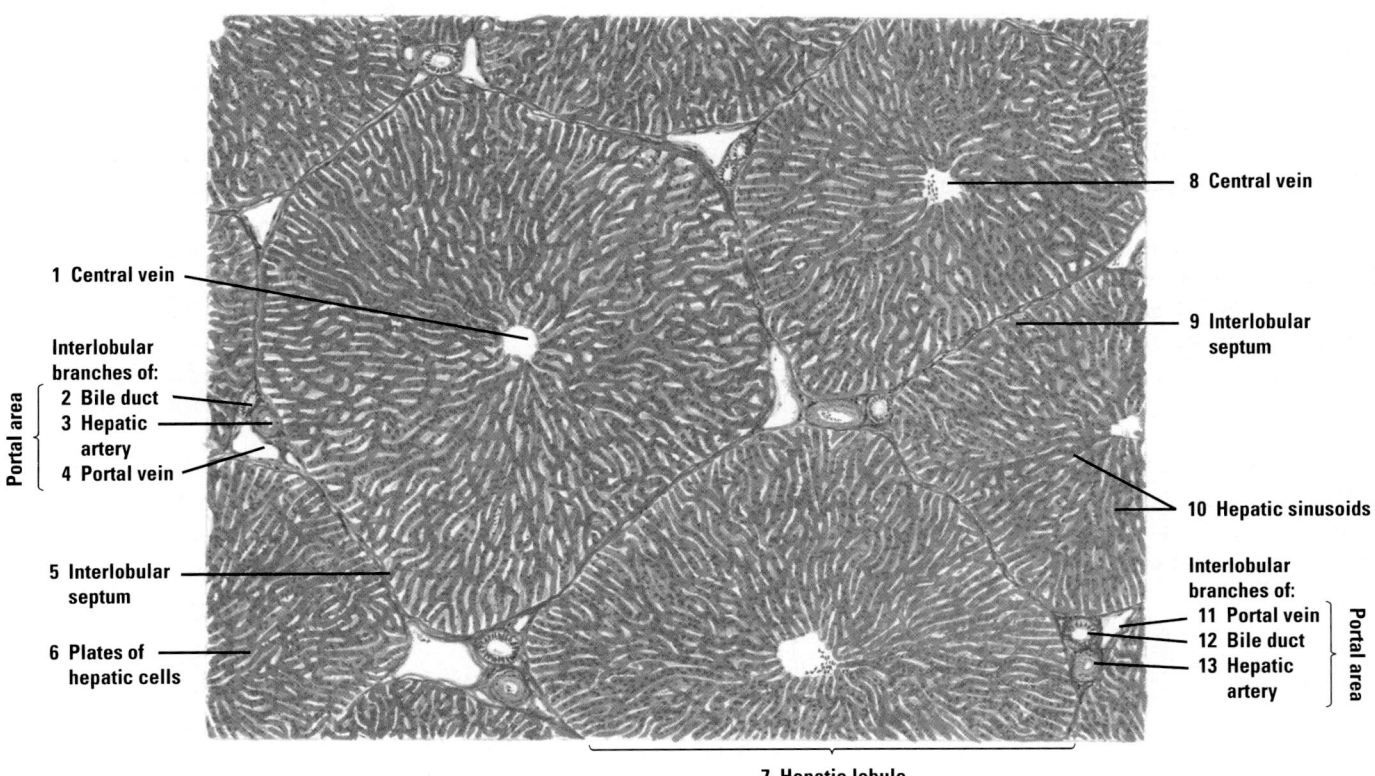

1 Central vein

Interlobular branches of:
  2 Bile duct
  3 Hepatic artery
  4 Portal vein

Portal area

5 Interlobular septum

6 Plates of hepatic cells

8 Central vein

9 Interlobular septum

10 Hepatic sinusoids

Interlobular branches of:
  11 Portal vein
  12 Bile duct
  13 Hepatic artery

Portal area

7 Hepatic lobule

Fig. 13-1   Pig's Liver (panoramic view, transverse section). Stain: Mallory-azan. Low magnification.

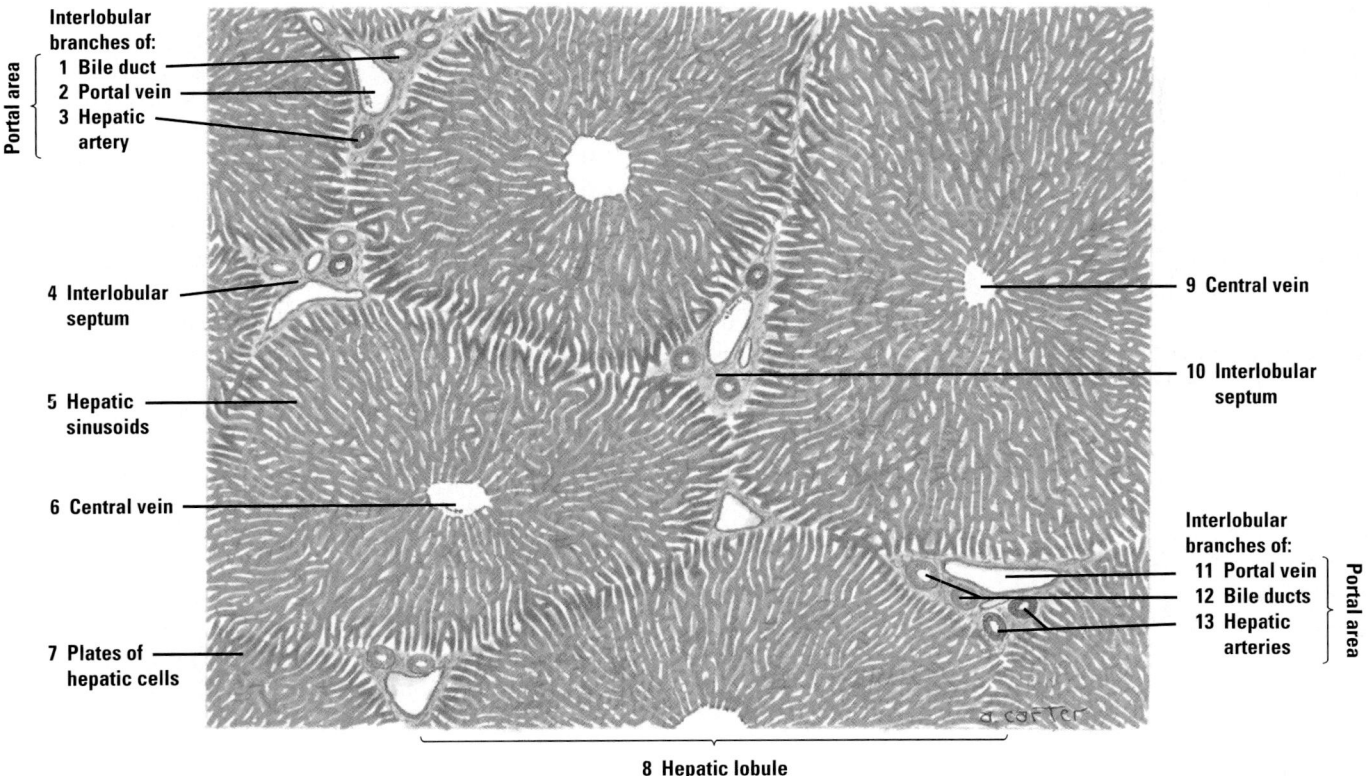

Interlobular branches of:
  1 Bile duct
  2 Portal vein
  3 Hepatic artery

Portal area

4 Interlobular septum

5 Hepatic sinusoids

6 Central vein

7 Plates of hepatic cells

9 Central vein

10 Interlobular septum

Interlobular branches of:
  11 Portal vein
  12 Bile ducts
  13 Hepatic arteries

Portal area

8 Hepatic lobule

Fig. 13-2   Primate Liver (panoramic view, transverse section). Stain: hematoxylin-eosin. Low magnification.

Figure 13-3   Hepatic (Liver) Lobule (sectional view, transverse section)

A portion of a hepatic lobule between the **central vein (1)** and the peripheral **interlobular septum (9)** is illustrated in greater detail and higher magnification than in Figure 13-2.

The central vein (1) is a venule lined with **endothelium (3).** At the periphery of the lobule is the **interlobular septum (9)** with the portal area, which consists of a **branch of portal vein (8),** two **branches of the hepatic artery (6, 12),** four sections of the **bile duct (7, 14)** and a **lymphatic vessel (13).**

The hepatic lobule consists of **plates of hepatic cells (11).** These plates branch and anastomose within the lobule. At the periphery of the lobule, the hepatic cells form a solid **limiting plate (10),** which separates the hepatic plates and sinusoids from the interlobular connective tissue septum (9). The portal venules and hepatic arterioles penetrate the connective tissue to form the **sinusoids (2, 5).**

The hepatic cells (11) are polygonal, vary in size, contain a large, round vesicular nucleus, and may occasionally be binucleate. The cells have a granular acidophilic cytoplasm which varies with their functional state (see also Fig. 13-4).

The **sinusoids (2, 5)** are situated between plates of hepatic cells, and follow their branchings and anastomoses. The sinusoids (2, 5) are lined with a discontinuous type of endothelium (3). Also present in the sinusoid wall are fixed macrophages, the Kupffer cells (see Fig. 13-4). The blood in the sinusoids, containing **erythrocytes (4)** and leukocytes, drains into the central vein (1).

Figure 13-4   Liver: Kupffer Cells (India Ink preparation)

To demonstrate the phagocytic system in the **sinusoids (2)** of the liver, a rabbit liver was intravenously injected with India ink. The **Kupffer cells (1, 5),** because of their phagocytosis of carbon particles, appear prominent in the sinusoids between the **hepatic cells (4).** The phagocytic Kupffer cells (1, 5) are large with several processes, and exhibit an irregular or stellate outline. Because of the increased phagocytosis, the nucleus is obscured by the accumulation of ingested carbon particles. **Endothelial cells (3)** are also visible in the sinusoids (2); they are smaller and usually only the nucleus is visible.

Figure 13-5   Liver: Bile Canaliculi (Osmic Acid preparation)

A section of liver was fixed in osmic acid and the sections prepared and stained with hematoxylin-eosin. Osmic acid fixation reveals the **bile canaliculi (2, 8),** which are minute channels between individual cells in the **hepatic plates (2, 6).** The canaliculi follow an irregular course between the **hepatic cells (1)** and branch freely within the hepatic plates (1, 6). In this figure, some canaliculi (8) are illustrated in a transverse plane.

The **sinusoids (4, 5)** are lined by **endothelial cells (7)** with small nuclei and a **Kupffer cell (9)** with a larger nucleus and branched cytoplasm. Also illustrated is a sinusoid (4, upper leader) opening into a **central vein (3).**

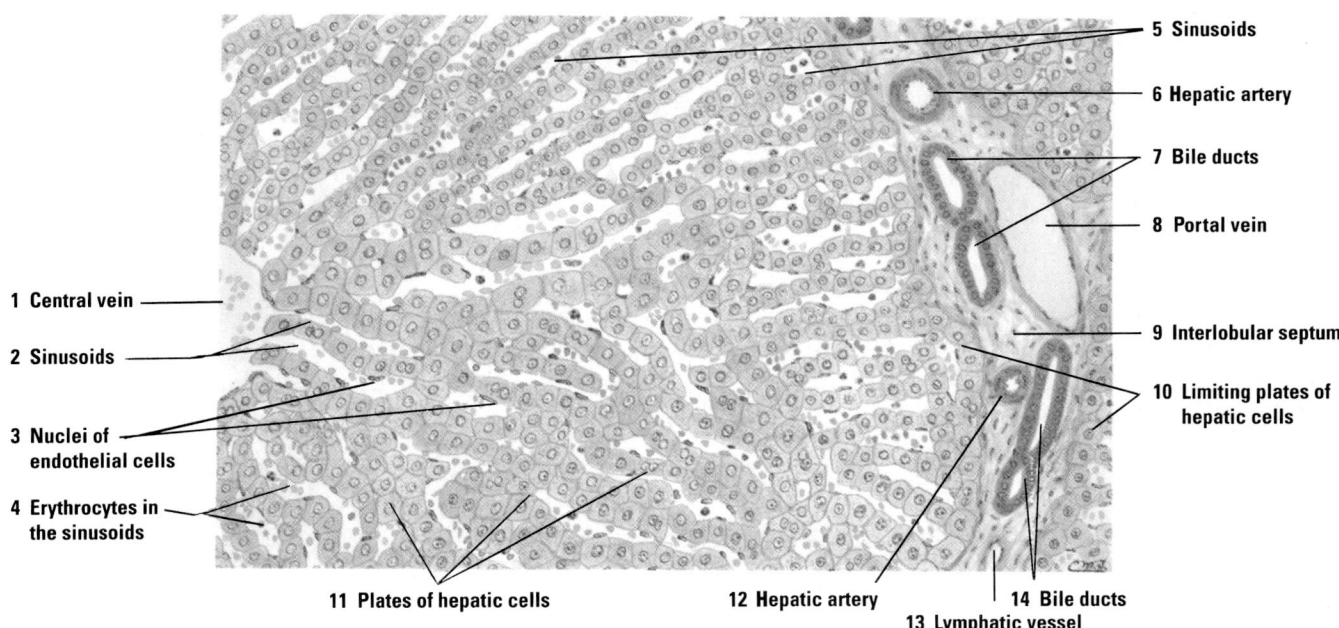

1 Central vein

2 Sinusoids

3 Nuclei of endothelial cells

4 Erythrocytes in the sinusoids

5 Sinusoids

6 Hepatic artery

7 Bile ducts

8 Portal vein

9 Interlobular septum

10 Limiting plates of hepatic cells

11 Plates of hepatic cells

12 Hepatic artery

13 Lymphatic vessel

14 Bile ducts

Fig. 13-3   Hepatic (Liver) Lobule (sectional view, transverse section). Stain: hematoxylin-eosin. High magnification.

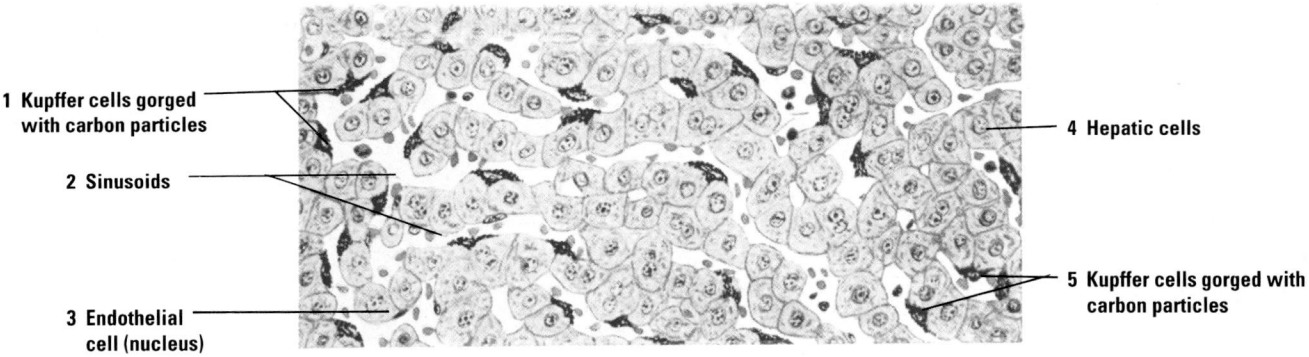

1 Kupffer cells gorged with carbon particles

2 Sinusoids

3 Endothelial cell (nucleus)

4 Hepatic cells

5 Kupffer cells gorged with carbon particles

Fig. 13-4   Liver: Kupffer Cells (India Ink preparation). Stain: hematoxylin-eosin. High magnification.

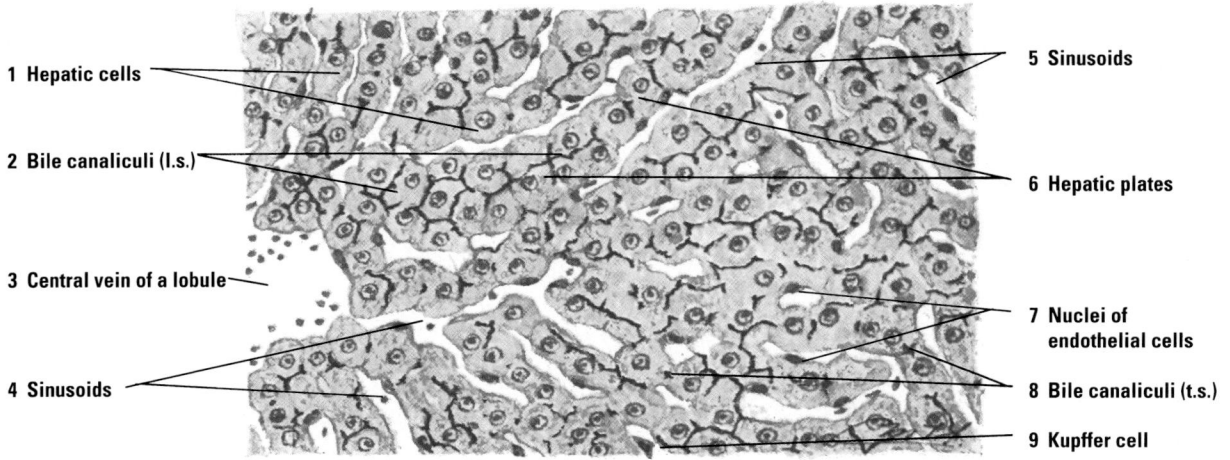

1 Hepatic cells

2 Bile canaliculi (l.s.)

3 Central vein of a lobule

4 Sinusoids

5 Sinusoids

6 Hepatic plates

7 Nuclei of endothelial cells

8 Bile canaliculi (t.s.)

9 Kupffer cell

Fig. 13-5   Liver: Bile Canaliculi (Osmic Acid preparation). Stain: hematoxylin-eosin. High magnification.

Figure 13-6   Mitochondria (red) and Fat Droplets (blue) in Liver Cells

This liver section was fixed in potassium bichromate and osmic acid, and then stained with acid fuchsin and picric acid. This preparation stains **mitochondria (2)** red. The **fat droplets (1)** usually stain black after osmic acid fixation, but in this preparation stain blue.

Figure 13-7   Glycogen in Liver Cells

Staining the liver sections with alcohol and ammonia solution of carmine demonstrates **glycogen (1)** as red granules that exhibit an irregular distribution within the cytoplasm. If the sections are previously stained with Meyer's hemalum, the nuclei appear violet.

Figure 13-8   Reticular Fibers in a Hepatic Lobule

The Del Rio Hortega modification of ammonium silver carbonate method for silver impregnation demonstrates the fine fibrillar structure of the liver stroma. The reticular fibers stain black and the liver cells pale violet.

The reticular fibers form most of the supporting connective tissue of the liver. They line the liver **sinusoids (1)** between the hepatocytes and the discontinuous endothelial cells, and form a dense network of **fibers (3)** around the **central vein (2).**

The collagen fibers in the dense irregular connective tissue of the **interlobular septa (4)** stain dark brown; the reticular fibers merge with these fibers.

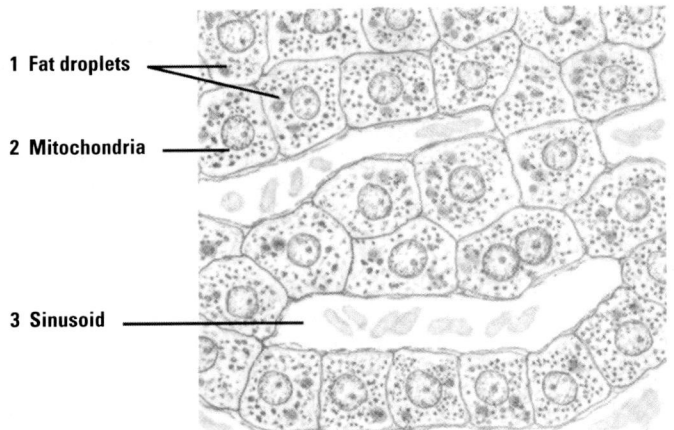

1 Fat droplets

2 Mitochondria

3 Sinusoid

Fig. 13-6   Mitochondria (red) and Fat Droplets (blue) in Liver Cells. Stain: Altmann's. Fixation in Champy's fluid. Oil immersion.

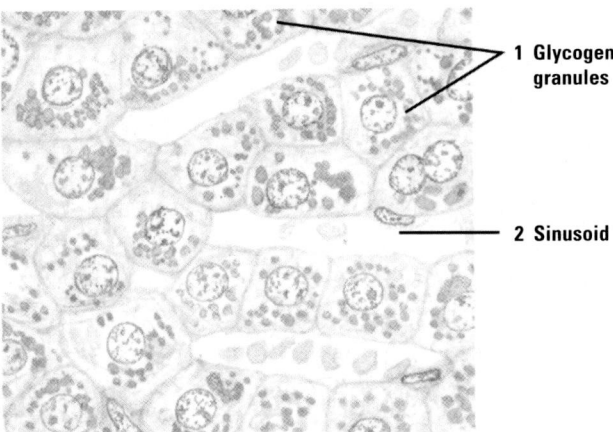

1 Glycogen granules

2 Sinusoid

Fig. 13-7   Glycogen in Liver Cells. Stain: Best's carmine. Oil immersion.

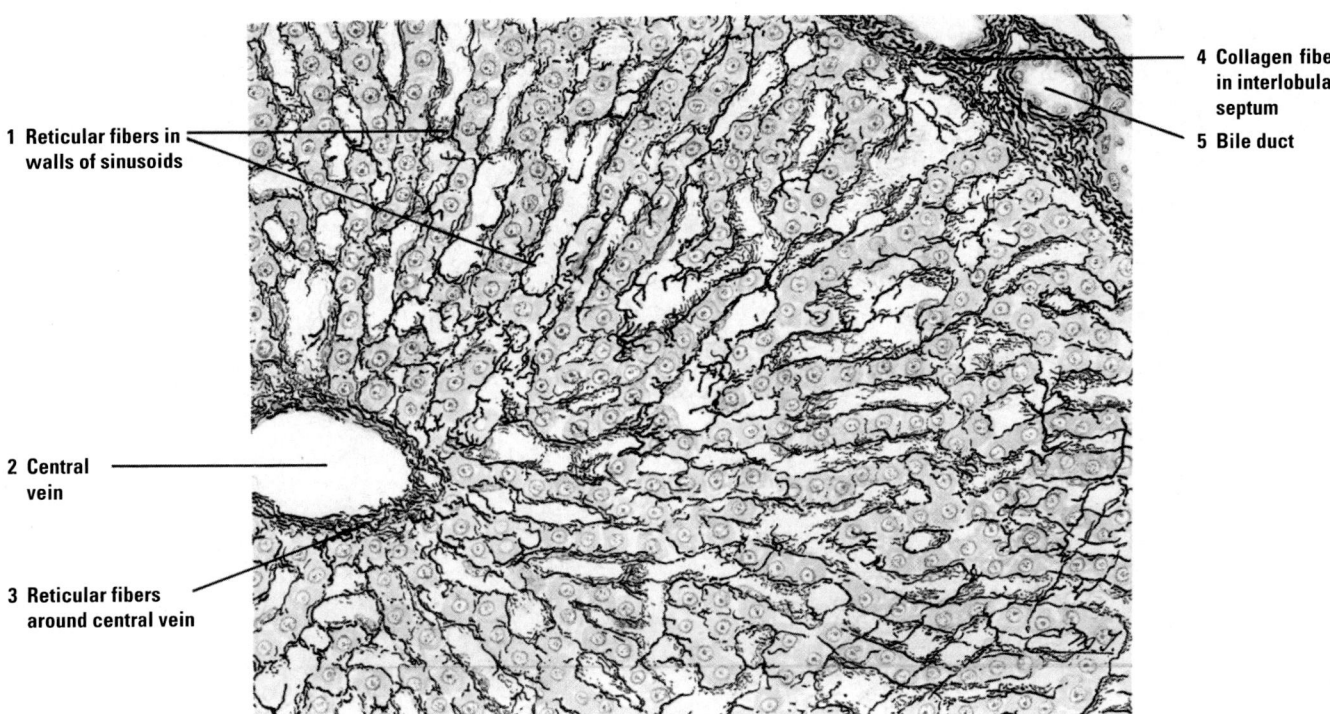

1 Reticular fibers in walls of sinusoids

2 Central vein

3 Reticular fibers around central vein

4 Collagen fibers in interlobular septum

5 Bile duct

Fig. 13-8   Reticular Fibers in a Hepatic Lobule. Stain: Del Rio Hortega. High magnification.

Figure 13-9   Gallbladder (panoramic view)

The wall of the gallbladder consists of a **mucosa (3, 4, 5)**, a **fibromuscular layer (2)**, a perimuscular **connective tissue layer (1, 10)**, and a **serosa (6)** on all of its surface except the hepatic, where an adventitia attaches it to the liver.

The mucosa exhibits temporary **folds (15)**, which disappear when the gallbladder is distended with bile. These folds resemble the villi in the small intestine; however, they vary in size, shape and irregular arrangement. The **crypts** or **diverticula (16)** between the folds often form deep indentations in the mucosa. In cross section, these **diverticula (18)** in the lamina propria resemble tubular glands; however, there are no glands in the gallbladder proper (except in the neck region).

The **lining epithelium (5, 14, 20)** is a simple tall columnar epithelium with lightly stained cytoplasms and basal nuclei. The **lamina propria (4, 17)** contains loose connective tissue and some diffuse lymphatic tissue.

The **smooth muscle fibers (7)** in the fibromuscular layer (2) are interspersed within the layers of loose connective tissue that are rich in **elastic fibers (8)**. In contrast to other organs in which a serosa or adventitia covers the muscular layer, the gallbladder has a wide layer of perimuscular loose connective tissue (1, 10), which contain **blood vessels (11, 13)**, lymphatics, and **nerves (12)**; serosa (6) is the outermost layer and covers all of these structures.

■ Functional Correlations–Gallbladder

The primary functions of the gallbladder are to store, concentrate, and expel **bile,** when needed for digestion. Sodium is actively transported through the simple columnar epithelium of the gallbladder into the extracellular connective tissue. Water and chloride ions follow passively, thus concentrating bile.

In response to the entrance of dietary **fats** into the proximal duodenum, a hormone called **cholecystokinin (CCK)** is released into the blood stream by the **enteroendocrine cells** located in the intestinal mucosa. CCK is carried in the blood to the gallbladder, where it causes rhythmic contractions of the **smooth muscles** in its wall. At the same time, the **sphincter muscles** around the neck of the gallbladder relax. This combined action forces the bile to enter the duodenum by way of the **common bile** duct. The function of bile in digestive process was mentioned earlier with the liver function.

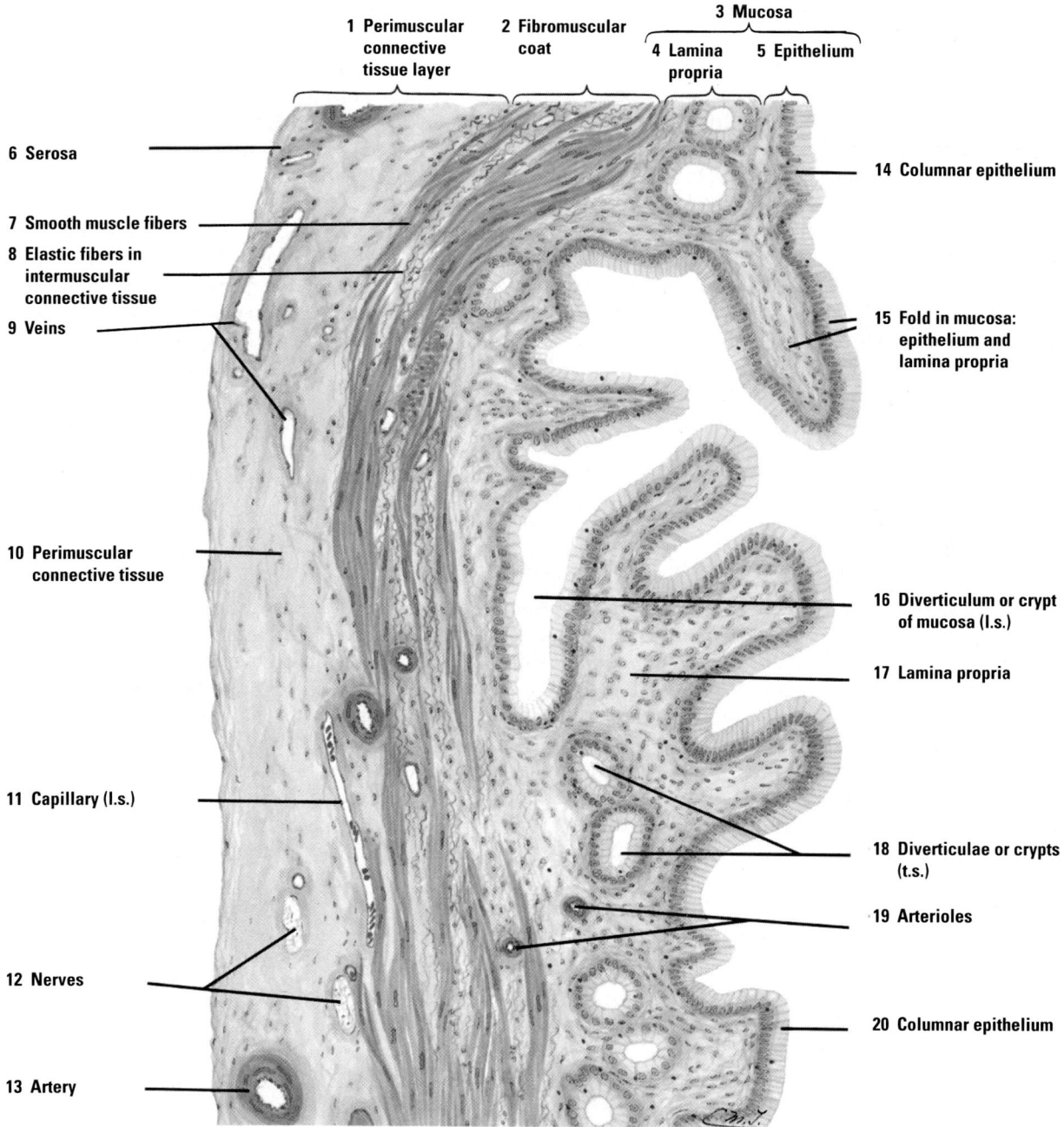

1 Perimuscular connective tissue layer

2 Fibromuscular coat

3 Mucosa

4 Lamina propria

5 Epithelium

6 Serosa

7 Smooth muscle fibers

8 Elastic fibers in intermuscular connective tissue

9 Veins

10 Perimuscular connective tissue

11 Capillary (l.s.)

12 Nerves

13 Artery

14 Columnar epithelium

15 Fold in mucosa: epithelium and lamina propria

16 Diverticulum or crypt of mucosa (l.s.)

17 Lamina propria

18 Diverticulae or crypts (t.s.)

19 Arterioles

20 Columnar epithelium

Fig. 13-9   Gallbladder (panoramic view). Stain: hematoxylin-eosin. Medium magnification.

Figure 13-10   Pancreas (sectional view)

The pancreas has both endocrine and exocrine components, which form the majority of the gland. The exocrine pancreas consists of closely packed secretory **serous acini (1)** arranged into numerous small lobules. The lobules are surrounded by thin intralobular and **interlobular connective tissue septa (4, 13)** with their corresponding **blood vessels (5), ducts (12)**, nerves, and occasional **Pacinian corpuscle (11).** Within the masses of serous acini (1) are found the isolated **pancreatic islets (islets of Langerhans) (3, 7).** These islets represent the endocrine portion of the pancreas and are its characteristic features.

A pancreatic acinus **(1)** consists of pyramidal-shaped, protein-secreting **zymogenic cells (1)** surrounding a small central lumen. The excretory ducts extend into individual acini and are visible as pale-staining **centroacinar cells (6, 10)** within their lumina. The secretory products from the acini are drained by the narrow **intercalated (intralobular) ducts (2).** These ducts (2) exhibit small lumina and low cuboidal epithelium. The centroacinar cells (6, 10) are continuous with the epithelium of the intercalated ducts (2). The intercalated ducts (2) then drain into **interlobular ducts (12)** that are found in the connective tissue septa (4, 13) that extend between the lobules. The small interlobular ducts (12) are lined by a simple cuboidal epithelium, which becomes taller and stratified in larger ducts.

The **pancreatic islets (3, 7)** are round masses of endocrine cells of varying size that are demarcated from the surrounding exocrine acinar tissue by thin layer of reticular fibers. The pancreatic islets (3, 7) are normally larger than the acini and appear as compact clusters of epithelial cells permeated by numerous **capillaries (8).** The cellular composition of individual pancreatic islets (3, 7) are illustrated at higher magnification in Figures 13-11 and 13-12.

■ Functional Correlations–Exocrine Pancreas

The pancreatic functions are performed by distinct population of cells. Because pancreas is both an endocrine and an exocrine organ, it produces numerous digestive enzymes and hormones. Pancreatic secretions are regulated by both hormones and vagal stimulation. Two intestinal hormones, **secretin** and **cholecystokinin,** secreted by the **enteroendocrine (APUD)** cells of the duodenal mucosa into the blood stream, regulate the pancreatic secretions. Pancreas produces an alkaline fluid and numerous digestive enzymes that break down proteins, fats, and carbohydrates into smaller molecules for absorption in the small intestine.

In response to the presence of acidic chyme in the small intestine (duodenum), secretin release stimulates the pancreatic cells to secrete large amounts of watery fluid rich in **sodium bicarbonate ions.** This fluid, which has little or no enzymatic activity, is produced primarily by the **centroacinar cells** and the cells that line the smaller **intercalated ducts.** The function of this fluid is to neutralize the acidic chyme and create an optimal environment for the activity of the pancreatic enzymes.

In response to the presence of fats and proteins in the small intestine, cholecystokinin release stimulates the acinar cells in the pancreas to secrete large amounts of different digestive enzymes. The pancreatic enzymes that are produced in the acinar cells enter the duodenum in an inactive form and are then activated by a hormone secreted by intestinal mucosa.

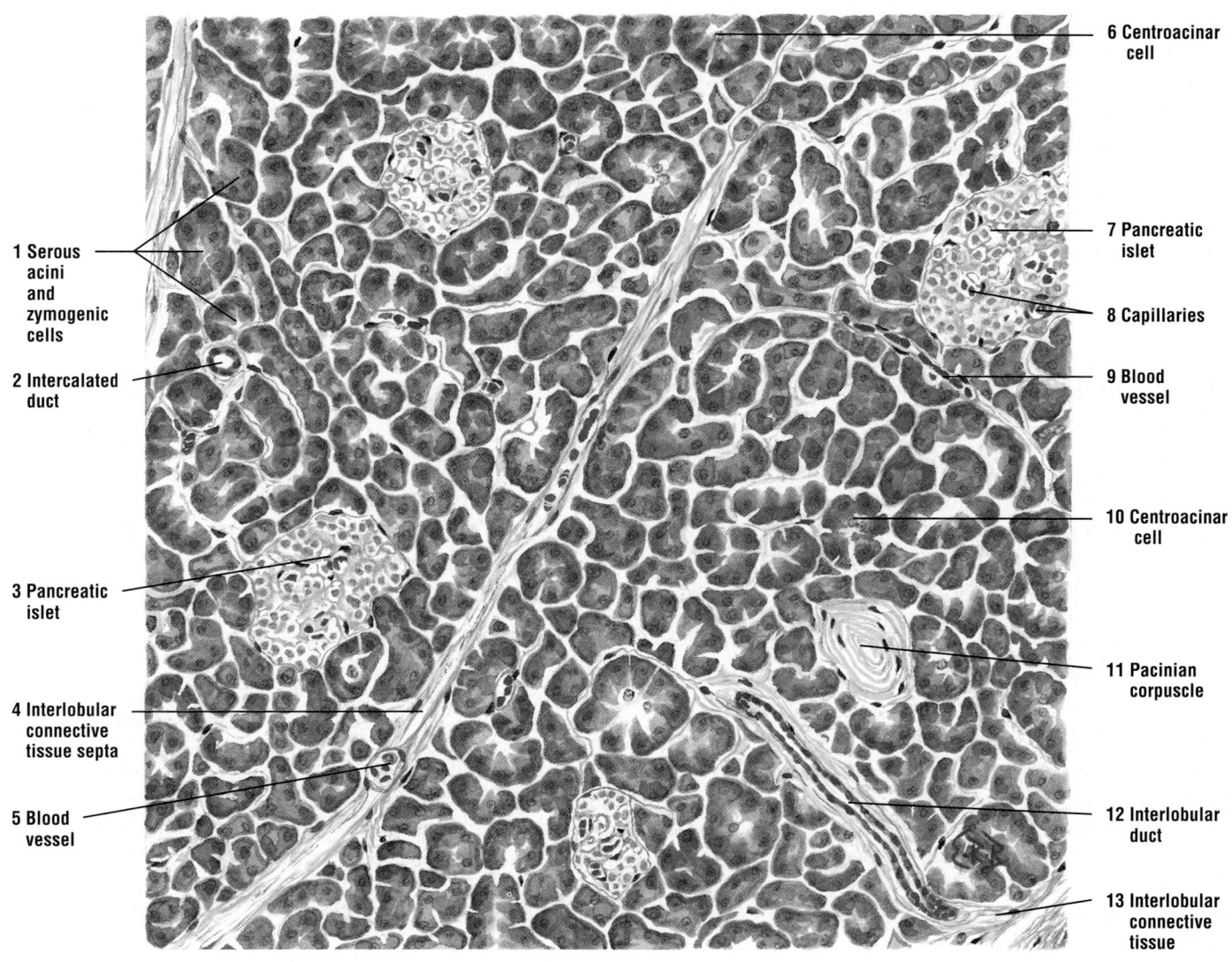

Fig. 13-10   Pancreas (sectional view). Stain: hematoxylin-eosin. Low magnification.

Figure 13-11   Pancreatic Islet

A pale-staining, spherical **pancreatic islet (islet of Langerhans) (2)** is illustrated at a higher magnification. The endocrine cells of the islet (2) are arranged in cords and clumps, between which are found delicate connective tissue fibers and a rich **capillary (3)** network. A thin **connective tissue capsule (4)** separates the endocrine pancreas from the dark-staining exocrine **serous acini (5)**. In some of the serous acini (5) are seen the pale-staining **centroacinar cells (5)**. These cells are part of the duct system that conduct the secretory products of the acini (5) into the **intercalated ducts (1)**. Myoepithelial cells do not surround the secretory acini in the pancreas.

The pancreatic islets contain several hormone-secreting cells; however, with routine histological preparations, individual cells cannot be identified and the islets must be prepared with special stains.

Figure 13-12   Pancreatic Islet (special preparation)

This pancreatic islet has been prepared with special stain to distinguish the glucagon-secreting **alpha (A) cells (1)** from the insulin-secreting **beta (B) cells (3)**. The cytoplasm of the alpha cells (1) stain pink while the cytoplasm of the beta cells (3) stain blue. Generally, the alpha (1) cells are situated more peripherally in the islet and the beta cells (3) deeper or more in the center of the islet. Also, the beta cells (3) are the predominant cell type of the pancreatic islets and constitute approximately 70% of their mass. The delta (D) cell (not illustrated) is also present in the islets. These cells are least abundant, have variable cell shape, and may occur anywhere in the pancreatic islet.

Numerous **capillaries (2)** are clearly visible around the different endocrine cells, demonstrating the rich viscularity of the pancreatic islets. The islet cells are separated from the **serous acini (6)** by a thin **connective tissue capsule (4)**. **Centroacinar cells (5)** are clearly visible in some of the surrounding acini.

■ Functional Correlations–Endocrine Pancreas

Pancreas secrete two major hormones that have a major effect on blood glucose levels and its metabolism. The **alpha cells** of the pancreatic islets produce the hormone **glucagon,** which is released in response to low levels of glucose in the body. The main physiological function of glucagon is to increase glucose levels in the blood. This function is primarily accomplished by accelerating the conversion of glycogen, amino acids, and fatty acids in the liver into glucose; these conversions elevate the sugar levels in the blood.

The **beta cells** of the pancreatic islets produce the hormone **insulin,** whose release is stimulated by the elevation of blood glucose right after a meal. The main physiological function of insulin is to lower the glucose levels in the blood by accelerating membrane transport of glucose into liver, muscle, and adipose cells. Insulin also accelerates the conversion of glucose into glycogen in the liver. The effects of insulin on the levels of blood glucose levels are just the opposite to that of glucagon.

The **delta** cells secrete the hormone **somatostatin.** It decreases and inhibits the secretory activities of both alpha (glucagon secreting) and beta (insulin secreting) cells through local action within the pancreatic islets.

To date, little is known about the function of F cells.

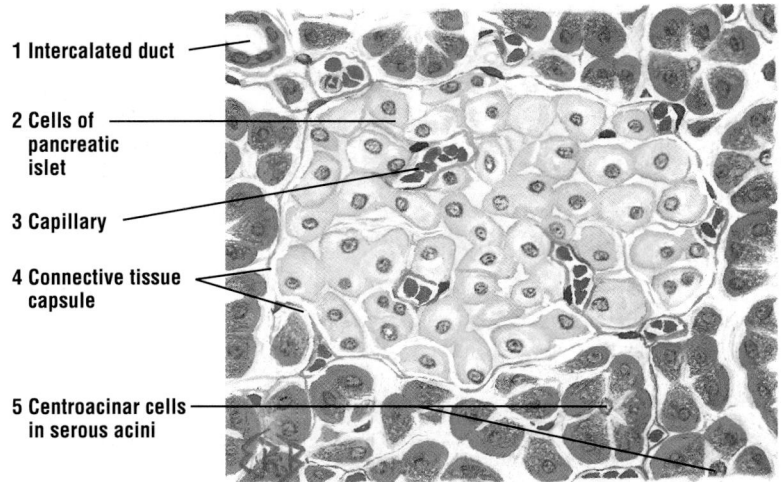

1 Intercalated duct

2 Cells of pancreatic islet

3 Capillary

4 Connective tissue capsule

5 Centroacinar cells in serous acini

Fig. 13-11   Pancreatic Islet. Stain: hematoxylin-eosin. High magnification.

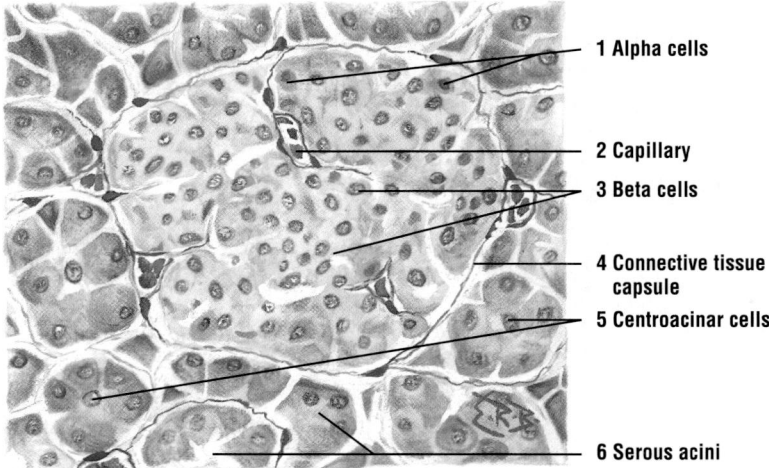

1 Alpha cells

2 Capillary

3 Beta cells

4 Connective tissue capsule

5 Centroacinar cells

6 Serous acini

Fig. 13-12   Pancreatic Islet (special preparation). Stain: Gomori's chrome alum hematoxylin-phloxine. High magnification.

Figure 13-13   Bovine Liver: Liver Lobule (transverse section)

A lower magnification photomicrograph of a bovine liver illustrates a central region of one classical hepatic (liver) lobule and peripheral regions of adjacent hepatic lobules. The periphery of the hepatic lobule, the portal area, contains the terminal branches of the **portal vein (5), hepatic artery (6),** and normally a bile duct, which is not seen in this illustration. In the center of each hepatic lobule is a **central vein (1),** from which radiate **plates of hepatic cells (2)** toward the lobule periphery. Located between the plates of hepatic cells (2) are the blood channels called **sinusoids (3).** These sinusoids (3) deliver blood from the portal vein (5) and hepatic artery (6) in the portal area to the central vein (1) of each hepatic lobule. Both the central vein (1) and the sinusoids (3) are lined by **endothelium (4),** which is of the discontinuous type in the sinusoids.

Figure 13-14   Pancreas: Endocrine (Pancreatic Islet) and Exocrine Regions

A higher magnification photomicrograph of the pancreas illustrates both its exocrine and endocrine regions. In the middle of the illustration is the light-staining endocrine **pancreatic islet (3).** A thin **connective tissue capsule (2)** surrounds the pancreatic islet (3) and separates it from the rest of pancreatic cells. The pancreatic islet (3) is highly vascularized by numerous blood vessels and **capillaries (6).** The exocrine portion, which constitutes the bulk of the pancreas, is a compound, tubuloacinar gland. Each exocrine **secretory acinius (5)** consist of pyramidal-shaped cluster of cells arranged around a small lumen. In the centers of most secretory acini (5) are seen one or more light-staining **centroacinar cells (4).** These cells represent the terminal lining cells of the excretory duct system. The smallest excretory ducts in the pancreas are the **intercalated ducts (1)** and they are lined by simple cuboidal epithelium.

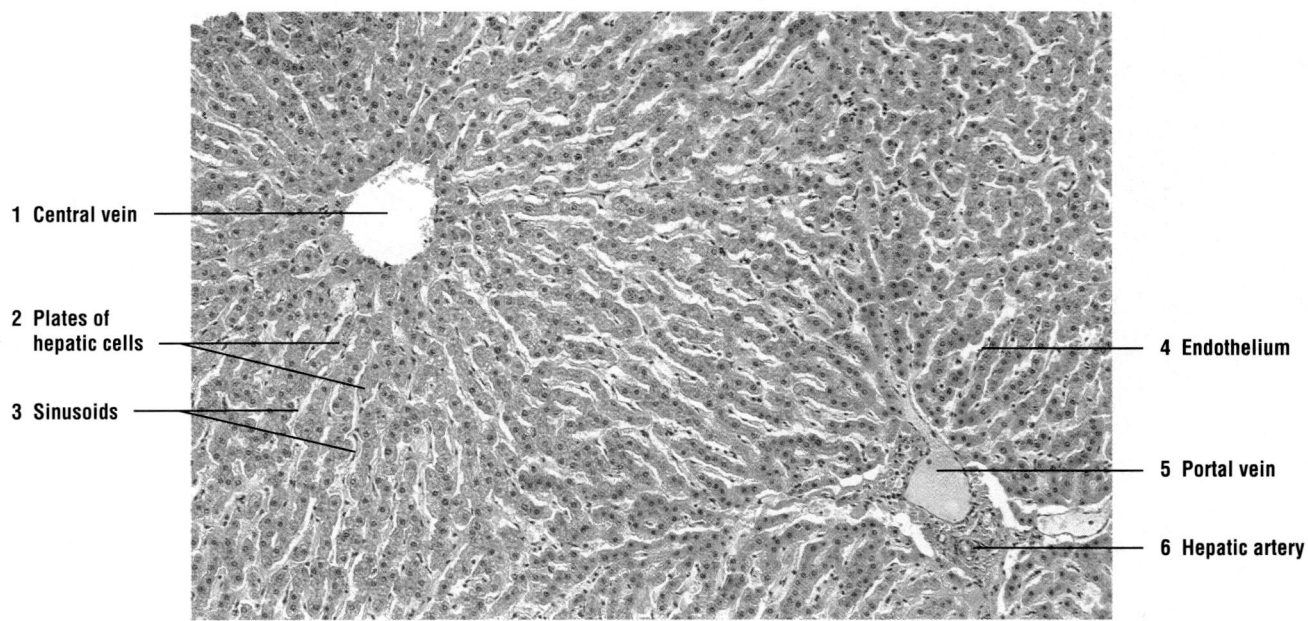

1 Central vein

2 Plates of
  hepatic cells

3 Sinusoids

4 Endothelium

5 Portal vein

6 Hepatic artery

Fig. 13-13   Bovine Liver: Liver Lobule (transverse section). Stain: hematoxylin-eosin. 30×

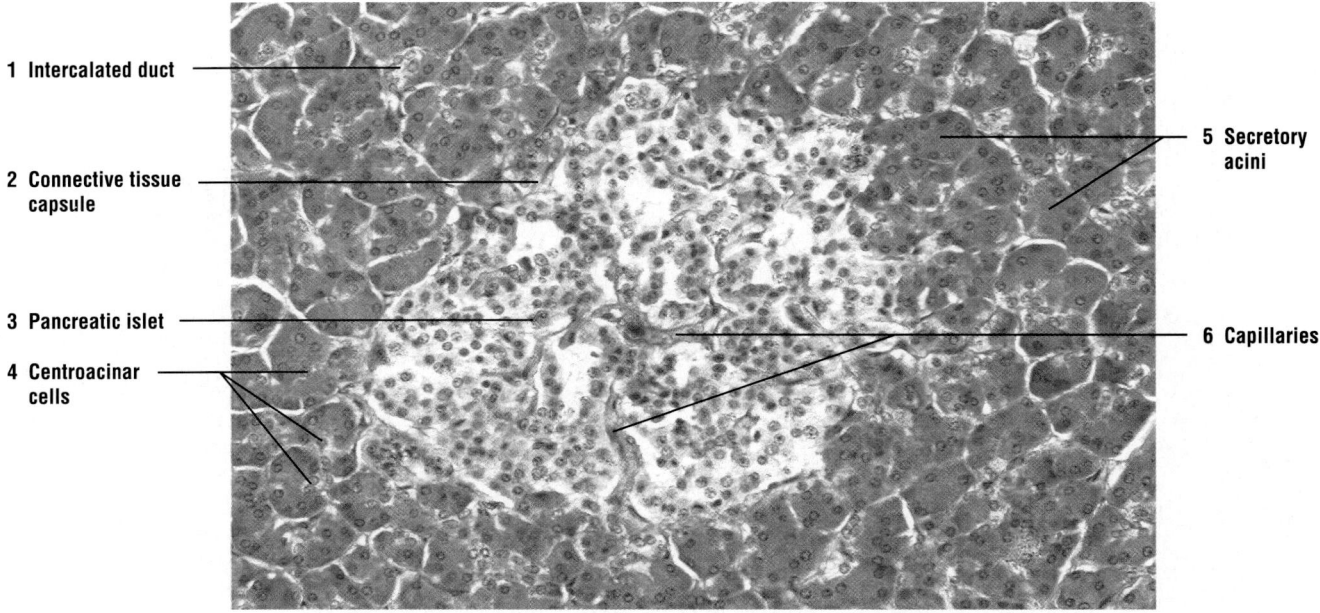

1 Intercalated duct

2 Connective tissue
  capsule

3 Pancreatic islet

4 Centroacinar
  cells

5 Secretory
  acini

6 Capillaries

Fig. 13-14   Pancreas: Endocrine (Pancreatic Islet) and Exocrine Regions. Stain: PAS and hematoxylin. 80×

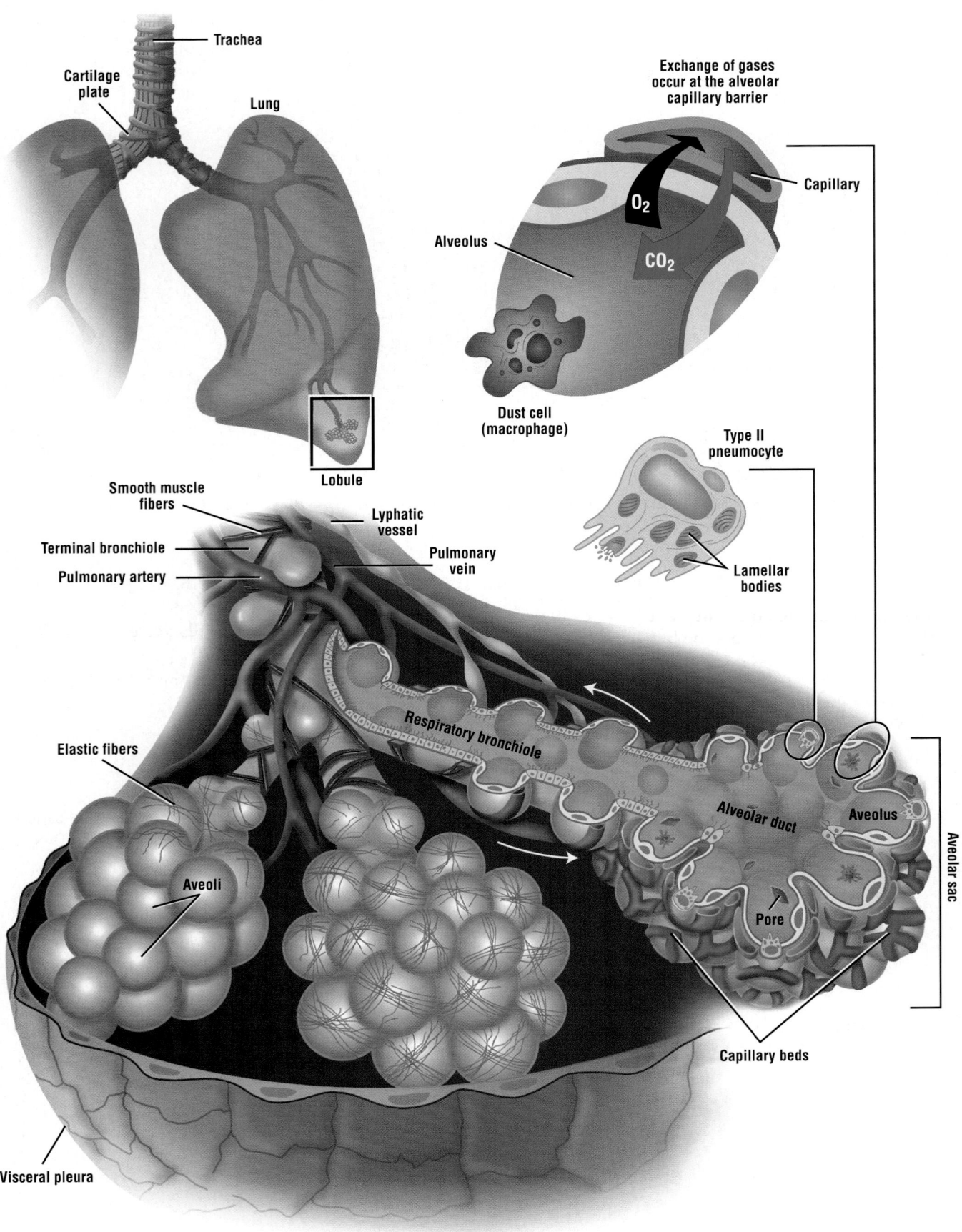

Trachea

Cartilage plate

Lung

Exchange of gases occur at the alveolar capillary barrier

Capillary

Alveolus

O₂

CO₂

Dust cell (macrophage)

Type II pneumocyte

Lamellar bodies

Smooth muscle fibers

Lyphatic vessel

Terminal bronchiole

Pulmonary artery

Pulmonary vein

Respiratory bronchiole

Elastic fibers

Alveolar duct

Aveolus

Aveoli

Aveolar sac

Pore

Visceral pleura

Capillary beds

Lobule

Respiratory System

COMPONENT PARTS OF THE RESPIRATORY SYSTEM

The respiratory system consists of two **lungs** and numerous **air passages** or **tubes** of various sizes that lead to and from each lung. The air passages consist of a conducting portion and respiratory portion. The **conducting portions** are the solid air passages outside as well as inside the lung that conduct air to the lungs for respiration. The **respiratory portion** are air passages within the lungs where respiration or gaseous exchange takes place. The epithelium in the extrapulmonary passages (outside of lungs), trachea, bronchi, and larger bronchioles is **pseudostratified ciliated epithelium** with numerous **goblet cells.** The diameter of the air passages in the lungs become progressively smaller and smaller. Similarly, there is also a gradual decrease in the height of the lining epithelium, amount of cilia, and the number of goblet cells in these tubules. Gaseous exchanges can only take place in the **alveoli,** the terminal air spaces of the respiratory system. Here, the lining epithelium is **simple squamous** and the goblet cells are absent. The air that enters the lungs also passes an epithelium in the nasal cavity that is specialized to detect odor; this is the olfactory epithelium.

OLFACTORY EPITHELIUM

The roof or the superior region of the **nasal cavity** contains a highly specialized epithelium for detection and transmission of odors or smell. This is the **olfactory epithelium** and it consists of three cell types: supportive (sustentacular), basal, and olfactory. The **olfactory cells,** distributed among the supportive cells, are the **sensory bipolar neurons;** these cells end at the surface of the olfactory epithelium as small olfactory bulbs. Radiating from each olfactory bulb are long, nonmotile olfactory **cilia** that lie flat on the epithelial surface in the overlying mucus and function as odor receptors. There are no goblet cells or motile cilia in the olfactory epithelium. In the connective tissue below the olfactory epithelium are found **olfactory nerves** and **olfactory glands (Figs. 14-1, 14-2, 14-13).**

CONDUCTING PORTION OF THE RESPIRATORY SYSTEM

The **conducting portion** of the respiratory system consists of nasal cavities; pharynx; larynx; trachea; extrapulmonary bronchi; and a series of intrapulmonary bronchi and bronchioles with decreasing diameters, culminating in the **terminal bronchioles.** To ensure that the larger air passageways are always patent (open), **hyaline cartilage** provides the structural support. Incomplete C-shaped **hyaline cartilage rings** encircle the **trachea.** As the trachea further divides into smaller

bronchi and the bronchi enter the lungs, the hyaline cartilage rings are replaced by **hyaline cartilage plates.** As the bronchi branch and become smaller, the cartilage plates are reduced in size and number. When the diameter of the bronchioles is reduced to about 1 mm, cartilage plates completely disappear from the conducting air passageways. The final conducting air passageways are the **terminal bronchioles,** with diameter sizes that range from 0.5 mm to 1.0 mm **(Figs. 14-5–4-7, 14-10, 14-14).** The epithelium height also changes with the decreasing diameter of the tubules. The larger bronchioles are lined by **ciliated pseudostratified epithelium** that is similar to that of trachea and bronchi. This epithelium gradually decreases in height to **simple ciliated epithelium.** Large bronchioles still contain **goblet cells** in their epithelium, but these gradually decrease in number, and are no longer found in the terminal bronchioles. Smaller bronchioles are lined by only **simple cuboidal epithelium.** Also, the terminal bronchioles are lined by non-ciliated cuboidal cells called **Clara cells;** these cells increase in number in the terminal bronchioles as the ciliated cells decrease **(Fig. 14-8).**

RESPIRATORY PORTION OF THE RESPIRATORY SYSTEM

The respiratory portion is the distal continuation of the conducting portion and consists of those air passageways where actual respiration or gaseous exchange occurs. The **terminal bronchioles** of the conducting system give rise to **respiratory bronchioles,** which are tubules characterized by thin-walled outpocketings called **alveoli.** The respiratory bronchioles represent the **transitional zone** between the air conduction and respiration or air exchange. Respiration can only occur in alveoli because the barrier between inspired air in the alveoli and the venous blood in the capillaries is extremely thin. The other intrapulmonary structures where respiration occurs are the **alveolar ducts, alveolar sacs,** and **alveoli.** Thus, the functional units of the lungs are the alveoli **(Figs. 14-8, 14-11, 14-14).**

The lung contains different cell types. In the lung alveoli are found two types of cells. The most abundant are the **squamous alveolar cells (type I pneumocytes).** These thin cells line all alveolar surfaces. The other cells, interspersed among the squamous alveolar cells either singly or in small groups, are the **great alveolar cells (type II pneumocytes). Alveolar macrophages (dust cells),** derived from the circulating blood monocytes, are found both in the connective tissue of the interalveolar septa (alveolar macrophages) between adjacent alveoli and in the alveoli (dust cells). Also, in the interalveolar septa are found extensive capillary networks, pulmonary arteries, pulmonary veins, lymphatic ducts, and nerves.

Figure 14-1   Olfactory Mucosa and Superior Concha (panoramic view)

The **olfactory mucosa (2, 5)** is illustrated on the surface of the **superior concha (1),** one of the bony shelves in the nasal cavity.

The respiratory epithelium in the nasal cavity is pseudostratified ciliated columnar epithelium with goblet cells. The **olfactory epithelium (2, 5;** Fig. 14-2) is specialized for reception of smell and therefore differs from the respiratory epithelium; it is pseudostratified tall columnar epithelium without goblet cells. The olfactory epithelium is found in the roof of each nasal cavity, on each side of the septum, and in the upper nasal conchae.

The underlying **lamina propria (2)** contains the branched tubuloacinar **olfactory glands (Bowman's glands) (3, 6).** These glands produce a serous secretion, in contrast to the mixed mucous and serous secretions produced by glands in the rest of the nasal cavity. Numerous small nerves found in the connective tissue of the lamina propria are the olfactory nerves or **fila olfactoria (4, 7).** These nerves represent the aggregated axons of the olfactory cells. The lamina propria (2) merges with the periosteum of the bone.

Figure 14-2   Olfactory Mucosa: Detail of a Transitional Area

This illustration depicts a transitional area between the **olfactory (1)** and **respiratory epithelia (9).** In this region, the histologic differences between these two important epithelia become obvious. The olfactory epithelium (1) is tall, pseudostratified columnar epithelium, composed of three different cell types: supportive, basal, and neuroepithelial olfactory cells. The individual cell outlines are difficult to distinguish in a routine histologic preparation; however, the location and shape of nuclei allow some identification of the cell types that comprise the olfactory epithelium.

The **supportive,** or **sustentacular cells (3)** are elongated, with oval nuclei situated more apically or superficially in the epithelium than the nuclei of the **olfactory cells (4).** The apical surfaces of the olfactory cells contain slender microvilli that protrude into the overlying layer of surface **mucus (2);** basally, the cells are slender.

The olfactory cells (4) have oval or round nuclei that occupy a region in the epithelium that is somewhat between the nuclei of the supportive cells (3) and **basal cells (5).** The apices of the olfactory cells (4) are slender and pass to the epithelial surface. Extending from the slender cell bases are axons that pass into the underlying connective tissue, or **lamina propria (6),** where they aggregate into small bundles of unmyelinated olfactory nerves, the **fila olfactoria (14).** These nerves ultimately leave the nasal cavity and pass into the olfactory bulbs at the base of the brain. The **basal cells (5)** are short, small cells located at the base of the epithelium between the bases of supportive (3) and olfactory cells (4).

The transition from the olfactory epithelium (1) to the respiratory epithelium (9) is abrupt. In this illustration, the respiratory epithelium (9) is pseudostratified columnar epithelium with distinct surface **cilia (10)** and an abundance of **goblet cells (11);** the goblet cells are not present in the olfactory epithelium (1). Also, in the transition area, the height of the respiratory epithelium appears similar to that of the olfactory; however, in other regions of the respiratory tract, the epithelial height is much reduced in comparison to olfactory epithelium.

Beneath the olfactory epithelium (1) is the lamina propria (6), containing a rich supply of capillaries, lymphatic vessels, **arterioles (8),** and **venules (13).** In addition to olfactory nerves (14), the lamina propria also contains branched, tubuloacinar **olfactory glands (Bowman's glands) (7).** These serous glands deliver their secretions through narrow **ducts (12),** which penetrate the olfactory epithelium (1) and open onto the surface. The secretions from these glands moisten the olfactory mucosa and provide the solvent necessary to dissolve odoriferous substances and stimulate the olfactory receptor cells (3).

■ Functional Correlations–Olfactory Epithelium

In order to detect odors, the odoriferous substances must first be dissolved. The dissolved odor molecules bind to receptor proteins on the **olfactory cilia** and stimulate the **receptors cells** in the olfactory epithelium. For this reason, the olfactory epithelium is always kept moist by a thin, watery secretion produced by serous tubuloacinar **olfactory (Bowman's) glands** located below the epithelium in the lamina propria. The watery secretion from these glands is delivered to the olfactory epithelium via ducts. The secretion constantly washes over the surface of the olfactory epithelium and, in this manner, allows the receptor cells to continuously detect and respond to new odors. The unmyelinated afferent axons of the sensory olfactory cells leave the olfactory epithelium and join to form small **olfactory nerve** bundles in the lamina propria. From here, these nerves pass through the ethmoid bone in the skull to synapse in the olfactory bulbs of the brain.

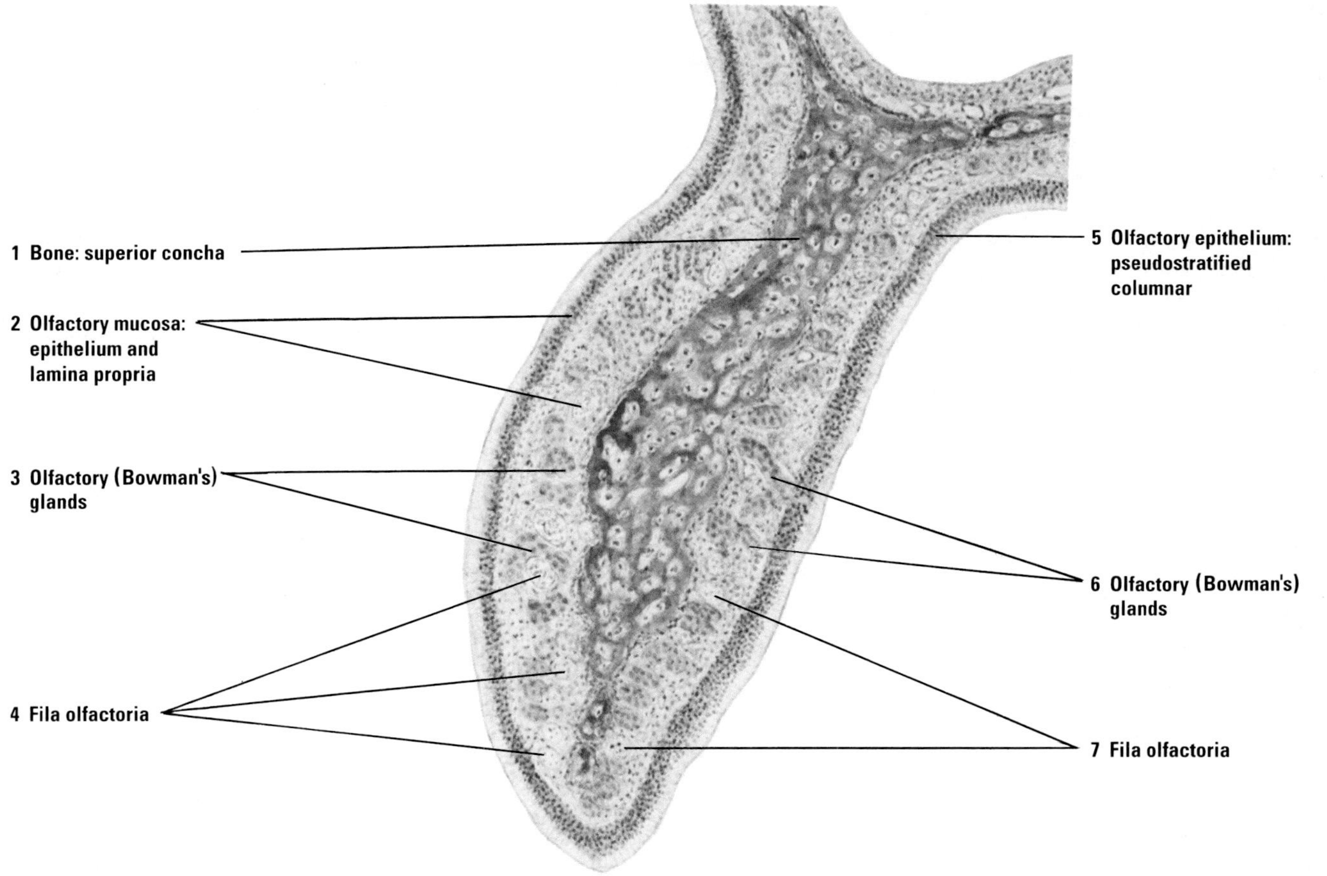

1 Bone: superior concha

2 Olfactory mucosa:
  epithelium and
  lamina propria

3 Olfactory (Bowman's)
  glands

4 Fila olfactoria

5 Olfactory epithelium:
  pseudostratified
  columnar

6 Olfactory (Bowman's)
  glands

7 Fila olfactoria

Fig. 14-1   Olfactory Mucosa and Superior Concha (panoramic view). Stain: hematoxylin-eosin. Low magnification.

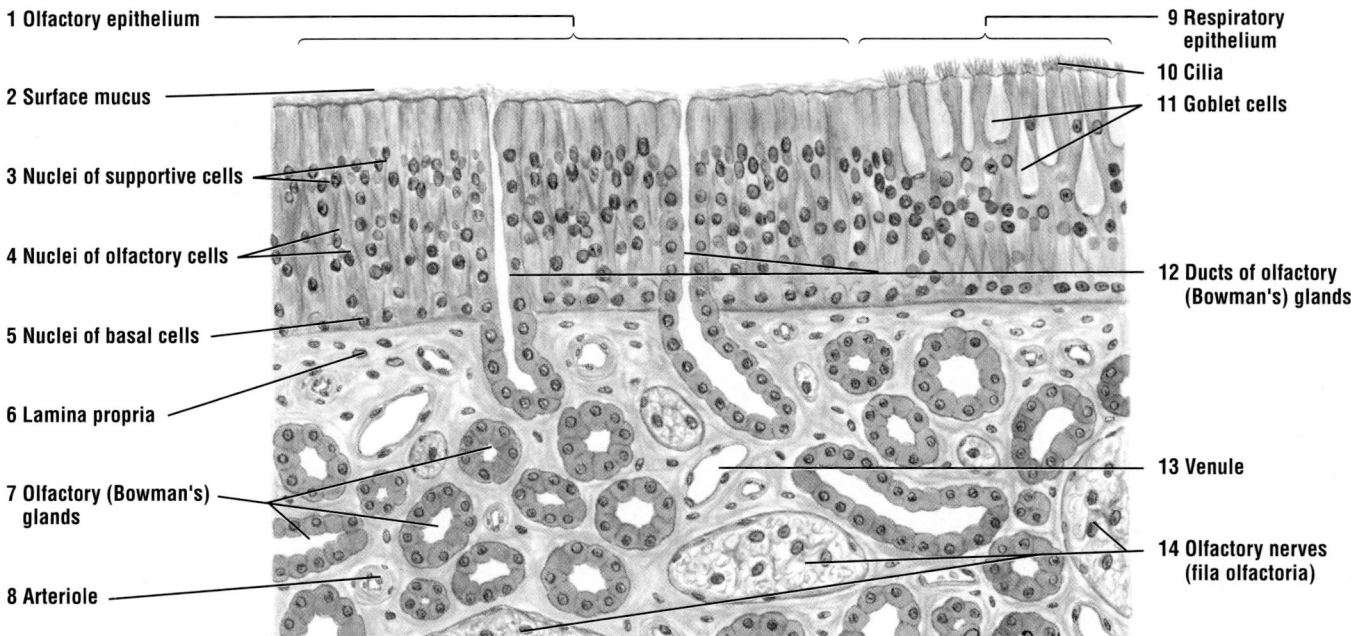

1 Olfactory epithelium

2 Surface mucus

3 Nuclei of supportive cells

4 Nuclei of olfactory cells

5 Nuclei of basal cells

6 Lamina propria

7 Olfactory (Bowman's)
  glands

8 Arteriole

9 Respiratory
  epithelium

10 Cilia

11 Goblet cells

12 Ducts of olfactory
   (Bowman's) glands

13 Venule

14 Olfactory nerves
   (fila olfactoria)

Fig. 14-2   Olfactory Mucosa: Detail of a Transitional Area. Stain: hematoxylin-eosin. High magnification.

Figure 14-3   Epiglottis (longitudinal section)

The epiglottis is the superior portion of the larynx; it projects upward from the larynx's anterior wall as a flat flap.

A central **epiglottic (elastic) cartilage (7)** forms the framework of the epiglottis. Its **anterior** or **lingual surface (6)** is covered with a noncornified **stratified squamous epithelium (9).** The underlying **lamina propria (4)** merges with the **perichondrium (8)** of the epiglottic cartilage (7).

The anterior, or lingual, mucosa (6) covers the apex of the epiglottis and more than half of the posterior or **laryngeal surface (2).** The **stratified squamous epithelium (3),** however, is lower; the connective tissue papillae disappear, and a transition is made to a respiratory epithelium, which is **pseudostratified ciliated columnar epithelium (5)** with goblet cells.

Tubuloacinar mucous, serous, or mixed glands are present in the lamina propria (4). Occasional **taste buds (1)** are seen in the epithelium. Solitary lymphatic nodules may be present in the lingual (6) or laryngeal mucosa (2).

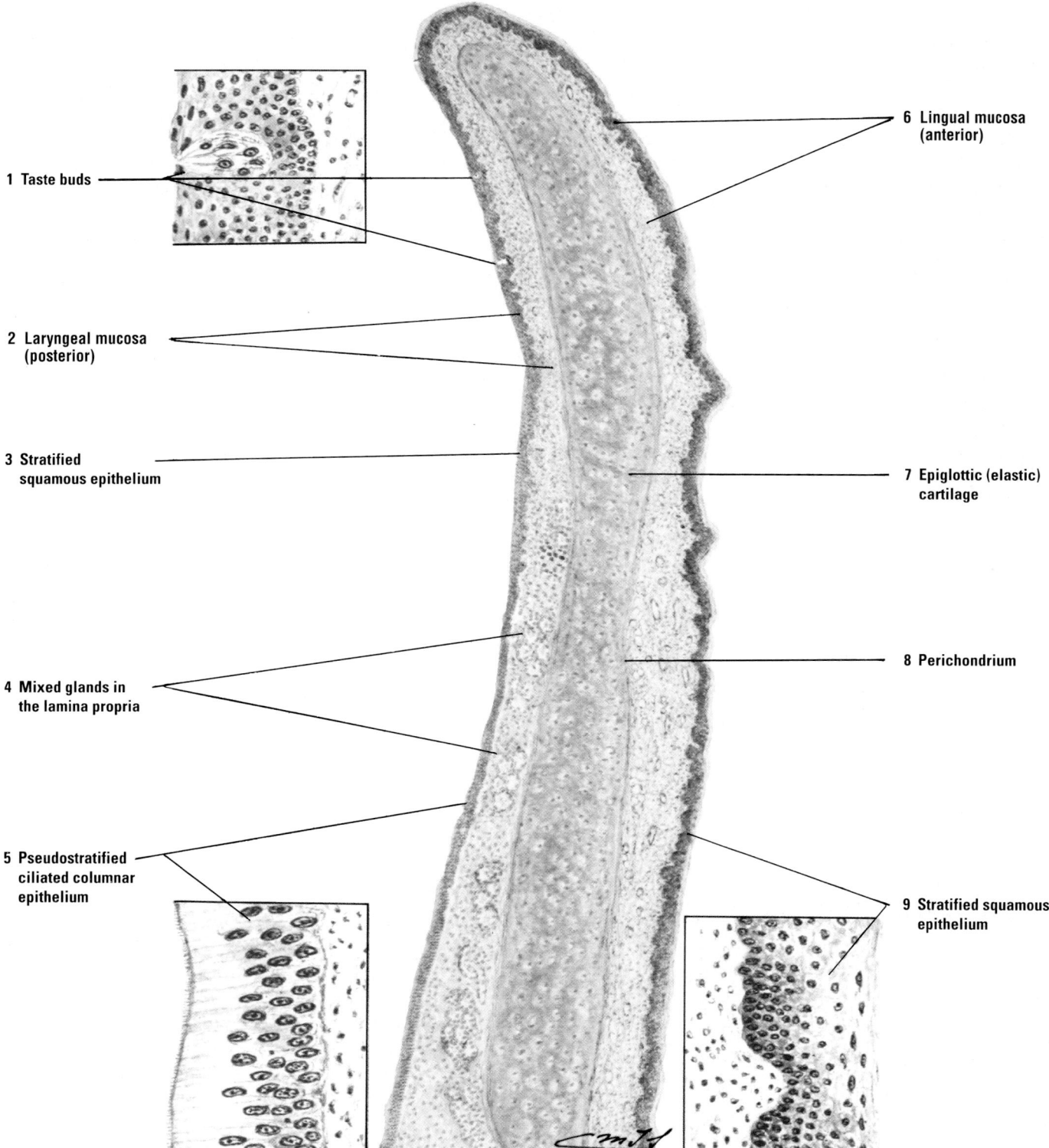

1 Taste buds

2 Laryngeal mucosa (posterior)

3 Stratified squamous epithelium

4 Mixed glands in the lamina propria

5 Pseudostratified ciliated columnar epithelium

6 Lingual mucosa (anterior)

7 Epiglottic (elastic) cartilage

8 Perichondrium

9 Stratified squamous epithelium

Fig. 14-3 Epiglottis (longitudinal section). Stain: hematoxylin-eosin. Low magnification. Insets: High magnification.

Figure 14-4   Larynx (frontal section)

A vertical section through the larynx shows the two prominent **vocal folds (13, 18–20)**, supporting **cartilages (8, 11)**, and **muscles (10, 20)**.

The **superior, or false, vocal fold (13)** of the larynx is formed by the mucosa and is continuous with the **posterior surface of the epiglottis (12)**. The lining epithelium is **pseudostratified ciliated columnar epithelium (14)** with goblet cells. Visible below the epithelium, in the **lamina propria (3)**, are **mixed glands (15)**, which are predominantly mucous. **Excretory ducts (16)**, which open onto the epithelial surface, are visible among the acini of the glands (15). **Lymphatic nodules (7)** are located in the lamina propria (3) on the ventricular side of the vocal fold.

The **ventricle (17)** is a deep indentation and recess separating the false vocal fold (13) from the **true vocal fold (18–20)**. The mucosa in the **lateral wall (3, 4, 5, 6)** of the ventricle (17) is similar to that of the false vocal fold (13). Lymphatic nodules are more numerous in this area and are sometimes called the **"laryngeal tonsils" (7)**. The lamina propria (3) blends with the **perichondrium (9)** of the **thyroid cartilage (8)**; there is no distinct submucosa. The lower wall of the ventricle makes the transition to a true vocal fold (18–20).

The mucosa of the true vocal fold (18–20) consists of noncornified, **stratified squamous epithelium (18)** and a thin, dense lamina propria devoid of glands, lymphatic tissue, or blood vessels. At the apex of the true vocal fold is the **vocal ligament (19)**, consisting of dense elastic fibers that spread out into the adjacent lamina propria and the skeletal **vocalis muscle (20)**. The skeletal **thyroarytenoid muscle (10)** and the **thyroid cartilage (8)** comprise the remaining wall.

The epithelium in the lower larynx changes to **pseudostratified ciliated columnar epithelium (21)**, and the underlying lamina propria contains **mixed glands (22)**. The **cricoid cartilage (11)** is the lowermost cartilage of the larynx.

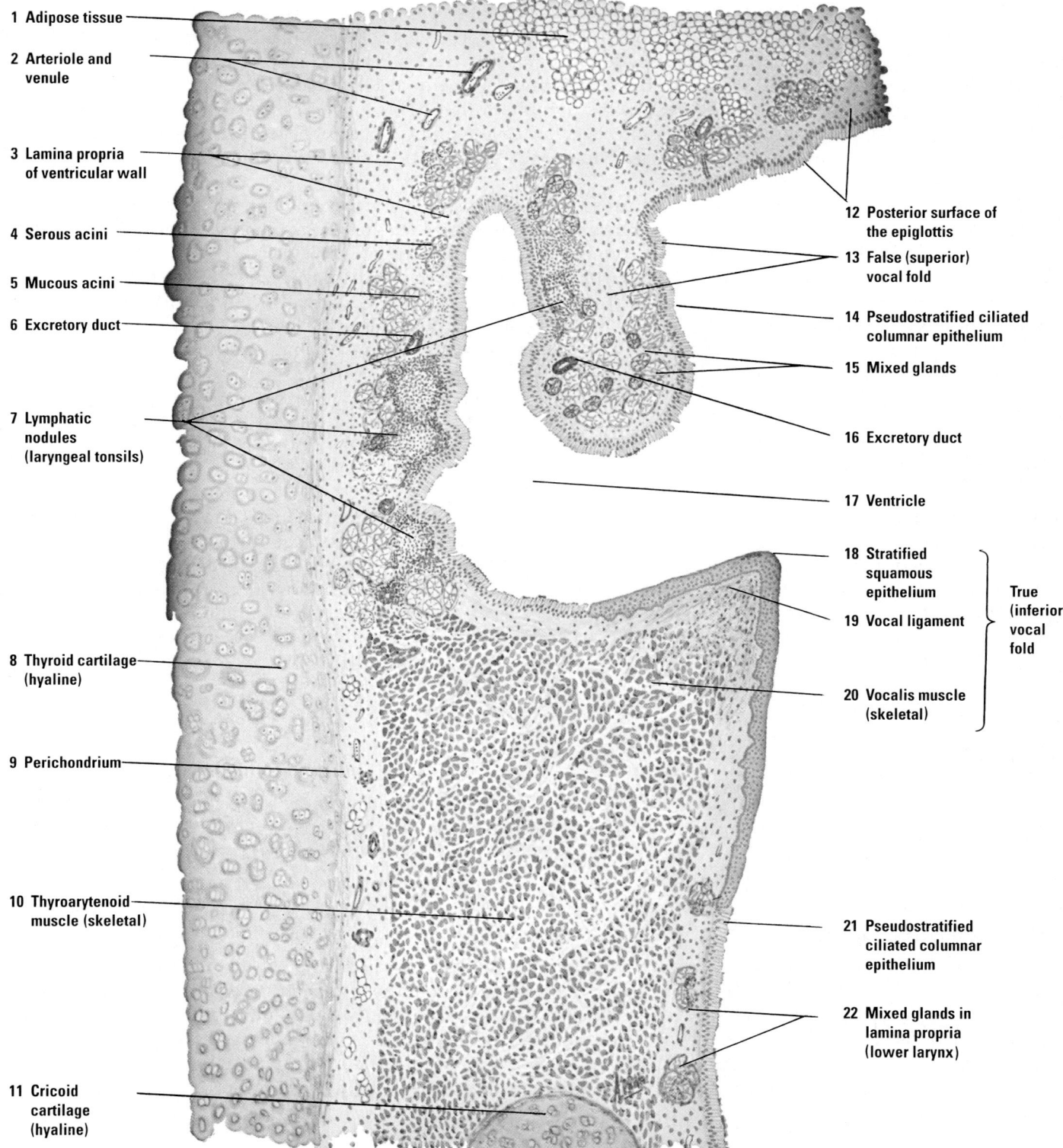

1 Adipose tissue

2 Arteriole and venule

3 Lamina propria of ventricular wall

4 Serous acini

5 Mucous acini

6 Excretory duct

7 Lymphatic nodules (laryngeal tonsils)

8 Thyroid cartilage (hyaline)

9 Perichondrium

10 Thyroarytenoid muscle (skeletal)

11 Cricoid cartilage (hyaline)

12 Posterior surface of the epiglottis

13 False (superior) vocal fold

14 Pseudostratified ciliated columnar epithelium

15 Mixed glands

16 Excretory duct

17 Ventricle

18 Stratified squamous epithelium

19 Vocal ligament

20 Vocalis muscle (skeletal)

True (inferior) vocal fold

21 Pseudostratified ciliated columnar epithelium

22 Mixed glands in lamina propria (lower larynx)

Fig. 14-4   Larynx (frontal section). Stain: hematoxylin-eosin. Low magnification.

Figure 14-5   Trachea (panoramic view, transverse section)

The wall of the trachea consists of mucosa, submucosa, hyaline cartilage, and adventitia. The cartilage in the trachea is a series of C-shaped rings between whose ends lies the smooth **trachealis muscle (9).**

The mucosa consists of **pseudostratified ciliated columnar epithelium (13)** with goblet cells. The **lamina propria (11, 14)** contains fine connective tissue fibers, diffuse **lymphatic tissue (14),** and occasional solitary lymphatic nodules. Deep in the lamina propria (11), the elastic fibers form a longitudinal **elastic membrane (15).** In the loose connective tissue of the **submucosa (16)** are mixed **tubuloacinar glands (4, 5)** whose **ducts (10, 17)** pass through the lamina propria (11) to the tracheal lumen.

The **hyaline cartilage (3)** is surrounded by dense connective tissue, the **perichondrium (2),** which merges with the submucosa (16) on one side and the **adventitia (1)** on the other side. Numerous **blood vessels and nerves (6)** course in the adventitia (1) and provide smaller branches to the outer layers.

The **mucosa (12)** exhibits folds along the posterior wall of the trachea where the cartilage is absent. The trachealis muscle (9) lies deep to the elastic membrane (15) of the mucosa and is embedded in the fibroelastic tissue that occupies the area between the ends of the cartilage rings. Most of the trachealis muscle fibers (9) insert into the perichondrium of the cartilage (2, upper leader). **Mixed glands (8)** are present in the submucosa; these can intermingle with the muscle fibers and extend into the adventitia.

Figure 14-6   Trachea (sectional view)

A small section of trachea is illustrated at a higher magnification to show details of the wall. The pseudostratified surface epithelium contains **ciliated (5)** and **goblet cells (10)** with irregularly located nuclei. Note the thickened **basement membrane (6).** A longitudinal **elastic membrane (7)** is visible in the deeper region of the lamina propria; in this illustration, the fibers are cut in transverse plane. Also seen in the lamina propria are a group of **mucous acini (9)** of the tracheal glands and their **duct (8).** In the adjacent **cartilage (2),** the larger lacunae and **chondrocytes (3)** in the interior become progressively flatter toward the **perichondrium (1)** while the matrix gradually blends with the connective tissue.

Figure 14-7   Trachea: Elastic Fiber Stain (sectional view)

This section of the trachea has been stained with Gallego's method to visualize **elastic fibers (8)** in the elastic membrane, which stain red with carbolfuchsin. Collagen fibers stain blue with aniline blue and provide a contrast where they intermix with the elastic fibers. Collagen fibers are also visible in the **perichondrium (1, lower leader), submucosa (3),** and **superficial lamina propria (9).**

■ Functional Correlations–Conducting Portion

The conducting portion of the respiratory system conditions and delivers air from the external environment to the respiratory portion in the lungs. **Mucus** plays an important role in conditioning the inspired air. It is continuously produced by the **goblet cells** in the respiratory epithelium and **mucous glands** in the lamina propria; a mucus layer covers the luminal surfaces in most of the conducting tubes. As a result, the **moist mucosa** in the conducting portion of the respiratory system humidifies, filters, and cleans the air of particulate matter, infectious microorganisms, or other airborne matter. In addition, a rich **capillary network** beneath the epithelium in the connective tissue warms the inspired air.

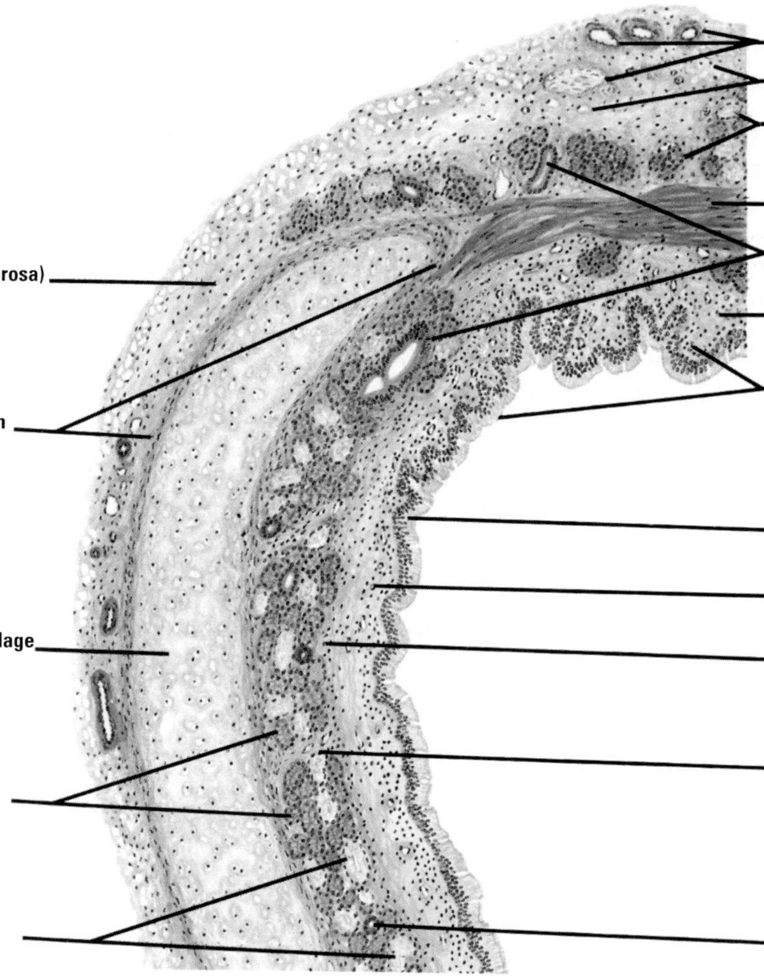

1 Adventitia (fibrosa)

2 Perichondrium

3 Tracheal cartilage
(hyaline)

4 Serous acini

5 Mucous acini

6 Arteriole, venule and nerve

7 Adipose cells in adventitia

8 Tracheal glands: mucous
and serous acini

9 Trachealis muscle (smooth)

10 Ducts of tracheal glands

11 Lamina propria

12 Folds in tracheal mucosa

13 Epithelium: pseudostratified
ciliated columnar with
goblet cells

14 Lamina propria with diffuse
lymphatic tissue

15 Elastic membrane

16 Submucosa with tracheal
glands

17 Duct of tracheal glands

Fig. 14-5   Trachea (panoramic view, transverse section). Stain: hematoxylin-eosin. Low magnification.

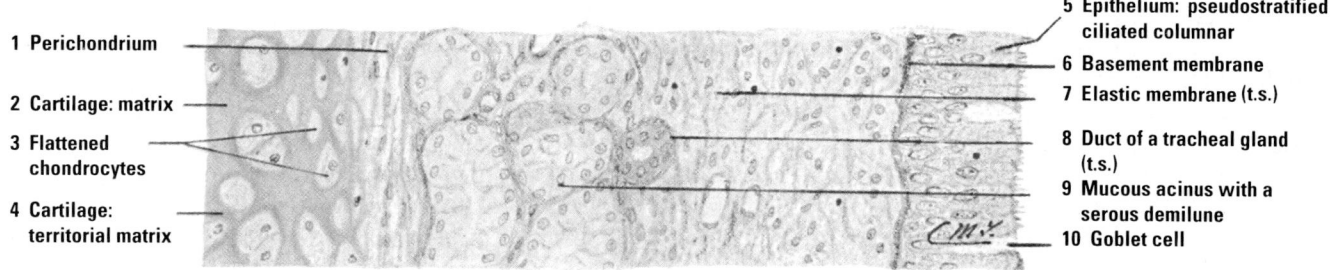

1 Perichondrium

2 Cartilage: matrix

3 Flattened
chondrocytes

4 Cartilage:
territorial matrix

5 Epithelium: pseudostratified
ciliated columnar

6 Basement membrane

7 Elastic membrane (t.s.)

8 Duct of a tracheal gland
(t.s.)

9 Mucous acinus with a
serous demilune

10 Goblet cell

Fig. 14-6   Trachea (sectional view). Stain: hematoxylin-eosin. Medium magnification.

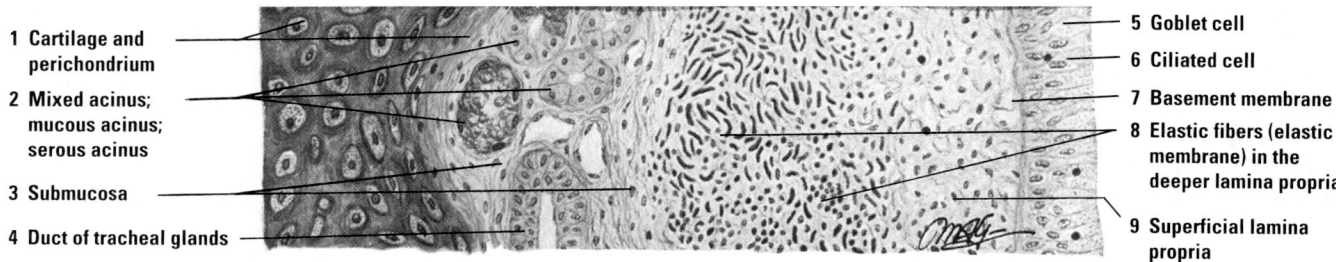

1 Cartilage and
perichondrium

2 Mixed acinus;
mucous acinus;
serous acinus

3 Submucosa

4 Duct of tracheal glands

5 Goblet cell

6 Ciliated cell

7 Basement membrane

8 Elastic fibers (elastic
membrane) in the
deeper lamina propria

9 Superficial lamina
propria

Fig. 14-7   Trachea: Elastic Fiber Stain (sectional view). Stain: Gallego's method for elastic fibers.
Medium magnification.

Figure 14-8   Lung (panoramic view)

The respiratory system, consisting of the lungs and the air passages, is divided into conducting and respiratory portions. The conducting portion consists of the nasal cavity, nasopharynx, larynx, trachea, bronchi, bronchioles, and terminal bronchioles. The respiratory portion consists of the respiratory bronchioles, alveolar ducts, alveolar sacs, and alveoli. The characteristic features of the lung are illustrated in this panoramic view. Figures 14-9 through 14-12 illustrate the histology of these divisions in greater detail and higher magnification. All cartilage in the lung is hyaline.

The histology of the extrapulmonary bronchi is similar to that of the trachea. In the intrapulmonary bronchi, the C-shaped cartilage rings are replaced by cartilage plates that encircle the bronchi. The smooth muscle spreads out from the trachealis muscle to surround the lumina of the bronchi.

The **intrapulmonary bronchus (33)** is normally identified by several **cartilage plates (30)** located in close proximity to each other. The **epithelium (32)** is pseudostratified columnar ciliated epithelium with goblet cells. The rest of the wall consists of a thin lamina propria, a narrow layer of **smooth muscle (31),** a submucosa with scattered bronchial glands, hyaline cartilage plate (30), and adventitia.

As the intrapulmonary bronchi branch and become smaller bronchi, the epithelial height and the amount of cartilage decreases. Farther down the airway tube, only occasional small pieces of cartilage are seen. In bronchi that are about 1 mm in diameter, cartilage is no longer visible.

In **bronchioles (16),** the epithelium is low, pseudostratified columnar ciliated epithelium with occasional goblet cells. The mucosa is normally folded and the smooth muscle surrounding the lumen is prominent. Glands and cartilage plates are no longer present, and adventitia surrounds these structures.

The **terminal bronchioles (6, 12)** exhibit a wavy mucosal lining and columnar ciliated epithelium; goblet cells are lacking in the terminal bronchioles. Still present, however, are a thin lamina propria, a layer of smooth muscle, and an adventitia.

The **respiratory bronchioles (5, 8, 17, 23, 26, 27)** are directly connected to the alveolar ducts and alveoli. In these bronchioles, the epithelium is low columnar or cuboidal (5, 8) and may be ciliated in the proximal portion of the tubules. A minimal amount of connective tissue supports the band of intermixed smooth muscle, the elastic fibers of the lamina propria, and the accompanying blood vessels. Individual **alveoli (25)** appear in the wall of the respiratory bronchioles (26) as small outpockets. Alveoli increase in number distally in the tubules. The epithelium and smooth muscle in the distal respiratory bronchioles appear as small, intermittent areas between the openings of the numerous alveoli (5, upper leader; 17, 23, 24, 25).

The terminal portion of each respiratory bronchiole branches into several **alveolar ducts (2, 15, 22);** in histologic sections only one such alveolar duct may be seen (2 and 5, lower leaders; 22, middle leader; 23, upper leader). The walls of the alveolar ducts (2, 15, 22) are formed by a series of alveoli situated adjacent to each other. A cluster of alveoli that open into an alveolar duct is called an **alveolar sac (14, 20).** The **alveoli (4, 21, 25)** form the parenchyma of the lung, giving it the appearance of fine lace (see Fig. 14-12 for details). In this illustration, a plane of section shows a continuous passageway from the terminal bronchiole (6) to the respiratory bronchiole (5, 26, 27) into the alveolar duct (2, lowest leader; 22, middle leader).

The **pulmonary artery (28)** branches repeatedly to accompany the divisions of the bronchial tree. Large pulmonary vein branches also accompany the bronchi and bronchioles; numerous small branches of the vein are seen in the lung **trabeculae (3).** Pulmonary arterioles (7, 10) supply the walls of various bronchi, bronchioles, (6, 12) and other areas of the lung. Small **bronchial veins (29)** may be seen in the walls of the larger **bronchi (33).**

The **visceral pleura (1)** adheres closely to lungs. It is composed of a thin layer of pleural **connective tissue (19)** and **pleural mesothelium (18).**

■ Functional Correlations–Different Lung Cells

The alveoli are lined by extremely thin, **simple squamous alveolar cells** (type I pneumocytes). These cells are in close contact with the endothelial lining of the capillaries and form the **blood–air barrier** for respiration. In addition, the alveoli also contain the **great alveolar cells** (type II pneumocytes). These cells are secretory and contain **lamellar bodies** in their cytoplasm. Great alveolar cells synthesize and secrete a phospholipid-rich product called pulmonary **surfactant.** Surfactant spreads over the alveolar cell surfaces, moistens them, and lowers the alveolar **surface tension.** In this manner, surfactant stabilizes alveolar diameters and prevents their collapse during respiration by minimizing the collapsing forces. During fetal development, sufficient surfactant is secreted by great alveolar cells during the last weeks (28 to 32) of gestation. In addition to producing surfactant, the great alveolar cells can divide and serve as **stem cells** for squamous alveolar cells.

Monocytes also enter the pulmonary connective tissue and become **alveolar macrophages.** The primary function of the these macrophages is protection: they clean the alveoli of invading microorganisms and inhaled particulate matter by **phagocytosis.**

1 **Visceral pleura**

2 **Alveolar ducts (l.s.)**

3 **Trabecula with pulmonary vein**

4 **Alveolus (t.s.)**

5 **Respiratory bronchiole (distal and proximal portions)**

6 **Terminal bronchiole**

7 **Pulmonary arteriole**
8 **Respiratory bronchiole (t.s.)**
9 **Alveolar duct (t.s.)**

10 **Pulmonary arteriole**
11 **Lymphatic nodule**
12 **Terminal bronchiole**

13 **Smooth muscle**

14 **Alveolar sac**

15 **Alveolar duct (l.s.)**

16 **Bronchiole**

17 **Respiratory bronchiole (distal portion, l.s.)**

18 **Pleural mesothelium**
19 **Pleural connective tissue**

20 **Alveolar sac**

21 **Alveoli**

22 **Alveolar ducts (l.s.)**

23 **Respiratory bronchioles (distal)**

24 **Simple columnar epithelium**
25 **Alveoli in distal respiratory bronchiole**
26 **Respiratory bronchiole (proximal)**
27 **Respiratory bronchiole (t.s.)**

28 **Pulmonary artery**

29 **Bronchial vein**

30 **Cartilage plates (hyaline)**

31 **Smooth muscle**
32 **Pseudostratified columnar ciliated epithelium**
33 **Intrapulmonary bronchus**

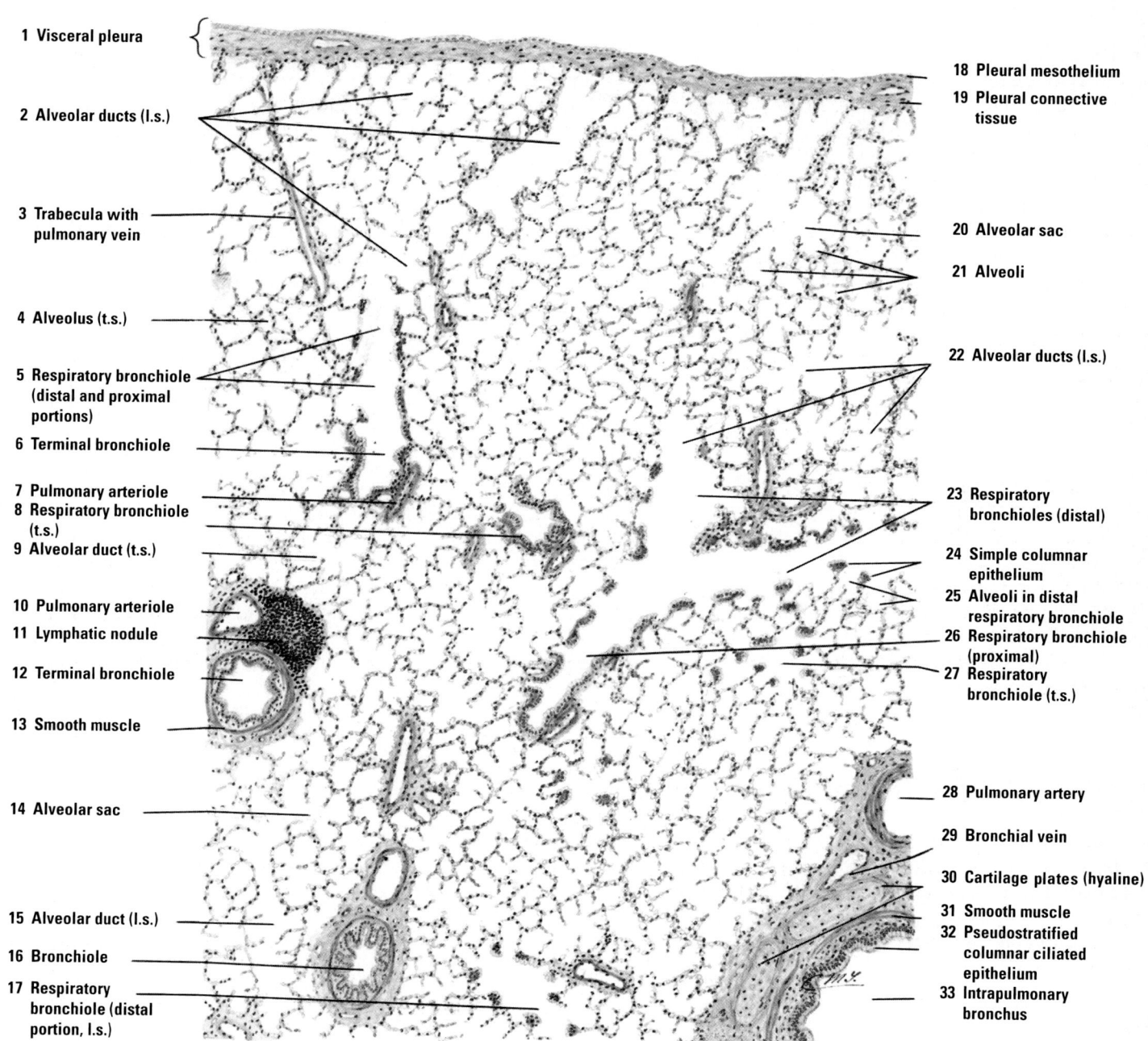

Fig. 14-8   Lung (panoramic view). Stain: hematoxylin-eosin. Low magnification.

Figure 14-9   Intrapulmonary Bronchus

The primary, or extrapulmonary, bronchi divide and give rise to a series of smaller intrapulmonary bronchi. Such bronchi are lined by pseudostratified columnar ciliated **epithelium (12),** a thin **lamina propria (13)** of fine connective tissue with many elastic fibers (not illustrated), and a few lymphocytes. **Ducts (2)** from the submucosal **bronchial glands (5, 8, 10)** pass through lamina propria (13) to open into the bronchial lumen. A thin layer of **smooth muscle (6)** surrounds the lamina propria (13). The submucosa contains glands of either **serous (5, 8),** mucous, or **mucoserous acini (10).** In the mixed glands, serous demilunes may be seen.

The **cartilage plates (4)** are distributed close together around the periphery of the bronchus; the plates become smaller and farther apart as the bronchi continue to divide and their size continues to decrease. Between the **cartilage plates (4),** the submucosal connective tissue blends with the well-developed **adventitia (3).**

The accompanying branch of the **pulmonary artery (15)** is located either adjacent to the bronchi or in the outer adventitia (14). A smaller branch of another **pulmonary artery (7)** probably accompanies a small bronchus or bronchiole located in another plane of section.

Bronchial vessels visible in the connective tissue of the bronchus include an **arteriole (16),** a **venule (11),** and **capillaries (9).**

Figure 14-10   Terminal Bronchiole

The terminal bronchioles have small diameters, about 1 mm or less. **Mucosal folds (4)** are prominent and the epithelium is low pseudostratified columnar ciliated with few goblet cells. In the terminal bronchioles, the **epithelium (5)** is columnar ciliated and the goblet cells are absent. A well-developed **smooth muscle (3)** layer surrounds the thin lamina propria which is, in turn, surrounded by the **adventitia (2).** Cartilage plates, glands, and goblet cells are absent.

Adjacent to the bronchiole is a small branch of the **pulmonary artery (6);** the bronchiole is surrounded by the **alveoli (7)** of the lung.

Figure 14-11   Respiratory Bronchiole

The wall of the respiratory bronchiole is lined with cuboidal **epithelium (4).** Cilia may be present in the epithelium of the proximal portion but disappear in the distal portion of the respiratory bronchiole. **Smooth muscle (3)** is located adjacent to the epithelium. A small branch of the **pulmonary artery (5)** accompanies the respiratory bronchiole.

An **alveolar duct (2)** arises from the respiratory bronchiole and numerous **alveoli (1)** open into the **alveolar duct (2).**

Figure 14-12   Alveolar Walls: Interalveolar Septa

The oval **alveoli (5)** are lined by simple squamous epithelium, which is not very obvious at this magnification. Adjacent alveoli share a common **interalveolar septum (4).** Located in the thin septum (4) are **capillary plexuses (1, 3)** supported by fine connective tissue fibers, fibroblasts, and other cells. As a result of the thin interalveolar septum (4) and its contents, the capillaries are in close proximity to the squamous cells of the adjacent alveoli, separated from the epithelium only by the sparse connective tissue. In routine preparation of lung tissue, it is difficult to distinguish between the nuclei of squamous cells in the alveoli (5), endothelial cells in the **blood vessels (capillaries) (1, 3),** and the **fibroblasts (6)** in the interalveolar septum (4).

At the free ends of the interalveolar septa (4) and around the open ends of the alveoli are narrow bands of **smooth muscle (2),** which is a continuation from the muscle layer of the respiratory bronchiole.

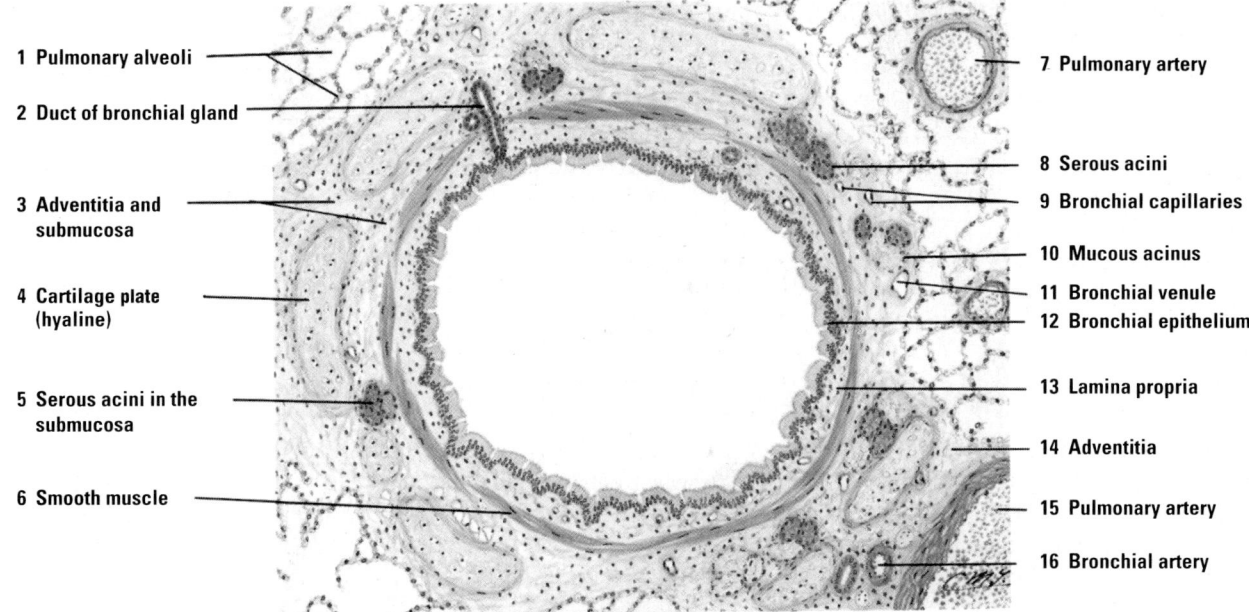

1 Pulmonary alveoli

2 Duct of bronchial gland

3 Adventitia and
   submucosa

4 Cartilage plate
   (hyaline)

5 Serous acini in the
   submucosa

6 Smooth muscle

7 Pulmonary artery

8 Serous acini

9 Bronchial capillaries

10 Mucous acinus

11 Bronchial venule

12 Bronchial epithelium

13 Lamina propria

14 Adventitia

15 Pulmonary artery

16 Bronchial artery

Fig. 14-9   Intrapulmonary Bronchus. Stain: hematoxylin-eosin. Low magnification.

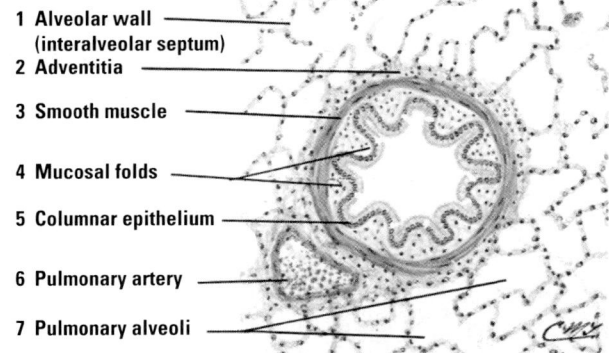

1 Alveolar wall
   (interalveolar septum)

2 Adventitia

3 Smooth muscle

4 Mucosal folds

5 Columnar epithelium

6 Pulmonary artery

7 Pulmonary alveoli

Fig. 14-10   Terminal Bronchiole. Stain: hematoxylin-eosin. Low magnification.

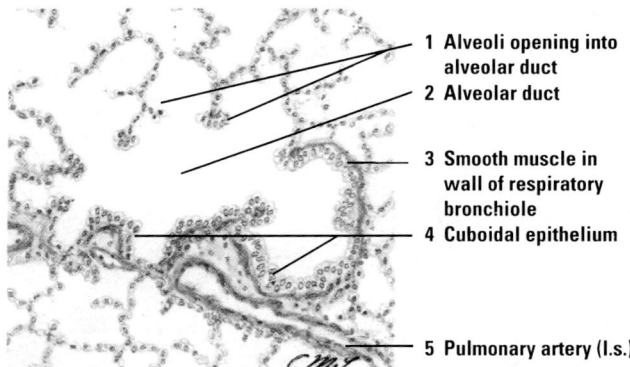

1 Alveoli opening into
   alveolar duct

2 Alveolar duct

3 Smooth muscle in
   wall of respiratory
   bronchiole

4 Cuboidal epithelium

5 Pulmonary artery (l.s.)

Fig. 14-11   Respiratory Bronchiole. Stain: hematoxylin-eosin. Low magnification.

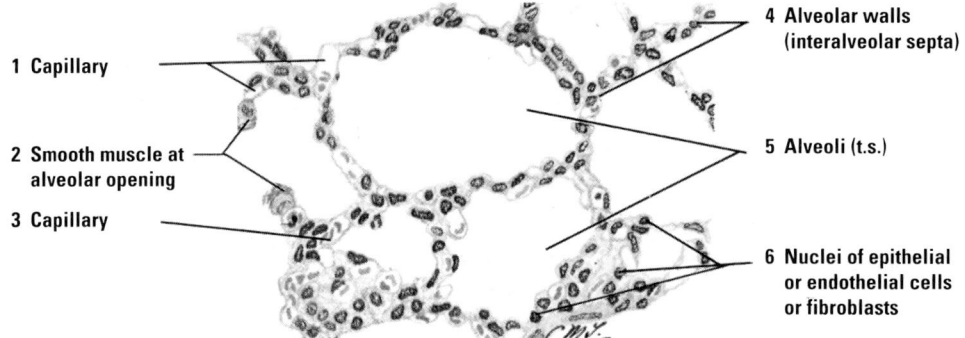

1 Capillary

2 Smooth muscle at
   alveolar opening

3 Capillary

4 Alveolar walls
   (interalveolar septa)

5 Alveoli (t.s.)

6 Nuclei of epithelial
   or endothelial cells
   or fibroblasts

Fig. 14-12   Alveolar Walls: Interalveolar Septa. Stain: hematoxylin-eosin. Oil immersion.

Figure 14-13   Olfactory Mucosa in the Nose: Transition Area

In the superior region of the nasal cavity, the **respiratory epithelium** changes abruptly into **olfactory epithelium.** This higher power photomicrograph shows a transition area between the two types of epithelia. The respiratory epithelium is lined by motile **cilia (1)** and contains numerous **goblet cells (2).** The olfactory epithelium lacks the cilia (1) and goblet cells (2). Instead, it exhibits nuclei of **supportive cells (5),** located near the epithelial surface, nuclei of odor receptive **olfactory cells (6),** located more in the middle of the epithelium, and the **basal cells (7),** located close to the **basement membrane (3).** Below the olfactory epithelium in the connective tissue **lamina propria (4)** are the **blood vessels (9), olfactory nerves (10),** and **olfactory (Bowman's) glands (8).**

Figure 14-14   Lung: Terminal Bronchiole, Respiratory Bronchiole, and Alveoli

In this photomicrograph, a section of the lung shows the smallest conducting passage, the **terminal bronchiole (1)** and an adjacent **blood vessel (7).** Both of these structures are surrounded on all sides by the lung **alveoli (2, 5, 8).** Each terminal bronchiole (1), in turn, divides and gives rise to thinner tubes, the **respiratory bronchioles (4, 9),** whose wall are characterized by numerous individual alveoli (2, 5, 8). Each respiratory bronchiole (4, 9) further divides into **alveolar ducts (3),** which continue into **alveolar sacs (6).**

Respiratory epithelium   Olfactory epithelium

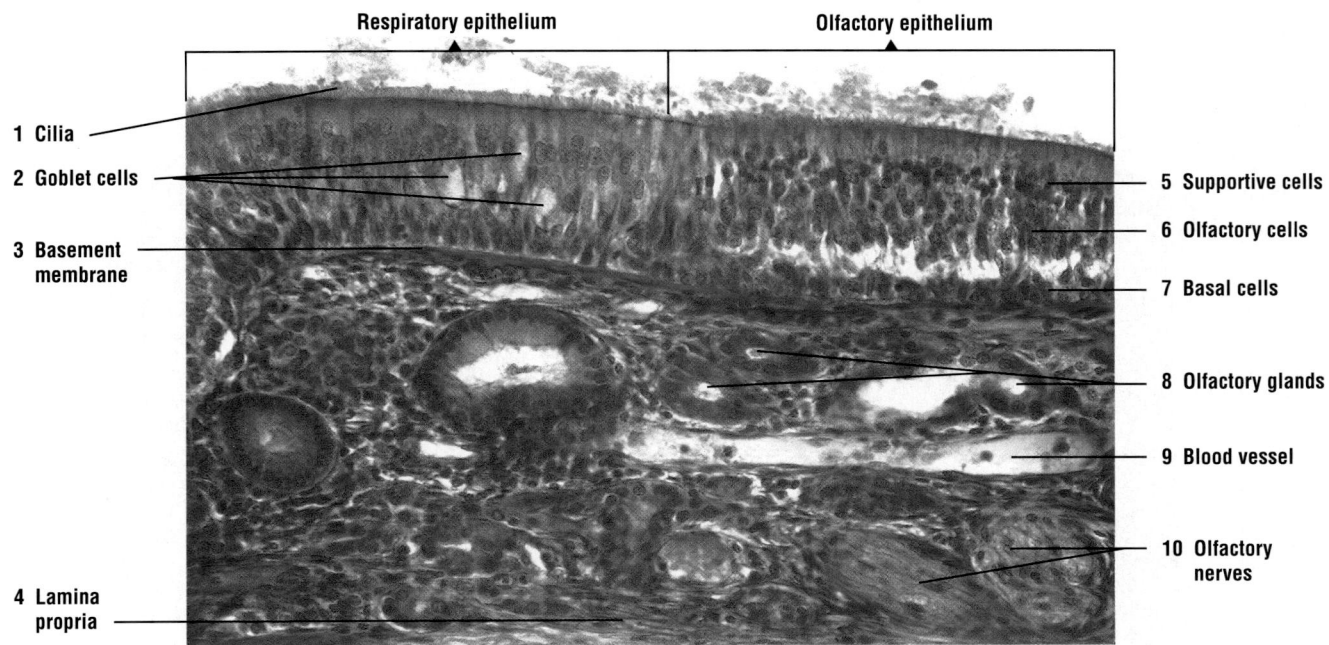

1 Cilia

2 Goblet cells

3 Basement
  membrane

4 Lamina
  propria

5 Supportive cells

6 Olfactory cells

7 Basal cells

8 Olfactory glands

9 Blood vessel

10 Olfactory
   nerves

Fig. 14-13   Olfactory Mucosa in the Nose: Transition Area. Stain: Mallory-azan. 80×

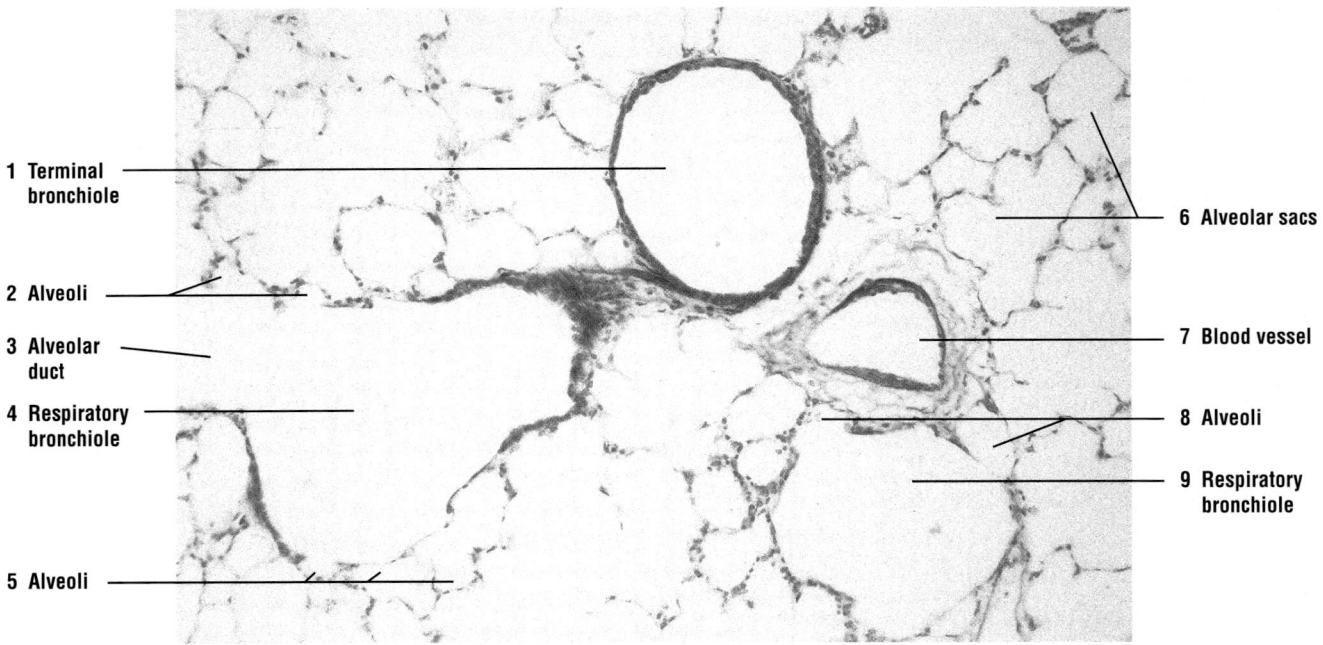

1 Terminal
  bronchiole

2 Alveoli

3 Alveolar
  duct

4 Respiratory
  bronchiole

5 Alveoli

6 Alveolar sacs

7 Blood vessel

8 Alveoli

9 Respiratory
  bronchiole

Fig. 14-14   Lung: Terminal Bronchiole, Respiratory Bronchiole, and Alveoli. Stain: Mallory-azan. 40×

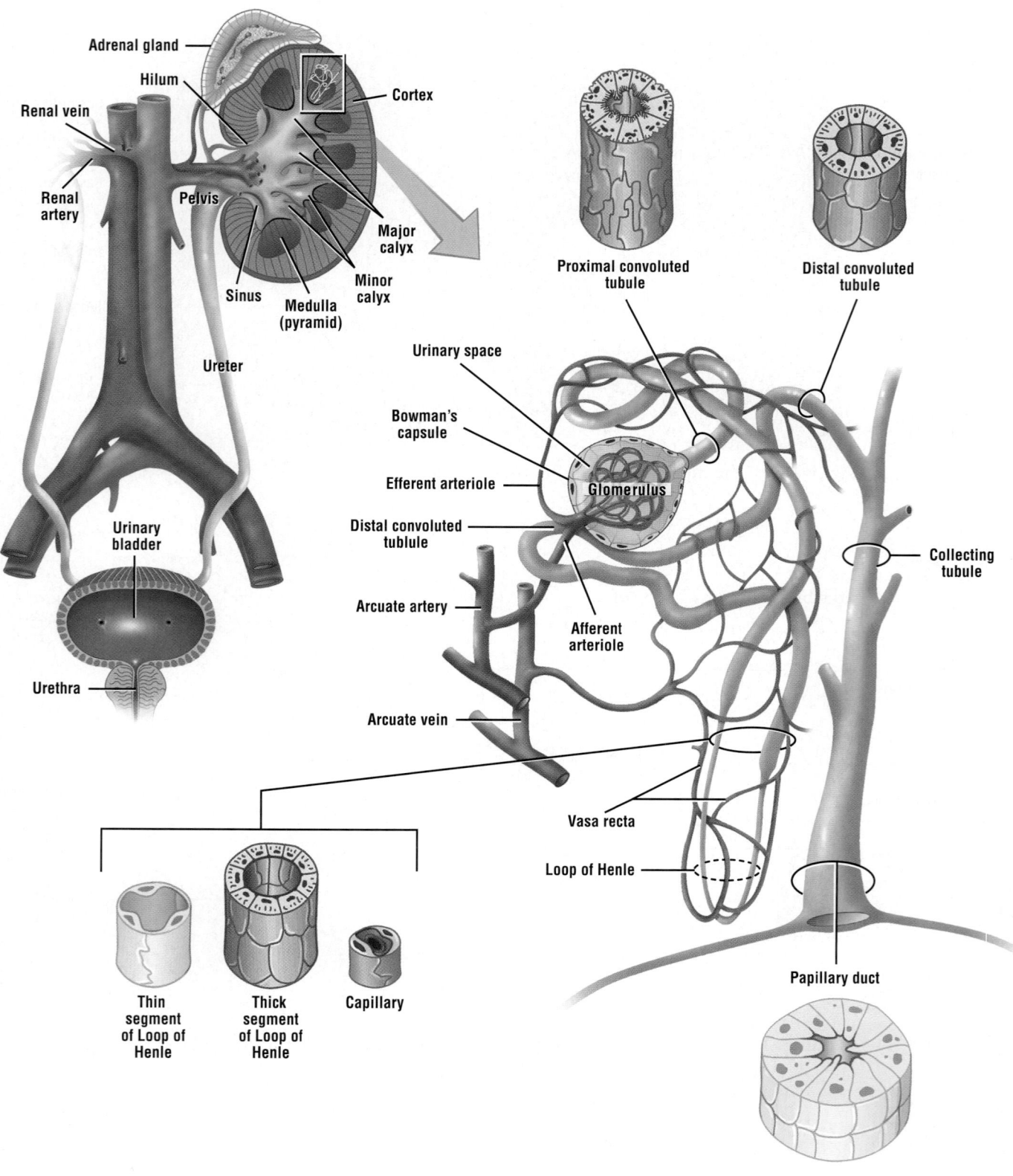

Adrenal gland

Hilum

Renal vein

Renal
artery

Pelvis

Cortex

Major
calyx

Sinus

Medulla
(pyramid)

Minor
calyx

Ureter

Urinary
bladder

Urethra

Proximal convoluted
tubule

Distal convoluted
tubule

Urinary space

Bowman's
capsule

Efferent arteriole

Glomerulus

Distal convoluted
tublule

Arcuate artery

Afferent
arteriole

Arcuate vein

Vasa recta

Loop of Henle

Collecting
tubule

Papillary duct

Thin
segment
of Loop of
Henle

Thick
segment
of Loop of
Henle

Capillary

Urinary System

THE KIDNEY

The urinary system consists of two kidneys and two ureters, which lead to a single urinary bladder, from which a single urethra opens to the exterior. Kidneys are large, bean-shaped organs located retroperitoneally on the posterior body wall. Superior to each kidney is the adrenal gland that is embedded in the renal connective tissue. The concave, medial border of the kidney is the **hilum,** in which are seen three large structures, the **renal artery, renal vein,** and the funnel-shaped **renal pelvis.** A sagittal section through the kidney reveals a darker, outer **cortex** and a lighter, inner **medulla,** which consists of conical-shaped **renal pyramids.** Downward extensions of the cortex between the pyramids forms the **renal columns.** The base of each pyramid is continuous with the cortex. The round apex of each pyramid, called the **renal papilla,** is surrounded by a funnel-shaped **minor calyx.** The minor calyces join to form a **major calyx,** which, in turn, join to form the funnel-shaped renal pelvis. Each renal pelvis leaves the kidney through the hilus, narrows to become a **ureter,** and descends toward the bladder on each side of the posterior body wall **(Fig. 15-1).**

THE URINIFEROUS TUBULES AND NEPHRONS OF THE KIDNEY

The functional unit of each kidney is the **uriniferous tubule,** which consists of a **nephron** and a **collecting duct** into which empty the filtered contents of the nephron. Located in each kidney cortex are millions of nephrons. The nephron, in turn, is subdivided into two components, the **renal corpuscle** and the **renal tubule.** The renal corpuscle consists of a tuft of capillaries called the **glomerulus** surrounded by a double layer of epithelial cells called the **glomerular [Bowman's] capsule.** The inner **visceral layer** of the capsule consists of highly modified, branching epithelial cells called **podocytes** that are adjacent to and completely invest the glomerular capillaries. The outer layer of the capsule is the **parietal layer** and it consists of simple squamous epithelial cells **(Figs. 15-2–15-3, 15-10).**

There are two types of nephrons in the kidney. The **cortical nephrons** are located in the cortex of the kidney. The **juxtamedullary nephrons** are situated near the junction of the cortex and medulla of the kidney. All nephrons participate in the process of urine formation. The juxtamedullary nephrons produce a hypertonic environment in the interstitium of the kidney medulla, a condition that is necessary for the production of concentrated (hypertonic) urine.

The **renal corpuscle** is the initial segment of each nephron. Here, blood is filtered through the capillaries of the glomerulus and the filtrate drains into the **capsu-lar (urinary) space** that is located between the parietal and visceral cell layers of the glomerular capsule. Each renal corpuscle has a **vascular pole,** where the arterial blood vessels of the glomerulus enter and exit. On the opposite end is the **urinary pole,** where the proximal convoluted tubule arises. Filtration of blood is facilitated by the glomerular endothelium. This endothelium is **porous** (fenestrated) and highly permeable to many substances in the blood but not to the formed elements or plasma proteins. Thus, the glomerular filtrate that enters the capsular space is similar to plasma, except for the absence of proteins **(Fig. 15-3, 15-10).**

THE KIDNEY TUBULES

The glomerular filtrate leaves the **renal corpuscle** and flows through the different parts of the nephron before reaching the collecting tubule. From the glomerular capsule, the filtrate first enters the **renal tubule,** which extends from the glomerular capsule to the collecting tubule. The renal tubule has several distinct histologic and functional regions. The renal tubule that starts at the renal corpuscle is the highly tortuous **proximal convoluted tubule.** This tubule is located in the cortex and then descends into the medulla to become continuous with the **loop of Henle.** The loop of Henle comprises a thick, descending portion of the proximal convoluted tubule, a thin descending and a thin ascending segment, and a thick, ascending portion of the **distal convoluted tubule.** The distal convoluted tubule is shorter and less convoluted than the proximal convoluted tubule. Glomerular filtrate flows from the distal convoluted tubule to the **collecting tubule.** The collecting tubule is not part of the nephron. A number of collecting tubules join to form the larger straight collecting ducts called the **papillary** ducts, which empty their contents into the minor calyx. In the juxtamedullary nephrons, the loop of Henle is long; it descends from the cortex of the kidney deep into the medulla and then loops back to ascend into the cortex **(Figs. 15-2, 15-4, 15-5, 15-11).**

THE JUXTAGLOMERULAR APPARATUS

Adjacent to the renal corpuscle and the distal convoluted tubule lie a special group of cells called the **juxtaglomerular apparatus.** This apparatus consists of **juxtaglomerular cells** and **macula densa.** The juxtaglomerular cells are a group of modified **smooth muscle cells** that are located in the wall of the **afferent arteriole** just before it enters the glomerular capsule to form the glomerulus. The macula densa is a group of modified cells of the distal convoluted tubule situated adjacent to the afferent arteriole with the juxtaglomerular cells. The juxtaglomerular cells and macula densa are functionally integrated for proper kidney function **(Fig. 15-3, 15-10).**

Figure 15-1   Kidney: Cortex and Pyramid (panoramic view)

The kidney is subdivided into an outer region, the **cortex (20)** and an inner region, the **medulla (21)**. Externally, the cortex is covered with a connective tissue **capsule (19)** and the perirenal connective and **adipose tissues (18)**.

In the cortex **convoluted tubules (3), glomeruli (2, 8), straight tubules (4),** and **medullary rays (5)** are found.

The cortex also contains renal corpuscles (glomerular [Bowman's] capsules and glomeruli), adjacent proximal and distal **convoluted tubules (3)** of the nephrons, **interlobular arteries (6)** and **interlobular veins (7)**. The **medullary rays (5)** contain straight portions of nephrons and collecting tubules. Medullary rays do not extend to the kidney capsule because of a narrow zone of **convoluted tubules (1)**.

The medulla comprises a number of renal pyramids. Each pyramid is situated with its **base (11)** adjacent to the cortex (20) and its apex directed inward. The apices of renal pyramids form the **papilla (16),** which projects into a **minor calyx (14)**. The medulla also contains the loops of Henle (straight or descending proximal tubules, thin segments, and straight or ascending distal tubules) and collecting tubules. The collecting tubules join in the medulla to form large papillary ducts (Figs. 15-4 and 15-5).

The papilla (16) usually is covered with a simple **columnar epithelium (12)**. As this epithelium reflects on to the outer wall of the calyx, it becomes **transitional epithelium (13)**. A thin layer of connective tissue and smooth muscle (not illustrated) is found under this epithelium, which then merges with the connective tissue of the **renal sinus (17)**.

In the renal sinus (17), between the pyramids, are branches of the renal artery and vein, the **interlobar vessels (15)**. These vessels enter the kidney and then arch over the base of the pyramid at the corticomedullary junction as the **arcuate vessels (9)**. The arcuate vessels give rise to smaller, **interlobular arteries and veins (6, 7, 10)**. The arcuate arteries (9) pass radially into the kidney cortex (20) and extend numerous afferent glomerular arteries to the glomeruli.

■ Functional Correlations–Kidney

The kidneys are vital organs for maintaining **homeostasis** of the body. They regulate blood pressure, blood composition, and fluid volume of the body; produce urine; and maintain acid–base balance. In addition, the cells of the kidney produce two important hormones, renin and erythropoietin. **Renin** regulates blood pressure to maintain proper filtration pressure for the kidneys. **Erythropoietin,** believed to be released by the endothelium of the peritubular capillary network, promotes red blood cell formation in the red bone marrow. Urine formation in the kidney involves **filtration, reabsorption,** and **secretion.** Approximately 99% of the glomerular filtrate produced by the kidneys is reabsorbed into the system in the nephron and only approximately 1% is voided as urine.

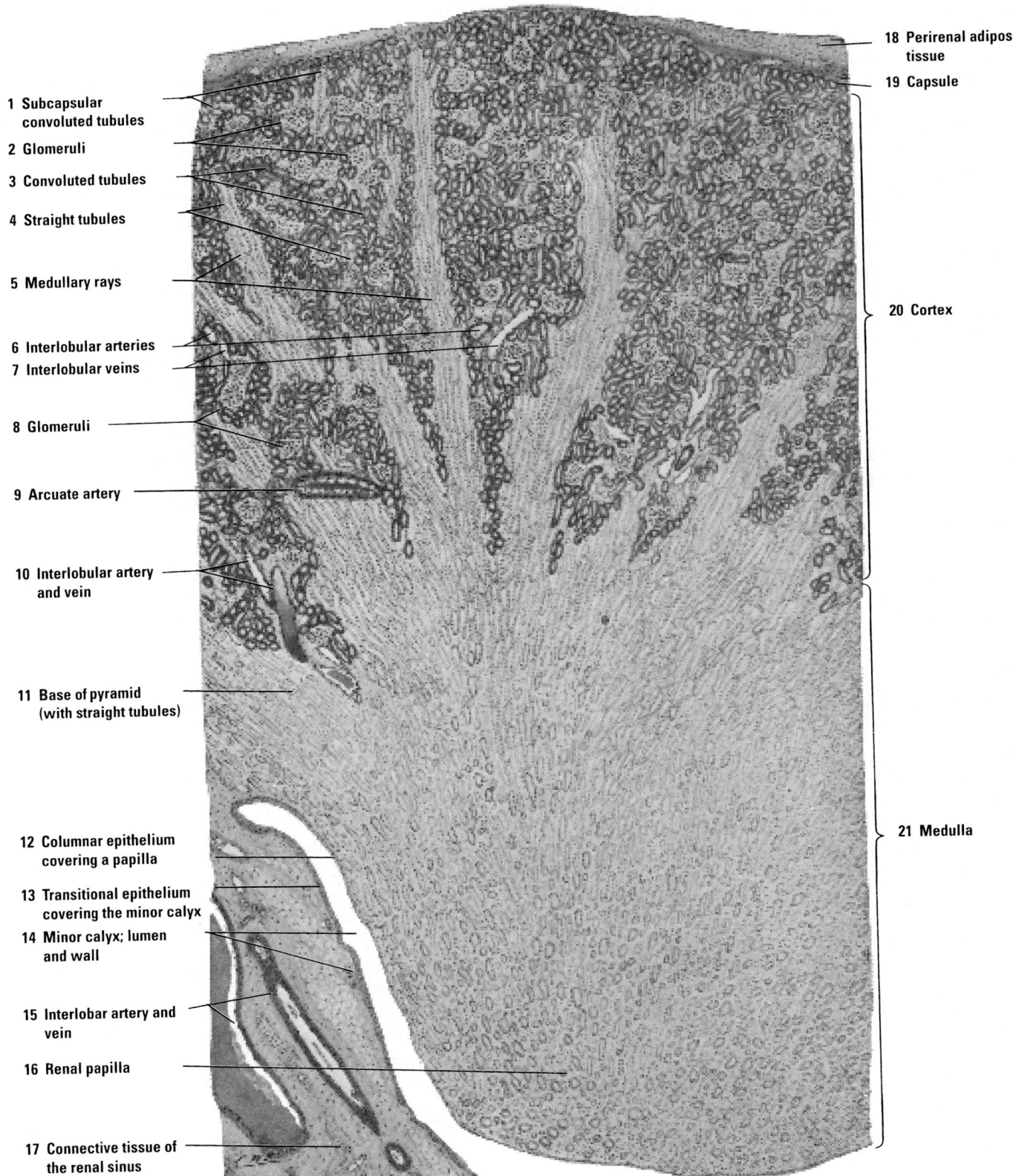

18 Perirenal adipose tissue

19 Capsule

1 Subcapsular convoluted tubules

2 Glomeruli

3 Convoluted tubules

4 Straight tubules

5 Medullary rays

6 Interlobular arteries

7 Interlobular veins

8 Glomeruli

9 Arcuate artery

10 Interlobular artery and vein

11 Base of pyramid (with straight tubules)

12 Columnar epithelium covering a papilla

13 Transitional epithelium covering the minor calyx

14 Minor calyx; lumen and wall

15 Interlobar artery and vein

16 Renal papilla

17 Connective tissue of the renal sinus

20 Cortex

21 Medulla

Fig. 15-1   Kidney: Cortex and Pyramid (panoramic view). Stain: hematoxylin-eosin. Low magnification.

Figure 15-2   Kidney: Deep Cortical Area and Outer Medulla

A higher magnification of the kidney cortex reveals greater details of the renal corpuscle. Each corpuscle consists of a **glomerulus (3)** and a **glomerular (Bowman's) capsule (2, 17).** The glomerulus (3) is a tuft of capillaries formed from the afferent glomerular arterioles and supported by fine connective tissue.

The **visceral layer (17)** of the glomerular capsule consists of modified epithelial cells called the podocytes. These cells closely follow the contours of the glomerulus and invest the capillary tufts. At the vascular pole, the visceral epithelium reflects to become the **parietal layer (17)** of the glomerular capsule. The space between the visceral and parietal layers of the capsule is the capsular space, which becomes continuous with the lumen of the proximal convoluted tubule at the urinary pole (see Fig. 15-3). At the urinary pole, the squamous epithelium of the parietal layer changes to cuboidal epithelium of the **proximal convoluted tubule (9).**

Numerous tubules, sectioned in various planes, lie adjacent to the renal corpuscles. The tubules are primarily of two types, the **proximal convoluted (4, 10, 15, 21)** and **distal convoluted (1, 14, 21);** these tubules are the initial and terminal segments of the nephron, respectively. The proximal convoluted tubules are numerous in the cortex, exhibit a small, uneven lumen, and contain a single layer of large cuboidal cells with intensely eosinophilic, granular cytoplasm. The well-developed **brush borders (15)** are present but are not always well preserved in sections.

Distal convoluted tubules (14) are fewer in number and exhibit a larger lumen with smaller, cuboidal cells. The cytoplasm stains less intensely and the brush borders are not present (14, compare with 15).

Renal corpuscles and their associated tubules constitute the kidney cortex. The cortex surrounds the medullary rays, which are composed of straight portions of the nephrons and collecting tubules. The medullary rays include three types of tubules: straight (descending) segments of the **proximal tubules (6),** straight (ascending) segments of the **distal tubules (11, 20),** and **collecting tubules (5, 19).** The straight segments of the proximal tubules are similar to the proximal convoluted tubules and the straight segments of the distal tubules are similar to distal convoluted tubules. Collecting tubules are distinct because of lightly stained cuboidal cells and visible cell membranes.

The medulla contains only straight portions of tubules and thin segments of loops of Henle. Illustrated in the outer medullary region are thin segments of **loops of Henle (13, 23)** lined with squamous epithelium, straight segments of distal tubules (20), and collecting tubules (12, 22).

■ Functional Correlations–Kidney Tubules

As the filtrate enters the **proximal convoluted tubule,** all of **glucose** and **amino acids,** and approximatley 75 to 80% of water and sodium chloride ions, are absorbed from the glomerular filtrate into the interstitium and the capillaries. This reabsorption takes place by means of the microvilli in the brush border that cover the cells of the proximal convoluted tubules. In addition, the proximal convoluted tubule secretes certain metabolites, dyes, and drugs such as penicillin from the body into the glomerular filtrate. Such metabolic waste products as urea and uric acid remain in the proximal convoluted tubule and are eliminated from the body in the urine.

The **loop of Henle** is necessary for the production of **hypertonic urine.** Sodium chloride and urea are concentrated in the interstitial tissue of the kidney medulla by means of a complex countercurrent multiplier system. The hypertonicity (high osmotic pressure) of the extracellular fluid in the medulla produced by this process removes the water from the glomerular filtrate as it flows through these tubules. The long loops of Henle in the juxtaglomerular nephrons assist in maintaining this osmotic gradient.

The **distal convoluted tubule** is shorter and less convoluted than the proximal tubule. The cells of the distal convoluted tubule actively resorb sodium ions from the glomerular filtrate into the intestitium. This resorptive activity is coupled with excretion of hydrogen or potassium ions into the filtrate or tubular urine. Sodium reabsorption in the distal convoluted tubule is controlled by the hormone **aldosterone** secreted by the adrenal cortex. In response to this hormone, the cells of the distal convoluted tubule actively absorb sodium from the filtrate. The functions of the distal convoluted tubules are vital for maintaining a proper acid–base balance of the body fluids.

1 Distal convoluted
  tubules

2 Glomerular (Bowman's)
  capsule

3 Glomerulus

4 Proximal convoluted
  tubules

5 Collecting tubules

6 Straight (descending)
  segment of a
  proximal tubule

7 Interlobular vein

8 Glomerular arteriole
  (t.s.)

9 Junction of glomerular
  capsule with
  proximal tubule

10 Proximal convoluted
   tubules

11 Straight (ascending)
   segments of distal
   tubules

12 Collecting tubules

13 Thin segments of
   loops of Henle

14 Distal convoluted tubules

15 Proximal convoluted
   tubules with brush
   borders

16 Glomerular arteriole (l.s.)

17 Visceral and parietal
   layers of glomerular
   capsule

18 Interlobular artery
   sectioned obliquely:
   wall and lumen

19 Collecting tubules

20 Straight (ascending)
   segments of distal tubules

21 Proximal and distal
   convoluted tubules

22 Collecting tubules

23 Thin segments of
   loops of Henle

24 Capillaries

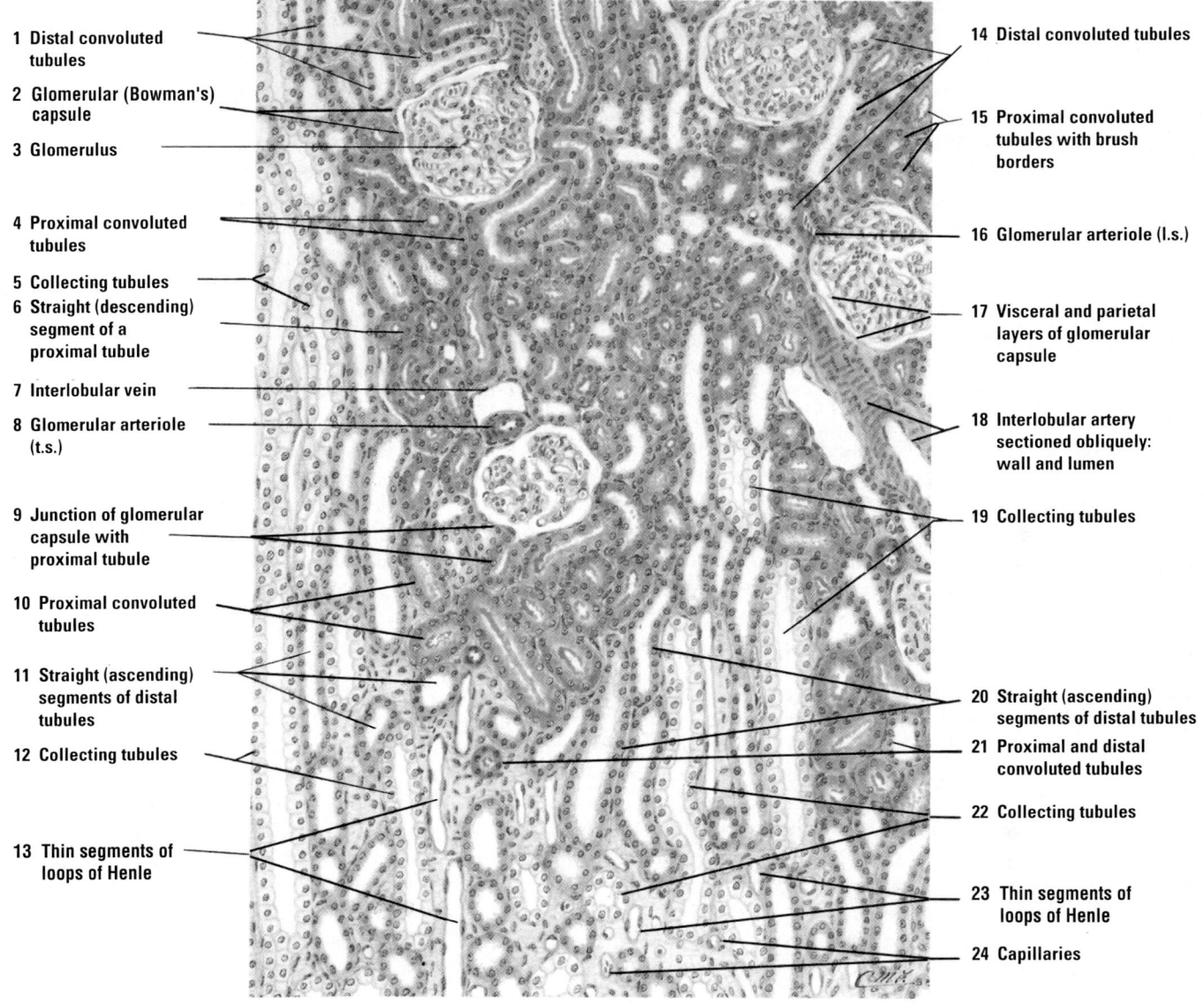

Fig. 15-2   Kidney: Deep Cortical Area and Outer Medulla. Stain: hematoxylin-eosin. Low magnification.

Figure 15-3   Kidney Cortex: Juxtaglomerular Apparatus

A still higher magnification of a small area of the kidney cortex illustrates the renal corpuscle, adjacent tubules, and juxtaglomerular apparatus.

The renal corpuscle exhibits the **glomerular capillaries (2), parietal (10a)** and **visceral (10b)** epithelium of **glomerular (Bowman's) capsule (10),** and the **capsular space (13).** Conspicuous brush borders and acidophilic cells distinguish the **proximal convoluted tubules (6, 14)** from the **distal convoluted tubules (1, 15),** whose smaller, less intensely stained cells lack brush borders. The cells of the **collecting tubules (8)** are cuboidal with distinct cell outlines and clear, pale cytoplasm. Distinct **basement membranes (9)** surround these tubules.

Each renal corpuscle exhibits a vascular pole on one side where the **afferent glomerular arterioles (12)** enter and efferent glomerular arterioles exit. On the opposite side of the corpuscle is the **urinary pole (11),** where the capsular space (13) becomes continuous with the lumen of the proximal convoluted tubule (6, 14). The plane of section through the renal corpuscle illustrated in this figure is seen only occasionally in the kidney cortex; however, illustration of both vascular and urinary poles represents an important structural association of the renal corpuscle with the region of blood filtration, glomerular filtrate accumulation, and initial stages of filtrate modification in urine formation.

At the vascular pole, smooth muscle cells in the tunica media of the afferent glomerular arteriole (12) are replaced by highly modified epithelioid cells with cytoplasmic granules. These are the **juxtaglomerular cells (4).** In the adjacent segment of the distal convoluted tubules, the cells that border the juxtaglomerular area are narrow and more columnar than elsewhere in the tubules. This area of darker, more compact cell arrangement is called the **macula densa (5).** The juxtaglomerular cells in the afferent glomerular arteriole (12) and the macula densa (5) cells in the distal convoluted tubule together constitute the juxtaglomerular apparatus.

■ Functional Correlations–Juxtaglomerular Apparatus

The **juxtaglomerular apparatus** performs an important role in maintaining normal blood pressure. The juxtaglomerular cells monitor changes in the **systemic blood pressure** by responding to stretching in the wall of the afferent arteriole. The cells in the macula densa probably respond to changes in the sodium chloride concentration and volume of the glomerular filtrate as it flows past them in the distal convoluted tubule.

A decrease in systemic blood pressure induces the juxtaglomerular cells to release the hormone **renin** into the blood stream. Renin converts the plasma protein **angiotensinogen** to **angiotensin I,** which in turn is converted to **angiotensin II** by enzyme present in the **endothelial cells** of the **lung.** Angiotensin II is an active hormone and a powerful **vasoconstrictor** that initially produces arterial constriction, thereby increasing the systemic blood pressure. In addition, angiotensin II stimulates release of the hormone **aldosterone** from the adrenal cortex. Aldosterone acts primarily on the cells of the distal convoluted tubules in the kidney to increase their reabsorption of sodium and chloride ions from the glomerular filtrate. As water follows sodium chloride osmotically, fluid volume in the circulatory system increases. This raises the systemic blood pressure and increases the glomerular filtration rate in the kidney.

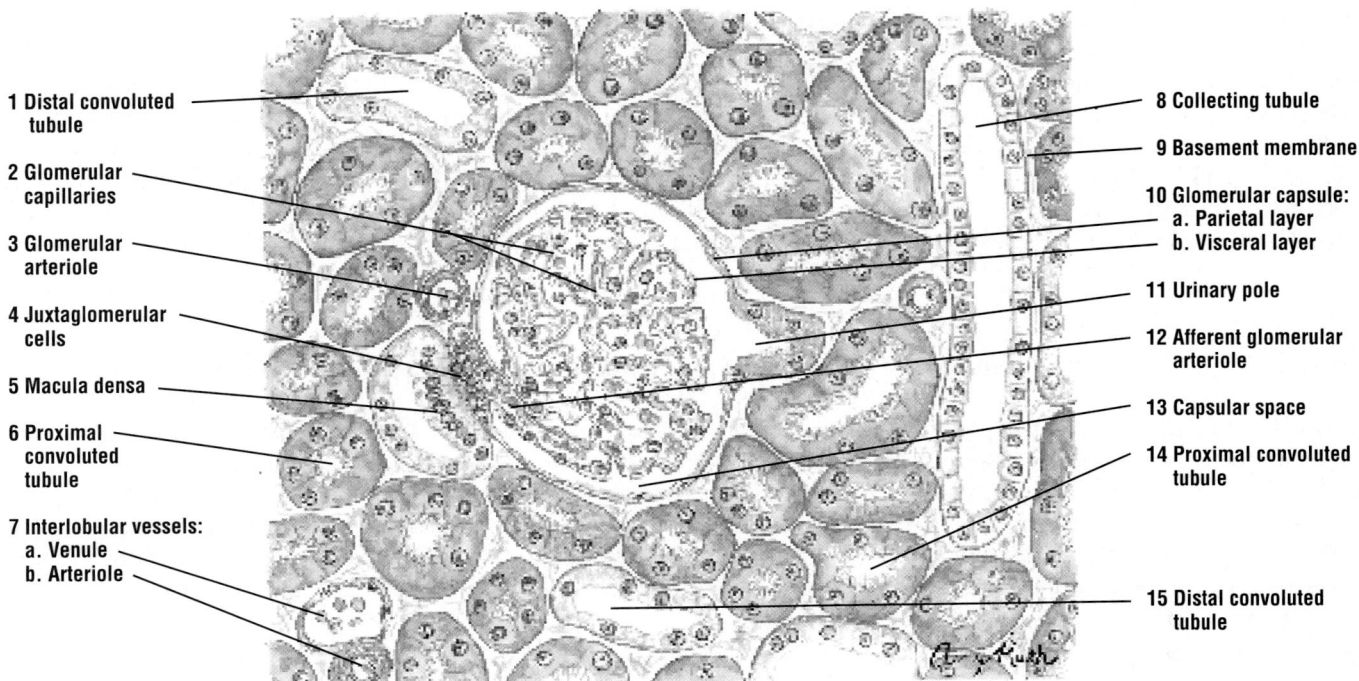

1 Distal convoluted
  tubule

2 Glomerular
  capillaries

3 Glomerular
  arteriole

4 Juxtaglomerular
  cells

5 Macula densa

6 Proximal
  convoluted
  tubule

7 Interlobular vessels:
  a. Venule
  b. Arteriole

8 Collecting tubule

9 Basement membrane

10 Glomerular capsule:
   a. Parietal layer
   b. Visceral layer

11 Urinary pole

12 Afferent glomerular
   arteriole

13 Capsular space

14 Proximal convoluted
   tubule

15 Distal convoluted
   tubule

Fig. 15-3 Kidney Cortex: Juxtaglomerular Apparatus. Stain: periodic acid-Schiff and hematoxylin. Medium magnification.

Figure 15-4   Kidney Medulla: Papilla (transverse section)

The papilla of the kidney contains the terminal portions of the collecting tubules, the **papillary ducts (2, 5, 6)**. These ducts have large diameters and wide lumina and are lined by tall, pale-staining columnar cells. Also seen in this region are cross sections of the thin segments of the **loops of Henle (3, 8)** and the ascending straight portions of the **distal tubules (7)**. **Connective tissue (10)** is more abundant in this region than elsewhere in the kidney, and the collecting tubules are not as close together. Numerous small **blood vessels (4, 9)** are also present. The thin segments of loops of Henle (3, 8) in cross section resemble capillaries or venules (4, 9).

Figure 15-5   Kidney Medulla: Papilla Adjacent to a Calyx (longitudinal section)

Several collecting tubules merge in the medulla to form large, straight tubules called **papillary ducts (5)**, which open at the tip of the papilla. Their numerous openings on the surface of the papilla produce a sievelike appearance; this is the area cribrosa. In this illustration, the papilla is covered by a **stratified cuboidal epithelium (8)**. At the area cribrosa, however, the covering epithelium usually is a simple columnar epithelium continuous with the lining of the papillary ducts. Also illustrated are thin segments of **loops of Henle (3, 4, 6)** and ascending straight portion of the **distal tubule (1)**. Abundant **connective tissue (7)** and many **capillaries (2)** are also seen.

■ **Functional Correlations**–Collecting Tubules and Antidiuretic Hormone

Glomerular filtrate flows from the distal convoluted tubule to the **collecting tubule;** this tubule normally is not permeable to water. During certain conditions, however, an **antidiuretic hormone (ADH)** is released from the posterior lobe (neurohypophysis) of the pituitary gland in response to decreased water intake in the body. As a result of ADH presence in the system, the epithelium of the collecting tubule becomes highly permeable to water. Consequently, as the glomerular filtrate in the collecting tubule flows through the medulla, water is drawn from the filtrate because of increased tubular permeability and high osmotic pressure created by the hypertonic extracellular fluid. The retained water in the extracellular region is then returned to the general circulation via the blood vessels (capillaries), and the glomerular filtrate in the collecting tubules becomes hypertonic (concentrated) urine. In the absence of circulating ADH, water does not leave the collecting tubule because the epithelium remains impermeable to water. As a result, the expelled filtrate is a dilute urine, containing more water.

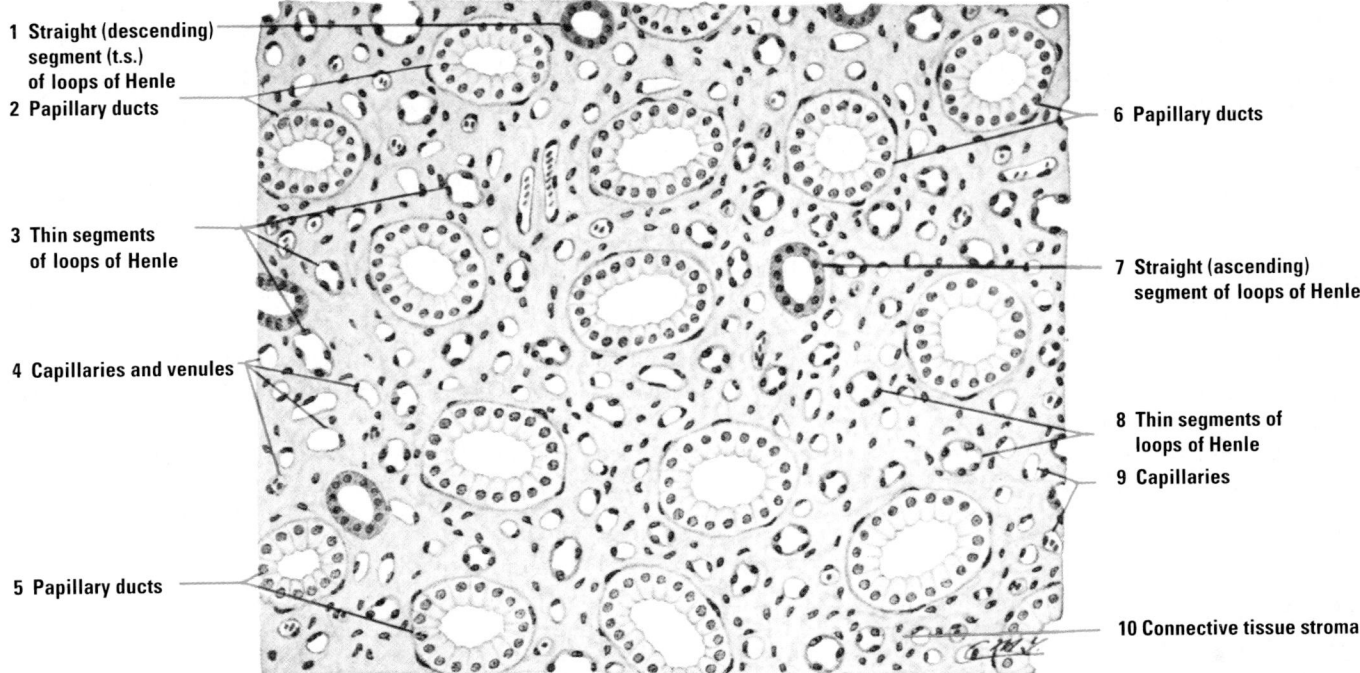

1 Straight (descending)
  segment (t.s.)
  of loops of Henle
2 Papillary ducts

3 Thin segments
  of loops of Henle

4 Capillaries and venules

5 Papillary ducts

6 Papillary ducts

7 Straight (ascending)
  segment of loops of Henle

8 Thin segments of
  loops of Henle
9 Capillaries

10 Connective tissue stroma

Fig. 15-4   Kidney Medulla: Papilla (transverse section). Stain: hematoxylin-eosin. Medium magnification.

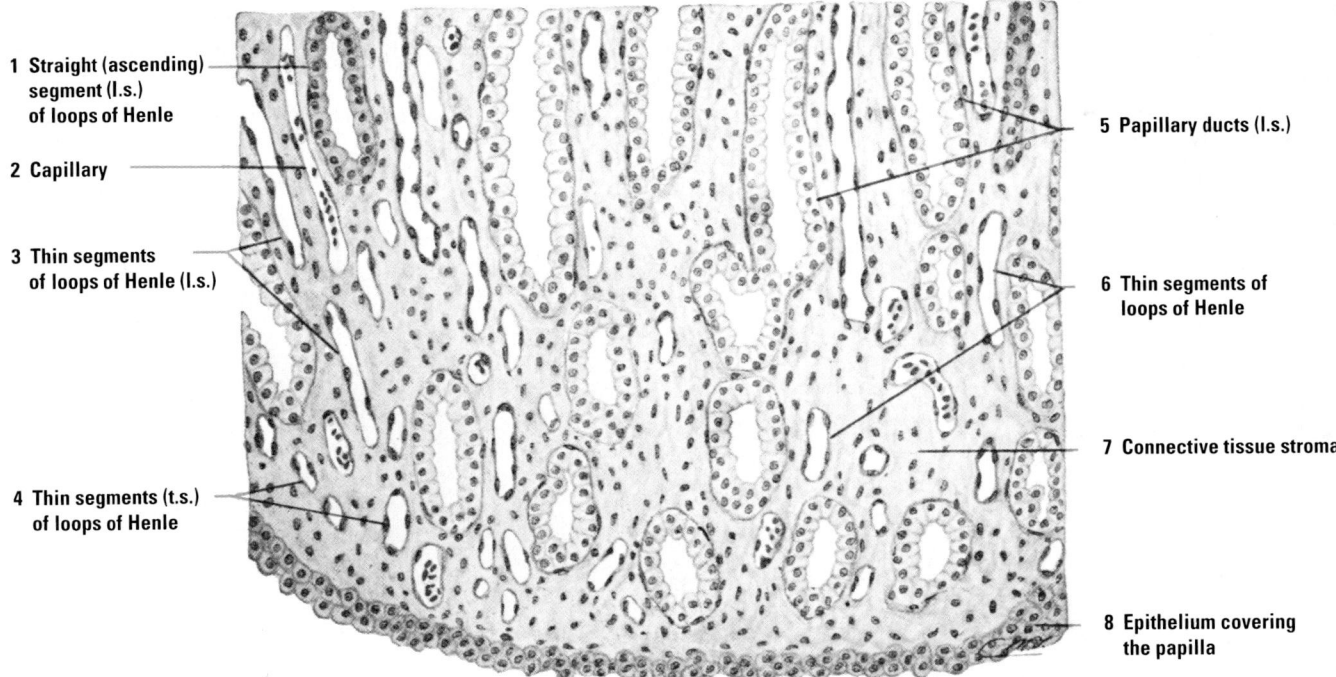

1 Straight (ascending)
  segment (l.s.)
  of loops of Henle

2 Capillary

3 Thin segments
  of loops of Henle (l.s.)

4 Thin segments (t.s.)
  of loops of Henle

5 Papillary ducts (l.s.)

6 Thin segments of
  loops of Henle

7 Connective tissue stroma

8 Epithelium covering
  the papilla

Fig. 15-5   Kidney Medulla: Papilla Adjacent to a Calyx (longitudinal section). Stain: hematoxylin-eosin. Medium magnification.

Figure 15-6   Ureter (transverse section)

An undistended ureter exhibits a convoluted lumen, formed by the longitudinal mucosal folds. The wall of the ureter consists of mucosa, muscularis, and adventitia.

The mucosa consists of **transitional epithelium (9, 10)** and a wide **lamina propria (5).** The transitional epithelium has several cell layers, the outermost layer characterized by large cuboidal cells (9). The intermediate cells are polyhedral in shape, whereas the basal cells are low columnar or cuboidal (10). The basal surface of the epithelium is smooth and there are no indentations by the connective tissue papillae.

The lamina propria (5) contains fibroelastic connective tissue, which is denser with more fibroblasts under the epithelium and looser near the muscularis. Diffuse lymphatic tissue and occasional small lymphatic nodules may be observed in the lamina propria.

In the upper ureter, the muscularis consists of an inner **longitudinal (3)** smooth muscle layer and an outer **circular (2)** smooth muscle layer; these layers are not always distinct. An additional outer longitudinal layer of smooth muscle is found in the lower third of the ureter.

The **adventitia (6)** blends with the surrounding fibroelastic **connective tissue** and **adipose tissue (1, 12),** which contain numerous **arteries (8), venules (11),** and small **nerves (7).**

Figure 15-7   Ureter Wall (transverse section)

A higher magnification of the ureter wall illustrates greater structural details and layers. The transitional epithelium (8, 9, 10) exhibits the same cell layers as described in Figure 15-6. The outermost cells often stain deeper than the remaining cells. The surface membrane, illustrated as a narrow acidophilic band (9), serves as an osmotic barrier between urine and tissue fluids.

In the **lamina propria (12),** fibroblasts are more numerous in the connective tissue under the epithelium than in the deeper region.

The **muscularis layer (7, 11)** often appears as loosely arranged smooth muscle bundles surrounded by abundant connective tissue, as illustrated in the inner **longitudinal layer (11).**

The **adventitia (5)** merges with the **connective tissue (6)** of the posterior abdominal wall in which the ureter is embedded.

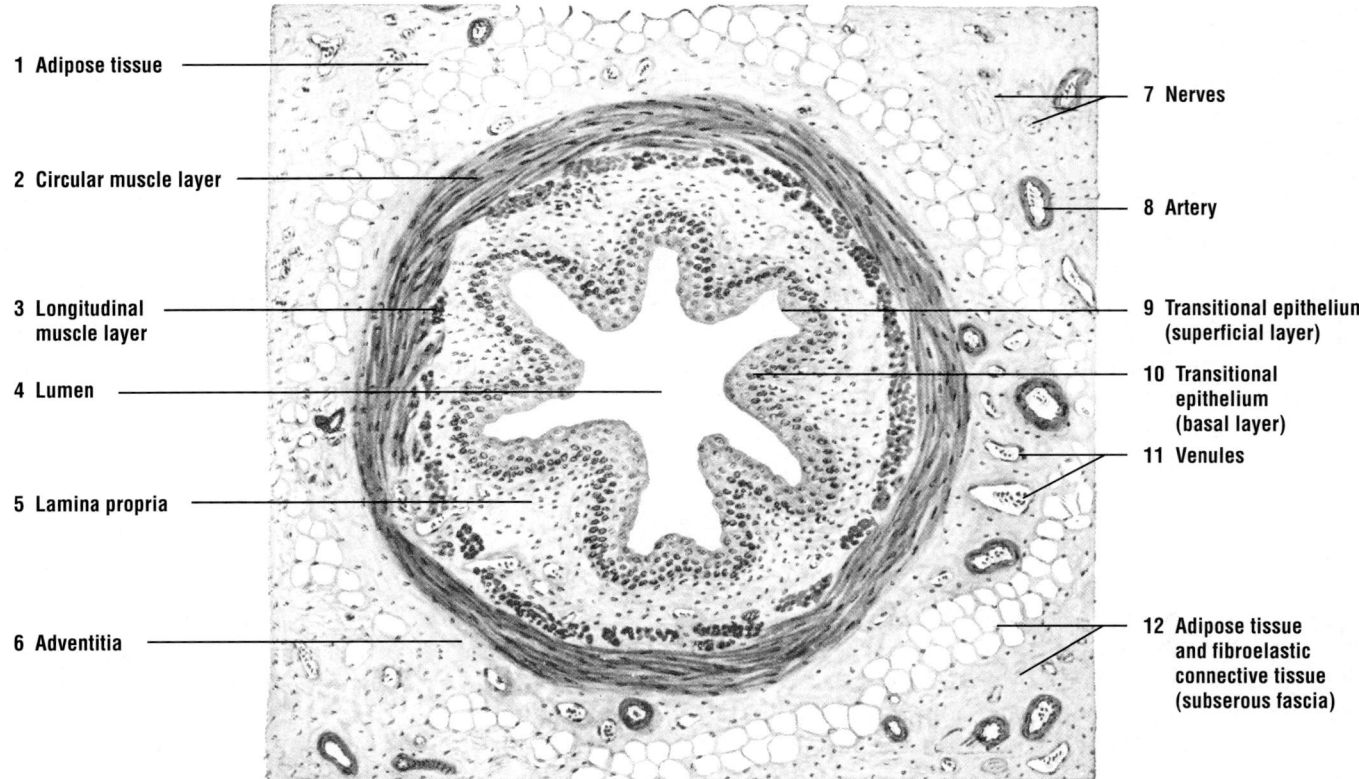

1 Adipose tissue

2 Circular muscle layer

3 Longitudinal
  muscle layer

4 Lumen

5 Lamina propria

6 Adventitia

7 Nerves

8 Artery

9 Transitional epithelium
  (superficial layer)

10 Transitional
   epithelium
   (basal layer)

11 Venules

12 Adipose tissue
   and fibroelastic
   connective tissue
   (subserous fascia)

Fig. 15-6   Ureter (transverse section). Stain: hematoxylin-eosin. Low magnification.

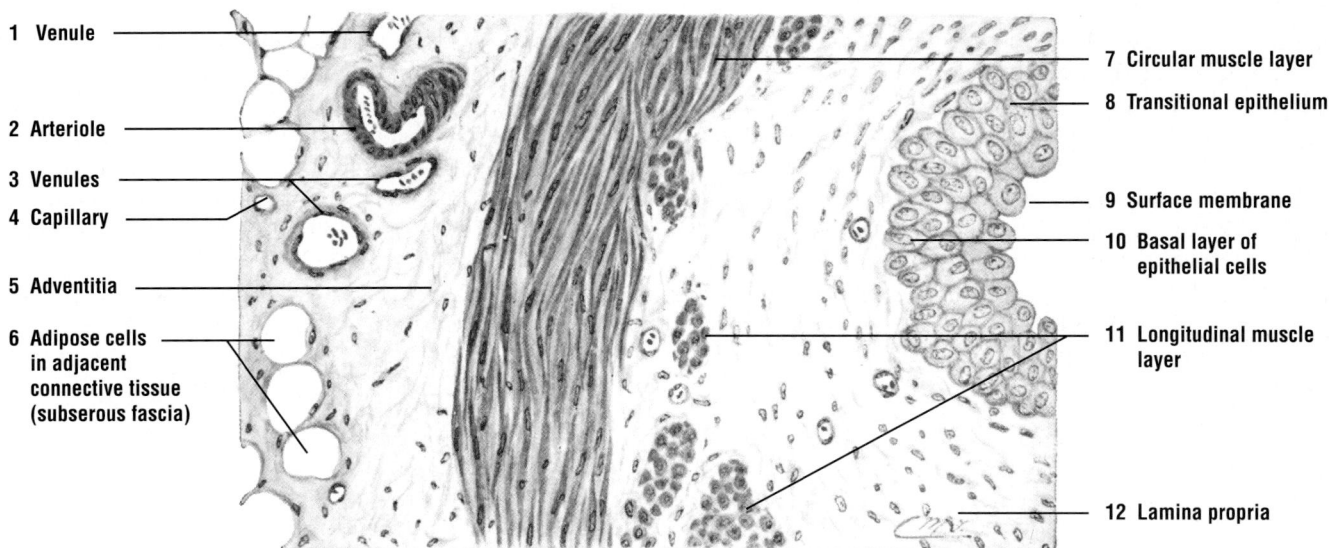

1 Venule

2 Arteriole

3 Venules

4 Capillary

5 Adventitia

6 Adipose cells
  in adjacent
  connective tissue
  (subserous fascia)

7 Circular muscle layer

8 Transitional epithelium

9 Surface membrane

10 Basal layer of
   epithelial cells

11 Longitudinal muscle
   layer

12 Lamina propria

Fig. 15-7   Ureter Wall (transverse section). Stain: hematoxylin-eosin. Medium magnification.

Figure 15-8   Urinary Bladder: Wall (transverse section)

The **smooth muscle (1)** layers in the bladder wall are similar to those in the ureter except for their thickness. The bladder wall consists of a **mucosa (6, 7, 8)**, a **muscularis (1, 9)**, and a **serosa (4, 5)** on the superior surface of the bladder. The inferior surface of the bladder is covered by adventitia, which merges with the connective tissue of adjacent structures.

The mucosa in an empty bladder exhibits numerous **folds (6)**; however, these folds disappear during bladder distension. The **transitional epithelium (7)** contains more cell layers and the **lamina propria (8)** is wider than in the ureter. The loose connective tissue in the deeper zone contains more elastic fibers.

The muscularis (1, 9) is thick, and the three layers in the neck of the bladder are arranged in anastomosing bundles (1) between which is found **loose connective tissue (2)**. In this section, muscle bundles are visible in various planes of section (1) and the three distinct muscle layers are difficult to distinguish. The interstitial connective tissue merges with the connective tissue of the serosa (4); **mesothelium (5)** is the outermost layer.

Figure 15-9   Urinary Bladder: Mucosa (transverse section)

The mucosa of the bladder is illustrated at a higher magnification.

In an empty bladder, the superficial cells of the **transitional epithelium (5)** are low **cuboidal** or **columnar (6)**. When the bladder is full and the transitional epithelium is stretched, cells exhibit a **squamous (9)** appearance. The acidophilic surface **membrane (7)** of the superficial cells may be prominent. The deeper layers of cells in the epithelium are round (5) and basal cells are more columnar (see also Figure 1-9).

In the **lamina propria (2)** are two zones, as in the ureter, but more pronounced. The subepithelial region is denser with fine fibers and numerous fibroblasts (2, upper leader). The deeper zone (2, lower leader) typically contains loose or moderately dense irregular connective tissue, which extends between the muscle fibers as interstitial connective tissue.

■ Functional Correlations–Urinary Bladder

The urinary bladder is a hollow organ whose main function is the storage of urine. The lumen of the bladder is lined by a **transitional epithelium,** which allows the organ to stretch or enlarge (change shape) as it fills with urine. The superficial cells may be round and large with scalloped appearance when the bladder is empty. These cells appear flat when the bladder wall is stretched to accomodate urine. The change in these cell shapes is due to the presence of unique thickened regions in the plasma membrane of the transitional epithelium called **plaques.** These plaques are connected to thinner, shorter, and more flexible **interplaque regions.** In an empty bladder, the interplaque regions allow the cell membrane to fold. When the bladder is filled and the cells are streched, these folds disappear.

The exposed cell membrane of the superficial cells in the transitional epithelium is somewhat thicker. In addition, the cells are attached to each other by desmosomes and occluding junctions. These properties of the transitional epithelium provide an effective **osmotic barrier** between the urine in the bladder and the underlying connective tissue.

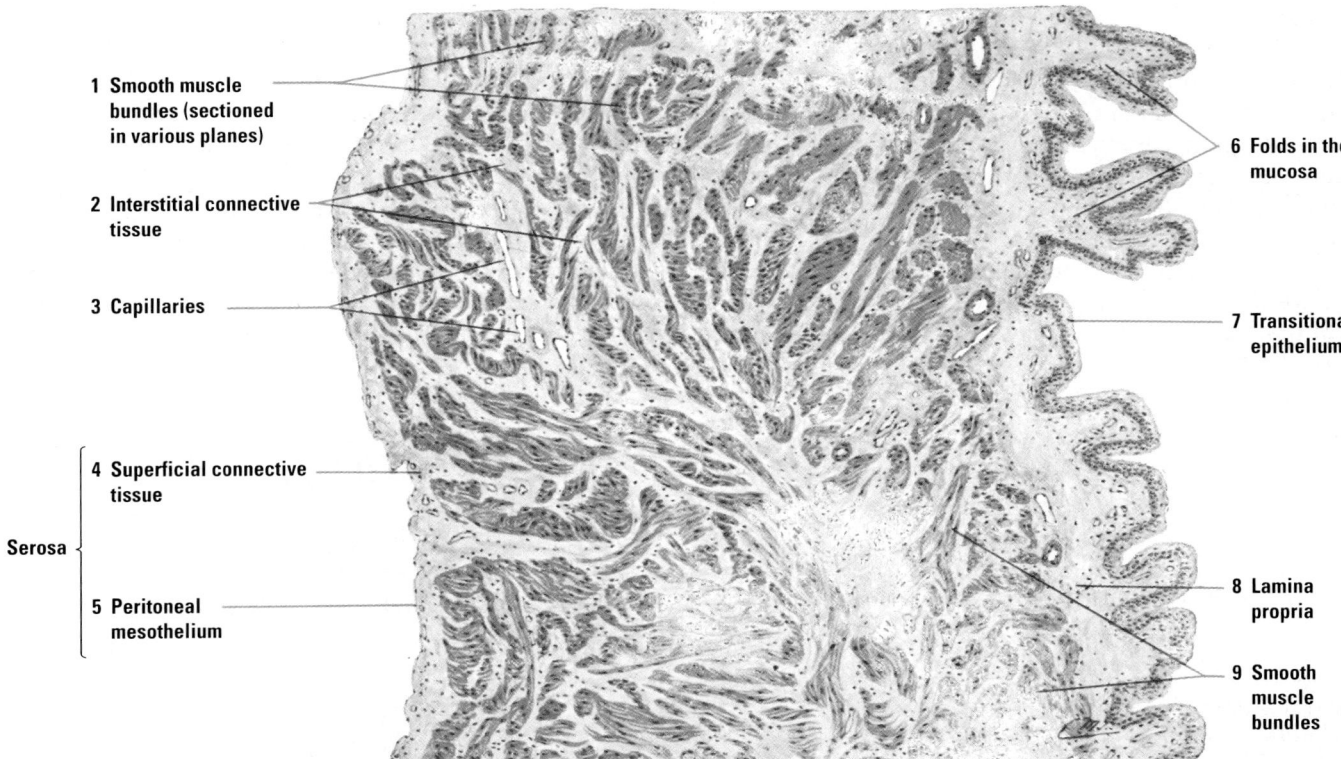

1 Smooth muscle bundles (sectioned in various planes)

2 Interstitial connective tissue

3 Capillaries

4 Superficial connective tissue

5 Peritoneal mesothelium

Serosa

6 Folds in the mucosa

7 Transitional epithelium

8 Lamina propria

9 Smooth muscle bundles

Fig. 15-8   Urinary Bladder: Wall (transverse section). Stain: hematoxylin-eosin. Low magnification.

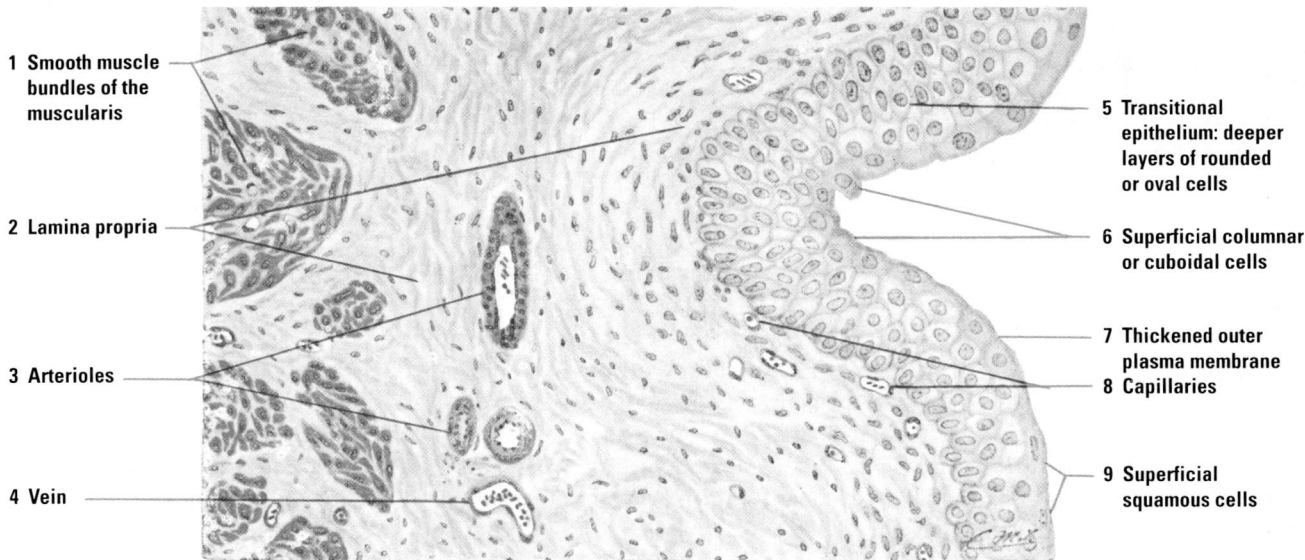

1 Smooth muscle bundles of the muscularis

2 Lamina propria

3 Arterioles

4 Vein

5 Transitional epithelium: deeper layers of rounded or oval cells

6 Superficial columnar or cuboidal cells

7 Thickened outer plasma membrane

8 Capillaries

9 Superficial squamous cells

Fig. 15-9   Urinary Bladder: Mucosa (transverse section). Stain: hematoxylin-eosin. Medium magnification.

Figure 15-10   Kidney: Renal Corpuscle and Juxtaglomerular Apparatus

The kidney cortex consists of blood filtering units and different types of tubules. In the middle of this high magnification photomicrograph is a renal corpuscle and the surrounding tubules. The renal corpuscle consists of a capillary tuft **glomerulus (1)** and a **glomerular capsule (2)** with its two layers, the **parietal layer (2a)** and **visceral layer (2b)**. Between these two capsular layers is the **capsular space (3)**. On the right side of the renal corpuscle is the **vascular pole (5)** where blood vessels enter and leave this structure. Near the vascular pole (5) is the **juxtaglomerular apparatus (6)**. This apparatus consists of modified smooth muscle cells of the afferent arteriole in the vascular pole (5), the **juxtaglomerular cells (6a),** and the **macula densa (6b),** a region of the distal convoluted tubule that contains a dense aggregation of tubule cells. Surrounding the renal corpuscle are numerous, darker-staining **proximal convoluted tubules (4)** and a few **distal convoluted tubules (8)**. Between the tubules are found numerous **blood vessels (7).**

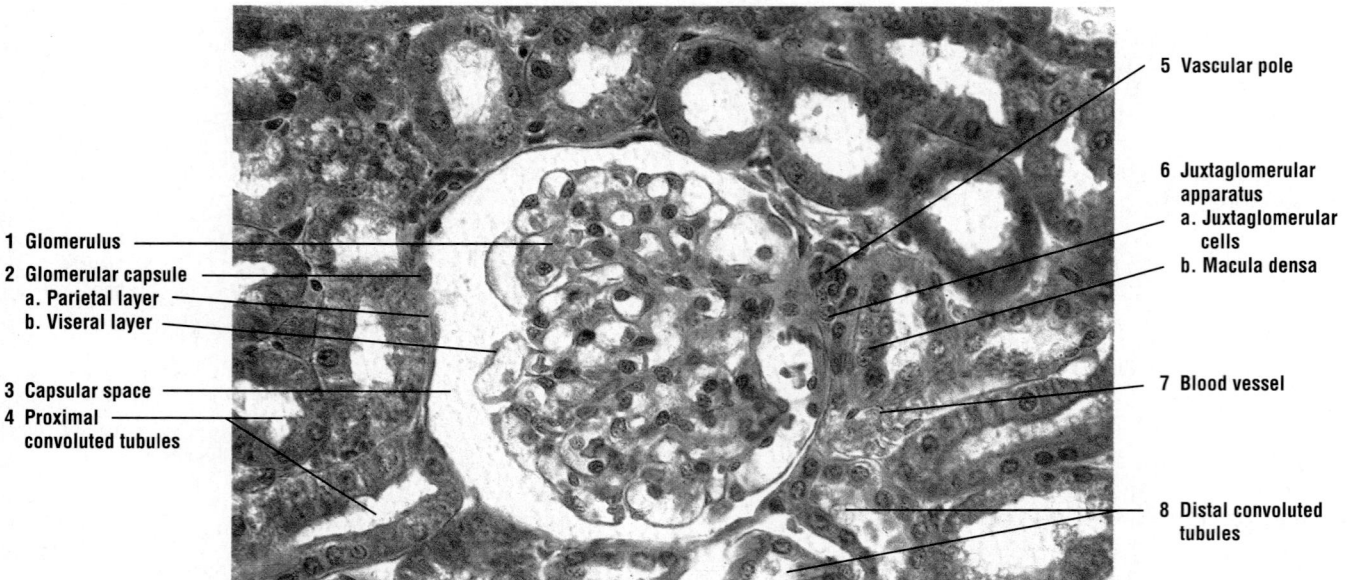

Fig. 15-10   Kidney: Renal Corpuscle and Juxtaglomerular Apparatus. Stain: Masson's Trichrome. 130×

Figure 15-11   Kidney: Ducts of Medullary Region (longitudinal section).

The medullary region of the kidney consists primarily of various-sized tubules, larger ducts, and blood vesses of the vesa recta. In this photomicrograph, different kidney tubules and blood vessels have been sectioned in a longitudinal plane. The tubules with large, light-staining cuboidal cells are the **collecting tubules (1)**. Adjacent to the collecting tubules (1) are tubules with darker-staining, cuboidal cells. These are the **thick segments of the loop of Henle (2).** Between the tubules are blood vessels of the **vesa recta (4)** and the **thin segments of the loop of Henle (3).** Blood vessels of the vesa recta (4) can be distinguished from the thin segments of the loop of Henle (3) by the presence of blood cells in their lumina.

Figure 15-12   Ureter (transverse section)

The ureter is a thick, muscular tube that conveys urine from the kidneys to the bladder. This low magnification photomicrograph shows an entire ureter in a transverse section. The mucosa of the ureter is highly folded and is lined by a thick, **transitional epithelium (1)**. Below it is the connective tissue **lamina propria (2)**. The muscularis of the ureter contains two smooth muscle layers, an **inner longitudinal muscle layer (3)** and a **middle circular muscle layer (4)**. A third, an outer longitudinal muscle layer, is added to the wall in lower third of the ureter. Surrounding the muscular wall of the ureter is the connective tissue **adventitia (6)**. Also present in the adventitia (6) and in its vicinity are numerous **blood vessels (5)** and **adipose tissue (7)**.

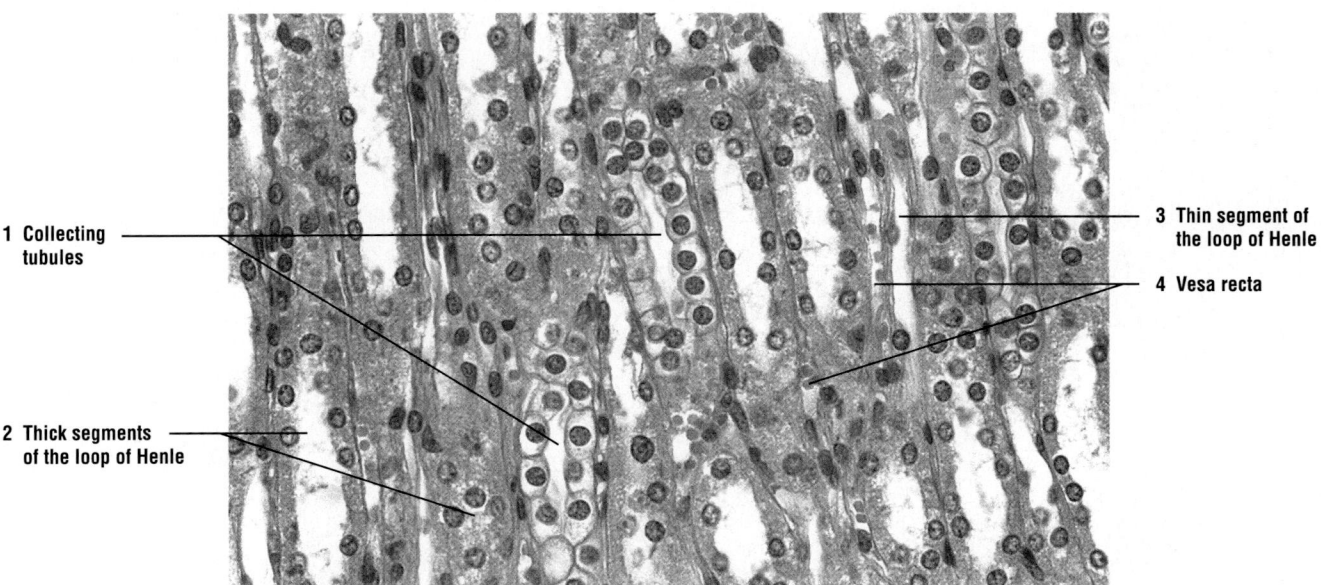

1 Collecting tubules

2 Thick segments of the loop of Henle

3 Thin segment of the loop of Henle

4 Vesa recta

Fig. 15-11   Kidney: Ducts of Medullary Region (longitudinal section). Stain: hematoxylin-eosin. 130×

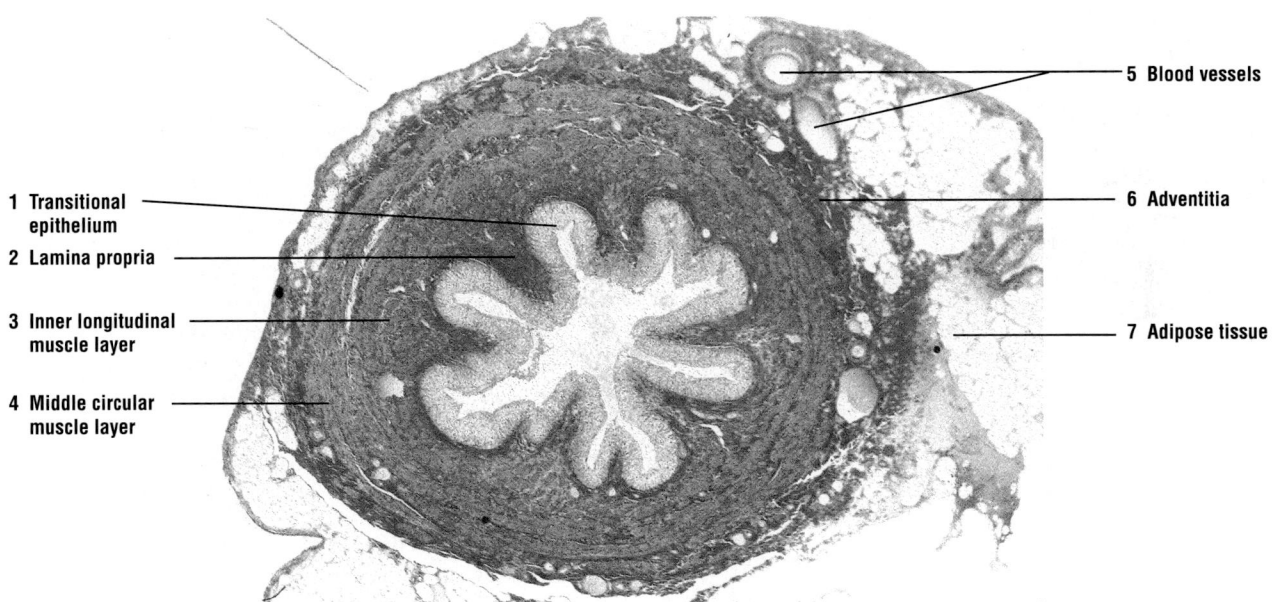

1 Transitional epithelium

2 Lamina propria

3 Inner longitudinal muscle layer

4 Middle circular muscle layer

5 Blood vessels

6 Adventitia

7 Adipose tissue

Fig. 15-12   Ureter (transverse section). Stain: iron hematoxylin and alcian blue (IHAB). 10×

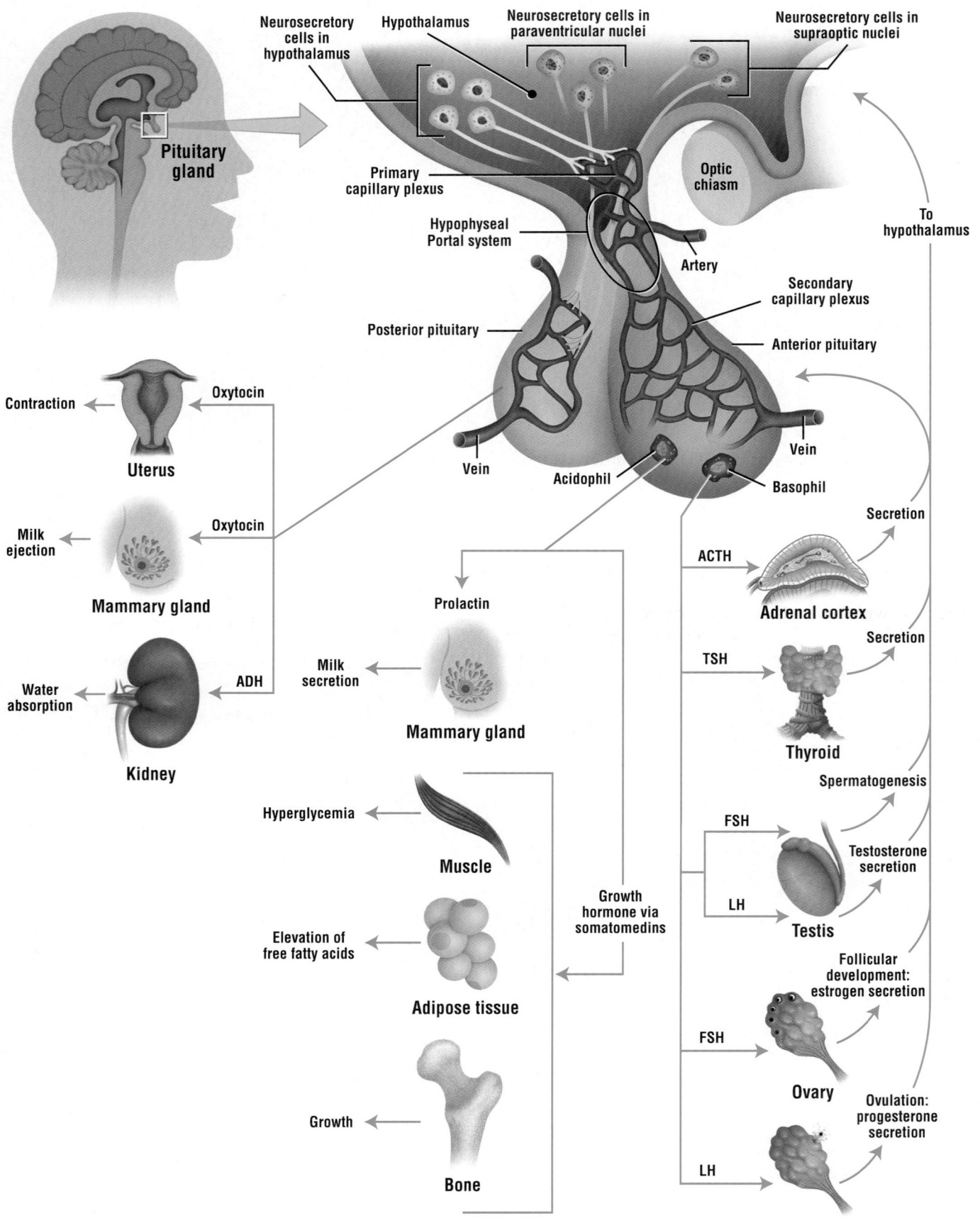

Pituitary gland

Neurosecretory cells in hypothalamus
Hypothalamus
Neurosecretory cells in paraventricular nuclei
Neurosecretory cells in supraoptic nuclei

Primary capillary plexus
Optic chiasm

Hypophyseal Portal system
Artery
To hypothalamus

Secondary capillary plexus

Posterior pituitary
Anterior pituitary

Vein
Vein

Acidophil
Basophil

Contraction
Oxytocin
Uterus

Milk ejection
Oxytocin
Mammary gland

Secretion
ACTH
Adrenal cortex

Water absorption
ADH
Kidney

Prolactin
Milk secretion
Mammary gland

Secretion
TSH
Thyroid

Hyperglycemia
Muscle

Spermatogenesis
FSH

Elevation of free fatty acids
Adipose tissue

Growth hormone via somatomedins

Testosterone secretion
LH
Testis

Growth
Bone

Follicular development: estrogen secretion
FSH
Ovary

Ovulation: progesterone secretion
LH

Endocrine System

SECTION 1
Hypophysis (Pituitary Gland)

The endocrine system consists of cells, tissues, and organs that synthesize and secrete **hormones** directly into the blood and lymph capillaries. As a result, the endocrine glands/organs are ductless, that is, they do not have excretory ducts. Furthermore, the cells in most endocrine organs are arranged into **cords** and **clumps,** and surrounded by an extensive **capillary network.** The hormones produced by the endocrine organs include peptides, proteins, steroids, and amino acid derivatives, including catecholamines. The hormones enter the blood vessels directly and are then transported in blood to distant **target organs,** where, via specific receptors, they influence the structure and function of their cells and tissues. The hormone receptors can be located either on the plasma membrane, cytoplasm, or nucleus of target cells.

There are also numerous exocrine organs that are associated with individual endocrine cells or endocrine tissues. Such mixed (endocrine-exocrine) organs are pancreas, kidneys, reproductive organs of both sexes, placenta, and gastrointestinal tract. Endocrine cells and tissues are discussed with the exocrine organs in their respective chapters. There are also distinct endocrine organs in the body. These include the **hypophysis,** or **pituitary gland** (described below), **thyroid gland, adrenal (suprarenal) glands,** and **parathyroid glands** (described in Section 2).

HYPOPHYSIS (PITUITARY GLAND): EMBRYOLOGIC ORIGIN AND ORGANIZATION

The structure and function of the hypophysis reflect its dual embryologic origin. During development, the epithelium of **pharyngeal roof** (oral cavity) forms an outpocketing, the **hypophyseal (Rathke's) pouch,** which later detaches from the oral cavity and becomes the cellular or glandular portion of the hypophysis, the **adenohypophysis (anterior pituitary).** At the same time, the downgrowth from the developing brain forms the neural portion of the hypophysis, the **neurohypophysis (posterior pituitary).** These two structures then unite to form the hypophysis, which remains attached to the base of the brain by a short **infundibular (neural) stalk.**

The adenohypophysis has three subdivisions, **pars distalis, pars tuberalis,** and **pars intermedia,** a thin cell layer of the hypophyseal pouch that is located between pars distalis and neurohypophysis. Pars intermedia is rudimentary in humans. The neurohypophysis also consists of three parts. **Median eminence** is at the base of the hypothalamus, **infundibulum (infudibular stalk)** extends down from the median eminence, and **pars nervosa (Figs. 16-1, 16-2, 16-9).**

The adenohypophysis establishes a vascular connection with the **hypothalamus** via the **hypophyseal portal system. Superior hypophyseal arteries** from the internal carotid artery supply pars tuberalis and infundibulum of the hypophysis, and form the **primary capillary plexus** in the median eminence of the hypothalamus. Secretory neurons in the hypothalamus produce hormones that influence cell functions in the adenohypophysis. The axons of these neurons terminate on the primary capillary plexus. Small venules drain primary capillary plexus and deliver the blood to the **secondary capillary plexus** in pars distalis. The venules that connect the primary capillary plexus with the secondary capillary plexus form the hypophyseal portal system. The capillaries in these plexuses are fenestrated.

Neurohypophysis remains connected to the brain by numerous unmyelinated axons, whose cell bodies are located in the **supraoptic** and **paraventruclar nuclei** of the hypothalamus. These axons form the **hypothalamohypophyseal tract** and the bulk of neurohypophysis. The neurosecretory cells in the hypothalamus synthesize the hormones that travel to the terminal ends of these axons to be stored as **Herring bodies** in the neurohypophysis or released into the blood stream.

CELLS OF THE HYPOPHYSIS

The cells of the adenohypophysis were classified as **chromophobes** and **chromophils,** based on the affinity of their cytoplasmic granules for specific stains. The pale-staining chromophobes are believed to be either degranulated chromophils or undifferentiated stem cells. The chromophils are further subdivided into **acidophils** and **basophils** because of their staining properties. Immunocytochemical techniques now identify these cells on the basis of their specific hormones. Thus, there are two types of acidophils, **somatotrophs** and **mammotrophs,** and three types of basophils, **gonadotrophs, thyrotrophs,** and **corticotrophs,** respectively **(Figs. 16-2–16-4,16-9).** These cells produce the hormones that are released from the adenohypophysis and carried in the blood target organs. Here, they bind to specific receptors that influence the structure and function of the affected cells. Once the target cells are activated, a feedback mechanism (positive or negative) controls further the synthesis and release of the hormone.

The neurohypophysis does not contain secretory neurons. Instead, it consists of supporting neuroglial cells, the **pituicytes,** and unmyelinated axons, whose cell bodies are located in the supraoptic and paraventricular nuclei of the hypothalamus **(Figs. 16-1, 16-2, 16-9).** The hormones released from the neurohypophysis are first synthesized in the hypothalamus, stored in the neurohypophysis as Herring bodies until needed, and then released from the axon terminals into the blood stream.

Figure 16-1   Hypophysis (panoramic view, sagittal section)

The hypophysis (pituitary gland) consists of two major subdivisions, the adenohypophysis and neurohypophysis. The adenohypophysis is further subdivided into **pars distalis (anterior lobe) (5), pars tuberalis (9),** and **pars intermedia (10).** The neurohypophysis is divided into **pars nervosa** or **infundibular process (11), infundibular (neural) stalk (8),** and tuber cinerum of the median eminence (not illustrated). The pars tuberalis (9) of the adenohypophysis surrounds the infundibular stalk (8) and is, therefore, visible above and below the stalk in a sagittal section; it extends higher on the anterior surface than the posterior surface of the hypophysis. The infundibular stalk (8) connects the hypophysis with the central nervous system (base of the brain).

The pars distalis (5) is the largest of the four divisions of the hypophysis and contains two main types of cells, **chromophobe cells (1)** and chromophil cells. The **chromophils** are subdivided into **acidophils (alpha cells) (3)** and **basophils (beta cells) (4).** (These are illustrated at a higher magnification in Fig. 16-2 below.)

The pars nervosa (11) is the second largest of the four divisions. Pars intermedia (10) and pars nervosa (11) form the posterior lobe of the hypophysis, which consists primarily of unmyelinated nerve fibers and supporting cells (pituicytes). The **connective tissue septa (12)** that arise from the surrounding capsule penetrate into the gland.

The pars intermedia (10) is situated between the pars distalis and the pars nervosa. This region contains colloid-filled cysts lined by different cells, with basophils predominating.

Figure 16-2   Hypophysis (sectional view)

Under higher magnification, numerous **sinusoidal capillaries (6)** and cell types are visible in the pars distalis. **Chromophobe cells (4)** exhibit a light-staining, homogeneous cytoplasm. They are normally smaller than the chromophils and are found in groups. The cytoplasm of chromophils stains red in **acidophils (3)** and blue in **basophils (5).**

The pars intermedia contains colloid-filled cysts or **vesicles (7)** lined by low columnar cells; some cells in these vesicles contain basophilic granules while others do not exhibit any granules in their cytoplasm. Follicles lined with **basophils (8)** are often seen in pars intermedia, with some cells exhibiting secretory granules in their cytoplasm (8, lower leader).

Also illustrated is a portion of **pars nervosa (9).** This region is characterized by unmyelinated axons and cytoplasmic processes of the **pituicytes (9, 10),** both of which stain lightly. Oval nuclei of the pituicytes are seen (10), but not the scanty cytoplasm.

■ Functional Correlations–Hypophysis

The synthesis and release of specific hormones from the adenohypophysis are directly influenced by hormones produced in the **hypothalamus.** Specific **releasing hormones (factors)** are produced for each hormone that is released by the hypophysis. In addition, **inhibitory hormones (factors)** are produced for growth hormone and prolactin. The releasing or inhibitory hormones that are released from the hypothalamus are carried to the adenohypophysis by way of the **hypophyseal portal system.** On reaching the adenohypophysis, releasing hormones bind to receptors and stimulate certain cells to secrete and release specific hormones into the circulation.

Neurohypophysis also releases hormones. The neurons in the **supraoptic** and **paraventricular nuclei** of the **hypothalamus** secrete two hormones, **oxytocin** and **vasopressin** (antidiuretic hormone or ADH). These hormones are transported along the microtubules in the unmyelinated axons to neurohypophysis, where they are stored in the axon terminals as **Herring bodies.** These hormones are then released from axon terminals into the blood vessels that drain the neurohypophysis, as needed.

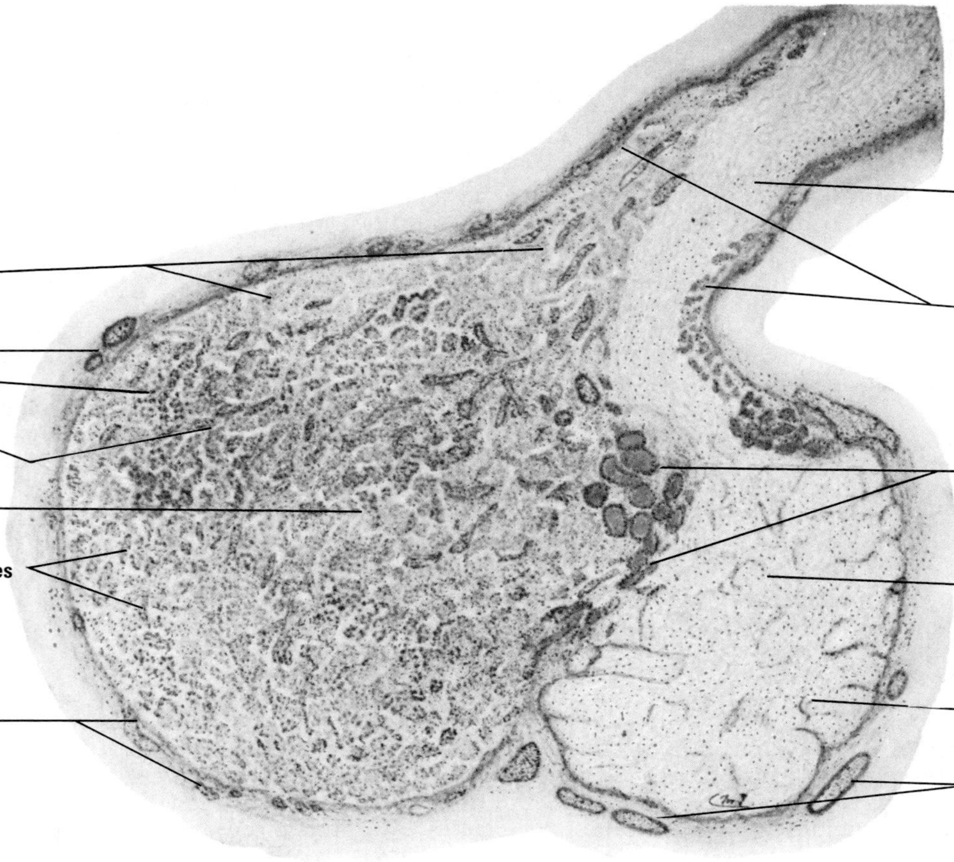

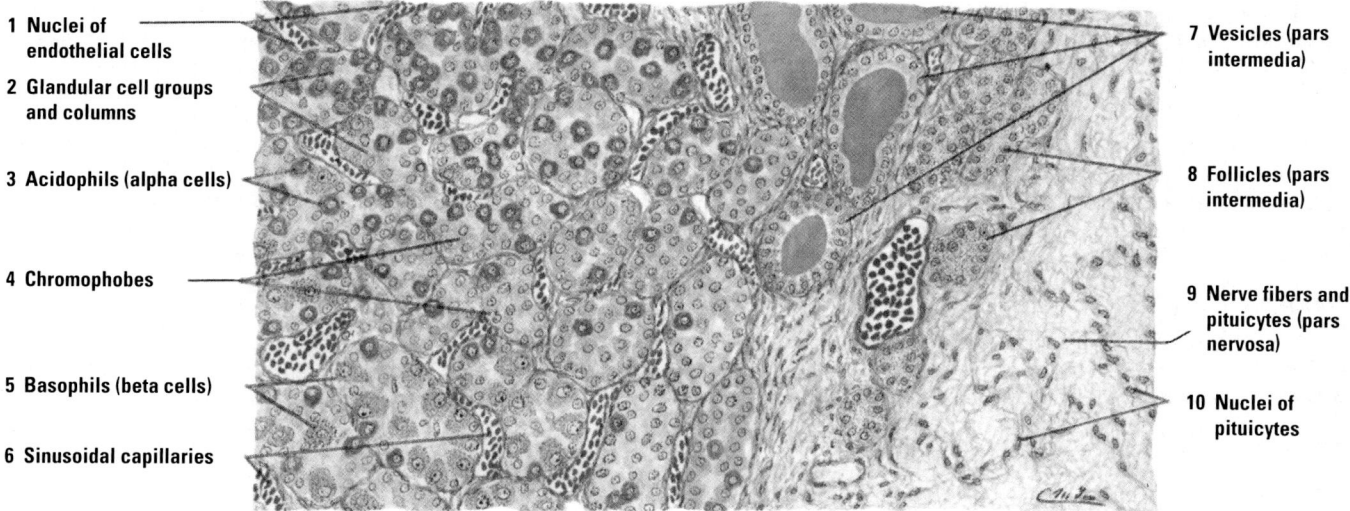

1 Chromophobes

2 Capsule
3 Cell group with predominance of acidophilic cells
4 Cell group with predominance of basophilic cells
5 Pars distalis
6 Sinusoidal capillaries
7 Veins

8 Infundibular stalk
9 Pars tuberalis
10 Pars intermedia with colloid vesicles
11 Pars nervosa (infundibular process)
12 Connective tissue septum
13 Blood vessels in the capsule

Fig. 16-1   Hypophysis (panoramic view, sagittal section). Stain: hematoxylin-eosin. Low magnification.

1 Nuclei of endothelial cells
2 Glandular cell groups and columns
3 Acidophils (alpha cells)
4 Chromophobes
5 Basophils (beta cells)
6 Sinusoidal capillaries

7 Vesicles (pars intermedia)
8 Follicles (pars intermedia)
9 Nerve fibers and pituicytes (pars nervosa)
10 Nuclei of pituicytes

Fig. 16-2   Hypophysis (sectional view). Stain: hematoxylin-eosin. Medium magnification.

Figure 16-3   Hypophysis: Pars Distalis (sectional view)

Various cell types in the pars distalis can readily be identified following special fixation and/or staining. In the illustration, the hypophysis was fixed with a corrosive sublimate mixture, and the section stained with azocarmine and differentiated with aniline oil. Phosphotungstic acid was then used to destain the connective tissue, followed by cytoplasmic staining with aniline blue and orange G. The cytoplasmic granules stain red, orange or blue, depending on their respective affinities; the nuclei of all cells stain orange.

Chromophobes (3) usually stain lightly after any stain. Their nuclei stain pale, the cytoplasm stains pale orange, and the cell outlines are poorly defined. The aggregation of chromophobes in groups or clumps is apparent in this illustration.

Two types of acidophils (1, 6) can be distinguished by their staining reaction (although not as clearly as after other specific stains); cells with coarse granules stain red with azocarmine (1) and those with smaller granules stain with orange G (6).

The basophils (2, 5) are readily recognized by blue-stained granules, but the different types of basophils are not distinguishable. The degree of granularity and the stain density vary in different cells.

Figure 16-4   Hypophysis: Various Cell Groups

Various cell types of the hypophysis are illustrated at higher magnification after azan staining. Nuclei of all cells are stained orange-red.

In the chromophobes (a), the light orange stain of the cytoplasm indicates that they are nongranular and their cell boundaries are indistinct. The cytoplasmic granules of acidophils (b) stain intense red and the cell outlines are distinct. A sinusoid capillary is visible in close proximity to the acidophils.

The basophils (c) exhibit variable round, polyhedral, or angular shapes. The blue granules vary in size and are not as compact as in the acidophils.

The pituicytes (d) of pars nervosa exhibit variable shape and size of the cells and nuclei (1). The small, orange-stained cytoplasm has diffuse cytoplasmic processes (2).

■ Functional Correlations–Hormones of Adenohypophysis

Acidophils

Somatotrophs secrete somatotropin (growth hormone or GH), which stimulates general body growth, uptake of amino acids, and protein synthesis. Somatotropin also stimulates the liver to produce somatomedins, which cause proliferation of cartilage cells in the epiphyseal plates of developing or growing long bones.

Mammotrophs produce the lactogenic hormone prolactin to stimulate the development of mammary glands during pregnancy. Following parturition (birth), prolactin maintains milk production in the mammary glands during lactation.

Basophils

Thyrotrophs secrete the thyroid-stimulating hormone (thyrotropin or TSH). TSH stimulates synthesis and secretion of the thyroid gland hormones thyroxin and triiodothyronine from the thyroid gland.

Gonadotrophs secrete follicle-stimulating hormone (FSH) and luteinizing hormone (LH). In females, FSH promotes estrogen secretion, and growth and maturation of ovarian follicles. In males, FSH stimulates spermatogenesis and secretion into the seminiferous tubules of the testes of androgen-binding protein by the Sertoli cells.

In females, LH in association with FSH, induces ovulation, promotes final maturation of the ovarian follicles, and formation of the corpus luteum following ovulation. LH also promotes secretion of estrogen and progesterone from corpus luteum. In males, LH maintains and stimulates the interstitial cells (of Leydig) in the testes to produce the hormone testosterone. As a result, LH is sometimes called interstitial cell-stimulating hormone (ICSH).

Corticotrophs secrete adrenocorticotropic hormone (ACTH). ACTH influences the function of cells in the adrenal cortex. ACTH also stimulates the synthesis and release of glucocorticoids from the zona fasciculata and zona reticularis of the adrenal cortex.

Pars Intermedia

In lower vertebrates (amphibians and fishes), pars intermedia is well developed and produces melanocyte-stimulating hormone (MSH). In these animals, MSH increases pigmentation of the skin by causing dispersion of the melanin granules. In humans and most other mammals, this region of the hypophysis is rudimentary.

HORMONES OF THE NEUROHYPOPHYSIS

Oxytocin

During labor of pregnancy, oxytocin is released from neurohypophysis; it induces strong contractions of smooth muscles in the uterus, resulting in childbirth. When nursing, the suckling action of the infant on the nipple activates the milk-ejection reflex in the lactating mammary glands. This action releases oxytocin, which stimulates the contraction of myoepithelial cells that surround the secretory alveoli and ducts in the mammary glands. This action causes milk ejection into the excretory ducts of the mammary gland and the nipple.

Vasopressin (ADH)

Release of vasopressin into the blood stream contracts smooth muscles in small arteries and arterioles. This action constricts their lumina and raises the blood pressure. The main action of vasopressin, however, is to increase water permeability in the distal convoluted tubules and collecting tubules of the kidney. This allows more water to be resorbed by the kidney tubules into the interstitium and retained in the body, while at the same time, increasing the concentration of urine.

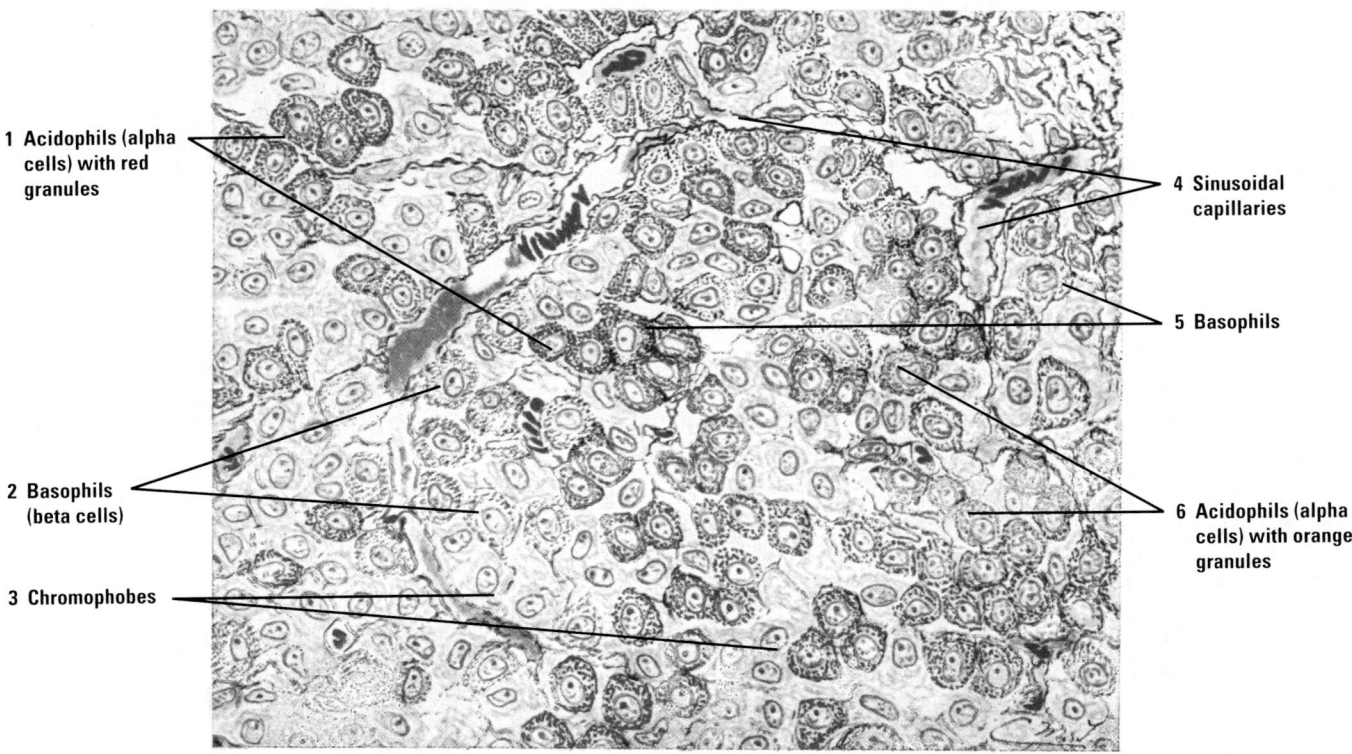

1 Acidophils (alpha cells) with red granules

2 Basophils (beta cells)

3 Chromophobes

4 Sinusoidal capillaries

5 Basophils

6 Acidophils (alpha cells) with orange granules

Fig. 16-3   Hypophysis: Pars Distalis (sectional view). Stain: azan (nuclei: orange; cytoplasmic granules of alpha cells: red or orange; cytoplasmic granules of beta cells: deep blue; collagen and reticular fibers: blue; erythrocytes: bright red; hemolyzed blood: deep yellow). High magnification.

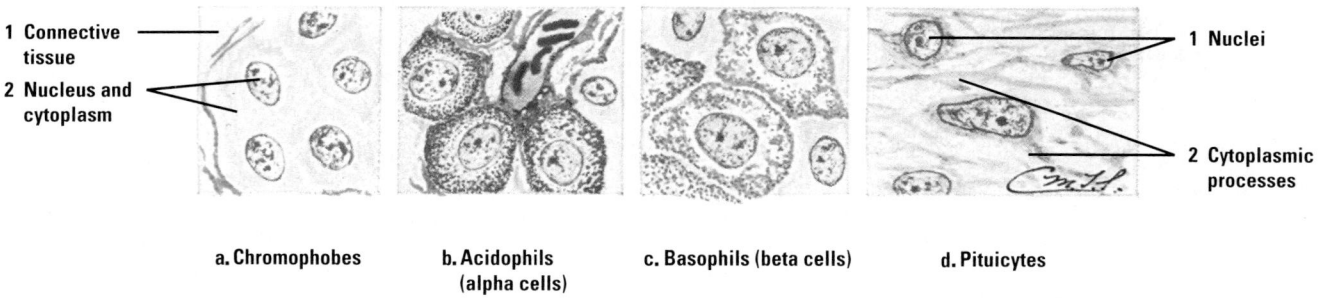

1 Connective tissue

2 Nucleus and cytoplasm

1 Nuclei

2 Cytoplasmic processes

a. Chromophobes   b. Acidophils (alpha cells)   c. Basophils (beta cells)   d. Pituicytes

Fig. 16-4   Hypophysis: Various Cell Groups. Stain: azan (see detailed explanation of stain above). Oil immersion.

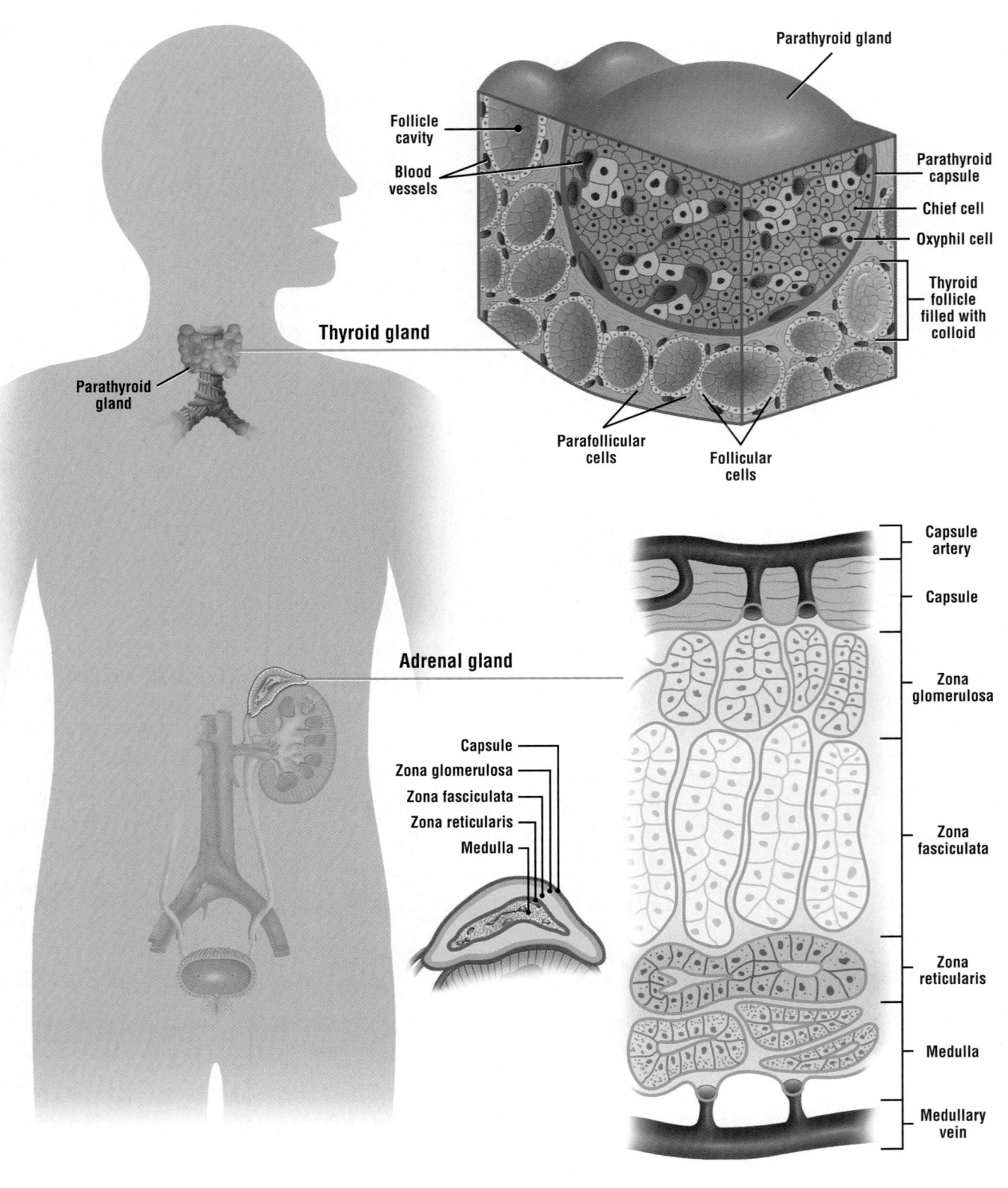

Parathyroid gland

Follicle cavity

Blood vessels

Thyroid gland

Parathyroid gland

Parathyroid capsule

Chief cell

Oxyphil cell

Thyroid follicle filled with colloid

Parafollicular cells

Follicular cells

Parathyroid gland

Adrenal gland

Capsule

Zona glomerulosa

Zona fasciculata

Zona reticularis

Medulla

Capsule artery

Capsule

Zona glomerulosa

Zona fasciculata

Zona reticularis

Medulla

Medullary vein

SECTION 2
Thyroid Gland, Parathyroid Glands, and Adrenal Gland

THYROID GLAND

The **thyroid gland** is located inferior to the larynx. It is one gland that consists of right and left lobes, connected in the middle by an isthmus. Cell of most endocrine organs store their secretory products within their cytoplasm. The thyroid gland is a unique endocrine organ in that its cells are arranged into spherical structures called **follicles,** instead of the normal cell cords and clusters. The cells that surround the follicles, the **follicular cells,** secrete and store their product extracellularly in the lumen of the follicles as a gelatinous substance called **colloid.** The colloid is composed of **thyroglobulin,** a glycoprotein containing several iodinated amino acids. The hormones of the thyroid gland are stored in the follicles as colloid bound to thyroglobulin. As a result, the follicles are the structural and functional units of the thyroid gland **(Figs. 16-5–16-7, 16-10).** In addition to the follicular cells, larger **parafollicular** cells are also present in the thyroid gland. They are either found within the follicular epithelium of the thyroid follicle or within the interfollicular spaces. Increased vascularity around the follicles allows for easy entrance of the hormones into the blood stream.

PARATHYROID GLANDS

Mammals generally have four **parathyroid glands.** These small glands are situated on the posterior surface of the thyroid gland, but separated from the thyroid gland by a thin connective tissue **capsule.** Normally, one parathyroid gland is located on superior and inferior pole of each lobe of the thyroid gland. In contrast to the thyroid gland and the follicles, the cells of the parathyroid glands are arranged into cords or clumps. There are two type of cells in the parathyroid glands, the functinal **chief cells** and the **oxyphil cells.** Oxyphil cells are larger and less numerous than the chief cells. On rare occasions, small colloid-filled follicles can be seen in the parathyroid glands **(Figs. 16-7, 16-10).**

ADRENAL (SUPRARENAL) GLANDS

The **adrenal glands** are paired organs that are situated near the superior pole of the kidneys. Each gland is surrounded by a dense connective tissue capsule and embedded in adipose tissue. Adrenal glands consists of an outer **cortex** and an inner **medulla.** Although these two regions of the adrenal gland are in one organ and linked by a common blood supply, they have distinct embryologic origin, structure, and function.

Cortex. The adrenal cortex exhibits three concentric zones: **zona glomerulosa, zona fasciculata,** and **zona reticularis.** The cells of these zones in the adrenal cortex produce three classes of hormones: **mineralocorticoids, glucocorticoids,** and **sex hormones (Figs. 16-8, 16-11).**

Medulla. The medulla lies in the center of the adrenal gland. The cells of adrenal medulla are modified postganglionic sympathetic neurons that secrete **catecholamines** (primarily epinephrine and norepinephrine). Their release from the adrenal medulla is under the direct control of the autonomic nervous system. The effects of these catecholamines are similar to those produced by stimulation of the sympathetic division of the autonomic nervous system **(Figs. 16-8, 16-11).**

Figure 16-5   Thyroid Gland: Canine (general view)

The thyroid gland is characterized by numerous spherical **follicles (2, 12),** with variable diameters, that are filled with an acidophilic **colloid** (2, 12) material. The follicles are usually lined by a simple cuboidal epithelium consisting of **follicular** or **principal cells (3, 7).** Follicles sectioned tangentially (4) do not exhibit a lumen. The follicular cells (3, 7) synthesize and secrete thyroid hormones. In routine histologic preparations, colloid often retracts from the follicular wall (12).

In addition to the follicular cells (3, 7), the thyroid gland contains another secretory cell type, the **parafollicular cells (1, 8).** They occur as single cells or in clumps on the periphery of the follicles. They stain lightly and are clearly visible in this illustration of canine thyroid. Parafollicular cells (1, 8) synthesize and secrete the hormone calcitonin.

The **connective tissue septa (5, 9)** from the thyroid gland capsule extend into the gland's interior, dividing it into lobules (9). Extensive distribution of blood vessels, **arterioles (6), venules (10),** and **capillaries (13)** is seen within the connective tissue septa (5, 9) and around the individual follicles (2, 12). Relatively little **interfollicular connective tissue (11)** is found between individual follicles.

Figure 16-6   Thyroid Gland Follicles: Canine (sectional view)

A higher magnification of the thyroid gland shows the detailed structure of individual **follicles (2, 9).** The height of **follicular cells (5, 11)** varies among follicles, depending on their state of activity. In highly active follicles, the epithelium is mainly cuboidal (9) whereas in less active follicles, the epithelium appears flattened (5). All follicles (2, 9) are filled with **colloid (2),** some of which show retraction (12) from the follicular wall or distortion (12) due to histologic preparation.

The **parafollicular cells (1, 10)** are situated within the follicular epithelium (1) or in small clumps (10) adjacent to the follicles (2, 9) but within their basement membrane. The parafollicular cells (1, 10), however, do not border directly on the follicular lumen. Instead, they are separated from the lumen by the processes of neighboring follicular cells (5, 11). The parafollicular cells (1, 10) are larger, oval or varied in shape, and exhibit cytoplasm that is lighter staining than that of the follicular cells (5, 11).

Surrounding the follicles (2, 9) is a thin **interfollicular connective tissue (3, 8),** in which are found numerous **blood vessels** (6) and **capillaries (4),** closely associated with the follicular (5, 11) and parafollicular cells (1, 10).

■ Functional Correlations–Thyroid Gland

The secretory functions of the **follicular cells** in the thyroid gland are controlled by the **thyroid-stimulating hormone (TSH)** of the adenohypophysis. This highly complex activity includes the synthesis of the thyroglobulin, iodination of the thyroglobulin, temporary storage of the thyroglobulin in the follicular lumen, and release of the thyroid hormones into general circulation when the need arises. In response to the secretory stimulus, follicular cells in the thyroid gland engulf and hydrolyze the iodinated thyroglobulin, and then release thyroid hormones at the cell base into the blood stream.

The thyroid hormones are **thyroxine (T4)** and **triiodothyronine (T3).** Their release into general circulation accelerates the metabolic rate of the body and increases cell metabolism, growth, differentiation, and development throughout the body. In addition, the thyroid hormones increase the rate of protein, carbohydrate, and fat metabolism.

The thyroid gland also contains the **parafollicular** cells. These cells appear on the periphery of the follicular epithelium as single cells or as clusters of cells between the follicles. The parafollicular cells synthesize and secrete the hormone **calcitonin (thyrocalcitonin).** The function of this hormone is to lower blood calcium levels in the body. This is accomplished primarily by reducing the number of **osteoclasts** in the bones and decreasing their activity, thus reducing bone resorption and calcium release. While the production and release of thyroid hormone depends on the pituitary gland hormone TSH, secretion and release of calcitonin by the parafollicular cells is directly controlled by blood calcium levels.

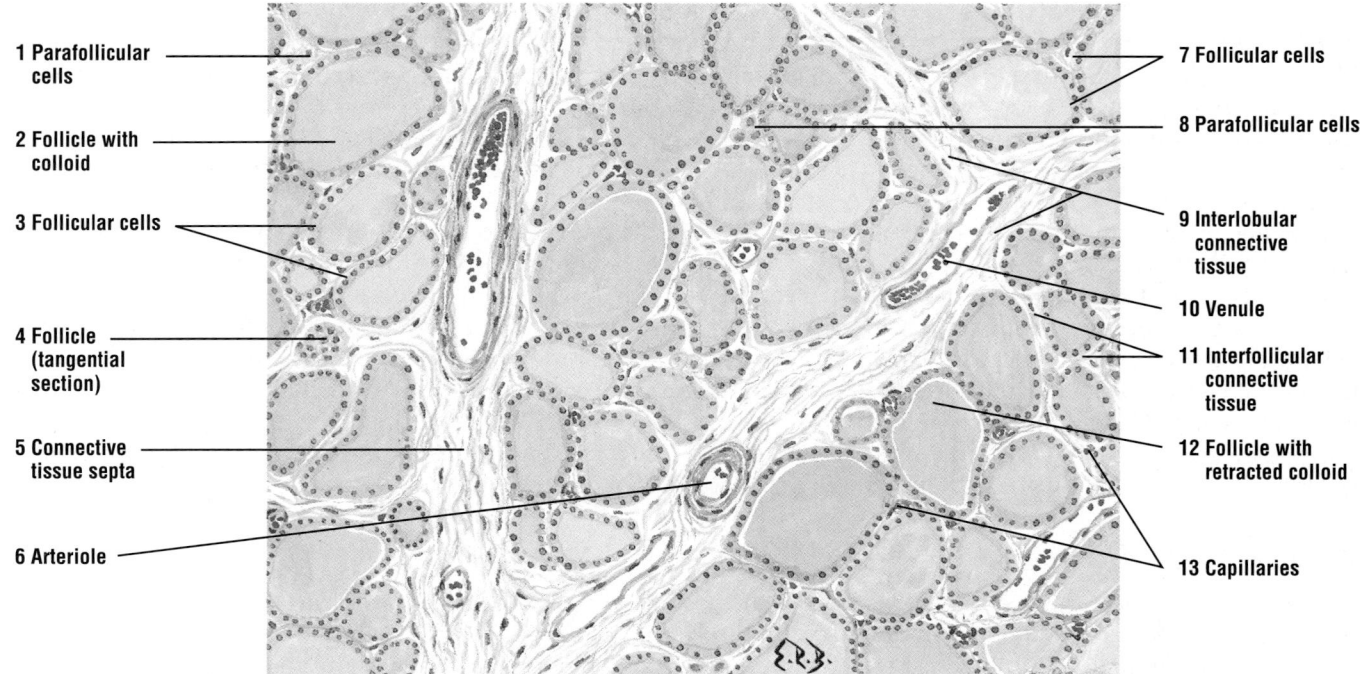

1 Parafollicular cells

2 Follicle with colloid

3 Follicular cells

4 Follicle (tangential section)

5 Connective tissue septa

6 Arteriole

7 Follicular cells

8 Parafollicular cells

9 Interlobular connective tissue

10 Venule

11 Interfollicular connective tissue

12 Follicle with retracted colloid

13 Capillaries

Fig. 16-5   Thyroid Gland: Canine (general view). Stain: hematoxylin-eosin. Low magnification.

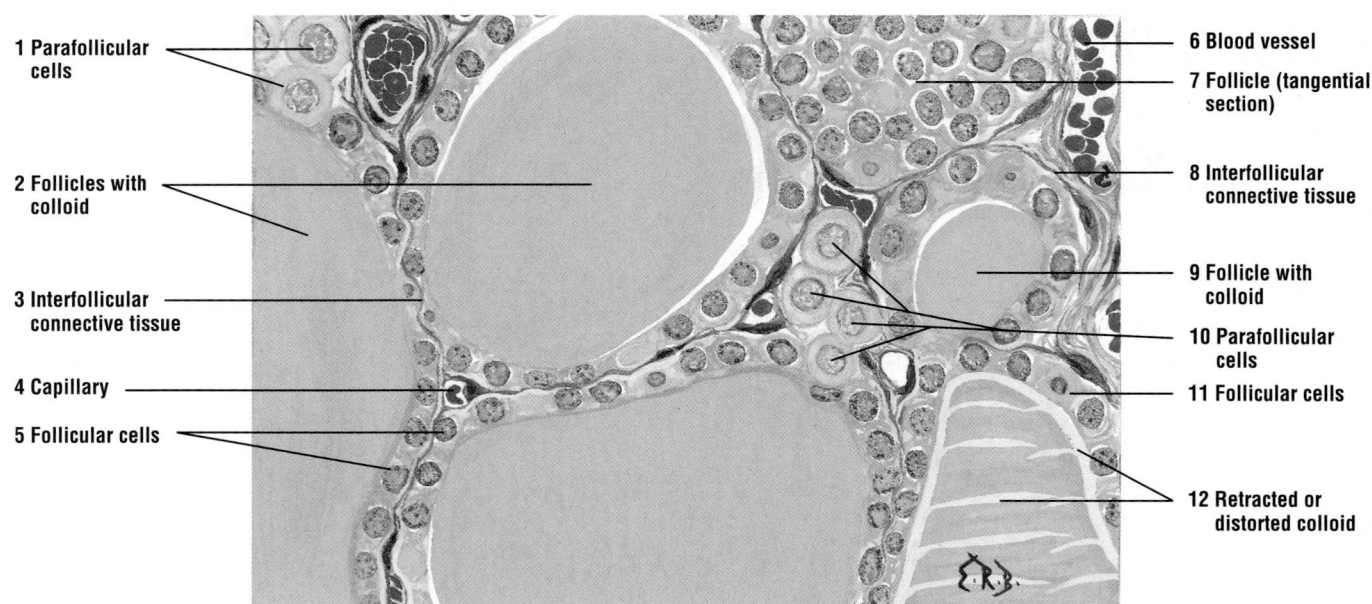

1 Parafollicular cells

2 Follicles with colloid

3 Interfollicular connective tissue

4 Capillary

5 Follicular cells

6 Blood vessel

7 Follicle (tangential section)

8 Interfollicular connective tissue

9 Follicle with colloid

10 Parafollicular cells

11 Follicular cells

12 Retracted or distorted colloid

Fig. 16-6   Thyroid Gland Follicles: Canine (sectional view). Stain: hematoxylin-eosin. High magnification.

Figure 16-7   Thyroid and Parathyroid Glands: Canine (sectional view)

The **thyroid gland (1)** is closely associated with the **parathyroid gland (3)**. A thin **connective tissue capsule (2)** with a rich **capillary plexus (9)** and **blood vessels (8)** separates the thyroid gland (1) from the parathyroid gland (3). Connective tissue **trabeculae (6)** from the capsule (2) extend into the parathyroid gland (3) and bring larger blood vessels (8) into the interior of the gland. These blood vessels then branch into an extensive capillary (9) network around the parathyroid cells.

The cells in the parathyroid gland (3) are arranged into anastomosing cords and clumps, instead of the **follicles with colloid (4)**, as seen in the thyroid gland (1). The parathyroid gland (3) contains two types of cells, **chief (principal) cells (7)** and **oxyphil cells (10)**. The chief cells (7) are the most numerous cells; they are round and exhibit a pale, slightly acidophilic cytoplasm. The oxyphil cells (10) are larger and less numerous than the chief cells (7), and exhibit a denser acidophilic cytoplasm with smaller, darker-staining nuclei (10). The oxyphil cells (10) are distributed as single cells or in small clumps. In humans, the oxyphil cells (10) are not normally present in the parathyroid glands of children under four years of age.

The follicles with colloid (4) seen in the thyroid gland (1) are not a characteristic feature of the parathyroid glands (3). However, occasionally an isolated small follicle with colloid material may be observed in the gland.

■ Functional Correlations–Parathyroid Glands

The **chief cells** of the parathyroid glands produce the **parathyroid hormone (parahormone),** whose main function is to maintains proper calcium level in the body fluids. This is accomplished by raising calcium levels in the blood, an action that is opposite or antagonistic to that of thyroid gland's calcitonin. The parathyroid hormone stimulates the activity and increases the proliferation of the **osteoclasts** in the bones. As a result of the increased osteolytic activities of the osteoclasts, more calcium is released into the blood, thereby maintaining normal calcium levels.

Parathyroid hormone also targets the kidneys and the intestines. The distal convoluted tubules in the kidneys increase their resorption of calcium from glomerular filtrate and the elimination of phosphate, sodium, and potassium ions into the urine. Parathyroid hormone also influences the kidneys to form the hormone **calcitriol,** the active form of vitamin D; calcitriol increases calcium absorption from the gastrointestinal tract into the blood.

The secretion and release of parathyroid hormone depends primarily on the concentration of calcium levels in the blood and not on the pituitary hormones. Because the parathyroid hormone maintains optimal levels of calcium in the blood, parathryoid glands are essential to life.

The function of the other type of cells found in the parathyroid glands, the **oxyphil cells,** is presently not known.

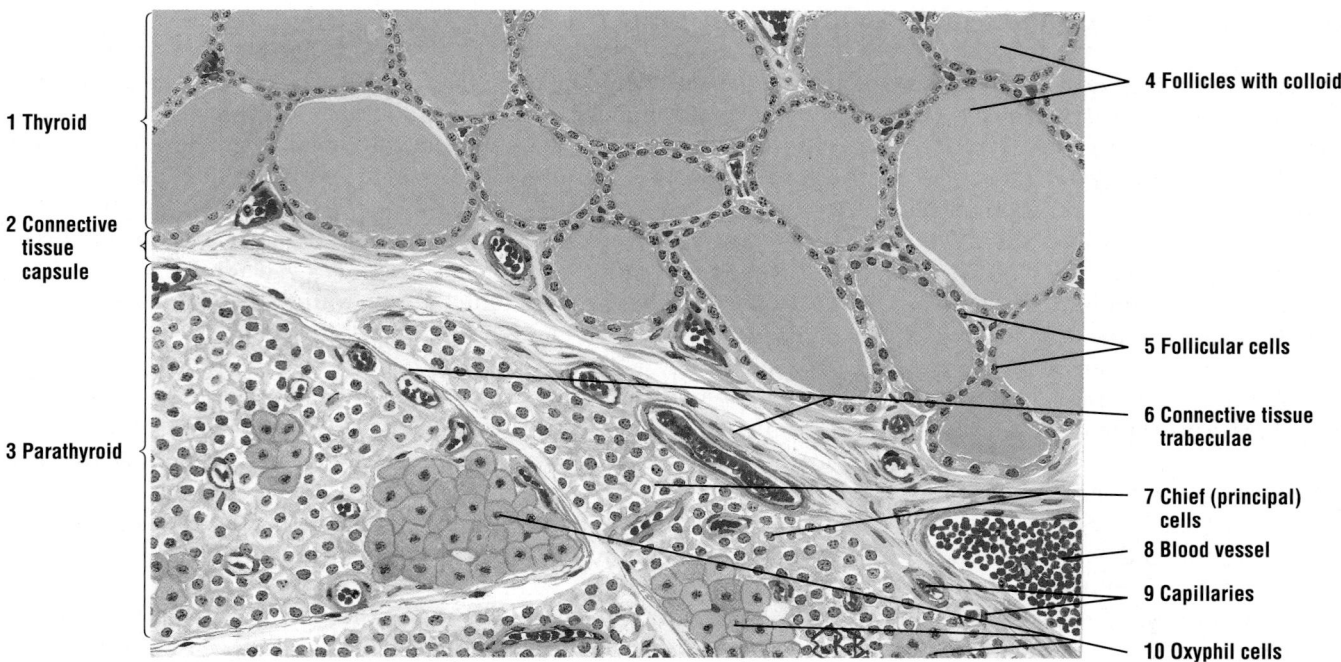

1 Thyroid

2 Connective tissue capsule

3 Parathyroid

4 Follicles with colloid

5 Follicular cells

6 Connective tissue trabeculae

7 Chief (principal) cells

8 Blood vessel

9 Capillaries

10 Oxyphil cells

Fig. 16-7   Thyroid and Parathyroid Glands: Canine (sectional view). Stain: hematoxylin-eosin. Low magnification.

Figure 16-8   Adrenal (Suprarenal) Gland

The adrenal (suprarenal) gland consists of an outer **cortex (2)** and an inner **medulla (3).** The gland is surrounded by a thick connective tissue **capsule (1)** in which are found branches of the main adrenal arteries, veins, **nerves (5)** (largely unmyelinated), and lymphatics. **Connective tissue trabeculae (4)** from the capsule pass into the cortex of the gland and the larger trabeculae carry **arteries (4)** to the medulla (3). **Sinusoidal capillaries (7, 9)** are found throughout the cortex (2) and medulla (3).

The adrenal cortex (2) is subdivided into three concentric zones that are not sharply demarcated from each other. Directly under the connective tissue capsule (1) is the first or the outermost cell layer of the adrenal gland cortex; this is the **zona glomerulosa (2a).** The **cells (6)** in this zone are arranged into ovoid groups. The cytoplasm of these cells (6) contains sparse lipid droplets. In hematoxylin-eosin preparations, the lipid droplets appear as vacuoles while their nuclei stain dark.

The middle cell layer is the **zona fasciculata (2b),** whose **cells (8)** are arranged into columns or plates with radial arrangement. An increased amount of lipid droplets in the cytoplasm gives the cells of zona fasciculata (8) a vacuolated appearance following a normal histologic preparation. The nuclei of these cells are vesicular. **Sinusoidal capillaries (9)** between the cell columns follow a similar radial course.

The third cell layer, the **zona reticularis (2c, 15),** borders the adrenal medulla. The **cells (10)** of this layer form anastomosing cords and are frequently filled with dark-staining, lipofuscin **pigment (11).** The capillaries in this layer exhibit an irregular arrangement.

The **medulla (3)** is not sharply demarcated from the cortex. The cells that constitute the majority of the medulla (3, 14) are arranged in groups. With normal histologic preparation of the adrenal gland, the cytoplasm in these cells appears clear (14). After tissue fixation in potassium bichromate, however, fine brown granules become visible in the cells of the medulla. This cellular alteration is termed the chromaffin reaction and indicates the presence of the catecholamines epinephrine and norepinephrine in the granules. The medulla also contains **sympathetic ganglion cells (13),** seen singly or in small groups. They exhibit the characteristic vesicular nucleus, prominent nucleolus, and a small amount of peripheral chromatin. Sinusoidal capillaries are also present in the medulla and drain its contents into the **medullary veins (12).**

■ Functional Correlations–Adrenal Gland Cortex and Adrenal Medulla

The cells of the **zona glomerulosa** produce **mineralocorticoid hormones,** of which **aldosterone** is the most potent. Aldosterone influences fluid and electrolyte balance in the body by increasing sodium resorption from the glomerular filtrate by distal tubules of the kidney and potassium excretion in urine. Water follows sodium, therefore this action increases fluid volume in the circulation, restores normal electrolyte balance, and raises blood pressure. Aldosterone secretion is initiated via the **renin-angiotensin** pathway in response to a decreased arterial blood pressure and plasma levels of sodium, as detected by the **juxtaglomerular apparatus** in the kidney cortex.

The cells of the zona fasciculata—and probably those of the zona reticularis—secrete **glucocorticoids,** of which **cortisol** and **cortisone** are the most important. Glucocorticoid secretion is an important bodily response to stress. It effects protein, fat, and carbohydrate metabolism, especially in increasing blood sugar levels. Glucocorticoids also suppress inflammatory responses by arresting mitotes in the lymphoid tissues and decreasing their production of antibodies. Although the cells of the zona reticularis are believed to produce sex steroids, the amount of the hormones produced are of little physiological significance. Glucocorticoid secretion and the secretory functions of the zona fasciculata and the zona reticularis are regulated by the pituitary gland adenocorticotropic hormone (ACTH).

The functions of adrenal medulla are controlled by the hypothalamus. The activation of cells in medulla in response to fear or acute stress results in increased release of catecholamines **epinephrine** and **norepinephrine.** This prepares the individual for a "fight" or "flight," resulting in increased heart rate, cardiac output, increased blood flow, and surge of glucose into the blood from the liver for added energy.

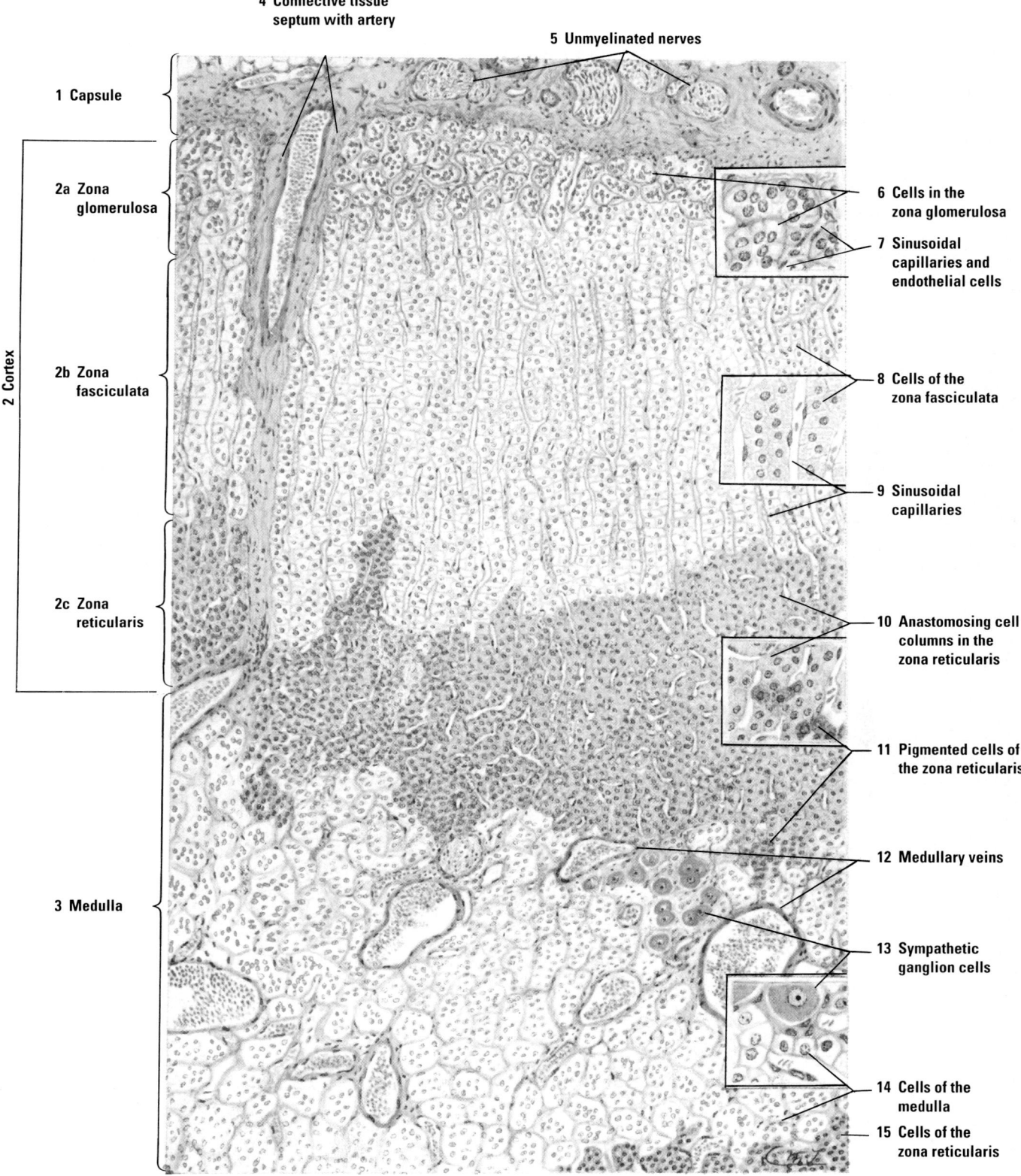

4 Connective tissue septum with artery

5 Unmyelinated nerves

1 Capsule

2a Zona glomerulosa

2 Cortex

2b Zona fasciculata

2c Zona reticularis

3 Medulla

6 Cells in the zona glomerulosa

7 Sinusoidal capillaries and endothelial cells

8 Cells of the zona fasciculata

9 Sinusoidal capillaries

10 Anastomosing cell columns in the zona reticularis

11 Pigmented cells of the zona reticularis

12 Medullary veins

13 Sympathetic ganglion cells

14 Cells of the medulla

15 Cells of the zona reticularis

Fig. 16-8   Adrenal (Suprarenal) Gland. Stain: hematoxylin-eosin. Medium magnification (insets: high magnification).

Figure 16-9   Hypophysis: Pars Distalis, Pars Intermedia, and Pars Nervosa (Human)

A higher power photomicrograph illustrates the dark-staining, cellular pars distalis of adenohypophysis, pars intermedia, and the light-staining neural pars nervosa of the hypophysis. With this stain, different cell types can be identified in pars distalis. The red-staining or eosinophilic cells in pars distalis are the **acidophils (5).** The cells that exhibit bluish cytoplasm are the **basophils (4).** The light, unstained cells scattered among the acidophils (5) and basophils (4) are the **chromophobes (7).** The pars intermedia region of the hypophysis exhibits small cysts or **vesicles (6)** that are filled with secretory colloid material. The pars nervosa contains non-myelinated, light-staining axons of secretory cells, whose cell bodies are located in the hypothalamus. Most of the red-staining nuclei in pars nervosa belong to the supportive cells **pituicytes (2).** Accumulations of neurosecretory material at the end of the axon terminals in pars nervosa are visible as irregular-shaped, red-staining structures called **Herring bodies (3).** These bodies are usually closely associated with capillaries and **blood vessels (1).** Surrounding the secretory cells and axons terminals in the hypophysis are numerous blood vessels (1) and fenestrated capillaries

Figure 16-10   Thyroid Gland and Parathryoid Gland

The parathyroid glands are embedded in the thyroid gland. This photomicrograph shows a section of parathyroid gland adjacent to the thyroid gland. A thin **connective tissue septa (3)** separates the two glands from each other. Different size **follicles** filled with **colloid (1)** and lined by **follicular cells (2)** characterize the thyroid gland parenchyma. The parathyroid gland parenchyma is characterized by the presence of two types of cells, instead of follicles that are seen in the thyroid gland. **Chief cells (4)** are smaller and more numerous. On the other hand, the **oxyphil cells (5)** are larger, less numerous, and their cytoplasm stains highly eosinophilic. Numerous **blood vessels (6)** surround the secretory cell in both endocrine organs.

Figure 16-11   Adrenal (Suprarenal) Gland: Cortex and Medulla

A lower magnification photomicrograph illustrates a section of the adrenal gland. The outer cortex is surrounded by a dense connective tissue **capsule (1).** In the cortex are visible three histological zones. Beneath the capsule (1) is the **zona glomerulosa (2),** whose cells are arranged in irregular ovoid clumps. The intermediate and the widest zone is the **zona fasciculata (3).** In this zone, the cells are arranged into light-staining, narrow cords, between which are found numerous capillaries and fine connective tissue fibers. The innermost zone of the adrenal cortex is the **zona reticularis (4).** The cells in this zone are arranged into irregular groups of branching cords and clumps. The adrenal **medulla (5)** is located adjacent to the zona reticularis (4). In the medulla, the cells are also arranged into clumps and are larger than the cells in zona reticularis (4). In addition, large **blood vessels (6)** (veins) are present in the medulla (5).

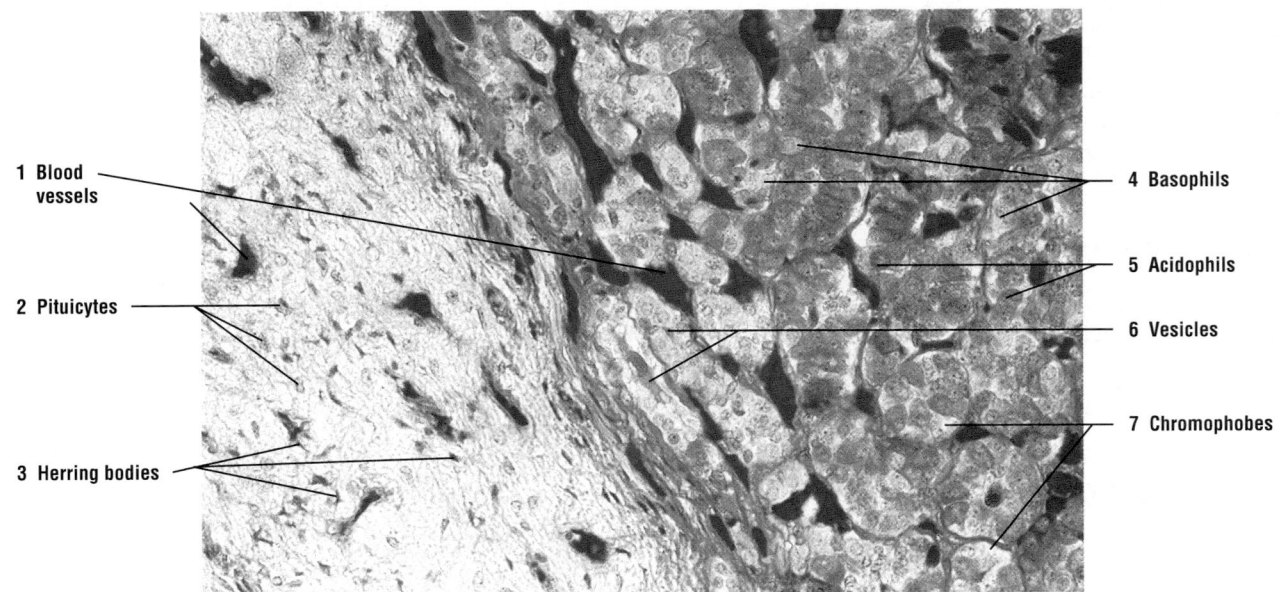

1 Blood vessels

2 Pituicytes

3 Herring bodies

4 Basophils

5 Acidophils

6 Vesicles

7 Chromophobes

Fig. 16-9   Hypophysis: Pars distalis, Pars Intermedia, and Pars Nervosa (Human). Stain: Mallory-azan and orange G. 80×

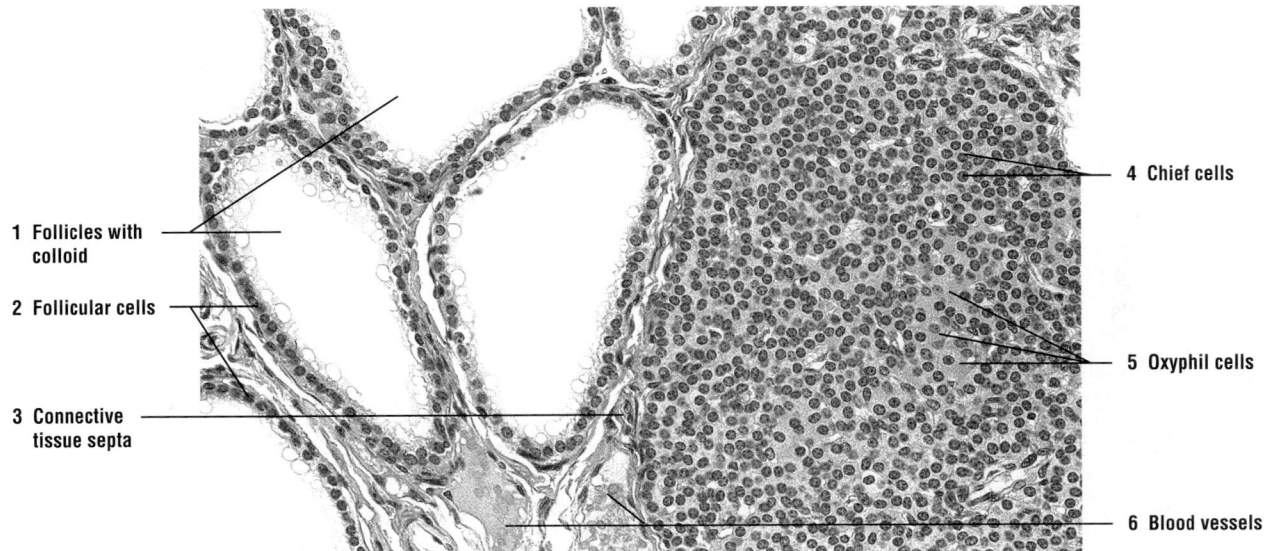

1 Follicles with colloid

2 Follicular cells

3 Connective tissue septa

4 Chief cells

5 Oxyphil cells

6 Blood vessels

Fig. 16-10   Thyroid Gland and Parathryoid Gland. Stain: hematoxylin-eosin. 80×

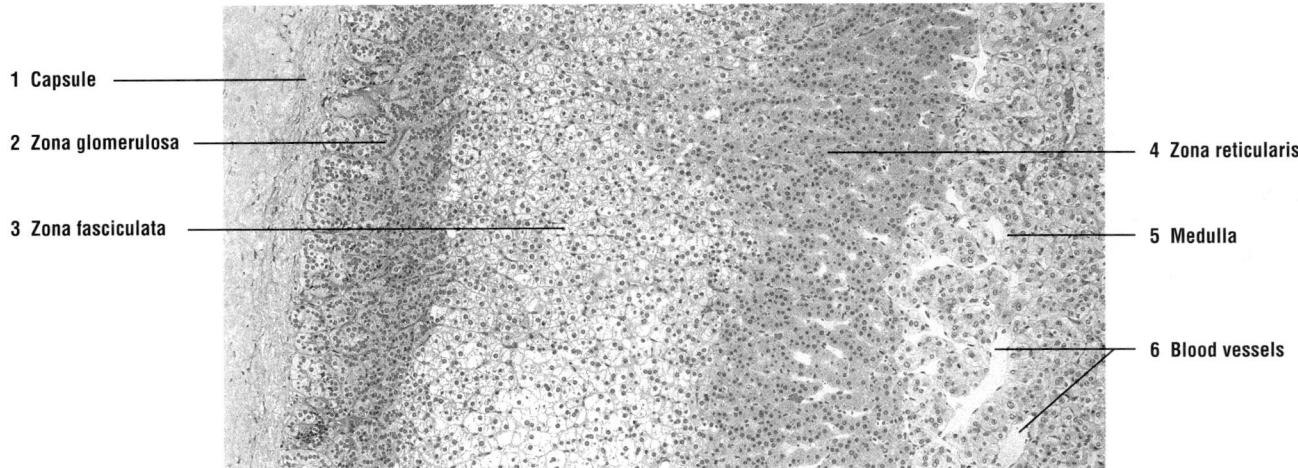

1 Capsule

2 Zona glomerulosa

3 Zona fasciculata

4 Zona reticularis

5 Medulla

6 Blood vessels

Fig. 16-11   Adrenal (Suprarenal) Gland: Cortex and Medulla. Stain: hematoxylin-eosin (plastic section). 25×

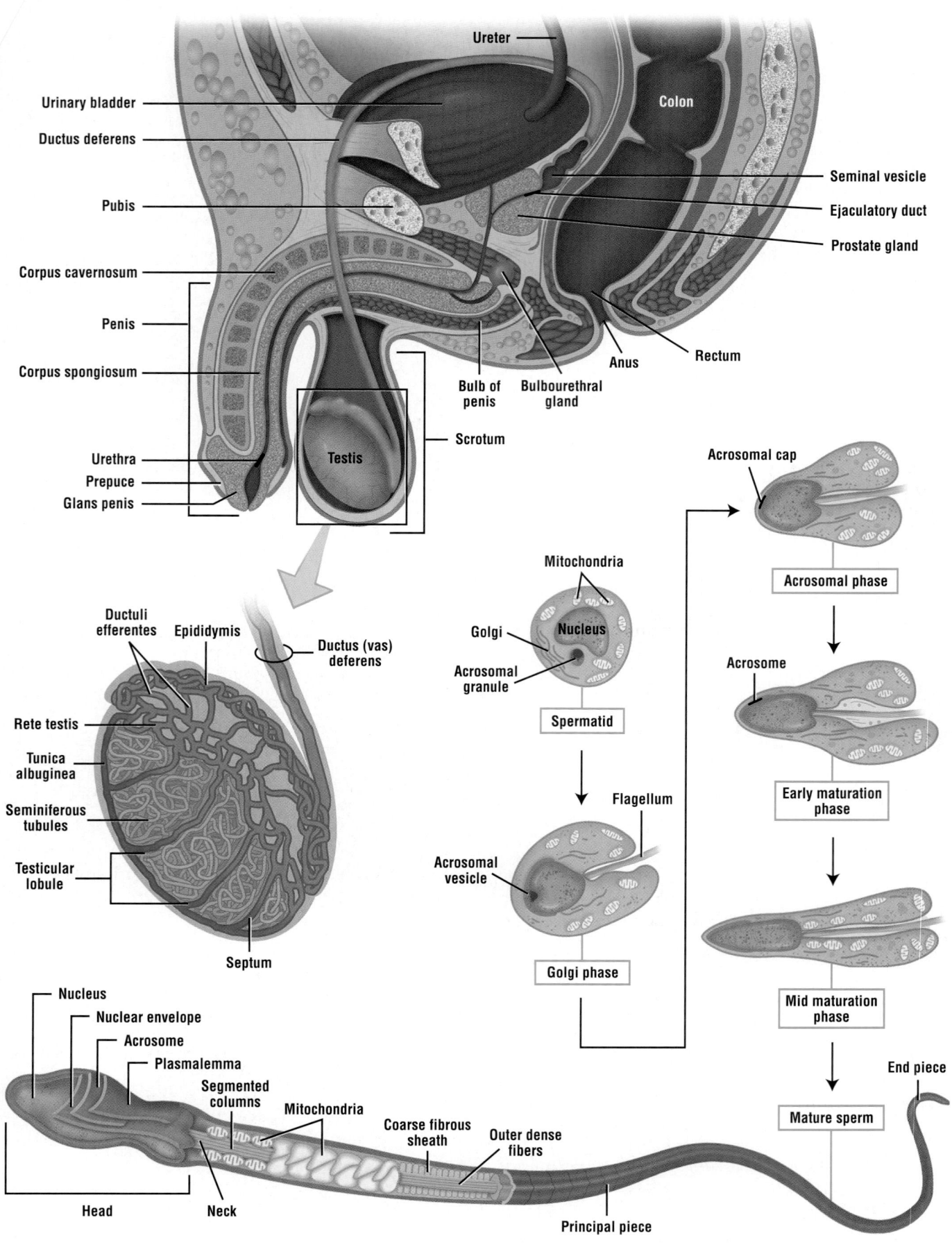

Ureter

Urinary bladder

Ductus deferens

Pubis

Corpus cavernosum

Penis

Corpus spongiosum

Urethra

Prepuce

Glans penis

Colon

Seminal vesicle

Ejaculatory duct

Prostate gland

Anus

Rectum

Bulb of penis

Bulbourethral gland

Scrotum

Testis

Ductuli efferentes

Epididymis

Ductus (vas) deferens

Rete testis

Tunica albuginea

Seminiferous tubules

Testicular lobule

Septum

Mitochondria

Golgi

Nucleus

Acrosomal granule

Spermatid

Acrosomal vesicle

Flagellum

Golgi phase

Acrosomal cap

Acrosomal phase

Acrosome

Early maturation phase

Mid maturation phase

Mature sperm

End piece

Nucleus

Nuclear envelope

Acrosome

Plasmalemma

Segmented columns

Mitochondria

Coarse fibrous sheath

Outer dense fibers

Head

Neck

Principal piece

Male Reproductive System

COMPONENT PARTS

The male reproductive system consists of reproductive organs, excretory ducts, and accessory glands. The major reproductive organs are the paired gonads or **testes.** Because lower body temperature is needed for sperm production, the testes are located in the **scrotum.** The testes continuously produce spermatozoa, which leave the testes and enter the epididymis for storage. The sperm leave the epididymis via the ductus (vas) deferens and exit through the penile **urethra.** The accessory glands are the paired **seminal vesicles,** paired **bulbourethral glands,** and a single **prostate gland.** Secretions from these glands are added to sperm to form **semen.** Penis serves as the copulatory organ. The penile urethra serves as a passageway for urine or semen.

TESTES

A thick, connective tissue capsule, the **tunica albugenia,** surrounds each testis. Posteriorly, the connective tissue extends inward into each testis and forms the **mediastinum testis.** Thin connective tissue **septa** from the mediastinum testis subdivide each testis into about 250 compartments or **testicular lobules,** each containing one to four coiled **seminiferous tubules.** Each seminiferous tubule is lined by the stratified **germinal epithelium,** containing the proliferating **spermatogenic (germ) cells** and nonproliferating **supporting (sustentacular)** or **Sertoli cells.** Here, the maturing spermatogenic cells transform into sperm. Surrounding each seminiferous tubule are fibroblasts, muscle-like cells, nerves, blood vessels, and lymphatic vessels. Between seminiferous tubules are clusters of epithelioid cells, the **interstitial cells (of Leydig),** which produce **testosterone (Figs. 17-1–17-4, 17-15).**

EXCRETORY DUCTS

Sperm from the seminiferous tubules pass first into **straight tubules** (tubuli recti) and then into **rete testis,** the epithelial-lined spaces in the **mediastinum testis.** From rete testis, the sperm enter the head of the **epididymis** via the **ductuli efferentes** (efferent ducts). During ejaculation, strong **smooth muscle** contractions around the epididymal tubules expel the sperms into the **ductus (vas) deferens,** which then conducts them to the urethra **(Figs. 17-2, 17-5–17-9, 17-16).**

ACCESSORY REPRODUCTIVE GLANDS

The **seminal vesicles** are located posterior to the bladder and superior to the prostate gland. Excretory duct of each seminal vesicle joins the dilated terminal part of each ductus (vas) deferens, the **ampulla,** to form the **ejaculatory ducts.** These penetrate the prostate gland and open into the **prostatic urethra (Figs. 17-8, 17-9, 17-11).**

The **prostate gland** is located inferior to the bladder. The **urethra** exits the bladder and passes through the prostate gland as **prostatic urethra.** Ejaculatory ducts and the excretory ducts of prostatic glands enter the prostatic urethra **(Figs. 17-9, 17-10, 17-17).**

The **bulbourethral glands** are small, pea-sized glands located at the root of the **penis** and embedded in the skeletal muscles of the urogenital diaphragm; their excretory ducts terminate in the proximal portion of the **penile urethra (Fig. 17-12).**

The **penis** consists of **erectile tissues,** the paired dorsal **corpora cavernosa** and a single ventral **corpus spongiosum** (urethrae), which expands distally as the **glans penis.** Penile urethra extends through the center of corpus spongiosum. Each erectile body is surrounded by dense connective tissue layer **tunica albugenia.** The erectile tissues consist of irregular vascular spaces lined by vascular endothelium. The trabeculae between these spaces contain collagen and elastic fibers, and smooth muscles. Blood enters the vascular spaces via the **dorsal artery** and **deep arteries of the penis** and is drained by different veins **(Figs. 17-13–17-14).**

■ Functional Correlations of Testes

Spermatogonia

The testes produce the **sperm** and **testosterone,** a hormone that is essential for male sexual characteristics and the accessory reproductive glands. The spermatogenic cells in the **seminiferous tubules** divide, differentiate, and produce sperm by **spermatogenesis.** This involves three phases: (1) **mitotic divisions** of spermatogonia to **spermatocytes;** (2) two **meiotic divisions,** to reduce chromosome numbers by half to form the **spermatids;** and (3) **spermiogenesis,** a morphological transformation of spermatids into sperm.

Sertoli Cells

The **Sertoli cells** perform numerous functions, among which are: (1) **support, protection,** and **nutrition** of the developing sperm (spermatids); (2) **phagocytosis** of excess cytoplasm (residual bodies) of the developing spermatids; (3) release of mature sperm, **spermiation,** into the seminiferous tubules; (4) secretion of **testicular fluid** for nourishment and transport of sperm; and (5) produciton of **androgen-binding protein (ABP)** and the hormone **inhibin.**

Blood-Testis Barrier

The Sertoli cells join laterally by **tight junctions** to form the **blood–testis barrier** that subdivides the seminiferous tubules into **basal** and **adluminal compartments.** This barrier keeps harmful substances in the blood from entering the germinal epithelium and restricts the passage of membrane **antigens** from developing sperm into the blood and the immune system. This prevents an autoimmune response to the individual's own sperm, antibody formation, and induction of sterility.

Hormones

The **follicle-stimulating hormone (FSH)** from the **adenohypophysis** controls the secretion of ABP by the Sertoli cells. The ABP concentrates testosterone in the seminiferous tubules for proper spermatogenesis. The hormone inhibin suppresses or inhibits the production of FSH by the pituitary gland.

Figure 17-1   Testis (sectional view)

Each testis is enclosed in a thick, connective tissue capsule, the **tunica albuginea (1).** Internal to this capsule is a vascular layer of loose connective tissue, the **tunica vasculosa (2, 8).** A loose connective tissue extends inward from the tunica vasculosa (2, 8) and forms the **interstitial connective tissue (3, 12)** of the testis. This connective tissue (3, 12) surrounds, binds, and supports the **seminiferous tubules (4, 6, 9).** Also, extending from the mediastinum testis (Fig. 17-2 below) toward the tunica albuginea (1) are thin fibrous **septa (7, 10).** These septa (7, 10) divide the testis into numerous compartments called lobules. Each lobule contains one to four seminiferous tubules (4, 6, 9). Because the septa are not complete, the lobules intercommunicate. Located in the interstitial connective tissue (3, 12) around the seminiferous tubules (4, 6, 9) are numerous **blood vessels (13),** various loose connective tissue cells, and clusters of epithelial **interstitial cells (of Leydig) (5, 11).** The interstitial cells (5, 11) are the endocrine cells of the testis and secrete the male sex hormone testosterone into the blood stream.

The **seminiferous tubules (4, 6, 9)** are long, highly convoluted tubules in the testis that are normally observed cut in transverse (4), longitudinal (6), or in tangential (9) planes of section. The seminiferous tubules (4, 6, 9) are lined with a specialized stratified epithelium called the **germinal epithelium (14),** which consists of two types of cells, the spermatogenic cells that give rise to the spermatozoa and the supportive Sertoli cells that nourish the developing spermatozoa. These cells rest on the basement membrane of the seminiferous tubules (4, 6, 9) and are illustrated in greater detail in Figures 17-3 and 17-4.

Figure 17-2   Seminiferous Tubules, Straight Tubules, Rete Testis, and Ductuli Efferentes (Efferent Ductules)

In the posterior region of the testis, the connective tissue of tunica albuginea (see the figure above) extends into the testis as the mediastinum testis. In this low magnification illustration, the plane of section passes through a small portion of the **seminiferous tubules (3, 5)** of the testis, the connective tissue and blood vessels of the **mediastinum testis (10, 16),** and the excretory ducts of the testis, the **ductuli efferentes (efferent ductules) (9, 13).** These structures are illustrated below in greater detail as three separate inserts.

A few **seminiferous tubules (3, 5)** are visible on the left side of the illustration; these are lined with spermatogenic epithelium and the sustentacular (Sertoli) cells. The **interstitial connective tissue (4)** of the testis contains the steroid (testosterone) producing **interstitial cells (of Leydig) (1)** and is continuous with the connective tissue of the mediastinum testis (10, 16). In the mediastinum testis (10, 16), the seminiferous tubules (3, 5) of each testicular lobule terminate and form **straight tubules (2, 6).** The straight tubules (2, 6) are short, narrow ducts lined with cuboidal or low columnar epithelium that are devoid of spermatogenic cells.

The straight tubules (2, 6) continue into **rete testis (7, 8, 12)** located in the connective tissue of the mediastinum testis (10, 16). The rete testis (7, 8, 12) are irregular, anastomosing network of tubules with wide lumina lined by a single layer of squamous to low cuboidal or low columnar epithelium; these tubules become wider near the **ductuli efferentes (efferent ductules) (9, 13)** into which they empty. The ductuli efferentes (9, 13) are straight; however, as they continue into the head of the epididymis, they become highly convoluted (see Fig. 17-5). The ductuli efferentes (9, 13) serve as connecting channels from rete testis (7, 8, 12) to the epididymis (see Fig. 17-5). In some of the rete testis (12) and ductuli efferentes (9, 13) are seen aggregations of **sperm (11, 14).**

The epithelium of ductuli efferentes (9, 13) is distinctive because it consists of groups of tall columnar cells that alternate with groups of shorter cuboidal cells. Because of the alterations in the cell heights, the lumina of the ductuli efferentes exhibit an uneven contours. The tall cells in these tubules generally exhibit apical **cilia (15)** while the cuboidal cells exhibit a brush-like border of microvilli.

■ Functional Hormonal Correlations-Male Reproductive Organs

Normal spermatogenesis depends on proper levels of both the **luteinizing hormone (LH)** and **follicle stimulating hormone (FSH),** hormones produced by the **gonadotrophs** in the **adenohypophysis** of the pituitary gland. LH stimulates the production of **testosterone** by the **interstitial cells.** FSH stimulates the **Sertoli cells** to produce the **androgen-binding protein;** high levels of testosterone are needed in the seminiferous tubules for normal spermatogenesis. In addition, the structure and function of all accessory reproductive glands, as well as development and maintenance of male secondary sexual characteristics are dependent on proper testosterone levels. In addition to hormones, proper **temperature** in the testes is crucial for spermatogenesis, which is normally approximately 2 to 3°C cooler than the core body temperature. Location of the testes in the scrotum provides some of this cooling. Also, a venous **pampiniform plexus** surrounds **testicular arteries** and provides for a countercurrent **heat-exchange.** Blood in the testicular arteries that flows into the testes is cooled and blood in the veins that returns to the body is warmed.

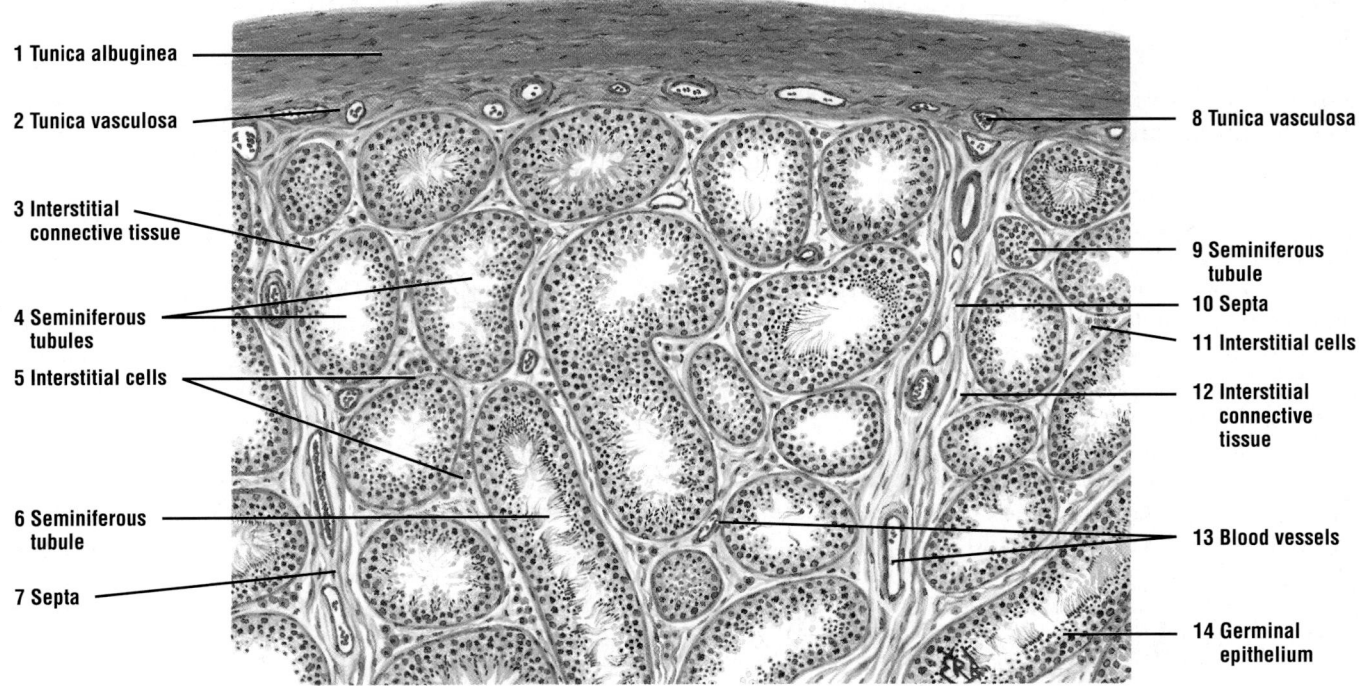

1 Tunica albuginea

2 Tunica vasculosa

3 Interstitial connective tissue

4 Seminiferous tubules

5 Interstitial cells

6 Seminiferous tubule

7 Septa

8 Tunica vasculosa

9 Seminiferous tubule

10 Septa

11 Interstitial cells

12 Interstitial connective tissue

13 Blood vessels

14 Germinal epithelium

Fig. 17-1   Testis (sectional view). Stain: hematoxylin-eosin. Low magnification.

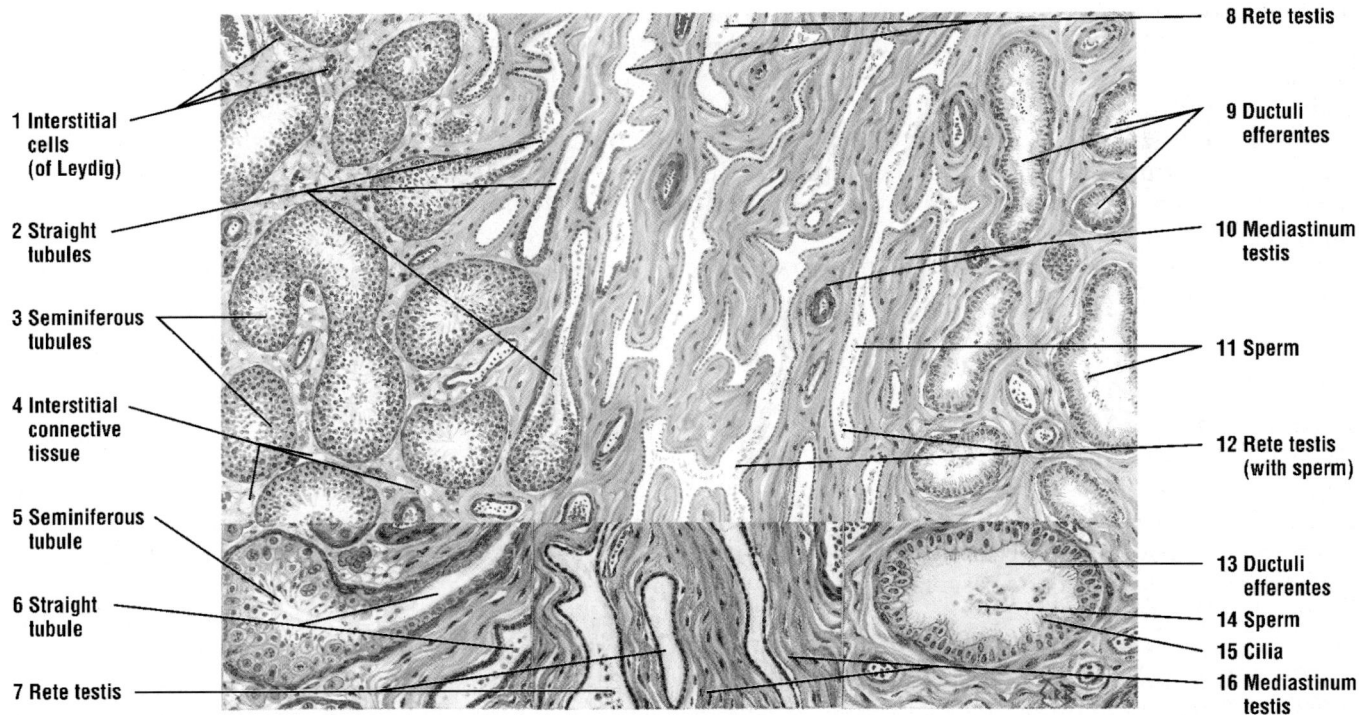

1 Interstitial cells (of Leydig)

2 Straight tubules

3 Seminiferous tubules

4 Interstitial connective tissue

5 Seminiferous tubule

6 Straight tubule

7 Rete testis

8 Rete testis

9 Ductuli efferentes

10 Mediastinum testis

11 Sperm

12 Rete testis (with sperm)

13 Ductuli efferentes

14 Sperm

15 Cilia

16 Mediastinum testis

Fig. 17-2   Seminiferous Tubules, Straight Tubules, Rete Testis, and Ductuli Efferentes (Efferent Ductules). Stain: hematoxylin-eosin. Low magnification (inset: high magnification).

Figure 17-3   Primate Testis: Spermatogenesis in Seminiferous Tubules (transverse section)

Different stages of spermatogenesis are illustrated in various **seminiferous tubules (3)**. Each tubule (3) is surrounded by an outer layer of connective tissue with **fibroblasts (1)** and an inner **basement membrane (2)**. Between the tubules is the interstitial tissue, consisting of **fibroblasts (18), blood vessels (10)**, nerves, and lymphatics. Also prominent between the seminiferous tubules (3) are the **interstitial cells (of Leydig) (11, 15)**.

The stratified germinal epithelium of the seminiferous tubules consists of the **supporting** or **Sertoli cells (6, 7, 14)** and the **spermatogenic cells (5, 9, 12)**. The Sertoli cells (6, 7, 14) are slender, elongated cells with irregular outlines extending from the basement membrane to the lumen of the seminiferous tubule (3). The nucleus of the Sertoli cells (6, 7, 14) is generally ovoid or elongated and contains fine, sparse chromatin. A distinct nucleolus in the Sertoli cells (6, 7, 14) distinguishes them from the spermatogenic cells (5, 9, 12), which are arranged in rows between and around the Sertoli cells. In different sections, the spermatogenic cells often appear superimposed on Sertoli cells (6, 7, 14), obscuring their cytoplasm.

The immature spermatogenic cells, the **spermatogonia (12)**, are situated adjacent to the basement membrane (2) of the seminiferous tubules (3). The spermatogonia (12) divide mitotically to produce several generations of cells. Three types of spermatogonia are usually recognized. The **pale type A spermatogonia (12a)** have a light-staining cytoplasm and a round or ovoid nucleus with pale, finely granular chromatin. The **dark type A spermatogonia (12b)** appear similar, but the chromatin stains darker. In type B spermatogonia (not illustrated), the chromatin granules in the spherical nucleus are variable and the nucleolus is centrally located.

Type A spermatogonia (12a) serve as stem cells of the germinal epithelium and give rise to other type A and type B spermatogonia. The final mitosis of type B spermatogonia produces **primary spermatocytes (5, 16)**. The nuclei of these cells have variable appearances because of different states of activity of the chromatin. These cells promptly enter the first meiotic division and the representative meiotic figures are prevalent in the seminiferous tubules (3).

Primary spermatocytes (5, 16) are the most obvious and largest germ cells in the seminiferous tubules (3) and occupy the middle region of the germinal epithelium. Their cytoplasm contains large nuclei with coarse clumps or thin threads of chromatin. The first meiotic division of the primary spermatocytes (Fig. 17-4 I, 5) produces smaller secondary spermatocytes with less dense nuclear chromatin (Fig. 17-4 I, 3). The secondary spermatocytes (Fig. 17-4 I, 3) undergo second meiotic division shortly after their formation and are therefore not frequently seen in sections of the seminiferous tubules (3).

Completion of the second meiotic division produces **spermatids (4, 8, 9, 13, 17)**, which are smaller cells than the primary or secondary spermatocytes (Fig. 17-4 I, 2, 3, 5). These cells lie in groups in the adluminal portion of the seminiferous tubule in close association with the Sertoli cells (6, 13, 14). In this environment, the spermatids (4, 8, 9, 13, 17) differentiate into spermatozoa by a process called spermiogenesis. The small, dark-staining heads of the maturing spermatids (4, 8) lie embedded in the cytoplasm of the Sertoli cells (6, 7, 14), and their tails extend into the lumen of the seminiferous tubule (3).

Figure 17-4   Primate Testis: Stages of Spermatogenesis

Three different stages of spermatogenesis are illustrated in greater detail. In the **left illustration (I)**, the **primary spermatocytes (5)** are undergoing meiotic division to form the **secondary spermatocytes (3)**, which in turn undergo rapid division to form the **spermatids (1, 2)**. In this stage, the spermatids (1) are embedded deep in the **Sertoli cell (4)** cytoplasm. Adjacent to the basement membrane are the **type A spermatogonia (6)**.

In the **middle illustration (II)**, the **spermatids (7)** are located peripherally near the lumen of the seminiferous tubule prior to being released. Also visible are clumps of round **spermatids (8)** and **primary spermatocytes (9)** in close association with the **Sertoli cells (10)**. Near the base of the tubule are found **spermatogonia (11)**.

In the **right illustration (III)**, the mature sperm have been released (spermiation) into the seminiferous tubule and the germinal epithelium contains only **spermatids (8), primary spermatocytes (9), spermatogonia (11)**, and the supporting **Sertoli cells (10)**.

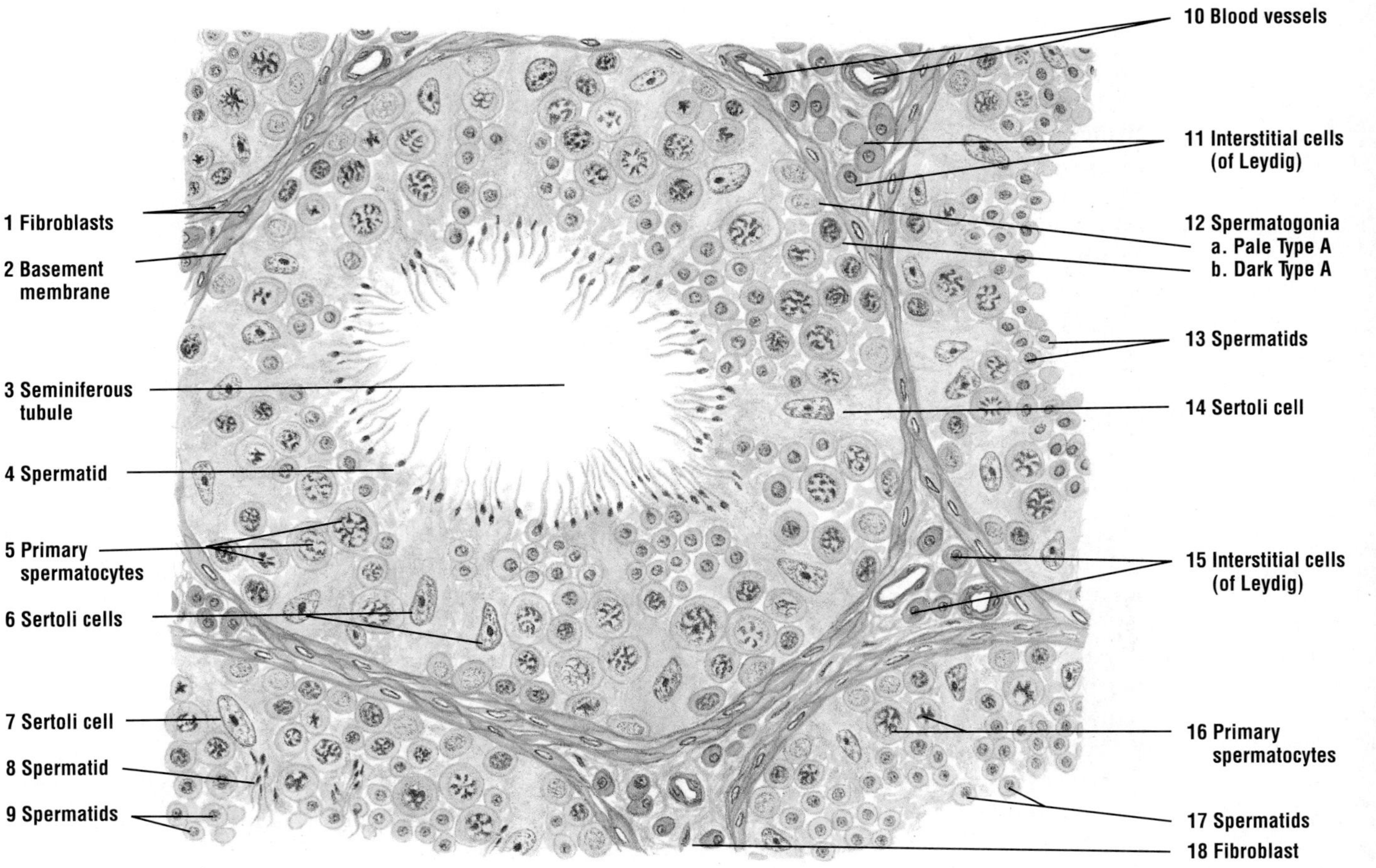

10 Blood vessels

11 Interstitial cells
(of Leydig)

1 Fibroblasts

2 Basement
membrane

12 Spermatogonia
a. Pale Type A
b. Dark Type A

3 Seminiferous
tubule

13 Spermatids

14 Sertoli cell

4 Spermatid

5 Primary
spermatocytes

6 Sertoli cells

15 Interstitial cells
(of Leydig)

7 Sertoli cell

8 Spermatid

16 Primary
spermatocytes

9 Spermatids

17 Spermatids

18 Fibroblast

Fig. 17-3   Primate Testis: Spermatogenesis in Seminiferous Tubules (transverse section). Stain: hematoxylin-eosin. Medium magnification.

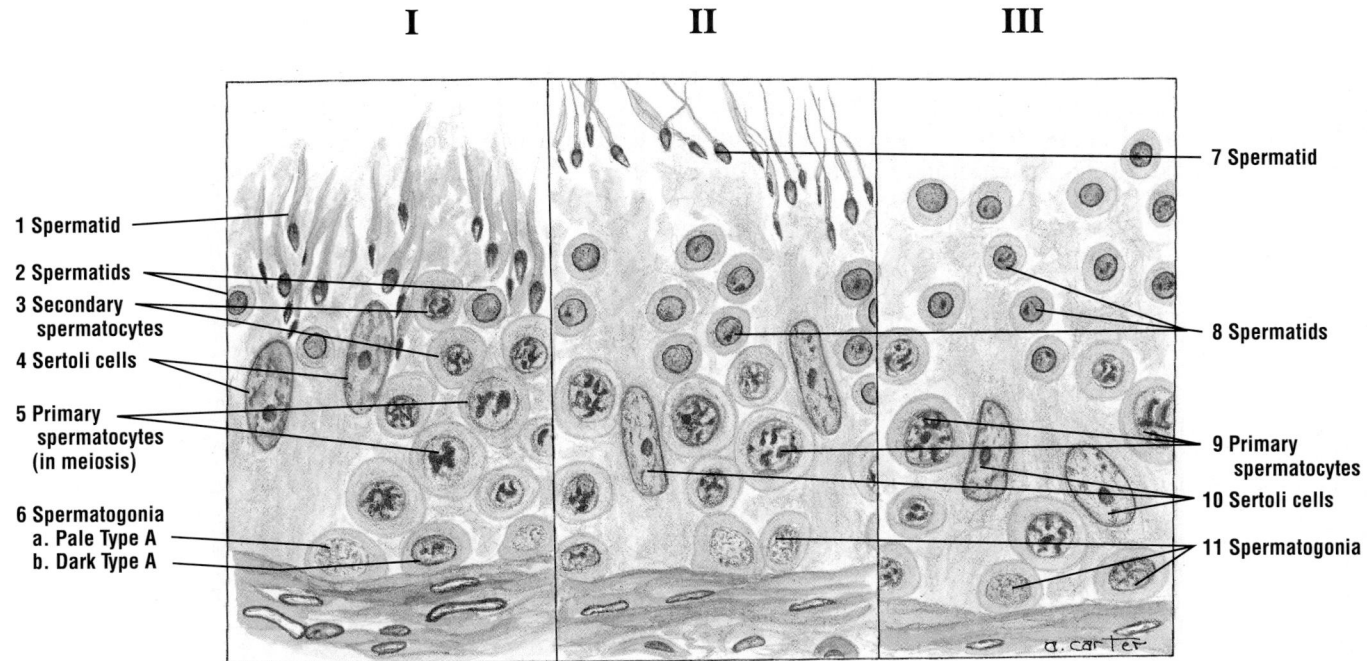

I   II   III

1 Spermatid

7 Spermatid

2 Spermatids

3 Secondary
spermatocytes

4 Sertoli cells

5 Primary
spermatocytes
(in meiosis)

8 Spermatids

6 Spermatogonia
a. Pale Type A
b. Dark Type A

9 Primary
spermatocytes

10 Sertoli cells

11 Spermatogonia

a. carter

Fig. 17-4   Primate Testis: Stages of Spermatogenesis. Stain: hematoxylin-eosin. High magnification.

Figure 17-5   Ductuli Efferentes and Transition to Ductus Epididymis

The ductuli efferentes (1, 4, 5) or efferent ductules emerge from the mediastinum on the posterior-superior surface of the testis and connect the rete testis with the ductus epididymis. The ductuli efferentes are located in the **connective tissue (2)** and form a portion of the head of the **epididymis (7).** Because of the tortuous, spiral course of the tubules, they are seen as isolated tubules cut in various planes of section (1, 5).

The lumina of the ducts exhibit a characteristic irregular contour. The lining epithelium is simple, consisting of alternating groups of tall **ciliated** and shorter **nonciliated cells (4),** which are believed to be absorptive. Occasional basal cells may be present, giving the epithelium a pseudostratified appearance. The basal surface of the tubules has a smooth contour. Located under the basement membrane is a thin layer of connective tissue containing a thin layer of circularly arranged **smooth muscle fibers (3).**

The distal ends of the tubules near the epididymis are lined with columnar cells only **(6),** and the lumina exhibit an even contour. As the ductuli efferentes terminate in the ductus epididymis, there is an abrupt transition of the epithelium to the tall pseudostratified columnar type of the **epididymis (7).**

Figure 17-6   Ductus Epididymis

The ductus epididymis is a long, highly convoluted tubule surrounded by the **connective tissue (1).** A transverse section through the epididymis shows the **convoluted tubules (2, 5, 6)** in highly varied forms. The individual tubules are surrounded by **smooth muscle fibers (7)** and **connective tissue (1).** Both the internal and external surfaces of the tubules have smooth contours.

The tubular epithelium of ductus epididymis is **pseudostratified (4, 9),** consisting of tall **columnar principal cells (9)** with long, nonmotile **stereocilia (8)** and small **basal cells (10).** The function of the columnar principal cells (9) with stereocilia (8) is primarily absorption of the tubular fluid; the function of the basal cells is not known. The stereocilia (8) are long, branched microvilli.

The **basement membrane (3)** that surrounds each tubule is distinct. The lamina propria with the circularly arranged smooth muscle fibers (7) is thin and more pronounced than in the ductuli efferentes. Mature spermatozoa are seen in the lumina of some of the tubules.

■ Functional Correlations–Excretory Ducts

The motile cilia in the **ductuli efferentes** assist in transporting the sperm from the seminiferous tubules to the ductus **epididymis.** The cuboidal nonciliated cells absorb some of the testicular fluid that was produced in the seminiferous tubules by the Sertoli cells. In addition, the **principal cells** that are lined with **stereocilia** in the ducts of the epididymis also absorb testicular fluid during the passage of sperm. The principal cells also **phagocytose** remaining residual bodies that were not removed by the Sertoli cells in the seminiferous tubules and any degenerating sperm cells. The highly coiled ducts of the epididymis function as sites for **accumulation, storage,** and **maturation** of sperm. Here, the sperm acquire the motility and ability to fertilize an egg. The principal cells also produce a glycoprotein that **inhibits capacitation** of the sperms until they are deposited in the female reproductive tract.

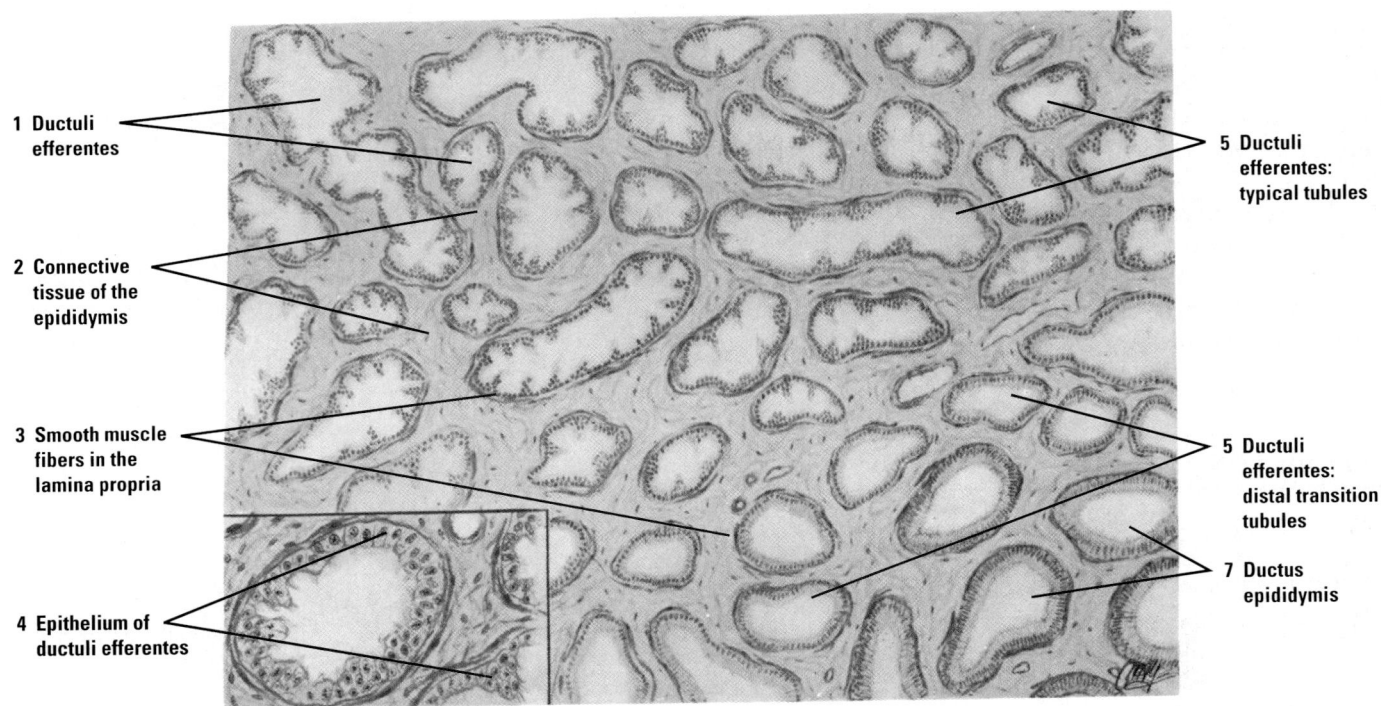

1 Ductuli efferentes

2 Connective tissue of the epididymis

3 Smooth muscle fibers in the lamina propria

4 Epithelium of ductuli efferentes

5 Ductuli efferentes: typical tubules

5 Ductuli efferentes: distal transition tubules

7 Ductus epididymis

Fig. 17-5 Ductuli Efferentes and Transition to Ductus Epididymis. Stain: hematoxylin-eosin. Low magnification (inset: medium magnification).

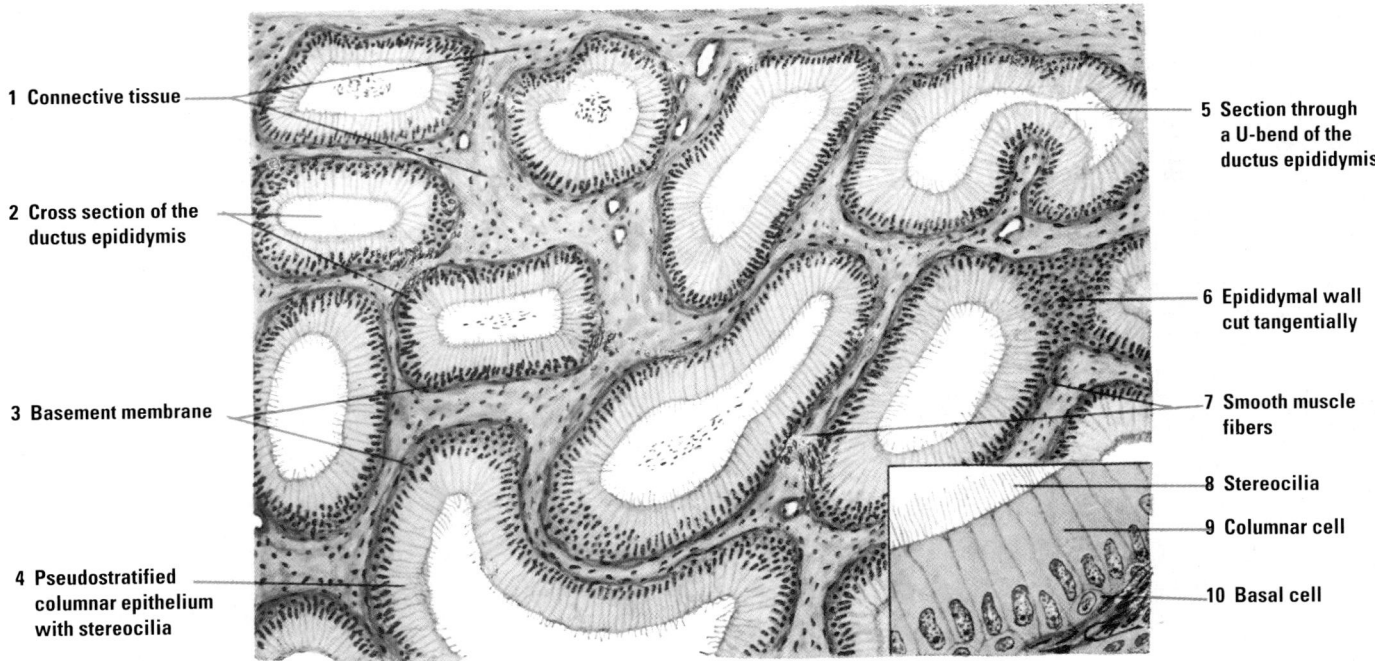

1 Connective tissue

2 Cross section of the ductus epididymis

3 Basement membrane

4 Pseudostratified columnar epithelium with stereocilia

5 Section through a U-bend of the ductus epididymis

6 Epididymal wall cut tangentially

7 Smooth muscle fibers

8 Stereocilia

9 Columnar cell

10 Basal cell

Fig. 17-6 Ductus Epididymis. Stain: hematoxylin-eosin. Low magnification (inset: high magnification).

Figure 17-7   Ductus Deferens (transverse section)

The ductus deferens exhibits a narrow, irregular lumen, a thin mucosa, a thick muscularis, and adventitia. The irregular outline of the lumen is caused by longitudinal folds of the **lamina propria (5, 6),** which in transverse section appear as crests or papillae (6). The thin lamina propria (5, 6) consists of compact collagen fibers and fine elastic network.

The **epithelium** is **pseudostratified columnar (7)** but is somewhat lower than the epithelium lining the ductus epididymis. The epithelium rests on a thin basement membrane and stereocilia is usually seen on the cell apices.

The muscularis consists of a thin **inner longitudinal layer (3),** a thick **middle circular layer (2),** and a thin **outer longitudinal smooth muscle layer (1).** The muscularis is surrounded by **adventitia (4),** which contains abundant blood vessels and nerves. The adventitia (4) merges with the connective tissue surrounding the spermatic cord.

Figure 17-8   Ampulla of the Ductus Deferens (transverse section)

The terminal portion of ductus deferens enlarges into an ampulla. The ampulla differs from the ductus deferens mainly in the structure of its mucosa.

The lumen of the ampulla is larger and the mucosa exhibits numerous thin, irregular, branching **folds (6)** with diverticula or **glandular crypts (5, 9)** located between them. The epithelium lining the lumen and the crypts is simple **columnar** or **cuboidal (7)** and is secretory in nature.

The muscularis is similar to the ductus deferens. It consists of a thin **outer longitudinal layer (3),** a thick **middle layer (2),** and a thin **inner longitudinal smooth muscle layer (1)** adjacent to the **lamina propria (8).**

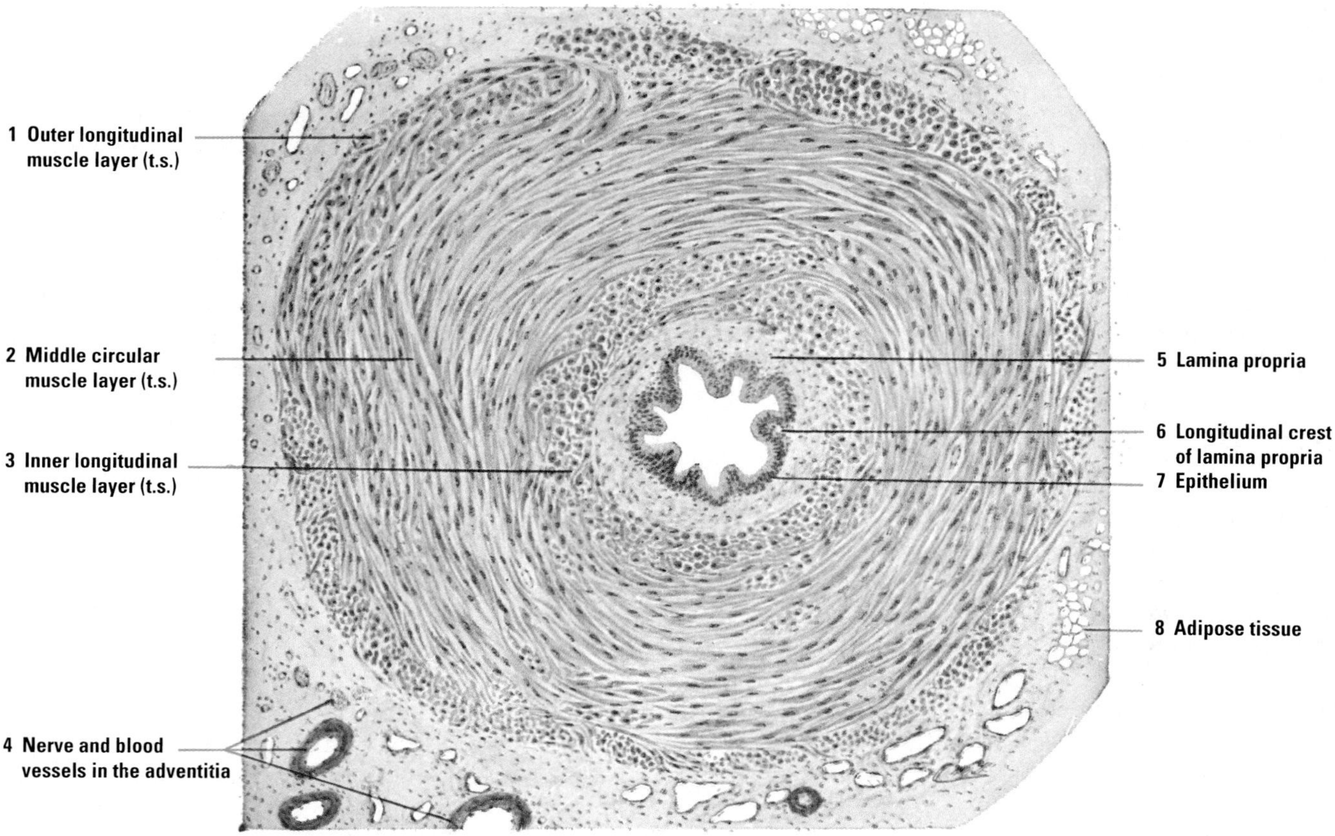

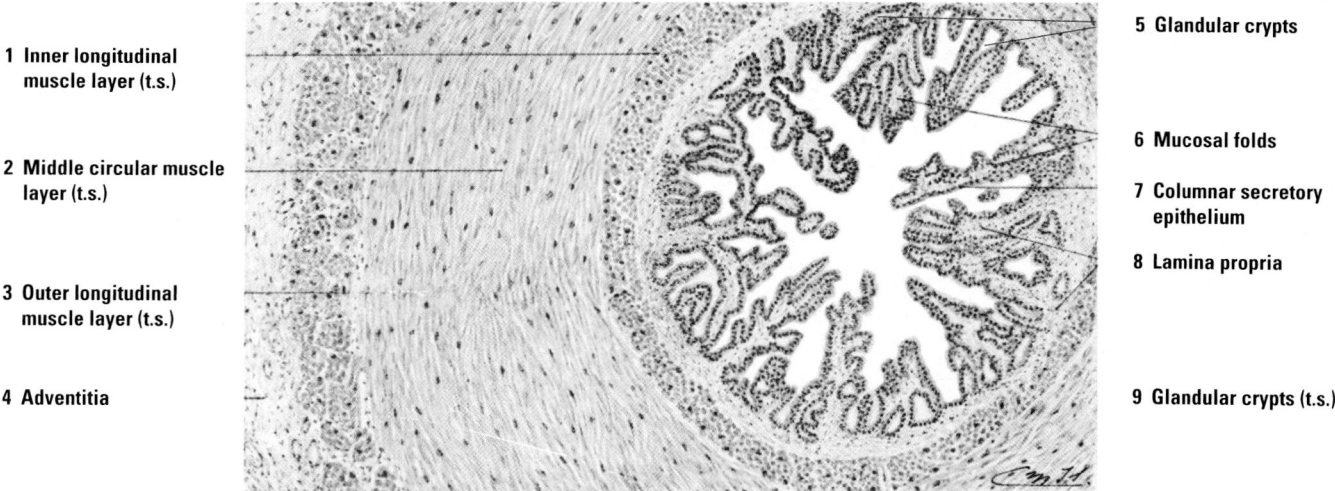

1 Outer longitudinal muscle layer (t.s.)

2 Middle circular muscle layer (t.s.)

3 Inner longitudinal muscle layer (t.s.)

4 Nerve and blood vessels in the adventitia

5 Lamina propria

6 Longitudinal crest of lamina propria

7 Epithelium

8 Adipose tissue

Fig. 17-7   Ductus Deferens (transverse section). Stain: hematoxylin-eosin. Low magnification.

1 Inner longitudinal muscle layer (t.s.)

2 Middle circular muscle layer (t.s.)

3 Outer longitudinal muscle layer (t.s.)

4 Adventitia

5 Glandular crypts

6 Mucosal folds

7 Columnar secretory epithelium

8 Lamina propria

9 Glandular crypts (t.s.)

Fig. 17-8   Ampulla of the Ductus Deferens (transverse section). Stain: hematoxylin-eosin. Low magnification.

Figure 17-9   Prostate Gland With Prostatic Urethra

In the prostate gland, the secretory **acini (4, 5)** are part of the many small, irregularly branched tubuloacinar glands; the acini (4, 5) vary in size. The larger-sized acini exhibit wide, irregular lumina (4) and variable epithelium (see Fig. 17-10). The glands are embedded in a characteristic, **fibromuscular stroma (3)** in which strands of **smooth muscle (6)**, collagen, and elastic fibers are oriented in various directions.

The **prostatic urethra (1)** is as a crescent-shaped structure with small **diverticula (8)** in its lumen; the diverticula are especially prominent in the **urethral recesses (9).** The epithelium in the prostatic urethra (1) is usually transitional and a fibromuscular stroma surrounds the urethra (3); however, a thin lamina propria may be present.

A ridge of dense fibromuscular stroma without glands, the **colliculus seminalis (2),** protrudes into the urethral lumen (1), giving it a crescent shape. The **prostatic utricle (7, 10)** is situated in the mass of the colliculus seminalis (2) and is often dilated at its distal end before entering the urethra. Its thin mucous membrane is typically folded, and the epithelium is usually of the simple secretory or pseudostratified columnar type.

Figure 17-10   Prostate Gland (sectional view, prostatic glands)

A small section of the prostate gland from Figure 17-9 is illustrated with more detail and at a higher magnification.

The size of **glandular acini (1)** is variable. Their lumina are wide and typically irregular because of the protrusion of the epithelium-covered connective **tissue folds (5).** A characteristic feature in the acini of the prostate gland are the spherical **prostatic concretions (8)** that are formed by concentric layers of condensed prostatic secretions. The number of prostatic concretions increases with the age of the individual, and they may become calcified.

Although the **glandular epithelium (4)** is usually simple columnar or pseudostratified and the cells are light-staining in the distal regions, there is considerable variation. In some regions, the epithelium may be squamous or cuboidal.

The **ducts (7)** of the glands may resemble the acini and it is often difficult to distinguish the difference between the two structures. In the terminal portions of the ducts (7), the epithelium is usually columnar and stains darker before entering the urethra.

The **fibromuscular stroma (6)** is a characteristic feature of the prostate gland. **Smooth muscle fibers (3)** and the **connective tissue fibers (9)** can, at times, be distinguished; however, they blend together in the **stroma (6)** and are distributed throughout the gland.

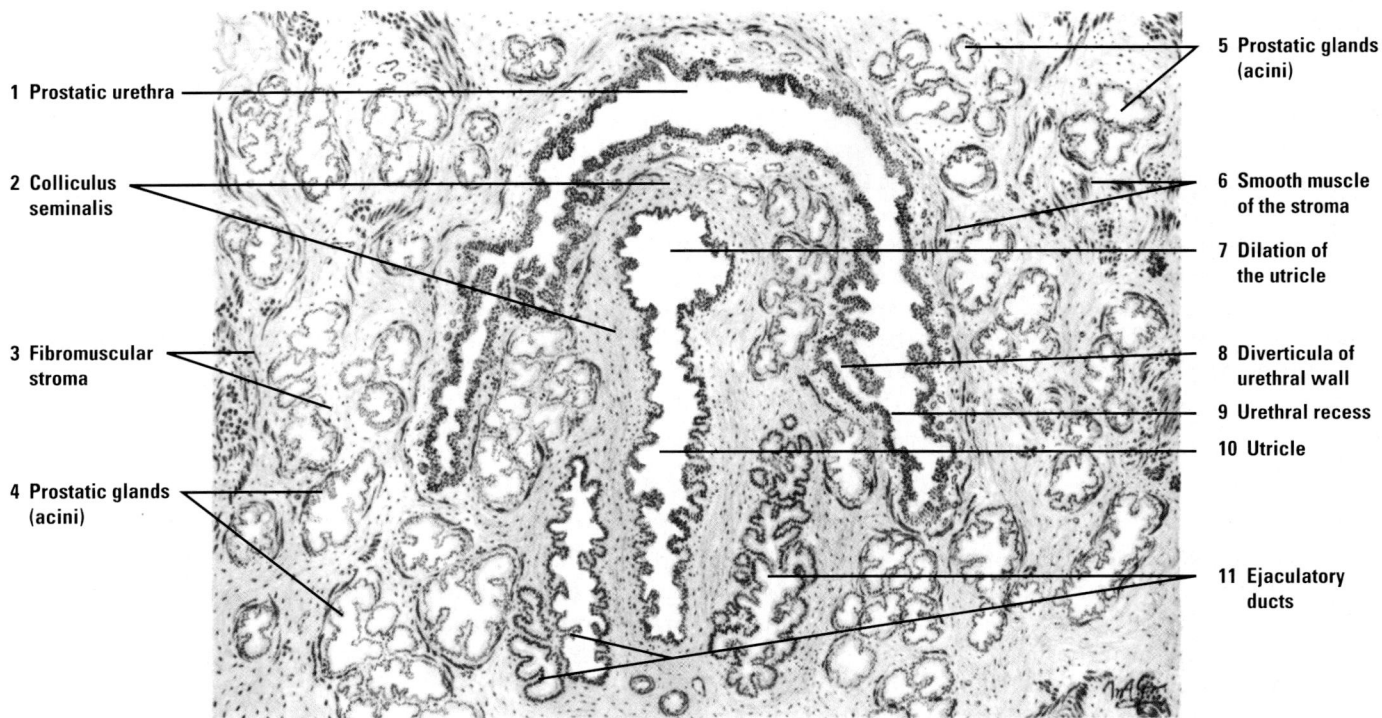

1 Prostatic urethra

2 Colliculus seminalis

3 Fibromuscular stroma

4 Prostatic glands (acini)

5 Prostatic glands (acini)

6 Smooth muscle of the stroma

7 Dilation of the utricle

8 Diverticula of urethral wall

9 Urethral recess

10 Utricle

11 Ejaculatory ducts

Fig. 17-9   Prostate Gland With Prostatic Urethra. Stain: hematoxylin-eosin. Low magnification.

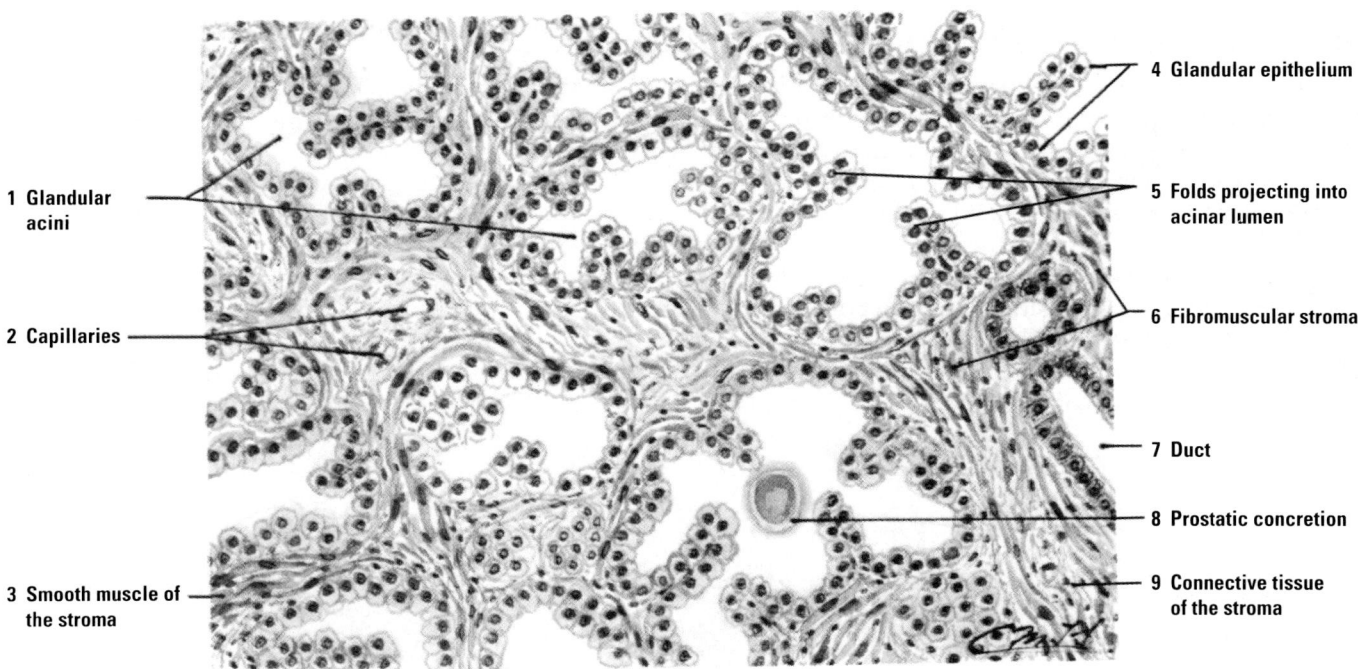

1 Glandular acini

2 Capillaries

3 Smooth muscle of the stroma

4 Glandular epithelium

5 Folds projecting into acinar lumen

6 Fibromuscular stroma

7 Duct

8 Prostatic concretion

9 Connective tissue of the stroma

Fig. 17-10   Prostate Gland (sectional view, prostatic glands). Stain: hematoxylin-eosin. Medium magnification.

Figure 17-11   Seminal Vesicle

The paired seminal vesicles are elongated bodies or sacs with highly convoluted and irregular lumina. A cross section through the gland illustrates the complexity of the **primary folds (5).** These folds branch into numerous **secondary folds (6)** which frequently anastomose, forming **crypts (1)** and cavities. The **lamina propria (7)** projects and forms the core of the larger primary folds (5) and thin stroma of smaller secondary folds (6). These folds extend far into the lumen of the seminal vesicle.

The **glandular epithelium (4)** of the seminal vesicles varies in appearance but is usually of the low pseudostratified type with basal cells and low columnar or cuboidal secretory cells.

The **muscularis (2)** consists of inner circular and outer longitudinal smooth muscle layers. This arrangement of the muscles is often difficult to observe because of the complex folding of the mucosa. The **adventitia (3)** surrounds the muscularis and blends with the connective tissue.

Figure 17-12   Bulbourethral Gland (sectional view)

This is a compound tubuloacinar gland. One lobule and portions of other lobules of the gland are illustrated in the figure. The bulbourethral gland is surrounded by **skeletal muscle (2)** and **connective tissue (1).** The skeletal muscle and some smooth muscle fibers are also present in the **interlobular septa (3).**

The secretory units vary in structure and size. Most of the units have **acinar (4)** shape and others exhibit **tubular (5)** or variable other shapes. The secretory product is primarily mucus (4). The secretory cells are cuboidal, low columnar or squamous, and light-staining. Interspersed among the secretory cells are darker-staining acidophilic cells.

Smaller excretory ducts may be lined with secretory cells, whereas the larger **excretory ducts (6)** exhibit pseudostratified or stratified columnar epithelium.

■ Functional Correlations–Accessory Reproductive Glands

The secretory products of seminal vesicles, the prostate gland, and bulbourethral glands, mixed with sperm, constitute **semen.** Semen provides the sperm with transport medium and nutrients, while neutralizing the acidity of the male urethra and vaginal canal, and activating the sperm after ejaculation.

The **seminal vesicles** produce a yellowish, viscous fluid that contains a high concentration of **fructose,** the main carbohydrate of the semen. Fructose is metabolized by the sperm and serves as a source of energy for the sperm's motility. Seminal vesicles produce most of the fluid found in the semen.

The **prostate gland** produces a thin, watery, slightly acidic fluid rich in citric acid, acid phosphatase, and amylase. The enzyme fibrinolysin in the fluid liquefies the congealed semen after ejaculation.

The **bulbourethral glands** produce a clear, viscid, mucus-like secretion that, during erotic stimulation, is released and serves as a lubricant for the penile urethra. During ejaculation, the secretions from bulbourethral glands precede other components of the semen.

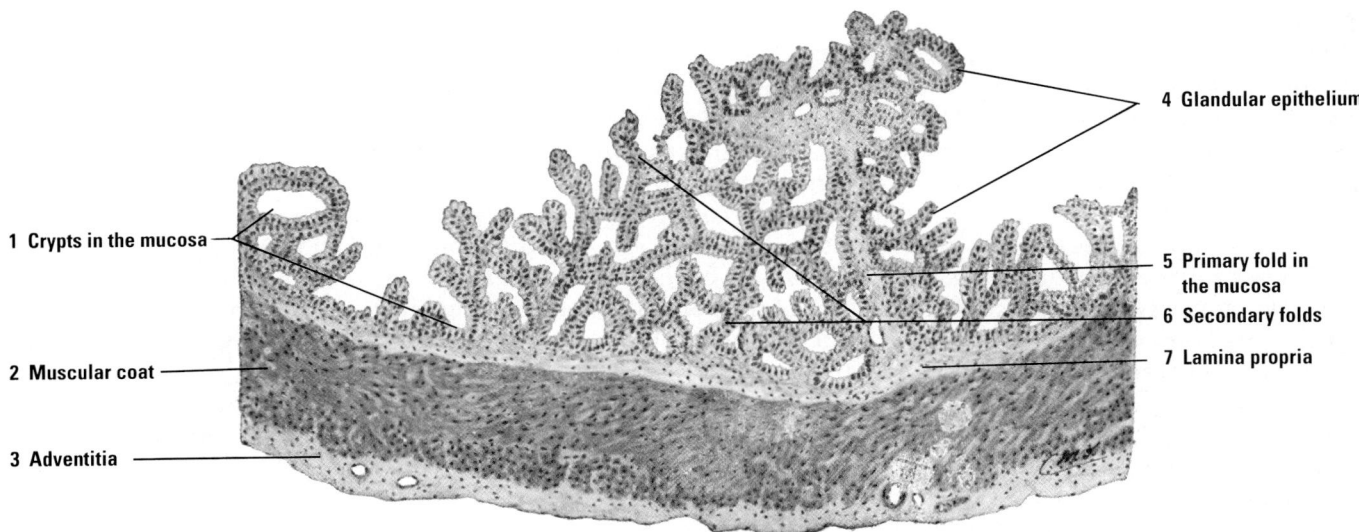

1 Crypts in the mucosa

2 Muscular coat

3 Adventitia

4 Glandular epithelium

5 Primary fold in
the mucosa

6 Secondary folds

7 Lamina propria

Fig. 17-11   Seminal Vesicle. Stain: hematoxylin-eosin. Low magnification.

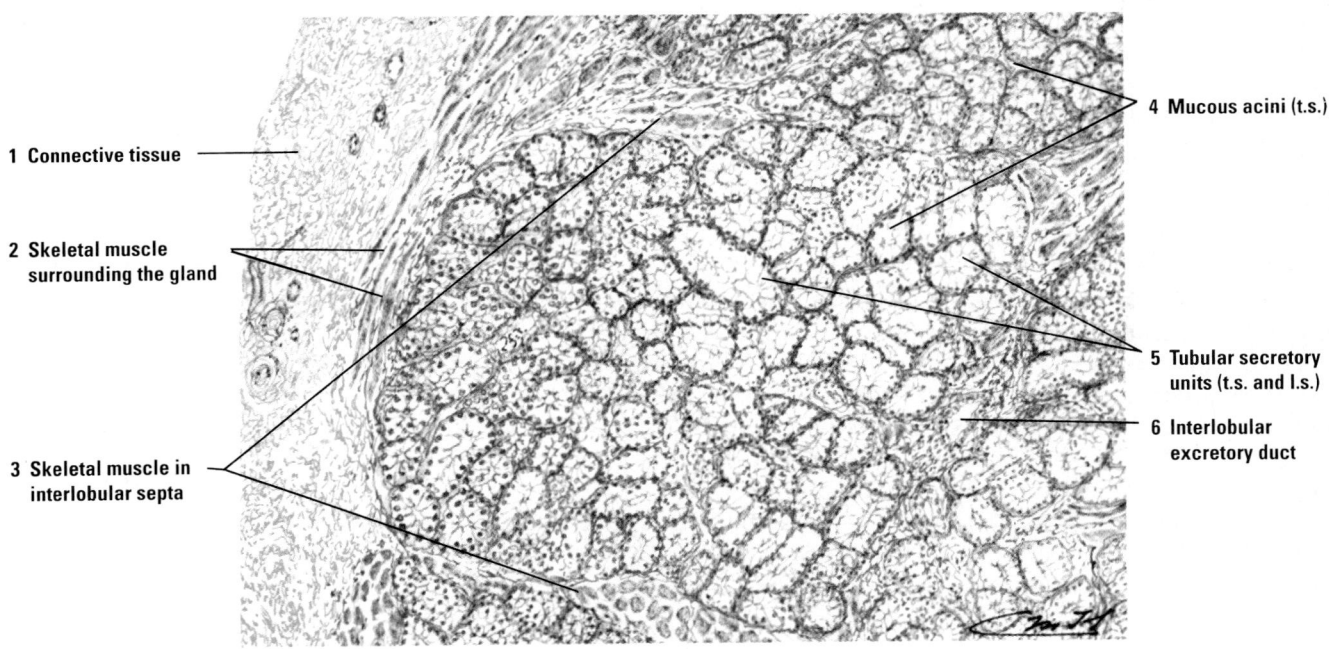

1 Connective tissue

2 Skeletal muscle
surrounding the gland

3 Skeletal muscle in
interlobular septa

4 Mucous acini (t.s.)

5 Tubular secretory
units (t.s. and l.s.)

6 Interlobular
excretory duct

Fig. 17-12   Bulbourethral Gland (sectional view). Stain: Masson's. High magnification.

Figure 17-13   Penis (transverse section)

A cross section of the penis (human) illustrates the three cavernous bodies: the two adjacent **corpora cavernosa (9)** and a single **corpus spongiosum (16)**, through which passes the **urethra (15)**. Surrounding the corpora cavernosa (9) of the penis is a thick, fibrous connective tissue capsule, the **tunica albuginea (5)**; it also extends between the two bodies as the **median septum (10)**. This septum is better developed at the posterior end of the penis than at the anterior end. The **tunica albuginea (6)** surrounding the **corpus spongiosum** (corpus cavernosa urethrae) **(16)** is thinner than that around the corpora cavernosa **(9)** and contains smooth muscle and elastic fibers.

All three cavernous bodies are surrounded by loose connective tissue, the deep **penile** (Buck's) **fascia (4)** which, in turn, is surrounded by the connective tissue of the **dermis (2)** that is located immediately under the **epidermis (1)**. Strands of smooth muscle, the **dartos tunic (3)**, and an abundance of peripheral blood vessels are located in the dermis (2). **Sebaceous glands (7)** are present in the dermis on the ventral side of the penis.

The core of each corpus cavernosum (9) is occupied by numerous **trabeculae (14),** which consist of collagenous, elastic, and smooth muscle fibers. The trabeculae (14) surround the cavernous cavities or **sinuses (veins) (12)** of the corpora cavernosa (9). Nerves and blood vessels are present in the trabeculae (14). The cavernous cavities or sinuses (12) of the corpora cavernosa (9) are lined with endothelium and receive blood from the **dorsal (8)** and **deep arteries (11)** of the penis. Smaller branches from the deep arteries (11) open into the cavernous cavities (12) of the corpora cavernosa (9). The corpus spongiosum (16) receives its blood supply largely from the bulbourethral artery, a branch of the internal pudendal artery. Blood that leaves the cavernous cavities exits mainly through the **superficial veins (13)** in the dermis (2) and the deep dorsal vein.

The urethra (15) is designated as the spongiosa or cavernous urethra. At the base of the penis, the urethra (15) is lined with pseudostratified or stratified columnar epithelium; however, at the external orifice, the epithelium becomes stratified squamous. The urethra also exhibits numerous small but deep invaginations in its mucous membrane. These are the urethral lacunae (of Morgagni) with mucous cells. Branched tubular urethral glands (of Littre) open into these recesses. The lacunae and the urethral glands are not visible at this magnification (see Fig. 17-14).

Figure 17-14   Cavernous Urethra (transverse section)

A section of the **cavernous urethra (4)** is illustrated with pseudostratified or **stratified columnar epithelium (5)** lining. A thin **lamina propria (3)** merges with the surrounding connective tissue of the corpus spongiosum.

Numerous various-sized mucosal outpockets or the **urethral lacunae** (of Morgagni) **(9)** give the **urethral lumen (4)** an irregular form. Some of these urethral lacunae (9) contain mucous cells. The deeper urethral lacunae (9) are connected with the branched **urethral glands (of Littre) (7)** located in the lamina propria of the corpus spongiosum (7, lowest leader). The urethral glands (7) are lined with the same type of epithelium that lines the lumen of the cavernous urethra (4) (stratified columnar in this illustration).

The **corpus spongiosum (1)** surrounds the urethra (4); its internal structure is similar to that of the corpora cavernosa described in Figure 17-13. In the illustration are seen the characteristic **trabeculae (1, 11)** of connective tissue and smooth muscle between the **cavernous veins (2, 8, 10)**.

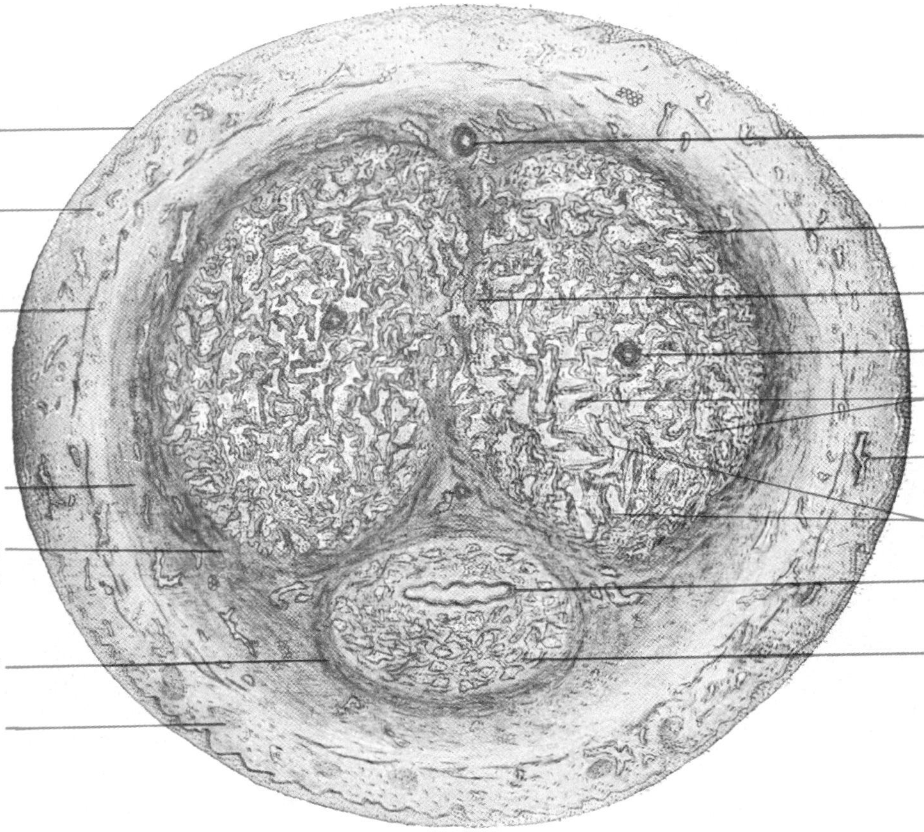

1 Epidermis

2 Dermis

3 Dartos tunic

4 Deep penile fascia

5 Tunica albuginea of corpus cavernosum

6 Tunica albuginea of corpus spongiosum

7 Sebaceous gland in dermis

8 Dorsal artery

9 Corpus cavernosum

10 Median septum

11 Deep artery

12 Cavities (cavernous veins) of corpus cavernosum

13 Superficial vein

14 Trabeculae

15 Cavernous urethra

16 Corpus spongiosum

Fig. 17-13   Penis (transverse section). Stain: hematoxylin-eosin. Low magnification.

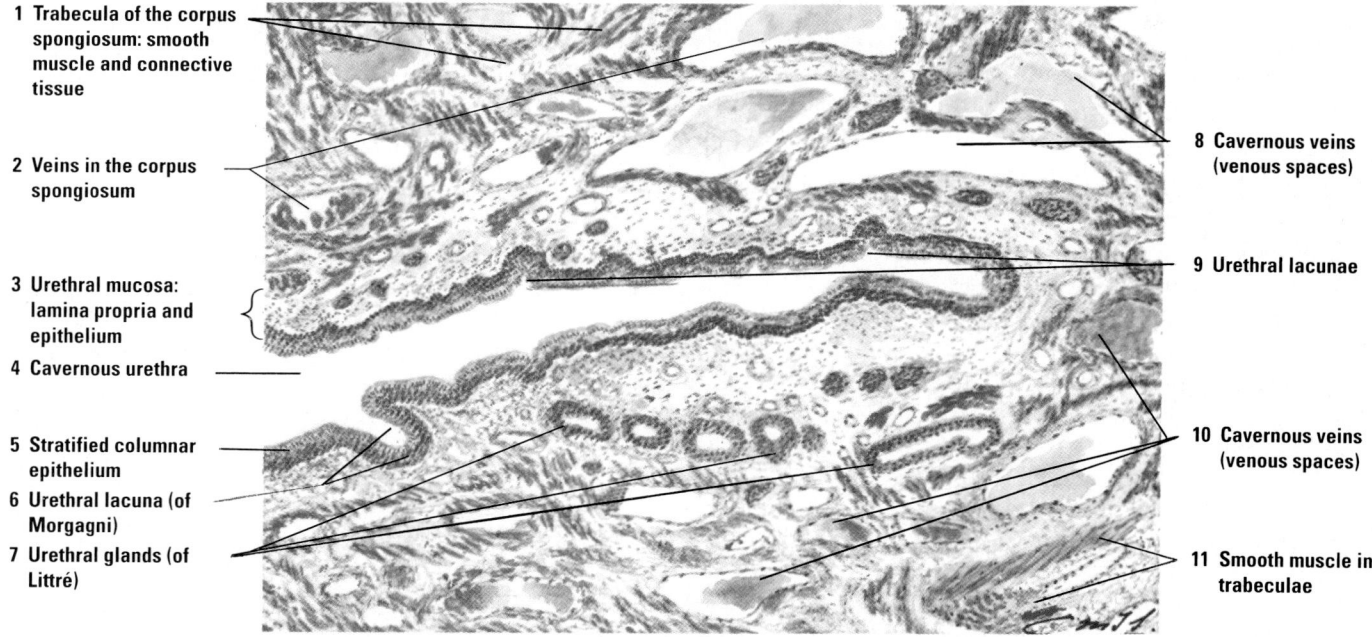

1 Trabecula of the corpus spongiosum: smooth muscle and connective tissue

2 Veins in the corpus spongiosum

3 Urethral mucosa: lamina propria and epithelium

4 Cavernous urethra

5 Stratified columnar epithelium

6 Urethral lacuna (of Morgagni)

7 Urethral glands (of Littré)

8 Cavernous veins (venous spaces)

9 Urethral lacunae

10 Cavernous veins (venous spaces)

11 Smooth muscle in trabeculae

Fig. 17-14   Cavernous Urethra (transverse section). Stain: hematoxylin-eosin. Low magnification.

Figure 17-15   Testis: Seminiferous Tubules (transverse section)

This photomicrograph illustrates a complete **seminiferous tubule (5)** and parts of adjacent seminiferous tubules of the testis cut in a transverse plane. A thick, multilayered germinal epithelium lines each active seminiferous tubule (5), which contains proliferating spermatogenic cells and the supportive Sertoli cells. The immature spermatogenic cells, the **spermatogonia (1)** are located in the basal region of the tubule. There are two types of spermatogonia (1), **dark Type A (1a)** and **pale Type B (1b).** The more mature **primary spermatocytes (2)** and **spermatids (7)** in different stages of maturation are visible in the germinal epithelium closer to the lumen. The tails of the more mature spermatids (7) protrude into the lumen of the seminiferous tubules (5). Located throughout the germinal epithelium are the supportive **Sertoli cells (6),** characterized by their ovoid nucleus and a prominent nucleolus. Each seminiferous tubule is surrounded by a fibromuscular interstitial **connective tissue (3).** Between the seminiferous tubules (5) in the interstitial connective tissue are found the **interstitial cells (4).** These cells secrete the male hormone testosterone.

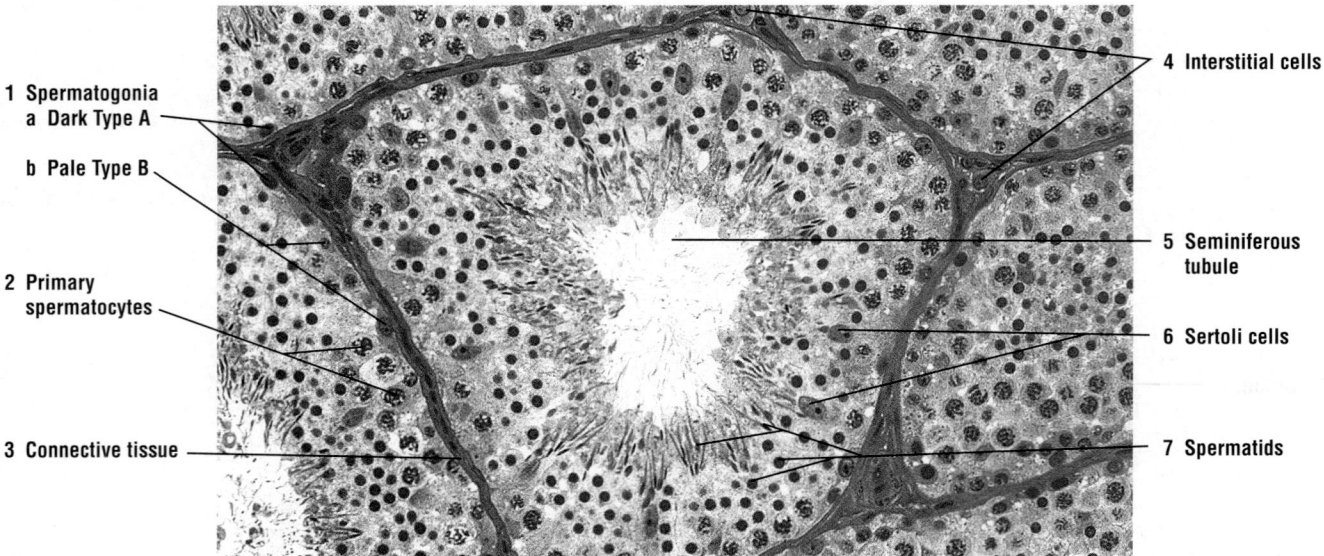

Fig. 17-15   Testis: Seminiferous Tubules (transverse section). Stain: hematoxylin-eosin (plastic section). 80×

Figure 17-16   Tubules of the Ductus Epididymis (transverse section)

The ductus epididymis is a long, highly convoluted tube. This photomicrograph illustrates numerous tubules of the ductus epididymis, some of which are filled with a concentration of **sperm (1).** The tubules are lined by **pseudostratified epithelium (2),** which consist of two cell types, the principal cells and basal cells. The **principal cells (2a)** are tall columnar and are lined with **stereocilia (5),** which are long, branching microvilli. The **basal cells (2b)** are small and spherical, and are situated near the base of the epithelium. A thin layer of **smooth muscle (3)** surrounds each tubule. Adjacent to the smooth muscle layer (3) are cells and fibers of the **connective tissue (4).**

Figure 17-17   Prostate Gland: Prostatic Glands With Prostatic Concretions

The parenchyma of the prostate gland consists of numerous, individual **prostatic glands (3)** that vary in size and shape. The glandular epithelium also varies from simple cuboidal or **columnar (2)** to pseudostratified epithelium. In older individuals, the secretory material of the prostatic glands (3) precipitates to form the characteristic dense staining **prostatic concretions (1, 5)** of various sizes. The prostate gland is also characterized by the presence of **fibromuscular stroma (4).** In this photomicrograph, the **smooth muscle fibers (4a)** of the prostate gland are stained red and the **connective tissue fibers (4b)** are stained blue.

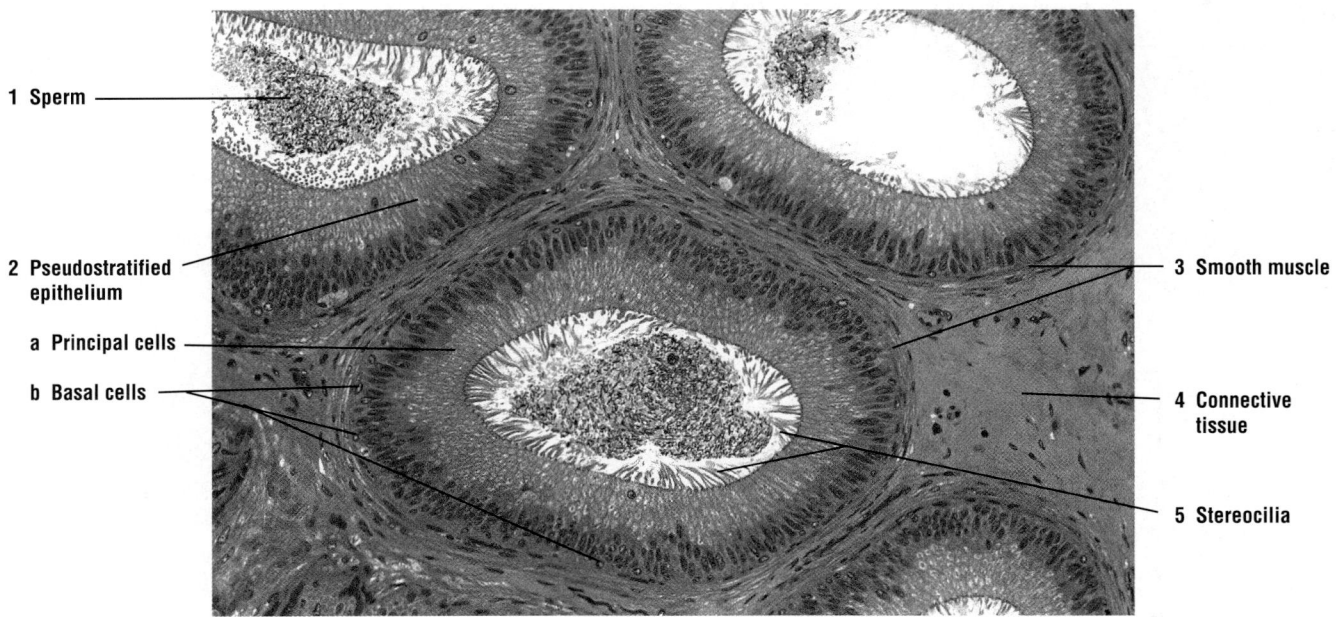

1 Sperm

2 Pseudostratified epithelium

a Principal cells

b Basal cells

3 Smooth muscle

4 Connective tissue

5 Stereocilia

Fig. 17-16 Tubules of the Ductus Epididymis (transverse section). Stain: hematoxylin-eosin (plastic section). 50×

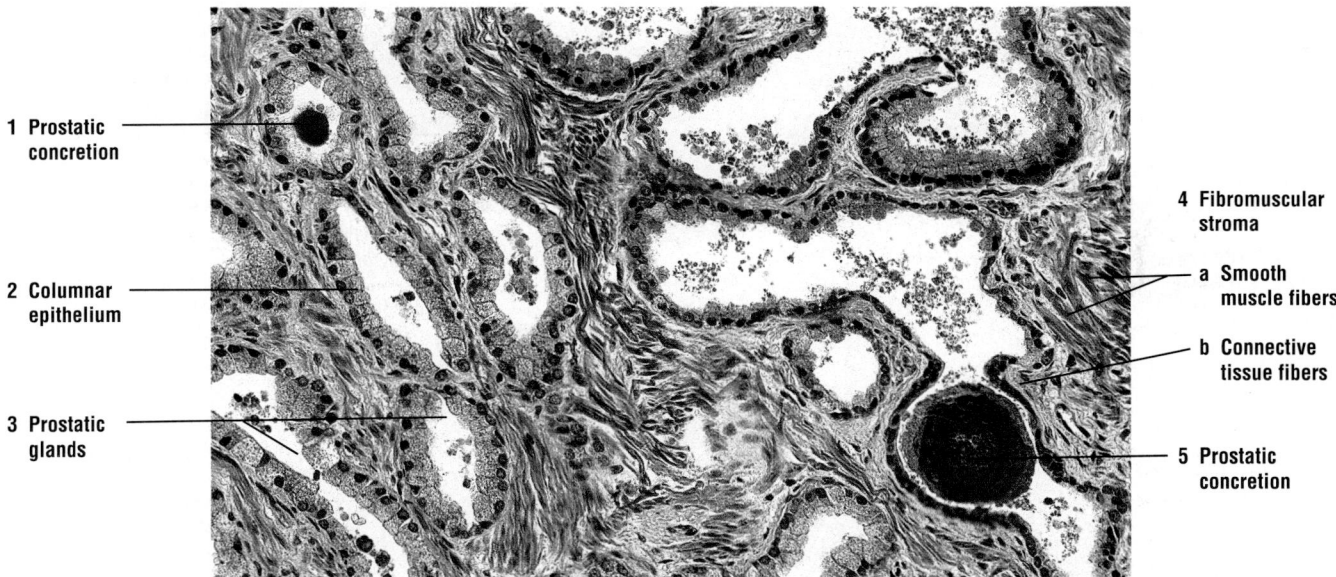

1 Prostatic concretion

2 Columnar epithelium

3 Prostatic glands

4 Fibromuscular stroma

a Smooth muscle fibers

b Connective tissue fibers

5 Prostatic concretion

Fig. 17-17 Prostate Gland: Prostatic Glands With Prostatic Concretions. Stain: Masson's trichrome. 64×

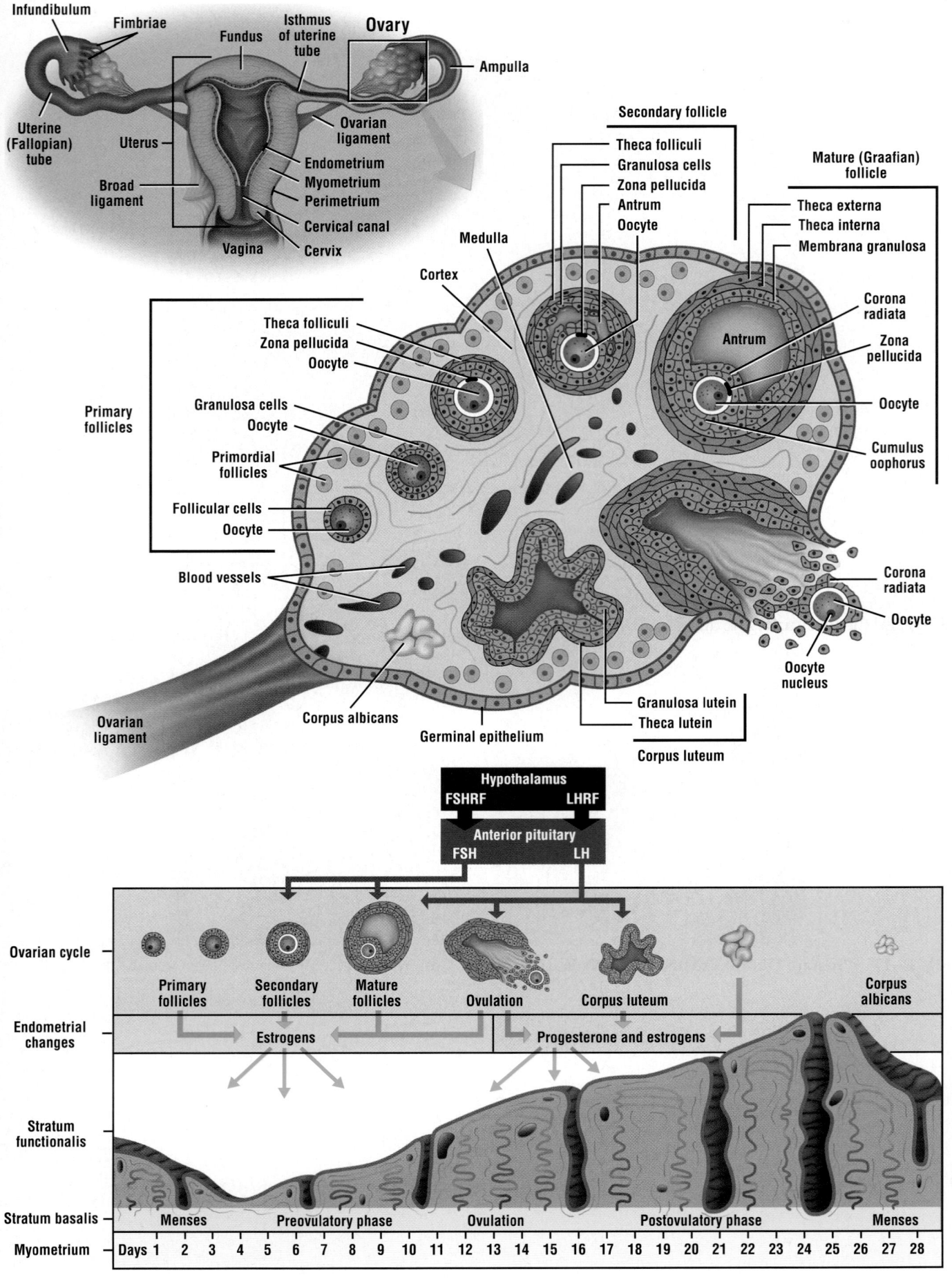

Female Reproductive System

SECTION 1
Ovaries, Uterine Tubes, and Uterus

COMPONENT PARTS

The reproductive system of a human female consists of paired internal **ovaries** and paired **uterine tubes (oviducts)** that provide a passageway from the ovaries to the **uterus.** Adjacent to the uterus and separated by **cervix** is a **vagina.** Because **mammary glands** are associated with the female reproductive system, their histologic structure and function are included in this chapter.

During reproductive life of the female, the reproductive organs exhibit cyclical monthly changes in both structure and function. In humans, these changes are called **menstrual cycles.** The menstrual cycle is primarily controlled by the adenohypophyseal (pituitary gland) hormones, the **follicle stimulating hormone (FSH)** and the **luteinizing hormone (LH),** and the ovarian hormones **estrogen** and **progesterone.** The individual organs of the female reproductive system perform numerous important functions, including secreting female sex hormones (estrogen and progesterone), producing ova, providing a suitable environment for fertilization of the oocyte, transporting and implanting blastocysts, development of the fetus during pregnancy, and nutrition of the newborn.

OVARIES

Each ovary is a flattened, ovoid structure that is located deep in the pelvic cavity. One section of the ovary is attached to the **broad ligament** by a peritonal fold called **mesovarium** and another section to the uterine wall by an **ovarian ligament.** The ovarian surface is covered by a layer of cells called the **germinal epithelium,** which overlies the dense, irregular connective tissue **tunica albuginea.** Located inferior to the tunica albuginea is the **cortex** of the ovary. Deep to the ovarian cortex is the highly vascularized, connective tissue core of the ovary, the **medulla.** There is no distinct boundary line between the cortex and medulla, and these two regions blend together **(Fig. 18-1).**

The cortex is normally filled with numerous **ovarian follicles** in various stages of development, including the large, **mature follicles** that extend deep into the medulla. In addition, there may be a large **corpus luteum** of an ovulated follicle, **corpus albicans** of a degenerated corpus luteum, and degenerataing **atretic follicles** in various stages of development **(Figs. 18-1–18-6, 18-13).**

UTERINE TUBES (OVIDUCTS)

Each uterine tube is approximately 12 cm in length and extends from the ovaries to the uterus. One end of the uterine tube opens into the uterus, and the other end opens into the peritoneal cavity near the ovary. The uterine tubes are normally divided into four continuous regions. The first region, which is close to the ovary, is the funnel-shaped **infundibulum.** Extending from the infudibulum are slender, finger-like processes called **fimbriae** that are located close to the ovary. Continuous with the infundibulum is the second region **ampulla.** This is the widest and longest portion. The **isthmus** is short and narrow and joins the uterine tube to the uterus. The last portion of the uterine tube is **interstitial (intramural) region.** It passes through the thick uterine wall to open into the uterine cavity **(Figs. 18-7–18-9, 18-14).**

UTERUS

The human uterus is pear-shaped organ with a thick wall. The **body,** or **corpus,** is the major portion of the uterus. The rounded upper portion of the uterus that extends above the entrance of the uterine tubes is the **fundus.** The lower, narrower, and the terminal portion of the uterus below the body or corpus region is the **cervix.** Cervix protrudes and opens into the vagina.

The wall of the uterus has three layers: an outer **perimetrium** (serosa or adventitia), a thick middle layer **myometrium** that consists of smooth muscle, and an inner **endometrium** (epithelium, uterine glands, and lamina propria).

The endometrium is normally subdivided into two layers, the luminal **stratum functionalis** and the basal **stratum basalis.** In a nonpregnant female, the superficial functionalis layer is sloughed off or shed monthly during menstruation, leaving intact the deeper basalis layer—the source of cells for regeneration of a new functionalis layer. The arterial supply to the endometrium plays an important role during the menstrual phase of the menstrual cycle.

Uterine arteries in the broad ligament give rise to the **arcuate arteries,** which penetrate and assume a circumferential course in the myometrium. These vessels divide into **straight** and **spiral arteries** that supply blood to the endometrium. The straight arteries are short and supply the basalis layer of the endometrium, whereas the spiral arteries are long and coiled, and pass to the surface (functionalis) layer of the endometrium. In contrast to the straight arteries, the spiral arteries are highly sensitive to altered levels of hormones (estrogen and progesterone) during the menstrual cycle **(Figs. 18-10–18-12, 18-15).**

Figure 18-1   Ovary: Dog (panoramic view)

The ovarian surface is covered by a single layer of low cuboidal or squamous cells, called the **germinal epithelium (1, 12).** This layer is continuous with the **mesothelium (14)** of the visceral peritoneum. Beneath the germinal epithelium is a dense, connective tissue layer, the **tunica albuginea (2).**

The ovary has a peripheral **cortex (8)** and a central **medulla (24).** The cortex (8) occupies the greater part of the ovary; its connective tissue stroma contains large, spindle-shaped fibroblasts. Compact collagen and reticular fibers course in all directions in the cortex (8).

The medullary stroma (24) is a typical dense irregular connective tissue, which is continuous with that of the **mesovarium (13).** Numerous **blood vessels (10)** in the medulla distribute smaller vessels to all parts of the cortex. The mesovarium (13) is covered by ovarian germinal epithelium (12) and by peritoneal mesothelium (14).

Numerous **ovarian follicles (3, 4, 7, 9, 16–20, 22, 25, 28, 29)** in various stages of development are located in the stroma of the cortex (8). The detailed structure of some of these follicles is illustrated in Figures 18-2 and 18-3. The most numerous follicles are the **primordial (3, 29, lower leader),** located in the periphery of the cortex (8) and under the tunica albuginea (2); these follicles are the smallest and simplest in structure. The largest of the ovarian follicles is the **mature follicle (16–20).** Its various parts are the **theca interna** and **theca externa (16),** the **granulosa cells (17),** a large **antrum (18)** filled with liquor folliculi (follicular fluid), and the **cumulus oophorus (19),** which contains the **primary oocyte (20).** The smaller follicles with stratified granulosa cells around the oocyte are the **growing follicles (4, lower leader).** Larger follicles with antral cavities of various sizes are called **secondary** or **antral follicles (7, 9, 28).** These larger follicles are situated deeper in the cortex and are surrounded by modified stromal cells, the **theca folliculi (6).** These cells differentiate into an inner secretory **theca interna (16, upper leader)** and an outer connective tissue **theca externa (16, lower leader).** Most of the illustrated large follicles contain a **primary oocyte (6, 20, 28)** and its nucleus. In the primordial follicles, the oocyte is small, but it gradually increases in size in the primary, growing, and vesicular follicles.

Most follicles never attain maturity and undergo degeneration (atresia) at various stages of growth, thus becoming **atretic follicles (11, 21, 26, 30; see also Fig. 18-4);** these follicles are gradually replaced by the stroma.

After ovulation the follicle collapses, its wall exhibits numerous folds, and the corpus luteum is formed (see Fig. 18-4). Successive stages in corpus luteum **regression** are indicated **(5, 15, 23, 27).** Figures 18-4 and 18-5 illustrate these changes at a higher magnification.

■ Functinal Correlations–Ovaries

During the reproductive life of the individual, the ovaries exhibit structural and functional changes during a menstrual cycle. These changes are seen as **follicular growth** and **maturation, ovulation,** and formation and degeneration of **corpus luteum.** The first half of the menstrual cycle involves growth of the ovarian follicles. During follicular growth, **FSH** is the principal circulating gonadotrophic hormone. FSH influences the growth and maturation of **ovarian follicles,** and stimulates the **theca interna cells** of the follicles to produce **androgens,** which are then converted by granulosa cells into **estrogens.** As circulating levels of estrogen rise, they inhibit the gondotropin-releasing hormone from the hypothalamus and the release of FSH from the pituitary gland. In addition, a hormone called **inhibin** is produced by granulosa cells in the ovarian follicles, which further inhibits the release of FSH from the pituitary gland.

At midcycle or shortly before ovulation, estrogen secretion reaches a peak. This causes a surge of **LH** release and a concomitant smaller release of FSH from the adenohypophysis of the pituitary gland. The increased levels of LH and FSH cause the following: the final **maturation** of the ovarian follicle and its **ovulation** (rupture); completion of the **first meiotic division** and liberation of a **secondary oocyte** into the uterine tube; and luteinization of the ovulated follicle and formation of **corpus luteum.** Final maturation of the secondary oocyte occurs only at fertilization, when the sperm penetrates the ovum. The liberated egg remains viable for approximately 24 hours in the female reproductive tract.

1 Germinal epithelium

2 Tunica albuginea

3 Primordial follicles

4 Follicular cells of a
   primary and a small
   growing follicle

5 Corpus albicans
   (residue of a corpus
   luteum)

6 Secondary
   follicle: theca folliculi

7 Antrum
   (follicular cavity)
   with fluid

8 Cortex

9 Vesicular (secondary)
   follicle: granulosa cells

10 Blood vessels in the
   medulla

11 Atretic follicles

12 Ovarian germinal
   epithelium

13 Mesovarium

14 Peritoneal
   mesothelium

15 Regressing corpus
   luteum

16 Thecae: interna
   and extrema

17 Granulosa cells

18 Antrum

19 Cumulus
   oophorus

20 Oocyte

21 Atretic follicle

Large mature follicle

22 Growing follicle

23 Regressing corpus
   luteum

24 Medulla

25 Follicle sectioned
   near its surface (tg. s.)

26 Atretic follicle

27 Regressing corpus
   luteum

28 Oocyte in a
   secondary follicle

29 Primary and primordial
   follicles

30 Atretic follicle

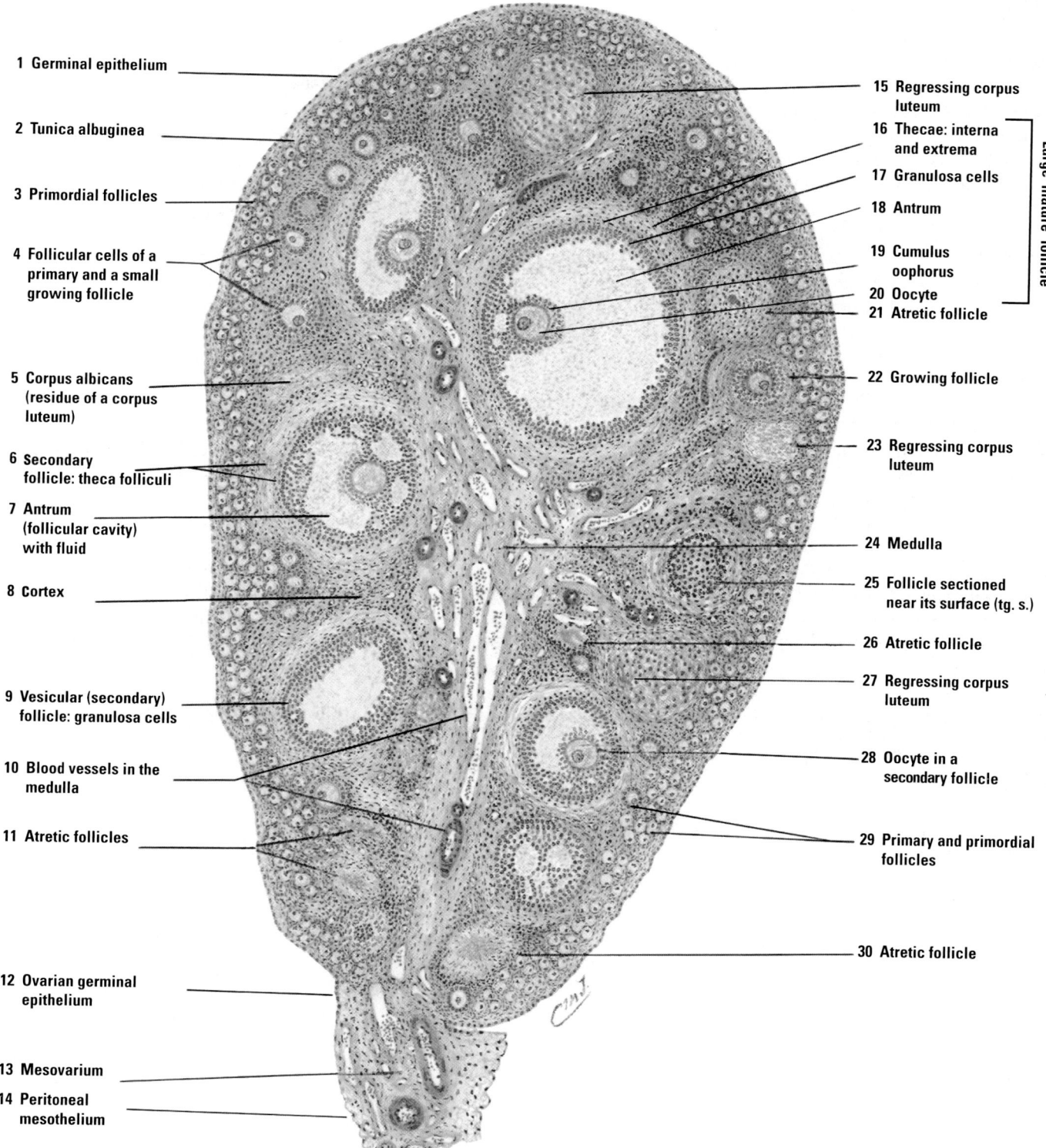

Fig. 18-1   Ovary: Dog (panoramic view). Stain: hematoxylin-eosin. Low magnification.

Figure 18-2   Ovary: Ovarian Cortex, Primary and Growing Follicles

The cuboidal **germinal epithelium (1)** lines the ovarian surface. Beneath the surface epithelium is a layer of dense connective tissue, the **tunica albuginea (2)**. Numerous **primordial follicles (5, 6)** are located immediately below the tunica albuginea (2). Each primordial follicle (5, 6) consists of a **primary oocyte (5)** surrounded by a single layer of squamous **follicular cells (6)**. In larger follicles, the **follicular cells (7)** change to cuboidal or low columnar.

In **growing follicles (4)**, the follicular cells proliferate by **mitotis (3)**, form layers of cuboidal cells called the **granulosa cells (10)**, and surround the **primary oocyte (4, 11)**. The innermost layer of the granulosa cells surrounding the oocyte form the **corona radiata (13)**; these cells are more columnar than the other granulosa cells. Between the corona radiata (13) and surrounding oocyte is the noncellular glycoprotein layer, the **zona pellucida (12)**. Stromal cells surrounding the follicular cells differentiate into the **theca interna (9)**; at this stage of follicular development the theca externa—the cell layer outside of the theca interna (9)—has not differentiated. The developing oocyte (4) has a large eccentric **nucleus (11)** with a conspicuous nucleolus.

A degenerating **atretic follicle (15)** is illustrated in the lower right corner of the illustration.

Figure 18-3   Ovary: Wall of a Mature Follicle

This figure illustrates a portion of the mature follicle with an **oocyte (11)**. The area represented in this figure is comparable to the area in Figure 18-1 that illustrates the mature follicle, **cumulus oophorus** with its **oocyte** and the different **thecae layers** (Fig. 18-1, **16, 19, 20)**.

Granulosa cells (6) enclose the central cavity or **antrum (8)** of the follicle. The antrum (8) is filled with follicular fluid that has been secreted by the surrounding granulosa cells (6). Smaller isolated accumulations of the **follicular fluid (14)** may also occur among the **granulosa cells (6)**. Some of these fluid accumulations appear as clear or faintly acidophilic **vacuoles (3, 7)**; their origin and function are not known.

A local thickening of the granulosa cells on one side of the mature follicle encloses the mature **oocyte (11)** and projects into the antrum (8), forming a hillock called the **cumulus oophorus (12)**. The oocyte is surrounded by a prominent, acidophilic-staining **zona pellucida (10)** and a single layer of radially arranged **corona radiata (9)** cells that are attached to the zona pellucida (10).

The basal row of granulosa cells rests on a **thin basement membrane (5)**. Adjacent to the basement membrane is the **theca interna (4),** an inner layer of vascularized, secretory cells. Surrounding the theca interna cells (4) is the **theca externa (2),** a layer of connective tissue cells.

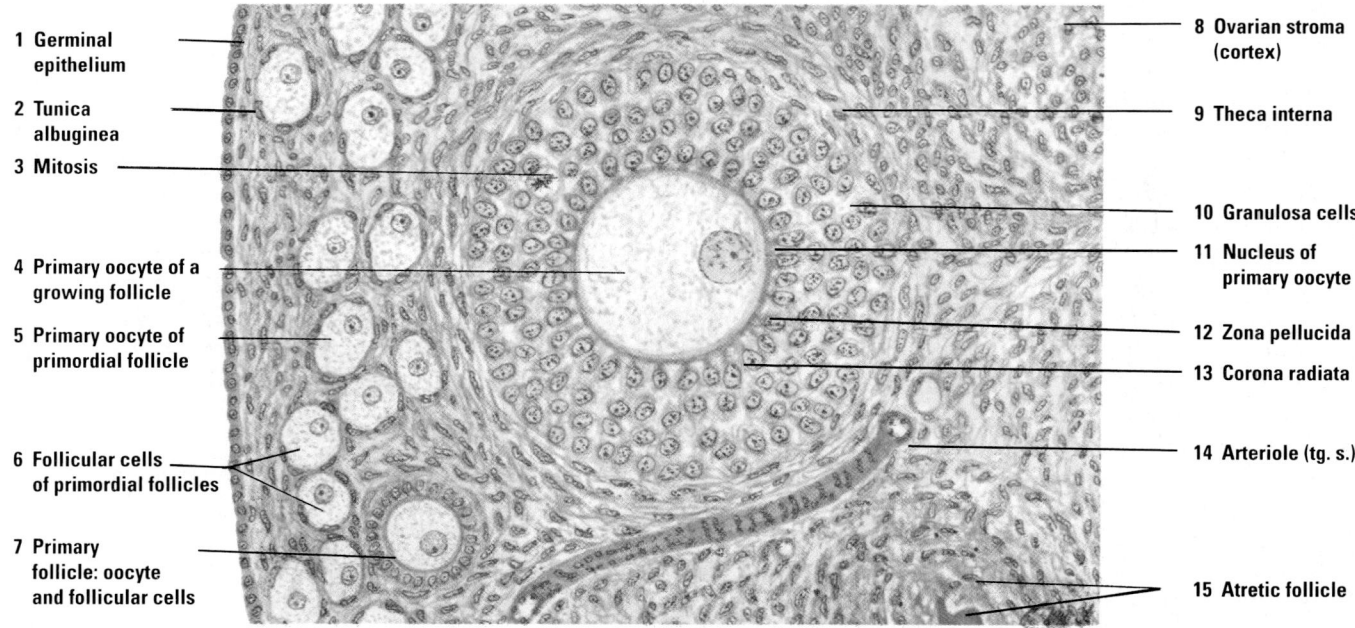

1 Germinal epithelium

2 Tunica albuginea

3 Mitosis

4 Primary oocyte of a growing follicle

5 Primary oocyte of primordial follicle

6 Follicular cells of primordial follicles

7 Primary follicle: oocyte and follicular cells

8 Ovarian stroma (cortex)

9 Theca interna

10 Granulosa cells

11 Nucleus of primary oocyte

12 Zona pellucida

13 Corona radiata

14 Arteriole (tg. s.)

15 Atretic follicle

Fig. 18-2   Ovary: Ovarian Cortex, Primary and Growing Follicles. Stain: hematoxylin-eosin. High magnification.

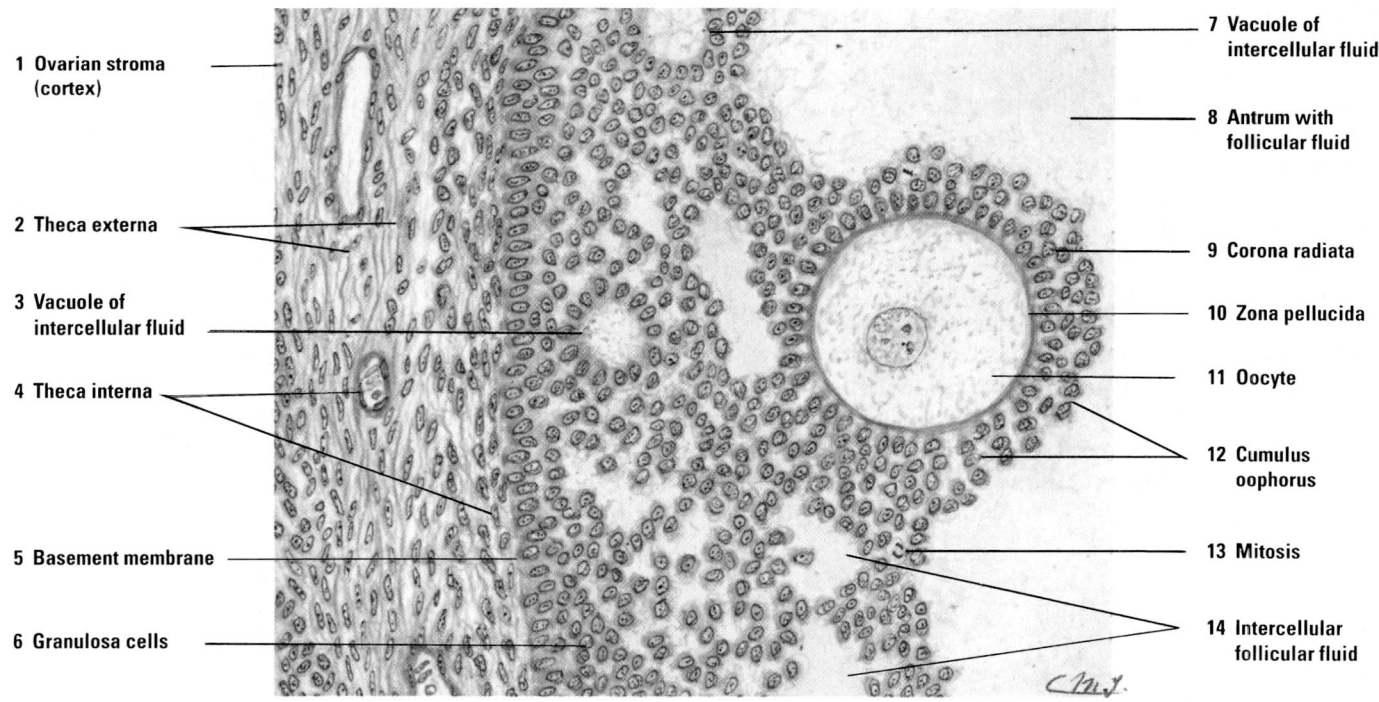

1 Ovarian stroma (cortex)

2 Theca externa

3 Vacuole of intercellular fluid

4 Theca interna

5 Basement membrane

6 Granulosa cells

7 Vacuole of intercellular fluid

8 Antrum with follicular fluid

9 Corona radiata

10 Zona pellucida

11 Oocyte

12 Cumulus oophorus

13 Mitosis

14 Intercellular follicular fluid

Fig. 18-3   Ovary: Wall of a Mature Follicle. Stain: hematoxylin-eosin. High magnification.

Figure 18-4   Human Ovary: Corpora Lutea and Atretic Follicles

This figure illustrates a newly formed corpus luteum, corpora lutea in various stages of regression, and several stages of follicular atresia.

The ovarian surface is covered by a single layer of **germinal epithelium (1)**. Lying directly underneath this layer is a connective tissue layer, the tunica albuginia. The **cortex (2, 18)** constitutes the greater portion of the ovary and contains the follicles and corpora lutea. The **medulla (7)** occupies the central region of the ovary. In the medulla (7) are found larger blood vessels that branch and supply the cortical region (2, 18) of the ovary.

The newly formed **corpus luteum (3)** is a large structure. It is formed after the rupture of the mature follicle and the collapse of its walls. The thin zone of **theca lutein cells (4)**, formed from the theca interna cells of the follicle, is located on the periphery of the corpus luteum (3) and in the contours of its folds. (See Figs. 18-5 and 18-6 for higher magnification and more details.) The mass of the corpus luteum wall (3) is formed from the **granulosa lutein cells (5)**, which are the hypertrophied granulosa cells of the follicle. The **connective tissue (6)** from the theca externa proliferates, forms the stroma for the blood vessels and capillaries in the wall of corpus luteum, and fills the former follicular cavity (6).

Also illustrated in the ovary is a portion of **corpus luteum in moderate regression (10)** with the plane of section passing through its outer wall. The granulosa lutein cells are smaller, the **nuclei pyknotic (10a)**, and larger **blood vessels (10b)** are growing in from the stroma. The theca lutein cells are not visible.

A later stage of **corpus luteum regression (16)** indicates further shrinkage of lutein cells, pyknosis of their **nuclei (16b)**, and a **fibrous central core (16a)**. Connective tissue invades the regressing luteal cells and replaces them as they degenerate. The stroma forms a **capsule (16c)** around the regressing corpus luteum; however, this is not a constant feature. Replacement by the connective tissue of all lutein cells leaves a fibrous, hyalinized scar, the **corpus albicans (15)**.

A large, normal **follicle (17)** exhibits the **theca interna (17a)** and the thick **granulosa cell layer (17b)**, separated by a thin basement membrane. The **cumulus oophorus (17d)** contains a normal **oocyte (17e)**; the **antrum (17c)** is filled with follicular fluid.

Numerous follicles undergo degenerative changes called atresia at any time before reaching maturity. Atresia in large follicles is gradual; however, serial changes of degeneration can be recognized by noting follicles in different stages of atresia. A follicle in an early stage of **atresia (14)** is illustrated. The **theca interna (14a)** and the **granulosa cells (14b)** are intact; however, some of the cells are beginning to slough off into the **antrum (14e)**, which still contains **follicular fluid (14d)**. Also, cumulus oophorus has been disrupted and degeneration of the oocyte is advanced. A remnant of the oocyte, surrounded by thickened **zona pellucida (14c)**, is visible in the antrum.

A follicle in **later atresia (13)** is also illustrated. The **theca interna (13a)** is still visible; however, the cells appear somewhat hypertrophied. The granulosa cells are no longer present; all of the cells have sloughed off and been resorbed. The basement membrane between these two layers has thickened and folded and is now called the **hypertrophied glassy membrane (13b)**. Loose connective tissue is growing in from the **stroma (13e)** and has partially filled the reduced **follicular cavity (13d)**, in which **follicular fluid (13c)** is still present.

With **further atresia (9)**, connective tissue **stroma replaces the theca interna cells (9a)**. The **hypertrophied glassy membrane (9b)** becomes thicker and more folded and the loose connective tissue with small blood vessels **fills the former antrum (9c)**. In the **last stages of atresia (11)**, the entire follicle is replaced by connective tissue; the hypertrophied and folded glassy membrane (11) remains for some time as the only indication of a follicle.

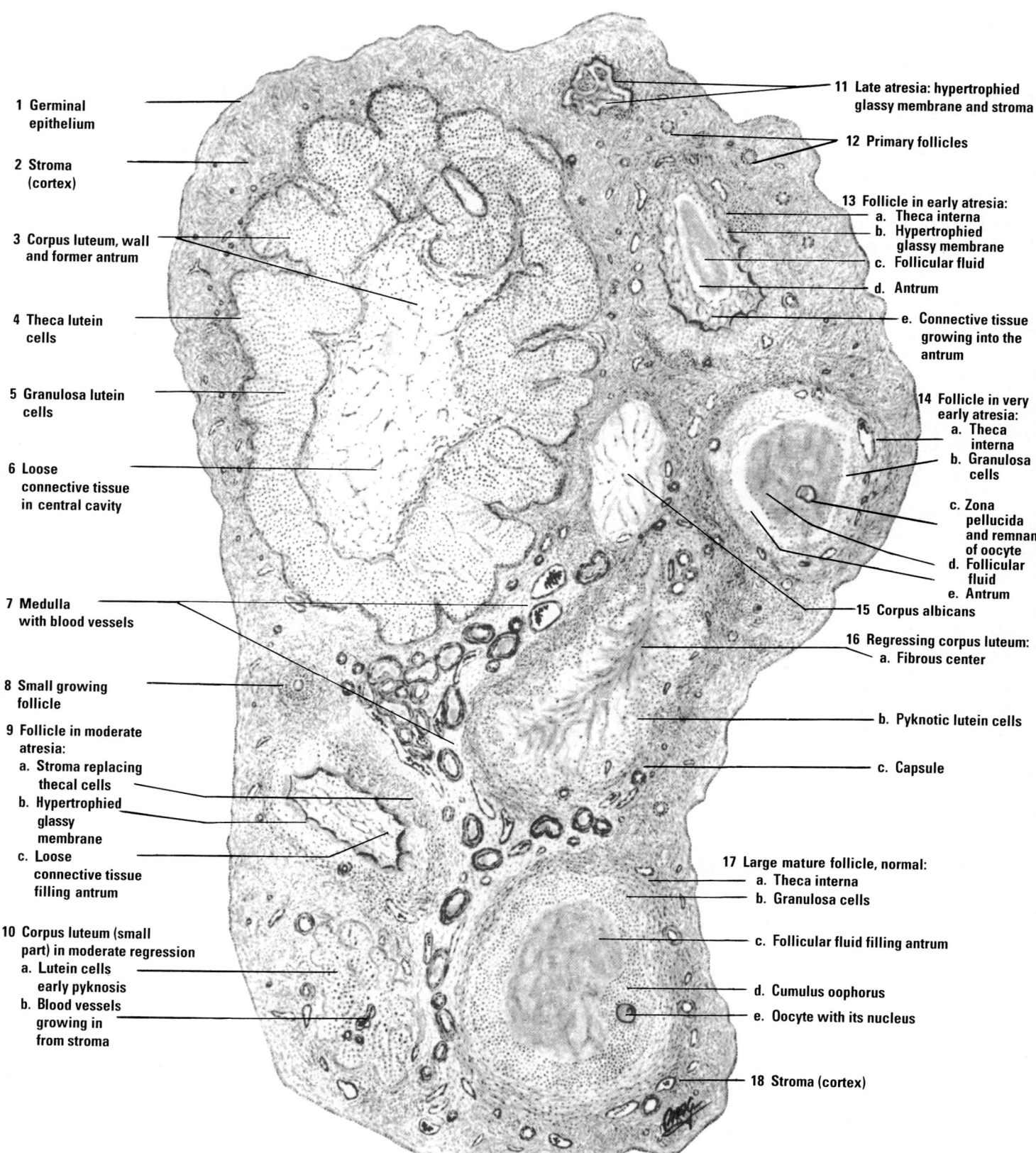

1 Germinal
  epithelium

2 Stroma
  (cortex)

3 Corpus luteum, wall
  and former antrum

4 Theca lutein
  cells

5 Granulosa lutein
  cells

6 Loose
  connective tissue
  in central cavity

7 Medulla
  with blood vessels

8 Small growing
  follicle

9 Follicle in moderate
  atresia:
  a. Stroma replacing
     thecal cells
  b. Hypertrophied
     glassy
     membrane
  c. Loose
     connective tissue
     filling antrum

10 Corpus luteum (small
   part) in moderate regression
   a. Lutein cells
      early pyknosis
   b. Blood vessels
      growing in
      from stroma

11 Late atresia: hypertrophied
   glassy membrane and stroma

12 Primary follicles

13 Follicle in early atresia:
   a. Theca interna
   b. Hypertrophied
      glassy membrane
   c. Follicular fluid
   d. Antrum
   e. Connective tissue
      growing into the
      antrum

14 Follicle in very
   early atresia:
   a. Theca
      interna
   b. Granulosa
      cells
   c. Zona
      pellucida
      and remnant
      of oocyte
   d. Follicular
      fluid
   e. Antrum

15 Corpus albicans

16 Regressing corpus luteum:
   a. Fibrous center

   b. Pyknotic lutein cells

   c. Capsule

17 Large mature follicle, normal:
   a. Theca interna
   b. Granulosa cells

   c. Follicular fluid filling antrum

   d. Cumulus oophorus
   e. Oocyte with its nucleus

18 Stroma (cortex)

Fig. 18-4   Human Ovary: Corpora Lutea and Atretic Follicles. Stain: hematoxylin-eosin. Low magnification.

Figure 18-5   Corpus Luteum (panoramic view)

At higher magnification, the corpus luteum appears as a highly folded, thick mass of **glandular epithelium (3)**, consisting primarily of **granulosa lutein cells (3, upper leader)** and peripheral **theca lutein cells (3, lower leader)**, which extend along the connective tissue **septa (2, 7)**. The theca externa cells form a poorly defined **capsule (1)** around the developing corpus luteum that also extends inward between the folds (2, 7). The central core of the corpus luteum (the former follicular cavity) contains remnants of follicular fluid, serum, occasional blood cells, and loose **connective tissue (8, 9)** from the theca externa, which has proliferated and penetrated the layers of the glandular tissue. The connective tissue also covers the inner surface of the luteal cells (8) and then spreads throughout the core of the corpus luteum (9).

The **ovarian stroma (4)** around the corpus luteum is highly vascular **(5)**.

Figure 18-6   Corpus Luteum: Peripheral Wall

The **granulosa lutein cells (7)** constitute the mass of the corpus luteum. These cells are the hypertrophied former granulosa cells of the mature follicle. The granulosa cells are large, and have large vesicular nuclei. These cells stain lightly because of lipid inclusions. The **theca lutein cells (2)** (the former theca interna cells) remain external to the granulosa lutein cells on the periphery of the corpus luteum and in the depressions between the folds. Theca lutein cells (2) are smaller than granulosa lutein cells (7); their cytoplasm stains deeper and their nuclei are smaller and darker.

Numerous **capillaries (4, 8)** and fine connective tissue **septa (6)** from the theca externa are visible between the anastomosing columns of lutein cells.

The connective tissue **capsule (5)** around the corpus luteum is poorly defined and the surrounding **stroma (1, 3, 4)** remains highly vascular.

■ Functional Correlations–Corpus Luteum

After ovulation of the mature follicle, the ovary enters the **luteal phase.** During this phase, LH transforms the granulosa and theca interna cells of the ruptured ovarian follicle into the **granulosa lutein** and **theca lutein cells** of the **corpus luteum.** LH then stimulates the lutein cells to secrete **estrogen** and large amounts of **progesterone.** High levels of these hormones stimulate further development of the uterus and mammary glands in anticipation of pregnancy.

The development and functional activity of the corpus luteum depends on LH. Rising level of progesterone produced by the corpus luteum, however, inhibits further release of LH by influencing both the hypothalamus and gonadotrophs in the adenohypophysis. If the ovulated oocyte is not fertilized, the corpus luteum eventually regresses into a nonfunctional scar tissue called **corpus albicans.** Estrogen and progesterone levels then decline and menstruation follows. With the regression of the corpus luteum, the inhibitory effects of its hormones on the pituitary gland and hypothalamus are removed. This causes a release of FSH from the adenohypophysis and an initiation of a new ovarian cycle of follicular development.

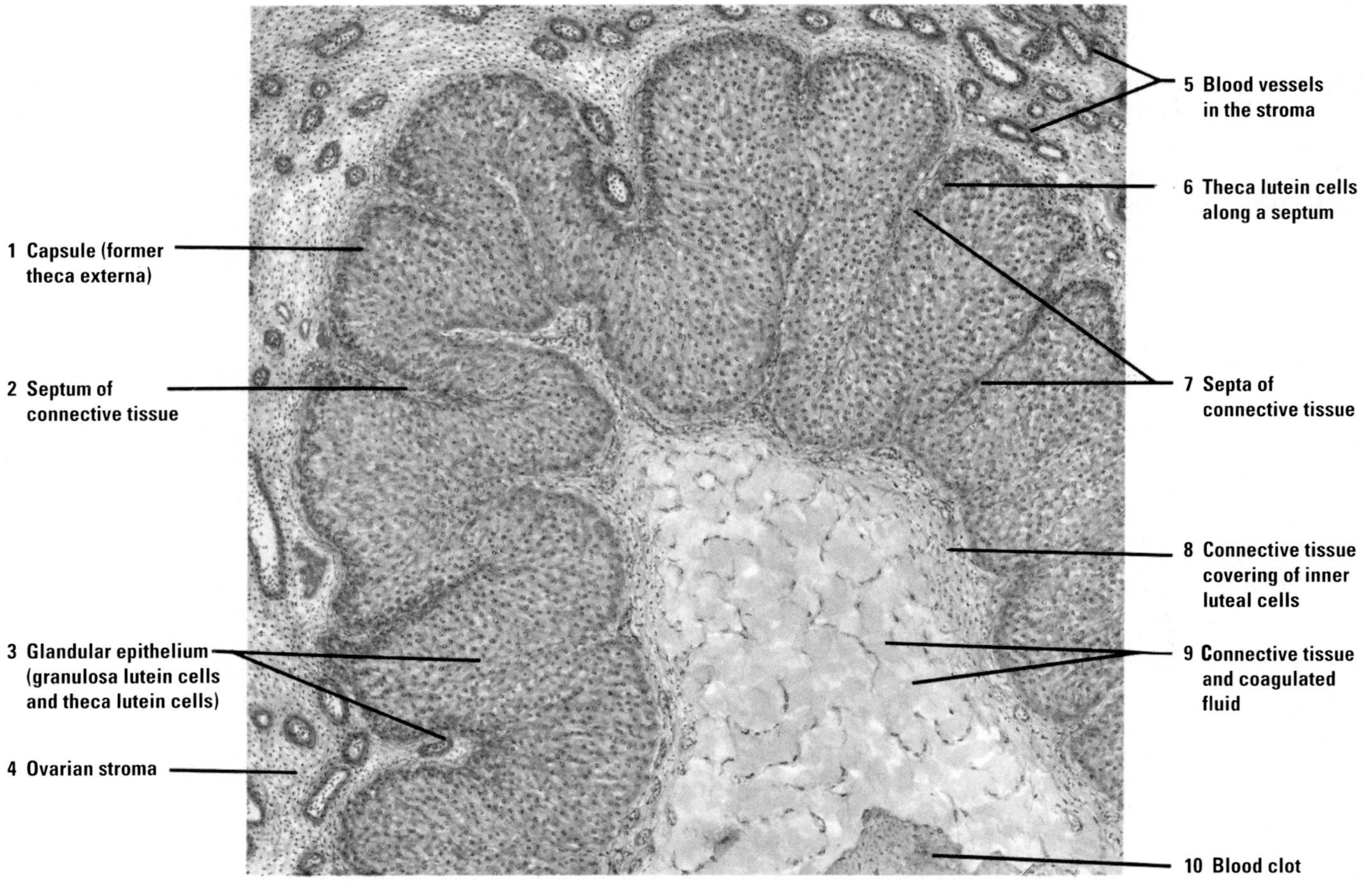

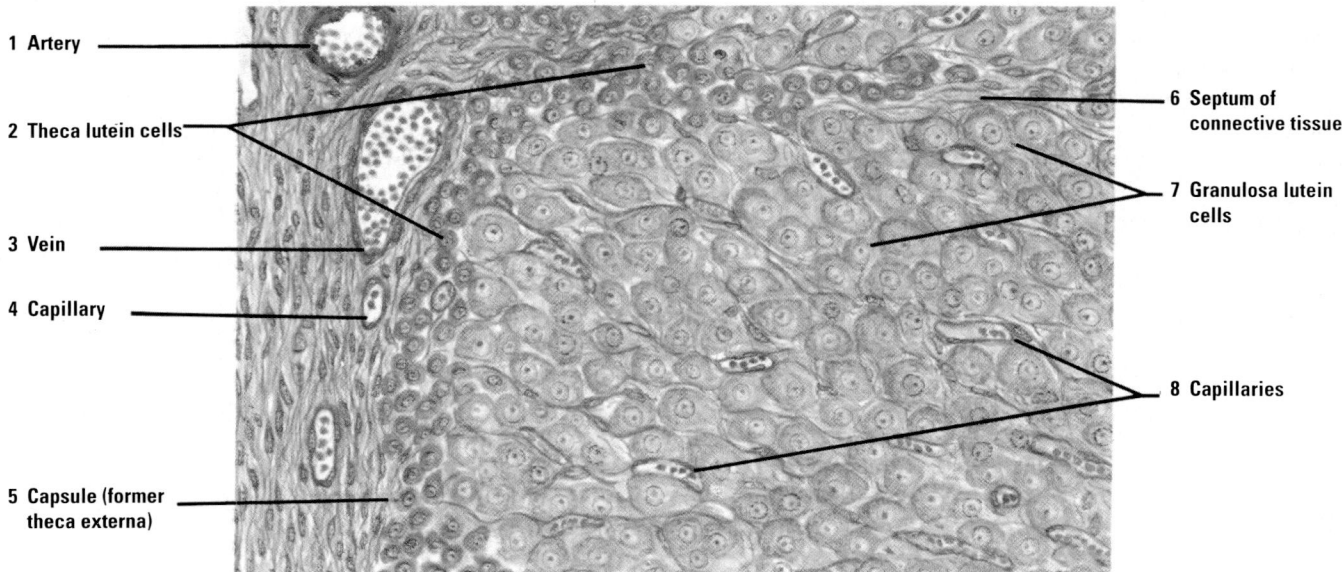

1 Capsule (former theca externa)

2 Septum of connective tissue

3 Glandular epithelium (granulosa lutein cells and theca lutein cells)

4 Ovarian stroma

5 Blood vessels in the stroma

6 Theca lutein cells along a septum

7 Septa of connective tissue

8 Connective tissue covering of inner luteal cells

9 Connective tissue and coagulated fluid

10 Blood clot

Fig. 18-5   Corpus Luteum (panoramic view). Stain: hematoxylin-eosin. Medium magnification.

1 Artery

2 Theca lutein cells

3 Vein

4 Capillary

5 Capsule (former theca externa)

6 Septum of connective tissue

7 Granulosa lutein cells

8 Capillaries

Fig. 18-6   Corpus Luteum: Peripheral Wall. Stain: hematoxylin-eosin. High magnification.

Figure 18-7   Uterine Tube: Ampulla (panoramic view, transverse section)

Extensive ramification of tall **mucosal folds (9)** forms an irregular lumen in the uterine (fallopian) tube. The lumen extends between the mucosal folds (9) and forms deep grooves in the tube. The lining **epithelium (10)** is simple columnar and the **lamina propria (8)** is a well vascularized, loose connective tissue. The muscularis consists of two smooth muscle layers, an inner **circular layer (1)** and an outer **longitudinal layer (6).** The interstitial **connective tissue (2)** is abundant and, as a result, the smooth muscle layers—especially the outer layer—are not distinct. The **serosa (7)** forms the outermost layer on the uterine tube.

Figure 18-8   Uterine Tube: Mucosal Folds (Early Proliferative Phase)

The lining epithelium is simple but may appear pseudostratified. It consists of **ciliated cells (1)** and nonciliated peg (secretory) cells. During the early proliferative phase of the menstrual cycle, the ciliated cells hypertrophy, exhibit cilia growth, and become predominant. Secretory activity in nonciliated cells increases. The epithelium of the uterine tube shows cycle changes and the proportion of ciliated and nonciliated cells varies with the stages of the menstrual cycle.

The **lamina propria (2)** is a highly cellular, loose connective tissue with fine collagen and reticular fibers.

Figure 18-9   Uterine Tube: Mucosal Folds (Early Pregnancy)

During the luteal phase of the menstrual cycle and early pregnancy, **peg** or **secretory cells (2)** predominate. These cells appear slender, with elongated nuclei and apices that protrude into tubular lumina. The secretory cells (2) intermix with **ciliated cells (3)** in the uterine tube.

■ Functional Correlations–Uterine Tubes

The uterine tubes perform several important functions. At ovulation, the **fimbria** of the infundibulum sweep the surface of the ovary to capture and conduct the **oocyte** through the uterine tube toward the **uterus.** This function is accomplished by the gentle peristaltic action of the smooth muscles in the uterine wall and fimbriae. In addition, the heavily ciliated cells on the fimbriae surfaces create a current that guides the oocyte into the infundibulum of the uterine tube.

The epithelium of the uterine tube consists of **ciliated** and **nonciliated (peg) cells.** Most of the cilia beat toward the uterus and, together with muscular contractions in the uterine tube wall, transport the captured oocyte or fertilized egg through the tube to the uterus. The nonciliated cells in the uterine tube are secretory and contribute important nutritive material for the initial development of the embryo. The uterine tubes also provide sites of **fertilization** for the egg, which normally occurs in the upper region of the **ampulla** of the tube.

The uterine tube epithelium exhibits cyclic changes that are associated with the ovarian cycles. The height of the epithelium in the uterine tubes is greatest during the follicular phase, at which time the ovarian follicles are maturing and circulating levels of estrogen are high.

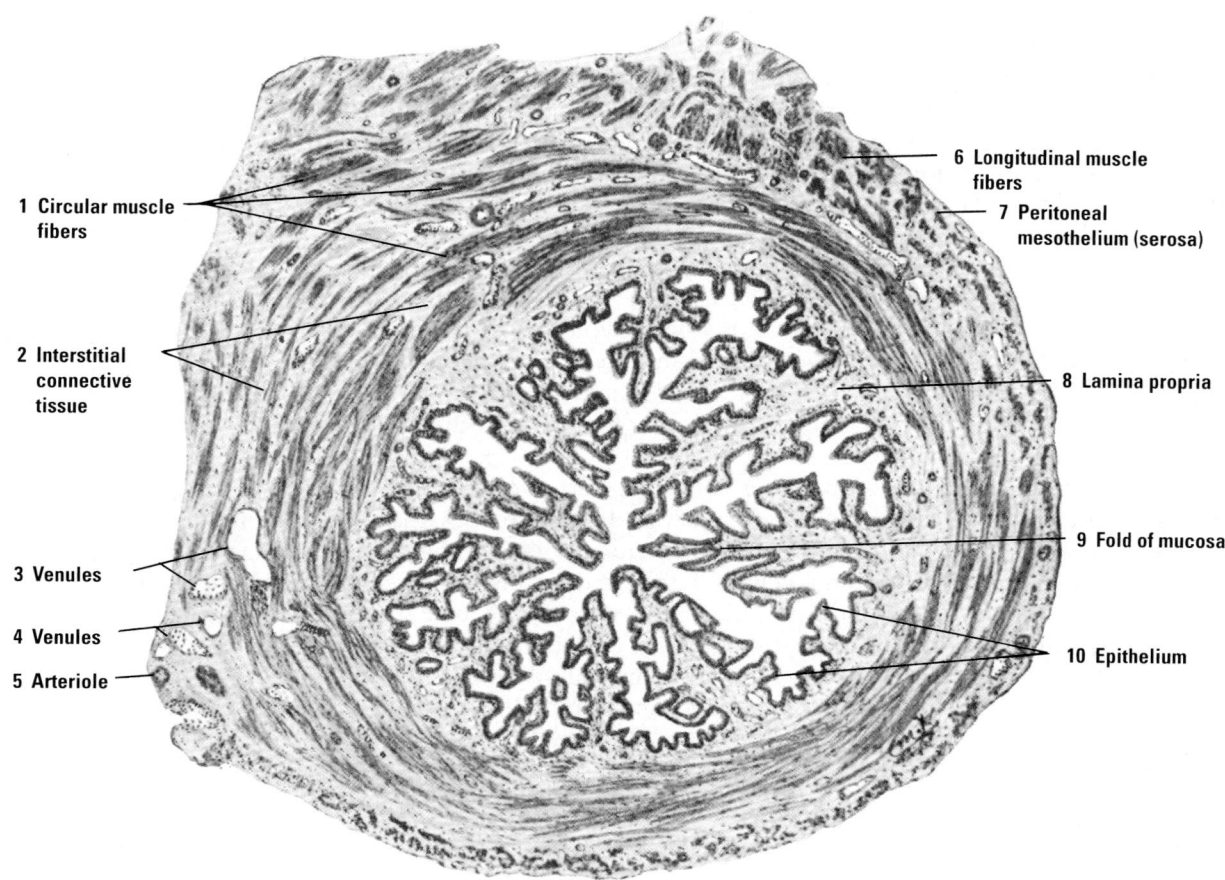

1 Circular muscle fibers

2 Interstitial connective tissue

3 Venules

4 Venules

5 Arteriole

6 Longitudinal muscle fibers

7 Peritoneal mesothelium (serosa)

8 Lamina propria

9 Fold of mucosa

10 Epithelium

Fig. 18-7   Uterine Tube: Ampulla (panoramic view, transverse section). Stain: hematoxylin-eosin. Low magnification.

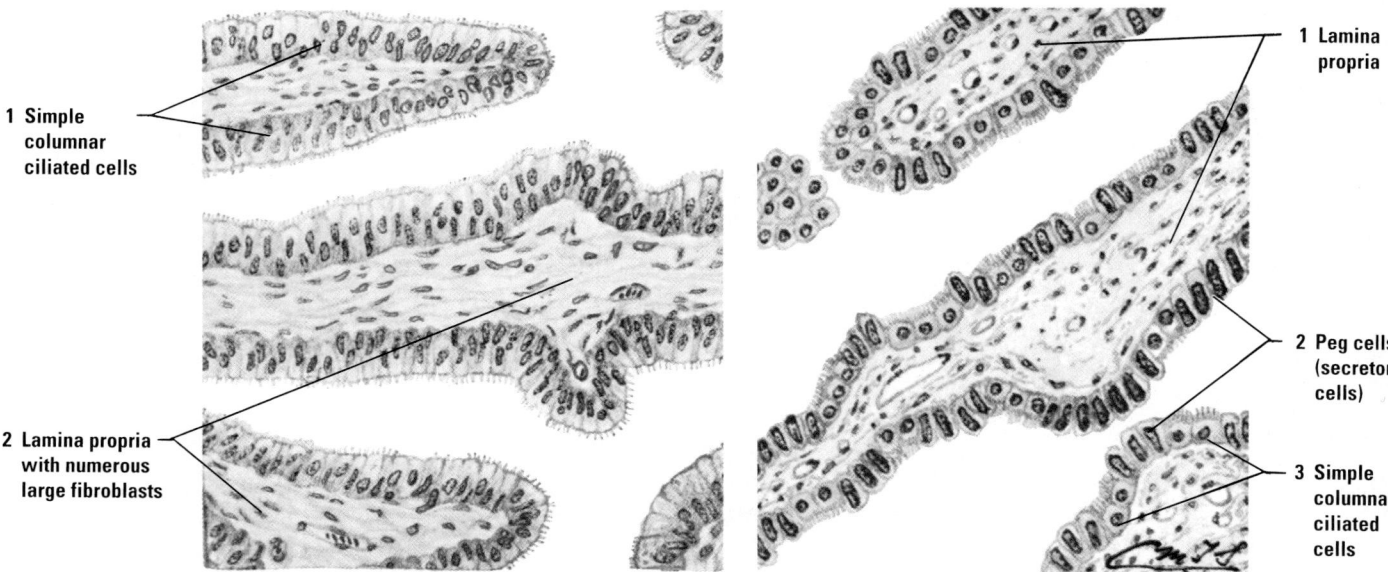

1 Simple columnar ciliated cells

2 Lamina propria with numerous large fibroblasts

Fig. 18-8   Uterine Tube: Mucosal Folds (Early Proliferative Phase). Stain: hematoxylin-eosin. High magnification.

1 Lamina propria

2 Peg cells (secretory cells)

3 Simple columnar ciliated cells

Fig. 18-9   Uterine Tube: Mucosal Folds (Early Pregnancy). Stain: hematoxylin-eosin. High magnification.

Figure 18-10   Uterus: Proliferative (Follicular) Phase

During a normal menstrual cycle, the endometrium exhibits a sequence of changes that are closely correlated with ovarian function. Cyclic activities in a nonpregnant uterus are divided into three distinct phases: a proliferative (follicular) phase, a secretory (luteal) phase, and a menstrual phase. The characteristic features of the endometrium during each of these phases are illustrated in detail in Figures 18-10, 18-11, and 18-12, respectively.

The uterine wall consists of three layers: the inner **endometrium (1, 2, 3, 4)**; a middle muscular layer **myometrium (5, 6)**; and the outer serous membrane, the perimetrium (not illustrated). The endometrium is further subdivided into two zones or layers: a narrow, deep **basalis layer (8)** adjacent to the myometrium (5) and the **functionalis layer (7)**, a wider, superficial layer above the basalis layer (8) that extends to the lumen of the uterus.

The surface of the endometrium is lined with a simple columnar **epithelium (1)** overlaying the thick **lamina propria (2)**. The surface epithelium (1) extends down into the connective tissue of the lamina propria (2) to form numerous long, tubular **uterine glands (4)**. The uterine glands (4) are usually straight in the superficial portion of the endometrium, but may exhibit branching in the deeper regions near the myometrium. As a result, numerous uterine glands (4) are seen in cross sections.

During the proliferative phase of the cycle, **coiled (spiral) arteries (3)** in cross section are seen primarily in the deeper regions of the endometrium. As this stage (proliferative phase), the coiled arteries (3) do not normally extend into the superficial third portion of the endometrium, which, at this time, contains veins and capillaries. The lamina propria (2) of the endometrium is cellular and resembles mesenchymal tissue. The branching fibroblasts are found in the network of reticular and fine collagen fibers of the ground substance. The connective tissue is more compact in the **basilis layer (8)** and appears somewhat darker in this illustration.

The endometrium is firmly attached to the underlying, highly **vascular (10)** myometrium (5, 6). This layer consists of compact bundles of **smooth muscle (5, 6)** separated by thin strands of **interstitial connective tissue (9)**. The bundles of muscle are seen in cross, oblique, and longitudinal sections.

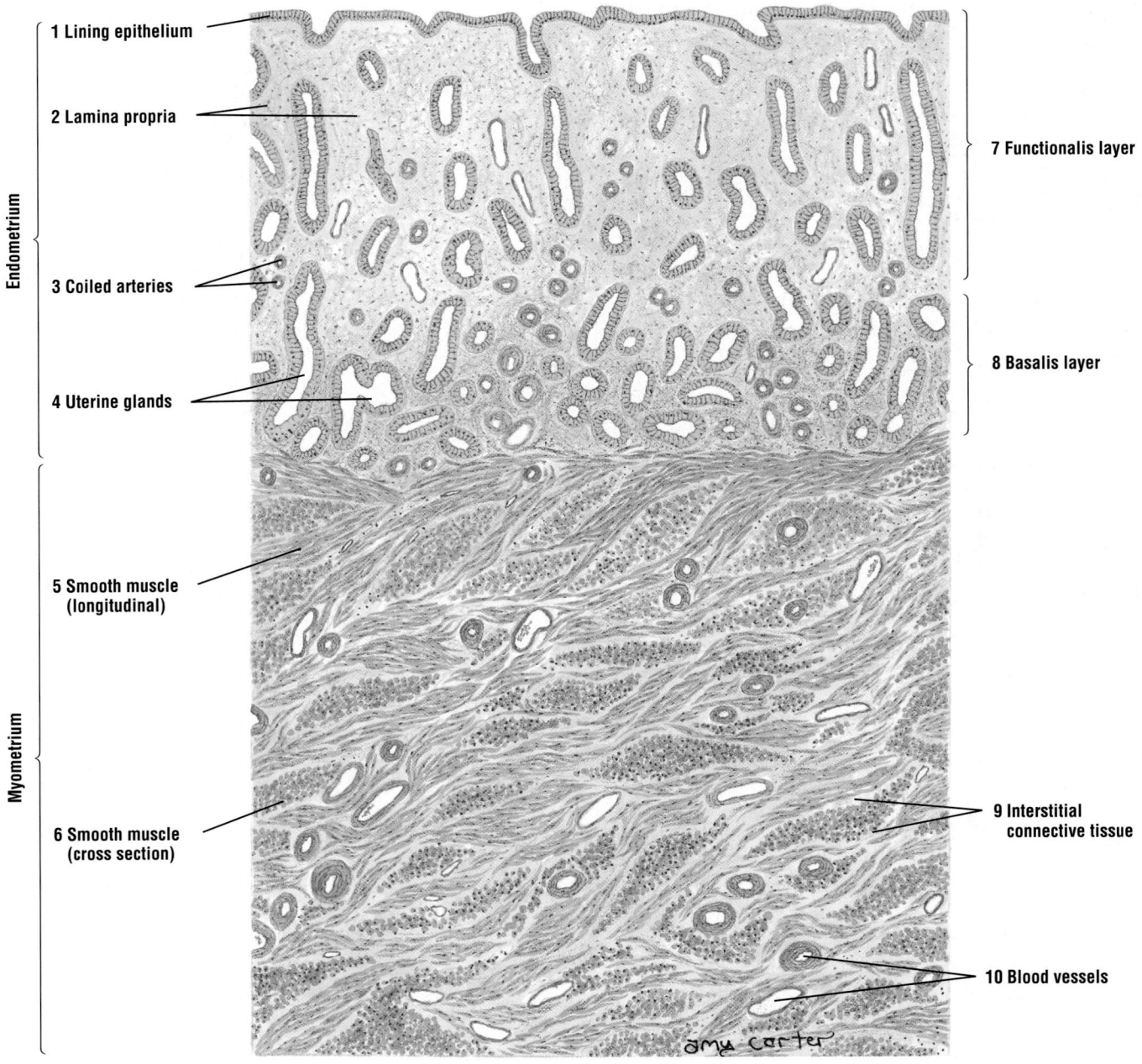

1 Lining epithelium

2 Lamina propria

Endometrium

3 Coiled arteries

4 Uterine glands

7 Functionalis layer

8 Basalis layer

Myometrium

5 Smooth muscle
(longitudinal)

6 Smooth muscle
(cross section)

9 Interstitial
connective tissue

10 Blood vessels

amy carter

Fig. 18-10   Uterus: Proliferative (Follicular) Phase. Stain: hematoxylin-eosin. Low magnification.

Figure 18-11 Uterus: Secretory (Luteal) Phase

During the secretory (luteal) phase of the menstrual cycle, the **functionalis layer (1)** and **basalis layer (2)** of the endometrium become thicker because of increased **glandular secretion (5)** and edema in the **lamina propria (6)**. The epithelium of the **uterine glands (5, 8)** hypertrophies because of the accumulation of large quantities of secretory product (5, 8). The uterine glands (5, 8) become highly tortuous and their lumina become dilated and filled with nutritive **secretory material (5)** that is rich in carbohydrates. The **coiled arteries (7)** now extend into the upper portion of the endometrium (functionalis layer) (1). These blood vessels (7) become prominent in the uterine sections because of their thicker walls.

The alterations in the surface **columnar epithelium** (4), uterine glands (5), and lamina propria (6) characterize the functionalis layer (1) of the endometrium during the secretory or luteal phase of the menstrual cycle. The basalis layer (2) exhibits minimal changes. Below the basalis layer is the prominent **myometrium (3)**, composed of **smooth muscle bundles (10)** sectioned in both longitudinal and transverse planes, and numerous **blood vessels (9)**.

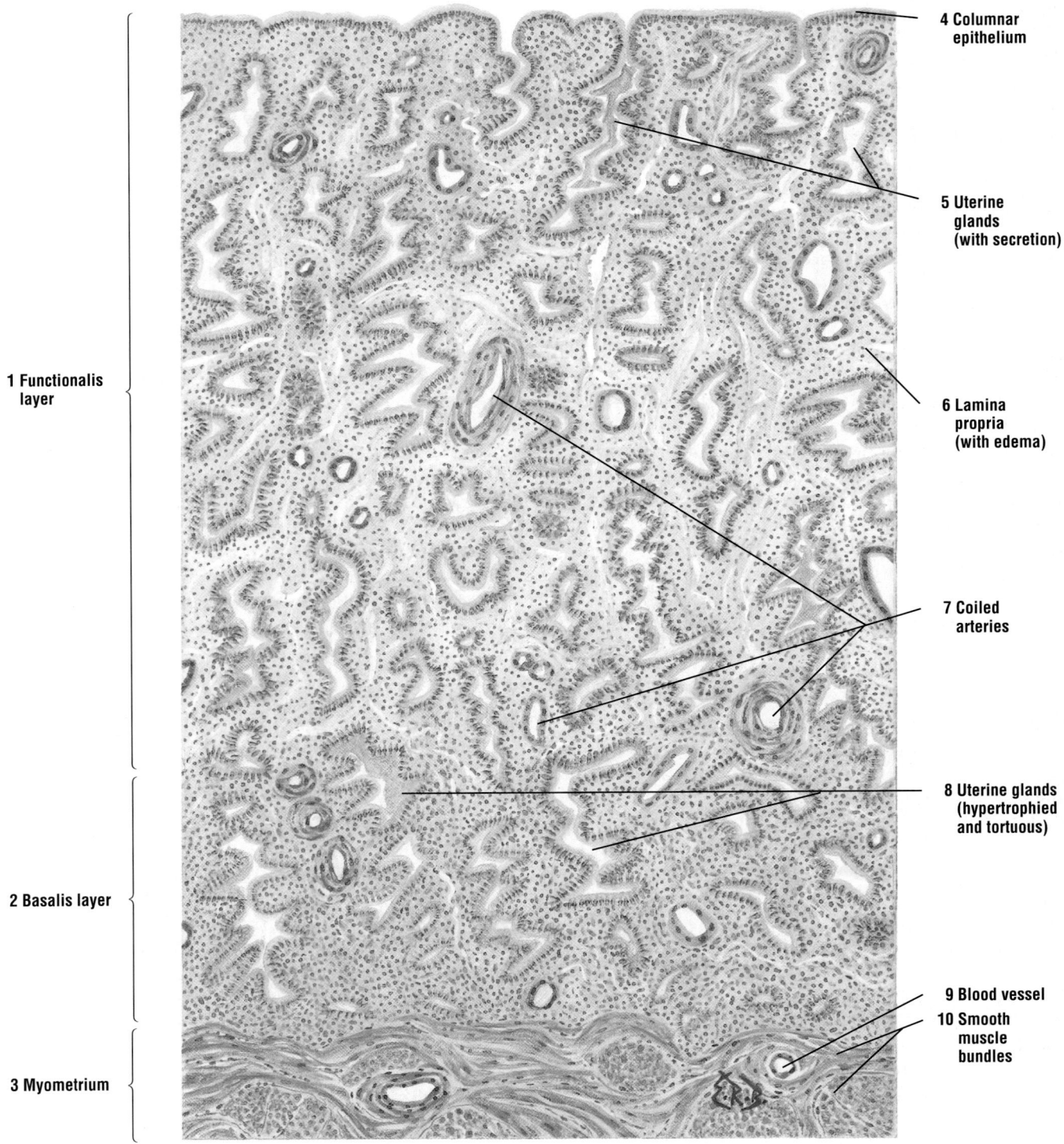

1 Functionalis layer

4 Columnar epithelium

5 Uterine glands (with secretion)

6 Lamina propria (with edema)

7 Coiled arteries

8 Uterine glands (hypertrophied and tortuous)

2 Basalis layer

9 Blood vessel

10 Smooth muscle bundles

3 Myometrium

Fig. 18-11   Uterus: Secretory (Luteal) Phase. Stain: hematoxylin-eosin. Low magnification.

Figure 18-12   Uterus: Menstrual Phase

During every menstrual cycle, the endometrium (1) in the functionalis layer is sloughed off during the menstrual phase. The endometrium that is shed contains **fragments of disintegrated stroma (6), blood clots (7),** and uterine glands. Some of the intact **uterine glands (2)** are filled with blood. In the deeper layers of the endometrium, the **basalis layer (4),** the **bases of the uterine glands (9)** remain intact during the menstrual flow.

The endometrial stroma of most of the functionalis layer contains aggregations of **erythrocytes (8);** these have been extruded from the torn and disintegrating blood vessels. In addition, endometrial stroma (6) exhibits moderate infiltration of lymphocytes and neutrophils.

The basalis layer (4) of the endometrium remains usually unaffected during this phase. The distal (superficial) portions of the **coiled arteries (3)** become necrotic and the deeper parts of these vessels remain intact.

■ Functional Correlations–Uterus

During pregnancy, the uterus provides the site for **implantation** of the blastocyst, formation of the placenta, and a suitable environment for the development of the fetus. The endometrium exhibits cyclic changes in structure and function in response to the ovarian hormones **estrogen** and **progesterone.** These changes prepare the uterus for implantation and nourishment of the embryo and fetus. If implantation does not occur, the blood vessels in the endometrium deteriorate and rupture, and a portion of the endometrium is shed during menstruation.

During each menstrual cycle, the endometrium goes through three continuous phases, each phase gradually passing into the next. The **preovulatory (proliferative, follicular) phase** is characterized by rapid growth and development of the endometrium. This phase starts at the end of the menstrual phase, approximately day 5, and continues to day 14 of the cycle. Increased mitotic activity of cells in the **lamina propria** and in the remnants of **uterine glands** in the **basalis layer** begin to cover the raw surface of the mucosa that was denuded during menstruation. As the functionalis layer of the endometrium thickens, the uterine glands proliferate, lengthen, and become closely packed. The **spiral arteries** begin to grow toward the endometrial surface and show only slight coiling. The growth of the endometrium during the proliferative phase closely coincides with the growth of the **ovarian follicles** and their increased secretion of **estrogen.**

The **postovulatory (secretory, luteal) phase** begins shortly after ovulation on approximately day 15 and continuous to approximately day 28 of the cycle. This phase is dependent on the secretion of **progesterone** (primarily by granulosa lutein cells) and **estrogen** (by theca lutein cells) of the functional corpus luteum of the ovary, which forms after ovulation. During this phase, the endometrium continues to thicken and to accumulate fluid, becoming **edematous.** In addition, the uterine glands hypertrophy and become tortuous, and their lumina become filled with secretory products that are rich in **nutrients,** especially **glycogen.** The spiral arteries in the endometrium lengthen, become more coiled, and extend almost to the surface of the endometrium.

The **menstrual (menses) phase** begins when fertilization and implantation fail to occur. Reduced levels of circulating progesterone (and estrogen), due to regressing corpus luteum, initiate this phase. Decreased levels of estrogen and progesterone cause the spiral arteries in the functionalis layer of the endometrium to constrict in an intermittent fashion. This action deprives the functionalis layer of oxygenated blood and produces transitory **ischemia,** necrosis, and its shrinkage. After extended periods of vascular constriction, the spiral arteries dilate and their walls rupture, leading to hemorrhage into the stroma. The necrotic functionalis layer is then exfoliated and shed in the **menstrual flow.** Blood, uterine fluid, stromal cells, secretory material, and epithelial cells from the functionalis layer mix to form the vaginal discharge. The shedding of the endometrium continues until only the raw surface of the basalis layer is left. The rapid proliferation of cells from the basalis layer, under the influence of rising levels of estrogen, restores the lost endometrial surface as the next phase of the menstrual cycle begins.

1 Superficial
  endometrium
  without epithelium

2 Glandular lumen
  filled with blood

3 Coiled arteries

4 Interglandular
  lamina propria
  of basal region

5 Smooth muscle
  fibers (myometrium)

6 Fragments of
  disintegrated stroma

7 Blood clots

8 Erythrocytes in
  lamina propria

9 Intact bases of
  uterine glands

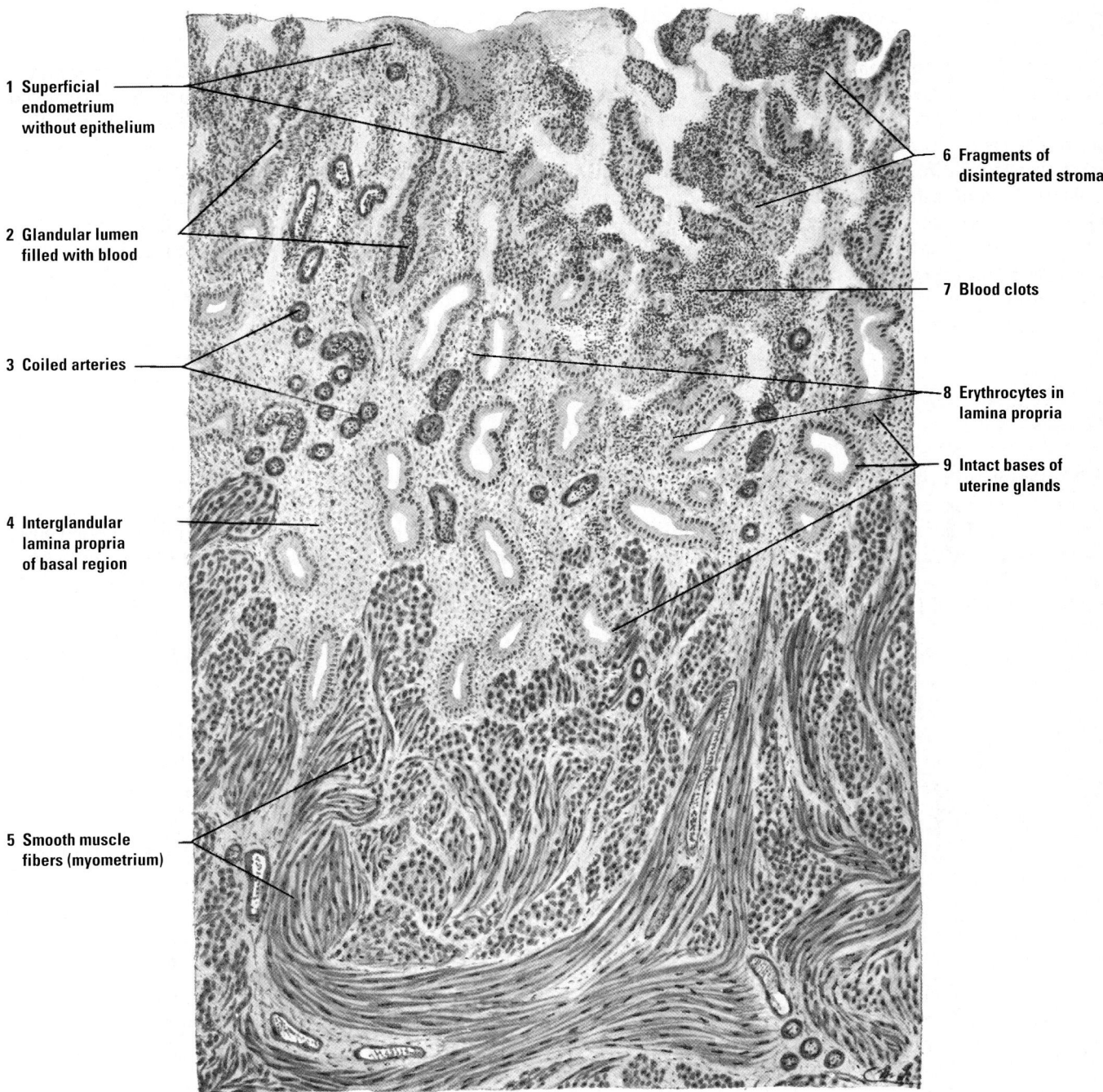

Fig. 18-12   Uterus: Menstrual Phase. Stain: hematoxylin-eosin. Low magnification.

Figure 18-13   Ovary: Primordial and Primary Follicles

A healthy and mature mammalian ovary is normally filled with a variety of developing follicles. This photomicrograph shows the follicular contents in an ovarian cortex. The undeveloped, immature follicles are the **primordial follicles (2).** Each primordial follicle (2) consists of a primary **oocyte (3)** surrounded by a layer of squamous **follicular cells (1, 7).** As the primordial follicles (2) grow to become **primary follicles (4),** the layer of squamous follicular cells around the oocyte change to a cuboidal layer. In a larger, more mature **primary follicle (8),** the follicular cells have proliferated into a stratified cell layer around the oocyte called **granulosa cells (11).** In addition, a prominent layer of glycoprotein, the **zona pellucida (10),** develops between the granulosa cells (11) and the larger **oocyte (9).** The cells around the developing follicles also organize into two distinct cell layers, the inner hormone-secreting **theca interna (12)** and the connective tissue outer **theca externa (13).** These cell layers are separated from the granulosa cells (11) by a thin but distinct **basement membrane (6).** Surrounding all of the follicles in the ovarian cortex are cells and fibers of the **connective tissue (5).**

Figure 18-14   Uterine Tube: Lining Epithelium

A higher magnification photomicrograph illustrates a section of the uterine tube wall. The uterine tube exhibits numerous complex mucosal folds that are lined by a **simple columnar epithelium (2).** The luminal epithelium consists of two cell types, the **ciliated cells (5)** and nonciliated **peg cells (6),** whose apical bulges extend above the cilia. A thin **basement membrane (1)** separates the luminal epithelium (2) from the underlying vascularized **connective tissue (4)** that forms the core of the folds. A portion of the **inner circular smooth muscle (3)** layer that surrounds the uterine tube is visible in the periphery of the illustration.

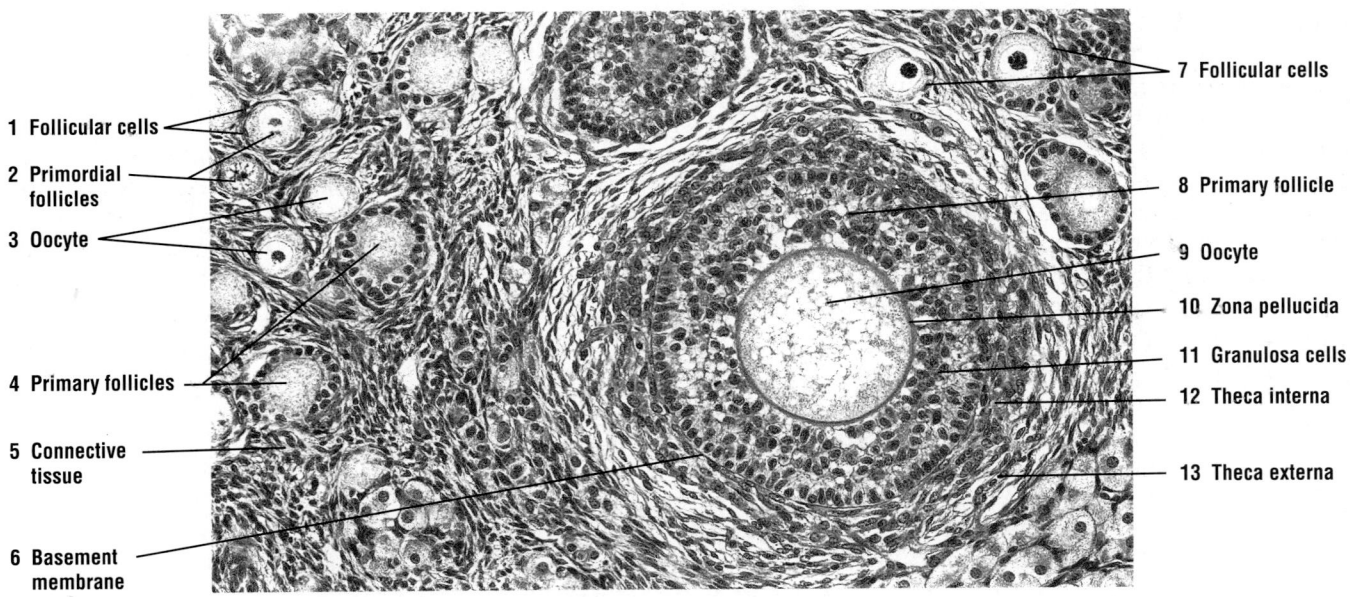

1 Follicular cells
2 Primordial follicles
3 Oocyte
4 Primary follicles
5 Connective tissue
6 Basement membrane

7 Follicular cells
8 Primary follicle
9 Oocyte
10 Zona pellucida
11 Granulosa cells
12 Theca interna
13 Theca externa

Fig. 18-13   Ovary: Primordial and Primary Follicles. Stain: hematoxylin-eosin. 64×

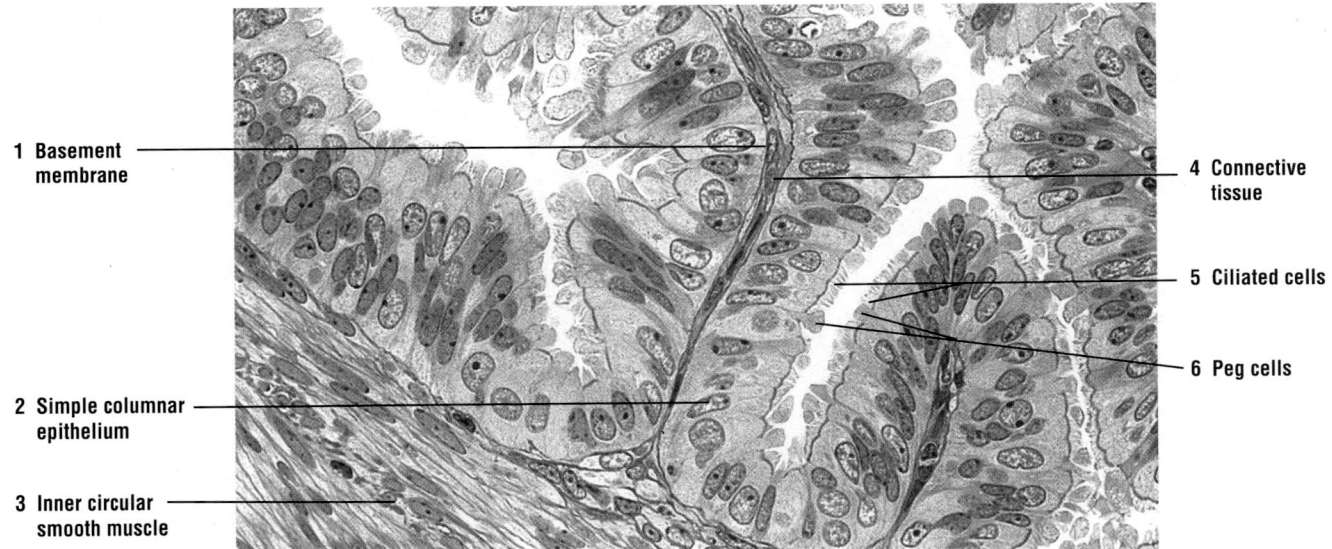

1 Basement membrane
2 Simple columnar epithelium
3 Inner circular smooth muscle

4 Connective tissue
5 Ciliated cells
6 Peg cells

Fig. 18-14   Uterine Tube: Lining Epithelium. Stain: hematoxylin-eosin (plastic section). 130×

Figure 18-15   Uterine Wall (Endometrium): Secretory (Luteal) Phase

A low power magnification illustrates a section of the uterine wall, the endometrium, during the secretory or luteal phase of the menstrual cycle. The thick, lighter area of the endometrium represents the **stratum functionalis (1).** The **uterine glands (3)** during this phase appear tortuous and secrete glycogen-rich nutrient material into their lumina. The darker, deeper region of the endometrium is the **stratum basalis (2).** Surrounding the uterine glands (3) is the highly cellular **connective tissue (4)** layer. The light, empty spaces in the connective tissue (4) layer are due to increased edema in the endometrium. Below the stratum basalis (2) is visible a portion of the smooth muscle layer of the uterine wall, the **myometrium (5).**

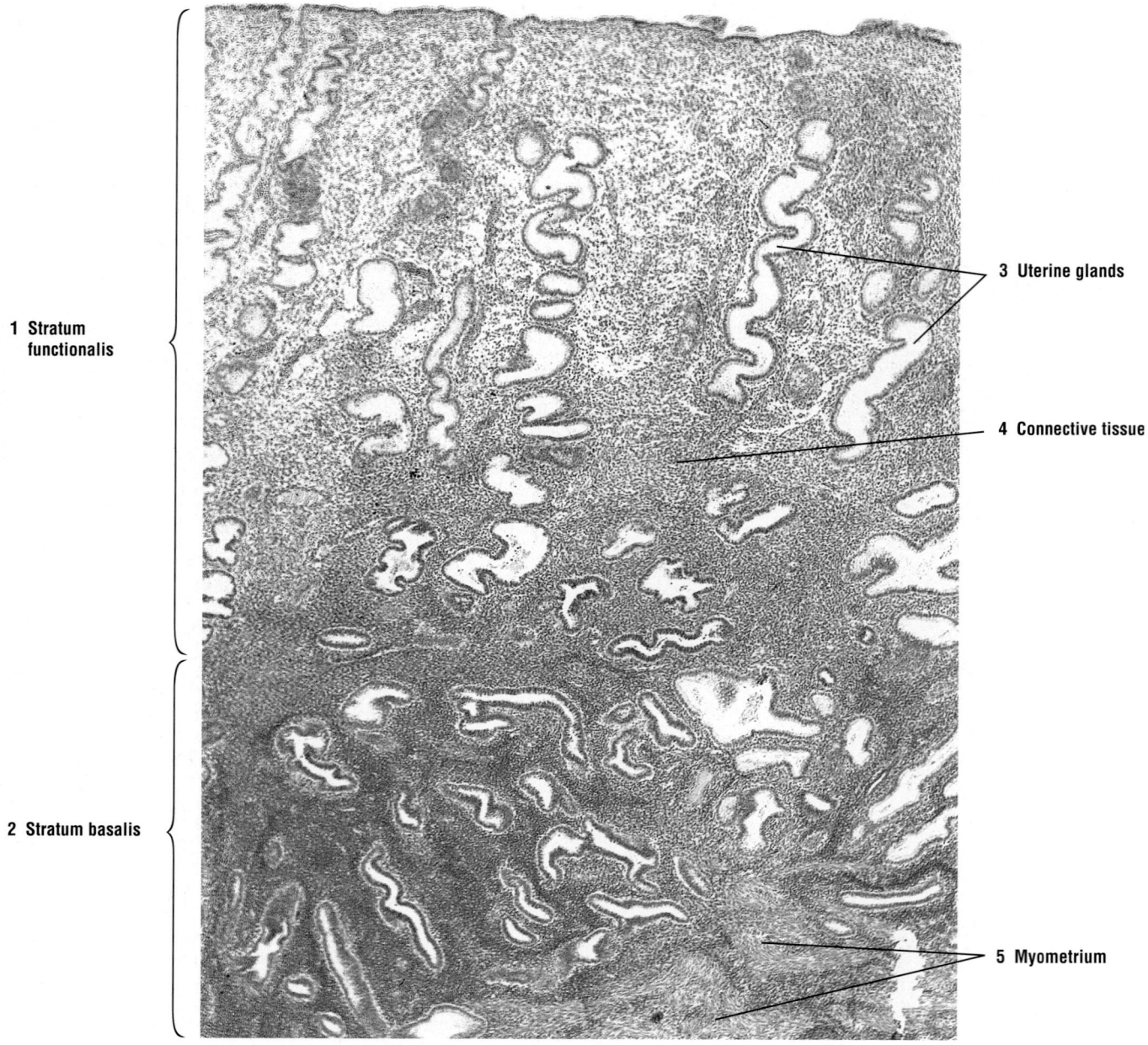

Fig. 18-15   Uterine Wall (Endometrium): Secretory (Luteal) Phase. Stain: hematoxylin-eosin. 10×

SECTION 2
Cervix, Vagina, Placenta, and Mammary Glands

CERVIX AND VAGINA

Cervix is the lower part of the uterus that projects into vaginal canal as **portio vaginalis.** A narrow **cervical canal** passes through the cervix. The opening of the cervical canal that communicates with the uterus is the **internal os** and with the vagina is the **external os.** Unlike the functionalis layer of the uterine endometrium, the cervical mucosa undergoes minimal changes and is not shed during menstruation. The cervix does, however, contain numerous branched **cervical glands,** and these exhibit altered secretory activities during the different phases of menstrual cycle **(Fig. 18-16, 18-27).** The amount and type of mucus secreted by the cervical glands change during the menstrual cycle due to different ovarian hormones.

The **vagina** is a fibromuscular tube that extends from the cervix to the vestibule of the external genitalia. Its wall has numerous folds and consists of an inner **mucosa,** a middle **muscular layer,** and an outer connective tissue **adventitia.** The vagina does not have any glands in its wall. The vaginal canal is lined by **stratified squamous epithelium** and lubricated by **mucus** produced by the **cervical glands** of the cervix. Loose fibroelastic connective tissue and rich vasculature compose the lamina propria, and smooth muscle fibers compose the muscular layer of the organ. Like the cervical epithelium, the vaginal lining is not shed during menstrual flow **(Figs. 18-17–18-19, 18-27).**

PLACENTA

During pregnancy, the fertilized ovum implants in the endometrium of the uterus and forms a **placenta.** The placenta consists of a **fetal portion,** formed by the **chorionic plate** and its **branching chorionic villi,** and a **maternal portion,** formed by the **decidua basalis** of the endometrium. Fetal and maternal blood come into close proximity in the villi of the placenta. Exchange of nutrients, electrolytes, hormones, antibodies, gaseous products, and waste metabolites takes place as the blood passes over the villi. Fetal blood enters the placenta through a pair of **umbilical arteries,** passes into the villi, and returns through a single **umbilical vein (Figs. 18-20–18-22).**

MAMMARY GLANDS

The adult mammary gland is a compound **tubuloalveolar gland** that consists of approximately 20 lobes. All lobes are connected to **lactiferous ducts** that open at the **nipple.** The lobes are separated by connective tissue partitions and adipose tissue. The resting or inactive mammary glands are small, consist primarily of **ducts,** and do not exhibit any developed or secretory alveoli. Inactive mammary glands also exhibit slight cyclic alterations during the course of the menstrual cycle. Under estrogenic stimulation, the secretory cells increase in height. Lumina appear in the ducts as a small amount of secretory material is accumulated **(Figs. 18-23–18-26, 18-28).**

Figure 18-16   Cervix, Cervical Canal, and Vaginal Fornix (longitudinal section)

The cervix is the lower part of the uterus. This figure illustrates a longitudinal plane of section through the cervix, the endocervix or **cervical canal (5),** a portion of the **vaginal fornix (8),** and the **vaginal wall (10).** The cervical canal (5) is lined with tall, mucus-secreting columnar **epithelium (2).** This epithelium differs from the uterine epithelium with which it is continuous. Similar epithelium also lines the numerous highly branched and tubular **cervical glands (3)** which extend at an oblique angle to the cervical canal (5) deep into the wide **lamina propria (12).** Some of these cervical glands may become occluded and develop into small **cysts (4).** The connective tissue in the lamina propria (12) of the cervix is more fibrous than in the uterus. Blood vessels, nerves, and occasional **lymphatic nodules (11)** may be seen.

The lower end of the cervix, the **os cervix (6),** bulges into the lumen of the **vaginal canal (13).** The columnar epithelium (2) of the cervical canal (5) at the lower end abruptly changes to nonkeratinized stratified squamous epithelium. This epithelium lines the vaginal portion of the cervix, called the **portio vaginalis (7),** as well as the external surface of the vaginal fornix (8). At the base of the fornix the epithelium (7) of the vagina cervix reflects back to become the **vaginal epithelium (9)** of the vaginal wall (10). The details of the vaginal wall are illustrated in greater detail in Figures 18-14 and 18-15.

The smooth muscle of the **muscularis (1)** layer in the cervix is not as compact as in the body of the uterus; however, both the muscularis (1) and the lamina propria (12) are well vascularized.

■ Functional Correlations–Cervix

During the **proliferative phase** of the menstrual cycle, the secretion of the cervical glands is thin and watery. This type of secretion allows for an easier passage of sperm through the cervical canal into the uterus. On the other hand, during the **luteal phase** of the menstrual cycle and **pregnancy,** the cervical gland secretions becomes highly viscous and form a **mucus plug** in the cervical canal. This hinders the passage of sperm and/or microorganisms from the vagina into the uterus.

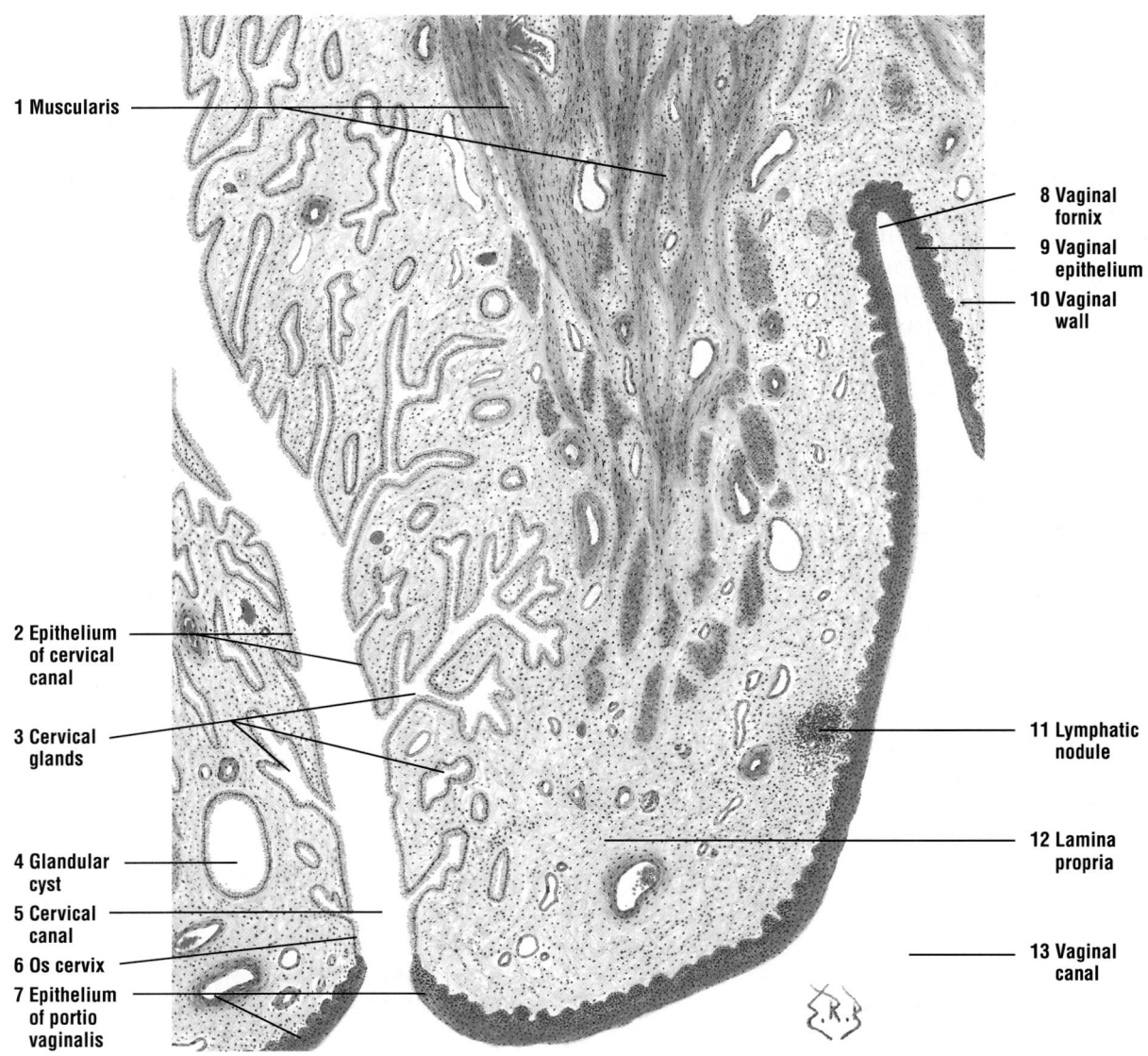

1 Muscularis

8 Vaginal fornix

9 Vaginal epithelium

10 Vaginal wall

2 Epithelium of cervical canal

3 Cervical glands

11 Lymphatic nodule

4 Glandular cyst

5 Cervical canal

12 Lamina propria

6 Os cervix

7 Epithelium of portio vaginalis

13 Vaginal canal

Fig. 18-16   Cervix, Cervical Canal, and Vaginal Fornix (longitudinal section). Stain: hematoxylin-eosin. Low magnification.

Figure 18-17   Vagina (longitudinal section)

The vaginal mucosa is highly irregular and exhibits numerous folds (1). The epithelium lining the surface of the vaginal canal is noncornified **stratified squamous (2).** Connective tissue **papillae (3)** below the epithelium are prominent and vary in height.

The wide **lamina propria (7)** contains moderately dense, irregular connective tissue that is rich in elastic fibers. Fibers from the lamina propria extend down and pass into the muscularis layer as **interstitial fibers (10).** Diffuse **lymphatic tissue (8), lymphatic nodules (4),** and numerous small **blood vessels** (arterioles and venules) **(9)** are usually observed in the lamina propria (7).

The muscularis consists predominantly of **longitudinal (5a)** and oblique bundles of smooth muscle fibers. The **transverse muscle fibers (5b)** are less numerous but more frequently found in the inner layers. The interstitial connective tissue (10) is rich in elastic fibers and the **adventitia (6, 12)** contains **blood vessels (11)** and nerve bundles.

Figure 18-18   Glycogen in Human Vaginal Epithelium

Glycogen is a prominent component of the vaginal epithelium except in the deepest layers, where it is minimal or lacking. During the follicular phase of the menstrual cycle, glycogen accumulates in the vaginal epithelium, reaching its maximum level before ovulation. Glycogen can be demonstrated by iodine vapor or iodine solution in mineral oil (Mancini's method); glycogen stains a reddish purple.

The vaginal specimens in illustrations **(A)** and **(B)** were fixed in absolute alcohol and formaldehyde. The amount of glycogen in the vaginal epithelium during the interfollicular phase of the cycle is illustrated in (A). During the follicular phase, glycogen content increases in the cells of the intermediate and the more superficial layers (B).

The tissue sample illustrated in **(C)** is from the same specimen as in (B), but was fixed by the Altmann-Gersch method (freezing and drying in a vacuum). This method produces less tissue shrinkage and illustrates abundant glycogen during the follicular phase, and its diffuse distribution throughout the vaginal epithelium.

■ Functional Correlations–Vagina

The vaginal epithelium does exhibit some cyclic changes during the menstrual cycle. During the follicular phase and estrogenic stimulation, the vaginal epithelium thickens. The vaginal cells synthesize and accumulate increased amounts of **glycogen** as they migrate toward and are desquamated into the lumen. Bacteria in the vagina metabolize the glycogen to **lactic acid,** thereby increasing the acidity of the vaginal canal.

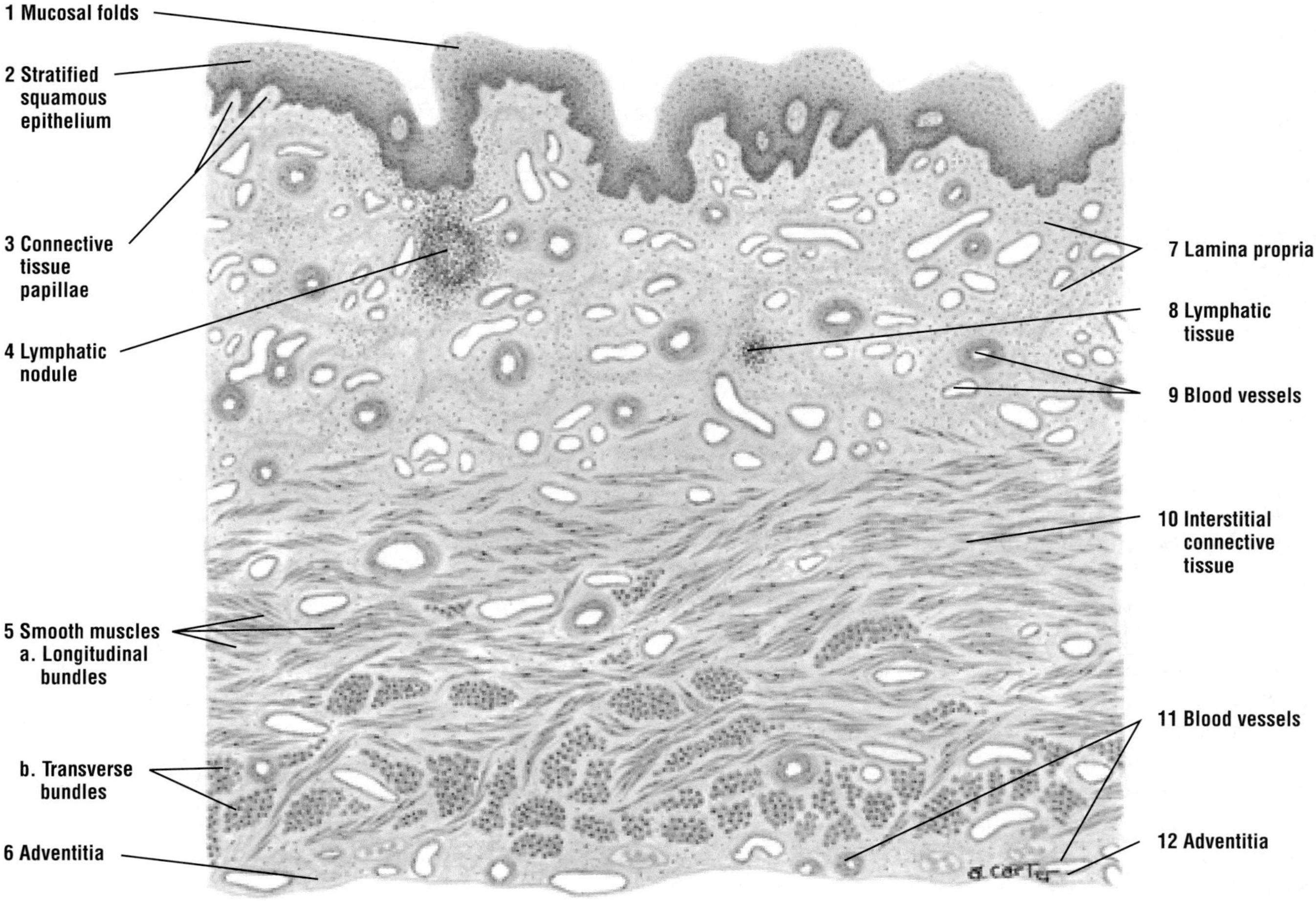

1 Mucosal folds

2 Stratified
squamous
epithelium

3 Connective
tissue
papillae

4 Lymphatic
nodule

7 Lamina propria

8 Lymphatic
tissue

9 Blood vessels

10 Interstitial
connective
tissue

5 Smooth muscles
a. Longitudinal
bundles

b. Transverse
bundles

6 Adventitia

11 Blood vessels

12 Adventitia

a. carter

Fig. 18-17   Vagina (longitudinal section). Stain: hematoxylin-eosin. Low magnification.

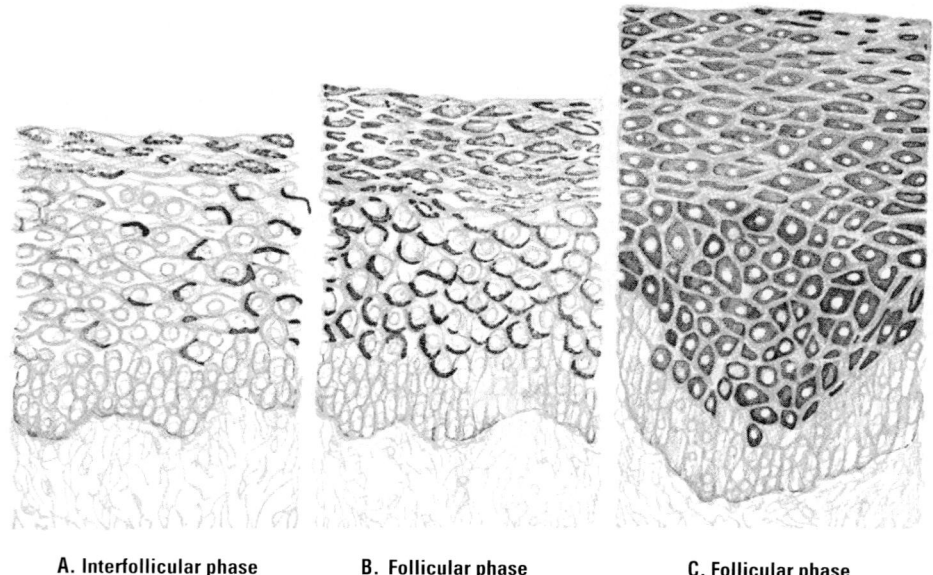

A. Interfollicular phase   **B. Follicular phase**   **C. Follicular phase**

Fig. 18-18   Glycogen in Human Vaginal Epithelium. Stain: Mancini's iodine technique. Medium magnification.

Figure 18-19   Vaginal Smears During Various Reproductive Phases

This figure illustrates cells in vaginal smears obtained from normal woman during the menstrual cycle, early pregnancy, and menopause. The Shorr's trichrome stain (Bierbrich scarlet, orange G, and fast green) plus Harris' hematoxylin facilitates recognition of different cell types.

Figure G illustrates individual cell types observed in a normal vaginal smear. The superficial **acidophilic cell (a)** of the vaginal mucosa appears flat and somewhat irregular in outline, measures from 35 to 65 μm in diameter, exhibits a small nucleus, and contains cytoplasm stained light orange. Adjacent to the acidophilic cell (a) is a similar **superficial basophilic cell (b)** with blue-green cytoplasm. Illustration **(c)** is a cell from the **intermediate stratum** of the vaginal epithelium. It is flattened like the superficial cells but is smaller, measuring 20 to 40 μm in diameter, and has a basophilic blue-green cytoplasm. The nucleus is somewhat larger than that of the superficial cells, and is often vesicular. Illustration **(d)** depicts **intermediate cells** in profile, characterized by their elongated form with folded borders and elongated, eccentric nucleus. Illustration **(e)** depicts **basal cells,** the cells of the internal basal layers of the vaginal epithelium. The larger cells are from the external portion of the basal layers. The smaller **parabasal cells** are from the more superficial portion of the basal layers. All basal cells are oval, measure from 12 to 15 μm in diameter, and exhibit a large nucleus with a prominent chromatin. Most of these cells exhibit basophilic staining.

Figure A illustrates a vaginal smear taken during the fifth day of the menstrual cycle (postmenstrual phase). The **intermediate cells (1)** from the outer layers of the intermediate layer (transitions to the deeper superficial cells) are predominant. A few **superficial acidophilic and basophilic (2)** cells and leukocytes are present.

Figure B represents a vaginal smear collected during the ovulatory phase (14th day) of the menstrual cycle. This phase is characterized by predominance of large superficial **acidophilic cells (8),** the scarcity of superficial **basophilic cells (10)** and **intermediate cells (9),** and the absence of leukocytes. This smear is characteristic of the high estrogenic stimulation normally observed before ovulation and is called the "follicular smear." The superficial cells (8) "mature" with increased estrogen levels and become acidophilic. A similar type of smear can be obtained from a menopausal woman treated with high doses of estrogen.

Figure C represents a vaginal smear taken during the luteal (progestational) phase (21st day of the menstrual cycle). This phase is indicative of increased levels of progesterone. Predominant are large cells from the **intermediate layers (3)** (precornified superficial cells) with folded borders that aggregate into clumps. Superficial **acidophilic cells (4),** superficial **basophilic cells (5),** and leukocytes are scarce.

The cells in Figure D represent the vaginal smear during the premenstrual phase (28th day of the menstrual cycle). This stage is characterized by a great predominance of grouped **intermediate cells (13, 14)** with folded borders, an increase of **neutrophilic cells (12),** a scarcity of **superficial cells (11),** and an abundance of mucus, which blurs the preparations.

Figure E illustrates a vaginal smear taken from a 3-month pregnancy, illustrating predominantly cells from the intermediate layers, many with **folded borders (6).** These cells typically form dense groups or **conglomerations (7).** Cells from superficial layers and neutrophilic cells are scarce.

The vaginal smear during menopause (Figure F) is different from all other phases. In a typical "atrophic" smear, the predominant cells are the oval **basal cells (17)** of various sizes. Cells from the **intermediate layers (15)** are scarce, whereas the **neutrophilic cells (16)** are abundant. Menopausal smears vary according to the stage of menopause and estrogen levels.

Vaginal exfoliate cytology is closely correlated with the ovarian cycle. Understanding its characteristic features permits recognition of follicular activity during normal menstrual phases or after estrogenic and other therapy. Also, exfoliate cytology provides important information (together with cells from the endocervix) for detecting regional pathologic or malignant conditions.

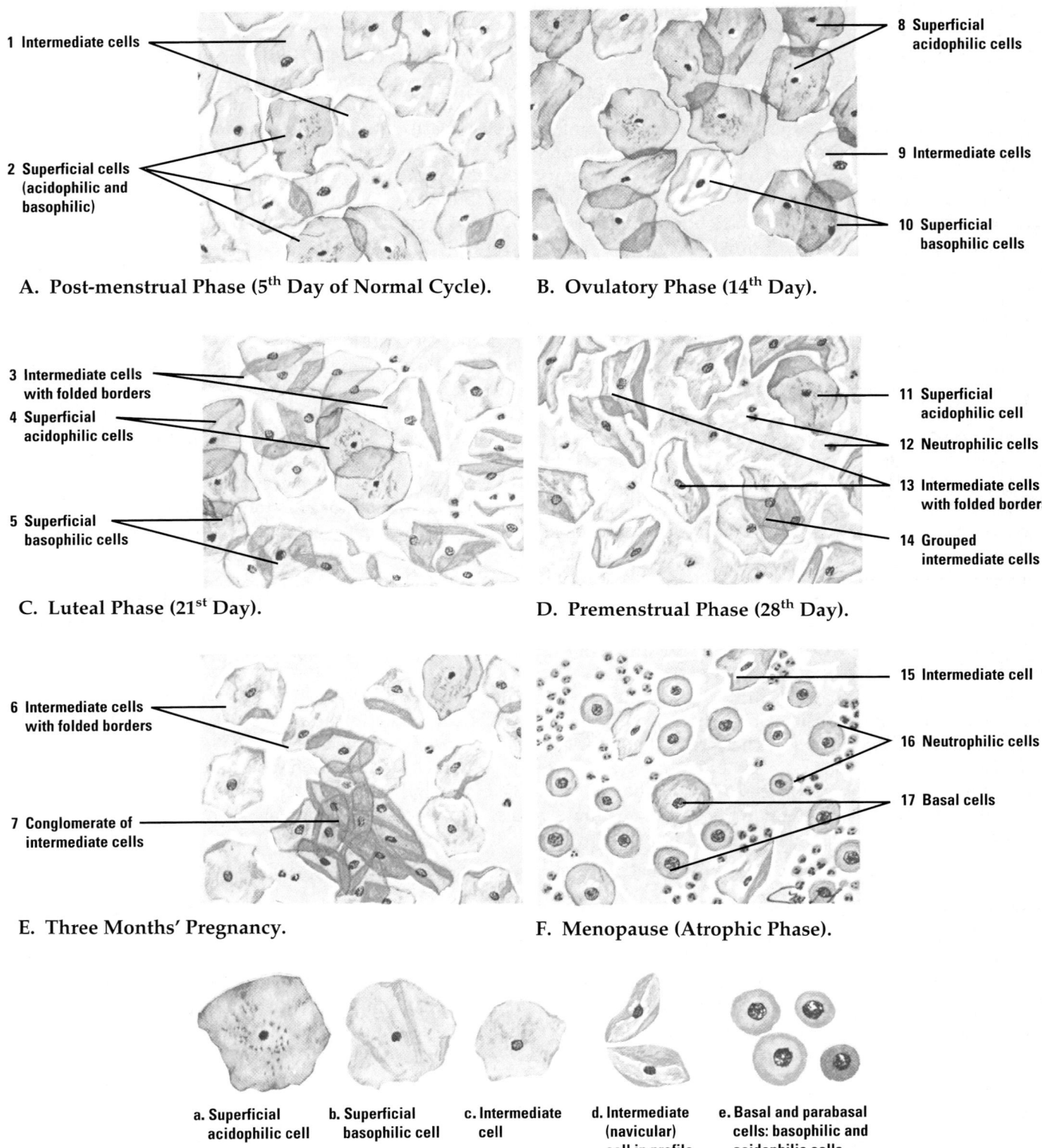

1 Intermediate cells

2 Superficial cells
(acidophilic and
basophilic)

8 Superficial
acidophilic cells

9 Intermediate cells

10 Superficial
basophilic cells

A. Post-menstrual Phase (5th Day of Normal Cycle).   B. Ovulatory Phase (14th Day).

3 Intermediate cells
with folded borders
4 Superficial
acidophilic cells

5 Superficial
basophilic cells

11 Superficial
acidophilic cell

12 Neutrophilic cells

13 Intermediate cells
with folded borders

14 Grouped
intermediate cells

C. Luteal Phase (21st Day).   D. Premenstrual Phase (28th Day).

6 Intermediate cells
with folded borders

7 Conglomerate of
intermediate cells

15 Intermediate cell

16 Neutrophilic cells

17 Basal cells

E. Three Months' Pregnancy.   F. Menopause (Atrophic Phase).

a. Superficial
acidophilic cell

b. Superficial
basophilic cell

c. Intermediate
cell

d. Intermediate
(navicular)
cell in profile

e. Basal and parabasal
cells: basophilic and
acidophilic cells

G. Detail of Individual Cells (high magnification).

Fig. 18-19   Vaginal Smears During Various Reproductive Phases. Stain: Shorr's trichrome. Medium magnification.

Figure 18-20   Placenta at 5 Months (panoramic view)

The upper region in the figure illustrates the fetal portion of the **placenta (10, 11)**. This includes the **chorionic plate (10)** and the **villi (4, 5, 7)** arising from it. The maternal placenta is the **decidua basalis (8)** and includes the functionalis layer of the **endometrium (12, 13, 14)**, which lies directly beneath the fetal placenta (10, 11). Below this region is the basalis layer of the endometrium, containing the basal parts of the **uterine glands (15)**; this region is not shed during parturition. A portion of the **myometrium (17)** is visible in the lower right field of the figure.

The surface of the **amnion (1)** is lined by the squamous epithelium. The underlying layer represents the merged **connective tissue (2)** of the amnion and chorion. Below the connective tissue layer (2) is the **trophoblast of the chorion (3, 10)**, details of which are not distinguishable at this magnification. The trophoblast (3, 10) and the underlying connective tissue (2) form the chorionic plate (10).

The **anchoring villi (4, 7)** arise from the chorionic plate (10), extend to the uterine wall, and embed in the decidua basalis (8). This continuity is not seen in this illustration; however, larger units in the fetal placenta probably represent sections of the anchoring villi (4, lower leader). These increase in size and complexity during pregnancy.

Numerous **floating villi (chorion frondosum) (5, 11)** are seen, sectioned in various planes because of their outgrowth in all directions from the anchoring villi (7). These villi "float" in the **intervillous spaces (6)**, which are bathed in maternal blood. (The structures of these villi are illustrated in detail in Figures 18-21, 18-22).

The maternal portion of the placenta, the decidua basalis (8), contains embedded anchoring villi (7), groups of large **decidual cells (8)**, and typical stroma. Also seen in the decidua basalis (8) are the distal portions of the uterine glands (14) in various stages of regression, and **maternal blood vessels (9)**, recognizable by their size or by red blood cells in their lumina. A maternal blood vessel opening into an **intervillous space (13)** is visible.

Coiled arteries (16) and basal portions of the **uterine glands (15)** are present deep in the endometrium. **Fibrin deposits (12)** appear on the surface of the decidua basalis (8) and increase in volume and extent as the pregnancy continues.

Figure 18-21   Chorionic Villi: Placenta at 5 Months

Several chorionic villi are illustrated at a higher magnification from a placenta at 5 months of pregnancy. The trophoblast epithelium consists of an outer layer of syncytial cells, the **syncytiotrophoblast (1)**, and an inner layer of cells, the **cytotrophoblast (2)**. The core of the villus contains **embryonic connective tissue (3)** and **fetal blood vessels (5)**, which are branches of umbilical arteries and veins; both nucleated and nonnucleated erythrocytes may be present. The **intervillous spaces (4)** are bathed by maternal blood and the erythrocytes are nonnucleated. One of the illustrated villi is **attached to the endometrium (6)** and several **decidual cells (7)** are seen in the stroma.

Figure 18-22   Chorionic Villi: Placenta at Term

Several chorionic villi are illustrated from a placenta at term. In contrast to the villi in Figure 18-14, the chorionic epithelium in these villi is observed only as **syncytiotrophoblast (1)**; its syncytial character is more pronounced than in Figure 18-14. The **connective tissue (2)** is more differentiated, illustrating more fibers, fewer typical fibroblasts, and numerous large, round **macrophages (Hofbauer cells) (4)**. **Fetal blood vessels (3)** are numerous, having increased in complexity during pregnancy.

■ Functional Correlations–Placenta

The placenta also serves as a temporary—yet major—**endocrine organ** that produces essential hormones for the maintenance of pregnancy. **Placental cells (syncytial trophoblasts)** secrete the hormone **chorionic gonadotropin** shortly after implantation of the fertilized egg. Chorionic gonadotropin is similar to luteinizing hormone (LH) in structure and function, and it maintains the **corpus luteum** during the early stages of pregnancy. Chorionic gonadotropin also stimulates the **corpus luteum** to produce **estrogen** and **progesterone**, the two hormones that are essential for maintaining the pregnancy. As pregnancy proceeds, the placenta takes over production of estrogen and progesterone from the corpus luteum and produces sufficient amounts of progesterone to maintain pregnancy until birth. Placenta also produces **relaxin**, a hormone that softens the fibrocartilage in the pubic symphysis to widen the pelvic canal for impending birth. In some mammals, placenta also secretes **placental lactogen**, a hormone that promotes growth and development of the maternal mammary glands.

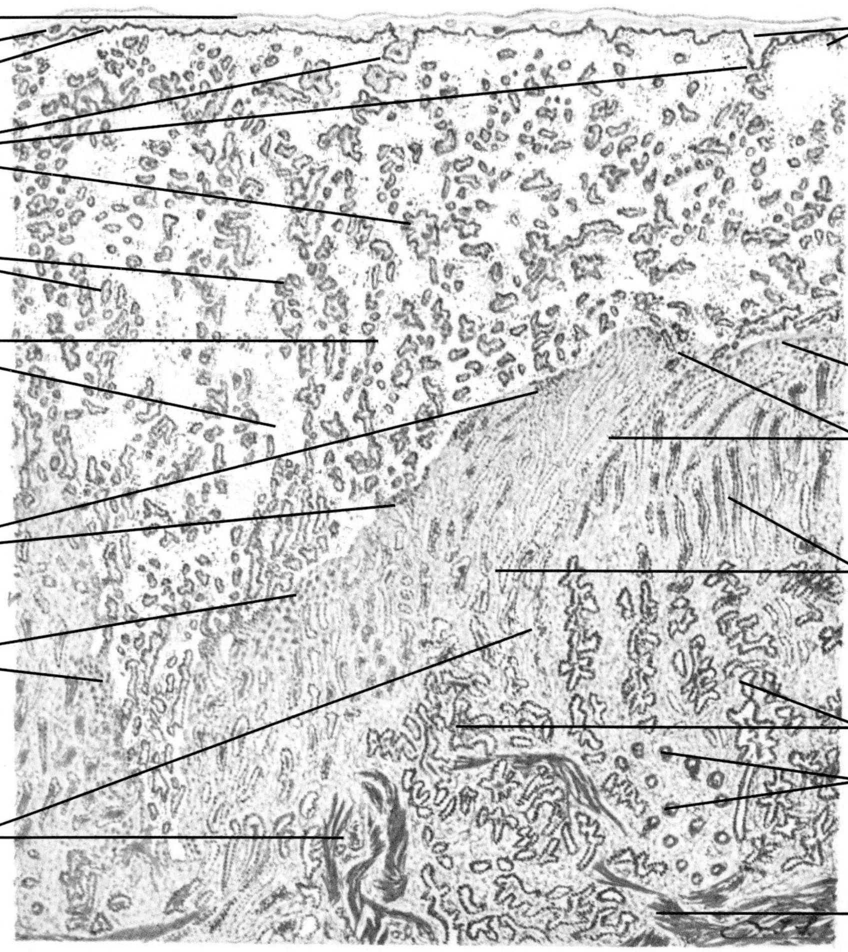

1 **Epithelium of amnion**
2 **Connective tissue**
3 **Trophoblast**
4 **Anchoring villi**
5 **Floating villi**
6 **Intervillous blood spaces**
7 **Anchoring villi**
8 **Decidual cells in the decidua basalis**
9 **Maternal blood vessels**

10 **Chorionic plate (connective tissue and trophoblast)**
11 **Chorion frondosum**
12 **Fibrin deposits**
13 **Blood vessel opening into intervillous space**
14 **Uterine glands (compressed or regressing)**
15 **Basal uterine glands**
16 **Coiled arteries**
17 **Myometrium**

Fig. 18-20   Placenta at 5 Months (panoramic view). Stain: hematoxylin-eosin. Low magnification.

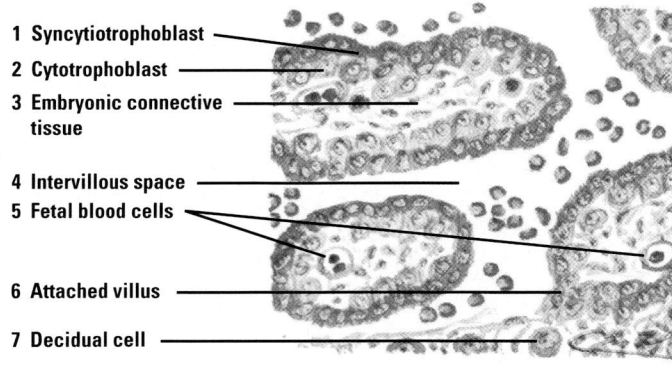

1 **Syncytiotrophoblast**
2 **Cytotrophoblast**
3 **Embryonic connective tissue**
4 **Intervillous space**
5 **Fetal blood cells**
6 **Attached villus**
7 **Decidual cell**

Fig. 18-21   Chorionic Villi: Placenta at 5 Months. Stain: hematoxylin-eosin. High magnification.

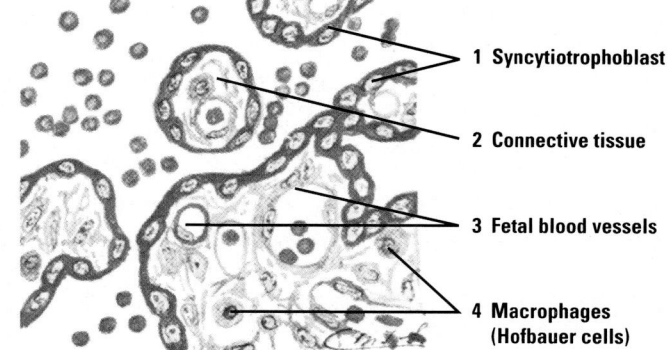

1 **Syncytiotrophoblast**
2 **Connective tissue**
3 **Fetal blood vessels**
4 **Macrophages (Hofbauer cells)**

Fig. 18-22   Chorionic Villi: Placenta at Term. Stain: hematoxylin-eosin. High magnification.

Figure 18-23   Mammary Gland, Inactive

The mammary gland (breast) consists of 15 to 25 lobes, each of which is an individual compound tubulo-alveolar type of gland (see Figure 1-11 and accompanying text). Each glandular lobe is separated by interlobar stroma and has its own lactiferous duct, which emerges independently onto the surface of the nipple. The interlobar stroma consists of dense connective tissue and varying amounts of **fat (11).** Each lobe contains **interlobular connective tissue (2, 4)** between individual lobules. One complete mammary gland lobule and a **portion of another lobule (1)** are illustrated here.

The inactive mammary gland is characterized by an abundance of connective tissue and a minimum of glandular elements. The lobule contains groups of small **tubules (3, 10)** that are lined with cuboidal or low columnar epithelium. These tubules resemble ducts and remain in this state as long as the mammary gland remains inactive. Some cyclic changes may be seen in the mammary gland; however, these regress at the end of the menstrual cycle. Occasionally a more defined tubule is seen, such as a small **intralobular duct (6)** or a large **intralobular excretory duct (8)** that emerges from the lobule to join the interlobular duct. Potential tubules may be present as undifferentiated solid **cords of cells (5).**

The excretory tubules are surrounded by a loose, fine connective tissue, the intralobular connective tissue (4), which contains fibroblasts, lymphocytes, plasma cells, and eosinophils. Surrounding this region is the dense interlobular connective tissue (2) and **adipose tissue (11).**

Figure 18-24   Mammary Gland During First Half of Pregnancy

The mammary gland exhibits extensive structural changes in preparation for lactation. During the first half of the pregnancy, the intralobular ducts undergo rapid proliferation and form terminal buds, which differentiate into **alveoli (2, 6).** Most of the alveoli are empty; however, some may contain a **secretory product (5).** At this stage of mammary gland development, it is difficult to distinguish between small **intralobular excretory ducts (9)** and alveoli (2, 6). The ducts appear more regular in outline and have a more distinct epithelial lining **(9).**

The glandular lobules contain numerous alveoli (2, 6) and the **loose intralobular connective tissue (7)** appears reduced. On the other hand, there is an increased infiltration of lymphocytes and other cells. The **interlobular dense connective tissue (3)** appears as septa between the developing lobules (1). The **interlobular excretory ducts (4)** that are lined with taller columnar cells course in the interlobular septa (3) and empty into the large **lactiferous ducts (8),** which are usually lined with low pseudostratified columnar epithelium. Each lactiferous duct (8) collects the secretory product of a lobe and transports it to the nipple.

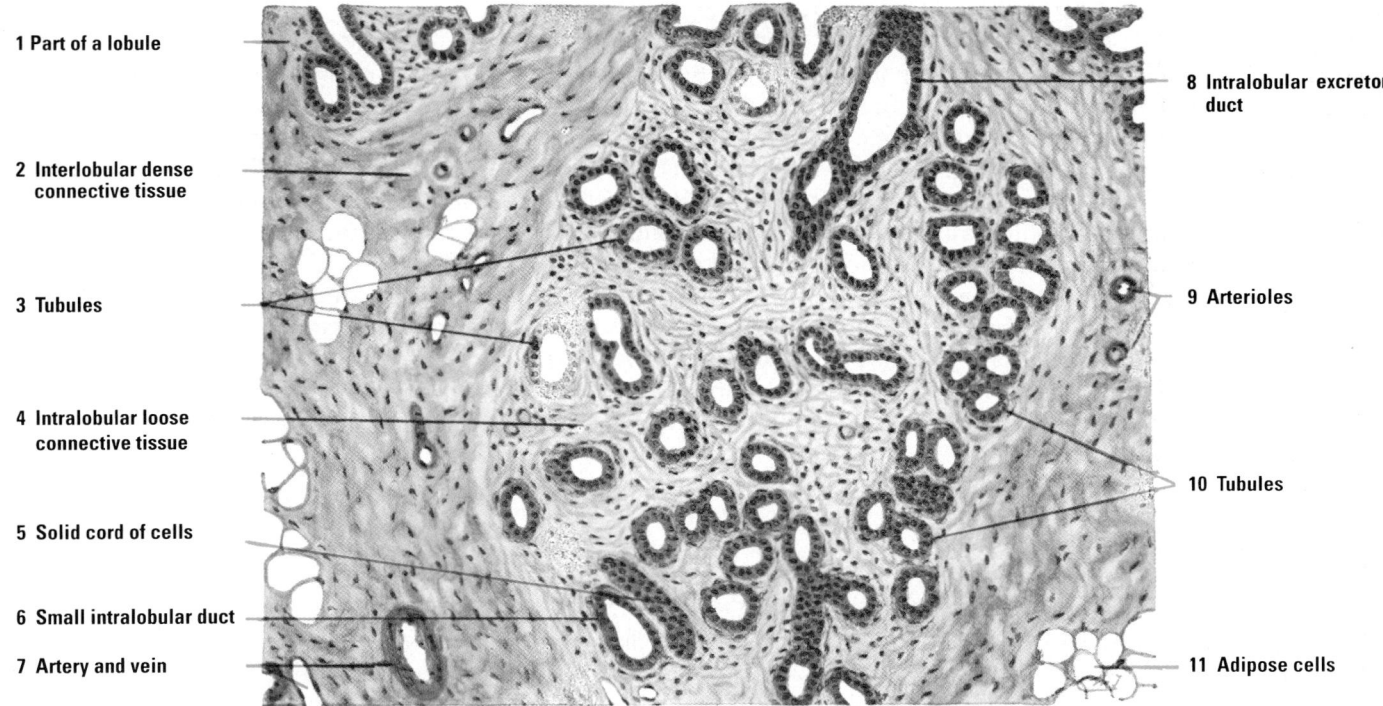

1 Part of a lobule

2 Interlobular dense connective tissue

3 Tubules

4 Intralobular loose connective tissue

5 Solid cord of cells

6 Small intralobular duct

7 Artery and vein

8 Intralobular excretory duct

9 Arterioles

10 Tubules

11 Adipose cells

Fig. 18-23   Mammary Gland, Inactive. Stain: hematoxylin-eosin. Medium magnification.

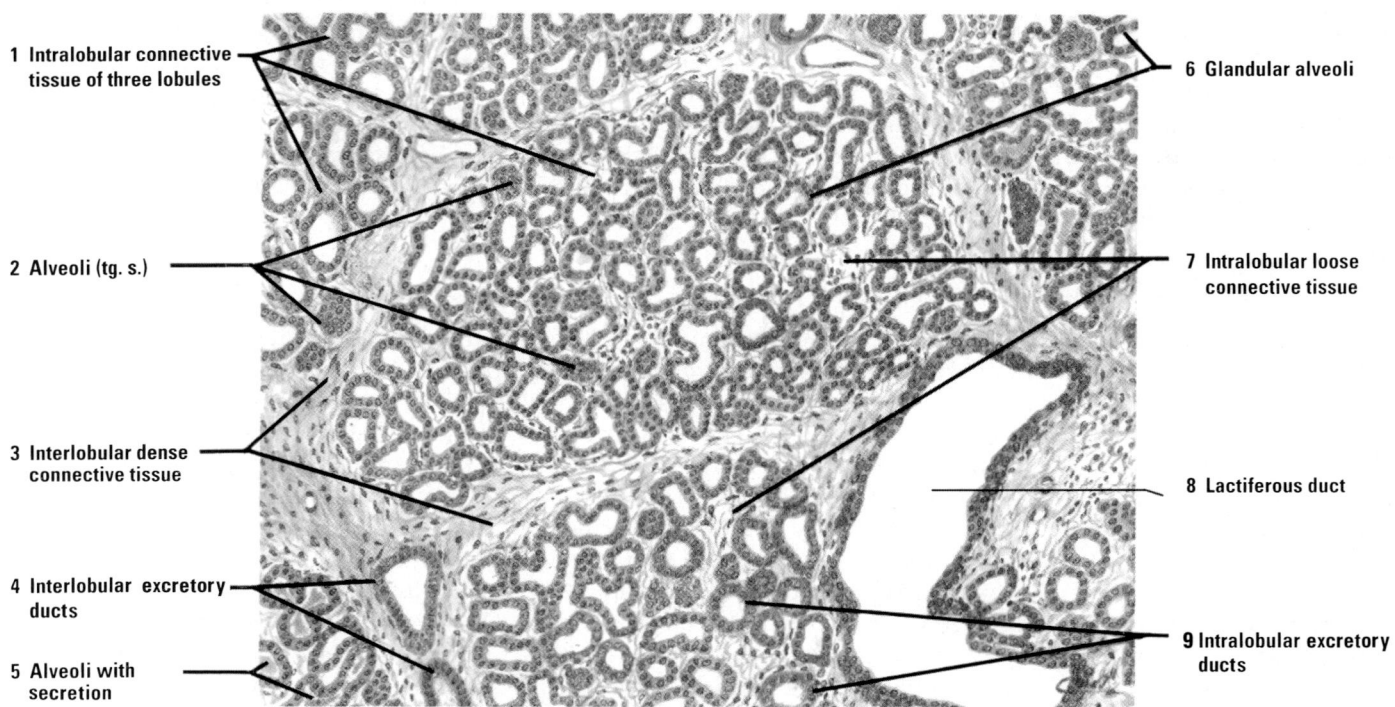

1 Intralobular connective tissue of three lobules

2 Alveoli (tg. s.)

3 Interlobular dense connective tissue

4 Interlobular excretory ducts

5 Alveoli with secretion

6 Glandular alveoli

7 Intralobular loose connective tissue

8 Lactiferous duct

9 Intralobular excretory ducts

Fig. 18-24   Mammary Gland During First Half of Pregnancy. Stain: hematoxylin-eosin. Medium magnification.

Figure 18-25   Mammary Gland During Late Pregnancy

A small section of mammary gland with lobules, connective tissue, and excretory ducts is illustrated at lower (left) and higher (right) magnification during pregnancy. At this stage of development, the glandular epithelium is being prepared for lactation; the **alveoli (2, 8)** and **ducts (1, 7, 13)** enlarge, and the alveolar cells become secretory. Some of the alveoli (2) contain secretory product (2, upper leader) that is rich in protein. However, the secretion of milk by the mammary gland does not begin until after parturition (birth). (The histology of a lactating mammary gland is illustrated in Figure 18-23.) Because the **intralobular excretory ducts** (1) of the mammary gland also contain secretory material, the distinction between the alveoli and ducts remains difficult.

As pregnancy progresses, there is a relative reduction in the amount of **intralobular connective tissue (4, 11)** compared to the amount of **interlobular connective tissue (3, 9).** This is because of the enlargement of glandular tissue. Surrounding the alveolar cells are flattened **myoepithelial cells (10, 12);** these are more visible at the higher magnification on the right. Located in the interlobular connective tissue (3, 9) are the **interlobular excretory ducts (7, 13), lactiferous ducts (14)** with secretory product in their lumina, various types of **blood vessels (5),** and **adipose cells (6).**

Figure 18-26   Mammary Gland During Lactation

This figure depicts a lactating mammary gland at lower (left) and higher (right) magnification. The depicted structures are generally similar to those in Figure 18-22.

The major difference in the lactating mammary gland is the presence of a large number of distended alveoli filled with milk secretion (2) and showing irregular **branching patterns (3).** Also, there is a reduction of **interlobular connective tissue septa (4).**

During lactation, the histology of individual alveoli varies; all of the alveoli do not exhibit the same state of secretory activity. The active alveoli (2) are lined by low epithelium and their lumina are filled with milk; milk appears as eosinophilic material with large vacuoles of dissolved **fat droplets (2, 9).** Some alveoli accumulate secretory product in their **cytoplasm (8),** and their apices appear vacuolated because of the removal of fat during the routine tissue preparation. Other alveoli appear **inactive (6, 11)** with empty lumina and taller epithelium.

In the mammary gland, the myoepithelial cells (not illustrated) are present between the alveolar cells and the basal lamina (see Figures 10-12–10-14). The contraction of the myoepithelial cells assists in expelling milk from the alveoli into the excretory ducts. The **interlobular excretory ducts (5, 7)** are embedded in the connective tissue septa, which contain numerous **adipose cells (1, 12).**

■ Functinal Correlations–Mammary Glands

During pregnancy, activation and growth of the mammary gland ducts and alveoli are promoted by the continuous and prolonged production of **estrogen** and **progesterone.** These hormones are initially produced by the corpus luteum of the ovary, and later by the placenta. In addition, further growth of the mammary glands depends on the pituitary hormone **prolactin, placental lactogen,** and adrenal corticoids. These hormones stimulate the intralobular ducts of the mammary glands to proliferate rapidly, branch, and form numerous **alveoli.** The contractile **myoepithelial cells** surround the secretory alveoli. The alveoli then hypertrophy and become active sites of **milk secretion** during lactation. At the end of pregnancy, the alveoli produce a fluid called **colostrum;** it is rich in proteins, vitamins, minerals, and antibodies. Unlike milk, however, colostrum contains little lipid.

After parturition (birth), hormones that inhibited milk secretion decrease and the mammary glands begin active secretion of milk, which is promoted by the pituitary hormone prolactin. During feeding, the tactile stimulation of the nipple area by the suckling infant promotes further release of prolactin, and milk production is prolonged. In addition, tactile stimulation of the nipple initiates the **milk ejection reflex.** This reflex causes the release of the hormone **oxytocin** from the neurohypophysis of the pituitary gland. Oxytocin induces the contraction of myoepithelial cells around the secretory alveoli and excretory ducts in the mammary glands, causing ejection of the accumulated milk from the mammary glands toward the nipple. Decreased nursing and suckling by the infant soon results in the cessation of milk production and eventual regression of the mammary glands to an inactive state.

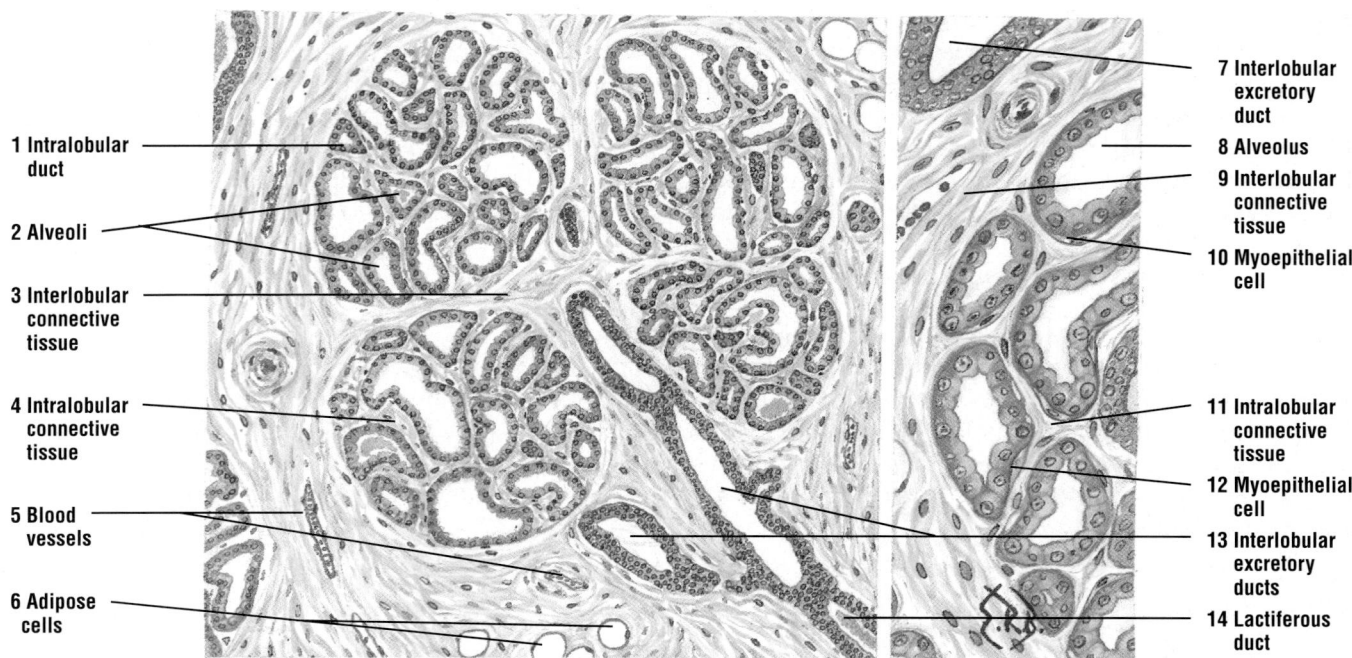

1 Intralobular duct
2 Alveoli
3 Interlobular connective tissue
4 Intralobular connective tissue
5 Blood vessels
6 Adipose cells

7 Interlobular excretory duct
8 Alveolus
9 Interlobular connective tissue
10 Myoepithelial cell
11 Intralobular connective tissue
12 Myoepithelial cell
13 Interlobular excretory ducts
14 Lactiferous duct

Fig. 18-25   Mammary Gland During Late Pregnancy. Stain: hematoxylin-eosin. Left: low magnification. Right: high magnification.

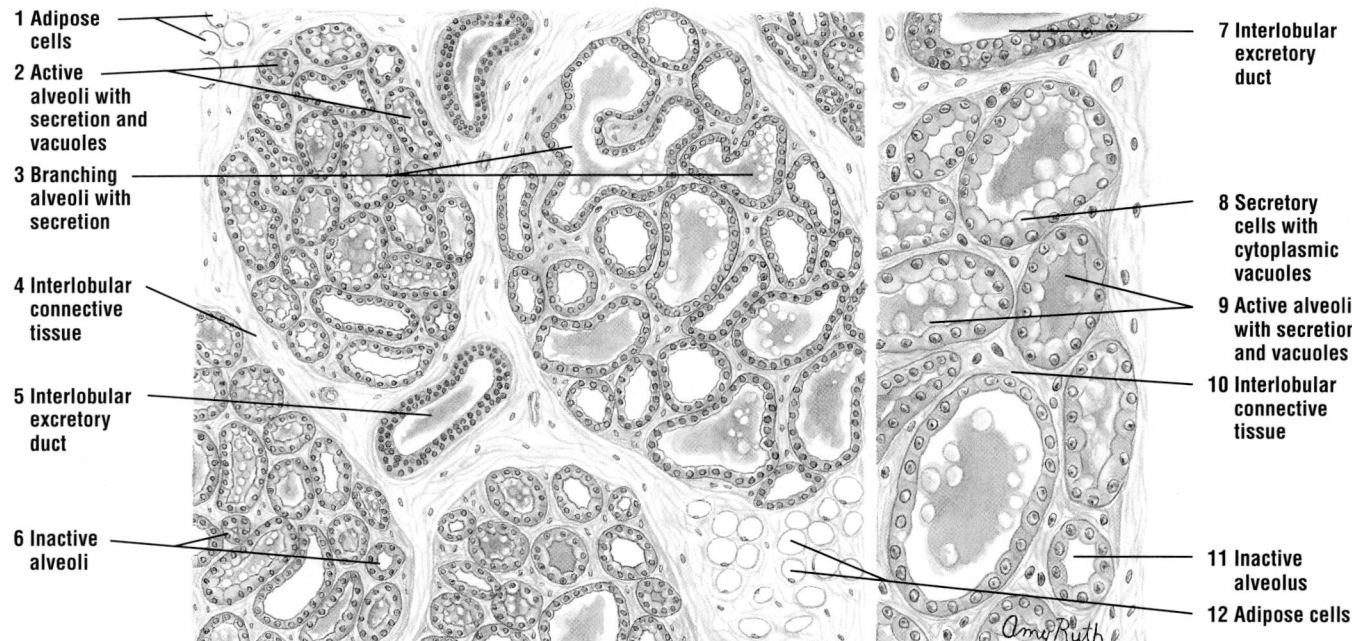

1 Adipose cells
2 Active alveoli with secretion and vacuoles
3 Branching alveoli with secretion
4 Interlobular connective tissue
5 Interlobular excretory duct
6 Inactive alveoli

7 Interlobular excretory duct
8 Secretory cells with cytoplasmic vacuoles
9 Active alveoli with secretion and vacuoles
10 Interlobular connective tissue
11 Inactive alveolus
12 Adipose cells

Fig. 18-26   Mammary Gland During Lactation. Stain: hematoxylin-eosin. Left: low magnification. Right: high magnification.

Figure 18-27   Vagina: Surface Epithelium

This higher magnification photomicrograph illustrates the vaginal epithelium and the underlying connective tissue. The surface epithelium of the vagina is **stratified squamous nonkeratinized (1).** Most of the cells in vaginal epithelium appear empty. This is due primarily to the accumulation of glycogen in their cytoplasm and its extraction by different chemicals during the histologic preparation of the organ. The **lamina propria (2)** is composed of dense, irregular connective tissue. It lacks glands, but it contains numerous **blood vessels (4)** and **lymphocytes (3).**

Figure 18-28   Mammary Gland During Lactation

This photomicrograph illustrates a lobule of a lactating mammary gland separated from adjacent lobule by a thin layer of **connective tissue (3).** A lactating mammary gland is characterized by the presence of numerous **alveoli (1)** that are distended with **secretory product (4)** milk and separated by thin connective tissue septa. Some of the alveoli (1) are single, while others are **branching alveoli (2).** All of the alveoli eventually drain into an excretory duct (see Figures 18-25 and 18-26).

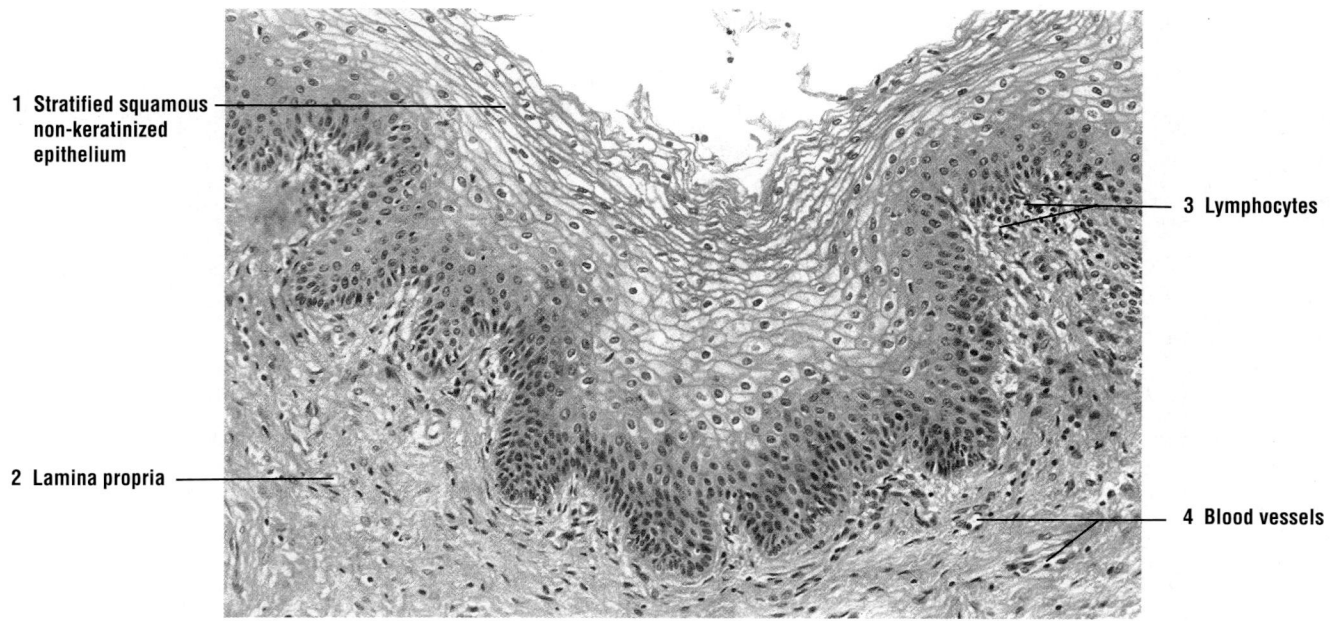

1 Stratified squamous non-keratinized epithelium

3 Lymphocytes

2 Lamina propria

4 Blood vessels

Fig. 18-27   Vagina: Surface Epithelium. Stain: hematoxylin-eosin. 50×

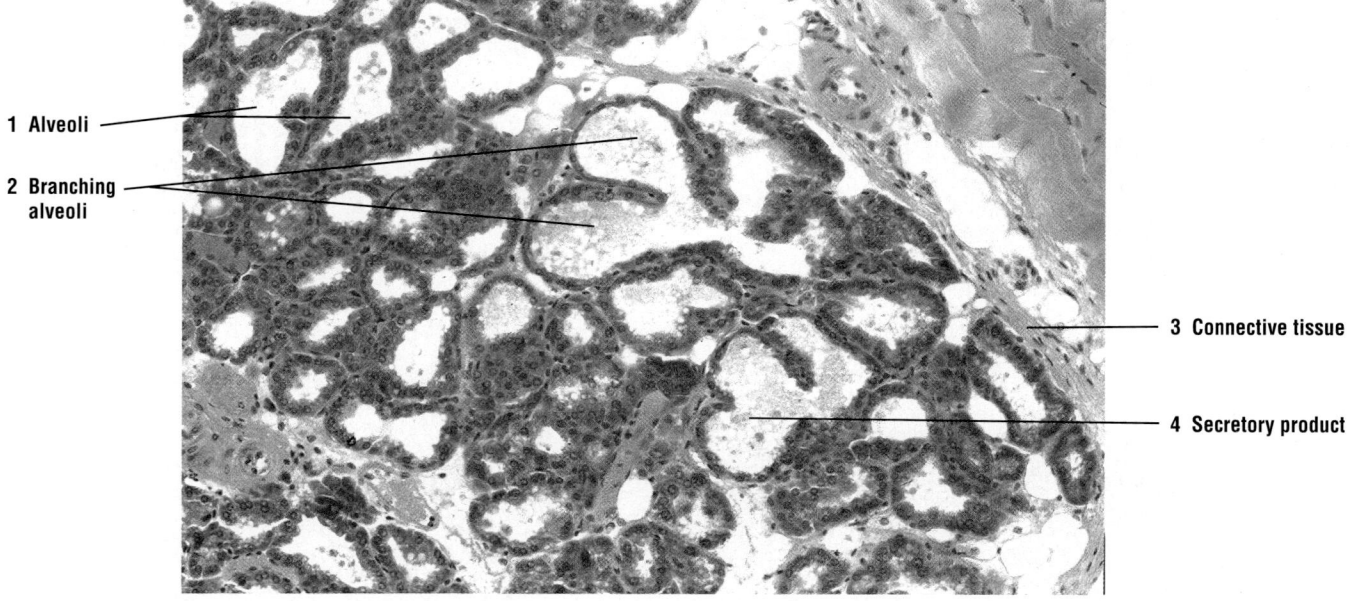

1 Alveoli

2 Branching alveoli

3 Connective tissue

4 Secretory product

Fig. 18-28   Mammary Gland During Lactation. Stain: hematoxylin-eosin. 50×

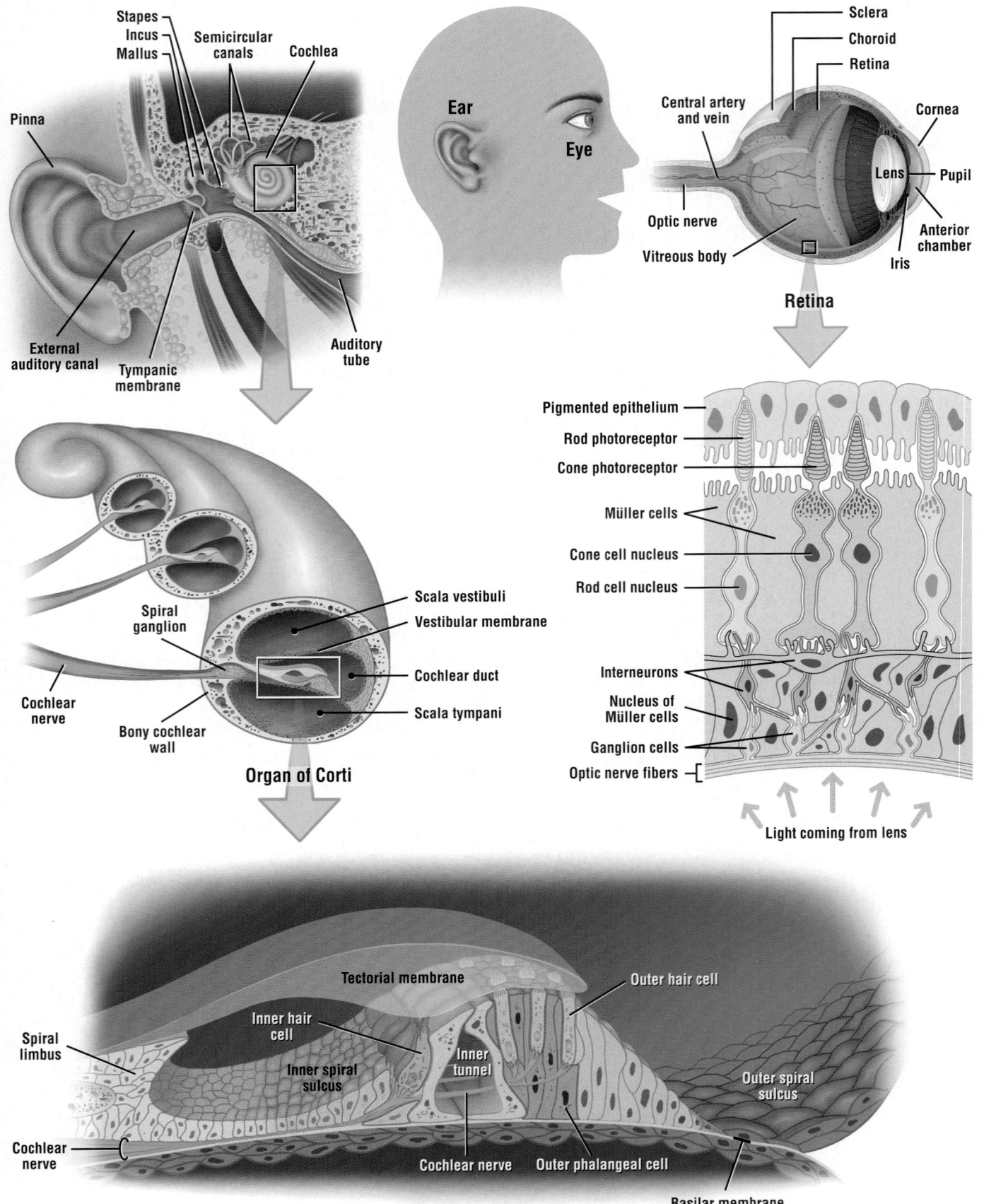

Ear

Stapes
Incus
Mallus
Semicircular canals
Cochlea
Pinna
External auditory canal
Tympanic membrane
Auditory tube

Spiral ganglion
Scala vestibuli
Vestibular membrane
Cochlear duct
Scala tympani
Cochlear nerve
Bony cochlear wall

Organ of Corti

Eye

Central artery and vein
Sclera
Choroid
Retina
Cornea
Lens
Pupil
Optic nerve
Anterior chamber
Vitreous body
Iris

Retina

Pigmented epithelium
Rod photoreceptor
Cone photoreceptor
Müller cells
Cone cell nucleus
Rod cell nucleus
Interneurons
Nucleus of Müller cells
Ganglion cells
Optic nerve fibers
Light coming from lens

Spiral limbus
Tectorial membrane
Outer hair cell
Inner hair cell
Inner tunnel
Inner spiral sulcus
Outer spiral sulcus
Cochlear nerve
Cochlear nerve
Outer phalangeal cell
Basilar membrane

Organs of Special Senses

STRUCTURE OF THE EYE
(Figures 19-2–19-6, 19-9)

The eye is a highly specialized sense organ for vision and photoreception. Each eyeball is surrounded by three distinct layers. The outer layer is the **sclera,** an opaque layer of dense connective tissue. Anteriorly the sclera is modified into a transparent **cornea,** through which light enters the eye. Internal to the sclera is a densely pigmented layer called the **choroid.** Located in the choroid are numerous blood vessels that nourish the photoreceptor cells in the retina and the structures of the eyeball. The innermost lining of the eye is the photosensitive **retina;** it lines the posterior three-quarters of the eye. The photosensitive cells of the retina terminate at a region called the **ora serrata.** Anterior to ora serrata, the retina is not photosensitive.

The eye also contains three chambers: the **anterior chamber,** situated between the cornea and the iris; the **posterior chamber,** situated between the iris and the lens; and the large **vitreous chamber** that contains the gelatinous **vitreous body,** situated between the lens and the retina. The anterior and posterior chambers are filled with a watery fluid called the **aqueous humor.** This fluid, continually produced by the **ciliary process** located behind the iris, circulates from the posterior to the anterior chamber, where it is then drained by way of veins.

The retina contains a layer of **photoreceptor cells (rods** and **cones)** that are sensitive light rays light that pass through the **lens.** Leaving the retina are **afferent** (sensory) **nerves** that conduct the light impulses from the photoreceptors via the **optic nerve** to the brain for visual interpretation.

The posterior region of the eye contains a yellowish pigmented spot called the **macula lutea.** In the center of macula lutea is a depression called the **fovea centralis.** The center of the fovea centralis is devoid of photoreceptive rods and blood vessels, but contains a dense condensation of cones.

STRUCTURE OF THE EAR
(Figures 19-7, 19-8, 19-10)

The ear is highly specialized for hearing, balance, and maintenance of equilibrium. The **auditory system** is composed of three parts: the external ear, the middle ear, and the inner ear.

The auricle or **pinna** of the **external ear** collects sound waves and directs them through the **external auditory canal** to the **tympanic membrane,** or ear drum, which separates the external auditory canal from the **middle ear.** The middle ear is a small, air-filled cavity, the **tympanic cavity,** that is located in and protected by the **temporal bone** of the skull. In the middle ear three very small bones, the **auditory ossicles** (stapes, incus, and malleus) and the auditory or **eustachian tube** that continues from the middle ear inferiorly to the nasopharynx region of the head.

The **inner ear** lies deep in the temporal bone. It consists of small, interconnected compartments and canals. Its sensory components are found in its semicircular canals and cochlea. The semicircular canals contain receptor cells that are responsible for maintaining **balance** and **equilibrium;** these function independently of the external ear and middle ear.

The **cochlea** constitutes the auditory portion of the inner ear and is specialized for sound reception. The cochlea is a spiral bony canal that resembles a snail's shell. It makes three turns on itself around a central bony pillar called the **modiolus.** The chochlea is partitioned into three channels, **scala vestibuli, scala tympani,** and **cochlear duct** (scala media). Located within the cochlear duct on its **basilar membrane** is the **organ of Corti,** which consists of numerous auditory receptor cells or **hair cells** and several types of supporting cells. The auditory stimuli (sound) are carried away from the receptor cells via the cochlear nerve to the brain for interpretation.

Figure 19-1   Eyelid (sagittal section)

The exterior layer of the eyelid is the thin skin (left side). The **epidermis (4)** consists of a stratified squamous epithelium with papillae. In the underlying **dermis (6)** are found **hair follicles (1, 3)** with their associated **sebaceous glands (3).** Also seen in the dermis are the **sweat glands (5).**

The interior layer of the eyelid is a mucous membrane, the **palpebral conjunctiva (15);** it lies adjacent to the eyeball. The lining epithelium of the palpebral conjunctiva (15) is a low stratified columnar type with a few goblet cells. The stratified squamous epithelium (4) of the skin continues over the margin of the eyelid and then transforms into the stratified columnar type of the palpebral conjunctiva (15). The thin lamina propria of the palpebral conjunctiva (15) contains elastic and collagen fibers. Beneath the lamina propria is a plate of dense, collagenous connective tissue, the **tarsus (16).** This region contains large, specialized sebaceous glands, the **tarsal (Meibomian) glands (17).** The secretory acini of these glands open into a long **central duct (19),** which runs parallel to the palpebral conjunctiva (15) and opens at the eyelid margin.

The free end of the eyelid contains **eyelashes (10),** which arise from large, long **hair follicles (9).** Associated with the eyelashes (10) are small **sebaceous glands (11).** Between the hair follicles of the eyelashes are large **sweat glands (of Moll) (18).**

The eyelid contains three sets of muscles: the extensive palpebral portion of the skeletal muscle, the **orbicularis oculi (8);** the skeletal **ciliary muscle (of Roilan) (20)** in the region of the hair follicles of the eyelashes (10) and tarsal glands (17); and, in the upper region of the eyelid, strands of the smooth muscle, the **superior tarsal muscle (of Müller (12).**

The **connective tissue (7)** of the eyelid also contains **adipose tissue (2), blood vessels (14),** and **lymphatic tissue (13).**

■ Functional Correlations–Eye

Associated with each eyeball are thin **eyelids** that cover the anterior surface of the eye and fine hairs, the **eyelashes,** which are located on the margins of the eyelids. These structures protect the eyes from foreign objects and excessive light. Situated above the eye is a secretory **lacrimal gland** that continually produces **lacrimal secretion (tears).** Blinking spreads the lacrimal secretion across the eyeball and the inner surface of the eyelid. The lacrimal secretion contains mucus, salts, and the antibacterial enzyme lysozyme. Its function is to clean, protect, moisten, and lubricate the surface of the eye.

The **aqueous humor** that fills the anterior and posterior chambers of the eye bathes the avascular **cornea** and **lens,** and supplies nutrients and oxygen to these structures. The vitreous chamber that is located behind the lens contains a gelatinous mass called the **vitreous body.** This substance transmits light, contributes to the intraocular pressure of the eyeball, and holds the retina in place against the pigmented layer of the eyeball.

The retina is photosensitive and contains three types of neurons: photoreceptive **rods** and **cones, bipolar cells,** and **ganglion cells.** The rods and cones synapse with the bipolar cells, which then connect the receptor cells with the ganglion cells. The axons that leave the ganglion cells converge posteriorly at the **optic papilla** (optic disk) and leave the eye as the **optic nerve.** The optic papilla is also called the blind spot because this area lacks photoreceptor cells. Because the rods and cones are situated next to the **choroid layer,** light rays must first pass through the ganglion and bipolar cell layers in order to reach and activate the photosensitive cells. The **pigmented layer** of the choroid next to the retina absorbs light rays and prevents them from reflecting back through the retina.

The rods are highly sensitive to light and function best under dim or **low light** conditions, such as at dusk or at night. The cones are less sensitive to low light and respond best to **bright light;** they function as sensors for high visual acuity and color vision (red, green, or blue). In the fovea centralis, light rays fall directly on and stimulate the tightly packed cones. As a result, fovea centralis region of the eye produces the greatest **visual acuity** and the sharpest **color discrimination.**

1 Hair follicle

2 Adipose cells

3 Sebaceous gland
(of hair follicle)

4 Epidermis

5 Sweat glands

6 Dermis

7 Connective tissue

8 Orbicularis oculi

9 Hair follicle (of eyelash)

10 Eyelashes

11 Sebaceous gland (of eyelash)

12 Superior tarsal
muscle (of Müller)

13 Lymphatic tissue

14 Blood vessels

15 Palpebral conjunctiva

16 Tarsus

17 Tarsal glands (Meibomian)

18 Sweat glands (of Moll)

19 Central duct (of tarsal glands)

20 Ciliary muscle (of Roilan)

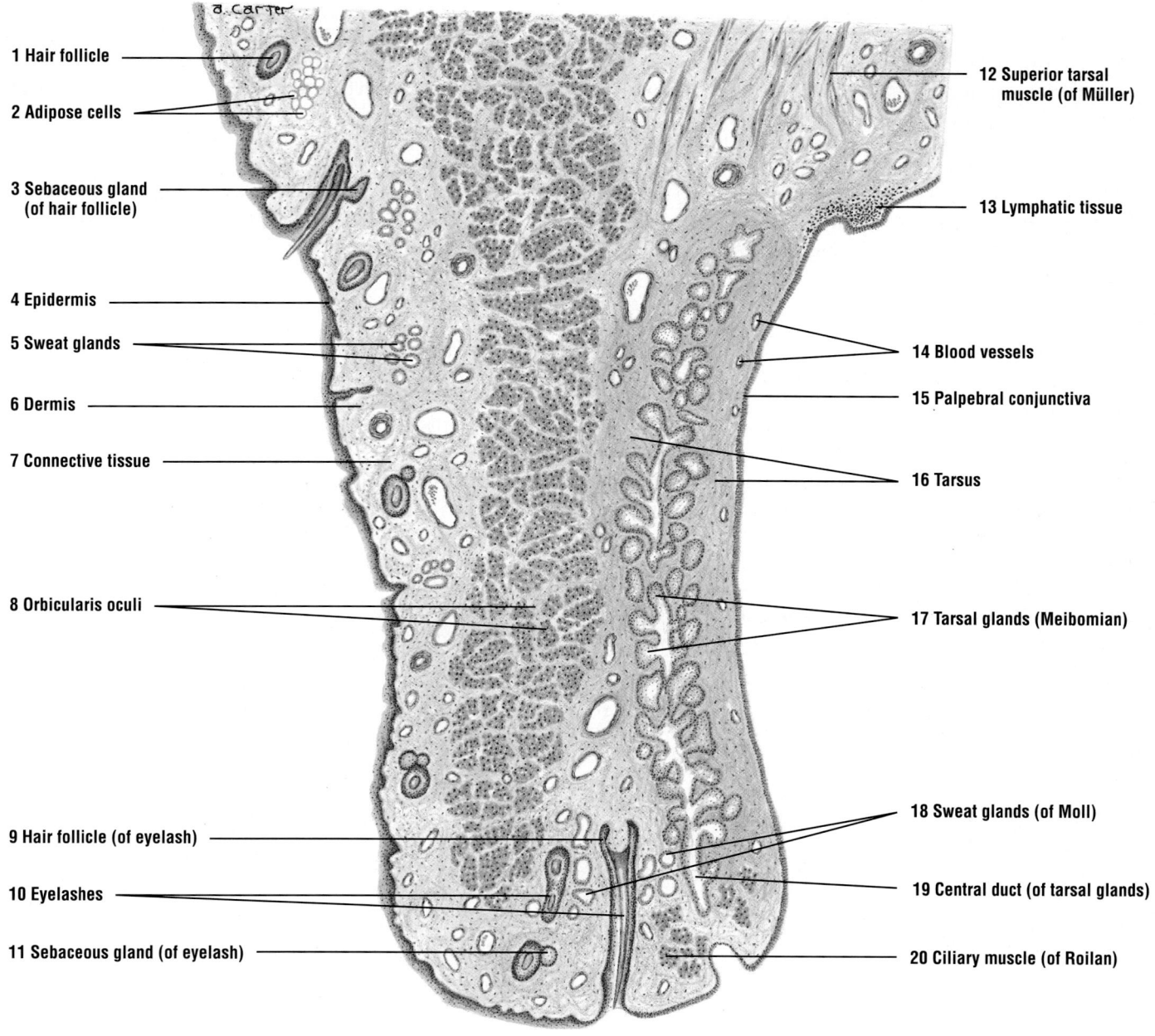

Fig. 19-1   Eyelid (sagittal section). Stain: hematoxylin-eosin. Low magnification.

Figure 19-2   Lacrimal Gland

The lacrimal gland secretes tears and is composed of several tubuloacinar glands. The secretory **acini (1, 8)** vary in size and shape and resemble the serous type; however, their lumina are larger. Some acini may exhibit irregular **outpocketings of cells (5)** in the lumina. The **acinar cells (1, 8)** are more columnar than pyramidal, contain large secretory granules and lipid droplets, and stain lightly. **Myoepithelial cells (3)** surround individual acini.

The smaller intralobular **excretory ducts (2, lower leader)** are lined with simple cuboidal or columnar epithelium. The larger intralobular ducts **(2, upper leader)** and the **interlobular ducts (7, 11)** are lined with two layers of low columnar cells or pseudostratified epithelium.

The **intralobular connective tissue (9)** is sparse; however, **interlobular connective tissue (4)** is abundant and may contain adipose cells.

Figure 19-3   Cornea (transverse section)

The anterior surface of the cornea is covered with nonpapillated, stratified squamous nonkeratinized **epithelium (1, 6, 7)**. The lowest (basal) cell layer is columnar and rests on a thin basement membrane (not illustrated). Beneath the corneal epithelium is a thick, homogeneous **anterior limiting membrane (Bowman's membrane) (2)**, which is derived from the underlying **corneal stroma (substantia propria) (3)**. The corneal stroma forms the body of the cornea. It consists of parallel bundles of collagen fibrils that form thin **lamellae (9)** and layers of flat, branching fibro-blasts, the **keratocytes (8)**, between the collagen fibers. The corneal keratocytes (8) are modified fibroblasts.

The posterior surface of the cornea is covered with a low cuboidal epithelium, the **posterior epithelium (5, 10)**, which is also the corneal endothelium. The **posterior limiting membrane (Descemet's membrane) (4)** is wide and constitutes the basement membrane of the posterior corneal epithelium (5, 10). It rests on the posterior portion of the corneal stroma (3).

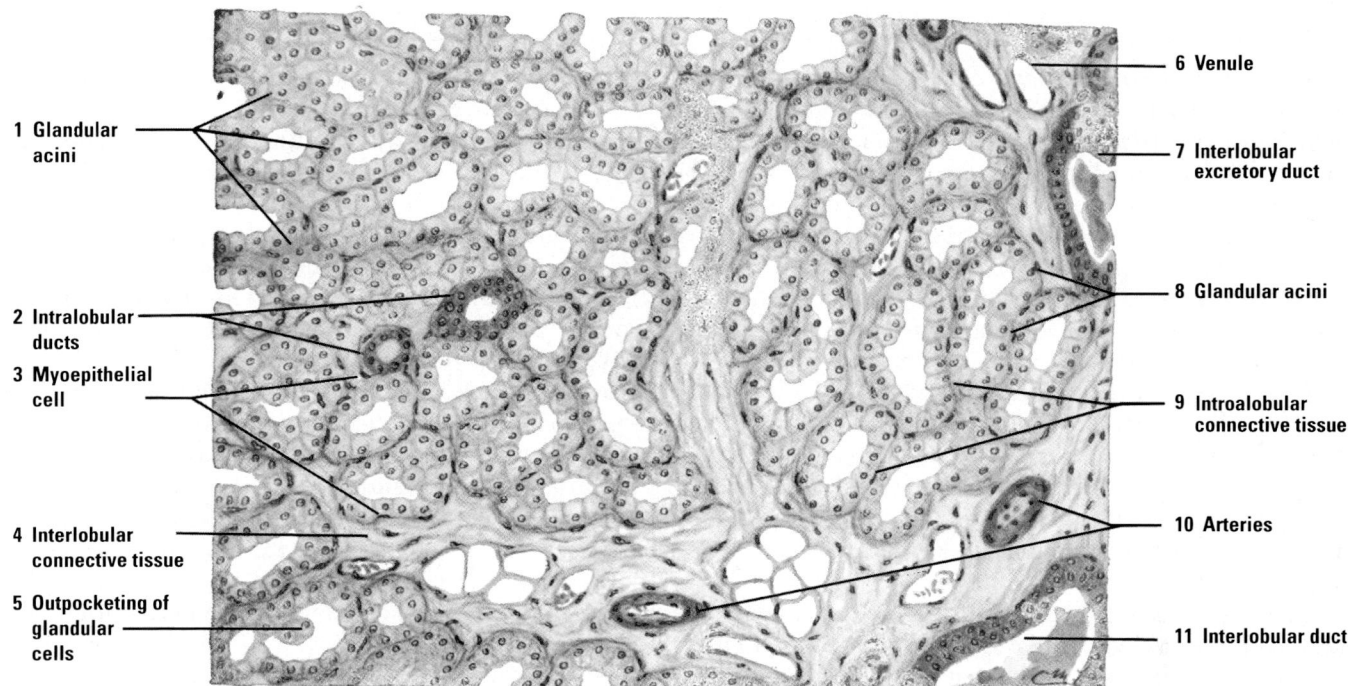

1 Glandular acini

2 Intralobular ducts

3 Myoepithelial cell

4 Interlobular connective tissue

5 Outpocketing of glandular cells

6 Venule

7 Interlobular excretory duct

8 Glandular acini

9 Introalobular connective tissue

10 Arteries

11 Interlobular duct

Fig. 19-2 Lacrimal Gland. Stain: hematoxylin-eosin. Medium magnification.

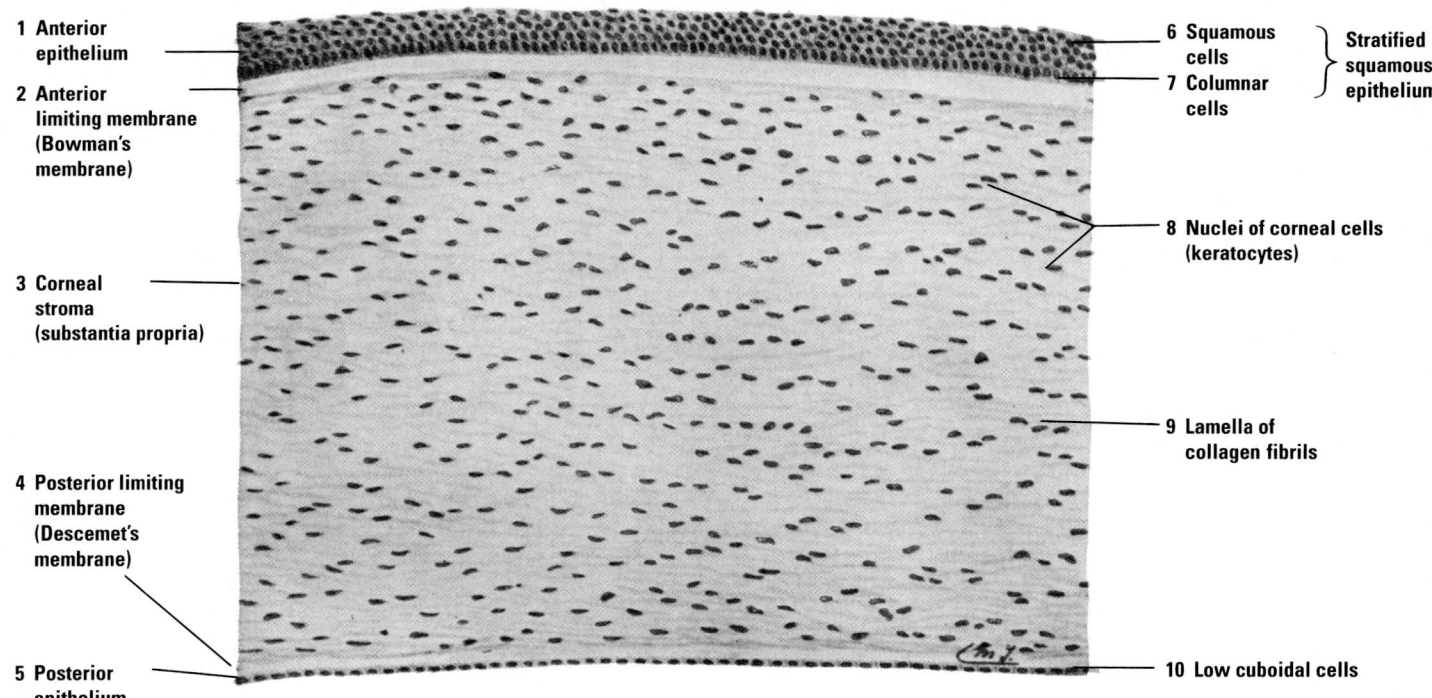

1 Anterior epithelium

2 Anterior limiting membrane (Bowman's membrane)

3 Corneal stroma (substantia propria)

4 Posterior limiting membrane (Descemet's membrane)

5 Posterior epithelium

6 Squamous cells

7 Columnar cells

} Stratified squamous epithelium

8 Nuclei of corneal cells (keratocytes)

9 Lamella of collagen fibrils

10 Low cuboidal cells

Fig. 19-3 Cornea (transverse section). Stain: hematoxylin-eosin. Medium magnification.

Figure 19-4   Whole Eye (sagittal section)

The eyeball is surrounded by three major concentric layers: an outer, tough, fibrous tissue layer composed of **sclera (18)** and **cornea (1);** a middle layer or uvea composed of the highly vascular, pigmented **choroid (7),** the **ciliary body (consisting of ciliary processes and ciliary muscle) (4, 14, 15),** and the **iris (13);** and the innermost layer composed of the photosensitive nerve tissue, the **retina (8).** The histology of the cornea (1) is illustrated in greater detail in Figure 19-3.

The sclera (18) is a white, opaque, and tough connective tissue layer composed of densely woven collagen fibers. It aids in maintaining rigidity of the eyeball and appears as the "white" of the eye. The junction between the cornea and sclera occurs at the transition area called the **limbus (12),** located in the anterior region of the eye. In the posterior region of the eye, where the **optic nerve (10)** emerges from the ocular capsule, is the transition site between the sclera (18) of the eyeball and the connective tissue **dura mater (23)** of the central nervous system.

The choroid (7) and the ciliary body (4, 14, 15) are situated adjacent to the sclera (18). In a sagittal section of the eyeball, the ciliary body (4, 14, 15) appears triangular in shape. It is composed of the **ciliary muscle (14)** and the **ciliary processes (4, 15).** The ciliary muscle (14) is a smooth muscle; its fibers are arranged longitudinally, circularly, and radially. The folded and highly vascular extensions of the ciliary body constitute the ciliary processes (4, 15). These processes attach to the equator of the **lens (16)** by the suspensory ligament or **zonular fibers (5)** of the lens. Contraction of the ciliary muscle reduces tension on the suspensory ligament and allows the lens (16) to assume a convex shape.

The **iris (13)** partially covers the lens and is the colored portion of the eye. The circular and radial distribution of the smooth muscle fibers forms a round opening in the iris called the **pupil (11).**

The interior portion of the eye located in front of the lens is subdivided into two compartments. The **anterior chamber (2)** is situated between the iris (13) and the cornea (1), and **the posterior chamber (3)** lies between the iris (13) and lens (16). Both the anterior (2) and posterior (3) chambers are filled with a watery fluid, the aqueous humor. The large posterior compartment in the eyeball located behind the lens is the **vitreous body (19).** It is filled with a gelatinous material, the transparent vitreous humor.

The inner layer or retina (8) of the eyeball is the photosensitive region of the eye; however, not all retina is photosensitive. Behind the ciliary body (4, 14, 15) is the **ora serrata (6, 17),** the sharp, anteriormost boundary of the photosensitive portion of the retina. Anterior to the ora serrata (6, 17) lies the nonphotosensitive region of the retina, which continues forward in the eyeball to form the inner lining of the ciliary body (4, 14, 15) and posterior part of the iris (13). Posterior to the ora serrata (6, 17) is the photosensitive optic retina (8). It consists of numerous cell layers, one of which contains the light-sensitive cells, the rods and cones. The histology of the retina is presented in greater detail in Figures 19-5 and 19-6.

The posterior wall of the eye contains the **macula lutea (20)** and the **optic papilla (9)** or optic disk. The macula lutea (20) is a small, yellow-pigmented spot in whose center is a shallow depression called the **fovea (20).** This region represents the area of greatest visual acuity in the eye. The center of the fovea (20) is devoid of rod cells and blood vessels. This region contains only cone cells.

The optic papilla (9) is the area where the **optic nerve (10)** leaves the eyeball. The optic papilla lacks both rods and cones, and thus constitutes the "blind spot" of the eye.

The outer sclera is adjacent to the orbital tissue, which contains loose connective tissue, **adipose cells (21)** of the orbital fatty tissue, nerve fibers, **blood vessels (22),** lymphatics, and glands.

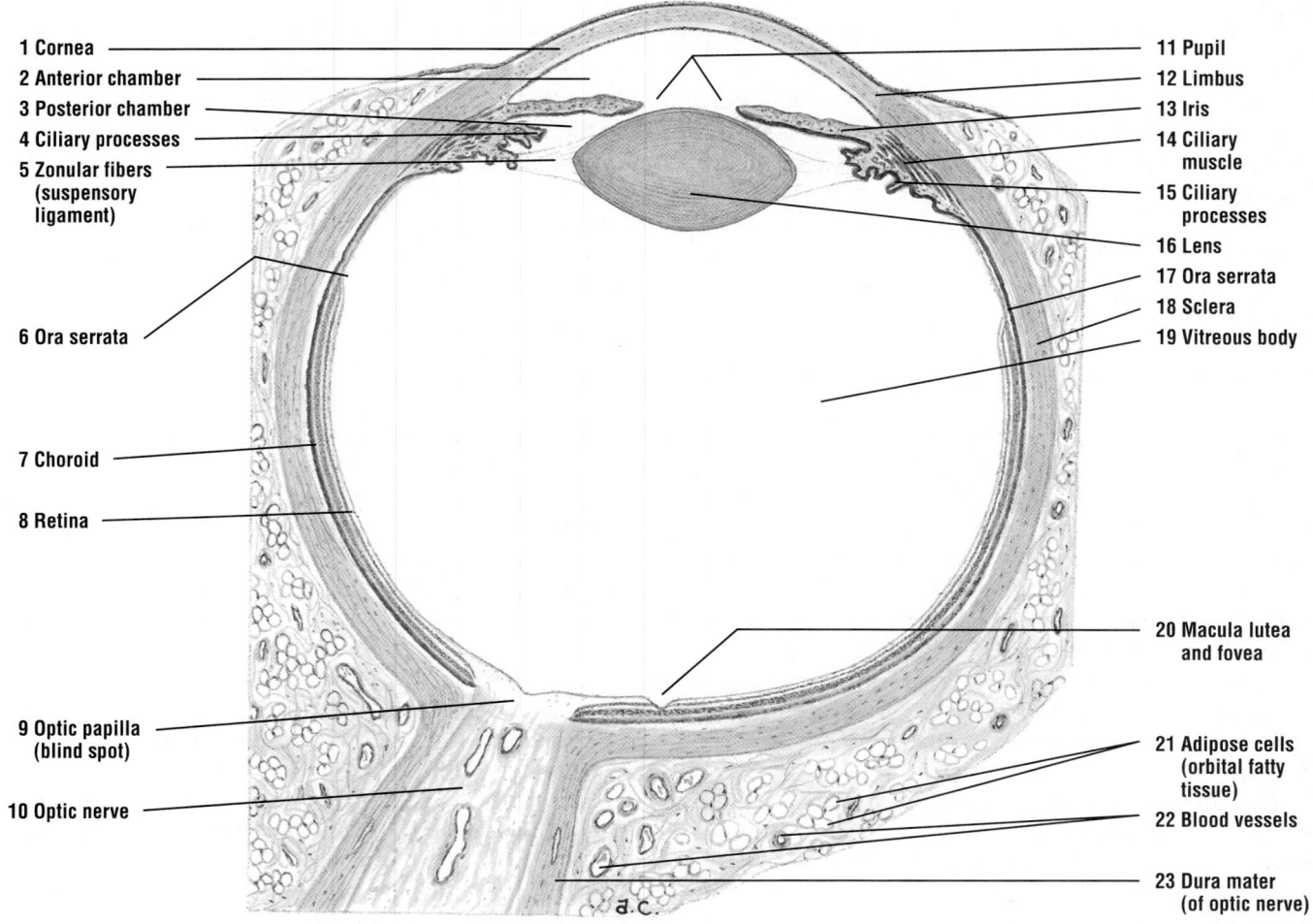

1 Cornea
2 Anterior chamber
3 Posterior chamber
4 Ciliary processes
5 Zonular fibers
   (suspensory
   ligament)

6 Ora serrata

7 Choroid

8 Retina

9 Optic papilla
   (blind spot)

10 Optic nerve

11 Pupil
12 Limbus
13 Iris
14 Ciliary
   muscle
15 Ciliary
   processes
16 Lens
17 Ora serrata
18 Sclera
19 Vitreous body

20 Macula lutea
   and fovea

21 Adipose cells
   (orbital fatty
   tissue)
22 Blood vessels

23 Dura mater
   (of optic nerve)

Fig. 19-4   Whole Eye (sagittal section). Stain: hematoxylin-eosin. Low magnification.

Figure 19-5   Retina, Choroid, and Sclera (panoramic view)

The wall of the eyeball is composed of the **sclera (1)**, **choroid (2)**, and **retina (3)**. The retina contains the photosensitive receptor cells. In this figure only the deeper portion of the sclera is illustrated. The stroma of the sclera (1) is composed of dense **collagen fibers (4),** which course parallel to the surface of the eyeball. Between the collagen bundles is a delicate network of elastic fibers. Flattened or elongated fibroblasts are present throughout the sclera (1), and **melanocytes (5)** are found in the deepest layer.

The layers of the choroid (2) and retina (3) are illustrated in this figure, and are shown in greater detail and higher magnification in Figure 19-6.

Figure 19-6   Layers of the Choroid and Retina (detail)

The choroid is subdivided into several layers: **the suprachoroid lamina (17), the vascular layer (18), the choriocapillary layer (19),** and the transparent limiting membrane, or glassy membrane (Bruch's membrane).

The suprachoroid lamina (17) consists of lamellae of fine collagen fibers, a rich network of elastic fibers, fibroblasts, and numerous large melanocytes. The vascular layer (18) contains numerous medium-sized and large **blood vessels (1).** In the loose connective tissue layer between the blood vessels (1) are numerous large flat **melanocytes (2),** which give this layer its characteristic dark color. The choriocapillary layer (19) contains a network of capillaries with large lumina in a stroma of fine collagen and elastic fibers. The innermost layer of the choroid, the glassy membrane, lies adjacent to the **pigment cells (3)** of the retina.

The outermost layer of the retina is the pigment epithelium (3); its basement membrane forms the innermost layer of the glassy membrane of the choroid. The cuboidal pigment cells (3) contain melanin (pigment) granules in apical regions of their cytoplasm, while their **processes (20)** with pigment granules extend between the **rods and cones (21, 22)** of the retina.

Adjacent to the pigment cells (3) is a photosensitive layer composed of slender **rods (4, 22)** and thicker **cones (5, 21).** These are situated next to the **outer limiting membrane (6, 23),** which is formed by the processes of the neuroglial cells, the **Müller's cells (30).**

The **outer nuclear layer (7, 8)** contains **nuclei of the rods (8, 25)** and **cones (7, 24)** and the **outer processes of Müller's cells (26).** In the **outer plexiform layer (9),** the axons of rods and cones synapse with the dendrites of **bipolar cells (28)** and **horizontal cells (27).** The **inner nuclear layer (10)** contains the nuclei of **bipolar (29),** horizontal, **amacrine (31),** and neuroglial Müller's cells (30). The horizontal and amacrine cells are association cells. In the **inner plexiform layer (11),** the axons of bipolar cells (29) synapse with the dendrites of the ganglion and amacrine cells.

The **ganglion cell layer (12)** contains the cell bodies of **ganglion cells (33)** and neuroglial cells. Dendrites from the ganglion cells synapse in the inner plexiform layer (11, 32, 33).

The **optic nerve fiber layer (13, 14, 15)** contains the axons of the ganglion cells (14) and the inner **fiber network of Müller's cells (13, 37). Axons of ganglion cells (14, 33)** converge toward the optic disk and form the optic nerve. The terminations of the inner fibers of Müller's cells (13, 37) expand to form the **inner limiting membrane (15, 36)** of the retina.

Blood vessels of the retina course in the optic nerve fiber layer (13, 14) and penetrate as far as the **inner nuclear layer (10).** Sections in various planes of some of the vessels can be seen in this layer (unlabeled).

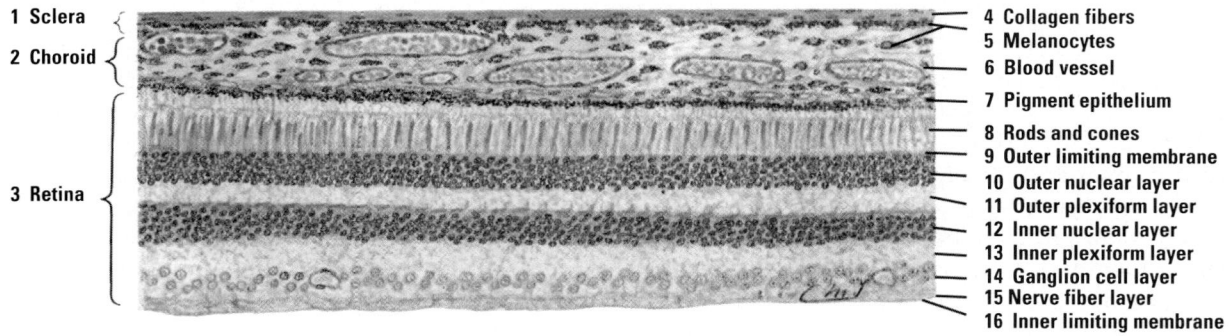

1 Sclera
2 Choroid
3 Retina

4 Collagen fibers
5 Melanocytes
6 Blood vessel
7 Pigment epithelium
8 Rods and cones
9 Outer limiting membrane
10 Outer nuclear layer
11 Outer plexiform layer
12 Inner nuclear layer
13 Inner plexiform layer
14 Ganglion cell layer
15 Nerve fiber layer
16 Inner limiting membrane

Fig. 19-5   Retina, Choroid, and Sclera (panoramic view). Stain: hematoxylin-eosin. Medium magnification.

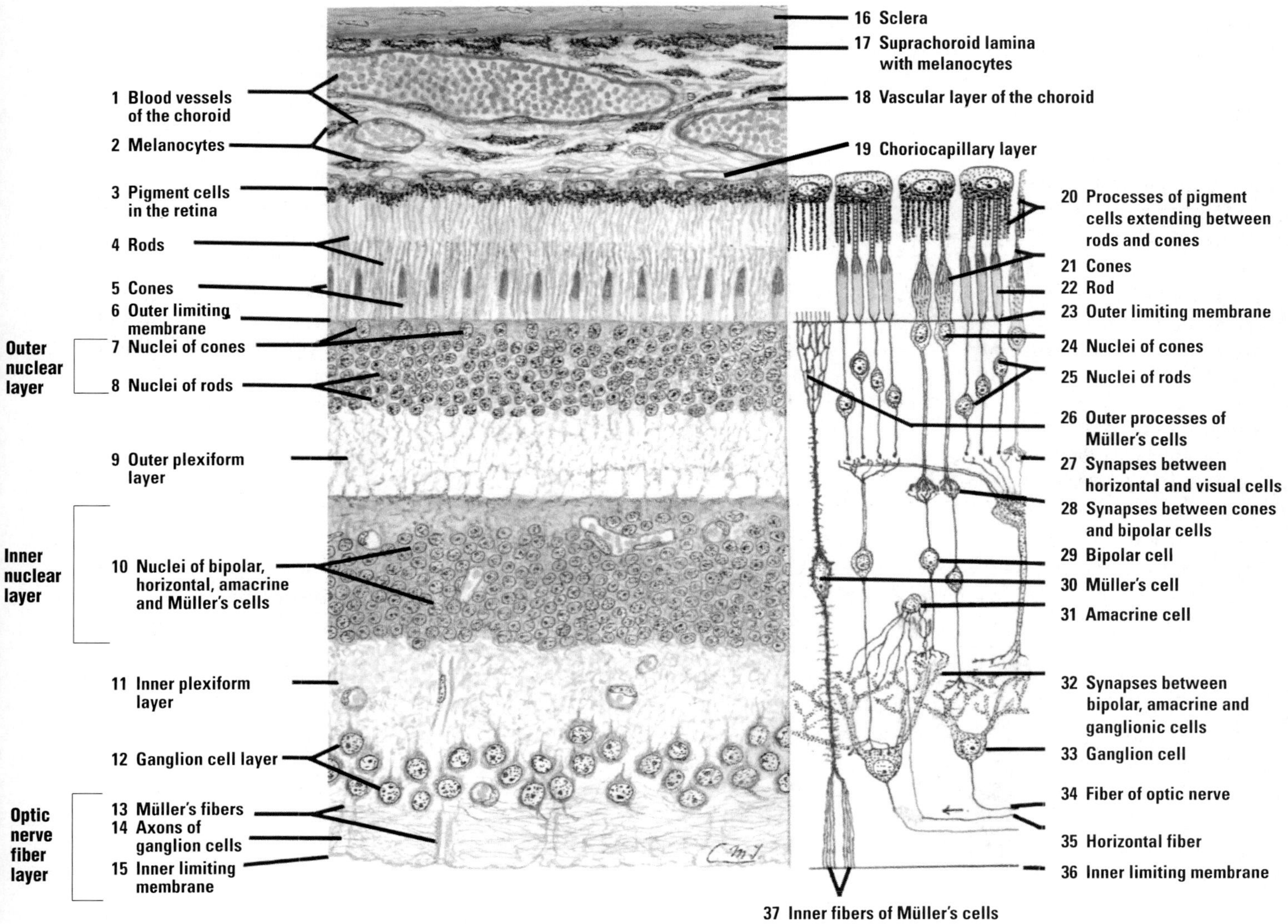

1 Blood vessels
   of the choroid
2 Melanocytes
3 Pigment cells
   in the retina
4 Rods
5 Cones
6 Outer limiting
   membrane

Outer nuclear layer
7 Nuclei of cones
8 Nuclei of rods

9 Outer plexiform
   layer

Inner nuclear layer
10 Nuclei of bipolar,
   horizontal, amacrine
   and Müller's cells

11 Inner plexiform
   layer

12 Ganglion cell layer

Optic nerve fiber layer
13 Müller's fibers
14 Axons of
   ganglion cells
15 Inner limiting
   membrane

16 Sclera
17 Suprachoroid lamina
   with melanocytes
18 Vascular layer of the choroid
19 Choriocapillary layer
20 Processes of pigment
   cells extending between
   rods and cones
21 Cones
22 Rod
23 Outer limiting membrane
24 Nuclei of cones
25 Nuclei of rods
26 Outer processes of
   Müller's cells
27 Synapses between
   horizontal and visual cells
28 Synapses between cones
   and bipolar cells
29 Bipolar cell
30 Müller's cell
31 Amacrine cell
32 Synapses between
   bipolar, amacrine and
   ganglionic cells
33 Ganglion cell
34 Fiber of optic nerve
35 Horizontal fiber
36 Inner limiting membrane
37 Inner fibers of Müller's cells

Fig. 19-6   Layers of the Choroid and Retina (detail). Stain: hematoxylin-eosin. High magnification.

Figure 19-7   Inner Ear: Cochlea (vertical section)

The osseous (bony) labyrinth of the **cochlea (16, 18)** spirals around a central axis of a spongy bone, the **modiolus (17).** Embedded within the modiolus is the **spiral ganglion (14),** which is composed of bipolar afferent neurons. Long axons from these bipolar cells join to form the **cochlear nerve (9);** shorter dendrites innervate the hair cells in the hearing apparatus, the **organ of Corti (13).**

The bony labyrinth is divided into two major cavities by the **osseous spiral lamina (8)** and the **basilar membrane (7).** The osseous spiral lamina (8) projects from the modiolus about halfway into the lumen of the cochlear canal. The basilar membrane (7) continues from the osseous spiral lamina (8) to the **spiral ligament (6),** which is a thickening of the periosteum on the **outer bony wall (5)** of the cochlear canal. The cochlear canal is subdivided into two large compartments, the lower **scala tympani (4)** and the upper **scala vestibuli (2).** Both compartments pursue a spiral course to the apex of the cochlea, where they communicate through a small opening called the **helicotrema (1).**

The **vestibular (Reissner's) membrane (10)** separates the scala vestibuli (2) from the **cochlear duct (scala media) (3)** and forms the roof of the cochlear duct (3). The sensory cells specialized for receiving sound vibrations and transmitting them as nerve impulses to the brain are located in the organ of Corti (13); this organ rests on the basilar membrane (7) on the floor of the cochlear duct (3). A **tectorial membrane (12)** overlies the cells in the organ of Corti (13).

Figure 19-8   Inner Ear: Cochlear Duct (Scala Media)

The **cochlear duct (9),** the **organ of Corti (12),** and associated cells are illustrated at higher magnification and in greater detail.

The outer wall of the cochlear duct (9) is formed by a vascular area called the **stria vascularis (16).** The stratified epithelium covering the stria vascularis is unique in that it contains an intraepithelial capillary network formed from the vessels that supply the connective tissue of the **spiral ligament (17).** The lamina propria in this region is the **spiral ligament (17, 19);** it consists of collagen fibers, pigmented fibroblasts, and numerous blood vessels.

The roof of the cochlear duct (9) is formed by the **vestibular (Reissner's) membrane (6),** which separates it from the **scala vestibuli (7).** The vestibular membrane (6) extends from the spiral ligament (17) of the outer wall of the cochlea, located at the upper extent of the stria vascularis (**15,** 16), to the thickened **periosteum of the osseous spiral lamina (4)** near the **spiral limbus (5).**

The spiral limbus (5) forms part of the floor of the **cochlear duct (9).** The limbus (5) is a thickened mass of periosteal connective tissue (4) of the **osseous spiral lamina (1)** that extends into the cochlear duct (9). It is supported by a lateral extension of the osseous spiral lamina (1). The limbus (5) is covered by an epithelium that appears columnar. The lateral extracellular extension of this epithelium beyond the limbus is the **tectorial membrane (10).** The tectorial membrane overlies the **internal spiral sulcus (8)** and a portion of the **organ of Corti (12),** including its **hair cells (11).**

The **basilar membrane (13)** consists of vascularized connective tissue underlying a thinner plate of basilar fibers. The organ of Corti (12), resting on these basilar fibers, extends from the spiral limbus (5) to the spiral ligament (17, 19). The highly specialized sensory or hair cells (11), several types of supporting cells, and spaces and tunnels constitute the organ of Corti (12).

Peripheral (afferent) processes (2) from the bipolar cells of the **spiral ganglion (3)** course through the channels in the osseous spiral lamina (1) and synapse with hair cells (11) in the organ of Corti (12).

■ Functional Correlations–Ear

Sound waves that enter the ear through the **external auditory canal** vibrate the **tympanic membrane.** These vibrations activate the three **ossicles** in the middle ear, which then transmit the vibrations across the air-filled **middle ear** or **tympanic cavity** to the fluid-filled **inner ear.** These vibrations eventually stimulate the sensitive **hair cells** in the **organ of Corti.** The organ of Corti then converts the mechanical vibrations in the inner ear into **nerve impulses.** The impulses for sound then pass along the axons, or nerve processes, of the **ganglion cells** located in the **spiral ganglia** of the inner ear. The axons from the spiral ganglia join to form the **auditory or cochlear nerve,** which carries the impulses from the cells in the organ of Corti of the inner ear to the brain for sound interpretation.

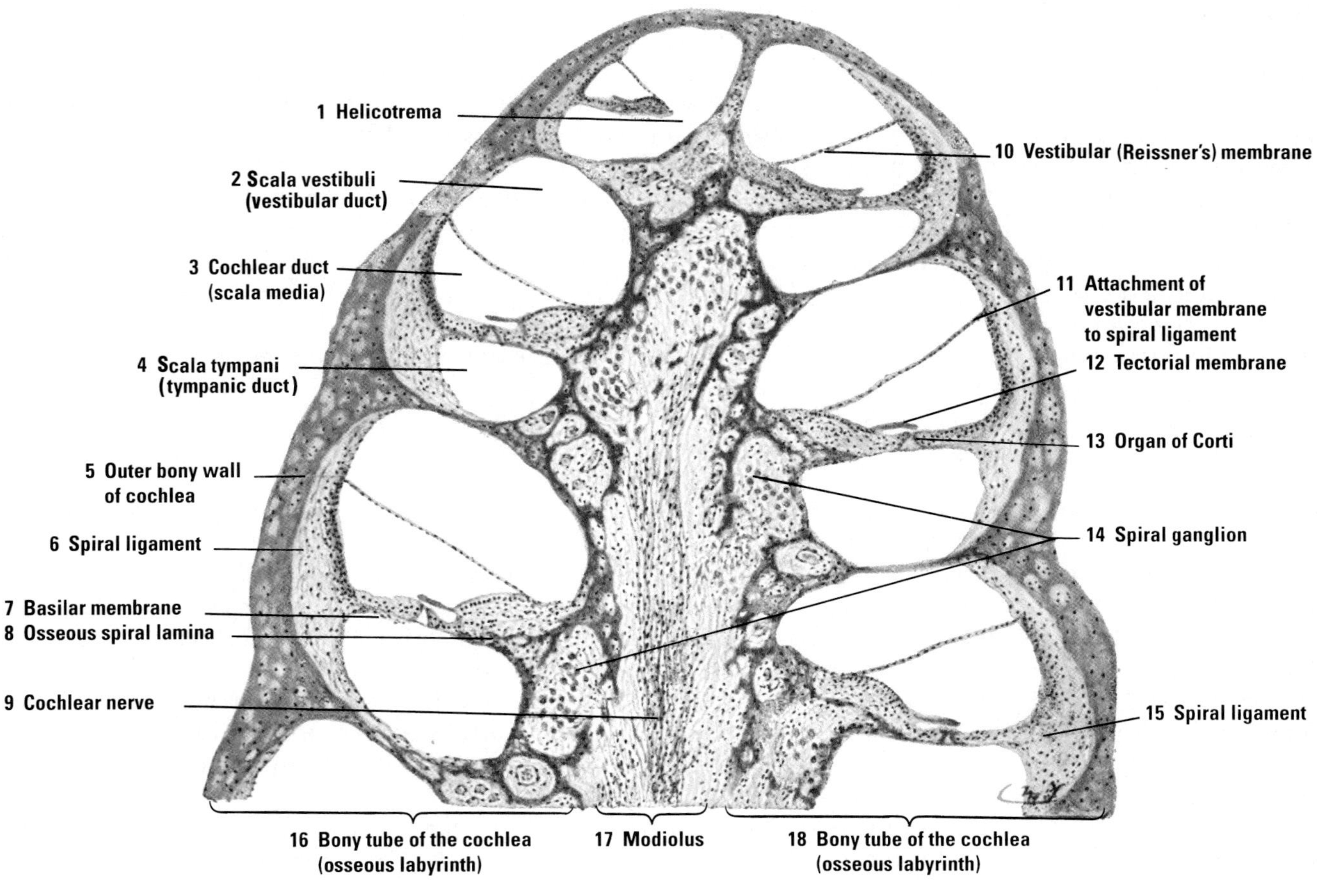

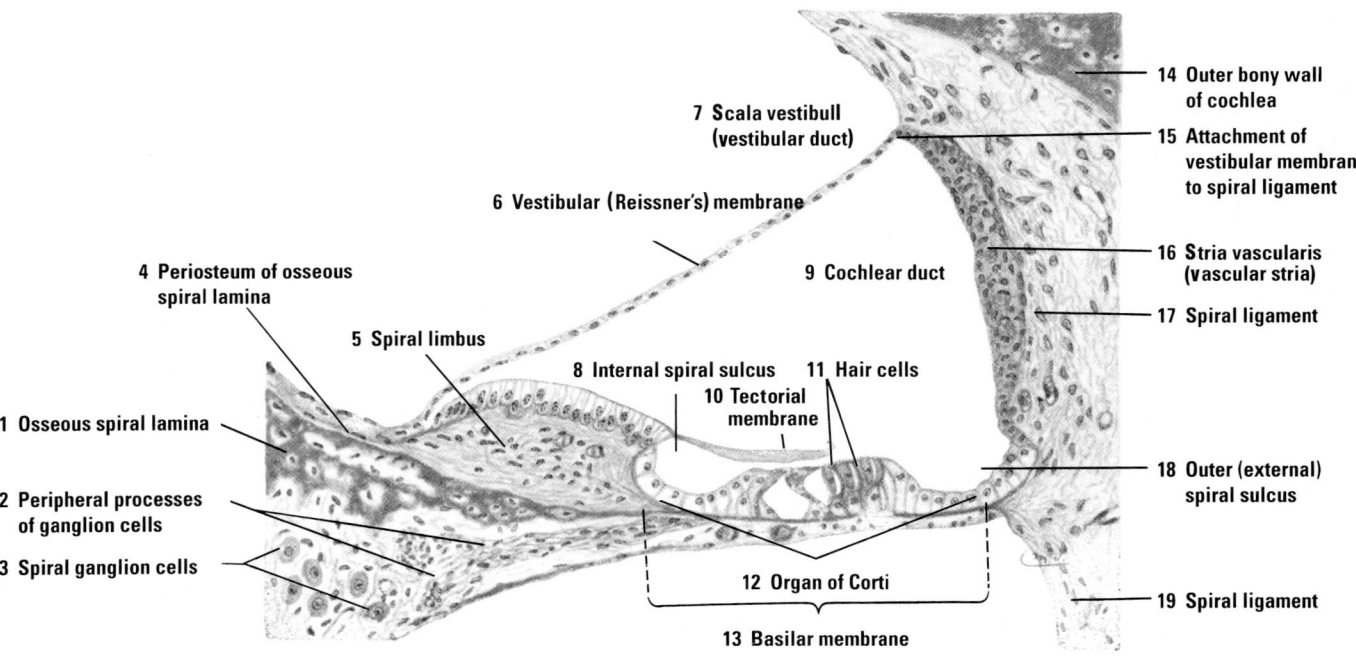

Fig. 19-7 Inner Ear: Cochlea (vertical section). Stain: hematoxylin-eosin. Low magnification.

1 Helicotrema
2 Scala vestibuli (vestibular duct)
3 Cochlear duct (scala media)
4 Scala tympani (tympanic duct)
5 Outer bony wall of cochlea
6 Spiral ligament
7 Basilar membrane
8 Osseous spiral lamina
9 Cochlear nerve
10 Vestibular (Reissner's) membrane
11 Attachment of vestibular membrane to spiral ligament
12 Tectorial membrane
13 Organ of Corti
14 Spiral ganglion
15 Spiral ligament
16 Bony tube of the cochlea (osseous labyrinth)
17 Modiolus
18 Bony tube of the cochlea (osseous labyrinth)

Fig. 19-8 Inner Ear: Cochlear Duct (Scala Media). Stain: hematoxylin-eosin. Medium magnification.

1 Osseous spiral lamina
2 Peripheral processes of ganglion cells
3 Spiral ganglion cells
4 Periosteum of osseous spiral lamina
5 Spiral limbus
6 Vestibular (Reissner's) membrane
7 Scala vestibull (vestibular duct)
8 Internal spiral sulcus
9 Cochlear duct
10 Tectorial membrane
11 Hair cells
12 Organ of Corti
13 Basilar membrane
14 Outer bony wall of cochlea
15 Attachment of vestibular membrane to spiral ligament
16 Stria vascularis (vascular stria)
17 Spiral ligament
18 Outer (external) spiral sulcus
19 Spiral ligament

Figure 19-9   Eye: Layers of Retina and Choroid

A high power photomicrograph illustrates a section of the photosensitive part of the eye, the retina, with its distinct histologic layers. The **choroid (1)** is a vascular outer layer that contains loose connective tissue and numerous pigmented melanocytes. The choroid (1) layer is situated adjacent to the outermost retinal layer, the single, **pigment epithelium (2)** layer. The light-sensitive **rods** and **cones (3)** form the next layer, which is separated from the dense **outer nuclear layer (4)** by a thin **outer limiting membrane (5)**. Deep to the outer nuclear layer (4) is a clear area of synaptic connections. This is the **outer plexiform layer (6)**. The dense layer of cell bodies of the integrating neurons form the next layer, the **inner nuclear layer (7)**, which is adjacent to a clear area, the **inner plexiform layer (8)**. In this layer, the axons of the integrating neurons form synaptic connections with fibers of the neurons that form the optic tract. The cell bodies of the optic tract neurons form **ganglion cell layer (9)** and their afferent axons form the light staining optic **nerve fiber layer (10)**. The innermost layer of the retina is the **inner limiting membrane (11)**, which separates the retina from the vitreous body of the eyeball.

Figure 19-10   Inner Ear: Cochlear Duct and the Organ of Corti

A higher magnification photomicrograph illustrates the inner ear with its cochlear canal and the hearing organ of Corti, enclosed in a **bony cochlea (1, 9)**. The cochlear canal is divided into three compartments, **scala vestibuli (10)**, **cochlear duct** (scala media) **(3)**, and **scala tympani (14)**. A thin, **vestibular membrane (2)** separates the cochlear duct (3) from the scala vestibuli (10). Another membrane, the **basilar membrane (7)**, separates the cochlear duct (3) from the scala typani (14). The basilar membrane (7) extends from the connective tissue **spiral ligament (6)** to a thickened **spiral limbus (11)**. The basilar membrane (7) supports the **organ of Corti (8)**, its sensory **hair cells (5)** and its different types of supportive cells. Extending from the spiral limbus (7) is the **tectorial membrane (4)**; it overlies a portion of the organ of Corti (8) and its hair cells (5). Surrounded by the bony cochlea (1, 9) are the sensory bipolar **spiral ganglion cells (13)**. Axons from these ganglion cells (13) travel through the **osseous spiral lamina (12)** and synapse with the hair cells (5) in the organ of Corti (8).

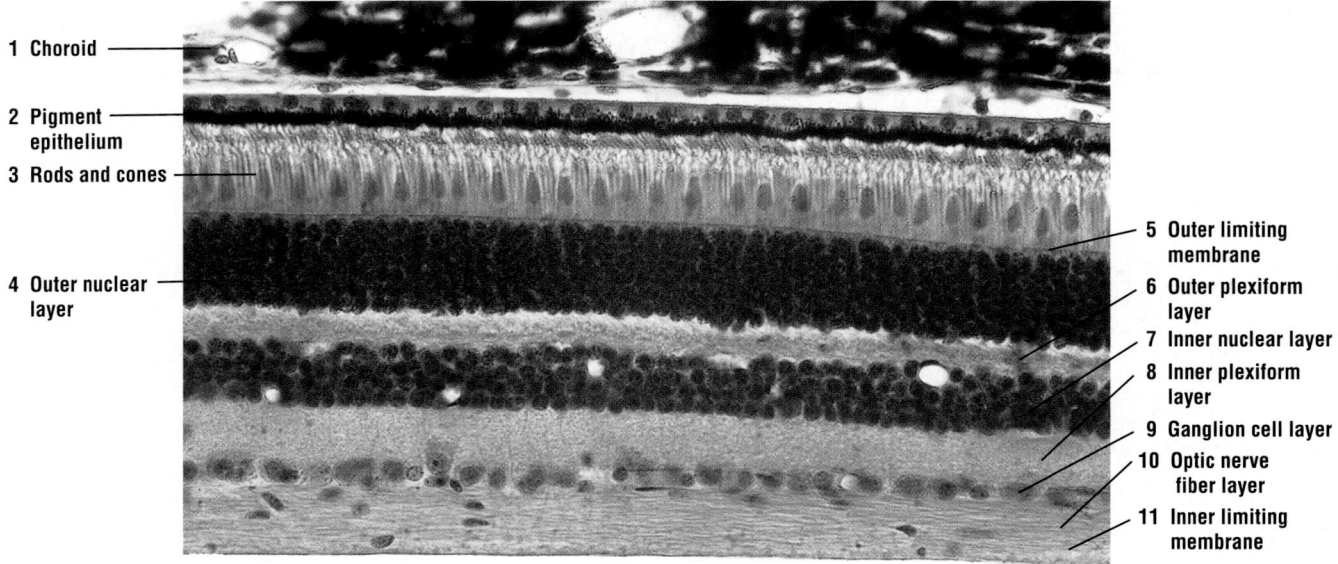

1 Choroid

2 Pigment epithelium

3 Rods and cones

4 Outer nuclear layer

5 Outer limiting membrane

6 Outer plexiform layer

7 Inner nuclear layer

8 Inner plexiform layer

9 Ganglion cell layer

10 Optic nerve fiber layer

11 Inner limiting membrane

Fig. 19-9   Eye: Layers of Retina and Choroid. Stain: Masson's trichrome. 100×

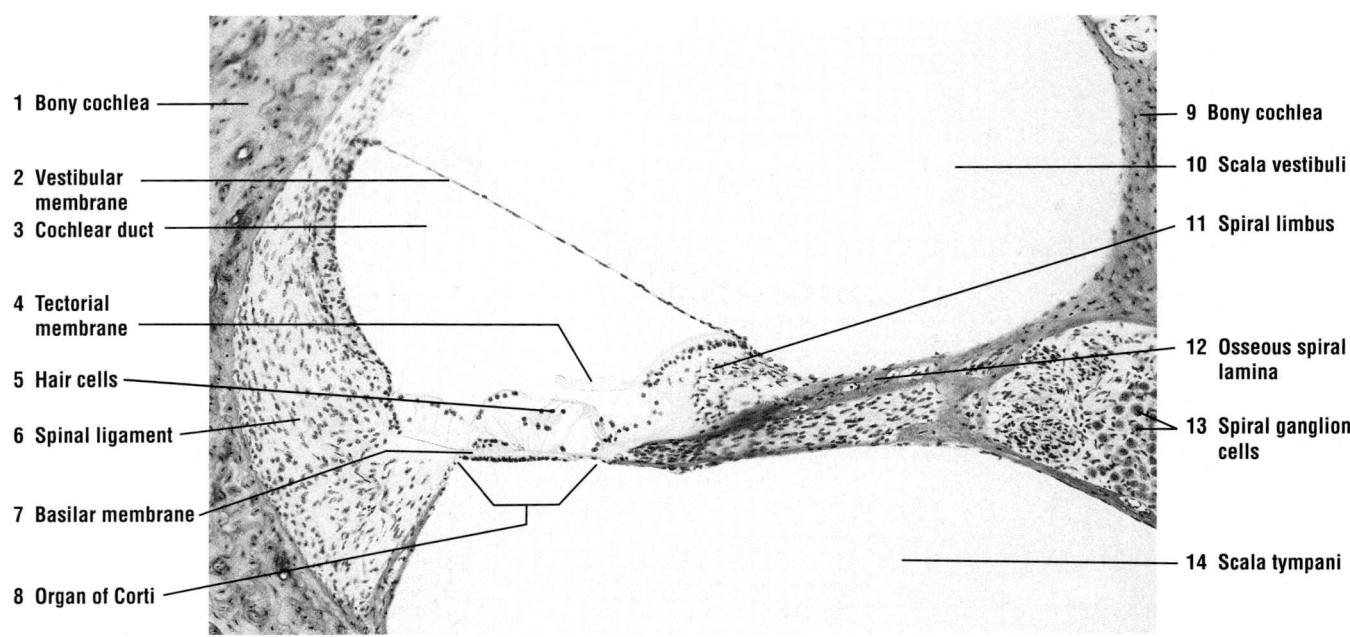

1 Bony cochlea

2 Vestibular membrane

3 Cochlear duct

4 Tectorial membrane

5 Hair cells

6 Spinal ligament

7 Basilar membrane

8 Organ of Corti

9 Bony cochlea

10 Scala vestibuli

11 Spiral limbus

12 Osseous spiral lamina

13 Spiral ganglion cells

14 Scala tympani

Fig. 19-10   Inner Ear: Cochlear Duct and the Organ of Corti. Stain: hematoxylin-eosin. 30×

Index

In this index, page numbers in *italic* designate figures; (*see also*) cross-references refer to related topics or more detailed topic breakdowns. Compound terms are listed under the noun; for example "connective tissue" may be found under Tissue(s): connective.

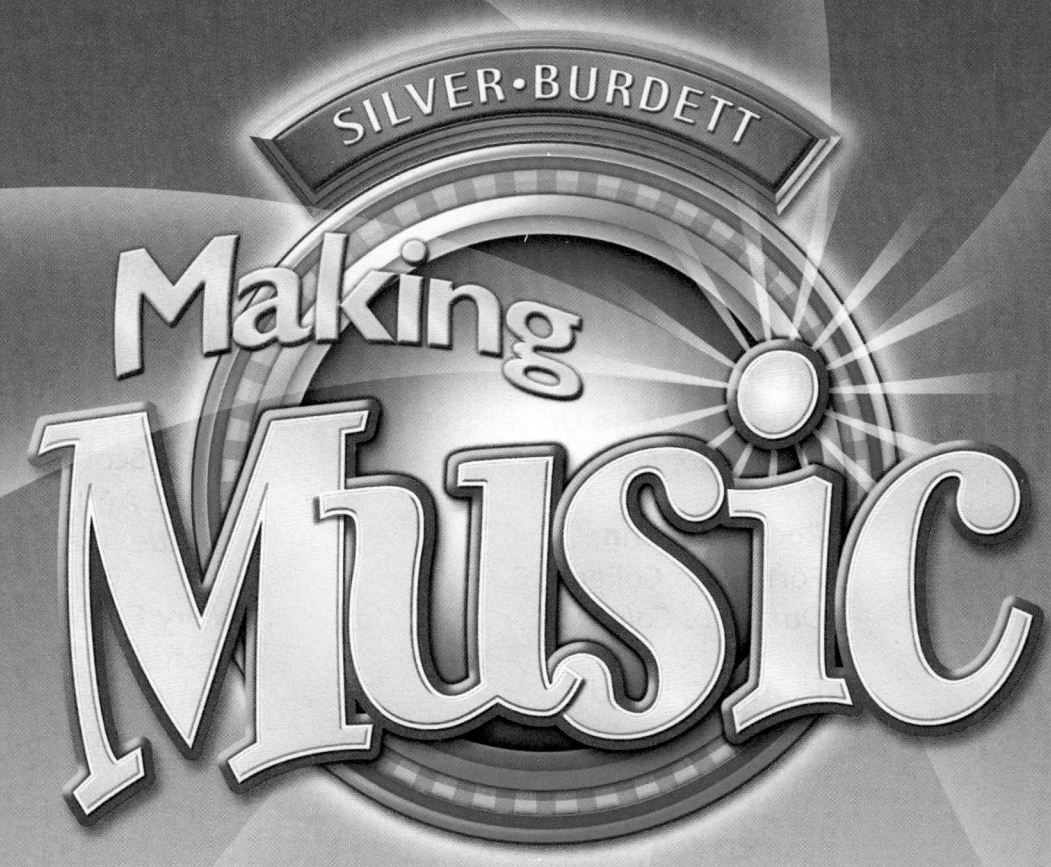

SILVER·BURDETT

Making Music

Teacher's Edition
Part One
Grade 6

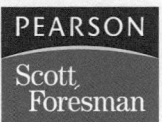

PEARSON

Scott
Foresman

Editorial Offices: Glenview, Illinois • Parsippany, New Jersey • New York, New York
Sales Offices: Needham, Massachusetts • Duluth, Georgia • Glenview, Illinois
Coppell, Texas • Sacramento, California • Mesa, Arizona

ISBN: 0-382-36596-8

Copyright © 2005 Pearson Education, Inc.

All Rights Reserved. Printed in the United States of America. This publication is protected by Copyright, and permission should be obtained from the
publisher prior to any prohibited reproduction, storage in a retrieval system, or transmission in any form by any means, electronic, mechanical,
photocopying, recording, or likewise. For information regarding permission(s), write to:
Permissions Department, Scott Foresman, 1900 East Lake Avenue, Glenview, Illinois 60025.

5 6 7 8 9 10 V064 13 12 11 10 09 08 07 06

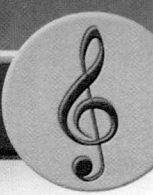

Authors

PROGRAM AUTHORS

Jane Beethoven
Music Author/Consultant
Westport, Connecticut

Susan Brumfield
Texas Tech University
Lubbock, Texas

Patricia Shehan Campbell
University of Washington
Seattle, Washington

David N. Connors
California State University
at Los Angeles
Los Angeles, California

Robert A. Duke
University of Texas at Austin
Austin, Texas

Judith A. Jellison
University of Texas at Austin
Austin, Texas

Rita Klinger
Cleveland State University
Cleveland, Ohio

Rochelle Mann
Fort Lewis College
Durango, Colorado

Hunter C. March
University of Texas at Austin
Austin, Texas

Nan L. McDonald
San Diego State University
San Diego, California

Marvelene C. Moore
University of Tennessee
Knoxville, Tennessee

Mary Palmer
University of Central Florida
Orlando, Florida

Konnie Saliba
University of Memphis
Memphis, Tennessee

Will Schmid
Professor Emeritus
University of Wisconsin—
Milwaukee
Milwaukee, Wisconsin

Carol Scott-Kassner
Music Author/Consultant
Seattle, Washington

Mary E. Shamrock
Professor Emeritus, California
State University at Northridge
Minneapolis, Minnesota

Sandra L. Stauffer
Arizona State University
Tempe, Arizona

Judith Thomas
Music Education Consultant
West Nyack, New York

Jill Trinka
University of St. Thomas
St. Paul, Minnesota

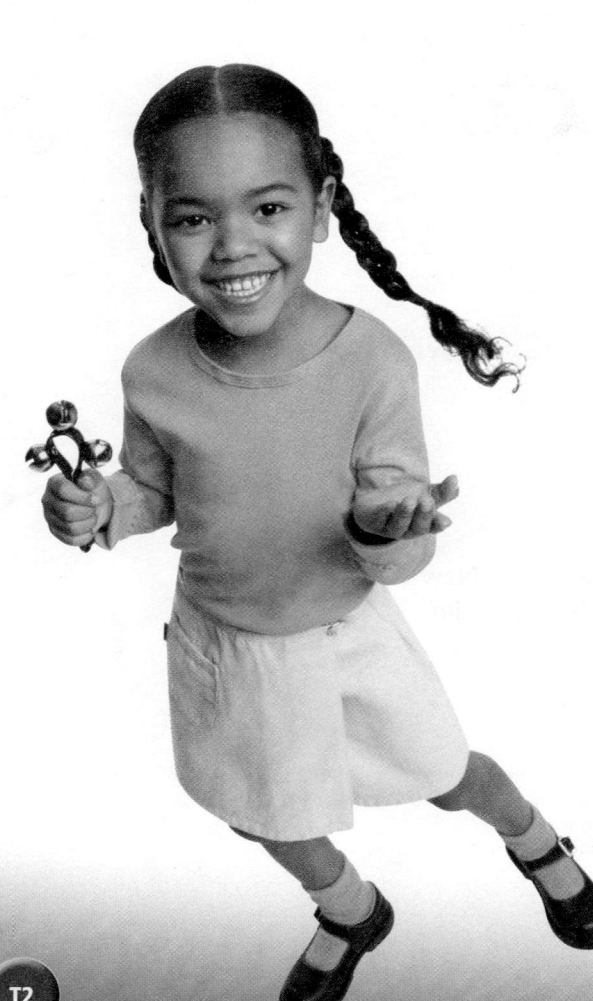

CONTRIBUTING AUTHORS

Audrey A. Berger
University of Rhode Island
Kingston, Rhode Island

Roslyn Burrough
Clinician/Consultant
Brooklyn, New York

J. Bryan Burton
West Chester University
West Chester, Pennsylvania

Jeffrey E. Bush
Arizona State University
Tempe, Arizona

John M. Cooksey
University of Utah
Salt Lake City, Utah

Shelly C. Cooper
University of Arizona
Tucson, Arizona

Alice-Ann Darrow
Florida State University
Tallahassee, Florida

Scott Emmons
University of Wisconsin—
Milwaukee
Milwaukee, Wisconsin

Debra Erck
Austin Independent
School District
Austin, Texas

Anne M. Fennell
Vista Unified School District
Vista, California

Doug Fisher
San Diego State University
San Diego, California

Carroll Gonzo
University of St. Thomas
St. Paul, Minnesota

Larry Harms
University of Southern California
Los Angeles, California

Martha F. Hilley
University of Texas at Austin
Austin, Texas

Debbie Burgoon Hines
Consultant
DeSoto, Texas

Mary Ellen Junda
University of Connecticut
Storrs, Connecticut

Donald Kalbach
Consultant
Bound Brook, New Jersey

Shirley E. Lacroix
Rhode Island College
Providence, Rhode Island

Henry Leck
Butler University
Indianapolis, Indiana

Sanna Longden
Clinician/Consultant
Evanston, Illinois

Glenn A. Richter
University of Texas at Austin
Austin, Texas

Carlos Xavier Rodriguez
University of Iowa
Iowa City, Iowa

Kathleen D. Sanz
District School Board of
Pasco County
Tampa, Florida

Julie K. Scott
Southern Methodist University
Dallas, Texas

Gwyn Spell
Clinician/Consultant
Marietta, Georgia

Barb Stevanson
Austin Independent
School District
Austin, Texas

Kimberly C. Walls
Auburn University
Auburn, Alabama

Jackie Wiggins
Oakland University
Rochester, Michigan

Maribeth Yoder-White
Appalachian State University
Boone, North Carolina

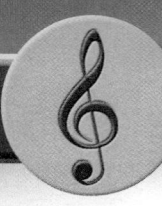

Program Contributors

LISTENING MAP CONTRIBUTING AUTHORS

Patricia Shehan Campbell
Seattle, Washington

Jackie Chooi-Theng Lew
Salisbury, Maryland

Ann Clements
Federal Way, Washington

Kay Edwards
Oxford, Ohio

Scott Emmons
Milwaukee, Wisconsin

Sheila Feay-Shaw
Shoreline, Washington

Kay Greenhaw
Austin, Texas

David Hebert
Seattle, Washington

Hunter C. March
Austin, Texas

Will Schmid
Milwaukee, Wisconsin

Carol Scott-Kassner
Seattle, Washington

Mary E. Shamrock
Minneapolis, Minnesota

Sandra L. Stauffer
Tempe, Arizona

MOVEMENT CONTRIBUTING AUTHORS

Judy Lasko
New York, New York

Marvelene C. Moore
Knoxville, Tennessee

Dixie Piver
New York, New York

Wendy Taucher
New York, New York

Susan Thomasson
Demarest, New Jersey

Judith Thompson-Barthwell
Detroit, Michigan

TEACHER ADVISORY PANEL

Kathryn Amshoff
Humble, Texas

Bevra L. Carruth
Midland, Texas

Rebekah Dykhuis
Austin, Texas

Gwendolyn J. Farris
DeSoto, Texas

Richard Gabrillo
Georgetown, Texas

Maria Yolanda Garza
San Antonio, Texas

Mary Lee Gilliland
Memphis, Tennessee

Jacque Hall
Arlington, Texas

Shari Hazell
Canton, Michigan

Lynette Hubler
Bondurant, Iowa

Tracy Walsh Juarez
El Paso, Texas

Barbara Keaton
Arlington, Texas

Jim Lovell
Plano, Texas

Scott Mahaffey
San Antonio, Texas

Laura L. McGregor
Sugar Land, Texas

Carol Moeller
Carmel, Indiana

Sue Niemi
*Downingtown,
Pennsylvania*

Kathy Lee Peinado
El Paso, Texas

Domingo Porras
Edinburg, Texas

Joseph Puzzo
Washington, D.C.

Pam Ramirez
Brownsville, Texas

Emily Roden
Denton, Texas

Beth Russell
Noblesville, Indiana

Chrissie Horany Seligson
Arlington, Texas

Tanya Seslar
Denver, Colorado

Donna Shortal
Winter Park, Florida

Barb Stevanson
Austin, Texas

Roseanne Stuetz
Maywood, New Jersey

Cathy Warnock
Mesquite, Texas

Wendy Weeks
Abilene, Texas

Barbara White
Williamsville, New York

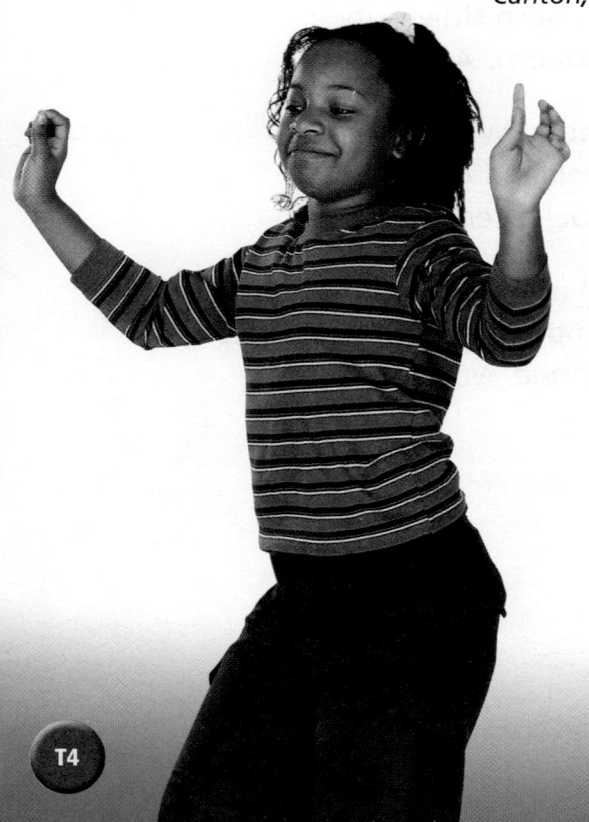

CRITIC READERS

Leon Adams
Little Rock, Arkansas

Barbara Alvarez
Muncie, Indiana

Elaine Bartee
Jonesboro, Arkansas

Patsy Biedenfield
Houston, Texas

Patricia A. Bourne
Bothell, Washington

Shaunda B. Butler
Pine Bluff, Arkansas

Kip Caton
Apex, North Carolina

Mary Cawley
Manasquan, New Jersey

Brenda Chapman
Jacksonville, Florida

Scott Chappell
*North Augusta,
South Carolina*

Craig Combs
New York, New York

Joyce W. Culwell
Aurora, Colorado

Shannon M. Daniels
Wichita Falls, Texas

Gloria Day
Tucson, Arizona

Don Doyle
Pasadena, California

Roger Dutcher
Plainfield, Indiana

Lana Dye
Sioux City, Iowa

Kay Edwards
Oxford, Ohio

Sue A. Fordtran
Corpus Christi, Texas

Elaine B. Gabriel
Houston, Texas

Lona George
Madison, Wisconsin

Laura R. Hancock
Tampa, Florida

Ann H. Hastings
Spring, Texas

Noreen Hofmann
Charlotte, North Carolina

Marianne Holland
Pickens, South Carolina

Ramona Holmes
Seattle, Washington

Mary Jeanette Howle
Jacksonville, Florida

Christine Jordanoff
Pittsburgh, Pennsylvania

Brenda Kimble
Champaign, Illinois

Janice R. Lancaster
Brandon, Florida

Anne M. Lanier
Columbia, South Carolina

Beverly M. Naumann
Chesterfield, Missouri

Marcus L. Neiman
Medina, Ohio

Shirley Neugebauer-Luebke
Sioux City, Iowa

Carol Nicolucci
Newton, Massachusetts

Sandra Nicolucci
Wellesley, Massachusetts

Dan Norris
Foley, Alabama

Leora Osborn
Wichita, Kansas

Johnnie R. M. Patton
Tyler, Texas

Teresa Pearl
Gastonia, North Carolina

Josephine Y. Poelinitz
Chicago, Illinois

Karen M. Renton
Topsham, Maine

Cecilia Riddell
Pasadena, California

Colleen Riddle
Spring, Texas

Cynthia A. Ripley
Hamburg, New York

Marc Schneider
Stamford, Connecticut

Lynn Schroeder
Apopka, Florida

Constance Shelengian
Scarsdale, New York

Pattie Simbulan
Burke, Virginia

Lisa Stern
Maitland, Florida

Lonnie W. Tanner
Houston, Texas

Nancy Ash Vondra
Omaha, Nebraska

Vanja Y. Watkins
Salt Lake City, Utah

Alejandro Ybarra
Mission, Texas

Penny E. Zaugg
Des Moines, Iowa

CULTURAL ADVISORS

CP Language Institute
New York, New York

Doreen Ackom, Zohar Azolay, Iris Bar-Ziv, Kveta Bendl,
Yvonne Bernardo, Marco Bertellini, Vadim Besprozranny,
Charlotte Cohen, Adrienne Cooper, Janna Deikan,
Rajesh Dhameliya, Victor Douger, Christine Dunoyer,
Sudkamol Ekkul, Joe Elias, Naomi Finkelstein, Judy Fixler,
Mel Gionson, Michal Guterman, Solange Habib, Trina Hedegaard,
Dr. Kim Huichin, Chang Huichin Wang, Marija Jaramoxovic,

Jacek Jarkowsky, Rebecca Johnson, Mikaela Kull, Edwin Lugo,
Yana Manovschi, Herand Markariann, Zahra Meigani,
Claudia Mejia, Iveta Mozsnyakova, Deborah Mullens,
Fidelma Murphy, Kazuha Okuchi, Gloria Ospina,
Andrea Philogene, Thierry Pomies, Virginia Rambal,
Wladyslaw Roczniak, Rackelle Roden, Martha Ruiz, Yuki Saito,
Esperanza Salazar, Sarah Smith, Eleonore Speckents,
Carime Triana, Ilian Troya, Huichin Wang,
Cathi Witkowski-Changanaqui, Dieter Wolthoff,
Wendy Wu, Bing Yang

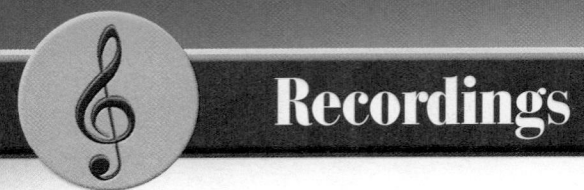

Recordings

RECORDING PERSONNEL

Executive Producer

Buryl Red, BR Productions

Associate Producers for Vocals

Bill and Charlene James, Tom Moore, J. Douglas Pummill, Michael Rafter, Robert Spivak, Jeanine Tesori, Linda Twine

Associate Producers for Instrumentals

Rick Baitz, Rick Bassett, Joseph Joubert, Bryan Louiselle, Michael Rafter, Buddy Skipper, Jeanine Tesori

Arrangers/Orchestrators

Rick Baitz, Rick Bassett, Jack Cortner, Bruce Coughlin, Cathy Elliott, Ned Ginsberg, Joseph Joubert, Dick Lieb, Bryan Louiselle, Chris McDonald, Gustavo Moretta, Valerie Naranjo, Janet Pummill, William Pursell, Buryl Red, Mick Rossi, Steve Shapiro, Buddy Skipper, Jeff Steinberg, Jeff Talman, Jeanine Tesori, David Thomas, Linda Twine, Dale Wilson, Ovid Young

Technical Engineering Staff

Jonathan Duckett, *supervisor*, Dave Darlington, Chris Miller, Tim Polashek, Amy Pummill, Patrick Pummill, Mick Rossi, Dan Rudin, William Santamaria, Bob Schaper, Ted Spencer, Jeff Talman, Tony Zimmerman

Instrumental Conductors

Bryan Louiselle, Michael Rafter, Buryl Red, Jeanine Tesori, Linda Twine

CHOIRS

Children's Choir Conductors and Choirs

Debbie Beinhorn
Beinhorn Singers

D. Shawn Berry
Bak Middle School of the Arts Boys Choir, Bak Middle School of the Arts Mixed Choir

Darrell Bledsoe
Darrell Bledsoe Children's Voices, Darrell Bledsoe Men's Chorus, Darrell Bledsoe Singers, Houston Vocal Edition, Richland Singers, Singing Boys of Houston, Spring Singers, Varsity Girls, Varsity Singers

Linda Bradberry
The Augusta Children's Choir

Madeline Bridges
The Nashville Children's Choir

Gregg Bunn
Lone Star Kids

Lori Casteel
Kidstyle Singers

Wayne Causey
The Cumberland Singers

Victor Cook
Victor Cook Singers

Debra Crowe
Debra Crowe Singers

David Czervinske
David Czervinske Children's Choir, David Czervinske Singers

Jerri Davidson
The Daggett Choir

Connie Drosakis
Bak Middle School of the Arts 6th Grade Treble Choir

Lynne Gackle
Miami Girls Choir

Ned Ginsburg
The Broadway Kids

Charlotte Greeson
Richland Singers

Joan Gregoryk
Chevy Chase Elementary Singers

Cathy Guajardo
Cathy Guajardo Singers

Jacque Hall
The Mary Moore Singers

Moses Hogan
The Moses Hogan Singers Youth Ensemble

Sandy Holland
The Charlotte Children's Choir

Eugenia Huanca
Eugenia Huanca Group

Laurie Jenschke
Eastman Children's Choir, Voices of Fredericksburg, Texas Children's Chorale

Brenda Jewell
The Nashville Children's Choir

Doug Jewett
The Smokey Mountain Children's Choir

Rebecca Johnson
The Sunshine Singers

Joseph Joubert
Joseph Joubert Singers

Mary Ellen Junda
The Treblemakers Children's Choir of the University of Connecticut

Jan Juneau
Woodland Singers

Henry Leck
The Indianapolis Children's Choir

Jeanine Tesori
Jeanine Tesori Singers

Carol Lockhart
The Carol Lockhart Singers

Chester Mahooty
American Indian Dance Theater

Albert McNeil
Albert McNeil Jubilee Singers

Jo Morris
Jo Morris Singers

Cynthia Nott
The Children's Chorus of Greater Dallas

Celia Ong
Asian American Youth Chorale

Rosalyn Payne
Step Chillin'

Ted Polk
Carrollton Singers

Douglas Pummill
Booker T. Washington Singers, Cantamos!, Children of the Heartland, The Dulcet Singers, Fiesta Americana, Heartland Youth, Heritage Children's Choir, Heritage Youth Choir, The New Horizons Show Choir, The North Texas Hispanic Choir, The Pan American Children's Choir, The Pan American Youth Choir, The Pan Asian Children's Choir, The Rainbow Children's Choir, The Rainbow Youth Choir, United in Youth

Eddie Quaid
Cypress Singers

Lynn Redmond
The Gwinnette Young Singers

Steve Roddy
The Houston Children's Choir, Steve Roddy Boys' Choir

Kenny Rodgers
Kenny Rodgers Singers

Betty Roe
McCullough Singers, Betty Roe Children's Choir

Reggie Royal
Calypso Royals

Sally Schott
South Houston Singers

Marilyn Shadinger
The Nashville Children's Choir

Martha Shaw
The Spivey Hall Children's Choir Chamber Ensemble

Kay Sherrill
Judson High School Chorale

Mark Slaughter
The Owensboro Children's Choir

Steve Stevens
The Seattle Boys Choir, The Seattle Children's Choir

Cameron Sullenburger
Wilson Middle School Varsity Boys Choir, Wilson Middle School Varsity Girls Choir, Wilson Middle School Varsity Mixed Choir

Sheryl Tallant
Kidstyle Singers

Barry Talley
Barry Talley Singers, Deer Park Singers

Julia Thorn
DeKalb County Children's Choir

Judy Tisch
Bammell Singers

Marie Tomlinson
Clitheroe Young Singers

Darryl Tookes
The Darryl Tookes Singers

Walter Turnbill
The Boys Choir of Harlem

Linda Twine
55th Street Jazz Singers, Linda Twine Singers

Tim Vaughn
La Porte Singers

Walt Whitman
The Soul Children of Chicago, The Walt Whitman Atlanta Singers, Walt Whitman's Soul Children

Linda Williams
Sundance Academy Singers, Westwind Singers

Judith Willoughby
The Temple University Children's Choir

Cheryl Wilson
Garland High School A cappella Choir, Garland High School A cappella Men, Garland High School A cappella Women

Janet Wilson
Janet Wilson Singers, Kid Connection

Karen Wolff
Cincinnati Children's Choir

Patrinell Wright
Total Experience Gospel Choir

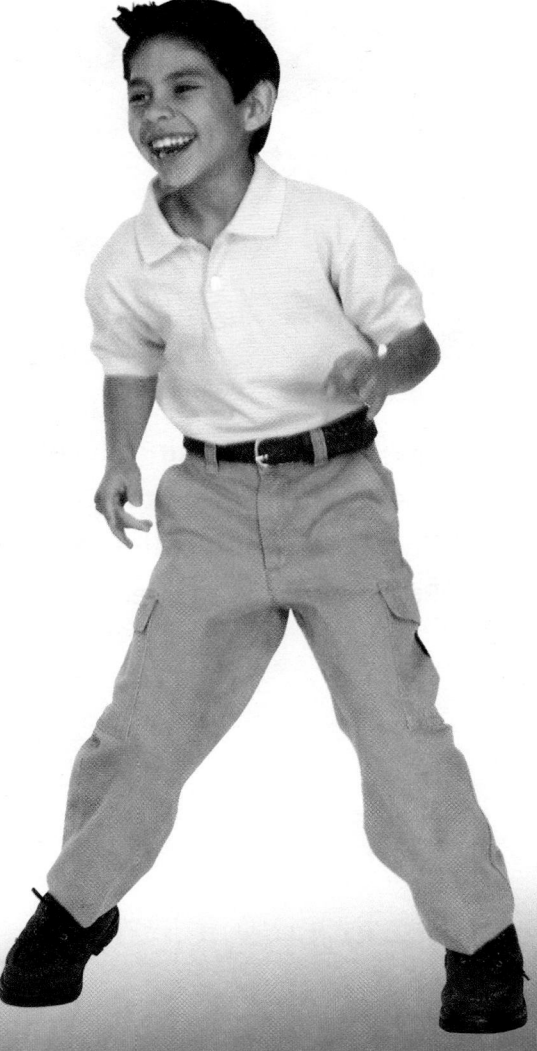

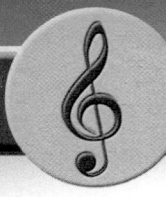
Welcome music educators!

Silver Burdett MAKING MUSIC is an active, balanced, and comprehensive music program. It provides both sequential teaching of music elements and skills as well as theme-based instruction for music educators and students.

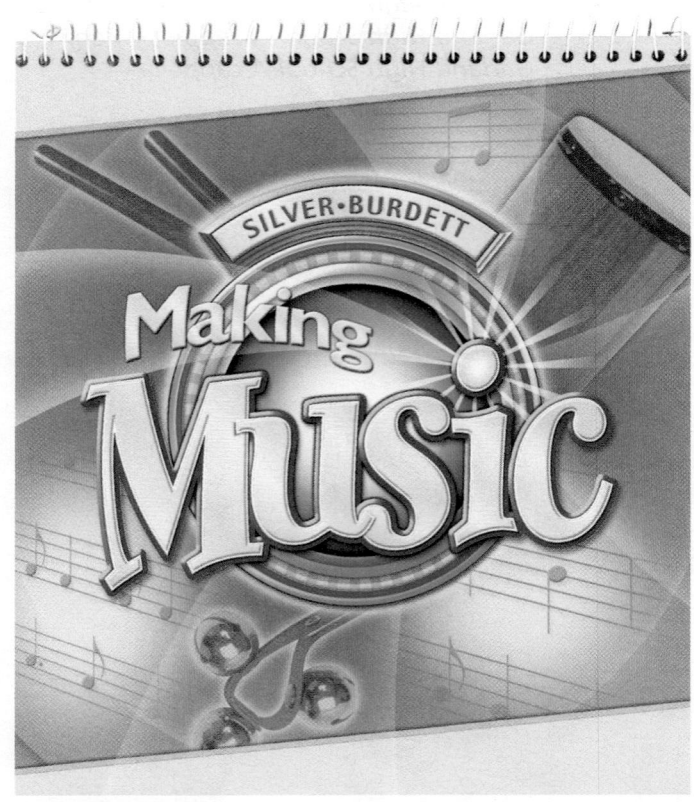

Kindergarten Big Book

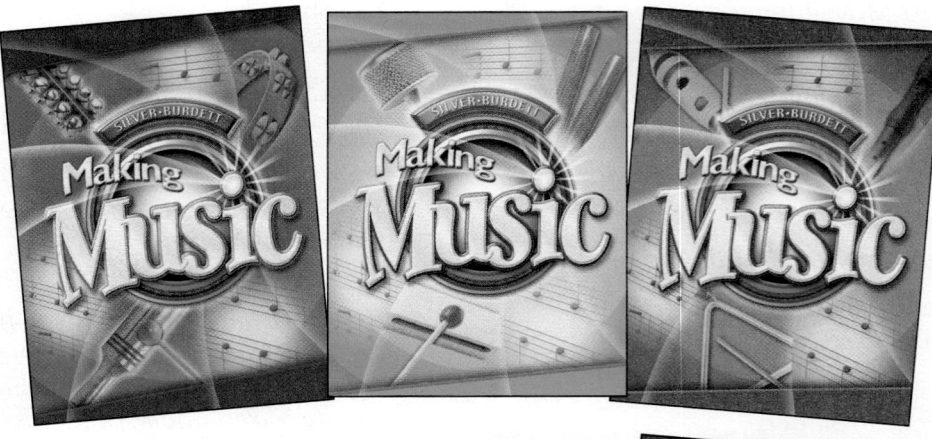

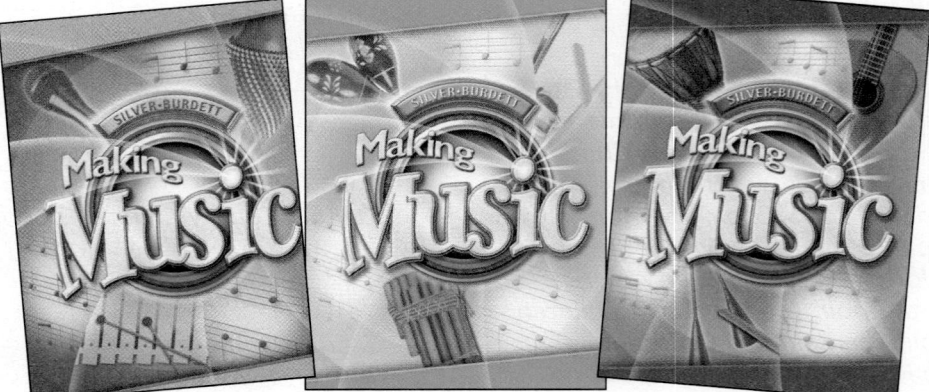

Student Editions, Grades 1–6

- **Active music making** develops musical knowledge and skills.
- **Exceptional song literature and recordings** provide a strong foundation for instruction.
- **Balanced organization** presents a comprehensive music curriculum.
- **Proven content** reflects the National Standards for Music Education.

Active music making that supports your teaching

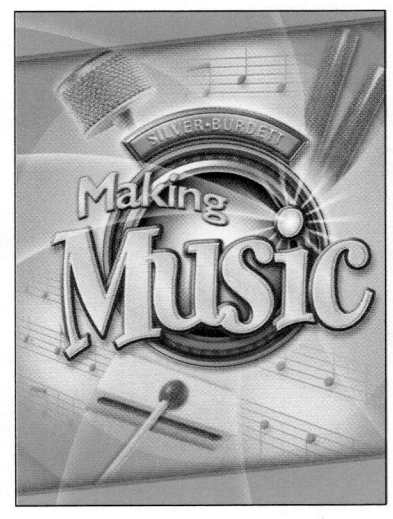

Student Editions

- Dynamic repertoire of song literature
- Opportunities to sing, listen to music, play instruments, read music, move to music, and connect to other disciplines

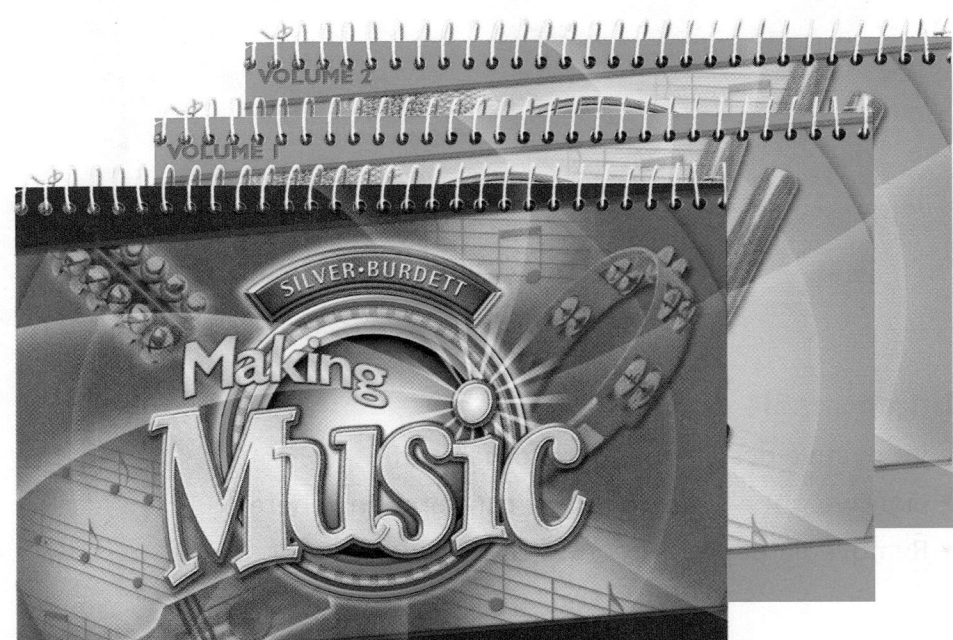

Grades 1 and 2

Big Books

- Big, bold, colorfully illustrated lessons
- Great for small-group and classroom instruction
- Many different musical experiences
- Sturdy easel for easy display
- One volume, Grades K–1; two volumes, Grade 2

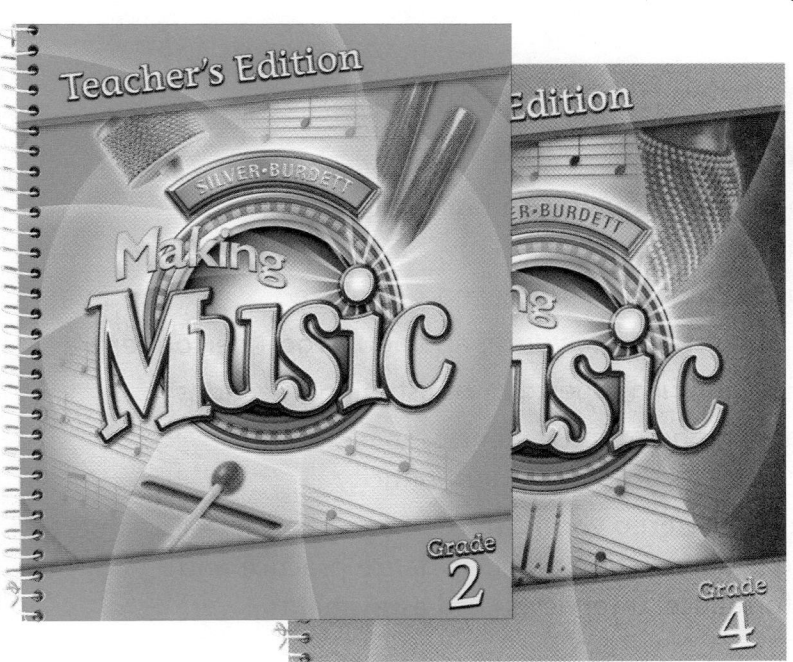

Teacher's Editions

- Sequential instruction in Units 1–6
- Theme-based instruction in Units 7–12
- National Standards integrated throughout
- Consistent, three-step lesson plan

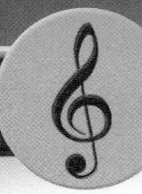
Recordings you'll want to carry everywhere

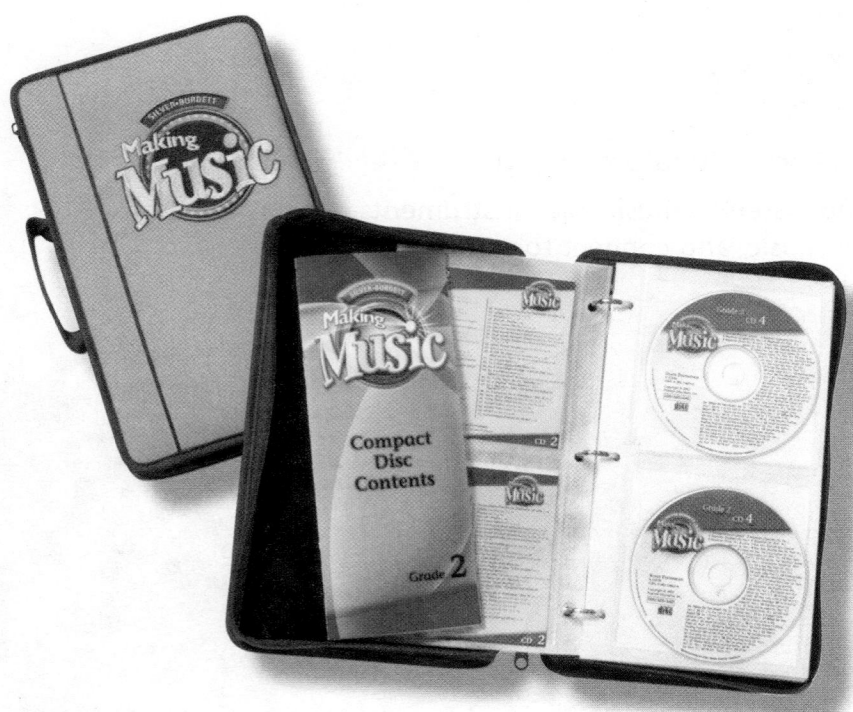

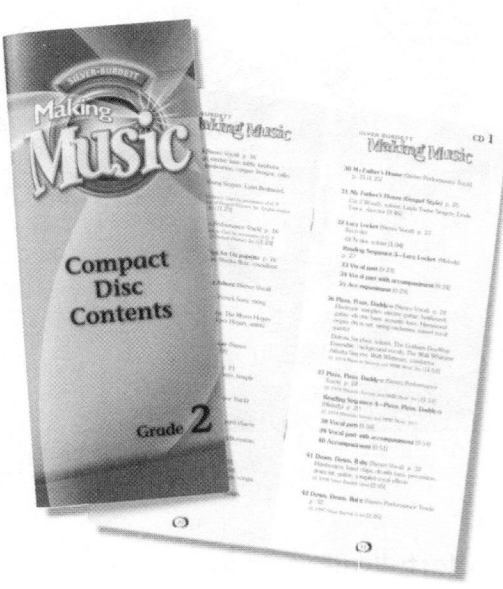

Ultraportable CD Cases

- Innovative design keeps you organized
- Lightweight and small so you can carry anywhere
- Removable pages for greater flexibility

Audio CD Booklets

- Quick, easy guide for each grade-level Audio CD package
- Comprehensive list of recorded tracks; includes information on performing groups, instrumentation, track length, page references, and special recorded features

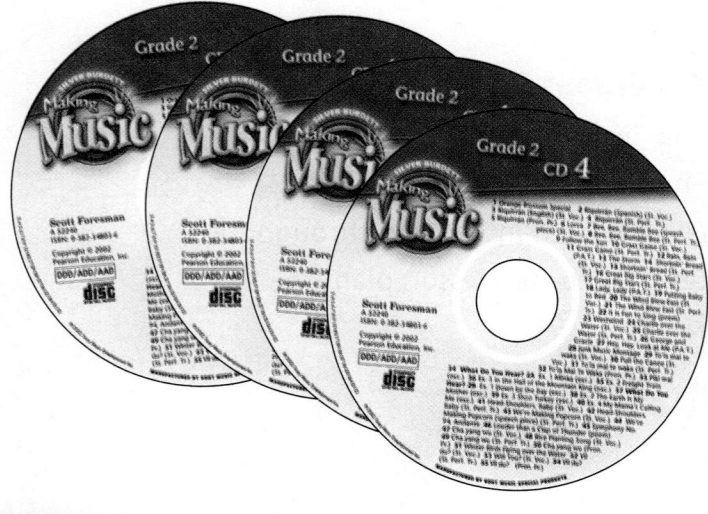

Professional Recordings

- Superb sound quality—a higher standard in educational recordings
- Artists that people know and recognize
- Variety of children, youth, and adult vocal performers
- Varied and rich repertoire of listening selections
- Widest range of music genres, styles, and cultures—recorded with authenticity
- Tracks for stereo vocals, stereo performance, teach-a-part, sung pronunciation practice, dance practice and performance, interviews, and assessments

Resources that enhance your music teaching

Keyboard Accompaniments

- Keyboard accompaniments for classroom use and performances
- Easy-to-use, spiral-bound book—hard-back cover stays upright on any keyboard stand

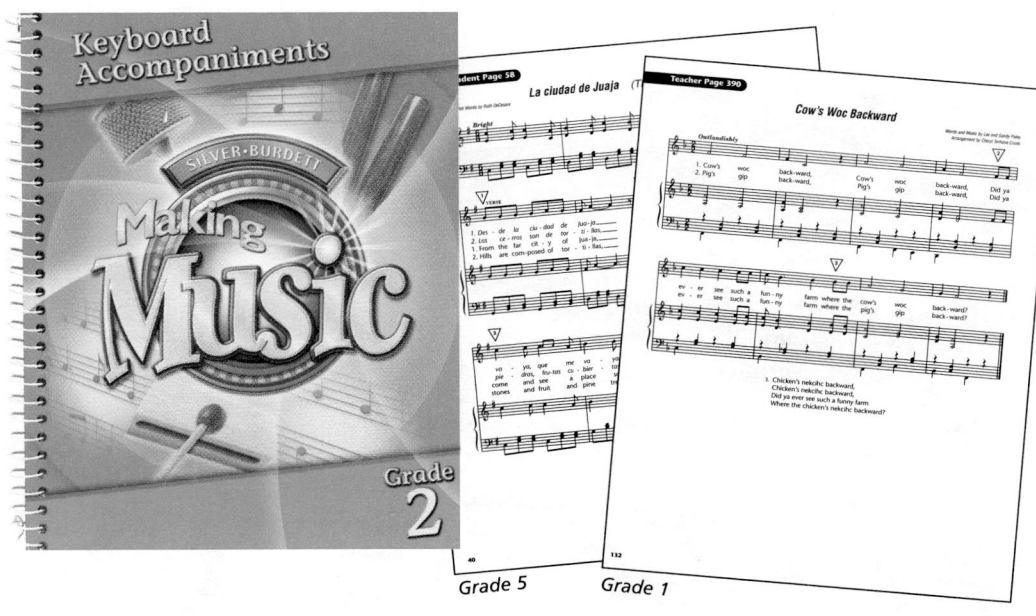

Grade 5   Grade 1

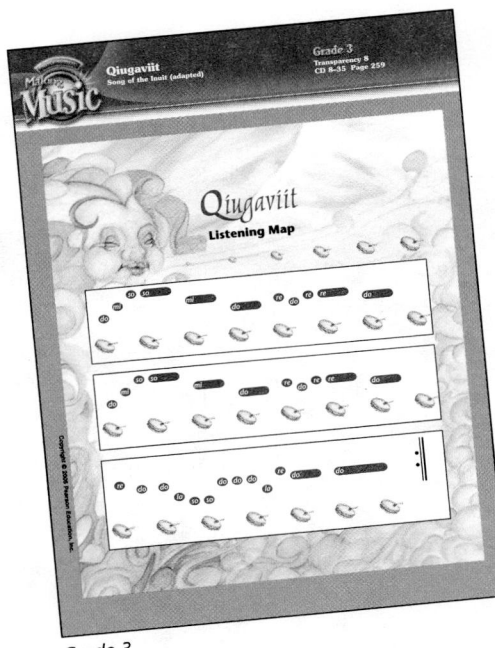

Grade 3

Listening Map Transparency Package

- Visual guides for listening selections
- Easy-to-follow graphics that build skills in listening and understanding music
- Reproducible masters to support instruction

Resource Books

Reproducible masters are available to support the following:

- Pronunciation Practice Guides
- Graphic Organizers
- Assessments and Rubrics
- Music Reading Worksheets
- Music Reading Practice (1–6)
- Orff Arrangements
- Signing Activities
- Keyboard (2–6)
- Recorder (3–6)
- Activity Masters

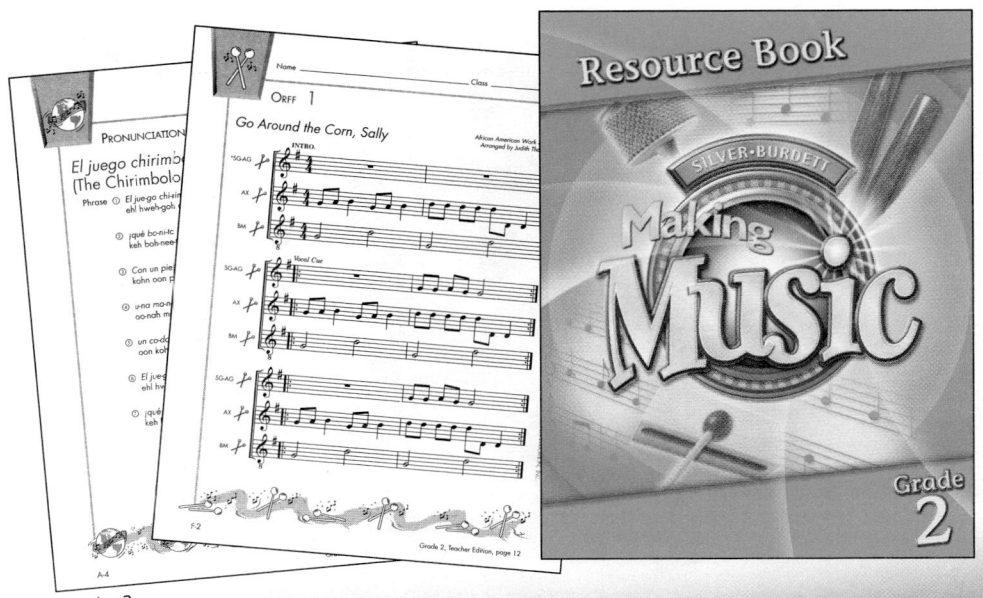

Grade 2

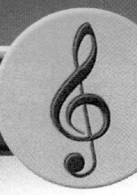

Teacher Support

More resources for music instruction

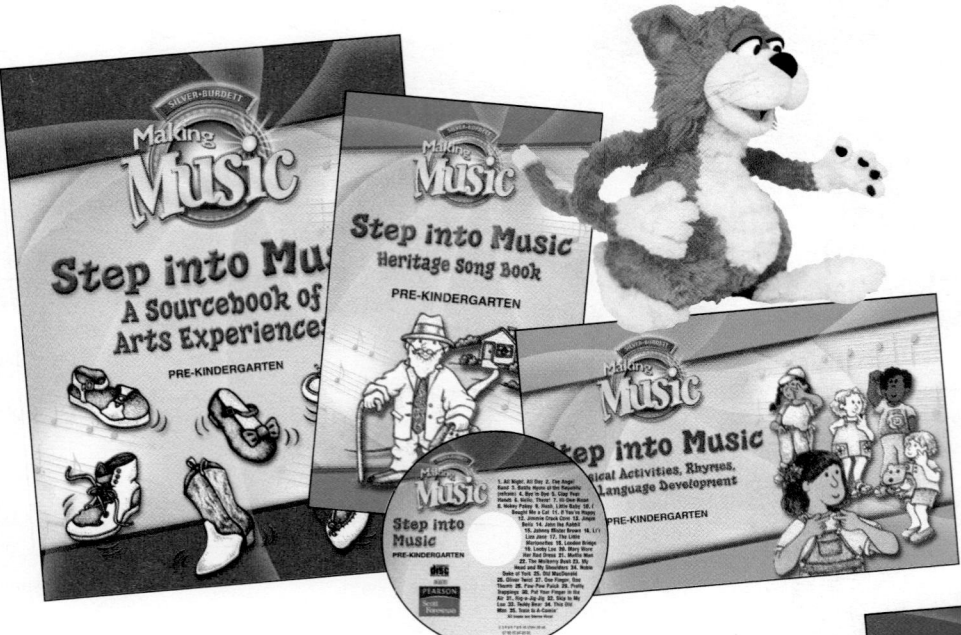

Step into Music, Pre-Kindergarten

- Complete fine arts program that builds early music literacy and language skills
- Effective support for children's physical, emotional, social, and cognitive development

Silver Burdett MAKING MUSIC, Grades 7–8

- Modular organization for maximum teaching flexibility
- Active music-making experiences
- Comprehensive music instruction
- National Standards integrated throughout

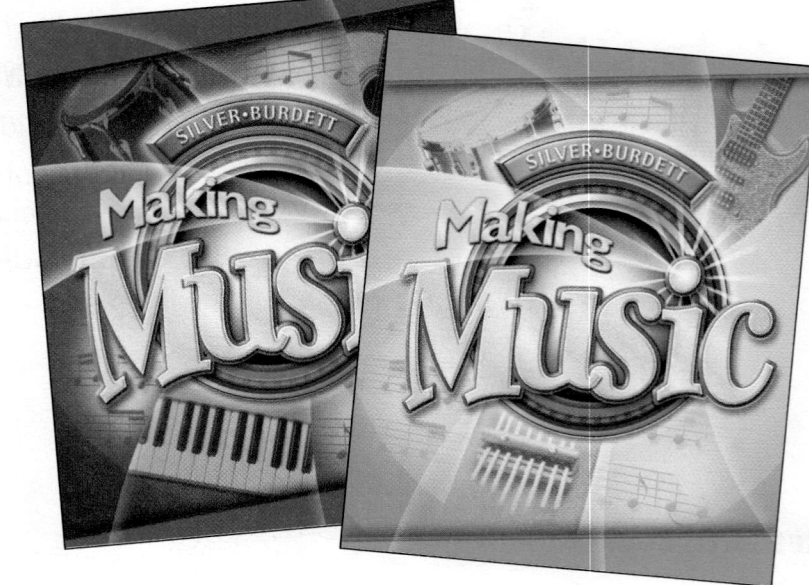

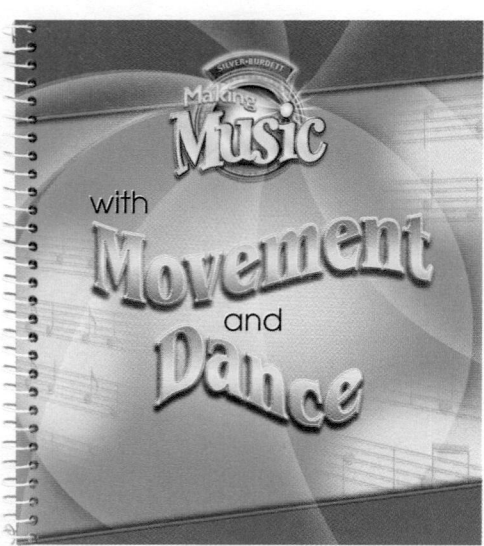

MAKING MUSIC with Movement and Dance

- Easy-to-follow guide for movement and dance activities
- Folk dances, ethnic dances, and creative movement
- One volume—all grade levels

¡A cantar!

- Traditional and contemporary songs in Spanish
- Theme and element connections
- Recorded pronunciation practice
- Two CDs with all songs and literature
- Primary and Intermediate Levels

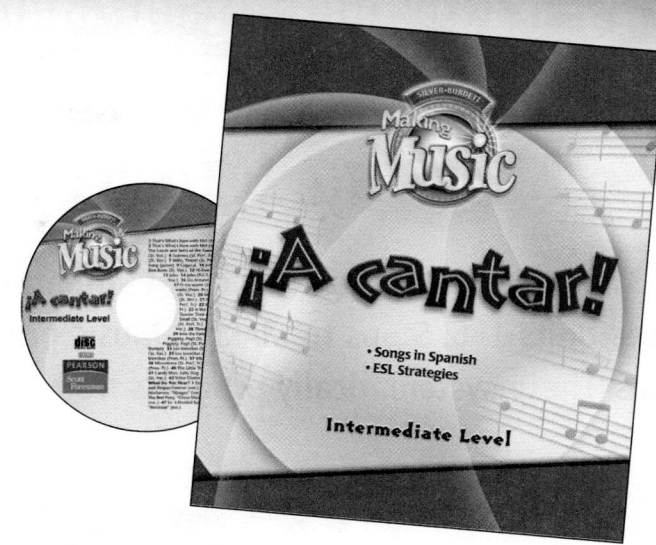

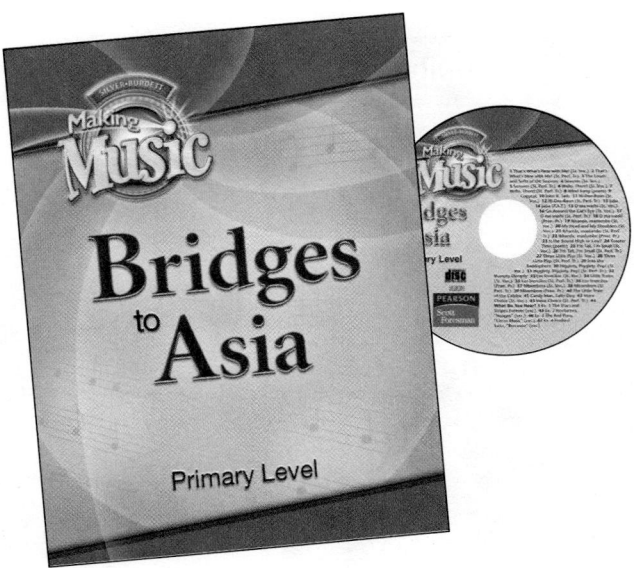

Bridges to Asia

- Additional lessons to explore the rich musical heritage of Asia
- Pronunciation practice for each song
- Four CDs with all songs and literature
- Primary and Intermediate Levels

New Activities for the Substitute Teacher

- Songs and activities for substitute teachers
- Song lyrics, teaching strategies, reproducible activity masters, and audio CD
- Integrated activities for all grade levels

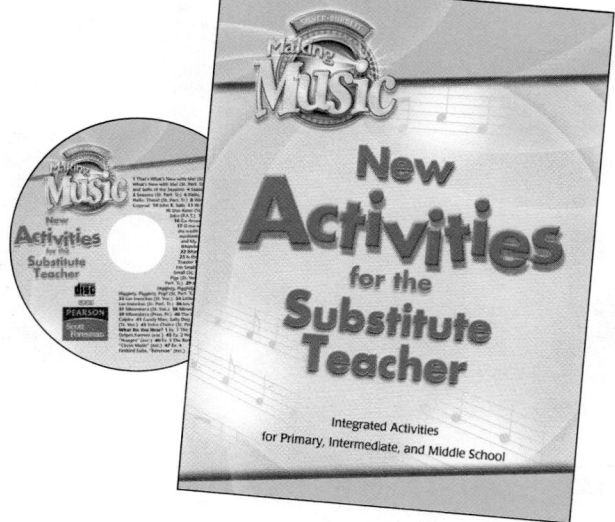

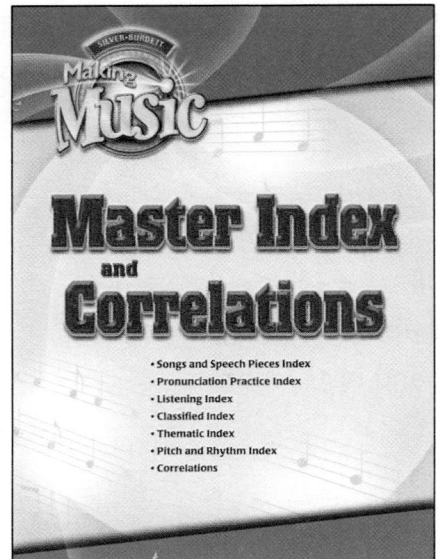

Master Index and Correlations

- Comprehensive reference to simplify planning
- Grades K–8 index of all songs, speech pieces, listening selections, and more
- Pitch and Rhythm Index
- Thematic Index
- Reading and Phonics Correlations

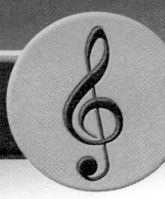

Steps to MAKING MUSIC for sequential instruction

Silver Burdett MAKING MUSIC has a balanced, two-part organization. Part 1 is Steps to MAKING MUSIC, which comprises Units 1–6. Steps to MAKING MUSIC provides sequential instruction using elements, skills, and connections. These systematically progress from unit to unit and grade to grade.

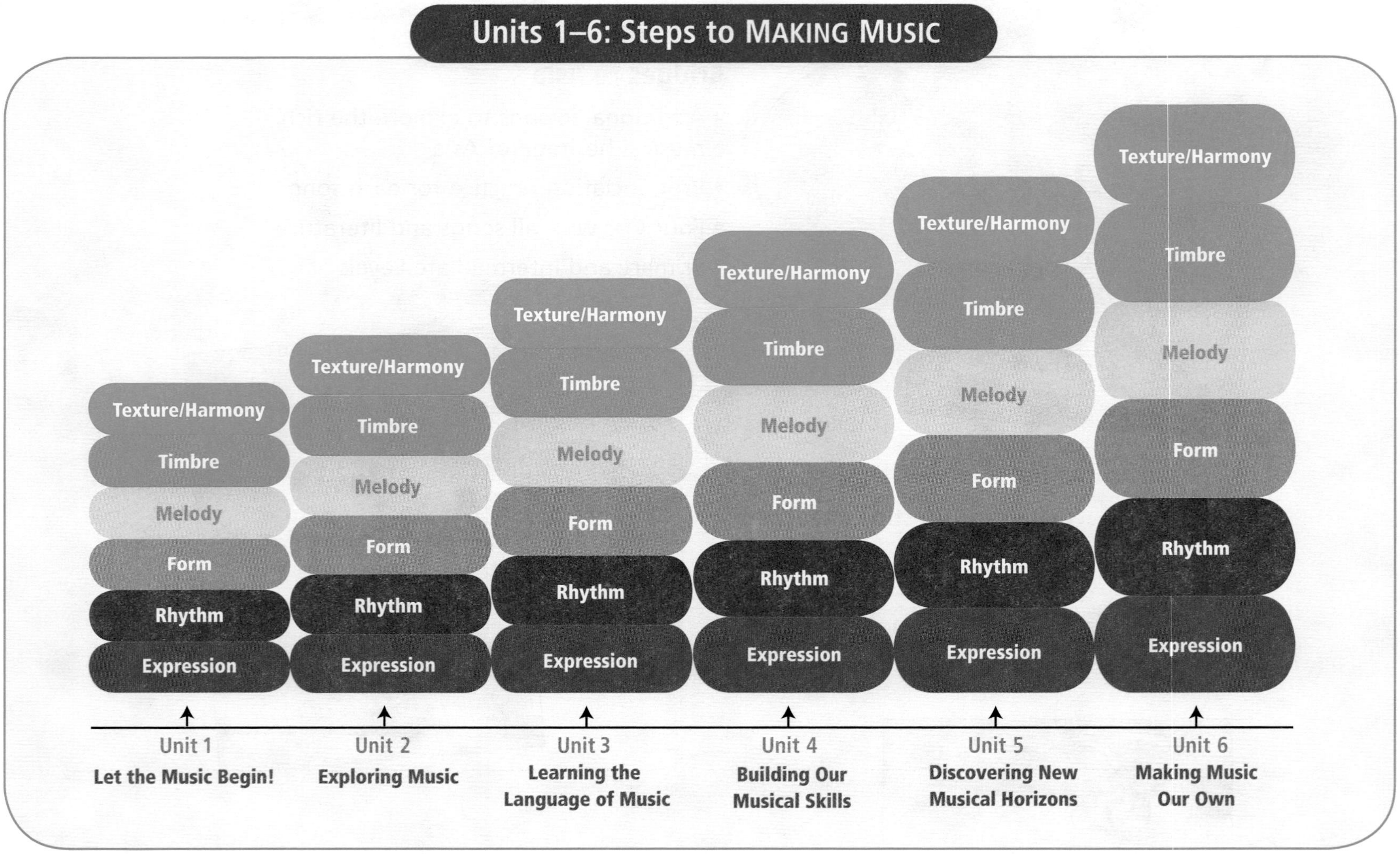

Units 1–6: Steps to MAKING MUSIC

Unit 1	Unit 2	Unit 3	Unit 4	Unit 5	Unit 6
					Texture/Harmony
				Texture/Harmony	Timbre
			Texture/Harmony	Timbre	Melody
		Texture/Harmony	Timbre	Melody	
	Texture/Harmony	Timbre	Melody		Form
Texture/Harmony	Timbre	Melody		Form	
Timbre	Melody		Form		Rhythm
Melody		Form	Form	Form	
Form	Form	Form		Rhythm	
		Rhythm	Rhythm	Rhythm	
Rhythm	Rhythm				
Expression	Expression	Expression	Expression	Expression	Expression
Let the Music Begin!	**Exploring Music**	**Learning the Language of Music**	**Building Our Musical Skills**	**Discovering New Musical Horizons**	**Making Music Our Own**

Units 1–6: Steps to MAKING MUSIC

- Sequenced instruction to help students learn music elements and skills
- Gradual increase in skill levels that allows students to assimilate and apply learning
- 72 total music lessons—36 weekly core lessons plus 36 lessons to expand instruction

Paths to MAKING MUSIC for theme explorations

Paths to MAKING MUSIC is Part 2 of the program and includes Units 7–12. This section increases your students' music knowledge and skills through theme-based activities and lessons. The themes are coordinated from grade to grade so that all students can share related instruction.

Units 7–12: Paths to MAKING MUSIC

6	Exploring America's Music	Say It with Drums	Be a Star!	Sound Waves	Strike Up the Chorus	Celebrate the Day
5	Building America in Song	Music Around the World	In the Pop Style	Keepers of the Earth	We Sing!	Holidays in Song
4	Going Places U.S.A.	Bring Your Passport	Chasing a Dream	Earth, Sea, and Sky	Sing Out!	Sing and Celebrate
3	Singing America	Our World of Music	Fun and Games	This Beautiful Planet	Tuneful Tales	Holidays to Share
2	Music–U.S.A.	Home and Away	Creature Feature	Our Planet Earth	Perform a Story	Celebrate the Season
1	Making Music at School	My Family and Me	Adventures with Friends	The Great Outdoors	Imagination Station!	Days to Celebrate
K	All About Me	My Neighbors and Me	Imagine That!	Nature Walk	Look What I Can Do!	Celebrate with Me!
	Unit 7 America Makes Music	Unit 8 From Home to the World	Unit 9 Expanding the Boundaries	Unit 10 Garden of the Earth	Unit 11 The Power of Performance	Unit 12 The Joy of Celebration

Units 7–12: Paths to MAKING MUSIC

- Thematic units aligned with themes commonly found in social studies, reading, science, and other curricular areas
- Terrific opportunities to make connections and present performances

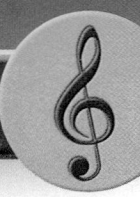

Easy-to-teach, flexible, and inspiring lessons

Objective Bar focuses your students' learning. The yellow burst highlights the assessed item.

Lesson at a Glance lists critical information to streamline planning.

CD References make it easy to access your audio collection.

More Music Choices provide options for further practice.

Footnotes support your instruction and help you make connections.

Building Skills Through Music connects music learning to other curricular areas.

LESSON **Core 4**

LESSON AT A GLANCE

Element Focus   **RHYTHM**   ♩ ♫ ♬ and ♬ ♫

Skill Objective   **PLAYING** Play sixteenth-note patterns

Connection Activity   **SOCIAL STUDIES** Investigate the historical context of a railroad song

MATERIALS
• "Drill, Ye Tarriers"   **CD 3-16**
   Recording Routine: Intro (4 m.); v. 1; refrain; interlude (4 m.); v. 2; refrain; interlude (4 m.); v. 3, refrain; coda
• **Music Reading Practice, Sequence 6**   **CD 3-18**
• **Dance Directions** for "Drill, Ye Tarriers" p. 554
• *Symphony No. 9*, Movement 1 (excerpt)   **CD 3-22**
• **Resource Book** p. E-7, F-6, I-6
• selected classroom percussion instruments

VOCABULARY
symphony   movement

◆ ◆ ◆ **National Standards** ◆ ◆ ◆
1b Sing easy pieces with technical accuracy
2b Perform easy instrumental pieces with technical accuracy
5a Read quarter, eighth, sixteenth notes in duple meter
5d Use standard notation to record musical ideas
6a Listen and describe events in music using appropriate terms
8b Identify ways music relates to social studies

MORE MUSIC CHOICES
For more experience with sixteenth-note patterns: "Camptown Races," p. 270

1 INTRODUCE

Have students listen to "Drill Ye Tarriers" **CD 3-16** and discuss the lyrics. Use the suggestions in Across the Curriculum below to engage students in a discussion of railroads.

Footnotes

MOVEMENT

▶ **Patterned Dance** Dancing is a natural part of Irish culture. It is said that when two Irishmen meet at a crossroad, they do a little jig. When the Irishmen who worked on the railroad had time to relax, they sang and danced. There were not many women at the railroad camps, so the men danced with each other, just as American cowboys and Argentine sailors did. See p. 554 for a movement pattern to accompany "Drill, Ye Tarriers."

BUILDING SKILLS THROUGH MUSIC

▶ **Math** Divide the class into two groups, with one group clapping the rhythm of the verse, the second group clapping a steady beat. Ask students to identify beats with one or more notes. Each beat will equal one [whole]. Review the fractions for 1/2 and 1/4. Have students identify fractions for each note. For example, an eighth note would equal 1/2; a sixteenth note would equal 1/4. Add the fractions for each beat, then for each measure.

54   Reading Sequence 6, p. 492

Grade 5

LESSON **4**   **Element: RHYTHM**   **Skill: PLAYING**   **Connection: SOCIAL STU**

Work to the Rhythm

In the 1880s, many different groups of immigrants helped to build American railroads. One of these groups was the Irish. **Sing** "Drill, Ye Tarriers," a song that tells of the hardships and injustices the railroad workers faced.

Listen for some clues in the text about what tarriers do.

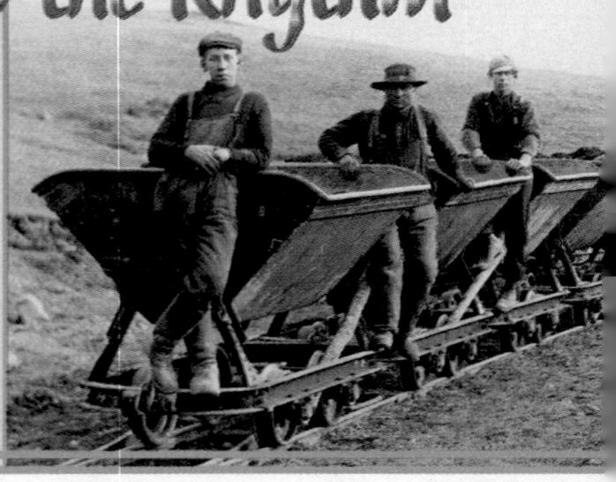

CD 3-16

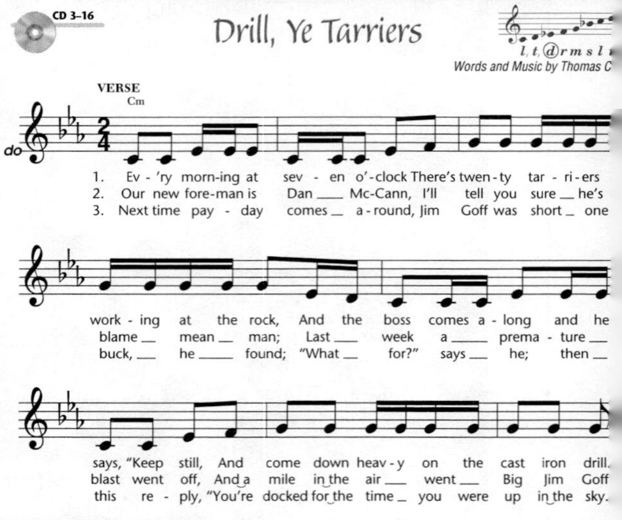

Drill, Ye Tarriers

l t @ r m s l
Words and Music by Thomas C

VERSE
Cm

do

1. Ev - 'ry morn-ing at sev - en o'-clock There's twen-ty tar - ri - ers
2. Our new fore-man is Dan ___ Mc-Cann, I'll tell you sure ___ he's
3. Next time pay - day comes ___ a - round, Jim Goff was short ___ one

work - ing at the rock, And the boss comes a - long and he
blame ___ mean ___ man; Last ___ week a ___ prema - ture ___ and
buck, ___ he ___ found; "What ___ for?" says ___ he; then ___

says, "Keep still, And come down heav - y on the cast iron drill.
blast went off, And a mile in the air ___ went ___ Big Jim Goff
this re - ply, "You're docked for the time ___ you were up in the sky.

54   Reading Sequence 6

ACROSS THE CURRICULUM

8b ▶ **Social Studies** Students may enjoy reading and then cre-ating a short historical-fact introduction to "Drill, Ye Tarriers" for performances. For interesting facts about the building of railroads across the United States, suggest they read *Ten Mile Day: And the Building of the Transcontinental Railroad* by Mary Ann Fraser (Henry Holt, 1996). This fascinating account of the build-ing of the Transcontinental Railroad in 1869 explores the histori-cal highlights and engineering feats, lives of the many ethnic groups who served as railroad workers, and the effects of the railroads on Native Americans.

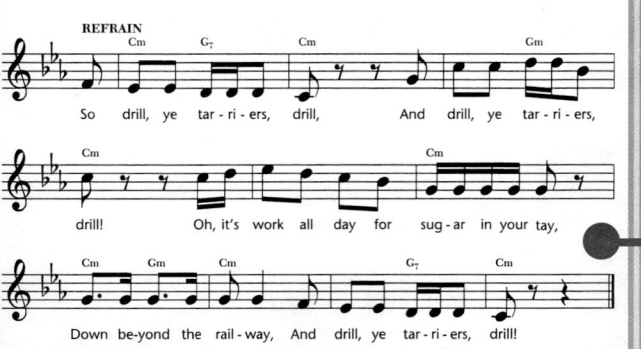

REFRAIN

So drill, ye tar - ri - ers, drill, And drill, ye tar - ri - ers,

drill! Oh, it's work all day for sug - ar in your tay,

Down be - yond the rail - way, And drill, ye tar - ri - ers, drill!

Railroad Rhythms

Find the 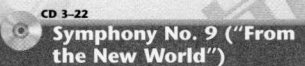 and ♩♩♩ patterns in the song.

Sing the song again, and when one of these patterns comes along, sing the rhythm syllables instead of the words. Good luck!

Play the rhythm parts below with the refrain of "Drill, Ye Tarriers."

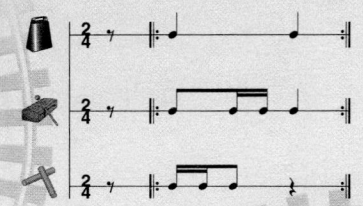

Listen to the  pattern in this excerpt.

CD 3–22
🔵 **Symphony No. 9 ("From the New World")**

Movement 1
by Antonín Dvořák
The name of this symphony, "From the New World," refers to the United States. Czech composer Antonín Dvořák [an-toh-NEEN d'VOHR-zhahk] wrote it at about the same time railroad workers were singing "Drill, Ye Tarriers."

Unit 2 55

---

2 DEVELOP

Reading
Ask volunteers to write three rhythms on the board:

 Set a steady beat and then have students
- Read each rhythm with rhythm syllables.
- Look at the notation for "Drill, Ye Tarriers" and count how many times each sixteenth-note rhythm appears in the song. Then read the verse of the song with rhythm syllables.

For more practice performing sixteenth-note rhythms, see Music Reading Practice, Sequence 6 on p. 492 and Resource Book p. E-6.

Creating
Add two beamed eighth notes, a quarter note, and a quarter rest to the rhythms on the board. Draw four blanks (two measures) on the board. Have students

- Decide how to fill in the blanks, using the patterns on the board. (The quarter note and quarter rest can be used only once.)
- Use standard symbols to notate rhythm in simple patterns and perform them using rhythm syllables. Then say their patterns one after another without silent beats in between.

Playing
Invite students to perform the instrumental parts on p. 55 with the refrain "Drill, Ye Tarriers."

Listening
Play the excerpt from *Symphony No. 9* **CD 3-22** and ask students to listen for the *tiri-ti* rhythm.

3 CLOSE

Element: RHYTHM ⟩ **ASSESSMENT**

 Performance/Observation Have students play their rhythm patterns, or those on p. 55, on selected percussion instruments as ostinatos, while singing "Drill, Ye Tarriers." Observe for rhythmic accuracy.

Systematic Instruction follows a consistent, three-step plan.

Song Notation on a white background improves readability.

National Standards at point of use identify your instructional goals.

Assessment allows you to monitor students' understanding.

SKILLS REINFORCEMENT 🎼

▶ **Recorder** To give students additional experience with rhythm patterns that use eighth and sixteenth notes, have them compose a rhythmic piece to play on their recorders. Invite students to create and notate four, two-beat measures using quarter, eighth, and sixteenth notes. Using their recorders, have them play their compositions to accompany the verse of "Drill, Ye Tarriers" by playing their composition on G. They will need to repeat their four-measure pieces or have a friend play the second set of four measures.

Another time, have students play the rhythm of the words on the note G during the verse of the song. Make sure they say *daah* on each note so the rhythm is articulated clearly.

A countermelody for "Drill, Ye Tarriers" can be found on Resource Book p. I-6.

CHARACTER EDUCATION 🎖

▶ **Collaboration** To promote students' understanding of the skills necessary to collaborate with others, discuss singing and professional partnerships. Singing in a group requires vocal control and careful listening to achieve appropriate balance and blend. Individuals often must adjust their performance to benefit the group. Ask students what other situations require that individuals sacrifice control to help the group. (Accept various answers including team sports and medical teams.)

TECHNOLOGY/MEDIA LINK 💻

Notation Software Have students notate their rhythm patterns from this lesson and print them before playing them.

Unit 2 *Exploring Music* 55

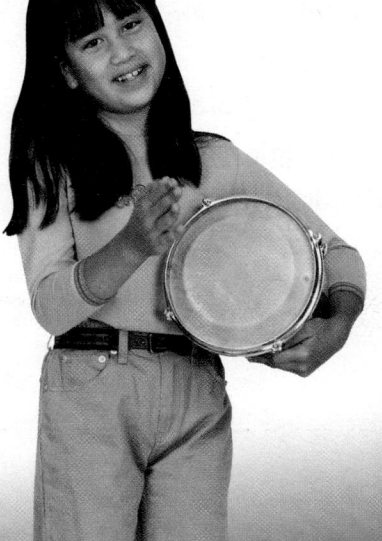

T17

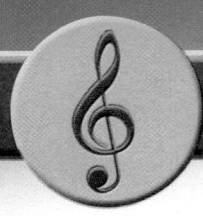

The best music, the widest selection

Favorite songs, award-winning songs, exciting originals! Silver Burdett MAKING MUSIC provides quality song literature of lasting value. An exciting mix of songs and recordings supports every type of music-making experience—singing, playing instruments, moving, listening, creating, reading, and notating.

Music that models and instructs

Children's voices provide vocal modeling and adult voices demonstrate style, expression, and cultural authenticity.

- Student soloists
- Student vocal ensembles
- Student choirs
- Adult soloists
- Adult choirs
- Adult vocal ensembles

Music that represents diverse genres and styles

Your students experience, perform, and evaluate the most diverse range of music.

- Folk
- Traditional
- Multicultural
- Popular
- Contemporary
- Patriotic
- Seasonal
- Holiday

Recordings that support music learning

- Listening selections
- Dances
- Instrumental sound banks
- Montages
- Recorded poems and stories
- Recorded interviews
- Recorded assessments

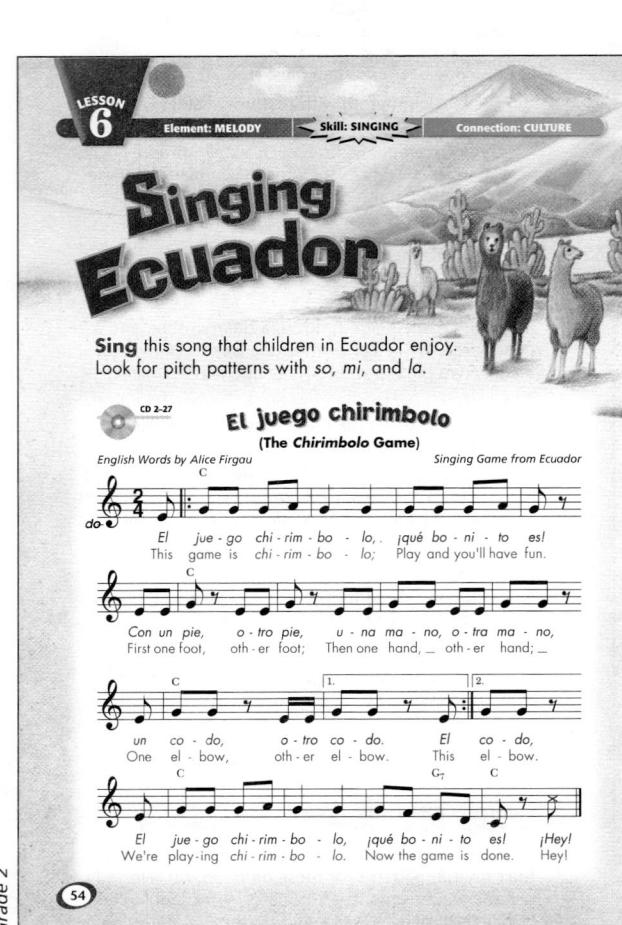

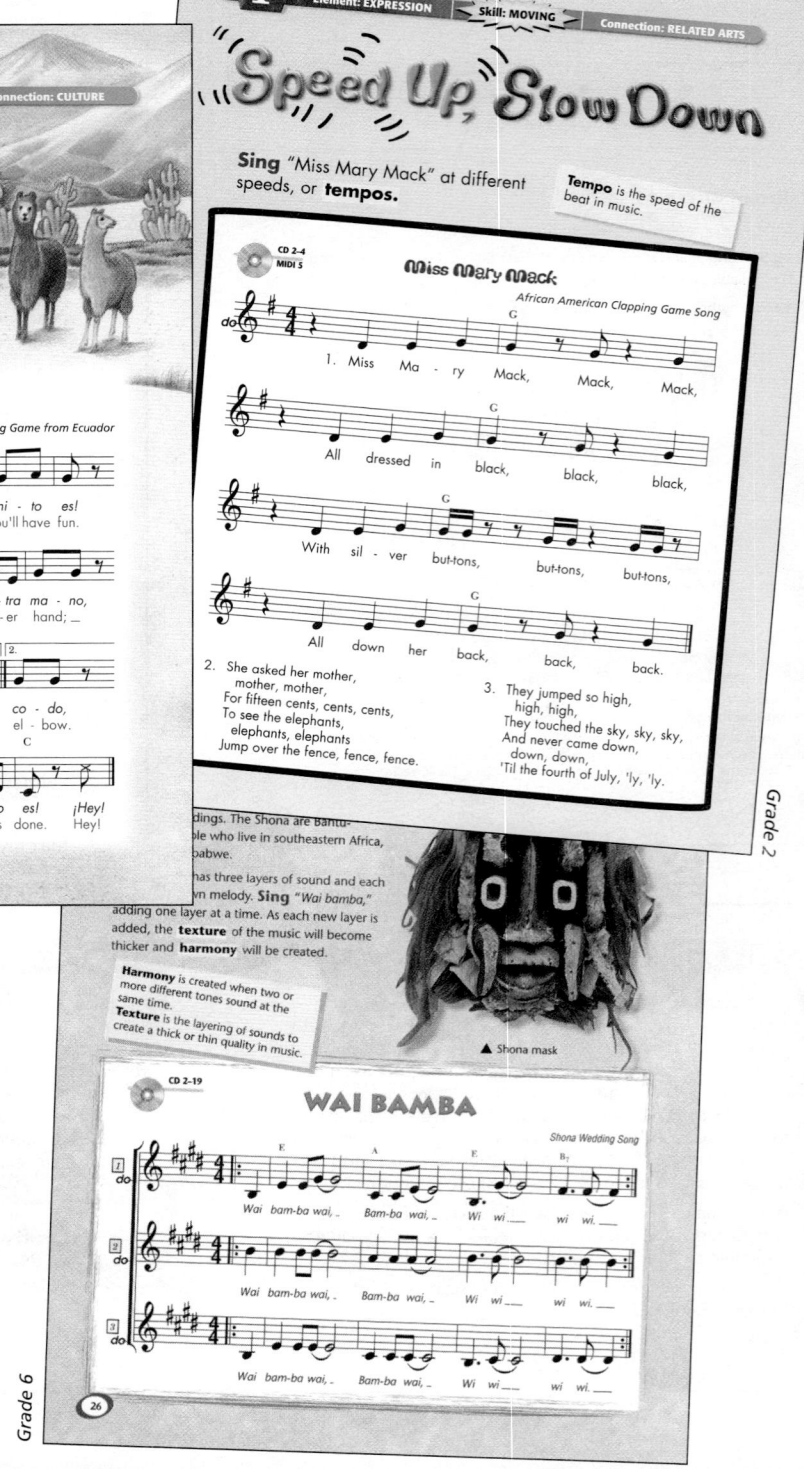

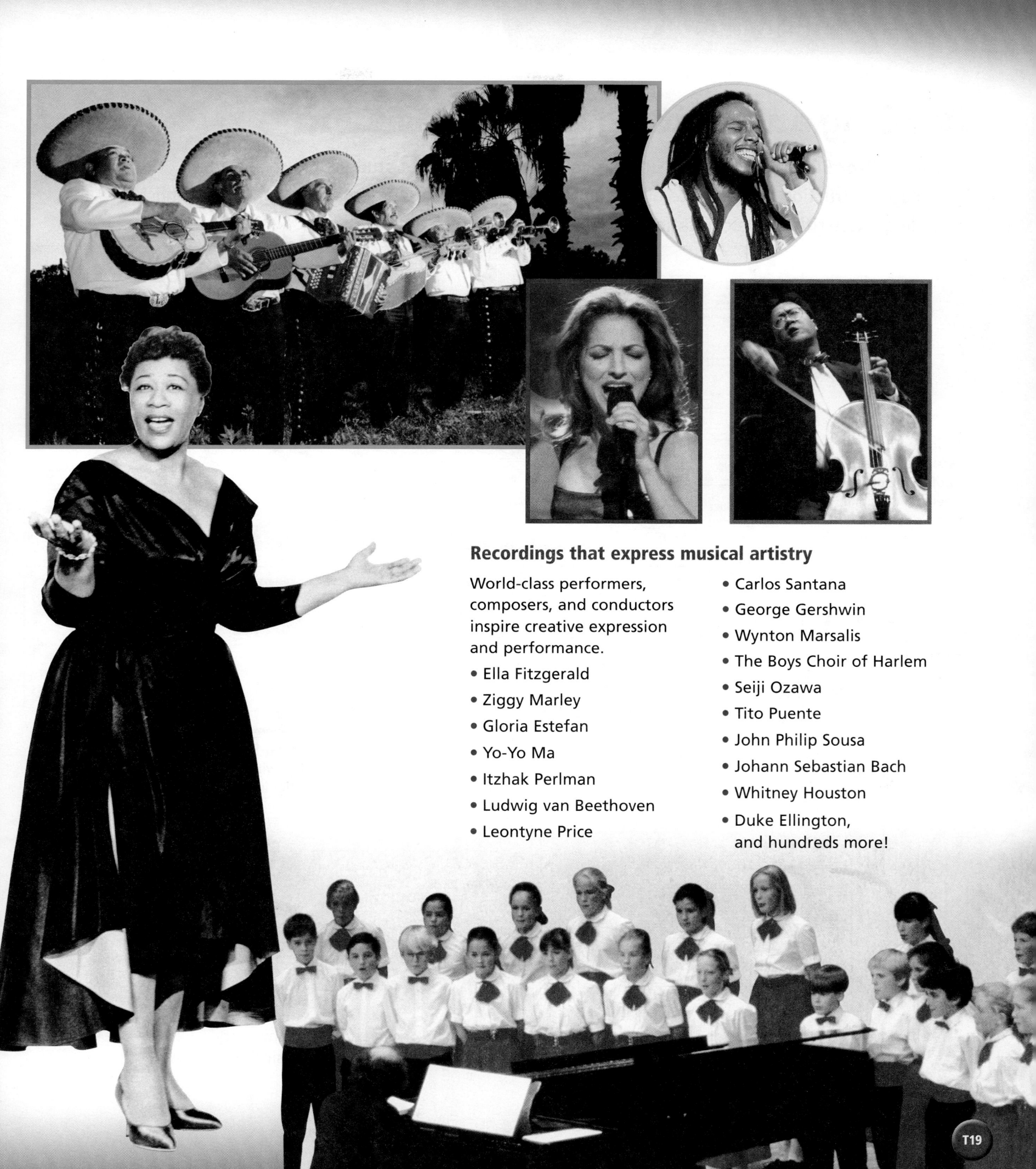

Recordings that express musical artistry

World-class performers, composers, and conductors inspire creative expression and performance.

- Ella Fitzgerald
- Ziggy Marley
- Gloria Estefan
- Yo-Yo Ma
- Itzhak Perlman
- Ludwig van Beethoven
- Leontyne Price
- Carlos Santana
- George Gershwin
- Wynton Marsalis
- The Boys Choir of Harlem
- Seiji Ozawa
- Tito Puente
- John Philip Sousa
- Johann Sebastian Bach
- Whitney Houston
- Duke Ellington, and hundreds more!

Reading and writing music notation

A goal of Silver Burdett MAKING MUSIC is to help you develop your students' music literacy. Systematic instruction and practice opportunities permit all your students to become accomplished at reading and writing music notation.

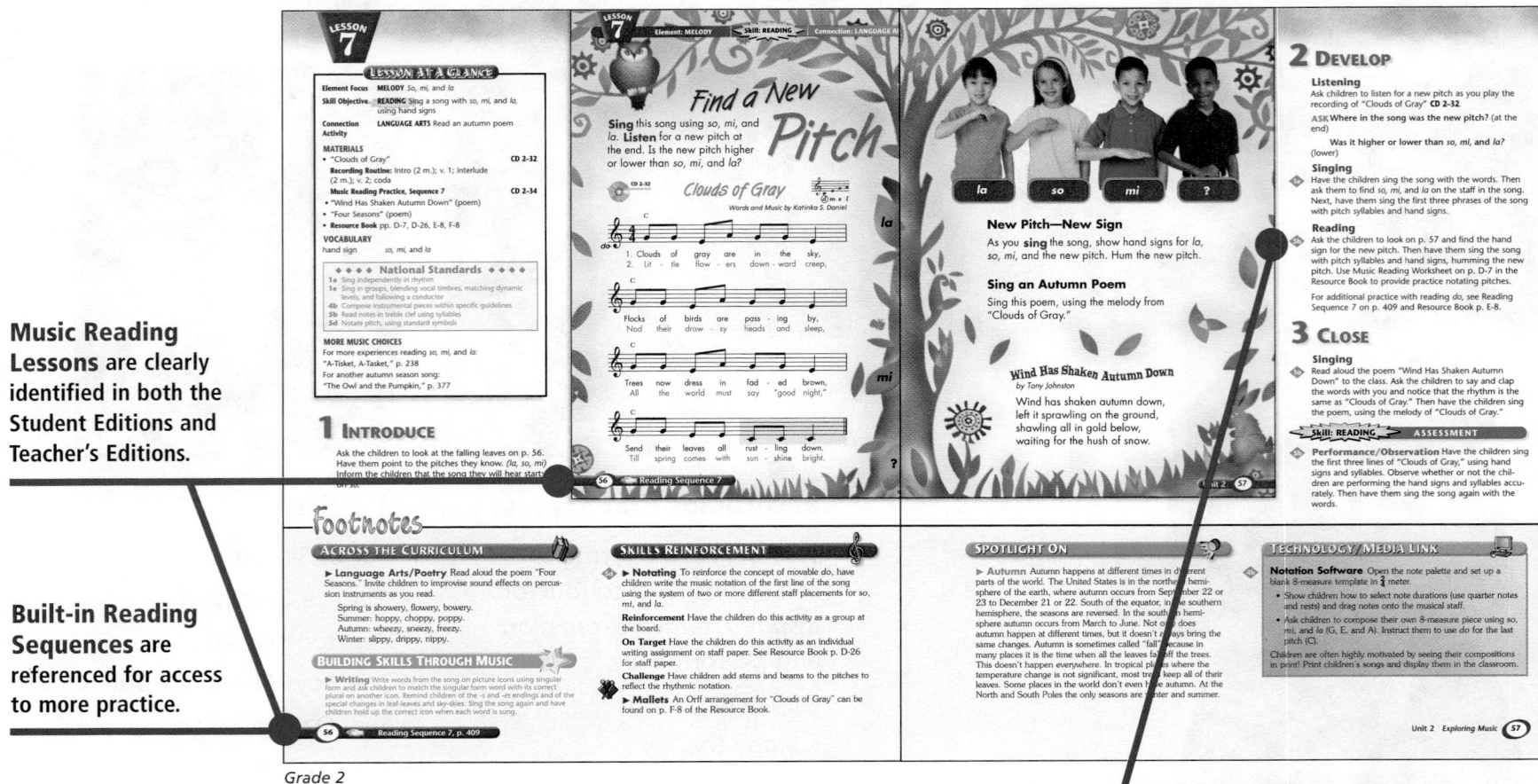

Music Reading Lessons are clearly identified in both the Student Editions and Teacher's Editions.

Built-in Reading Sequences are referenced for access to more practice.

Grade 2

Instructional Strategies for Reading Music align with National Standards to meet your specific curricular goals.

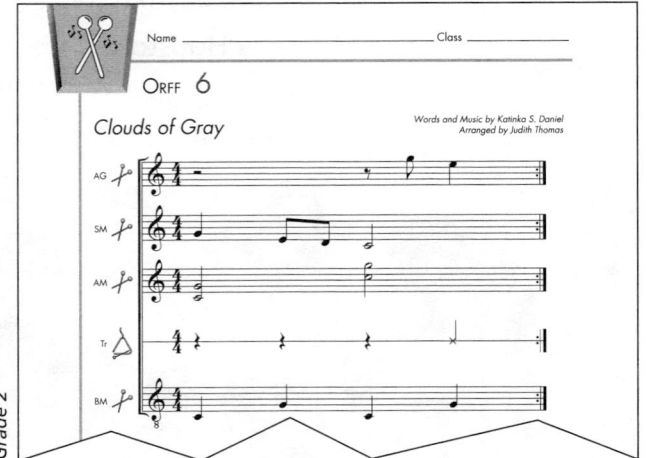

Orff Accompaniments add enrichment to many reading lessons.

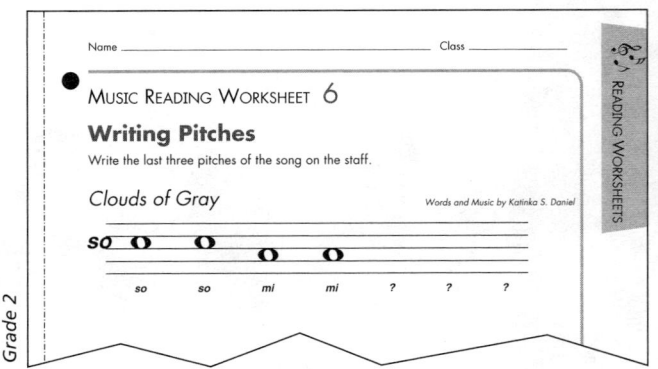

Music Reading Worksheets accompany every lesson to reinforce and extend music literacy.

Music Reading Practice Section reinforces melodic and rhythmic literacy. The section contains 24 Reading Sequences at each grade level for ample practice.

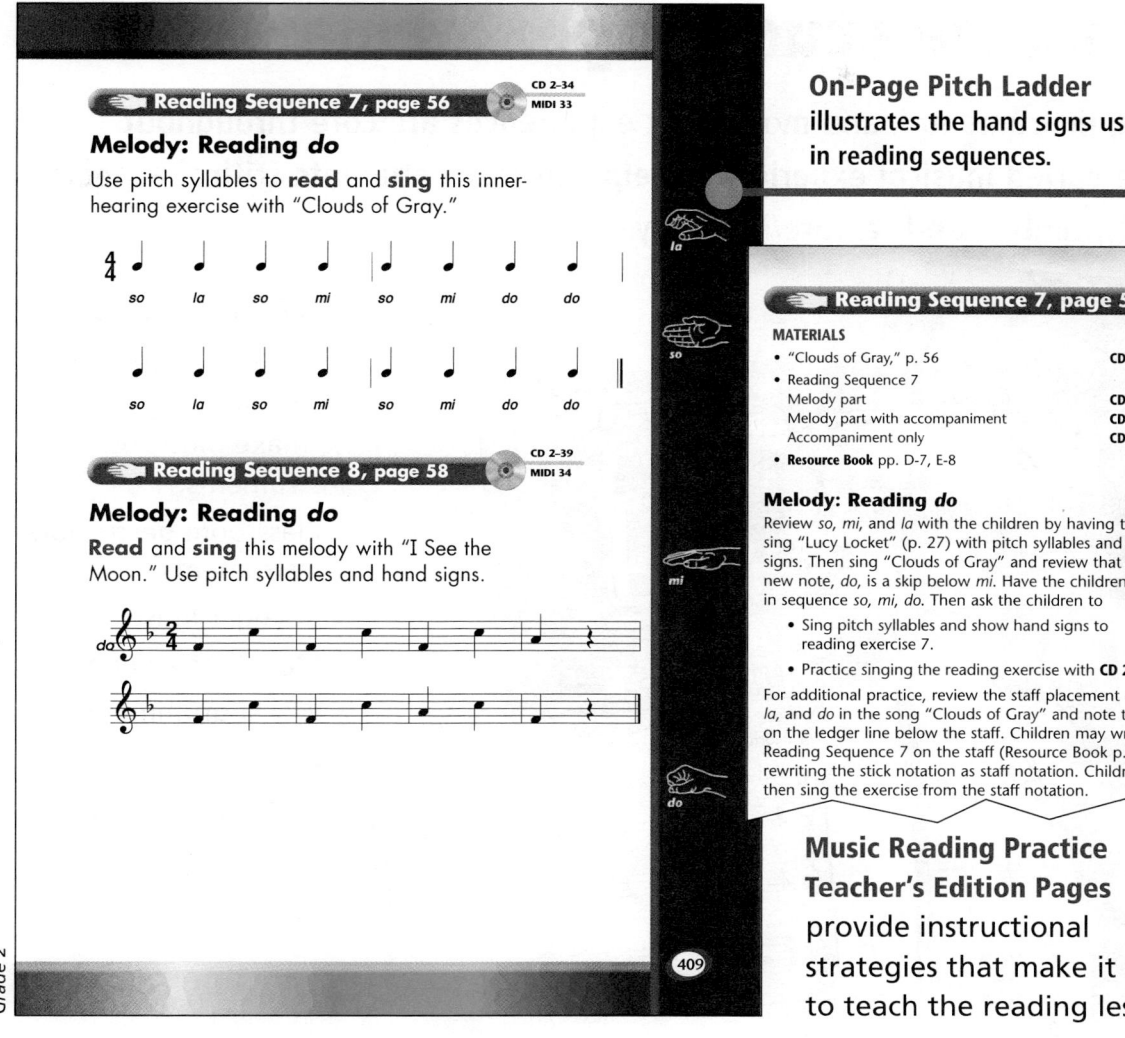

On-Page Pitch Ladder illustrates the hand signs used in reading sequences.

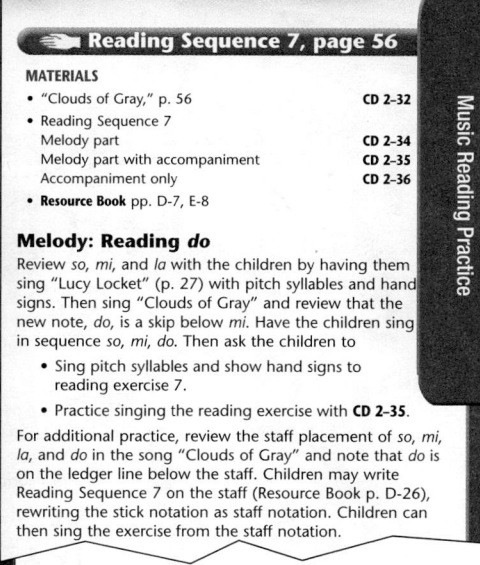

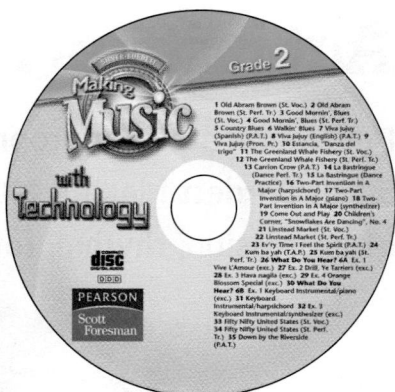

MIDI Tracks are provided for every Reading Sequence, allowing your students to practice individual parts at various tempos and keys.

Music Reading Practice Teacher's Edition Pages provide instructional strategies that make it easy to teach the reading lessons.

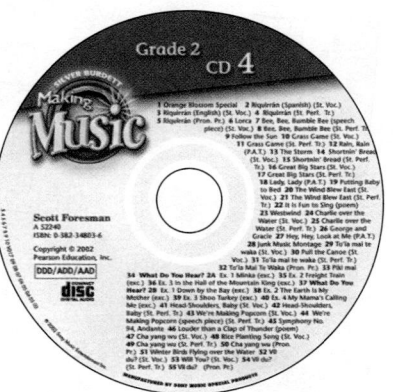

Audio CDs include both individual vocal and instrumental parts, as well as accompaniment tracks for each Reading Sequence.

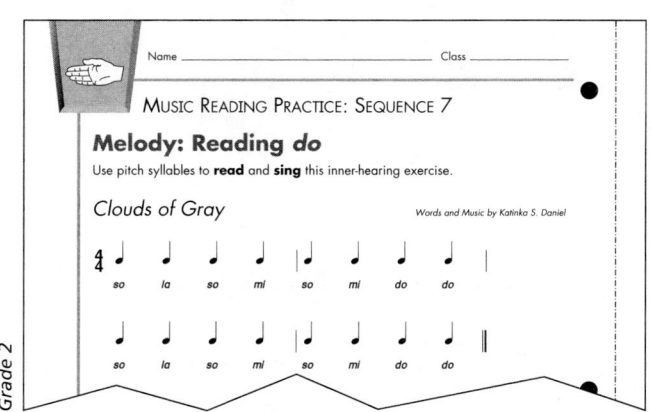

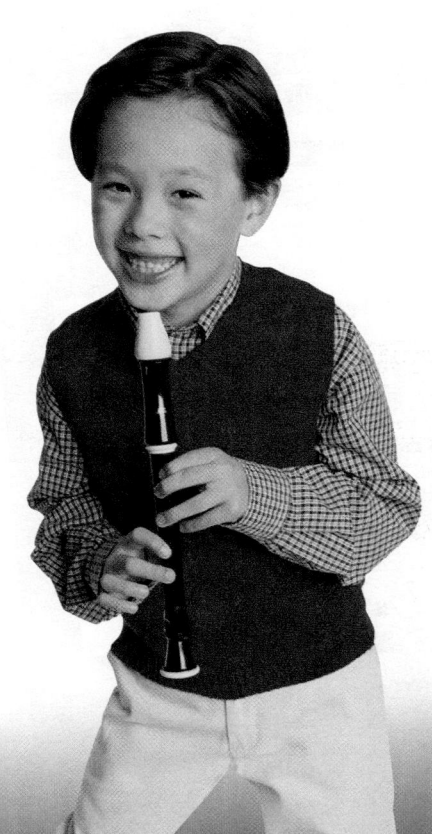

Music Reading Practice Worksheets support each Reading Sequence. Use the worksheets to create overhead transparencies for group instruction.

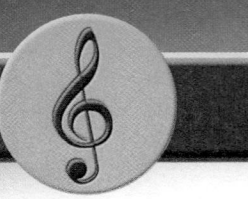

Activities for creative student performances

Developmentally appropriate vocal, instrumental, and movement experiences are core throughout Silver Burdett MAKING MUSIC. These varied musical experiences help you teach students critical aspects of expression, rhythm, form, melody, timbre, and texture/harmony.

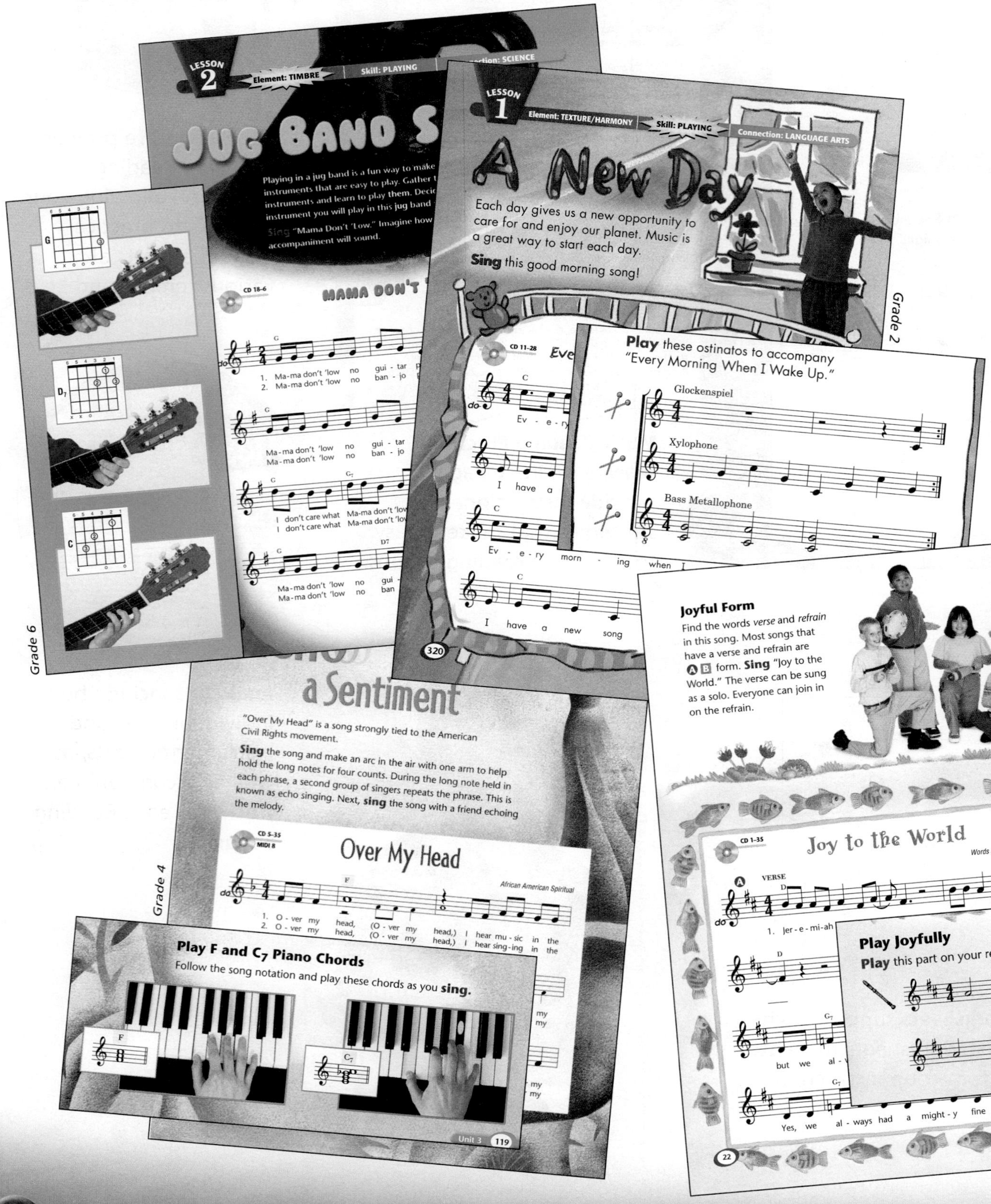

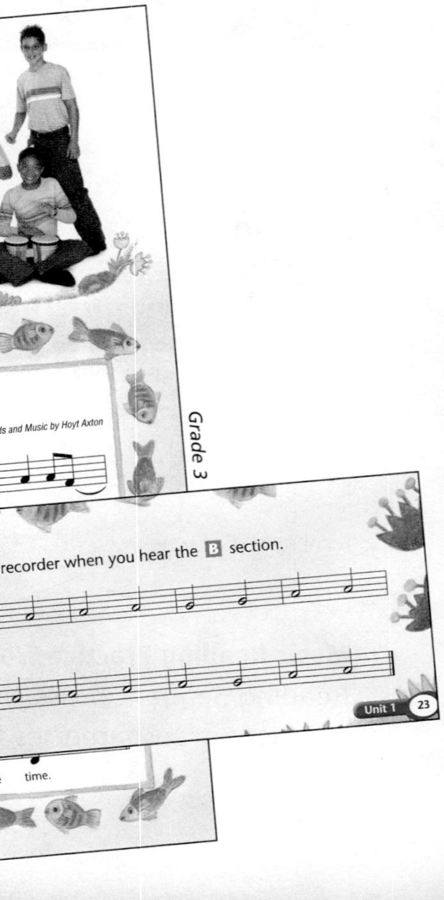

Playing instruments

Frequent opportunities encourage your students to make music using instruments.

- Classroom percussion instruments
- Keyboard instruments
- Mallet instruments
- World drumming
- Recorder (3–6)
- Guitar (4–6)

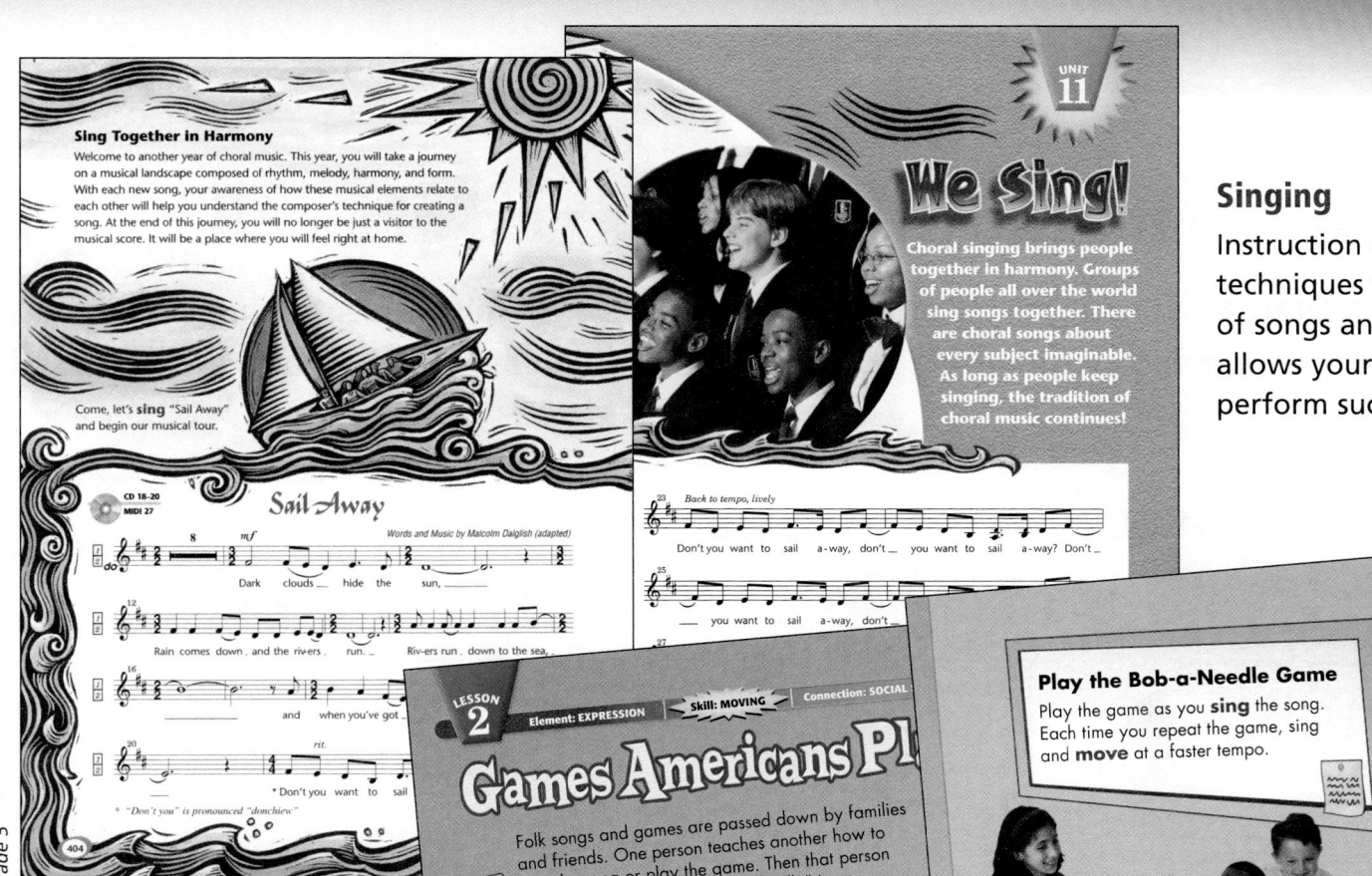

Singing

Instruction on good singing techniques through a variety of songs and choral literature allows your students to perform successfully.

Moving

A wide variety of movement activities helps you teach rhythmic patterns and develop students' creative expression.

- Body percussion
- Conducting
- Creative and interpretive movement
- Dramatizing/pantomimes
- Finger plays
- Folk and patterned dances
- Game songs (singing and rhythm games)
- Hand jives
- Locomotor movements
- Nonlocomotor movements
- Play-parties
- Popular dance
- Signing

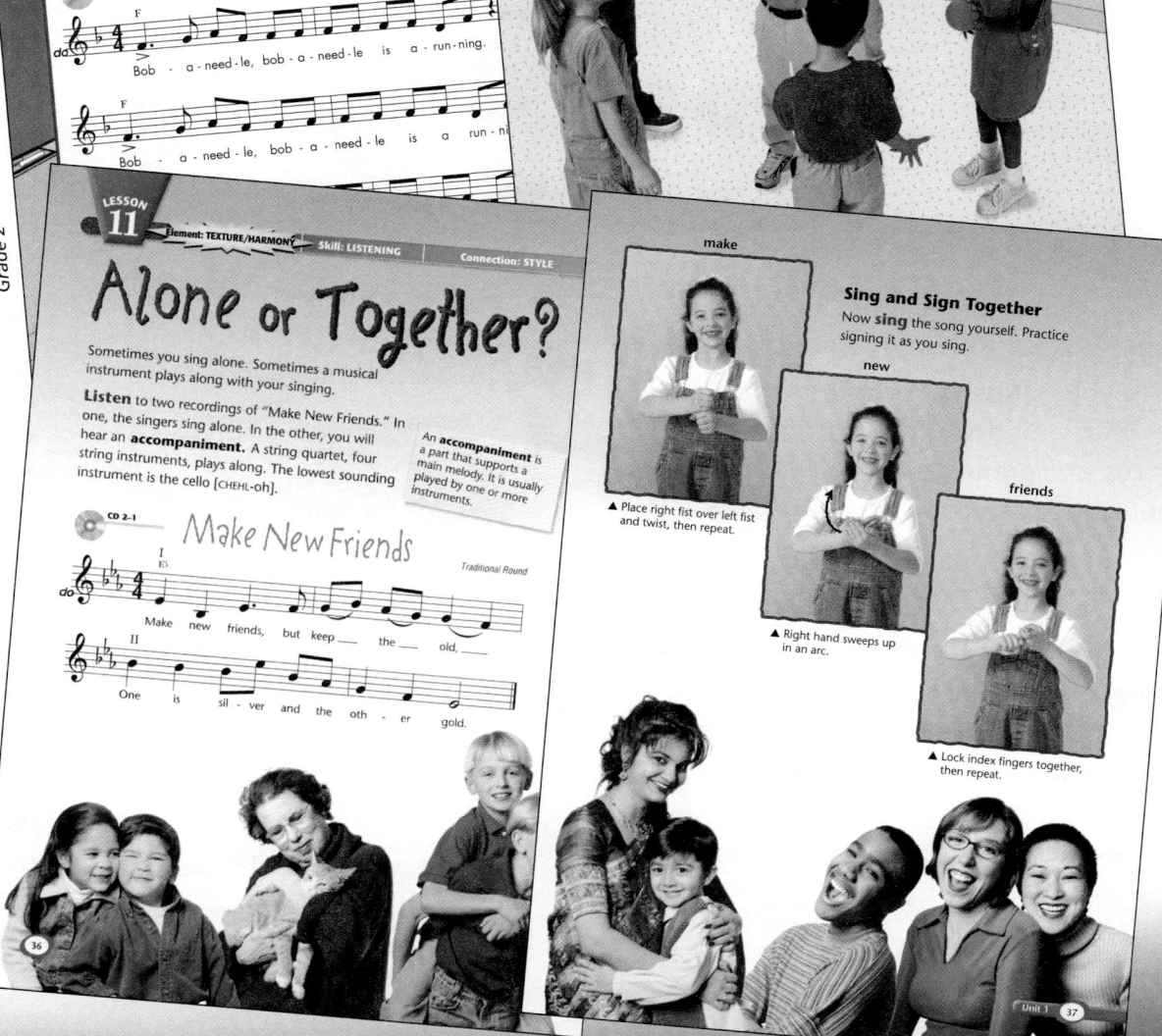

Assessment to monitor learning and growth

Silver Burdett MAKING MUSIC provides a variety of tools to help you assess your students' music knowledge and skills. Choose from performance, written, and oral assessments according to your specific teaching style and instructional needs.

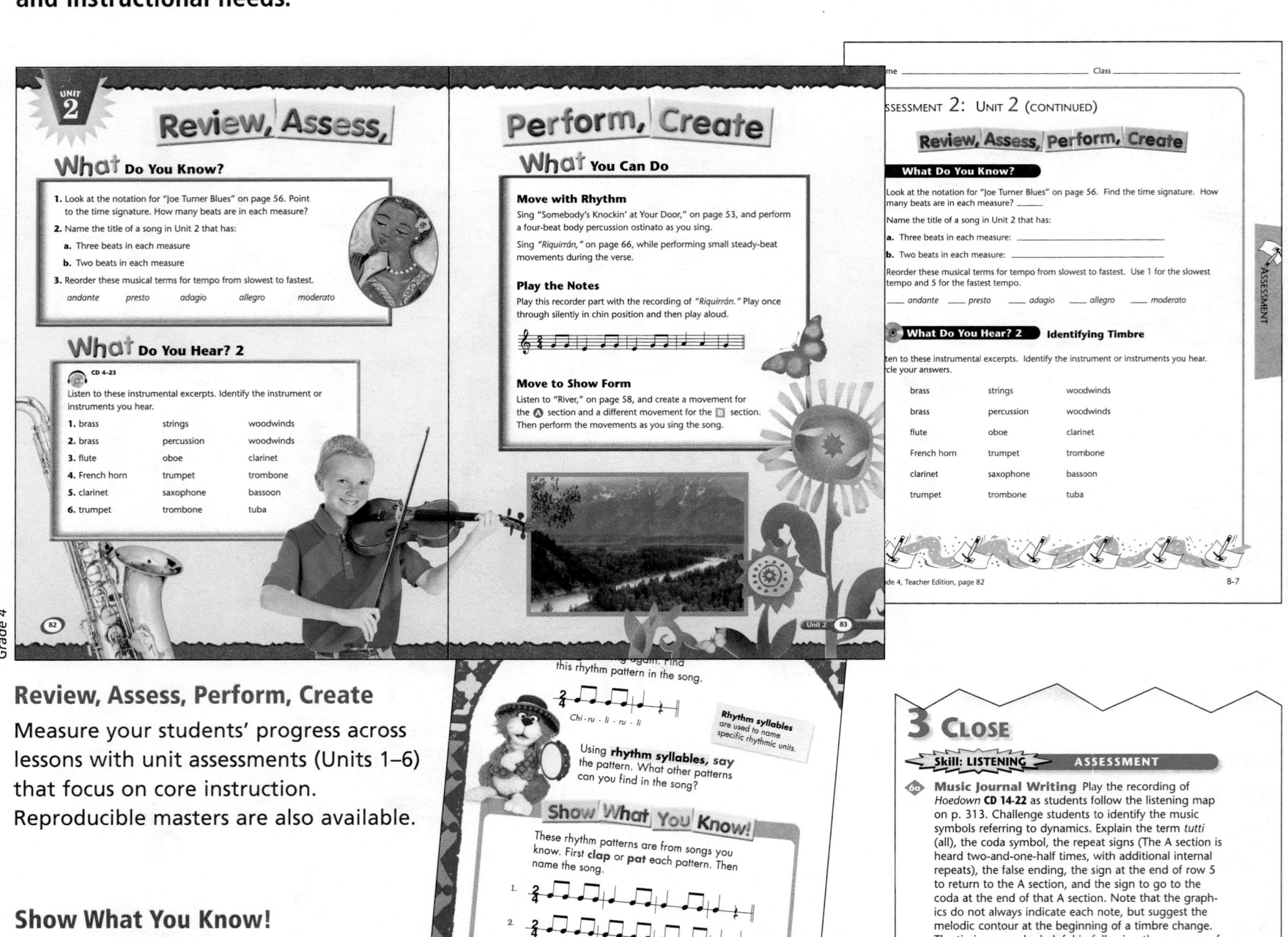

Review, Assess, Perform, Create

Measure your students' progress across lessons with unit assessments (Units 1–6) that focus on core instruction. Reproducible masters are also available.

Show What You Know!

Assessments take place midway through each unit (Units 1–6) to gauge your students' melodic and rhythmic skills. Reproducible masters are also available.

End-of-Lesson Assessment

Every lesson is designed to assess your students' understanding of a critical music element, skill, or connection.

National Standards Correlation for easy planning

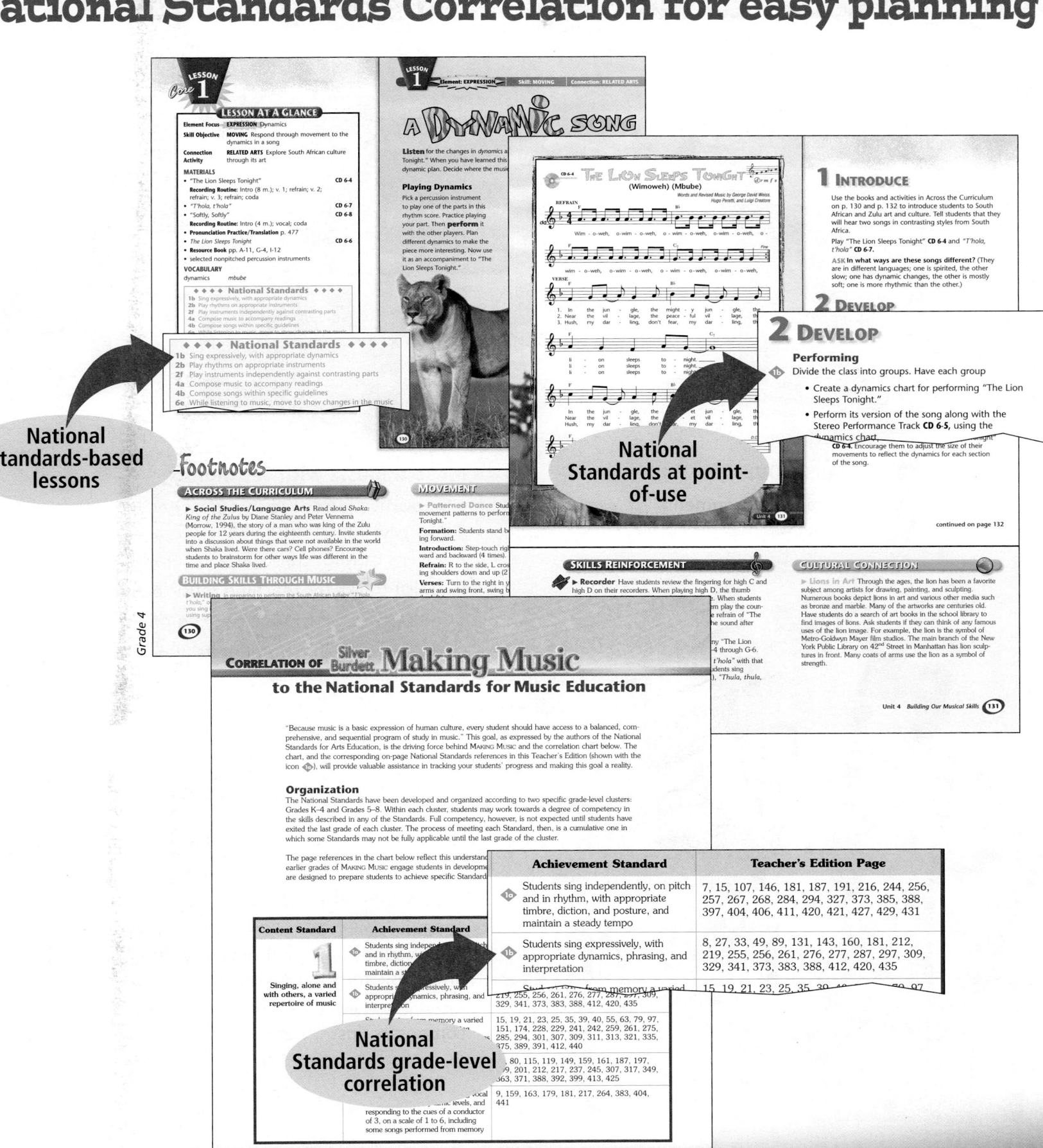

National Standards-based lessons

National Standards at point-of-use

National Standards grade-level correlation

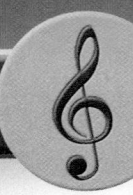

Dynamic tools to motivate and engage students

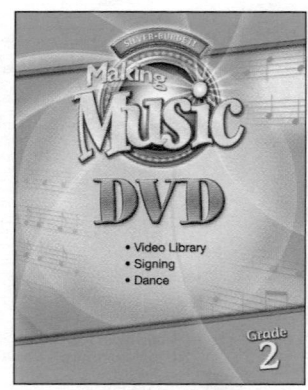

MAKING MUSIC DVD

- Instructional video segments
- Signing activities
- Dances

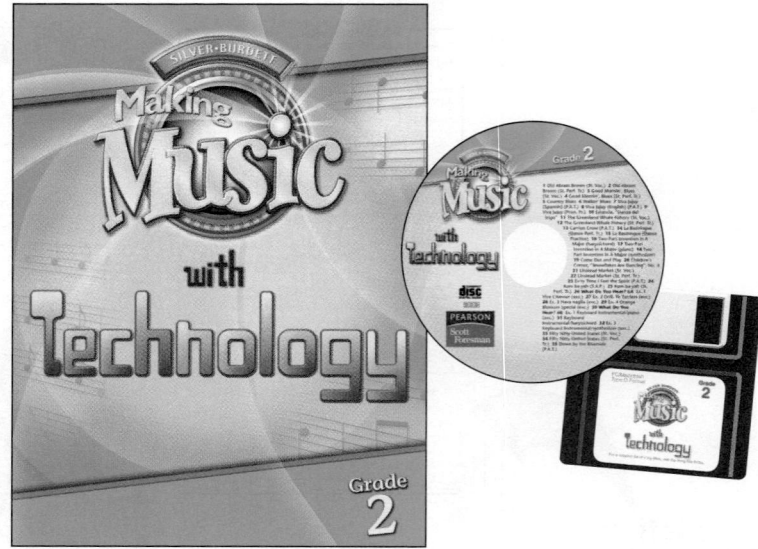

MAKING MUSIC with Technology

- Innovative lessons to integrate technology into your music curriculum
- Dozens of MIDI tracks at each grade level
  - MIDI tracks for teaching music elements
  - MIDI tracks for music reading practice
  - MIDI tracks for choral units (4–6)

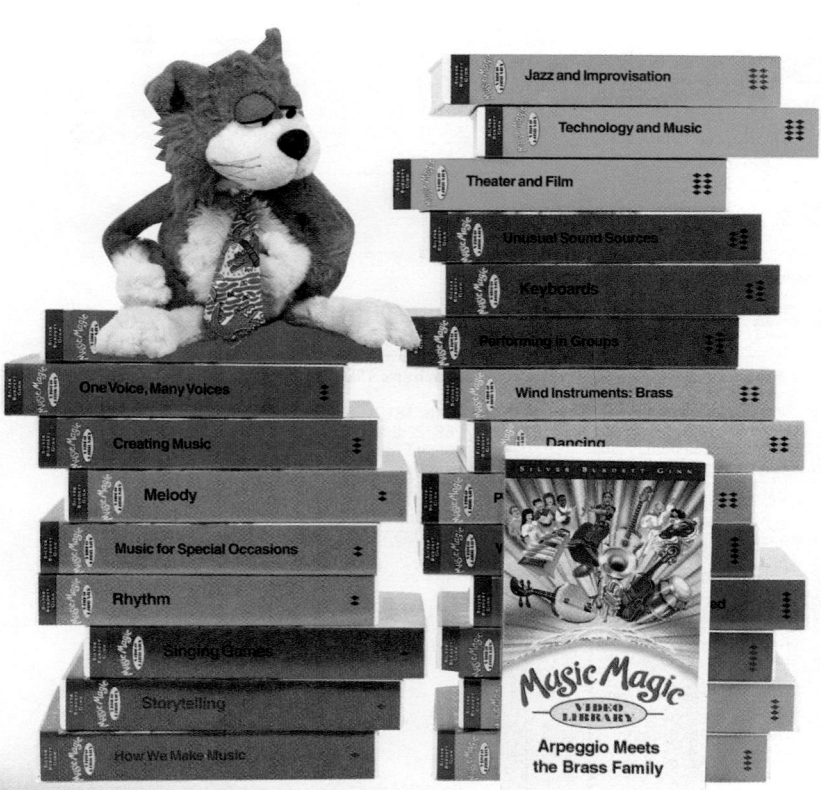

Music Magic Video Library

- Versatile collection of 25 videos on topics ranging from melody and rhythm to keyboards, dancing, and music for special occasions
- Interviews with world-leading musicians, composers, instrument makers, and dancers

An online work center that revolutionizes teaching

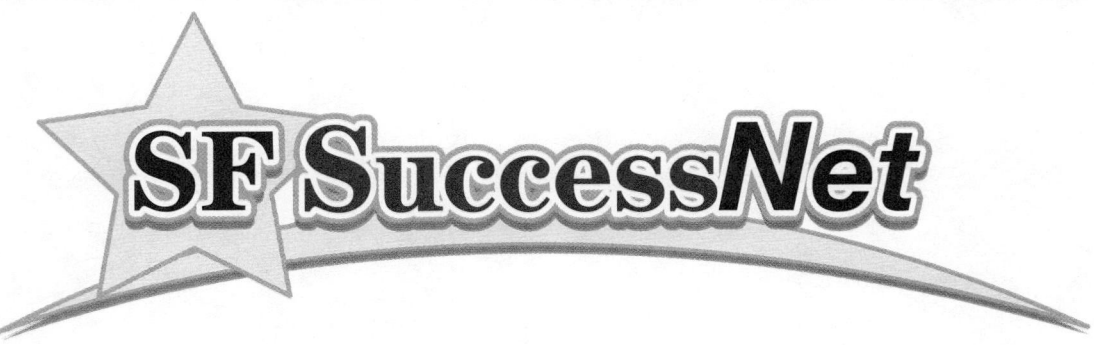

Online Lesson Planner and Teacher's Edition

Scott Foresman SuccessNet is a next-generation work center for Silver Burdett MAKING MUSIC teachers. It's a place where teachers can go to plan their lessons, streamline their work, and access standards-based instruction.

- Access instructional notes
- Create custom lesson plans
- Schedule lessons
- Organize resources
- Block out holidays
- Assign dates and times
- Save/edit lessons from year to year
- Print day, week, or monthly views

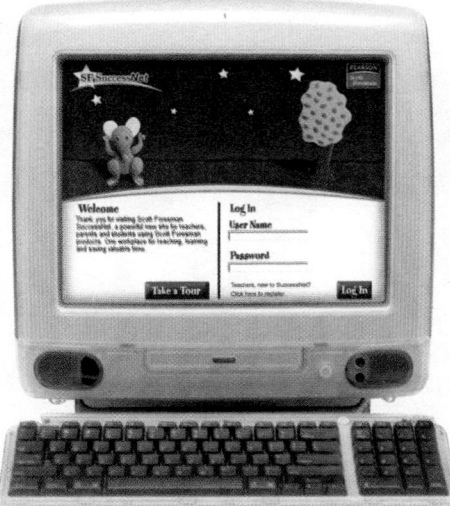

Online Resources for Teachers and Students

Take It to the NET at *www.sfsuccessnet.com* provides access to an entire collection of music resources.

- Theme musicals
- Grades K–8 index of all songs, listening selections, and more
- Standards-based practice
- Music reference articles
- Adaptations for meeting individual needs
- Rubrics—plus more!

Register Today!

To access Take It to the NET, follow three simple steps.

1. Go to *www.sfsuccessnet.com*
2. Click on the link to register
3. Enter the code **MakingMusic** (no spaces)

Note: You must register your students for **Take It to the NET** to access music reference articles.

T27b

Contents
Steps to Making Music

= Core Lesson
= Music Reading Lesson

Unit 3   Learning the Language of Music

Unit 4   Building Our Musical Skills

= **Core Lesson**

= **Music Reading Lesson**

= Core Lesson

= Music Reading Lesson

Paths to Making Music

Unit 7 Making America's Music

Unit 8 Say It with Drums

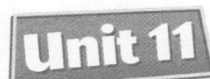

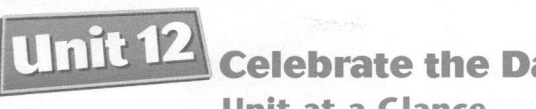

Unit 12 Celebrate the Day

Music Resources and Indexes

T33a

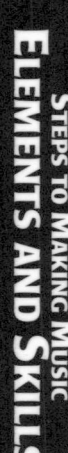

STEPS TO MAKING MUSIC
ELEMENTS AND SKILLS

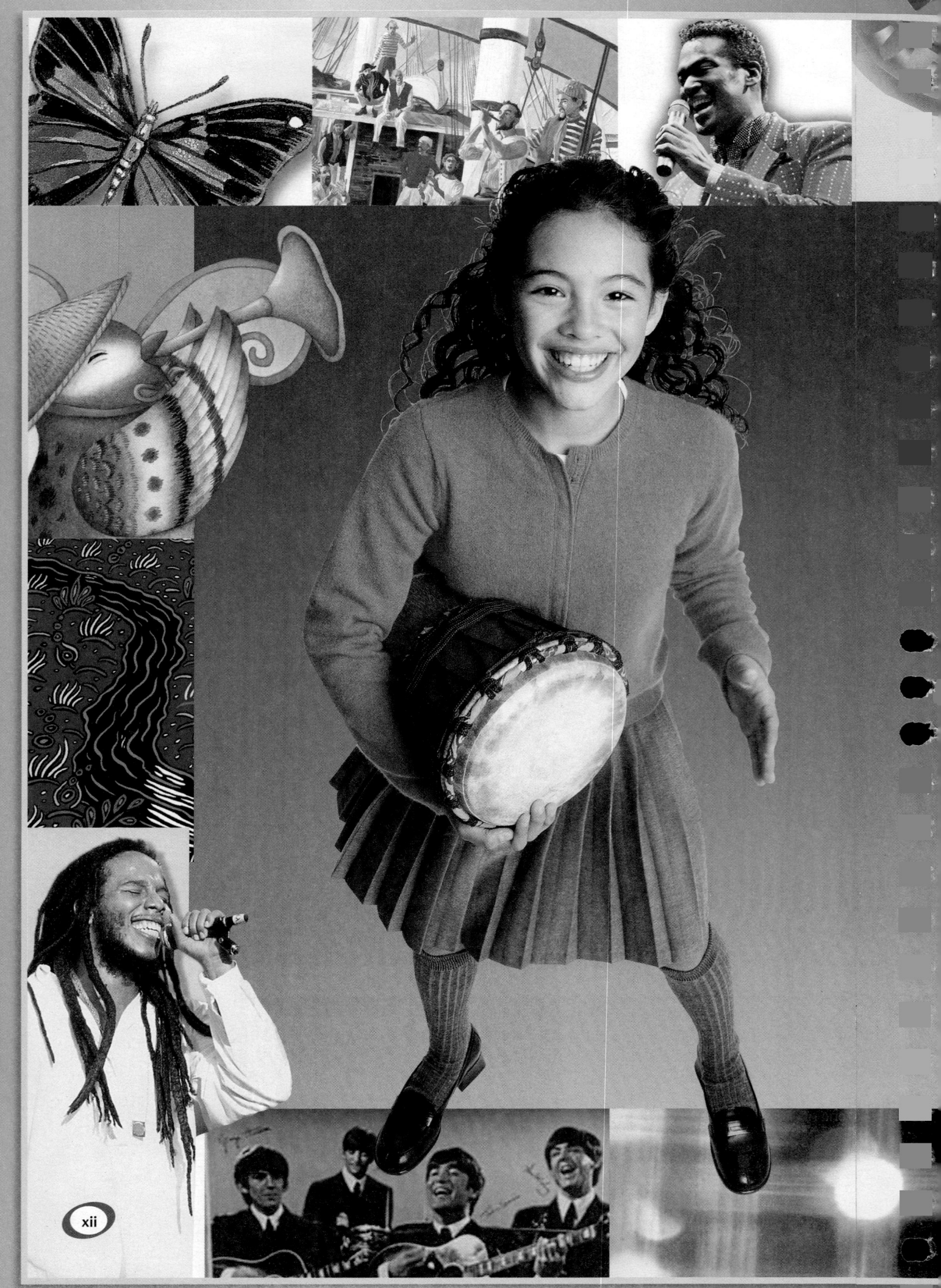

PATHS TO MAKING MUSIC

THEME-BASED LESSONS

221b

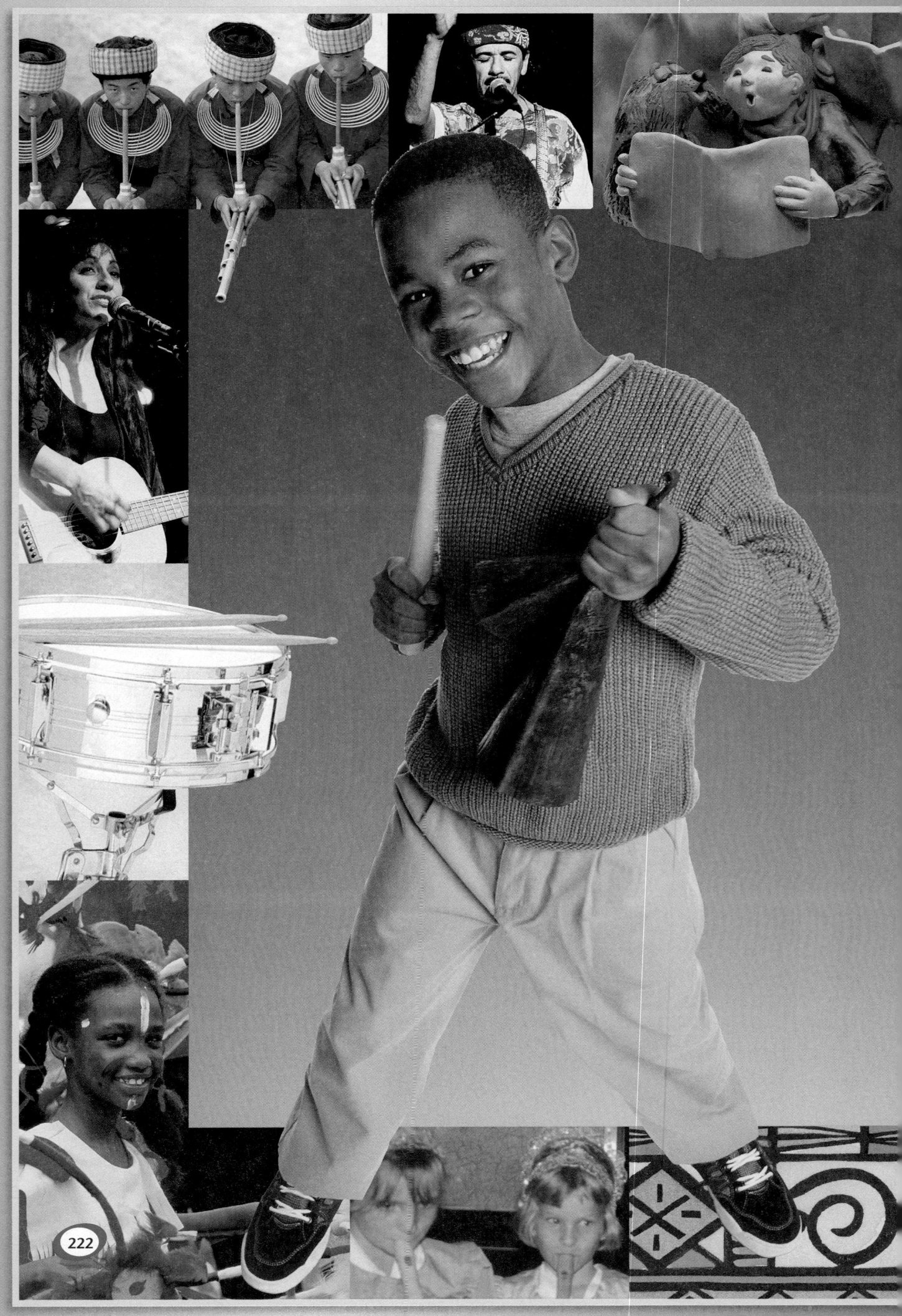

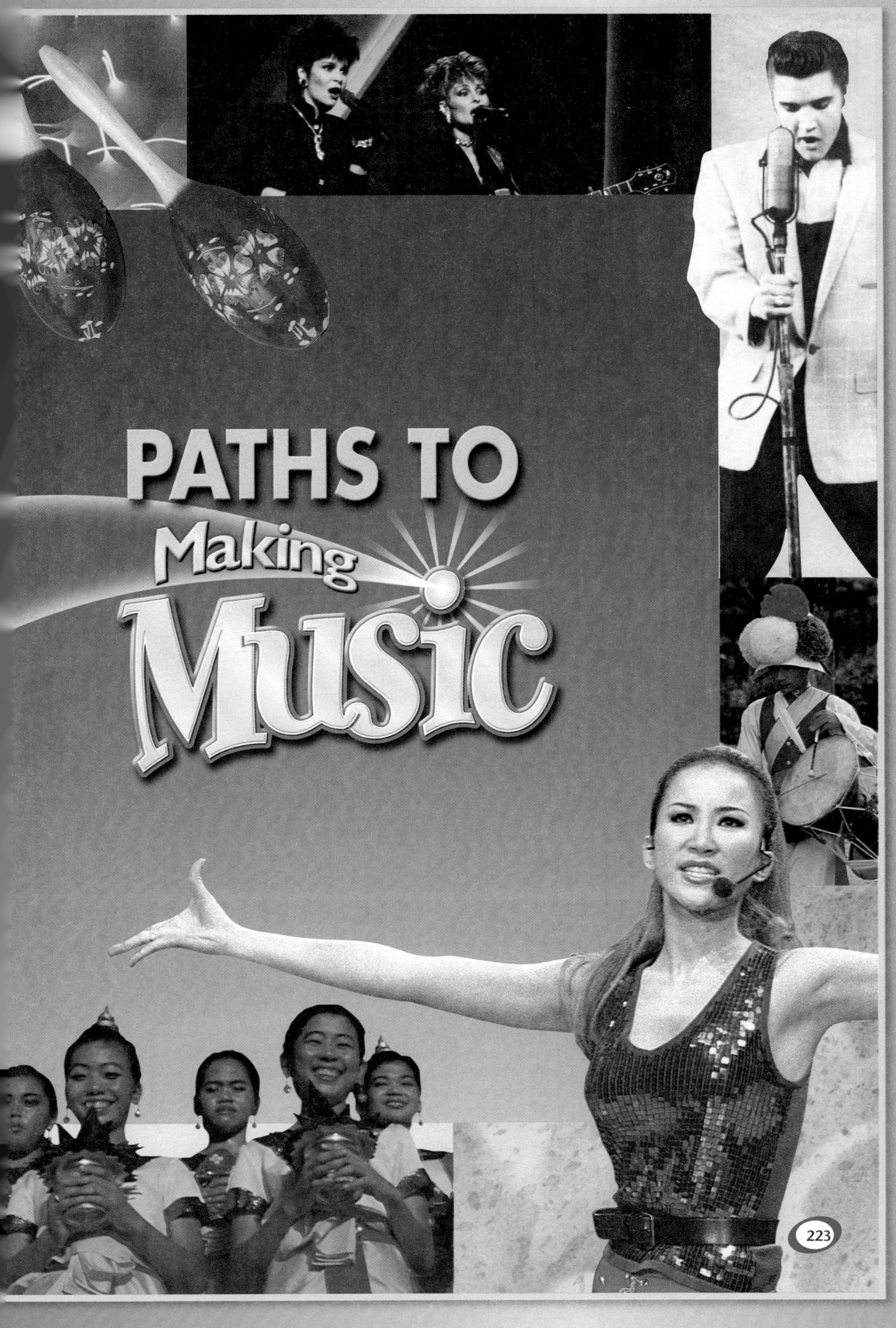

PATHS TO Making Music

Lesson	Elements	Skills

LESSON 1

A New World

pp. 228–231

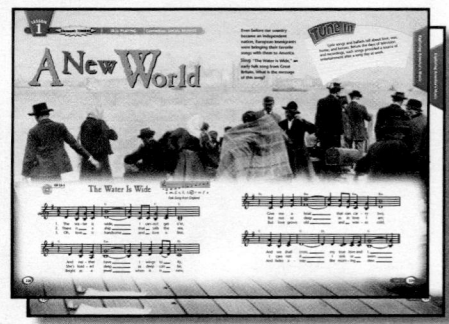

Element: Timbre
Concept: Instrumental
Focus: Percussion sounds from West Africa

Secondary Element
Texture/Harmony: harmony in sixths

National Standards
1d   2c   4b   4c   6b   8b   9b

Skill: Playing
Objective: Play rhythm patterns to accompany a song from West Africa

Secondary Skills
- **Reading** Read pitch syllables
- **Singing** Sing two-part harmony
- **Playing** Play call-and-response rhythm patterns; play West African rhythm ensemble accompaniment

SKILLS REINFORCEMENT
- **Creating** Create a vocal descant
- **Guitar** Play a finger-style guitar accompaniment
- **Mallets** Learn an Orff accompaniment

LESSON 2

Spiritual and Gospel

pp. 232–235

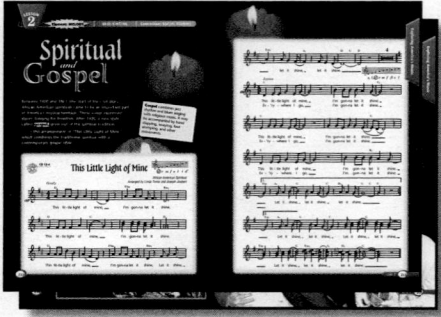

Element: Melody
Concept: Pitch and direction
Focus: Melodic contour

Secondary Element
Expression: dynamics, style, and tempo

National Standards
1c   2d   3b   6a   6b   8b   9c

Skill: Singing
Objective: Perform a traditional spiritual in contemporary gospel style

Secondary Skills
- **Listening** Listen to a spiritual; listen to a gospel choir sing a spiritual
- **Analyzing** Discuss musical elements that can change style
- **Creating** Create new lyrics for a spiritual

SKILLS REINFORCEMENT
- **Guitar** Play a guitar accompaniment to a spiritual
- **Recorder** Learn a recorder descant for a song

LESSON 3

Timbre on the Move

pp. 236–239

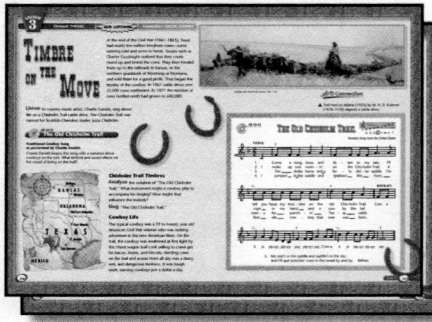

Element: Timbre
Concept: Instrumental
Focus: Cowboy music

Secondary Element
Instrument timbres associated with cowboy music

National Standards
1c   2a   2d   6b   8a   8b

Skill: Listening
Objective: Identify and discern the timbres of instruments in cowboy ballads and dance tunes

Secondary Skills
- **Analyzing** Familiarize students with the region in which cowboys worked
- **Listening** Allow students to hear the different timbres of cowboy instruments
- **Playing** Play a simple accompaniment on guitar

SKILLS REINFORCEMENT
- **Listening** Listen to country music and identify different types of guitars
- **Using a Guitar Capo** Learn the purpose of and how to use a capo

Connections

Music and Other Literature

Connection: Social Studies
Activity: Explore the influence of immigrants from Europe and West Africa

- **TEACHER TO TEACHER** **Bulletin Board Idea** Create a bulletin board on the influence of immigrants on American music
- **CULTURAL CONNECTION** **Ellis Island** Facts on Ellis Island and immigration
- **SPOTLIGHT ON**
  The English Ballad Ballads from England
  Nigeria Facts on the country
  JuJu Style Musical style from West Africa
- **ACROSS THE CURRICULUM** **Social Studies** Read about an immigrant's migration to the United States
- **BUILDING SKILLS THROUGH MUSIC** **Language** Identify emotion in lyrics

Songs
"The Water Is Wide"
"Ise oluwa"

More Music Choices:
"Scarborough Fair," p. 95
"Take Time in Life," p. 292

ASSESSMENT
Performance/Music Journal Writing Play a rhythm pattern to accompany a song from West Africa and write timbre descriptions of African drum accompaniment

TECHNOLOGY/MEDIA LINK
Web Site Learn more about African drumming and vocal styles

Connection: Social Studies
Activity: Discuss the historical roots of the spiritual and gospel musical traditions

- **CULTURAL CONNECTION**
  Freedom Songs Song about freedom from slavery
  Gospel Music Gospel's beginnings in the 1920s
- **ACROSS THE CURRICULUM**
  Language Arts Share a book on early African Americans
  Social Studies Read about the beginnings of the Fisk Jubilee Singers
- **CHARACTER EDUCATION** **Caring** Find inspiration through spirituals
- **SPOTLIGHT ON**
  African American Spirituals Early History of spirituals
  The Golden Gate Quartet Facts on how this quartet started
- **SCHOOL TO HOME CONNECTION** **Gospel Scrapbook** Locate local gospel choirs and ask members about their favorite spirituals
- **BUILDING SKILLS THROUGH MUSIC** **Social Studies** Show the development of musical styles through history

Song "This Little Light of Mine"

Listening Selections
The Battle of Jericho
Swing Low, Sweet Chariot
Jonah
M·U·S·I·C M·A·K·E·R·S
The Fisk Jubilee Singers
The Golden Gate Quartet

More Music Choices
"Ain't Gonna Let Nobody Turn Me 'Round," p. 85
"Glory, Glory, Hallelujah," p. 52
"Peace Like a River," p. 190

ASSESSMENT
Performance/Interview Sing new melodies and lyrics for "This Little Light of Mine"

TECHNOLOGY/MEDIA LINK
Video Library View video on solo and choral gospel singing

Connection: Social Studies
Activity: Learn about the historical heyday of the cowboys that followed the Civil War

- **CULTURAL CONNECTION** **Singing Movie Cowboys** Find out about about singing cowboy actors
- **ACROSS THE CURRICULUM**
  Social Studies Learn more about cowboys
  Visual Arts Discover young western artists
- **SPOTLIGHT ON**
  Cowboy Instruments Learn about instruments cowboys played
  Lawrence "Larry" Chittenden Facts about the poet-rancher
- **BUILDING SKILLS THROUGH MUSIC** **Reading** Identify what lyrics describe

Songs
"The Old Chisholm Trail"
"Cowboys' Chrstmas Ball"

Listening Selections
The Old Chisholm Trail
Cowboys' Christmas Ball

More Music Choices
"Bury Me Not on the Lone Prairie," p. 19
"El payo," p. 145

ASSESSMENT
Observation Find other recordings of, and identify instruments featured in cowboy songs

TECHNOLOGY/MEDIA LINK
Electronic Keyboard Explore electronic keyboard sounds for a cowboy song

Lesson	Elements	Skills	

LESSON 4 — The Blues Feeling
pp. 240–243

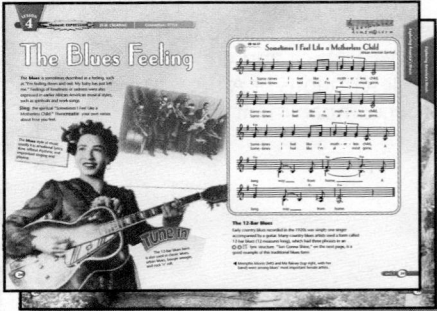

Element: Expression
Concept: Tempo
Focus: Blues style

Secondary Element
Form: aab

National Standards
1b 1d 2a 2d 4a 6b 9a

Skill: Creating
Objective: Create new verses for a blues song

Secondary Skills
- **Singing** Sing two songs in the blues style
- **Creating** Create new song lyrics
- **Moving** Perform and create movements to reflect lyrics
- **Analyzing** Discuss the rhyme scheme of song
- **Reading** Read the notation of a blues song
- **Playing** Play various instrumental accompaniments to blues songs

SKILLS REINFORCEMENT
- **Keyboard** Play broken chords as accompaniment
- **Recorder** Play the stylized recorder part
- **Creating** Create 12-bar blues lyrics
- **Guitar** Use rhythm-and-blues strumming
- **Singing** Sing a blues song

LESSON 5 — You "Got Country"
pp. 244–249

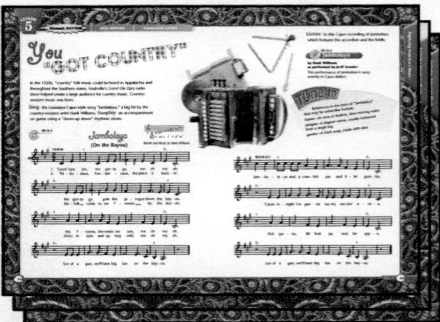

Element: Rhythm
Concept: Pattern
Focus: Quarter-note/eighth-note pattern

Secondary Element
Form: verse-refrain form

National Standards
1c 5a 6b 8b 9a

Skill: Moving
Objective: Move to the Cajun two-step

Secondary Skills
- **Singing** Sing a Cajun-style song; sing a country and western song; sing a sentimental song
- **Playing** Play accompaniment on various instruments to Cajun and country and western songs
- **Listening** Listen to instruments in a Cajun band; listen to a melody in a country and western song; listen to a contemporary country group
- **Moving** perform a Cajun two-step

SKILLS REINFORCEMENT
- **Signing** Learn sign language for a song
- **Mallets** Learn an Orff arrangement
- **Recorder** Play a harmonic accompaniment to a Cajun song on the recorder

LESSON 6 — Jazz: Made in America
pp. 250–253

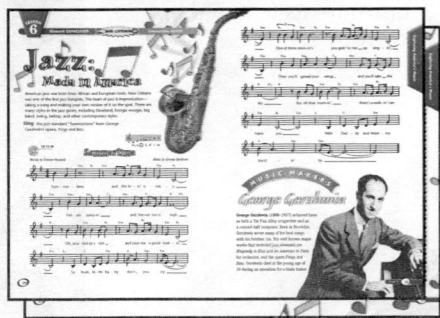

Element: Expression
Concept: Articulation
Focus: Solo improvisation

Secondary Element
Texture/Harmony: major, minor, and seventh chords

National Standards
1c 2c 3b 3c 8a 9b

Skill: Listening
Objective: Listen to and evaluate individual examples of jazz improvisation

Secondary Skills
- **Singing** Sing an American classic with a recording or accompaniment
- **Playing** Play and improvise on the E-minor pentatonic scale
- **Listening** Listen to a recording of a blues legend's version of an American classic

SKILLS REINFORCEMENT
- **Improvising** Learn about improvisational techniques

Connections

Music and Other Literature

Connection: Style

Activity: Discover how the blues gave voice to the African American experience in the twentieth century

ACROSS THE CURRICULUM **Social Studies** Learn about the origins of African American blues style

CULTURAL CONNECTION **Switching Cultures** Explain that jazz is a cultural performance style and category of music

SPOTLIGHT ON
Country Blues Learn about delta blues
Classic Blues Learn about the blues in the 1920s
Urban Blues Learn about 1950s "R&B"

MOVEMENT **Patterned Dance** Perform a 12-bar blues movement routine

BUILDING SKILLS THROUGH MUSIC **Social Studies** Create a concept map

Songs
"Sometimes I Feel Like a Motherless Child"
"Sun Gonna Shine"
"Key to the Highway"

Listening Selection *Key to the Highway*

More Music Choices
"Birthday," p. 90
"Rock and Roll Is Here to Stay," p. 36
"Worried Man Blues," p. 371

ASSESSMENT

Self-Assessment/Music Journal Writing Create personal renditions of blues songs

TECHNOLOGY/MEDIA LINK

CD-ROM Improvise over a 12-bar-blues background on *Band-in-a-Box*

Connection: Genre

Activity: Explore elements of country and western music

ACROSS THE CURRICULUM
Social Studies Discuss the historical beginnings of country music
Science Learn about the importance of crayfish in New Orleans cooking

SPOTLIGHT ON
Country and Western Geographic regions of country music
The Songwriter Facts about Hank Williams
Non-Traditional Instruments Triangle and washboard accompaniment
Guitars Steel-string and dreadnought guitars

CULTURAL CONNECTION
Glossary for "Jambalaya" Learn various Cajun terms
Cajuns of Louisiana Facts on Cajun culture

MEETING INDIVIDUAL NEEDS
Learning Foreign Terms Useful aids to learning terms
Including Everyone Use singing and playing activities for students

BUILDING SKILLS THROUGH MUSIC **Writing** Write a short story

Songs
"Jambalaya"
"You Are My Sunshine"
"Green, Green Grass of Home"

Listening Selection
Jambalaya
You Are My Sunshine
Don't Look Down
M·U·S·I·C M·A·K·E·R·S
Sweethearts of the Rodeo

More Music Choices
"Bury Me Not on the Lone Prairie," p. 19
"Down in the Valley," p. 375
"Red River Valley," p. 11

ASSESSMENT

Performance/Observation Observe students' mastery of Cajun rhythms

TECHNOLOGY/MEDIA LINK

Video Library Show a video featuring country singer Pam Tillis

---

Connection: Genre

Activity: Understand jazz as an expression of an era, as well as a musical style

MOVEMENT **Creative Movement** Use movement to illustrate abstract ideas

SPOTLIGHT ON
The Opera About *Porgy and Bess*
The Performer About Miles Davis

ACROSS THE CURRICULUM **Language Arts** Research jazz artists and create a bulletin board with their

MEETING INDIVIDUAL NEEDS **English Language Learners** Teach English words in a game of charades

TEACHER TO TEACHER **Classroom Management** Provide clear guidelines for students to know what is expected of them

BUILDING SKILLS THROUGH MUSIC **Language** Discuss metaphors

Song "Summertime"

Listening Selection *Summertime*
M·U·S·I·C M·A·K·E·R·S
George Gershwin

More Music Choices
"Hit Me with a Hot Note and Watch Me Bounce," p. 112
"I Got Rhythm," p. 101
"Scattin' A-Round," p. 160

ASSESSMENT

Performance/Self-Assessment Play students' recordings of, and have them assess their improvisations

TECHNOLOGY/MEDIA LINK

CD-ROM Improvise over chords for "Summertime" while using *Band-in-a-Box*

Transparency Display the listening map transparency for *Summertime*

Lesson	Elements	Skills	

LESSON 7 — Let's Rock!
pp. 254–259

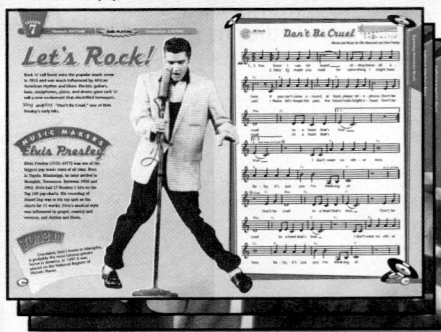

Element: Rhythm
Concept: Pattern
Focus: Rock rhythms

Secondary Element
Timbre: rock drum set (trap set)

National Standards
2a 3c 4c 6a 8b 9a

Skill: Playing
Objective: Perform examples of rock 'n' roll shuffle and even rock patterns

Secondary Skills
- **Singing** Sing an early American rock classic; sing a British 1960s rock hit
- **Listening** Listen to a Buddy Holly rock classic and a British rock hit
- **Moving** Invent dance steps for two rock 'n' roll beats
- **Creating** Explore different rock styles through composition

SKILLS REINFORCEMENT
- **Keyboard** Play a chord accompaniment on keyboard
- **Playing** Play straight eighth-note rock rhythms on percussion

LESSON 8 — The Surfin' Sound
pp. 260–261

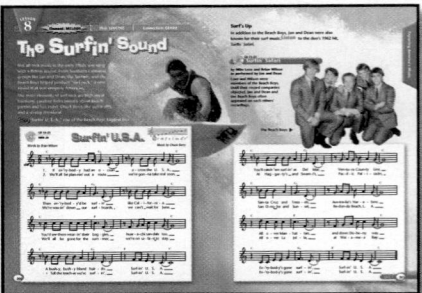

Element: Melody
Concept: Tonality
Focus: Flatted-seventh blues note

Secondary Element
Timbre: rock ensembles

National Standards
1c 2d 4c 6a 6b 8b

Skill: Singing
Objective: Sing a "surf rock" hit song with a flatted-seventh blues note

Secondary Skills
- **Reading** Read notation of a surf rock song
- **Listening** Listen to a surf rock recording

SKILLS REINFORCEMENT
- **Singing** Sing and improvise vocal backups
- **Playing** Improvise a chord progression with a flatted-seventh

LESSON 9 — Latin Pop Is Hot!
pp. 262–267

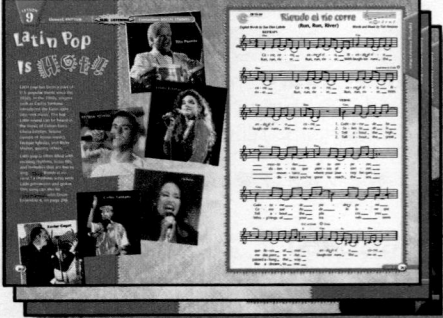

Element: Rhythm
Concept: Pattern
Focus: Latin Rhythm patterns

Secondary Element
Form: verse-refrain form

National Standards
1c 2c 4c 5a 6a 8b 9a

Skill: Listening
Objective: Listen for specific rhythm patterns in Latin pop music

Secondary Skills
- **Singing** Sing a *Tejano* song in English and Spanish
- **Playing** Learn and perform guitar chords and percussion accompaniments to Latin music
- **Moving** Progressively create movements to a *Tejano* song; learn basic *salsa* movements

- **Creating** Create a Latin pop song or dance arrangement

SKILLS REINFORCEMENT
- **Guitar** Play an accompaniment to a Latin song
- **Playing** Use percussion ensemble for accompaniment
- **Listening** Listen to music with themes based on rivers

LESSON 10 — World Music
pp. 268–271

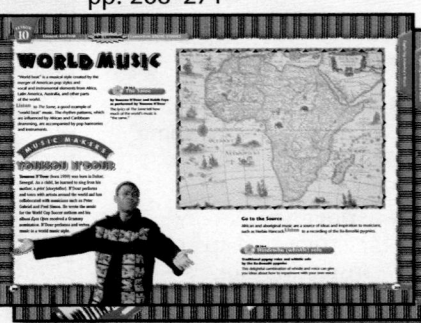

Element: Rhythm
Concept: Pattern
Focus: World beat

Secondary Element
Timbre: instrumental

National Standards
6a 6b 8b 9a 9c

Skill: Listening
Objective: Listen for specific stylistic features in world beat

Secondary Skills
- **Listening** Listen to and discuss and compare various styles, influences, and renditions of world music
- **Playing** Improvise and play world beat rhythm patterns; play an Afro-pop rhythm pattern

SKILLS REINFORCEMENT
- **Listening** Listen to world music selections in a "drop-the-needle" game

Connections | Music and Other Literature

Connection: Culture

Activity: Explore British and American pop culture of the 1950s and 1960s

- **ACROSS THE CURRICULUM**
  Language Arts Read about Elvis Presley; read about the Beatles
  Related Arts Explore historical facts on the British invasion
- **SPOTLIGHT ON**
  The Entertainer Facts on Elvis Presley
  The Performers Information on the Beatles, Buddy Holly, Chubby Checker
- **CULTURAL CONNECTION** Teen Idols; A Friendly Invasion
- **MEETING INDIVIDUAL NEEDS** **Classroom Management** Boys and drums
- **AUDIENCE ETIQUETTE** **Specific Venues/Genres** Concerts
- **SCHOOL TO HOME CONNECTION** Rock in the '50s and '60s
- **BUILDING SKILLS THROUGH MUSIC** **Social Studies** Categorize rhythms

Songs
"Don't Be Cruel"; "Downtown"

Listening Selections
That'll Be the Day; Penny Lane
Let's Twist Again; Interview with Petula Clark
M·U·S·I·C M·A·K·E·R·S
  Elvis Presley; Petula Clark

More Music Choices
"Birthday," p. 90
"Rock and Roll Is Here to Stay," p. 36
"Surfin' U.S.A," p. 260

ASSESSMENT

Performance/Self-Assessment Play the shuffle and even rock rhythms on percussion instruments and self-assess performance

TECHNOLOGY/MEDIA LINK

CD-ROM Explore rock 'n' roll styles with *Band-in-a-Box*

Connection: Genre

Activity: Explore the history and stylistic elements of surf rock

- **SPOTLIGHT ON** **The Performers** Facts on the Beach Boys
- **CULTURAL CONNECTION** **The Surf Scene** The 1960s California surf scene
- **BUILDING SKILLS THROUGH MUSIC** **Writing** Write about a favorite sport

Song "Surfin' U.S.A."

Listening Selection *Surfin' Safari*

More Music Choices
"Birthday," p. 90
"Rock and Roll Is Here to Stay," p. 36

ASSESSMENT

Performance/Observation Sing major scales and scales with a flatted-seventh; sing a surf rock song with a flatted-seventh

TECHNOLOGY/MEDIA LINK

MIDI/Sequencing Software Manipulate and transpose a melody

Connection: Social Studies

Activity: Latin American music and Caribbean and Mexican traditions

- **CULTURAL CONNECTION**
  Tejano *Tejano* music facts
  Music of the Caribbean European and West African hybrid
  Salsa The origins and background of salsa music
- **SPOTLIGHT ON** **Latin Music Legends** Puente, Santana, Selena
- **ACROSS THE CURRICULUM** **Language Arts** Latin pop; **Science** Rivers
- **MOVEMENT** **Nonlocomotor Movement; Patterned Dance** *Salsa*
- **SCHOOL TO HOME CONNECTION** **Latin Influence**
- **BUILDING SKILLS THROUGH MUSIC** **Language** Outline information

Song *"Riendo el río corre"* ("Run, Run, River")

Listening Selections
Ayer; Si tú no estás (excerpt)
M·U·S·I·C M·A·K·E·R·S
  Tish Hinojosa
  Franco de Vita

More Music Choices
"El payo," p. 145
"Má Teodora," p. 301
"Magnolia," p. 16
"O lê lê O Bahía," p. 165

ASSESSMENT

Music Journal Writing Listen to Latin music selections and write about its style, instruments, and rhythm

TECHNOLOGY/MEDIA LINK

CD-ROM Use *Band-in-a-Box* to explore Latin styles
Web Site Discover information on Latin pop stars

Connection: Social Studies

Activity: Relate music from around the world to their culture of origin

- **SPOTLIGHT ON**
  World Beat Music Around the World Artists whose music reflects the influence of world beats
  The Performer Background on CoCo Lee
- **ACROSS THE CURRICULUM** **Related Arts** A world music bulletin board
- **CULTURAL CONNECTION**
  Ba-Benzélé Pygmies Facts on pygmies
  Aborigines of Australia Facts on aborigines
- **TEACHER TO TEACHER** **Make a Didgeridoo**
- **BUILDING SKILLS THROUGH MUSIC** **Writing** Write about transportation and communication

Listening Selections
The Same (excerpt)
Hindewhu (whistle) solo
Watchers of the Canyon
Watermelon Man (excerpt)
Colours of the World
Brolga (excerpt)
M·U·S·I·C M·A·K·E·R·S
  Youssou N'Dour

More Music Choices
Evening Samba, p. 297
Gidden riddum, p. 299
"Give a Little Love," p. 140

ASSESSMENT

Music Journal Writing Listen to world music selections and write on the influence of other styles, paying special attention to rhythm

TECHNOLOGY/MEDIA LINK

CD-ROM Use *Band-in-a-Box* to explore world music styles

INTRODUCING THE UNIT

From schools to concert halls to streets and beyond, America makes music! People from all over the world have brought their music with them to America. Through the years, their music has combined to create musical styles unique to the United States. In Unit 7, students will see and hear the many elements that helped define American music.

UNIT PROJECT

This unit on Exploring America's Music presents an opportunity to focus on how America received the musical gifts that came with immigrants from Europe, Africa, and other parts of the world; then it took those gifts and forged unique American musical styles.

Ask students to create a musical presentation. Have students

- Learn to sing the songs. Feature soloists or small groups on some verses.
- Add instruments such as guitars, Autoharps, keyboards, electric basses, and drums wherever possible.
- Develop a narration between songs. Include quotes from pop music stars or historical figures.
- Add dances or theatrical skits to the songs.
- Develop simple costumes or props like hats.
- Present a gallery of photo images as a background.
- Invite parents or prominent community members to be part of the presentation.
- Video record the presentation.

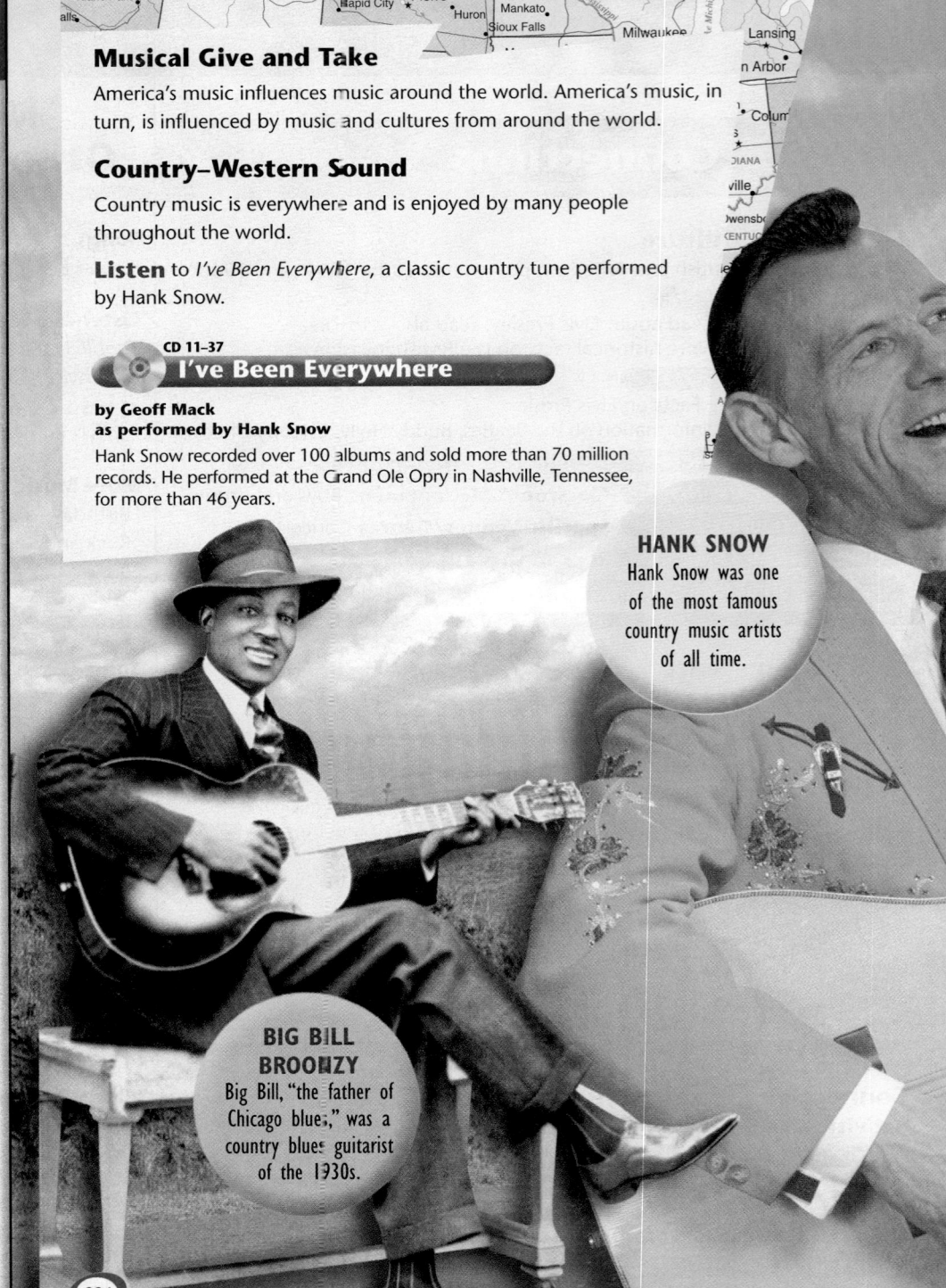

Musical Give and Take

America's music influences music around the world. America's music, in turn, is influenced by music and cultures from around the world.

Country–Western Sound

Country music is everywhere and is enjoyed by many people throughout the world.

Listen to *I've Been Everywhere*, a classic country tune performed by Hank Snow.

CD 11–37
I've Been Everywhere

by Geoff Mack
as performed by Hank Snow

Hank Snow recorded over 100 albums and sold more than 70 million records. He performed at the Grand Ole Opry in Nashville, Tennessee, for more than 46 years.

HANK SNOW
Hank Snow was one of the most famous country music artists of all time.

BIG BILL BROONZY
Big Bill, "the father of Chicago blues," was a country blues guitarist of the 1930s.

224

ACROSS THE CURRICULUM

Unit Highlights The following interdisciplinary activities in this unit are related to the music elements presented in the lessons and are intended to enhance student learning. For a more detailed topical description, see the Unit at a Glance, pp. 223a–223f.

▶ LANGUAGE ARTS

- Read about African Americans before the Civil War (p. 232)
- Read about jazz musicians and create a bulletin board with their pictures (p. 251)
- Read about the life of Elvis Presley (p. 254)
- Read a book about the Beatles (p. 257)
- Create a journal on Latin pop stars (p. 263)

▶ RELATED ARTS

- Explore historical facts on the "British Invasion" (p. 257)
- Design a world music bulletin board (p. 268)

▶ SOCIAL STUDIES

- Read about an immigrant's journey to the United States (p. 230)
- Read about the beginnings of the Fisk Jubilee Singers (p. 234)
- Learn more about cowboys (p. 236)
- Learn about the origins of African American blues style (p. 240)
- Discuss the historical origins of country music (p. 244)

▶ SCIENCE

- Learn about the science behind New Orleans cooking (p. 247)
- Discover facts about rivers (p. 264)

▶ VISUAL ARTS

- Discover young western artists (p. 238)

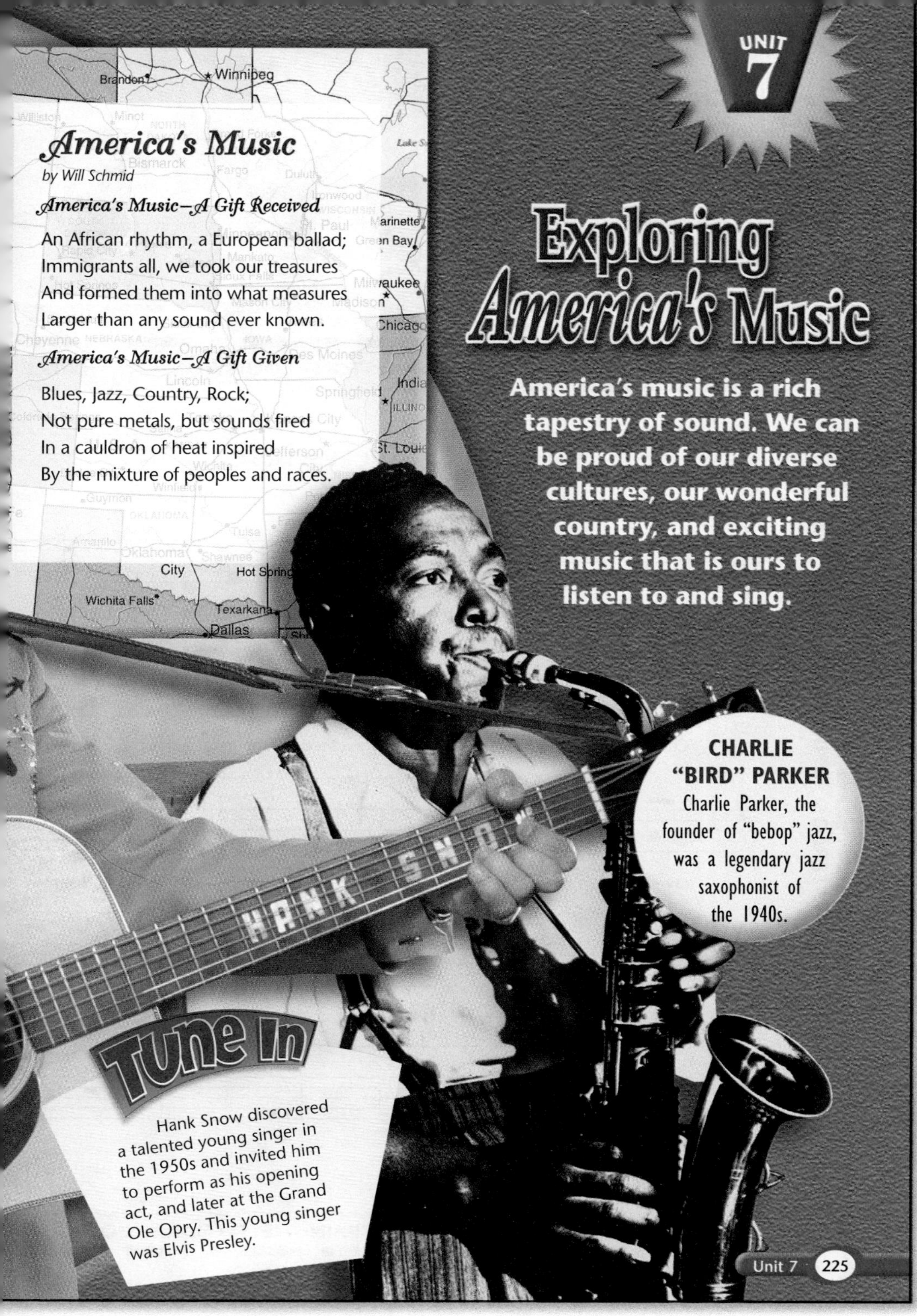

UNIT 7

America's Music
by Will Schmid

America's Music—A Gift Received

An African rhythm, a European ballad;
Immigrants all, we took our treasures
And formed them into what measures
Larger than any sound ever known.

America's Music—A Gift Given

Blues, Jazz, Country, Rock;
Not pure metals, but sounds fired
In a cauldron of heat inspired
By the mixture of peoples and races.

Exploring America's Music

America's music is a rich tapestry of sound. We can be proud of our diverse cultures, our wonderful country, and exciting music that is ours to listen to and sing.

CHARLIE "BIRD" PARKER
Charlie Parker, the founder of "bebop" jazz, was a legendary jazz saxophonist of the 1940s.

Tune In
Hank Snow discovered a talented young singer in the 1950s and invited him to perform as his opening act, and later at the Grand Ole Opry. This young singer was Elvis Presley.

Unit 7   **225**

MUSIC SKILLS
ASSESSED IN THIS UNIT

Reading Music: Rhythm
- Play a rhythm accompaniment to "Ise oluwa" (p. 231)

Reading Music: Pitch
- Listen to, sing, and identify pairs of scales in which one is major and the other contains a flatted-seventh (p. 261)

Performing Music: Playing
- Play the rhythm of a melody on a non-pitched instrument (p. 249)
- Practice drum set patterns and assess personal ability (p. 259)

Listening to Music
- Find recordings of instruments also featured on cowboy song recordings and identify the featured instruments (p. 239)
- Listen to and assess other students' improvisations on "Summertime" (p. 253)
- Listen to Latin music selections and identify what was learned (p. 267)
- Listen to world music selections and write, in a journal, descriptions of their musical influences (p. 271)

Moving to Music
- Do the Cajun two-step (p. 249)

Creating Music
- Create and sing melodies for "This Little Light of Mine (p. 235)
- Write verses to "Sometimes I Feel Like a Motherless Child" (p. 243)

CULTURAL CONNECTION

Unit Highlights   The musical literature in this unit provides opportunities for students to explore a variety of American music influences. A more detailed description of the resources and activities can be found in the Unit at a Glance on pp. 223a–223f

▶ AFRICAN/AFRICAN AMERICAN
- Learn about the history of freedom songs (p. 232)
- Explore the history of the gospel choir movement (p. 234)
- Learn more about the Ba-Benzélé Pygmies (p. 269)

▶ AMERICAN REGIONAL
- Find out facts on Ellis Island and immigration (p. 228)
- Learn about singing cowboy actors (p. 236)
- Discover how jazz is both a cultural performance style as well as a category of music (p. 240)

- Explore facts about Cajun culture (p. 247)
- Find out about the "British Invasion" (p. 258)
- Learn about the surf culture (p. 261)

▶ ASIAN; AUSTRALIAN
- Find out about the Aborigines of Australia (p. 270)

▶ CARIBBEAN
- Explore Caribbean music's roots (p. 264)

▶ LATIN AMERICAN
- Learn about the roots of *Tejano* music (p. 262)
- Find out where *salsa* dancing originated (p. 266)

▶ MANY CULTURES
- Learn about teen idols of the 1950s and 1960s (p. 255)

OPENING ACTIVITIES

MATERIALS
- "I've Been Everywhere" **CD 11–38**
  Recording Routine
  Intro (4 m.); refrain; interlude (2 m.); v.1; refrain;
  interlude (2 m.); v. 2; refrain; interlude (2 m.); v. 3;
  refrain; interlude (2 m.); v. 3; refrain; interlude (2 m.);
  v. 4; refrain
- *I've Been Everywhere* **CD 11–37**

Listening

Have students read the poem "America's Music" on p. 225, and discuss where immigrants came from.

Then share with students the concept that each of the styles to be studied in this unit represents an interesting recipe of mixed ingredients from these various cultures.

Invite students to listen to "I've Been Everywhere" **CD 11–38**, as they follow the song notation on p. 226.

Explain to students that the styles found in Unit 7 represent America making music, even though these styles are from all over the globe. Unit 7 styles include English ballads, *Juju* (West African), Spirituals, Gospel, Cowboy, Blues, Country and Western, Cajun, Opera, Jazz, Rock 'n' Roll, Surf Rock, *Tejano,* Latin, Caribbean, *Salsa,* Venezuelan folk, World beat, and Aboriginal Australian.

Reading

Ask students to look for the following things in the music:
- Key signatures and keynote (tonic). (F major)
- Flatted-third blue notes (A♭). This blues addition to country music is a perfect illustration of how African American music influenced other styles.

Singing

Have students learn to sing the main melody of the first section. Focus on the difference between the A and the A♭ pitches.

Work out the semi-spoken place names in the second section.

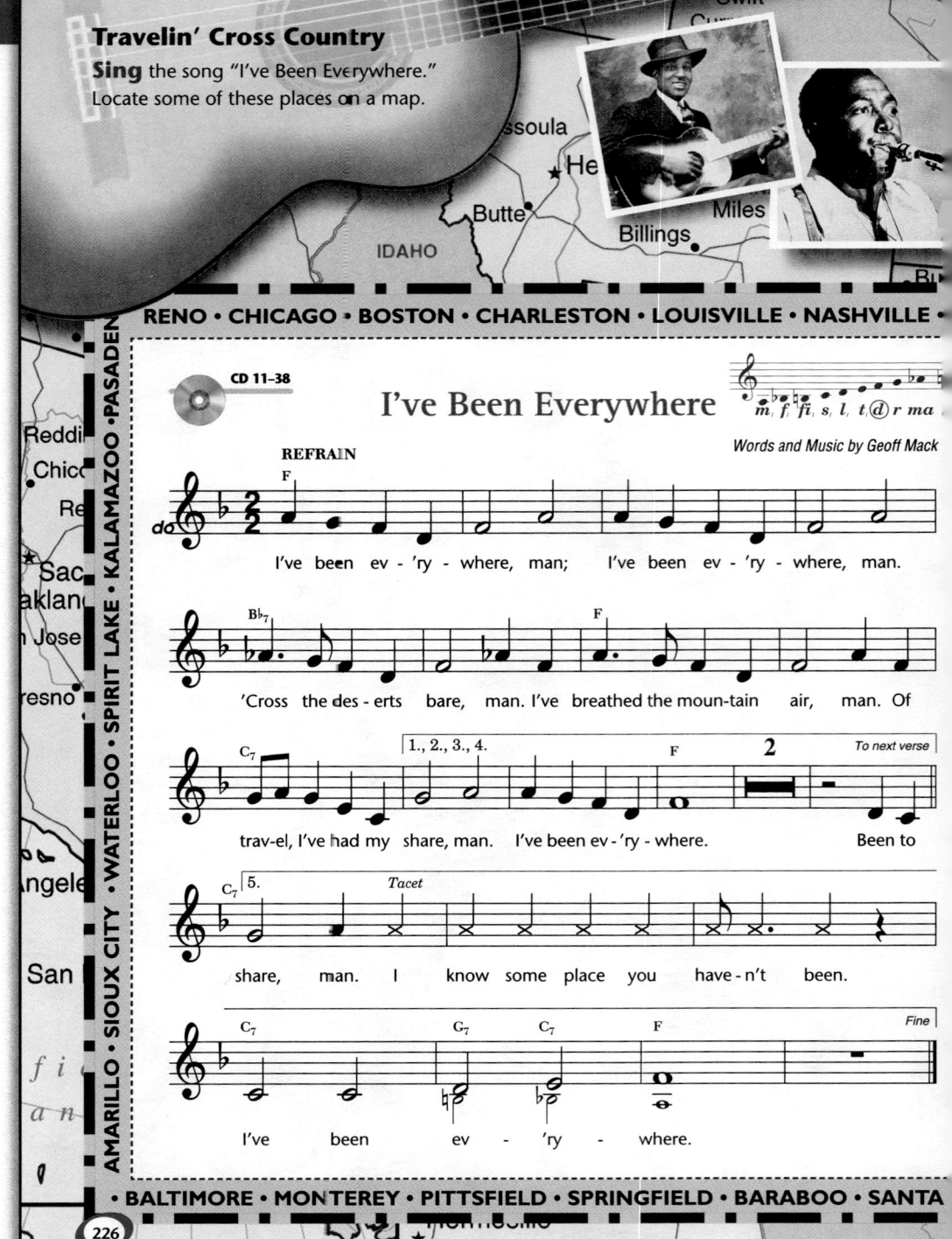

Travelin' Cross Country

Sing the song "I've Been Everywhere."
Locate some of these places on a map.

RENO • CHICAGO • BOSTON • CHARLESTON • LOUISVILLE • NASHVILLE •

CD 11–38

I've Been Everywhere

Words and Music by Geoff Mack

• BALTIMORE • MONTEREY • PITTSFIELD • SPRINGFIELD • BARABOO • SANTA

226

ASSESSMENT

Unit Highlights The lessons in this unit were chosen and developed to support the theme "Exploring America's Music." Each lesson, as always, presents a clear element focus, a skill objective, and an end-of-lesson assessment. The overall sequence of lessons, however, is organized according to this theme, rather than concept or skill development. In this context, formal assessment strategies, such as those presented in Units 1–6, are no longer applicable.

▶ **RUBRICS**

Visit *www.sfsuccessnet.com* for rubrics to assess students' achievement in music skills.

▶ **INFORMAL ASSESSMENTS**

At the close of each Teacher's Edition lesson in this unit, one of the following types of assessments is used to evaluate the learning of the key element focus or skill objective.

- Journal Writing (pp. 267, 271)
- Observation (p. 239)
- Performance/Interview (p. 235)
- Performance/Music Journal Writing (p. 231)
- Performance/Observation (pp. 249, 261)
- Performance/Self-Assessment (pp. 253, 259)
- Self-Assessment/Music Journal Writing (p. 243)

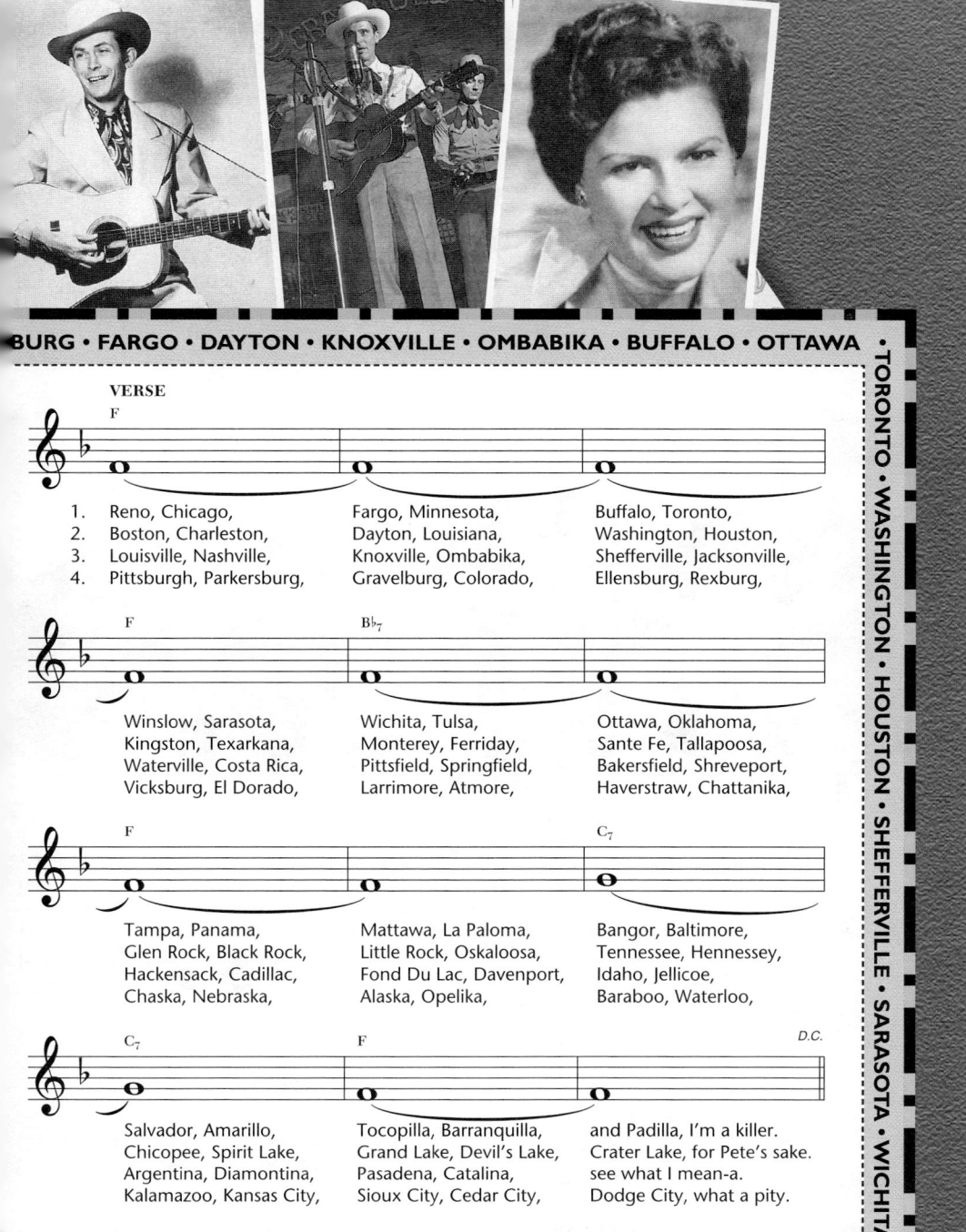

ASK What other style uses spoken text, rhythmically chanted to the music's beat? (Rap)

Tell students that there were some blues songs that also had chanted, even spoken, passages.

Moving

Invite students to work out a movement routine on the verses where they take turns standing up and rhythmically saying the place names.

Creating

Use the place names in the verses as an opportunity to study a map of your own state.

Have students

* Refer to a detailed map of your state and make lists of interesting sounding place names—cities, rivers, lakes, or regions.
* Study the lists and have small groups put together their own new verses to the song "I've Been Everywhere."

Assign each of the styles presented in this unit to a pair or students. Encourage groups to find pictures representing each style and use them to create a bulletin board. Feature the pictures of each style as you study it in the unit.

INNOVATIVE TEACHER SUPPORT FOR THIS UNIT

* **MAKING MUSIC DVD, Grade 6** contains video segments that support lessons, including signing and movement.
* **MAKING MUSIC with Movement and Dance** provides more opportunities for large group activities in music or physical education classes.
* **MAKING MUSIC with Technology** provides lesson plans for many technology applications; includes MIDI files.
* *¡A cantar!* features recorded songs and lessons from around the Spanish-speaking world; includes strategies for bilingual classes and for English-speaking teachers working with Spanish-speaking students.
* **Bridges to Asia** features recorded songs and lessons from Asian and Pacific region cultures.
* *www.sfsuccessnet.com* provides an online lesson planner to conveniently create lesson plans at school or at home. Includes rubrics for assessment, lesson modifications to meet the needs of all students, performance musicals based on program content, and more.

TECHNOLOGY/MEDIA LINK

Unit Highlights The following components are used in this unit to reinforce and expand student's understanding of music elements and related themes.

▶ **CD-ROM**

* Improvise over a 12-bar-blues background on *Band-in-a-Box* (p. 243)
* Improvise over chords for "Summertime" while using *Band-in-a-Box* (p. 253)
* Explore rock 'n' roll styles in *Band-in-a-Box* (p. 259)
* Use *Band-in-a-Box* to create Latin songs and dances (p. 267)
* Use *Band-in-a-Box* to explore world music styles (p. 271)

▶ **ELECTRONIC KEYBOARD**

* Explore MIDI keyboard sounds for a cowboy song (p. 239)

▶ **MIDI/SEQUENCING SOFTWARE**

* Manipulate and transpose melody (p. 261)

▶ **TRANSPARENCY**

* Display the listening map transparency for "Summertime" (p. 253)

▶ **VIDEO LIBRARY/DVD**

* View video on solo and choral gospel singing (p. 235)
* Show a video featuring country singer Pam Tillis (p. 249)

▶ **WEB SITE**

* Learn more about African drumming and vocal styles (p. 231)
* Discover information on Latin pop stars (p. 267)

LESSON AT A GLANCE

Element Focus **TIMBRE** Percussion sounds from West Africa

Skill Objective **PLAYING** Play rhythm patterns to accompany a song from West Africa

Connection Activity **SOCIAL STUDIES** Explore the influence of immigrants from Europe and West Africa

MATERIALS

- "The Water Is Wide"   **CD 12–1**
  Recording Routine: Intro (4 m.); v. 1; interlude (4 m.); v. 1; interlude (4 m.); v. 2; interlude (4 m.); v. 3; coda
- "*Ise oluwa*"   **CD 12–3**
  Recording Routine: Intro (12 m.); vocal; instrumental; vocal; coda
- **Pronunciation Practice/Translation** p. 531
- **Resource Book** pp. A-19, F-22
- selected classroom instruments
- double bell, rattles, hand drums
- a world map

VOCABULARY

ballad   call and response

◆ ◆ ◆ National Standards ◆ ◆ ◆

1d Sing music written in two and three parts
2c Perform instrumental music from diverse cultures
4b Arrange pieces for voices
4c Arrange, using electronic media
6b Listen and analyze uses of timbre in music from diverse cultures
8b Identify ways music relates to social studies
9b Classify high-quality musical works by style

MORE MUSIC CHOICES

For more songs from England and West Africa:
"Scarborough Fair," p. 95
"Take Time in Life," p. 292

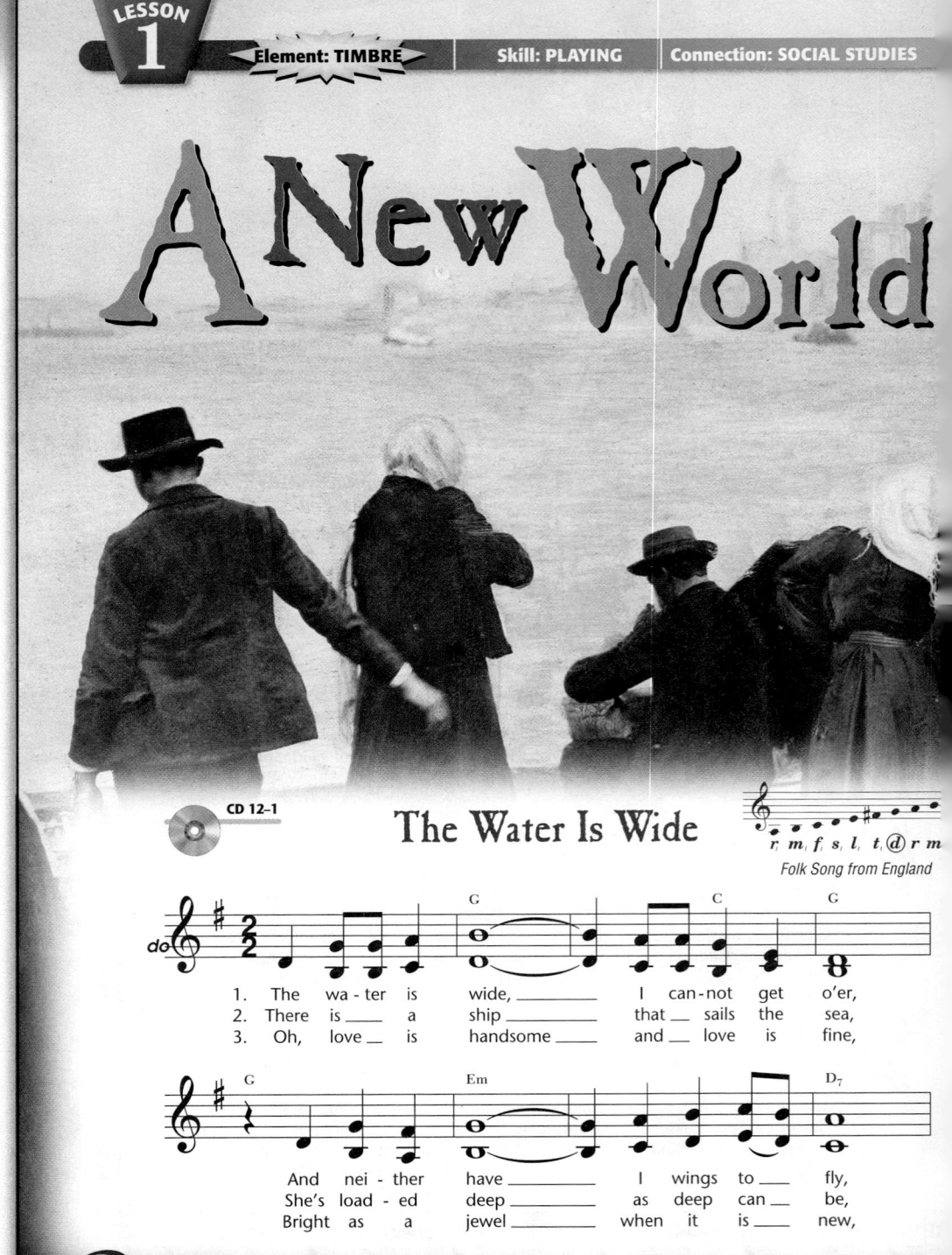

A New World

CD 12–1
The Water Is Wide

r, m, f, s, l, t, d, r m

Folk Song from England

1. The wa-ter is wide, _____ I can-not get o'er,
2. There is ____ a ship _____ that ____ sails the sea,
3. Oh, love __ is handsome _____ and __ love is fine,

And nei - ther have _____ I wings to ____ fly,
She's load - ed deep _____ as deep can ____ be,
Bright as a jewel _____ when it is ____ new,

228

Footnotes

TEACHER TO TEACHER

▶ **Bulletin Board Idea** Create a bulletin board that reflects the progression of this unit. Start with the music of England and West Africa in Lesson 1 and gradually add the other American music traditions covered in the unit. Ask students to help find appropriate visuals and artwork for the display.

BUILDING SKILLS THROUGH MUSIC

▶ **Language** Have students identify the words or phrases that reflect optimism in the lyrics of "The Water is Wide," and then identify the words or phrases that reflect despair or sadness.

CULTURAL CONNECTION

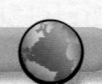

▶ **Ellis Island** A 27-acre island, near the Statue of Liberty in New York harbor, was the main processing center for immigrants who arrived in the United States from 1892 to 1954. The new-comers, after their long journey of sometimes three months or more, were examined for illnesses, for deportation, or for admittance into the country. Over 12 million people came to the United States through Ellis Island. Many had their foreign names Americanized by the immigration officers.

In 1990 the restored main building was opened as the Ellis Island Immigration Museum. Many pictures and stories, as well as a wall of chiseled names, are displayed there.

Even before our country became an independent nation, European immigrants were bringing their favorite songs with them to America.

Sing "The Water Is Wide," an early folk song from Great Britain. What is the message of this song?

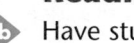

Lyric songs and ballads tell about love, war, home, and heroes. Before the days of television and recordings, such songs provided a source of entertainment after a long day at work.

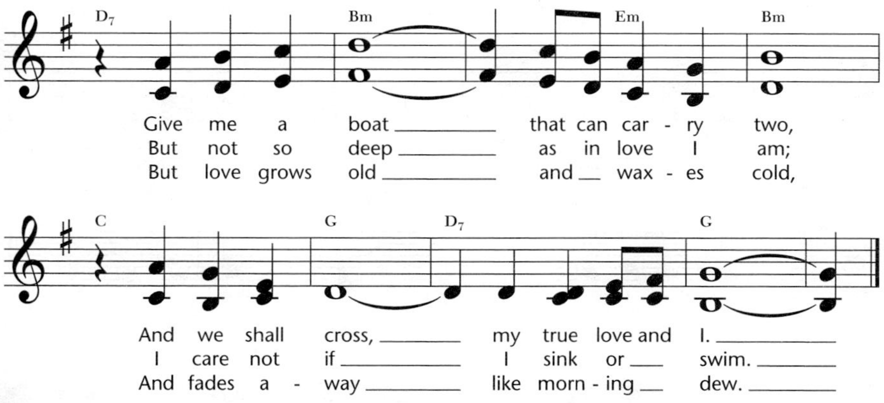

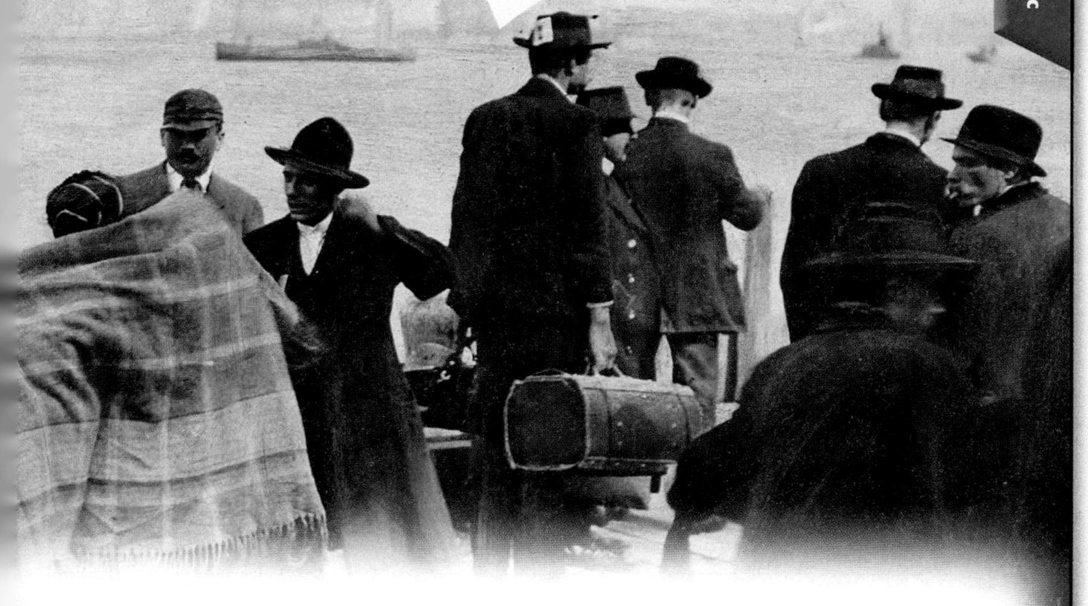

D₇   Bm   Em   Bm

Give me a boat _____ that can car - ry two,
But not so deep _____ as in love I am;
But love grows old _____ and __ wax - es cold,

C   G   D₇   G

And we shall cross, _____ my true love and I. _____
I care not if _____ I sink or __ swim. _____
And fades a - way _____ like morn - ing __ dew. _____

Unit 7 **229**

1 INTRODUCE

Explain that this lesson begins a classroom celebration of two of the many "root" musical traditions (European and African) that have helped produce the "tree" that is American music. For a wealth of information and activities related to the influence of these traditions on American culture, see Teacher to Teacher and Cultural Connection, p. 228; Spotlight On, below and p. 231; and Across the Curriculum, p. 230

2 DEVELOP

Reading

8b Have students locate England on a map, then echo sing the melody of "The Water Is Wide." Invite students to follow the music and sing "The Water Is Wide" **CD 12–1.**

ASK What is the home tone (do), or tonic note, in this song? (G)

Using pitch syllables, how would you describe the range of the melody, from low to high? (so₁ to so)

Share the information about Ellis Island in Cultural Connection on p. 228 and discuss the photo on pp. 228 and 229.

ASK In what ways did the early immigrants affect the music of this country? (Immigrants brought music from their own cultures with them, influencing and creating new musical styles.)

Point out to students that this is an ongoing process, which continues to this day.

continued on page 230

SPOTLIGHT ON

▶ **The English Ballad** Toward the end of the nineteenth century, Francis James Child collected five volumes of ballads under the title *English and Scottish Popular Ballads*. These volumes have become the standard collection of ballads from the British Isles and have spun off other collections based on them, such as Bertrand Bronson's *The Traditional Tunes of the Child Ballads*. Today many familiar ballads, such as "Barb'ry Allen" (Child #84) and "The Golden Vanity" (Child #286), are known by their numbers in the Child collection.

SKILLS REINFORCEMENT

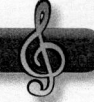

4b ▶ **Creating** After students are familiar with the song "The Water Is Wide," have them create a vocal descant for the song.

Reinforcement Pair students that have good singing and creative ability with students that may have difficulty creating an original vocal part. Ask the advanced student to guide his or her partner through the same tasks as the main class.

On Target Ask students to create a vocal descant, using the syllable *ooh*. Suggest that students change the note with every chord change in the song. Have students listen carefully to assure that their notes fit into the harmony of the chord changes.

4c **Challenge** Invite students to create a countermelody using a MIDI keyboard, or sequencing software. Ask students to select appropriate timbres for their musical line and to perform their countermelody as the class sings the song.

Unit 7 *Exploring America's Music* **229**

Singing

 1d Encourage students to sing "The Water Is Wide" **CD 12–1** in two-part harmony.

Playing

2c Encourage students to learn the melody of "The Water Is Wide" on recorder, xylophone, resonator bells, keyboard, or guitar and then play it as an echo in two sections.

Singing

Have students

8b • Locate Nigeria on a map of Africa.

• Learn the translation of the Yoruba words of the song "Ise oluwa." ("God's work cannot be undone.")

• Learn the pronunciation with Pronunciation Practice **CD 12–5** and the Pronunciation Practice Guide on Resource Book p. A-19.

1d • Learn the two parts of the response by echoing the teacher. (Point out that this technique reflects the African oral tradition, in which stories and songs are passed down from one generation to the next.)

• Sing, from the notation, both parts of the response with the recording **CD 12–3**.

• Learn to sing the call; then sing it with the recording.

Divide the class into two sections. Have one section sing the *call* and the other section the two- and three-part *response*. Have sections switch parts.

Songs of West Africa

West Coast Africans from countries like Ghana, Ivory Coast, Sierra Leone, and Nigeria brought their songs and their rhythms with them to America. These songs often took the form of **call and response.**

Listen to and then **sing** the Nigerian song "Ise oluwa" in the call-and-response style. What instruments do you hear on the recording?

> **Call and response** is a style of performance in which a leader sings a call and a group responds.

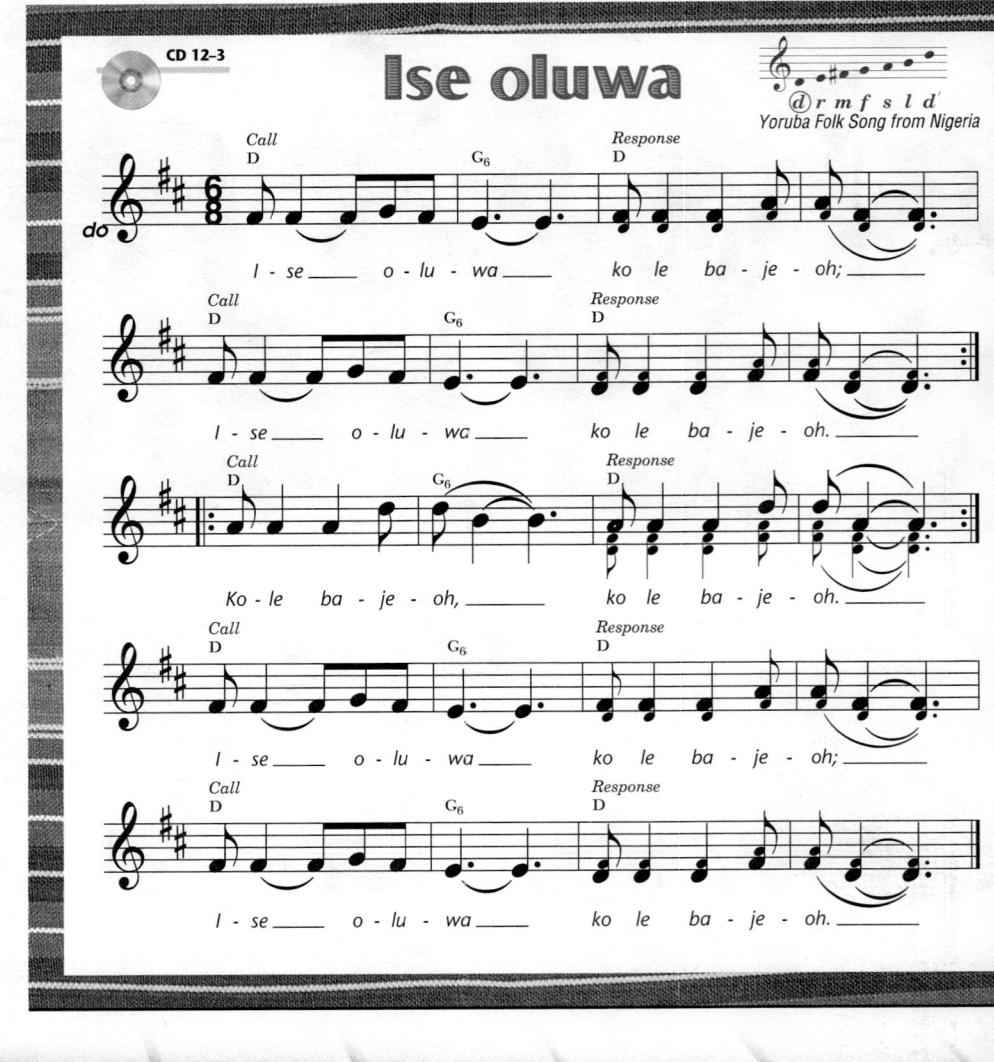

CD 12–3

Ise oluwa

Yoruba Folk Song from Nigeria

I - se o - lu - wa ko le ba - je - oh;

I - se o - lu - wa ko le ba - je - oh.

Ko - le ba - je - oh, ko le ba - je - oh.

I - se o - lu - wa ko le ba - je - oh;

I - se o - lu - wa ko le ba - je - oh.

Footnotes

SKILLS REINFORCEMENT

 ▶ **Guitar** This finger-style guitar part can be played with "Ise oluwa."

2c The D chord is played in the usual position, and the G₆ chord is played by pressing the third finger on the sixth string at fret 5 (strings 4 through 1 are open).

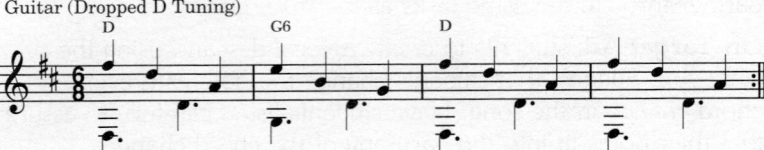
Guitar (Dropped D Tuning)

 ▶ **Mallets** Students may enjoy playing the Orff arrangement of "The Water Is Wide" on Resource Book p. F-22.

ACROSS THE CURRICULUM

8b ▶ **Social Studies** Invite students to read *When Jessie Came Across the Sea* by Amy Hest (Candlewick, 1997), an endearing story of a young immigrant's journey to the United States in the early 1900s. Engage students in a discussion about differences between the 1900s and now. Who are the immigrants coming to the United States today? What are the challenges they face? Do students know people who have recently immigrated to the United States? Are any students recent immigrants?

Sounds of West Africa

Play the following rhythm accompaniment for *"Ise oluwa."*

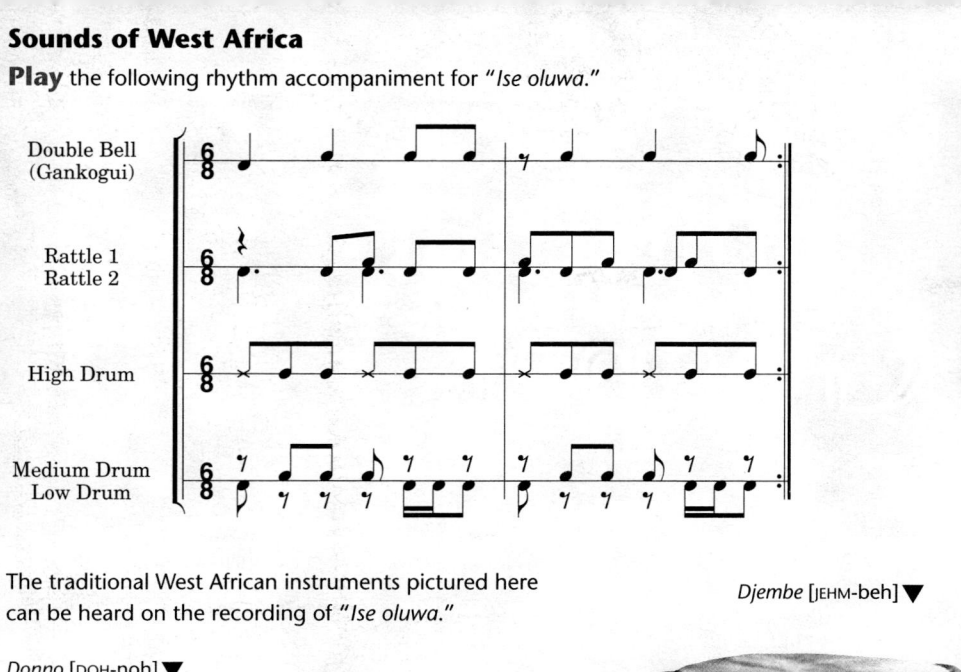

The traditional West African instruments pictured here can be heard on the recording of *"Ise oluwa."*

Donno [DOH-noh] ▼

Gankogui [gahn-KOH-gwee] ▼

Djembe [JEHM-beh] ▼

Shekere [sheh-KEE-reh] ▼

CD-ROM Use *Band-in-a-Box* to create an arrangement of *Ise oluwa* using the African style.

Unit 7 **231**

Playing

Have students

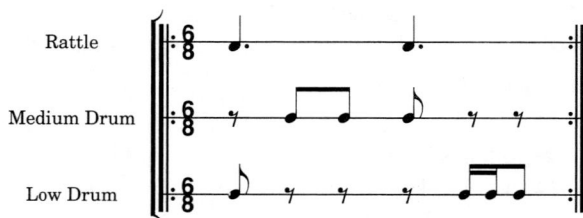

- Listen to the recording of *"Ise oluwa"* **CD 12–3.** (See Spotlight On below for related style information.)
- Learn the rhythm parts shown on this page or the following easier alternative.

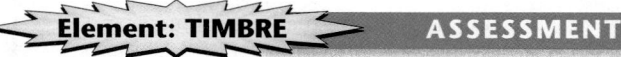

- Perform either rhythm accompaniment with *"Ise oluwa."*

Invite students to play the guitar accompaniment for *"Ise oluwa"* as shown in Skills Reinforcement on p. 230. Have them use the finger style part for D and G_6 chords. To tune the guitar to a "dropped D" tuning, lower the sixth string (E) one whole step to D.

Listening

Invite students to listen to recordings of the *donno, shekere,* and *djembe* found in the Sound Bank, starting on p. 512.

3 CLOSE

Element: TIMBRE   **ASSESSMENT**

6b **Performance/Music Journal Writing** Have students play the rhythm accompaniment on p. 231 with *"Ise oluwa."* Then ask students to write a description of the changes in tone color of *"Ise oluwa"* when the double bell, rattles, and drums are added as accompaniment.

SPOTLIGHT ON

▶ **Nigeria** Nigeria, named after the Niger River, has the largest population of any country in Africa. A former British colony, Nigeria became independent in 1960. The country's most important economic resource is petroleum. The Niger River and its tributary, the Benue River, form a "Y" that divides the country into three regions. Nigeria has over 250 ethnic groups. The principal tribes are the *Fulani, Hausa, Ibo,* and *Yoruba.*

9b ▶ **Juju Style** *"Ise oluwa"* is performed in both the traditional West African style and in the contemporary *juju* musical style. This style, which evolved in Nigeria in the 1970s, adds electric guitars and Western percussion to the traditional mix of West African instruments. See Unit 8 (*"Nana Kru,"* "Take Time in Life," "Everybody Loves Saturday Night") and have students listen to and describe these West African pop music styles.

CHARACTER EDUCATION

▶ **Character Traits** Ask students what character traits must immigrants to a new country possess (strength, courage, commitment, perseverance, patience)? What emotions would an immigrant to a new country likely feel (excitement, apprehension, fear, relief)? These emotions may be some of the same emotions experienced by people who are new to our school. What traits do we expect from those who immigrate to our country (loyalty, industriousness, law-abiding, patriotism)?

TECHNOLOGY/MEDIA LINK

Web Site Visit *www.sfsuccessnet.com* to learn more about West African drumming and vocal styles.

LESSON AT A GLANCE

Element Focus ◀ **MELODY** Melodic contour

Skill Objective **SINGING** Perform a traditional spiritual in contemporary gospel style

Connection Activity **SOCIAL STUDIES** Discuss the historical roots of the spiritual and gospel musical traditions

MATERIALS

- "This Little Light of Mine"   **CD 12–6**
  Recording Routine: Intro (4 m.); vocal; interlude (4 m.); vocal
- *The Battle of Jericho*   **CD 12–8**
- *Swing Low, Sweet Chariot*   **CD 12–9**
- *Jonah*   **CD 12–10**
- **Resource Book** p. I-19
- guitars, keyboards, recorders

VOCABULARY

spiritual   gospel

◆ ◆ ◆ ◆ National Standards ◆ ◆ ◆ ◆

1c Sing music from diverse genres
2d Perform simple accompaniments by ear
3b Improvise melodic embellishments on given melodies
6a Listen and describe events in music using appropriate terms
6b Listen and analyze uses of pitch in music from diverse genres
8b Identify ways music relates to social studies
9c Compare, in several cultures, functions music serves

MORE MUSIC CHOICES

For more practice singing African American spirituals and gospel songs:

"Ain't Gonna Let Nobody Turn Me 'Round," p. 85

"Glory, Glory, Hallelujah," p. 52

"Peace Like a River," p. 190

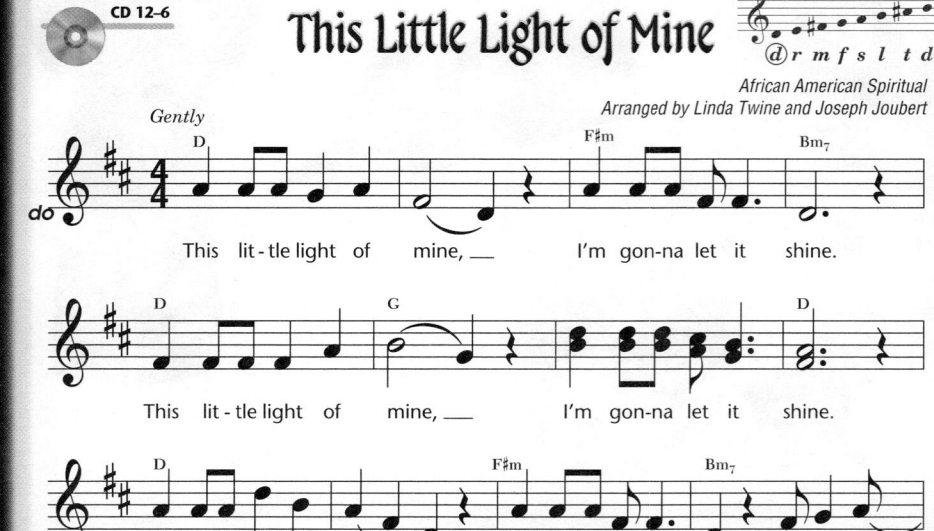

Spiritual *and* Gospel

Between 1800 and 1861 (the start of the Civil War), African American spirituals came to be an important part of America's musical heritage. These songs expressed slaves' longing for freedom. After 1920, a new style, called **gospel**, grew out of the spiritual tradition.

Sing this arrangement of "This Little Light of Mine," which combines the traditional spiritual with a contemporary gospel style.

Gospel combines jazz rhythm and blues singing with religious music. It may be accompanied by hand clapping, swaying, foot stomping, and other movements.

CD 12–6

This Little Light of Mine

d r m f s l t d'

African American Spiritual
Arranged by Linda Twine and Joseph Joubert

Gently

This lit-tle light of mine, ___ I'm gon-na let it shine.

This lit-tle light of mine, ___ I'm gon-na let it shine.

This lit-tle light of mine, ___ I'm gon-na let it shine, Let it shine, ___

232

Footnotes

CULTURAL CONNECTION

8b ▶ **Freedom Songs** Like many spirituals, "This Little Light of Mine" symbolizes the hope African Americans had for their freedom from oppression and slavery. This song has been sung for generations as a source of inspiration for civil rights efforts. After introducing the song, develop with students a list of additional reasons why people today might sing this song (for example, disability rights, homelessness issues).

BUILDING SKILLS THROUGH MUSIC

▶ **Social Studies** Have students outline the information in the footnotes about spirituals, freedom songs, and gospel music. Include the information from Music Makers on p. 234. Ask them to develop a time line to show the order in which these musical styles were developed.

ACROSS THE CURRICULUM

▶ **Language Arts** To discover more about the heroic efforts and achievements of African Americans before the Civil War, students can read *Nightjohn* by Gary Paulsen (Dell, 1995).

CHARACTER EDUCATION

▶ **Caring** Tell students spirituals served many purposes, including providing inspiration and boosting morale. "This Little Light of Mine" speaks of letting your *light shine*. Ask what can you do to let your *light shine* and why is it important? Have students share examples of people they know who have let their *light shine*. Discuss their behaviors and how their willingness to share themselves with others has made for a better world.

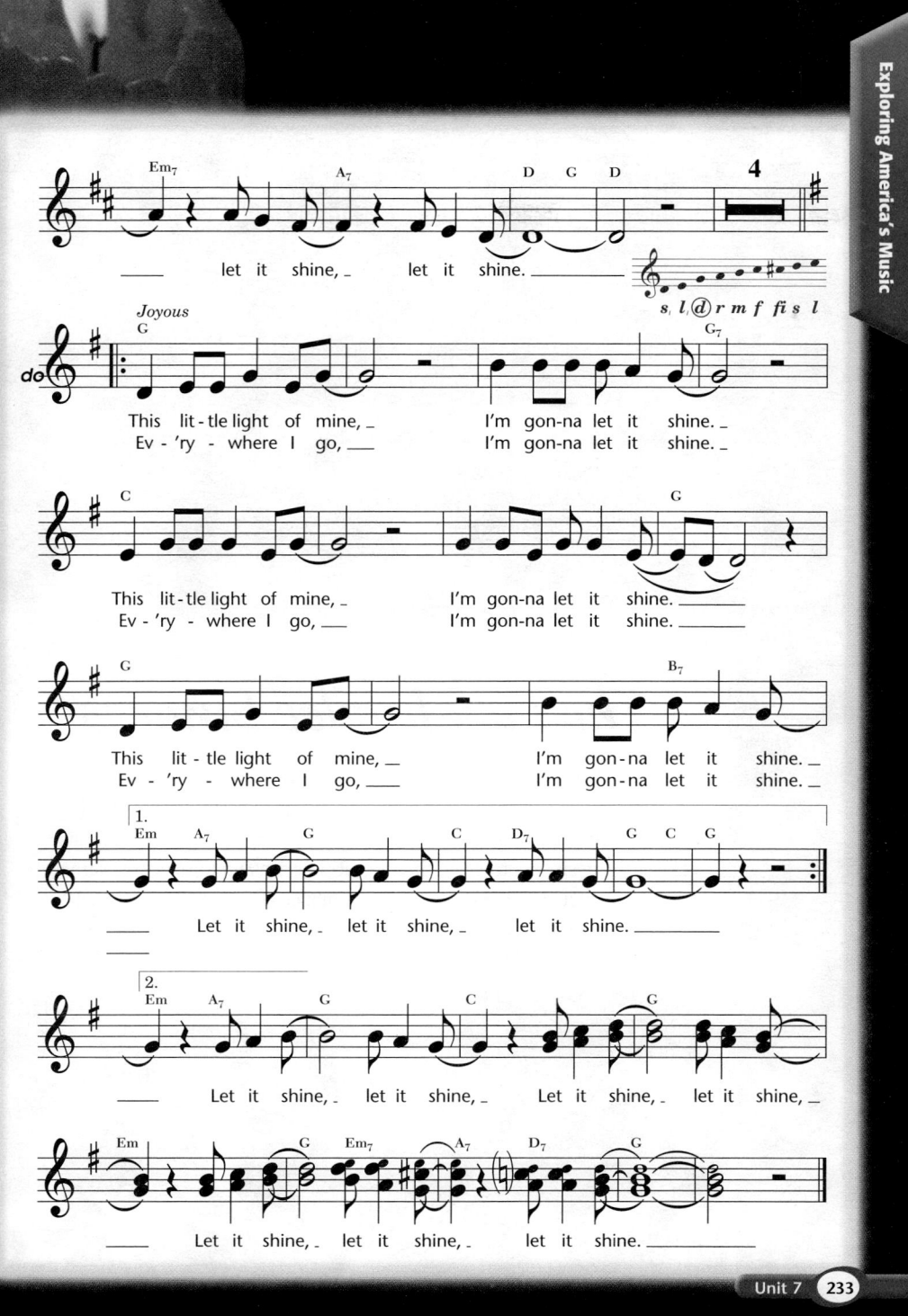

let it shine, _ let it shine. _____

s, l, (d) r m f fis l

Joyous

do
This lit-tle light of mine, _ I'm gon-na let it shine. _
Ev - 'ry - where I go, ___ I'm gon-na let it shine. _

This lit-tle light of mine, _ I'm gon-na let it shine.
Ev - 'ry - where I go, ___ I'm gon-na let it shine.

This lit-tle light of mine, _ I'm gon-na let it shine. _
Ev - 'ry - where I go, ___ I'm gon-na let it shine. _

1.
____ Let it shine, _ let it shine, _ let it shine. _____

2.
____ Let it shine, _ let it shine, _ Let it shine, _ let it shine, _

____ Let it shine, _ let it shine, _ let it shine. _____

Unit 7 233

1 INTRODUCE

9c Share with students the historical information, found in Spotlight On below and Cultural Connection on pp. 232 and 234, about African American spiritual and gospel traditions. Explain that spirituals spread through America after the Civil War and served as a foundation for the later style called gospel. In this lesson, students will experience one of the great African American spirituals, "This Little Light of Mine."

2 DEVELOP

Listening

SAY Listen for a change in style, tempo, dynamics, and timbre.

Have students

- Listen to "This Little Light of Mine" **CD 12–6.**

1c
- Sing the song with the recording or other accompaniment, such as guitar or keyboard.

ASK In what style does this song begin? (traditional spiritual)

At what point in the music does the style change? (at the end of line 4)

How does the musical style change? (The style moves from a traditional spiritual to the newer, gospel style.)

Analyzing

6a Discuss with students the changes in the musical elements that contribute to the change in style. (tempo: gets faster; dynamics: get louder; timbre: solo changes to unison chorus, and new instruments are introduced)

6b Help students focus on the melody in each section of the song.

ASK What happens to the home tone *(do)* **at the beginning of line 5?** (It moves from D to G.)

continued on page 234

SKILLS REINFORCEMENT

▶ **Guitar** This arrangement of "This Little Light of Mine," as printed on pp. 232 and 233, has two sections, each in a different key. The second of these sections is in the key of G and does not require barred chords, so it is quite manageable for beginning guitar players. There are two chord changes that will need some attention. The first is the change from G to C. For convenience and to produce a pleasing sound, guitarists will sometimes "merge" the two chords. The other chord change, from B₇ to Em, is made easier by keeping the second finger on the fifth string as the change is executed. (Note that in the recording, this section of the song modulates to A♭ on the repeat.)

▶ **Recorder** For a recorder descant for "This Little Light of Mine," see Resource Book p. I-19.

SPOTLIGHT ON

9c ▶ **African American Spirituals** African American spirituals are songs that were created by slaves and passed on by oral tradition in America before the Civil War (1861–1865). The spirituals often contained secret messages that made reference to the Underground Railroad or other means of escaping slavery. Common themes of spirituals are identification with the enslaved Israelites of the Old Testament (for example, "Go Down Moses," "Joshua Fought the Battle of Jericho," "Ezekiel Saw the Wheel") and judgment day (for example, "Wade in the Water").

Lesson 2 Continued

Ask students to compare the basic melodic contour of each phrase in the "spiritual" section of the song with the corresponding phrases in the "gospel" section.

Creating

 Have students create new verses for "This Little Light of Mine," using lines 2–5 on p. 233. (Encourage students to improvise on, or embellish, the printed melody. Explain that this is a common practice in gospel style.)

Singing

Have students

 • Sing several examples of their new verses as models. ("Right here in [name city or school], We're gonna let it shine." "We've got the light of freedom, We're gonna let it shine.")

• Collect the verses to sing selected examples as a class.

Listening

 Have students listen to the Moses Hogan Chorale sing the traditional spiritual *The Battle of Jericho* **CD 12–8.**

ASK How does this performance differ from the arrangement of "This Little Light of Mine"? (*The Battle of Jericho* is sung in traditional concert spiritual style, not in gospel style.)

Have students listen to the Fisk Jubilee Singers' version of *Swing Low, Sweet Chariot* **CD 12–9.**

ASK How does this version differ from the later gospel style of music you have heard? (It sounds much more formal; it is in a concert style.)

Have students listen to the Golden Gate Quartet sing *Jonah* **CD 12–10.**

ASK What do you hear in this recording that sounds like pop music? (syncopation, backup singers, rhythmic repetition)

Spirituals Live On

Listen to another African American spiritual, performed in gospel style.

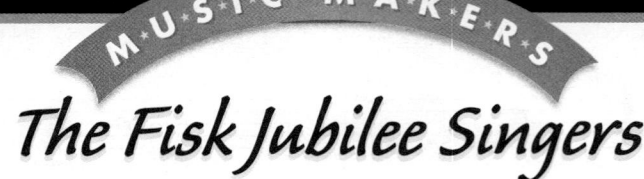

CD 12–8
The Battle of Jericho

**African American Spiritual
as performed by the Moses Hogan Chorale**

The Moses Hogan Chorale is one of the premier choirs in the nation. They specialize in singing traditional African American spirituals and contemporary gospel arrangements.

Read about the Fisk Jubilee Singers below and then listen to this early historical recording of another spiritual.

CD 12–9
Swing Low, Sweet Chariot

**African American Spiritual
as performed by the Fisk Jubilee Singers**

The "scratches" you hear on the recording are from old vinyl records that have been played many times.

M·U·S·I·C M·A·K·E·R·S

The Fisk Jubilee Singers

The Fisk Jubilee Singers were organized in 1871 at Fisk University in Nashville, Tennessee. They were named after the biblical "year of jubilee," a time when all slaves were freed. (All of the original singers were former slaves.) The singers traveled throughout America and Europe and were a star attraction at the 1872 World Peace Jubilee. Their concert included both popular songs of the day and spirituals. As a permanent institution at Fisk, the current Jubilee Singers are continuing this vital choral tradition.

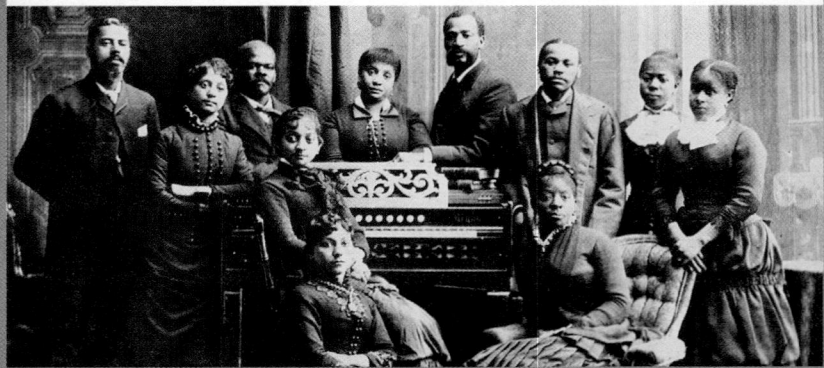

234

Footnotes

CULTURAL CONNECTION

 ▶ **Gospel Music** The gospel choir movement started in the 1920s when Thomas A. Dorsey began writing spirituals with a more modern sound ("Precious Lord, Take My Hand"). In addition to gospel choirs, gospel vocal quartets such as the Golden Gate Quartet were common in the 1930s. Besides black gospel, white gospel music also flourished during the same period. Spirituals and gospel are similiar in that they were both created by African Americans, and they often have religious themes. Gospel music is a newer type of spiritual.

ACROSS THE CURRICULUM

 ▶ **Social Studies** Fisk University, in Nashville, Tennessee, was founded in 1865 and incorporated in 1867 to train African American teachers. In its early years, the university was able to survive only through the fund-raising efforts of the Fisk Jubilee Singers. In a series of extensive (and exhausting) concert tours, the singers popularized African American spirituals among both white and black audiences in the United States and in Europe during the period from 1867 to 1900. Students may be interested in exploring the history of other African American colleges and universities in this country. To learn more about the Fisk Jubilee Singers, invite students to read *A Band of Angels* by Deborah Hopkinson (Atheneum, 1999).

Golden Gospel

Listen to *Jonah*, a gospel song about the man who was swallowed by a whale.

CD 12–10
Jonah

Traditional Gospel Song
as performed by the Golden Gate Quartet

Gospel quartet singing was popular in the 1930s and 1940s. It laid the foundation for many African American popular styles that emerged after World War II.

MUSIC MAKERS

The Golden Gate Quartet

The **Golden Gate Quartet** was a gospel/pop quartet of the 1930s and 1940s. Their smooth harmonies allowed them to cross over into pop music as well. They began recording for RCA/Victor in 1937. This was followed by national radio broadcasts. An appearance on a 1938 "Spirituals to Swing" concert at Carnegie Hall made them coast-to-coast favorites.

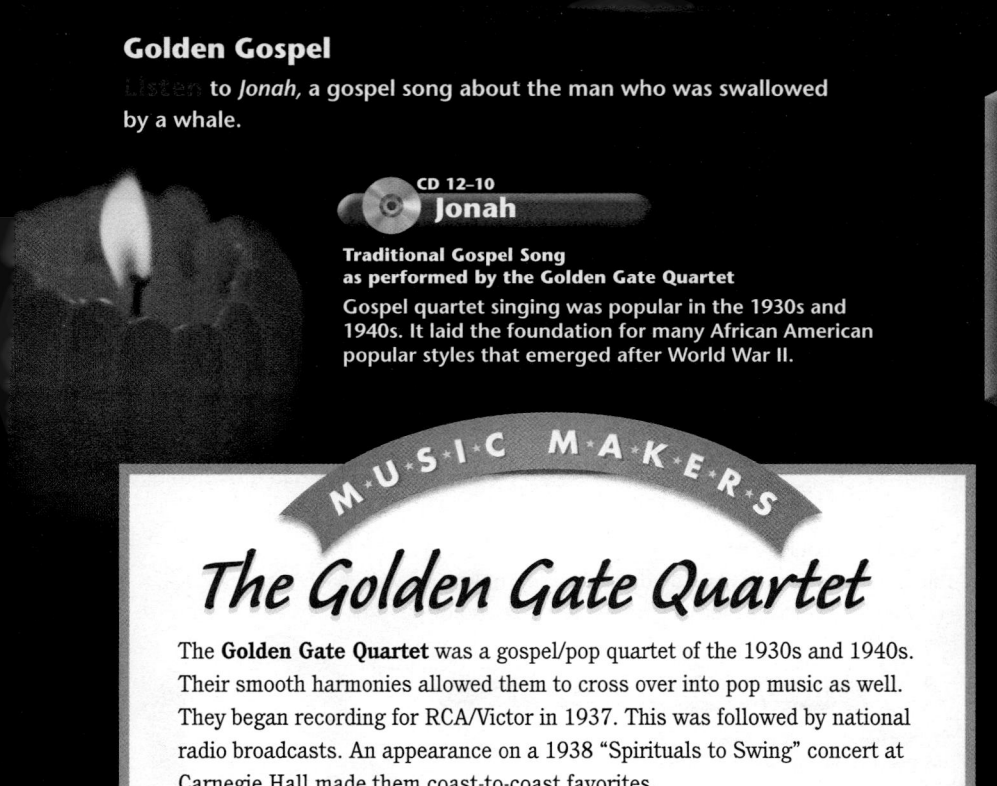

▲ The Golden Gate Quartet and guitar accompanist

Unit 7 **235**

---

3 CLOSE

Element: MELODY ASSESSMENT

6b **Performance/Interview** Ask students to create and sing their own melodies for the new verses of "This Little Light of Mine." Tell them to create their melodies in G-pentatonic. As selected examples are performed for the class, have students interview the performers to discuss and compare the melodic contour of the new melodies with the original melody in lines 5–8 of the song. Have the class discuss the singing styles that are appropriate to gospel music.

SPOTLIGHT ON

8b ▶ **The Golden Gate Quartet** The Golden Gate Quartet began in the 1930s at a barbershop outside Norfolk, Virginia. Members wanted to sing gospel music in the new, looser, more rhythmic "jubilee" style that was popular in Virginia churches. By 1937, with several personnel changes, they had gained a strong regional reputation and were noticed by Bluebird Records talent scout and producer Eli Oberstein. Soon after, their hit "Golden Gate Gospel Train" brought them immediate recognition, and the quartet's highly successful recording career was on its way. Between 1938 and 1941, the quartet gained a national reputation, appearing at Carnegie Hall and at President Franklin Delano Roosevelt's inaugural gala at Constitution Hall.

SCHOOL TO HOME CONNECTION

▶ **Gospel Scrapbook** Ask students to locate gospel choirs in the area and ask the choir members to name which spirituals they most enjoy singing. Students could include the history and sheet music for each favorite song in a scrapbook.

TECHNOLOGY/MEDIA LINK

Video Library The following videos may be used to compare and discuss solo gospel style and gospel choir style.

• *Whitney Houston* singing the "Star-Spangled Banner"
• *The Total Experience Gospel Choir*

LESSON AT A GLANCE

Element Focus   **TIMBRE** Instrument timbres associated with cowboy music

Skill Objective   **LISTENING** Identify and discern the timbres of instruments in cowboy ballads and dance tunes

Connection Objective   **SOCIAL STUDIES** Learn about the historical heyday of the cowboy that followed the Civil War

MATERIALS

- "The Old Chisholm Trail"   **CD 12–12**
  Recording Routine: Intro (4 m.); v. 1; refrain; interlude (1 m.); v. 2; refrain; interlude (1 m.); v. 3; refrain; interlude (1 m.); v. 4; refrain; instrumental; v. 5; refrain; coda
- "Cowboys' Christmas Ball"   **CD 12–15**
  Recording Routine: Intro (9 m.); v. 1; interlude (4 m.); v. 2; interlude (4 m.); v. 3; interlude (4 m.); v. 4; coda
- *The Old Chisholm Trail*   **CD 12–11**
- *Cowboys' Christmas Ball*   **CD 12–14**
- guitars, Autoharps, keyboards (optional)
- map of Texas, Oklahoma, and Kansas

VOCABULARY

cattle drive

◆ ◆ ◆ National Standards ◆ ◆ ◆

1c Sing music from diverse genres
2a Play instruments accurately alone
2d Perform simple accompaniments
6b Listen and analyze uses of timbre in music from diverse genres
8a Show how different arts portray the same emotion in unique ways
8b Identify ways music relates to social studies and language arts

MORE MUSIC CHOICES . . .

For more practice in singing cowboy songs:
"Bury Me Not on the Lone Prairie," p. 19
"El payo," p. 145

TIMBRE ON THE MOVE

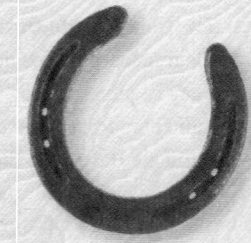

At the end of the Civil War (1861–1865), Texas had nearly five million longhorn cows—some running wild and some in herds. Texans such as Charles Goodnight realized that they could round up and brand the cows. They then herded them up to the railroads in Kansas, or the northern grasslands of Wyoming or Montana, and sold them for a good profit. Thus began the heyday of the cowboy. In 1867 cattle drives sent 35,000 cows northward. By 1871 the number of cows herded north had grown to 600,000.

Listen to country music artist, Charlie Daniels, sing about life on a Chisholm Trail cattle drive. The Chisholm Trail was named for Scottish-Cherokee trader, Jesse Chisholm.

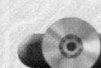
CD 12–11
The Old Chisholm Trail

Traditional Cowboy Song
as performed by Charlie Daniels

Charlie Daniels begins this song with a narrative about cowboys on the trail. What timbres and sound effects set the mood of being on the trail?

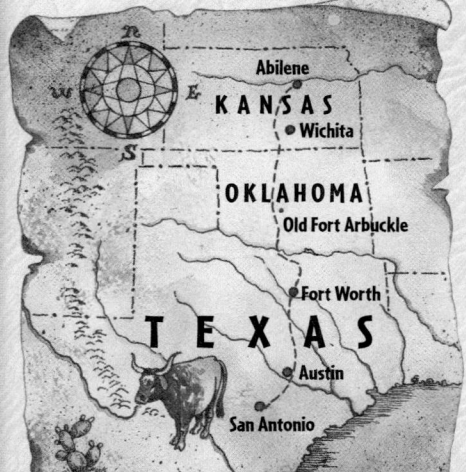

Chisholm Trail Timbres

Analyze the notation of "The Old Chisholm Trail." What instrument might a cowboy play to accompany his singing? How might that influence the melody?

Sing "The Old Chisholm Trail."

Cowboy Life

The typical cowboy was a 19 to twenty year old American Civil War veteran who was seeking adventure in the new American West. On the trail, the cowboy was awakened at first light by the chuck wagon trail cook yelling to come get his bacon, beans, and biscuits. Herding cows on the trail and across rivers all day was a dusty, wet, and dangerous business. It was tough work, earning cowboys just a dollar a day.

Footnotes

CULTURAL CONNECTION

▶ **Singing Movie Cowboys** One of the first singing movie cowboys was the "Father of Country Music," Jimmie Rodgers (1897–1933). Rodgers, known as the "yodeling brakeman," helped establish yodeling in the cowboy singer's repertoire. During the 1930s and 1940s, singer-guitar players Gene Autry, Roy Rogers and Dale Evans, Rex Allen, and many others starred in movies that often featured their songs.

BUILDING SKILLS THROUGH MUSIC

▶ **Reading** Have students read the lyrics of "Cowboys' Christmas Ball" and analyze what the author chose to describe (the landscape, the instruments, the participants, and the dancing) and the order in which he described them.

ACROSS THE CURRICULUM

8b ▶ **Social Studies** Students may read *The Cowboys* from *The Old West* series published by Time-Life Books (1973) for additional information about and outstanding photos of the cowboy era from the Civil War (1865) to the turn of the century.

Invite students to explore these other important cattle trails:

- Shawnee Trail (from Brownsville, Texas to Kansas City and St. Louis)
- Western Trail (from San Antonio, Texas to Dodge City, Kansas and on to Montana and the Dakotas)
- Goodnight-Loving Trail (from West Texas through Colorado to Cheyenne, Wyoming)

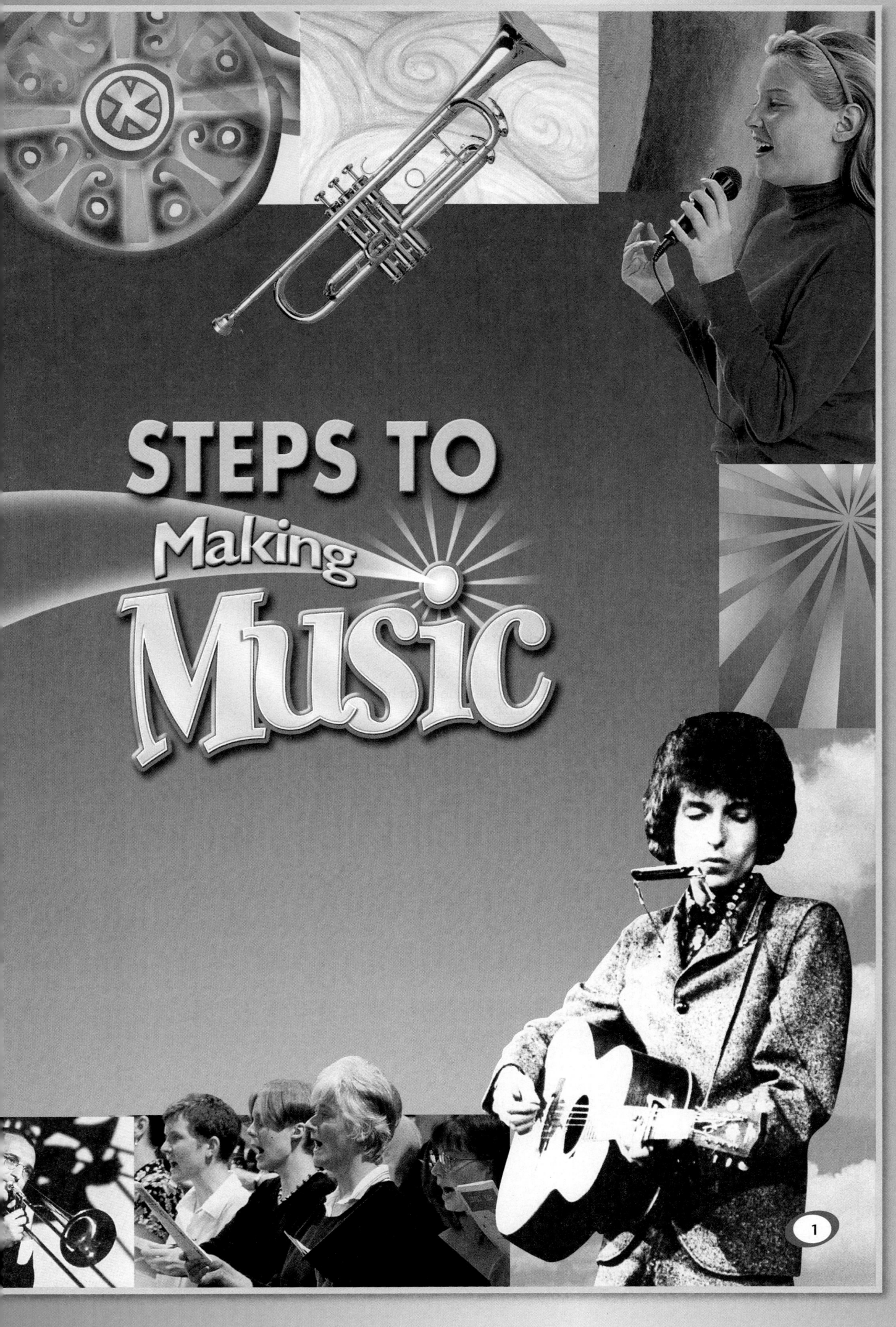

STEPS TO Making Music

1

Lesson	Elements	Skills	

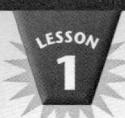

LESSON 1

CORE
Express Yourself
pp. 6–9

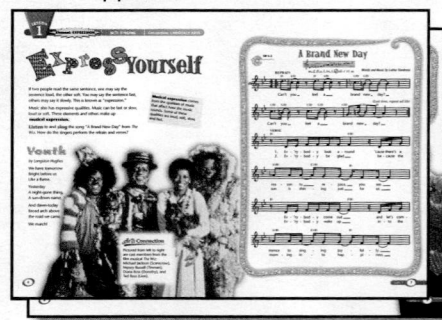

Element: Expression
Concept: Dynamics
Focus: Changes in Dynamics

Secondary Element
Rhythm: tie

National Standards
1a 1b 6a 6b 8b

Skill: Singing
Objective: Sing a song, using dynamic inflection to create expressive effects

Secondary Skills
• **Listening** Listen for excitement expressed; describe music as lively, loud and having a strong beat
• **Singing** Sing a song with proper dynamics
• **Moving** Create movements to show expressive elements of a song
• **Listening** Listen for changes in dynamics and tempo

SKILLS REINFORCEMENT
• **Vocal Development** Tips for proper vocal technique; be aware of changes in voice
• **Keyboard** Review keyboard skills

LESSON 2

Lonesome Cowboy Rhythms
pp. 10–11

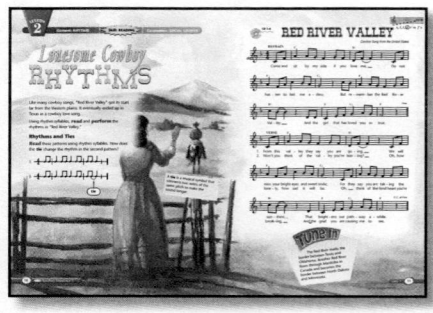

Reading Sequence 1, p. 488

Element: Rhythm
Concept: Duration
Focus: Tie, pickup, and basic note values

Secondary Element
Melody: pentatonic, diatonic scales

National Standards
1a 5a 5b 6a 8b

Skill: Reading
Objective: Read from notation and sing a song that includes ties and pickups

Secondary Skills
• **Listening** Listen to a cowboy song and conduct in meter in 4
• **Reading** Identify rhythmic characteristics of a cowboy song
• **Singing** Sing the song using hand signs and pitch syllables

SKILLS REINFORCEMENT
• **Vocal Development** Use vocal warm-up patterns
• **Recorder** Learn a soprano or alto recorder countermelody
• **Reading** Review rhythms

LESSON 3

CORE
Listen to Lele Bird
pp. 12–13

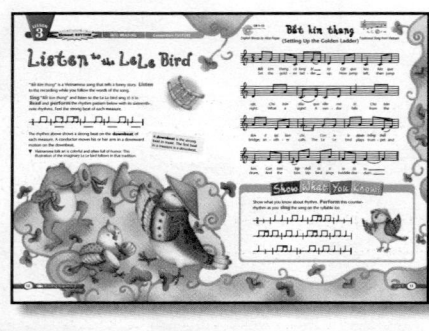

Reading Sequence 2, p. 488

Element: Rhythm
Concept: Patterns
Focus: Dotted-note and sixteenth-note rhythm patterns, and anacrusis

Secondary Element
Melody: pentatonic scale

National Standards
1c 5a 6b 9a

Skill: Reading
Objective: Read and sing from notation a song that includes dotted notes, sixteenth notes, and anacruses

Secondary Skills
• **Listening** Listen to a Vietnamese song and perform a pat-snap ostinato
• **Reading** Speak rhythm syllables while conducting
• **Singing** Identify the pitch set of a song; sing and conduct

SKILLS REINFORCEMENT
• **Reading** Sing a countermelody to a Vietnamese song
• **Singing** Sing other pentatonic song from other cultures
• **Notating** Write bar lines, a pitch set, and a pentatonic melody

Connections

Music and Other Literature

Connection: Language Arts

Activity: Discuss the similarities between expressive devices in poetry and music

CULTURAL CONNECTION
The Wiz Discuss this African American version of *The Wizard of Oz*
Greetings Explore the multitude of greetings in the world

SPOTLIGHT ON
The Poet Discuss Langston Hughes
"A Brand New Day" Discuss this song featured in *The Wiz*

ACROSS THE CURRICULUM
Language Arts Read a poem by Japanese poet Matsuhito
Literature Read *The Wonderful Wizard of Oz*
Art Make "Trold Haugen" trolls

CHARACTER EDUCATION **Freedom** Help students understand freedom

BUILDING SKILLS THROUGH MUSIC **Language** Identify words or phrases that express hope

Song "A Brand New Day"

Listening Selection *Wedding Day at Troldhaugen*
Poems
"Youth"
"I Like You"
M·U·S·I·C M·A·K·E·R·S
Luther Vandross

More Music Choices
"Green, Green Grass of Home," p. 248
"Summertime," p. 250
"This Little Light of Mine," p. 232

ASSESSMENT

Performance/Observation
Sing using dynamic inflection

TECHNOLOGY/MEDIA LINK
Video Library View a performance of a pop singer and discuss the apparent influences

---

Connection: Social Studies

Activity: Discuss ways in which folk music is transmitted beyond its place of origin

MOVEMENT **Patterned Dance** Learn a traditional American dance

ACROSS THE CURRICULUM **Social Studies** Learn geographical background of "Red River Valley"

BUILDING SKILLS THROUGH MUSIC **Math** Solve a music related math problem

Song "Red River Valley"

More Music Choices
"Bury Me Not on the Lone Prairie," p. 19
"Gonna Build a Mountain," p. 21
"*Wai bamba,*" p. 26

ASSESSMENT

Performance/Observation
Sing and conduct a song using hand signs and pitch syllables, then lyrics, while conducting

TECHNOLOGY/MEDIA LINK
MIDI/Sequencing Software Create a multiple-track composition for MIDI drum sounds

---

Connection: Culture

Activity: Read about and discuss the cultural context of traditional Vietnamese melodies

TEACHER TO TEACHER **Teaching Non-English Language Songs** Use Pronunciation Practice track to teach the lyrics of a Vietnamese song

CULTURAL CONNECTION **Vietnamese Music** Background information on Vietnamese music

CHARACTER EDUCATION **Open-mindedness/Respect** Create a recipe for a good listener

BUILDING SKILLS THROUGH MUSIC **Social Studies** Document Vietnam and Vietnamese music

Song "*Bát kim thang*" ("Setting up the Golden Ladder")

More Music Choices
"America, the Beautiful," p. 485
"*Siyahamba,*" p. 212

ASSESSMENT

Performance/Observation
Read and clap a counter-rhythm; sing a song with the counter-rhythm

TECHNOLOGY/MEDIA LINK
Web Site Learn more about the music and culture of Vietnam and other Southeast Asian countries

Lesson	Elements	Skills

LESSON 4

CORE
Building a Song
pp. 14–15

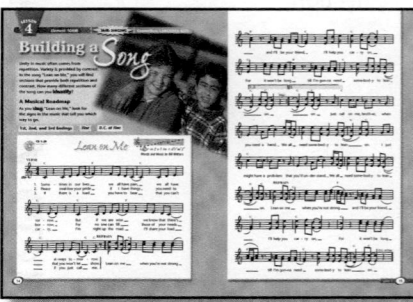

Element: Form
Concept: Form
Focus: Repetition and contrast

Secondary Element
Harmony: harmony in thirds and sixths

National Standards
1c 1d 6a

Skill: Singing
Objective: Sing a song song that illustrates repetition and contrast

Secondary Skills
- **Singing** Sing a song with a recording; learn a harmony part
- **Analyze** Identify contrasting sections of a song

SKILLS REINFORCEMENT
- **Recorder** Play a countermelody on soprano recorder

LESSON 5

Musical Building Blocks
pp. 16–17

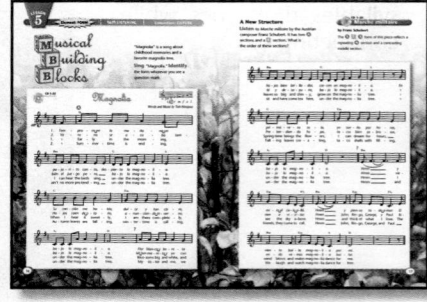

Element: Form
Concept: Form
Focus: ABA and AAB forms

Secondary Element
Timbre: symphony orchestra

National Standards
1c 4a 6a

Skill: Listening
Objective: Identify and describe the differences between contrasting sections of a listening selection

Secondary Skills
- **Singing** Sing a song and identify its form
- **Listening** Listen for contrasting sections, dynamics, and instrumental timbres in a classical piece
- **Creating** Create compositions with AAB or ABA form

SKILLS REINFORCEMENT
- **Creating** Create an AAB or ABA compositions in groups
- **Recorder** Learn a recorder part
Secondary Skills
- **Singing** Sing and analyze a song with sections
- **Creating** Create an AAB or ABA composition

LESSON 6

CORE
Melodic Roundup
pp. 18–19

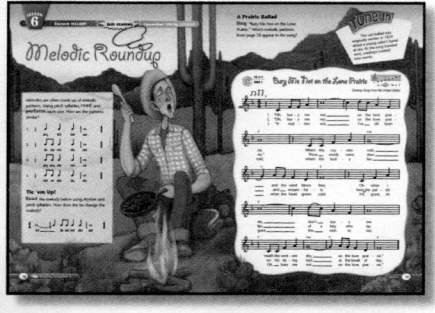

Element: Melody
Concept: Patterns
Focus: Melodic patterns

Secondary Element
Form: phrases

National Standards
1a 2a 5a 5c 6b 6c

Skill: Reading
Objective: Read from notation and sing a pentatonic song

Secondary Skills
- **Reading** Review the tie and pickup
- **Singing** Sing pitch syllables and perform hand signs for melodic patterns; identify the scale used

SKILLS REINFORCEMENT
- **Recorder** Accompany a song with a countermelody
- **Reading** Work with meter in four, ties, and pickups
- **Mallets** Learn an Orff accompaniment
- **Keyboard** Review keyboard skills

Reading Sequence 3, p. 489

Connections

Music and Other Literature

Connection: Language Arts

Activity: Discuss the meaning of lyrics that express ideas about friendship

MEETING INDIVIDUAL NEEDS **Including Everyone** Use small-group activities to build positive relationships

MOVEMENT **Patterned Dance** Learn a dance in pairs

SCHOOL TO HOME CONNECTION
Repetition and Contrast Find local examples of repetition and contrast in visual art and architecture
Family Anecdotes Ask friends and family about a time when someone helped them

BUILDING SKILLS THROUGH MUSIC **Language** Discuss the meaning of lyrics

Song "Lean on Me"

More Music Choices
"Bridges," p. 86
"El cóndor pasa," p. 46
"Free at Last," p. 468

ASSESSMENT

Self-Assessment Sing a song in section

TECHNOLOGY/MEDIA LINK
Electronic Keyboard Create an ABA composition

Connection: Culture

Activity: Discuss aspects of Tejano culture

MEETING INDIVIDUAL NEEDS **English Language Learners** Provide a word bank for students

SPOTLIGHT ON
"Magnolia" and Tejano Music Background on Tejano music, the song, and the composer
The Composer Discuss Austrian composer Franz Schubert

BUILDING SKILLS THROUGH MUSIC **Social Studies** Identify artworks or events that demonstrate the blending of cultures

Song "Magnolia"

Listening Selection *Marche militaire,* p.51, No.1

More Music Choices
"Bridges," p. 86
"Riendo el río corre," p. 263

ASSESSMENT

Written Assessment Listen to a piece and write a comparison of its A and B sections

TECHNOLOGY/MEDIA LINK
Multimedia Create a slide show to accompany a song

Connection: Social Studies

Activity: Read and discuss the lyrics of a song about life as a cowboy in the American West of the late 1800s

ACROSS THE CURRICULUM **Language Arts** Read and dramatize poetry on Old West themes

BUILDING SKILLS THROUGH MUSIC **Language** Create new lyrics for a song

Song "Bury Me Not on the Lone Prairie"

More Music Choices
"Bắt kim thang," p. 13
"Glory, Glory Hallelujuah," p. 54

ASSESSMENT

Performance/Observation Read and sing a song using pitch syllables and hand signs

TECHNOLOGY/MEDIA LINK
MIDI/Sequencing Software Create an accompaniment for a song using a bass part and arpeggiated harmonies
Video Library Introduce MIDI technology with a video

Lesson	Elements	Skills

LESSON 7

Reach for the Sky!

pp. 20–21

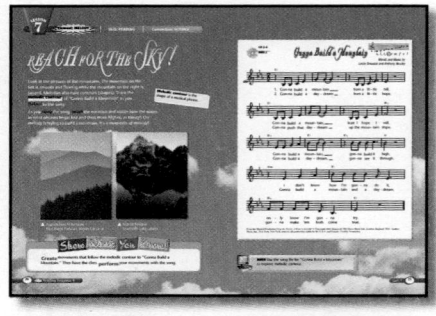

Reading Sequence 4, p. 489

Element: Melody
Concept: Pitch and Direction
Focus: Melodic contour, diatonic melody

Secondary Element
Rhythm: 2/2 meter

National Standards
1a 5b 5c 6b 6c

Skill: Reading
Objective: Read and sing ascending and descending melodic contours

Secondary Skills
- **Listening** Listen to and read a song; trace the melodic contour of the melody
- **Reading** Identify the pitch set of two sections of a song
- **Singing** Conduct and say rhythm syllables, then show hand signs and sing pitch syllables

---

SKILLS REINFORCEMENT
- **Vocal Development** Develop breath support

LESSON 8

Musical Shapes

pp. 22–23

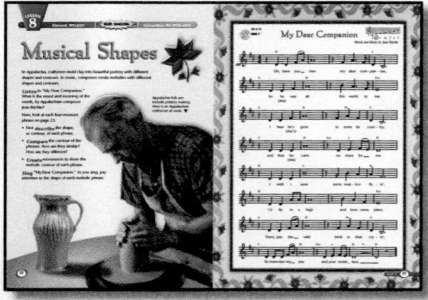

Element: Melody
Concept: Pattern
Focus: Melodic contour

Secondary Element
Melody: pentatonic scale

National Standards
1a 1b 7b 8b

Skill: Singing
Objective: Sing a song with phrases that have similar melodic countour

Secondary Skills
- **Listening** Listen to melodic characteristics of a song
- **Singing** Sing an Appalachian song with a recording and draw the shape of each melody heard
- **Create** Create a dance for an Appalachian song

SKILLS REINFORCEMENT
- **Movement** Create a dance for a song

LESSON 9

CORE
Vocal Timbres

pp. 24–25

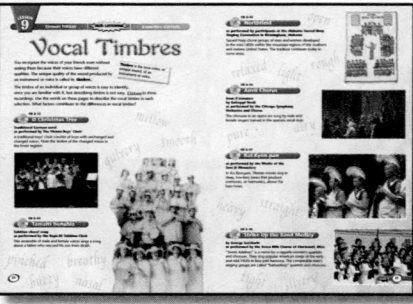

Element: Timbre
Concept: Texture
Focus: Vocal timbre (choral)

Secondary Element
Timbre: folk instruments

National Standards
6b 7a 9b

Skill: Listening
Objective: Listen to vocal choral timbres from diverse cultures

Secondary Skills
- **Analyzing** Describe vocal timbre and determine texture
- **Listening** Understand how vocal timbre may be influenced by culture and region

---

Connections

Music and Other Literature

Connection: Science

Activity: Investigate the processes through which mountains are created

ACROSS THE CURRICULUM **Science** Research plate tectonics and mountains

MEETING INDIVIDUAL NEEDS **Composing** Compose a melody that follows the contour of a given pattern

BUILDING SKILLS THROUGH MUSIC **Social Studies** List mountain ranges of the United States

Song "Gonna Build a Mountain"

More Music Choices
"Bury Me Not on the Lone Prairie," p. 19
"My Dear Companion," p. 23

ASSESSMENT

Performance/Observation Sing phrases and first show the contour of each, then use pitch syllables and hand signs

TECHNOLOGY/MEDIA LINK

MIDI/Sequencing Software Use the graphic editor to examine melodic contour

---

Connection: Related Arts

Activity: Explore folk arts and crafts of Appalachia

ACROSS THE CURRICULUM **Related Arts** Discuss background information on the film "The Songcatcher"

MOVEMENT **Movement** Create a dance for an Appalachian song

CULTURAL CONNECTION **Music of Southern Appalachia** Discuss Appalachian music expert Jean Ritchie

BUILDING SKILLS THROUGH MUSIC **Reading** Identify the mood of lyrics

Song "My Dear Companion"

More Music Choices
"Gonna Build a Mountain," p. 21
"Vive l'amour," p. 176

ASSESSMENT

Performance/Observation Sing a song and trace the shape of the melody

TECHNOLOGY/MEDIA LINK

MIDI/Sequencing Software Sing and record an improvised melody and harmony using a digital audio program

Web Site Learn more about Appalachian music and instruments

Connection: Culture

Activity: Explore diverse cultures and their styles of choral music

TEACHER TO TEACHER **Unusual Vocal Sounds** Discuss what vocal sounds make people laugh

CULTURAL CONNECTION
Tahiti Discuss European influence on the indigenous vocal timbre of this island
Tibetan Monasteries Discuss chant abilities of Tibetan monks

SPOTLIGHT ON
Il Trovatore and the Anvil Chorus Discuss this famous Italian opera
Sacred Harp Singing Facts about the style's history

SCHOOL TO HOME CONNECTION **Timbre** Search Strengthen sensitivity to different timbre

BUILDING SKILLS THROUGH MUSIC **Language** Complete a Semantic Feature Analysis

Listening Selections
O Christmas Tree
Tamaiti hunania
Northfield
Anvil Chorus
Kui.Kyon.pan
Strike Up the Band Medley

More Music Choices
"Key to the Highway," p. 243
"Mr. Tambourine Man," p. 148
"It Don't Mean a Thing," p. 386

ASSESSMENT

Music Journal Writing Describe various vocal timbres

TECHNOLOGY/MEDIA LINK

Video Library Watch the video *Bobby McFerrin* to see a master of vocal timbre

Lesson	Elements	Skills

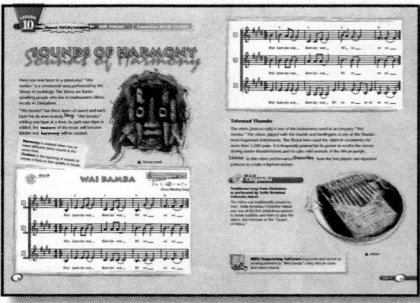

LESSON 10
Sounds of Harmony

pp. 26–27

Element: Texture/Harmony
Concept: Texture
Focus: Layered ostinatos

Secondary Element
Timbre: folk instruments

National Standards
1a 1c 4c 6a 6b

Skill: Singing
Objective: Sing a song using layered parts

Secondary Skills
- **Listening** Listen for the number of voices in a song; listen for and discuss the *mbira*
- **Singing** Sing a song in three ostinato layers

SKILLS REINFORCEMENT
- **Playing** Accompany an African song with percussion

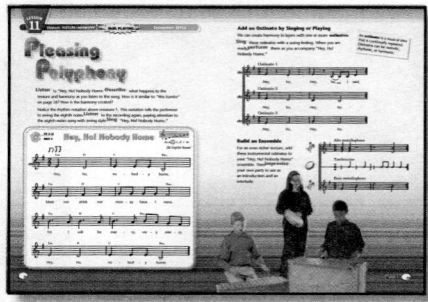

LESSON 11
CORE
Pleasing Polyphony

pp. 28–29

Element: Texture/Harmony
Concept: Texture
Focus: Layering (density, ostinatos)

Secondary Element
Timbre: folk instruments

National Standards
1a 2a 4b 4c

Skill: Playing
Objective: Play an accompaniment using layered ostinatos

Secondary Skills
- **Listening** Listen to layered ostinatos
- **Singing** Sing a melody with a recording; count the number of ostinatos used in the accompaniment
- **Playing** Create and play ostinatos as accompaniment

SKILLS REINFORCEMENT
- **Mallets** Learn an Orff accompaniment
- **Keyboard** Play an ostinato accompaniment
- **Signing** Learn the signing for an Old English round

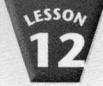

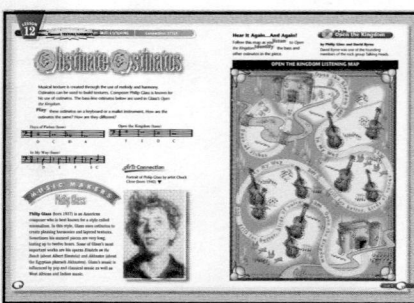

LESSON 12
Obstinate Ostinatos

pp. 30–31

Element: Texture/Harmony
Concept: Texture
Focus: Changes in density

Secondary Element
Timbre: individual vocal

National Standards
4a 6b 9b

Skill: Listening
Objective: Identify changes in the texture of a listening selection

Secondary Skills
- **Listening** Listen and recognize characteristics of a minimalist piece
- **Analyzing** Recognize patterns and changing textures in a minimalist piece
- **Playing** Play ostinatos

SKILLS REINFORCEMENT
- **Creating** Create a collective minimalist composition using eight-beat percussive ostinatos

Connections

Music and Other Literature

Connection: Social Studies

Activity: Explore the history and culture of the Shona farmers of southeast Africa

SPOTLIGHT ON *Mbira* Share information about this African percussion instrument

ACROSS THE CURRICULUM

Social Studies Learn more about celebrations from around the world

Language Arts Learn about the *mbira's* role in ceremonial events

TEACHER TO TEACHER **The Changing Voice** Singing ostinatos with a narrow range will be easier for those with changing voices

BUILDING SKILLS THROUGH MUSIC **Social Studies** List songs utilized in celebrations or events

Song *"Wai bamba"*

Listening Selection
Chigamba

More Music Choices
"Banuwa," p. 294
"Gloria, Gloria," p. 459
"Let Us Sing Together," p. 156

ASSESSMENT

Performance/Self-Assessment Perform a song in three parts

TECHNOLOGY/MEDIA LINK

MIDI/Sequencing Software Use African sounds on a MIDI device to improvise melodic and rhythmic patterns

---

Connection: Style

Activity: Discover what makes "swing" notes different from other rhythms

MOVEMENT **Patterned Dance** Perform a movement for an Old English round

TEACHER TO TEACHER **The Changing Voice** Singing ostinatos with a narrow range will be easier for those with changing voices

BUILDING SKILLS THROUGH MUSIC **Visual Arts** Represent musical textures with visual art

Song *"Hey, Ho! Nobody Home"*

More Music Choices
"Dona nobis pacem," p. 125
"Scattin' A-Round," p. 160

ASSESSMENT

Performance/Self-Assessment Perform a round with layered ostinatos

TECHNOLOGY/MEDIA LINK

MIDI/Sequencing Software Use a MIDI file to create multiple-track percussion arrangements of a round

---

Connection: Style

Activity: Experience minimalist style and the use of ostinatos

ACROSS THE CURRICULUM **Visual Arts** Create a "laser" show for a selection using flashlights

SPOTLIGHT ON **Minimalism** Discuss characteristics of minimalism

BUILDING SKILLS THROUGH MUSIC **Language** Experiment with minimalism in writing

Listening Selection *Open the Kingdom* (excerpt)

M•U•S•I•C M•A•K•E•R•S
Philip Glass

Listening Map *Open the Kingdom*

More Music Choices
"Fais do do," p. 403
"Free at Last," 468
"Ise oluwa," p. 230

ASSESSMENT

Observation Identify the number of layers in the texture of a minimalist piece

TECHNOLOGY/MEDIA LINK

Transparency Use listening map to follow ostinatos

Web Site Learn more about minimalism in music and painting

INTRODUCING THE UNIT

Unit 1 presents the first step in a sequenced approach to understanding musical elements. Using the musical skills of Performing, Listening, Reading, Moving, and Creating, the students will review musical concepts and elements as they develop their musical skills and appreciation of music. A brief overview of the skills assessed in this unit can be found on p. 3. Unit highlights are on pp. 4–5 and curricular experiences are listed in the footnotes. Students will enjoy their journey to a lifetime of musical enjoyment as they *Let the Music Begin.*

UNIT PROJECT

Ask students to read the Enjoy Life paragraph on p. 2.

Tell students the lyrics to John Mellencamp's song, "Your Life Is Now," present an opportunity to have students envision their future life and how it might be different from their parents' or grandparents' lives.

Have students respond to any of the following questions:

- If I could be anything I wanted, I would be a . . .
- Some of the people who make real contributions to the lives of others in our communities are . . .
- People I admire the most are . . .
- Opportunities that I have that my parents did not have are . . .

Student responses could come in many forms:

- A written description.
- A photograph of that kind of person.
- A drawing or painting.
- A description from a book or magazine.

Invite students to create a bulletin board display on the theme of Your Life is Now, using the materials they gather from above. Expand the bulletin board with *musical* ideas that can enrich their lives as they progress through Unit 1.

Enjoy Life

Congratulations, you're in the sixth grade!
You're on your way to bigger and better things.

Being in the sixth grade is not always easy. After all, you still have homework and tests. Part of learning to succeed is knowing how to balance your responsibilities (school) and your personal life (having fun, we hope).

In his song "Your Life Is Now," John Mellencamp reminds us to make the most of each day. Be responsible, and remember to enjoy yourself, your family, your friends, and life.

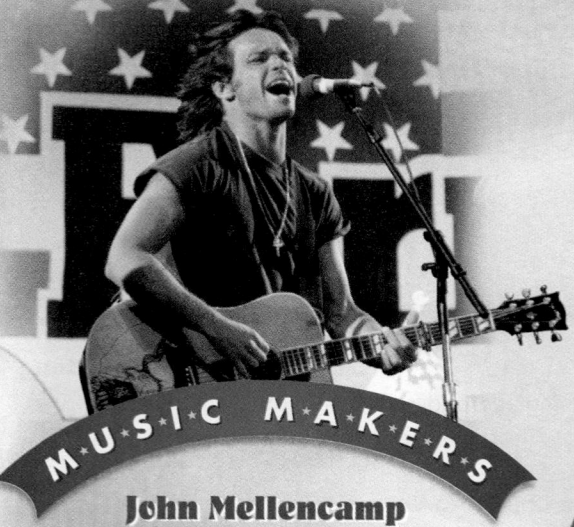

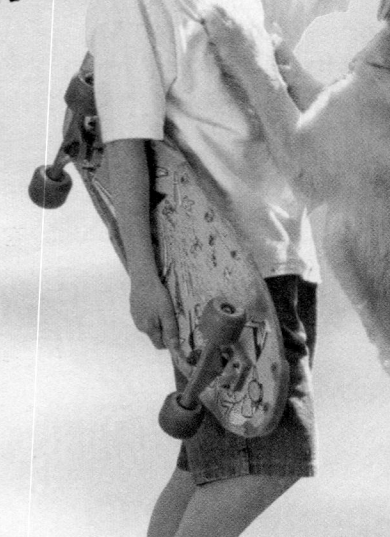

MUSIC MAKERS

John Mellencamp

John Mellencamp (born 1951) joined his first band when he was in the fifth grade. Since then, he has had an extensive and successful musical career, selling over 25 million albums in the U.S. alone. He has over 36 gold, platinum, and multi-platinum awards and has been nominated for 11 Grammy awards. Mellencamp has given several concerts for Farm Aid and has devoted much of his time to helping autistic children.

2

ACROSS THE CURRICULUM

Unit Highlights The following interdisciplinary activities in this unit are related to the music elements presented in the lessons and are intended to enhance student learning. For a more detailed topical description, see the Unit at a Glance on pp. 1a–1h.

▶ **ART/DRAMA**

- Create a "Troldhaugen" troll using a variety of media (p. 8)
- See a film about and learn about musicologists and Appalachian mountain songs (p. 22)
- Create a laser show based on musical ostinatos (p. 30)

▶ **LANGUAGE ARTS**

- Read an eighth-century Japanese poem (p. 7)
- Read a book that inspired the musical *The Wiz* (p. 8)
- Read and dramatize poems about cowboys (p. 18)
- Read a book about the African *mbira* (p. 27)

▶ **SOCIAL STUDIES**

- Trace the historical movement of a cowboy song (p. 11)
- Read about celebrations around the world (p. 27)

▶ **SCIENCE**

- Investigate the science of mountain building (p. 20)

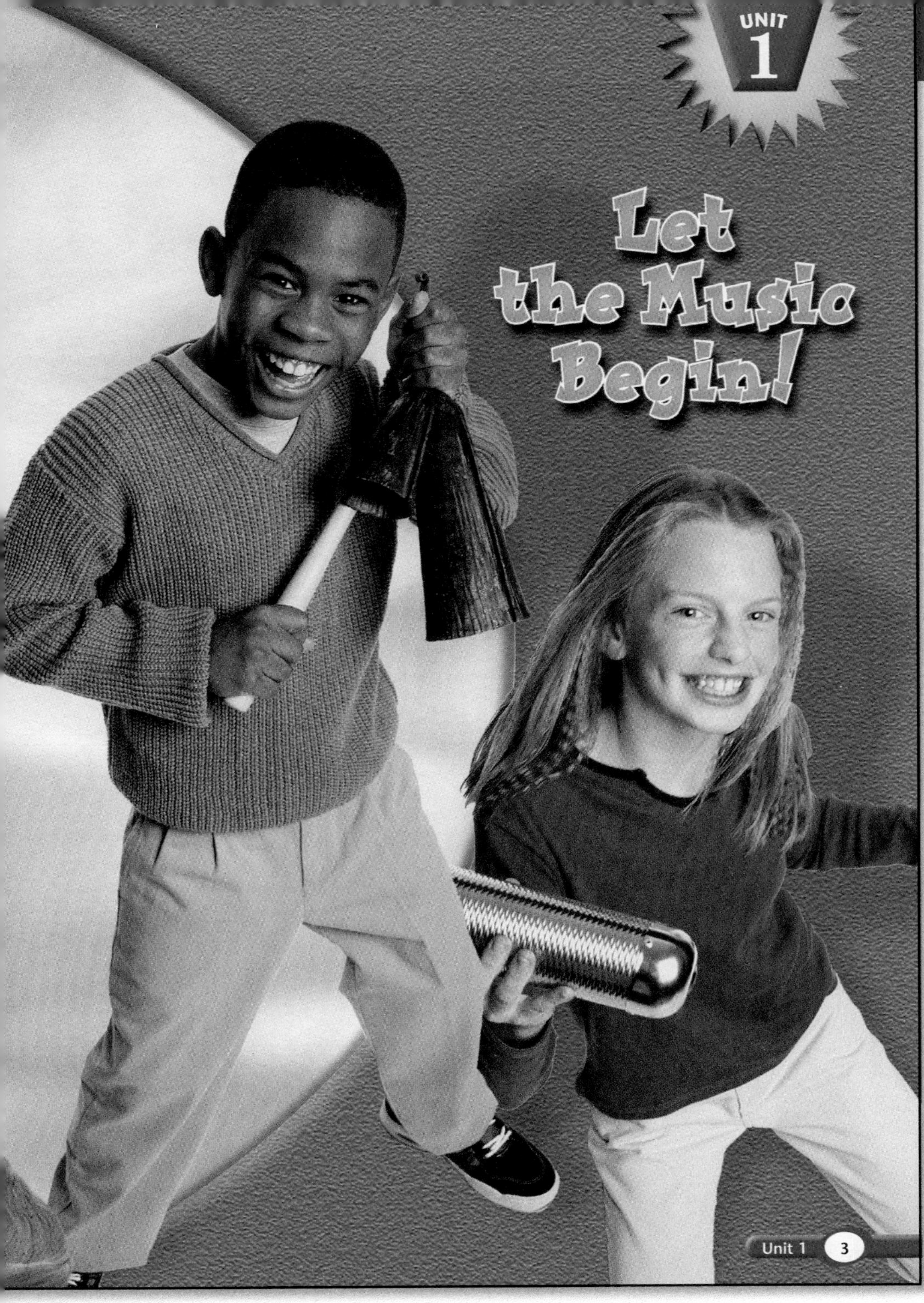

Let the Music Begin!

Unit 1 ③

MUSIC SKILLS
ASSESSED IN THIS UNIT

Reading Music: Rhythm

- Read and sing from notation that includes ties and pickups (p. 10)
- Read and sing from notation that includes dotted-note rhythms and anacrusis (p. 12)

Reading Music: Pitch

- Read and sing a pentatonic song (p. 18)
- Read and sing "Gonna Build a Mountain," demonstrating melodic contour (p. 20)

Performing Music: Singing

- Sing "A Brand New Day," using dynamic inflections to create expression (p. 6)
- Sing "Lean on Me," illustrating repetition and contrast (p. 14)
- Sing *Wai bamba"* in layered parts (ostinatos) (p. 26)

Performing Music: Playing

- Play a percussion accompaniment (p. 28)
- Play an ostinato accompaniment (p. 28)

Listening to Music

- Listen to *March militaire,* identifying A and B sections (p. 16)
- Listen to and identify vocal timbres from diverse cultures (p. 24)
- Identify changes in ostinato textures (p. 30)

Moving to Music

- Perform a movement, using repetition and contrast (p. 14)
- Trace the melodic contours for "My Dear Companion," as students sing (p. 22)

Creating Music

- Create a chant in AAB or ABA form (p. 16)
- Create an eight-beat rhythmic ostinato (p. 30)

CULTURAL CONNECTION

Unit Highlights The musical literature in this unit provides many opportunities for students to explore a variety of world cultures. A more detailed description of the resources and activities listed below can be found in the Unit at a Glance on pp. 1a–1h.

▶ AFRICAN AMERICAN

- Learn about the African American version of *The Wizard of Oz* (p. 6)

▶ AMERICAN

- Discover the many ways people greet each other (p. 8)
- Discover facts about Appalachian songwriter Jean Ritchie (p. 22)

▶ ASIAN

- Learn about Vietnamese melodies (p. 12)
- Learn facts about Tibetan chants (p. 24)

▶ SOUTH PACIFIC

- Discover facts about Tahiti and its choral music (p. 24)

OPENING ACTIVITIES

MATERIALS

- "Your Life Is Now," p. 4   **CD 1-1**

    Recording Routine:
    Intro (4 m.); v. 1; refrain; interlude (2 m.); v. 2; refrain; interlude (10 m.); refrain; coda

Listening

Have students read the Music Makers feature on John Mellencamp on p. 2. Invite students to listen to "Your Life Is Now" **CD 1-1**, as they follow along in their books.

Reading

Direct students to the notation of "Your Life Is Now." Ask students to look for and analyze the following:

- Lyrics. Discuss what students think is the meaning of *Your father's days are lost to you,* or all of verse 2.
- Key signature and keynote (F major; F)
- What notes are used in this song? (F G A C D C♯)
- Repeated melodic motives or phrases. (phrases 1 and 2 are similar; many motives using pitches A, F, and G)
- Syncopations. (The refrain is full of good examples.)

Singing

Have students work out small sections of the melody in the following order:

- Refrain: mm. 1–4; 5–10; last 5 measures
- Entire refrain
- Verse 1: first two phrases, then remainder
- Verse 2

Sing the entire song with the Stereo Performance track **CD 1-2.**

Moving

Invite students to feel the eighth-note subdivision of the beat by having them

- First, tap the four beats of each measure on their thighs with their dominant hand.

Enjoy Music

Sing "Your Life Is Now."
Enjoy the song. Enjoy life now!

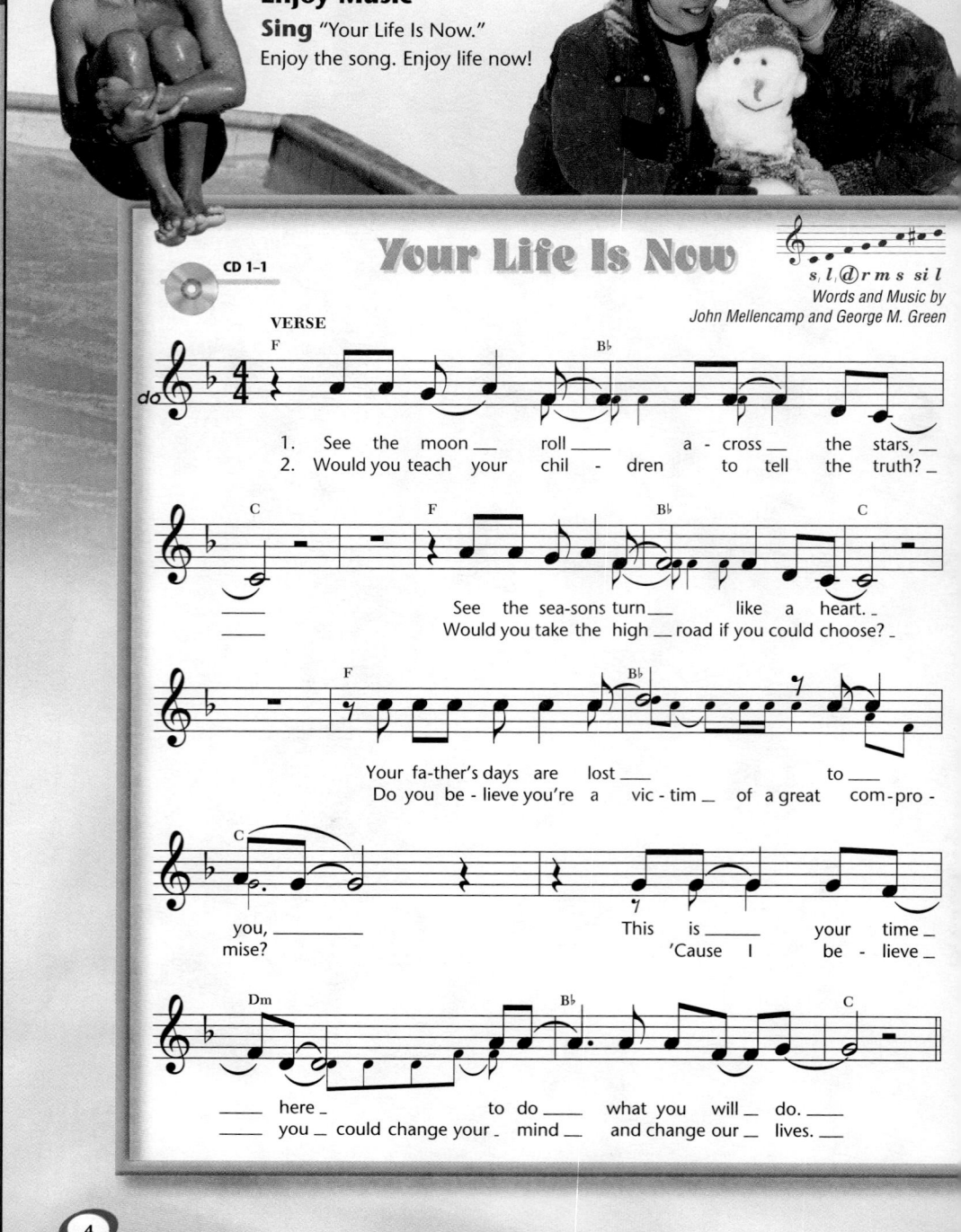

CD 1–1

Your Life Is Now

s l ⓐ *r m s s i l*
Words and Music by John Mellencamp and George M. Green

VERSE

1. See the moon __ roll __ a - cross __ the stars,
2. Would you teach your chil - dren to tell the truth? __

See the sea-sons turn __ like a heart. __
Would you take the high __ road if you could choose? __

Your fa-ther's days are lost __ to __
Do you be - lieve you're a vic - tim __ of a great com-pro-

you, __ This is __ your time __
mise? 'Cause I be - lieve __

___ here __ to do __ what you will __ do. __
___ you __ could change your __ mind __ and change our __ lives. __

4

ASSESSMENT

Unit Highlights This unit includes a variety of strategies and methods, described below, to track students' progress and assess their understanding of lesson objectives. Reproducible masters for Show What You Know! and Review, Assess, Perform, Create can be found in the Resource Book.

▶ **FORMAL ASSESSMENTS**

The following assessments, using written language, cognitive aware-ness, and performance skills, help teachers and students conceptual-ize the learning that is taking place.

- **Show What You Know!** Element-specific assessments, on the student page, for Rhythm (p. 13) and Melody (p. 20).
- **Review, Assess, Perform, Create** This end-of-unit activity (pp. 32–33) can be used for review and to assess students' learning of the core lessons in this unit.

▶ **INFORMAL ASSESSMENTS**

At the close of each Teacher's Edition lesson in this unit, one of the following types of assessments is used to evaluate the learning of the key element focus or skill objective.

- Music Journal Writing (p. 25)
- Observation (p. 31)
- Performance/Observation (pp. 9, 11, 13, 19, 21, 23)
- Performance/Self-Assessment (p. 15, 27, 29)
- Written Assessment (p. 17)

▶ **RUBRICS**

Visit *www.sfsuccessnet.com* for rubrics to assess students' achievement in music skills.

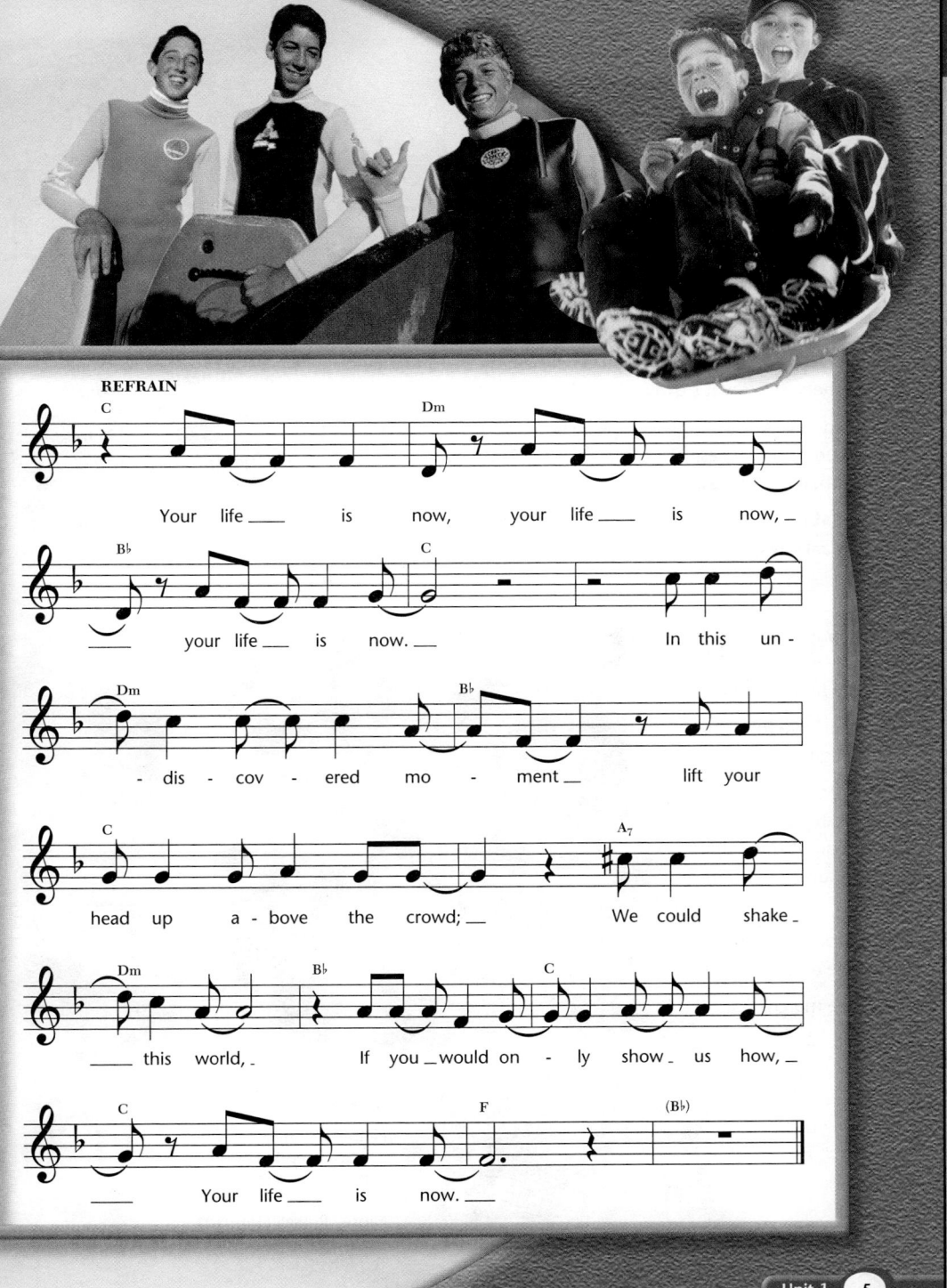

REFRAIN

Your life ___ is now, your life ___ is now, ___

___ your life ___ is now. ___ In this un-

- dis - cov - ered mo - ment ___ lift your

head up a - bove the crowd; ___ We could shake ___

___ this world, ___ If you ___ would on - ly show ___ us how, ___

Your life ___ is now. ___

Unit 1   **5**

- Next, hold their other hand about six inches above their thigh while the tapping continues.
- Tap their thighs (down) on the beat and their other hand (up) on the offbeat.
- Count *1 and 2 and 3 and 4 and.*
- Realize that the up-beats are where the syncopations come.
- Continue tapping while they say the refrain phrase, *In this undiscovered moment.* (All syllables except *In* are on the up-beat.)

Creating

Have students improvise on the F major pentatonic (F G A C D) against the chord background of the first four measures.

Use *Band-in-a-Box* to provide the background chords, or have some students play the chords on keyboards, guitars (capo 3: play D, G, A), or Autoharps.

Start the improvisation using only the notes F, G, and A; then add the C and D when ready.

Instruments that work well for the improvisation include Resonator bells; Recorder; Xylophone; Guitar; and Keyboard.

INNOVATIVE TEACHER SUPPORT FOR THIS UNIT

- **MAKING MUSIC DVD, Grade 6** contains video segments that support lessons, including signing and movement.
- **MAKING MUSIC with Movement and Dance** provides more opportunities for large group activities in music or physical education classes.
- **MAKING MUSIC with Technology** provides lesson plans for many technology applications; includes MIDI files.
- *¡A cantar!* features recorded songs and lessons from around the Spanish-speaking world; includes strategies for bilingual classes and for English-speaking teachers working with Spanish-speaking students.
- **Bridges to Asia** features recorded songs and lessons from Asian and Pacific region cultures.
- *www.sfsuccessnet.com* provides an online lesson planner to conveniently create lesson plans at school or at home. Includes rubrics for assessment, lesson modifications to meet the needs of all students, performance musicals based on program content, and more.

TECHNOLOGY/MEDIA LINK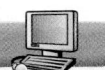

Unit Highlights The following components are used in this unit to reinforce and expand students' understanding of music.

▶ **ELECTRONIC KEYBOARD**

- Create an ABA composition, using an electronic keyboard (p. 15)

▶ **MIDI/SEQUENCING SOFTWARE**

- Create a multiple-track for MIDI drum sounds (p. 11)
- Sequence bass and harmony parts (p. 19)
- Explore the melodic contour, using a graphic editor (p. 21)
- Improvise and record a vocal harmony (p. 23)
- Explore African sounds on a MIDI keyboard (p. 27)
- Create a drum composition for "Hey, Ho! Nobody Home" (p. 29)

▶ **MULTIMEDIA**

- Create a multimedia slide show of Mexican or *Tejano* art and photos to accompany the song "Magnolia" (p. 17)

▶ **TRANSPARENCY**

- Display the listening map for *Open the Kingdom* (p. 31)

▶ **VIDEO LIBRARY/DVD**

- Show the video *Whitney Houston* (p. 9)
- Watch *Using MIDI in the Elementary Music Classroom* (p. 19)
- See a video about Bobby McFerrin and his voice (p. 25)

▶ **WEB SITE/DVD**

- Learn more about Vietnamese culture and music (p. 13)
- Learn more about Appalachian music and instruments (p. 23)
- Learn about minimalism in music and painting (p. 31)

LESSON AT A GLANCE

Element Focus	**EXPRESSION** Changes in dynamics
Skill Objective	**SINGING** Sing a song, using dynamic inflection to create expressive effects
Connection Activity	**LANGUAGE ARTS** Discuss the similarities between expressive devices in poetry and music

MATERIALS

- "A Brand New Day" **CD 1-3**
  Recording Routine: Intro (4 m.); refrain; v. 1; refrain; v. 2; refrain
- *Wedding Day at Troldhaugen* **CD 1-5**
- "Youth" (poem)
- "I Like You" (poem)
- **Resource Book** pp. H-2–H-6

VOCABULARY

expression   dynamics   tempo

◆ ◆ ◆ ◆ National Standards ◆ ◆ ◆ ◆

1a Sing accurately in small and large ensembles
1b Sing easy pieces with expression
6a Listen and describe events in music using appropriate terms
6b Listen and analyze uses of dynamics in music from diverse genres
8b Identify ways music relates to language arts

MORE MUSIC CHOICES

For more practice with expression:
"Green, Green Grass of Home," p. 248
"Summertime," p. 250
"This Little Light of Mine," p. 232

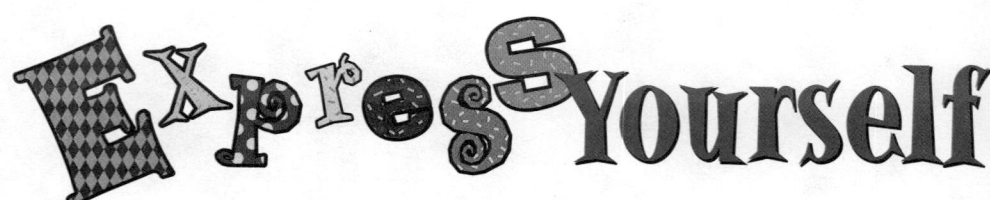

Express Yourself

If two people read the same sentence, one may say the sentence loud, the other soft. You may say the sentence fast, others may say it slowly. This is known as "expression."

Music also has expressive qualities. Music can be fast or slow, loud or soft. These elements and others make up **musical expression.**

Listen to and **sing** the song "A Brand New Day" from *The Wiz.* How do the singers perform the refrain and verses?

> **Musical expression** comes from the qualities of music that affect how the music sounds. Some of these qualities are loud, soft, slow, and fast.

Youth

by Langston Hughes

We have tomorrow
Bright before us
Like a flame.

Yesterday
A night-gone thing,
A sun-down name.

And dawn-today
Broad arch above
the road we came.

We march!

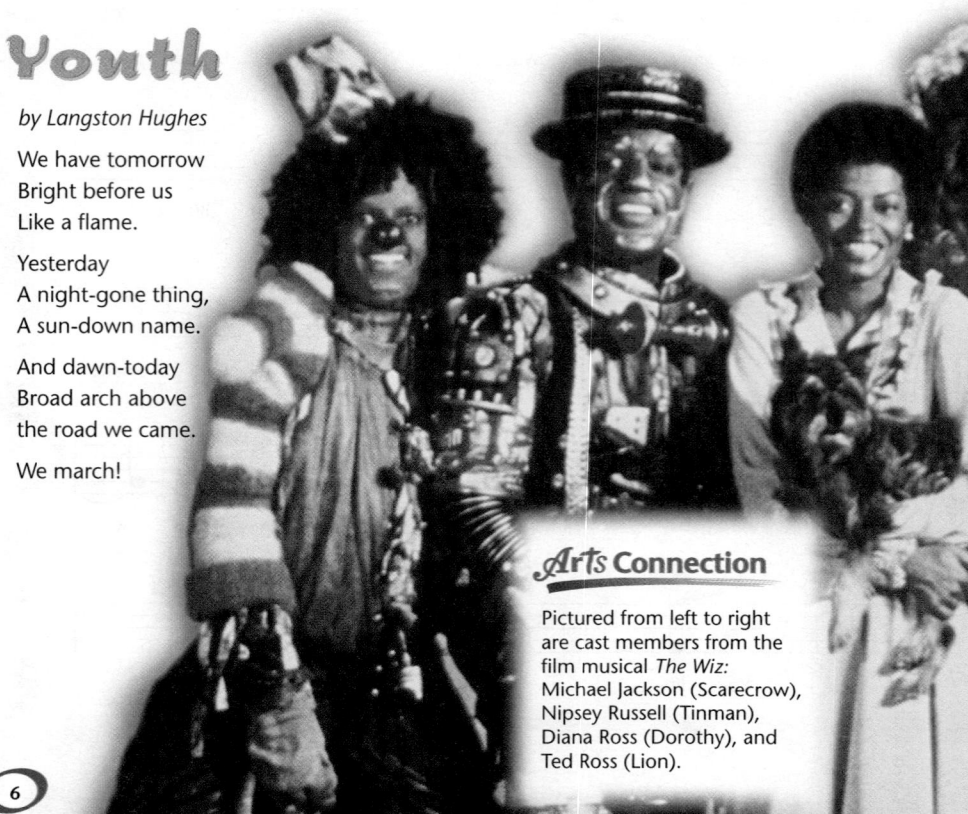

Arts Connection

Pictured from left to right are cast members from the film musical *The Wiz:* Michael Jackson (Scarecrow), Nipsey Russell (Tinman), Diana Ross (Dorothy), and Ted Ross (Lion).

6

Footnotes

CULTURAL CONNECTION

▶ **The Wiz** This updated African American version of the popular movie classic *The Wizard of Oz* is set in an inner city neighborhood and includes characters with an urban-culture flair. Quincy Jones scored the film and William Brown wrote the story.

▶ *Troldhaugen* Literally, "Hill of the Trolls." It is the name of Edvard Grieg's home in Bergen, Norway.

BUILDING SKILLS THROUGH MUSIC

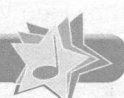

▶ **Language** Have students identify the words or phrases that express hope or optimism in the lyrics of "A Brand New Day." Ask them how Langston Hughes expresses hope in the poem "Youth." Have them compare the differences and effectiveness of each.

SPOTLIGHT ON

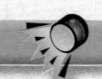

▶ **The Poet** Langston Hughes (1902–1967), one of the greatest African American authors of the twentieth century, was born in Joplin, Missouri. After his parents divorced, Hughes and his mother moved to Kansas. Hughes also lived with his father for a short time in Mexico. He returned to the United States and began writing poetry when he was in high school. Hughes was also an excellent writer of fiction and drama. Most of his work is about African American culture. Hughes is still considered one of the most versatile and prolific of modern American authors.

▶ **"A Brand New Day"** This song was featured in the movie version of *The Wiz,* although it did not appear in the Broadway musical. Your students might enjoy watching *The Wiz* on video to see how "A Brand New Day" fits into the plot.

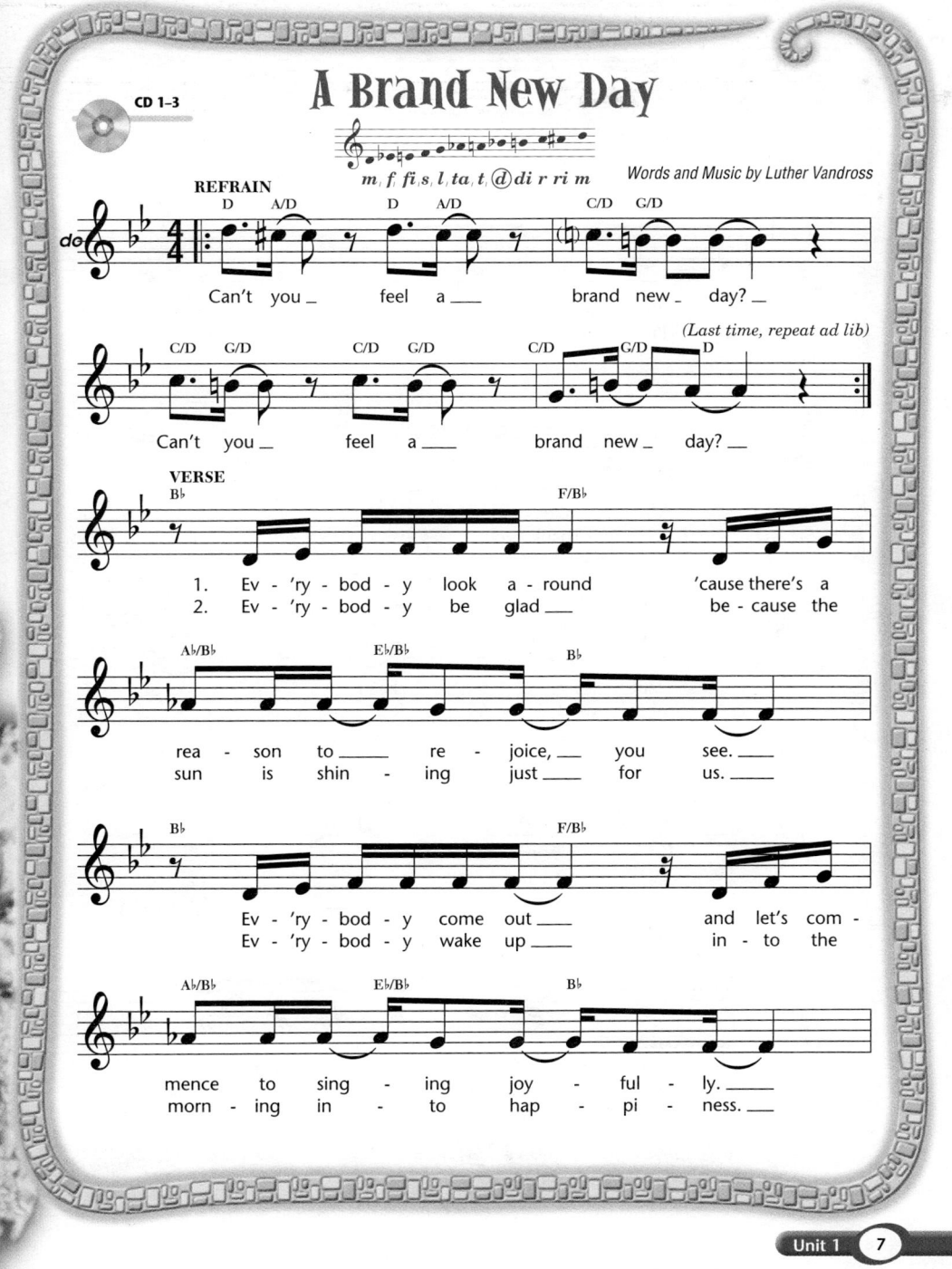

A Brand New Day

Words and Music by Luther Vandross

REFRAIN

Can't you __ feel a __ brand new __ day? __

(Last time, repeat ad lib)

Can't you feel a __ brand new __ day? __

VERSE

1. Ev - 'ry - bod - y look a - round 'cause there's a
2. Ev - 'ry - bod - y be glad ___ be - cause the

rea - son to _____ re - joice, ___ you see.
sun is shin - ing just _____ for us.

Ev - 'ry - bod - y come out _____ and let's com -
Ev - 'ry - bod - y wake up _____ in - to the

mence to sing - ing joy - ful - ly. _____
morn - ing in - to hap - pi - ness. _____

Unit 1 7

---

continued on page 8

1 INTRODUCE

Invite students to

- Read the poem "Youth" from the student text.
- Discuss the meaning of the poem. (It is about forgetting the past, living for today, and planning for the future.)

As students take turns reading the poem, help them discover that each student reads the poem differently. (Some read it louder than others, some read faster, and different words may be stressed.)

8b Ask students to read about expression in music, on p. 6 in their books.

Share with students the poem "I Like You," found in Across the Curriculum below, and discuss the similarities and relationships between expressive devices in poetry and music. For example, ask students how dynamics would affect expression in music, and in poetry.

2 DEVELOP

Listening

Invite students to listen to "A Brand New Day" **CD 1-3.** As they listen, students should think about why the music is exciting.

Help students discover that both the poem and the lyrics of the song celebrate today rather than the past.

ASK How do the singers seem to feel about this new day? (The singers are excited.)

6a How does the music express their excitement? (The music is lively, loud, and has a strong beat.)

Is one section of the song louder than the other? (The refrain is performed louder than the verses.)

ACROSS THE CURRICULUM

▶ **Language Arts** Share a poem from the eighth-century Japanese poet Matsuhito in *A Poem a Day* by Helen H. Moore (Scholastic, 1997). Have students take turns reading the poem with different kinds of expression.

I Like You

Although I saw you
The day before yesterday,
And yesterday, and today,
This much is true—
I want to see you tomorrow, too!

SKILLS REINFORCEMENT

1a ▶ **Vocal Development** Help students' vocal needs by singing vocalises and songs in varied keys. Aim for a uniform vocal quality in all registers. Add harmony parts so that all may participate. Familiarize students with vocal change concepts.

At the start of each class, review the following. Posture: sit and stand to allow proper breathing. Breathing: exhale on *sss*—start at eight counts, build to twenty. Placement: hum "whirlies" in each vocal register. Range: sing three-note (*mi–re–do*) and five-note (*do–re–mi–fa–so*) vocalises, from A4 to G5. Intonation: sing major chords (B♭–G), major scales, and arpeggios.

▶ **Keyboard** Use Resource Book pp. H-2–H-6 to review keyboard skills used throughout this book.

Unit 1 *Let the Music Begin!* 7

Lesson 1 Continued

Singing

Invite students to

- Sing the song, reminding them to sing the refrain louder than the verses.

- Volunteer as soloists or in small groups to sing each phrase of the verses, with the entire class singing the refrain.

Help students discover that adding and deleting voices or instruments is one way of making music louder or softer.

ASK What is another way to make music louder? (Sing with more volume.)

SAY The music term for "volume" is *dynamics*.

Moving

Encourage students to create movements that reflect the expressive elements in "A Brand New Day." Then have them perform their movements with the song.

Inform students that "A Brand New Day" was composed by Luther Vandross and encourage them to read about him in the Music Makers feature on p. 9 in their books.

Listening

Have students listen to *Wedding Day at Troldhaugen* **CD 1-5** and raise their hands whenever they hear a change in dynamics.

ASK What methods did the composer use to create loud and soft dynamics? (Dynamic changes are created primarily through the type and number of instruments playing.)

Did anything else change in the music? (Yes, there are changes in tempo.)

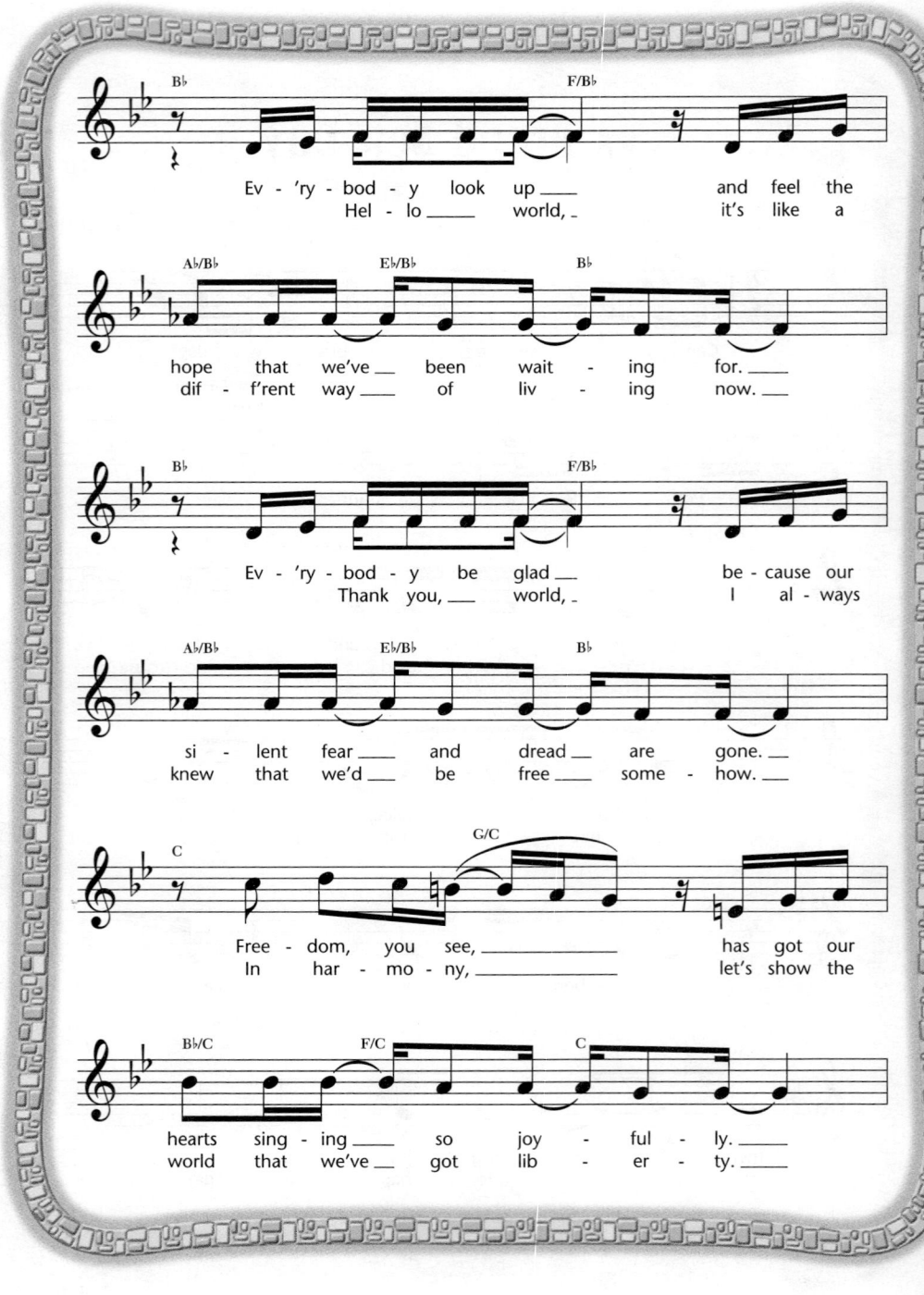

⑧

Footnotes

CULTURAL CONNECTION

▶ **Greetings** "A Brand New Day" deals with greeting the day and new beginnings. Brainstorm with students the many possibilities of greetings.

Ask students

- How do we greet each other with words? With movements?

- How do young people today greet each other?

- How did people greet each other in earlier times?

- How do people greet someone who is very important?

- Are there different greetings in different cultures?

- Do special groups, such as sports teams and scouting organizations, have specific greetings?

ACROSS THE CURRICULUM

▶ **Literature** Encourage students to read the book *The Wonderful Wizard of Oz*. Written by L. Frank Baum in 1900, it is the inspiration for *The Wiz* and the movie *The Wizard of Oz*.

▶ **Art** Invite students to create their own "Troldhaugen" trolls. They might draw, paint, sculpt, or create a fabric troll.

CHARACTER EDUCATION

▶ **Freedom** To help students understand freedom and its responsibilities, ask them to list the decisions and choices they are free to make. Then have them make a list of choices they are not free to make. Ask them, why can't they make these choices right now? Which of these choices can they make as they get older?

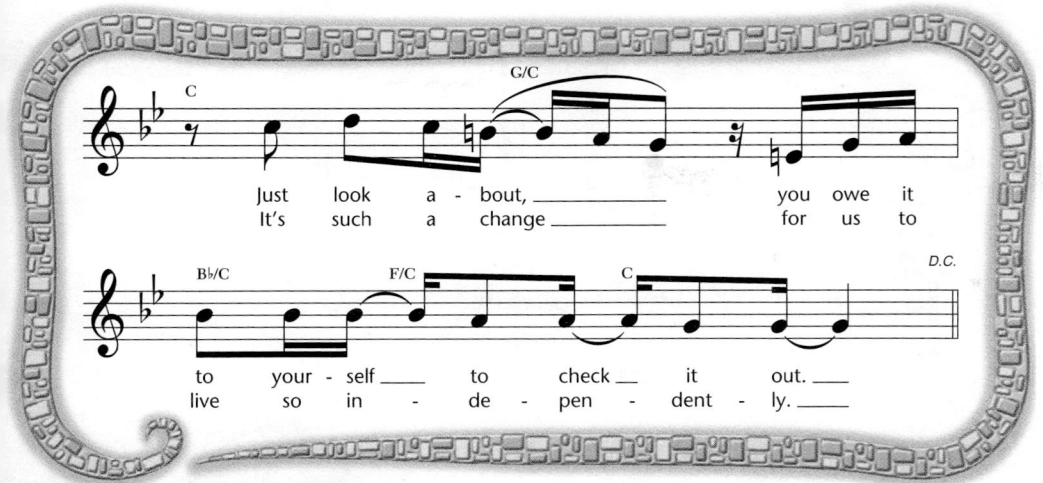

Just look a - bout, _____ you owe it
It's such a change _____ for us to

to your - self ___ to check __ it out.
live so in - de - pen - dent - ly. ___

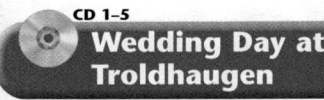

Luther Vandross

Luther Vandross (born 1951) is a performer and a composer. Vandross began playing piano at age three and started his professional career singing jingles and backup for other performing artists. His songwriting breakthrough came in 1972 when "A Brand New Day" was included in the hit musical *The Wiz*. Vandross has written songs for Whitney Houston, Ringo Starr, and Aretha Franklin. His albums typically go platinum.

A Musical Story

Expressive elements are found in all styles of music.
Listen to *Wedding Day at Troldhaugen*. What expressive elements do you hear?

CD 1–5
Wedding Day at Troldhaugen

from *Lyric Suite*, **Op. 65, No. 6**
by Edvard Grieg

Wedding Day at Troldhaugen uses Norwegian melodies. Troldhaugen, Grieg's home, means Troll's Hill. Do you know what trolls are?

Unit 1 **9**

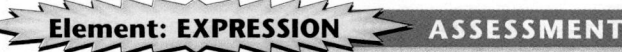

3 CLOSE

Element: EXPRESSION | **ASSESSMENT**

Performance/Observation Have students

 • Sing "A Brand New Day" **CD 1-3**, using dynamic inflection to convey the feelings expressed in the song text.

• Sing the song again, with small groups singing the verse and the entire class singing the refrain.

Observe whether the students perform the song with the appropriate dynamic inflections.

SKILLS REINFORCEMENT

▶ **Vocal Development** When boys are around 12 years old, their voices typically begin to change. Some sixth-grade boys will have a two-octave singing range, while others may lose the ability to sing comfortably in the middle or upper registers.

Female vocal change is less dramatic. Signs of a girl's vocal change include huskiness in the speaking voice and breathiness in the singing voice. Teachers may refer to *Teaching Kids to Sing* by Kenneth Phillips (Wadsworth Publishing, 1996) for more information on this subject.

SCHOOL TO HOME CONNECTION

▶ **Goals** Ask students to make a list of their hopes and dreams. Next to each idea, students can write one thing they could do now to reach their goal. If a student expresses the desire to go to college, for example, he or she can write, "I will work hard in school and do all my assignments on time."

TECHNOLOGY/MEDIA LINK

Video Library Have students view a video of another popular singer, Whitney Houston. Ask them to discuss the popular and gospel influences on her singing style.

LESSON AT A GLANCE

Element Focus   **RHYTHM** Tie, pickup, and basic note values

Skill Objective   **READING** Read from notation and sing a song that includes ties and pickups

Connection Activity   **SOCIAL STUDIES** Discuss ways in which folk music is transmitted beyond its place of origin

MATERIALS

- "Red River Valley"   **CD 1-6**
  Recording Routine: Intro (2 m.); refrain; v. 1; refrain; interlude (4 m.); v. 2; refrain; coda
- Music Reading Practice, Sequence 1   **CD 1-8**
- Resource Book pp. E-2, I-3
- Dance Directions for "Red River Valley," p. 554

VOCABULARY

anacrusis   tie   pickup   diatonic

> ◆ ◆ ◆ ◆ **National Standards** ◆ ◆ ◆ ◆
>
> **1a** Sing accurately in large ensembles
> **5a** Read quarter and eighth notes in duple meter
> **5d** Use standard notation to record musical ideas
> **6a** Listen and describe events in music using appropriate terms
> **8b** Identify ways music relates to social studies

MORE MUSIC CHOICES. . .

For more practice with ties:
"Bury Me Not on the Lone Prairie," p. 19
"Gonna Build a Mountain," p. 21
"Wai bamba," p. 26

1 INTRODUCE

Lead students in a discussion of the American cowboy song tradition and the westward expansion of the nineteenth century. See Across the Curriculum on p. 11 for information to share with students.

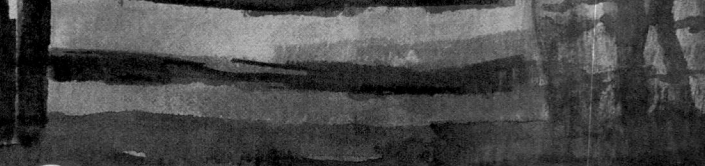

Lonesome Cowboy RHYTHMS

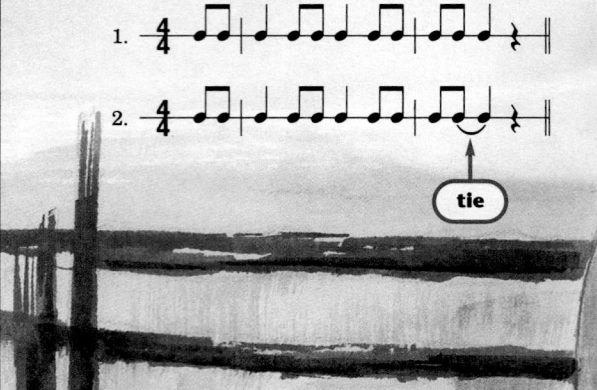

Like many cowboy songs, "Red River Valley" got its start far from the Western plains. It eventually ended up in Texas as a cowboy love song.

Using rhythm syllables, **read** and **perform** the rhythms in "Red River Valley."

Rhythms and Ties

Read these patterns using rhythm syllables. How does the **tie** change the rhythm in the second pattern?

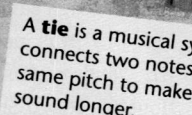

A **tie** is a musical sym connects two notes same pitch to make t sound longer.

tie

Footnotes

MOVEMENT

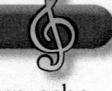

▶ **Patterned Dance** See Dance Directions, beginning on p. 554, for the "Red River Valley" progressive trio dance. This American folk dance has been a traditional favorite for decades.

Use the Dance Practice Track **CD 1-12** for additional help in learning the routine. Use Dance Performance Track **CD 1-11** when performing the dance routine.

BUILDING SKILLS THROUGH MUSIC

▶ **Math** Have students solve the following problem. If a = the number of times the rhythm on p. 10 appears in the verse, and b = the number of times that rhythm appears in the refrain, formulate an equation for how many times that rhythm will occur when singing the entire song (both verses and following the D.C. al Fine). (Ans. $2a + 3b = x$)

SKILLS REINFORCEMENT

1a ▶ **Vocal Development** Here are some vocal warm-up echo patterns to use for reading "Red River Valley."

mi–re–do   re–do–la₁–so₁–do

do–mi–so–fa–mi   so–fa–mi–re–do–re–mi–so–fa

fa–mi–do–la₁   fa–la₁

fa–la₁–so₁–la₁–ti₁–do   fa–la₁–so₁–ti₁–do–re–mi–re–do

▶ **Recorder** Resource Book p. I-3 offers a countermelody that can be played on recorder with the verse of "Red River Valley."

▶ **Reading** Lead students in a review of time signature, number of beats per measure, and quarter-note, quarter-rest, eighth-note, and half-note rhythms. See p. 488, or Resource Book p. E-2, for additional Music Reading Practice.

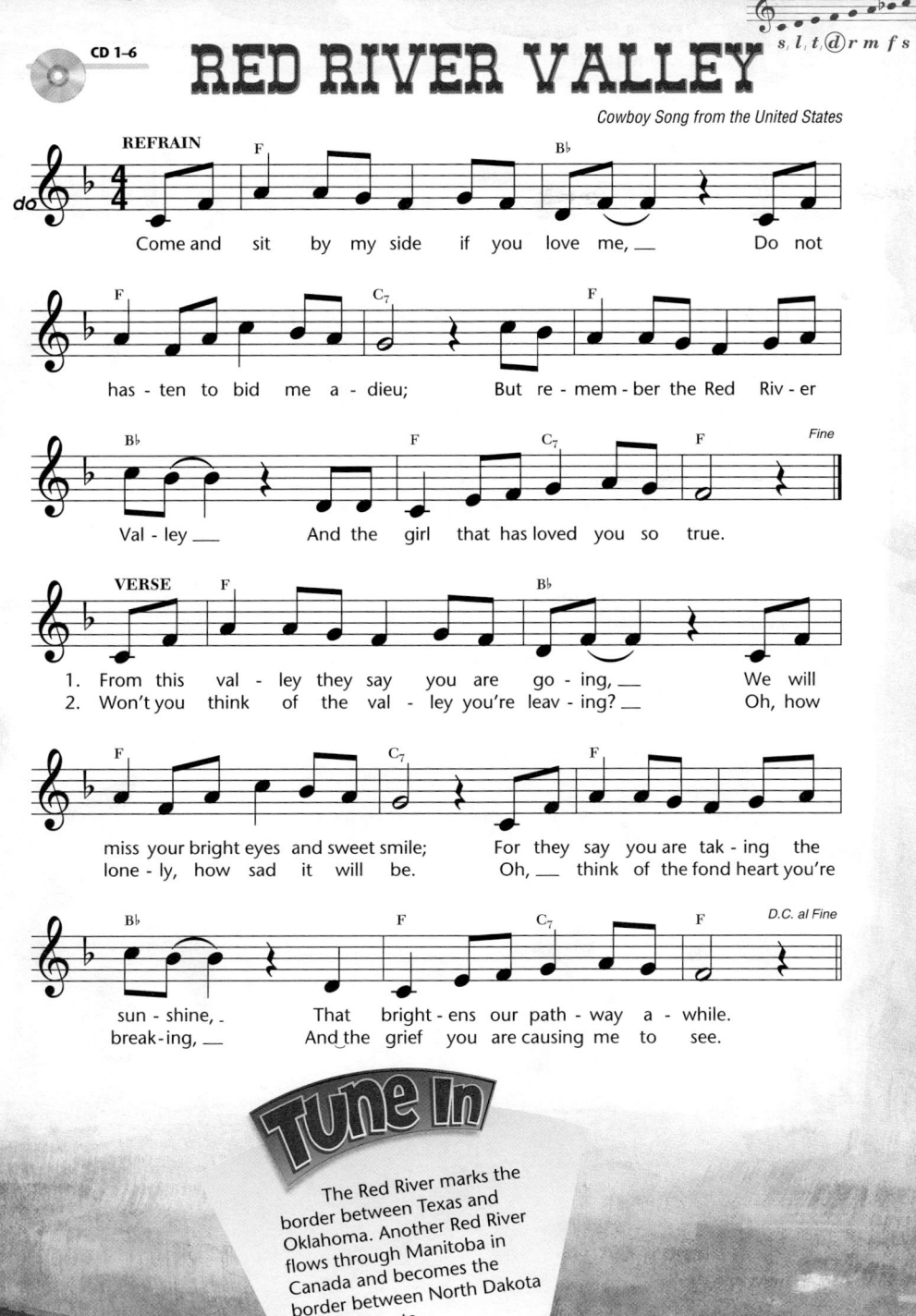

RED RIVER VALLEY

s l t (d) r m f s

CD 1–6

Cowboy Song from the United States

REFRAIN

Come and sit by my side if you love me, — Do not has-ten to bid me a-dieu; But re-mem-ber the Red Riv-er Val-ley — And the girl that has loved you so true.

VERSE

1. From this val-ley they say you are go-ing, — We will miss your bright eyes and sweet smile; For they say you are tak-ing the sun-shine, — That bright-ens our path-way a-while.
2. Won't you think of the val-ley you're leav-ing? — Oh, how lone-ly, how sad it will be. Oh, — think of the fond heart you're break-ing, — And the grief you are caus-ing me to see.

Fine

D.C. al Fine

Tune In

The Red River marks the border between Texas and Oklahoma. Another Red River flows through Manitoba in Canada and becomes the border between North Dakota and Minnesota.

2 DEVELOP

Listening

6a Have students listen to "Red River Valley" **CD 1-6** and conduct in meter in 4. Have them identify that the first refrain is a slow introduction.

Reading

ASK What rhythmic features are in measure 2 that are not in measure 1? (tie, quarter rest)

5a Have students locate all ties in the song, then

- Conduct and say the rhythm syllables for the rhythms on p. 10.
- Find rhythm pattern 2 in the notation on p. 11.

SAY A pickup is the pitch or group of pitches before the first downbeat. A pickup is also called an anacrusis.

ASK How many pickups are in "Red River Valley?" (8)

What is different about the last pickup? (It is a quarter note.)

Singing

5d Lead students in singing the F-*do* diatonic scale with hand signs and pitch syllables. Have the students arrange the pitches in "Red River Valley" from lowest to highest on a staff.

- Sing the scale with hand signs and pitch syllables.

5a - Read and sing "Red River Valley" using pitch syllables.

3 CLOSE

Skill: READING　　　　**ASSESSMENT**

5a **Performance/Observation** Have students read and sing "Red River Valley" from the notation, using hand signs and pitch syllables. Observe their ability to accurately read and sing from the notation.

ACROSS THE CURRICULUM

8b ▶ **Social Studies** Folk music is transmitted from one area to another when people move from one area to another and take their favorite music with them. In the 1800s, cowboys from Manitoba (a central province in Canada) sang about their Red River Valley. Have students locate the province and river on a map. The cowboys gradually moved down as far as Texas in the 1880s and kept singing their song. There is another Red River that marks the boundary of Oklahoma and Texas, and people in these states may think of this river when they sing the song. Have students locate this Red River on a map. Ask them to find information about early settlers of these Red River Valleys, including Native Americans, Spanish settlers, and pioneers from the eastern United States and Europe.

TECHNOLOGY/MEDIA LINK

MIDI/Sequencing Software Prepare the computer to be used as a learning center. In small groups, students will create a multiple-track composition for MIDI drum sounds. Have students

- Set keyboard for percussion sounds.
- Experiment with percussion sounds.
- Perform and record several tracks of whole-, half-, quarter-, and eighth-note rhythms, using various percussion sounds.
- Play compositions back for other small groups.

LESSON AT A GLANCE

Element Focus	**RHYTHM** Dotted-note and sixteenth-note rhythm patterns, and anacrusis
Skill Objective	**READING** Read and sing from notation a song that includes dotted notes, sixteenth notes, and anacrusis
Connection Activity	**CULTURE** Read about and discuss the cultural context of traditional Vietnamese melodies

MATERIALS

- "Bắt kim thang" — CD 1-13
  Recording Routine: Intro (free tempo); instrumental; vocal
- **Pronunciation Practice/Translation** p. 521
- **Music Reading Practice, Sequence 2** — CD 1-17
- **Resource Book** pp. A-2, B-2, C-4, D-3, E-3

VOCABULARY

downbeat   upbeat   anacrusis   pickup   bar lines

♦ ♦ ♦ ♦ **National Standards** ♦ ♦ ♦ ♦

1c Sing music from diverse cultures
5a Read quarter and eighth notes in duple meter
6b Listen and analyze uses of rhythm in music from diverse cultures
9a Describe characteristics of music styles from a variety of cultures

MORE MUSIC CHOICES

For more practice with duple meter with one-beat pickups:
"America, the Beautiful," p. 485
"Siyahamba," p. 212

1 INTRODUCE

Discuss with students the information on Vietnamese music in Cultural Connection, below, and invite them to read the suggested books that give a cultural context to the music.

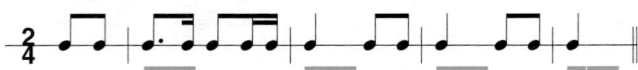
Element: RHYTHM | Skill: READING | Connection: CULTURE

Listen to the LeLe Bird

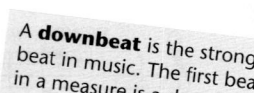

"Bắt kim thang" is a Vietnamese song that tells a funny story. **Listen** to the recording while you follow the words of the song.

Sing "Bắt kim thang" and listen to the Le Le bird sing tò tí te.
Read and **perform** the rhythm pattern below with its sixteenth-note rhythms. Feel the strong beat of each measure.

The rhythm above shows a strong beat on the **downbeat** of each measure. A conductor moves his or her arm in a downward motion on the downbeat.

▼ Vietnamese folk art is colorful and often full of humor. This illustration of the imaginary Le Le bird follows in that tradition.

> A **downbeat** is the strong beat in music. The first beat in a measure is a downbeat.

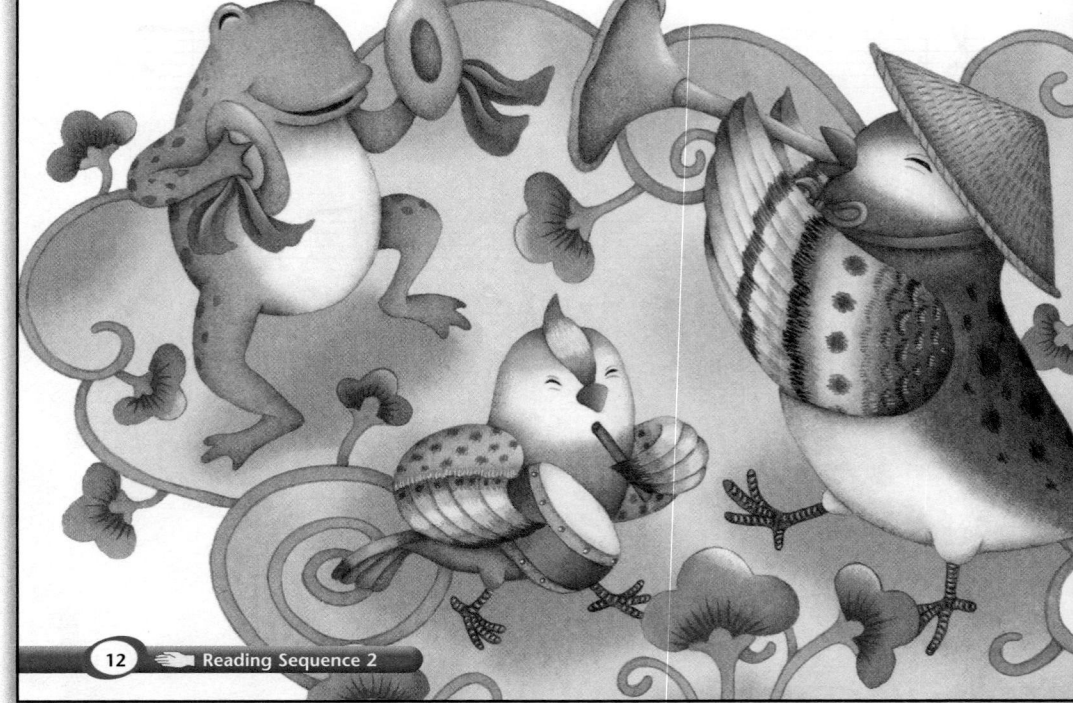

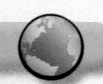

Footnotes

TEACHER TO TEACHER

▶ Teaching Non-English-Language Songs

To give students an opportunity to hear a native speaker sing "Bắt kim thang" in Vietnamese, play the Pronunciation Practice Track **CD 1-16.** Then distribute copies of Resource Book p. A-2, the Pronunciation Practice Guide, and use the Pronunciation Practice/Translation on p. 521 to teach the Vietnamese version.

BUILDING SKILLS THROUGH MUSIC

▶ **Social Studies** Have students use a KWHL Chart (Resource Book p. C-4) to document what the class knows about Vietnam and Vietnamese music, generate questions they want to answer, and brainstorm ways to research the answers. On another day the students can report their new knowledge to the class to complete the chart.

CULTURAL CONNECTION

9a ▶ **Vietnamese Music** Traditional Vietnamese melodies are mostly pentatonic but may also include passing tones, equivalent to the Western fa and ti scale degrees. Vietnamese performers often ornament melodies. This is known as hoa lá, "adding flowers and leaves." Many Vietnamese people emigrated to the United States in the last several decades, so Vietnamese music is becoming part of America's cultural heritage. Students may enjoy hearing examples of Vietnamese music found in Patricia Shehan Campbell's *Sounds of the World, Music of Southeast Asia: Lao, Hmong, Vietnamese* (Music Educators National Conference, 1986) and Campbell and Nguyen's *From Rice Paddies and Temple Yards: Traditional Music of Vietnam* (World Music Press, 1996).

Bắt kim thang
s l ⓓ r m

English Words by Alice Firgau
(Setting Up the Golden Ladder)
Traditional Song from Vietnam

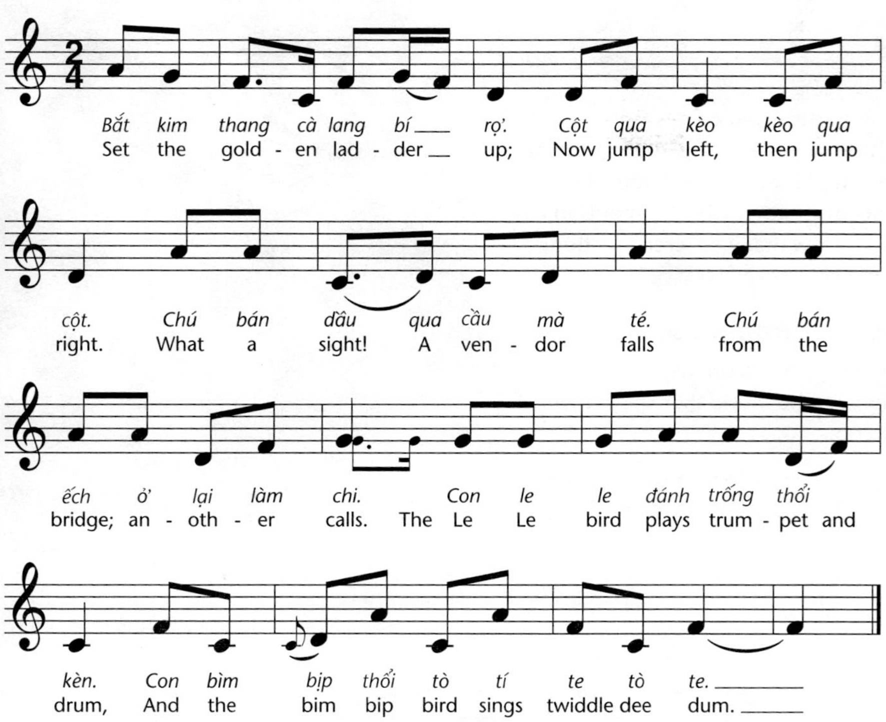

Bắt kim thang cà lang bí___ rọ'. Cột qua kèo kèo qua
Set the gold - en lad - der___ up; Now jump left, then jump

cột. Chú bán dầu qua cầu mà té. Chú bán
right. What a sight! A ven - dor falls from the

ếch ở' lại làm chi. Con le le đánh trống thổi
bridge; an - oth - er calls. The Le Le bird plays trum - pet and

kèn. Con bìm bịp thổi tò tí te tò te.___
drum, And the bim bip bird sings twiddle dee dum.___

Show What You Know!

Show what you know about rhythm. **Perform** this counter-rhythm as you **sing** the song on the syllable *loo*.

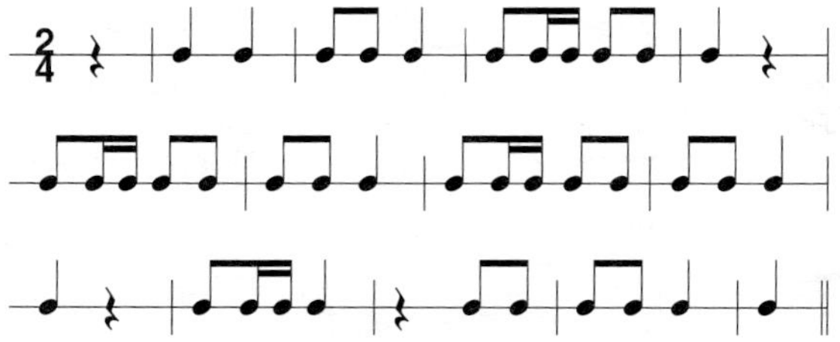

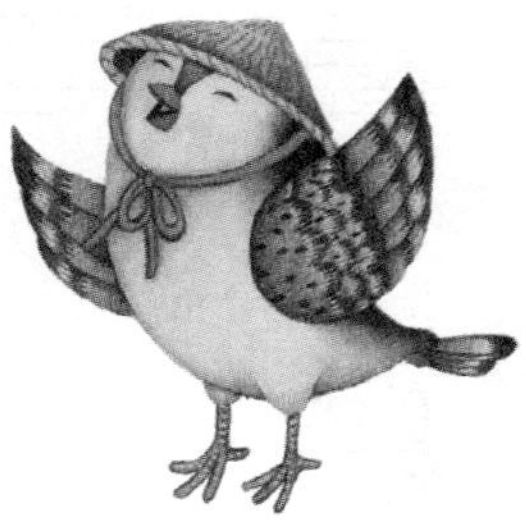

Unit 1　13

2 DEVELOP

Listening

6b Discuss with students that strong beats are called *downbeats,* and weak beats are *upbeats.* Show students how to conduct downbeats and upbeats in 2/4 time.

Have students listen to *"Bắt kim thang"* **CD 1-13** as they perform a pat-snap ostinato, identifying the arrangement of stronger and weaker beats.

ASK What is the arrangement of strong and weak beats in this song? (weak-strong, weak-strong)

Reading

5a **ASK If bar lines are placed before the downbeat, where should the first bar line be placed?** (after the first two notes)

See Skills Reinforcement below for a related activity.

Have students say the rhythm syllables while conducting and then tap the beat of the example on p. 12 while speaking the rhythm syllables.

Singing

9a Help students discover the pitch set of the song (F-*do* pentatonic) before they sing and conduct it with the
1c recording of *"Bắt kim thang."*

3 CLOSE

Element: RHYTHM　**ASSESSMENT**

5a **Performance/Observation** Have students clap the Show What You Know! rhythm on p. 13. Divide the class into two groups. Have one group sing *"Bắt kim thang"* **CD 1-13** as the other group claps the Show What You Know! as a counter-rhythm. Then switch parts. Observe students' ability to perform the rhythms and anacrusis accurately. See p. B-2 in the Resource Book for the corresponding worksheet.

SKILLS REINFORCEMENT

▶ **Reading** Invite students to sing a countermelody to *"Bắt kim thang"* in Music Reading Practice on p. 488, or Resource Book p. E-3.

▶ **Singing** Students may enjoy singing *"Bắt kim thang"* as well as other pentatonic songs from diverse cultures such as *"Asadoya"* on p. 303, *"Skye Boat Song"* on p. 372, and *"New Hungarian Folk Song"* on p. 196.

▶ **Notating** Invite students to write the bar lines for *"Bắt kim thang"* on Music Reading Worksheet D-3. They may also write the pitch set for the song and notate a pentatonic melody. After students complete Music Reading Worksheet D-3, have them notate their own rhythms, placing bar lines correctly for meter in 2.

CHARACTER EDUCATION

▶ **Open-mindedness/Respect** To encourage students to listen to different types of music with respect, invite them to create a recipe for a good listener. The ingredients in the recipe will be characteristics evident in an open-minded, respectful person. For example, acceptance of varied types of music would be an essential ingredient. Discuss similarities between recipes and the characteristics of an open-minded person.

TECHNOLOGY/MEDIA LINK

Web Site Visit *www.sfsuccessnet.com* to learn more about the music and culture of Vietnam. Teachers may also search the Internet for information about other Southeast Asian countries to share with students.

LESSON AT A GLANCE

Element Focus	**FORM** Repetition and contrast
Skill Objective	**SINGING** Sing a song that illustrates repetition and contrast
Connection Activity	**LANGUAGE ARTS** Discuss the meaning of lyrics that express ideas about friendship

MATERIALS
- "Lean on Me" **CD 1-20**
  Recording Routine: Intro (8 m.); v. 1; refrain; v. 2; refrain; bridge; refrain; v. 3; refrain; coda
- **Resource Book** p. G-2

VOCABULARY
repetition and contrast   1st and 2nd Ending
D.C. al Fine   Fine

◆ ◆ ◆ ◆ **National Standards** ◆ ◆ ◆ ◆
1c Sing music from diverse genres
1d Sing music written in two parts
6a Listen and describe events in music using appropriate terms

MORE MUSIC CHOICES
For more practice in identifying repetition and contrast:
"Bridges," p. 86
"El cóndor pasa," p. 46
"Free at Last," p. 468

1 INTRODUCE

Invite students to think about what makes their best friend special, in what ways they are alike and different, and how they lean on each other. See Meeting Individual Needs below.

Have students silently read the lyrics of "Lean on Me." Lead a discussion of the meaning of the lyrics and how communicating needs to others is important.

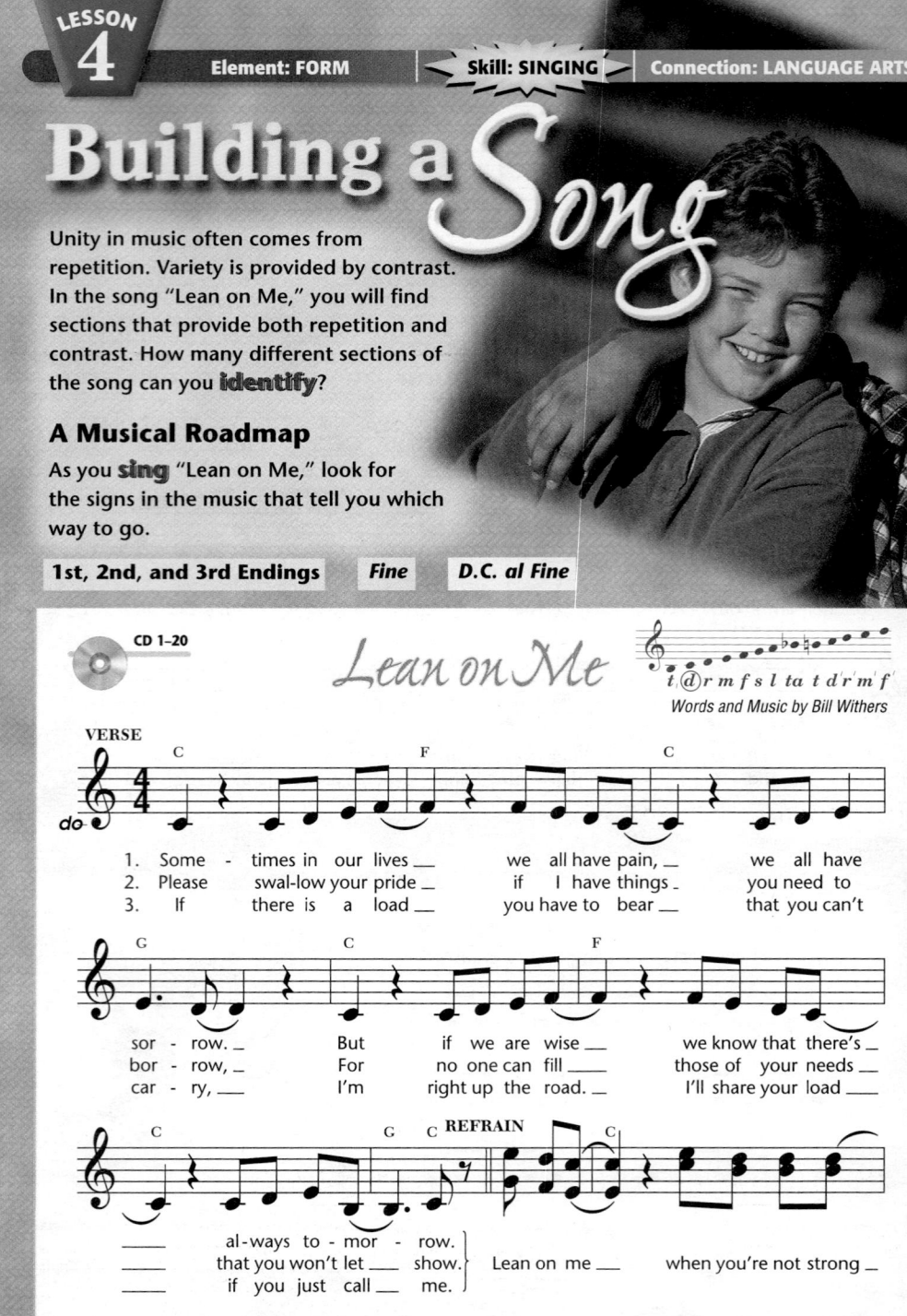

Building a Song

Unity in music often comes from repetition. Variety is provided by contrast. In the song "Lean on Me," you will find sections that provide both repetition and contrast. How many different sections of the song can you **identify**?

A Musical Roadmap
As you **sing** "Lean on Me," look for the signs in the music that tell you which way to go.

1st, 2nd, and 3rd Endings	Fine	D.C. al Fine

Footnotes

SKILLS REINFORCEMENT

▶ **Recorder** After students are familiar with the form of "Lean on Me," have them play this countermelody for soprano recorder on the verses. Review playing leaps from G up to C, and C down to G, reminding students to move their fingers together.

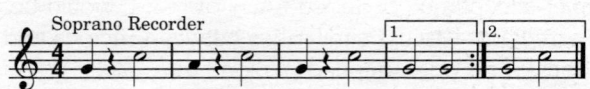

BUILDING SKILLS THROUGH MUSIC

▶ **Language** After students have silently read the lyrics of "Lean on Me," lead them in a discussion of the meaning of the words. Direct them to write a brief paragraph describing how someone helped them or how they have helped someone else. Ask for volunteers to share their writing.

MEETING INDIVIDUAL NEEDS

▶ **Including Everyone** Guide students with disabilities to build friendships and positive relationships with non-disabled peers.

Reinforcement Help students build positive relationships through enjoyable small-group activities. Emphasize to students that it is acceptable to ask others if they need help, and to ask for help for yourself.

On Target Lead students in a discussion of the ideas presented in the introduction. Have students form small groups and ask each group member to suggest one way to be helpful to others.

Challenge Invite students to discuss the importance of volunteers to local communities, hospitals, and charitable organizations. Can individuals make a difference to society?

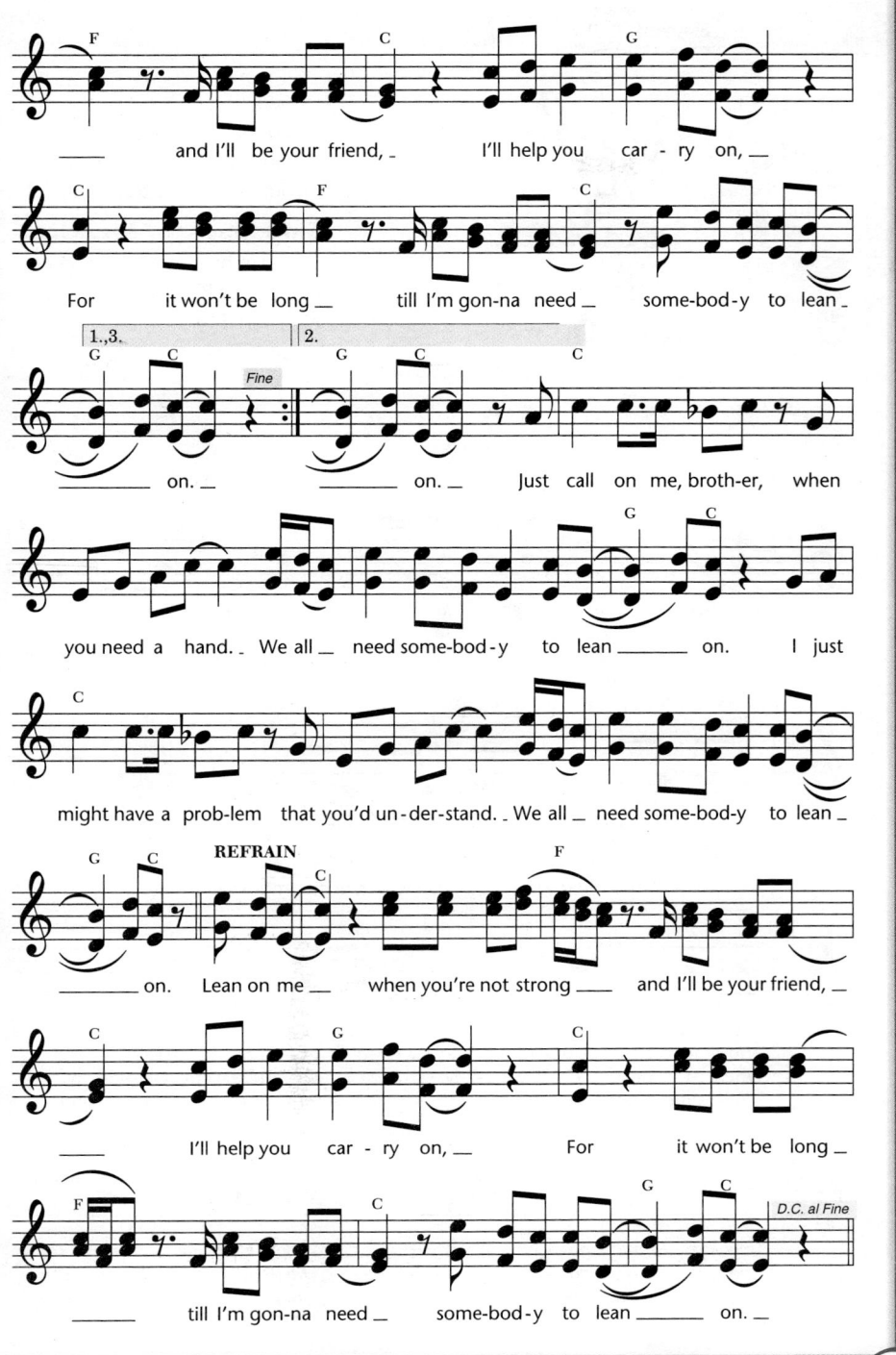

and I'll be your friend, _ I'll help you car - ry on, _

For it won't be long _ till I'm gon-na need _ some-bod-y to lean _

1., 3. | 2.

Fine

on. _ on. _ Just call on me, broth-er, when

you need a hand. _ We all _ need some-bod-y to lean _____ on. I just

might have a prob-lem that you'd un-der-stand. _ We all _ need some-bod-y to lean _

REFRAIN

_____ on. Lean on me _ when you're not strong _____ and I'll be your friend, _

I'll help you car - ry on, _ For it won't be long _

D.C. al Fine

till I'm gon-na need _ some-bod-y to lean _____ on. _

2 DEVELOP

Singing

Have students

 • Sing the melody of "Lean on Me" **CD 1-20** along with the recording. (Lower or changing voices may have to sing the higher melody notes an octave lower.)

 • Learn to sing the harmony part, one section at a time.

Analyzing

Have students

• Locate the different sections of the song.

• Follow the song's road map with their finger as they pay attention to the musical road signs.

ASK Which sections of the song are repeated? (The first section repeats in verses 2 and 3; the refrain section repeats after each verse, and again on p. 15; phrases repeat within the larger sections.)

How does the refrain contrast with the verses? (The vocal range in the refrain is higher; it is in two parts.)

Moving

Help students perform the movement routine for "Lean on Me." (See Movement, below.) Point out to students that the movements illustrate the repetition and contrast present in the song.

3 CLOSE

Skill: SINGING   **ASSESSMENT**

Self-Assessment Organize the class into three groups and assign each group to sing one section of "Lean on Me." Each group should sing its repeated and contrasting parts at the appropriate time. Ask students to assess their performance and understanding of repetition and contrast.

MOVEMENT

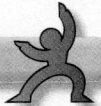

▶ **Patterned Dance** For "Lean on Me," place students in pairs around the room. During sections A and C they stand side by side. During section B they stand back to back.

Section A: Move alone, side to side:
                L-step, R-close behind, L-step, R-close (1-2-3-4).

Section B: Move with a friend, back to back:
                Step forward, together, step back, together (1-2-3-4).

Section C: Move side to side:
                L-step, R-together, R-step, L-together (1-2-3-4).

▶ **Signing** A sign interpretation for "Lean On Me" can be found on Resource Book p. G-2.

SCHOOL TO HOME CONNECTION

▶ **Repetition and Contrast** Ask students to find examples of visual art and architecture in their neighborhood that use repetition and contrast. How does repetition in an artwork create a feeling of unity?

▶ **Family Anecdotes** Invite students to ask family members and friends about a time when someone helped them. Students should ask permission before sharing the anecdote with the class.

TECHNOLOGY/MEDIA LINK

Electronic Keyboard Have students create an ABA composition for electronic keyboard. Students will gain experience in using repetition and contrast to make sections clear.

LESSON AT A GLANCE

Element Focus — **FORM** ABA and AAB forms

Skill Objective — **LISTENING** Identify and describe the differences between contrasting sections of a listening selection

Connection Activity — **CULTURE** Discuss aspects of Tejano culture

MATERIALS

- *"Magnolia"* (Spanish) — **CD 1-22**
- *"Magnolia"* (English) — **CD 1-23**
  Recording Routine: Intro; (4 m.); v. 1; interlude (2 m.), v. 2; coda
- *Pronununciation Practice/Translation* p. 521
- *Marche militaire,* Op. 51, No. 1 — **CD 1-26**
- **Resource Book** pp. A-3, I-4

VOCABULARY

unity	variety	A section	B section
Tejano	coda		

◆ ◆ ◆ ◆ National Standards ◆ ◆ ◆ ◆

1c Sing music from diverse cultures
4a Compose short pieces, demonstrating unity and variety through music
6a Listen and describe events in music using appropriate terms

MORE MUSIC CHOICES

For more practice with identifying A and B sections:
"Bridges," p. 86
"Riendo el río corre," p. 263

1 INTRODUCE

Discuss aspects of *Tejano* culture by sharing the information in Spotlight On, p. 17, with students.

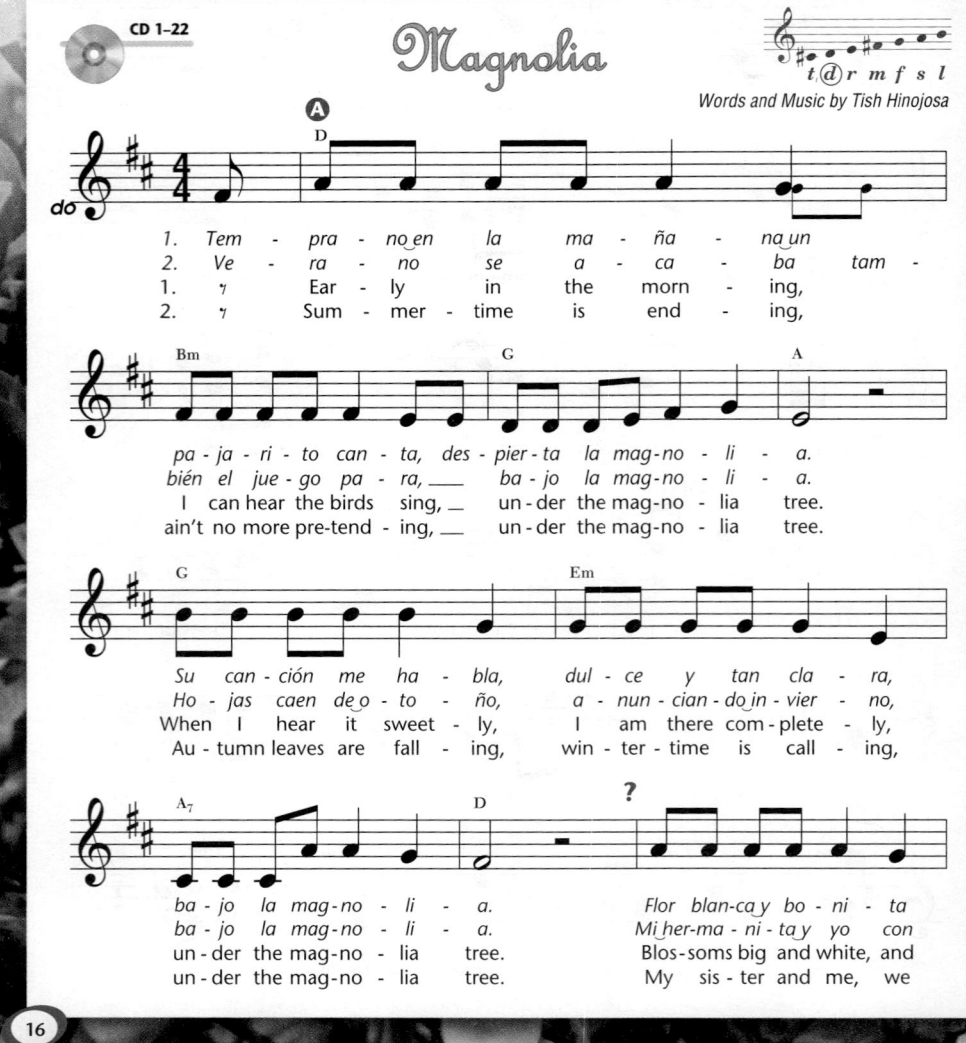

"Magnolia" is a song about childhood memories and a favorite magnolia tree.

Sing *"Magnolia."* **Identify** the form by choosing a section letter (A or B) when you see a question mark.

Footnotes

MEETING INDIVIDUAL NEEDS

▶ **English Language Learners** For students learning English, you may want to pre-select a number of topics for the Skills Reinforcement activity, at right. As you select the topics, you may also want to create a list of related words that could be used in the assignment. This word bank would allow all students to participate in the activity. Students can add their own words to the word bank as well.

BUILDING SKILLS THROUGH MUSIC

▶ **Social Studies** Have students identify artworks or events in their community that demonstrate the blending of cultures. Ask them to list the cultures in their community.

SKILLS REINFORCEMENT

4a ▶ **Creating** Have students form small groups to create a piece in AAB or ABA sectional form and perform it. Have students use a section of newspaper, a map, or a favorite subject for ideas and select and list 10 to 30 words with interesting rhythms.

Students may create section A by selecting one or two words. Have several members of the group speak them as an ostinato. (Other members of the group will chant words from the list over the ostinato.) Students may create section B by choosing a contrasting tempo or dynamic or using another idea based on different words from the list.

▶ **Recorder** Have students learn the recorder part for *"Magnolia"* on Resource Book p. I-4 and play it as the class sings the song.

A New Structure

Listen to *Marche militaire* by the Austrian composer Franz Schubert. It has two sections and a **B** section. What is the order of these sections?

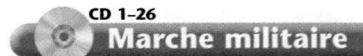
Marche militaire
by Franz Schubert

The form of this piece reflects a repeating section and a contrasting middle section.

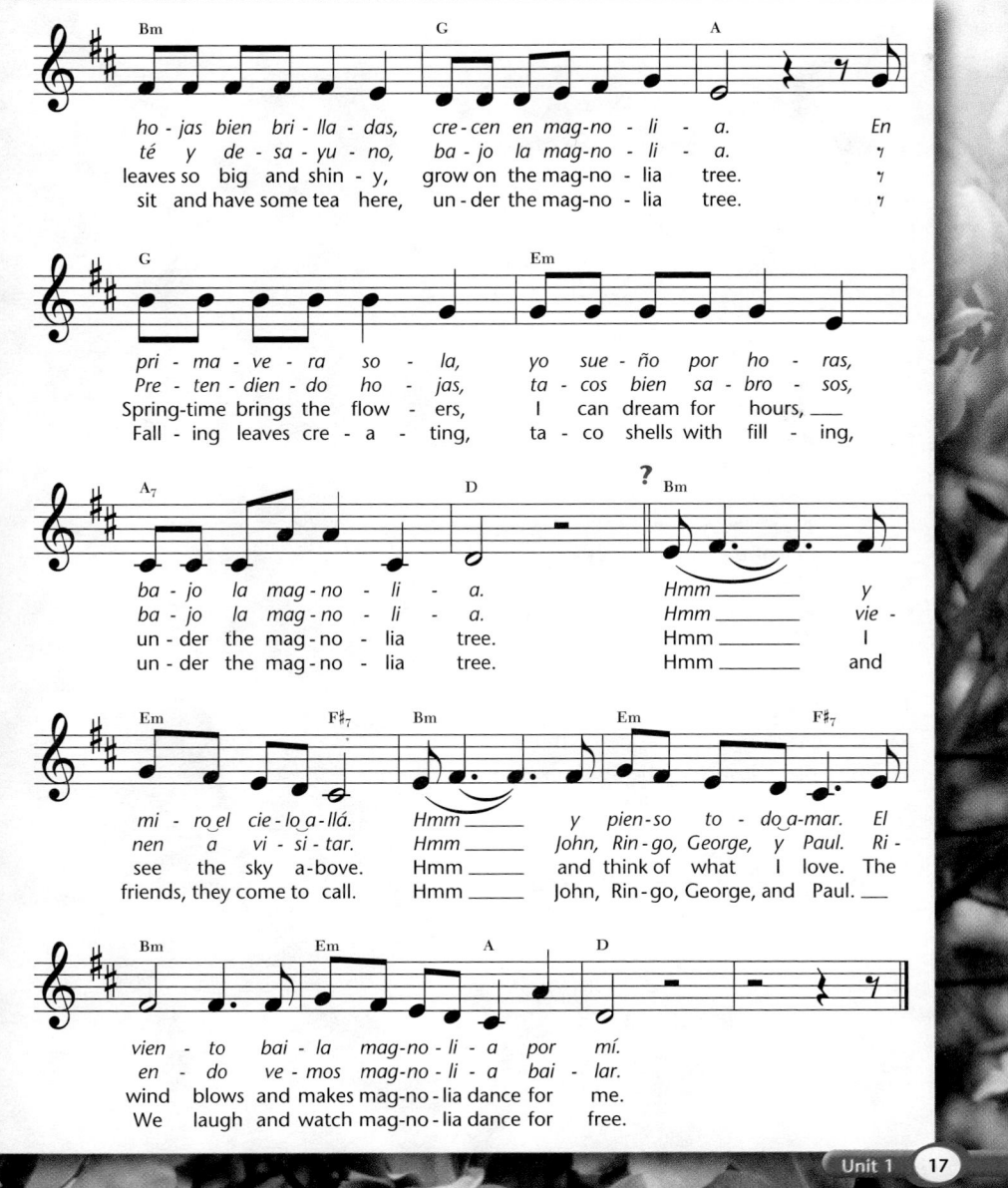

ho - jas bien bri - lla - das, cre - cen en mag-no - li - a. En
té y de - sa - yu - no, ba - jo la mag-no - li - a.
leaves so big and shin - y, grow on the mag-no - lia tree.
sit and have some tea here, un - der the mag-no - lia tree.

pri - ma - ve - ra so - la, yo sue - ño por ho - ras,
Pre - ten - dien - do ho - jas, ta - cos bien sa - bro - sos,
Spring-time brings the flow - ers, I can dream for hours,
Fall - ing leaves cre - a - ting, ta - co shells with fill - ing,

ba - jo la mag-no - li - a. Hmm_____ y
ba - jo la mag-no - li - a. Hmm_____ vie -
un - der the mag-no - lia tree. Hmm_____ I
un - der the mag-no - lia tree. Hmm_____ and

mi - ro el cie - lo a - llá. Hmm_____ y pien-so to - do a-mar. El
nen a vi - si - tar. Hmm_____ John, Rin-go, George, y Paul. Ri -
see the sky a-bove. Hmm_____ and think of what I love. The
friends, they come to call. Hmm_____ John, Rin-go, George, and Paul.__

vien - to bai - la mag-no - li - a por mí.
en - do ve - mos mag-no - li - a bai - lar.
wind blows and makes mag-no - lia dance for me.
We laugh and watch mag-no - lia dance for free.

---

2 DEVELOP

Singing

Have students

 1c
- Sing *"Magnolia"* **CD 1-23** with the recording.

6a
- Analyze the notation to decide whether the question marks found in the score should be A (a repeated section) or B (a contrasting section).

Use the Pronunciation Practice Track **CD 1-25** for the correct pronunciation of the Spanish lyrics of *"Magnolia."* Refer to the Pronunciation Practice Guide on Resource Book p. A-3.

Listening

6a
Have students listen for contrasting sections, dynamics, and instrumental timbres in Schubert's *Marche militaire* **CD 1-26.**

ASK What does Schubert do to contrast the A and B sections? (The B section is more lyrical, smoother *[legato]*, and softer; some passages are in minor, with no trumpets or timpani.)

Is the last A section exactly the same as the first A section? (No; it is shorter, with an added *coda*.)

Creating

4a
Have students form small groups to create their own compositions using AAB or ABA sectional forms. See Skills Reinforcement on p. 16. Listen for clear contrast between the A and B sections. Have students listen to other compositions and decide whether the form is AAB or ABA.

3 CLOSE

Element: FORM   ASSESSMENT

Written Assessment Ask students to listen to *Marche militaire* **CD 1-26** and write brief descriptions of the differences between the A and B sections of the piece.

SPOTLIGHT ON

▶ **"Magnolia" and Tejano Music** *"Magnolia"* was written by Tejana singer-songwriter Tish Hinojosa [ee-noh-HOH-sah]. Born in San Antonio, Texas, Hinojosa began playing guitar, singing, and writing her own songs while still a teenager. *Tejano* music is a popular style that blends Mexican culture with other Texas cultures. It has elements of Caribbean, Mexican American *conjunto,* and country music, and is usually bilingual (Spanish and English).

▶ **The Composer** Franz Schubert (1797–1828) was an Austrian composer. He was a chorister at the Imperial Chapel in Vienna as a boy and started composing at age 13. He wrote many works for voice, piano, chorus, and symphony orchestra. *Marche militaire,* Op. 51, No. 1, was originally written for one piano, four hands.

TECHNOLOGY/MEDIA LINK

Multimedia Assign pairs of students to find examples of Mexican art or photos of *Tejano* artists and then save the graphics as computer files. To create a slide show, type *"Magnolia"* on the first slide. Then create a button that will play an audio file of *"Magnolia"* and advance to the next slide. On the second slide, add graphics and a button that goes to the third slide. On the third slide, add other graphics and a button that goes back to the second slide.

Have students practice presenting their slide shows. Slide 2 should be shown during the repeated sections of *"Magnolia"*; slide 3 should be shown during the contrasting section.

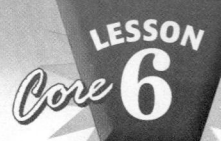

LESSON AT A GLANCE

Element Focus	**MELODY** Melodic patterns	
Skill Objective	**READING** Read from notation and sing a pentatonic song	
Connection Activity	**SOCIAL STUDIES** Read and discuss the lyrics of a song about life as a cowboy in the American West of the late 1800s	

MATERIALS

* "Bury Me Not on the Lone Prairie" **CD 2-1**
  Recording Routine: Intro (4 m.); v. 1; interlude (4 m.); v. 2; interlude (8 m.); v. 3; coda
* Music Reading Practice, Sequence 3 **CD 2-3**
* **Resource Book** pp. D-4, E-4, F-2, H-7
* available percussion instruments

VOCABULARY

pentatonic anacrusis pickup tie diatonic

> ◆ ◆ ◆ ◆ **National Standards** ◆ ◆ ◆ ◆
>
> **1a** Sing accurately in large ensembles
> **2a** Play instruments accurately alone
> **5a** Read quarter and eighth notes in duple meter
> **5c** Identify standard notation symbols for pitch
> **6b** Listen and analyze uses of pitch in music
> **6c** Understand and use basic principles of tonality in music

MORE MUSIC CHOICES

For more practice with F-*do* pentatonic songs:
"Bắt kim thang," p. 13
"Glory, Glory Hallelujah," p. 52

1 INTRODUCE

Play the recording of "Bury Me Not on the Lone Prairie" **CD 2-1.** Then discuss the sentiment of this folk song with students.

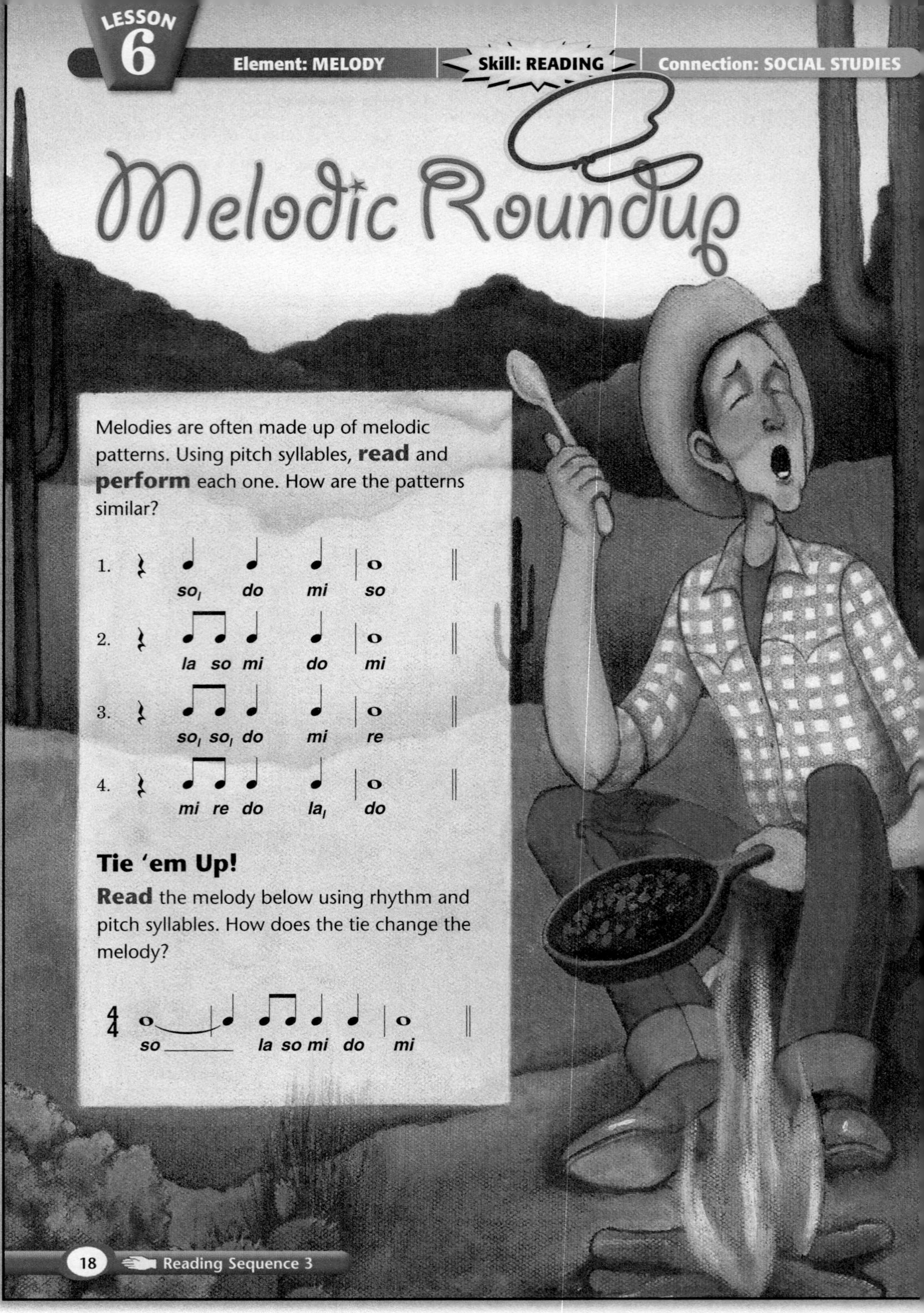

Melodic Roundup

Melodies are often made up of melodic patterns. Using pitch syllables, **read** and **perform** each one. How are the patterns similar?

1. so͵ do mi so
2. la so mi do mi
3. so͵ so͵ do mi re
4. mi re do la͵ do

Tie 'em Up!

Read the melody below using rhythm and pitch syllables. How does the tie change the melody?

4/4 so ___ la so mi do mi

Footnotes

ACROSS THE CURRICULUM

▶ **Language Arts** Invite students to read poetry on Old West themes in *Singing Our Way West: Songs and Stories of America's Westward Expansion* by Jerry Silverman (Millbrook, 1998) and *Home on the Range—Cowboy Poetry* selected by Paul Janeczko (Dial, 1997).

Students could read or dramatize one of these poems or stories as an introduction to "Bury Me Not on the Lone Prairie."

BUILDING SKILLS THROUGH MUSIC

▶ **Language** Have students read the lyrics to "Bury Me Not on the Lone Prairie." Have the class discuss the text, then read the Tune In on p. 19. Working in small groups, have students create new lyrics that would be appropriate for a young sailor's burial at sea.

SKILLS REINFORCEMENT

▶ **Recorder** When students can play C, D, F, and G on the alto recorder, have them add this countermelody while others sing "Bury Me Not on the Lone Prairie." Check student hand position: LH on top and RH below, with right thumb behind the fourth and fifth holes and RH fingers curved over the holes.

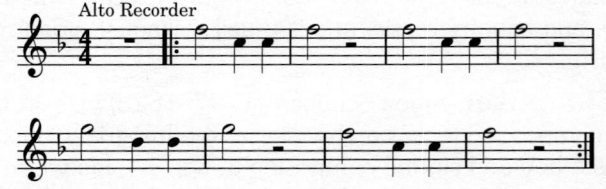

Alto Recorder

A Prairie Ballad

Sing "Bury Me Not on the Lone Prairie." Which melodic patterns from page 18 appear in the song?

Tune In

This sad ballad was originally written in 1839 about a young sailor's burial at sea. As the song traveled west, cowboys created new words.

CD 2–1 MIDI 1

Bury Me Not on the Lone Prairie

s, l, (d) r m s l

Cowboy Song from the United States

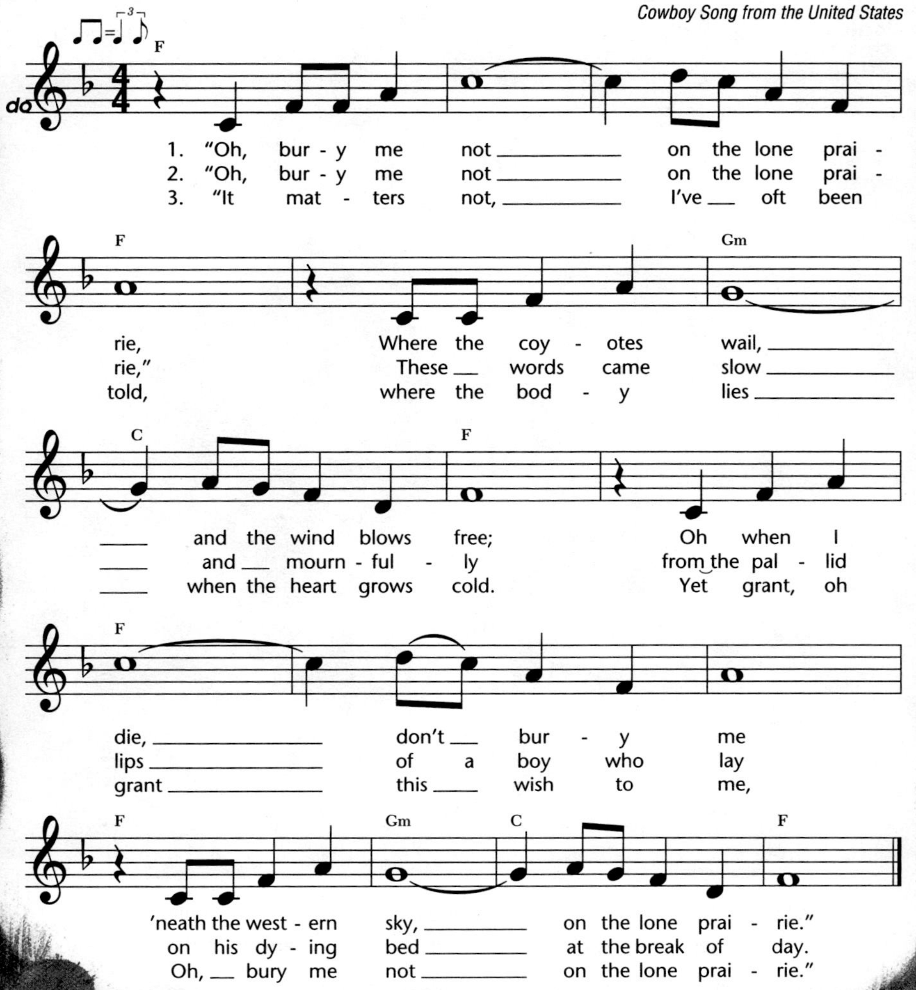

do

1. "Oh, bur-y me not _____ on the lone prai-
2. "Oh, bur-y me not _____ on the lone prai-
3. "It mat-ters not, _____ I've ___ oft been

rie, Where the coy-otes wail, _____
rie," These ___ words came slow _____
told, where the bod-y lies _____

_____ and the wind blows free; Oh when I
_____ and ___ mourn-ful-ly from the pal-lid
_____ when the heart grows cold. Yet grant, oh

die, _____ don't ___ bur-y me
lips _____ of a boy who lay
grant _____ this ___ wish to me,

'neath the west-ern sky, _____ on the lone prai-rie."
on his dy-ing bed _____ at the break of day.
Oh, ___ bur-y me not on the lone prai-rie."

Unit 1 19

---

2 DEVELOP

Reading

5a Review the tie and pickup. Have students say rhythm syllables for "Bury Me Not on the Lone Prairie." Use Reading Music Worksheet D-4 for additional practice.

Singing

5c Direct students to p. 18 of the Student Edition. For each melody pattern, have them

• Sing pitch syllables and show hand signs.
• Sing pitch syllables and point to hand-staff positions.

6b Divide the class into small groups of 2–3 students. Have the groups determine in what order they will sing the patterns. Invite the groups to perform their patterns.

6c Using standard symbols, have students notate all pitches in the song from lowest to highest on a staff, using correct spacing between *la,* and *do* and between *mi* and *so.* Have them use hand signs as they sing pitch syllables, ascending and descending.

ASK **What kind of scale is used in the song "Bury Me Not on the Lone Prarie?"** (pentatonic)

How is this scale different from the diatonic scale we identfied for the song "Red River Valley?" (no *fa*; no *ti*)

Add the pitches for *fa* and *low ti* on the staff and have the students now sing the diatonic scale using pitch syllables and handsigns. Erase the *fa* and *low ti* from the staff and have students sing the pentatonic scale.

3 CLOSE

Skill: READING   ASSESSMENT

1a **Performance/Observation** Have students read
5c and sing "Bury Me Not on the Lone Prairie," using hand signs and pitch syllables. Observe students' ability to read and sing from notation, using hand signs and pitch syllables.

SKILLS REINFORCEMENT

▶ **Reading** For more practice with meter in four, ties, and pickups, use Music Reading Worksheet p. D-4 in the Resource Book.

For additional reading practice, invite students to sing a countermelody to "Bury Me Not on the Lone Prairie" on p. 489, or Resource Book p. E-4.

 ▶ **Mallets** Invite students to learn to play the Orff accompaniment for "Bury Me Not on the Lone Prairie" found on Resource Book p. F-2.

 ▶ **Keyboard** Students may enjoy playing the keyboard part for the song found on Resource Book p. H-7.

TECHNOLOGY/MEDIA LINK

MIDI/Sequencing Software Open the MIDI song file of the melody of "Bury Me Not on the Lone Prairie." Have students select an empty track and assign it a bass patch (sound). Then sequence a bass part using the roots and fifths of the chords. Have them select a sound for the harmony track that they think is appropriate for a cowboy song and record chord arpeggios in repeating rhythms. Play the sequences one at a time to accompany the song.

Video Library The video *Using MIDI in the Elementary Music Classroom* will provide a general introduction to the benefits this technology offers.

LESSON AT A GLANCE

Element Focus **MELODY** Melodic contour, diatonic melody

Skill Objective **READING** Read and sing ascending and descending melodic contours

Connection Activity **SCIENCE** Investigate the processes through which mountains are created

MATERIALS

- "Gonna Build a Mountain"　　　　　　**CD 2-6**
  Recording Routine: Intro (8 m.); v. 1; instrumental; v. 2; coda
- **Music Reading Practice, Sequence 4**　**CD 2-8**
- **Resource Book** pp. D-5, E-5
- mallet instruments

VOCABULARY

melodic contour　　ascending　　descending
phrase　　diatonic

◆ ◆ ◆ **National Standards** ◆ ◆ ◆

1a Sing accurately in large ensembles
5b Sightread melodies in treble clef
5c Identify standard notation syllables for pitch
6b Listen and analyze uses of pitch in music
6c Understand and use basic principles of tonality in music

MORE MUSIC CHOICES

For more practice with melodic contour designs:
"Bury Me Not on the Lone Prairie," p. 19
"My Dear Companion," p. 23

1 INTRODUCE

Direct students to the photos of the mountains, the text about melodic contour and the song notation on p. 21.

ASK Which mountain best resembles the contour of the melody? Why ? (Smooth mountains; the melody gradually ascends and descends.)

See Across the Curriculum below for additional geology topics.

REACH FOR THE SKY!

Look at the pictures of the mountains. The mountain on the left is smooth and flowing while the mountain on the right is jagged. Melodies also have contours (shapes). Trace the **melodic contour** of "Gonna Build a Mountain" as you **listen** to the song.

> **Melodic contour** is the shape of a musical phrase.

As you **sing** the song, **read** the notation and notice how the notes in most phrases begin low and then move higher, as though the melody is trying to build a mountain. It's a mountain of melody!

▲ Appalachian Mountains
Blue Ridge Parkway, North Carolina

▲ Mount Reagan
Sawtooth Lake, Idaho

Show What You Know!

Create movements that follow the melodic contour to "Gonna Build a Mountain." Then have the class **perform** your movements with the song.

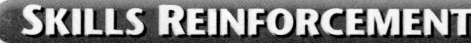
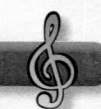
20　Reading Sequence 4

Footnotes

ACROSS THE CURRICULUM

▶ **Science** Interested students might like to investigate the theory of plate tectonics and the geological process by which mountains are created. Encourage students to locate and research the two mountain ranges in the photos on p. 20—the Appalachian Mountains ("Blue Ridge" of North Carolina) and the Sawtooth Mountains (central Idaho).

BUILDING SKILLS THROUGH MUSIC

▶ **Social Studies** Ask students to list the mountain ranges in the United States. Then, have students locate the mountains closest to where they live, using a map, globe, or atlas.

SKILLS REINFORCEMENT

1a ▶ **Vocal Development** Have students sing the final phrase of "Gonna Build a Mountain" in one breath.

To help develop breath support, have students

- Assume correct posture, with both feet on the floor, one slightly ahead of the other, shoulders slightly back and down, and head held level and high.
- Take a deep breath without moving their shoulders.
- Release the breath in a slow, steady hiss.
- Slowly but forcefully, blow the air at a candle or pinwheel.

▶ **Reading** For additional reading practice, see Music Reading Sequence 4 on p. 489, or Resource Book p. E-5.

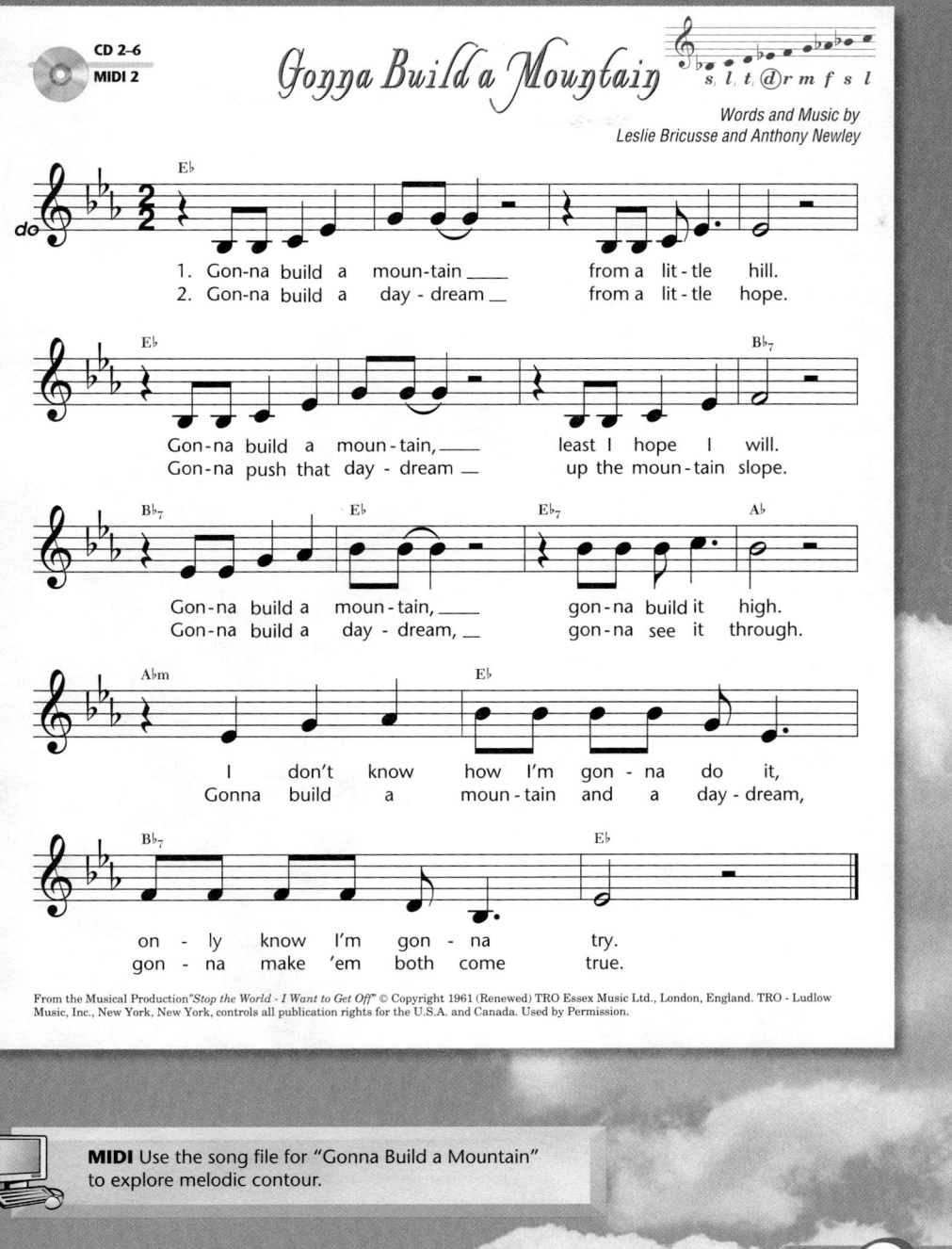

Gonna Build a Mountain

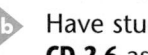
s, l, t, @ r m f s l

*Words and Music by
Leslie Bricusse and Anthony Newley*

1. Gon-na build a moun-tain____ from a lit-tle hill.
2. Gon-na build a day-dream__ from a lit-tle hope.

Gon-na build a moun-tain,____ least I hope I will.
Gon-na push that day-dream__ up the moun-tain slope.

Gon-na build a moun-tain,____ gon-na build it high.
Gon-na build a day-dream,__ gon-na see it through.

I don't know how I'm gon-na do it,
Gonna build a moun-tain and a day-dream,

on-ly know I'm gon-na try.
gon-na make 'em both come true.

From the Musical Production *"Stop the World - I Want to Get Off"* © Copyright 1961 (Renewed) TRO Essex Music Ltd., London, England. TRO - Ludlow Music, Inc., New York, New York, controls all publication rights for the U.S.A. and Canada. Used by Permission.

MIDI Use the song file for "Gonna Build a Mountain" to explore melodic contour.

Unit 1 **21**

2 DEVELOP

Listening

Have students listen to "Gonna Build a Mountain" **CD 2-6** as they read the song notation and trace the melodic contour of the melody.

Help students discover that each melody pattern in phrases 1–3 ascends.

ASK How is the melodic contour of phrase 4 different? (It ascends and descends.)

Reading

Have students identify the final pitch of the song as *do*, and then place all pitches used in mm.1-8 on a staff, from lowest to highest (B-flat *do*).

ASK Is this pitch set pentatonic? (yes)

Have students place the remaining pitches on the staff.

ASK Did the pitch set stay pentatonic? (no)

What kind of scale is used in the song "Gonna Build a Mountain?" (diatonic)

Have students use hand signs and pitch syllables to sing the diatonic scale.

Singing

Direct students to Resource Book, p. D-5. Have them conduct and say rhythm syllables, show hand signs and sing pitch syllables, then sing the lyrics.

ASK What is the relationship of Resource Book, p. D-5 to the song "Gonna Build a Mountain" on p. 21? (The Resource Book notation is a skeletal version.)

3 CLOSE

Element: MELODY   ASSESSMENT

Performance/Observation Have students read and sing "Gonna Build a Mountain," first showing melodic contour, then using pitch syllables and hand signs. Observe students' ability to accurately show contour and hand signs.

MEETING INDIVIDUAL NEEDS

▶ **Composing** Ask students to compose a melody that follows the contour of the lines above each pattern in Resource Book, p. D-5. Then encourage students to play their compositions on mallet instruments.

Reinforcement Students having motor difficulty with writing or performing may create arm or full-body movements that illustrate the ascending and descending melodic contour of the song.

On Target Many students will enjoy working with a composing partner for this project.

Challenge Invite students to compose their composition using **MIDI File 2** for "Gonna Build a Mountain." Challenge students to select pitches that complement the song's melody. Then create a bass track for the song.

TECHNOLOGY/MEDIA LINK

MIDI/Sequencing Software Using the MIDI song file for "Gonna Build a Mountain," have students

- Select the software program's graphic editor. Examine the contour of the melody and the other tracks.

- Explore graphic editing features (for example: deleting, entering, and changing the pitch and length of notes).

- Discuss ways melodic contour can be changed.

- Turn off accompaniment tracks and play back several alterations of the melody.

LESSON AT A GLANCE

Element Focus	**MELODY** Melodic contour
Skill Objective	**SINGING** Sing a song with phrases that have similar melodic contours
Connection Activity	**RELATED ARTS** Explore folk arts and crafts of Appalachia

MATERIALS
- "My Dear Companion"   **CD 2-11**
  Recording Routine: Intro (3 m.); vocal; interlude (7 m.); vocal; coda

VOCABULARY
melodic contour   ascending   descending   pentatonic

◆ ◆ ◆ ◆ National Standards ◆ ◆ ◆ ◆
1a Sing accurately with good breath control
1b Sing easy pieces with technical accuracy
7b Students use specific criteria for evaluating their own performances
8b Identify ways music relates to school subjects

MORE MUSIC CHOICES
For more practice singing melodic contours:
"Gonna Build a Mountain," p. 21
"Vive l'amour," p. 176

1 INTRODUCE

Appalachian craftspeople create pottery with different shapes. In music, melodies also have shapes (contours). Melodic contour can influence the lyrics, mood, and meaning of a song. Have students read the song lyrics as they listen to "My Dear Companion" **CD 2-11**. Encourage them to think about what the song means and how contour is used in the melody.

ASK What is the mood of the singer? (sad, lonely)

Why do you think the singer wants to be "some swallow flyin'?" (to fly away from sadness)

Musical Shapes

In Appalachia, craftsmen mold clay into beautiful pottery with different shapes and contours. In music, composers create melodies with different shapes and contours.

Listen to "My Dear Companion." What is the mood and meaning of the words, by Appalachian composer Jean Ritchie?

Now, look at each four-measure phrase on page 23.

- First **describe** the shape, or contour, of each phrase.
- **Compare** the contour of the phrases. How are they similar? How are they different?
- **Create** movements to show the melodic contour of each phrase.

Sing "My Dear Companion." As you sing, pay attention to the shape of each melodic phrase.

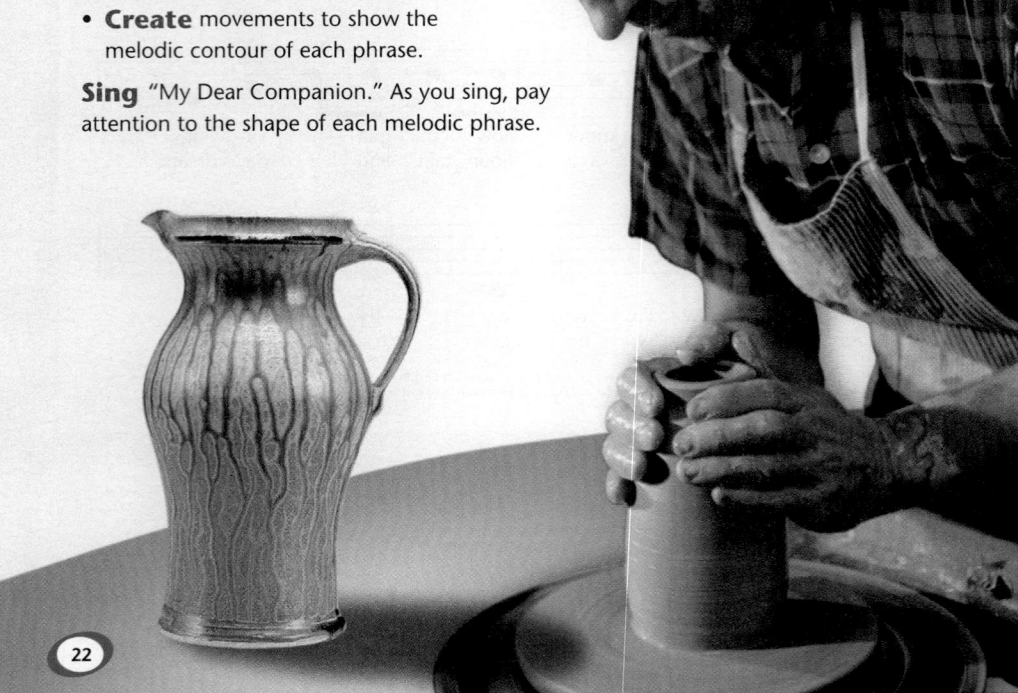

Appalachia folk arts include pottery making. Here is an Appalachian craftsman at work. ▼

 22

Footnotes

ACROSS THE CURRICULUM

▶ **Related Arts** The film, "The Songcatcher," is about a female musicologist's work in the early 1900s. She recorded Appalachian mountain songs and their history. The film includes authentic Appalachian folk singing, instruments, culture, and dance.

8b Musicologists Cecil Sharp and Maud Karpeles collected southern Appalachian English folk songs. They traced these mountain melodies to their oral musical and historical connections in original English folk songs of the 17th and 18th centuries.

BUILDING SKILLS THROUGH MUSIC

▶ **Reading** Since mood is the feeling writers create through the language they use, have students identify the words or phrases in the lyrics that give this piece its mood.

SKILLS REINFORCEMENT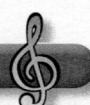

▶ **Movement** Invite students to work in small groups to create a dance for the song, "My Dear Companion." Ask students to think of how to move their whole bodies in the shape of the melody lines of this song. Ask them: How will they move to show the melodic contour of each line? (in upward, then sustained, then downward patterns) What is the mood of the created dance? (sad, lonely) Why? (The singer has lost his or her dear companion.)

Once students have begun to think of movement ideas, visit each group and encourage students to stay on-task as they create a dance to perform for the entire class. Encourage students to practice their dance several times and to sing as they move.

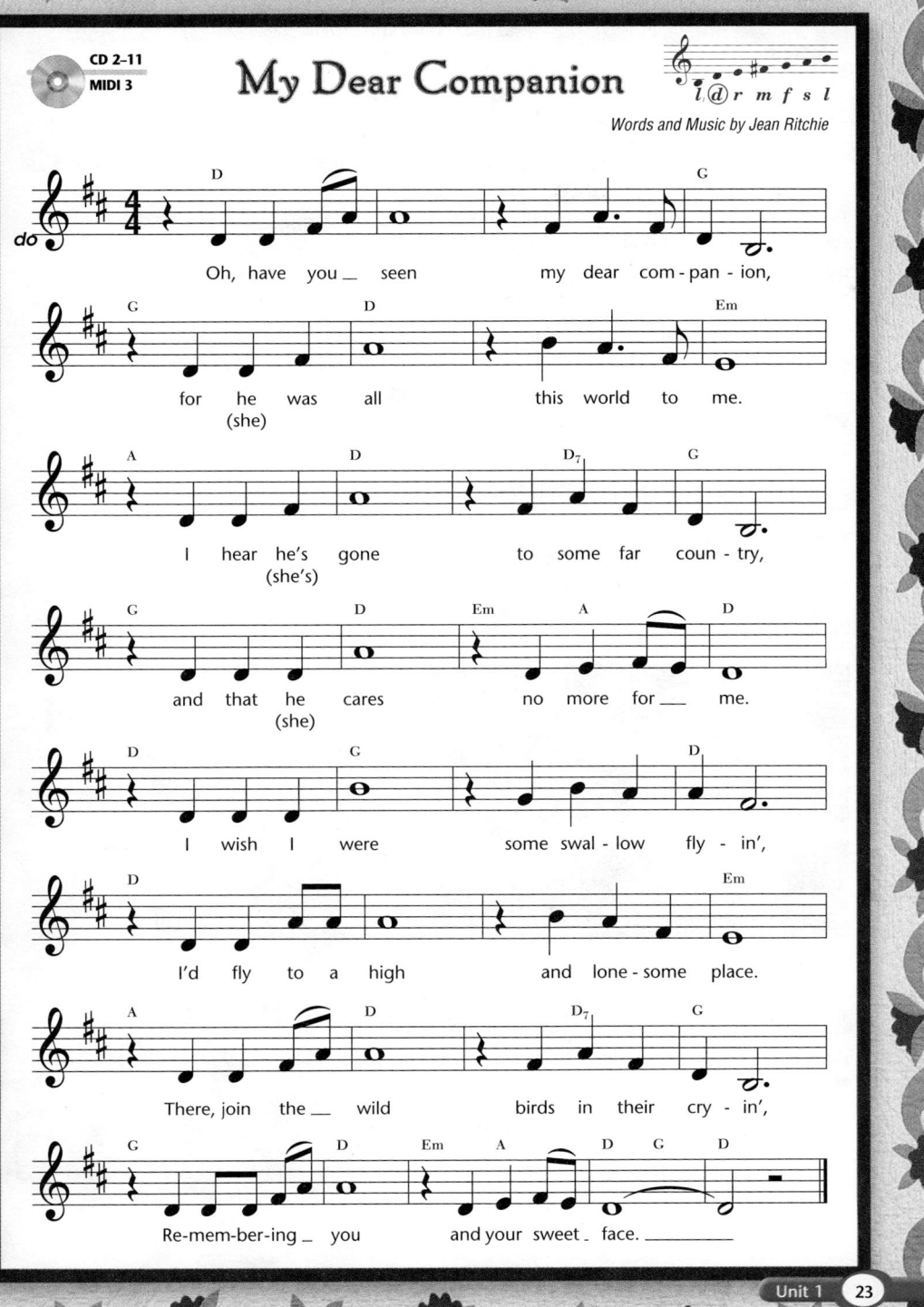

My Dear Companion

Words and Music by Jean Ritchie

Oh, have you seen my dear com-pan-ion,
for he was all this world to me.
(she)
I hear he's gone to some far coun-try,
(she's)
and that he cares no more for me.
(she)
I wish I were some swal-low fly-in',
I'd fly to a high and lone-some place.
There, join the wild birds in their cry-in',
Re-mem-ber-ing you and your sweet face.

2 DEVELOP

Listening

1b Have students listen again to "My Dear Companion" **CD 2-11.** Ask students to look at the melodic contour of each line (a four measure phrase) of this song. Have them answer the following:

ASK Can you identify the melodic scale? (pentatonic)

Are the lines similar in shape? (yes)

How are they similar? (Each line ascends the first two measures, has a whole note, a rest, then descends the second two measures.)

What does each line have in common? (ascending, descending patterns; similar rhythmic values; sustained notes; placement of rests)

Singing

Invite students to sing the song with the recording and draw the shape of each melody line on paper with a pencil. Then, have them trace the contour with their hand as they sing (left to right) in space. Be sure the students use longer symbols and movements for sustained note values.

Create

Using the Skills Reinforcement on p. 22, invite students to create a dance for "My Dear Companion" that uses whole body movements to illustrate the melodic contour of each phrase.

3 CLOSE

Skill: SINGING   **ASSESSMENT**

1a **Performance/Observation:** Have students sing "My Dear Companion" and trace the shape of the melody as they sing. Observe their ability to correctly sing and map the melodic contour of each phrase.

CULTURAL CONNECTION

8b ▶ **Music of Southern Appalachia** Singer and composer Jean Ritchie has given the world an insight into the music of Southern Appalachia. Ritchie grew up in Viper, Kentucky, learning a rich variety of hymns, traditional love songs, ballads, and Stephen Foster songs. When she moved to New York, she sang the songs mainly to entertain the children who were in the Henry Street Settlement, where she worked. Eventually, she was asked to perform professionally. Read more about Jean Ritchie in her book *Singing Family of the Cumberlands* (University Press of Kentucky, 1988).

Because of the influence of the Old Regular Baptist Church in Southern Appalachia in the late nineteenth century, most people there felt that singing only *melody* was acceptable; *harmony* was considered "frivolous."

TECHNOLOGY/MEDIA LINK

7b **MIDI/Sequencing Software** Record improvised vocal harmony, using a digital audio program. Open the MIDI song file for "My Dear Companion." Save the file, using a different name. Students may sing and record the melody in one track, then record the harmony part in another track. Have students individually evaluate whether or not

1. Melody is sung in time to the accompaniment.

2. Melody uses correct notes and rhythms.

3. Harmony is sung in time to the accompaniment and uses correct notes and rhythms.

Web Site For more about Appalachian music and instruments, visit *www.sfsuccessnet.com.*

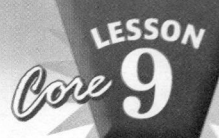

LESSON Core 9

LESSON AT A GLANCE

Element Focus   **TIMBRE** Vocal timbre (choral)

Skill Objective   **LISTENING** Listen to vocal choral timbres from diverse cultures

Connection Activity   **CULTURE** Explore diverse cultures and their styles of choral music

MATERIALS

O Christmas Tree	**CD 2-13**
Tamaiti hunahia	**CD 2-14**
Northfield	**CD 2-15**
Anvil Chorus	**CD 2-16**
Kui.Kyon.pan	**CD 2-17**
Strike Up the Band Medley	**CD 2-18**

• **Resource Book** p. C-5

VOCABULARY

timbre   SATB   overtone   barbershop

> ◆ ◆ ◆ ◆ **National Standards** ◆ ◆ ◆ ◆
>
> **6b** Listen and analyze uses of timbre and harmony in music from diverse cultures
> **7a** Create standards for evaluating performances
> **9b** Describe the characteristics of high-quality musical works

MORE MUSIC CHOICES

For more experience with varied vocal timbres:
"Key to the Highway," p. 243
"Mr. Tambourine Man," p. 150
It Don't Mean a Thing, p. 386

1 INTRODUCE

Tell students that the human voice has the flexibility to sound a great many different ways. Tell them they will use the timbre words printed on pp. 24–25 to describe the vocal timbres they hear from choral groups around the world.

Element: TIMBRE   **Skill: LISTENING**   **Connection: CULTURE**

Vocal Timbres

You recognize the voices of your friends even without seeing them because their voices have different qualities. The unique quality of the sound produced by an instrument or voice is called its **timbre.**

> **Timbre** is the tone color, or unique sound, of an instrument or voice.

The timbre of an individual or group of voices is easy to identify, once you are familiar with it, but describing timbre is not easy. **Listen** to these recordings. Use the words on these pages to describe the vocal timbre in each selection. What factors contribute to the differences in vocal timbre?

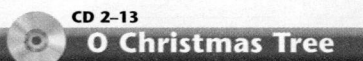

CD 2–13 O Christmas Tree

Traditional German carol as performed by The Vienna Boys' Choir

A traditional boys' choir consists of boys with unchanged and changed voices. Note the timbre of the changed voices in the lower register.

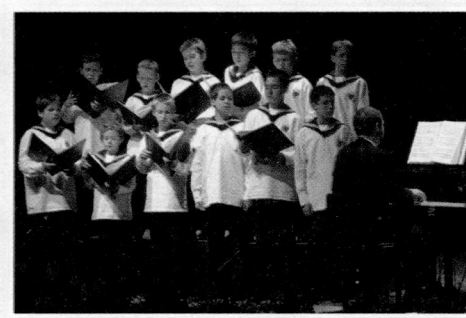

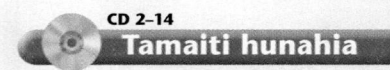

CD 2–14 Tamaiti hunahia

Tahitian choral song as performed by the Rapa Iti Tahitian Choir

This ensemble of male and female voices sings a song about a father who rescued his son from death.

mellow   smoot   quivery   pinched   breathy   buzzy   nasal

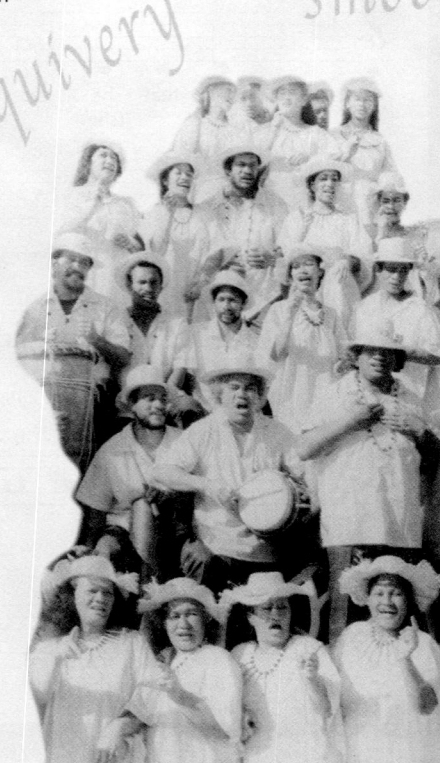

24

Footnotes

TEACHER TO TEACHER

▶ **Unusual Vocal Sounds** Different and unusual vocal sounds often will provoke laughter. Lead a discussion with students on the kinds of voice sounds that make them laugh. Explain to students that every culture has vocal sounds that it likes; these sounds may be related to the language that is spoken. Other sounds (timbres) may seem strange and even funny to that culture. Remind students that in a concert setting, they should exhibit proper etiquette and be informed listeners with music of all types.

BUILDING SKILLS THROUGH MUSIC

▶ **Language** Have students complete a Semantic Feature Analysis (Resource Book, p. C-5). Include all the descriptor words of vocal timbre and the vocal styles heard in class, putting checks in the boxes that apply to each piece of music.

CULTURAL CONNECTION

▶ **Tahiti (ta-HEE-tee)** Tahiti is the largest of the Society Island group in the South Pacific. Missionaries, traders, and settlers visited Tahiti bringing with them European culture, including choral music. *Tamaiti hunahia* demonstrates integration of European part singing with indigenous vocal timbre.

▶ **Tibetan Monasteries** Monks dedicated to the practice of Tibetan Buddhism develop the unique ability to chant in very low tones with a resonance that allows an overtone that is 2 octaves and a third above it to "ring" along with the low tone (for example, for a low C, the overtone is E). Tibetan Buddhism is practiced today outside of Tibetan China, notably in India.

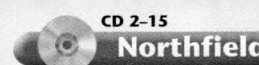

Northfield
CD 2–15

as performed by participants at the Alabama Sacred Harp Singing Convention in Birmingham, Alabama

Sacred Harp choral groups of men and women developed in the mid-1800s within the mountain regions of the southern and eastern United States. The tradition continues today in some areas.

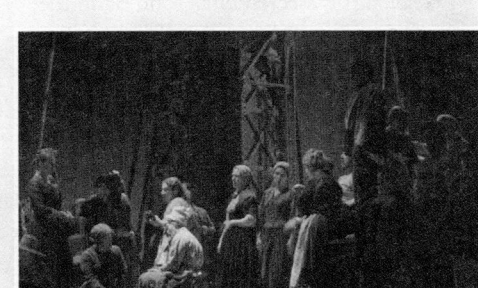

Anvil Chorus
CD 2–16

**from *Il trovatore*
by Guiseppi Verdi
as performed by the Chicago Symphony Orchestra and Chorus**

The choruses in an opera are sung by male and female singers trained in the operatic vocal style.

Kui.Kyon.pan
CD 2–17

as performed by the Monks of the Sera Jé Monastery

In *Kui.Kyon.pan*, Tibetan monks sing in deep, low-bass tones that produce overtones, or harmonics, above the bass tones.

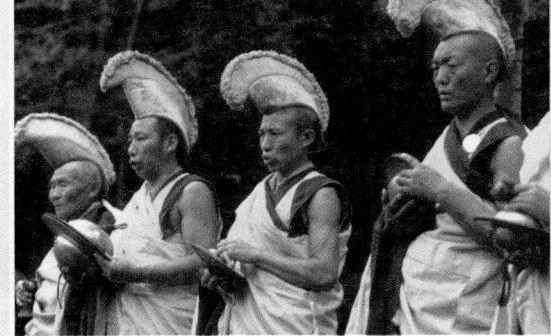

Strike Up the Band Medley
CD 2–18

**by George Gershwin
as performed by the Seven Hills Chorus of Cincinnati, Ohio**

"Sweet Adelines" is a name for *a cappella* women's quartets and choruses. They sing popular American songs of the early and mid-1900s in four-part harmony. The comparable men's singing groups are called "barbershop" quartets and choruses.

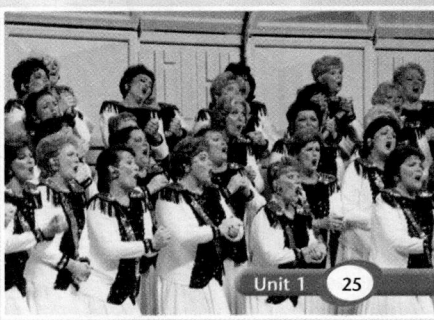

 Unit 1 **25**

relaxed light rough
pure airy
heavy straight
tight silvery

2 DEVELOP

Analyzing

6b For each listening example have students

- Describe the aurally-presented music and the vocal timbre of these diverse cultures.
- Determine the vocal texture. (unison or parts)

Listening

Guide students to understand how vocal timbre may be influenced by culture and region.

7a **1** Austria; a traditional boys' choir. Ask students what vocal timbres they hear. (boys, men) The boys' choir sound is important to this timbre. (SATB: soprano, alto, tenor, and bass) (timbre: light, airy, pure, silvery, smooth, mellow, relaxed, and quivery)

2 Tahiti. Tahitian choral singing was learned from Europeans. The Tahitians applied their own unique vocal timbre. (SATB) (timbre: heavy, and rough)

3 Southern Appalachia region of the eastern United States. These groups sing hymns reading from shape notes. (SATB) (timbre: heavy, rough, nasal, pinched)

9b **4** Italy; an opera house. The chorus is on stage, in costume, singing this song as part of the opera story. (SATB) (timbre: quivery, heavy, smooth, and open)

5 Tibet. The monks of the Sera Jé Buddhist Monastery produce extremely low-pitched sounds, with an overtone ringing above. (timbre: rough, heavy, buzzy, quivery, breathy, and pinched)

6b **6** United States; a Sweet Adelines competition (timbre: open, smooth, straight)

3 CLOSE

Element: LISTENING ━ **ASSESSMENT**

Music Journal Writing Play a brief excerpt of each example. Have students write two descriptive words that best identifies each timbre. Observe students understanding of vocal timbre.

SPOTLIGHT ON

▶ ***Il Trovatore* and the "Anvil Chorus"** First performed in Rome, Italy, in 1853, Giuseppe Verdi's *Il Trovatore* is among the most famous of all operas. The "Anvil Chorus," with its trademark anvil sound, is one of the most recognized opera melodies of all time.

▶ **Sacred Harp Singing** In the mid-1800s, many people in the rural eastern and southern mountain areas were taught to read music by "shape notes"—circles, triangles, squares, and diamonds that represented the tones *fa, sol, la,* and *mi* (repeated to form a complete scale). The repertoire consisted of Christian hymns written in four-part arrangements, with the melody in the tenor part. The most important and popular collection was called *The Sacred Harp*; the entire style of singing eventually became to be known by this name.

SCHOOL TO HOME CONNECTION

▶ **Timbre Search** Strengthen sensitivity to timbre by having students go on a "timbre search" for sounds at school, home, and in their community. Have students share their sounds with the class.

TECHNOLOGY/MEDIA LINK

Video Library See the video *Bobby McFerrin* to see a master at using his voice to produce a wide variety of vocal timbres. He uses his voice to imitate various instruments in classical music as well as to sing songs. Some of his CDs are: 1) *YoYo Ma and Bobby McFerrin*; 2) *Paper Music*; 3) *The Mozart Sessions*; and 4) *Circlesongs*. McFerrin's song "Don't Worry, Be Happy" won a Grammy for Song of the Year in 1988.

LESSON AT A GLANCE

Element Focus **TEXTURE/HARMONY** Layered ostinatos

Skill Objective **SINGING** Sing a song using layered parts

Connection Activity **SOCIAL STUDIES** Explore the history and culture of the Shona farmers of southeast Africa

MATERIALS

- "Wai bamba" **CD 2-19**

  Recording Routine: Intro (4 m.); vocal (unison); interlude (4 m.); vocal (3-part round); coda
- Chigamba **CD 2-21**
- alto and bass metallophone, tambourine

VOCABULARY

harmony   mbira

◆ ◆ ◆ ◆ **National Standards** ◆ ◆ ◆ ◆

1a Sing accurately in large ensembles
1c Sing music from diverse cultures
4c Arrange, using electronic media
6a Listen and describe events in music using appropriate terms
6b Listen and analyze uses of harmony in music from diverse genres

MORE MUSIC CHOICES

For more practice with layered harmonies:

"Banuwa," p. 294

"Gloria, Gloria," p. 459

"Let Us Sing Together," p. 156

1 INTRODUCE

Direct students to the Shona mask and *mbira* on pp. 26–27. Invite students to discuss each Shona artifact. (See Spotlight On, below.)

ASK What do these artifacts tell us about the people who created them? (Both are made using mostly natural materials. Both are highly decorated, suggesting skilled craftsmanship.)

SOUNDS OF HARMONY

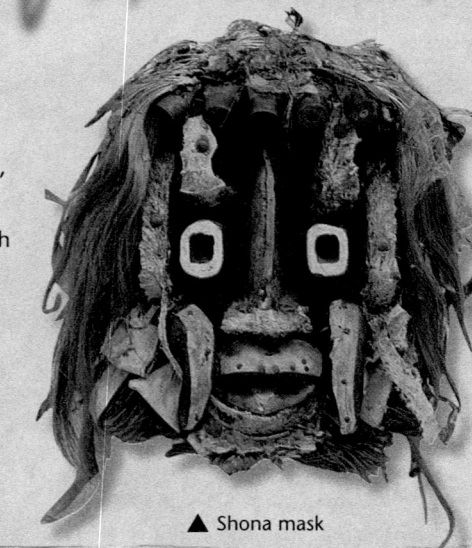

Have you ever been to a ceremony? "Wai bamba" is a ceremonial song performed by the Shona at weddings. The Shona are Bantu-speaking people who live in southeastern Africa, mostly in Zimbabwe.

"Wai bamba" has three layers of sound and each layer has its own melody. **Sing** "Wai bamba," adding one layer at a time. As each new layer is added, the **texture** of the music will become thicker and **harmony** will be created.

Harmony is created when two or more different tones sound at the same time.
Texture is the layering of sounds to create a thick or thin quality in music.

▲ Shona mask

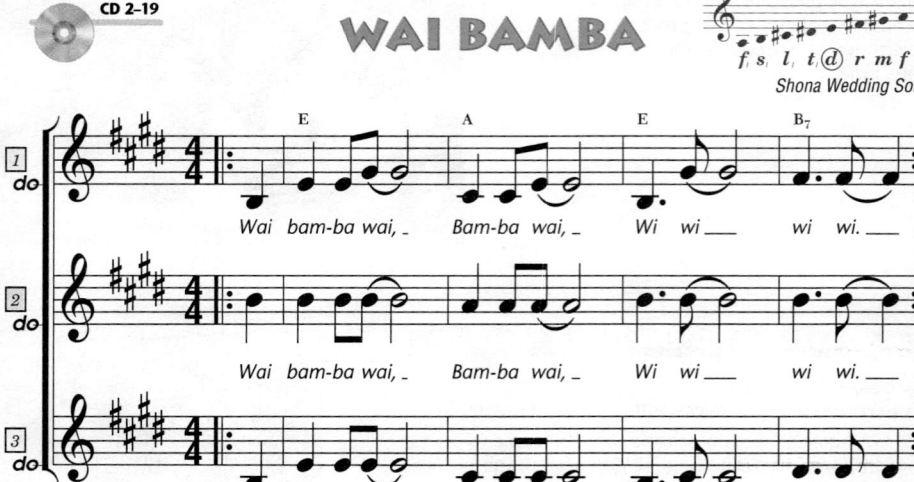

CD 2–19

WAI BAMBA

f s, l, t @ r m f s
Shona Wedding Song

1 do
Wai bam-ba wai, _ Bam-ba wai, _ Wi wi ___ wi wi.

2 do
Wai bam-ba wai, _ Bam-ba wai, _ Wi wi ___ wi wi.

3 do
Wai bam-ba wai, _ Bam-ba wai, _ Wi wi ___ wi wi.

26

Footnotes

SPOTLIGHT ON

▶ **Mbira** The *mbira* is a unique African percussion instrument. It consists of a gourd resonator or wooden box, often with sound holes. To this is attached very thin strips of metal, wood, or cane. The pitch of each strip can be changed by adding wax to its free end or by increasing or decreasing its length. Jingles or beads are often added to the keys to create a rich, buzzing tone. The performer plays the instrument by plucking the strips with the thumbs and fingers.

BUILDING SKILLS THROUGH MUSIC

▶ **Social Studies** Ask students to read the information on p. 26, then share with them the information from Across the Curriculum on p. 27. Ask students to list songs that are used in celebrations, or events. Guide them to determine the culture, describing some traits, in which the songs are used.

SKILLS REINFORCEMENT

2a ▶ **Playing** Encourage interested students to accompany the vocal parts of "Wai bamba" with the following percussion arrangement. Students should create a routine that emphasizes the layering effect of the sung parts.

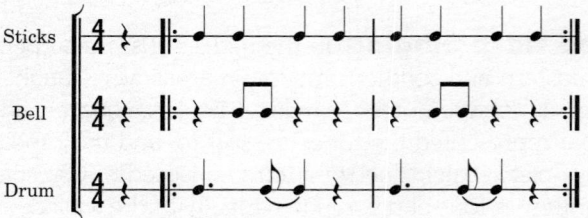

Sticks

Bell

Drum

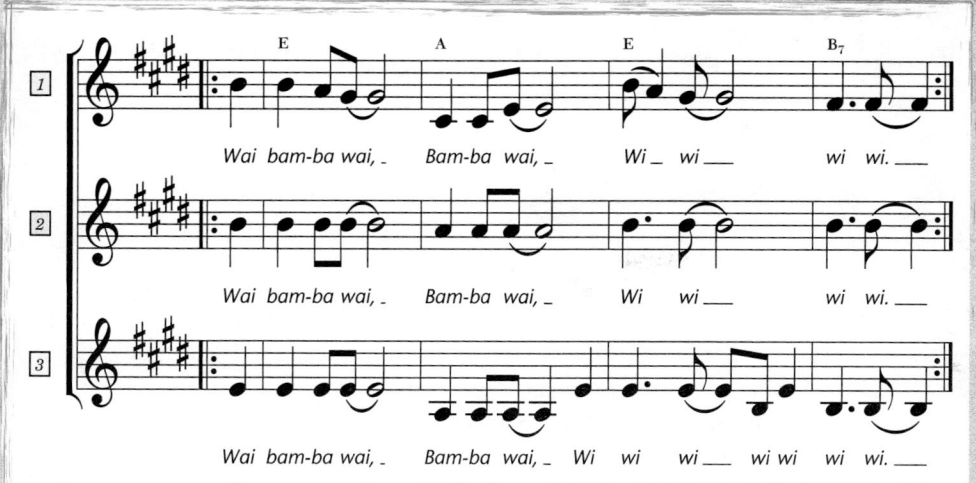

Wai bam-ba wai, _ Bam-ba wai, _ Wi wi _ wi wi. _

Wai bam-ba wai, _ Bam-ba wai, _ Wi wi _ wi wi. _

Wai bam-ba wai, _ Bam-ba wai, _ Wi wi wi _ wi wi wi wi. _

Talented Thumbs

The *mbira* [mm-BEE-rah] is one of the instruments used to accompany "*Wai bamba*." The *mbira*, played with the thumb and forefingers, is one of the Shona's most important instruments. The Shona have used the *mbira* in ceremonies for more than 1,000 years. It is frequently praised for its power to soothe the nerves during severe thunderstorms and to calm wild animals of the African jungle.

Listen to this *mbira* performance. **Describe** how the two players use repeated patterns to create a layered texture.

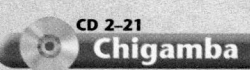 CD 2–21
Chigamba

Traditional song from Zimbabwe as performed by Stella Rambisai Chiweshe Nekati

The *mbira* was traditionally played by men. Stella Rambisai Chiweshe Nekati was one of the first Zimbabwe women to break tradition and learn to play the *mbira*. She is known as the "Queen of Mbira."

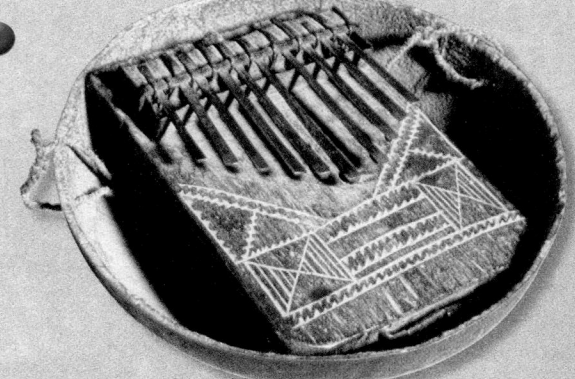

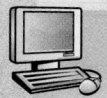 **MIDI/Sequencing Software** Improvise and record an accompaniment to "*Wai bamba*" using African drum and *mbira* sounds.

▲ Mbira

2 DEVELOP

Listening

6a Sing or play Part 1 of "*Wai bamba*" **CD 2-19.** Invite students to follow the part as they listen.

ASK How many voice parts were added to the melody you were following? (2)

6b Help students understand that layering voices on top of one another creates harmony.

Singing

1a
1c Divide the class into three groups. Assign each group one layer of "*Wai bamba*." Have students

- Sing each layer separately with the recording.
- Sing the entire song in parts, beginning with layer 1 and adding layers 2 and 3 at the appropriate time.

ASK How did the music change when we added layers? (The texture became thicker.)

Listening

6a Invite students to listen for the *mbira* featured in *Chigamba* **CD 2-21** and in the Sound Bank **CD 23-32.**

ASK How would you describe the timbre of the *mbira*? (Accept all answers–metallic sound; percussive rattling; resonating tones.)

6b Ask students to read the information about the *mbira* on p. 27. Tell them that *mbira* music relies on layering simple parts on top of one another and can be used to accompany singing.

3 CLOSE

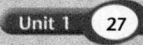
Element:TEXTURE/HARMONY ← **ASSESSMENT**

Performance/Self-Assessment Have students perform all parts of "*Wai bamba*" without the recording. Allow students to evaluate their understanding of layered ostinatos and whether they successfully created the layering effect in their singing.

ACROSS THE CURRICULUM

▶ **Social Studies** Encourage students to learn more about special occasions from around the world in *Celebrations! Children Just Like Me* by Barnabas and Anabel Kindersley (DK Publishing, 1997). As students read more about other children's experiences, they will be able to relate to the specific music of other cultures in a more meaningful way.

▶ **Language Arts** Ceremonial events of the Shona people of Africa are usually celebrated with the *mbira* in ensembles of up to 20 instruments. African people brought *mbiras* to the Caribbean and to North, South, and Central America. In the United States, the instrument is known as the thumb piano. Read *The Soul of Mbira: Music and Traditions of the Shona People of Zimbabwe* by Paul Berliner (University of Chicago Press, 1994) for detailed information about the *mbira*.

TECHNOLOGY/MEDIA LINK

4c **MIDI/Sequencing Software** Have students listen to "*Wai bamba*" **CD 2-19** and list African folk instruments that can be used to accompany the recording (drums, *mbira*). Then have students

- Locate and explore African sounds on their MIDI keyboard.
- Improvise melody patterns using the *mbira* sound.
- Improvise rhythm patterns using the drum sounds.
- Use sequencing software to record their accompaniment.
- Record new tracks to create additional layers of texture, harmony, melody, and rhythm.

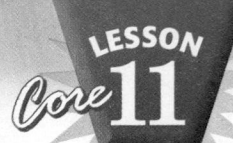

LESSON AT A GLANCE

Element Focus	**TEXTURE/HARMONY** Layering (density, ostinatos)
Skill Objective	**PLAYING** Play an accompaniment using layered ostinatos
Connection Activity	**STYLE** Discover what makes "swing" notes different from other rhythms

MATERIALS

- "Hey, Ho! Nobody Home"   **CD 2-22**
  Recording Routine: Intro (4 m.); ostinatos (12 m.); vocal; interlude (8 m.); vocal; interlude (8 m.); coda
- **Resource Book** pp. F-3, G-4, H-8
- Pitched and nonpitched classroom instruments

VOCABULARY

ostinato

◆ ◆ ◆ ◆ National Standards ◆ ◆ ◆ ◆

1a Sing accurately in large and small ensembles
2a Play instruments accurately alone and in small ensembles
4b Arrange pieces for instruments
4c Compose, using electronic media

MORE MUSIC CHOICES

For more practice playing or singing ostinatos:
"Dona nabis pacem," p. 125
"Scattin' A-Round," p. 160

1 INTRODUCE

Invite students to echo-clap a four-beat rhythm pattern of your choosing. Divide the class into four groups. Give each group its own rhythm and gesture (clap, patsch, snap, or tap) to perform. Begin with one group, then layer each group's patterns on top, one at a time. Ask students how texture is created. (by layering short patterns)

Pleasing Polyphony

Listen to "Hey, Ho! Nobody Home." **Describe** what happens to the texture and harmony as you listen to the song. How is it similar to *"Wai bamba"* on page 26? How is the harmony created?

Notice the rhythm notation above measure 1. This notation tells the performer to swing the eighth notes. **Listen** to the recording again, paying attention to the eighth notes sung with swing style. **Sing** "Hey, Ho! Nobody Home."

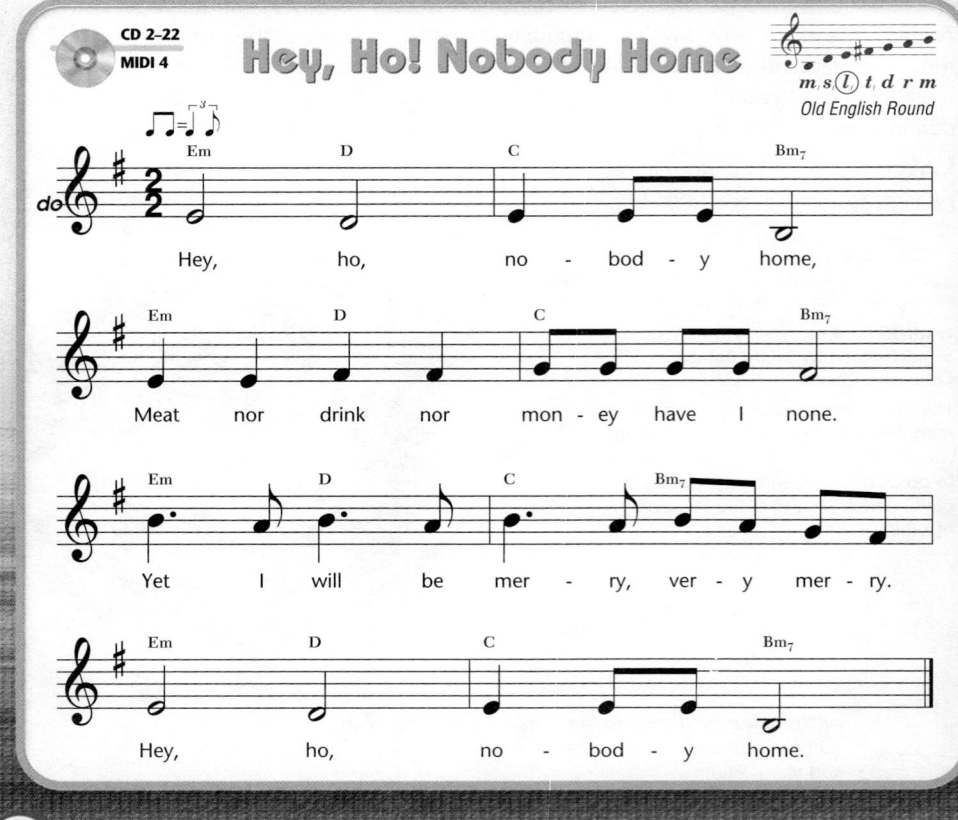

Hey, Ho! Nobody Home

CD 2–22 MIDI 4

Old English Round

Hey, ho, no - bod - y home,

Meat nor drink nor mon - ey have I none.

Yet I will be mer - ry, ver - y mer - ry.

Hey, ho, no - bod - y home.

28

Footnotes

SKILLS REINFORCEMENT

▶ **Mallets** Invite students to learn the Orff accompaniment for "Hey, Ho! Nobody Home" on Resource Book p. F-3.

▶ **Keyboard** Have students play an ostinato accompaniment to "Hey, Ho! Nobody Home," on Resource Book p. H-8.

▶ **Signing** Students may be interested in learning the signing to "Hey, Ho! Nobody Home" on Resource Book p. G-4.

BUILDING SKILLS THROUGH MUSIC

▶ **Visual Arts** Divide students into groups and have them create ostinatos for the song "Hey, Ho! Nobody Home." Then, have them create a visual representation of the texture used in their performance. Have the groups share their pictures and perform their ostinatos. Ask the class to compare the aural and visual representation of the texture, expressing ideas based on their observations.

MOVEMENT

▶ **Patterned Dance** Invite students to perform this movement routine with "Hey, Ho! Nobody Home."

Formation: Stand in four horizontal lines across the room.

Measure 1: Step forward on left, step forward on right.

Measure 2: Place hands on chest, then away (to represent "no").

Measure 3: Move left arm, with palm up, to left side.

Measure 4: Move right arm, with palm up, to right side.

Measure 5: Sway left, sway right.

Measure 6: Twirl in a circle.

Measure 7: Repeat measure 1.

Measure 8: Repeat measure 2.

Add an Ostinato by Singing or Playing

We can create harmony in layers with one or more **ostinatos**.

Sing these ostinatos with a swing feeling. When you are ready, **perform** them as you accompany "Hey, Ho! Nobody Home."

> An **ostinato** is a musical idea that is continually repeated. Ostinatos can be melodic, rhythmic, or harmonic.

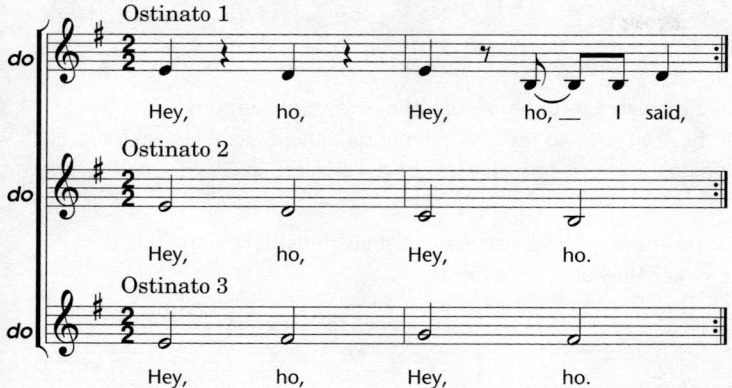

Ostinato 1
do — Hey, ho, Hey, ho, — I said,

Ostinato 2
do — Hey, ho, Hey, ho.

Ostinato 3
do — Hey, ho, Hey, ho.

Build an Ensemble

For an even richer texture, add these instrumental ostinatos to your "Hey, Ho! Nobody Home" ensemble. Then **improvise** your own parts to use as an introduction and an interlude.

Alto metallophone

Tambourine

Bass metallophone

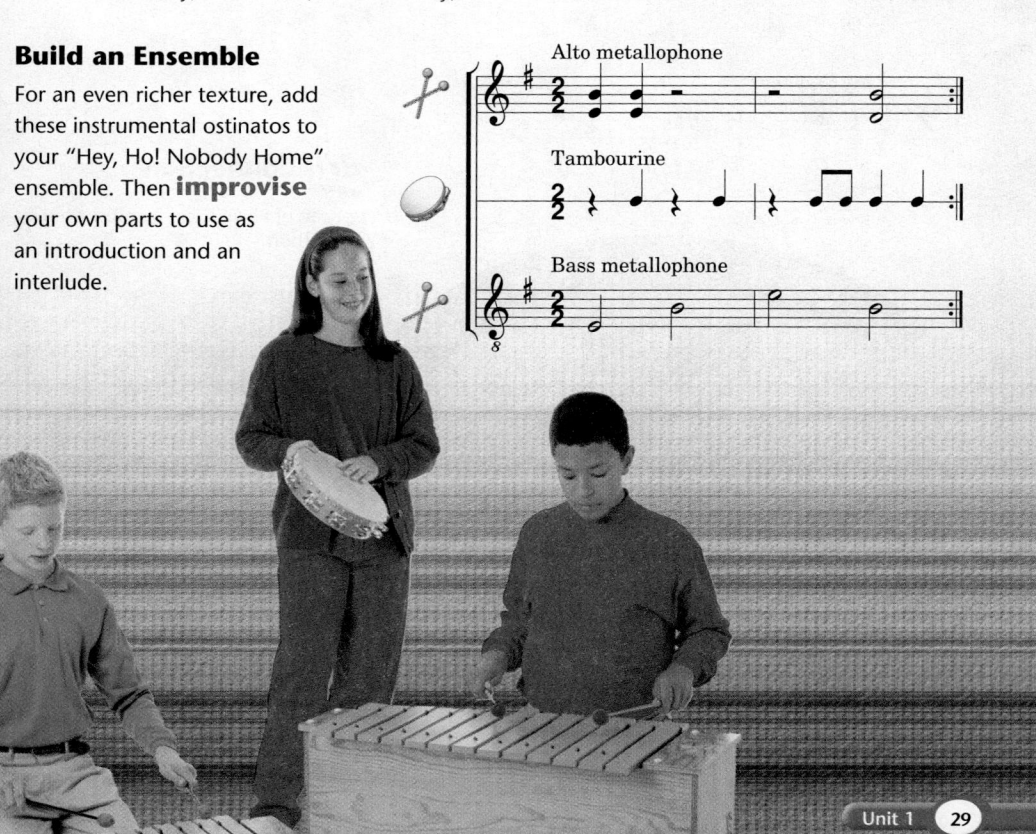

Unit 1 **29**

Listening

Have students listen to "Hey, Ho! Nobody Home" **CD 2-22** as they follow the layered ostinatos.

Singing

1a Invite students to sing the melody of "Hey, Ho! Nobody Home" with the recording. Have them count the number of ostinatos used for accompaniment. (3)

Have students

- Practice the melody and each ostinato.
- Sing the entire song, starting with Ostinato 1; then, in order, add Ostinatos 2 and 3, and, finally, the melody. (Each part will sing four measures before the next part enters.)

ASK **Which parts have rhythms that fall on the beat?** (parts 2, 3) **Off the beat?** (part 1)

Point out that the rhythm also includes "swing" eighth notes, as indicated above the first line of the melody.

Playing

2a

4b Divide the class into groups of four. Have each group

- Play one ostinato from the vocal parts, then instrumental parts, written on p. 29.
- Create and play two original ostinatos. (Remind students that each part is two measures long.)
- Sing the melody of "Hey, Ho! Nobody Home" with the instrumental accompaniment.

3 CLOSE

Skill: PLAYING   **ASSESSMENT**

Performance/Self-Assessment Have each group perform the ostinatos for "Hey, Ho! Nobody Home." Have students evaluate if the layered ostinatos were performed accurately and in time with one another.

TEACHER TO TEACHER

▶ **The Changing Voice** Some sixth-grade boys may be entering the first phase of voice change. They may experience difficulty singing songs having a wide range. These singers are often limited to a few pitches they can sing well and in tune. Ostinatos, especially ostinatos within a narrow range, provide opportunities for them to be successful at singing in harmony. The chances for success will be greater if these students are assigned to parts that best match their present vocal range.

TECHNOLOGY/MEDIA LINK

4c **MIDI/Sequencing Software** Ask students to work in small groups to create rhythmic phrases for a multiple-track composition for MIDI drum sounds. Have students

- Play back the MIDI song file for "Hey, Ho! Nobody Home."
- Experiment with percussion sounds.
- Compose and record several phrases, layering the rhythm tracks and using various percussion sounds.
- Perform rhythm arrangements for classmates.

LESSON AT A GLANCE

Element Focus **TEXTURE/HARMONY** Changes in density

Skill Objective **LISTENING** Identify changes in the texture of a listening selection

Connection Activity **STYLE** Experience minimalist style and the use of ostinatos

MATERIALS

• *Open the Kingdom*   **CD 2-24**

VOCABULARY

minimalism   ostinato

◆ ◆ ◆ ◆ National Standards ◆ ◆ ◆ ◆

4a Compose short pieces, demonstrating balance through music
6b Listen and analyze uses of texture in music from diverse genres
9b Classify high-quality musical works by composer

MORE MUSIC CHOICES

For more practice with changing textures:

"Fais do do," p. 403
"Free at Last," p. 468
"Ise oluwa," p. 230

1 INTRODUCE

Ask students to describe musical texture (1) when there is a melody only; (2) when there is a melody plus accompaniment; and (3) when there are two or more melodies happening at once.

ASK What happens to the music when more melodies are added in layers? (The texture becomes thicker.)

9b Share with students the information about minimalism as a musical style. See Spotlight On on p. 30.

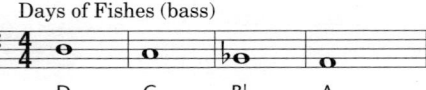
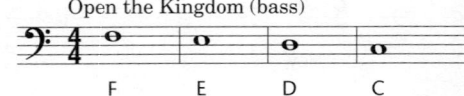

Obstinate Ostinatos

Musical texture is created through the use of melody and harmony. Ostinatos can be used to build textures. Composer Philip Glass is known for his use of ostinatos. The bass-line ostinatos below are used in Glass's *Open the Kingdom.*

Play these ostinatos on a keyboard or a mallet instrument. How are the ostinatos the same? How are they different?

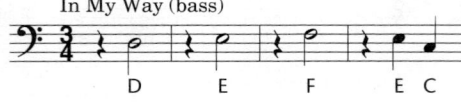

Days of Fishes (bass)
D   C   B♭   A

Open the Kingdom (bass)
F   E   D   C

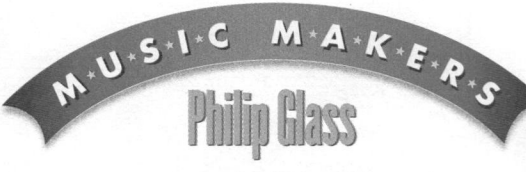

In My Way (bass)
D   E   F   E C

Arts Connection

Portrait of Philip Glass by artist Chuck Close (born 1940) ▼

MUSIC MAKERS
Philip Glass

Philip Glass (born 1937) is an American composer who is best known for a style called minimalism. In this style, Glass uses ostinatos to create pleasing harmonies and layered textures. Sometimes his musical pieces are very long, lasting up to twelve hours. Some of Glass's most important works are his operas *Einstein on the Beach* (about Albert Einstein) and *Akhnaten* (about the Egyptian pharaoh Akhnaten). Glass's music is influenced by pop and classical music as well as West African and Indian music.

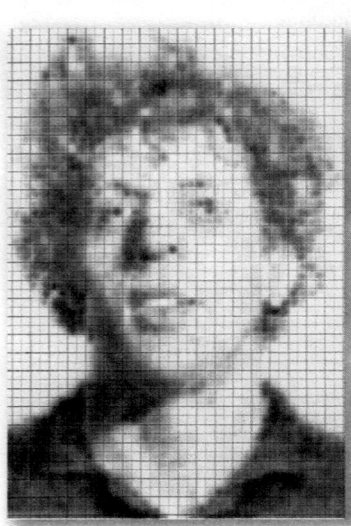

30

Footnotes

ACROSS THE CURRICULUM

▶ **Visual Arts** Invite students to create an *Open the Kingdom* "laser" show, using five flashlights. Cover each lens with a different-colored theater gel. Assign one color to the vocal melody, and a different color to each ostinato. Encourage students to experiment with their lasers to find a visual pattern that fits their assigned part. Then, have students synchronize their lasers with the music on the recording.

BUILDING SKILLS THROUGH MUSIC

▶ **Language** Share the information from Spotlight On below, with students. Invite them to experiment with minimalism in writing. Have them begin with a basic sentence, then repeat it over and over with small changes, that grow gradually over time. Tell students this can become a performance piece by overlapping the many variations.

SPOTLIGHT ON

▶ **Minimalism** Minimalism emerged as a musical style in the 1970s. A group of young composers wanted to create music with the smallest possible amount of musical material.

Minimalists take a musical idea and repeat it over and over with only small changes. These changes are very gradual and occur over a period of time. The effect is sometimes hypnotic. Minimalist composers include Philip Glass, John Adams, Steve Reich, Terry Riley, and Lamont Young.

Minimalism can also be found in the work of sculptors and other visual artists of this era. Their work is usually a simple object, often geometric, stripped of human receptiveness. Frank Stella, Anne Truitt, Ellsworth Kelly, Carl Andre, and Donald Judd are some of the artists who worked in minimalist style.

Hear It Again...And Again!

Follow this map as you **listen** to *Open the Kingdom*. **Identify** the bass and other ostinatos in the piece.

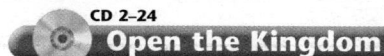

CD 2–24

Open the Kingdom

by Philip Glass and David Byrne
David Byrne was one of the founding members of the rock group Talking Heads.

OPEN THE KINGDOM LISTENING MAP

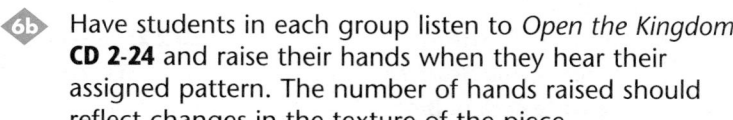

Unit 1 **31**

---

2 DEVELOP

Listening

Invite students to

- Read about the composer Philip Glass.
- Look at the listening map for *Open the Kingdom*.

ASK Do you expect the music to be performed by instruments or voices? (both)

Invite students to listen to *Open the Kingdom* **CD 2-24** as they follow the listening map.

ASK How is the melody performed? (by a singer)

What did you notice about the accompaniment? (It has four different layers, or patterns.)

Analyzing

Divide the class into five groups. Assign each group either the melody or one of the ostinato-like patterns on p. 30.

6b Have students in each group listen to *Open the Kingdom* **CD 2-24** and raise their hands when they hear their assigned pattern. The number of hands raised should reflect changes in the texture of the piece.

Playing

Invite students to play the ostinatos on p. 30.

3 CLOSE

Element:TEXTURE/HARMONY — ASSESSMENT

Observation Ask students to

- Listen to *Open the Kingdom* **CD 2-24** with their eyes closed.
- Hold up one, two, three, four, or five fingers to indicate how many different parts they hear as the piece progresses.

Observe students' ability to perceive changes in musical texture by indicating the number of parts they hear.

SKILLS REINFORCEMENT

4a ▶ **Creating** Divide the class into several groups and assign each group a color. Invite each group to create an eight-beat rhythm, using body percussion. Give each group five to eight sheets of paper in its color. Place eight sheets of white paper in a horizontal line on a wall to represent a total of eight measures. Assign each group a horizontal line under the white markers and allow students to choose in which measures they will perform their ostinato. Have them indicate this by placing a sheet of their "group color" paper beneath the appropriate white measure markers. (They will not have enough papers to fill every measure.) After all the groups have attached their paper to the wall, have students perform the composition, observing their ability to perform it accurately. Encourage students to watch and listen to the textural changes in their composition.

TECHNOLOGY/MEDIA LINK

Transparency Display the listening map transparency for *Open the Kingdom*. Invite students to trace the progress of the song with a finger on the map in their books as you trace on the overhead projection.

Web Site Visit *www.sfsuccessnet.com* to learn more about minimalism in music and painting.

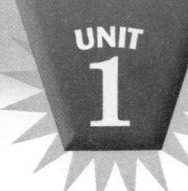

UNIT 1 — Review and Assessment

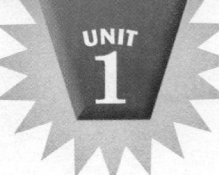 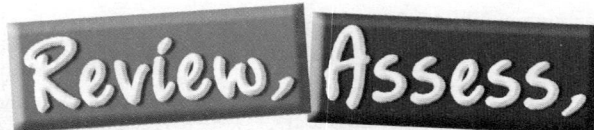

WHAT DO YOU KNOW?

MATERIALS
- **Resource Book** p. B-3

Review with students musical expression on pp. 6–9 (What Do You Know? 1) and downbeat and anacrusis on pp. 12–13. (What Do You Know? 2)

When ready, students may answer questions 1 and 2 in What Do You Know?, using Resource Book p. B-3.

WHAT DO YOU HEAR?

MATERIALS
- *What Do You Hear? 1A*   **CD 2-25 to 2-30**
- *What Do You Hear? 1B*   **CD 2-31**
- **Resource Book** p. B-4

Review vocal styles and timbre on pp. 24–25. Have students listen to the vocal selections on p. 32. (*What Do You Hear? 1A* **CD 2-25 to CD 2-30**) Ask them to select the correct vocal performance for each listening selection.

Review the concept of form on pp. 14–15. Then, play the recording of "Lean on Me" **CD 2-31**. Have students identify the correct form of the song using form symbols (**A**, **B**, and so on).

Students may mark their answers on the worksheet on Resource Book p. B-4.

What Do You Know?

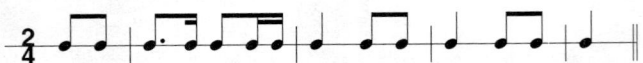

1. For each term on the left, identify the type of musical expression.

Performance	Musical Expression
a. fast	• dynamics
b. loud	• tempo
c. soft	
d. slow	

2. Point to the downbeats in this rhythm. How many downbeats are there? Point to the pickups (anacrusis) in this rhythm. How many pickups are there?

What Do You Hear? 1A

CD 2–25

Vocal Timbre

Listen to these recordings of vocal timbres. Identify the correct vocal performance for each selection.

Excerpt	Vocal Performance
1. _____	**a.** opera chorus
2. _____	**b.** women's "barbershop" chorus
3. _____	**c.** Tibetan monks of Central Asia
4. _____	**d.** boys' choir
5. _____	**e.** men's and women's chorus of Tahiti
6. _____	**f.** sacred harp singing

32

Footnotes

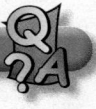

ANSWER KEY

▶ What Do You Know?

1. a. tempo

   b. dynamics

   c. dynamics

   d. tempo

2. There are four downbeats.
The pickup is the first two eighth notes of the rhythm.
There is one pickup.

▶ What Do You Hear? 1A

1. b. women's barbershop chorus

2. e. men's and women's chorus of Tahiti

3. f. sacred harp singing

4. d. boys' choir

5. c. Tibetan monks of Central Asia

6. a. opera chorus

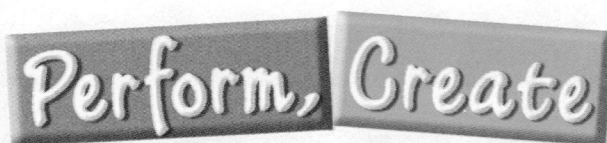

Perform, Create

What Do You Hear? 1B

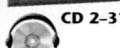
CD 2–31

Form

Listen to the recording of "Lean on Me." Using the form symbols on the right, identify the correct form for the selection.

Form	Form Symbols
a. ABBA	• **A** Verse
b. BABA	• **B** Refrain
c. ABAB	

What You Can Do

Sing Melodic Patterns

Using pitch syllables, read and perform these melodic patterns.

1. so₁ do mi so

2. la so mi do mi

3. so₁ so₁ do mi re

4. mi re do la₁ do

Play and Create Textures with Ostinatos

Select and perform one of the ostinatos for "Hey, Ho! Nobody Home" on page 29. Then, create a new ostinato to accompany the song. When ready, perform your ostinato as a new texture to the song.

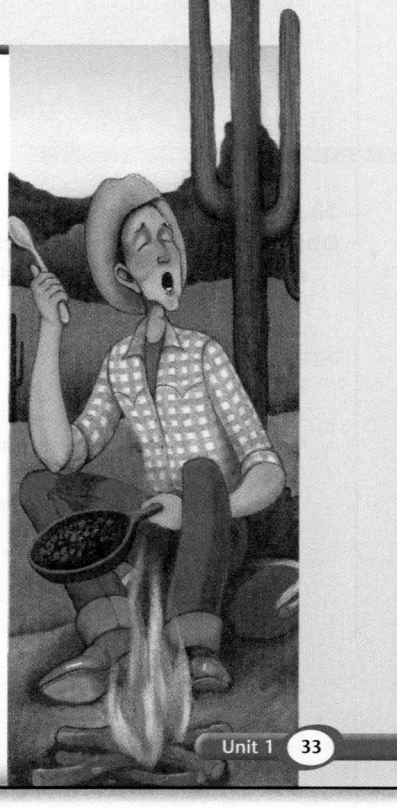

Unit 1　33

WHAT YOU CAN DO

> **MATERIALS**
> • **Resource Book** p. B-5
> • alto metallophone, bass metallophone, tambourine, nonpitched percussion instruments

Sing Melody Patterns

Review the melody patterns in "Bury Me Not on the Lone Prairie" on p. 19, using pitch syllables. Then, lead students in a review of how to sing the notation and syllables found on p. 33, where students must sing the pitch and rhythm accurately from just the syllables. Allow students to practice the patterns. When ready, ask students to sing the melody patterns on p. 33 with pitch syllables, using the worksheet on Resource Book p. B-5.

Play and Create Textures with Ostinatos

Review the vocal and instrumental ostinatos for "Hey, Ho! Nobody Home" on p. 29. Invite students to create a new ostinato to accompany the song, using the worksheet on Resource Book p. B-5. When ready, have students perform their ostinato as an accompaniment, and a new texture, to the song.

▶ **What Do You Hear? 1B**

Form: c. ABAB (Verse, Refrain, Verse, Refrain)

TECHNOLOGY/MEDIA LINK

▶ Rubrics

Visit *www.sfsuccessnet.com* for rubrics to assess students' achievement in music skills.

Lesson	Elements	Skills	
LESSON 1 **CORE** **Soft to Loud!** pp. 38–41 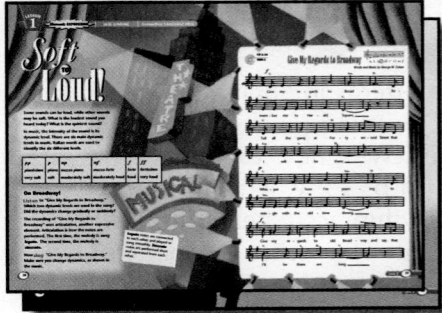	**Element: Expression** **Concept:** Dynamics/articulation **Focus:** Dynamics and articulation **Secondary Element** Form: abac **National Standards** 4c 6b 8a 8b	**Skill: Singing** **Objective:** Sing using dynamic changes to create expressive effects **Secondary Skills** • **Listening** Identify changes in dynamics • **Singing** Sing a song; pay close attention to articulation and dynamics • **Creating** Create a nonpitched percussion accompaniment for a poem and use vocal dynamics in reading it • **Listening** Listen to a musical setting of a poem	**SKILLS REINFORCEMENT** • **Keyboard** Perform a keyboard arrangement of a song • **Listening** Listen to a song and focus on its form • **Recorder** Play a recorder part
LESSON 2 **CORE** **Signs of Time** pp. 42–43 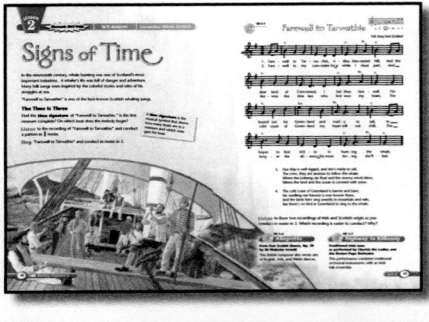 **Reading Sequence 5, p. 490**	**Element: Rhythm** **Concept:** Meter **Focus:** Meter in 3 **Secondary Element** Form: question-and-answer phrases **National Standards** 2a 4c 5a 5d 6b	**Skill: Reading** **Objective:** Read and perform rhythm patterns in triple meter while conducting the beat **Secondary Skills** • **Listening** Listen to a Scottish folk song and conduct to find the upbeat • **Singing** Sing a Scottish folk song while showing the melodic contour of the phrase • **Moving** Move to the rhythm of a song with a meter in 3	**SKILLS REINFORCEMENT** • **Recorder** Play a countermelody on a soprano recorder • **Reading** Practice working with meter in 3, upbeats, and rhythmic dictation • **Mallets** Learn an Orff accompaniment for a song
LESSON 3 **Ballad Rhythms** pp. 44–45 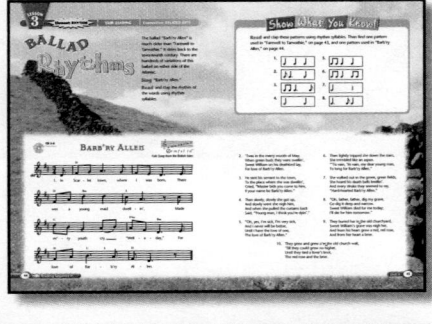 **Reading Sequence 6, p. 490**	**Element: Rhythm** **Concept:** Meter **Focus:** Meter in 3 **Secondary Element** Form: abcd **National Standards** 5a 6b 8b 9a	**Skill: Reading** **Objective:** Read and perform rhythms **Secondary Skills** • **Listening** Identify time signature and story of a ballad • **Reading** Clap the rhythm and conduct phrases of a ballad • **Listening** Identify phrases of a song and how singers express stories in songs	**SKILLS REINFORCEMENT** • **Mallets** Learn an Orff accompaniment for a ballad • **Reading** Practice working with pitch set and rhythms of a ballad • **Singing** Demonstrate understanding of narrative and dialogue exchanges

Connections

Music and Other Literature

Connection: Language Arts

Activity: Explore dynamics and articulation in interpreting a poem

TEACHER TO TEACHER **School Musicals** Read a book about how to produce a successful musical

SPOTLIGHT ON
The Poet Facts about Robert Frost
The Composer Facts about Randall Thompson

MOVEMENT **Patterned Dance** Perform a dance routine

MEETING INDIVIDUAL NEEDS **Including Everyone** Use a poem to help students discover activity in speech

ACROSS THE CURRICULUM **Language Arts/Poetry** Read poems and listen to choral settings of Frostiana

CHARACTER EDUCATION **Expression** Help students understand the importance of nonverbal and verbal expression

SCHOOL TO HOME CONNECTION **Interview** Favorite musicals

BUILDING SKILLS THROUGH MUSIC **Writing** Rewrite a story from a different point of view

Song "Give My Regards to Broadway"

Poem "Stopping by Woods on a Snowy Evening"

Listening Selection "Stopping by Woods on a Snowy Evening" from *Frostiana*

More Music Choices
"Goin' to Boston," p. 433
"Run! Run! Hidel," p. 340
"This Little Light of Mine," p. 232

ASSESSMENT
Performance/Observation Sing using vocal dynamics and *legato* and *stacatto* articulations

TECHNOLOGY/MEDIA LINK
MIDI/Sequencing Software Experiment with changing dynamics

Connection: Social Studies

Activity: Discuss interesting facts and stories about the lives of whalers

TEACHER TO TEACHER **Question-and-Answer Form** Analyze the melodic contour of question-and-answer form

ACROSS THE CURRICULUM **Social Studies** Discuss facts and stories about whalers in the late nineteenth century

BUILDING SKILLS THROUGH MUSIC **Science** Investigate the decline in the whaling industry

Song "Farewell to Tarwathie"

Listening Selection
"Allegretto" from *Four Scottish Dances*, Op. 59
Highway to Kilkenny

More Music Choices
"America," p. 484
"*Fais do do,*" p. 403

ASSESSMENT
Performance/Observation Read and sing a Scottish folk song while conducting meter in 3

TECHNOLOGY/MEDIA LINK
MIDI/Sequencing Software Create an ostinato accompaniment and a countermelody for a song
Web Site Learn more about the music of Scotland

Connection: Related Arts

Activity: Dramatize a ballad

ACROSS THE CURRICULUM **Related Arts** Perform a dramatized ballad

SPOTLIGHT ON **The Lyrics** Additional verses of a ballad

BUILDING SKILLS THROUGH MUSIC **Reading** Analyze the literary elements of a song

Song "Barb'ry Allen"

Listening Selection *Sellenger's Round*

More Music Choices
"*Gloria, Gloria,*" p. 459
Waltz of the Flowers, p. 325

ASSESSMENT
Performance/Observation Read and perform rhythms in meter in 3 using rhythm syllables

TECHNOLOGY/MEDIA LINK
Multimedia Create graphic illustrations of selected verses of a ballad

Lesson	Elements	Skills

LESSON 4 — CORE

A Favorite Form

pp. 46–49

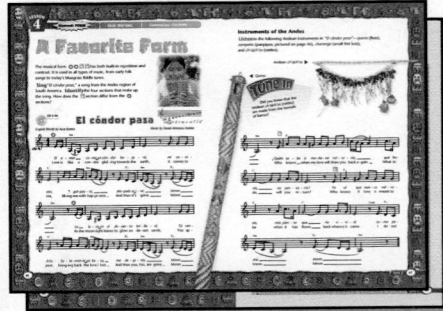

Element: Form
Concept: aabb form
Focus: aabb form

Secondary Element
Timbre: folk instruments

National Standards
1c 6b 8a 8b

Skill: Moving
Objective: Perform movement to illustrate the form of a song

Secondary Skills
- **Listening** Identify the aabb form of a melody; identify aabb form in a melody
- **Analyzing** Analyze the notation of an Andean song
- **Singing** Sing an Andean song with Spanish lyrics
- **Singing** Sing a song and identify the sections

SKILLS REINFORCEMENT
- **Recorder** Play a countermelody to accompany a song
- **Mallets** Learn an Orff accompaniment
- **Guitar** Learn a song with first-position chords on a guitar

LESSON 5

Playing with Form

pp. 50–51

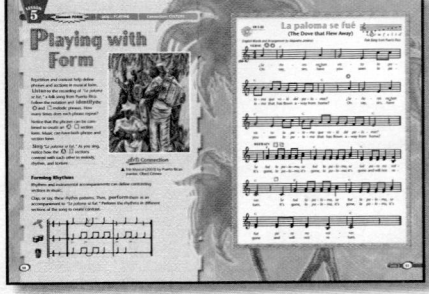

Element: Form
Concept: phrase form
Focus: aabb phrase form, AB section form

Secondary Element
ostinato

National Standards
1a 1c 2b 2e 4c 6b

Skill: Playing
Objective: Perform ostinato patterns to accompany a song

Secondary Skills
- **Listening** Listen for and identify the large A and B forms in a Puerto Rican folk song
- **Singing** Sing a Puerto Rican folk song with English and Spanish lyrics
- **Playing** Perform percussion ostinatos

SKILLS REINFORCEMENT
- **Mallets** Learn an Orff accompaniment to a Puerto Rican folk song

LESSON 6

Glorious Gospel

pp. 52–53

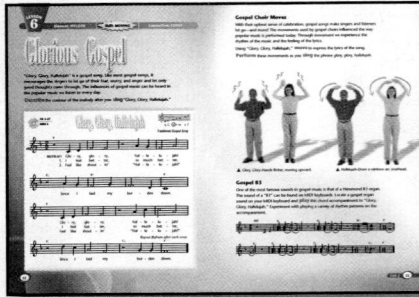

Element: Melody
Concept: Pitch and direction
Focus: Melodic contour

Secondary Element
Timbre: small vocal ensemble

National Standards
1a 2a 4c 8a

Skill: Moving
Objective: Move to express the lyrics of a song and show melodic contour

Secondary Skills
- **Singing** Identify the melodic contour of a song
- **Movement** Create and perform movements to a gospel song

SKILLS REINFORCEMENT
- **Vocal Development** Sing in small ensembles to develop good vocal tone quality

Connections

Music and Other Literature

Connection: Culture
Activity: Discuss the musical and cultural history of Elizabethan England

CULTURAL CONNECTION
Andean Instruments Discuss facts about Andean Instruments
Sixteenth-Century Elizabethan England Discuss sixteenth-century Elizabethan England

AUDIENCE ETIQUETTE **At School Assemblies** Practice and enforce audience behavior

ACROSS THE CURRICULUM
Social Studies Introduce students to the Andes mountains
Visual Arts Find visuals that show aabb form

MEETING INDIVIDUAL NEEDS **Gifted and Talented** Create panpipes to explore how length of pipes affects pitch

SCHOOL TO HOME CONNECTION **Research** Research the indigenous people of the Andes region of South America

BUILDING SKILLS THROUGH MUSIC **Science** Use bottles to experiment with pitch

Songs
"El cóndor pasa"
"Greensleeves"

More Music Choices
"Alumot" (aabb), p. 306
"Everybody Loves Saturday Night" (aaba), p. 296
"Sun Gonna Shine" (aab), p. 242

ASSESSMENT

Performance/Music Journal Writing Complete and present an integrated art project to show understanding of aabb form

TECHNOLOGY/MEDIA LINK
Video Library Watch a video about the *charango*

Connection: Culture
Activity: Discuss the cultural heritage of the native peoples of Puerto Rico

CULTURAL CONNECTION **Puerto Rico's Music** Discuss the music and instruments of Puerto Rico

ACROSS THE CURRICULUM **Social Studies** Learn about explorer Christopher Columbus and his discovery of the Taíno people

BUILDING SKILLS THROUGH MUSIC **Writing** Write a description of a composition

Song *"La paloma se fué"* ("The Dove that Flew Away")

More Music Choices
"Greensleeves," p. 49
"El cóndor pasa," p. 46

ASSESSMENT

Performance/Self-Assessment Create a rhythmic composition in aabb phrase form

TECHNOLOGY/MEDIA LINK
Electronic Keyboard Create an aabb rhythmic composition for electronic keyboard

---

Connection: Genre
Activity: Explore the gospel genre with regard to movement and spirit of the lyrics

MEETING INDIVIDUAL NEEDS **Including Everyone** Use smaller gestures to allow students with muscular disabilities to synchronize with the beat

CULTURAL CONNECTION **A Crossover Tune** Discuss two songs that use the same melody

BUILDING SKILLS THROUGH MUSIC **Social Studies** Discuss the influences of gospel music

Songs
"Glory, Glory Hallelujah"
"Will the Circle Be Unbroken" (lyrics only)

More Music Choices
The Battle of Jericho, p. 234
Jonah, p. 235
"This Little Light of Mine," p. 232

ASSESSMENT

Performance/Self-Assessment Perform a gospel song with movements

TECHNOLOGY/MEDIA LINK
MIDI/Sequencing Software Explore melodic contour using graphic editing features

Lesson	Elements	Skills	
LESSON 7 **Go with the Melody** pp. 54–55 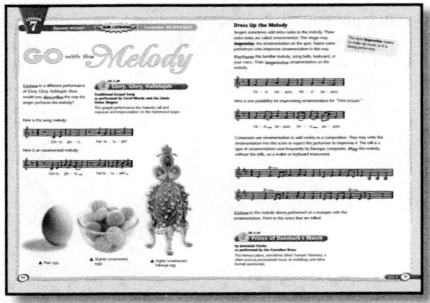	**Element: Melody** **Concept:** Pitch and direction **Focus:** Melodic ornamentation **Secondary Element** Timbre: trumpet **National Standards** 1c 3b 6a 8a	**Skill: Listening** **Objective:** Listen for, identify, and describe ornamentation in brass music **Secondary Skills** • **Listening** Listen to an ornamented version of a gospel song • **Analyzing** Describe the way a singer performs a melody by discussing ornamentation • **Singing** Sing along with an ornamented version of a song • **Playing** Perform a song with ornamentation on melodic instruments	**SKILLS REINFORCEMENT** • **Reading** Look for "skeleton melody" when reading music
LESSON 8 **CORE** **A Singing "Tonic"** pp. 56–57 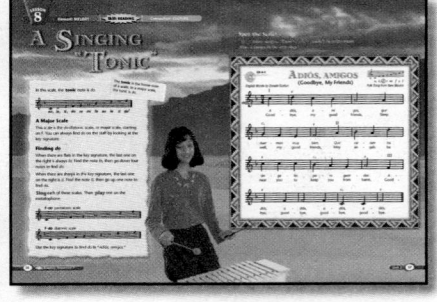 🖐 Reading Sequence 7, p. 491	**Element: Melody** **Concept:** Tonality **Focus:** Major scale **Secondary Element** Texture: rounds **National Standards** 1c 5b 5c 6b	**Skill: Reading** **Objective:** Read the major diatonic scale **Secondary Skills** • **Reading** Identify a pentatonic scale; find do with sharp and flat key signatures • **Singing** Identify the key of and sing a New Mexican folk song from notation	**SKILLS REINFORCEMENT** • **Reading** Sing a countermelody for a New Mexican folk song • **Signing** Learn the signing for a New Mexican folk song • **Analyzing** Analyze scales to develop analytical and problem-solving skills
LESSON 9 **Migrate to Minor** pp. 58–59 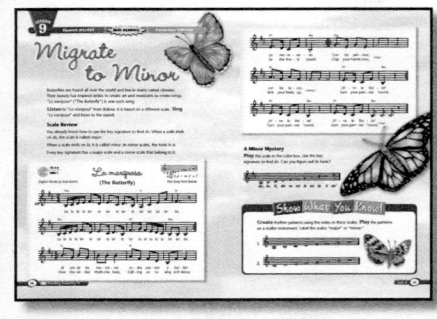 🖐 Reading Sequence 8, p. 491	**Element: Melody** **Concept:** Tonality **Focus:** Minor Scales **National Standards** 1c 2a 5b 6b	**Skill: Reading** **Objective:** Read *la* diatonic scales **Secondary Skills** • **Reading** Identify the key of a Bolivian folk song • **Playing** Play rhythmic ostinato accompaniments to a Bolivian folk song • **Singing** Sing a Bolivian folk song in Spanish • **Moving** Learn and perform a Bolivian folk dance	**SKILLS REINFORCEMENT** • **Guitar** Play an accompaniment to a Bolivian folk song • **Reading** Practice reading scores • **Playing** Play percussion ostinatos

Connections

Music and Other Literature

Connection: Related Arts

Activity: View and discuss ornamentation in visual art

ACROSS THE CURRICULUM **Related Arts** Discover facts about Fabergé eggs

SPOTLIGHT ON
Prince of Denmark's March Background on *Prince of Denmark's March*
The Canadian Brass Background on the brass quintet

SCHOOL TO HOME CONNECTION **Gospel Performers** Listen to gospel artists

BUILDING SKILLS THROUGH MUSIC **Writing** Elaborate on a simple sentence using prepositional phrases

Listening Selections
"Glory, Glory Hallelujah"
Glory, Glory, Hallelujah (Gospel)
Prince of Denmark's March

More Music Choices
Watermelon Man, p. 270
L'union, p. 487

ASSESSMENT

Observation Listen for, identify, and describe instrumental ornamentation

TECHNOLOGY/MEDIA LINK
Video Library View a gospel choir performance

Connection: Culture

Activity: Discuss the purpose of lullabies

ACROSS THE CURRICULUM **Science** Examine the harmonic series in a discussion of diatonic scales

TEACHER TO TEACHER **Instrument Tips** Have B-flat, F-sharp, and C-sharp bars available in this lesson for mallet instruments

BUILDING SKILLS THROUGH MUSIC **Writing** Create new lyrics

Song *"Adiós, amigos"* ("Goodbye, My Friends")

More Music Choices
"Red River Valley," p. 11
"Give a Little Love," p. 140

ASSESSMENT

Performance/Observation Play diatonic major and minor scales on keyboard or barred instruments

TECHNOLOGY/MEDIA LINK
CD-ROM Explore *Major Scales* in *Alfred's Essentials of Music Theory (Vol. 2)* music software

---

Connection: Culture

Activity: Perform a Bolivian folk dance

CULTURAL CONNECTION **Andean Instruments** Learn about Andean instruments

MOVEMENT **Patterned Dance** Learn a Bolivian folk dance

BUILDING SKILLS THROUGH MUSIC **Science** Determine the effect of size instrument on pitch

Song *"La mariposa"* ("The Butterfly")

More Music Choices
"I Walk the Unfrequented Road," p. 179
"El cóndor pasa," p. 46

ASSESSMENT

Performance/Observation Read the major and minor diatonic scales using pitch syllables and hand signs

TECHNOLOGY/MEDIA LINK
MIDI/Sequencing Software Experiment with altering melodies
Video Library Show a video of a Bolivian *charango* ensemble

Lesson	Elements	Skills	
LESSON 10 **Shades of Sound** pp. 60–61 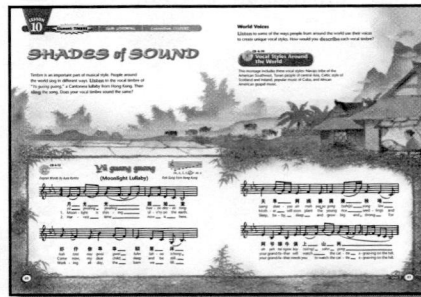	**Element: Timbre** **Concept:** Vocal **Focus:** Vocal timbres of several cultures **Secondary Element** Texture: ostinatos **National Standards** 1c 5a 6b 9a	**Skill: Listening** **Objective:** Describe different vocal timbres **Secondary Skills** • **Singing** Explore vocal timbre; sing a Cantonese song with a recording • **Listening** Discuss various vocal timbres • **Playing** Play a pattern from a Cantonese song on rhythm instruments	
LESSON 11 CORE **Musical Colors** pp. 62–65 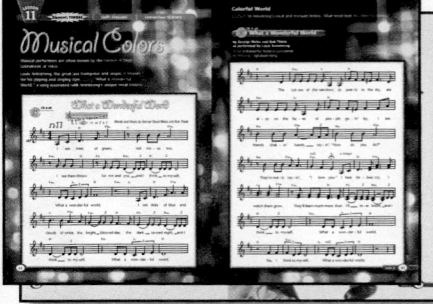	**Element: Timbre** **Concept:** Vocal **Focus:** Vocal timbre **Secondary Element** Form: aaba **National Standards** 3b 4c 6b 8b	**Skill: Singing** **Objective:** Sing and discuss vocal timbres and scat singing **Secondary Skills** • **Reading** Visually identify form of a song • **Singing** Sing a traditional song and then sing the same song using scat syllables • **Listening** Describe the vocal timbres in three recordings of the same song • **Create** Create scat syllables to a melody	**SKILLS REINFORCEMENT** • **Recorder** Play a countermelody in D major • **Listening** Pat a steady beat to a recording of a jazz tune
LESSON 12 CORE **Partners for Peace** pp. 66–69 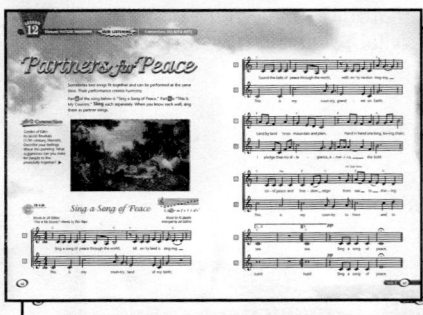	**Element: Texture/Harmony** **Concept:** Texture **Focus:** Combining independent melodies **Secondary Element** Melody: major/minor **National Standards** 1b 1d 2c 2d 6a	**Skill: Listening** **Objective:** Discern when two melodies are performed together to create harmony **Secondary Skills** • **Describing** Verbalize reactions to a painting • **Listening** Listen to a discuss the theme of a song; follow a listening map through a classical piece • **Singing** Sing partner songs that are unrelated but share the same harmony • **Playing** Play altered melodies together as a partner song	**SKILLS REINFORCEMENT** • **Keyboard** Play a chordal accompaniment for a song • **Movement** Create a movement routine with different interpretations for a song • **Recorder** Learn a recorder duet accompaniment for a song • **Playing** Discuss and perform altered melodies

Connections

Music and Other Literature

Connection: Culture

Activity: Explore ways of celebrating cultural diversity

CULTURAL CONNECTION **A World Food Fest** Host a potluck dinner with food from around the world

SPOTLIGHT ON **Diversity** Discuss individual and cultural differences

ACROSS THE CURRICULUM **Social Studies** Facts about the first Chinese immigration to the United States

BUILDING SKILLS THROUGH MUSIC **Social Studies** Discuss the influence of Chinese immigration in the West

Song *"Yü guang guang"* ("Moonlight Lullaby")

Listening Selection *Vocal Styles Around the World*

More Music Choices
"Kelo aba w'ye," p. 290
"Vem kan segla?" p. 417

ASSESSMENT

Music Journal Writing Write brief descriptions of different vocal timbres

TECHNOLOGY/MEDIA LINK

Video Library Present a variety of vocal timbres

Connection: Science

Activity: Explore how the physics of sound (acoustics) determines timbre

ACROSS THE CURRICULUM
Science Experiment with recording instruments to identify their sound envelope
Related Arts Illustrate ideas in a song in color

SPOTLIGHT ON
Eva Cassidy Discuss the life of Eva Cassidy
Joey Ramone Discuss the life of Joey Ramone
Louis Armstrong and the Hot Five Discuss this studio ensemble

MEETING INDIVIDUAL NEEDS **Including Everyone** Give students the chance to scat and improvise with instruments

SCHOOL TO HOME CONNECTION **Our Wonderful World** Make a list of the things that make the world wonderful

BUILDING SKILLS THROUGH MUSIC **Language** Develop and describe an opinion using support statements

Song "What a Wonderful World"

Listening Selection *What a Wonderful World*

M·U·S·I·C   M·A·K·E·R·S
Louis Armstrong

More Music Choices
"It's Time," p. 274
"Jambalaya," p. 244
"Just a Snap-Happy Blues," p. 388
"Scattin' A-Round," p.160

ASSESSMENT

Performance/Music Journal Writing Perform a song with attention to vocal timbre; describe and contrast different vocal timbres

TECHNOLOGY/MEDIA LINK

Electronic Keyboard Use the auto-accompaniment function on your keyboard to accompany a song

---

Connection: Related Arts

Activity: Describe a fine arts piece

ACROSS THE CURRICULUM
Social Studies Discuss countries' efforts to achieve world peace
Language Arts Read a book and work creatively to share ideas about world peace

TEACHER TO TEACHER **Tips** Helpful tips for less confident singers

CHARACTER EDUCATION **Peace** Help students consider their role in promoting a peaceful world

AUDIENCE ETIQUETTE **A Museum Visit** Create a set of behavior guidelines for a visit to a museum

SPOTLIGHT ON **The Composer** Discuss the nineteenth-century French composer Georges Bizet

SCHOOL TO HOME CONNECTION **Need for Peace** Follow the news to determine where peace is needed in the world

BUILDING SKILLS THROUGH MUSIC **Math** Graph polled data of the class

Song "Sing a Song of Peace"

Listening Selection "Farandole" from *L'Arlésienne Suite, No. 2*
Listening Map *Farandole*

More Music Choices
"Angels on the Midnight Clear," p. 423
"Going upon the Mountain," p. 105
Jesu, Joy of Man's Desiring, p. 87

ASSESSMENT

Music Journal Writing Listen to determine when two melodies are played together and describe the effect

TECHNOLOGY/MEDIA LINK

Transparency Follow a listening map while listening to a recording

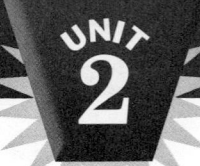

INTRODUCING THE UNIT

Exploring Music is a lifelong journey in which students will find endless possibilities for musical enjoyment. As students begin their travel, Unit 2 will take them on a tour from the Andes in South America to New York's Broadway, from panpipes to jazz trumpet, from ballads to aabb form, and from the sixteenth century to the present century. Students will enjoy *Exploring Music* as they begin their journey by traveling back to the 1950s in the United States.

UNIT PROJECT

Exploring Music can begin with students examining the time line and pictures on pp. 34–35. List the names of each person on the board. Invite students to

- Raise their hands for names they recognize as you point to the list.
- Discuss what they know about each person. (Refer to the text for hints.)
- Identify the #1 songs for certain years, using pp. 34–35. (Point out that most of the #1 songs were performed by solo artists.)

ASK What will be the #1 song this year? Who will be the #1 artist this year? (List student answers on the board.)

Encourage students to research individual names and events listed on pp. 34–35. Throughout the unit, begin lessons with mini-reports by students. Assign a topic to each student and post a schedule showing when each student is responsible for presenting information. Ask students to present only three facts about each person or event. Students may wish to create a time line bulletin board from materials gathered in their research on this unit.

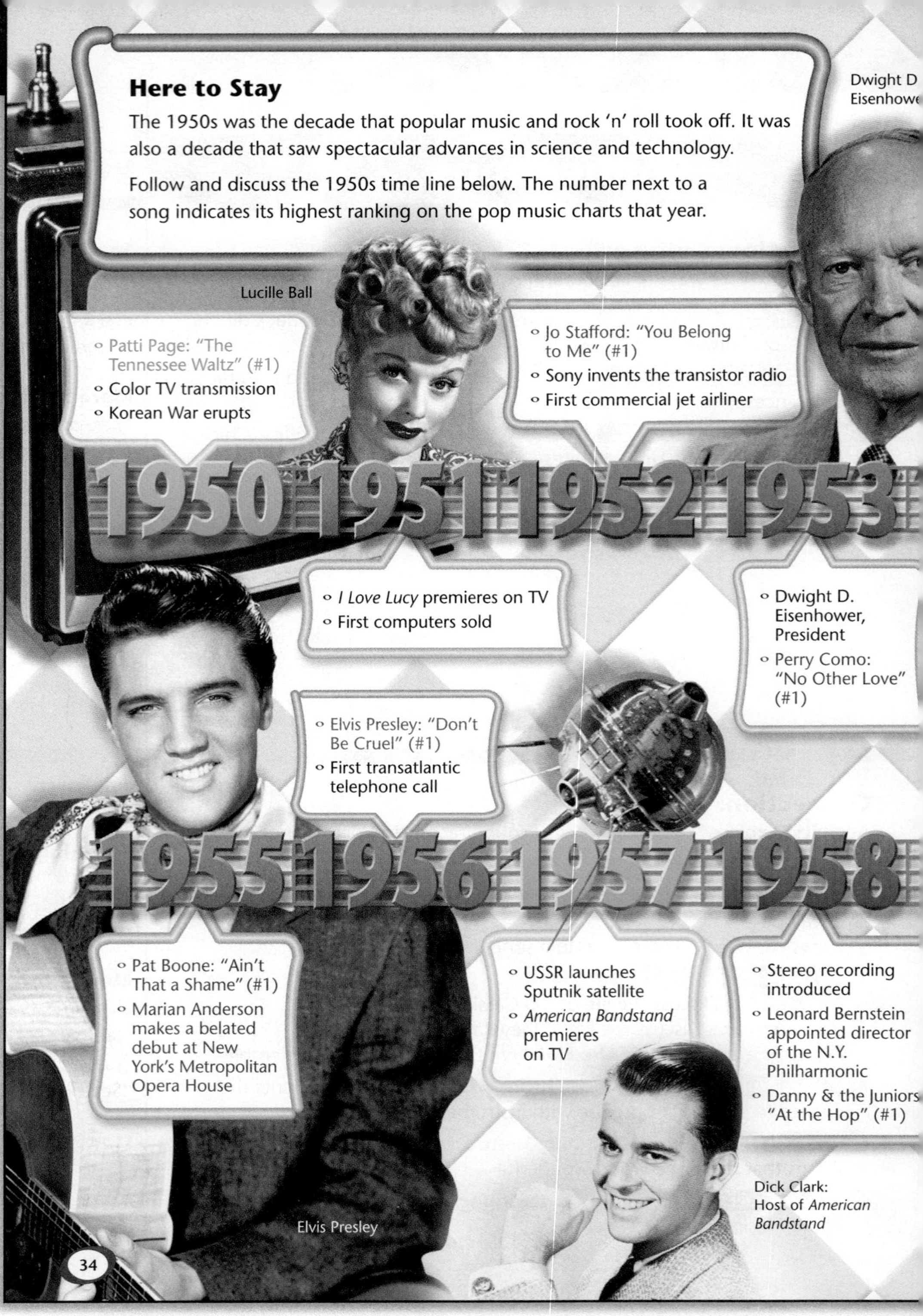

Here to Stay

The 1950s was the decade that popular music and rock 'n' roll took off. It was also a decade that saw spectacular advances in science and technology.

Follow and discuss the 1950s time line below. The number next to a song indicates its highest ranking on the pop music charts that year.

Dwight D. Eisenhower

Lucille Ball

- Patti Page: "The Tennessee Waltz" (#1)
- Color TV transmission
- Korean War erupts

- Jo Stafford: "You Belong to Me" (#1)
- Sony invents the transistor radio
- First commercial jet airliner

1950 1951 1952 1953

- *I Love Lucy* premieres on TV
- First computers sold

- Dwight D. Eisenhower, President
- Perry Como: "No Other Love" (#1)

- Elvis Presley: "Don't Be Cruel" (#1)
- First transatlantic telephone call

1955 1956 1957 1958

- Pat Boone: "Ain't That a Shame" (#1)
- Marian Anderson makes a belated debut at New York's Metropolitan Opera House

- USSR launches Sputnik satellite
- *American Bandstand* premieres on TV

- Stereo recording introduced
- Leonard Bernstein appointed director of the N.Y. Philharmonic
- Danny & the Juniors "At the Hop" (#1)

Dick Clark: Host of *American Bandstand*

Elvis Presley

34

ACROSS THE CURRICULUM

Unit Highlights The following interdisciplinary activities in this unit are related to the music elements presented in the lessons and are intended to enhance student learning. For a more detailed topical description, see the Unit at a Glance on pp. 33a–33h.

▶ **ART/DRAMA**

- Dramatize a seventeenth-century ballad (p. 44)
- Find visual art that demonstrates aabb form (p. 48)
- Learn facts about Fabergé eggs (p. 54)
- Illustrate the imagery in a classic jazz song (p. 63)

▶ **LANGUAGE ARTS**

- Read a book about making the world a better place (p. 69)

▶ **LITERATURE**

- Read poems by an American poet set to music (p. 40)

▶ **SOCIAL STUDIES**

- Learn about the history of whaling (p. 43)
- Share two books about the Andes mountains (p. 47)
- Discover facts about the Taíno people and Columbus (p. 51)
- Locate two Chinese cities on a map and discuss Chinese immigration to the United States in the 1850s (p. 61)
- Discuss partnerships by countries for peace (p. 66)

▶ **SCIENCE**

- Examine the harmonic (overtone) series (p. 56)
- Conduct an acoustics experiment using digital recordings (p. 62)

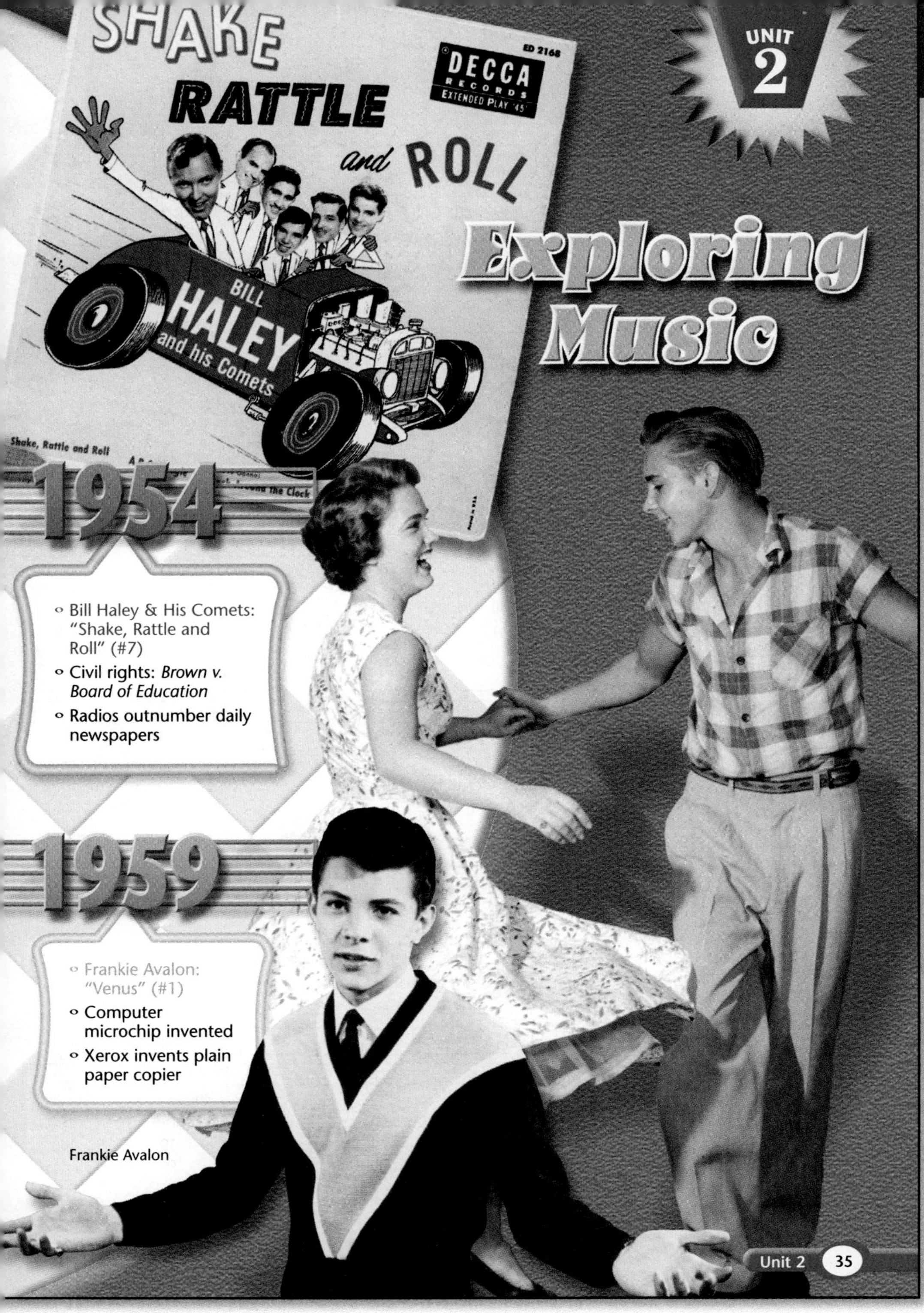

Exploring Music

1954

○ Bill Haley & His Comets: "Shake, Rattle and Roll" (#7)

○ Civil rights: *Brown v. Board of Education*

○ Radios outnumber daily newspapers

1959

○ Frankie Avalon: "Venus" (#1)

○ Computer microchip invented

○ Xerox invents plain paper copier

Frankie Avalon

Unit 2 **35**

MUSIC SKILLS
ASSESSED IN THIS UNIT

Reading Music: Rhythm

• Read and perform rhythms in meter in 3 (p. 42)
• Read and perform rhythms in triple meter using rhythm syllables (p. 44)

Reading Music: Pitch

• Read and sing F-*do* and D-*do* diatonic scales (p. 56)
• Read and sing a *la*-diatonic and *do*-diatonic scale (p. 58)

Performing Music: Singing

• Sing a song expressively, using dynamic changes and articulations (p. 38)
• Sing a song with various timbres (p. 62)

Performing Music: Playing

• Play a piece in aabb or AB form (p. 50)
• Play a keyboard accompaniment to "Glory, Glory, Hallelujah" (p. 52)

Listening to Music

• Describe melodic ornamentation (p. 54)
• Identify independent melodies (p. 66)
• Follow a listening map for *Farandole* and indicate changes in texture (p. 66)

Moving to Music

• Perform an original dance in aabb form (p. 46)
• Perform gospel choir movements to demonstrate melodic contour (p. 52)

Creating Music

• Create and perform a dance in aabb form (p. 46)
• Create a rhythm composition in aabb or AB form (p. 50)

CULTURAL CONNECTION

Unit Highlights The musical literature in this unit provides many opportunities for students to explore a variety of world cultures. A more detailed description of the resources and activities listed below can be found in the Unit at a Glance on pp. 33a–33h.

▶ **AFRICAN AMERICAN**

• Learn about the melody of "Glory, Glory, Hallelujah" (p. 52)

▶ **ASIAN**

• Celebrate cultural diversity by hosting a world food fest (p. 60)

▶ **CARIBBEAN**

• Explore Puerto Rico's music and instruments (p. 50)

▶ **EUROPEAN**

• Learn about sixteenth-century Elizabethan England (p. 48)
• Learn about the melody of "Will the Circle Be Unbroken" (p. 52)

▶ **SOUTH AMERICAN**

• Explore the Andean instruments in *"El condor pasa"* (p. 46)
• Discover facts about Andean instruments (p. 58)

OPENING ACTIVITIES

MATERIALS

- "Rock and Roll Is Here to Stay," p. 36   **CD 2-32**

  Recording Routine:
  Intro (8 m.) v. 1; refrain; interlude (6 m.); v. 2, refrain;
  interlude (4 m.); v. 3; refrain; coda

Listening

Invite students to listen to "Rock and Roll Is Here to Stay"
CD 2-32.

ASK What instruments do you hear? (List answers on the
board.) Point out that electric guitars were just becoming
popular when this song was written, so people were not
used to hearing them.

Discuss what instruments are used in today's pop music.

Reading

Write a G major scale on the board using notation and letter names underneath (G A B C D E F♯ G). Invite students to
name the notes used in the melody. Notate and write the
letter names on a new staff as they are called out. Help students discover that the B♭ in the melody is different from
the scale. Identify it as a blue note, or lowered scale
degree.

Singing

Choose soloists to sing the first 12 measures of each verse.
Have the entire class join in for the last four measures of the
verses. Everyone sings the chorus together each time.

Moving

Invite students to perform these movements to "Rock and
Roll Is Here to Stay."

Verse: Students walk to a steady beat around the room.

Refrain: Students stop where they are and make up their
own movements.

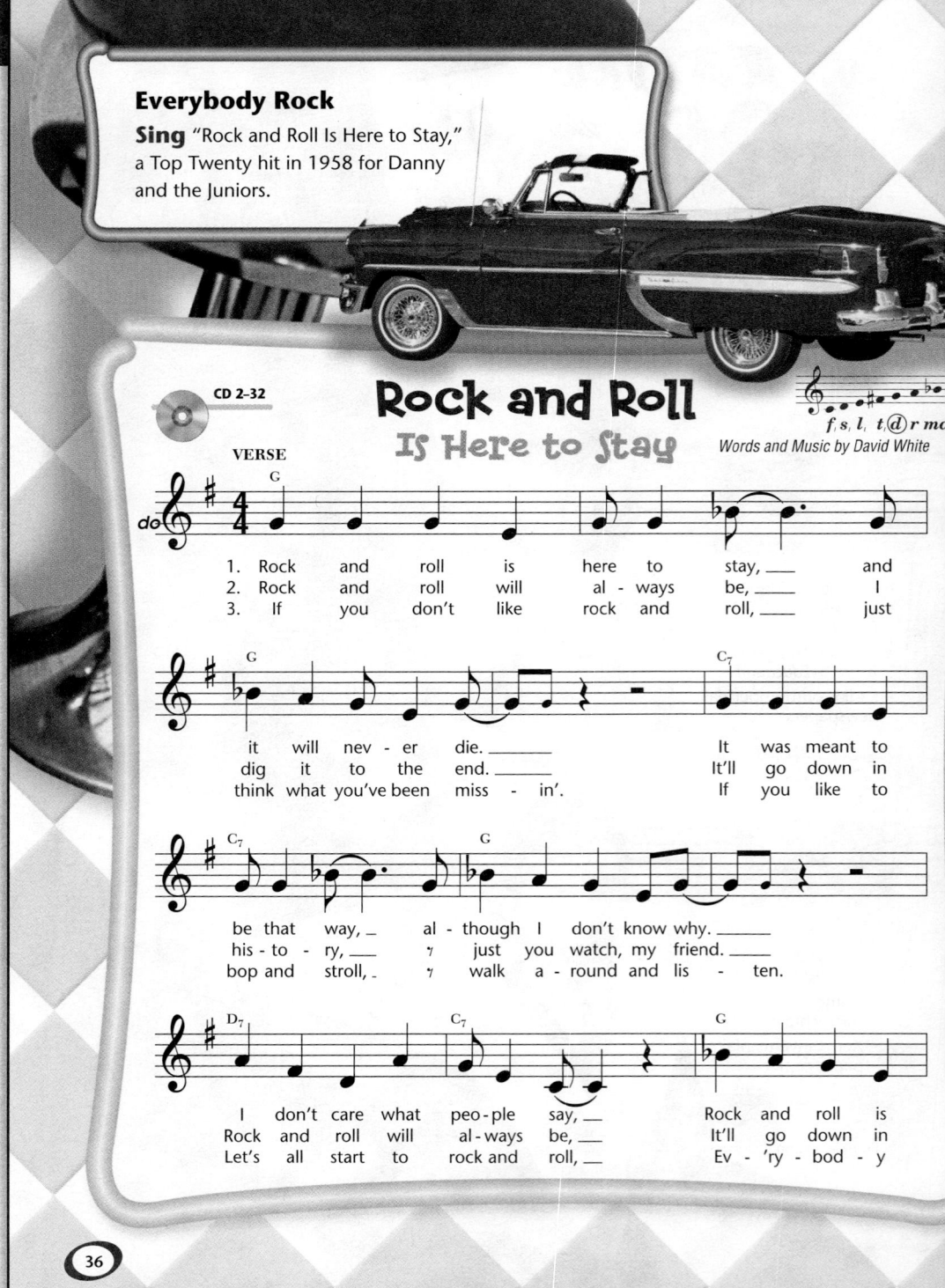

Everybody Rock

Sing "Rock and Roll Is Here to Stay,"
a Top Twenty hit in 1958 for Danny
and the Juniors.

36

ASSESSMENT

Unit Highlights This unit includes a variety of strategies and
methods, described below, to track students' progress and assess their
understanding of lesson objectives. Reproducible masters for Show
What You Know! and Review, Assess, Perform, Create can be found
in the Resource Book.

▶ **FORMAL ASSESSMENTS**

The following assessments, using written language, cognitive, and
performance skills, help teachers and students conceptualize the
learning that is taking place.

- **Show What You Know!** Element-specific assessments, on the
  student page, for Rhythm (p. 45) and Melody (p. 59)
- **Review, Assess, Perform, Create** This end-of-unit activity
  (pp. 70–71) can be used for review and to assess students' learning
  of the core lessons in this unit.

▶ **INFORMAL ASSESSMENTS**

At the close of each Teacher's Edition lesson in this unit, one of the
following types of assessments is used to evaluate the learning of the
key element focus or skill objective.

- Music Journal Writing (p. 61, 69)
- Observation (p. 55)
- Performance/Observation (pp. 41, 43, 45, 57, 59)
- Performance/Music Journal Writing (p. 49, 65)
- Performance/Self-Assessment (p. 51, 53)

▶ **RUBRICS**

Visit *www.sfsuccessnet.com* for rubrics to assess students'
achievement in music skills.

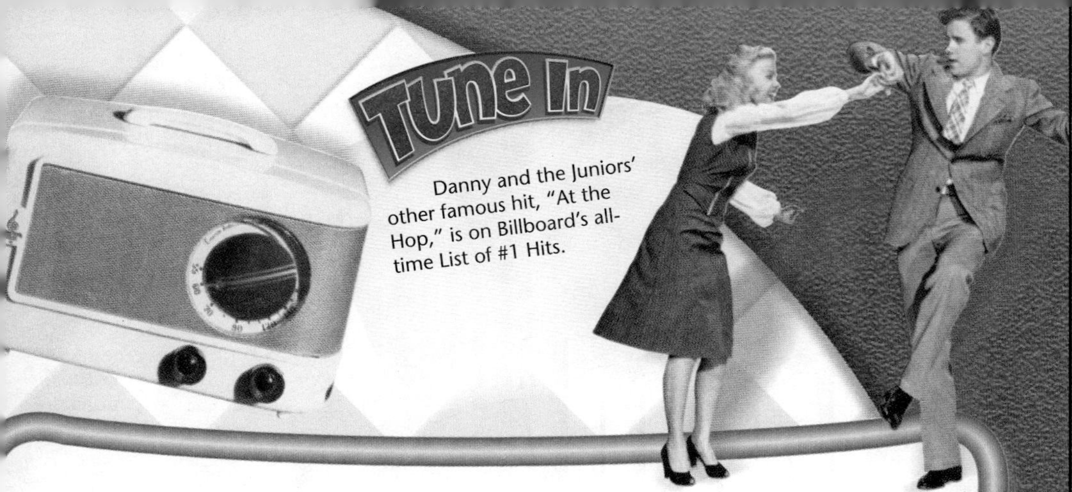

Tune In

Danny and the Juniors' other famous hit, "At the Hop," is on Billboard's all-time List of #1 Hits.

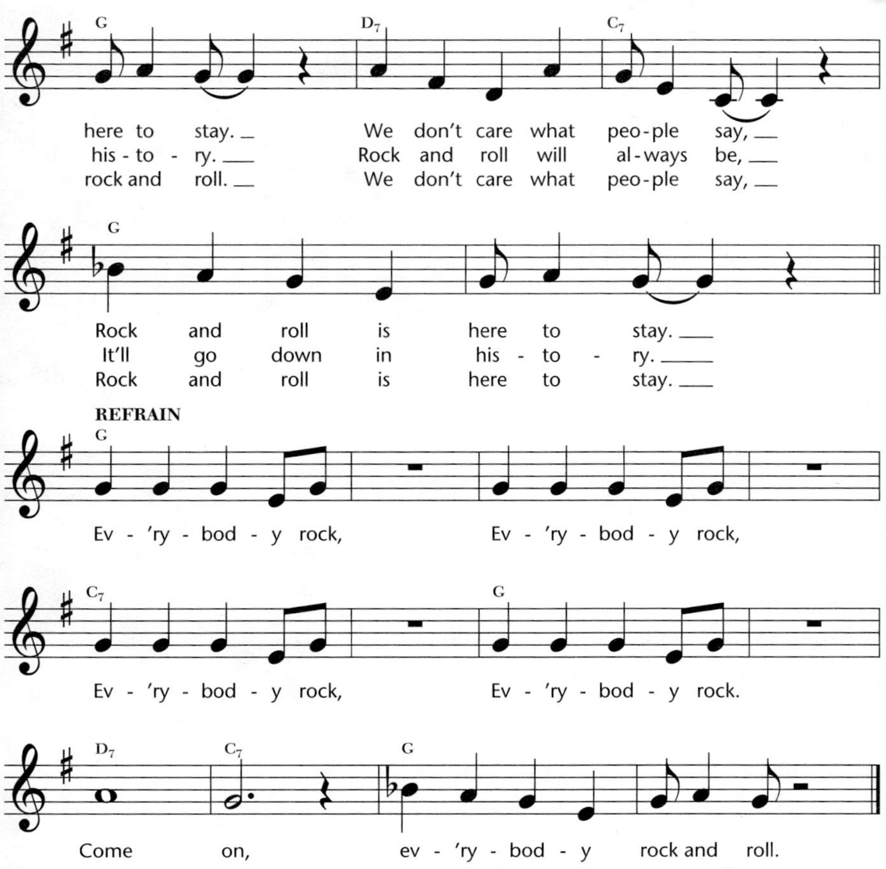

here to   stay. __   We   don't care what   peo-ple say, __
his - to - ry. __   Rock and   roll   will   al-ways be, __
rock and   roll. __   We   don't care what   peo-ple say, __

Rock   and   roll   is   here   to   stay. __
It'll   go   down   in   his - to - ry. __
Rock   and   roll   is   here   to   stay. __

REFRAIN

Ev - 'ry - bod - y rock,   Ev - 'ry - bod - y rock,

Ev - 'ry - bod - y rock,   Ev - 'ry - bod - y rock.

Come   on,   ev - 'ry - bod - y   rock and   roll.

Unit 2   **37**

Try this as students are first entering classroom. Their last position could be standing in front of their chairs.

Invite students to make up their own movements or dance to sections of the song.

Creating

Students may be interested in creating an improvisation in a variety of styles and genres.

Divide the class into small groups. Ask each group to think of a new style for a performance of "Rock and Roll Is Here to Stay." Let each group try their idea first, then invite the class to join in. Examples could include

- Rap.
- Reading as poetry.
- Singing in triple meter.
- "Boy band" style ('N Sync, Backstreet Boys) complete with choreography.

INNOVATIVE TEACHER SUPPORT FOR THIS UNIT

- **MAKING MUSIC DVD, Grade 6** contains video segments that support lessons, including signing and movement.
- **MAKING MUSIC with Movement and Dance** provides more opportunities for large group activities in music or physical education classes.
- **MAKING MUSIC with Technology** provides lesson plans for many technology applications; includes MIDI files.
- *¡A cantar!* features recorded songs and lessons from around the Spanish-speaking world; includes strategies for bilingual classes and for English-speaking teachers working with Spanish-speaking students.
- **Bridges to Asia** features recorded songs and lessons from Asian and Pacific region cultures.
- *www.sfsuccessnet.com* provides an online lesson planner to conveniently create lesson plans at school or at home. Includes rubrics for assessment, lesson modifications to meet the needs of all students, performance musicals based on program content, and more.

TECHNOLOGY/MEDIA LINK

Unit Highlights The following components are used in this unit to reinforce and expand students' understanding of music elements and related themes.

▶ **CD-ROM**

- Use *Alfred's Essentials of Music Theory* to explore scales (p. 57)

▶ **ELECTRONIC KEYBOARD**

- Create composition using repetition and contrast (p. 51)
- Select a style and perform an auto-accompaniment (p. 65)

▶ **MIDI/SEQUENCING SOFTWARE**

- Change the dynamics of MIDI song files (p. 41)
- Notate a melody and compose an accompaniment (p. 43)
- Examine the melodic contours of a MIDI song file (p. 53)

- Alter the melody of a MIDI song file (p. 59)

▶ **MULTIMEDIA**

- Create a slide show of illustrations and photos (p. 45)

▶ **TRANSPARENCY**

- Display the listening map transparency for *Farandole* (p. 69)

▶ **VIDEO LIBRARY/DVD**

- Watch a video featuring a South American *charango* (p. 49)
- See a gospel choir in *Total Experience Gospel Choir* (p. 55)
- Show the video *Charango and Ensemble* (p. 59)
- Show the videos *Whitney Houston, Bobby McFerrin, Pam Tillis, and Total Experience Gospel Choir* (p. 61)

▶ **WEB SITE**

- Learn more about the music of Scotland (p. 43)

LESSON AT A GLANCE

Element Focus   **EXPRESSION** Dynamics and articulation

Skill Objective   **SINGING** Sing using dynamic changes to create expressive effects

Connection Activity   **LANGUAGE ARTS** Explore dynamics and articulation in interpreting a poem

MATERIALS
- "Give My Regards to Broadway"   CD 2-34
  Recording Routine: Intro (8 m.); vocal; interlude (6 m.); vocal; coda
- "Stopping by Woods on a Snowy Evening" (poem)   CD 2-36
- "Stopping by Woods on a Snowy Evening" from *Frostiana*   CD 2-37
- **Resource Book** pp. H-9, I-5, J-4
- keyboard, selected pitched and nonpitched classroom percussion instruments (claves, temple blocks, woodblock, sleigh bells, rain stick, hand drum), picture cards

VOCABULARY

dynamics   articulation   *legato*   *staccato*

◆ ◆ ◆ National Standards ◆ ◆ ◆
4c Compose, using non-traditional sound sources
6b Listen and analyze uses of dynamics, form, and rhythm in music from diverse genres
8a Show how different arts portray the same scene in unique ways
8b Identify ways music relates to language arts

MORE MUSIC CHOICES
For more practice with dynamics and articulation:
"Goin' to Boston," p. 433
"Run! Run! Hide!" p. 340
"This Little Light of Mine," p. 232

Soft TO Loud!

Some sounds can be loud, while other sounds may be soft. What is the loudest sound you heard today? What is the quietest sound?

In music, the intensity of the sound is its dynamic level. There are six main dynamic levels in music. Italian words are used to identify the six different levels.

pp	*p*	*mp*	*mf*	*f*	*ff*
pianissimo	*piano*	*mezzo piano*	*mezzo forte*	*forte*	*fortissimo*
very soft	soft	moderately soft	moderately loud	loud	very loud

On Broadway!

Listen to "Give My Regards to Broadway." Which two dynamic levels are used in the song? Did the dynamics change gradually or suddenly?

The recording of "Give My Regards to Broadway" uses articulation, another expressive element. Articulation is how the notes are performed. The first time, the melody is sung **legato**. The second time, the melody is **staccato**.

Now **sing** "Give My Regards to Broadway." Make sure you change dynamics, as shown in the music.

Legato notes are connected to each other and played or sung smoothly. **Staccato** notes are performed short and separated from each other.

38

Footnotes

TEACHER TO TEACHER

▶ **School Musicals** For information on how to produce your own successful school musicals, read *Junior Broadway: How to Produce Musicals with Children 9 to 13* by Beverly B. Ross and Jean B. Durgin (McFarland, 1983). This is a comprehensive guide to selecting appropriate scripts, casting, lighting, set design, staging, choreography, costuming, publicity, and other important details.

BUILDING SKILLS THROUGH MUSIC

▶ **Writing** Using the poem, "Stopping by Woods on a Snowy Evening" on p. 41, have students sketch out all the events of the evening, and then write the story from the horse's point of view. Invite them to include as many details as they can support from the poem itself.

SPOTLIGHT ON

▶ **The Songwriter** George M. Cohan (1878–1942) is a legendary figure in American popular entertainment. He was a performer, songwriter, stage director, and Broadway producer. He is best known for his trend-setting musicals. Cohan was born on July 4, 1878. His parents performed in vaudeville. He joined them on stage when he was very young and soon began writing scripts for them. Cohan published his first song when he was ten years old. He loved America and wrote many songs that have become patriotic standards. He received the Congressional Medal of Honor for his famous World War I song, "Over There." Cohan wrote the book, music, and lyrics for 20 musicals during his lifetime and starred in many of his own shows. He composed "Give My Regards to Broadway" in 1904 for his very first show. The song remains one of his most popular.

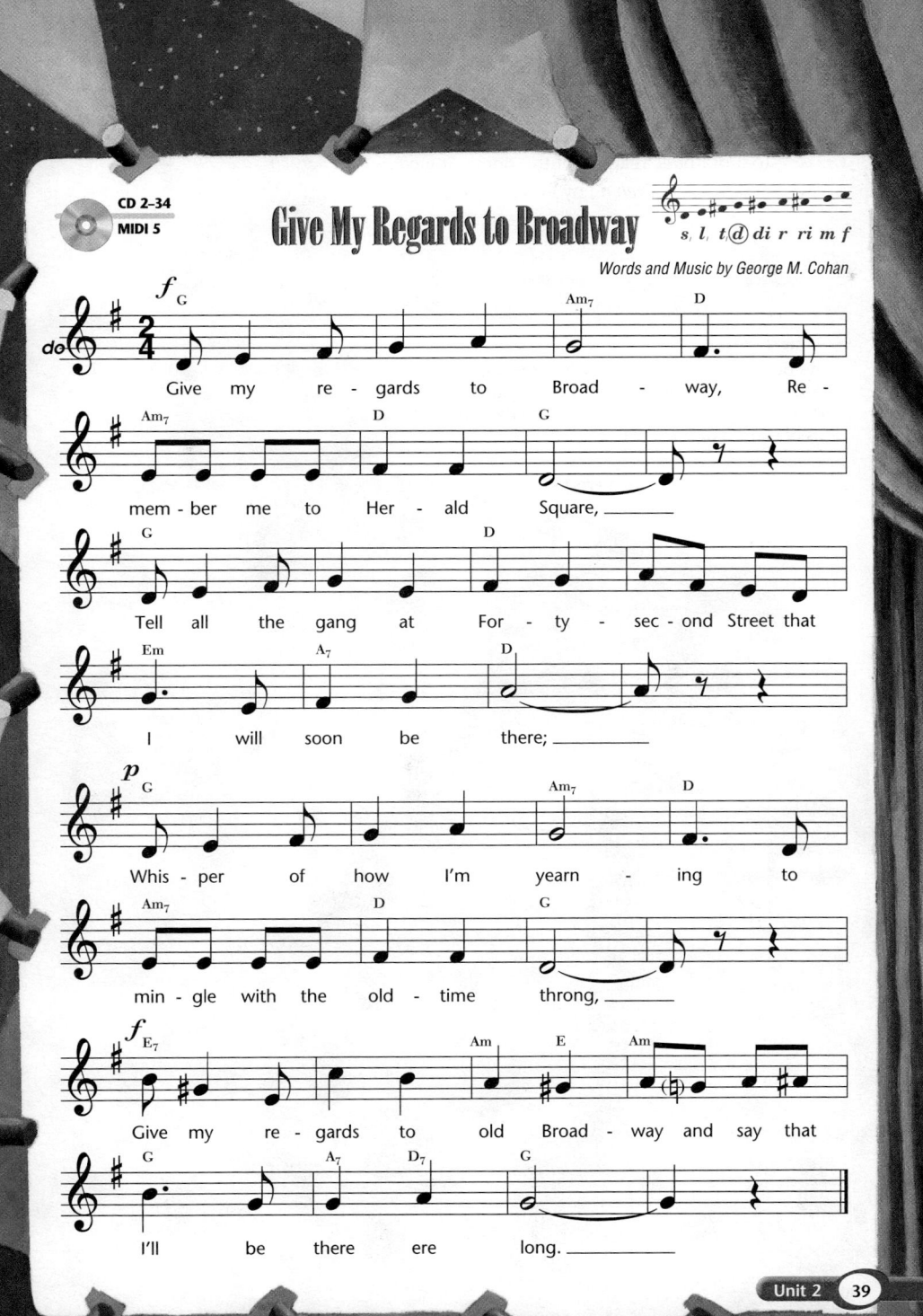

Give My Regards to Broadway

Words and Music by George M. Cohan

CD 2–34 / MIDI 5

1 INTRODUCE

Invite students to

- Read the text at the top of p. 38.
- Identify environmental sounds that would fit the different dynamic levels presented in the chart below the text.
- Complete the dynamics chart in the Activity Master 3 worksheet on Resource Book p. J-4.

2 DEVELOP

Listening

Have students follow the music as they listen for dynamic levels in "Give My Regards to Broadway" **CD 2-34.**

6b **ASK** **How many different dynamic levels did you hear?** (two: *forte* and *piano*)

Did the dynamic levels change gradually or suddenly? (suddenly)

SAY When the dynamics become suddenly softer, the change is *subito piano.*

Help students identify and interpret where the articulation changes from *legato* to *staccato.*

Singing

Have students

- Sing "Give My Regards to Broadway" **CD 2-34** with the recording.
- **6b** Observe the changes in dynamics and articulation as they sing the song.
- Discuss the effects that the changes in dynamics and articulation have on the performance of the song.

continued on page 40

SKILLS REINFORCEMENT

▶ **Keyboard** Have students learn a keyboard arrangement of "Give My Regards to Broadway" in Resource Book, p. H-9.

6b ▶ **Listening** Play the recording of "Give My Regards to Broadway" **CD 2-34** and ask students to focus on form. Help students discover the less common abac phrase form of this song. Ask students to identify a rhythm pattern that appears in the same place in each phrase.

(Each phrase begins with 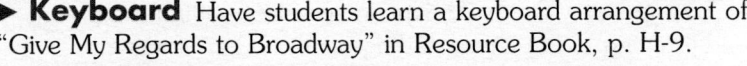)

▶ **Recorder** Invite students to play the recorder part for "Give My Regards to Broadway" on Resource Book p. I-5.

MOVEMENT

▶ **Patterned Dance** Invite students to perform this routine with "Give My Regards to Broadway."

Arm Position: R arm high, L arm low, elbows bent, hands waving.

Mm. 1–4: Move forward on R diagonal—step R, step L, step R, kick L. Move backward to starting place—step L, step R, step L, touch R.

Mm. 5–8: Repeat above on L diagonal; switch arm positions.

Mm. 9–16: In place—Cross-step R in front of L, then L in front of R. Step R, step L, in place. Repeat four times.

Mm. 17–24: Stand, hands on bent knees; bounce to the beat.

Mm. 25–32: Move forward—stomp R, high kick L, stomp L, high kick R. Perform pattern three times; then, beginning on the word *long,* take four steps back to place—R, L, R, L.

Creating

Invite students to

- Read about the use of expression in poetry on p. 40.
- Describe how expression in poetry and the fine arts relate to music concepts.
- Read Robert Frost's poem "Stopping by Woods on a Snowy Evening" on p. 41.
- Ask students to read Frost's poem aloud, as a group, with expression.

Share with students information about Robert Frost in Spotlight On on p. 41.

Divide the class into small groups. Have each group

- Experiment with different vocal dynamics and articulations to determine which levels and articulations best fit the text of the poem.
- **4c** Create an accompaniment for the poem, using pitched and nonpitched classroom percussion instruments and non-traditional sound sources to accompany a reading of the poem.

Have the class identify appropriate criteria and constructively evaluate each group's performance. Help students begin to develop criteria by discussing these points:

- Were the vocal dynamics and articulations used effectively to enhance the poem?
- Was the percussion accompaniment appropriate to the mood of the poem?
- Did the reading of the poem sound natural?

Invite students to listen to "Stopping by Woods on a Snowy Evening" **CD 2-36** and discuss this reading of the poem with regard to expressive elements, and how those expressive elements are similar to those used in music. (dynamics, articulation, tempo, timbre)

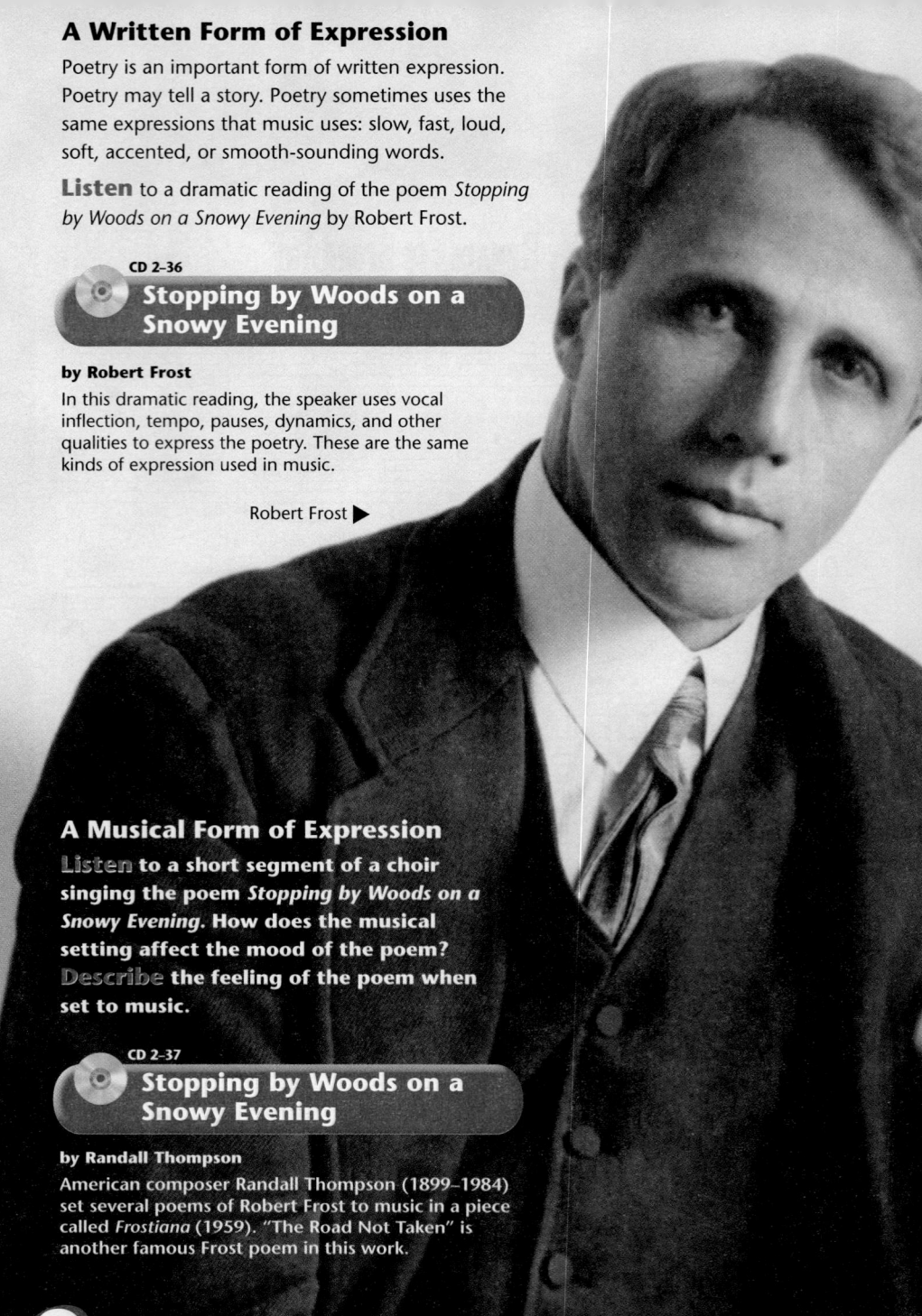

A Written Form of Expression

Poetry is an important form of written expression. Poetry may tell a story. Poetry sometimes uses the same expressions that music uses: slow, fast, loud, soft, accented, or smooth-sounding words.

Listen to a dramatic reading of the poem *Stopping by Woods on a Snowy Evening* by Robert Frost.

> **CD 2-36**
> **Stopping by Woods on a Snowy Evening**

by Robert Frost

In this dramatic reading, the speaker uses vocal inflection, tempo, pauses, dynamics, and other qualities to express the poetry. These are the same kinds of expression used in music.

Robert Frost ▶

A Musical Form of Expression

Listen to a short segment of a choir singing the poem *Stopping by Woods on a Snowy Evening*. How does the musical setting affect the mood of the poem? **Describe** the feeling of the poem when set to music.

> **CD 2-37**
> **Stopping by Woods on a Snowy Evening**

by Randall Thompson

American composer Randall Thompson (1899–1984) set several poems of Robert Frost to music in a piece called *Frostiana* (1959). "The Road Not Taken" is another famous Frost poem in this work.

40

Footnotes

MEETING INDIVIDUAL NEEDS

▶ **Including Everyone** Guide students to discover activities using the poem "Stopping by Woods on a Snowy Evening."

8a **Reinforcement** For English language learners, supplement the text of "Stopping by Woods on a Snowy Evening" with pictures that support the meaning of the poem. Help students create a picture story, using a series of illustrations.

8b **On Target** Short examples of dynamics (expression) that might occur in everyday speech may help students understand that text in poems and music can determine the dynamics for performance. Invite students to create a dialogue on a topic utilizing dynamic expression in their dialogue.

Challenge Invite students to select a new poem and to read the poem to the class, improvising the use of dynamics to create expression in the reading.

ACROSS THE CURRICULUM

8b ▶ **Language Arts** Students may enjoy reading the poems and listening to the choral settings of the other works in *Frostiana*, including "The Road Not Taken," "The Pasture," "The Telephone," and "Choose Something Like a Star."

CHARACTER EDUCATION

▶ **Expression** Help students understand the importance of nonverbal and verbal expression. In pairs, one person shares important information with their partner while the partner listens intently. Reverse roles, but with the listener responding inappropriately. Discuss how various responses made the speaker and the listener feel. How did they know something was or was not important to their partner? Why is it important to consider both verbal and nonverbal expression when communicating?

Stopping by Woods on a Snowy Evening

by Robert Frost

Whose woods these are I think I know.
His house is in the village though;
He will not see me stopping here
To watch his woods fill up with snow.
My little horse must think it queer
To stop without a farmhouse near
Between the woods and frozen lake
The darkest evening of the year.
He gives his harness bells a shake
To ask if there is some mistake.
The only other sound's the sweep
Of easy wind and downy flake.
The woods are lovely, dark, and deep.
But I have promises to keep,
And miles to go before I sleep,
And miles to go before I sleep.

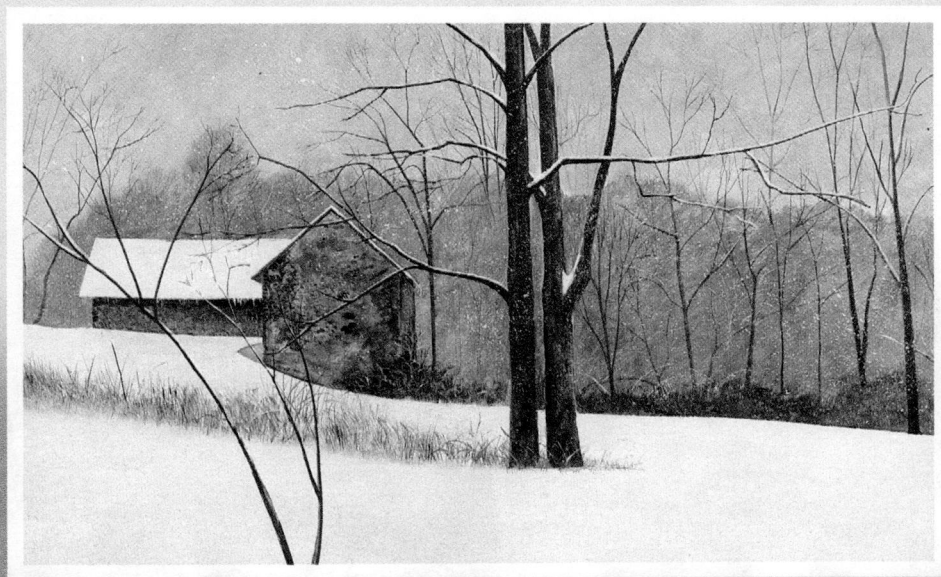

Arts Connection

▲ *Snow Pa.ace* (1986) is a painting by Karl J. Kuerner III. The Kuerner family, from Pennsylvania's Brandywine Valley, lived near another famous American artist, Andrew Wyeth.

Unit 2 **41**

3 CLOSE

Listening

Inform students that Randall Thompson, an American composer, set Robert Frost's poem to music. Share with students information in Spotlight On below.

Invite students to listen to Thompson's setting of *Stopping by Woods on a Snowy Evening* **CD 2-37.** Help students to listen closely for the all-male vocal timbre and the use of harp and low, quiet clarinets, bassoons, flute, and low brass.

Ask students to

 • Describe the feeling of the poem when set to music. (sad, quiet, lonely, melancholy, thoughtful)

 • Write a review of the music for their journals. (Their reviews should evaluate the composer's use of dynamics and articulation in interpreting the text of Robert Frost's poem.)

Creating

Offer students the challenge of creating their own melodies for the first four lines of *Stopping by Woods on a Snowy Evening.* Suggest to students that they use Thompson's setting (minor key, melody) as a start. Using headphones, allow students to imitate a melody line on keyboard from what they hear on the recording, and then modify the melody in new ways. Students may notate their melodies on paper.

Play or sing the new original melodies for the class.

Element: EXPRESSION   ASSESSMENT

Performance/Observation Have students perform "Give My Regards to Broadway" **CD 2-34,** identifying and singing the dynamics indicated by symbols in the music and using *legato* articulations the first time and *staccato* articulations the second time. In a subsequent performance, ask students to incorporate more subtle dynamic inflection in each phrase to create an expressive performance. Observe students' ability to perform the song with correct dynamics and articulations.

SPOTLIGHT ON

▶ **The Poet** Robert Frost (1874–1963) was a highly honored American poet of the twentieth century. He was born in San Francisco. His father was a newspaper editor and his mother was a teacher. Frost published his first poem in his high school newspaper. During his life, Frost received literary, academic, and public honors, including four Pulitzer Prizes. In 1961, at his inauguration as President of the United States, John F. Kennedy declared Frost poet laureate.

▶ **The Composer** Randall Thompson (1899–1984) was born in New York City. He taught at several universities, including Harvard, where Leonard Bernstein became one of his students. Thompson is best known for his choral works. *Frostiana* (1959), a choral setting of seven well-known poems by Robert Frost, is characteristic of his work.

SCHOOL TO HOME CONNECTION

▶ **Interview** Write a short list of famous musicals (or movies) on the board (e.g. *Oklahoma, West Side Story, The Sound of Music*). Ask students to interview family and relatives about the musicals they remember and why they were memorable.

TECHNOLOGY/MEDIA LINK

MIDI/Sequencing Software Encourage students to

• Select several of their favorite songs on the MIDI song files.

• Experiment with changing the dynamics of the songs and note the effects dynamic changes have on the songs.

LESSON AT A GLANCE

Element Focus   **RHYTHM** Meter in 3

Skill Objective   **READING** Read and perform rhythm patterns in triple meter while conducting the beat

Connection Activity   **SOCIAL STUDIES** Discuss interesting facts and stories about the lives of whalers

MATERIALS

• "Farewell to Tarwathie"   **CD 3-1**
  Recording Routine: Intro (4 m.); v. 1–4, with interludes (4 m.); coda
• **Music Reading Practice, Sequence 5**   **CD 3-3**
• "Allegretto" from *Four Scottish Dances*, Op. 59   **CD 3-6**
• *Highway to Kilkenny*   **CD 3-7**
• **Resource Book** pp. D-6, E-6, F-4
• soprano recorders

VOCABULARY

time signature   meter in 3   upbeat

◆ ◆ ◆ ◆ National Standards ◆ ◆ ◆ ◆

2a Play instruments accurately alone and in small ensembles
4c Arrange, using electronic media
5a Read quarter notes, eighth notes, dotted notes, and half notes in triple meter
5d Use standard notation to record musical ideas
6b Listen and analyze uses of rhythm and form in music from diverse cultures

MORE MUSIC CHOICES

For more practice with meter in 3:
"America," p. 484
"*Fais do do,*" p. 403

1 INTRODUCE

Have students read the first paragraph on p. 42 aloud, then turn to "Farewell to Tarwathie." Share the books in Across the Curriculum, p. 43, which offer interesting facts and stories about the lives of whalers. Discuss the reasons for the decline of the whaling industry.

Signs of Time

In the nineteenth century, whale hunting was one of Scotland's most important industries. A whaler's life was full of danger and adventure. Many folk songs were inspired by the colorful stories and tales of his struggles at sea.

"Farewell to Tarwathie" is one of the best-known Scottish whaling songs.

The Time Is Three

Find the **time signature** of "Farewell to Tarwathie." Is the first measure complete? On which beat does the melody begin?

Listen to the recording of "Farewell to Tarwathie" and conduct a pattern in ¾ meter.

Sing "Farewell to Tarwathie" and conduct in meter in 3.

> A **time signature** is the musical symbol that shows how many beats are in a measure and which note gets the beat.

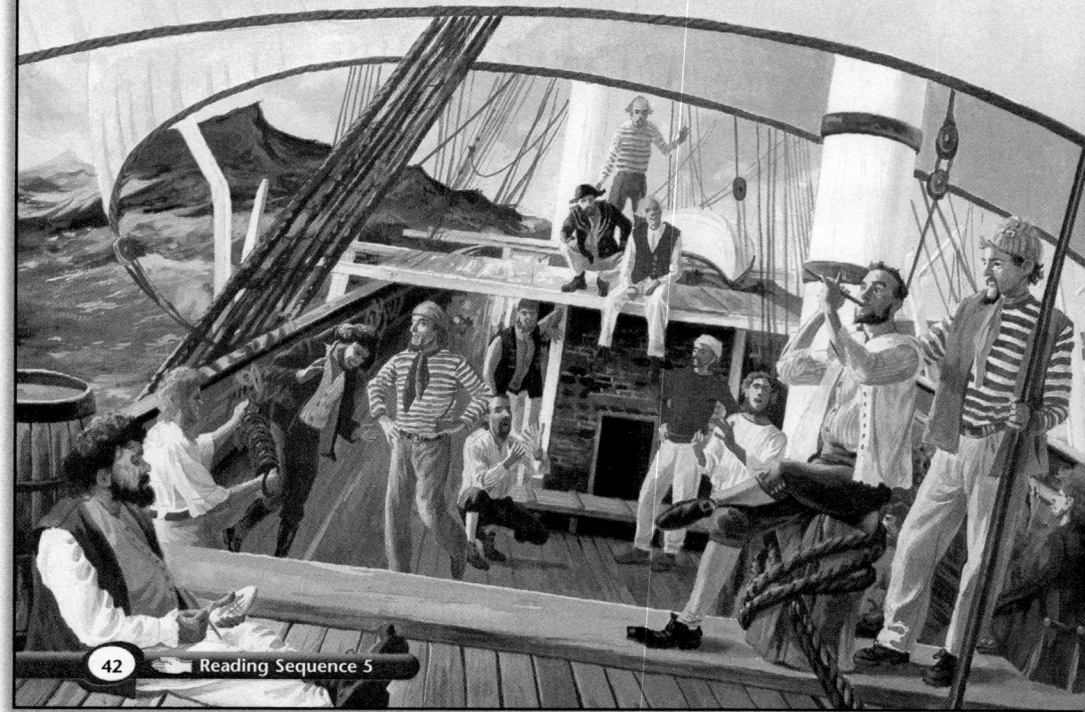

42   Reading Sequence 5

Footnotes

TEACHER TO TEACHER

6b ▶ **Question-and-Answer Form** To help students review melodic question-and-answer form, draw the melodic contour of phrases 1 and 2 of "Farewell to Tarwathie" on the board. Identify for students that the first phrase is a melodic question (the melodic statement goes up at the end and it does not end on the tonic, or home tone *do*). The second phrase is a melodic answer (the melodic statement descends at the end and rests on the tonic, or home tone *do*).

BUILDING SKILLS THROUGH MUSIC

▶ **Science** Invite students to imagine they were scientists who needed to research the reasons for the decline in the whaling industry. Ask them to describe the plan for their investigation, the questions they would ask, and their hypotheses. Ask them what methods or technology might they use to find the answers?

SKILLS REINFORCEMENT

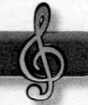

▶ **Recorder** The melody below can be played on the soprano recorder by some students while others sing "Farewell to Tarwathie." When playing notes in the lower register, students should whisper *daah* gently as they play.

2a

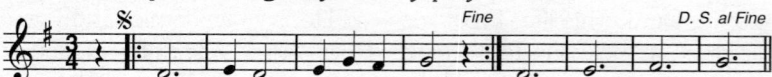

5d ▶ **Reading** Distribute Reading Music Worksheet p. D-6 for more practice with meter in 3, upbeats, and rhythmic dictation. See Resource Book p. E-6, or p. 490, for additional Music Reading Practice.

▶ **Mallets** See Resource Book p. F-4 for an Orff arrangement of "Farewell to Tarwathie."

Farewell to Tarwathie

s l @ d r m s l

Folk Song from Scotland

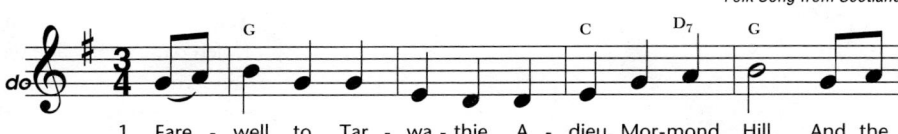

1. Fare - well to Tar - wa - thie, A - dieu Mor - mond Hill, And the
2. Fare - well to my com - rades for a while I must part, And ___

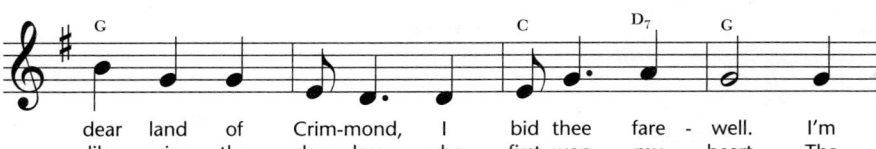

dear land of Crim - mond, I bid thee fare - well. I'm
like - wise the dear lass who first won my heart, The

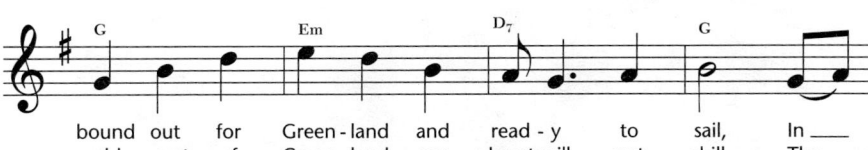

bound out for Green - land and read - y to sail, In ___
cold coast of Green - land my heart will not chill, The ___

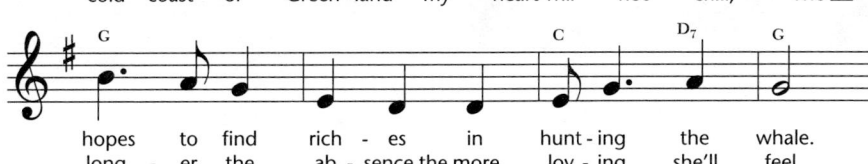

hopes to find rich - es in hunt - ing the whale.
long - er the ab - sence the more lov - ing she'll feel.

3. Our ship is well rigged, and she's ready to sail,
The crew, they are anxious to follow the whale.
Where the icebergs do float and the stormy winds blow,
Where the land and the ocean is covered with snow.

4. The cold coast of Greenland is barren and bare,
No seedling nor harvest is ever known there,
And the birds here sing sweetly in mountain and vale,
But there's no bird in Greenland to sing to the whale.

Listen to these two recordings of Irish and Scottish origin as you conduct in meter in 3. Which recording is easier to conduct? Why?

CD 3-6
Allegretto

from *Four Scottish Dances*, Op. 59
by Sir Malcolm Arnold

This British composer also wrote sets of English, Irish, and Welsh dances.

CD 3-7
Highway to Kilkenny

Traditional Irish tune
as performed by Cherish the Ladies and
the Boston Pops Orchestra

This performance combines traditional orchestral instruments with an Irish folk ensemble.

Unit 2 **43**

2 DEVELOP

Reading

ASK What is the time signature for "Farewell to Tarwathie"? ($\frac{3}{4}$)

5a Ask students to find the number of beats in a measure (three), the beat note (quarter), and the meter (in 3).

Listening

6b Play "Farewell to Tarwathie" **CD 3-1** and have students identify the upbeat for each phrase by conducting in meter in 3. Then play *Allegretto* **CD 3-6** as students conduct in meter in 3. Finally, play *Highway to Kilkenny* **CD 3-7** as they conduct in meter in 3.

ASK Which recordings were easier to conduct? Why? (*Highway to Kilkenney* was the easiest to conduct because it was slower. *Allegretto* is more difficult with its *rubato* tempo. "Farewell to Tarwathie" is in a fast three and may be easier to conduct in meter in 1.)

Singing

Have students sing "Farewell to Tarwathie" **CD 3-1**, showing the melodic contour of phrases as they sing. Have them identify the melodic form of the first two phrases as question-and-answer. (See Teacher to Teacher, p. 42.)

Moving

Play *Highway to Kilkenny* **CD 3-7**. Ask students to move to the rhythm of the music, demonstrating meter in 3 by making stronger movements on the first beat of each measure.

3 CLOSE

Element: RHYTHM **ASSESSMENT**

Performance/Observation Have students read and sing "Farewell to Tarwathie" **CD 3-1** while conducting meter in 3. Observe their ability to independently read and perform rhythm patterns in meter in 3 with accuracy.

ACROSS THE CURRICULUM

▶ **Social Studies** To prepare for a discussion of interesting facts and stories about whalers in the late nineteenth century, students may enjoy reading the following books.

- *Thar She Blows! Whaling in the 1860s* by Sue Kassirer (Soundprints, 1997). This book and cassette recording tell about a young girl who visits a whaling exhibit at the Museum of Natural History. During her visit, she finds herself suddenly transported back in time to the deck of a nineteenth-century whaling ship.

- *Arctic Whales & Whaling* by Bobbie Kalman (Crabtree, 1988). The author gives a realistic account of the history of whaling, from Inuit hunters to modern whaling operations.

TECHNOLOGY/MEDIA LINK

4c **MIDI/Sequencing Software** Have students use the notation tool to enter the melody of "Farewell to Tarwathie" on one track. On another track, they should use the pitches G, A, B, D, and E (G-*do* pentatonic) to compose an ostinato accompaniment. On a third track, they might compose a countermelody, or descant, with the same notes. They should choose appropriate sounds for each track.

Have the class select the best sequence for a performance of the song.

Web Site Have students visit *www.sfsuccessnet.com* to learn more about the music of Scotland.

LESSON AT A GLANCE

Element Focus	**RHYTHM** Meter in 3
Skill Objective	**READING** Read and perform rhythms in triple meter
Connection Activity	**RELATED ARTS** Dramatize a ballad

MATERIALS

- "Barb'ry Allen"   **CD 3-8**
  Recording Routine: No intro; v. 1–14 (a cappella)
- Music Reading Practice, Sequence 6   **CD 3-9**
- *Sellenger's Round*   **CD 3-14**
- **Dance Directions** for *Sellenger's Round* p. 554
- **Resource Book** pp. B-6, C-7, D-7, F-5

VOCABULARY

upbeat   ballad   time signature   phrase

◆ ◆ ◆ ◆ National Standards ◆ ◆ ◆ ◆

5a Read quarter notes, eighth notes, and dotted notes in triple meter

6b Listen and analyze uses of rhythm and form in music from diverse genres

8b Identify ways music relates to language arts

9a Describe characteristics of music genres from a variety of cultures

MORE MUSIC CHOICES

For more practice with meter in 3:

"Gloria, Gloria," p. 459

Waltz of the Flowers, p. 325

1 INTRODUCE

9a Tell students that they will be listening to and singing a ballad (a song that tells a story) from England and that this song also exists in many versions in the United States. Point out that traditional ballads can be classified by the type of story told, such as a humorous, love, religious, historical, or tragic story.

BALLAD Rhythms

The ballad "Barb'ry Allen" is much older than "Farewell to Tarwathie." It dates back to the seventeenth century. There are hundreds of variations of this ballad on either side of the Atlantic.

Sing "Barb'ry Allen."

Read and clap the rhythm of the words using rhythm syllables.

CD 3–8

BARB'RY ALLEN

Folk Song from the British Isles

@ r m f s l t d'

1. In Scar-let town, where I was born, There was a young maid dwell-in', Made ev'-ry youth cry, _____ "Well-a-day," For love of Bar-b'ry Al-len.

44   Reading Sequence 6

Footnotes

ACROSS THE CURRICULUM

8b ▶ **Related Arts** "Barb'ry Allen" could easily be performed as a dramatized ballad. Decide which of the song's verses, or lines within verses, could be sung by soloists, which could be sung just by boys or just by girls, and which verses could be sung by all students. Ask students to dramatize selected verses. As part of this experience, refer to the Dance Directions on p. 554 for a folk dance (*Sellenger's Round* **CD 3-14**).

BUILDING SKILLS THROUGH MUSIC

▶ **Reading** Using the Story Map graphic organizer (Resource Book, p. C-7), have students analyze the story, plot, setting, characters, problem, and resolution as they are presented in the song, "Barb'ry Allen."

SPOTLIGHT ON

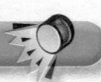

▶ **The Lyrics** Additional verses for "Barb'ry Allen":

(Between verses 5 and 6)

"Oh, ken ye not in yonder town, In the place where you were dwellin', / You gave a toast to the ladies all, But you slighted Barb'ry Allen." / "Oh yes, I ken, I ken it well, In the place where I was dwellin', / I gave a toast to the ladies all, But my love to Barb'ry Allen."

(Between verses 7 and 8)

Her eyes looked east, her eyes looked west, She saw his pale corpse comin', / She cried, "Bearers, bearers, put him down, That I may look upon him." / The more she looked, the more she grieved, Until she burst out cryin'; / She cried, "Bearers, bearers, take him off, for I am now a-dyin'!"

Show What You Know!

Read and clap these patterns using rhythm syllables. Then find one pattern used in "Farewell to Tarwathie," on page 43, and one pattern used in "Barb'ry Allen," on page 44.

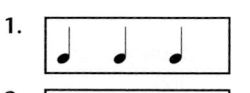
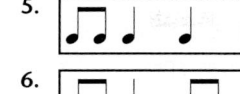
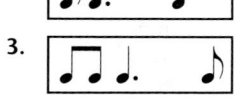
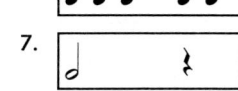

2. 'Twas in the merry month of May,
   When green buds they were swellin',
   Sweet William on his deathbed lay,
   For love of Barb'ry Allen.

3. He sent his servant to the town,
   To the place where she was dwellin',
   Cried, "Master bids you come to him,
   If your name be Barb'ry Allen."

4. Then slowly, slowly she got up,
   And slowly went she nigh him,
   And when she pulled the curtains back
   Said, "Young man, I think you're dyin'."

5. "Oh, yes, I'm sick, I'm very sick,
   And I never will be better,
   Until I have the love of one,
   The love of Barb'ry Allen."

6. Then lightly tripped she down the stairs,
   She trembled like an aspen.
   "'Tis vain, 'tis vain, my dear young man,
   To long for Barb'ry Allen."

7. She walked out in the green, green fields,
   She heard his death bells knellin'.
   And every stroke they seemed to say,
   "Hard-hearted Barb'ry Allen."

8. "Oh, father, father, dig my grave,
   Go dig it deep and narrow.
   Sweet William died for me today;
   I'll die for him tomorrow."

9. They buried her in the old churchyard,
   Sweet William's grave was nigh her,
   And from his heart grew a red, red rose,
   And from her heart a brier.

10. They grew and grew o'er the old church wall,
    'Till they could grow no higher,
    Until they tied a lover's knot,
    The red rose and the brier.

2 DEVELOP

Singing

6b **8b** Play "Barb'ry Allen" **CD 3-8** and have students identify the time signature by ear (3/4), and summarize the story. Ask students to sing the song.

ASK What happened to the characters in this ballad? (It is a sad love story between William and Barb'ry Allen.)

See Across the Curriculum on p. 44 for a dramatization.

Reading

5a Have students look at the notation of "Barb'ry Allen" as they

- Listen to the recording **CD 3-8** and conduct in meter in 3.
- Tap the beat and say the rhythm syllables.
- Conduct phrases 1 and 3 and clap the rhythm for phrases 2 and 4 as they sing the first verse.
- Switch to clapping the rhythm for phrases 1 and 3 and conducting phrases 2 and 4.

Listening

6b Play "Barb'ry Allen" **CD 3-8** and have students

- Show the phrases and identify that each phrase begins with a single eighth-note upbeat.
- Identify the phrase form as abcd.

ASK Does the singer always perform the rhythm and melody exactly as notated? (no)

3 CLOSE

Element: RHYTHM **ASSESSMENT**

5a **Performance/Observation** Direct students to the rhythms in Show What You Know! or in the Resource Book p. B-6. Have students read and perform the rhythms using rhythm syllables. Observe students' ability to read the rhythms in meter in 3 with accuracy.

SKILLS REINFORCEMENT

▶ **Mallets** Invite some students to learn the Orff accompaniment for "Barb'ry Allen," on Resource Book p. F-5. Students may play the accompaniment as the class sings the song.

▶ **Reading** To give students more practice with the pitch set and rhythms of "Barb'ry Allen," distribute copies of Resource Book p. D-7.

For more practice using standard symbols to notate rhythm, have students complete the activities for "Barb'ry Allen" found on p. 490 and on Resource Book p. D-7.

▶ **Singing** Have students demonstrate their understanding of the narrative and dialogue exchanges by having girls sing the "Barb'ry Allen" lines and boys sing the "Sweet William" lines.

TECHNOLOGY/MEDIA LINK

Multimedia Ask interested students to create graphic illustrations of selected verses of "Barb'ry Allen." Use a digital camera to photograph the results. Import the drawings or photos, one per slide, into a slide show program such as *Powerpoint, iPhoto,* or other slide show or photo program. Have students advance the slide show as the class sings the ballad. If a digital camera is not available, scan the illustrations into the slide show.

LESSON AT A GLANCE

Element Focus   **FORM** aabb form

Skill Objective   **MOVING** Perform movement to illustrate the form of a song

Connection Activity   **CULTURE** Discuss the musical and cultural history of Elizabethan England

MATERIALS

- *"El cóndor pasa"* (Spanish)   **CD 3-16**
- *"El cóndor pasa"* (English)   **CD 3-17**
  Recording Routine: Intro (free tempo); instrumental; vocal; instrumental
- **Pronunciation Practice/Translation** p. 523
- **"Greensleeves"**   **CD 3-20**
  Recording Routine: Intro (4 m.); v. 1; interlude (2 m.); v. 2; coda
- **Resource Book** pp. A-6, F-6
- tubes, soprano recorders, guitars

VOCABULARY

unity   contrast   aabb form   anacrusis

◆ ◆ ◆ ◆ National Standards ◆ ◆ ◆ ◆

1c Sing music from diverse genres and cultures

6b Listen and analyze uses of form, harmony, and timbre in music from diverse genres and cultures

8a Show how different arts portray the same idea in unique ways

8b Identify ways music relates to social studies, language arts, science, and the visual arts

MORE MUSIC CHOICES

For more practice with song form:

"Alumot" (aabb), p. 306

"Everybody Loves Saturday Night" (aaba), p. 296

"Sun Gonna Shine" (aab), p. 242

A Favorite Form

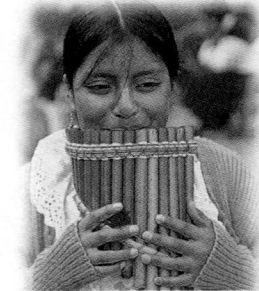

The musical form **a a b b** has both built-in repetition and contrast. It is used in all types of music, from early folk songs to today's bluegrass fiddle tunes.

Sing *"El cóndor pasa,"* a song from the Andes region of South America. **Identify** the four sections that make up the song. How does the **b** section differ from the **a** sections?

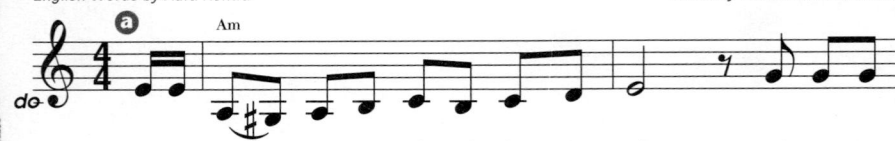

El cóndor pasa

English Words by Aura Kontra   *Music by Daniel Almonica Robles*

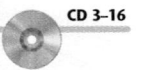

El a - mor   co - mo un cón - dor ba - ja - rá,   mi co - ra -
Love is like a con - dor glid - ing towards the earth,   It comes to

zón,   gol - pea - rá, _____ des - pués se i - rá. _____ Mmm _____
me,   fill - ing me with hap - pi - ness. _ And then it's gone. ____ Mmm ____

La _ lu - na en el de - sier - to bri - lla - rá   Tú ven -
As the moon - light leaves its glow on de - sert sands,   You ap -

drás. So - la - men - te un be - so, _ me de - ja - rás. ____ Mmm ____
pear, bring - ing back the love I lost. _ And then you, too, are gone. _ Mmm ____

Footnotes

CULTURAL CONNECTION

▶ **Andean Instruments** Notice that this recording of *"El cóndor pasa"* features Andean folk instruments. Listen for the *charango* [cha-RAHNG-go] (a small guitarlike instrument with an armadillo shell back) and guitar in the introduction. The *charango* provides a rhythmically-strummed accompaniment. The *zampoña* [zham-POH-nyah] (panpipes) plays the melody after the singers sing the song. The *zampoña* is played by blowing air over the ends of the tubes, as if blowing air over the top of a bottle to make a sound.

BUILDING SKILLS THROUGH MUSIC

▶ **Science** Using beverage bottles with graduated amounts of water, have students blow across the bottles to sound pitches. Then, have them chart the results, showing the size of the bottle (its possible volume), the amount of water in the bottle, and the pitch it produces. Compare the data with the students' current knowledge of the properties of how pitch is produced and changed.

AUDIENCE ETIQUETTE

▶ **At School Assemblies** In each school year, students may attend performances in assemblies, such as performances of the school choir, band, visiting performers, or groups. School assemblies provide excellent opportunities for practicing and reinforcing audience behaviors. Encourage students to

- Be attentive to your personal space. Respect the space of others.
- Use good eye contact and look attentively at the speakers or performers.
- Be active listeners. Concentrate and think about what you hear.
- Show appreciation by clapping.

Instruments of the Andes

Listen to the following Andean instruments in *"El cóndor pasa"*—*quena* (flute), *zampoña* (panpipes; pictured on page 46), *charango* (small fret lute), and *ch'ajch'as* (rattles).

Andean *ch'ajch'as* ▶

◀ *Quena*

Tune In

Did you know that the Andean *ch'ajch'as* (rattles) are made from the toenails of llamas?

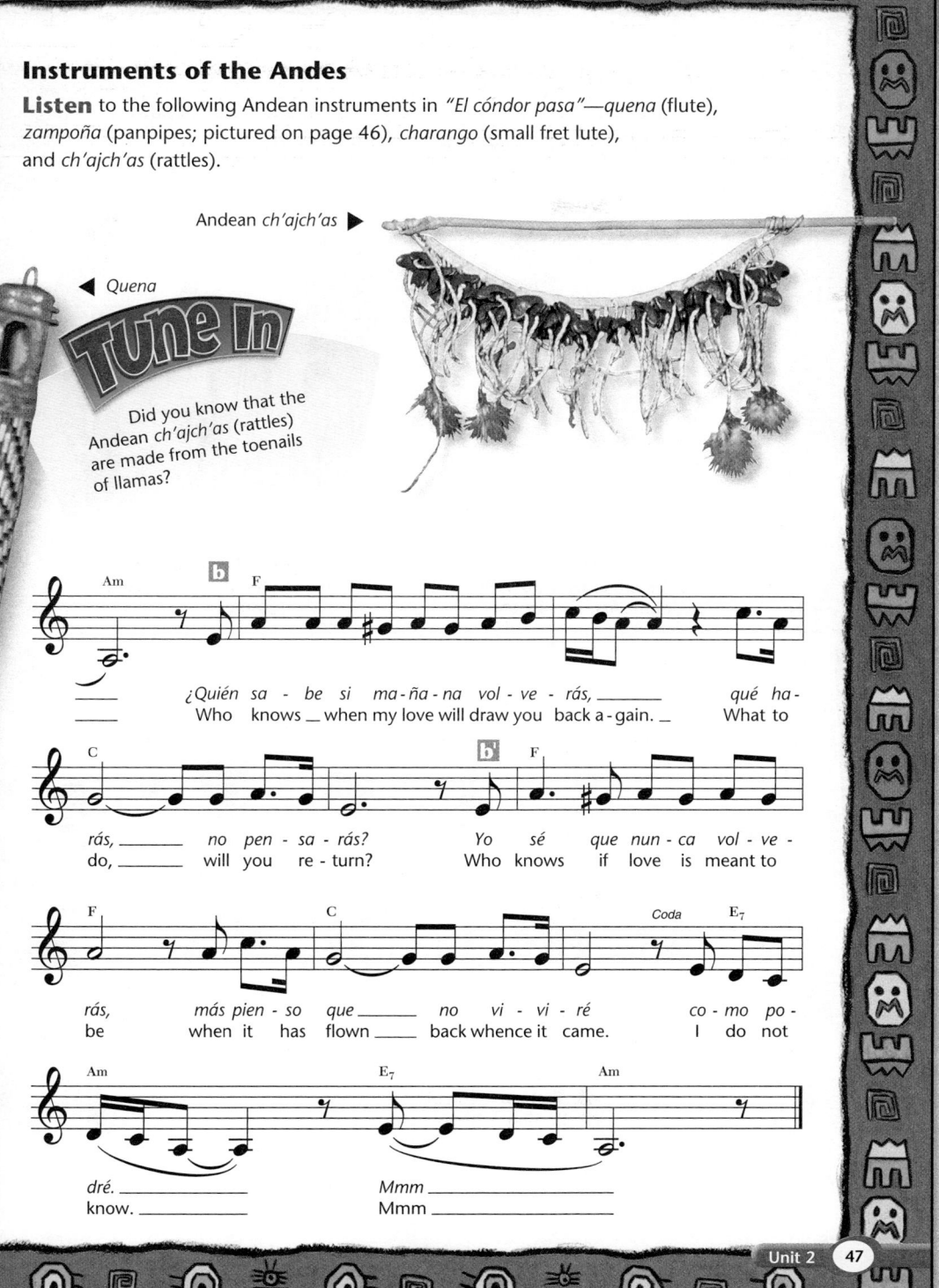

¿Quién sa - be si ma-ña-na vol-ve - rás, _____ qué ha-
Who knows _ when my love will draw you back a-gain. _ What to

rás, _____ no pen - sa - rás? Yo sé que nun-ca vol-ve-
do, _____ will you re-turn? Who knows if love is meant to

rás, más pien - so que_____ no vi-vi - ré co-mo po-
be when it has flown ____ back whence it came. I do not

dré. Mmm _____
know. _____ Mmm _____

Unit 2 **47**

1 INTRODUCE

Ask students to think about how they are the same as or different from a sibling or a friend, and to describe those similarities and differences in the context of musical form (a, a', b). Write a, a', and b on the board and tell students to use these terms when discussing the following. Have students

- Discuss how they could be similar to someone else (a).
- Discuss how they could be slightly different (a').
- Discuss how they could be very different (b).

Tell students they will now analyze the form of a song, using these phrase labels. Guide students to understand that the prime character (') is used to denote a similar, but slightly different version of the phrase.

2 DEVELOP

Listening

6b Play the recording of *"El cóndor pasa"* **CD 3-16**. Ask students to identify the elements of form such as

- The aabb phrases of the melody. (a = mm. 1–6; a = mm. 7–12; b = mm. 13–16; b = mm. 17–22)
- The anacrusis, or upbeat, that begins each phrase.

Analyzing

Have students sing *"El cóndor pasa"* **CD 3-17** with the English lyrics. Ask students to analyze the song notation.

6b **ASK Is the music of the second "a" phrase almost exactly the same as the first?** (yes)

Is the music of the second "b" phrase exactly the same as the first? No; the second b phrase is slightly different and has an added ending, two measures long. The form, therefore, is aabb'.

Tell students that the form may be analyzed as aabb or aabb', both of which would be correct. When discussing form, the general form (aabb) is most commonly used.

continued on page 48

ACROSS THE CURRICULUM

▶ **Social Studies** Introduce students to the Andes mountains by sharing *This Place Is High* by Vicki Cobb (Walker & Co., 1993). This book describes the Andes and the animals and people who live there. Also, recommend the Newbery Award book *Secret of the Andes* by Ann Nolan Clark (Puffin, 1976). This is the story of an Incan boy who raises llamas and learns the secrets of his ancestors.

MEETING INDIVIDUAL NEEDS

8b ▶ **Gifted and Talented** Ask students to make their own panpipes. (1/2-inch PVC plastic plumbing pipe is excellent.) Arrange them in graduated lengths that will produce the pitches they need (diatonic scale, pentatonic scale, for example). Corks or other stoppers may be used to close off the lower end of a tube.

SKILLS REINFORCEMENT

▶ **Recorder** Have students play the melody below to accompany "Greensleeves" on p. 49.

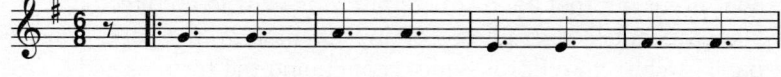

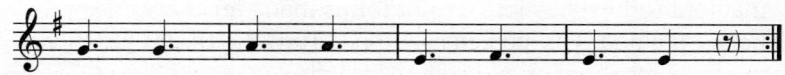

▶ **Mallets** Have students learn the Orff arrangement of *"El cóndor pasa,"* found on Resource Book p. F-6.

Singing

1c Use the Pronunciation Practice Track **CD 3-19** to help students learn to sing *"El cóndor pasa"* with the Spanish lyrics. Refer to Resource Book p. A-6 for the Pronunciation Practice Guide.

Moving

Explain to students that a condor is a large vulture found in the higher elevation of the Andes mountains in South America, and that it is an endangered species in the United States, under government protection. Refer students to p. 48 and invite them to

- Show the form of *"El cóndor pasa,"* using smooth gliding movements like the soaring of a condor.
- Make their movements for the b phrases contrast with those of the a phrases.

Listening

6b Have students

- Read about and discuss the Andean instruments featured on pp. 46–47. See Cultural Connection, on p. 46.
- Listen to *"El cóndor pasa"* **CD 3-16**, which features the following instruments: *bombo* [BOHM-boh], *chajchas* [CHA-chaz], guitar, *charango* [cha-RAHNG-go], *quena* [KEH-nah], and *zampoña* [zham-POH-nah].

Move with *"El cóndor pasa"*

You can **move** to show the form of *"El cóndor pasa."* You will use smooth, gliding movements. Practice and then **perform** the movements.

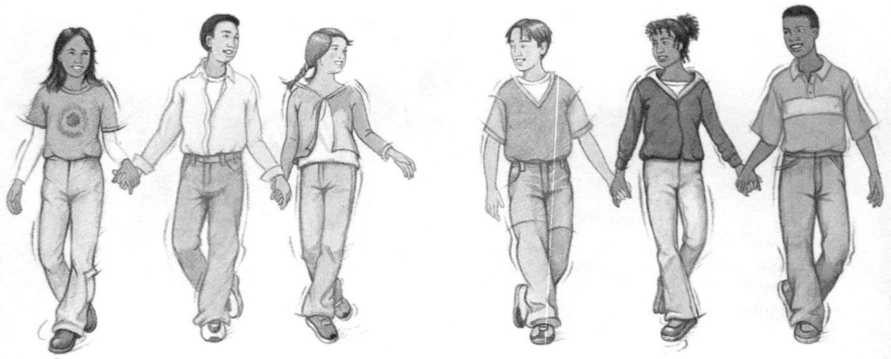

▲ **Section** **a** In a circle formation, move to the left, using a cross-step pattern, for the first six measures of the song.

▲ Move to the right, using a cross-step pattern, for the next six measures.

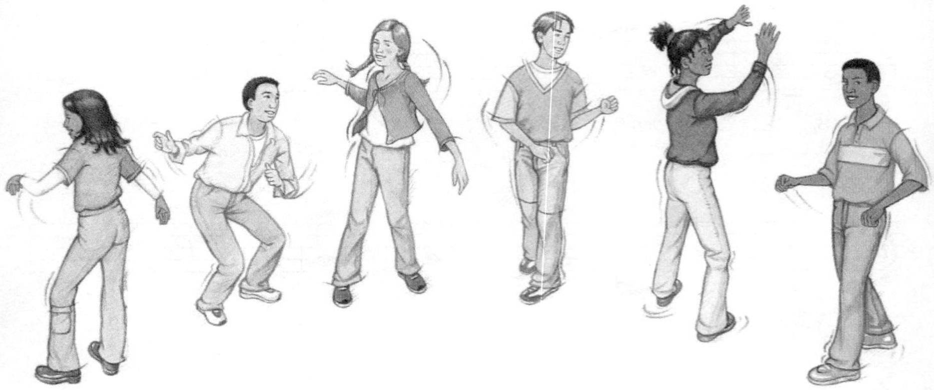

▲ **Section** **b** In place, create smooth, flowing patterns, using your whole body.

48

Footnotes

ACROSS THE CURRICULUM

8b ▶ **Visual Arts** Ask students to find examples of visual art works that use aabb form. Ask them if this form is as common as aba. Point out that aabb structural forms exist in architecture. Have students collect photos of any variation on the aabb principal in architecture (for instance, continuing the form as ccdd). You may opt to turn this into a hunt for as many architecture variations on a and b as students can find. Turn the results into a visual computer show or a bulletin board display.

CULTURAL CONNECTION

8b ▶ **Sixteenth-Century Elizabethan England** Elizabeth I, who reigned as queen of England from 1558 to 1603, brought England to enormous power and influence in Europe. Following are some of the high points of this period.

- Sir Francis Drake circumnavigated the globe, 1577–1580.
- England became a major seafaring nation and defeated the Spanish Armada in 1588.
- William Shakespeare wrote his famous plays and sonnets.
- Popular musical instruments of the period included the virginal (a harpsichordlike instrument), the lute, viol (an early version of the violin family with frets), and recorder. Queen Elizabeth was very proficient on both the virginal and the lute.

Greatest Hits of the 1500s

Sing "Greensleeves," a sixteenth-century melody also known as the English carol "What Child Is This?" "Greensleeves" also uses form. Notice that the second **a** and **b** phrases are slightly different. One way of showing this is **a a′ b b′**.

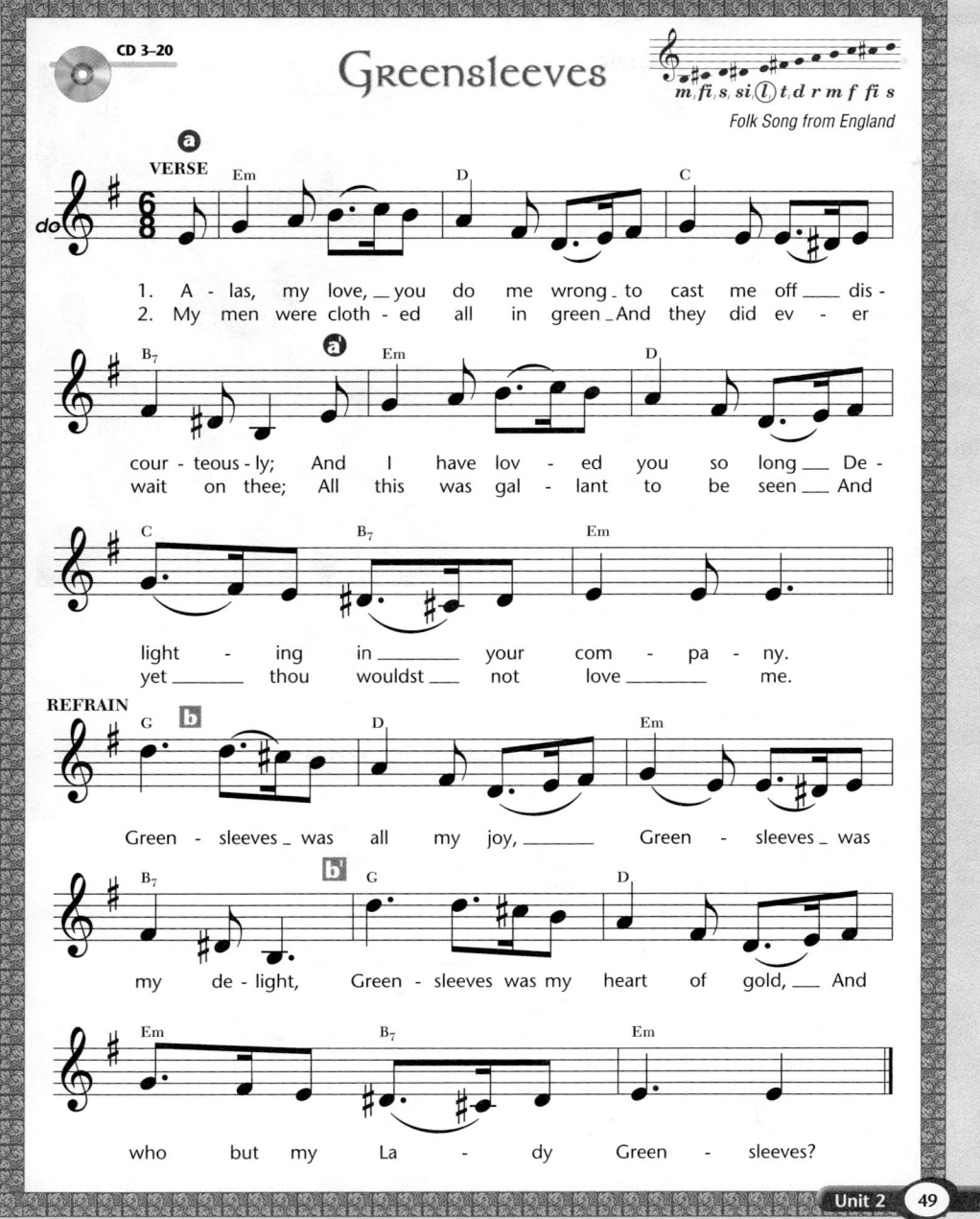

CD 3–20

Greensleeves

Folk Song from England

a VERSE

Em · D · C

1. A - las, my love, you do me wrong to cast me off dis -
2. My men were cloth - ed all in green And they did ev - er

a B₇ · Em · D

cour - teous - ly; And I have lov - ed you so long De -
wait on thee; All this was gal - lant to be seen And

C · B₇ · Em

light - ing in your com - pa - ny.
yet thou wouldst not love me.

REFRAIN **b** G · D · Em

Green - sleeves was all my joy, Green - sleeves was

b′ B₇ · G · D

my de - light, Green - sleeves was my heart of gold, And

Em · B₇ · Em

who but my La - dy Green - sleeves?

Listening

6b Have students

- Listen to "Greensleeves" **CD 3-20.**
- Identify the overall form of the melody. (aabb)

ASK How is this song similar to *"El cóndor pasa"*? (Both are in aabb phrase form.)

Singing

1c Have students sing "Greensleeves" with **CD 3-20.**

6b ASK Is the music of the second "a" phrase the same as the first? (No; it has a different ending.)

Is the music of the second "b" phrase the same as the first? (No; this phrase, too, ends differently. The form, therefore, is aa′bb′.)

Have students read the paragraph describing "Greensleeves" as a sixteenth-century carol. Explain to students that since the song credit describes it as an English folk song and that it is from the sixteenth century, it is from Elizabethan England. Discuss with students the musical and cultural history of Elizabethan England. Use Cultural Connection on p. 48 for topics and information.

3 CLOSE

Element: FORM ASSESSMENT

8a Performance/Music Journal Writing As a way of augmenting students' understanding of aabb form, ask them to do one of the following integrated art projects.

- Create a short dance in aabb form.
- Create a visual arts piece in aabb form.
- Create a sound piece in aabb form.

After students present or perform their projects, ask them to describe the process they used and record it in their music journals.

SKILLS REINFORCEMENT

▶ **Guitar** "Greensleeves" is part of the basic beginning repertoire for guitarists because it uses only first-position chords, yet requires frequent changes and playing of all three lower bass strings. These characteristics can be used as a strategy for learning the song on guitar. Have students

- Use a simple thumb strum, two to a measure.
- Finger the chords without playing in rhythm or up to tempo, but just to get a feel for the many chord changes; then try it in rhythm, fingering chords silently.
- Finger the chords, sounding only the proper bass strings. (This will be harder than it seems here.)
- Play the song with chords and strum, monitoring correct bass notes and chord changes.

SCHOOL TO HOME CONNECTION

▶ **Research** Challenge students to research information about and collect photos of the people and arts of the Andes region of South America. Invite students to share what they find with the class. Use this information to design a bulletin board.

TECHNOLOGY/MEDIA LINK

Video Library Invite students to watch the video, *Charango and Ensemble,* to see and listen to the *charango,* a popular instrument from the Andes region of South America.

LESSON AT A GLANCE

Element Focus — **FORM** aabb phrase form, AB section form

Skill Objective **PLAYING** Perform ostinato patterns to accompany a song

Connection Activity **CULTURE** Discuss the cultural heritage of the native peoples of Puerto Rico

MATERIALS
- "La paloma se fué"   **CD 3-22**
- "The Dove that Flew Away"   **CD 3-23**

  Recording Routine: Intro (4 m.); vocal; interlude (4 m.); vocal; coda
- **Pronunciation Practice/Translation** p. 524
- **Resource Book** p. A-7, F-8
- mallet instruments, bongos, selected rhythm instruments

VOCABULARY

contrast   aabb form   AB form   syncopation   ostinato

◆ ◆ ◆ National Standards ◆ ◆ ◆

1a Sing accurately in small ensembles
1c Sing music from diverse cultures
2b Perform easy instrumental pieces with technical accuracy
2e In instrumental ensembles, perform moderately easy pieces accurately
4c Arrange, using electronic media
6b Listen and analyze uses of form in music from diverse genres

MORE MUSIC CHOICES . . .

For more aabb forms:

"Greensleeves," p. 49

"El cóndor pasa," p. 46

1 INTRODUCE

"La paloma se fué" is in aabb phrase form. Ask students to describe things that are alike. For example, two boys could be aa, and two girls bb. What other things in the room represent this form? (two pencils/pens; two pairs of shoes)

Playing with Form

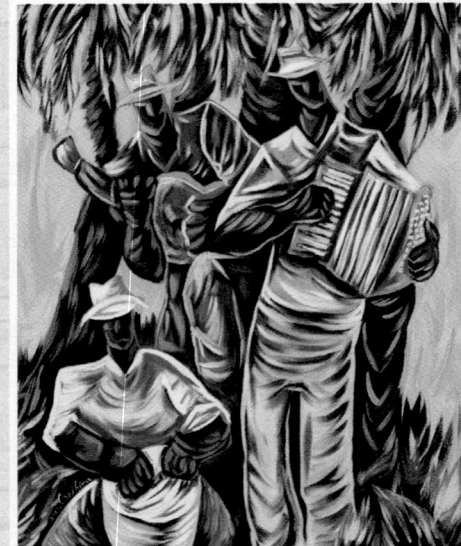

Repetition and contrast help define phrases and sections in musical form. **Listen** to the recording of "La paloma se fué," a folk song from Puerto Rico. Follow the notation and **identify** the **a** and **b** melodic phrases. How many times does each phrase repeat?

Notice that the phrases can be combined to create an **A** **B** section form. Music can have both phrase and section form.

Sing "La paloma se fué." As you sing, notice how the **A** **B** sections contrast with each other in melody, rhythm, and texture.

Arts Connection

▲ Trío Musical (2003) by Puerto Rican painter, Obed Gómez

Forming Rhythms

Rhythms and instrumental accompaniments can define contrasting sections in music.

Clap, or say, these rhythm patterns. Then, **perform** them as an accompaniment to "La paloma se fué." Perform the rhythms in different sections of the song to create contrast.

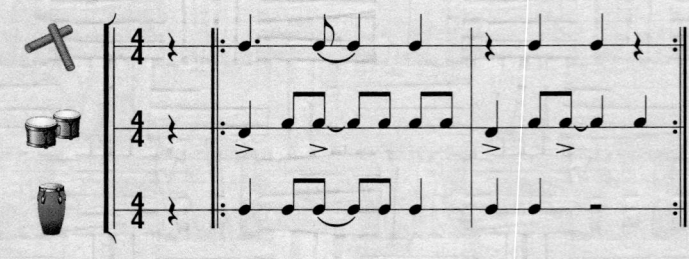

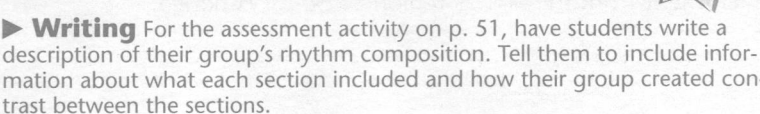
Footnotes

CULTURAL CONNECTION

▶ **Puerto Rico's Music** Puerto Rican music is among the predominant Caribbean music heard in the United States. Some of the instruments used in traditional Puerto Rican music originated with the Taíno people. Most noteworthy is the *güicharo*, or *güiro*, a notched hollowed-out gourd, which was adapted from pre-Columbian days. The musical traditions of the Spanish and Africans can also be heard in Puerto Rico's music.

BUILDING SKILLS THROUGH MUSIC

▶ **Writing** For the assessment activity on p. 51, have students write a description of their group's rhythm composition. Tell them to include information about what each section included and how their group created contrast between the sections.

SKILLS REINFORCEMENT

▶ **Mallets** Invite students to learn the Orff arrangement of "La paloma se fué" found on Resource Book p. F-8.

Reinforcement If students have difficulty playing a part in the arrangement, invite them to play a simplified bass xylophone part. Have them play a single whole note on each measure following the chord roots (C, F, G). Ask students to write this new part on manuscript paper.

On Target Guide students to learn their parts by playing slowly, repeating and learning each part, gradually bringing the parts up to tempo.

Challenge Two students may play each chord on the soprano and alto xylophone. Challenge and guide students to hold three mallets and play the complete chords by themselves.

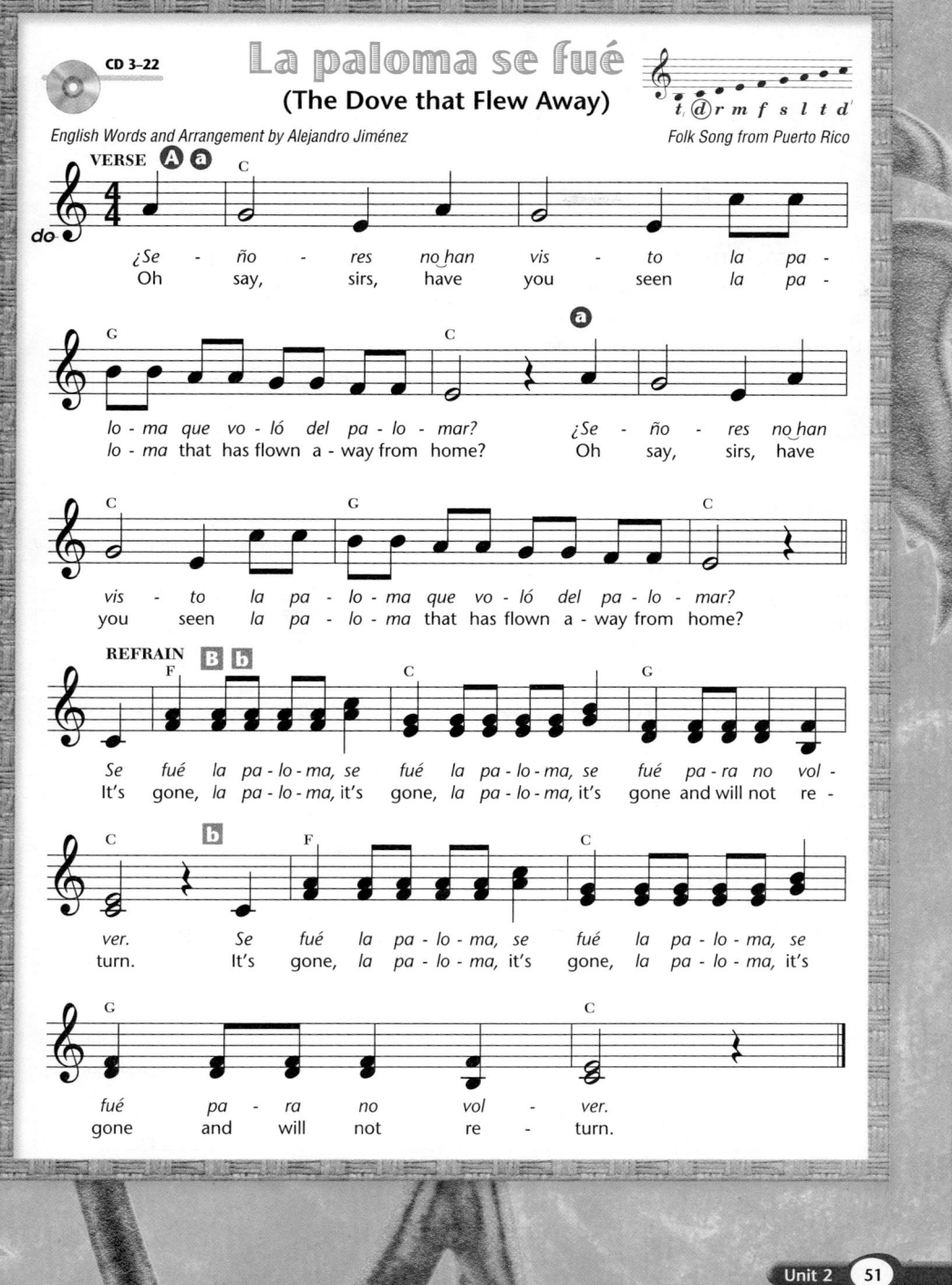

2 DEVELOP

Listening

6b Play "*La paloma se fué*" **CD 3-22** and ask students to listen for the a and b phrases. Guide students to see that the aa and bb phrases combine to form larger A and B sections. Form can be based on phrases (aabb), and sections (AB).

ASK How are the two large sections different? (They have different melodies, rhythms, and texture—the B section is in thirds.)

Invite students to perform the rhythms of the A and B sections, using contrasting body percussion on each section.

Singing

1a Have students sing "*La paloma se fué*" with English lyrics, with two groups singing the A and B sections.

1c Use the Pronunciation Practice Track **CD 3-25** to help students learn and sing the Spanish lyrics.

Playing

Ask students to perform the percussion ostinatos on p. 50. Assist students with the alternation between the left and right hands on the bongo part, and identify which hand plays the accents (left hand).

ASK Where are the syncopations? (between the second and third beats)

2e Invite students to perform the ostinatos on percussion instruments as the class sings "*La paloma se fué.*"

3 CLOSE

Element: FORM ‖ **ASSESSMENT**

2b **Performance/Self-Assessment** Invite groups to create a rhythm composition in aabb phrase form, showing contrast between the A and B sections. Have students assess their success at contrasting the A and B sections.

ACROSS THE CURRICULUM

▶ **Social Studies** When Columbus reached Hispaniola in 1492, he found the Taíno people, the most highly developed society in the Caribbean at that time. The islands throughout the Greater Antilles were dotted with Taíno communities nestled in valleys and along the rivers and coastlines. Some communities were inhabited by thousands of people. This first "new world" society that Columbus encountered was one of tremendous creativity and energy. The Taíno were talented and expressive in the arts of sculpture, ceramics, jewelry, weaving, dance, music, and poetry.

TECHNOLOGY/MEDIA LINK

4c ▶ **Electronic Keyboard** Have students create an aabb rhythm composition for electronic keyboard. Encourage them to be creative using repetition and contrast to clearly differentiate the sections. Invite students to explore the timbres of the electronic keyboard to help differentiate sections. If the electronic keyboard includes a MIDI sequencer, have students record their compositions into the sequencer for later playback.

LESSON 6

LESSON AT A GLANCE

Element Focus **MELODY** Melodic contour

Skill Objective **MOVING** Move to express the lyrics of a song and show melodic contour

Connection Activity **GENRE** Explore the gospel genre with regard to movement and spirit of the lyrics

MATERIALS
- "Glory, Glory, Hallelujah" **CD 3-27**
  Recording Routine: Intro (8 m.); refrain; v. 1; refrain; interlude (8 m.); refrain; v. 2; refrain
- "Will the Circle Be Unbroken" (lyrics only)
- piano or MIDI keyboard

VOCABULARY

melodic contour   genre   gospel style

◆ ◆ ◆ ◆ National Standards ◆ ◆ ◆ ◆
1a Sing accurately alone and in small ensembles
2a Play instruments accurately alone
4c Arrange, using electronic media
8a Show how different arts portray the same emotion in unique ways

MORE MUSIC CHOICES
For more experience with gospel style:
The Battle of Jericho, p. 234
Jonah, p. 235
"This Little Light of Mine," p. 232

1 INTRODUCE

8a **ASK What does your voice sound like when you feel good?** (Accept a variety of answers.)

Choose students to read the text of "Glory, Glory, Hallelujah" aloud using a variety of expressive techniques. (speak softly, shout, pronounce words slowly or fast) Encourage students to relate to music that helps lift their spirits and describe the music that changes their mood.

LESSON 6
Element: MELODY | Skill: MOVING | Connection: GENRE

Glorious Gospel

"Glory, Glory, Hallelujah" is a gospel song. Like most gospel songs, it encourages the singers to let go of their fear, worry, and anger and let only good thoughts come through. The influences of gospel music can be heard in the popular music we listen to every day.

Describe the contour of the melody after you **sing** "Glory, Glory, Hallelujah."

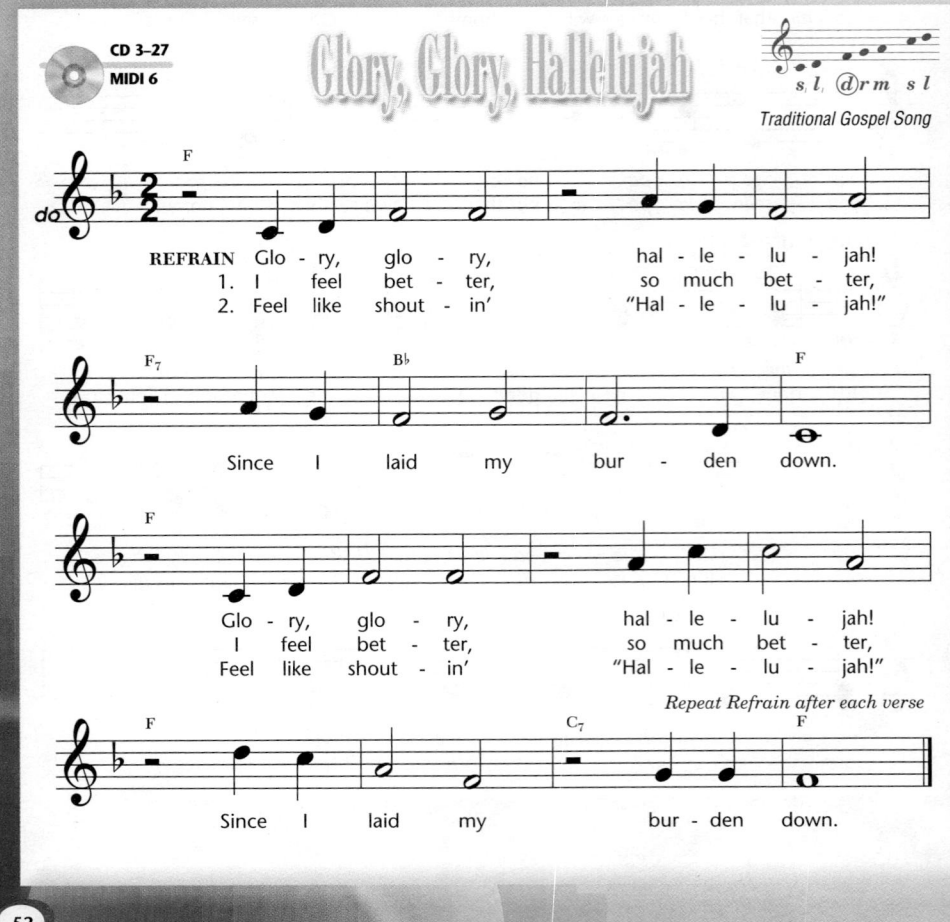

52

Footnotes

MEETING INDIVIDUAL NEEDS

▶ **Including Everyone** Students with a muscular disability will find it difficult to sway and move energetically to the gospel beat. Include those students by demonstrating smaller gestures that they are able to synchronize with the beat.

BUILDING SKILLS THROUGH MUSIC

▶ **Social Studies** Discuss with students the factors that contributed to the origins of gospel music. Extend the discussion to present-day society and the factors that support the continuation of gospel music.

CULTURAL CONNECTION

▶ **A Crossover Tune** The European American gospel song "Will the Circle Be Unbroken" uses the same melody as "Glory, Glory, Hallelujah." It has been recorded by many popular recording artists including Willie Nelson, Jerry Lee Lewis, the Jordanaires, and Tammy Wynette. Sing these words from "Will the Circle Be Unbroken" with the melody of "Glory, Glory, Hallelujah."

Will the circle be unbroken,
By and by, Lord, by and by?
There's a better home a-waiting
In the sky, Lord, in the sky.

Gospel Choir Moves

With their upbeat sense of celebration, gospel songs make singers and listeners let go—and move! The movements used by gospel choirs influenced the way popular music is performed today. Through movement we experience the rhythm of the music and the feeling of the lyrics.

Using "Glory, Glory, Hallelujah," **move** to express the lyrics of the song.
Perform these movements as you **sing** the phrase *glory, glory, hallelujah.*

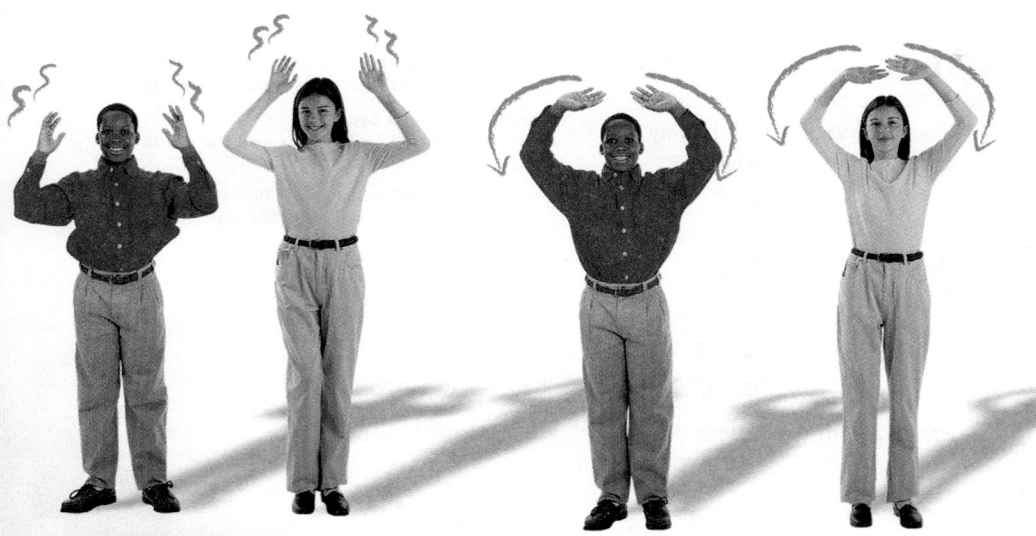

▲ *Glory, Glory*–Hands flicker, moving upward.   ▲ *Hallelujah*–Draw a rainbow arc overhead.

Gospel B3

One of the most famous sounds in gospel music is that of a Hammond B3 organ. The sound of a "B3" can be found on MIDI keyboards. Locate a gospel organ sound on your MIDI keyboard and **play** this chord accompaniment to "Glory, Glory, Hallelujah." Experiment with playing a variety of rhythm patterns on the accompaniment.

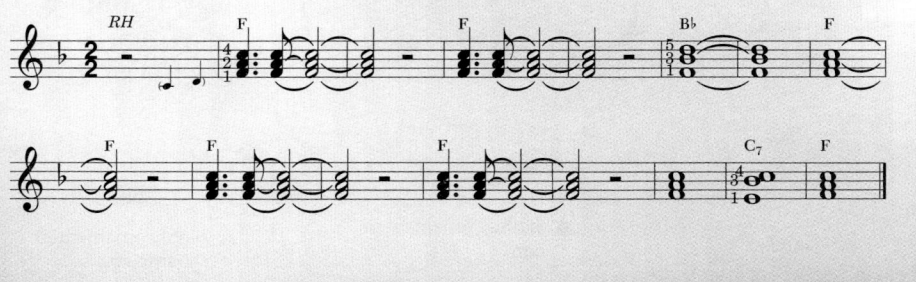

2 DEVELOP

Singing

Direct students to pp. 20–23 to review melodic contour.

1a Invite students to sing "Glory, Glory, Hallelujah" **CD 3-27** with the recording, tracing the contour of the melody.

ASK **Where does the high point of the melody occur?** (m. 13, on the word *Since*)

In which measures does the melody reflect the meaning of the words? (mm. 7 and 8, on the words *burden down*)

What do you think the intended feeling is for this song: meditative or joyful? (joyful)

Moving

8a Explain that gospel choirs often sway and clap on the offbeats while singing. Gospel music often inspires an emotional or physical reaction.

Allow students to practice the movements on p. 53. Invite students to create a motion for the words *Since I laid my burden down.*

1a Have students sing and perform their movements with the Stereo Performance Track **CD 3-28.**

Playing

2a Invite students to perform the keyboard accompaniment on p. 53 on piano or MIDI keyboard. Encourage them to experiment with different rhythm patterns.

3 CLOSE

Skill: MOVING   ASSESSMENT

Performance/Self-Assessment Invite students to perform their movements demonstrating melodic contour to "Glory, Glory, Hallelujah" as the class sings. Have students critique their own performance.

SKILLS REINFORCEMENT

1a ▶ **Vocal Development** Encourage students to sing alone or in small groups. These individual and small-group performances give you opportunities to listen to an individual singer's tone quality. During these performances, watch for signs of tension, such as a jutting neck or jaw. Make note of any problems and help students fix them later, during large-group performance. Commenting on a student's tone quality or concentrating on the singer's problems during individual or small-group performances might discourage the singer from wanting to sing again in small groups.

TECHNOLOGY/MEDIA LINK

4c **MIDI/Sequencing Software** Using the MIDI song file for "Glory, Glory, Hallelujah," have students

- Select the software program's graphic editor and examine the contour of the melody.
- Explore graphic editing features such as deleting, entering, and changing pitches.
- Turn off accompaniment tracks and play back several alterations of the melody.

LESSON AT A GLANCE

Element Focus   **MELODY** Melodic ornamentation

Skill Objective   **LISTENING** Listen for, identify, and describe ornamentation in brass music

Connection Activity   **RELATED ARTS** View and discuss ornamentation in visual art

MATERIALS

- "Glory, Glory, Hallelujah"   **CD 3-27**
- *Glory, Glory, Hallelujah* (version two)   **CD 3-29**
- *Prince of Denmark's March* (excerpt)   **CD 3-30**
- bells, keyboard, or other melodic instruments

VOCABULARY

ornamentation   improvisation   trill

◆ ◆ ◆ ◆ National Standards ◆ ◆ ◆ ◆

1c Sing music from diverse genres, with appropriate expression
3b Improvise melodic embellishments on given melodies
6a Listen and describe events in music using appropriate terms
8a Show how different arts portray the same idea in unique ways

MORE MUSIC CHOICES

For more experience with melodic ornamentation:
Watermelon Man, p. 270
L'union, p. 487

1 INTRODUCE

8a View and discuss with students the photos of plain and elaborately decorated, or ornamented, eggs. See Across the Curriculum below. Explain that performers and composers, like all artists, often use ornamentation in creating or interpreting works of art.

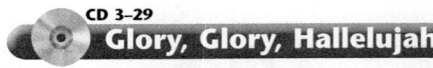

GO with the Melody

Listen to a different performance of *Glory, Glory, Hallelujah.* How would you **describe** the way the singer performs the melody?

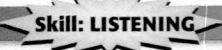 CD 3–29
Glory, Glory, Hallelujah

Traditional Gospel Song as performed by Carol Woods and the Linda Twine Singers

This gospel performance also features call and response and improvisation on the Hammond organ.

Here is the song melody:

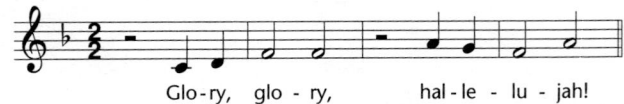

Glo-ry,   glo-ry,   hal-le - lu - jah!

Here is an ornamented melody:

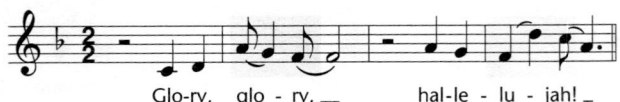

Glo-ry,   glo - ry, —   hal-le - lu - jah! _

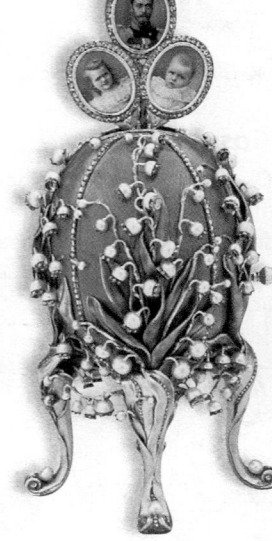

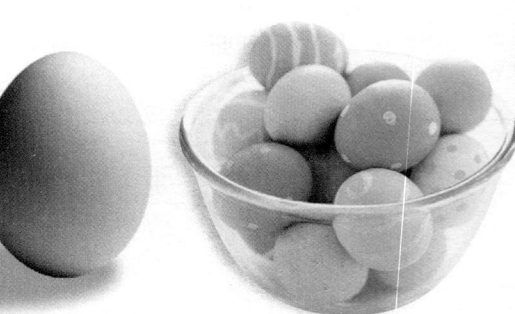

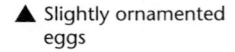

▲ Plain egg   ▲ Slightly ornamented eggs   ▲ Highly ornamented Fabergé egg

Footnotes

ACROSS THE CURRICULUM

8a ▶ **Related Arts** Carl Fabergé's ornamented eggs were introduced in 1884 when Alexander III, czar of Russia, commissioned one for his wife as an Easter gift. Each egg was different, took a year to create, and contained a surprise. The egg pictured on this page is titled *Lilies of the Valley*; it contains photos of Czar Nicholas and his daughters Olga and Tatyana.

BUILDING SKILLS THROUGH MUSIC

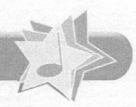

▶ **Writing** Just as music can be ornamented, so too can our writing. Invite students to begin with a simple sentence about an egg, then elaborate on that idea, using prepositional phrases. The new sentences should range from small ornamentations to very elaborate and complex descriptions.

SKILLS REINFORCEMENT

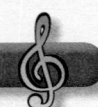

▶ **Reading** Teach students to look for the basic notes when reading a melody. This "skeleton melody," like the frame of a house, supports many fancy decorations and elaboration. This approach, utilizing pattern recognition, will help students learn and memorize songs faster, and is one of the keys to improving reading and improvising skills. Here is the skeleton melody for the first part of "Glory, Glory, Hallelujah."

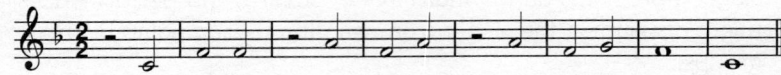

Dress Up the Melody

Singers sometimes add extra notes to the melody. These extra notes are called *ornamentation*. The singer may **improvise** the ornamentation on the spot. Name some performers who improvise ornamentation in this way.

> The term **improvise** means to make up music as it is being performed.

Perform this familiar melody, using bells, keyboard, or your voice. Then **improvise** ornamentation on the melody.

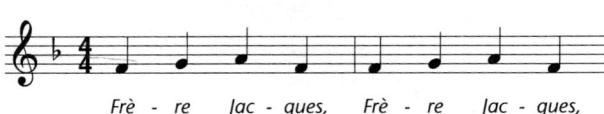

Frè - re   Jac - ques,   Frè - re   Jac - ques,

Here is one possibility for improvising ornamentation for *"Frère Jacques."*

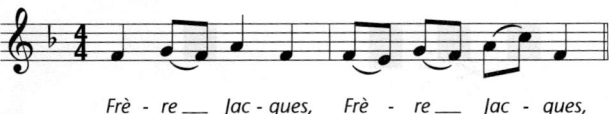

Frè - re ___ Jac - ques,   Frè - re ___ Jac - ques,

Composers use ornamentation to add variety to a composition. They may write the ornamentation into the score or expect the performer to improvise it. The trill is a type of ornamentation used frequently by Baroque composers. **Play** this melody, without the trills, on a mallet or keyboard instrument.

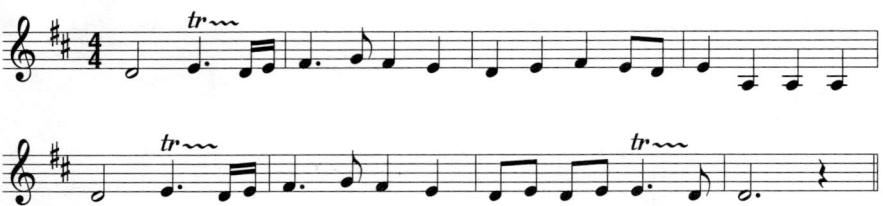

Listen to the melody above performed on a trumpet with the ornamentation. Point to the notes that are trilled.

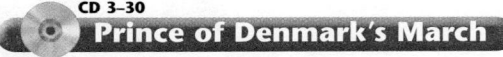
CD 3–30
Prince of Denmark's March

by Jeremiah Clarke
as performed by the Canadian Brass
This famous piece, sometimes titled *Trumpet Voluntary*, is often used as processional music at weddings and other formal ceremonies.

Unit 2   55

---

2 DEVELOP

Listening

1c Have students focus on the melodic contour as they listen to and sing "Glory, Glory, Hallelujah" **CD 3-27** on p. 52. Then, play the ornamented version of *Glory, Glory, Hallelujah* **CD 3-29**.

ASK How would you describe differences between the first recording of the song and the ornamented version? (In the second version, the singer ornaments the melody in gospel style by adding extra notes and improvises the melodic ornaments on the spot.)

Analyzing

6a Help students describe the way the singer performs the melody in the two recordings by discussing the similarities in the melodies, the ornamentation in the second example, and how the ornamentation changed the contour of the melody.

Singing

1c Have students sing along with the ornamented version of *Glory, Glory, Hallelujah* **CD 3-29**.

Playing

3b Ask students to perform the first two measures of *"Frère Jacques"* on a melody instrument, and then add the ornamentation. Students may then improvise ornamentation on the rest of the melody.

3 CLOSE

Skill: LISTENING   ASSESSMENT

6a **Observation** Familiarize students with the nonornamented version of the main theme from *Prince of Denmark's March* (see Spotlight On below). Then play the recording **CD 3-30**. Ask students to describe the ornamentation and indicate where in the melody it occurs.

SPOTLIGHT ON

▶ *Prince of Denmark's March* Once attributed to Henry Purcell (with the title *Trumpet Voluntary*), this popular piece featuring trumpet was composed by Jeremiah Clarke (c.1674–1707). Notated below is the main melody. Ornamentation is indicated with an asterisk.

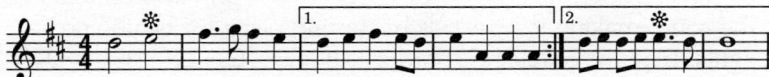

▶ **The Canadian Brass** This popular performing group has been together for more than 30 years. The musicians entertain audiences and demonstrate strong support for music education throughout the world with their unbeatable blend of virtuosity and humor. The selections on their many recordings range from Gabrieli to Gershwin.

SCHOOL TO HOME CONNECTION

▶ **Gospel Performers** Encourage students to listen to recordings of gospel style by such artists as Mahalia Jackson, André Crouch, Whitney Houston, and Aretha Franklin. Students can write reviews for their music journals.

TECHNOLOGY/MEDIA LINK

Video Library Students may be interested in viewing a gospel choir performance in the video, *Total Experience Gospel Choir*. They may also be interested in the video *Whitney Houston*, which shows the gospel influence on this popular singer.

LESSON AT A GLANCE

Element Focus **MELODY** Major scale

Skill Objective **READING** Read the major diatonic scale

Connection Activity **CULTURE** Discuss the purpose of lullabies

MATERIALS

- "Adiós, amigos"   **CD 4-1**
- "Goodbye, My Friends"   **CD 4-2**
  Recording Routine: Intro (4 m.); vocal (unison); interlude (4 m.); vocal (2x as 3-part round); coda
- **Music Reading Practice, Sequence 7**   **CD 4-5**
- **Pronunciation Practice/Translation** p. 524
- **Resource Book** pp. A-6, D-8, E-8, G-7
- mallet instruments or keyboard, rattles, drums, guitar

VOCABULARY

pitch set	diatonic	pentatonic	hexachordal
tonic	major scale	key signature	

◆ ◆ ◆ ◆ National Standards ◆ ◆ ◆ ◆

1c Sing music from diverse cultures
5b Sightread melodies in treble clef
5c Identify standard notation symbols for pitch
6b Listen and analyze uses of pitch in music from diverse cultures

MORE MUSIC CHOICES. . .

For more practice with major diatonic songs:
"Red River Valley," p. 11
"Give a Little Love," p. 140

1 INTRODUCE

Lead students to discover that *"Adiós, amigos"* is a lullaby, and that cultures around the world use lullabies to sing their children to sleep.

1c Play *"Adiós, amigos"* **CD 4-1** and explain to students that this song from Mexico is in meter in 3 and is based on a special scale.

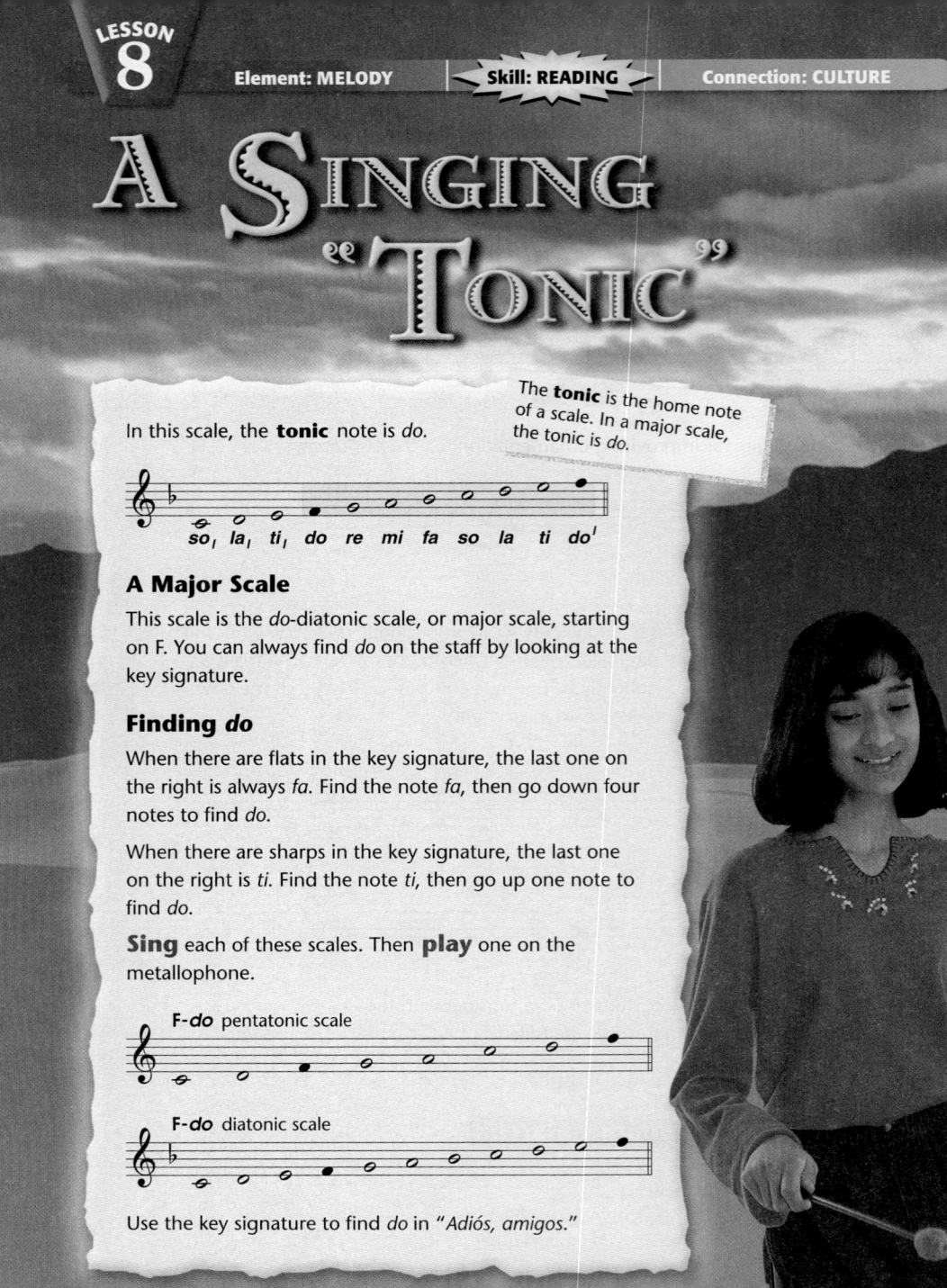

A SINGING "TONIC"

> The **tonic** is the home note of a scale. In a major scale, the tonic is *do*.

In this scale, the **tonic** note is *do*.

so₁ la₁ ti₁ do re mi fa so la ti do¹

A Major Scale

This scale is the *do*-diatonic scale, or major scale, starting on F. You can always find *do* on the staff by looking at the key signature.

Finding *do*

When there are flats in the key signature, the last one on the right is always *fa*. Find the note *fa*, then go down four notes to find *do*.

When there are sharps in the key signature, the last one on the right is *ti*. Find the note *ti*, then go up one note to find *do*.

Sing each of these scales. Then **play** one on the metallophone.

F-*do* pentatonic scale

F-*do* diatonic scale

Use the key signature to find *do* in *"Adiós, amigos."*

56 Reading Sequence 7

Footnotes

ACROSS THE CURRICULUM

▶ **Science** In a more in-depth discussion of diatonic scales, have students examine the harmonic series. The harmonic series follows the harmonics (overtones) that result from a vibrating string. A vibrating string vibrates in segments, or loops—whole string (1), 1/2, 1/3, 1/4, and so on—thus producing the overtones that give an instrument its timbre. The harmonic series also demonstrates the intervals—fundamental, octave, fifth, fourth, third, and so on.

BUILDING SKILLS THROUGH MUSIC

▶ **Writing** Invite students to write new lyrics for *"Adiós, amigos,"* following the same rhythm that is in the song. Brainstorm ideas for appropriate lullaby words, then modify them to fit the song.

TEACHER TO TEACHER

▶ **Instrument Tips** In playing the scales in this lesson on mallet instruments, you will need to have B♭ bars, F♯ bars, and C♯ bars available.

An easy guitar accompaniment for *"Adiós, amigos"* is possible by transposing it to the key of G. There are only two chords in the song, making it an excellent starting place for beginning students. Play the following chord substitutes.   F = G   C₇ = D₇

Spot the Scale!

Sing "Adiós, amigos." Then **identify** each F-do in the music. (One is shown in the color box.)

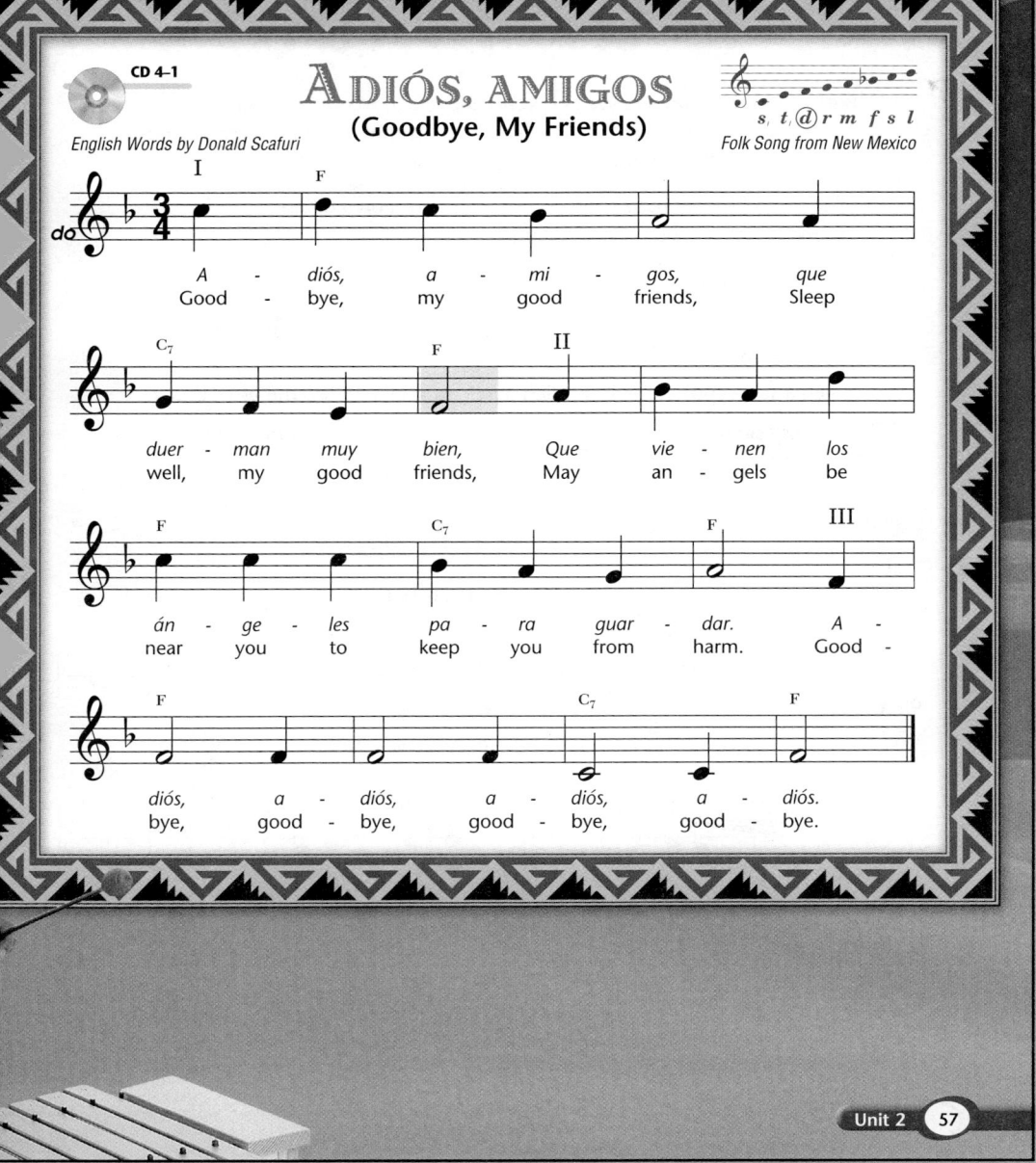

CD 4-1

ADIÓS, AMIGOS
(Goodbye, My Friends)

English Words by Donald Scafuri

Folk Song from New Mexico

s, t, (d) r m f s l

I
A - diós, a - mi - gos, que
Good - bye, my good friends, Sleep

II
duer - man muy bien, Que vie - nen los
well, my good friends, May an - gels be

III
án - ge - les pa - ra guar - dar. A -
near you to keep you from harm. Good -

diós, a - diós, a - diós, a - diós.
bye, good - bye, good - bye, good - bye.

2 DEVELOP

Reading

5c Write the F-pentatonic scale on the staff (C, D, F, G, A). Have students sing pitch syllables and use hand signs to identify the *do* pentatonic scale. Play the scale on a barred instrument or keyboard. See Teacher to Teacher on p. 56.

2a
6b Play "Adiós, amigos" **CD 4-1** and have students determine that the song does not use a pentatonic scale.

Singing

5b Direct students to p. 56. Have them sing the F-*do* scale using pitch syllables. Lead them to discover the major scale and how to find *do* when the key signature contains a flat. (The last flat is *fa;* count down a fourth to find *do.*) Have students

- Sing and play the scales on p. 56 on a mallet instrument or keyboard.
- Identify the scale of "Adiós, amigos" from the key signature.
- Read the notation of "Adiós, amigos" and sing pitch syllables.

1c Use the Pronunciation Practice Track **CD 4-4** to echo the Spanish words. Have students sing the song, first in unison then as a round.

Reading

5c Lead students to discover how to find *do* when there are sharps in the key signature. (The last sharp in the key signature is *ti;* go up one note to *do.*) Using Resource Book p. D-8, have students sing the D-*do* diatonic scale.

3 CLOSE

Skill: READING **ASSESSMENT**

Performance/Observation Use Music Reading Worksheet on p. D-8 to have students read the F-*do* and D-*do* diatonic scales using pitch syllables. Observe students' ability to read and sing the scales accurately.

SKILLS REINFORCEMENT

▶ **Reading** For additional reading practice, invite students to sing a countermelody to "Adiós, amigos" in the Music Reading Practice section on p. 491, or Resource Book p. E-8.

▶ **Signing** Invite students to learn the signing to "Adiós, amigos" on Resource Book p. G-7.

▶ **Analyzing** The process of analyzing scales (for example, comparing the differences between the F-*do* pentatonic and diatonic scales) develops analytical and problem-solving skills for the student. Use music theory tools, such as *Alfred's Essentials of Music Theory* CD-ROM, to further develop these musical and analytical skills.

TECHNOLOGY/MEDIA LINK

▶ **CD-ROM** *Alfred's Essentials of Music Theory.* Invite students to work in small groups to explore *Major Scales* in *Alfred's Essentials of Music Theory (Vol. 2)* music software. Allow students to share with the class the information that they learn.

LESSON AT A GLANCE

Element Focus   **MELODY** Minor scale

Skill Objective   **READING** Read *la* diatonic scales

Connection Activity   **CULTURE** Perform a Bolivian folk dance

MATERIALS

- "La mariposa"   **CD 4-8**
- "The Butterfly"   **CD 4-9**
   Recording Routine: Intro (4 m.); vocal; instrumental
- **Music Reading Practice, Sequence 8**   **CD 4-12**
- **Pronunciation Practice/Translation** p. 520
- **Resource Book** pp. A-9, B-6, D-9, E-9
- mallet instruments or keyboard, rattles, drums, guitar

VOCABULARY

minor scale   *la* pentachord   *la* hexachord

◆ ◆ ◆ ◆ **National Standards** ◆ ◆ ◆ ◆

1c Sing music from diverse cultures
2a Play instruments accurately in small ensembles
5b Sight-read melodies in treble clef
6b Listen and analyze uses of pitch in music from diverse genres

MORE MUSIC CHOICES

For more practice with minor diatonic songs:
"I Walk the Unfrequented Road," p. 79
"El condor pasa," p. 46

1 INTRODUCE

Tell students that they are about to learn a Bolivian folk song based on a special scale. Guide them to learn that the Andes mountain range is in Bolivia, and that folk instruments from this region are used in Bolivian folk music. Discuss with students the information on Andean instruments in Cultural Connection below.

Migrate to Minor

Butterflies are found all over the world and live in many varied climates. Their beauty has inspired artists to create art and musicians to create songs. *"La mariposa"* ("The Butterfly") is one such song.

Listen to "La mariposa" from Bolivia. It is based on a different scale. **Sing** "La mariposa" and listen to the sound.

Scale Review

You already know how to use the key signature to find *do*. When a scale ends on *do*, the scale is called *major*.

When a scale ends on *la*, it is called *minor*. In minor scales, the tonic is *la*.

Every key signature has a major scale and a minor scale that belong to it.

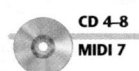
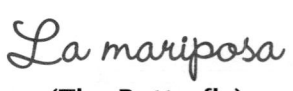
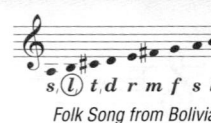

CD 4–8
MIDI 7

La mariposa
(The Butterfly)

English Words by Aura Kontra

Folk Song from Bolivia

s (l) t, d r m f s l

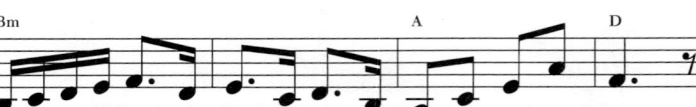
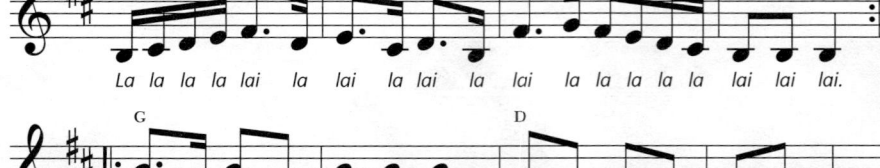

La la la la lai   la   lai   la lai   la   lai   lai lai lai   lai,

La la la la lai   la   lai   la la   lai   la la la la la   lai lai lai.

Al   son de   las   ma - tra - cas   to - dos can - tan   y   bai - lan
Hear   the rat - tles'   rhyth-mic beat,   Call - ing   us   to   sing and dance

Footnotes

CULTURAL CONNECTION

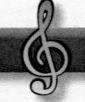

▶ **Andean Instruments** "La mariposa" features Andean folk instruments. The *charango* (a small guitarlike instrument with an armadillo shell back) plays a strummed accompaniment. The *zampoña* (panpipes made of two rows of several tubes of hollow reed tied together in graduated lengths) plays the melody. The *zampoña* is played by blowing over the ends of the tubes, as if blowing over the top of a bottle to make a sound.

BUILDING SKILLS THROUGH MUSIC

▶ **Science** Share with students the information on the *zampoña* in Cultural Connection above. Have students determine the effect of length on pitch using either a stringed instrument or panpipes (or narrow PVC cut to various lengths to imitate panpipes). Then, have them identify their hypothesis and the method they will use to collect the data.

SKILLS REINFORCEMENT

▶ **Guitar** The chords to "La mariposa" are easier to play on guitar by using a capo at fret 2. Play these chord substitutes:

2a

Bm = Am   A = G   D = C   F♯ = E   G = F   Em = Dm

▶ **Reading** For additional reading practice, see Music Reading Sequence 8 on p. 491, or Resource Book p. E-9.

▶ **Playing** Encourage students to play these ostinatos as they sing "La mariposa."

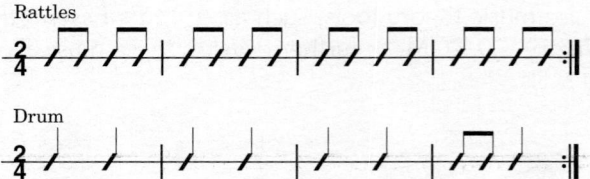

Rattles

Drum

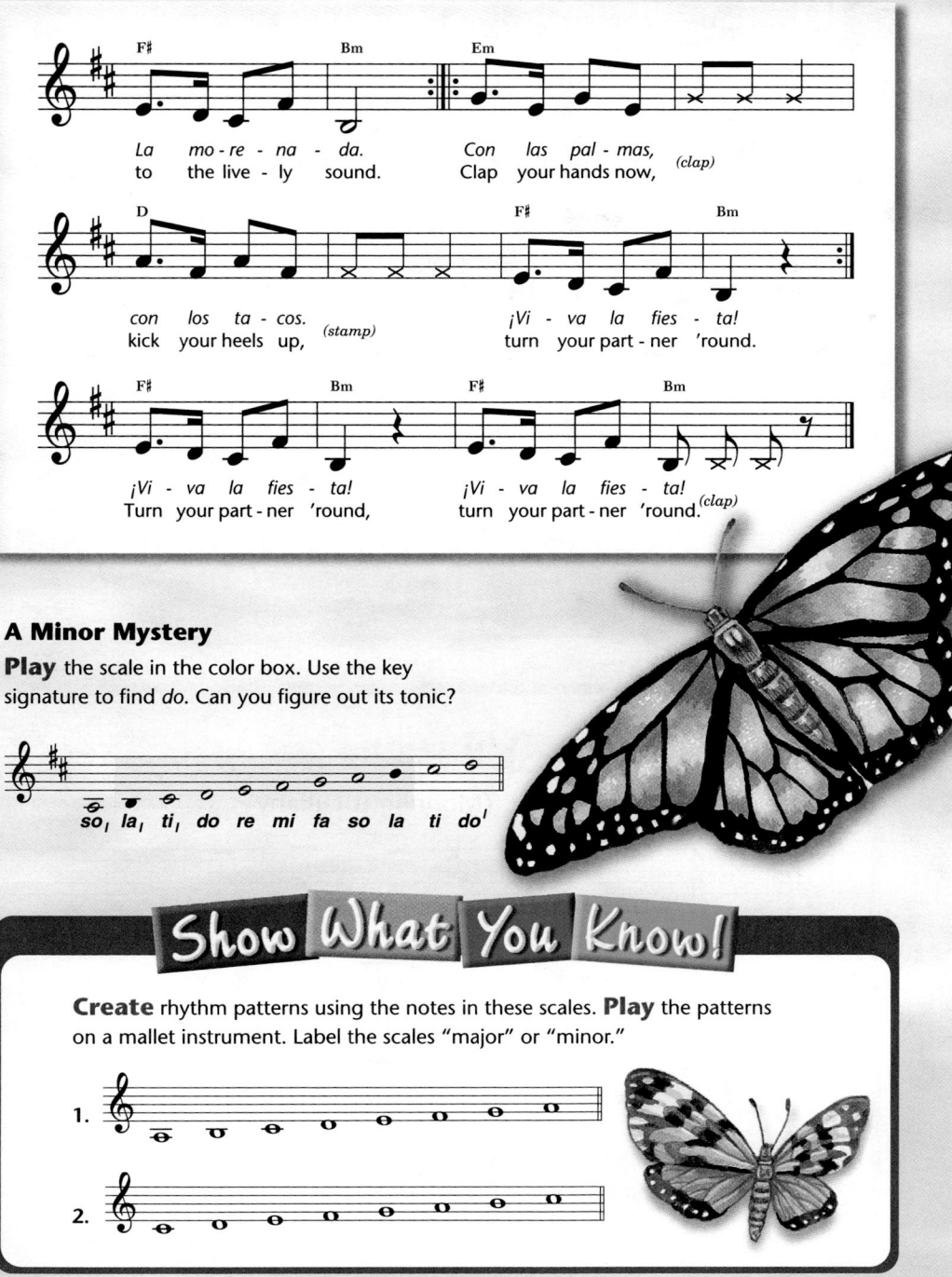

La mo-re-na-da. Con las pal-mas, *(clap)*
to the live-ly sound. Clap your hands now,

con los ta-cos. ¡Vi-va la fies-ta!
kick your heels up, *(stamp)* turn your part-ner 'round.

¡Vi-va la fies-ta! ¡Vi-va la fies-ta!
Turn your part-ner 'round, turn your part-ner 'round.*(clap)*

A Minor Mystery

Play the scale in the color box. Use the key signature to find *do*. Can you figure out its tonic?

so₁ la₁ ti₁ do re mi fa so la ti do¹

Show What You Know!

Create rhythm patterns using the notes in these scales. **Play** the patterns on a mallet instrument. Label the scales "major" or "minor."

1.
2.

2 DEVELOP

Listening

6b Have students listen to *"La mariposa"* **CD 4-8.**

ASK Is the scale of this song the same as the major diatonic scale for *"Adiós, amigos?"* (no, it is minor)

Reading

5b Direct students to p. 59. Have them compare the scale on the page to the scale on p. 56, name the B-*la* tonic, and name the minor scale (B-minor). Then, invite students to sing *"La mariposa"* at a slow tempo, using pitch syllables.

Playing

2a Have students play the rhythm ostinatos in Skills Reinforcement, p. 58, and Drum Ensemble 4, p. 298, with *"La mariposa"* **CD 4-8.**

Ask students to create rhythm patterns in Resource Book, p. B-6 and clap their rhythms with the recording.

Singing

1c Have students use the Pronunciation Practice Track **CD 4-11** to learn the Spanish words and sing *"La mariposa"* with the recording **CD 4-8.**

Moving

Encourage students to learn and perform a Bolivian folk dance to accompany *"La mariposa"* using the dance directions in Movement below.

3 CLOSE

Skill: READING   ASSESSMENT

5b **Performance/Observation** Have students read the major and minor diatonic scales in Show What You Know on p. 59, or Resource Book p. B-6, using pitch syllables and hand signs. Observe students' ability to accurately read, sing, and play these scales.

MOVEMENT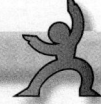

▶ **Patterned Dance** Help students learn this Bolivian dance. Wear rattles around the ankles to add an exciting timbre.

8-beat introduction: Circle formation.

Mm.1–8: Small running steps to the left; joined hands held down in V position. On repeat, move to right.

Mm. 9–14: Small running steps to left, with left hand on shoulder of person in front. On repeat, move to right, using right hand on shoulder.

Mm. 15–16: Small running steps to left/stop and clap.

Mm. 17–18: Small running steps to left/stop and stamp.

Mm. 19–20: Small running steps to left.

Repeat mm. 15–20 to right.

Mm. 21–22: Small running steps to left.

Mm. 23–24: Small running steps to right.

4-beat coda: Step, step, clap-clap-clap.

TECHNOLOGY/MEDIA LINK

MIDI/Sequencing Software Have students use the MIDI song file of *"La mariposa"* to experiment with altering the melody. For example,

• How could the melody be altered to make it major diatonic?

• What effect would this have on the overall sound of the song?

Video Library Show the video *Charango and ensemble* to your students to present a Bolivian *charango* ensemble in performance.

LESSON AT A GLANCE

Element Focus **TIMBRE** Vocal timbres of several cultures

Skill Objective **LISTENING** Describe different vocal timbres

Connection Activity **CULTURE** Explore ways of celebrating cultural diversity

MATERIALS

* "Yü guang guang" — CD 4-15
* "Moonlight Lullaby" — CD 4-16

  Recording Routine: Intro (2 m.); v. 1; interlude (2 m.); v. 2; coda
* **Pronununciation Practice/Translation** p. 520
* *Vocal Styles Around the World* — CD 4-19
* **Resource Book** p. A-10
* selected rhythm instruments

VOCABULARY

timbre   vibrato

◆ ◆ ◆ ◆ National Standards ◆ ◆ ◆ ◆

1c Sing music from diverse cultures
5a Read dotted notes in duple meter
6b Listen and analyze uses of timbre in music from diverse genres
9a Describe characteristics of music styles from a variety of cultures

MORE MUSIC CHOICES

For more experience with listening to different vocal timbres:

"Kelo aba w'ye," p. 290

"Vem kan segla?" p. 417

1 INTRODUCE

Lead a discussion about how we celebrate cultural diversity in the United States. Then use Cultural Connection and Spotlight On below to engage students in activities that celebrate diversity.

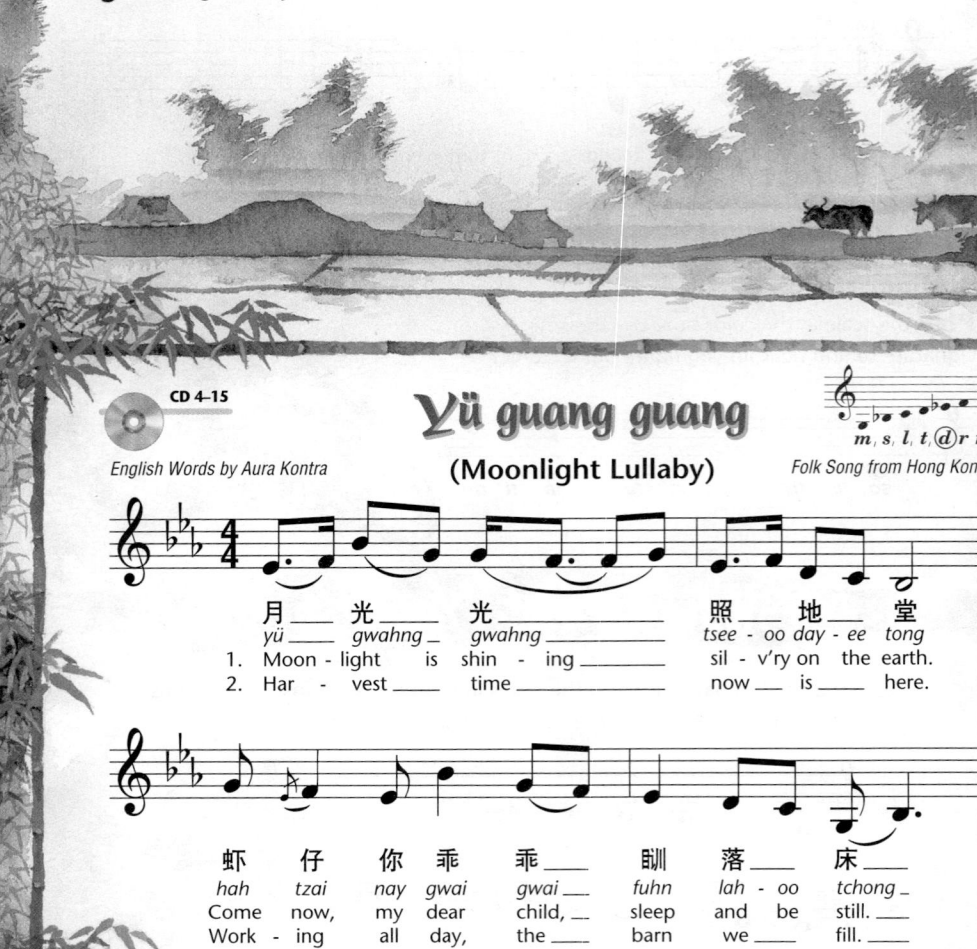

SHADES of SOUND

Timbre is an important part of musical style. People around the world sing in different ways. **Listen** to the vocal timbre of "Yü guang guang," a Cantonese lullaby from Hong Kong. Then **sing** the song. Does your vocal timbre sound the same?

CD 4-15

Yü guang guang
(Moonlight Lullaby)

English Words by Aura Kontra

Folk Song from Hong Kong

月 ___ 光 ___ 光 ___ gwahng ___   照 ___ 地 ___ 堂
yü ___ gwahng ___ gwahng ___   tsee - oo day - ee tong
1. Moon - light   is   shin - ing ___   sil - v'ry on the earth.
2. Har - vest ___   time ___   now ___ is ___ here.

虾 仔 你 乖 乖 ___ 瞓 落 ___ 床
hah tzai nay gwai gwai ___ fuhn lah - oo tchong ___
Come now, my dear child, ___ sleep and be still. ___
Work - ing   all day,   the ___ barn   we ___ fill. ___

60

Footnotes

CULTURAL CONNECTION

▶ **A World Food Fest** Celebrate cultural diversity by hosting an event where students invite their families to a potluck dinner of foods from around the world. Students may wish to share what they have learned about music from different cultures at the dinner. Students can also create a bulletin board, multimedia show, or video about our diverse world.

BUILDING SKILLS THROUGH MUSIC

▶ **Social Studies** Share with students the information in Across the Curriculum on p. 61. Ask students to research Chinese immigration to the United States in the mid-1880s and describe their work and significance to the gold rush and Transcontinental Railroad. Ask them how they contributed to the society, culture, and economy of the western states.

SPOTLIGHT ON

▶ **Diversity** Each individual is unique, with his or her own looks, talents, interests, and tastes. In the same way, individual cultures vary in their customs and lifestyles. Encourage students to discuss individual and cultural differences, such as

artistic expression	clothing	ways of raising children
types of houses	religions	dances
languages	calendars	books

This activity will help students move beyond tolerance to a genuine celebration of diversity.

World Voices

Listen to some of the ways people from around the world use their voices to create unique vocal styles. How would you **describe** each vocal timbre?

CD 4–19
Vocal Styles Around the World

This montage includes these vocal styles: Navajo tribe of the American Southwest, Tuvan people of central Asia, Celtic style of Scotland and Ireland, popular music of Cuba, and African American gospel music.

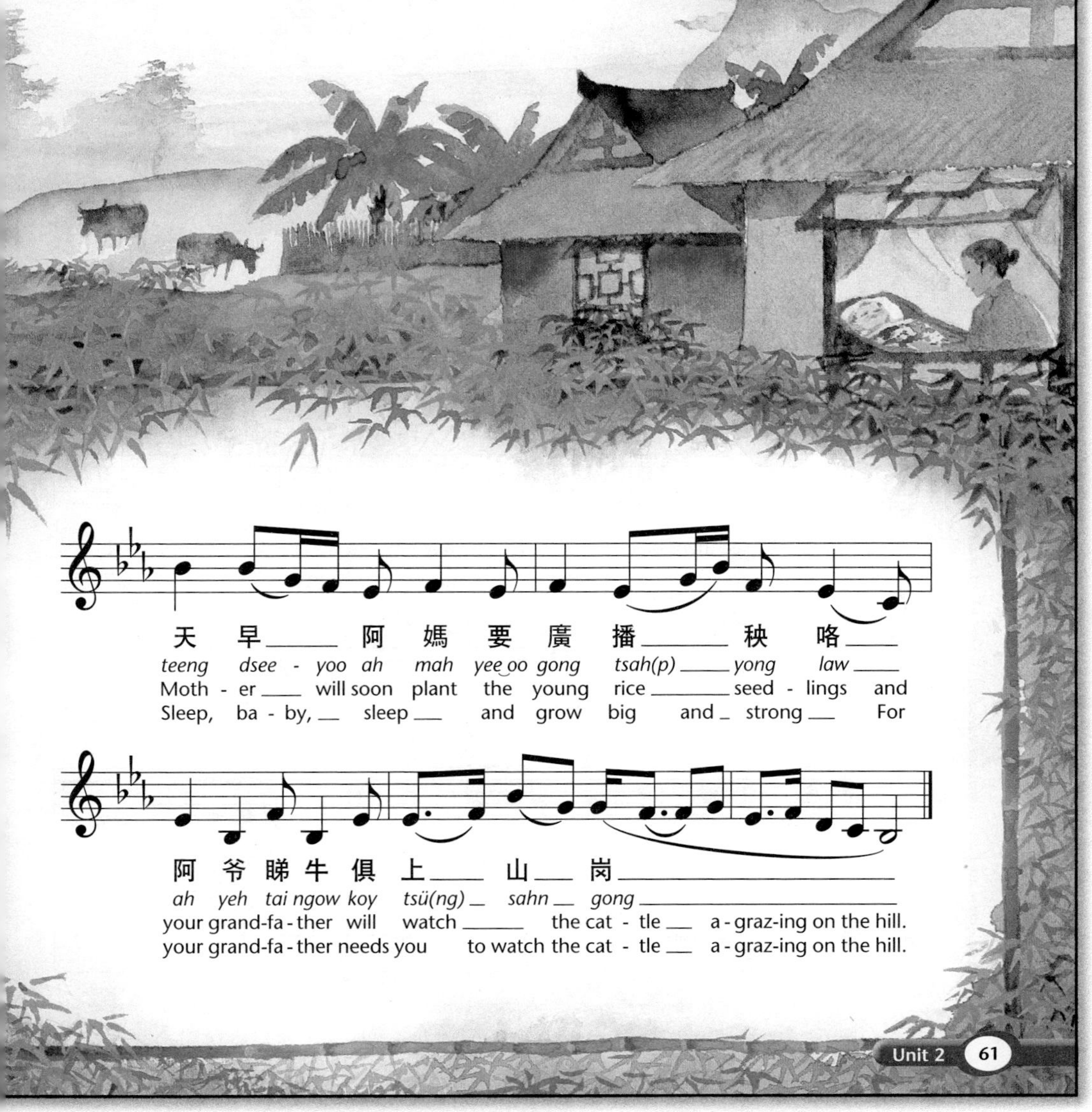

天　早＿＿　阿　媽　要　廣　播＿＿　秧　咯＿＿
teeng　dsee - yoo ah　mah　yee oo gong　tsah(p)＿＿ yong　law＿＿
Moth - er＿＿ will soon plant　the　young　rice＿＿ seed - lings　and
Sleep,　ba - by, ＿ sleep＿＿ and　grow　big　and ＿ strong＿＿ For

阿　爺　睇　牛　俱　上＿＿　山＿　崗＿＿＿＿＿
ah　yeh　tai ngow koy　tsü(ng) ＿　sahn＿　gong＿＿＿＿＿＿
your grand-fa - ther　will　watch＿＿＿ the cat - tle ＿ a - graz-ing on the hill.
your grand-fa - ther needs you　to watch the cat - tle ＿ a - graz-ing on the hill.

2 DEVELOP

Singing

SAY Just as we may learn about new and exciting foods or art from other lands, we can also be open to new vocal timbres.

1c Have students listen to and then sing "Moonlight Lullaby" **CD 4-16.**

6b **ASK How would you describe the timbre of the singers on the recording?** (open-throated, mellow; a "typical" vocal sound in English)

Have students

1c
- Learn the Cantonese words, using the *"Yü guang guang"* Pronunciation Practice Track **CD 4-18** and Resource Book p. A-10.
- Sing the song with the recording **CD 4-15** and individually demonstrate vocal timbre.

ASK How would you describe the vocal timbre of the Cantonese soloist? (nasal, reedy)

Listening

Have students listen to *Vocal Styles Around the World* **CD 4-19** and choose words from the list that describe each timbre in the montage.

Playing

Have students locate the pattern in *"Yü guang guang"* and play the pattern on rhythm instruments.

5a

3 CLOSE

Element: TIMBRE　ASSESSMENT

9a **Music Journal Writing** Have students write brief descriptions of the different vocal timbres heard on *Vocal Styles Around the World* **CD 4-19.** Each description should include at least three terms that describe the characteristics of each vocal timbre.

ACROSS THE CURRICULUM

▶ **Social Studies** Have students locate Guangzhou—the capital of Guangdong province—and Hong Kong on a map. Have them research the first Chinese emigration from the Guangzhou area to the United States to participate in the gold rush (1849) in California. The journey across the Pacific was very difficult, but the terrible famine in the Guangzhou area of China at that time caused many men to be brave enough to try it. Men came to work in the gold fields around Sacramento. Many later sent for their families and settled in San Francisco. There was a Chinese opera house in San Francisco, but it was destroyed by the 1906 earthquake. Many Chinese men also worked on the first transcontinental railroad in the United States in the 1860s.

TECHNOLOGY/MEDIA LINK

Video Library Show the videos *Whitney Houston, Bobby McFerrin, Pam Tillis,* and *Total Experience Gospel Choir* to students to present a variety of vocal timbres.

LESSON AT A GLANCE

Element Focus	**TIMBRE** Vocal timbre	
Skill Objective	**SINGING** Sing and discuss vocal timbres and scat singing	
Connection Activity	**SCIENCE** Explore how the physics of sound (acoustics) determines timbre	

MATERIALS

- "What a Wonderful World" **CD 4-20**
  Recording Routine: Intro (4 m.); vocal; coda
- *What a Wonderful World* (L. Armstrong) **CD 4-22**
- *What a Wonderful World* (E. Cassidy) **CD 4-23**
- *What a Wonderful World* (J. Ramone) **CD 4-24**
- *Hotter Than That* **CD 4-25**
- **Resource Book** p. I-6
- two tape recorders (optional)

VOCABULARY

timbre   tone color   scat singing
glissando   improvisation

◆◆◆◆ National Standards ◆◆◆◆

3b Improvise music from diverse cultures and melodic variations on given melodies
4c Arrange, using electronic media
6b Listen and analyze uses of form and timbre in music from diverse genres
8b Identify ways music relates to science

MORE MUSIC CHOICES

For more experience with different timbres:
"It's Time," p. 274
"Jambalaya," p. 244
For more experience with scat singing:
"Just a Snap-Happy Blues," p. 388
"Scattin' A-Round," p. 160

Musical Colors

Musical performers are often known by the timbre of their instrument or voice.

Louis Armstrong, the great jazz trumpeter and singer, is known for his playing and singing style. **Sing** "What a Wonderful World," a song associated with Armstrong's unique vocal timbre.

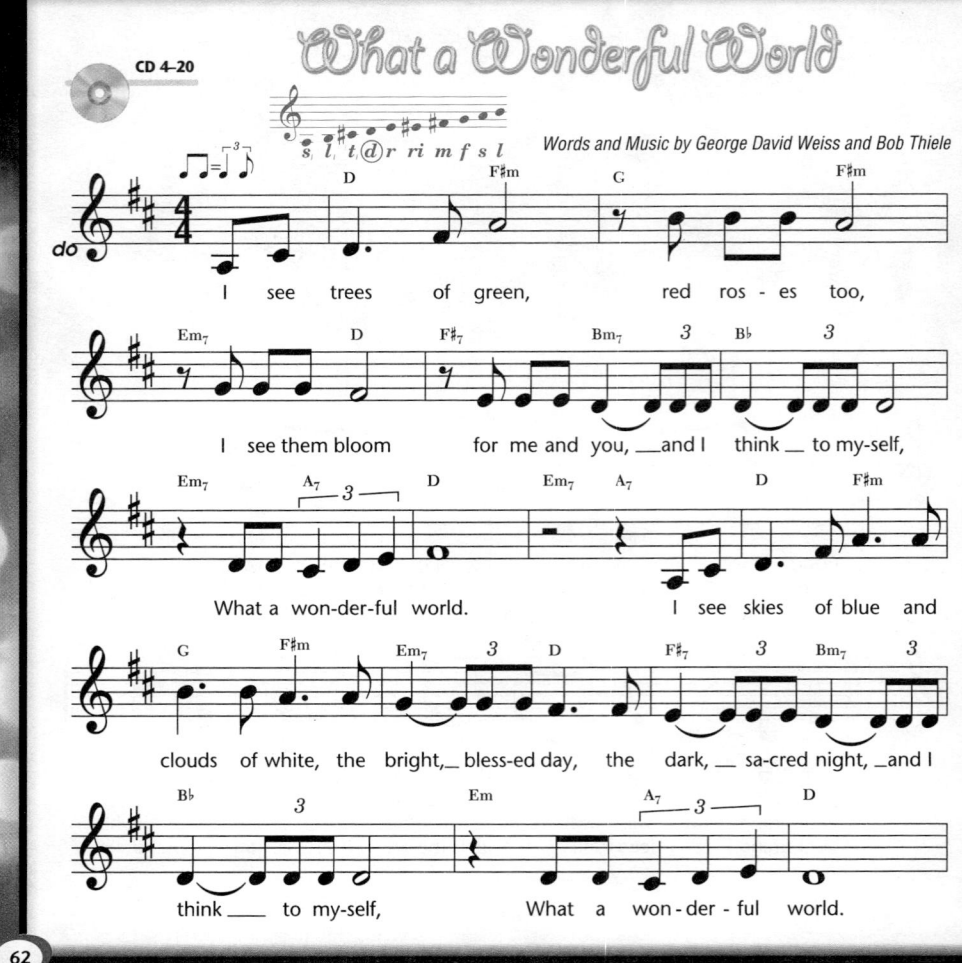

What a Wonderful World

Words and Music by George David Weiss and Bob Thiele

CD 4-20

I see trees of green, red ros-es too,
I see them bloom for me and you, ___and I think ___ to my-self,
What a won-der-ful world. I see skies of blue and
clouds of white, the bright,__ bless-ed day, the dark, ___ sa-cred night, ___and I
think ____ to my-self, What a won-der-ful world.

62

Footnotes

SKILLS REINFORCEMENT

▶ **Recorder** Invite students to learn the D-major scale on recorder and play a countermelody for "What a Wonderful World." These may be found on Resource Book p. I-6.

BUILDING SKILLS THROUGH MUSIC

▶ **Language** After students have listened to *What a Wonderful World* performed by Louis Armstrong, Eva Cassidy, and Joey Ramone, have them write a brief paragraph describing the version that they preferred, using supporting statements for their choice.

ACROSS THE CURRICULUM

8b ▶ **Science** Help students conduct an experiment in acoustics, the science of sound, using digital recording software.

- Digitally record (one at a time) a number of different musical instruments playing the same pitch for ten seconds. Play each sample and ask students to identify the instruments.
- Using your recording software, duplicate each sample. Then cut off the beginnings (*attack*) and endings (*decay*) of each sample. Change the order of the samples.
- Play the new samples of instruments without attacks or decays and ask students to identify the timbres. (This is difficult.)

This experiment shows that we identify instruments not only by their *wave forms*, but by the entire *sound envelope*, which includes the attack, the wave form, and the decay.

Colorful World

Listen to Armstrong's vocal and trumpet timbre. What word best describes his timbre?

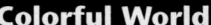

CD 4–22

What a Wonderful World

by George Weiss and Bob Thiele
as performed by Louis Armstrong

What a Wonderful World is considered Armstrong's signature song.

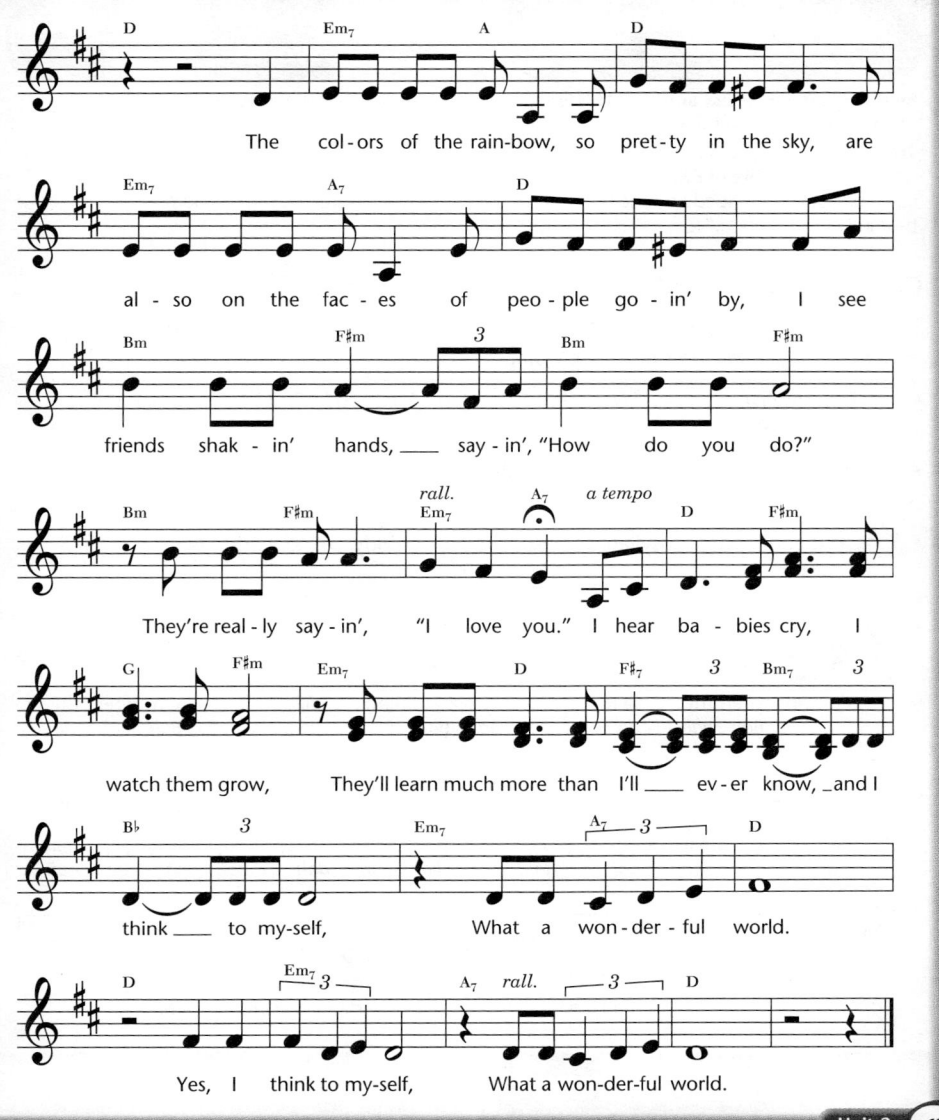

Unit 2 **63**

1 INTRODUCE

ASK When someone telephones you and says "Hi," how do you identify who it is? (You listen for the vocal timbre.)

Tell students that in this lesson they will explore vocal timbre by singing and listening to a classic song by one of the great performers of jazz, and by singing a jazz style called scat singing.

See Across the Curriculum on p. 62 for an experiment with timbre to share with students.

2 DEVELOP

Reading

Have students read the text on p. 62 and then listen to "What a Wonderful World" **CD 4-20** while following the notation.

 ASK What are the four main sections that make up the song? (1: mm. 1–7; 2: mm. 8–15; 3: mm. 16–24; 4: mm. 24–35)

What letters would you use to describe the form? (AABA)

Singing

Invite students to

- Sing the melody of each A section of "What a Wonderful World."
- Sing the B section, observing patterns.
- Sing the entire melody with **CD 4-20.**

Listening

Have students listen to Louis Armstrong singing *What a Wonderful World* **CD 4-22**, paying close attention to his vocal timbre.

 ASK How would you describe the timbre of Armstrong's voice? (raspy, scratchy, noisy, buzzy).

continued on page 64

ACROSS THE CURRICULUM

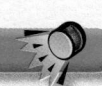

▶ **Related Arts** The song text of "What a Wonderful World" is full of imagery of a variety of beautiful things in life: trees, roses, blue skies, clouds, day, night, rainbows, faces of people, friends shaking hands, babies growing up, and so on. Invite students to form teams and to imagine that they are artists. Assign each team a section of song text to illustrate in color on large poster paper. After the posters are completed they may be used in a performance of the song, in which illustrations are held above students' heads at the appropriate time. For more ideas for illustrating the text of this song, see *What a Wonderful World* by George David Weiss and Bob Thiele (Simon and Schuster Children's, 1995).

SPOTLIGHT ON

▶ **Eva Cassidy** (1963–1996) A once rising young singer and guitarist, Eva Cassidy has been described as "one of the most beautiful voices of her generation," "the voice of an angel," and a "crystalline soprano." Cassidy's album, *Live at Blues Alley*, has posthumously sold over 1 million copies. She was comfortable singing jazz, folk, blues, spirituals, country, and pop. Eva Cassidy died of cancer at the age of 33.

▶ **Joey Ramone** (1951–2001) As lead vocalist of the punk rock band The Ramones, Joey Ramone sang with a unique electric power sound comprising drums, electric guitar, bass, and vocals. The Ramones' music appeared in the 1979 film *Rock 'n' Roll High School*. With 18 albums and over 2,263 performances to their credit, the choice to perform *What a Wonderful World* on his first solo album is a tribute to this classic song. Joey Ramone died of cancer at the age of 49.

Lesson 11 Continued

SAY Now I will play two new performances of *What a Wonderful World.* As you listen, describe the timbre of each performer.

- Play *What a Wonderful World* performed by Eva Cassidy **CD 4-23.**
- Play *What a Wonderful World* performed by Joey Ramone **CD 4-24.**

Discuss with students the differences in vocal timbre among the three performers they have heard singing the song. Ask how vocal timbre and style change the character and mood of the song.

Share with students the information in Spotlight On, p. 63.

Explain to students that the essence of jazz is improvisation—how a singer or player modifies the melody of a piece.

SAY Now we will sing and listen to an example of how vocal and instrumental timbres are used in jazz.

Singing

ASK When a song is sung with nonsense syllables and certain vocal effects are used, what is the style called? (scat)

Have students

- Sing through the regular words of "When the Saints Go Marching In."
- Sing the melody, using the scat syllables.

Creating

Invite students to create and perform their own scat syllables to the melody of "When the Saints Go Marching In."

Listening

Have students listen to Louis Armstrong and the Hot Five play the famous 1927 recording of *Hotter Than That* **CD 4-25.** Share with students the information in Spotlight On below.

Wonderful Timbres, Wonderful Styles

Popular hit songs are often rerecorded by artists using different timbres and styles of music.

Listen to singer Eva Cassidy perform the song *What a Wonderful World.* **Describe** the timbre of her voice.

Then **listen** to rock singer Joey Ramone perform his version of *What a Wonderful World.* Notice how Ramone and the band use a distorted guitar timbre along with **power chords** .

Power chords are chords containing only a root and fifth (no third), often used b... rock guitarists.

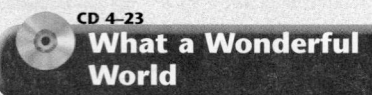
CD 4-23
What a Wonderful World

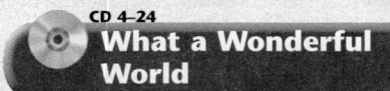
CD 4-24
What a Wonderful World

by George David Weiss and Bob Thiele as performed by Eva Cassidy
This live recording at *Blues Alley* features the smooth vocal timbre of Eva Cassidy, whose voice has been described as "one of the best in her generation."

by George David Weiss and Bob Thiele as performed by Joey Ramone
Joey Ramone was lead singer for the rock band The Ramones. *What a Wonderful World* is from his solo album.

Cool Cat Scat

Try your hand at scat singing, one of Louis Armstrong's trademarks, by following these simple steps:

- **Sing** a familiar song like "When the Saints Go Marching In," using the original words.
- **Sing** the same song in scat style by substituting syllables such as *bah* and *dah* for the words.
- **Create** your own scat syllables to go with the melody.

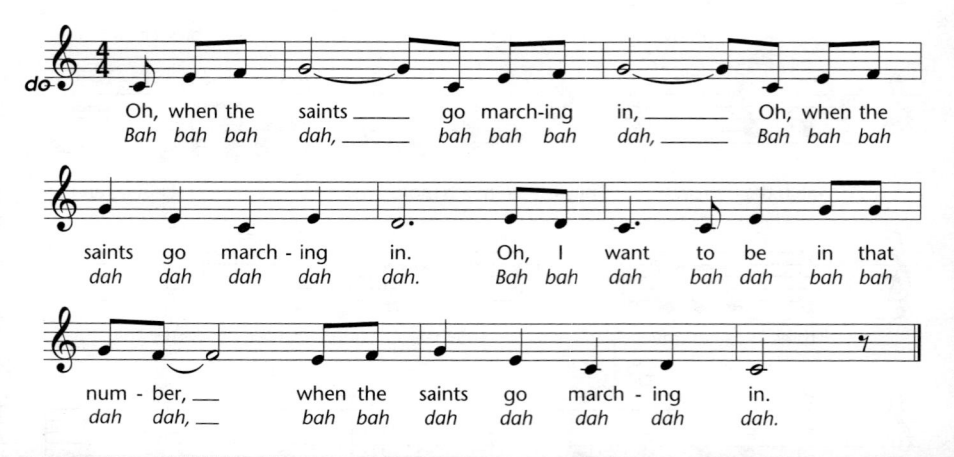

Oh, when the   saints _____ go march-ing in, _____ Oh, when the
Bah bah bah   dah, _____ bah bah bah   dah, _____ Bah bah bah

saints go   march - ing   in.   Oh, I   want   to   be   in that
dah   dah   dah   dah   dah.   Bah bah   dah   bah dah   bah bah

num - ber, ___   when the   saints   go   march - ing   in.
dah   dah, ___   bah bah   dah   dah   dah   dah   dah.

 Footnotes

SPOTLIGHT ON

▶ **Louis Armstrong and the Hot Five** Louis Armstrong's Hot Five and Hot Seven were groups of jazz musicians assembled solely for the purpose of making studio recordings in 1927 and 1928. Featured on *Hotter Than That* are Louis Armstrong (trumpet and vocal), Kid Ory (trombone), Johnny Dodds (clarinet), Lil Hardin Armstrong (piano and composer), Johnny St. Cyr (banjo), and Lonnie Johnson (guitar).

MEETING INDIVIDUAL NEEDS

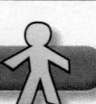

3b ▶ **Including Everyone** Give students opportunities to sing scat and also improvise on instruments. Have all students first practice (by tapping) two or three rhythm patterns that you point to while they sing or hum "When the Saints Go Marching In." Include at least one rhythm that can be performed successfully by most students, including students with disabilities. Each student may then perform (with the group or as a soloist) any of the three rhythms, "improvising" while others sing the song. Create a rhythm section (four or five students with and without disabilities) whose members will perform the three rhythms, as they individually choose, to accompany scat singers (a small group or the entire class).

Encourage students to develop their scat-singing skills by applying these techniques to other songs, such as "Blue Skies," p. 88.

Hot Cat

Listen to Louis Armstrong play *Hotter Than That*. Which instrument has the "buzzy" tone? What techniques do the Dixieland band instruments use to sound "jazzy"?

 CD 4–25
Hotter Than That

**by Lil Hardin Armstrong
as performed by Louis Armstrong
and the Hot Five**

This famous recording from 1927 features Armstrong's spectacular trumpet playing and his trademark "scat singing" solos.

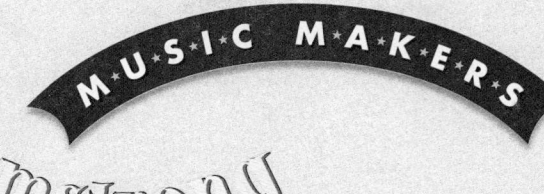
MUSIC MAKERS

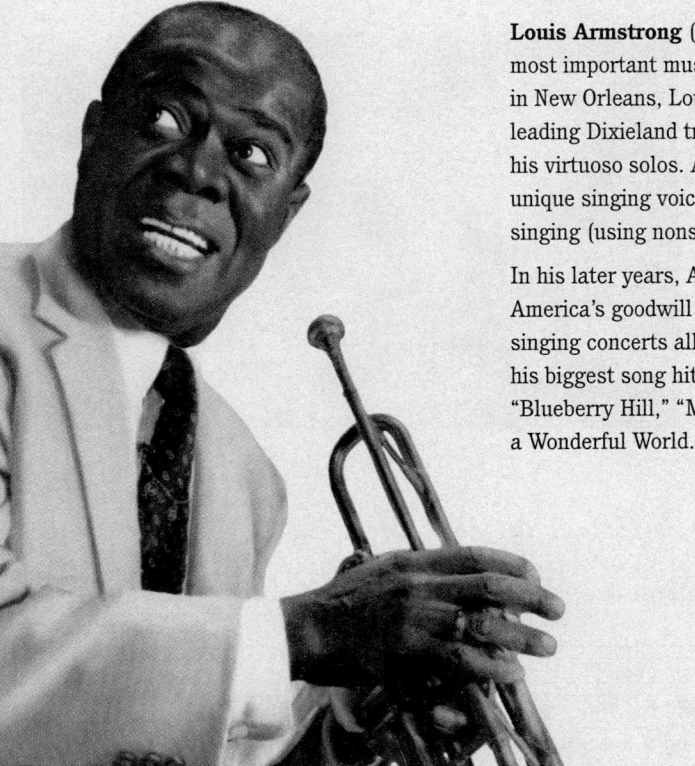
Louis Armstrong

Louis Armstrong (1901–1971) was one of the most important musicians in jazz history. Born in New Orleans, Louisiana, he became the leading Dixieland trumpet player, known for his virtuoso solos. Armstrong also had a unique singing voice, and he popularized scat singing (using nonsense syllables).

In his later years, Armstrong became America's goodwill ambassador, playing and singing concerts all over the world. Some of his biggest song hits were "Hello, Dolly," "Blueberry Hill," "Mack the Knife," and "What a Wonderful World."

Unit 2 **65**

Students may be interested in reading the Music Maker on Louis Armstrong on p. 65. Invite students to discuss the legacy of Louis Armstrong's influence on jazz.

6b **ASK Which instrument had the "buzziest" timbre?** (the muted trombone solo)

Play the recording again and discuss the following with students.

- The use of a guitar in a Dixieland band is highly unusual. The scat singing and guitar dialogue is one of the most interesting parts of this recording.
- The clarinet and trombone solos and their use of *glissando* (smearing) between pitches are true hallmarks of jazz style.

Ask students to describe the musical elements in a Dixieland band that are unique to its style and period. (Timbre: a Dixieland band generally uses the same instruments—clarinet, trumpet, trombone, banjo, piano, bass, and drums; Texture: consists of moving melodic parts; Melody: has a prominent melody; Style: instruments often take solos; clarinet and trombone glissandos.)

3 CLOSE

Element: TIMBRE   ASSESSMENT

Performance/Music Journal Writing Ask students to sing their choice of "What a Wonderful World," or "Cool Cat Scat," and to be aware of their vocal timbre as they sing. Have students write a description of their vocal timbre.

Students may also wish to write a short description of each of the recordings for *What a Wonderful World* performed by Louis Armstrong, Eva Cassidy, and Joey Ramone, comparing the vocal timbre of each performer.

SKILLS REINFORCEMENT

▶ **Listening** Invite students to listen to *Hotter Than That* **CD 4-25,** patting the steady beat. This is difficult to do during some of the improvised solos. Tell students to listen carefully to the drums and bass to hear the steady beat. Challenge students to continue patting as they listen to the scat vocal section where the band stops playing completely.

SCHOOL TO HOME CONNECTION

▶ **Our Wonderful World** Ask students to make a list of ten things that they think make the world wonderful and life beautiful. Invite students to make the list a family project.

TECHNOLOGY/MEDIA LINK

4c **Electronic Keyboard** Have students select an appropriate style for "What a Wonderful World" from the auto-accompaniment bank of a MIDI keyboard. Have a student perform the song accompaniment by playing the chord roots listed in the book while the class sings. (Use A_7 for the introduction.) After several performers have played, have students choose the best arrangement/performance for a concert.

LESSON AT A GLANCE

Element Focus   **TEXTURE/HARMONY** Combining independent melodies

Skill Objective   **LISTENING** Discern when two melodies are performed together to create harmony

Connection Activity   **RELATED ARTS** Describe a fine arts piece

MATERIALS

- "Sing a Song of Peace"   **CD 4-26**
  Recording Routine: Intro (6 m.); vocal (part 1); vocal (part 2); vocal (parts 1 and 2); coda
- "Farandole" from *L'Arlésienne Suite No. 2*   **CD 4-28**
- **Resource Book** p. I-7
- keyboard and other melody instruments

VOCABULARY

quodlibet

◆ ◆ ◆ ◆ National Standards ◆ ◆ ◆ ◆

1b Sing easy pieces with technical accuracy
1d Sing music written in two parts
2c Perform instrumental music from diverse genres
2d Perform simple accompaniments by ear
6a Listen and describe events in music using appropriate terms

MORE MUSIC CHOICES

For more practice with combining independent melodies:
"Angels On the Midnight Clear," p. 423
"Going upon the Mountain," p. 105
Jesu, Joy of Man's Desiring, p. 87

Partners for Peace

Sometimes two songs fit together and can be performed at the same time. Their performance creates harmony.

Part [1] of the song below is "Sing a Song of Peace." Part [2] is "This Is My Country." **Sing** each separately. When you know each well, sing them as partner songs.

Arts Connection

Garden of Eden by Jacob Bouttats (17th century, Flemish). Describe your feelings about this painting. What suggestions can you make for people to live peacefully together? ▶

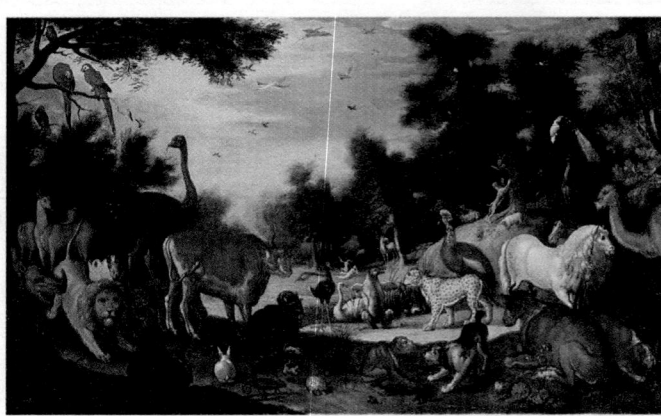

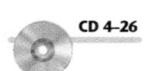 CD 4–26

Sing a Song of Peace

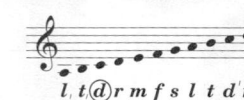

Words by Jill Gallina
"This Is My Country"–Words by Don Raye

Music by Al Jacobs
Arranged by Jill Gallina

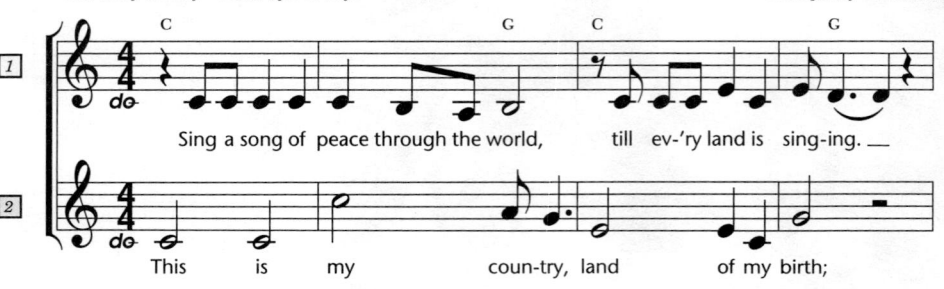

Sing a song of peace through the world,   till ev-'ry land is sing-ing. ___

This   is   my   coun-try, land   of my birth;

 66

Footnotes

ACROSS THE CURRICULUM

▶ **Social Studies** Have students discuss some of the new partnerships that countries are making, or have made in the last few years, to try to achieve a new peace among their neighbors and across the world.

BUILDING SKILLS THROUGH MUSIC

▶ **Math** Invite students to brainstorm all the partner songs that everyone in the class can identify. For each, poll the class members to see how many know each of them. Then, draw and compare different graphical representations (for example, circle graph, chart, table, sentence form) to determine which best represents the data.

TEACHER TO TEACHER

▶ **Tips** The range and melodic movement of part 1 of "Sing a Song of Peace" make this a more accessible choice for those students who may not be secure, confident singers.

CHARACTER EDUCATION

▶ **Peace** Help students consider their role in promoting a peaceful world. Ask them to list peaceful acts they can do each day. Include words and behaviors they can use at home, at school, and in the community to promote peace. Challenge students to select one act they will do consistently over the next few weeks. Have students discuss their progress in incorporating these peaceful acts. Were they able to act this way consistently? How did they feel? Was it difficult or easy?

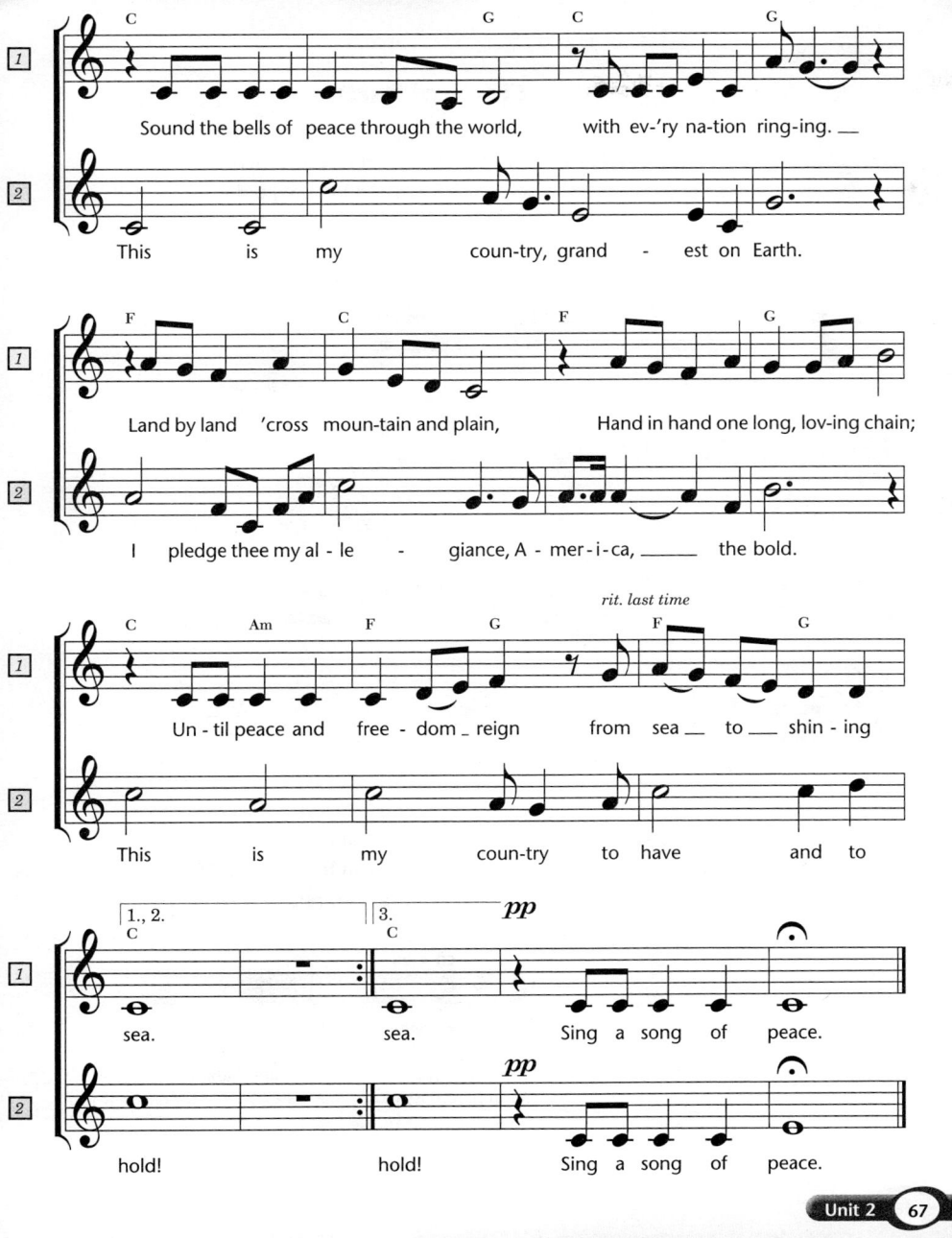

Sound the bells of peace through the world, with ev-'ry na-tion ring-ing. ___

This is my coun-try, grand - est on Earth.

Land by land 'cross moun-tain and plain, Hand in hand one long, lov-ing chain;

I pledge thee my al - le - giance, A - mer-i-ca, _____ the bold.

rit. last time

Un - til peace and free - dom _ reign from sea _ to _ shin - ing

This is my coun-try to have and to

1., 2.   3.   *pp*

sea.   sea.   Sing a song of peace.

pp

hold!   hold!   Sing a song of peace.

1 INTRODUCE

Ask students to relate times when they might have sung partner songs together—at camp, in youth groups, or in school. Invite them to name some of the partner songs that they remember.

2 DEVELOP

Describing

Have students

- Read the information on p. 66.
- Focus their attention on the painting *Garden of Eden* on p. 66 and verbalize their reactions to the painting.

Have students name and describe all of the animals they can find in the painting.

ASK Is it unusual for animals that are natural ene-mies to be peacefully assembled as in this scene? (yes)

How can people live peacefully together? (Answers will vary.)

Listening

Discuss with students the routine of "Sing a Song of Peace" **CD 4-26.** Have them

- Listen to the recording as they follow the music.
- Indicate by raising two fingers when the two melodies are sung together.

Engage students in a discussion of the theme of the song and their view of the theme of *Garden of Eden*.

continued on page 68

▶ **Keyboard** The three primary chords used in "Sing a Song of Peace" can be easily played on keyboard. Encourage students to follow the chord symbols in the music to accompany the song.

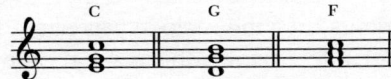

▶ **Movement** Encourage students to create a movement rou-tine for "Sing a Song of Peace" that uses different interpretations for each partner song.

▶ **Recorder** Encourage students to learn the recorder duet for "Sing a Song of Peace" on Resource Book p. I-7.

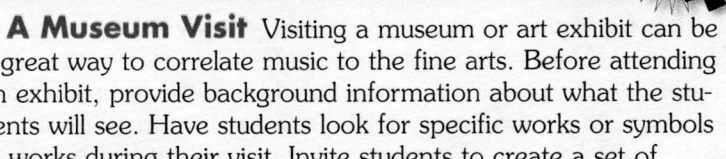

▶ **A Museum Visit** Visiting a museum or art exhibit can be a great way to correlate music to the fine arts. Before attending an exhibit, provide background information about what the stu-dents will see. Have students look for specific works or symbols in works during their visit. Invite students to create a set of behavior guidelines, such as

- Stay with your group and listen to the teacher or the guide.
- Wear comfortable clothes and shoes; leave backpacks at home.
- Don't touch the art. Art can be damaged by oil from hands.
- Discussing, analyzing, deliberating, and talking about art in the museum is encouraged, but be courteous to other viewers by keeping voices low.

Singing

ASK What makes it possible for these two songs to be sung at the same time? (Both songs can be performed with the same accompaniment; they share the same harmony.)

What do we call songs that can be performed at the same time and fit together because they have the same harmony? (partner songs)

SAY Sometimes the melodies for partner songs are intentionally composed to be sung together. In other instances partner songs result when two or more individual, unrelated songs that share the same harmony can be sung together.

Have students

- Sing part 1, "Sing a Song of Peace," with the recording **CD 4-26.**
- Sing part 2, "This Is My Country," with the recording.
- Learn each part thoroughly so as to maintain independence when singing in parts.

Divide the class into two groups. Assign one group to sing part 1 and the second group to sing part 2.

Have students sing "Sing a Song of Peace" as a partner song and then switch parts.

Classical Partners

Classical composers also combine different themes as partners. The French composer Georges Bizet [jorj bee-ZAY] did just that with the two melodies below.

Theme 1

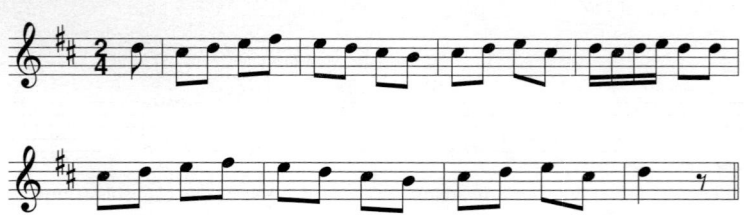

Theme 2

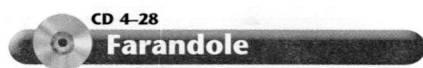

Listen to how the two melodies are used in *Farandole.* As you follow the listening map, locate the themes and the canon.

CD 4–28
Farandole

from *L'Arlésienne Suite No. 2***
by Georges Bizet**

Bizet uses the melody of a well-known Christmas tune and combines it with a second theme that is in sharp contrast to the first.

Footnotes

SPOTLIGHT ON

▶ **The Composer** Both parents of Georges Bizet (1838–1875) were lovers of music. In fact, he first learned about music from his parents, who supported his desire to become a musician. As a young man of 10, he began his formal music study at the Paris Conservatory and composed his first symphony at age 17. Although Bizet composed many compositions, he is best known for his opera *Carmen. Farandole* is one of 27 pieces Bizet composed to go with the play *L'Arlésienne.* The piece has two main themes: an old marchlike song called *"Marche de Turenne,"* which he borrowed from the Provence region of France, and a second theme that is more dancelike. Many people will recognize the first theme as the Christmas carol "The March of the Kings." Bizet died at age 37, just months after the first performance of *Carmen.*

SKILLS REINFORCEMENT

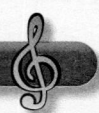

▶ **Playing** The first statement of theme 1 in Bizet's *Farandole* is in the key of D minor, as shown above. When paired with theme 2, the melody is altered and is heard in the parallel key of D major. (The meter is also "adjusted" to fit that of theme 2.) Discuss with students how the melody was altered (see below) and allow volunteers to perform this version on available instruments.

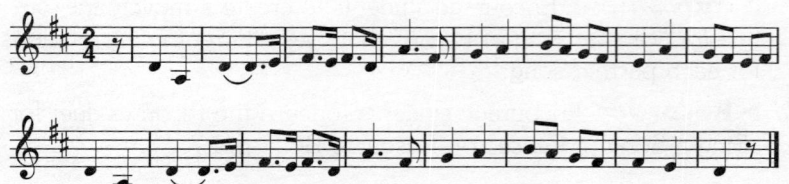

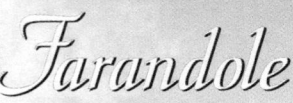

Farandole
LISTENING MAP

Theme 1

Theme 1 in canon

Theme 2

(continues . . .
then Theme 1 fast)

Themes 1 and 2
(2:40)

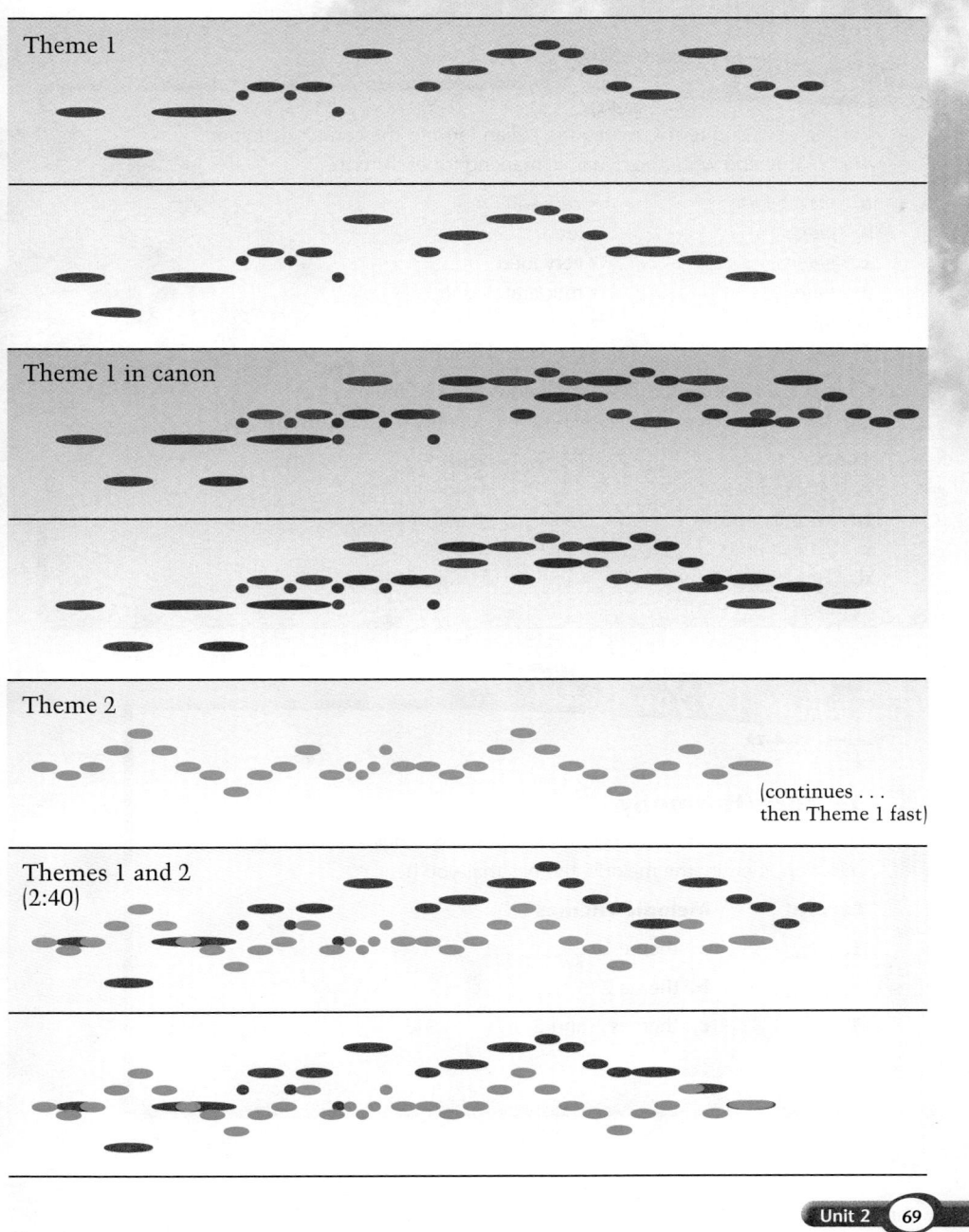

Playing

SAY Partner songs aren't just sung. Composers have been fitting melodies together in instrumental compositions for many years. One such example is *Farandole* from Georges Bizet's *L'Arlésienne Suite No. 2.*

Before students listen to *Farandole,* have them

- Play on a keyboard or other melody instrument each of the two themes from *Farandole,* notated on p. 68.

- Play theme 1 in D major, instead of D minor. (See Skills Reinforcement, p. 68.)

To play the melodies together as a partner song, play the modified theme 1 found in Skills Reinforcement on p. 68 with theme 2 on p. 68 in the student text. The modifications of meter and key to theme 1 assist in partnering the themes.

Singing

Invite students to sing theme 1 and theme 2 on p. 68 using pitch syllables. As they sing, guide students to realize that singing with pitch syllables will reinforce their understanding of major and minor.

Listening

Direct students' attention to the listening map. Play the recording of *Farandole* **CD 4-28** and guide students through the map. (See Technology/Media Link below.)

3 CLOSE

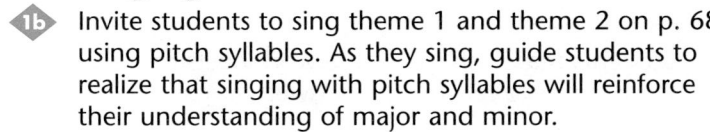
Skill: LISTENING   ASSESSMENT

Music Journal Writing Have students listen to *Farandole* once again and, without consulting the listening map, determine when the two themes are played together. Ask students to describe this effect in their music journals.

ACROSS THE CURRICULUM

▶ **Language Arts** Read aloud *The Day the Earth Was Silent* by Michael McGuffee (Inquiring Voice, 1996). This book describes how students can work together to change their world for the better. Invite students to create their own class book about peace and good will. As they do so, arrange for several adults to ask them, "Why are you trying?" and encourage students to articulate their views. Study people who have made a difference in achieving peace. *The Peace Seekers: The Nobel Peace Prize* by Nathan Aaseng (Lerner Pub., 1991) is a great resource for this.

SCHOOL TO HOME CONNECTION

▶ **Need for Peace** Students may or may not be aware of events and places in the world where conflicts, wars, and disagreements dominate the news. Ask students to follow the news media to determine where peace is needed. Is peace needed in situations within our own neighborhoods, schools, towns, and cities?

TECHNOLOGY/MEDIA LINK

Transparency Display the listening map transparency for *Farandole* as you play the recording. You may wish to point to each section of the piece on the first listening to help students follow along. On subsequent listenings, invite a student to point to the sections as the recording is played.

WHAT DO YOU KNOW?

MATERIALS
• **Resource Book** p. B-7

Review dynamic and expression markings found on p. 38. Then, have students read and answer the questions on p. 70 independently and check their answers with a partner before sharing answers with the rest of the class.

Review the song notation listed in What Do You Know? 2 for scale type and *do.* Then, have students identify the type of scale and pitch name for *do* for those selections on p. 70.

Students may wish to use the worksheets on Resource Book p. B-7 to record their answers.

WHAT DO YOU HEAR?

MATERIALS	
• *What Do You Hear?* 2A	**CD 4-29 to 4-34**
• *What Do You Hear?* 2B	**CD 4-35, 36**
• **Resource Book** pp. B-7, B-8	

Review the concepts of texture/harmony on pp. 66–69. Then, have students listen to the recording of *Farandole* (What Do You Hear? 2A) **CD 4-29 to 4-34.** Have students indicate the melodies they hear for each selection, using the worksheet on Resource Book p. B-7.

Review the concept of timbre on pp. 62–65. Then play the recordings of "What a Wonderful World" (What Do You Hear? 2B) **CD 4-35, 36.** Ask students to describe the vocal and instrumental timbres in the recordings by choosing appropriate words from the list on p. 71, using the worksheet on Resource Book p. B-8.

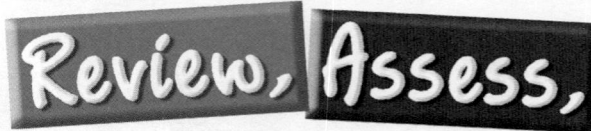
What Do You Know?

1. For the following terms, match the Italian term to the correct definition. Then name and write the dynamic marking for each term.

a. *mezzo forte*	• very soft	
b. *piano*	• loud	
c. *pianissimo*	• very loud	
d. *forte*	• moderately soft	
e. *mezzo piano*	• soft	
f. *fortissimo*	• moderately loud	

2. Look at the notation for the songs below. Point to the name of the scale on which each melody is based. Identify *do* in each song.

Song	Page	Scale	Do
a. "Adiós, amigos"	57	Major or Minor	____
b. "El cóndor pasa"	46	Major or Minor	____
c. "La mariposa"	58	Major or Minor	____
d. "Farewell to Tarwathie"	43	Major or Minor	____

What Do You Hear? 2A

 CD 4–29

Texture/Harmony

Listen to the two melodic themes of Bizet's *Farandole* on page 68. For each selection, identify the melodic themes that you hear.

Excerpt	Melodic Themes
1. _____	**a.** theme 1
2. _____	**b.** theme 2
3. _____	**c.** themes 1 and 2
4. _____	

Footnotes

ANSWER KEY

▶ What Do You Know?

1. Dynamic Term	Definition	Symbol
a. *mezzo forte*	moderately loud	*mf*
b. *piano*	soft	*p*
c. *pianissimo*	very soft	*pp*
d. *forte*	loud	*f*
e. *mezzo piano*	moderately soft	*mp*
f. *fortissimo*	very loud	*ff*

▶ What Do You Know?

2. Song	Scale	Do
a. "Adiós, amigos"	Major (F)	*do* = F
b. "El cóndor pasa"	Minor (A)	*do* = C
c. "La mariposa"	Minor (B)	*do* = D
d. "Farewell to Tarwathie"	Major (G)	*do* = G

▶ What Do You Hear? 2A

1. a. theme 1 (in minor)

2. c. themes 1 and 2

3. a. theme 1 (in canon)

4. b. theme 2

Perform, Create

What Do You Hear? 2B

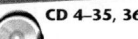
CD 4–35, 36

Timbre

Listen to two recordings of *What a Wonderful World.* As you listen, identify the words that describe the timbres of the voices and instruments on the recordings.

Excerpt	Timbre	
1. ____	**a.** smooth violins	**e.** buzzy voice
2. ____	**b.** piano	**f.** mellow drums
	c. trumpet	**g.** clear voice
	d. soft guitar	**h.** children's voices

What You Can Do

Move to Show Form

Analyze and describe the form of "*El cóndor pasa,*" page 46. Create two movements (**a** and **b**) that go with the song. Perform each movement with the corresponding section of the song.

Read and Play Rhythms in 3

Follow the notation of "Farewell to Tarwathie," page 43, and conduct the beat in 3. Play the rhythms in the song on a nonpitched rhythm instrument. Create new rhythms in 3 that can be performed with the song.

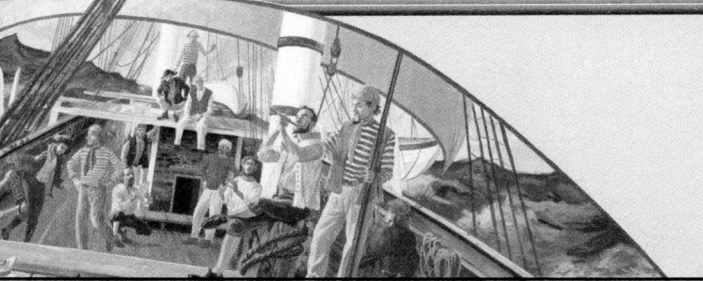

WHAT YOU CAN DO

MATERIALS	
• "*El cóndor pasa,*" p. 46	**CD 3-16**
• "Farewell to Tarwathie," p. 43	**CD 3-1**
• **Resource Book** p. B-8	
• nonpitched percussion instruments	

Move to Show Form

Invite students to listen to "*El cóndor pasa*" **CD 3-16** as they follow the notation on p. 43. Have them work in groups to write the phrase form using letters (aabb). Students may then create movements for "*El cóndor pasa.*" Tell them that contrasting phrases should have contrasting patterns of movement.

Read and Play Rhythms in Three

Play the recording of "Farewell to Tarwathie," p. 43, **CD 3-1** while students conduct in meter in 3. Then, have them first play the song rhythms on nonpitched percussion instruments. Finally, have students develop a rhythmic ostinato in 3 that they can perform with the song, using the worksheet on Resource Book p. B-8.

▶ **What Do You Hear? 2B**

1. a. smooth violins
  f. mellow drums
  g. clear voice(s)
  h. children's voices
2. b. piano
  d. soft guitar
  e. buzzy voice
  f. mellow drums

The word that best describes the timbre of Louis Armstrong's voice is *buzzy.*

▶ **What You Can Do**

Move to Show Form: The form for "*El cóndor pasa*" is aaba.

TECHNOLOGY/MEDIA LINK

▶ Rubrics

Visit *www.sfsuccessnet.com* for rubrics to assess students' achievement in music skills.

Lesson	Elements	Skills	

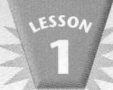

LESSON 1

CORE
Dynamics Bring Music to Life
pp. 76–79

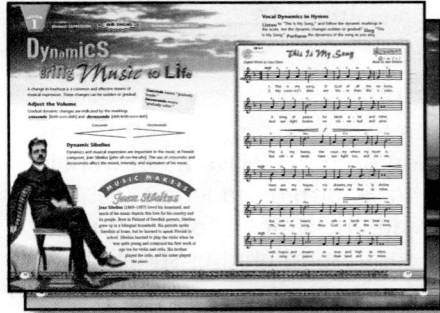

Element: Expression
Concept: Dynamics
Focus: Dynamic changes

Secondary Element
Melody: minor tonality

National Standards
1b 2a 4a 5c 6b

Skill: Singing
Objective: Sing two songs with dynamic changes

Secondary Skills
- **Listening** Listen to a song, paying particular attention to dynamics
- **Analyzing** Discuss the meaning of lyrics
- **Singing** Sing a song while performing dynamics correctly
- **Moving** Create a movement routine to accompany a piece of music
- **Creating** Create and perform a short rhythmic composition with dynamic changes

SKILLS REINFORCEMENT
- **Vocal Development** Gain control of performing crescendos and decrescendos; sing vocalises in minor
- **Recorder** Learn recorder countermelodies for a song

LESSON 2

CORE
Playing for Time
pp. 80–81

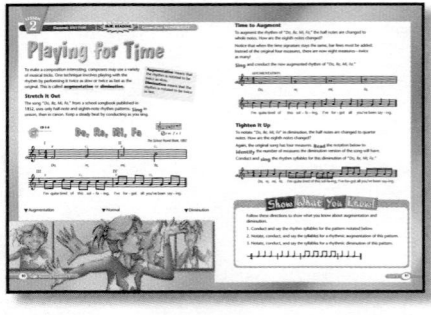 

Reading Sequence 9, p. 492

Element: Rhythm
Concept: Duration
Focus: Augmentation and diminution

Secondary Element
Form: abc

National Standards:
1d 5a 6c 8b

Skill: Reading
Objective: Read augmented and diminished song rhythms

Secondary Skills
- **Analyzing** Analyze and understand the nature of augmentation and diminution; analyze note values of augmented and diminished rhythms
- **Singing** Sing a diminished rhythm
- **Moving** Perform a movement routine for a song

SKILLS REINFORCEMENT
- **Recorder** Play a recorder ostinato with a song

LESSON 3

Joyful Rhythms
pp. 82–83

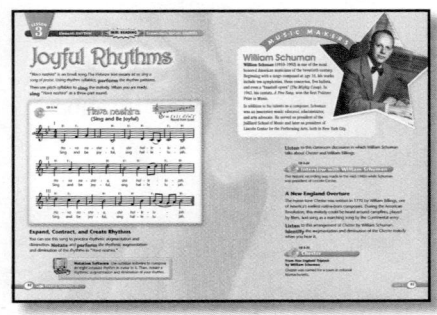

Reading Sequence 10, p. 492

Element: Rhythm
Concept: Duration
Focus: Augmentation and diminution

Secondary Element
Form: abc

National Standards:
1c 1d 5a 5b 6c

Skill: Reading
Objective: Read augmented and diminished song rhythms

Secondary Skills
- **Moving** Perform a movement routine for a song
- **Analyzing** Analyze and understand the nature of augmentation and diminution
- **Conducting** Conduct a quarter note beat
- **Singing** Sing a song in a round, in augmentation and in diminution
- **Listening** Listen to a piece of music and physically demonstrate the points of augmentation and diminution

SKILLS REINFORCEMENT
- **Singing** Play an ostinato on resonator bells
- **Reading** Practice with augmentation and diminution

Connections

Music and Other Literature

Connection: Science

Activity: Discuss how loud and quiet sounds relate to near and far sound sources

SPOTLIGHT ON
Jean Sibelius Facts on the composer Jean Sibelius
Kerenski Facts about the dance and music

ACROSS THE CURRICULUM Science Discover how the concept of near and far is related to dynamic changes

CULTURAL CONNECTION Finland Discover facts about Finland

CHARACTER EDUCATION Peace Encourage peace

MEETING INDIVIDUAL NEEDS English Language Learners Practice pronouncing song lyrics

SCHOOL TO HOME CONNECTION Ancestry Discuss folk music with family

BUILDING SKILLS THROUGH MUSIC Reading Infer with context clues

Songs
"This is My Song"
"I Walk the Unfrequented Road"

Listening Selections
Finlandia (excerpt)
Kerenski

M•U•S•I•C M•A•K•E•R•S
Jean Sibelius

More Music Choices
"A Brand New Day," p. 7
"Run! Run! Hide!" p. 340
"Summertime," p. 250

ASSESSMENT

Performance/Observation
Sing a song while observing dynamic markings

TECHNOLOGY/MEDIA LINK

Web Site Research folk music from Finland and elsewhere in Scandinavia

---

Connection: Mathematics

Activity: Explore multiplication and division with time

ACROSS THE CURRICULUM Math Discuss how math operations relate to augmentation and diminution of meter

MOVEMENT Locomotor Movement Move in canon with this activity

BUILDING SKILLS THROUGH MUSIC Math Work with augmentation

Song *"Do, Re, Mi, Fa"*

More Music Choices
"Dance for the Nations," p. 122
"Hava nashira," p. 82

ASSESSMENT

Performance/Observation
Read and sing a song in the original, augmented, and diminished versions while softly patting the steady beat

TECHNOLOGY/MEDIA LINK

Notation Software
Notate augmented and diminished rhythms

Connection: Social Studies

Activity: Discover historical facts on the music of Israel

MOVEMENT *"Hava nashira"* Learn the *"Hava nashira"* dance movements

SPOTLIGHT ON The Music Sight read a melody and listen to an interview with composer William Schuman

SCHOOL TO HOME CONNECTION Interview Have students ask adults to find a choral connection in their lives

BUILDING SKILLS THROUGH MUSIC Reading Recall information from text

Song *"Hava nashira"* ("Sing and Be Joyful")

Listening Selections
"Chester," from *New England Triptych*
Interview with William Schuman
M•U•S•I•C M•A•K•E•R•S
William Schuman

More Music Choices
"Scattin' A-Round," p. 160
"Do, Re, Mi, Fa," p. 80

ASSESSMENT

Performance/Observation
Read and sing a song in the original, augmented, and diminished versions while softly patting the steady beat

TECHNOLOGY/MEDIA LINK

Web Site Research the life and work of composer William Schuman and discover facts about Israel

Lesson	Elements	Skills	
LESSON 4 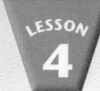 **Backbeat Rhythm** pp. 84–85 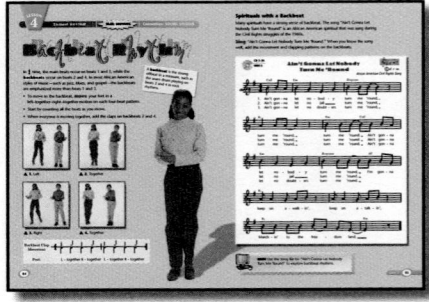	**Element: Rhythm** **Concept:** Beat **Focus:** Backbeat **Secondary Element** Texture: countermelody **National Standards:** 1c 1d 7a 8b 9a	**Skill: Moving** **Objective:** Move to and clap the backbeat of a song **Secondary Skills** • **Moving** Familiarize students with the backbeat through movement • **Singing** Sing a song while moving to the beat • **Listening** Identify the backbeat in music recordings • **Creating** Create new verses	**SKILLS REINFORCEMENT** • **Singing** Sing a song in harmony in thirds • **Recorder** Play a countermelody with a song • **Signing** Learn sign language for a song
LESSON 5 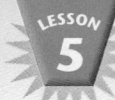 **CORE** **Musical Bridges** pp. 86–87 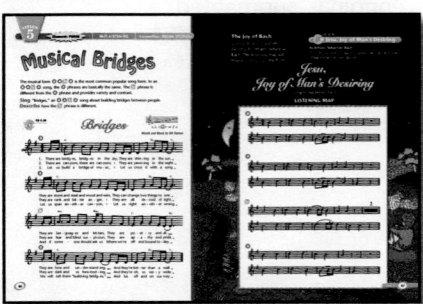 	**Element: Form** **Concept:** aaba/AABA **Focus:** aaba and AABA form **Secondary Element** Texture: countermelody **National Standards:** 2d 6c 8b 9b	**Skill: Listening** **Objective:** Listen to and identify aaba (phrases) and AABA (sections) form **Secondary Skills** • **Analyzing** Identify similar phrases in a song • **Singing** Sing a song and identify the contrasting section • **Playing** Accompany a song on a chordal instrument • **Listening** Listen for the aaba and the AABA form	**SKILLS REINFORCEMENT** • **Recorder** Play the alto and soprano recorder countermelodies for a song
LESSON 6 **Sing a Standard** pp. 88–89 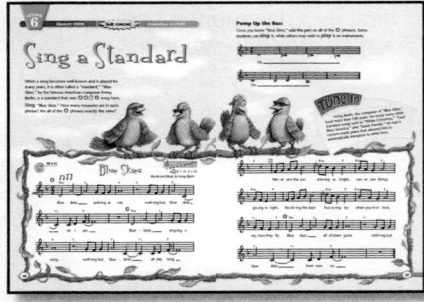 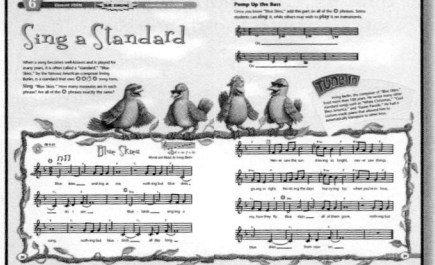	**Element: Form** **Concept:** aaba **Focus:** aaba form **Secondary Element** Melody: accidentals **National Standards** 1a 2d 6a 8b	**Skill: Singing** **Objective:** Sing a song in aaba song form **Secondary Skills** • **Analyzing** Identify the phrases in a song • **Singing** Sing a song with a chromatic line • **Playing** Play the chromatic line on an instrument while the class sings	**SKILLS REINFORCEMENT** • **Recorder** Play a recorder part for a song • **Keyboard** Play a keyboard countermelody during a song

Connections

Music and Other Literature

Connection: Social Studies
Activity: Discuss the role of music in the American Civil Rights movement

- SPOTLIGHT ON **Civil Rights Songs** Facts about songs of the civil rights movement
- CHARACTER EDUCATION **Commitment** Have students think about commitments they make and how they effect their lives
- BUILDING SKILLS THROUGH MUSIC **Language** Paraphrase lyrics

Song "Ain't Gonna Let Nobody Turn Me 'Round"

More Music Choices
"A Brand New Day," p. 7
"Lean On Me," p. 14

ASSESSMENT

Performance/Self-Assessment Rate one's own ability to perform a movement pattern and clap a backbeat while singing

TECHNOLOGY/MEDIA LINK
MIDI/Sequencing Software Record a new percussion track using the sequencing software

---

Connection: Social Studies
Activity: Discuss current social issues as conveyed by lyrics of a song

- ACROSS THE CURRICULUM **Social Studies** Read about and discuss stories of world peace and social justice
- SPOTLIGHT ON **The Composer** Facts of Johann Sebastian Bach
- BUILDING SKILLS THROUGH MUSIC **Language** Recognize metaphors in lyrics

Song "Bridges"

Listening Selections
Jesu, Joy of Man's Desiring
Listening Map: *Jesu, Joy of Man's Desiring*

More Music Choices
"Everybody Loves Saturday Night," p. 296
"What a Wonderful World," p. 62

ASSESSMENT

Performance/Observation Create and perform a rhythmic composition in aaba or AABA form

TECHNOLOGY/MEDIA LINK
Notation Software Notate a song and discuss the importance of repetition in music composition
Transparency Display the listening map for *Jesu, Joy of Man's Desiring*

Connection: Culture
Activity: Relate a standard pop song to the decade of its origin in the United States

- CULTURAL CONNECTION **The Roaring Twenties** Explore facts about American culture in the 1920s
- SPOTLIGHT ON **The Composer** Facts about Irving Berlin
- SCHOOL TO HOME CONNECTION **Conducting a Survey** Talk to friends and relatives about Irving Berlin
- BUILDING SKILLS THROUGH MUSIC **Math** Create a graph or table

Song "Blue Skies"

More Music Choices
"I Got Rhythm," p. 101
"What a Wonderful World," p. 62

ASSESSMENT

Performance/Observation Sing a song in aaba form, with good vocal quality, while following the notation

TECHNOLOGY/MEDIA LINK
Multimedia Create a slide show to visually represent a song

Lesson	Elements	Skills

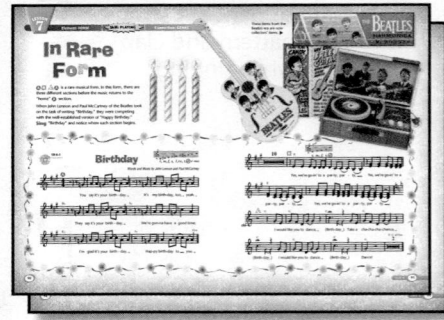

LESSON 7
In Rare Form
pp. 90–93

Element: Form
Concept: ABCA
Focus: ABCA form

Secondary Element
Melody: motive

National Standards:
2d 3c 5c 6b 7a 9b

Skill: Playing
Objective: Play 12-bar blues bass lines and a boogie-woogie bass line

Secondary Skills
- **Analyzing** Identify the sections of a song
- **Notating** Write and play triads and chords
- **Singing** Have students sing a bass line and melody simultaneously
- **Listening** Listen to boogie-woogie bass
- **Creating** Improvise a guitar or bass guitar line

SKILLS REINFORCEMENT
- **Singing** Identify notes that outline a major triad while singing a song
- **Keyboard** Have students learn an accompaniment using roots and thirds; use proper fingerings to play a bass line

---

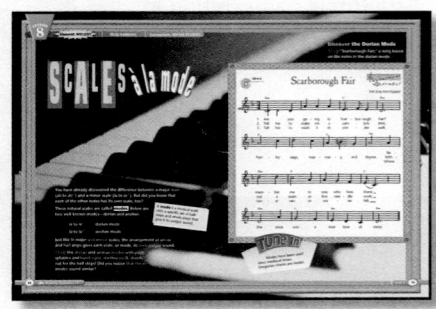

LESSON 8
Scales à la Mode
pp. 94–95

Reading Sequence 11, p. 493

Element: Melody
Concept: Tonality
Focus: Dorian and Aeolian modes

Secondary Element
Form: introduction

National Standards:
2a 3a 5b 5c 8b

Skill: Reading
Objective: Read and sing from notation a song in dorian mode

Secondary Skills
- **Reading** Introduce the word *mode;* Identify the key signature of a song
- **Listening** Identify the type of mode in a recording
- **Singing** Have students sing a dorian mode tone ladder with pitch syllables

SKILLS REINFORCEMENT
- **Creating** Create a four-measure introduction/interlude
- **Reading** Use pitch syllables and hand signs for various modes
- **Keyboard** Learn a "strumming" keyboard accompaniment

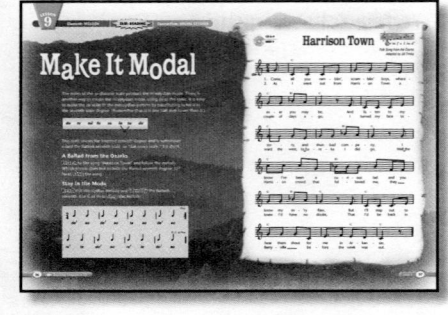

LESSON 9
CORE
Make It Modal
pp. 96–97

Reading Sequence 12, p. 493

Element: Melody
Concept: Tonality
Focus: Mixolydian mode

Secondary Element
Rhythm: $\frac{2}{4}$ meter

National Standards:
1a 4c 5a 5c 6a

Skill: Singing
Objective: Sing a song in mixolydian mode

Secondary Skills
- **Listening** Identify and sing in Ionian and mixolydian modes
- **Singing** Sing a mixolydian melody using pitch syllables

SKILLS REINFORCEMENT
- **Reading** Sign scales using hand signs and pitch syllables
- **Recorder** Play an alto recorder countermelody

Connections

Music and Other Literature

Connection: Genre

Activity: Apply knowledge of 12-bar blues to boogie-woogie game

TEACHER TO TEACHER **Celebrating Birthdays** Create a class birthday book and share family birthday traditions

SPOTLIGHT ON
The Musicians Read about Beatles memorabilia and trivia
The Performers Facts about Tommy and Jimmy Dorsey

SCHOOL TO HOME CONNECTION **Beatles Memorabilia** Have students explore their houses for Beatles memorabilia

CULTURAL CONNECTION
Pop Culture Research musical pop culture terms in use today

BUILDING SKILLS THROUGH MUSIC **Writing** Write verses of music

---

Song "Birthday"

Listening Selection *Boogie-Woogie*

More Music Choices
"Downtown," p. 258
"Surfin' U.S.A.," p. 260
"Key to the Highway," p. 243
"Sun Gonna Shine," p. 242

ASSESSMENT

Performance/Peer Critique Play 12-bar blues lines

TECHNOLOGY/MEDIA LINK
CD-ROM Create a blues or boogie-woogie accompaniment using *Band-in-a-Box*
Web Site Research the Beatles and their music

Connection: Social Studies

Activity: Discuss the black plague as the context for a ballad

ACROSS THE CURRICULUM **Social Studies** Explore facts about the black plague

TEACHER TO TEACHER **Tone Ladders** Write out the tone set for a song and identify the harmonic minor

BUILDING SKILLS THROUGH MUSIC **Math** Use logic to come to a conclusion

---

Song "Scarborough Fair"

More Music Choices
"Greensleeves" (melodic minor), p. 49
"Sometimes I Feel Like a Motherless Child" (harmonic minor), p. 241

ASSESSMENT

Performance/Observation Have students read a song from notation and observe their ability to sing in dorian mode

TECHNOLOGY/MEDIA LINK
Multimedia Create a slide show and display it as the class sings a ballad

---

Connection: Social Studies

Activity: Discuss the Ozarks region of the United States

SPOTLIGHT ON **The Ozark Mountains** Facts about the Ozarks and the people who live there

TEACHER TO TEACHER **Tone Ladders** Identify flatted tones in a tone ladder

BUILDING SKILLS THROUGH MUSIC **Social Studies** Discuss natural resources

---

Song "Harrison Town"

More Music Choices "Goin' to Boston," p. 433

ASSESSMENT

Performance/Observation Sing and change pitches to demonstrate understanding of the difference between the Ionian and mixolydian modes

TECHNOLOGY/MEDIA LINK
MIDI/Sequencing Software Alter the melody pitches of a song file to reflect Ionian, aeolian, and dorian modes

Lesson	Elements	Skills	

LESSON 10 — Melodic Motives
pp. 98–101

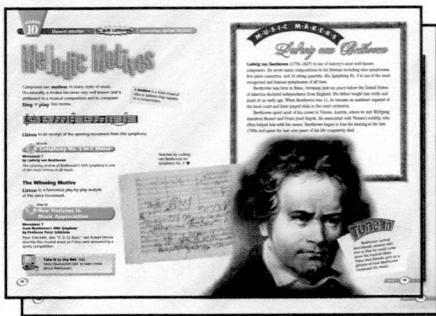

Element: Melody
Concept: Pattern
Focus: Melodic Motives

Secondary Element
Rhythm: syncopation

National Standards:
1a 2b 3b 6b 6c 8b

Skill: Listening
Objective: Aurally identify a melodic motive and its transposition

Secondary Skills
- **Listening** Listen to a symphony and identify motives; discuss harmonic treatment of motives and themes
- **Singing** Sing a song while clapping the half-note beat
- **Analyzing** Identify a motive in a song
- **Playing** Improvise on a motive

SKILLS REINFORCEMENT
- **Analyzing** Play a motive and its treatments on a melodic instrument
- **Keyboard** Play eighth-note subdivisions of a melody

LESSON 11 — CORE
Sounds of Strings
pp. 102–103

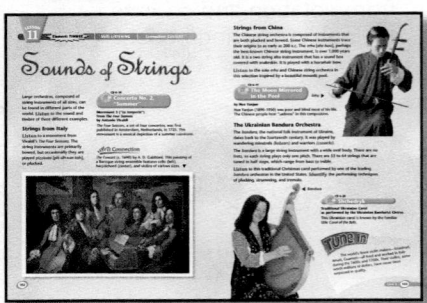

Element: Timbre
Concept: Instrumental
Focus: String instruments

Secondary Element
Expression: articulation

National Standards:
4c 6b 9a

Skill: Listening
Objective: Listen to recordings of string orchestras from different cultures and compare the tone qualities and playing techniques

Secondary Skills
- **Listening** Listen to different timbres offered by different instruments in the same family

SKILLS REINFORCEMENT
- **Listening** Identify string instruments and playing techniques in recordings
- **Sound Bank** Have students listen to various stringed instruments

---

LESSON 12 — CORE
Melody/Countermelody
pp. 104–107

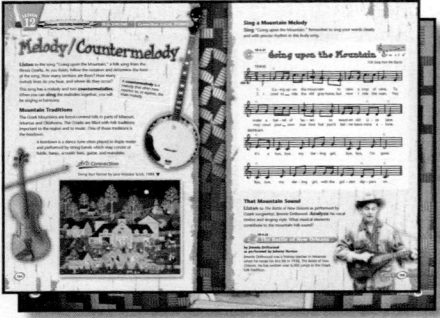

Element: Texture/Harmony
Concept: Texture
Focus: Countermelodies

Secondary Element Form: verse/refrain, coda

National Standards:
1d 2a 2c 5a 5b 8b

Skill: Singing
Objective: Sing a song with melody and countermelody

Secondary Skills
- **Playing** Clap a rhythmic pattern to accompany a song; perform in an ensemble
- **Listening** Listen to a folk song and describe the instruments
- **Analyzing** Read the notation of a song while listening to it and follow the countermelodies
- **Reading** Read and perform rhythms and melodies using rhythms and pitch syllables
- **Singing** Sing a song with and without countermelodies to discover harmony and texture
- **Moving** Perform a hoedown dance

SKILLS REINFORCEMENT
- **Keyboard** Practice a five finger position tune
- **Recorder** Learn and perform two countermelodies
- **Analyzing Mallet Parts** Analyze mallet parts for the refrain of a song

Connections

Music and Other Literature

Connection: Social Studies

Activity: Discuss the mood of the time of the American and French revolutions

ACROSS THE CURRICULUM
Social Studies/Drama Write a short play about Ludwig van Beethoven

SPOTLIGHT ON The "Musicalologist" Facts on Peter Schickele

TEACHER TO TEACHER **Character Motives** Have students learn that music is often connected to characters and actions of a movie

MEETING INDIVIDUAL NEEDS **Including Everyone** Practice singing a motive and its retrograde in pairs

CULTURAL CONNECTION Jazz and Jewish Folk Song Influences on George Gershwin's musical style

BUILDING SKILLS THROUGH MUSIC Language Set up a timeline

Song "I Got Rhythm"

Listening Selections
Symphony No. 5 in C Minor, Movement 1 (excerpt)
New Horizons in Music Appreciation, Movement 1 (excerpt)
M·U·S·I·C M·A·K·E·R·S
Ludwig van Beethoven

More Music Choices
"Peace Like a River," p. 190
"Gonna Build a Mountain," p. 21
"Ain't Gonna Let Nobody Turn Me 'Round," p. 85
"Birthday," p. 90

ASSESSMENT
Written Assessment Identify a motive and its permutations while listening to a recording

TECHNOLOGY/MEDIA LINK
CD-ROM Create and identify the section of an accompaniment using *Band-in-a-Box*
Web Site Research the life and music of Ludwig van Beethoven

Connection: Culture

Activity: Learn how diverse cultures use string instruments in different ways

TEACHER TO TEACHER **Comparing and Constructing Instruments** Explore different instruments from around the world

CULTURAL CONNECTION Chinese String Instruments Facts about Chinese orchestras

SCHOOL TO HOME CONNECTION **Community Strings** Be aware of local string ensembles

BUILDING SKILLS THROUGH MUSIC Language Develop a symantic feature analysis chart

Listening Selections
"Summer," *from Concerto No. 2, Movement 3*
The Moon Mirrored in the Pool
Shchedryk

More Music Choices
"Allegretto giovale," from *Lyric Suite*, p. 169
"Finale," from *Serenade for Strings in C, Op. 48*, (excerpt) p. 363

ASSESSMENT
Observation/Music Journal Writing Identify the timbre of string instruments in a recording

TECHNOLOGY/MEDIA LINK
Sequencing Software Record string sounds and identify techniques of making sounds with string instruments

---

Connection: Social Studies

Activity: Discover the geography and folk traditions of the Ozark Mountains

MEETING INDIVIDUAL NEEDS **Independent Singing** Practice common tone parts to prepare for moving countermelodies

SPOTLIGHT ON Jimmy Driftwood Facts about folk musician Jimmy Driftwood

ACROSS THE CURRICULUM **Social Studies** Learn about the Battle of New Orleans and the War of 1812

MOVEMENT The Hoedown Describes a hoedown

TEACHER TO TEACHER **Solid Singing** Put solid singers in both groups when dividing the class for singing
Double Mallets Have two sets of three mallet instruments to play verse and refrain parts

BUILDING SKILLS THROUGH MUSIC Writing Describe music through words

Song "Going upon the Mountain"

Listening Selections
The Battle of New Orleans

More Music Choices
"Eres tú," p. 473
"Sing a Song of Peace," p. 66

ASSESSMENT
Performance/Observation Sing a countermelody and melody in groups

TECHNOLOGY/MEDIA LINK
Sequencing Software Record an ensemble accompaniment
Digital Audio Recording Record instrumental parts using acoustic instruments

---

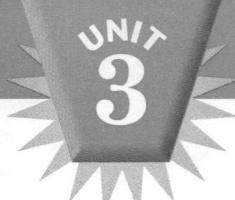
INTRODUCING THE UNIT

Learning the Language of Music allows students to better understand, enjoy, and appreciate music and improve their performance and listening skills. Unit 3 includes the musical language of dynamics, augmentation, diminution, aaba and ABCA forms, dorian and mixolydian modes, melodic motives, string timbres, and countermelodies. The skills assessed in this unit can be found on p. 73 with unit highlights listed in the footnotes. Students will enjoy learning the language of music.

UNIT PROJECT

Direct students to the definition of *recitative* on p. 74. Remind them that songs from musicals and opera use recitatives to forward the dialogue and action between songs *(arias).* Tell them they will write a recitative.

Ask students to write dialog about their everyday experiences and then create their own recitatives. Have them

- Form groups of two to four students.
- Understand that they are going to create a short amount of dialog about some everyday happening.
- Spend five minutes brainstorming something they could write about and sketch their ideas on paper, then choose the strongest idea for their group.
- Circulate among the groups and verify their ideas.
- Write about eight to ten sentences, in a dialogue, about their topic. This could be a single person talking (solo), a dialog between two people (duet), or a group discussion (ensemble).
- Sing the dialog with some kind of melody (similar to an opera or a musical). The results may be unusual, but it will nevertheless get across the idea.
- Perform their dialogs for the rest of the class (ask for volunteers).

Expressing History through Music

The musical *Evita* (1978), by composer Andrew Lloyd Webber and lyricist Tim Rice, tells the story of Argentina's Eva Perón. Eva ("Evita") rose from poverty to become a successful radio actress. She met and married Juan Perón, who became president of Argentina. Eva Perón was politically active alongside her husband and helped the women's political movement in Argentina.

The musical *Evita* was a tremendous success, with over 2,900 performances in London and 1,567 performances in New York. In 1996, *Evita* was made into a movie.

Patti LuPone played E▓ Perón in the 1979 stag▓ production of *Evita.*

72

ACROSS THE CURRICULUM

Unit Highlights The following interdisciplinary activities in this unit are related to the music elements presented in the lessons and are intended to enhance student learning. For a more detailed topical description, see the Unit at a Glance on pp. 71a–71h.

▶ **MATH**
- Relate augmentation and diminution to mathematics (p. 80)

▶ **SCIENCE**
- Relate the concepts of dynamic changes to science (p. 76)

▶ **SOCIAL STUDIES**
- Discuss how to build "bridges" to find peace (p. 86)
- Learn about the lyrics of "Scarborough Fair" in relation to its historical period (p. 94)
- Write a short play about Ludwig van Beethoven (p. 98)
- Learn facts about the Battle of New Orleans (p. 105)

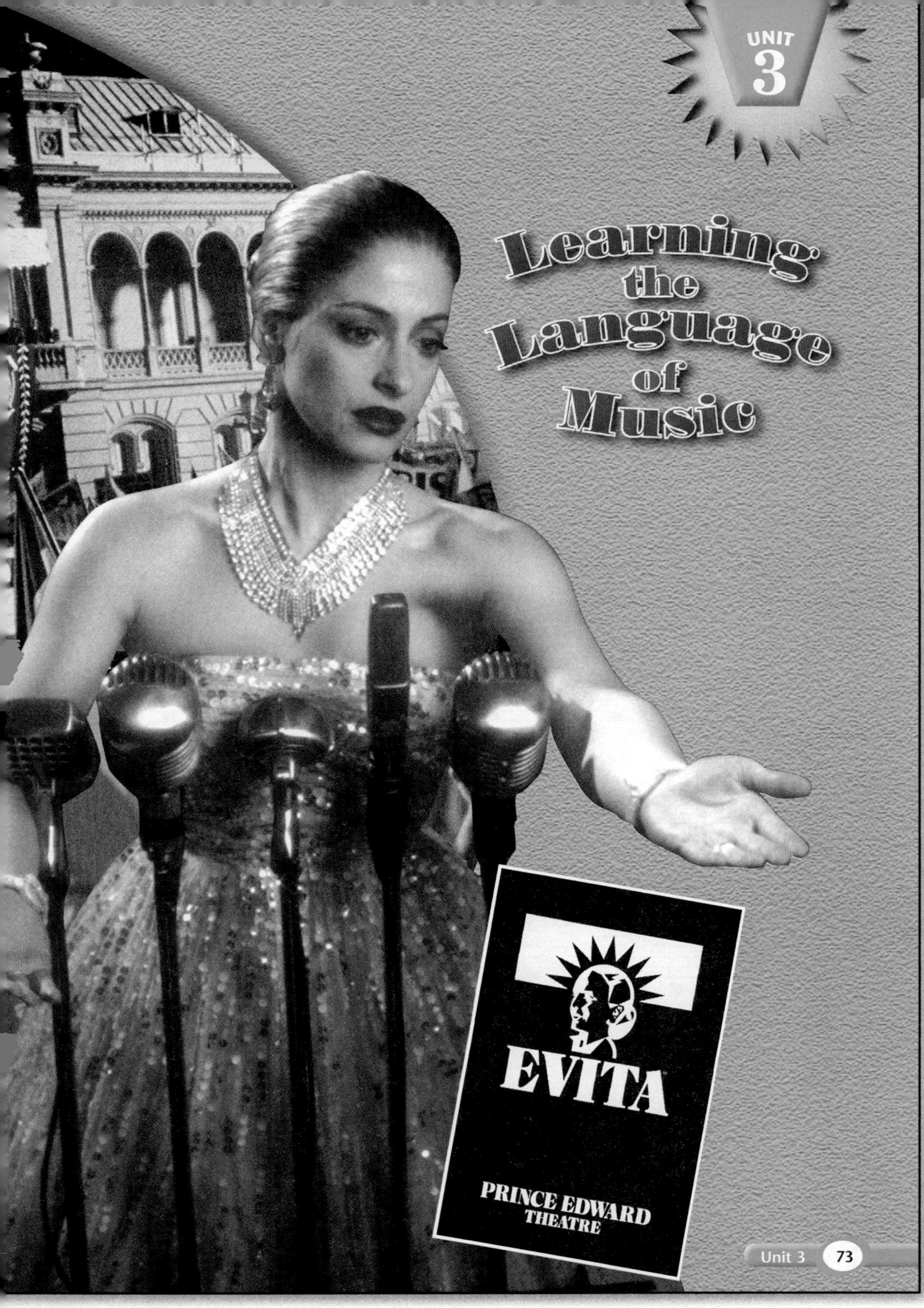

Learning the Language of Music

EVITA

PRINCE EDWARD THEATRE

Unit 3   **73**

MUSIC SKILLS
ASSESSED IN THIS UNIT

Reading Music: Rhythm

- Read and perform rhythms in augmentation and diminution (p. 81)
- Read *"Hava nashira"* in augmentation and diminution (p. 83)

Reading Music: Pitch

- Read and sing a song in dorian mode (p. 95)
- Read and sing a song in mixolydian mode (p. 97)

Performing Music: Singing

- Sing "This Is My Song" performing dynamics (p. 79)
- Sing a song, from notation, with good vocal quality (p. 89)
- Sing a countermelody in a song (p. 107)

Performing Music: Playing

- Play a 12-bar blues bass line on guitar or keyboard (p. 93)

Listening to Music

- Listen to an orchestra selection and identify a motive (p. 101)
- Listen to a string selection and identify *pizzicato* technique (p. 103)

Moving to Music

- Sing, move, and clap a backbeat in a song (p. 85)

Creating Music

- Create a rhythm composition in aaba form (p. 87)

CULTURAL CONNECTION

Unit Highlights   The musical literature in this unit provides many opportunities for students to explore a variety of world cultures. A more detailed description of the resources and activities listed below can be found in the Unit at a Glance on pp. 71a–71h.

▶ ASIAN

- Discover facts about Chinese string instruments (p. 102)

▶ EUROPEAN

- Learn facts about Finland (p. 77)

▶ UNITED STATES

- Learn about the decade of the Roaring Twenties (p. 88)
- Learn about the term boogie-woogie in the 1920s and the terms that might describe the pop culture of today (p. 92)
- Explore how jazz and Jewish folk song influenced George Gershwin (p. 101)

OPENING ACTIVITIES

MATERIALS

- "Don't Cry for Me, Argentina" **CD 4–37**

  Recording Routine: Intro (2 m.); recitative (15 m.); v. 1; refrain; v. 2; refrain; refrain; coda

- **Resource Book** p. I-32

- guitars, Autoharps, or keyboards

Listening

Have students read the text on p. 74. Invite students to listen to "Don't Cry for Me, Argentina," **CD 4–37,** as they follow the song notation.

Reading

Ask students to look for and discuss the following in the music:

- Lyrics. Discuss what students think Eva is saying about her rise from poverty to being alongside her husband as head of state in Argentina.

ASK Does this poverty-to-fame scenario happen in the United States? Can they think of examples? (Bill Clinton)

- Key signature and *do.* (D major; *do* = D)

ASK When does the first low D appear? (close to and at the end of the music)

ASK When does the recitative stop and the aria start? (refrain)

Singing

Begin by having the class sing the better-known melody of the refrain of "Don't Cry for Me, Argentina" **CD 4–37** with the recording. Then, have them try the recitative-like sections. Explain that flexible rhythm such as this is hard to do as a group since it is meant for an individual soloist.

Sing the entire song with the recording. When students know the melody to the refrain well, have them try to find a harmony part below the melody—a third below (except for the lyrics, *the truth is I never left you,* where they sing an A on the syllable, *nev*). Have them sing unison on the last phrase, *don't keep your distance.*

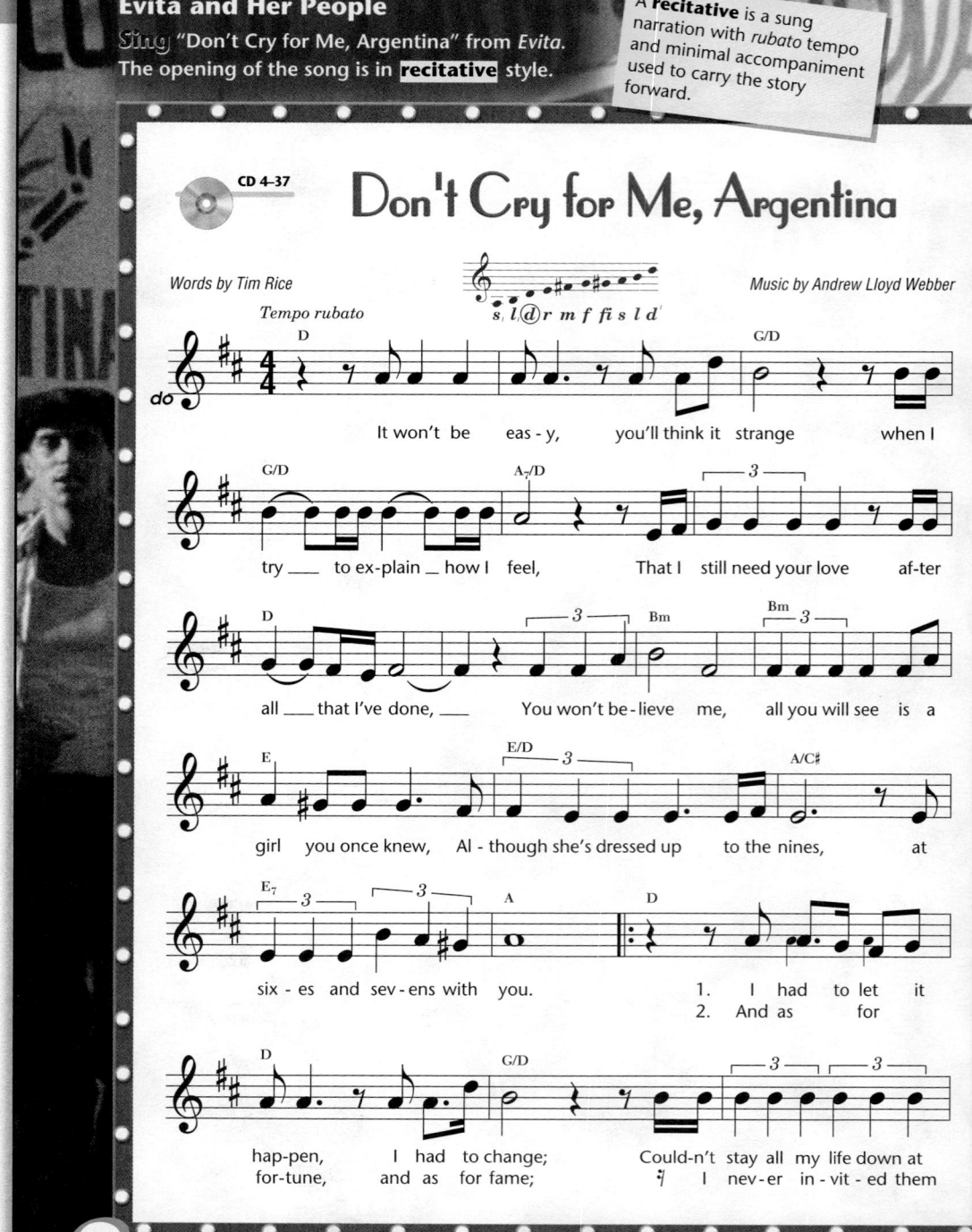

Evita and Her People

Sing "Don't Cry for Me, Argentina" from *Evita.* The opening of the song is in **recitative** style.

A **recitative** is a sung narration with *rubato* tempo and minimal accompaniment used to carry the story forward.

CD 4-37

Don't Cry for Me, Argentina

Words by Tim Rice

Music by Andrew Lloyd Webber

74

ASSESSMENT

Unit Highlights This unit includes a variety of strategies and methods, described below, to track students' progress and assess their understanding of lesson objectives. Reproducible masters for Show What You Know! and Review, Assess, Perform, Create can be found in the Resource Book.

▶ **FORMAL ASSESSMENTS**

The following assessments, using written language, cognitive, and performance skills, help teachers and students conceptualize the learning that is taking place.

- **Show What You Know!** Element-specific assessments, on the student page, for Rhythm (p. 81) and Melody (p. 100)
- **Review, Assess, Perform, Create** This end-of-unit activity (pp. 108–109) can be used for review and to assess students' learning of the core lessons in this unit.

▶ **INFORMAL ASSESSMENTS**

At the close of each Teacher's Edition lesson in this unit, one of the following types of assessments is used to evaluate the learning of the key element focus or skill objective.

- Observation/Music Journal Writing (p. 103)
- Performance/Observation (pp. 79, 81, 83, 87, 89, 95, 97, 107)
- Performance/Peer Critique (p. 93)
- Performance/Self-Assessment (p. 85)
- Written Assessment (p. 101)

▶ **RUBRICS**

Visit *www.sfsuccessnet.com* for rubrics to assess students' achievement in music skills.

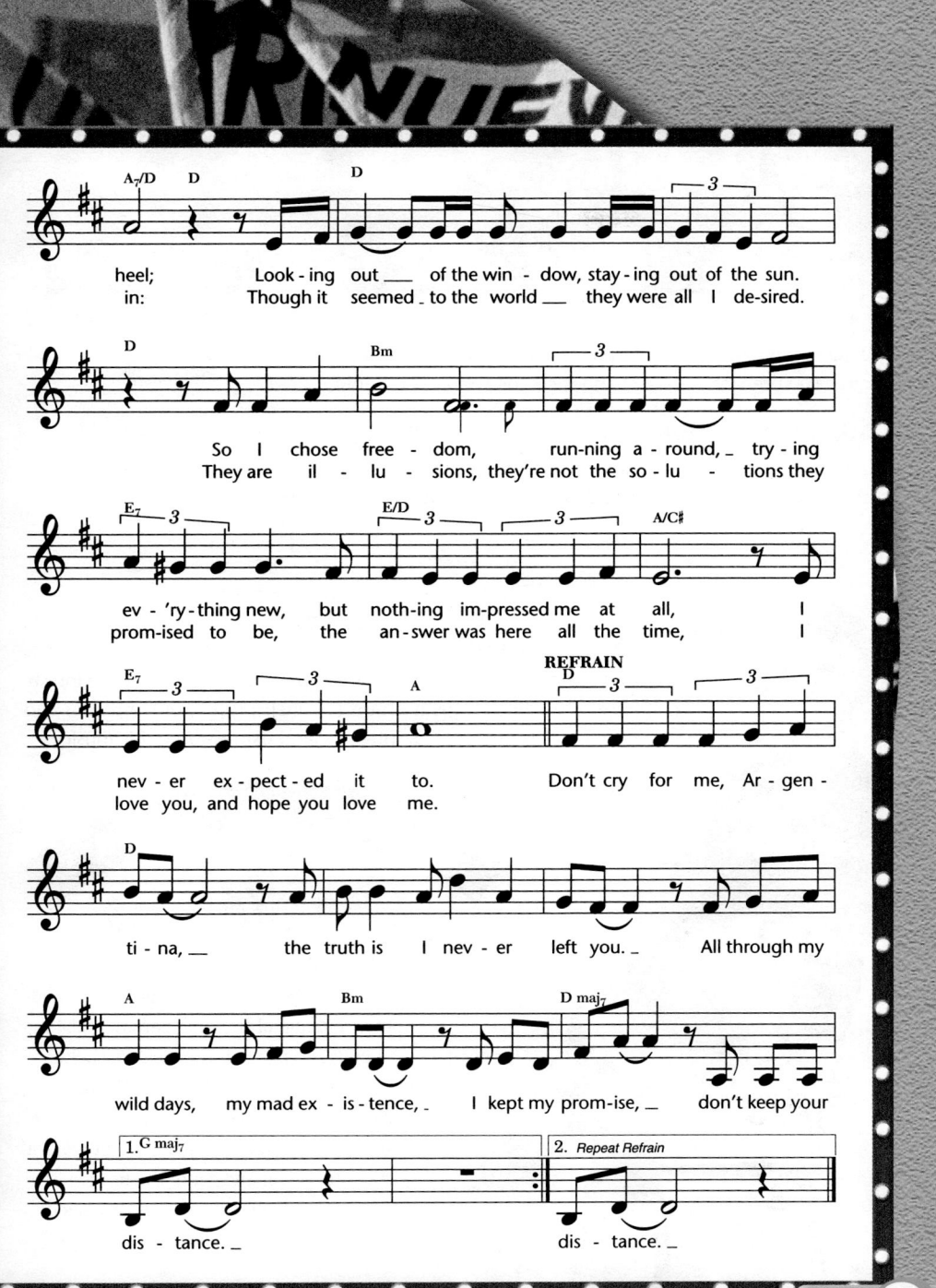

Moving

Invite students to feel the combination of a three-against-two rhythm:

- On their thighs, have them pat:

  R   R   R (3)

  L   L (against 2)

- Next ask them to tap their left foot along with their left hand.
- Students should be doing triplets with their right hand while the left hand and their toe is keeping the steady beat.
- Students may choose to use the opposite hands for this exercise.
- Explain that the three-against-two rhythm found in this song is a very important part of Latin American music.

Playing

The melody of the refrain is quite easily played on recorder. Play the last phrase up an octave.

Have students review the fingerings (D E F♯ G A B D) for soprano recorder on Resource Book p. I-32.

INNOVATIVE TEACHER SUPPORT FOR THIS UNIT

- **MAKING MUSIC DVD, Grade 6** contains video segments that support lessons, including signing and movement.
- **MAKING MUSIC with Movement and Dance** provides more opportunities for large group activities in music or physical education classes.
- **MAKING MUSIC with Technology** provides lesson plans for many technology applications; includes MIDI files.
- *¡A cantar!* features recorded songs and lessons from around the Spanish-speaking world; includes strategies for bilingual classes and for English-speaking teachers working with Spanish-speaking students.
- **Bridges to Asia** features recorded songs and lessons from Asian and Pacific region cultures.
- *www.sfsuccessnet.com* provides an online lesson planner to conveniently create lesson plans at school or at home. Includes rubrics for assessment, lesson modifications to meet the needs of all students, performance musicals based on program content, and more.

TECHNOLOGY/MEDIA LINK

Unit Highlights The following components are used in this unit to reinforce and expand students' understanding of music elements and related themes.

▶ **CD-ROM**

- Use *Band-in-a-Box* to create an accompaniment (p. 93)
- Enter a chord progression into *Band-in-a-Box* (p. 101)

▶ **DIGITAL AUDIO RECORDING**

- Record acoustic instruments, using digital audio (p. 107)

▶ **MIDI/SEQUENCING SOFTWARE**

- Add new percussion tracks to a MIDI file (p. 85)
- Use the graphic editor to change a MIDI file (p. 97)

▶ **MULTIMEDIA**

- Create a slide show to represent aaba form (p. 89)
- Photograph illustrations for a slide show (p. 95)

▶ **NOTATION SOFTWARE**

- Notate augmented and diminished rhythms (p. 81)
- Notate a and b phrases and create an aaba form (p. 87)

▶ **SEQUENCING SOFTWARE**

- Use digital audio to record and modify string sounds (p. 103)
- Create an accompaniment for a song (p. 107)

▶ **TRANSPARENCY**

- Display listening map for *Jesu, Joy of Man's Desiring* (p. 87)

▶ **WEB SITE**

- Research music of Finland and Scandinavia (p. 79)
- Learn more about William Schuman (p. 83)
- Learn more about the Beatles and their music (p. 93)
- Learn about Ludwig van Beethoven (p. 101)

LESSON AT A GLANCE

Element Focus	**EXPRESSION** Dynamic changes
Skill Objective	**SINGING** Sing two songs with dynamic changes
Connection Activity	**SCIENCE** Discuss how loud and soft sounds relate to near and far sound sources

MATERIALS

- "This Is My Song"   **CD 5-1**
  Recording Routine: Intro (4 m.); verse 1; interlude (4 m.); verse 2; coda
- "I Walk the Unfrequented Road"   **CD 5-6**
  Recording Routine: Intro (4 m.); v. 1; interlude (2 m.); v. 2; interlude (4 m.); v. 3; coda
- *Finlandia* (excerpt)   **CD 5-3**
- *Kerenski*   **CD 5-4**
- **Dance Directions** for *Kerenski* p. 555
- classroom percussion instruments
- **Resource Book** p. I-8

VOCABULARY

dynamics   crescendo   decrescendo   sforzando

mezzo piano   forte

◆ ◆ ◆ ◆ National Standards ◆ ◆ ◆ ◆

1b Sing easy pieces with expression
2a Play instruments accurately in small ensembles
4a Compose short pieces, demonstrating tension and release through music
5c Identify standard notation symbols for dynamics
6b Listen and analyze uses of dynamics in music from diverse genres

MORE MUSIC CHOICES

For more experience with dynamic changes:
"A Brand New Day," p. 7
"Run! Run! Hide!" p. 340
"Summertime," p. 250

DynamiCS
BriNg Music to Life

A change in loudness is a common and effective means of musical expression. These changes can be sudden or gradual.

> **Crescendo** means "gradually louder."
> **Decrescendo** means "gradually softer."

Adjust the Volume

Gradual dynamic changes are indicated by the markings **crescendo** [kreh-SHEN-doh] and **decrescendo** [deh-kreh-SHEN-doh].

Crescendo   Decrescendo

Dynamic Sibelius

Dynamics and musical expression are important in the music of Finnish composer, Jean Sibelius [jahn sih-BAY-lee-uhs]. The use of *crescendos* and *decrescendos* affect the mood, intensity, and expression of his music.

MUSIC MAKERS
Jean Sibelius

Jean Sibelius (1865–1957) loved his homeland, and much of his music depicts this love for his country and its people. Born in Finland of Swedish parents, Sibelius grew up in a bilingual household. His parents spoke Swedish at home, but he learned to speak Finnish in school. Sibelius learned to play the violin when he was quite young and composed his first work at age ten for violin and cello. His brother played the cello, and his sister played the piano.

76

Footnotes

SPOTLIGHT ON

▶ **Jean Sibelius** (1865–1957) is one of Finland's most prominent composers. Although Sibelius is considered to be a nationalist composer, he did not actually use Finnish folk music in his compositions. Rather, Sibelius often incorporated elements and stylistic features of Finnish folk music in his pieces. *Finlandia* is one of Sibelius's best-known works.

BUILDING SKILLS THROUGH MUSIC

▶ **Reading** Have students read about Sibelius in Music Makers on p. 76. Ask them who might have played Sibelius's first composition? (his family) Students should support their answer with text evidence.

ACROSS THE CURRICULUM

▶ **Science** Relate the concept of near and far to dynamic changes by walking around the classroom and playing a drum at a constant volume. Ask students what happens to the dynamic level as you approach them while playing the drum and what happens when you walk away from them while playing the drum. Encourage students to tell about experiences they may have had listening to the gradual dynamic changes of a jet passing overhead or a train approaching and passing them by. Students may have also noticed the change of pitch of a train whistle as the train sped past them.

Vocal Dynamics in Hymns

Listen to "This Is My Song," and follow the dynamic markings in the score. Are the dynamic changes sudden or gradual? **Sing** "This is My Song." **Perform** the dynamics of the song as you sing.

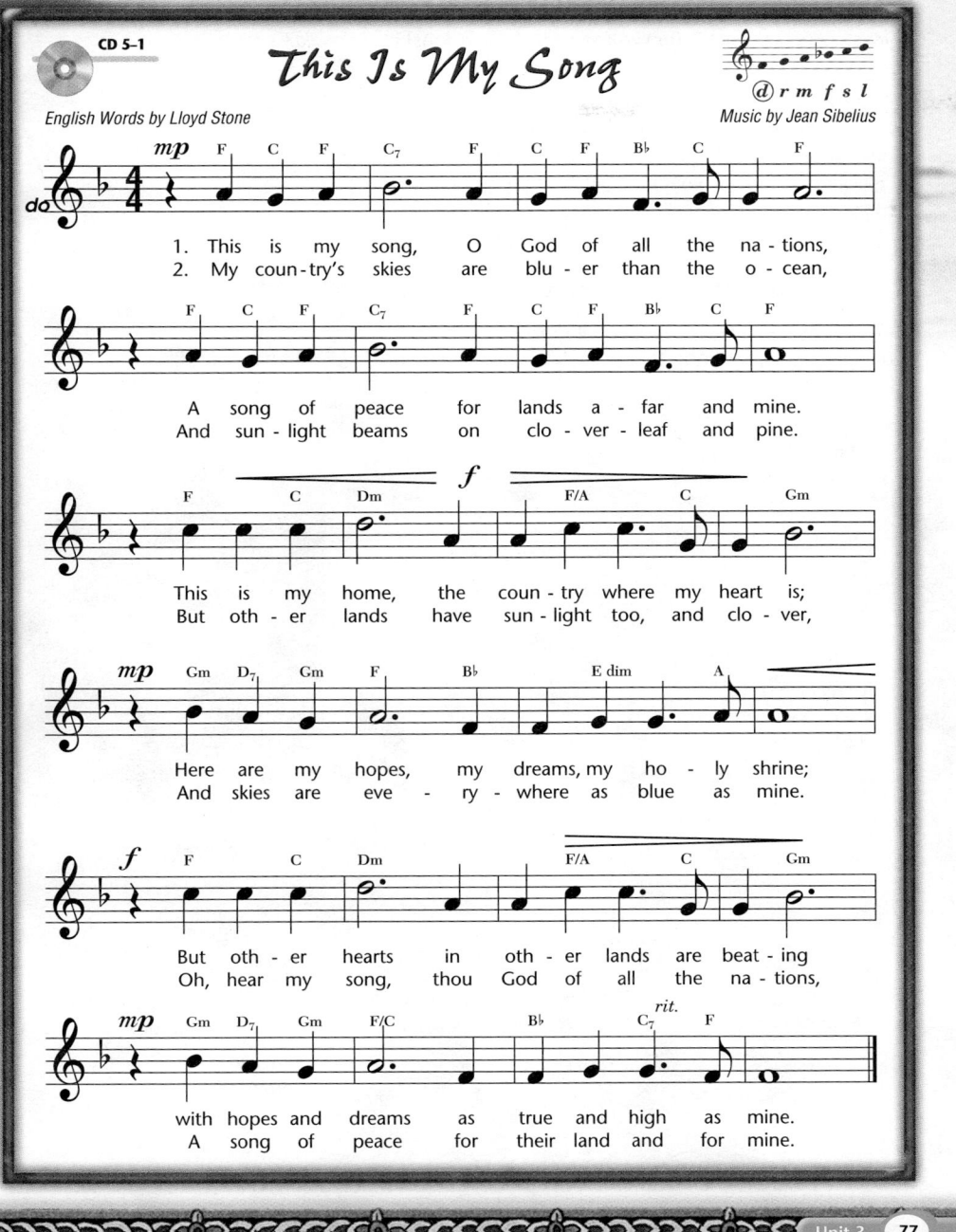

CD 5-1

This Is My Song

English Words by Lloyd Stone

Music by Jean Sibelius

d r m f s l

mp

1. This is my song, O God of all the na - tions,
2. My coun-try's skies are blu - er than the o - cean,

A song of peace for lands a - far and mine.
And sun - light beams on clo - ver - leaf and pine.

f

This is my home, the coun - try where my heart is;
But oth - er lands have sun - light too, and clo - ver,

mp

Here are my hopes, my dreams, my ho - ly shrine;
And skies are eve - ry - where as blue as mine.

f

But oth - er hearts in oth - er lands are beat - ing
Oh, hear my song, thou God of all the na - tions,

mp *rit.*

with hopes and dreams as true and high as mine.
A song of peace for their land and for mine.

Unit 3 77

continued on page 78

1 INTRODUCE

Engage students in a brief discussion of loud and soft environmental sounds that surround them daily.

See Across the Curriculum, p. 76, for activities that will take this discussion of loud and soft sounds and relate it to near and far sound sources.

ASK **How do you feel when a very long, loud sound stops?** (relieved)

How do you feel when a soft sound is interrupted by a loud sound? (startled)

Explain that

- Changes in dynamics contribute to the expressive qualities in music.
- Dynamic changes can be abrupt or they can be gradual.

2 DEVELOP

Listening

Invite students to listen to the recording of "This Is My Song" **CD 5-1**, paying attention to the dynamics.

6b **ASK** **Did the dynamic level remain the same throughout the performance?** (no)

How did the dynamics change? (Sometimes the music gradually became louder and sometimes it gradually became softer.)

5c Explain that in music

- The word *crescendo* means to become gradually louder.
- The word *decrescendo* means to become gradually softer.

Direct students to p. 77 in the Student Edition. Ask them to identify the dynamic markings that are used in "This Is My Song." (*mezzo piano* (*mp*); *forte* (*f*); *crescendo*; *decrescendo*) Ask students to identify the

---

SKILLS REINFORCEMENT

▶ **Vocal Development** Many young singers change the dynamics too quickly when performing crescendos and decrescendos. Help singers gain control by counting the numbers slowly as they practice identifying and interpreting the dynamic changes on a single pitch.

1	2	3	4	5	6	7	8	9	10	11	12	13	14	15
ppp	*pp*	*p*	*mp*	*mf*	*f*	*ff*	*fff*	*ff*	*f*	*mf*	*mp*	*p*	*pp*	*ppp*

▶ **Recorder** Invite students to learn the soprano and alto recorder countermelodies for "I Walk the Unfrequented Road," **2a** found on Resource Book p. I-8.

CULTURAL CONNECTION

▶ **Finland** Finland is located in northern Europe, between Sweden and Russia. A country of more than 5 million people, Finland is slightly smaller in size than the state of Montana and contains over 60,000 lakes. Finns have lived in what is now Finland since 3000 B.C. Finland is rightly known as the land of forests, since more than three-quarters of its surface is covered with trees. The extreme northern part of Finland is in darkness for about 51 days in winter, but the summer, sun shines continuously for about 73 days. In the summer, many boys and girls skate down the streets at midnight. The flag of Finland has a white background with a solid blue cross.

Lesson 1 Continued

dynamic changes as they listen to the recording **CD 5-1** again.

Analyzing

Have students locate the names of the composer (Jean Sibelius) and the text writer (lyricist, Lloyd Stone). Ask individuals to read the words to "This Is My Song" aloud. Discuss with students the meaning of the words.

Singing

 Invite students to sing "This Is My Song" **CD 5-1** with the recording. Remind students to identify music terms referring to dynamics (*mp*, *f*, *crescendo*, *decrescendo*) as notated in the music, and to interpret them correctly when performing as notated in the music.

Listening

Tell students that the melody of "This Is My Song" came from a piece titled *Finlandia* by Jean Sibelius. Ask them to listen for the familiar melody as they hear the piece.

Tell students that they will be "dynamic detectives" as they listen to *Finlandia* **CD 5-3**.

5c Have students use standard symbols to notate dynamics. Have them make cards showing a range of dynamics, one symbol per card, from *ppp* through *fff*.

Have students show the dynamics and dynamic changes they hear by holding up the appropriate card while listening.

Moving

Invite students to listen to *Kerenski* **CD 5-4** and perform the movement routine. See Dance Directions, p. 555. You may wish to use the Dance Practice **CD 5-5** to help students learn the routine.

Dynamics Used in Symphonic Music

Few composers before Beethoven (1770–1827) placed dynamic markings in their music. Since Beethoven's time, composers have used dynamic markings to create more expressive music.

As you **listen** to *Finlandia*, discover the changes in dynamic levels. Are there any **sforzandos** [sfohrt-SAHN-dohs] in *Finlandia*?

Sforzando is a sudden accent on a note or chord.

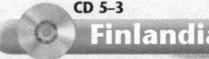
Finlandia
by Jean Sibelius

CD 5–3

Finlandia, written in 1899, is a tone poem. A tone poem is music that tells a story or describes an event. This music was later used in the movies *Die Hard 2* and *The Hunt for Red October*.

A Fine Finnish Folk Dance

The *kerenski* [keh-REHN-skee] was a popular folk dance in Finland during the 1920s and is still danced today.

Perform the dance, using movements modeled by your teacher.

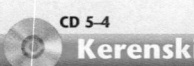
Kerenski
Folk Dance from Finland

CD 5–4

The Finnish version of this dance was named for Aleksandr Fyodorovich Kerensky (1881–1970), a premier of Soviet Russia.

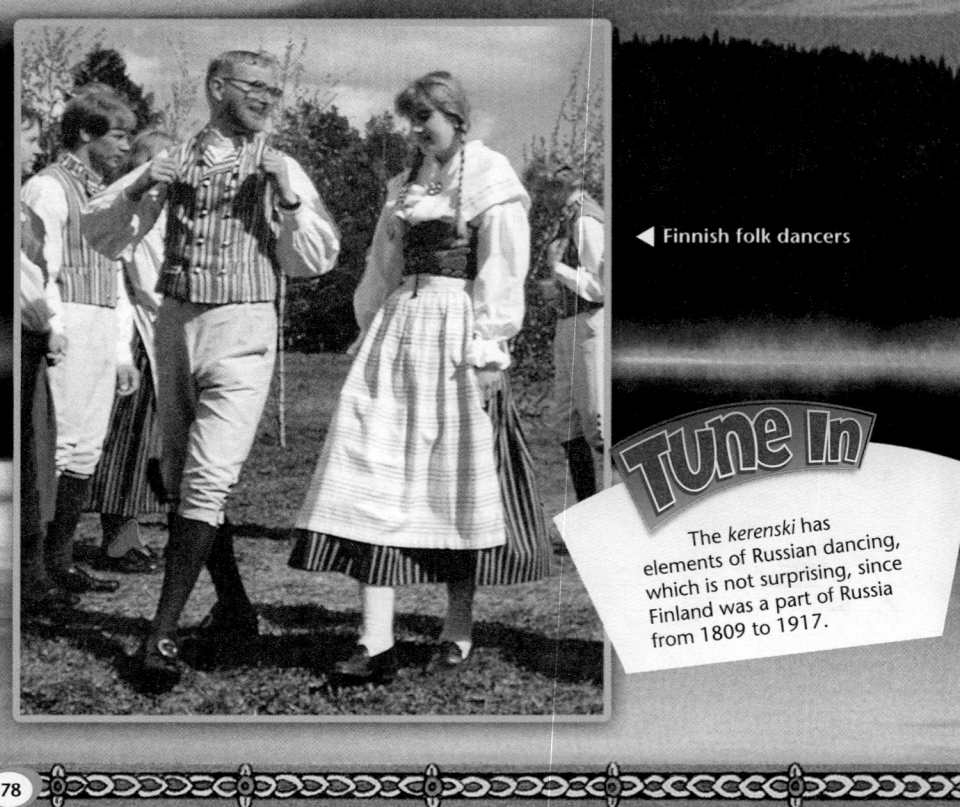

◀ Finnish folk dancers

The *kerenski* has elements of Russian dancing, which is not surprising, since Finland was a part of Russia from 1809 to 1917.

78

Footnotes

SKILLS REINFORCEMENT

▶ **Vocal Development** Encourage students to begin singing vocalises in minor. Begin with the pattern *(do–ti₁–la₁)* before attempting the five-note pattern *(mi–re–do–ti₁–la₁)*.

- Sing and have students echo the pattern *do–ti₁–la₁* in E minor (G-F♯-E).
- Sing G-G♯ on a neutral syllable to establish new tonality, and model the pattern in each key from E minor to A minor; students echo.
- Try the vocalise, using a neutral syllable such as *noo* or *moo*.
- Once students can model each pattern accurately, give the new starting pitch for each pattern but omit the model.
- Follow the same procedure for the five-note pattern.

SPOTLIGHT ON

▶ *Kerenski* According to sources from Finland, the real name of this dance is *Kerenskoi*. It is a very old dance. It is known in Luumäki and Vuokkiniemi, areas in Karelia, a region that was part of Finland before the Russians gained control.

CHARACTER EDUCATION

▶ **Peace** Both songs in this lesson are about peace. "This is My Song" reflects on peace between countries, while "I Walk the Unfrequented Road" focuses on personal peace. Guide students to understand the commonality in the message between the songs and encourage them to consider ways they can promote peace in their own lives. Encourage them to consider ways of promoting peace at home, at school, and in the community. Challenge students to select one means of promoting peace and adopt that behavior consistently.

Dynamic Travels

Listen to "I Walk the Unfrequented Road" and decide if the dynamic changes are sudden or gradual. **Sing** the song and show the dynamics as you sing.

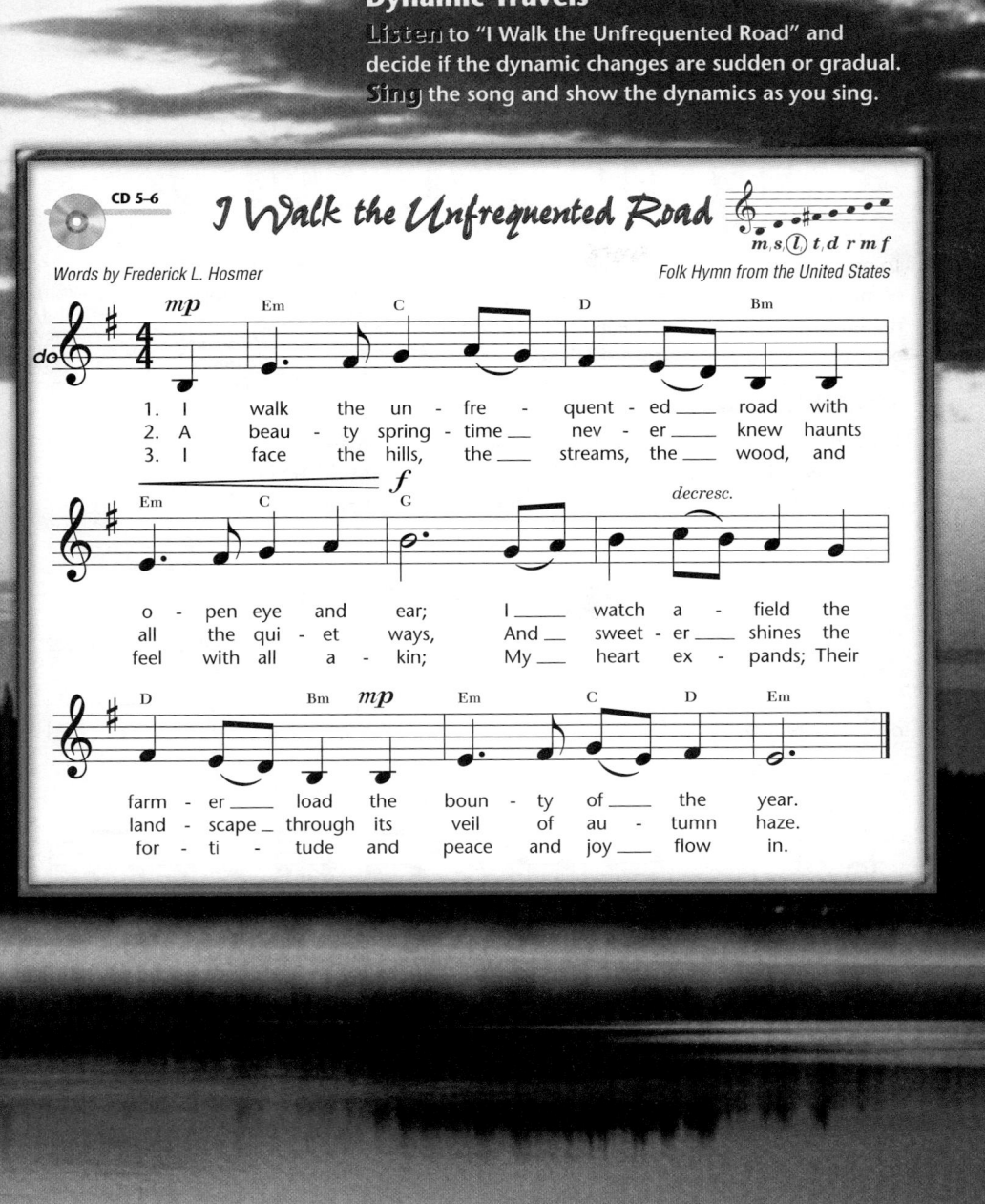

I Walk the Unfrequented Road

CD 5-6

Words by Frederick L. Hosmer

Folk Hymn from the United States

1. I walk the un - fre - quent - ed road with
2. A beau - ty spring - time nev - er knew haunts
3. I face the hills, the streams, the wood, and

o - pen eye and ear; I watch a - field the
all the qui - et ways, And sweet - er shines the
feel with all a - kin; My heart ex - pands; Their

farm - er load the boun - ty of the year.
land - scape through its veil of au - tumn haze.
for - ti - tude and peace and joy flow in.

Unit 3 **79**

Singing

1b Invite students to sing "I Walk the Unfrequented Road" **CD 5-6**, changing dynamics with the recording.

Direct students' attention to the musical symbols for *crescendo* and *decrescendo*.

After students sing the song with the recording a second time, encourage them to suggest where *crescendos* and *decrescendos* might be placed in the music on p. 79.

Creating

Explain that the notation for *sforzando* is *sfz*.

Divide the class into several small groups. Encourage each group to

4a
- Create and notate a short rhythmic composition with dynamic changes, using *crescendos, decrescendos,* and at least one *sforzando.*

- Perform its composition on classroom instruments.

5c
- Identify the dynamic changes performed by other groups, using the terms *crescendo, decrescendo,* and *sforzando.*

3 CLOSE

Skill: SINGING **ASSESSMENT**

Performance/Observation Invite students to sing "This Is My Song" again with the Stereo Performance track **CD 5-2.** Remind them to follow the dynamic markings in the music. Observe students' ability to perform the dynamics accurately as they sing the song.

MEETING INDIVIDUAL NEEDS

▶ **English Language Learners** The text of "I Walk the Unfrequented Road" provides a good opportunity for students to work on pronunciation. There are many different English speech sounds in the words of this song. You may want to have students pronounce all of the lyrics before singing. You may also wish to construct flash cards with selected words, such as *road, load, bounty, springtime, quiet, veil,* and *open*—words that may be difficult to pronounce.

SCHOOL TO HOME CONNECTION

▶ **Ancestry** Encourage students to ask family members about folk dances that may be in their family's background. Allow class time for reports.

TECHNOLOGY/MEDIA LINK

Web Site Go to *www.sfsuccessnet.com* to research other folk music from Finland and elsewhere in Scandinavia.

LESSON AT A GLANCE

Element Focus	**RHYTHM** Augmentation and diminution
Skill Objective	**READING** Read augmented and diminished song rhythms
Connection Activity	**MATHEMATICS** Explore multiplication and division with time

MATERIALS

* "Do, Re, Mi, Fa" **CD 5-8**
  Recording Routine: Intro (4 m.); vocal; interlude (4 m.); vocal (4-part round); coda
* **Music Reading Practice, Sequence 9** **CD 5-10**
* soprano and alto recorder
* pencils and blank sheets of paper
* **Resource Book** pp. D-10, E-10

VOCABULARY

augmented   augmentation   diminished   diminution

◆ ◆ ◆ ◆ **National Standards** ◆ ◆ ◆ ◆

1d Sing music written in three parts
5a Read eighth, quarter, half, and whole notes in duple meter
6c Understand and use basic principles of meter in music analysis
8b Identify ways music relates to math

MORE MUSIC CHOICES

For more practice reading and notating augmented and diminished rhythms:

"Dance for the Nations," p. 122

"Hava nashira," p. 82

1 INTRODUCE

1d Ask students to sing "Do, Re, Mi, Fa" **CD 5-8** using pitch syllables and hand signs. Have students sing the song in canon. Challenge students to sing the song first as a 3-part round, and then as a 4-part round.

Tell students they will learn how to change the rhythm of a song to be twice as slow, and twice as fast.

Playing for Time

To make a composition interesting, composers may use a variety of musical tricks. One technique involves playing with the rhythm by performing it twice as slow or twice as fast as the original. This is called **augmentation** or **diminution**.

Augmentation means that the rhythm is notated to be twice as slow.
Diminution means that the rhythm is notated to be twice as fast.

Stretch It Out

The song "Do, Re, Mi, Fa," from a school songbook published in 1852, uses only half-note and eighth-note rhythm patterns. **Sing** in unison, then in canon. Keep a steady beat by conducting as you sing.

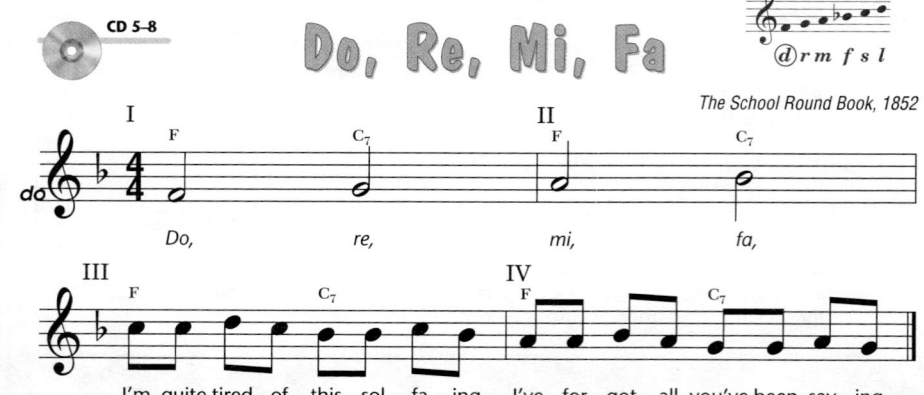

The School Round Book, 1852

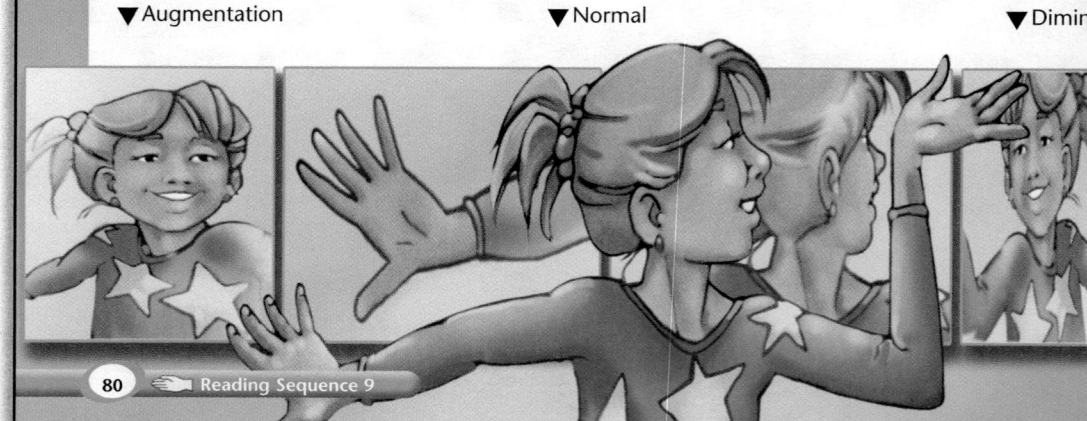

Do,   re,   mi,   fa,

I'm quite tired of this sol-fa-ing, I've for-got all you've been say-ing.

▼ Augmentation   ▼ Normal   ▼ Dimin

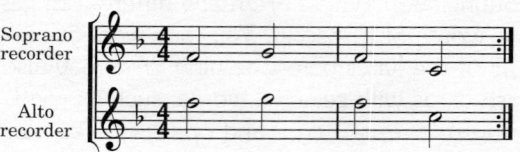

80   Reading Sequence 9

Footnotes

ACROSS THE CURRICULUM

8b ▶ **Math** Engage students in a discussion of the mathematical operations of multiplication, division, addition, and subtraction as they relate to augmentation and diminution. Invite students to time performances of a favorite song in the original version, the augmented version, and the diminished version. Help students maintain a consistent tempo for all three performances.

BUILDING SKILLS THROUGH MUSIC

▶ **Math** Ask students which of the following would be an augmentation of the series 2, 2, 4, 6, 2, 8? (A)

A: 4, 4, 8, 12, 4, 16.   Or B: 4, 4, 6, 8, 4, 10.

Ask them which of the following would be a diminution of the series? (D)

C: 1, 1, 3, 5, 1, 7.   Or D: 1, 1, 2, 3, 1, 4.

SKILLS REINFORCEMENT

▶ **Recorder** Invite students to play this ostinato for "Do, Re, Mi, Fa" on soprano recorder or alto recorder.

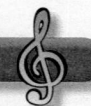

Soprano recorder

Alto recorder

▶ **Reading** For additional reading practice, invite students to perform a three-part rhythm accompaniment to "Do, Re, Mi, Fa" on p. 492, or Resource Book E-10.

Time to Augment

To augment the rhythm of "Do, Re, Mi, Fa," the half notes are changed to whole notes. How are the eighth notes changed?

Notice that when the time signature stays the same, bar lines must be added. Instead of the original four measures, there are now eight measures—twice as many!

Sing and conduct the new augmented rhythm of "Do, Re, Mi, Fa."

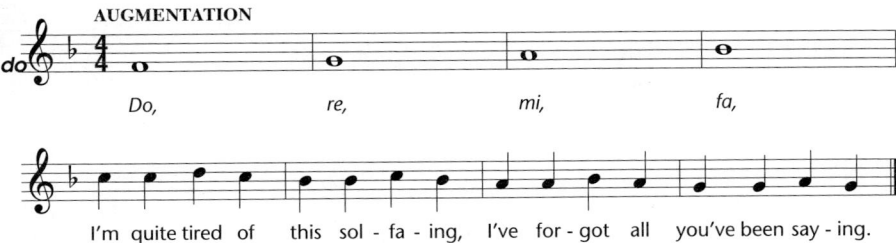

Do,　　re,　　mi,　　fa,

I'm quite tired of　this sol-fa-ing,　I've for-got all　you've been say-ing.

Tighten It Up

To notate "Do, Re, Mi, Fa" in diminution, the half notes are changed to quarter notes. How are the eighth notes changed?

Again, the original song has four measures. **Read** the notation below to **identify** the number of measures the diminution version of the song will have.

Conduct and **sing** the rhythm syllables for this diminution of "Do, Re, Mi, Fa."

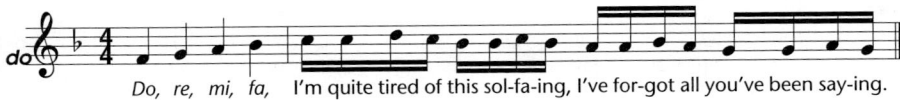

Do, re, mi, fa,　I'm quite tired of this sol-fa-ing, I've for-got all you've been say-ing.

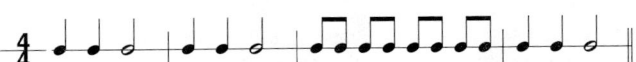

Follow these directions to show what you know about augmentation and diminution.

1. Conduct and say the rhythm syllables for the pattern notated below.
2. Notate, conduct, and say the syllables for a rhythmic augmentation of this pattern.
3. Notate, conduct, and say the syllables for a rhythmic diminution of this pattern.

---

2 DEVELOP

Analyzing

Invite students to tap the beat and follow the augmented notation on p. 81 as you sing the rhythm twice as slowly. Tell students that when a rhythm is performed twice as slowly, and the beat remains the same, the rhythm has been *augmented*.

6c **ASK** What kind of notes are needed to notate the first two measures of *"Do, Re, Mi, Fa"* to be twice as slow? (whole notes)

Have students tap the beat and follow the diminished notation on p. 81, as you sing the rhythm twice as fast. Tell them, the rhythm has been *diminished*.

6c **ASK** How does the diminished version of *"Do, Re, Mi, Fa"* compare to the original song notation? (it is two measures long, or one-half of the original song; all notes are one-half of the original note values)

8b See Across the Curriculum on p. 80 as to how augmentation and diminution relate to math operations.

Singing

Have students tap the quarter-note beat and sing the augmented version of *"Do, Re, Mi, Fa"* on p. 81.

Invite students to sing the diminished version of *"Do, Re, Mi, Fa"* on p. 81 as they tap the quarter-note beat.

Moving

Invite students to learn the movement routine for *"Do, Re, Mi, Fa."* (See Movement, on p. 81.)

3 CLOSE

Skill: READING　　　　　　**ASSESSMENT**

5a **Performance/Observation** Have students read
6c and sing *"Do, Re, Mi, Fa"* in the original, augmented, and diminished versions on pp. 80–81. Observe students' ability to accurately read and perform augmentation and diminution.

MOVEMENT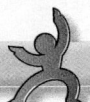

▶ **Locomotor Movement** Your students can move in canon with this routine while singing *"Do, Re, Mi, Fa."* Invite students to form four concentric circles, one for each voice of the canon. The innermost circle is voice I, the next circle out is voice II, and so on; the outer circle is voice IV.

Voice I Circle: Walk clockwise while singing the song.

Voice II Circle: Walk counterclockwise while singing; begin as voice I starts m. 2.

Voice III Circle: Walk clockwise while singing; begin as voice II starts m. 2.

Voice IV Circle: Walk counterclockwise while singing; begin as voice III starts m. 2.

TECHNOLOGY/MEDIA LINK

▶ **Notation Software** Have students notate augmented and diminished rhythms for *"Do, Re, Mi, Fa."*

Reinforcement Ask students to notate the melody and change the note values of the melody to demonstrate augmentation and diminution.

On Target Have students notate the original, augmented, and diminished versions of the melody into separate staves in the notation software.

Challenge Invite students to enter their melodies into the notation software using a MIDI keyboard. Have students "play" their augmented and diminished melodies into the software.

LESSON AT A GLANCE

Element Focus   **RHYTHM** Augmentation and diminution

Skill Objective   **READING** Read augmented and diminished rhythms

Connection Activity   **SOCIAL STUDIES** Discover historical facts on the music of Israel.

MATERIALS

- *"Hava nashira"*   CD 5-16
- *"Sing and be Joyful"*   CD 5-17
  Recording Routine: Intro (2 m.); vocal; vocal (3-part round)
- **Music Reading Practice, Sequence 10**   CD 5-19
- **Pronunciation Practice/Translation** p. 520
- *Interview with William Schuman*   CD 5-24
- *"Chester"* from *New England Triptych*   CD 5-25

Resource Handbook pp. A-11, D-11, E-11

- resonator bells

VOCABULARY

augmented   augmentation   diminished   diminution

◆ ◆ ◆ ◆ **National Standards** ◆ ◆ ◆ ◆

1c Sing music from diverse cultures
1d Sing music in three parts
5a Read eighth, quarter, half, and whole notes in duple meter
5b Sight-read melodies in treble clef
6c Understand and use basic principles of meter in music analysis

MORE MUSIC CHOICES . . .

For more practice in notating augmented and diminished rhythms:

"Scattin' A-Round," p. 158

"Do, Re, Mi, Fa," p. 80

1 INTRODUCE

Discuss the meaning of the title, *"Hava nashira"* (sing and be joyful).

Joyful Rhythms

"Hava nashira" is an Israeli song. The Hebrew text means *let us sing a song of praise.* Using rhythm syllables, **perform** the rhythm patterns.

Then use pitch syllables to **sing** the melody. When you are ready, **sing** *"Hava nashira"* as a three-part round.

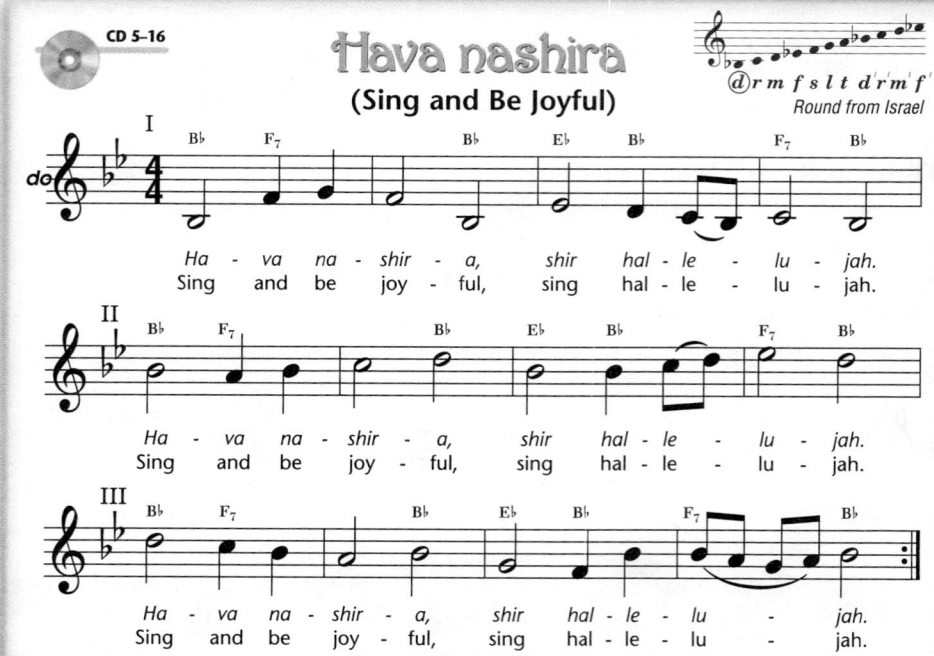

CD 5-16

Hava nashira
(Sing and Be Joyful)
Round from Israel

I
Ha - va na - shir - a,   shir hal - le - lu - jah.
Sing and be joy - ful, sing hal - le - lu - jah.

II
Ha - va na - shir - a,   shir hal - le - lu - jah.
Sing and be joy - ful, sing hal - le - lu - jah.

III
Ha - va na - shir - a,   shir hal - le - lu - jah.
Sing and be joy - ful, sing hal - le - lu - jah.

Expand, Contract, and Create Rhythms

You can use this song to practice rhythmic augmentation and diminution. **Notate** and **perform** the rhythmic augmentation and diminution of the rhythms in *"Hava nashira."*

Notation Software Use notation software to compose an eight measure rhythm in meter in 4. Then, notate a rhythmic augmentation and diminution of your rhythm.

Footnotes

MOVEMENT

▶ *"Hava nashira"* Students can perform this movement to *"Hava nashira."* Have students form three concentric circles. The innermost circle, Voice I, walks clockwise as they sing. When Voice I finishes the first phrase, the outermost circle, Voice II walks clockwise as they sing. When Voice II finishes phrase 1, the middle circle, Voice III walks counterclockwise as they sing. Voice I sings the round three times, then stops singing and moving. In turn, Voices II and III follow suit.

BUILDING SKILLS THROUGH MUSIC

▶ **Reading** Have students read the information about William Schuman on p. 83. Have them identify the four musical vocations mentioned and give an example of his position or accomplishment while in that position.

SKILLS REINFORCEMENT

▶ **Singing** Invite students to sing this ostinato for *"Hava nashira"* and play it on resonator bells as the class sings.

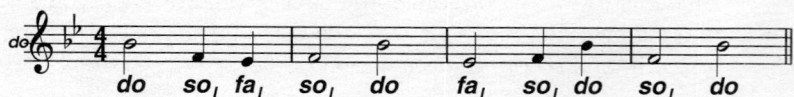

do so₁ fa₁ so₁ do   fa₁ so₁ do so₁ do

do   so, fa,   so,   do   fa,   so, do   so,   do

▶ **Reading** For more practice using standard symbols to notate rhythmic augmentation and diminution of *"Do, Re, Me, Fa"* and *"Hava nashira,"* see Resource Book p. D-11.

For additional reading practice, invite students to perform a two-part rhythm accompaniment to *"Hava nashira"* on p. 492, or Resource Book E-11.

William Schuman

William Schuman (1910–1992) is one of the most honored American musicians of the twentieth century. Beginning with a tango composed at age 16, his works include ten symphonies, three concertos, five ballets, and even a "baseball opera" (*The Mighty Casey*). In 1943, his cantata, *A Free Song*, won the first Pulitzer Prize in Music.

In addition to his talents as a composer, Schuman was an innovative music educator, administrator, and arts advocate. He served as president of the Juilliard School of Music and later as president of Lincoln Center for the Performing Arts, both in New York City.

Listen to this classroom discussion in which William Schuman talks about *Chester* and William Billings.

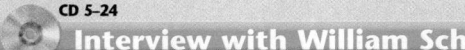

CD 5-24
Interview with William Schuman

This historic recording was made in the mid-1960s while Schuman was president of Lincoln Center.

A New England Overture

The hymn tune *Chester* was written in 1770 by William Billings, one of America's earliest native-born composers. During the American Revolution, this melody could be heard around campfires, played by fifers, and sung as a marching song by the Continental army.

Listen to this arrangement of *Chester* by William Schuman. **Identify** the augmentation and diminution of the *Chester* melody when you hear it.

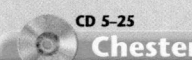

CD 5-25
Chester

from *New England Triptych*
by William Schuman
Chester was named for a town in colonial Massachusetts.

2 DEVELOP

Moving

6c Play *"Hava nashira"* **CD 5-16** and have students tap, then step, a quarter-note beat while listening to the song. Then tap, then step, a half-note beat.

Notating

6c Direct students to identify the rhythmic structure of the song (AAA') on p. 82. Have them identify the number of measures in the song (12). Help them discover that augmented notation of the song would have twice as many measures (24), and that diminished notation would have half the measures (6). (See Skills Reinforcement, on p. 82 for more practice with notation.)

Singing

1c Invite students to listen to *"Hava nashira"* **CD 5-16**. Use the Pronunciation Practice track **CD 5-18** and Resource Book p. A-11 to teach students the Hebrew pronunciation.

1d Have students sing *"Hava nashira"* in unison, then as a two-, then three-part round. Then, have students tap a steady quarter-note beat as they sing the song in augmentation, and then in diminution.

Listening

5b Discuss with students the information on William Schuman in Music Makers. Listen to *Interview with William Schuman* **CD 5-24** and discuss Schuman's comments about his own music.

6c Play the recording of *Chester* **CD 5-25**, and invite students to indicate when they hear augmentation and when they hear diminution. Direct students to the *Chester* theme in Spotlight On below, as they listen.

3 CLOSE

Skill: READING   **ASSESSMENT**

5a **Performance/Observation** Have students read and perform the original, augmented, and diminished notations of *"Hava nashira."* Observe students' ability to perform each version accurately.

SPOTLIGHT ON

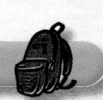

▶ **The Music** Write the theme of "Chester" (in C major) on the board and invite students to sight-read the melody as they listen to both the interview with William Schuman and the listening selection.

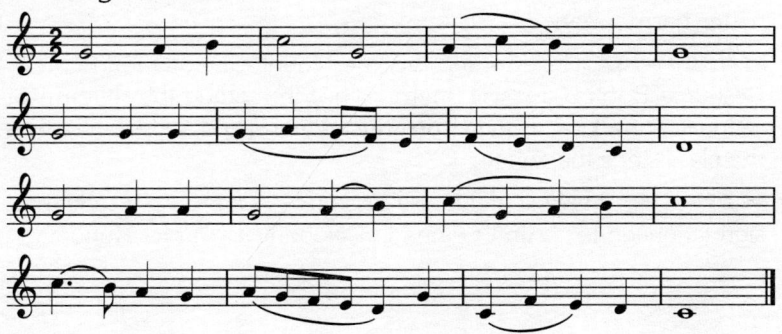

SCHOOL TO HOME CONNECTION

▶ **Interview** Invite students to interview older family members or friends to find a choral connection in their lives. Questions students may ask include: How were you taught to sing in school, in a community choir, or in a choir at a place of worship? What are your memories of performing in or listening to choral singing? What songs or choral pieces are your favorites?

TECHNOLOGY/MEDIA LINK

Web Site Ask students to visit *www.sfsuccessnet.com* to research further the life and work of composer William Schuman. Invite students to visit *www.sfsuccessnet.com* and discover historical facts on the music of Israel.

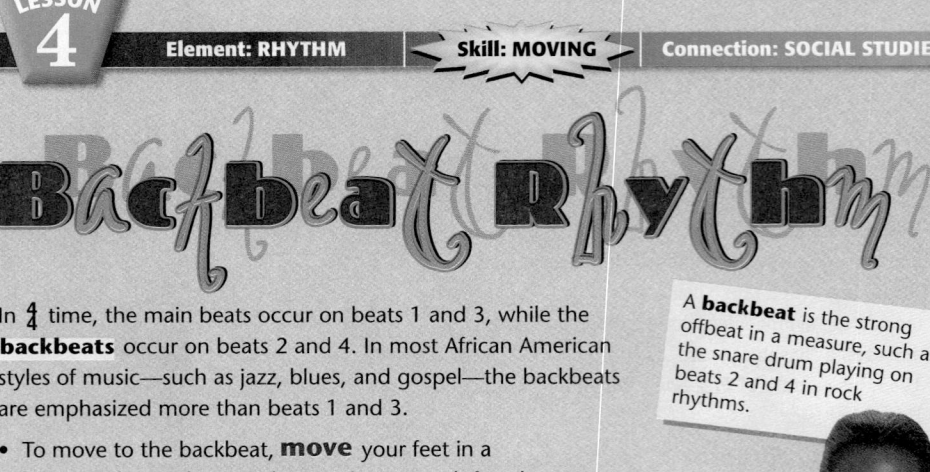

Backbeat Rhythm

LESSON AT A GLANCE

Element Focus **RHYTHM** Backbeat

Skill Objective **MOVING** Move to and clap the backbeat of a song

Connection Activity **SOCIAL STUDIES** Discuss the role of music in the American Civil Rights movement

MATERIALS

- "Ain't Gonna Let Nobody Turn Me 'Round" **CD 5-26**
  Recording Routine: Intro (4 m.); v. 1; interlude (4 m.); v. 2; interlude (10 m.); v. 3; coda
- **Resource Book** pp. G-9, I-9

VOCABULARY

backbeat

♦ ♦ ♦ ♦ National Standards ♦ ♦ ♦ ♦

1c Sing music from diverse cultures
1d Sing music written in two parts
7a Students evaluate the music they perform
8b Identify ways music relates to social studies
9a Describe characteristics of music styles from a variety of cultures

MORE MUSIC CHOICES

For more African American songs with a backbeat:
"A Brand New Day," p. 7
"Lean on Me," p. 14

1 INTRODUCE

8b Have the class read the lyrics of "Ain't Gonna Let Nobody Turn Me 'Round" in unison. Make a list with students of words that describe the tone of these lyrics. (brave, hopeful, strong, determined, positive) Explain that this is a song of the Civil Rights movement, and share the information in Spotlight On below. Tell students that *turn me 'round* means not going back to earlier times.

In $\frac{4}{4}$ time, the main beats occur on beats 1 and 3, while the **backbeats** occur on beats 2 and 4. In most African American styles of music—such as jazz, blues, and gospel—the backbeats are emphasized more than beats 1 and 3.

> A **backbeat** is the strong offbeat in a measure, such as the snare drum playing on beats 2 and 4 in rock rhythms.

- To move to the backbeat, **move** your feet in a left–together–right–together motion on each four-beat pattern.
- Start by counting all the beats as you move.
- When everyone is moving together, add the claps on backbeats 2 and 4.

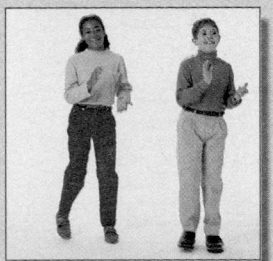

▲ **1.** Left

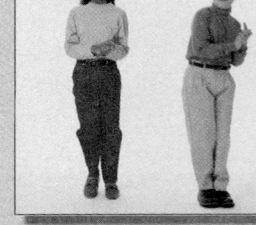

▲ **2.** Together

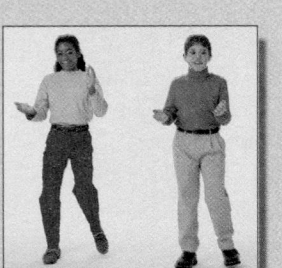

▲ **3.** Right

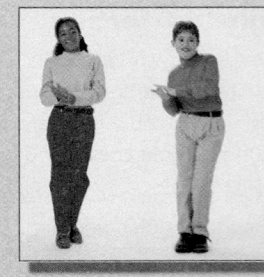

▲ **4.** Together

Backbeat Clap Movement

$\frac{4}{4}$

Feet: L - together R - together L - together R - together

84

Footnotes

SPOTLIGHT ON

8b ▶ **Civil Rights Songs** The Civil Rights movement of the 1950s and 1960s reworked many older African American spirituals and labor songs into topical songs used in marches, sit-ins, protests, and gatherings. "This Little Light of Mine," p. 232, is a good example of a modified spiritual, and "We Shall Overcome" is an example of a revamped labor song. Many of these songs are naturally conducive to participation by everyone, and new verses may easily be created by changing just a few words.

BUILDING SKILLS THROUGH MUSIC

▶ **Language** Have students read the lyrics of "Ain't Gonna Let Nobody Turn Me Around" on p. 85 and write a paragraph to paraphrase the lyrics of the song. Ask them to match the tone of the lyrics, but avoid using the exact same words.

SKILLS REINFORCEMENT

1d ▶ **Singing** Your students can learn to sing harmony for "Ain't Gonna Let Nobody Turn Me 'Round" by singing the notes a third lower than the melody notes. On the melody note E in an E-minor chord, have students sing the note B (a fourth lower) for better harmonization.

▶ **Recorder** The soprano recorder countermelody found on Resource Book p. I-9 will offer practice in reading the rhythms of "Ain't Gonna Let Nobody Turn Me 'Round" and add harmony as the class sings the song.

▶ **Signing** Have students use Resource Book p. G-9 to learn sign language for "Ain't Gonna Let Nobody Turn Me 'Round."

Spirituals with a Backbeat

Many spirituals have a strong sense of backbeat. The song "Ain't Gonna Let Nobody Turn Me 'Round" is an African American spiritual that was sung during the Civil Rights struggles of the 1960s.

Sing "Ain't Gonna Let Nobody Turn Me 'Round." When you know the song well, add the movement and clapping patterns on the backbeats.

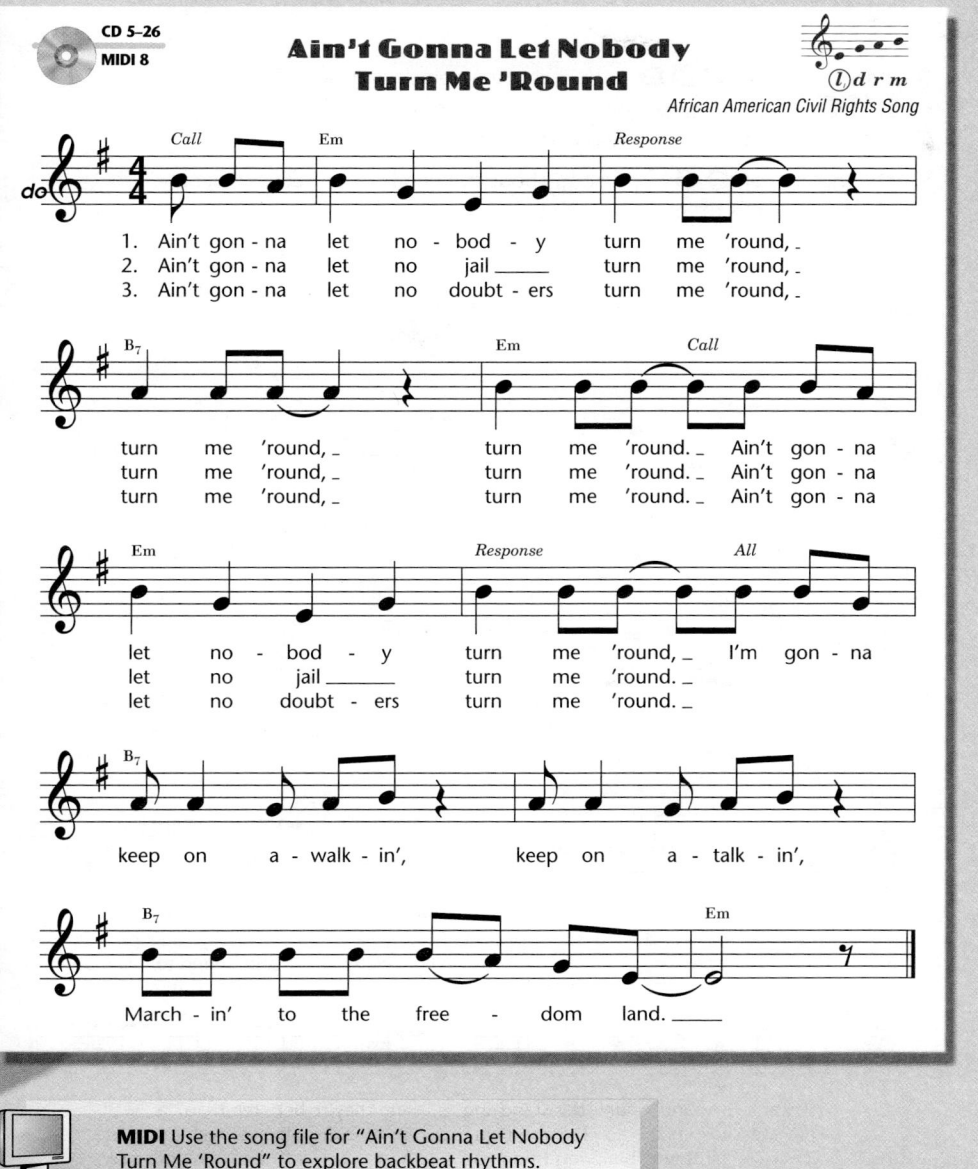

MIDI Use the song file for "Ain't Gonna Let Nobody Turn Me 'Round" to explore backbeat rhythms.

Unit 3 **85**

2 DEVELOP

Moving

Have students count 1-2-3-4 and clap on beats 1 and 3. Point out that these beats often get the most emphasis in music. In most African American musical styles, however, the accents come on the backbeats: beats 2 and 4.

Help students count the beats 1-2-3-4 as they step left–together–right–together, then clap on beats 2 and 4, as shown on p. 84.

Singing

Invite students to

- Take turns practicing the *call* part as soloists.
- Sing "Ain't Gonna Let Nobody Turn Me 'Round" **CD 5-26** with soloists singing the *call* and the class singing the *response*.
- Add the stepping movement while singing the song again.

Listening

Ask students to bring in other recordings that use a backbeat. See More Music Choices for two more songs that have a backbeat.

Creating

Have students fill in the blank to create a new verse for "Ain't Gonna Let Nobody Turn Me 'Round."

"Ain't gonna let _____ turn me 'round."

3 CLOSE

 Skill: MOVING **ASSESSMENT**

Performance/Self-Assessment Ask students to rate their ability to perform the movement pattern and clap the backbeat while singing "Ain't Gonna Let Nobody Turn Me 'Round" **CD 5-26.**

CHARACTER EDUCATION

▶ **Commitment** Tell students that the people who worked for the Civil Rights movement demonstrated great commitment to their beliefs. Ask students what it means to stand strong in their beliefs? How can they do this without offending others? Remind them commitment demands great perseverance and effort. Have them think about some commitments they make every day (making their bed every morning, telling the truth, turning in homework on time). Were they able to keep these commitments? If so, how did that make them feel? What gets in the way of keeping commitments? Have students write a commitment down on a piece of paper that they can keep for six weeks, along with the things that might prevent them from keeping the commitment. In six weeks, ask them to evaluate how well they were able to honor their commitments.

TECHNOLOGY/MEDIA LINK

MIDI/Sequencing Software Use the computer, keyboard, and MIDI sequencing software to play back the MIDI song file of "Ain't Gonna Let Nobody Turn Me 'Round." After students sing along with the MIDI accompaniment, invite them to

- Record a new percussion track.
- Find a bass drum and a snare drum keyboard setting.
- Practice playing the bass drum on beats 1 and 3 and the snare drum on beats 2 and 4.
- Turn off the prerecorded percussion track and rehearse a new track, using the above rhythms.

Students may work in pairs, if desired, one playing the snare drum part and one playing the bass drum part.

Unit 3 *Learning the Language of Music*

LESSON AT A GLANCE

Element Focus   **FORM** aaba and AABA form

Skill Objective   **LISTENING** Listen to and identify aaba (phrases) and AABA (sections) form

Connection Activity   **SOCIAL STUDIES** Discuss current social issues as conveyed by lyrics of a song

MATERIALS
- "Bridges"   CD 5-28
  Recording Routine: Intro (2 m.); v. 1; interlude (2 m.); v. 2; instrumental; v. 3; coda
- *Jesu, Joy of Man's Desiring*   CD 5-30
- **Resource Book** pp. I-10, I-11
- guitars, Autoharps, keyboards, or other chordal instruments
- various classroom percussion instruments

VOCABULARY
bridge   *obbligato*   chorale   cantata

◆ ◆ ◆ ◆ **National Standards** ◆ ◆ ◆ ◆
2d Perform simple accompaniments by ear
6c Understand and use basic principles of rhythm in music analysis
8b Identify ways music relates to social studies
9b Classify high-quality musical works by historical period

MORE MUSIC CHOICES
For more experience with aaba form:
"Everybody Loves Saturday Night," p. 296
"What a Wonderful World," p. 62

1 INTRODUCE

Explain to students that when discussing form, a lower-case letter represents a phrase (or small group of one or two phrases), and an uppercase letter represents a large section (containing multiple phrases).

Musical Bridges

The musical form **a a b a** is the most common popular song form. In an **a a b a** song, the **a** phrases are basically the same. The **b** phrase is different from the **a** phrase and provides variety and contrast.

Sing "Bridges," an **a a b a** song about building bridges between people.
Describe how the **b** phrase is different.

CD 5–28

Bridges

s l t d r m f s

Words and Music by Bill Staines

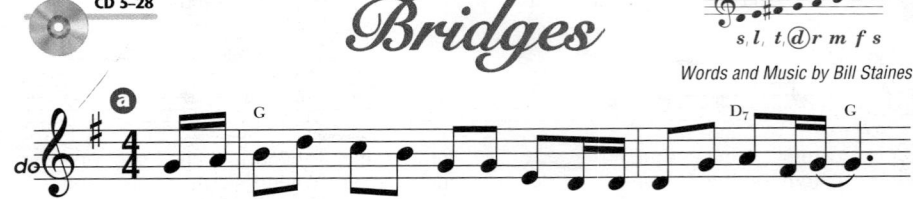

1. There are bridg-es, bridg-es in the sky, They are shin-ing in the sun.
2. There are can-yons, there are can-yons, They are yawn-ing in the night.
3. Let us build a bridge of mu-sic, Let us cross it with a song.

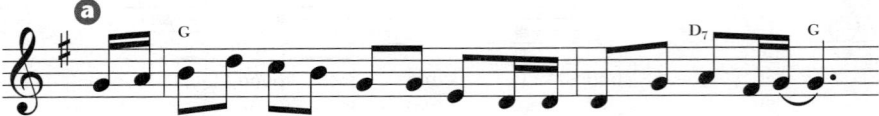

They are stone and steel and wood and wire, They can change two things to one.
They are rank and bit-ter an-ger, They are all de-void of light.
Let us span an-oth-er can-yon, Let us right an-oth-er wrong.

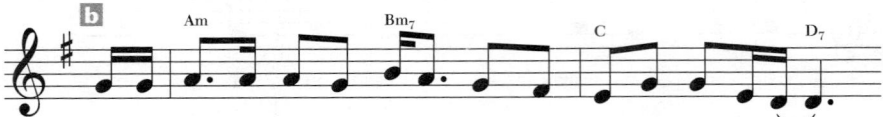

They are lan-guag-es and let-ters, They are po-et-ry and all.
They are fear and blind sus-pi-cion, They are ap-a-thy and pride,
And if some-one should ask us Where we're off and bound to-day,

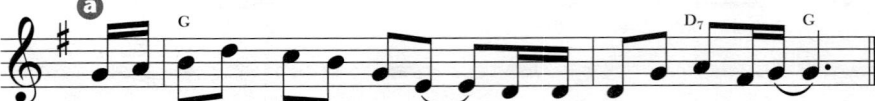

They are love and un-der-stand-ing, And they're bet-ter than a wall.
They are dark and so fore-bod-ing, And they're oh, so ver-y wide.
We will tell them "build-ing bridg-es," And be off and on our way.

86

Footnotes

SKILLS REINFORCEMENT

▶ **Recorder** Invite students to learn the alto and soprano recorder countermelodies for "Bridges" on Resource Book pp. I-10 and I-11. Students should practice whispering the sylla-ble *daah* as they begin each note to achieve a legato articulation.

BUILDING SKILLS THROUGH MUSIC

▶ **Language** Have students identify the metaphors used in the lyrics of "Bridges." Then ask them to list the words that expand upon and give [mean]ing to each metaphor.

ACROSS THE CURRICULUM

8b ▶ **Social Studies** Discuss the song text of "Bridges." What are some of the "canyons of darkness" we must bridge to help heal anger and suspicion in our world today? How do we begin to bridge these canyons and find peace and understanding with others?

Encourage students to read *The Day the Earth Was Silent* by Michael McGuffee (Inquiring Voices Press, 1996), a moving and thought-provoking story about young people working together to promote peace, cooperation, and social justice. In spite of being asked "Why try?" the children in the story find a way to make the world a better place.

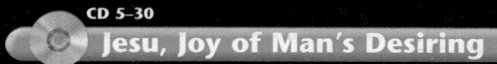
The Joy of Bach

Listen to *Jesu, Joy of Man's Desiring*, by Johann Sebastian Bach. The listening map will help you analyze the form.

by Johann Sebastian Bach

This chorale is from Bach's *Cantata No.147*. It is one of Bach's best-known pieces.

Jesu, Joy of Man's Desiring

Johann Sebastian Bach

LISTENING MAP

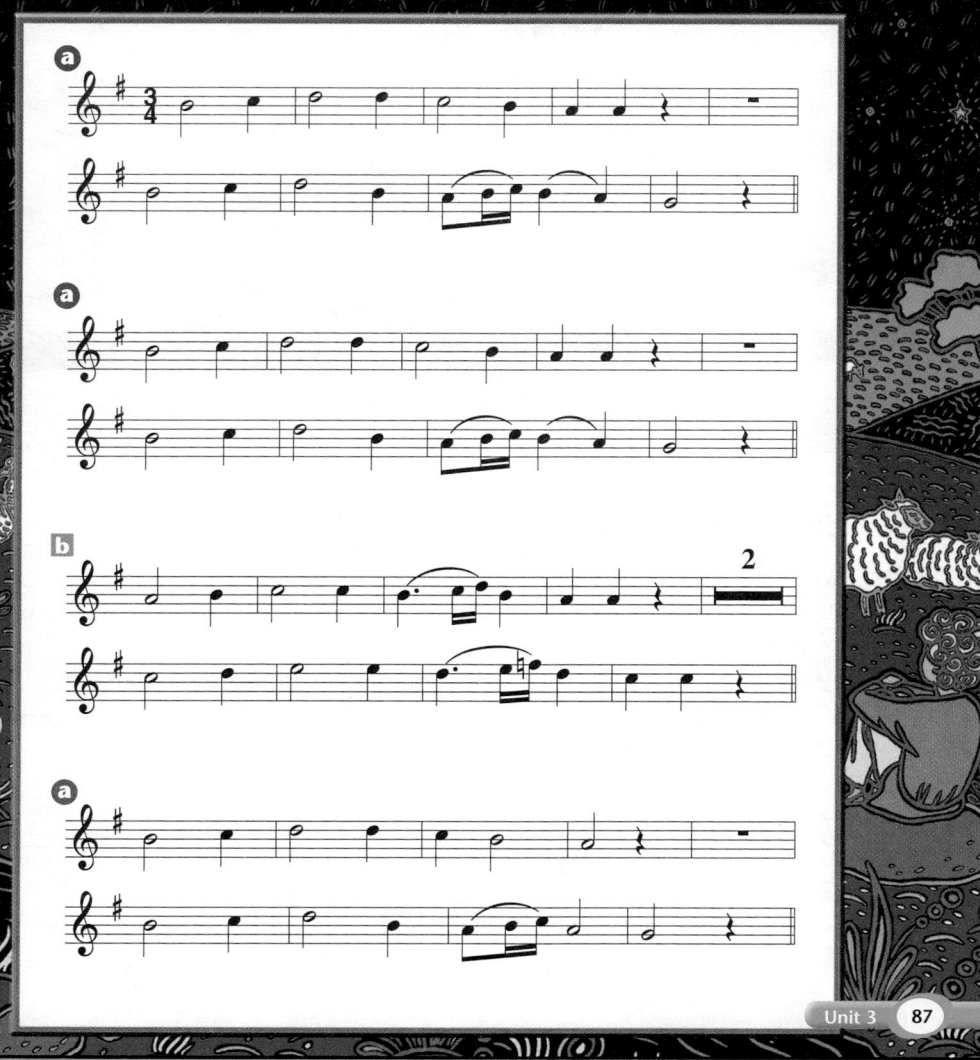

2 DEVELOP

Analyzing

Play the recording of "Bridges" **CD 5-28** and help students to follow the music, finding the phrases that are the same or very similar. (first, second, and fourth, labeled "a")

Singing

Have students sing "Bridges" along with the recording and raise a hand when they sing the contrasting melody. (third phrase, labeled "b")

8b **ASK** What is the social message of this song? (Answers will vary. See Across the Curriculum, p. 86.)

Playing

2d As the class sings "Bridges" again, invite students to accompany the song on a chordal instrument, such as guitar, keyboard, or Autoharp.

Listening

9b Help students identify music forms presented aurally. Have them

- Listen to *Jesu, Joy of Man's Desiring* **CD 5-30** while reading the chorale melody on the listening map and identify the aaba form.

- Listen again and focus on the *obbligato* (florid melody around the chorale). Tell students that combining the obbligato and chorale phrases as section (A) results in an AABA section form.

3 CLOSE

Element: FORM   **ASSESSMENT**

6c **Performance/Observation** Invite students to work in small groups to create a rhythm composition in aaba phrase form. Students may then perform their compositions for the class as their classmates listen and raise a hand when they hear the contrasting section.

SPOTLIGHT ON

▶ **The Composer** Johann Sebastian Bach (1685–1750) was one of the culminating figures of the Baroque period. Bach composed music for the professional positions he held as court composer and as church musician. In his work as organist, choir director, and composer for various churches, he composed a great many works, including nearly 300 cantatas and a book of chorale (meaning "hymn") settings for organ, called *Orgelbüchlein* ("Little Organ Book"), that were based on Lutheran chorales used during church services. He also composed chorale fantasias and preludes and fugues for organ. Bach's *Cantata 147*, from which *Jesu, Joy of Man's Desiring* is taken, was first performed in a church service in Leipzig in 1723. The title of the entire work is *Herz und Mund und Tat und Leben* ("Heart and Mouth and Deed and Life").

TECHNOLOGY/MEDIA LINK

6c **Notation Software** Invite students to find another song in aaba phrase form elsewhere in the book. Ask them to use the computer to notate the a and b phrases of the song. Then encourage students to

- Use the copy and paste functions to notate the whole song.

- Discuss the importance of repetition in music composition.

Transparency Display the listening map transparency for *Jesu, Joy of Man's Desiring*. Invite students to trace the progress of the selection with a finger on the map in their books as you trace on the overhead projection.

LESSON AT A GLANCE

Element Focus	**FORM** aaba song form
Skill Objective	**SINGING** Sing a song in aaba form
Connection Activity	**CULTURE** Relate a standard pop song to the decade of its origin in the United States

MATERIALS
- "Blue Skies" **CD 5-31**

  Recording Routine: Intro (4 m.); vocal; interlude (4 m.); vocal; coda
- guitar, electric bass, or keyboard; soprano recorders
- **Resource Book** p. H-11

VOCABULARY
standard   aaba form

◆ ◆ ◆ ◆ **National Standards** ◆ ◆ ◆ ◆

1a Sing accurately in large ensembles
2d Perform simple accompaniments by ear
6a Listen and describe events in music using appropriate terms
8b Identify ways music relates to social studies

MORE MUSIC CHOICES
For more aaba songs:
"I Got Rhythm," p. 101
"What a Wonderful World," p. 62

1 INTRODUCE

SAY Here is another song in aaba form. "Blue Skies" is a standard—a song that has been popular for years.

Share with students the information about the 1920s, when the song was written, found in Cultural Connection below.

Sing a Standard

When a song becomes well-known and is played for many years, it is often called a "standard." "Blue Skies," by the famous American composer Irving Berlin, is a standard that uses **a a b a** song form.

Sing "Blue Skies." How many measures are in each phrase? Are all of the **a** phrases exactly the same?

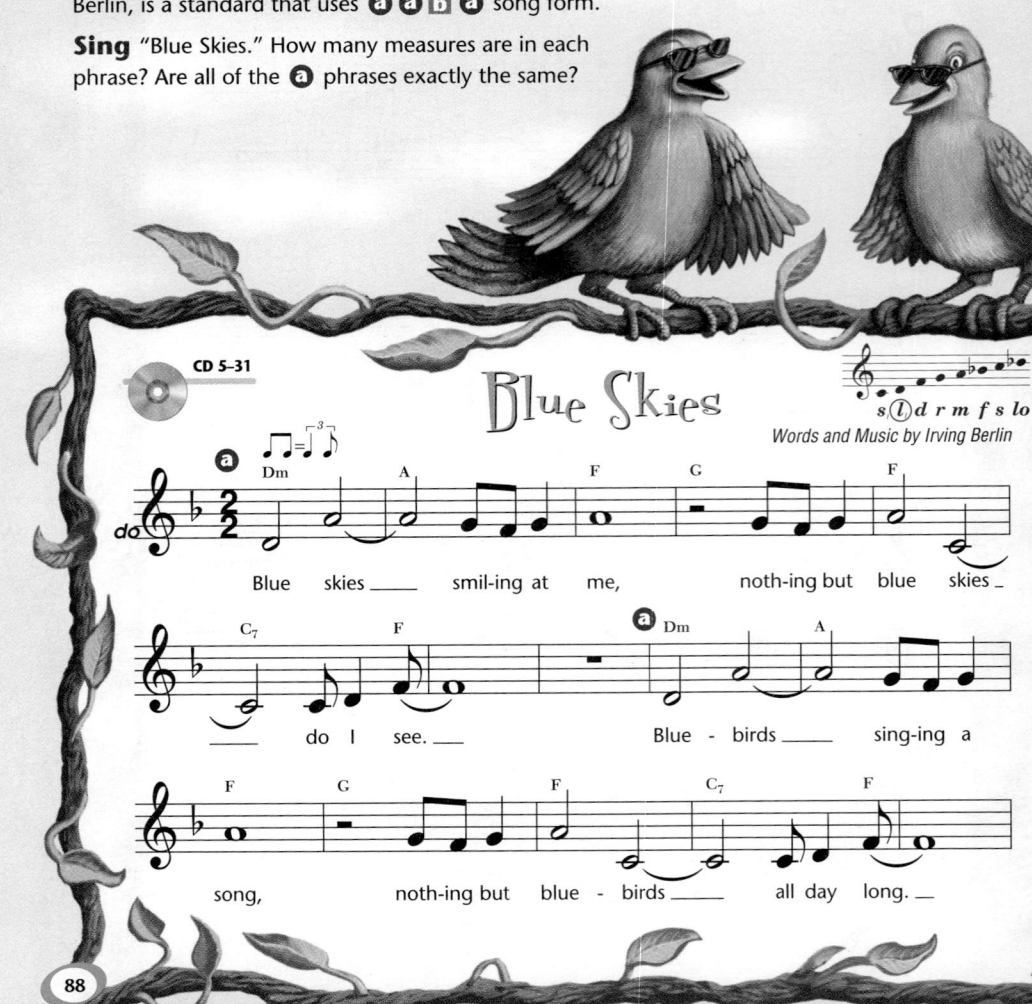

CD 5-31

Blue Skies

Words and Music by Irving Berlin

Blue skies ___ smil-ing at me, noth-ing but blue skies ___
do I see. ___ Blue - birds ___ sing-ing a
song, noth-ing but blue - birds ___ all day long. ___

88

Footnotes

CULTURAL CONNECTION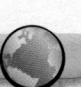

8b ▶ **The Roaring Twenties** "Blue Skies" was written in the decade from 1920 to 1930. This was a decade of important events: the Prohibition (1920); the birth of radio; silent movies; Babe Ruth's hitting 60 home runs (1927); the first talking movie, *The Jazz Singer* (1927), which featured "Blue Skies;" Charles Lindbergh's crossing the Atlantic Ocean in an airplane (1927); Mickey Mouse's debut (1928); and the stock market crash (1929).

BUILDING SKILLS THROUGH MUSIC

Math Have students gather survey information from School to Home ... 89. Ask students to include grandparents in their survey and ...esults. Ask them to create a graphical representation (circle ... or chart), which best shows the data.

87

SPOTLIGHT ON

▶ **The Composer** Russian-born songwriter Irving Berlin (1888–1989) was originally named Israel Baline. A printer's error on his first published song caused the name change, and he decided to keep it that way. Berlin's father was a solo singer in a synagogue in Russia, and when the family moved to New York City, young Irving became a singer as well, starting out as a street singer and a singing waiter. In 1910 he began singing songs he had written in Broadway musical revues. Before long Berlin was writing songs for smash hit Broadway revues and shows, and Hollywood movies. Some of his most famous songs include "God Bless America," "Easter Parade," "Alexander's Ragtime Band," "Puttin' on the Ritz," "White Christmas," and "There's No Business Like Show Business."

Pump Up the Bass

Once you know "Blue Skies," add this part on all of the ⓐ phrases. Some students can **sing** it, while others may wish to **play** it on instruments.

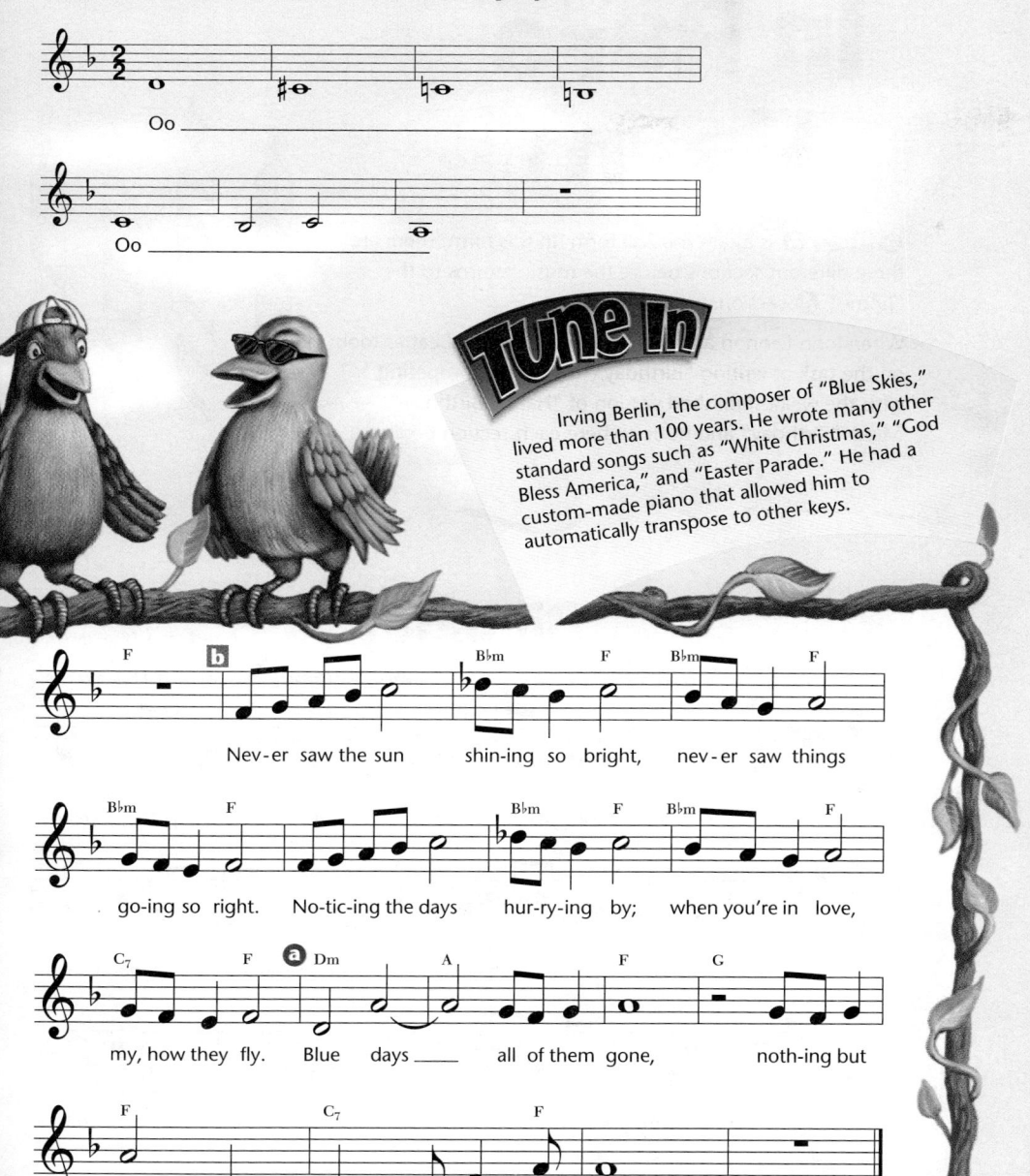

Unit 3 89

2 DEVELOP

Analyzing

Play the recording of "Blue Skies" **CD 5-31** and help students locate all of the phrases.

6a **ASK** How many measures are in each phrase? (eight)

Are all of the "a" phrases exactly the same, or are some slightly different? (the same)

How would you describe what happens to the "b" phrase of "Blue Skies"? (It repeats.)

Singing

Invite students to

- Sing the melody of "Blue Skies" **CD 5-31** with the recording.
- Learn the chromatic line on this page by singing it with pitch syllables.

Playing

2d Invite students to play the chromatic line during the a phrases on keyboard, guitar, or electric bass as the class sings "Blue Skies." Students may then learn and play the recorder part and keyboard countermelody (see Skills Reinforcement below) as the class sings the song.

3 CLOSE

Skill: SINGING ASSESSMENT

1a **Performance/Observation** Have students sing "Blue Skies" with good vocal quality while following the notation. Observe students' ability to sing this song accurately in aaba form.

SKILLS REINFORCEMENT

▶ **Recorder** To reinforce the aaba form of "Blue Skies," invite students to learn and play this recorder part with phrase a of the song. Be sure to review the fingerings for C, D, E, F, G, and A before playing. (See Playing the Recorder, p. 500.)

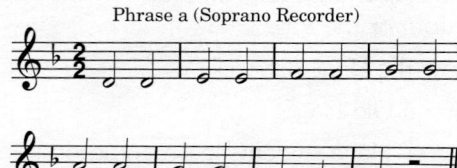

Phrase a (Soprano Recorder)

▶ **Keyboard** For more reinforcement of the form of "Blue Skies," have students learn the keyboard countermelody for the a phrase, found on p. H-11 in the Resource Book.

SCHOOL TO HOME CONNECTION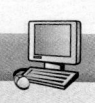

▶ **Conducting a Survey** Invite students to ask adult friends and relatives which songs by Irving Berlin they know. Encourage students to tabulate the results of their survey. (See Spotlight On, p. 88, for a partial list of songs.)

TECHNOLOGY/MEDIA LINK

Multimedia Have students create a slide show to visually represent the form of "Blue Skies." They may create three slides of the same image (labeled a) and another slide (labeled b) to show aaba form. Lead students to consider the lyrics and mood of the song when designing their slide images.

LESSON 7

LESSON AT A GLANCE

Element Focus	**FORM** ABCA form; 12-bar blues form	
Skill Objective	**PLAYING** Play a 12-bar blues bass line and a boogie-woogie bass line	
Connection Activity	**GENRE** Apply knowledge of 12-bar blues to boogie-woogie genre	

MATERIALS

- "Birthday"   **CD 6-1**
  Recording Routine: Intro (12 m.); vocal; interlude (10 m.); vocal; interlude (2 m.); vocal; coda
- *Birthday*   **CD 6-1**
- *Boogie-Woogie*   **CD 6-3**
- **Resource Book** p. H-12, J-5
- guitar, Autoharp, keyboard, or electric bass (optional)
- pencils and staff paper

VOCABULARY

triad	*D.C. al Fine*	chord progression
boogie-woogie	12-bar blues	

◆ ◆ ◆ ◆ National Standards ◆ ◆ ◆ ◆

2d Perform simple accompaniments by ear
3c Improvise unaccompanied melodies with consistent style, meter, and tonality
5c Identify standard notation symbols for pitch
6b Listen and analyze uses of form in music from diverse genres
7a Create standards for evaluating compositions
9b Classify high-quality musical works by genre

MORE MUSIC CHOICES

For more rock 'n' roll from the 1960s:
"Downtown," p. 258
"Surfin' U.S.A.," p. 260
For more experience with 12-bar blues songs:
"Key to the Highway," p. 243
"Sun Gonna Shine," p. 242

In Rare Form

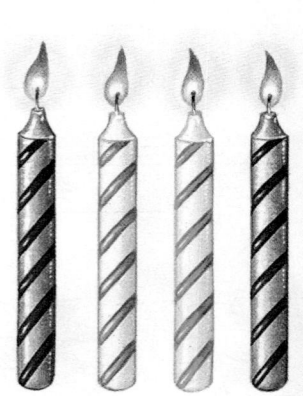

A B C A is a rare musical form. In this form, there are three different sections before the music returns to the "home" **A** section.

When John Lennon and Paul McCartney of the Beatles took on the task of writing "Birthday," they were competing with the well-established version of "Happy Birthday." **Sing** "Birthday" and notice where each section begins.

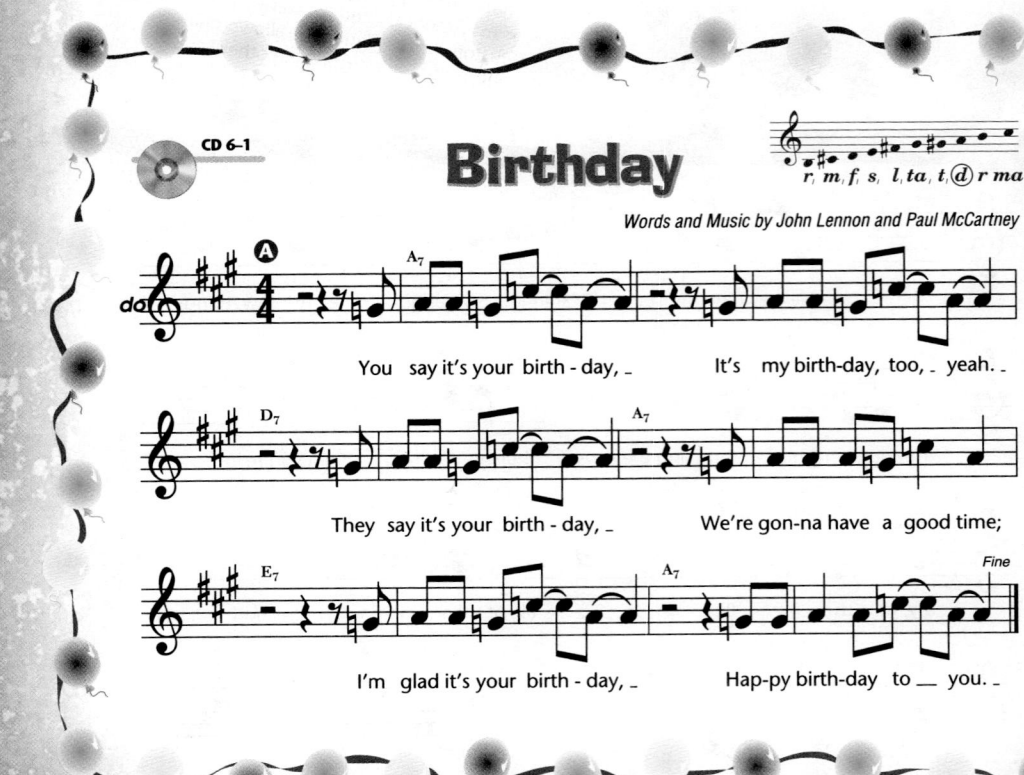

CD 6-1

Birthday

Words and Music by John Lennon and Paul McCartney

You say it's your birth-day, _ It's my birth-day, too, _ yeah.
They say it's your birth-day, _ We're gon-na have a good time;
I'm glad it's your birth-day, _ Hap-py birth-day to __ you.

90

Footnotes

TEACHER TO TEACHER

▶ **Celebrating Birthdays** Design a class Birthday Book in which each student's name and birthday are listed with space for classmates to write greetings and birthday wishes. Devote one page to each student. When a student's birthday arrives, encourage class members to write one nice thing about the person celebrating the birthday, allowing him or her to keep the birthday page. Encourage the birthday girl or boy to share family birthday traditions with the class.

BUILDING SKILLS THROUGH MUSIC

▶ **Writing** Have students write verses for the 12-bar blues form, using ... k p. J-5 as a guide. Encourage them to use literary devices such ... simile, and metaphor.

SKILLS REINFORCEMENT

6b ▶ **Singing** You may wish to reinforce aural identification and singing of major triads. Sing with students any of the songs listed here that they may know from memory and invite students to raise a hand when they hear (or realize they are singing) notes that outline a major triad. Explain that they may outline the triad from the bottom or the top.

"Michael, Row the Boat Ashore"

"You're a Grand Old Flag"

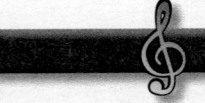 ▶ **Keyboard** Have students learn an accompaniment using roots and thirds for "Birthday" on Resource Book p. H-12.

Pump Up the Bass

Once you know "Blue Skies," add this part on all of the phrases. Some students can **sing** it, while others may wish to **play** it on instruments.

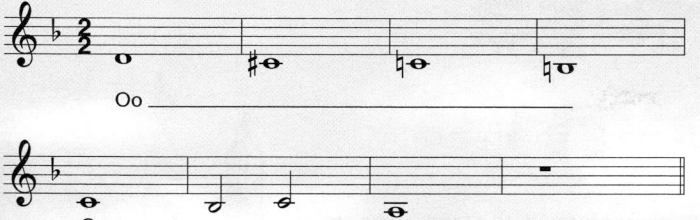

Oo _____

Oo _____

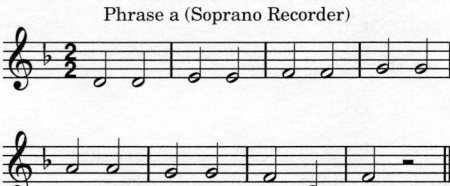

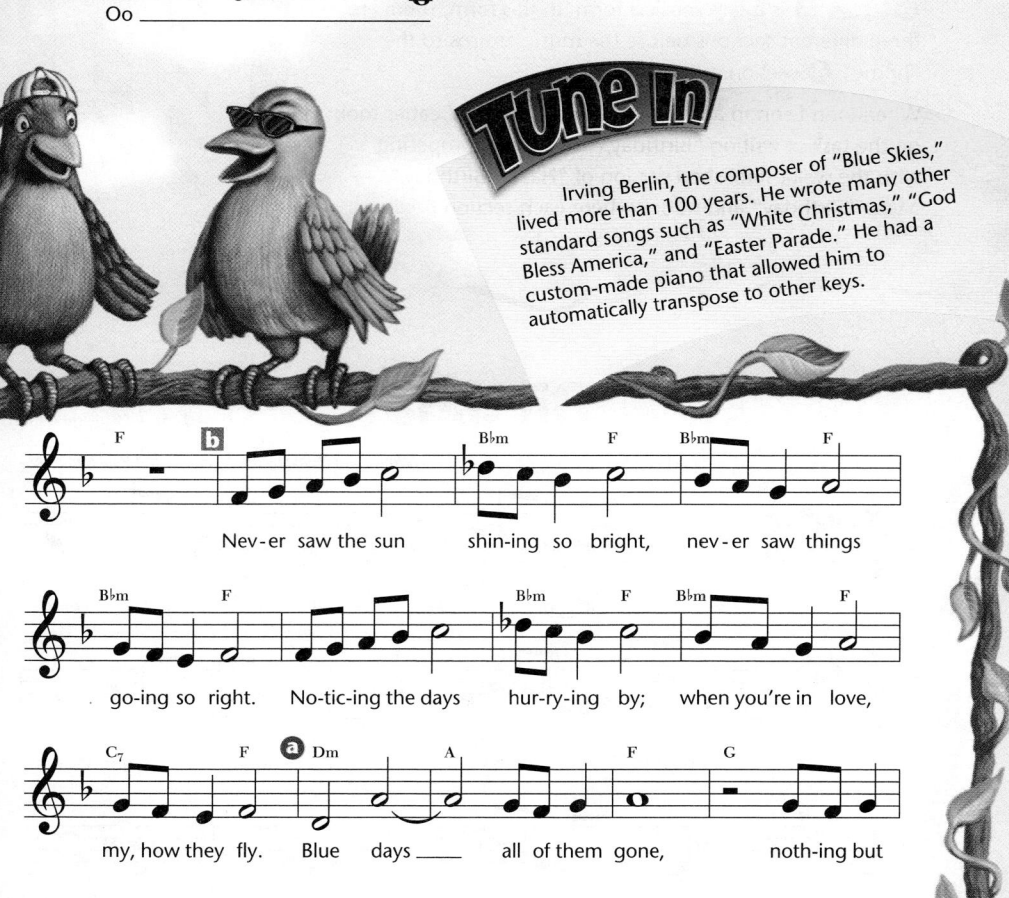

Nev-er saw the sun   shin-ing so bright,   nev-er saw things

go-ing so right.   No-tic-ing the days   hur-ry-ing by;   when you're in love,

my, how they fly.   Blue   days ___   all of them gone,   noth-ing but

blue   skies ___   from now   on. ___

Tune In

Irving Berlin, the composer of "Blue Skies," lived more than 100 years. He wrote many other standard songs such as "White Christmas," "God Bless America," and "Easter Parade." He had a custom-made piano that allowed him to automatically transpose to other keys.

Unit 3   89

---

2 DEVELOP

Analyzing

Play the recording of "Blue Skies" **CD 5-31** and help students locate all of the phrases.

6a **ASK** How many measures are in each phrase? (eight)

Are all of the "a" phrases exactly the same, or are some slightly different? (the same)

How would you describe what happens to the "b" phrase of "Blue Skies"? (It repeats.)

Singing

Invite students to

* Sing the melody of "Blue Skies" **CD 5-31** with the recording.
* Learn the chromatic line on this page by singing it with pitch syllables.

Playing

2d Invite students to play the chromatic line during the a phrases on keyboard, guitar, or electric bass as the class sings "Blue Skies." Students may then learn and play the recorder part and keyboard countermelody (see Skills Reinforcement below) as the class sings the song.

3 CLOSE

Skill: SINGING   **ASSESSMENT**

1a **Performance/Observation** Have students sing "Blue Skies" with good vocal quality while following the notation. Observe students' ability to sing this song accurately in aaba form.

SKILLS REINFORCEMENT

▶ **Recorder** To reinforce the aaba form of "Blue Skies," invite students to learn and play this recorder part with phrase a of the song. Be sure to review the fingerings for C, D, E, F, G, and A before playing. (See Playing the Recorder, p. 500.)

Phrase a (Soprano Recorder)

▶ **Keyboard** For more reinforcement of the form of "Blue Skies," have students learn the keyboard countermelody for the a phrase, found on p. H-11 in the Resource Book.

SCHOOL TO HOME CONNECTION

▶ **Conducting a Survey** Invite students to ask adult friends and relatives which songs by Irving Berlin they know. Encourage students to tabulate the results of their survey. (See Spotlight On, p. 88, for a partial list of songs.)

TECHNOLOGY/MEDIA LINK

Multimedia Have students create a slide show to visually represent the form of "Blue Skies." They may create three slides of the same image (labeled a) and another slide (labeled b) to show aaba form. Lead students to consider the lyrics and mood of the song when designing their slide images.

LESSON AT A GLANCE

Element Focus   **FORM** ABCA form; 12-bar blues form

Skill Objective   **PLAYING** Play a 12-bar blues bass line and a boogie-woogie bass line

Connection Activity   **GENRE** Apply knowledge of 12-bar blues to boogie-woogie genre

MATERIALS

- "Birthday"   **CD 6-1**

   Recording Routine: Intro (12 m.); vocal; interlude (10 m.); vocal; interlude (2 m.); vocal; coda

- *Birthday*   **CD 6-1**
- *Boogie-Woogie*   **CD 6-3**
- **Resource Book** p. H-12, J-5
- guitar, Autoharp, keyboard, or electric bass (optional)
- pencils and staff paper

VOCABULARY

triad   *D.C. al Fine*   chord progression

boogie-woogie   12-bar blues

◆ ◆ ◆ ◆ National Standards ◆ ◆ ◆ ◆

2d Perform simple accompaniments by ear

3c Improvise unaccompanied melodies with consistent style, meter, and tonality

5c Identify standard notation symbols for pitch

6b Listen and analyze uses of form in music from diverse genres

7a Create standards for evaluating compositions

9b Classify high-quality musical works by genre

MORE MUSIC CHOICES

For more rock 'n' roll from the 1960s:

"Downtown," p. 258

"Surfin' U.S.A.," p. 260

For more experience with 12-bar blues songs:

"Key to the Highway," p. 243

"Sun Gonna Shine," p. 242

In Rare Form

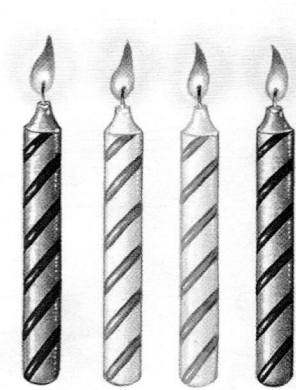

Ⓐ Ⓑ Ⓒ Ⓐ is a rare musical form. In this form, there are three different sections before the music returns to the "home" Ⓐ section.

When John Lennon and Paul McCartney of the Beatles took on the task of writing "Birthday," they were competing with the well-established version of "Happy Birthday." **Sing** "Birthday" and notice where each section begins.

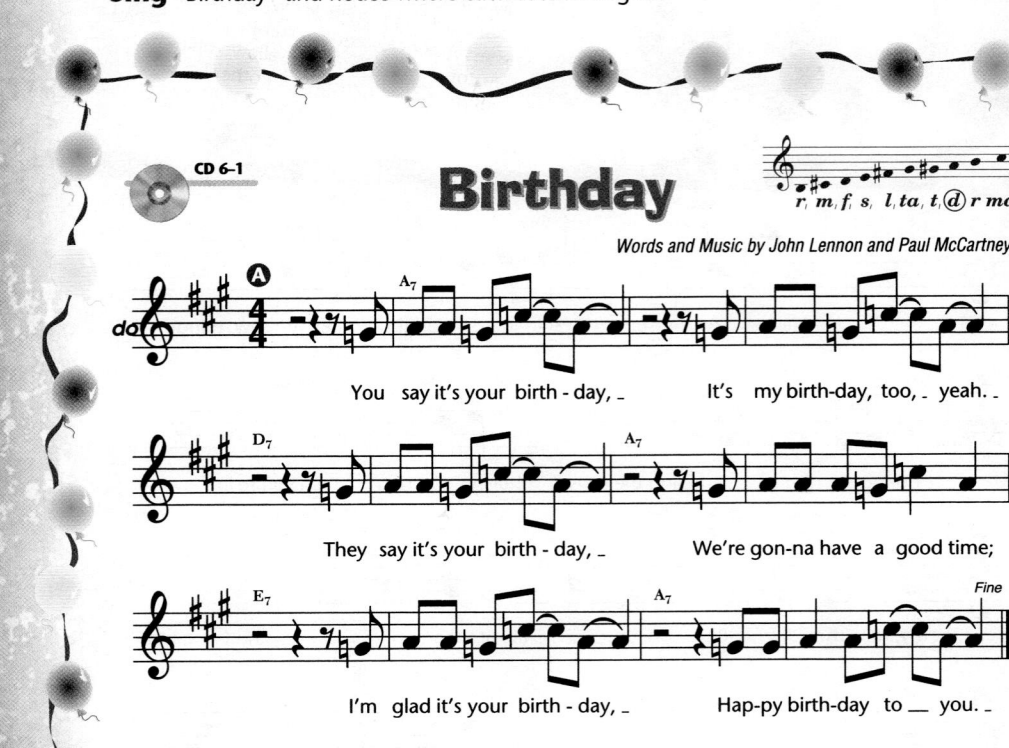

CD 6-1

Birthday

Words and Music by John Lennon and Paul McCartney

r, m, f, s, l, ta, t, (d) r ma

Ⓐ   A₇

You   say it's your birth - day, _   It's   my birth-day, too, _ yeah. _

D₇   A₇

They   say it's your birth - day, _   We're gon-na have a good time;

E₇   A₇   *Fine*

I'm glad it's your birth - day, _   Hap-py birth-day to __ you. _

Footnotes

TEACHER TO TEACHER

▶ **Celebrating Birthdays** Design a class Birthday Book in which each student's name and birthday are listed with space for classmates to write greetings and birthday wishes. Devote one page to each student. When a student's birthday arrives, encourage class members to write one nice thing about the person celebrating the birthday, allowing him or her to keep the birthday page. Encourage the birthday girl or boy to share family birthday traditions with the class.

BUILDING SKILLS THROUGH MUSIC

▶ **Writing** Have students write verses for the 12-bar blues form, using Resource Book p. J-5 as a guide. Encourage them to use literary devices such as symbolism, simile, and metaphor.

SKILLS REINFORCEMENT

6b ▶ **Singing** You may wish to reinforce aural identification and singing of major triads. Sing with students any of the songs listed here that they may know from memory and invite students to raise a hand when they hear (or realize they are singing) notes that outline a major triad. Explain that they may outline the triad from the bottom or the top.

"Michael, Row the Boat Ashore"

"You're a Grand Old Flag"

▶ **Keyboard** Have students learn an accompaniment using roots and thirds for "Birthday" on Resource Book p. H-12.

These items from the Beatles era are now collectors' items. ▶

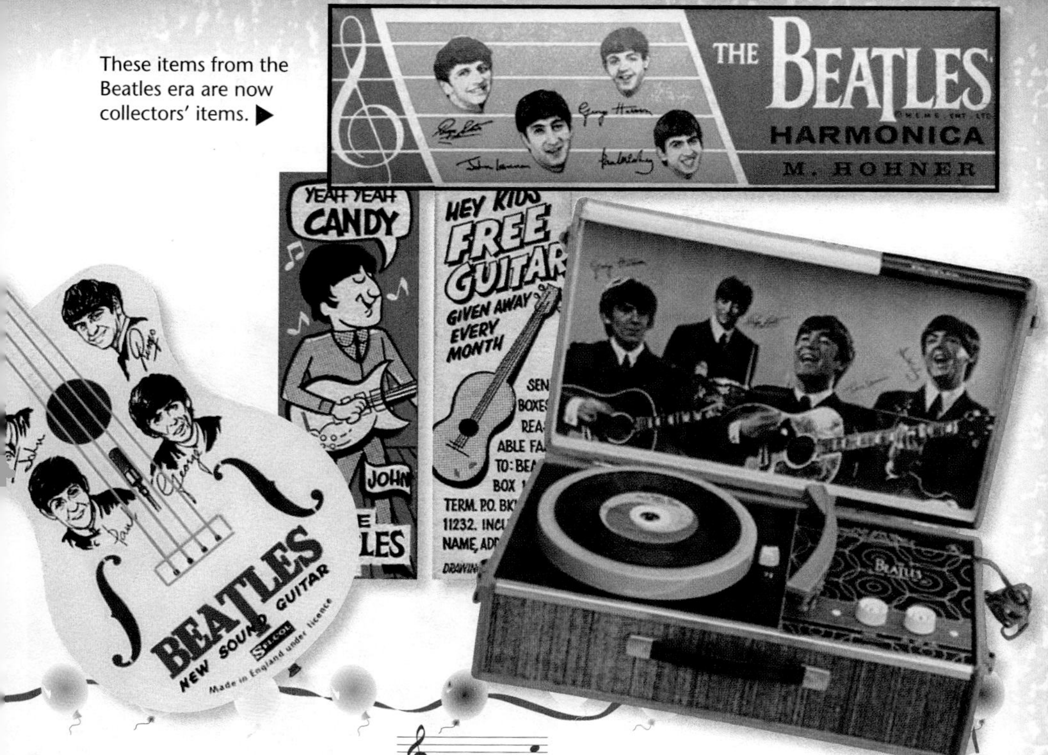

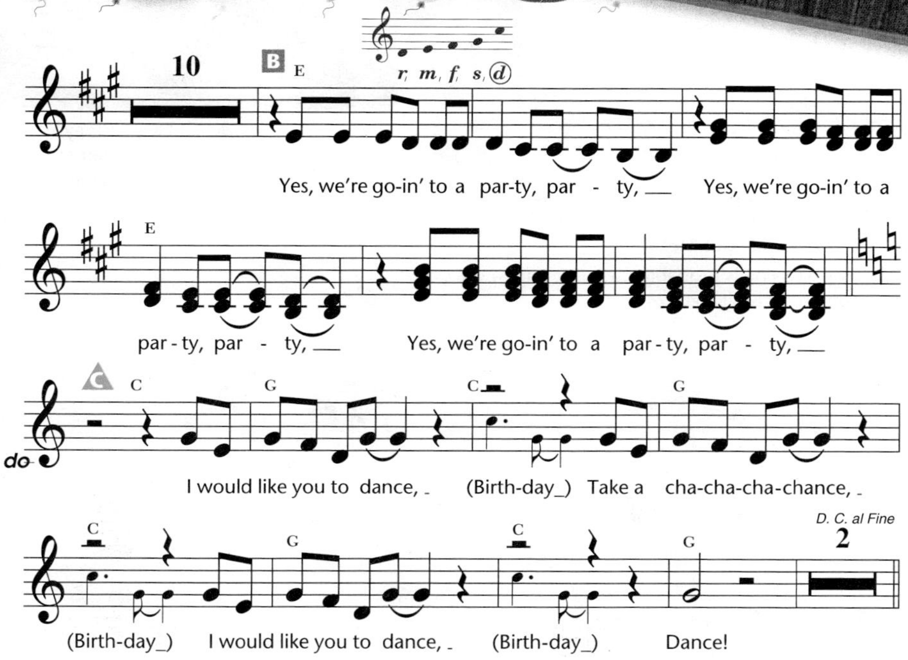

THE **BEATLES**
THEME, ENT., LTD.
HARMONICA
M. HOHNER

YEAH YEAH CANDY

HEY KIDS FREE GUITAR GIVEN AWAY EVERY MONTH

BEATLES NEW SOUND GUITAR
Made in England under license

10 🅱 E   r, m, f, s, (d)

Yes, we're go-in' to a par-ty, par - ty, ___ Yes, we're go-in' to a

E

par - ty, par - ty, ___ Yes, we're go-in' to a par-ty, par - ty, ___

🅲 C   G   C   G

do-   I would like you to dance, _   (Birth-day_)   Take a   cha-cha-cha-chance,

C   G   C   G   *D. C. al Fine*   **2**

(Birth-day_)   I would like you to dance, _   (Birth-day_)   Dance!

Unit 3 **91**

1 INTRODUCE

SAY Many hit songs are built around a good bass line. In this lesson we will look at bass lines for the 12-bar blues and the boogie-woogie.

ASK **How many of you have heard of "The Beatles"?** (Accept a show of hands.)

SAY "The Beatles" were a British pop group that created an international sensation in the 1960s. We will use their song "Birthday" to explore ABCA form, the 12-bar blues, and boogie-woogie.

Direct students to the Beatles memorabilia on p. 91 and share with students the information in Spotlight On and School to Home Connection on p. 91.

2 DEVELOP

Analyzing

Help students identify the ABCA form presented through the music notation for "Birthday."

Play **CD 6-1** as students read the music notation.

6b ASK **What happens in the A section melody?** (It repeats the same motive over and over.)

What happens in the B section melody? (It starts with a melody, then builds parallel layers of thirds, forming triads.)

What happens in the C section melody? (Like the A section, it repeats the motive over and over.)

Singing

Invite students to sing the melody of "Birthday" **CD 6-1** with the recording.

Notating

5c Invite students to write triads based on A, E, and D, with a key signature of three sharps, and label the notes *root*, *third*, and *fifth*. Tell students to label the root 1 and count up to find the third and fifth.

continued on page 92

SPOTLIGHT ON

▶ **The Musicians** Your students may enjoy reading more about Beatles memorabilia and trivia. Suggested reading:

The Beatles: Every Little Thing: A Compendium of Witty, Weird and Ever-Surprising Facts About the Fab Four by Maxwell MacKenzie (Morrow, 1998)

The Beatles: A Reference and Value Guide, 2nd ed., by Barbara Crawford, Michael Stern, Hollis Lamon (Collector Books, 1998)

The Beatles Memorabilia Price Guide, 3rd ed., by Jeff Augsberger et al. (Antique Trader, 1997)

Who Was Eleanor Rigby...: And 908 More Questions and Answers About the Beatles by Brandon Toropov (HarperCollins, 1996)

SCHOOL TO HOME CONNECTION

▶ **Beatles Memorabilia** Invite students to scour their homes for old Beatles albums (especially LPs), buttons, lunch boxes, songbooks, books, videos, or any other Beatles memorabilia. Students may bring items in to show the class. Explain to students that items like these, if in good condition, could be valuable.

Help students to

• Write the chords for A_7, D_7, and E_7, by adding the seventh to the chord, then sing each chord.

2d • Play the B-section chords on keyboard, guitar, or Autoharp while the class sings the song.

SAY We have explored the form of "Birthday" (ABCA) and how the A_7, D_7, and E_7 chords are used in the song. We will now look at how these chords are used in a 12-bar blues form, and in boogie-woogie.

ASK Do any of you play electric guitar, or electric bass, in a rock band? (Accept a show of hands.)

SAY At a band rehearsal, someone in the band might say, "Let's play a chord progression in the key of A." This is sometimes called "jamming."

ASK What chords do you think they might play in the key of A? (A_7, D_7, and E_7)

SAY This chord progression is called the 12-bar blues and is referred to as the 12-bar blues form. The 12-bar blues is used in rock, pop, blues, boogie-woogie, country, and other styles of music.

Direct students to p. 92 and help students discover how the harmonic functions of the chords (I_7, IV_7, V_7) are used in the 12-bar blues. Guide them to understand the importance of the bass guitar part in "Birthday."

Singing

5c Have students sing up and down the I_7, IV_7, and V_7 chords in the key of A, using pitch syllables.

ASK If you put letter names to these chords, what would they be? (A_7, D_7, and E_7; the same chords are at the start of "Birthday.")

Invite students to sing the bass part (p. 92) for *Birthday* **CD 6-1.** Split the class into two groups and invite one group to sing the bass part and the other to sing the melody of "Birthday" (p. 90) with the recording.

Blues Bass

The chord progression and bass line of the **A** section of *Birthday* are based on the 12-bar blues form. This form typically uses just three different chords. Here are the three chords in the key of A. Notice that all three include the 7th.

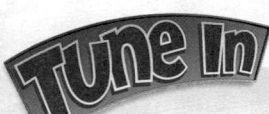

Birthday Blues

As you listen to *Birthday*, play the chords or the bass part below. Follow the color boxes and chord progression to help you **identify** the form as 12-bar blues.

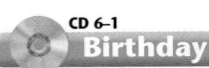

Notice the Roman numerals below the chords at the bottom of the page. They tell the step of the scale on which the chord is built. I means the first step of the scale. Rock players often say, "Let's play a I-IV-V progression in A."

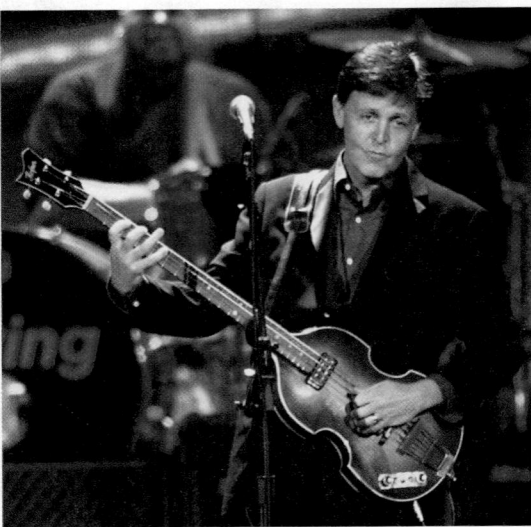

▲ Paul McCartney, playing a Hofner left-handed bass guitar.

CD 6–1
Birthday

by John Lennon and Paul McCartney
McCartney's bass line is probably the most important musical element in *Birthday*.

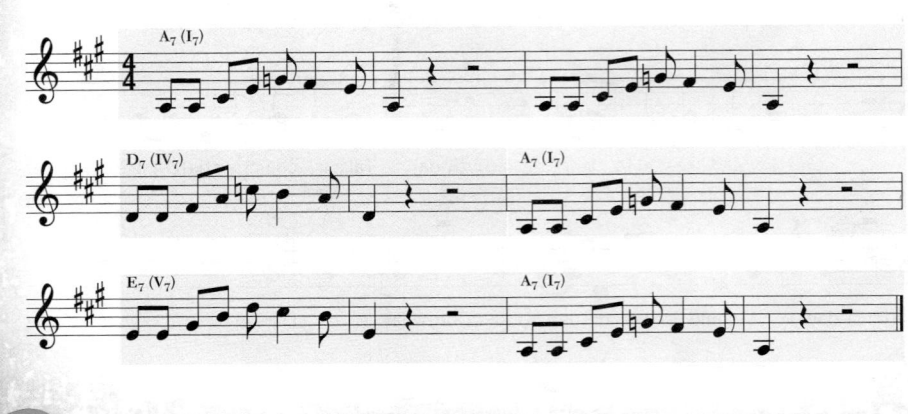

92

 Footnotes

CULTURAL CONNECTION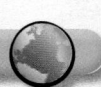

9b ▶ **Pop Culture** *Boogie-woogie* is a term created to describe a certain style of music and dance in a particular culture of the 1920s and 1930s. Ask students which words are used today to describe music of their popular culture. (Possible answers include hip-hop, rap, funk, bebop, cool jazz, world beat.) Invite students to research one or two of these cultural styles in their local library or record store and report their findings to the class.

SKILLS REINFORCEMENT

▶ **Keyboard** Help students to play the above bass lines to "Birthday" and *Boogie-Woogie* on keyboard.

2d For the two-bar patterns in "Birthday," have students use these fingerings.

If using the left hand: 5, 5, 3, 2, 1, 2, 1, 5.

Right hand: 1, 1, 2, 3, 5, 4, 3, 1.

For the two-bar patterns in *Boogie-Woogie,* have students use these fingerings.

Left hand: 5, 5, 3, 3, 1, 1, 2, 2, 1, 1, 2, 2, 1, 1, 3, 3.

Right hand: 1, 1, 2, 2, 3, 3, 4, 4, 5, 5, 4, 4, 3, 3, 2, 2.

To play along with the Tommy Dorsey recording, transpose the boogie-woogie patterns to the key of F.

Can You Boogie?

Another type of bass line that outlines chords is **boogie-woogie.** You can **play** this boogie-woogie on a keyboard instrument.

Boogie-woogie is a special blues chord progression that uses blues chords and swing rhythm. Boogie-woogie is sometimes called "eight-to-the-bar."

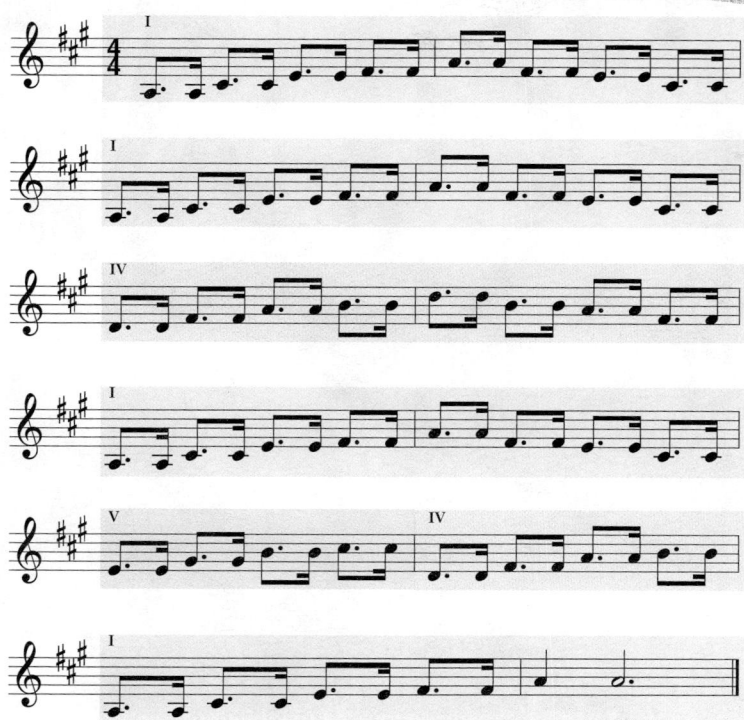

Listen to this classic example of boogie-woogie style.

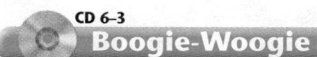

CD 6–3
Boogie-Woogie

by Pine Top Smith
as performed by the Tommy Dorsey Orchestra

Boogie-Woogie, recorded in 1938, was one of Dorsey's most successful arrangements.

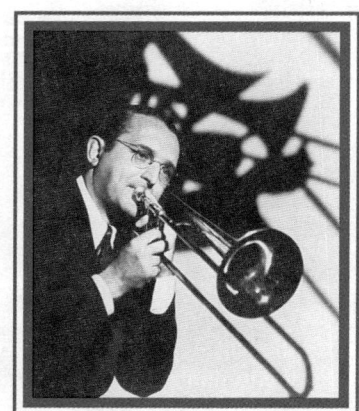

◀ Big band leader Tommy Dorsey

Encourage students to

- Play the "Birthday" bass line on keyboard with the recording.
- Play the boogie-woogie bass line on keyboard. See Skills Reinforcement, p. 92.

Listening

Have students listen to *Boogie-Woogie* **CD 6-3** to hear another example of boogie-woogie bass (in the key of F).

Creating

Encourage students to improvise a bass line on keyboard or guitar that fits the 12-bar blues form. Invite students to write their bass lines on staff paper. Then direct them to create a song using Activity Master 5 in Resource Book p. J-5.

3 CLOSE

Skill: PLAYING   **ASSESSMENT**

Performance/Peer Critique Have students play their 12-bar blues bass lines for the class on guitar or keyboard. As they play, invite each classmate to listen and evaluate each bass line and the performance of it for 12-bar blues form. Then have students take turns playing the boogie-woogie bass line and evaluating their peers' performances.

SPOTLIGHT ON

▶ **The Performers** Tommy Dorsey (1905–1956) and his brother, Jimmy (1904–1957), were born in Shenandoah, Pennsylvania, and each learned to play several instruments during childhood. Tommy gravitated toward brass and Jimmy specialized in woodwinds. Both loved jazz and popular music. The duo went to New York City in 1924 and started playing with some of the most prominent jazz players around town. They soon formed the Dorsey Brothers Orchestra and began making recordings. Sometime in 1935, however, they had some differences of opinion and split up as a musical team. Tommy started the Tommy Dorsey Orchestra (heard on *Boogie Woogie*), which featured prominent soloists and serious jazz innovators. Finally, Jimmy joined his brother's band in 1953. They had a hit TV series from 1955 to 1956.

TECHNOLOGY/MEDIA LINK

CD-ROM Have students type a blues progression into the *Band-in-a-Box* program and select a blues or boogie-woogie style to generate accompaniments. Under song settings they should uncheck *embellish chords*; accompaniment parts will contain basic chord tones. Students may solo the bass part and display notation view so they can inspect various bass line patterns. Help students to display the guitar window and click on B to show where the bass notes are located on the bass guitar fret board.

Web Site Visit *www.sfsuccessnet.com* to learn more about The Beatles and their music.

LESSON AT A GLANCE

Element Focus — **MELODY** Dorian and aeolian modes

Skill Objective **READING** Read and sing from notation a song in dorian mode

Connection Activity **SOCIAL STUDIES** Discuss the black plague as the context for a ballad

MATERIALS

- "Scarborough Fair" **CD 6-4**

  Recording Routine: Intro (4 m.); v. 1; interlude (4 m.); v. 2; interlude (4 m.); v. 3; coda

- **Music Reading Practice, Sequence 11** **CD 6-6**

- **Resource Book** pp. D-12, E-12, H-13

- keyboard, recorder, guitar

VOCABULARY

minor scale   aeolian mode   dorian mode   ionian mode

♦ ♦ ♦ ♦ **National Standards** ♦ ♦ ♦ ♦

2a Play instruments accurately alone
3a Improvise simple harmonic accompaniments
5b Sight-read melodies in treble clef
5c Identify standard notation symbols for pitch
8b Identify ways music relates to social studies

MORE MUSIC CHOICES

For practice comparing dorian mode with harmonic and melodic minor:

"Greensleeves" (melodic minor), p. 49

"Sometimes I Feel Like a Motherless Child" (harmonic minor), p. 241

1 INTRODUCE

Tell students that one-third of the population of Europe died from the black plague between 1347 and 1350. Share the information about the context of "Scarborough Fair" with students. See Across the Curriculum below.

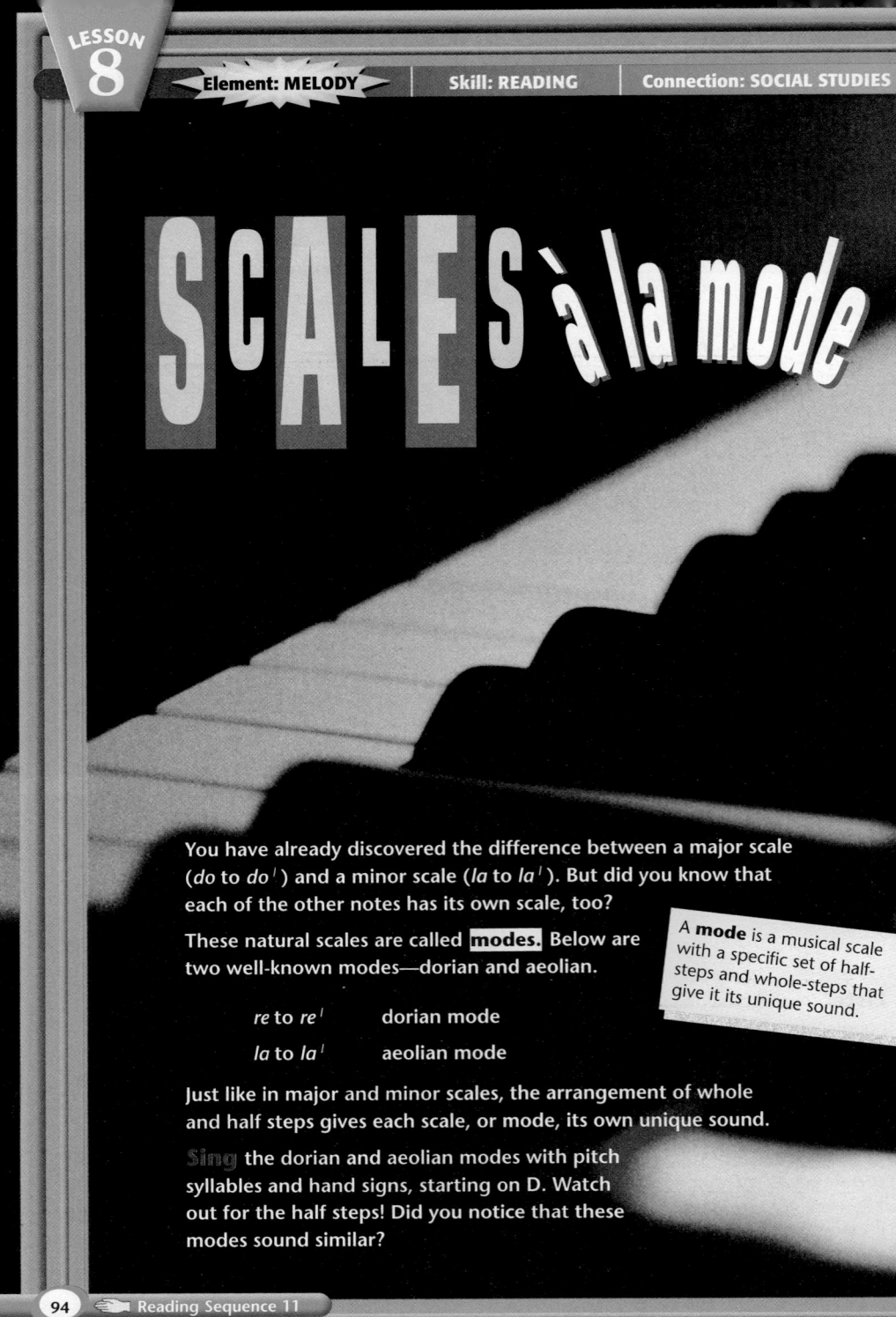

SCALES à la mode

You have already discovered the difference between a major scale (*do* to *do*¹) and a minor scale (*la* to *la*¹). But did you know that each of the other notes has its own scale, too?

These natural scales are called modes. Below are two well-known modes—dorian and aeolian.

> A **mode** is a musical scale with a specific set of half-steps and whole-steps that give it its unique sound.

| *re* to *re*¹ | dorian mode |
| *la* to *la*¹ | aeolian mode |

Just like in major and minor scales, the arrangement of whole and half steps gives each scale, or mode, its own unique sound.

Sing the dorian and aeolian modes with pitch syllables and hand signs, starting on D. Watch out for the half steps! Did you notice that these modes sound similar?

94 ◁ Reading Sequence 11

Footnotes

ACROSS THE CURRICULUM

8b ▶ **Social Studies** The seasonings mentioned in "Scarborough Fair" were used at the time of the plague to preserve dead bodies. Some say that the shirt in the song is burial clothing and that the singer feels he is dying and wishes to be remembered by a loved one. Encourage students to write a story that ends with the lyrics of the song. Have them imagine the setting for the story and illustrate it.

BUILDING SKILLS THROUGH MUSIC

▶ **Math** Tell students that at the start of the lesson, they were told that third the population of Europe died from the black plague. Ask students ermine what information they will need and what calculations they prove or disprove this statement.

Reading Sequence 11, p. 493

SKILLS REINFORCEMENT

2a
3a ▶ **Creating** Assign pairs of students to create a four-measure introduction or interlude for "Scarborough Fair" to establish dorian mode. Have one student play guitar and another play recorder.

▶ **Reading** Music Reading Worksheet D-12 in the Resource Book offers pitch syllables and hands signs for practice with the major and minor scales, and ionian, aeolian, and dorian modes.

For additional reading practice, invite students to sing a countermelody to "Scarborough Fair" on p. 493 or Resource Book E-12.

 ▶ **Keyboard** Invite students to learn to play the broken-chord keyboard accompaniment for "Scarborough Fair," on Resource Book p. H-13.

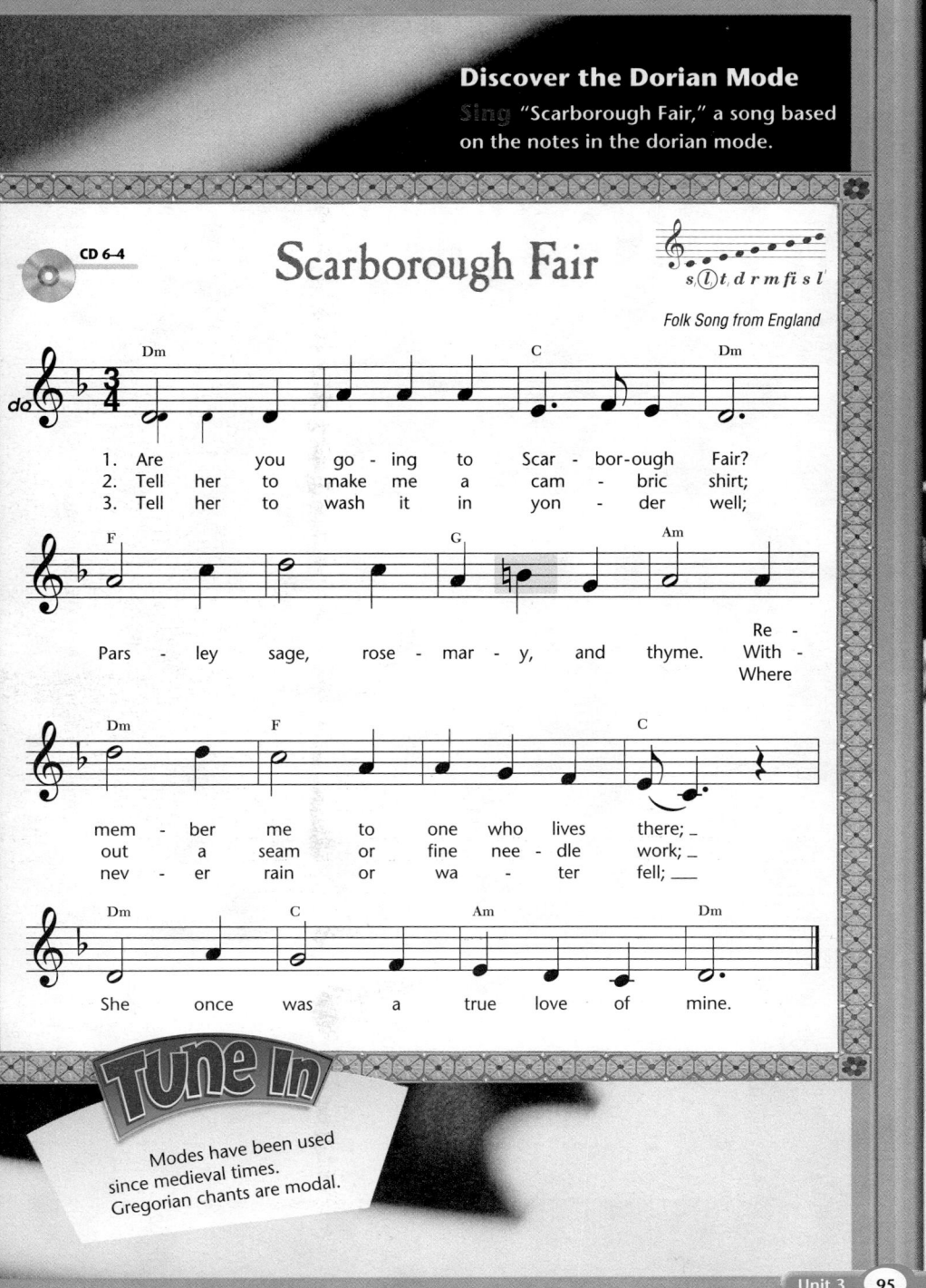

Discover the Dorian Mode

Sing "Scarborough Fair," a song based on the notes in the dorian mode.

CD 6-4

Scarborough Fair

s, (l,) t, d r m f s l

Folk Song from England

1. Are you go - ing to Scar - bor-ough Fair?
2. Tell her to make me a cam - bric shirt;
3. Tell her to wash it in yon - der well;

Pars - ley sage, rose - mar - y, and thyme. With - Where

mem - ber me to one who lives there; _
out a seam or fine nee - dle work; _
nev - er rain or wa - ter fell; ___

She once was a true love of mine.

Tune In

Modes have been used since medieval times. Gregorian chants are modal.

Unit 3 95

2 DEVELOP

Reading

5c Direct students' attention to p. 94 and introduce the term *mode* as another way musicians refer to scales.

SAY Scales can be built on each of the pitch syllables.

Have students discuss, using music terms, where the half steps in the major scale and ionian mode occur (between *mi-fa* and *ti-do*) and the pitch syllable name for the tonic (*do*).

Listening

Play the recording of "Scarborough Fair" **CD 6-4.**

ASK Is the tonality of this song major? (no)

SAY When a scale begins and ends on *la*, it is called the *la* scale, the natural minor scale, or the aeolian mode.

Reading

5c Help students use music terms to identify the key signature (one flat) and the major tonic (F-*do*). Direct attention to the final note in the song (D) and have them identify the minor tonic (*la*). Lead students to find the altered tone *fi* in measure 7. Have students sing the minor scale from *la,* to *la* with a raised *fa*. Teach the *fi* hand sign and identify this mode as the dorian mode.

Singing

Have students sing the aeolian and dorian modes on D–*la*. Then, invite students to sing "Scarborough Fair" **CD 6-4** with the recording.

Draw a dorian mode tone ladder and have students sing it, using pitch syllables. (See Teacher to Teacher below.)

3 CLOSE

Element: MELODY — ASSESSMENT

5b Performance/Observation Have students read and sing "Scarborough Fair" **CD 6-4** from the notation. Observe their ability to read from the notation and sing the song in dorian mode.

TEACHER TO TEACHER

▶ **Tone Ladders** When drawing a tone ladder with sharped tones, write the sharped tone to the right of the ladder, as shown below.

l
s
     fi
m
r
d
t
l

For more instruction in the minor scales, students may write out the tone set for *"El cóndor pasa,"* p. 46, and find that the *la* scale includes *si* (sharped *so*), making it the harmonic minor scale.

TECHNOLOGY/MEDIA LINK

Multimedia Use a digital camera to photograph the "Scarborough Fair" illustrations of the setting from the Across the Curriculum activity on p. 94. Import the drawings, one per slide, into a slide show file. Have students advance the slide show as the class sings the ballad. If a digital camera is not available, scan the illustrations into the slide show.

LESSON AT A GLANCE

Element Focus	**MELODY** Mixolydian mode
Skill Objective	**READING** Read a song in the mixolydian mode
Connection Activity	**SOCIAL STUDIES** Discuss the Ozarks region of the United States

MATERIALS

- "Harrison Town"   **CD 6-9**
  Recording Routine: Intro (4 m.); v. 1; interlude (4 m.); v. 2; coda
- **Music Reading Practice, Sequence 12**   **CD 6-11**
- **Resource Book** pp. D-14, E-13, I-12

VOCABULARY

ionian mode	mixolydian mode
aeolian mode	dorian mode

◆ ◆ ◆ ◆ **National Standards** ◆ ◆ ◆ ◆

1a Sing accurately in large ensembles
4c Arrange, using electronic media
5a Read sixteenth notes and dotted notes in duple meter
5c Identify standard notation symbols for pitch
6a Listen and describe events in music using appropriate terms

MORE MUSIC CHOICES

For more practice with mixolydian mode:
"Goin' to Boston," p. 433

1 INTRODUCE

Tell students that "Harrison Town" is a folk song from the Ozarks region of the United States. Use the information in Spotlight On below to start a discussion of this region.

Make It Modal

The notes of the *so* diatonic scale produce the mixolydian mode. There is another way to create the mixolydian mode, using *do* as the tonic. It is easy to make the *do* scale fit the mixolydian pattern by substituting *ta* for *ti* as the seventh scale degree. (Remember that *ta* is one half step lower than *ti*.)

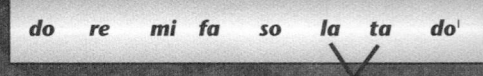
do   re   mi   fa   so   la   ta   do'

This scale shows the lowered seventh degree and is sometimes called the flatted-seventh scale, or "flat-seven scale," for short.

A Ballad from the Ozarks

Listen to the song "Harrison Town" and follow the melody. Which phrase does not include the flatted-seventh degree, *ta*? Next, **sing** the song.

Stay in the Mode

Read this mixolydian melody and **identify** the flatted-seventh. Use C as *do* to **sing** this melody.

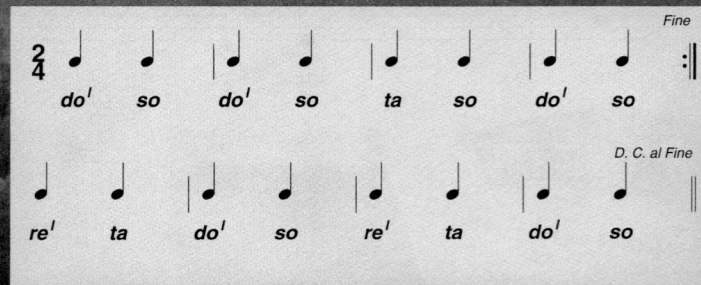

Fine

do'   so   do'   so   ta   so   do'   so

D. C. al Fine

re'   ta   do'   so   re'   ta   do'   so

96   Reading Sequence 12

Footnotes

SPOTLIGHT ON

▶ **The Ozark Mountains** Occupying about 50,000 square miles, the Ozark mountains are located in Missouri, northern Arkansas, southern Illinois, and southeastern Kansas. "Ozark," as a name, probably came from a French trading post in the region named *Aux Arc*. The area, which has many underground streams, is known for agriculture, timber, lead, and zinc. Folk music, featuring such instruments as the banjo, concertina, dulcimer, and harmonica, is popular.

BUILDING SKILLS THROUGH MUSIC

Social Studies Share the information from Spotlight On above. Have students describe the natural resources of the Ozarks and their effect on that economy.

SKILLS REINFORCEMENT

5a ▶ **Reading** Use Music Reading Worksheet on p. D-14 in the Resource Book for practice with ionian, mixolydian, dorian, and aeolian modes. Then review all of the scales and modes students have studied thus far by having them sing the scales using hand signs and pitch syllables (major diatonic scale–ionian mode, mixolydian mode, minor diatonic scale, natural minor scale–aeolian mode, dorian mode).

For additional reading practice, invite students to sing a countermelody to "Harrison Town" on p. 493, or Resource Book p. E-13.

▶ **Recorder** Encourage students to learn the alto recorder countermelody for "Harrison Town" on Resource Book p. I-12.

Reading Sequence 12, p. 493

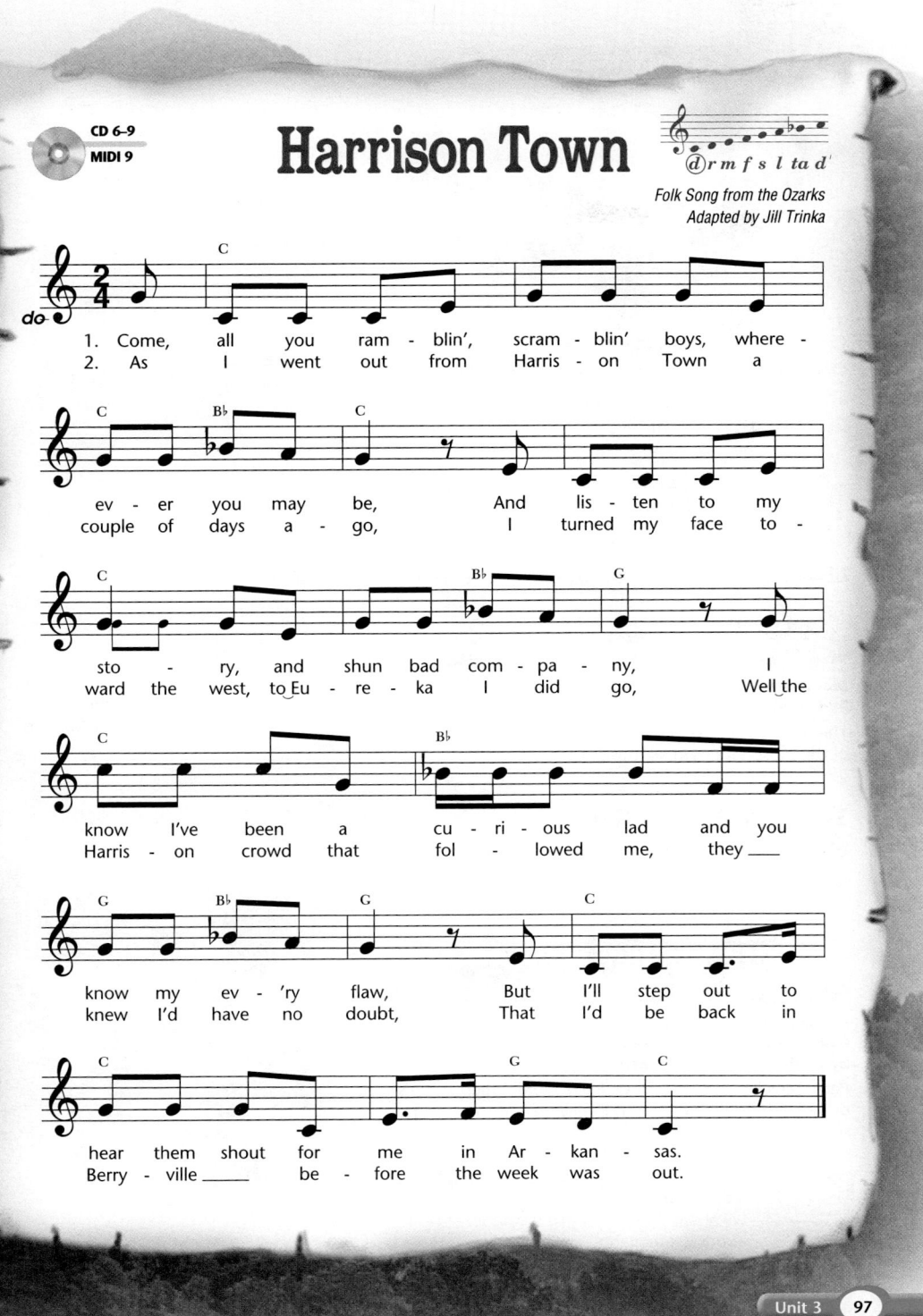

Harrison Town

Folk Song from the Ozarks
Adapted by Jill Trinka

1. Come, all you ram - blin', scram - blin' boys, where -
2. As I went out from Harris - on Town a

ev - er you may be, And lis - ten to my
couple of days a - go, I turned my face to -

sto - ry, and shun bad com - pa - ny, I
ward the west, to Eu - re - ka I did go, Well the

know I've been a cu - ri - ous lad and you
Harris - on crowd that fol - lowed me, they ___

know my ev - 'ry flaw, But I'll step out to
knew I'd have no doubt, That I'd be back in

hear them shout for me in Ar - kan - sas.
Berry - ville ___ be - fore the week was out.

2 DEVELOP

Listening

6a Play the major scale (ionian mode) on keyboard, using *C-do,* then the mixolydian mode. Ask students to iden- tify which pitch name is altered and how. (*ti;* lowered)

Play the melody of "Harrison Town." Ask students to raise their hands when they hear the lowered *ti's* (called *ta*). The ionian mode with a lowered *ti,* or *ta,* becomes a new mode called the mixolydian mode.

Have students practice singing the mixolydian mode with hand signs and pitch syllables. See Skills Reinforcement, p. 96.

Reading

5a Direct students' attention to the notation of "Harrison Town." Have students

5c • Find all of the patterns that use *do, mi,* and *so.* (mm. 1–2; 5–6; 13–14)

• Identify each lowered *ti* (*ta*). (mm. 3, 7, 10, 11)

• Sing the entire melody using pitch syllables.

Singing

1a Have students sing the mixolydian melody on p. 96 with hand signs and pitch syllables. Then have students sing "Harrison Town" **CD 6-9.**

3 CLOSE

Skill: READING   **ASSESSMENT**

5a **Performance/Observation** Have students use pitch syllables and hand signs to read the notation of "Harrison Town." Have students read the song again, but have them change each *ta* to *ti* to demonstrate their understanding of the difference between the ion- ian and mixolydian modes. Observe students' ability to accurately read a song in mixolydian mode.

TEACHER TO TEACHER

▶ **Tone Ladders** When drawing a tone ladder with flatted tones, write the flatted tone to the left of the ladder, as shown below.

	d
ta	
	l
	s
	f
	m
	r
	d

TECHNOLOGY/MEDIA LINK

4c **MIDI/Sequencing Software** Using the MIDI song file for "Harrison Town," have students arrange melodic phrases by

• Selecting the software program's graphic editor.

• Using the graphic editing features to alter the melody pitches to reflect the following modes: ionian, aeolian, dorian.

• Turning off accompaniment tracks and play back each version of the melody.

Unit 3   *Learning the Language of Mus*

LESSON AT A GLANCE

Element Focus   **MELODY** Melodic motives

Skill Objective   **LISTENING** Aurally identify a melodic motive and its transposition

Connection Activity   **SOCIAL STUDIES** Discuss the mood of the time of the American and French revolutions

MATERIALS

- "I Got Rhythm"   **CD 6-16**
  Recording Routine: Intro (4 m.); vocal; instrumental/vocal
- *Symphony No. 5 in C Minor,* Movement 1 (excerpt)   **CD 6-14**
- *New Horizons in Music Appreciation,* Movement 1 (excerpt)   **CD 6-15**
- **Resource Book** p. B-9
- keyboards or other melodic instruments
- sequencing software; VCR, TV, and rental movie (optional)

VOCABULARY

motive   transpose   retrograde   inversion

◆ ◆ ◆ ◆ National Standards ◆ ◆ ◆ ◆

1a Sing accurately in small ensembles
2b Perform easy instrumental pieces with technical accuracy
3b Improvise rhythmic variations on given melodies
6b Listen and analyze uses of pitch in music from diverse genres
6c Understand and use basic principles of intervals in music analysis
8b Identify ways music relates to social studies

MORE MUSIC CHOICES

For more experience with motives:
"Ain't Gonna Let Nobody Turn Me 'Round," p. 85
"Birthday," p. 90
For more practice in identifying melodic motives:
"Peace Like a River," p. 190
"Gonna Build a Mountain," p. 21

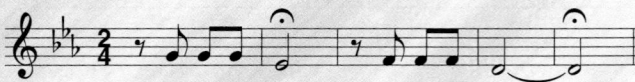

Melodic Motives

Composers use **motives** in many styles of music. Occasionally, a motive becomes very well known and is attributed to a musical composition and its composer. **Sing** or **play** this motive.

> A **motive** is a short musical idea or pattern that repeats in a composition.

Listen to an excerpt of the opening movement from this symphony.

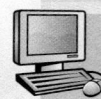
CD 6–14
Symphony No. 5 in C Minor

Movement 1
by Ludwig van Beethoven

The opening motive of Beethoven's *Fifth Symphony* is one of the most famous in all music.

The Winning Motive

Listen to a humorous play-by-play analysis of this same movement.

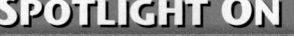
CD 6–15
New Horizons in Music Appreciation

Movement 1
from Beethoven's *Fifth Symphony*
by Professor Peter Schickele

Peter Schickele, alias "P. D. Q. Bach," and Robert Dennis describe this musical event as if they were announcing a sports competition.

 Take It to the Net Visit *www.sfsuccessnet.com* to learn more about Beethoven.

Sketches by Ludwig van Beethoven for *Symphony No. 5* ▼

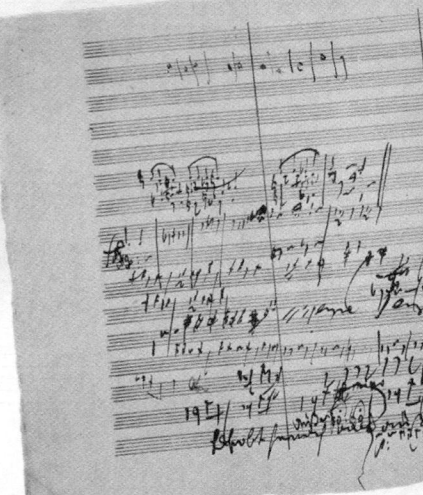

98

Footnotes

ACROSS THE CURRICULUM

8b ▶ **Social Studies** Ask students to write a short play about Ludwig van Beethoven, based on information they have read about his life, musical compositions, and times. The play could be entitled *A Visit with Beethoven* and could include an "interview" with the composer concerning his compositions and lifestyle. Suggest that students perform the play for younger children, using recordings of the famous composer's works.

BUILDING SKILLS THROUGH MUSIC

▶ **Language** Have students use the information on p. 99 to set up a [time]line of Beethoven's life, then use the article from *www.sfsuccessnet.com,* [othe]r sources, to fill in details about the life and work of Beethoven.

SPOTLIGHT ON

▶ **The "Musicalologist"** Peter Schickele (b. 1935) is a leading humorist in music. He studied composition with Roy Harris and Vincent Persichetti. Schickele received a Ford Foundation grant to work in the Los Angeles public schools as a composer-in-residence from 1960 to 1961 and then taught at Juilliard, his *alma mater.* He was not influenced just by classical music, however. Jazz, pop, rock, and theater music found a place in his work. When he invented the "composer" P.D.Q. Bach and began to present his "works," a new era began in musical humor. Pieces were "discovered" for such instruments as the double-reed slide music stand, the left-handed sewer flute, and viola four hands. On a more serious note, Schickele has written a large number of highly regarded classical compositions, and is a tireless promoter of music education.

Ludwig van Beethoven

Ludwig van Beethoven (1770–1827) is one of history's most well-known composers. He wrote many compositions in his lifetime including nine symphonies, five piano concertos, and 16 string quartets. His *Symphony No. 5* is one of the most recognized and famous symphonies of all time.

Beethoven was born in Bonn, Germany, just six years before the United States of America declared independence from England. His father taught him violin and piano at an early age. When Beethoven was 11, he became an assistant organist at the local court and later played viola in the court orchestra.

Beethoven spent most of his career in Vienna, Austria, where he met Wolfgang Amadeus Mozart and Franz Josef Haydn. He associated with Vienna's nobility, who often helped him with his career. Beethoven began to lose his hearing in the late 1790s and spent the last nine years of his life completely deaf.

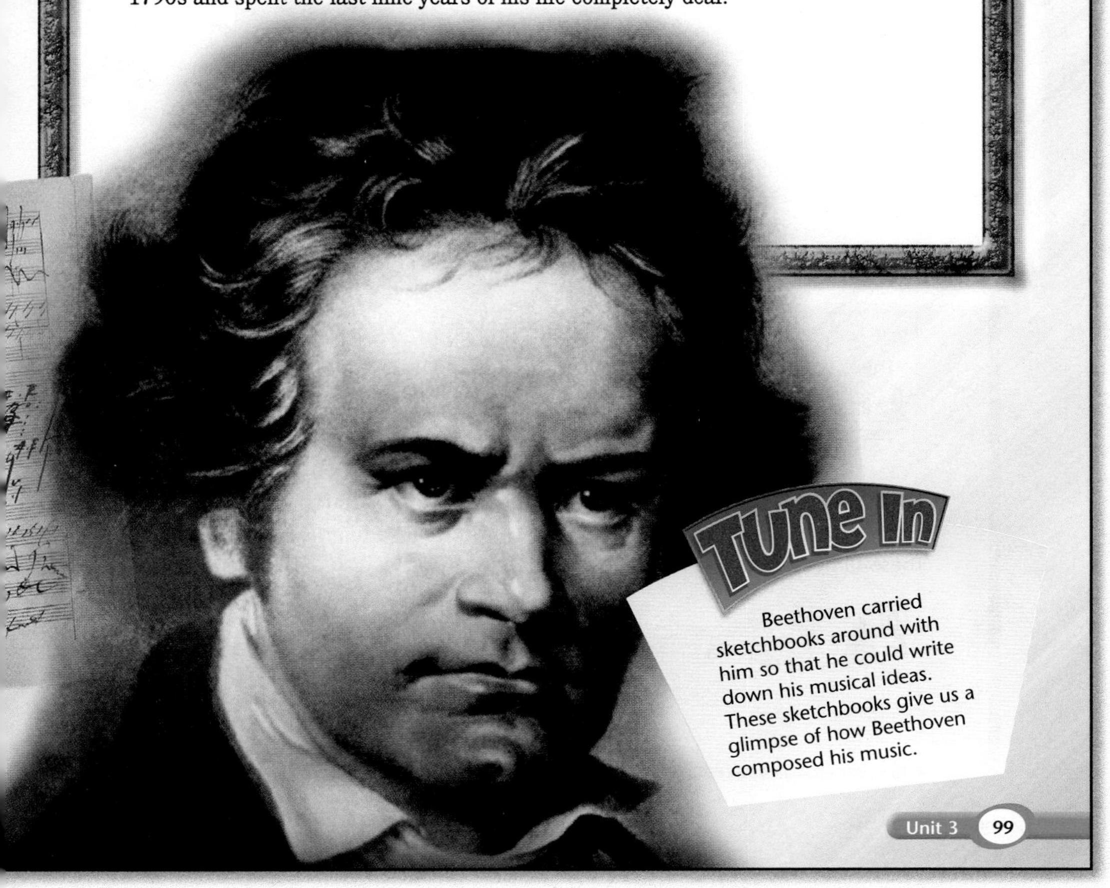

Tune In

Beethoven carried sketchbooks around with him so that he could write down his musical ideas. These sketchbooks give us a glimpse of how Beethoven composed his music.

Unit 3 **99**

1 INTRODUCE

8b Ask students to read the Music Makers information about Beethoven. Lead a discussion on the restless mood at the time of the American and French revolutions. Stress the restlessness of the working class in France and the hope for independence in America. Invite students to think about Beethoven's music as that of a revolutionary time.

2 DEVELOP

Listening

Explain that a motive is transposed when it appears at a different pitch level. (See Skills Reinforcement below for more permutation possibilities.)

6b Help students to

- Listen to the opening of *Symphony No. 5 in C Minor* **CD 6-14.**
- Identify the motive and realize that it is repeated at different pitch levels.
- Realize that the rhythmic motive usually stays the same on each repetition, but the melodic motive is usually transposed or is sometimes inverted.

Playing

Encourage students to sing, then play, the opening motive on a keyboard or other melodic instrument.

Listening

6b Have students listen to *New Horizons in Music Appreciation* **CD 6-15** and discuss humorous treatment of motives and themes.

Have students listen again and list the instrument families they hear playing the motive through the development. (orchestra, strings, orchestra, strings, brass, orchestra; development: brass, strings)

continued on page 100

SKILLS REINFORCEMENT

6c ▶ **Analyzing** A motive can be performed in retrograde, or in reverse. Beethoven transposed his motives. Invite students to play the following motive and its treatments (or permutations) on a melodic instrument.

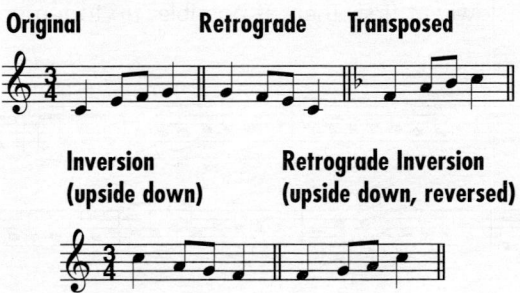

Original   **Retrograde**   **Transposed**

Inversion (upside down)   **Retrograde Inversion** (upside down, reversed)

TEACHER TO TEACHER

▶ **Character Motives** Have students discover that musical motives or themes are often connected to the characters and action of a movie. Select a movie appropriate to view in class (for example, *E.T. the Extra-Terrestrial*), along with a VCR and TV.

Reinforcement Guide students to identify the major characters of the movie. Then have them identify that a theme or motive repeats when a character is onscreen. (*E.T.'s Theme*)

On Target Ask students to select a theme and describe the onscreen events each time the theme occurs. Ask them if the theme changes from occurrence to occurrence (most often, yes).

Challenge Ask select students to notate a character theme or motive for a movie character of their choice.

Singing

Invite students to

- Listen to "I Got Rhythm" **CD 6-16**, clapping the half-note beat as they follow along in the book.
- Sing the song while clapping the half-note beat.

Analyzing

Invite students to look at the first line (phrase) of "I Got Rhythm." Help students understand that in the first phrase, the rhythm of the first two-measure motive is repeated in mm. 3–4, and the order of the pitches is reversed, that is, in retrograde.

ASK How many times does the first two-measure motive appear? (six times, including the repeat)

How is the motive used in the middle section? (The rhythm is the same, but the melody goes up and down, then is repeated a step lower.)

Playing

Help students to

- Play the motive of "I Got Rhythm" from the Show What You Know box on a melodic instrument, then play it in retrograde (mm. 3–4, p. 101). See Resource Book p. B-9 for a worksheet.
- Improvise rhythms, using the four pitches of the motive until they create a new motive they like.

SAY George Gershwin was a master of melody. One of his secrets was creating a catchy, short melodic idea, then repeating it in different ways. These short musical ideas are called motives. Share the information in Cultural Connection, p. 101, with students and discuss the influence of Gershwin's Russian Jewish cultural heritage on his music.

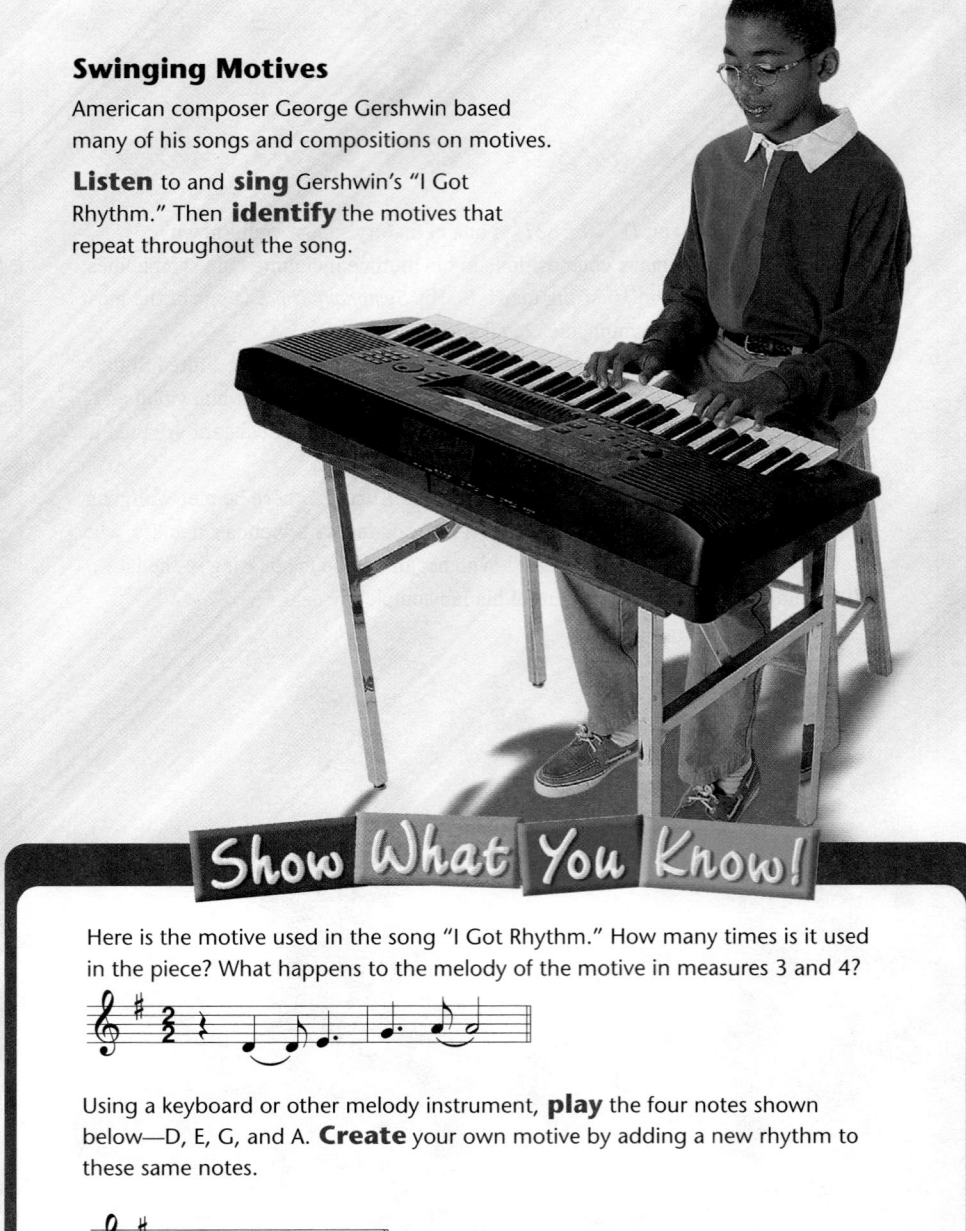

Swinging Motives

American composer George Gershwin based many of his songs and compositions on motives.

Listen to and **sing** Gershwin's "I Got Rhythm." Then **identify** the motives that repeat throughout the song.

Show What You Know!

Here is the motive used in the song "I Got Rhythm." How many times is it used in the piece? What happens to the melody of the motive in measures 3 and 4?

Using a keyboard or other melody instrument, **play** the four notes shown below—D, E, G, and A. **Create** your own motive by adding a new rhythm to these same notes.

D   E   G   A

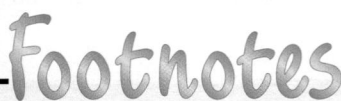

MEETING INDIVIDUAL NEEDS

▶ **Including Everyone** Visually scanning and searching printed music to find motives and retrogrades will be very difficult for some students. Have students work in pairs and practice singing (on neutral syllables) and playing (on pitched instruments) the first motive (D, E, G, A) and its retrograde. When both partners are successful, they should take turns, with one singing and the other tracing the notation. Have students share one book as they coordinate singing and tracing.

SKILLS REINFORCEMENT

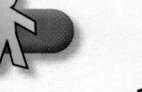

▶ **Keyboard** One way to tighten up the syncopated rhythms in "I Got Rhythm" is to break down the melody into subdivisions of eighth notes. Have students learn this eighth-note keyboard version of the melody for the first two lines of the song. Students should play it slowly at first, then, if possible, up to tempo with **CD 6-16.**

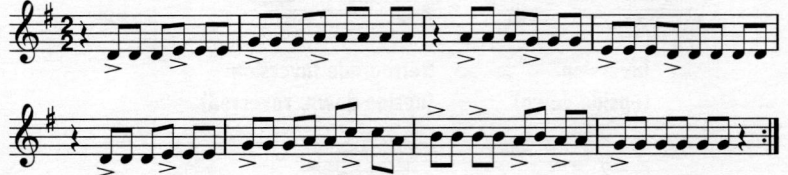

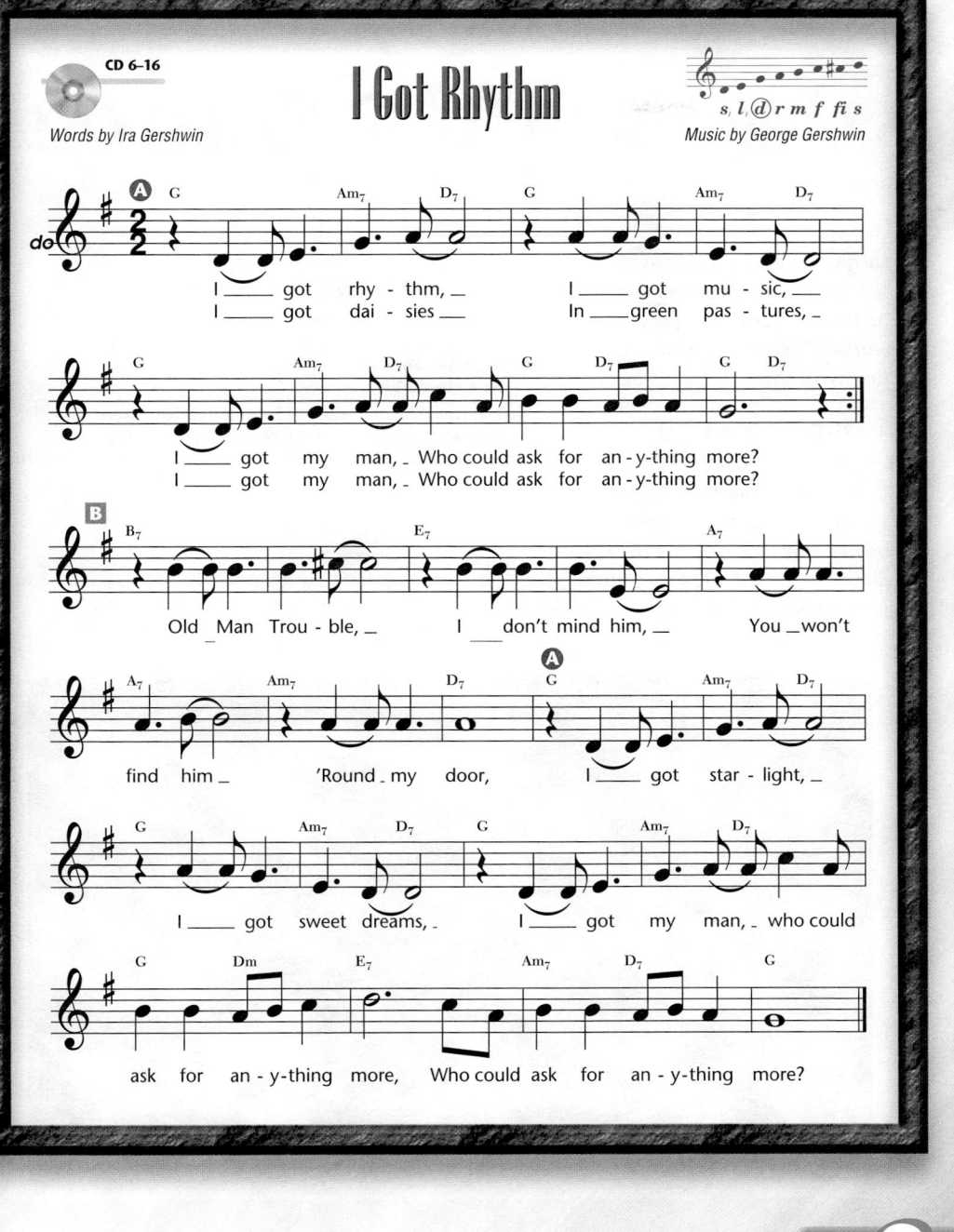

I Got Rhythm

CD 6–16

Words by Ira Gershwin

Music by George Gershwin

s l d r m f f i s

A G / Am7 / D7 / G / Am7 / D7

I ____ got rhy - thm, ____ I ____ got mu - sic, ____
I ____ got dai - sies ____ In ____ green pas - tures, ____

G / Am7 / D7 / G / D7 / G / D7

I ____ got my man, ____ Who could ask for an - y - thing more?
I ____ got my man, ____ Who could ask for an - y - thing more?

B B7 / E7 / A7

Old Man Trou - ble, ____ I ____ don't mind him, ____ You ____ won't

A7 / Am7 / D7 / **A** G / Am7 / D7

find him ____ 'Round ____ my door, I ____ got star - light, ____

G / Am7 / D7 / G / Am7 / D7

I ____ got sweet dreams, ____ I ____ got my man, ____ who could

G / Dm / E7 / Am7 / D7 / G

ask for an - y - thing more, Who could ask for an - y - thing more?

Students may be interested in discovering how musical motives and themes are used in movies and associated with movie characters. (See Teacher to Teacher on p. 99.)

3 CLOSE

Skill: LISTENING ASSESSMENT

6b Written Assessment Have students listen to the first 20 seconds (stop at the third *fermata*) of *Symphony No. 5 in C Minor* **CD 6-14** and write a 1 on a sheet of paper each time they hear the original motive or any of its permutations (13). Have students listen again to check their answers.

CULTURAL CONNECTION

▶ **Jazz and Jewish Folk Song** George Gershwin's musical style was influenced by the jazz that surrounded him in New York and by the melodies and dance rhythms of his own Jewish heritage. His parents were Jewish Russian immigrants. Gershwin often used the minor thirds of Jewish folk music as well as the rhythmic lilt of dances from the Jewish tradition. See p. 251 for more biographical information on George Gershwin.

TECHNOLOGY/MEDIA LINK

Web Site Visit *www.sfsuccessnet.com* to learn more about the life and music of Ludwig van Beethoven.

CD-ROM Have students enter the chord progression for "I Got Rhythm" into *Band-in-a-Box*. Help students find the form of the piece (AABA, 32-bar song form). As students sing along with the accompaniment, ask them to change to a different combo setting each time a new section of the form starts.

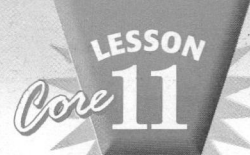

LESSON AT A GLANCE

Element Focus — **TIMBRE** String instruments

Skill Objective **LISTENING** Listen to recordings of string orchestras from different cultures and compare the tone qualities and playing techniques

Connection Activity **CULTURE** Learn how diverse cultures use string instruments in different ways

MATERIALS

- "Summer" from *Concerto No. 2*, Movement 3   **CD 6-18**
- *The Moon Mirrored in the Pool*   **CD 6-19**
- *Shchedryk*   **CD 6-20**
- **Resource Book** p. C-5
- violin and bow

VOCABULARY

pizzicato   tremolo   timbre

◆ ◆ ◆ ◆ **National Standards** ◆ ◆ ◆ ◆

4c Arrange, using electronic media
6b Listen and analyze uses of timbre in music from diverse cultures
9a Describe characteristics of music styles from a variety of cultures

MORE MUSIC CHOICES

For more experience with string timbre:
Lyric Suite, p. 169
Serenade for Strings, p. 363

1 INTRODUCE

SAY String instruments play an important role in the music of most cultures. Although most string instruments have much in common (they are bowed, plucked, or struck), they may be constructed in a variety of shapes and played in different ways.

Share with students the information in Teacher to Teacher and Cultural Connection below.

Sounds of Strings

Large orchestras, composed of string instruments of all sizes, can be found in different parts of the world. **Listen** to the sound and timbre of three different examples.

Strings from Italy

Listen to a movement from Vivaldi's *The Four Seasons.* The string instruments are primarily bowed, but occasionally they are played *pizzicato* [pit-sih-KAH-toh], or plucked.

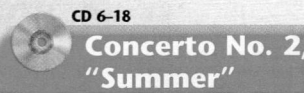

Concerto No. 2, "Summer"

CD 6-18

Movement 3 ("*La tempesta*") from *The Four Seasons* by Antonio Vivaldi

The Four Seasons, a set of four concertos, was first published in Amsterdam, Netherlands, in 1725. This movement is a musical depiction of a summer rainstorm.

Arts Connection

The Concert (c. 1690) by A. D. Gabbiani. This painting of a Baroque string ensemble features cello (left), harpsichord (center), and violins of various sizes. ▼

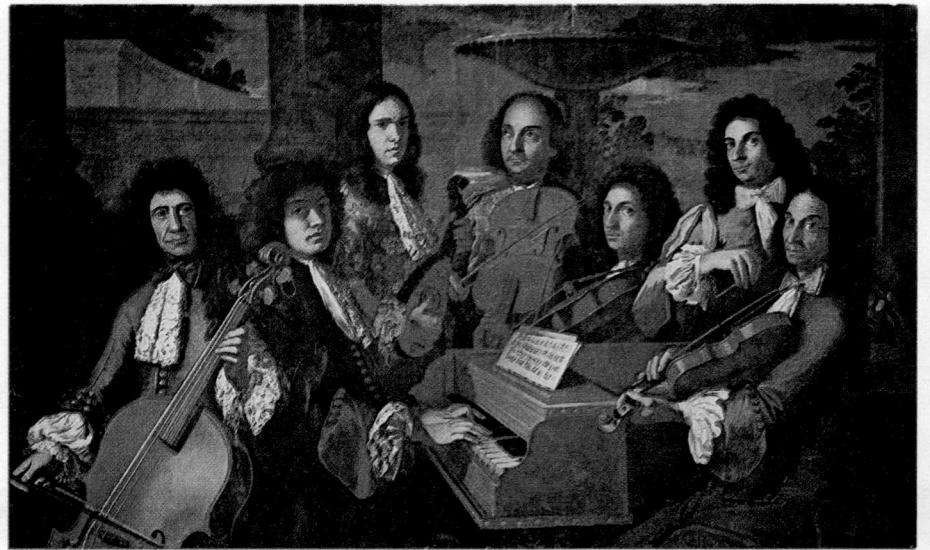

Footnotes

TEACHER TO TEACHER

▶ **Comparing and Constructing Instruments** Ask students to compare string instruments from around the world. The *erhu* from China is basically a spike fiddle. Make a simple spike fiddle by putting an old broomstick (neck) through a coffee can (resonator); then attach a string or wire at each end of the stick and run it over a bridge on the end of the can. Compare the *erhu* to the *bandura* which is a type of zither (strings stretched over a board) that is in the same family as the piano, Autoharp, and *koto.*

BUILDING SKILLS THROUGH MUSIC

▶ **Language** Share the information in the lesson on string instruments. Have students develop a semantic feature analysis chart, using Resource Book p. C-5, to analyze the information on the orchestral string instruments, *erhu,* and *bandura.*

CULTURAL CONNECTION

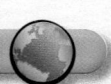

▶ **Chinese String Instruments** A typical Chinese orchestra contains a number of Chinese string instruments as well as some Western instruments, like the cello. Here is a list of the primary Chinese string instruments.

Bowed Strings

- *Erhu, banhu, goahu, zhonghu, gehu, bass gehu*

Plucked Strings

- *Pipa* (lute), *ruan* (moon lute), *sanxian* (relative of Japanese *shamisen*) *yuequin* (hammered dulcimer), *zheng* (zither)

Invite students to select any one of these instruments, research it in the local library, and present a report to the class.

Strings from China

The Chinese string orchestra is composed of instruments that are both plucked and bowed. Some Chinese instruments trace their origins to as early as 200 B.C. The *erhu* [ehr-hoo], perhaps the best-known Chinese string instrument, is over 1,000 years old. It is a two-string alto instrument that has a sound box covered with snakeskin. It is played with a horsehair bow.

Listen to the solo *erhu* and Chinese string orchestra in this selection inspired by a beautiful moonlit pool.

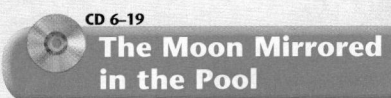

CD 6-19
The Moon Mirrored in the Pool
Erhu ▶

by Hua Yanjun
Hua Yanjun (1890–1950) was poor and blind most of his life. The Chinese people hear "sadness" in this composition.

The Ukrainian Bandura Orchestra

The *bandura*, the national folk instrument of Ukraine, dates back to the fourteenth century. It was played by wandering minstrels *(kobzars)* and warriors *(cossacks)*.

The *bandura* is a large string instrument with a wide oval body. There are no frets, so each string plays only one pitch. There are 55 to 64 strings that are tuned in half steps, which range from bass to treble.

Listen to this traditional Christmas carol performed by one of the leading *bandura* orchestras in the United States. **Identify** the performing techniques of plucking, strumming, and tremolo.

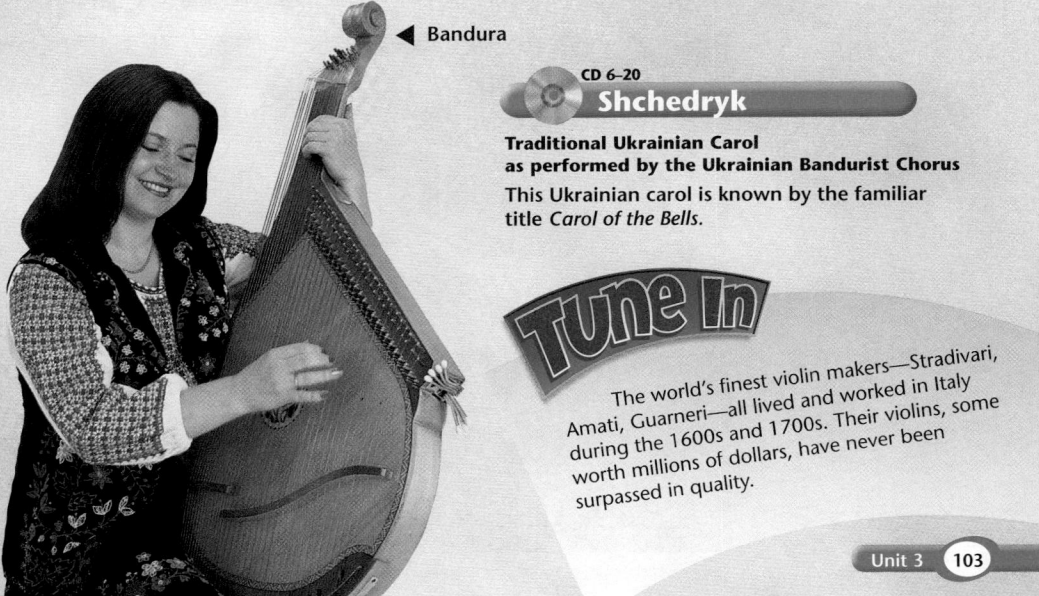

◀ Bandura

CD 6-20
Shchedryk
**Traditional Ukrainian Carol
as performed by the Ukrainian Bandurist Chorus**
This Ukrainian carol is known by the familiar title *Carol of the Bells*.

Tune In

The world's finest violin makers—Stradivari, Amati, Guarneri—all lived and worked in Italy during the 1600s and 1700s. Their violins, some worth millions of dollars, have never been surpassed in quality.

---

2 DEVELOP

Listening
Invite students to bow and pluck the strings on a violin.

6b **ASK** What is the Italian name for plucking a string? (*pizzicato*)

Have students listen to *Concerto No. 2* **CD 6-18** and discuss how Vivaldi used string instruments to depict a summer rainstorm.

9a **ASK** What are the differences between the *erhu* (on p. 103) and the violin? (see p. 355) (*erhu*: two strings, played vertically, cylinder shape; violin: four strings, played horizontally, hourglass shape)

6b Have students listen to *The Moon Mirrored in the Pool* **CD 6-19** and use music terms to discuss how the Chinese instruments sound different from violins.

9a **ASK** What American string instrument is somewhat like the Ukrainian *bandura*? (Autoharp)

How are the Ukrainian *bandura* and the piano alike and different? (Alike: both have many strings tuned in half steps; different: shapes; played with fingers vs. keys and hammers.)

Invite students to listen to *Shchedryk* **CD 6-20** and discuss the sound of a *bandura* orchestra and the effects of plucking, strumming, and tremolo. See Skills Reinforcement below for additional listening activities.

3 CLOSE

Element: TIMBRE   **ASSESSMENT**

6b **Observation/Music Journal Writing** Play the recording of *Concerto No. 2* **CD 6-18** and ask students to close their eyes. Observe them as they raise a hand to signal when they hear the timbre of a string instrument played *pizzicato*. Then, play **CD 6-19** and **CD 6-20** ask students to write comparisons in their music journals.

SKILLS REINFORCEMENT

6b ▶ **Listening** Have students listen to other examples of string instruments played in a variety of ways. One example is *What a Wonderful World* **CD 4-20**. Have students focus on the plucked arpeggios of the guitar in the accompaniment and the bowed violins in the accompaniment. Tell students that bowed string technique is called *arco*.

Sound Bank Invite students to listen to the *erhu* **CD 23–24**, *bandura* **CD 23–12**, violin **CD 23–48**, cello **CD 23–16**, and string bass **CD 23–40** found in the Sound Bank beginning on p. 512. The Sound Bank includes pictures, descriptions, and sound examples of selected instruments.

SCHOOL TO HOME CONNECTION

▶ **Community Strings** Encourage students to search newspapers and listen to the radio to become aware of upcoming performances of string groups in their community. If they attend a live performance, they can report on it to the class.

TECHNOLOGY/MEDIA LINK

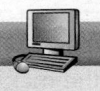

4c **Electronic Keyboard** Invite students to locate sounds for string instruments on their MIDI keyboards. (violin, viola, cello, bass, and so on) Ask students to select one of these string instrument sounds and create a short melody. Then have students perform their melodies and demonstrate articulations such as *pizzicato* or *legato*.

LESSON AT A GLANCE

Element Focus	**TEXTURE/HARMONY** Melody and counter-melody
Skill Objective	**SINGING** Sing a song with melody and countermelody
Connection Activity	**SOCIAL STUDIES** Discover the geography and folk traditions of the Ozark Mountains

MATERIALS

*   "Going upon the Mountain"   **CD 6-21**
    Recording Routine: Intro (4 m.); v. 1; refrain; interlude (4 m.); v. 2; refrain; interlude (16 m.); v. 1; refrain with countermelody 1; interlude (4 m.); v. 2; refrain with countermelody 2; coda
*   *The Battle of New Orleans*   **CD 6-23**
*   bass and alto xylophones, glockenspiel, double tone block, spoons

VOCABULARY

countermelody   Ozarks   hoedown

◆ ◆ ◆ ◆ National Standards ◆ ◆ ◆ ◆

1d Sing music written in two parts
2a Play instruments accurately in small ensembles
2c Perform instrumental music from diverse genres
5a Read half, quarter, and eighth notes in duple meter
5b Sight-read melodies in treble clef
8b Identify ways music relates to other school subjects

MORE MUSIC CHOICES...

For more songs with countermelodies:
"Eres tú," p. 473
"Sing a Song of Peace," p. 66

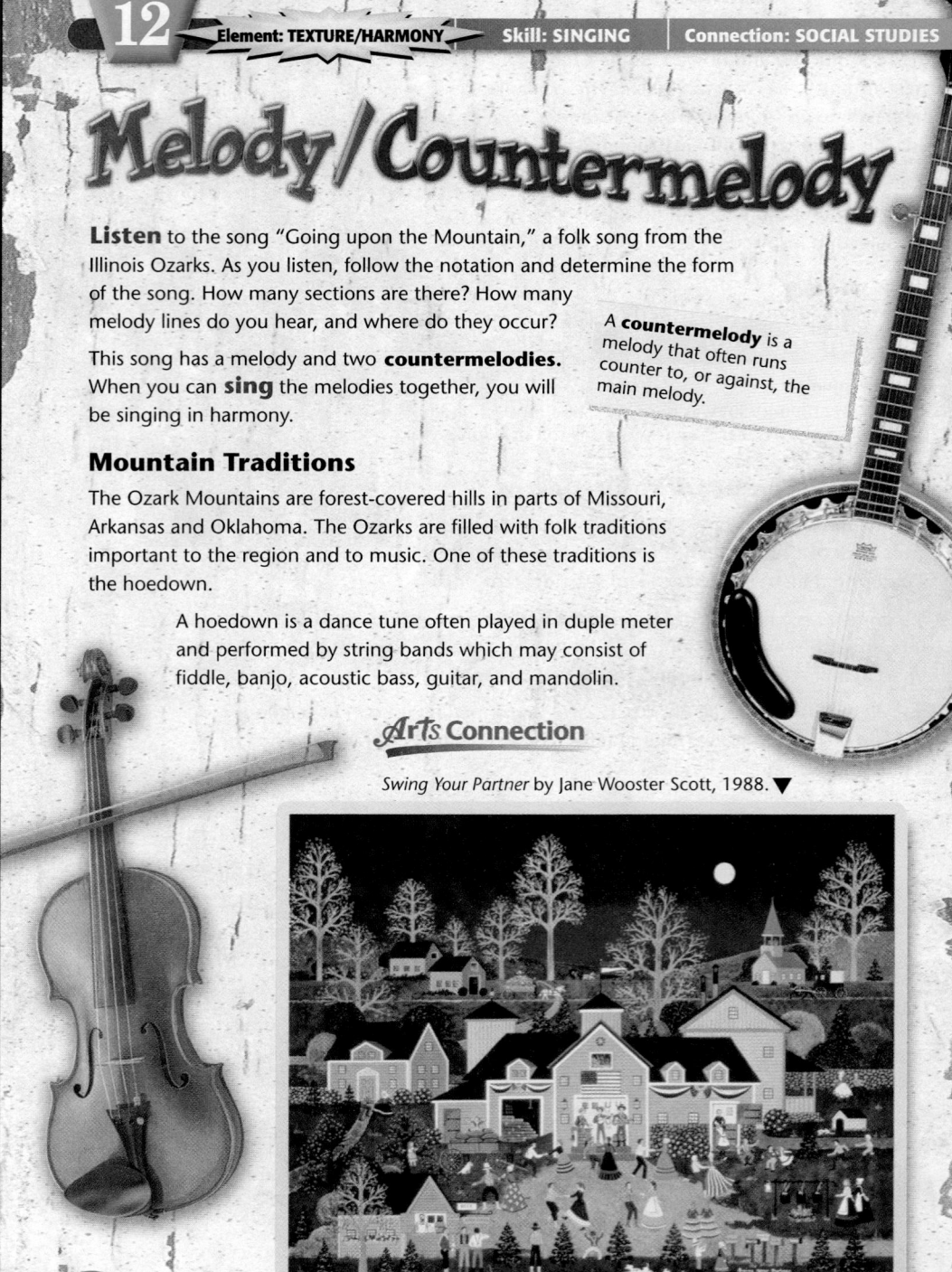

Melody/Countermelody

Listen to the song "Going upon the Mountain," a folk song from the Illinois Ozarks. As you listen, follow the notation and determine the form of the song. How many sections are there? How many melody lines do you hear, and where do they occur?

This song has a melody and two **countermelodies.** When you can **sing** the melodies together, you will be singing in harmony.

> A **countermelody** is a melody that often runs counter to, or against, the main melody.

Mountain Traditions

The Ozark Mountains are forest-covered hills in parts of Missouri, Arkansas and Oklahoma. The Ozarks are filled with folk traditions important to the region and to music. One of these traditions is the hoedown.

A hoedown is a dance tune often played in duple meter and performed by string bands which may consist of fiddle, banjo, acoustic bass, guitar, and mandolin.

Arts Connection

Swing Your Partner by Jane Wooster Scott, 1988. ▼

104

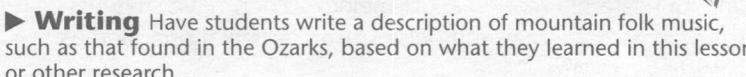
Footnotes

MEETING INDIVIDUAL NEEDS

▶ **Independent Singing** Students may find it difficult to sing an independent countermelody; the movement of the melody is too distracting. As preparation for the countermelody to "Going upon the Mountain," try a "common tone" part (this works in songs having only I and V chords). On the pitch G, have students sing half notes throughout; the text can be "So long, I'm gone." Once students can maintain this one tone while hearing the melody move, they are more prepared for the moving countermelodies.

BUILDING SKILLS THROUGH MUSIC

▶ **Writing** Have students write a description of mountain folk music, such as that found in the Ozarks, based on what they learned in this lesson or other research.

SKILLS REINFORCEMENT

2c ▶ **Keyboard** The refrain of "Going upon the Mountain" is an excellent "five finger position" tune for beginning keyboard players; once the tune is known as a song, students will be able to figure it out through experimentation. (Place thumb on middle C, use D, E, and G above it.)

▶ **Recorder** Invite students to learn and perform the two countermelodies on p. 106 for "Going upon the Mountain" on soprano recorders.

Sing a Mountain Melody

Sing "Going upon the Mountain." Remember to sing your words clearly and with precise rhythm in this lively song.

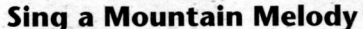

Going upon the Mountain

CD 6–21

d r m s l d'

Folk Song from the Ozarks

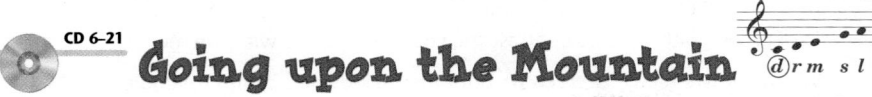

VERSE

1. Go-ing up-on the moun-tain to raise a crop of cane, To
2. I used to __ ride the old gray horse, but now I ride the roan, You

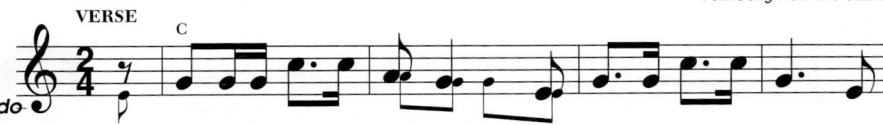

make a bar-rel of 'las-ses to sweet-en old Li - za Jane.
may court your __ own true love but you'd bet - ter leave mine a - lone.

REFRAIN

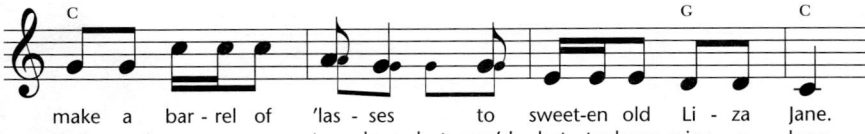

It's a bye, bye, my dar - ling girl, bye, bye, I'm gone.

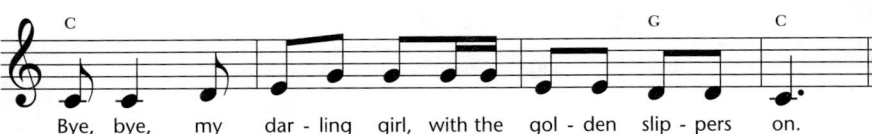

Bye, bye, my dar - ling girl, with the gol - den slip - pers on.

That Mountain Sound

Listen to *The Battle of New Orleans* as performed by Ozark songwriter, Jimmie Driftwood. **Analyze** his vocal timbre and singing style. What musical elements contribute to the mountain folk sound?

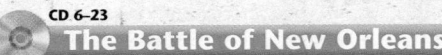

CD 6–23

The Battle of New Orleans

by Jimmie Driftwood
as performed by Johnny Horton

Jimmie Driftwood was a history teacher in Arkansas when he wrote his first hit in 1958, *The Battle of New Orleans*. He has written over 6,000 songs in the Ozark folk tradition.

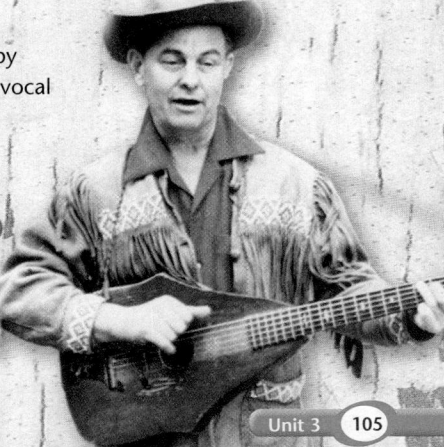

Unit 3   105

1 INTRODUCE

ASK From what geographical region does the song "Going upon the Mountain" come? (Illinois, Ozarks)

Invite students to read "Mountain Traditions" on p. 104. Ask them

- Where are the Ozarks? (forest-covered hills in parts of Missouri, Arkansas, Oklahoma, and Illinois)
- What is the name of the dance that accompanies this song? (hoedown)

Tell students that in this lesson, they will sing a song with a melody and countermelody and discover the hoedown.

2 DEVELOP

Playing

Invite students to echo you on an easy four-measure body percussion pattern in meter in 2. Ask them to independently perform the following with accurate rhythm to demonstrate fundamental skills.

- Clap pat clap-pat pat. *(ta ta ti-ti ta)* (two times)

Give students a second example to echo.

As you play "Going upon the Mountain" **CD 6-21**, have students

- Clap a pattern during the first four measures of the verse.
- Echo you on mm. 5–8 of the verse.
- Join you in clapping the beat during the refrain.

Listening

 Ask students to read "That Mountain Sound" on p. 105. Share with them the information on Jimmy Driftwood in Spotlight On and in Across the Curriculum below. To help students describe aurally-presented music representing diverse styles, play *The Battle of New Orleans* **CD 6-23**. Ask students to identify the instruments and describe the timbres that contribute to this folk style.

continued on page 106

SPOTLIGHT ON

▶ **Jimmy Driftwood** Beloved as a musician in the folk style, Jimmy Driftwood (born, James Corbett Morris) was born in Mountain View, Arkansas, in 1907. He became a teacher, and started setting poems to music for the purpose of teaching history. His folk-style songs attracted wider attention and he gained regional and national popularity as a performer and recording artist. His songs were about life and folklore of the Ozarks and of the United States. Driftwood sang and played the guitar his grandfather made for him. He also played his own version of the mouth bow, resembling a small shooting bow. The curved wood piece of the mouth bow is pressed against the mouth for resonance, and the string is "twanged."

ACROSS THE CURRICULUM

▶ **Social Studies** The Battle of New Orleans has come to be known as the decisive battle ending The War of 1812. Actually, it took place several weeks after the peace treaty had been signed in Europe, but this news had not reached the United States. In January 1815, a large, well-trained British fleet moved in from the West Indies with the goal of capturing New Orleans, important as a port city on the Mississippi River. General Andrew Jackson commanded the American forces. Though strongly outnumbered, Johnson's men significantly damaged the British in the first encounter; the British pulled back and never resumed fighting.

Analyzing

Play "Going upon the Mountain," **CD 6-21** and ask students to look at the song notation on p. 105 and follow the verse text. During the refrains, ask them to listen for the part that is not the melody and follow the notation on p. 106. Identify these as "countermelodies" ("counter," since they sometimes move in opposite direction from the melody). Tell them when a countermelody is combined with the melody, vocal harmony results.

Reading

5b Ask students to sight-read Countermelody 1 in treble clef and the key of C using pitch syllables and hand signs. Have them identify the key and meter, paying attention to *fa* and *ti*.

5a Have students read and perform the rhythms using rhythm syllables, then read and sing the melody using pitch syllables. Play the recording again, **CD 6-21**, and have students sing the lyrics for Countermelody 1. Stop the recording. Repeat the sight-reading procedure for Countermelody 2; play the recording again. Then have students sing both countermelodies using lyrics.

Singing

1d Independent Singing: Divide the class in half; have one group sing Countermelody 1 and the other half sing the refrain. Repeat, trading parts. Do the same with Countermelody 2. Reinforce the concept that this is vocal harmony. Use Meeting Individual Needs, p. 104, and Teacher to Teacher, p. 106, for assistance in developing independent singing.

When ready, have individual students independently perform the countermelodies with accurate intonation demonstrating fundamental skills.

Moving

SAY Now, we are going to create a hoedown dance using echoes. Have students

- Read the directions in Hoedown Dance on p. 106.
- Form a circle with a partner.
- When ready, perform the dance with the Stereo Performance track **CD 6-22.**

Counter that Melody

Look at these countermelodies. In which section are they performed? How do the melody and countermelodies contrast each other? **Sing** each countermelody. Experiment with ways to contrast the countermelodies with the melody.

When you are ready, **perform** both the melody and countermelodies to "Going upon the Mountain." **Sing** in the spirit of a festive hoedown.

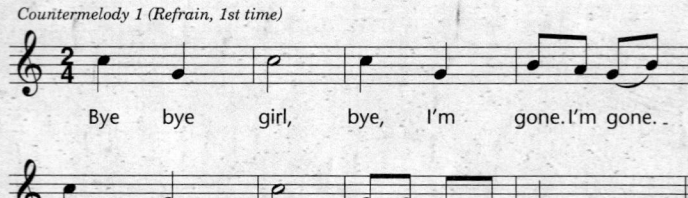

Countermelody 1 (Refrain, 1st time)

Bye   bye   girl,   bye,   I'm   gone. I'm gone.

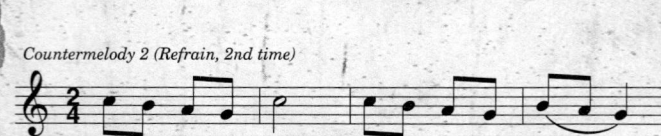

Bye   bye   girl,   gold-en slip-pers on.

Countermelody 2 (Refrain, 2nd time)

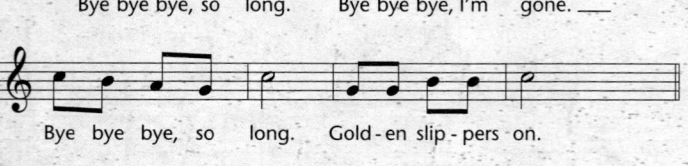

Bye bye bye, so long.   Bye bye bye, I'm   gone. ____

Bye bye bye, so long.   Gold-en slip-pers on.

Create a Hoedown Dance

Learn these movements for "Going upon the Mountain." Experiment with creating different body percussion rhythms for each verse. When ready, **perform** the movements with the song.

- **Starting position:** Partners form two large circles facing each other.
- **Verse:** As you sing, the inner circle partner creates a body percussion rhythm for four measures. The outer circle partner matches the body percussion rhythm on the next four measures.
- **Refrain:** Both circles turn to their right and move forward with a shuffle step. At the end of the refrain, new partners face each other and begin the body percussion movements on the verse.

106

Footnotes

MOVEMENT

▶ **The Hoedown** This term is probably best known as the identifying term for a rural social gathering at which dancing is the featured entertainment. The musicians play various types of folk tunes, including the "hoedown" represented here by "Going upon the Mountain." Typically these tunes have two sections (sometimes three); with repeats, these are played over and over to make an appropriately long dance accompaniment.

Remind students that the musical concepts of unity, sectional form, repeats, and variety are related and equally important to the art of dance as well.

TEACHER TO TEACHER

▶ **Solid Singing** Make sure there are some solid singers in both groups when you divide up melody and countermelody. Having both parts heard clearly *the first time* is important as an aural model.

▶ **Double Mallets** Students may have trouble remembering parts for both the verse and refrain of "Going upon the Mountain." Therefore, it is advisable to have two sets of the three mallet instruments needed for the accompaniment, so that one group of students can play the verse parts and a second group the refrain parts. If only one bass xylophone is available, two students can share if they have their own mallets, taking care to move quickly out of the way when their parts are finished.

Add an Ensemble

Learn these instrumental parts to accompany "Going upon the Mountain." How do the mallet parts contrast in each section? Add the percussion instruments once you have learned the mallet parts.

When you are ready, **perform** the ensemble as the class sings the song.

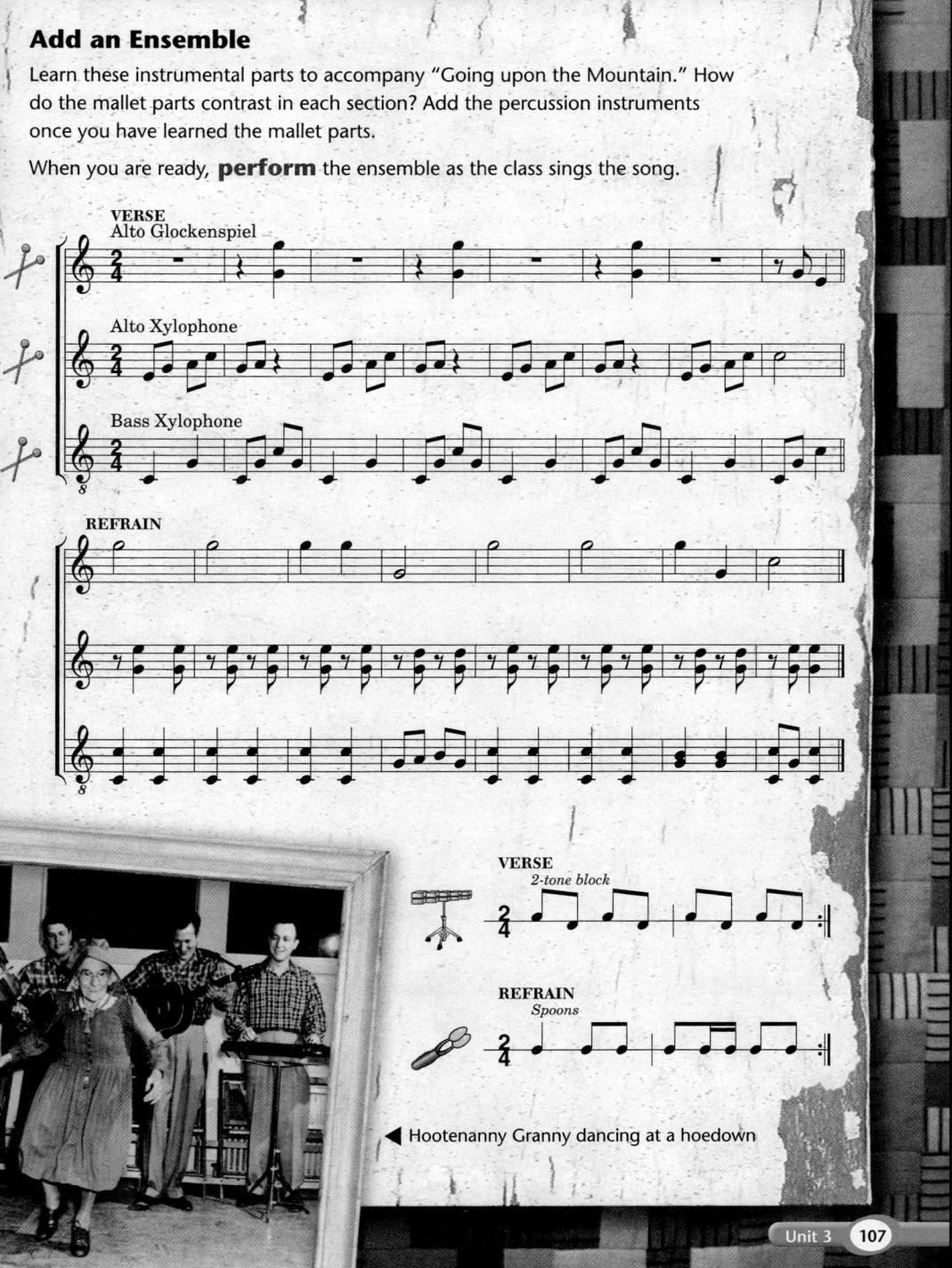

▲ Hootenanny Granny dancing at a hoedown

Tell students that the inside partner will perform the rhythm patterns during the first four measures; the outside partner will respond with the echo during mm. 5-8. For the refrain, both inside and outside partners turn to their right and walk around the circle with a shuffle step; they can also clap. At the end of the refrain they will face new partners and start over. This time, instead of walking on the refrain, students will stand in place and sing.

Playing

Help students analyze the ensemble notation on p. 107, using the following tips.

Verse

Glockenspiel: count 3 beats, on beat 4, play octave G's; do this three times. The fourth time, follow with "rest g-e."

Alto xylophone: the pattern is "L-R-L (crossing) R-L-R rest." This is done three times; the fourth time, replace the "g a" ending with just "c."

Bass xylophone: the mallet pattern is "L, R, L-R-L cross-R."

Use Skills Reinforcement below to analyze the refrain's mallet parts.

2a
2c When ready, have students perform the ensemble as an accompaniment to "Going upon the Mountain," using instruments. Add the small percussion parts. See Teacher to Teacher, p. 106, for improving mallet performance.

3 CLOSE

Element: TEXTURE/HARMONY — ASSESSMENT

1d **Performance/Observation** In small groups, have students sing either countermelody 1 or 2 to "Going upon the Mountain" as another group of 5–6 students sings the melody. Observe students' ability to independently sing a countermelody with accurate rhythm, demonstrating basic performance techniques.

SKILLS REINFORCEMENT

▶ **Analyzing Mallet Parts** Have students analyze the mallet parts for the refrain of "Going upon the Mountain."

Refrain

Glockenspiel: Have students sight-read the part while singing the pitches; then have them identify which patterns are repeated exactly and which patterns have changes.

Alto xylophone: Have students perform the rhythm. Then have them notice that only the right hand moves, with the following pattern: 6 E's, 2 D's, 4 E's, 2 D's, and ending with 2 E's. The left hand just plays along on G.

Bass xylophone: playing desktop, observe that there are 6 octave C's, then the little L-R-L-R pattern, then 4 more C's, two G/B's and the ending C's with the right hand moving to G.

TECHNOLOGY/MEDIA LINK

▶ **Sequencing Software** Have students use sequencing software to record the accompaniment on p. 107. Ask students to use timbres found in a string band to replace the mallet instruments. The bass xylophone can be plucked bass, the alto xylophone can be banjo or guitar, and the glockenspiel can be a fiddle. Students may record separate instrumental tracks by either playing the parts or by using the step-record feature. Have students "mix" the separate tracks and use them as accompaniment for "Going upon the Mountain."

▶ **Digital Audio Recording** Advance students may wish to use the digital recording features of the sequencing software to record the instrumental parts using acoustic instruments.

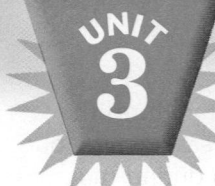
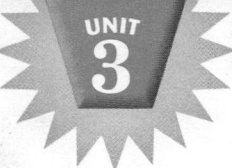 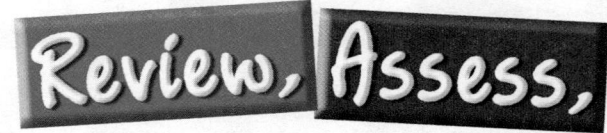

WHAT DO YOU KNOW?

MATERIALS
• **Resource Book** p. B-10

Have students review dynamic and expression terms on pp. 76–78. Then, have students select the correct definitions for the vocabulary words in question 1. Students may write the answers on the worksheet on Resource Book p. B-10.

Have students review augmentation and diminution on pp. 80–83. Ask students to read the rhythms for question 2 and select the rhythm from the right that is the augmentation of the shaded rhythm on the left.

Ask students to read the rhythms for question 3 and select the rhythm from the right that is the correct diminution of the shaded rhythm on the left.

WHAT DO YOU HEAR? 3

MATERIALS	
• *What Do You Hear? 3*	**CD 6-24 to 6-27**
• **Resource Book** p. B-11	

Have students refer to Resource Book p. B-11 for a chart like the one pictured on p. 109. If that is not available, they can make their own copy of the chart.

Play What Do You Hear? 3 **CD 6-24** through **6-27**. Have students listen carefully to each selection. As they identify which technique is being used to produce the sound in each selection, they can place a check mark in the appropriate column. Remind them that each selection may use more than one string technique.

What Do You Know?

1. Match the correct definition to the vocabulary word. On a separate piece of paper, draw the musical symbols for the dynamic terms.

Vocabulary	**Definition**
a. *crescendo*	• a short musical idea
b. *sforzando*	• gradually getting louder
c. *decrescendo*	• suddenly loud
d. motive	• gradually getting softer

2. Look at the rhythms below. Point to the rhythm on the right that is the augmentation of the rhythm in the left column.

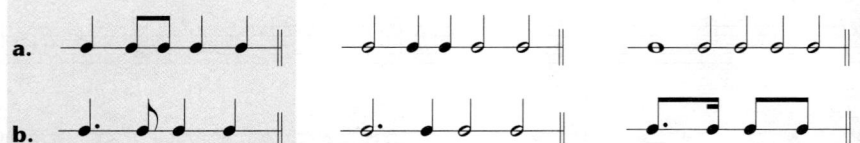

3. Look at the rhythms below. Point to the rhythm on the right that is the diminution of the rhythm in the left column.

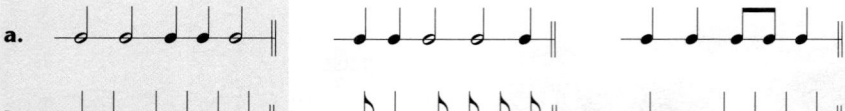

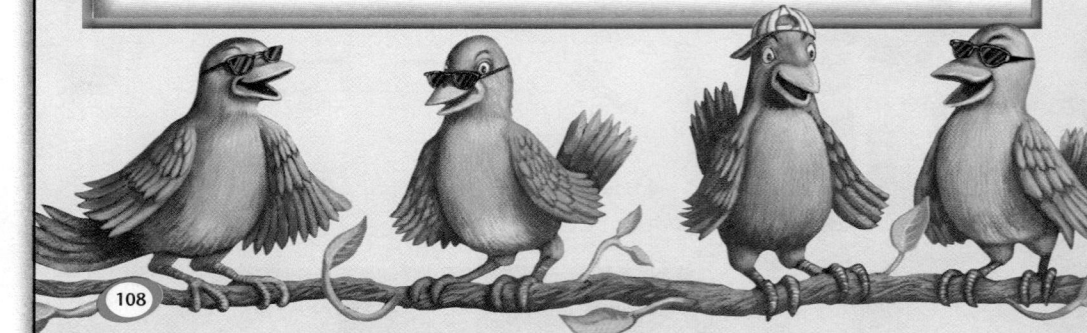

Footnotes

ANSWER KEY

▶ What Do You Know?

1. **a.** *crescendo* gradually getting louder
   b. *sforzando* suddenly loud
   c. *decrescendo* gradually getting softer
   d. motive a short musical idea

2. **a.** middle column
   b. middle column

3. **a.** right column
   b. middle column

▶ What Do You Hear? 3

1. bowing (*arco*)
2. bowing (*arco*), plucking (*pizzicato*), and tremolo
3. strumming, plucking (*pizzicato*), and tremolo
4. bowing (*arco*)

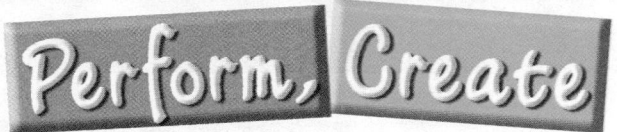
Perform, Create

What Do You Hear? 3

CD 6–24

Timbre

Listen to these examples of string instruments playing. For each selection, identify which techniques of producing sound are used. Selections may use more than one string technique.

STRING TECHNIQUES				
EXCERPT	BOWING (ARCO)	STRUMMING	PLUCKING (PIZZICATO)	TREMOLO
1. Symphony No. 5				
2. The Moon Mirrored in the Pool				
3. Shchedryk				
4. Concerto No. 2, "Summer"				

What You Can Do

Show Form with Movement

Listen to the song "Bridges," page 86. Identify the form of the song using the letters **a** and **b**. Create a movement for each letter and then perform the movements with the appropriate phrases of the song.

Sing Modes

Sing "Harrison Town" on page 97 using pitch syllables. Use *ta* to indicate the flatted seventh of the scale. Then, sing the song with lyrics using hand signs each time you sing the motive *ta-la-so.*

Sing Textures

As a class, sing "Going upon the Mountain" on page 105. Form small groups and perform the countermelodies as the class sings the song. As a challenge, sing "Harrison Town" as a countermelody to "Going upon the Mountain."

WHAT YOU CAN DO

MATERIALS	
• "Bridges," p. 86	**CD 5-28**
• "Harrison Town," p. 97	**CD 6-9**
• "Going upon the Mountain," p. 105	**CD 6-21**
• **Resource Book** p. B-12	

Show Form with Movement

Ask students to look at the notation for "Bridges" **CD 5-28** on p. 86 while you play the recording. Have them notice the form of the piece (aaba). Divide students into groups. Ask them to demonstrate the form by creating two movements, one to be performed during "a" phrases and a contrasting movement for the "b" phrase.

Sing Modes

Play the recording of "Harrison Town" **CD 6-9** while students follow the notation in their books, p. 97. Then, have them sing the song, using pitch syllables, paying particular attention to the *ta-la-so* motive. Ask students to notate *ta-la-so* in the key of C major on a staff, using Resource Book p. B-12. Create exercises using these syllables and have students use hand signs while singing them. Then, encourage students to use the same hand signs while singing the song.

Sing Textures

Have students sing "Going upon the Mountain" **CD 6-21**, p. 105. Invite a student to conduct the song as the class sings. Divide the class into groups to sing countermelodies to the song. As a further challenge, have them sing "Harrison Town" and "Going upon the Mountain" as partner songs.

▶ **What You Can Do**

Show Form with Movement

The form of "Bridges" is aaba (by phrase).

TECHNOLOGY/MEDIA LINK

▶ **Rubrics**

Visit *www.sfsuccessnet.com* for rubrics to assess students' achievement in music skills.

Lesson	Elements	Skills	
LESSON 1 **CORE** **Take Your Time** pp. 114–117 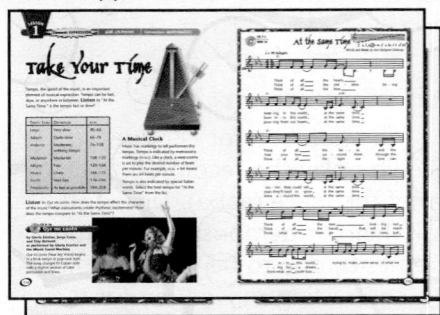	**Element: Expression** **Concept:** Tempo **Focus:** Tempo **Secondary Element** Rhythm: beat **National Standards** 1c 6c 7a 7b 8b	**Skill: Listening** **Objective:** Listen to a song at different tempos to illustrate how tempo affects a song's character **Secondary Skills** • **Singing** Sing a song while tapping at a steady tempo • **Listening** Listen to and compare different tempos of songs	**SKILLS REINFORCEMENT** • **Listening** Choose a tempo marking for a listening selection; check that marking by using a metronome • **Singing** Identify and list songs in the book with the same tempo markings
LESSON 2 **CORE** **Meter—The Foundation of Music** pp. 118–119 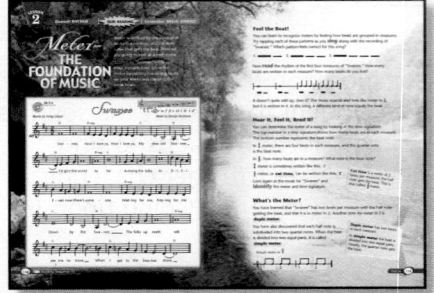 **Reading Sequence 13, p. 494**	**Element: Rhythm** **Concept:** Meter **Focus:** $\frac{2}{2}$ meter, cut time **Secondary Element** Melody: accidentals **National Standards** 4c 5a 5c 6b 6c 8b	**Skill: Reading** **Objective:** Read rhythms in $\frac{2}{2}$ meter **Secondary Skills** • **Listening** Listen to a song and tap rhythm patterns that best fit the song • **Reading** Understand various kinds of meter	**SKILLS REINFORCEMENT** • **Reading** Learn conducting patterns; sing a song with rhythm syllables • **Keyboard** Play a whole-note accompaniment
LESSON 3 **A Springtime Meter** pp. 120–121 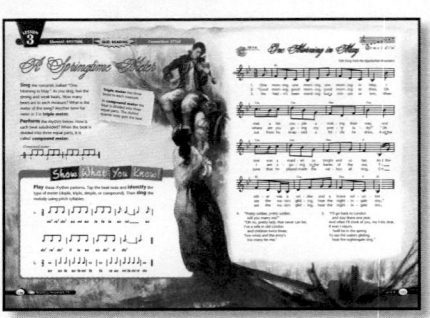 **Reading Sequence 14, p. 494**	**Element: Rhythm** **Concept:** Meter **Focus:** $\frac{3}{8}$ meter **Secondary Element** Timbre: vocal **National Standards** 5a 6a 6c 8b	**Skill: Reading** **Objective:** Read the rhythm of a song in $\frac{3}{8}$ meter **Secondary Skills** • **Analyze** Recognize $\frac{3}{8}$ meter; determine that the meter of a song is compound with one beat per measure • **Listening** Listen to a folk song ballad • **Singing** Sing a song with rhythm syllables	**SKILLS REINFORCEMENT** • **Reading** Read songs in $\frac{6}{8}$ meter and $\frac{3}{8}$ meter and compose melodies • **Mallets** Learn an Orff mallet accompaniment

Connections

Music and Other Literature

Connection: Mathematics

Activity: Relate math symbols to musical terms for tempo

TEACHER TO TEACHER   **Dividing the Class** Organize groups by fun topics

SPOTLIGHT ON   **Metronome** Facts about the metronome

MEETING INDIVIDUAL NEEDS
Learning a New Language Tips on how to teach Italian tempo terms
English Language Learners Write extension sentences

ACROSS THE CURRICULUM   **Math** Use multiplication and division to relate a variety of tempos

BUILDING SKILLS THROUGH MUSIC   **Reading** Determine the mood of lyrics

---

Songs "At the Same Time"

Listening Selections *Oye mi canto*

More Music Choices
"Jambalaya," p. 244
"Down in the Valley," p. 375

ASSESSMENT

Performance/Self-Assessment Perform and listen to a song in different tempos; decide which tempo is best for the expression of the song

TECHNOLOGY/MEDIA LINK

MIDI/Sequencing Software Experiment with changing the tempo of a song

---

Connection: Social Studies

Activity: Discuss the social and economic significance of rivers, lakes, and oceans

ACROSS THE CURRICULUM   **Social Studies** Discuss the significance of rivers, lakes, and oceans

MOVEMENT   **Conducting** Learn basic conducting patterns

BUILDING SKILLS THROUGH MUSIC   **Writing** Write a letter of persuasion

---

Song "Swanee"

More Music Choices
"Hey, Ho! Nobody Home," p. 28
"Lost My Gold Ring," p. 158
"You Are My Sunshine," p. 246

ASSESSMENT

Performance/Observation Read and sing the song with rhythm syllables and a steady beat in 2/2 meter

TECHNOLOGY/MEDIA LINK

Notation Software Compose and notate an accompaniment for a song

---

Connection: Style

Activity: Explore Appalachian ballad style

ACROSS THE CURRICULUM   **Language Arts** Relate word syllables to meter

CULTURAL CONNECTION   **Appalachian Style** Read an Appalachian tale

BUILDING SKILLS THROUGH MUSIC   **Language** Draw conclusions based on text

---

Song "One Morning in May"

More Music Choices
"Scarborough Fair," p. 95
"Skye Boat Song," p. 372

ASSESSMENT

Performance/Self-Assessment Read and tap a beat and rhythm patterns

TECHNOLOGY/MEDIA LINK

Notation Software Notate and change the meter of a song

Lesson	Elements	Skills

LESSON 4 CORE
A Famous Form

pp. 122–123

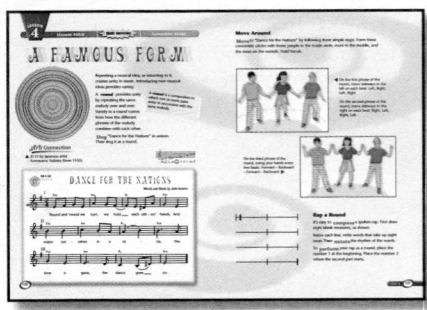

Element: Form
Concept: Round
Focus: Three-part round

Secondary Element
Harmony: three-part harmony

National Standards
◆1a ◆4a ◆4c ◆5a

Skill: Moving
Objective: Perform a circle dance while singing a three-part round

Secondary Skills
- **Listening** Listen for repetition and contrast of a round
- **Singing** Sing *a cappella*, in unison, and as a round
- **Playing** Play a keyboard accompaniment
- **Moving** Perform movement to song
- **Creating** Create a rap; perform it as a round

SKILLS REINFORCEMENT
- **Singing** Indicate raised and normal sevenths while singing part of a song
- **Keyboard** Play a left-handed ostinato part

LESSON 5
Canon Form

pp. 124–127

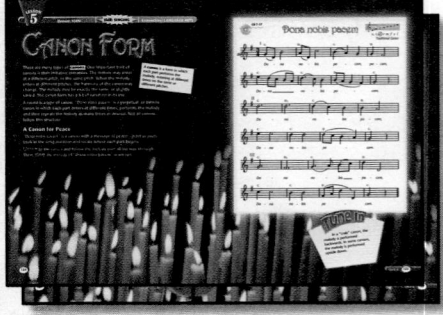
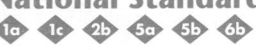

Element: Form
Concept: Canon
Focus: Canon

Secondary Element
Melody: melodic contour

National Standards
◆1a ◆1c ◆2b ◆5a ◆5b ◆6b

Skill: Singing
Objective: Sight-read and sing a song in three-part canon

Secondary Skills
- **Analyzing** Recognize characteristics of a round; analyze form
- **Singing** Sing, compare, and analyze three melodies
- **Playing** Play a metallophone accompaniment

SKILLS REINFORCEMENT
- **Singing** Sing a scale in a two-part canon
- **Extending the Vocal Range** Use warm up exercises to extend the upper range in student's voices

LESSON 6
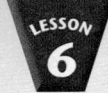
Fugue Form

pp. 128–129

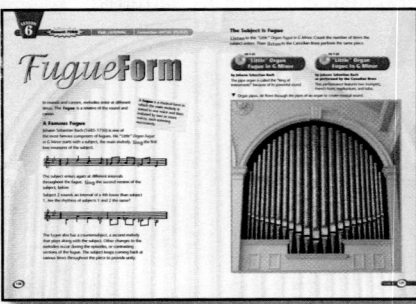

Element: Form
Concept: Fugue
Focus: Fugue

Secondary Element
Melody: tonality

National Standards
◆1a ◆5a ◆6a ◆6c ◆8b

Skill: Listening
Objective: Aurally identify the entrance of the subject in a fugue

Secondary Skills
- **Listening** Listen for the countersubjects in a fugue

SKILLS REINFORCEMENT
- **Singing** Teach and sing the intervals within a harmonic minor scale

Connections

Music and Other Literature

Connection: Genre
Activity: Demonstrate the characteristics of a round by creating a spoken round

MEETING INDIVIDUAL NEEDS **Inclusion** Avoid action that will set students apart as being "different"

ACROSS THE CURRICULUM **Language Arts** Read loud, dramatize, and create movements for a poem

BUILDING SKILLS THROUGH MUSIC **Math** Work with fractions

Songs
"Dance for the Nations"

Poem
"Celebration"

More Music Choices
"Gloria, Gloria," p. 459
"Let Us Sing Together," p. 156

ASSESSMENT

Performance/Peer Critique Perform a circle dance with the round to show form

TECHNOLOGY/MEDIA LINK
Sequencing Software Create a round by copying and pasting a melody into additional tracks

---

Connection: Language Arts
Activity: Discuss the use of the Latin language in the past and in the present

MEETING INDIVIDUAL NEEDS **Gifted and Talented** Find English words that have Latin Roots

SPOTLIGHT ON **Canon Versus Rounds** Distinguish the differences between canons and rounds

MOVEMENT **Locomotor Movement** Learn movements to accompany a song

TEACHER TO TEACHER **Playing I, IV, and V Chords on Mallet Instruments** Follow chosen mallet chords for best voice leading and hand position

CULTURAL CONNECTION
An Ancient Language Learn about Latin and its uses today and in the past
A Living Language Discuss the uses of Latin in modern society

BUILDING SKILLS THROUGH MUSIC **Language** Use inference to learn the meaning of words

Song *"Dona nobis pacem"*

Listening Selection
Canon for Violin and Cello

More Music Choices
"Hey, Ho! Nobody Home," p. 28
"Do, Re, Mi, Fa," p. 80
"Alleluia," p. 133

ASSESSMENT

Performance/Observation Identify the form of *"Dona nobis pacem"* and sing the song in three-part canon

TECHNOLOGY/MEDIA LINK
Sequencing Software Compose a canon
MIDI Keyboard Experiment with sounds that are appropriate to accompany the song

---

Connection: Social Studies
Activity: Discuss events in United States history that occurred during the lifetime of J.S. Bach

SPOTLIGHT ON **Johann Sebastian Bach and Pipe Organs** Facts about Bach and organs

ACROSS THE CURRICULUM
Social Studies Put the life of Bach into the context of U.S. history

BUILDING SKILLS THROUGH MUSIC **Science** Determine pitches of pipes by size

Listening Selections
"Little" Organ Fugue in G Minor (organ)
"Little" Organ Fugue in G Minor (brass)

More Music Choices
Jesu, Joy of Man's Desiring, p. 87
"Minuet" from *Orchestral Suite No. 2 in B Minor,* p. 192

ASSESSMENT

Observation Listen to identify a fugue subject

TECHNOLOGY/MEDIA LINK
MIDI/Sequencing Software Create a fugue using a pre-composed subject

Lesson	Elements	Skills	
LESSON 7 **Building Intervals** pp. 130–131 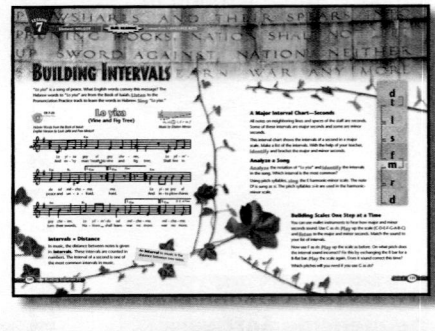 Reading Sequence 15, p. 495	**Element: Melody** **Concept:** Melodic Intervals **Focus:** Half steps, whole steps **Secondary Element** Melody: harmonic minor scales **National Standards** 1c 5e 6a 6b 6c	**Skill: Reading** **Objective:** Read and identify intervals in a harmonic minor song **Secondary Skills** • **Listening** Listen to a song and determine its key • **Analyzing** Compare the key signature of a song with a pitch set; identify intervals	**SKILLS REINFORCEMENT** • **Mallets** Play an Orff accompaniment • **Reading** Practice working with intervals • **Singing** Sing a canon
LESSON 8 **CORE** **Moving Motives** pp. 132–133 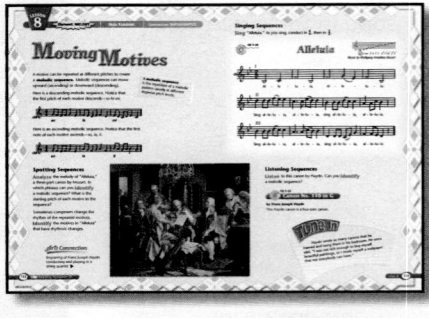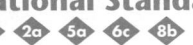 Reading Sequence 16, p. 495	**Element: Melody** **Concept:** Pattern **Focus:** Melodic Sequence **Secondary Element** Rhythm: meter **National Standards** 1d 2a 5a 6c 8b	**Skill: Reading** **Objective:** Read melodic sequences **Secondary Skills** • **Singing** Sing sequences with pitch syllables • **Reading** Locate a motive and sequence in a score • **Listening** Listen for a sequence	**SKILLS REINFORCEMENT** • **Notating** Notate a diatonic B-flat major scale, circle pitch set of a song, then transpose it
LESSON 9 **Sequence-It** pp. 134–135 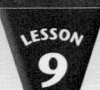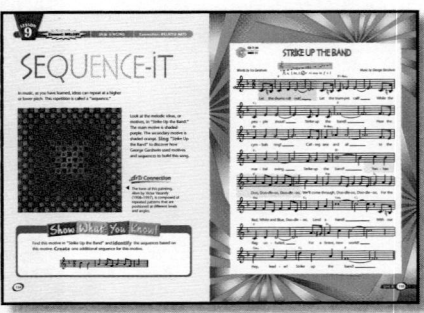	**Element: Melody** **Concept:** Pattern **Focus:** Sequences **Secondary Element** Rhythm: meter **National Standards** 1a 2a 4c 6c 8a	**Skill: Singing** **Objective:** Sing a song that employs sequences **Secondary Skills** • **Analyzing** Analyze sequences • **Movement** Create movements to represent melodic sequences	**SKILLS REINFORCEMENT** • **Recorder** Play a countermelody

Connections

Music and Other Literature

Connection: Language Arts

Activity: Identify Hebrew words and phrases in a song

TEACHER TO TEACHER **Interval Charts** Use creative methods to help understand intervals

ACROSS THE CURRICULUM **Language Arts** Share a book about working together to change the world for better

BUILDING SKILLS THROUGH MUSIC **Writing** Write a paragraph about changing the world

Song "Lo yisa" ("Vine and Fig Tree")

More Music Choices
"El cóndor pasa," p. 46
"Sometimes I Feel Like a Motherless child," p. 241

ASSESSMENT

Performance/Observation
Read the notation of a song and identify major and minor seconds

TECHNOLOGY/MEDIA LINK

Sequencing Software
Record the melody for a song and create two more tracks using copy and paste functions to create a three-part round

---

Connection: Mathematics

Activity: Examine a mathematical sequence in a word problem

SPOTLIGHT ON **The Composer** Facts about Franz Joseph Haydn

ACROSS THE CURRICULUM **Math** Explore a numerical sequence in a word problem; notate it in C major

CHARACTER EDUCATION **Cooperation** Discuss what things take cooperation and why is it important

BUILDING SKILLS THROUGH MUSIC **Language** Compare the lives of two composers

Songs "Alleluia"

Listening Selection
Canon No. 110 in G (excerpt)

More Music Choices
"Strike Up the Band," p. 135
"Hava nagila," p. 153

ASSESSMENT

Performance/Observation
Sing a countermelody while indicating a melodic sequence

TECHNOLOGY/MEDIA LINK

Notation Software
Notate and play back created sequences in canon

Connection: Related Arts

Activity: Compare sequences in visual art to sequences in music

SPOTLIGHT ON **Title Song** Facts about the song and the show it is from

ACROSS THE CURRICULUM **Visual Arts** Learn facts about Victor Vasarely; read a book containing imitative and sequential designs

BUILDING SKILLS THROUGH MUSIC **Writing** Use poetry to illustrate sequence

Song "Strike Up the Band,"

More Music Choices
"Goin' to Boston," p. 433
"Take Time in Life," p. 292

ASSESSMENT

Performance/Observation
Sing a song and move to show melodic sequences

TECHNOLOGY/MEDIA LINK

MIDI/Sequencing Software Add an electronic percussion part to song

Lesson	Elements	Skills

LESSON 10

CORE
Hear the Band!
pp. 136–139

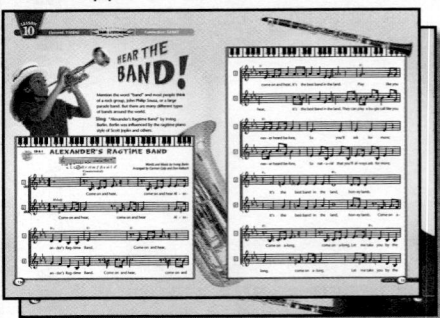

Element: Timbre
Concept: Instrumental
Focus: Band instrumentation

Secondary Element
Melody: motive

National Standards
1d 5a 6b 8b 9a

Skill: Listening
Objective: Listen for the differences between a big band and a concert band

Secondary Skills
- **Reading** Listen for rhythmic motives in a song
- **Singing** Sing and identify rhythmic motives from a song and sing the song
- **Listening** Explore instruments within the concert band

SKILLS REINFORCEMENT
- **Listening** Distinguish whole steps and half steps aurally

---

LESSON 11

CORE
Reggae Harmonies
pp. 140–143

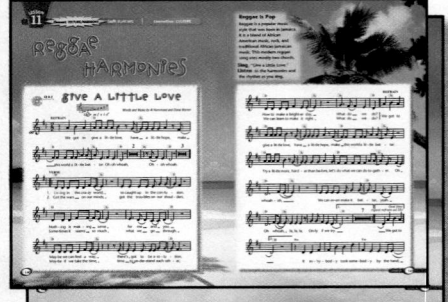
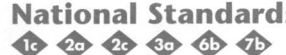

Element: Texture/Harmony
Concept: Texture
Focus: Chordal accompaniment

Secondary Element
Form: verse/refrain

National Standards
1c 2a 2c 3a 6b 7b

Skill: Playing
Objective: Plan an accompaniment in reggae style

Secondary Skills
- **Listening** Following the notation and identify the form of a song
- **Singing** Sing while accenting the strong beat of a song
- **Analyzing** Analyze beat, chord structure and frequency
- **Playing** Play chords for a song
- **Listening** Listen for changes in texture

SKILLS REINFORCEMENT
- **Recorder** Learn an accompaniment
- **Improvising** Improvise a drum part for a song
- **Singing** Sing songs from other cultures

LESSON 12

Guitar Textures
pp. 144–145

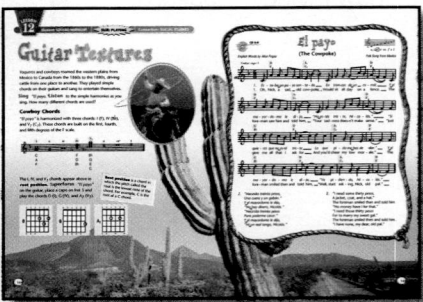

Element: Texture/Harmony
Concept: Texture
Focus: Homophonic texture

Secondary Element
Rhythm: $\frac{6}{8}$ meter

National Standards
1c 2a 5c 6c 8b

Skill: Playing
Objective: Accompany a song on the guitar or piano using the F, B-flat and C-seven chords

Secondary Skills
- **Singing** Sing a song with the recording in English and Spanish
- **Playing** Accompany a song with guitar and piano

SKILLS REINFORCEMENT
- **Mallets** Play an Orff accompaniment
- **Recorder** Play a soprano recorder accompaniment
- **Guitar** Accompany a song using a rhythm in the book

Connections

Connection: Genre

Activity: Understand the role and history of different kinds of bands

ACROSS THE CURRICULUM
Social Studies Learn about world events in the year 1911
Math Explore the overtone series with a bugle

SPOTLIGHT ON
The Concert Band Facts about concert bands
The Composer Morton Gould

CULTURAL CONNECTION
The British Brass Band Facts about British brass bands

TEACHER TO TEACHER **Listening** Write descriptions of instrumental and musical events

SCHOOL TO HOME CONNECTION **Interviews** Talk to family and friends about concert bands

BUILDING SKILLS THROUGH MUSIC **Social Studies** Create a timeline

Connection: Culture

Activity: Recognize that popular culture today is influenced by cultures from all over the world

MEETING INDIVIDUAL NEEDS **Syncopated Lyrics** Suggested activities for dealing with syncopation

SPOTLIGHT ON **Harmony** Construct the primary chords on scale tones

ACROSS THE CURRICULUM **Social Studies** Explore the geography and history of Jamaica

CHARACTER EDUCATION **Kindness and Social Responsibility** Discuss what students might do to make the world better

CULTURAL CONNECTION **Jamaican *Ska*** Facts about *ska* style

BUILDING SKILLS THROUGH MUSIC **Language** Create an outline

Connection: Social Studies

Activity: Explore the history of cowboy culture in the West

TEACHER TO TEACHER **Resonator Bells and Hand Chimes** Can be a substitute for the keyboard

SCHOOL TO HOME CONNECTION **Interview and Report** Interview friends and family who travel and have them report their findings

BUILDING SKILLS THROUGH MUSIC **Math** Create a chart

Music and Other Literature

Song "Alexander's Ragtime Band"

Listening Selections
"March" from *Suite No. 2 in F, Op. 28b*
Fanfare for Freedom
M·U·S·I·C M·A·K·E·R·S
Gustav Holst

More Music Choices
Variation on "The Carnival of Venice", p. 161
Galliard battaglia, p. 362
March militaire, Op. 51, No. 1, p.17

Song "Give a Little Love"

Listening Selection
Reggae Is Now
M·U·S·I·C M·A·K·E·R·S
Ziggy Marley

More Music Choices
"*Adiós, amigos*," p. 57
"Down in the Valley, p. 375

Song "*El payo*" ("The Cowpoke")

More Music Choices
"*Las mañanitas*," p. 481
"Red River Valley" p. 11

ASSESSMENT

Music Journal Writing Listen and write about the differences in timbre between a big band and a concert band

TECHNOLOGY/MEDIA LINK

Electronic Keyboard Create an accompaniment with a desired instrument sound found on a MIDI keyboard

ASSESSMENT

Performance/Peer Critique Sing a song in reggae style; perform a chordal accompaniment and a rhythm complex with the song and evaluate texture changes

TECHNOLOGY/MEDIA LINK

CD-ROM Try different accompaniments for a song

Web Site Learn more about the music of Jamaica

ASSESSMENT

Performance/Observation Sing a song while pairs of students play a chordal accompaniment

TECHNOLOGY/MEDIA LINK

Web Site Learn more about Mexican music and *mariachi* bands

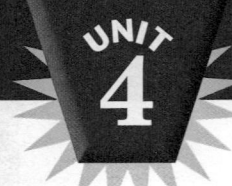

INTRODUCING THE UNIT

Unit 4, *Building Our Musical Skills,* provides students with the additional tools they need to be successful performers, listeners, and composers. Students will explore a variety of musical styles, genres, and musical elements as they build their musical skills. This unit features American jazz, folk songs, ballads; reggae and Mexican harmonies; canon and fugue form; and melodic intervals, motives, and sequences. Skills assessed in this unit can be found on p. 111. Unit highlights are listed in the footnotes.

UNIT PROJECT

Invite students to read the text on p. 110. Write these categories on the board: timbre, dynamics, melody, harmony, rhythm, and expression. Have students listen to *In the Mood* **CD 6–28.** Discuss what elements of the song are "hot," using the categories as a guide. (For example, the rhythm is syncopated and fast with surprising pauses; the timbre is bright and brassy.)

Discuss the different sounds made by the instruments pictured on pp. 110–111. Help students think of adjectives to describe each instrument. Guide them to understand that our ears can distinguish the differences in timbres between instruments.

Invite students to create movements for *In the Mood.* Assign half of the class to represent the woodwind timbre and half to represent the brass timbre. Have students perform a unique movement when they hear their instrument's timbre.

Jazz—Hot, Swing, and Big Band

American big band jazz of the 1930s is often categorized as both "swing" and "hot." These slang terms describe jazz that is fast, exciting, energetic, and rhythmic. The big band sound and improvised jazz solos added to the excitement.

The excitement of big band jazz is heard in music performed by Glenn Miller (1904–1944), an arranger and bandleader. The Glenn Miller Orchestra was one of the most popular bands of the 1930s and 1940s.

Listen to one of Glenn Miller's most famous big band pieces, *In the Mood.*

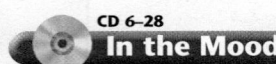

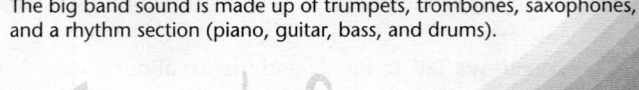
CD 6–28
In the Mood

by Joseph Garland
as performed by the Glenn Miller Orchestra

The big band sound is made up of trumpets, trombones, saxophones, and a rhythm section (piano, guitar, bass, and drums).

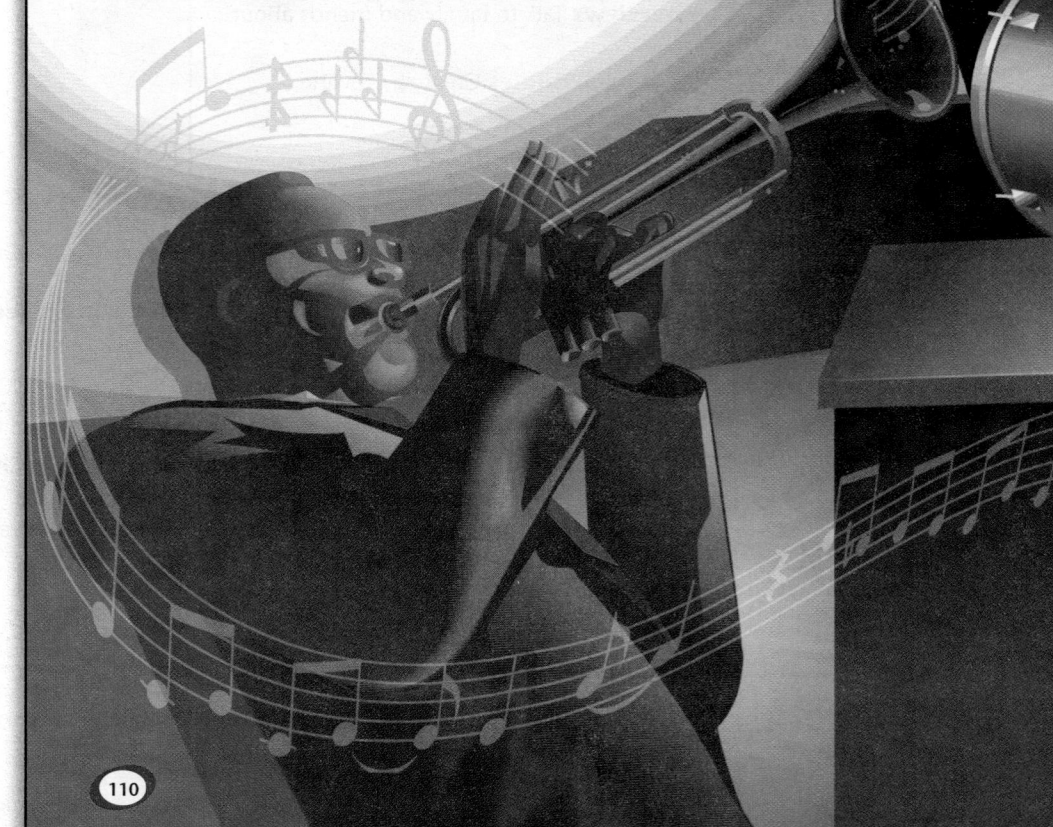

110

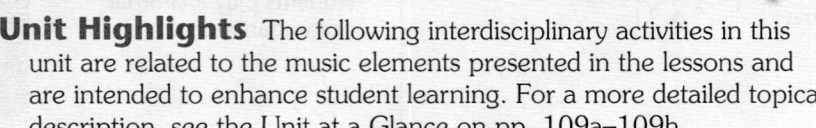

ACROSS THE CURRICULUM

Unit Highlights The following interdisciplinary activities in this unit are related to the music elements presented in the lessons and are intended to enhance student learning. For a more detailed topical description, see the Unit at a Glance on pp. 109a–109h.

▶ **LANGUAGE ARTS**
- Categorize words as simple and compound meter (p. 120)
- Read a poem, dramatize it and create movements (p. 122)
- Read a book about making the world a better place (p. 130)

▶ **MATH**
- Use math symbols to compare tempos (p. 116)
- Solve a word problem based on a mathematic series (p. 133)
- Explore the harmonic series of a B♭ bugle (p. 138)

▶ **SOCIAL STUDIES**
- Learn about the importance of rivers (p. 118)
- Learn facts about J. S. Bach and research other composers (p. 129)
- Share historical events from the year 1911 (p. 136)
- Discover information about Jamaica (p. 141)

▶ **VISUAL ARTS**
- Discover facts about artists Victor Vasarely and M. C. Escher (p. 134)

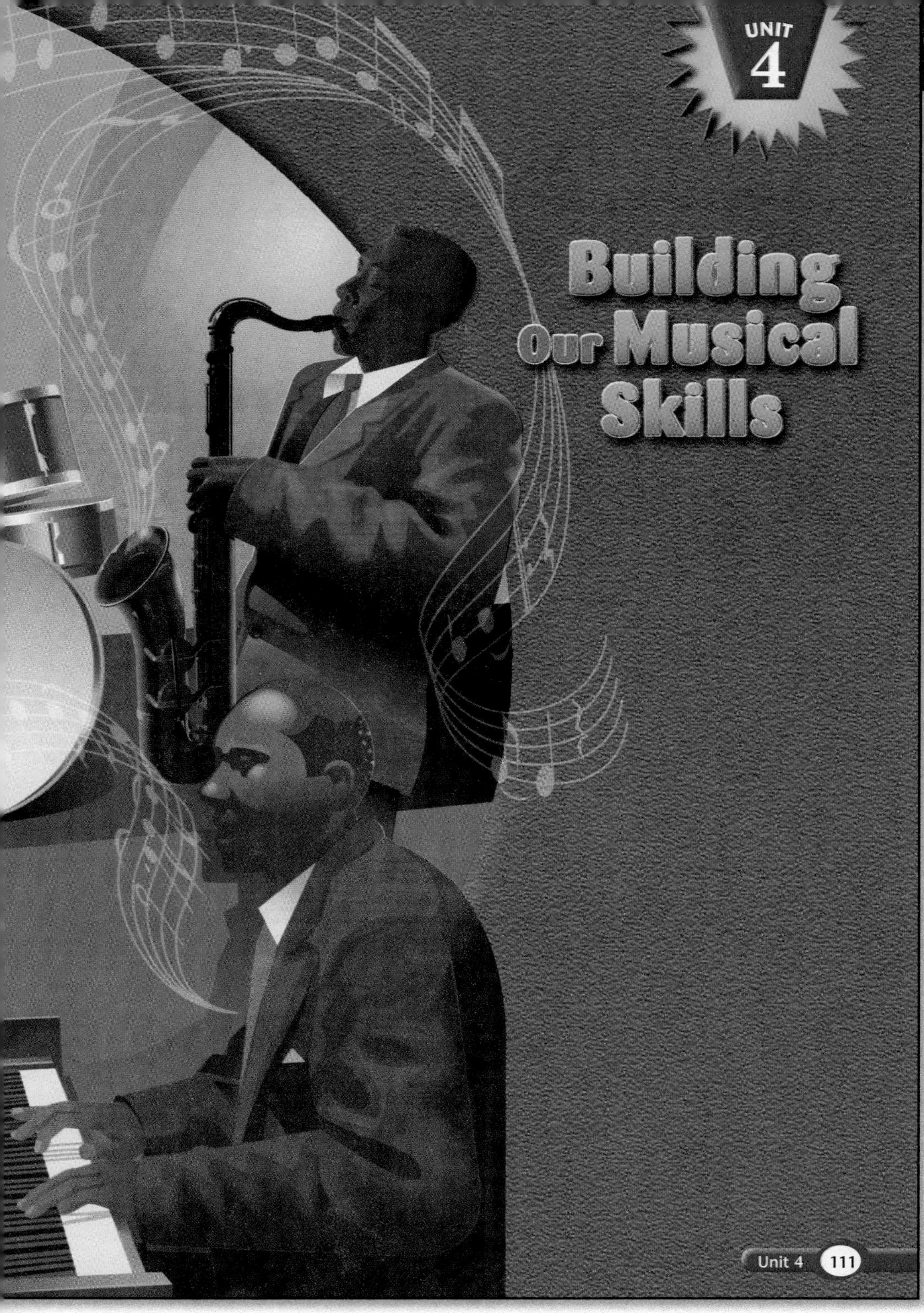

Building Our Musical Skills

MUSIC SKILLS ASSESSED IN THIS UNIT

Reading Music: Rhythm

- Read and perform rhythms in $\frac{2}{2}$ meter (p. 119)
- Read and perform rhythms in $\frac{3}{8}$ and $\frac{6}{8}$ meter (p. 121)

Reading Music: Pitch

- Read and identify the intervals of a major and minor second in a song (p. 131)
- Read and sing a countermelody using pitch syllables (p. 133)

Performing Music: Singing

- Sing "At the Same Time" with an appropriate tempo (p. 117)
- Sing the three-part canon *"Dona nobis pacem"* (p. 127)
- Sing a song and perform movements to show phrases and melodic sequences (p. 135)

Performing Music: Playing

- Perform chord and rhythm accompaniments to a reggae song (p. 143)
- Perform a chord accompaniment on guitar to *"El payo"* (p. 145)

Listening to Music

- Listen to a fugue and identify the subject (p. 129)
- Listen to and describe the instrumental timbre in several band selections (p. 139)

Moving to Music

- Sing and perform movements to "Dance for the Nations" (p. 123)

CULTURAL CONNECTION

Unit Highlights The musical literature in this unit provides many opportunities for students to explore a variety of world cultures. A more detailed description of the resources and activities listed below can be found in the Unit at a Glance on pp. 109a–109h.

▶ **CARIBBEAN**

- Explore the history and roots of Jamaican *ska* (p. 143)

▶ **EUROPEAN**

- Learn about the Latin language and its uses (p. 127)
- Discover facts about the British brass band (p. 137)

▶ **UNITED STATES**

- Read about and listen to Appalachian Mountain music (p. 121)

OPENING ACTIVITIES

MATERIALS

- "Hit Me with a Hot note and
  Watch Me Bounce"   **CD 6–29**

  Recording Routine: Intro (4 m.); vocal; coda

- **Dance Directions** for "Hit Me with a Hot Note
  and Watch Me Bounce," p. 556

- *In the Mood*   **CD 6–28**

- *Interview with Ann Hampton Callaway
  and Michael Rafter*   **CD 6–33**

- barred mallet instruments

Listening

Listen to the recorded interview of Ann Hampton Callaway and Michael Rafter **CD 6–33**, and discuss the differences and similarities of their musical careers.

Listen to "Hit Me With a Hot Note and Watch Me Bounce" **CD 6–29**.

Singing

Sing "Hit Me With a Hot Note and Watch Me Bounce" as a class. Assign individuals or small groups to sing the solo parts of the song. Encourage others to join in on parts marked "All."

Reading

Give students a primer in reading "Hit Me With a Hot Note and Watch Me Bounce." Guide them through the music, noting the following points. Have students discover

- An indication to swing the eighth notes, above the key signature. (Give an aural example.)
- *Do* is E♭.
- G♭ and F♯ are blue notes. Tell students the accidentals are notated because they are not in the key signature.
- The markings "Solo" and "All."

Bouncin' Along

Sing the jazz song "Hit Me with a Hot Note and Watch Me Bounce." After you know the song, snap your fingers on the offbeats as you sing. Be cool.

"Hit Me with a Hot Note and Watch Me Bounce" is a jazz classic by Duke Ellington. This song is featured in the Broadway musical *Swing*.

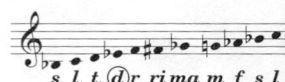

CD 6–29

Hit Me with a Hot Note and Watch Me Bounce

Words by Don George   Music by Duke Ellington

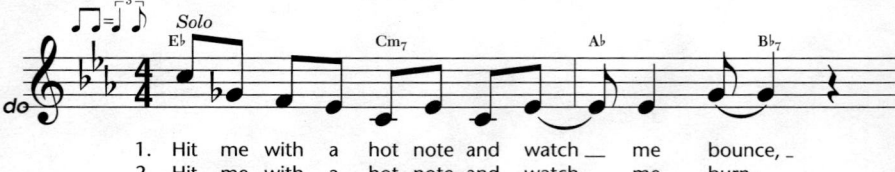

1. Hit me with a hot note and watch __ me bounce, _
2. Hit me with a hot note and watch __ me burn, _
3. Hit me with a hot note and watch __ me bounce, _

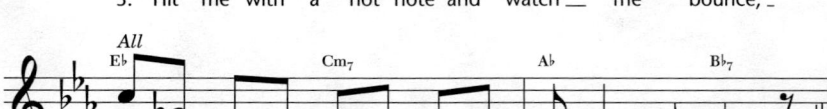

Hit me with a hot note and watch __ me bounce, _   When
Slap me down with rhy-thm from stem __ to stern, _   When
Knock me out with mu-sic in great __ a-mounts, _   Oh,

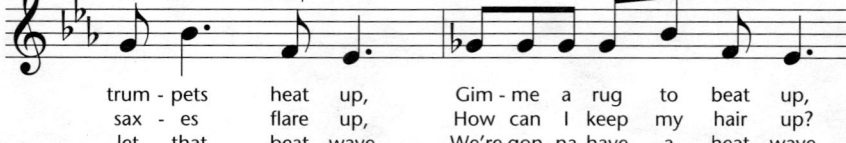

trum-pets heat up,   Gim-me a rug to beat up,
sax-es flare up,   How can I keep my hair up?
let that beat wave,   We're gon-na have a heat wave,

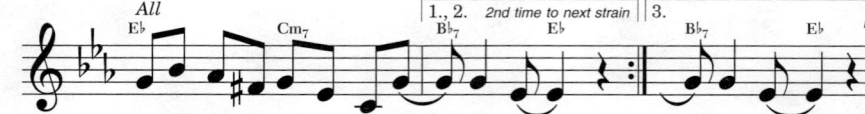

Hit me with a hot note and watch _ me bounce. _   _ me bounce. _
Hit me with a hot note and watch _ me bounce. _
Hit me with a hot note and watch _

(112)

ASSESSMENT

Unit Highlights This unit includes a variety of strategies and methods, described below, to track students' progress and assess their understanding of lesson objectives. Reproducible masters for Show What You Know! and Review, Assess, Perform, Create can be found in the Resource Book.

▶ FORMAL ASSESSMENTS

The following assessments, using written language, cognitive, and performance skills, help teachers and students conceptualize the learning that is taking place.

- **Show What You Know!** Element-specific assessments, on the student page, for Rhythm (p. 120) and Melody (p. 134)
- **Review, Assess, Perform, Create** This end-of-unit activity (pp. 146–147) can be used for review and to assess students' learning of the core lessons in this unit.

▶ INFORMAL ASSESSMENTS

At the close of each Teacher's Edition lesson in this unit, one of the following types of assessments is used to evaluate the learning of the key element focus or skill objective.

- Music Journal Writing (p. 139)
- Observation (p. 129)
- Performance/Observation (pp. 119, 127, 131, 133, 135, 145)
- Performance/Peer Critique (pp. 123, 143)
- Performance/Self-Assessment (pp. 117, 121)

▶ RUBRICS

Visit *www.sfsuccessnet.com* for rubrics to assess students' achievement in music skills.

MUSIC MAKERS

Ann Hampton Callaway and Michael Rafter

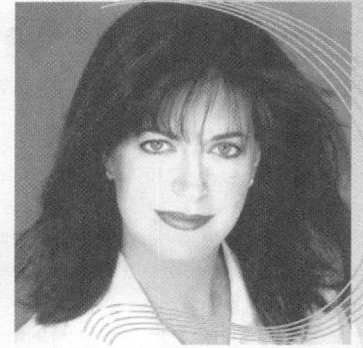

Ann Hampton Callaway is a jazz singer and songwriter. Born in Chicago, she began her career as a singer in Chicago jazz clubs, and later in New York cabarets. Callaway is well-known for her ballads and scat singing. As a songwriter, Callaway wrote "At the Same Time," page 115, which was recorded by Barbra Streisand. She also wrote the opening theme to the TV show *The Nanny.* Callaway has appeared in the Broadway musical *Swing,* and has toured internationally, performing songs from her acclaimed CD, *To Ella with Love.*

Michael Rafter is a conductor, music supervisor, producer, and an arranger. In addition to *Swing,* he has worked on the Broadway musicals *Les Misèrables, The King and I, Gypsy, The Sound of Music,* and *Thoroughly Modern Millie.* Rafter worked with Bette Midler in the TV movie *Gypsy,* which won an Emmy for Musical Direction. Rafter has worked as an arranger and recording producer for *Making Music.*

Listen to Ann Hampton Callaway and Michael Rafter discuss their careers in music.

CD 6–33
Interview with Ann Hampton Callaway and Michael Rafter

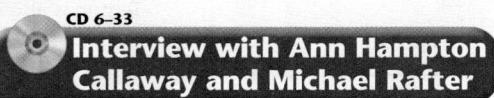

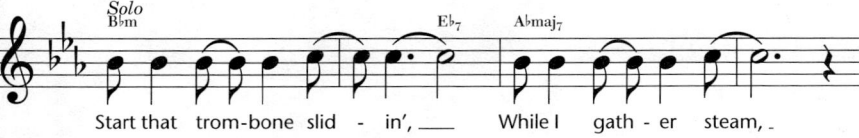

Start that trom-bone slid - in', ___ While I gath - er steam, _

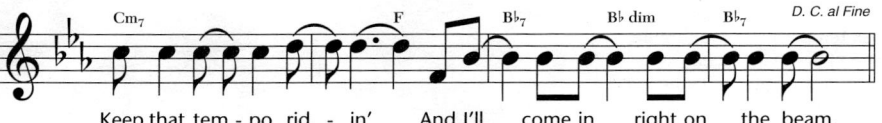

Keep that tem - po rid - in' ___ And I'll ___ come in ___ right on ___ the beam.

Unit 4 (113)

- The chord names written above the melody line. Tell them a piano player or guitarist can accompany the song using this notation.
- How to navigate the ends of phrases: There is a repeat at the end of the first verse; the second verse is followed by the B section on p. 113; *D. C. al Fine* means go back to the beginning and sing until the *Fine* sign (the end); and the third verse has its own ending.

Moving

Invite students to create jazz movements to the Dance Performance track of "Hit Me With a Hot Note and Watch Me Bounce" **CD 6–30.** See Dance Directions on p. 556 for movement instructions.

Improvising

Set up a variety of barred mallet instruments around the room to let students experiment with a blues scale. Take off bars as needed so each instrument has the following scale: E♭ F F♯ G A♭ B♭ C. Invite students to create a mini-melody, using these seven notes. Require each melody to use a blue note at least once.

INNOVATIVE TEACHER SUPPORT FOR THIS UNIT

- **MAKING MUSIC DVD, Grade 6** contains video segments that support lessons, including signing and movement.
- **MAKING MUSIC with Movement and Dance** provides more opportunities for large group activities in music or physical education classes.
- **MAKING MUSIC with Technology** provides lesson plans for many technology applications; includes MIDI files.
- *¡A cantar!* features recorded songs and lessons from around the Spanish-speaking world; includes strategies for bilingual classes and for English-speaking teachers working with Spanish-speaking students.
- **Bridges to Asia** features recorded songs and lessons from Asian and Pacific region cultures.
- *www.sfsuccessnet.com* provides an online lesson planner to conveniently create lesson plans at school or at home. Includes rubrics for assessment, lesson modifications to meet the needs of all students, performance musicals based on program content, and more.

TECHNOLOGY/MEDIA LINK

Unit Highlights The following components are used in this unit to reinforce and expand students' understanding of music elements and related themes.

▶ **CD-ROM**

- Use *Band-in-a-Box* to create different accompaniment styles for a reggae song (p. 143)

▶ **ELECTRONIC KEYBOARD**

- Perform a bass xylophone part on MIDI keyboard (p. 127)
- Play an accompaniment, using band timbres (p. 139)

▶ **MIDI/SEQUENCING SOFTWARE**

- Discover how tempo changes expression (p. 117)
- Enter fugue subjects and create a fugue (p. 129)
- Add an electronic accompaniment to a MIDI song file (p. 135)

▶ **NOTATION SOFTWARE**

- Compose and notate an accompaniment for a song (p. 119)
- Notate a rhythm in $\frac{3}{8}$ meter and change it to $\frac{6}{8}$ meter (p. 121)
- Notate and play back sequences in canon (p. 133)

▶ **SEQUENCING SOFTWARE**

- Enter a melody of a song and create a round (p. 123)
- Compose a canon, using sequencing software (p. 127)
- Record the melody of "Lo yisa" and create a round (p. 131)

▶ **WEB SITE**

- Learn more about the music of Jamaica (p. 143)
- Discover facts about *mariachi* style (p. 145)

LESSON AT A GLANCE

Element Focus	**EXPRESSION** Tempo
Skill Objective	**LISTENING** Listen to a song at different tempos and determine how tempo affects the character of a song
Connection Activity	**MATHEMATICS** Relate math symbols to musical terms for tempo

MATERIALS

- "At the Same Time" **CD 7-1**
  Recording Routine: Intro (2 m.); v. 1; v. 2; bridge; v. 3; coda
- *Oye mi canto* **CD 6-34**
- **Resource Book** p. C-6
- ticking timepiece, metronome

VOCABULARY

tempo	metronome	M.M.	*largo*
adagio	*andante*	*moderato*	*allegro*
vivace	*presto*	*prestissimo*	

◆ ◆ ◆ ◆ National Standards ◆ ◆ ◆ ◆

1c Sing music with appropriate expression
6c Understand and use basic principles of rhythm in music analysis
7a Students evaluate the music they hear
7b Students use specific criteria for evaluating their own performances
8b Identify ways music relates to math and social studies

MORE MUSIC CHOICES

For more practice exploring tempo:
"Jambalaya," p. 244
"Down in the Valley," p. 375

 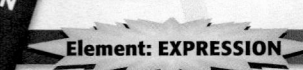
Take Your Time

Tempo, the speed of the music, is an important element of musical expression. Tempo can be fast, slow, or anywhere in between. **Listen** to "At the Same Time." Is the tempo fast or slow?

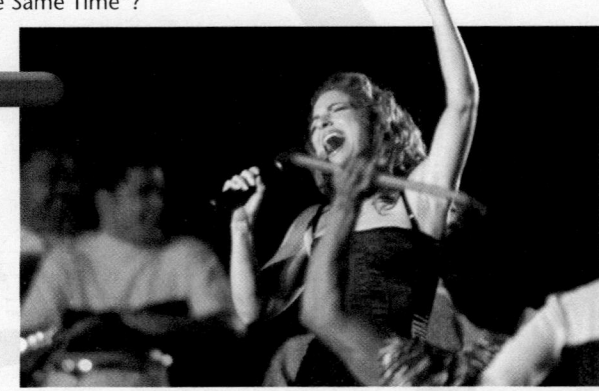

TEMPO TERM	DEFINITION	M.M.
Largo	Very slow	40–66
Adagio	Quite slow	66–76
Andante	Moderate, walking tempo	76–108
Moderato	Moderate	108–120
Allegro	Fast	120–168
Vivace	Lively	168–176
Presto	Very fast	176–184
Prestissimo	As fast as possible	184–208

A Musical Clock

Music has markings to tell performers the tempo. Tempo is indicated by metronome markings (M.M.). Like a clock, a metronome is set to play the desired number of beats per minute. For example, M.M. = 64 means there are 64 beats per minute.

Tempo is also indicated by special Italian words. Select the best tempo for "At the Same Time" from the list.

Listen to *Oye mi canto*. How does the tempo affect the character of the music? What instruments create rhythmic excitement? How does the tempo compare to "At the Same Time"?

 CD 6–34
Oye mi canto

**by Gloria Estefan, Jorge Casas, and Clay Ostwald
as performed by Gloria Estefan and the Miami Sound Machine**

Oye mi canto (Hear My Voice) begins in a brisk tempo in pop-rock style. The song changes to Cuban style with a rhythm section of Latin percussion and brass.

(114)

Footnotes

TEACHER TO TEACHER

▶ **Dividing the Class** Avoid the rut of dividing the class into groups by classroom location by using a variety of interesting and fun ways to split the class into groups. Try grouping students by topics such as the season of students' birthdays, colors worn by students on a given day, pet preferences, or favorite foods.

BUILDING SKILLS THROUGH MUSIC

▶ **Reading** Have students determine the mood of the lyrics of the song "At the Same Time." Let them use the semantic map on Resource Book, p. C-6, to document what the mood is and to show the phrases or words from the lyrics that support that answer.

SKILLS REINFORCEMENT

7a ▶ **Listening** Invite students to sharpen their listening skills with regard to tempo and knowing how each tempo sounds. Play listening selections from this book and have students write the Italian name for the tempo on a sheet of paper. After listening to each selection, invite a student volunteer to use a metronome to determine the beats per minute (the M.M. number) of the selection and find that tempo name in the chart on p. 114. Invite students to reveal the tempo name they chose while listening and why they chose it. You may wish to choose selections in which the tempo remains constant. Remind students to use standard music terminology for tempo names, as found in musical performance.

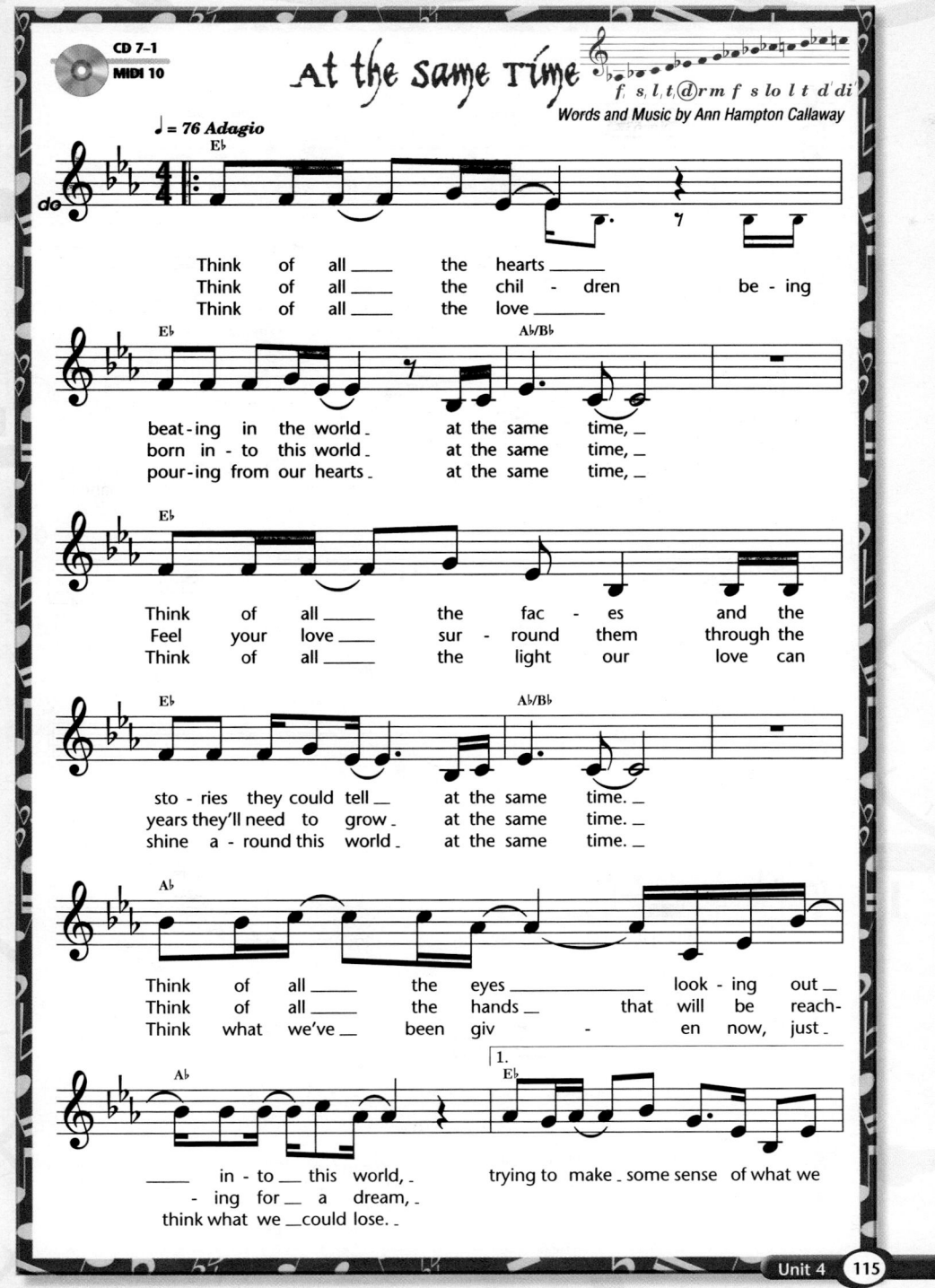

At the Same Time

CD 7-1
MIDI 10

Words and Music by Ann Hampton Callaway

♩ = 76 Adagio

Think of all ___ the hearts ___
Think of all ___ the chil - dren be - ing
Think of all ___ the love ___

beat-ing in the world ___ at the same time, ___
born in - to this world ___ at the same time, ___
pour-ing from our hearts ___ at the same time, ___

Think of all ___ the fac - es and the
Feel your love ___ sur - round them through the
Think of all ___ the light our love can

sto - ries they could tell ___ at the same time. ___
years they'll need to grow ___ at the same time. ___
shine a - round this world ___ at the same time. ___

Think of all ___ the eyes ___ look - ing out ___
Think of all ___ the hands ___ that will be reach-
Think what we've ___ been giv - en now, just ___

___ in - to ___ this world, ___
- ing for ___ a dream, ___
think what we ___ could lose. ___

trying to make ___ some sense of what we

Unit 4 **115**

1 INTRODUCE

Invite students to find their pulse and then tap the beat of their pulse on their desktops.

ASK Is your pulse steady or unsteady? (steady)

Encourage students to compare their pulse rate with a neighbor's rate and determine if the two pulses are beating at the same speed or at two different speeds.

Have students listen to the ticking of a timepiece and discover that its speed is 60 beats per minute.

Direct students' attention to the chart on p. 114.

6c **SAY** When M.M. equals a number, that number is the number of beats per minute. The marking indicates how fast the pulse, or beat, of the music should beat. The speed of the beat is the *tempo*.

ASK Which music term on the chart would indicate 60 beats per minute? *(largo)*

Explain to students that tempo is an important aspect of musical expression and that the musical terms and symbols indicating tempo tell the performing musician when to change tempo.

2 DEVELOP

Singing

1c Encourage students to interpret the tempo of "At the Same Time" **CD 7-1** by lightly tapping the steady beat on their desks as they sing the song with the recording.

ASK Was the tempo fast or slow? (slow)

Tell students that Italian words are used to describe the tempo and expressive character of a piece of music. The words give a general idea of how fast or slow a piece of music should be performed. Metronome markings are also used to indicate tempo and are more precise than the Italian terms. See Spotlight On below for more on the metronome.

continued on page 116

8b ▶ **The Metronome** The metronome is a device used to indicate the tempo of a piece of music by sounding regular beats at an adjustable speed. It was invented in 1812 by Dietrich Winkler and improved upon by Johann Maelzel, who added a scale of tempo divisions.

The nonelectronic metronome has a pendulum with a weight on each end and makes a ticking sound each time the pendulum changes direction. The weight at the top of the pendulum is movable. The pendulum's swing and the ticking sound become faster or slower when the weight is moved closer to or farther away from the axis. An M.M. (metronome marking) of 120 means that the pendulum oscillates from one side to the other 120 times per minute.

▶ **Learning a New Language** Frustration and withdrawal may occur for students who lack efficient strategies to quickly apply their learning of new words from a new language. Focus students' attention to this list of three distinct tempos that all have one-word meanings: *adagio* = slow, *moderato* = moderate, *allegro* = fast. Keep students' attention focused as you introduce each Italian word and its meaning. Point out the similarity between the words *moderate* and *moderato*. Invite students to sing phrases from familiar songs in each tempo and, with a partner, decide which is most appropriate for each song. Select a patient partner for any student who experiences difficulty using these new words.

ASK Which term best describes the tempo of "At the Same Time"? *(adagio)*

Listening

6c Invite students to determine the tempo marking for *Oye mi canto* **CD 6-34** as they listen to the recording.

ASK Is the tempo of *Oye mi canto* faster or slower than that of "At the Same Time"? *(faster)*

Which tempo marking would best fit the song? *(allegro or vivace)*

What would happen to the performance of this piece if it were played *largo*? (It would be unexciting and boring.)

SAY *Oye mi canto* was performed at a metronome marking of M.M. = 120, and you sang "At the Same Time" with the recording at a metronome marking of M.M. = 76. Let's find out what effect a faster tempo will have on "At the Same Time."

Invite students to sing "At the Same Time" with **CD 7-1**. Then, invite them to sing the song at M.M. = 120 without the recording.

Have students evaluate the effectiveness of tempo on musical performance.

7b **ASK** What happened when we changed the tempo to M.M. = 120? (The song became too fast to sing, and it lost its expressive quality.)

Explain to students that the Italian terms on p. 114 indicate not just tempo but the expressive character desired in performance. The literal meanings are:

- *largo* = broad
- *adagio* = at ease
- *andante* = walking
- *moderato* = moderately
- *allegro* = cheerful
- *vivace* = lively, vivacious

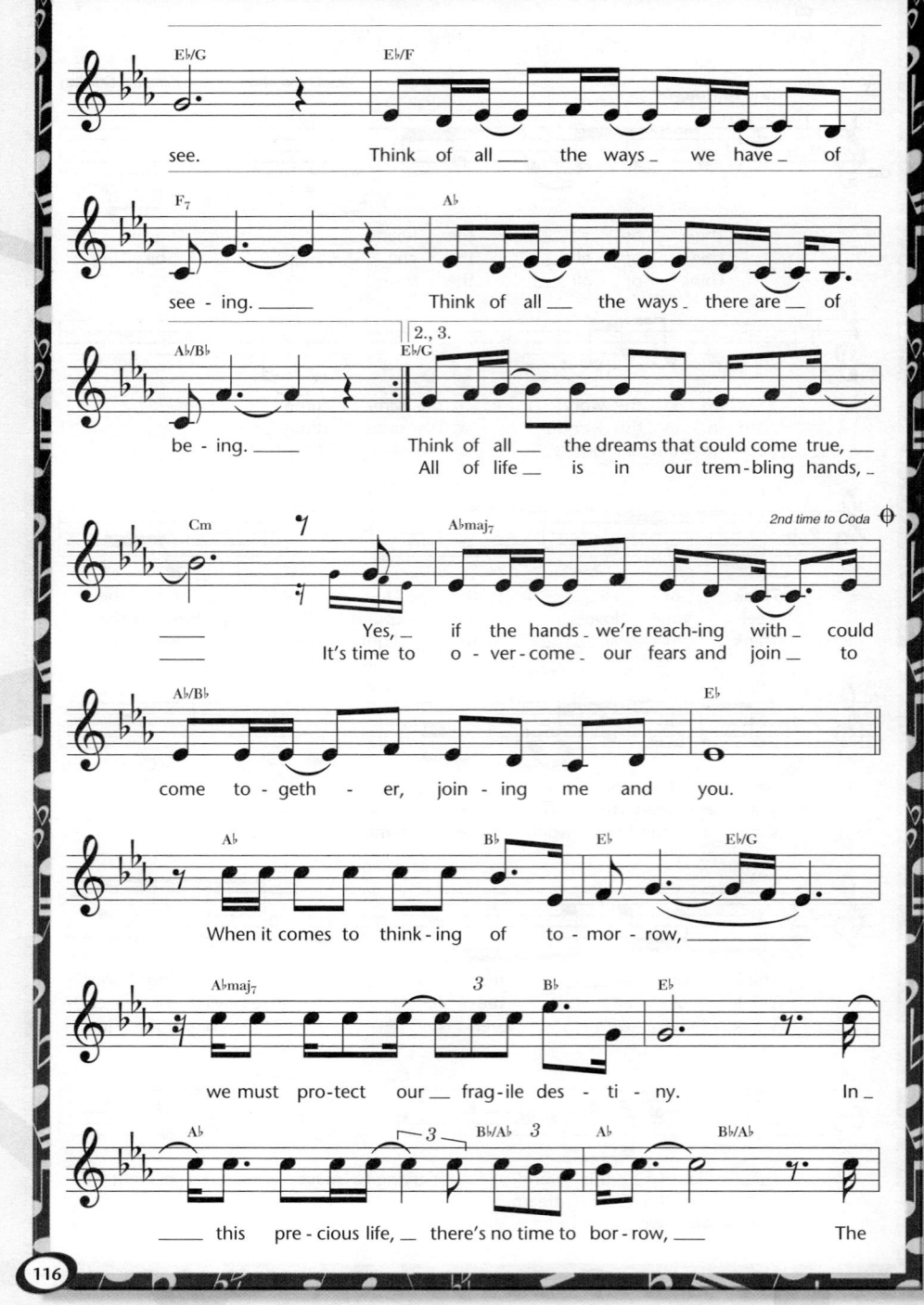

Footnotes

ACROSS THE CURRICULUM

8b ▶ **Math** Use the math symbols for greater than (>) and less than (<) to compare (relate) tempos as "faster than" and "slower than." Write pairs of tempo names on the board and have students write the correct math symbol between them; for example, *vivace > andante*, and *adagio < presto*. Have students

- Compare a *moderato* tempo of 120 to a *largo* tempo of 60: The *moderato* tempo has twice as many beats per minute as the *largo* ($120 = 2 \times 60$), so the *moderato* is twice as fast as the *largo*.

- Compare a *largo* tempo of 48 to an *allegro* tempo of 144: The *largo* tempo is three times slower than the *allegro*. ($48 = 144 \div 3$)

SKILLS REINFORCEMENT

6c ▶ **Singing** For each tempo listed on p. 114, have students look for at least one song from their books to illustrate it. Then do the following activity as a class.

Tell students that metronome and tempo markings are not indicated in many songs. They will need to determine tempos by singing and then approximating the correct tempo.

1c Make copies of the tempo chart found on p. 114. Identify ten of their favorite songs from the book. Sing each song with the recording to determine the tempo that best fits the expression of the song. Write the song title underneath the appropriate tempo marking. When the class has finished, make a composite list of songs that provides examples of each tempo marking.

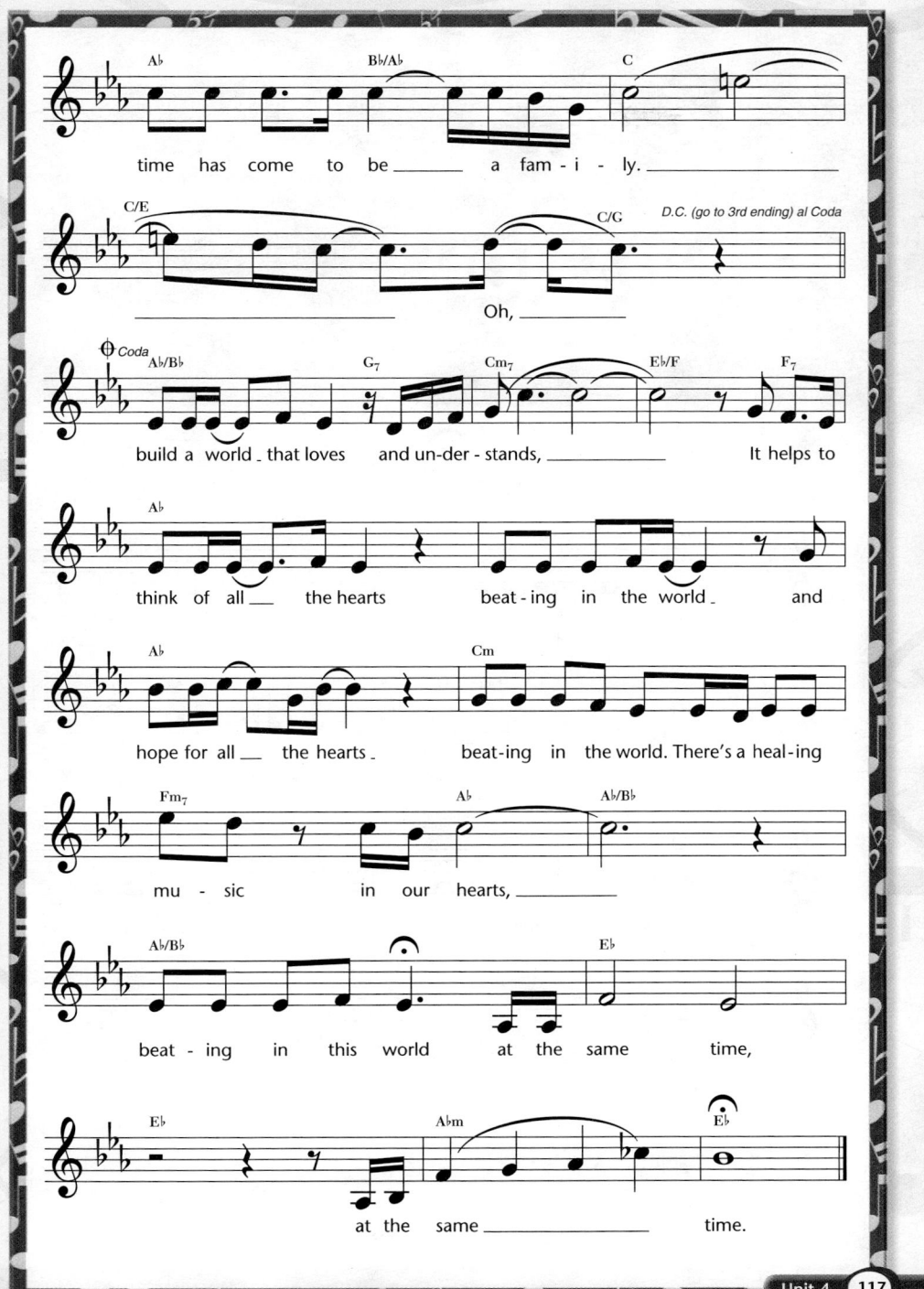

time has come to be ___ a fam-i-ly. ___

Oh, ___

build a world _ that loves and un-der-stands, ___ It helps to

think of all ___ the hearts beat-ing in the world _ and

hope for all ___ the hearts _ beat-ing in the world. There's a heal-ing

mu - sic in our hearts, ___

beat - ing in this world at the same time,

at the same ___ time.

- *presto* = very fast
- *prestissimo* = as fast as possible

See Across the Curriculum on p. 116 for ways of relat-ing tempos and math.

3 CLOSE

Element: EXPRESSION **ASSESSMENT**

 Performance/Self-Assessment Ask students, working in small groups, to decide the best tempo for "At the Same Time." Have students identify the follow-ing criteria for evaluating their performance.

Ask each group to sing the first verse without the recording. Encourage the class to decide if the tempo allowed the performers to sing words expressively with the rhythm.

If the class feels that the tempo was not effective, have the group experiment with another tempo and repeat the process until the tempo works well for the expres-sive qualities of the song.

The tempo may be different from that of the recording or what has been sung in class, but students should be ready to defend their chosen tempo.

MEETING INDIVIDUAL NEEDS

▶ **English Language Learners** The verses in this song provide an opportunity for students to write extension sentences, using a frame from the song text. Ask students to think about other things that many people are doing at the same time and invite them to write additional lines for the song. You may wish to write a frame like the following on the board.

   Think of all the _____ at the same time.

You may wish to suggest topics for students' consideration, such as meals being eaten at the same time, people going to work at the same time, or people laughing or crying at the same time. This activity will provide a fun extension and practice of English vocabulary.

TECHNOLOGY/MEDIA LINK

MIDI/Sequencing Software Open the MIDI song file for "At the Same Time." Invite students to experiment with changing the tempo of the song. Students may wish to make notes in their journals on the way the expressive quality of the song changes as the tempo gets faster and slower. Encourage students to report to the class, especially if they find a tempo that better suits the expression of the song than the tempo of the recording.

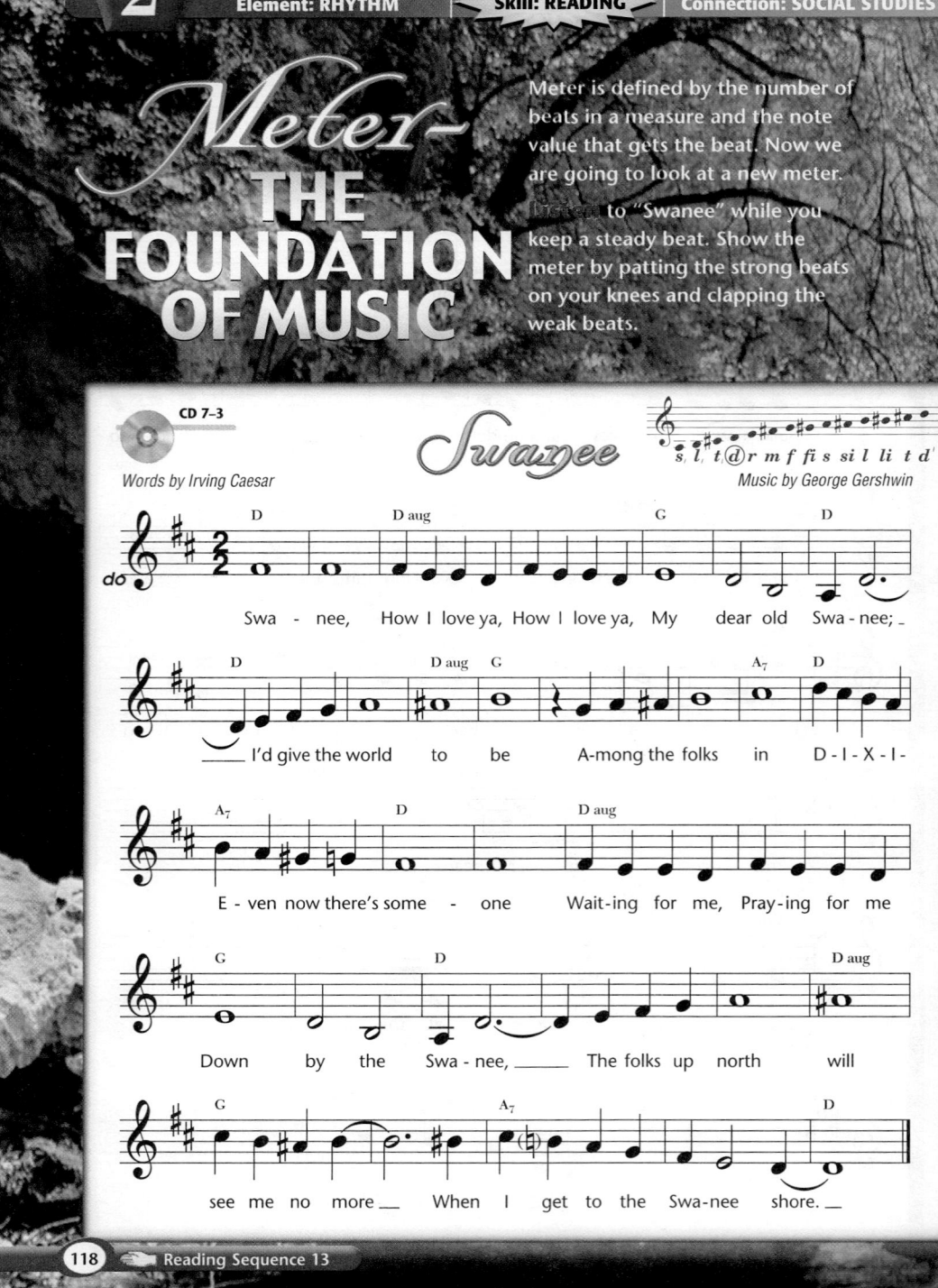

Core LESSON 2

LESSON AT A GLANCE

Element Focus	**RHYTHM** $\frac{2}{2}$ meter, cut time
Skill Objective	**READING** Read rhythms in $\frac{2}{2}$ meter
Connection Activity	**SOCIAL STUDIES** Discuss the social and economic significance of rivers, lakes, and oceans

MATERIALS
• "Swanee"   **CD 7-3**
  Recording Routine: Intro (4 m.); vocal; interlude (14 m.); partial vocal; coda
• **Music Reading Practice, Sequence 13**   **CD 7-5**
• **Resource Book** pp. D-16, E-14, H-14
• metronome

VOCABULARY
$\frac{4}{4}$ meter $\frac{2}{2}$ meter   ¢   cut time

◆ ◆ ◆ ◆ National Standards ◆ ◆ ◆ ◆
4c Compose, using electronic media
5a Read quarter notes and half notes in duple meter
5c Identify standard notation symbols for rhythm
6b Listen and analyze uses of rhythm in music from diverse cultures
6c Understand and use basic principles of meter in music analysis
8b Identify ways music relates to social studies

MORE MUSIC CHOICES
For more practice in cut time:
"Hey, Ho! Nobody Home," p. 28
"You Are My Sunshine," p. 246
For more practice reading simple duple meter:
"Lost My Gold Ring," p. 158

1 INTRODUCE

Tell students that "Swanee" is actually "Suwanee," a river located in southeast Georgia and northwest Florida. Lead a discussion about the social and economic importance of lakes and rivers. See Across the Curriculum below.

Footnotes

ACROSS THE CURRICULUM

8b ▶ **Social Studies** The title of the song "Swanee" represents a river in the southern United States. The lyrics imply that the singer has a loved one waiting back home in the South, by the shore of the Swanee. People who live by rivers, port cities, or lakeshores find that the body of water nearby is important to them in many ways. For some, the beauty of the water is enough. For others, the water is important for travel, shipping, fishing, or tourism.

BUILDING SKILLS THROUGH MUSIC

▶ **Writing** Share Across the Curriculum above with students. Ask students to select a body of water (lake, river, reservoir, ocean) near them and write a letter to someone to persuade them to move to its shores. Include at least three reasons why they should make the move.

SKILLS REINFORCEMENT

6c ▶ **Reading** Use Resource Book p. D-16 to teach students the conducting patterns for $\frac{2}{2}$, $\frac{3}{4}$, and $\frac{4}{4}$ meters. Tell students that the patterns for $\frac{2}{4}$ and $\frac{2}{2}$ will look the same. Then, have students interpret the metronome number markings for the examples and determine the tempo. (66=*adagio*, 132=*allegro*)

Tell students the metronome speed of the beat note is the same for examples 2 and 3 as they perform. Ask students to sing "Swanee" **CD 7-3** with rhythm syllables while conducting.

For more reading practice, invite students to perform a counter-rhythm for "Swanee" on p. 494, or Resource Book E-14.

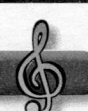 ▶ **Keyboard** Have students learn the whole-note keyboard acccompaniment in the Resource Book on p. H-14 for "Swanee."

Feel the Beat!

You can learn to recognize meters by feeling how beats are grouped in measures. Try tapping each of these patterns as you **sing** along with the recording of "Swanee." Which pattern feels correct for this song?

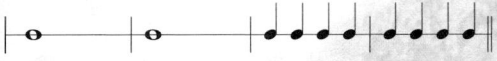

Now **read** the rhythm of the first four measures of "Swanee." How many beats are written in each measure? How many beats do you feel?

It doesn't quite add up, does it? The music sounds and feels like meter in 2, but it is written in 4. In this song, a different kind of note equals the beat.

Hear It, Feel It, Read It!

You can determine the meter of a song by looking at the time signature. The top number in a time signature shows how many beats are in each measure. The bottom number represents the beat note.

In $\frac{4}{4}$ meter, there are four beats in each measure, and the quarter note is the beat note.

In $\frac{2}{2}$, how many beats are in a measure? What note is the beat note?

$\frac{4}{4}$ meter is sometimes written like this. C

$\frac{2}{2}$ meter, or **cut time,** can be written like this. ¢

Look again at the music for "Swanee" and **identify** the meter and time signature.

> **Cut time** is a meter of 2 beats per measure; the half note gets the beat. This is also called $\frac{2}{2}$ meter.

What's the Meter?

You have learned that "Swanee" has two beats per measure with the half note getting the beat, and that it is in meter in 2. Another term for *meter in 2* is **duple meter.**

You have also discovered that each half note is subdivided into two quarter notes. When the beat is divided into two equal parts, it is called **simple meter.**

> **Duple meter** has two beats in each measure.
>
> In **simple meter** the beat is divided into two equal parts. Usually, the quarter note gets the beat.

Simple meter in $\frac{2}{4}$

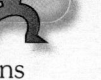

Unit 4 **119**

---

2 DEVELOP

Listening

Have students tap each pattern on p. 119 as they listen to and then sing "Swanee" **CD 7-3.**

6b **ASK** Which pattern feels correct for this song? (1) How many beats are in the pattern? (two) How many heavy beats? (one)

Reading

Help students to

5a
- Sight-read the first four measures of "Swanee" in the key of D in treble clef.

6c
- Use standard notation terminology and explain that the top number in the meter signature tells the number of beats in each measure and that the bottom number tells the beat note.

- Find that in $\frac{2}{2}$ meter there are two beats per measure and that the half note is the beat note.

- Understand that $\frac{2}{2}$ meter is also called cut time, shown by ¢.

5c
- Read the meter signature of "Swanee" and determine that there are two beats per measure and that the beat note is a half note.

- Compare examples of songs in $\frac{2}{2}$ and $\frac{2}{4}$ and lead students to discover that meter in 2 is duple meter, and that when the beat is divided into two equal parts, it is called simple meter.

See Skill Reinforcement, p. 118, and Movement below for additional activities.

3 CLOSE

Skill: READING ASSESSMENT

Performance/Observation Invite the class to pat the steady half-note beat in "Swanee" **CD 7-3** and read the notation with rhythm syllables. Observe students' ability to read the notation in $\frac{2}{2}$ meter.

MOVEMENT

5a ▶ **Conducting** Teach students the basic conducting patterns of $\frac{4}{4}$ (common time) and $\frac{2}{2}$ (cut time). As they listen to "Swanee" **CD 7-3,** have half the students conduct the $\frac{4}{4}$ pattern and the other half conduct the $\frac{2}{2}$ pattern at the same time, with the $\frac{4}{4}$ pattern being double the speed of the $\frac{2}{2}$ pattern. Tell the $\frac{4}{4}$ group members that they are conducting quarter notes in $\frac{4}{4}$ time and inform the $\frac{2}{2}$ group members that they are conducting half notes in $\frac{2}{2}$ time. Then reverse the roles.

TECHNOLOGY/MEDIA LINK

4c **Notation Software** Compose and notate an accompaniment for "Swanee." Notate the melody first, then add a staff for a bass part. Next choose an appropriate voice and notate half-note chord roots or chord roots and fifths. Then add another staff to notate half-note or quarter-note block chords. Students may then play back the file while singing the song.

LESSON AT A GLANCE

Element Focus   **RHYTHM** $\frac{3}{8}$ meter

Skill Objective   **READING** Read the rhythm of a song in $\frac{3}{8}$ meter

Connection Activity   **STYLE** Explore Appalachian ballad style

MATERIALS

- "One Morning in May"   **CD 7-8**
  Recording Routine: Intro (4 m.); v. 1; interlude (2 m.); v. 2; interlude (2 m.); v. 3; interlude (2 m.); v. 4; interlude (2 m.); v. 5; coda
- **Music Reading Practice, Sequence 14**   **CD 7-10**
- **Resource Book** pp. B-13, D-17, E-15, F-13

VOCABULARY

$\frac{6}{8}$ meter $\frac{3}{8}$ meter   ballad

◆ ◆ ◆ ◆ **National Standards** ◆ ◆ ◆ ◆

5a Read dotted quarter notes in $\frac{3}{8}$ meter
6a Listen and describe events in music using appropriate terms
6c Understand and use principles of meter in music analysis
8b Identify ways music relates to language arts

MORE MUSIC CHOICES

For more experience with ballads:
"Scarborough Fair," p. 95
For more practice in reading $\frac{6}{8}$ meter:
"Skye Boat Song," p. 372

1 INTRODUCE

8b Remind students that a ballad is a song with many verses that tells a story. Play "One Morning in May" **CD 7-8** and have students follow the story: A soldier plays his fiddle for a maiden. He plays so well she wants to marry him, however, he already has a wife. See Cultural Connection, p. 121, for another Appalachian story.

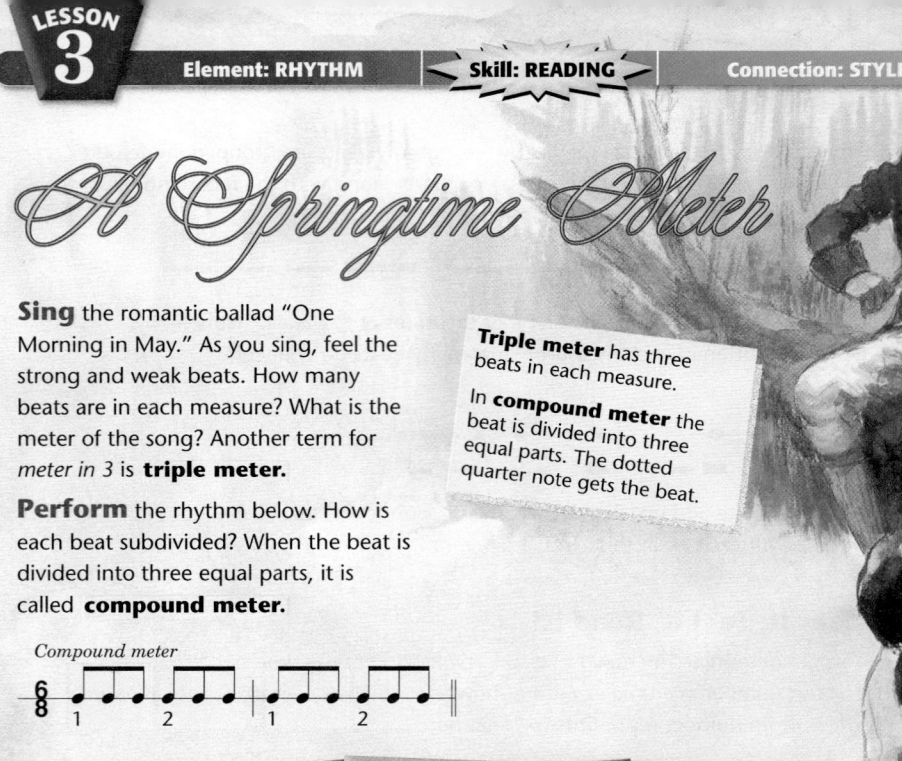

A Springtime Meter

Sing the romantic ballad "One Morning in May." As you sing, feel the strong and weak beats. How many beats are in each measure? What is the meter of the song? Another term for *meter in 3* is **triple meter.**

Perform the rhythm below. How is each beat subdivided? When the beat is divided into three equal parts, it is called **compound meter.**

> **Triple meter** has three beats in each measure.
>
> In **compound meter** the beat is divided into three equal parts. The dotted quarter note gets the beat.

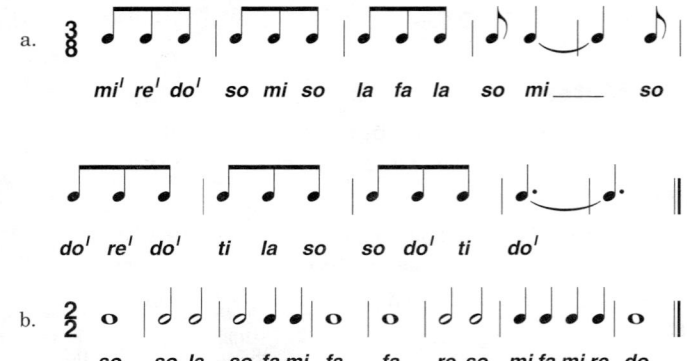

Compound meter

Show What You Know!

Play these rhythm patterns. Tap the beat note and **identify** the type of meter (duple, triple, simple, or compound). Then **sing** the melody using pitch syllables.

a.
mi¹ re¹ do¹ so mi so la fa la so mi____ so

do¹ re¹ do¹ ti la so so do¹ ti do¹

b.
so   so la so fa mi fa   fa   re so mi fa mi re do

Footnotes

ACROSS THE CURRICULUM

8b ▶ **Language Arts** Divide the class into two groups. Identify one group as compound meter and the other as simple meter. Select a category such as animals, fruits, or countries. With each word representing a beat note, ask students to produce words with syllables that fit their meter. For example, *elephant* could represent the three subdivisions of a beat in compound meter or two sixteenths and an eighth in simple meter.

BUILDING SKILLS THROUGH MUSIC

▶ **Language** Ask students to silently read the lyrics of "One Morning in May." Have them use the lyrics to draw a conclusion as to when this story may have taken place. Have them look for clues in the language used, as well as the events that took place.

SKILLS REINFORCEMENT

▶ **Reading** Encourage students to use Resource Book p. D-17 for practice in reading examples in $\frac{6}{8}$ meter and $\frac{3}{8}$ meter. Students will also benefit from conducting practice in these meters. Use the page to compose a *do*-pentatonic melody for the rhythm patterns and also a major diatonic melody for the rhythms.

Invite students to perform a two-part rhythm accompaniment for "One Morning in May" on p. 494, or Resource Book E-15.

▶ **Mallets** Have some students learn the Orff acccompaniment on Resource Book p. F-13 for "One Morning in May." Have students add standard symbols for dynamics on their copies of the notation. As some students play the accompaniment and others sing the song, have both groups follow the dynamics symbols.

One Morning in May

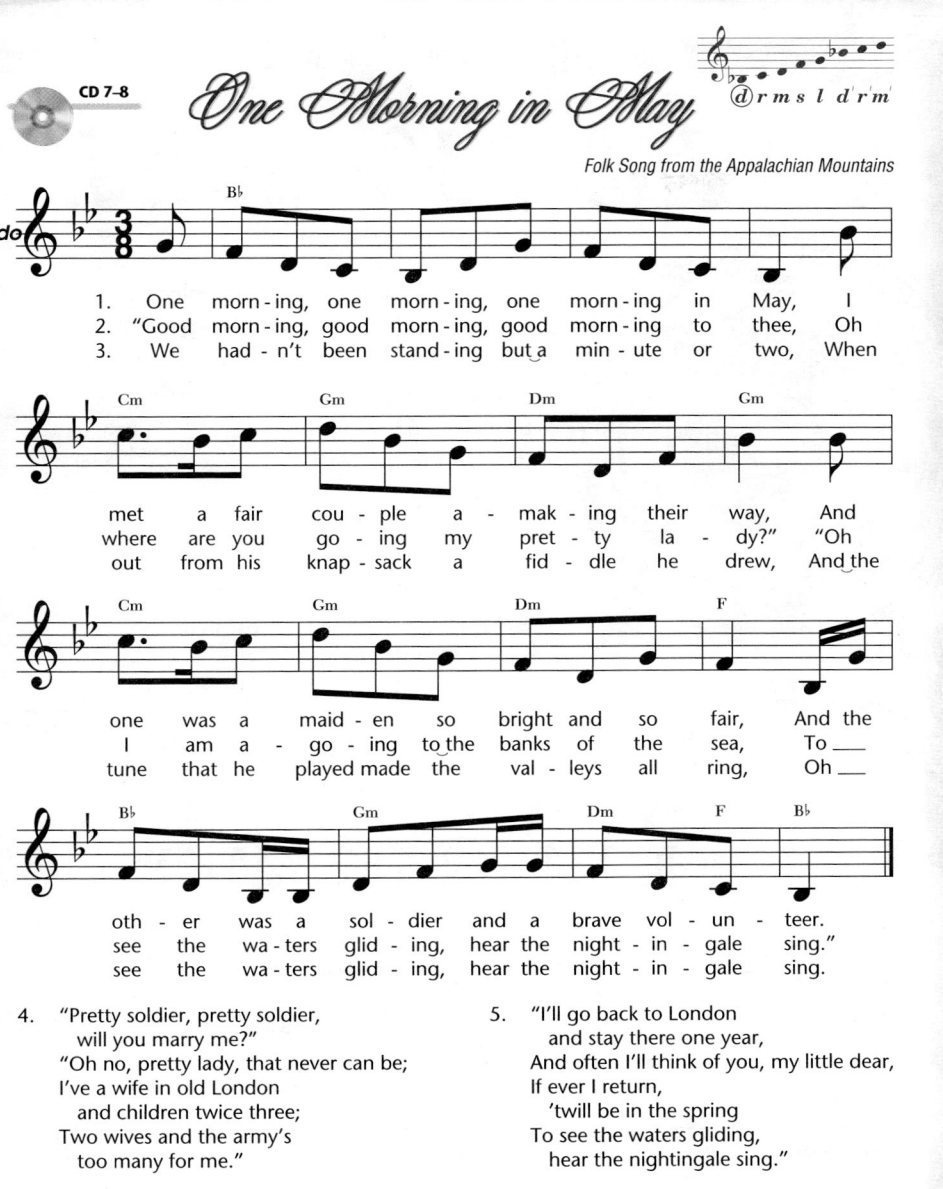

Folk Song from the Appalachian Mountains

1. One morn-ing, one morn-ing, one morn-ing in May, I
2. "Good morn-ing, good morn-ing, good morn-ing to thee, Oh
3. We had-n't been stand-ing but a min-ute or two, When

met a fair cou-ple a-mak-ing their way, And
where are you go-ing my pret-ty la-dy?" "Oh
out from his knap-sack a fid-dle he drew, And the

one was a maid-en so bright and so fair, And the
I am a-go-ing to the banks of the sea, To ___
tune that he played made the val-leys all ring, Oh ___

oth-er was a sol-dier and a brave vol-un-teer.
see the wa-ters glid-ing, hear the night-in-gale sing."
see the wa-ters glid-ing, hear the night-in-gale sing.

4. "Pretty soldier, pretty soldier,
   will you marry me?"
   "Oh no, pretty lady, that never can be;
   I've a wife in old London
   and children twice three;
   Two wives and the army's
   too many for me."

5. "I'll go back to London
   and stay there one year,
   And often I'll think of you, my little dear,
   If ever I return,
   'twill be in the spring
   To see the waters gliding,
   hear the nightingale sing."

2 DEVELOP

Analyzing

6a Have students read the notation of "One Morning in May" and identify that

- There are three eighth-note beats per measure.
- $\frac{3}{8}$ is a triple meter because the beats are grouped in threes.

Listening

6c Play "One Morning in May" **CD 7-8.** As students listen, have them tap one beat per measure. Lead students to discover that the performance feels more like one beat per measure than three beats per measure. The new beat note is the dotted quarter note.

Reading

5a Have students compare the difference between $\frac{3}{8}$ and $\frac{2}{2}$ meters by reading and performing the rhythms in the Show What You Know box on p. 120.

6c Use Resource Book pp. D-17 to lead students to discover that $\frac{6}{8}$ meter uses the dotted quarter note as the beat note and that when the beat note is divided into groups of three equal parts, the meter is a compound meter.

Singing

5a Invite students to

- Sing "One Morning in May" **CD 7-8** with rhythm syllables, tapping one beat note per measure.
- Sing all five verses of the song with the recording.

3 CLOSE

Skill: READING   **ASSESSMENT**

Performance/Self-Assessment Observe students' ability to read and perform $\frac{3}{8}$ and $\frac{6}{8}$ meter by having them tap the beat note and say rhythm syllables for the rhythms on Resource Book, p. D-17.

CULTURAL CONNECTION

▶ **Appalachian Style** Read aloud and listen to the authentic Appalachian Mountain music and read-along narration performed on an accompanying audiotape of *Melvin's Melons* by Sherry T. Vaughn (Overmountain Press, 1996). It tells the story of a 12-year-old boy who sets out to see the world. Set in the Appalachian Mountains, the modern-day fairy tale is full of regional colloquialisms and colorful descriptions of Melvin's adventures. A glossary helps readers understand the interesting Appalachian folk terms and dialect used within the story.

SCHOOL TO HOME CONNECTION

▶ **Folk Styles** Invite students to ask about any interesting folk music that may exist in their family's cultural background. Encourage students to learn a folk song from their own heritage or find a recording of a folk song they like to present to the class.

TECHNOLOGY/MEDIA LINK

Notation Software Invite students to notate the rhythm of "One Morning in May" using notation software in $\frac{3}{8}$ meter. Have students highlight all the measures and then change the meter to $\frac{6}{8}$ meter. Ask students if the meter change works for this song. (Yes, it does.)

LESSON AT A GLANCE

Element Focus **FORM** Three-part round

Skill Objective ▸**MOVING** Perform a circle dance while singing a three-part round

Connection Activity **GENRE** Demonstrate the characteristics of a round by creating a spoken round

MATERIALS

• "Dance for the Nations"   **CD 7-15**

 Recording Routine: Intro (4 m.); vocal; interlude (2 m.); vocal (three-part round); interlude (12 m.); vocal (three-part round twice); coda

• "Celebration" (poem)
• **Resource Book** p. H-15
• keyboards, Autoharp

VOCABULARY

round   imitative   melodic minor scale

◆ ◆ ◆ ◆ **National Standards** ◆ ◆ ◆ ◆

1a Sing accurately with good breath control
4a Compose short pieces, demonstrating unity and variety through music
4c Arrange, using electronic media
5a Read eighth, quarter, and dotted notes in duple meter

MORE MUSIC CHOICES

For more experience with rounds:
"Gloria, Gloria," p. 459
"Let Us Sing Together," p. 156

1 INTRODUCE

SAY In music, repetition creates unity, and contrast of new material creates variety. A round is a genre that has both repetition and contrast at the same time.

A FAMOUS FORM

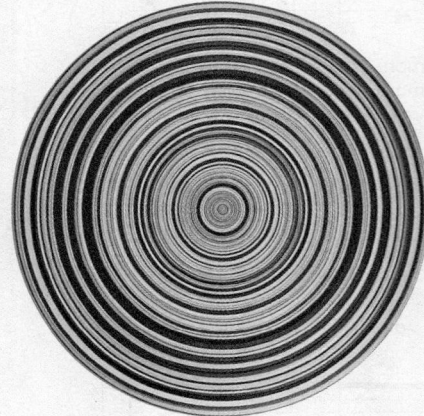

Repeating a musical idea, or returning to it, creates unity in music. Introducing new musical ideas provides variety.

A **round** provides unity by repeating the same melody over and over. Variety in a round comes from how the different phrases of the melody combine with each other.

> A **round** is a composition in which two or more parts enter in succession with the same melody.

Sing "Dance for the Nations" in unison. Then sing it as a round.

Arts Connection

▲ *B126* by Japanese artist Kuwayama Tadasky (born 1935)

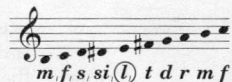

$m\ f, s, si\ \textcircled{l}\ t\ d\ r\ m\ f$

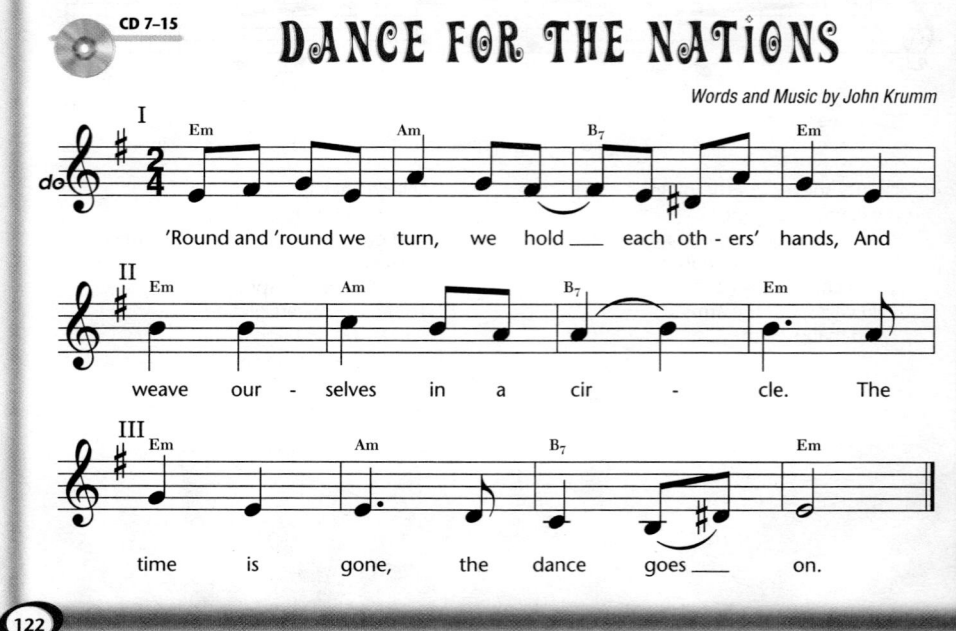

CD 7-15

DANCE FOR THE NATIONS

Words and Music by John Krumm

I
Em   Am   B₇   Em
'Round and 'round we turn, we hold ___ each oth - ers' hands, And

II
Em   Am   B₇   Em
weave our - selves in a cir - cle. The

III
Em   Am   B₇   Em
time is gone, the dance goes ___ on.

122

Footnotes

MEETING INDIVIDUAL NEEDS

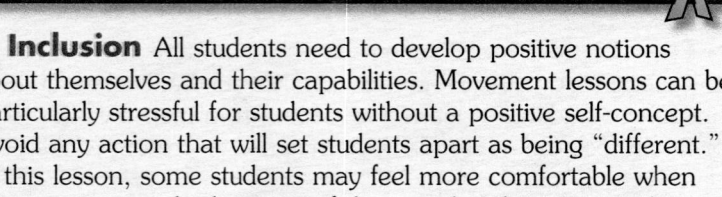

▸ **Inclusion** All students need to develop positive notions about themselves and their capabilities. Movement lessons can be particularly stressful for students without a positive self-concept. Avoid any action that will set students apart as being "different." In this lesson, some students may feel more comfortable when they are singing the last part of the round and moving in the out-side circle between two peers who are positive and supportive.

BUILDING SKILLS THROUGH MUSIC

▸ **Math** Ask students to solve this problem: Divide the class into three unequal groups for the movement activity on p. 123. Start with ____ (3/6) of the class in the outer circle. What fraction of the class should be in the middle circle? (2/6) What fraction of the class should be in the inner circle? (1/6) Ask them to remember that the three fractions must add up to one whole, and that they are unequal.

ACROSS THE CURRICULUM

▸ **Language Arts** Read aloud, dramatize, and create move-ments for "Celebration" by Alonzo Lopez from Tomie DePaola's *Book of Poems* (Putnam, 1988).

> I shall dance tonight.
> When the dusk comes crawling,
> There will be dancing and feasting.
> I shall dance with the others
>   in circles,
>   in leaps,
>   in stomps.
> Laughter and talk
>   will weave into the night,
> Among the fires of my people.
> Games will be played
> And I shall be a part of it.

Move Around

Move to "Dance for the Nations" by following these simple steps: Form three concentric circles with fewer people in the inside circle, more in the middle, and the most on the outside. Hold hands.

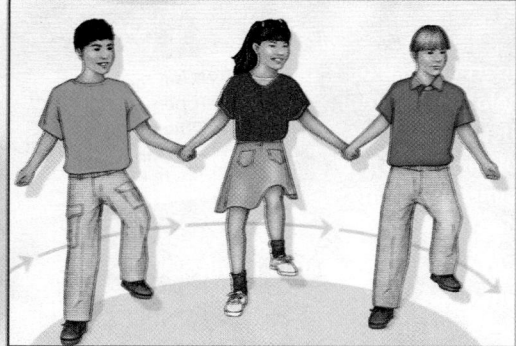

◄ On the first phrase of the round, move sideways to the left on each beat: Left, Right, Left, Right

On the second phrase of the round, move sideways to the right on each beat: Right, Left, Right, Left

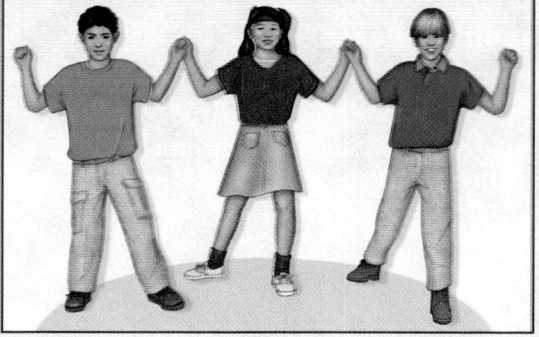

On the third phrase of the round, swing your hands every two beats: Forward – Backward – Forward – Backward ▶

Rap a Round

It's easy to **compose** a spoken rap. First draw eight blank measures, as shown.

Below each line, write words that take up eight beats. Then **notate** the rhythm of the words.

To **perform** your rap as a round, place the number 1 at the beginning. Place the number 2 where the second part starts.

---

2 DEVELOP

Listening

Invite students to listen to "Dance for the Nations" **CD 7-15** for the repetition and contrast the round offers. See Across the Curriculum, p. 122, for a Native American poem that also celebrates dancing.

Singing

Divide the class into three groups and invite students to perform "Dance for the Nations" *a cappella,* in unison, and with accurate intonation. Then sing it as a round, with each group entering as indicated and singing the melody once, demonstrating basic performance techniques.

Playing

Invite volunteers to play the keyboard part in Skills Reinforcement below while the class sings the song again with the recording **CD 7-15.**

Moving

Help students learn and perform the movement routine for "Dance for the Nations" **CD 7-15** as illustrated.

Creating

Divide the class into small groups. Invite each group to create rhythmic phrases in a rap style. Have students

- Write a four-line rap with eight beats per line.
- Mark *1* at the beginning and *2* at the fifth measure, where the second group starts.
- Practice their rap in unison and as a two-part round, and then perform it for the class.

3 CLOSE

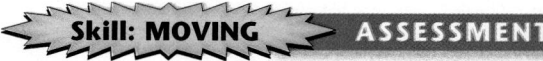

Skill: MOVING **ASSESSMENT**

Performance/Peer Critique As half the class sings and moves to the Stereo Performance track for "Dance for the Nations" **CD 7-15,** have the other half observe and critique the performance. Ask students to describe the form of the song. (round)

 SKILLS REINFORCEMENT

▶ **Singing** "Dance for the Nations" was composed in the melodic minor scale. This kind of scale uses a normal seventh *(so)* when descending, and a raised seventh *(si)* when ascending. Have students practice singing the last four measures of the song, holding hands out with palms down when they sing the normal seventh, and palms up when they sing the raised seventh.

 ▶ **Keyboard** Have some students learn the left-handed keyboard ostinato acccompaniment on Resource Book p. H-15 for "Dance for the Nations." They may then play the accompaniment while the class sings the song.

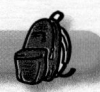 **SCHOOL TO HOME CONNECTION**

▶ **Music Festival** Create an International Music and Dance Festival at your school. Invite local music and dance groups to perform with student musicians and dancers. Feature invited groups in school musical performances and invite family and friends to attend.

 TECHNOLOGY/MEDIA LINK

 Sequencing Software Have students arrange the melodic phrases of "Dance for the Nations," using sequencing software. After students have sequenced the piece, they may create a round by copying and pasting the melody into additional tracks.

LESSON AT A GLANCE

Element Focus	**FORM**	Canon
Skill Objective	**SINGING**	Sight-read and sing a song in three-part canon
Connection Activity	**LANGUAGE ARTS**	Discuss the use of the Latin language in the past and in the present

MATERIALS

- *"Dona nobis pacem"*   **CD 7-17**
  Recording Routine: Intro (4 m.); vocal in unison; interlude (4 m.); vocal as canon (each part 1x); coda
  Pronunciation Practice/Pronunciation p. 526
- *Canon for Violin and Cello*   **CD 7-20**
- bass xylophones, bass metallophones

VOCABULARY

canon   round   *dona nobis pacem*   ostinato

◆ ◆ ◆ ◆ **National Standards** ◆ ◆ ◆ ◆

1a Sing accurately in small ensembles
1c Sing music from diverse genres
2b Perform easy instrumental pieces expressively
5a Read quarter, half, and dotted notes in triple meter
5b Sightread melodies in treble clef
6b Listen and analyze uses of form in music from diverse genres

MORE MUSIC CHOICES . . .

For more practice in singing canons and rounds:
"Hey, Ho! Nobody Home," p. 28
"Do, Re, Mi, Fa," p. 80
"Alleluia," p. 133

CANON FORM

There are many types of **canons.** One important trait of canons is their imitative entrances. The melody may enter at a different pitch, or the same pitch. When the melody enters at different pitches, the harmony of the canon may change. The melody may be exactly the same, or slightly varied. The canon form has a lot of variation in its use.

A round is a type of canon. *"Dona nobis pacem"* is a perpetual, or infinite, canon in which each part enters at different times, performs the melody, and then repeats the melody as many times as desired. Not all canons follow this structure.

> A **canon** is a form in which each part performs the melody, entering at different times on the same or different pitches.

A Canon for Peace

"Dona nobis pacem" is a canon with a message of peace—*grant us peace.* Look at the song notation and locate where each part begins.

Listen to the canon and follow the melody part all the way through. Then, **sing** the melody of "Dona nobis pacem" in unison.

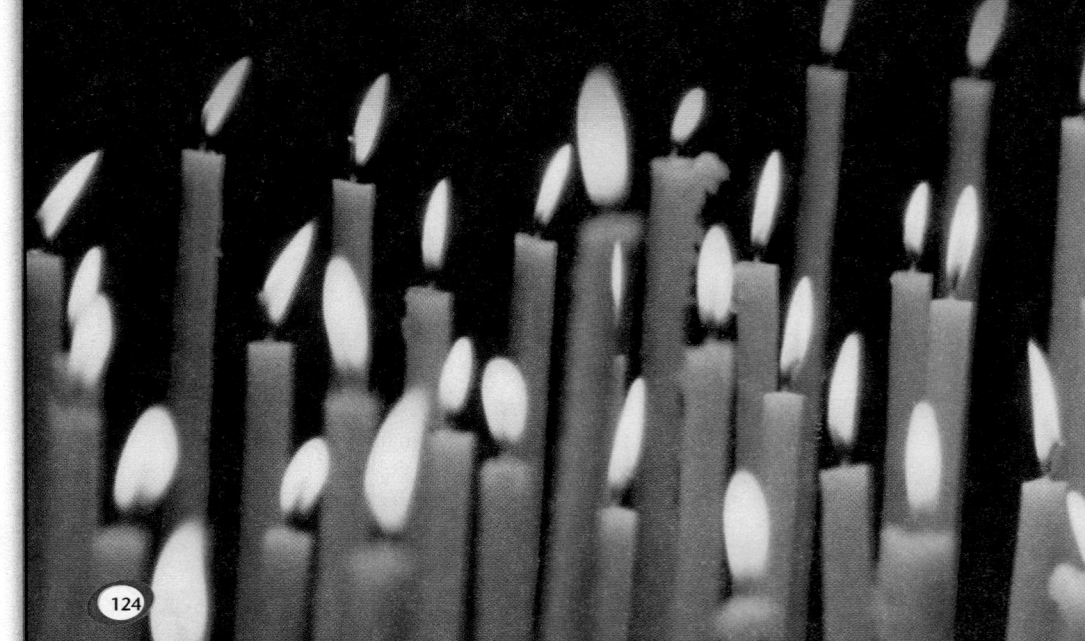

Footnotes

MEETING INDIVIDUAL NEEDS

▶ **Gifted and Talented** Invite students to go on a "word hunt" to find English words that have Latin roots. Ask students to look up and translate the following Latin terms and phrases. For best results, tell them to use an unabridged dictionary.

ad hoc	*ex post facto*	*et cetera* (etc.)
carpe diem	*Homo sapiens*	*semper fidelis*
et al	*id est* (i.e.)	*quid pro quo*

BUILDING SKILLS THROUGH MUSIC

▶ **Language** Share Spotlight On, p. 125, with students. Tell students that *"Dona nobis pacem"* is referred to as a perpetual canon. Ask students, based on the context of what they learned about rounds and canons in Spotlight On, what they think the word perpetual means.

SKILLS REINFORCEMENT

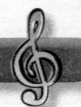

▶ **Singing** Have students sing this warm-up scale in a two-part (or four-part) canon. The second group will come in after two beats.

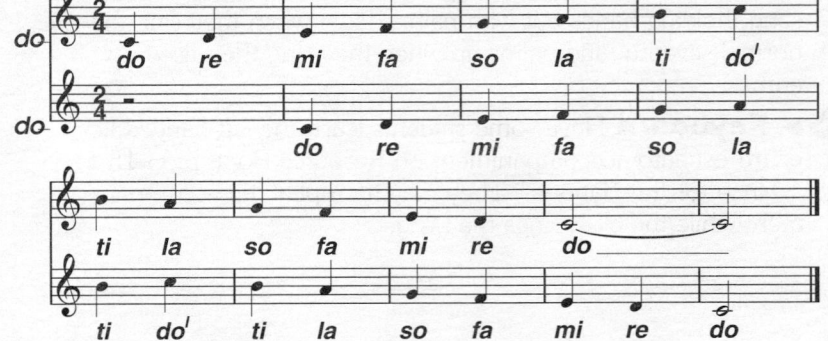

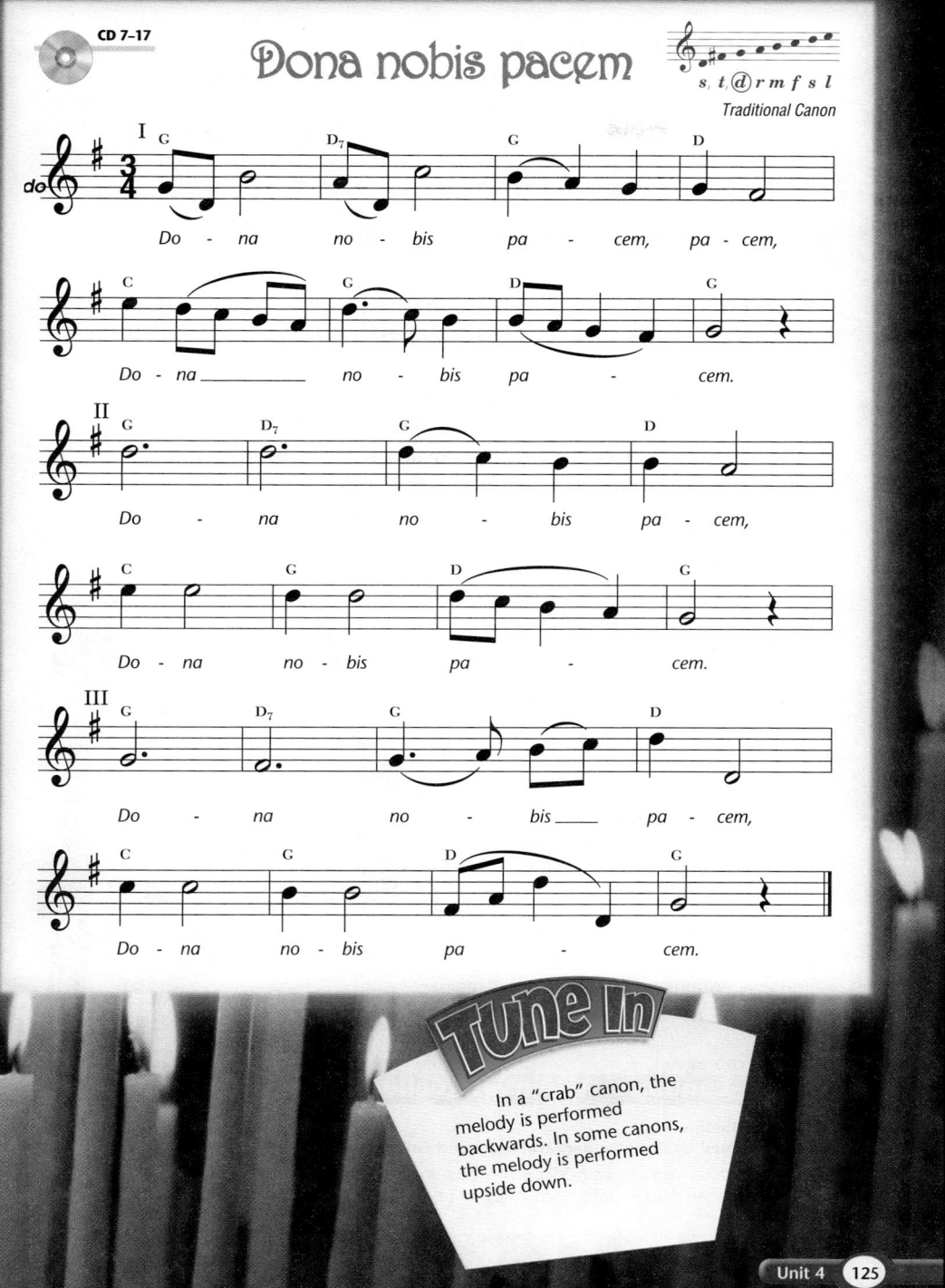

Dona nobis pacem

CD 7–17

s t d r m f s l

Traditional Canon

Do - na no - bis pa - cem, pa - cem,

Do - na no - bis pa - cem.

Do - na no - bis pa - cem,

Do - na no - bis pa - cem.

Do - na no - bis pa - cem,

Do - na no - bis pa - cem.

Tune In

In a "crab" canon, the melody is performed backwards. In some canons, the melody is performed upside down.

Unit 4 **125**

1 INTRODUCE

Ask students to identify the language of the lyrics in *"Dona nobis pacem,"* on p. 125. (Latin) Share with students the information in Cultural Connection on p. 127, and Meeting Individual Needs on p. 124. Lead a discussion on the importance of Latin in today's culture. Invite students to read the Arts Connection on p. 127 and relate its message of peace to the song.

Tell students they will sing a song in canon form and practice sight-reading skills.

2 DEVELOP

Analyzing

Review with the students the definition of a round on p. 122. Remind them that one group enters first, followed by other groups at specific time intervals.

ASK In the song notation on p. 125, what is the time interval at which each group enters? (8 m.)

ASK What is the pitch interval at which each group enters? (Each group enters at the same pitch, unison.)

Remind students that the terms canon and round are sometimes used interchangeably. Share with students the information in Spotlight On below.

Singing

 Tell students that they will sight-read a simple melody in the key of G major. Ask them to look at the melodic outline for the first phrase of *"Dona nobis pacem"* on p. 126. Using this melody, have students follow this procedure as they sight-read:

 • Name the key signature (G) and time signature. ($\frac{3}{4}$)

• Sing the scale silently, using pitch syllables. Then, perform the rhythm, using rhythm syllables.

• Sight-read and sing the melody without rhythm, using pitch syllables. Then, sing the melody in rhythm, using pitch syllables and hands signs.

continued on page 126

SPOTLIGHT ON

▶ **Canons Versus Rounds** Explain to students that the distinction between canons and rounds can be confusing, partly because these terms are often used interchangeably. A *round* is actually a type of canon known as a *perpetual* or *infinite* canon, so-called because each part can return to the beginning an indefinite number of times. The earliest known *perpetual canon* is *"Sumer is icumen in,"* which was written in the thirteenth century. Some of the most famous perpetual canons of today are "Row, Row, Row Your Boat" and *"Frère Jacques."* Another type of canon begins exactly like a round, but the ending is different. Instead of *rounding off,* all of the parts end simultaneously at a designated place in the music, creating a final chord. In instrumental canons, the parts usually enter at various pitch levels.

MOVEMENT

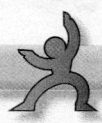

▶ **Locomotor Movement** Have students stand in a circle. Teach the following movements for *"Dona nobis pacem."*

1. Walk left around the circle for six beats, stepping quarter notes in three-beat patterns. ("Left, two, three, four, five, six.")

2. Repeat step 1 to the right. ("Right, two three, four, five, six.")

3. Walk into the circle for three beats, while lifting arms. Step back out of the circle for three beats, while lowering arms. ("In, two three, out, two, three.")

4. Each individual will turn in place in a clockwise circle for three beats, lifting arms. Then, stand in place and lower arms for three beats. ("Turn, two, three, stand, arms down.")

Have the students perform the movements three times as they sing *"Dona nobis pacem"* in unison.

Lesson 5 Continued

5b Have students sight-read this melody and use music terms to compare it to the melody on p. 126. (additional notes were added)

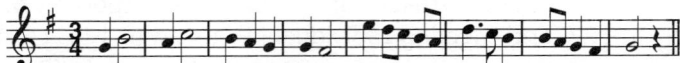

Finally, have students sing the entire first phrase of "*Dona nobis pacem*" on p. 125, using pitch syllables. Then, have students learn and sing the entire song.

Ask students to analyze and compare each melodic outline to the melody. Tell them that when they sight-read, they will create melodic outlines as they sing.

1a Invite students to sing a warm up, using Skills Reinforcement on p. 124. To extend the vocal ranges of students, see Skills Reinforcement, p. 126.

1c Have students use the Pronunciation Practice track **CD 7-19** to learn the Latin text.

Analyzing

6b Invite students to listen to "*Dona nobis pacem*" **CD 7-17** and use music terms to analyze its form. (unison, interlude, three-part canon) Ask them how the song ends. (Each group "rounds off" at the end.)

Singing

1a Divide the class into three groups. Have them sing "*Dona nobis pacem*" **CD 7-17** following the same form as the recording—unison, interlude, three-part canon.

Moving

Invite students to perform a movement for "*Dona nobis pacem*," using the instructions in Movement, below.

Listening

6b Tell students that canons are used in instrumental music. Play *Canon for Violin and Cello* **CD 7-20** on p. 126 and have students raise their hands each time they hear a canonic entrance of the violin or cello.

Singing a Canon by Sight

Learning to sing a melody the first time you read the music is a challenge. This skill is called **sight-reading.** The better you can sight-read, the easier it is to sing a melody and a canon.

> **Sight-reading** is the ability to read music accurately the first time.

Here are some general sight-reading tips.

- Determine the key of the song, then find and **sing** *do*. In this song, what pitch is *do*?

- **Sing** the scale of the song using pitch syllables. In this song, which scale do you sing? This puts the sound of the scale (key) in your head and helps you to hear the notes.

- Next, learn to recognize the important pitches of the melody as you sing them. Here is an example using the first phrase of "*Dona nobis pacem*." **Sing** this phrase using pitch syllables. Then, gradually add more notes to your melody until you are finally singing all of the pitches correctly.

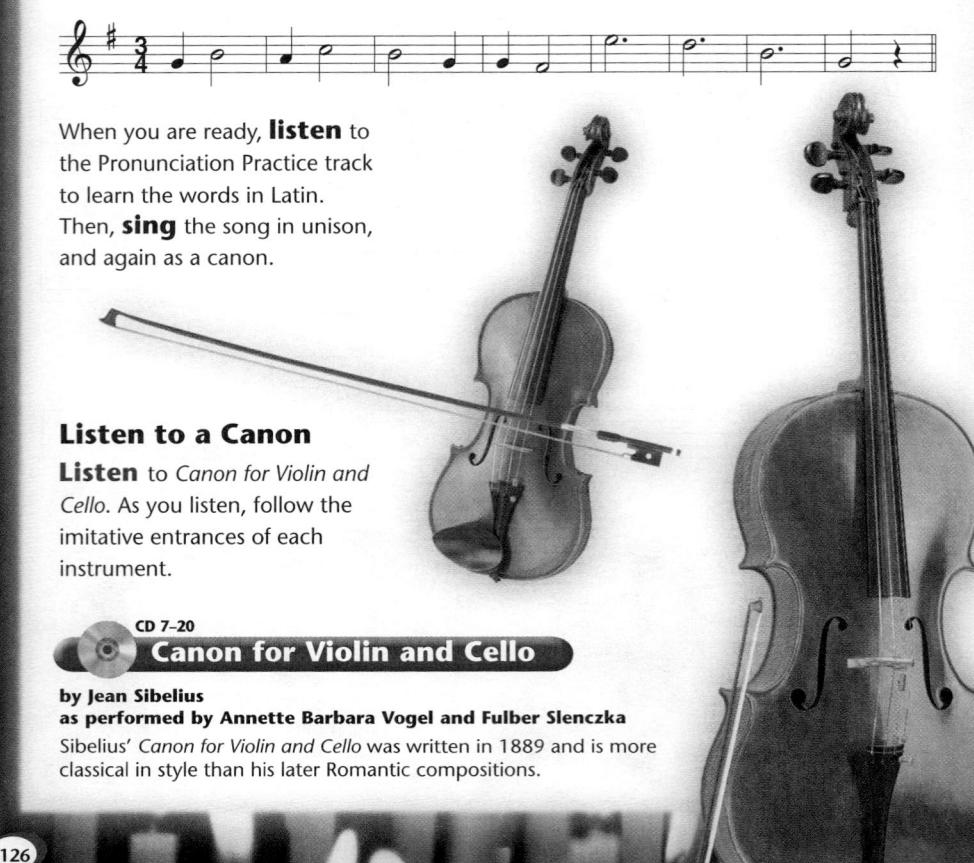

When you are ready, **listen** to the Pronunciation Practice track to learn the words in Latin. Then, **sing** the song in unison, and again as a canon.

Listen to a Canon

Listen to *Canon for Violin and Cello*. As you listen, follow the imitative entrances of each instrument.

 CD 7–20
Canon for Violin and Cello

**by Jean Sibelius
as performed by Annette Barbara Vogel and Fulber Slenczka**

Sibelius' *Canon for Violin and Cello* was written in 1889 and is more classical in style than his later Romantic compositions.

126

Footnotes

SKILLS REINFORCEMENT

▶ **Extending the Vocal Range** These warm-up exercises will help extend the upper range of students' voices.

- Echo *whoo, whoo, whoo.* Model a head voice and use a lot of breath as students move up the register.

- Have students use a pure *oh* when they sing *know.*

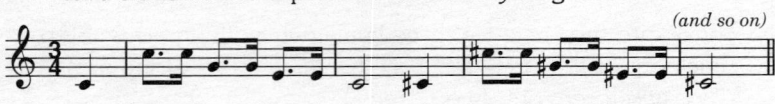

(and so on)

I know, I know, I know, I know.   I know, I know, I know, I know.

- Begin on middle C and move up to G. Have students *slide (glissando)* between the slurred notes.

(and so on)

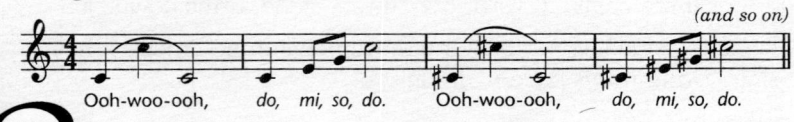

Ooh-woo-ooh,   do, mi, so, do.   Ooh-woo-ooh,   do, mi, so, do.

126

TEACHER TO TEACHER

▶ **Playing I, IV, and V Chords on Mallet Instruments** Mallet instruments can be played with two, three, or even four mallets. Most students will play with two mallets. Therefore, only two notes of a chord triad will be played. When teaching the chords for a melody, remind the students that the triads for the I, IV, and V chords are actually made up of three notes (1. Triads). The mallet chords chosen below (2. Mallet chords) are considered to be the best choices because of voice leading and hand position.

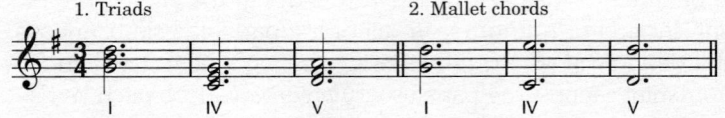

1. Triads   2. Mallet chords

I   IV   V   I   IV   V

Add a Bass Ostinato

One way to add interest to a canon is to add mallet instruments to the accompaniment. Learn this ostinato on a bass mallet instrument. When you are ready, **play** the accompaniment with the class as they sing "*Dona nobis pacem*" as a canon.

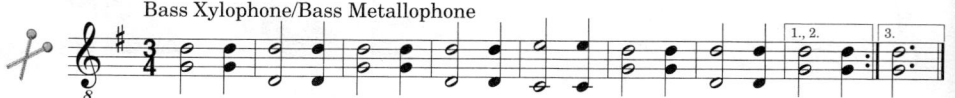
Bass Xylophone/Bass Metallophone

Latin Is the Language

The language of "*Dona nobis pacem*" is Latin, a language that is not spoken very much today. Why do schools teach Latin? In what famous place in Italy might you hear Latin? Do you know what professions write in Latin? What common objects have Latin words inscribed on them?

Art for Peace

Pablo Picasso (1881–1973) is recognized as one of the most influential artists of the 20th century. Born in Malaga, Spain, Picasso created over 22,000 works of art in his lifetime. He is known as one of the founders of *cubism*, a new style of art, in the early 1900s. Peace is one of the recurring themes found in his work.

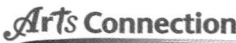 **Connection**

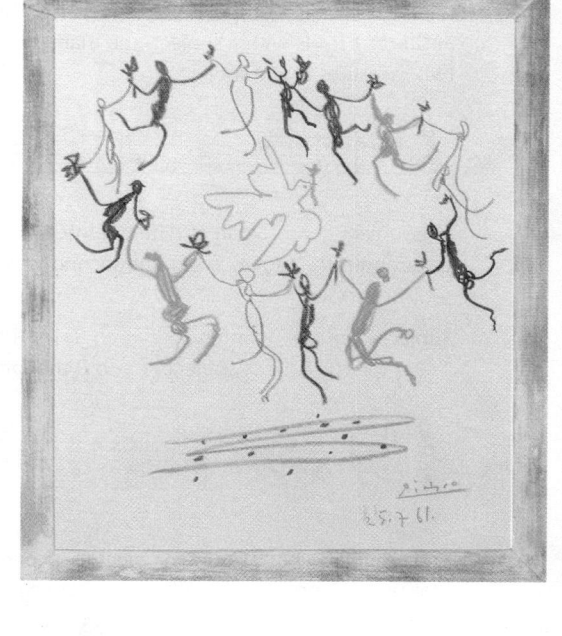

La Ronde by Pablo Picasso. This work is also titled as *Ronde de l'amitie, Circle of Friendship,* or *Circle of Youth.* ▶

Playing

Ask students to look at the song notation of "*Dona nobis pacem*" on p. 125. Ask them

- What chords are used to accompany the song? (G, C, D, D₇)
- In the key of G, what Roman numerals would you assign to each of these chords? (I, IV, V and V₇)

Using Teacher to Teacher on p. 126, guide students to see that the bass xylophone/bass metallophone part on p. 127 uses the I, IV, and V chords. Explain that chords on mallet instruments often use fewer notes than on a keyboard.

Using the mallet part on p. 127, have students

- Sing the bass line for the accompaniment part, using the chord numbers to help them memorize the chord progression.

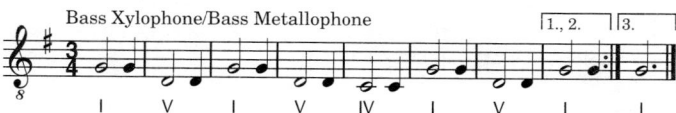
Bass Xylophone/Bass Metallophone

I V I V IV I V I I

- Play the bass line on the bass xylophones and bass metallophones. (Add contrabass bars, if available.)
- Identify the name of each upper note, then locate both notes on their mallet instruments.
- Play the two notes for each chord on their mallet instrument using the correct chord progression.

2b Select students to play the accompaniment as the rest of the class sings "*Dona nobis pacem*" in unison, then in a three-part canon. Remind the performers to end when Part III completes the canon.

3 CLOSE

Skill: SINGING   ASSESSMENT

1a **Performance/Observation** Have students identify the form of "*Dona nobis pacem*"(canon). Divide the class into three groups and invite students to sing "*Dona nobis pacem*" in unison, then in a three-part canon. Observe students' abilities to sing the three-part canon accurately.

CULTURAL CONNECTION

▶ **An Ancient Language** One of the most well-known uses of the Latin language is for the worship services of the Roman Catholic Church—the Mass. For many centuries, Latin was the language used in every Catholic church in the world. Priests were concerned that church members did not understand the Latin words in the Mass. Between 1962–1965, a conference called *Vatican Council II* decided that the Mass would be conducted in the vernacular—the language of the people. Today, all members of the Catholic Church can understand the Mass.

▶ **A Living Language** Latin is a language that is no longer spoken, yet it has a great influence on our lives. Have students discuss the use of Latin in science, law, medicine, and in everyday language. Ask them if they have come across any Latin words for plants or animal species in their science classes.

TECHNOLOGY/MEDIA LINK

▶ **Sequencing Software** Students can compose a canon by using sequencer software. Select a track, click on the Record button, and play an eight-measure melody, using the black notes of the keyboard. Click Stop to stop recording, then copy the melody. Paste it into a new track, starting in m. 3, then paste the melody into another new track, starting in m. 5. Play the three tracks together, and listen to the new canon.

▶ **MIDI Keyboard** Have students experiment with sounds on the MIDI keyboard that are appropriate to accompany "*Dona nobis pacem.*" Once they have found an appropriate timbre, let them take turns playing the bass xylophone part on p. 127 on the keyboard.

LESSON AT A GLANCE

Element Focus	**FORM** Fugue
Skill Objective	**LISTENING** Aurally identify the entrance of the subject in a fugue
Connection Activity	**SOCIAL STUDIES** Discuss events in United States history that occurred during the life-time of J. S. Bach

MATERIALS
- "*Little*" Organ Fugue in G Minor (organ) **CD 7-21**
- "*Little*" Organ Fugue in G Minor (brass) **CD 7-22**

VOCABULARY

fugue	subject
countersubject	counterpoint

◆ ◆ ◆ ◆ National Standards ◆ ◆ ◆ ◆
1a Sing accurately in large ensembles
5a Read quarter and eighth notes in duple meter
6a Listen and describe events in music using appropriate terms
6c Understand and use basic principles of tonality in music analysis
8b Identify ways music relates to social studies

MORE MUSIC CHOICES
For more experience with the music of J. S. Bach:
Jesu, Joy of Man's Desiring, p. 87
"Minuet" from *Orchestral Suite No. 2 in B Minor*, p. 192 (excerpt)

1 INTRODUCE

Explore with students the history of the United States from 1685 to 1750, to set the stage for a study of the life of J. S. Bach.

Have students do the research activity described in Across the Curriculum on p. 129 and display the time line on the bulletin board.

FugueForm

In rounds and canons, melodies enter at different times. The **fugue** is a relative of the round and canon.

> A **fugue** is a musical form in which the main melody is stated in one voice and then imitated by two or more voices, each entering successively.

A Famous Fugue

Johann Sebastian Bach (1685–1750) is one of the most famous composers of fugues. His "*Little*" Organ Fugue in G Minor starts with a subject, the main melody. **Sing** the first two measures of the subject.

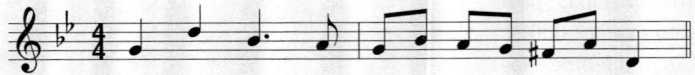

The subject enters again at different intervals throughout the fugue. **Sing** the second version of the subject, below.

Subject 2 sounds an interval of a 4th lower than subject 1. Are the rhythms of subjects 1 and 2 the same?

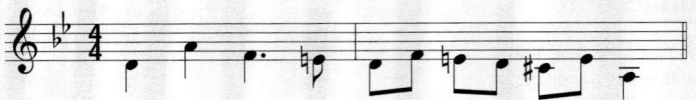

The fugue also has a countersubject, a second melody that plays along with the subject. Other changes to the melodies occur during the episodes, or contrasting sections of the fugue. The subject keeps coming back at various times throughout the piece to provide unity.

Footnotes

SKILLS REINFORCEMENT

1a ▶ **Singing** Use either numbers or pitch syllables to teach the intervals of the harmonic minor scale. First, review the intervals in *la*-pentatonic and add intervals in the minor scale: major second, *la-ti*; minor sixth, *la-fa*; major seventh, *la-si*. Next, have students sing the pitch syllable for each interval, then say the interval name. Divide the class into two groups and have each group sing the interval as a chord. Repeat with all of the intervals of the scale in order, from unison to the octave.

BUILDING SKILLS THROUGH MUSIC

▶ **Science** Have students look at the photograph of pipes from a pipe organ on p. 129. Ask them which pipes would have the highest pitch sounds and which would have the lowest? Have them explain why.

SPOTLIGHT ON

▶ **Johann Sebastian Bach and Pipe Organs** Share with students that in addition to writing fugues, toccatas, and sonatas for organ, J. S. Bach wrote 143 chorale preludes—organ pieces based on a chorale, or hymn.

Here are some facts about the parts of a pipe organ:

- Keyboards are called manuals. There are often three or more manuals on an organ.
- Pedals are played with the feet to produce bass notes.
- Stops are knobs that are pulled to control which pipes, and timbres, will sound.
- Pipes are metal tubes of various sizes that produce sound when air is pumped through them.

The Subject Is Fugue

Listen to the *"Little" Organ Fugue in G Minor.* Count the number of times the subject enters. Then **listen** to the Canadian Brass perform the same piece.

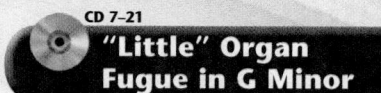

CD 7–21
"Little" Organ Fugue in G Minor

by Johann Sebastian Bach
The pipe organ is called the "king of instruments" because of its powerful sound.

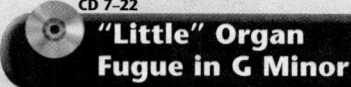

CD 7–22
"Little" Organ Fugue in G Minor

by Johann Sebastian Bach
as performed by the Canadian Brass
This performance features two trumpets, French horn, euphonium, and tuba.

▼ Organ pipes. Air flows through the pipes of an organ to create musical sound.

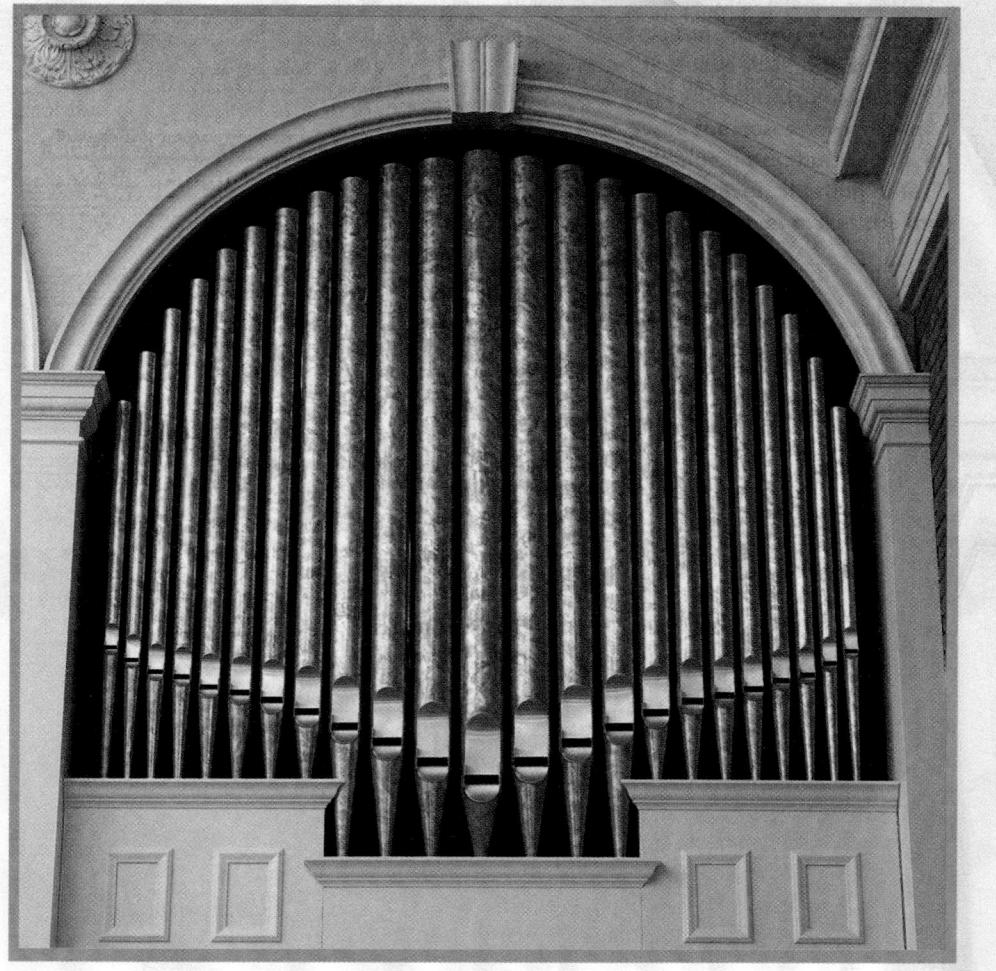

2 DEVELOP

Listening

Invite students to

5a • Listen to and read subject 1 as you play it.

1a • Sing subject 1 on a neutral syllable and again with a major third (B-natural).

6c Tell students that they will hear the subject in minor and major keys.

Have students listen to and read subject 2 as you play, then sing it with you.

6a **ASK How is the second entrance of the subject different from the first entrance?** (It is at a lower pitch.)

Is the rhythm of subject 2 the same as that of subject 1, or different? (the same)

Explain to students that they will hear a second melody, called a countersubject, played with the subject.

Have students listen to *"Little" Organ Fugue in G Minor,* first played on the organ **CD 7-21**, and then by the Canadian Brass **CD 7-22**. Ask them to raise a hand whenever they hear the entrance of the subject. After listening, have students describe this music, which is representative of the Baroque period.

3 CLOSE

Element: FORM **ASSESSMENT**

Observation Have students

• Listen to *"Little" Organ Fugue in G Minor* (organ) **CD 7-21**.

• Hold one fist against their chest (so classmates won't see) and raise their thumb each time they hear the subject.

• Describe the form of the selection. (fugue)

ACROSS THE CURRICULUM

▶ **Social Studies** For more information about J. S. Bach and other famous composers, encourage students to read *Lives of the Musicians: Good Times, Bad Times (and What the Neighbors Thought)* by Kathleen Krull (Harcourt, Brace, 1993).

8b Assist students in putting the life of J. S. Bach into the context of United States history. Explain that during Bach's lifetime, the French established settlements in America and carried on a vigorous fur trade. The English continued developing colonial America. The College of William and Mary (1693) and Yale (1701) were established. Have students continue this historical perspective by researching one topic of their choice on United States history from 1685 to 1750 and reporting to the class. Use their reports to develop a time line of important events.

TECHNOLOGY/MEDIA LINK

MIDI/Sequencing Software Invite students to enter subject 1 of *"Little" Organ Fugue in G minor* into one staff of the sequencing software program. Have them enter subject 2 into m. 4 of the second staff. Guide students to copy, paste, move, and transpose the segments (try an interval of a fifth down) to create the beginning of a small fugue, adding notes (using half notes and the notes of the Gm, D_7, Dm, A_7 chords) to fill out the melody lines. Ask students to play their fugues. Have them correct the notes that do not sound "right" by dragging the notes on each staff to new pitches that sound better. This is a challenging assignment, but one which will be a lot of fun.

Students may have a new-found respect for Johann Sebastian Bach after creating their own fugues.

| Element: MELODY | Skill: READING | Connection: LANGUAGE ARTS |

LESSON AT A GLANCE

Element Focus	**MELODY** Melodic intervals: half steps, whole steps
Skill Objective	**READING** Read and identify intervals in a harmonic-minor song
Connection Activity	**LANGUAGE ARTS** Identify Hebrew words and phrases in a song

MATERIALS

- *"Lo yisa"* — CD 7-23
- "Vine and Fig Tree" — CD 7-24
  Recording Routine: Intro (4 m.); vocal; instrumental; vocal; coda
- **Music Reading Practice, Sequence 15** — CD 7-27
- **Pronunciation Practice/Translation** p. 526
- **Resource Book** pp. A-12, D-18, E-16, F-14

VOCABULARY

| harmonic-minor scale | interval |
| major second | minor second |

◆ ◆ ◆ ◆ National Standards ◆ ◆ ◆ ◆

1c Sing music from diverse cultures
5e In performance classes sightread easy music accurately
6a Listen and describe events in music using appropriate terms
6b Listen and analyze uses of pitch in music from diverse cultures
6c Understand and use basic principles of tonality in music

MORE MUSIC CHOICES

For more practice with intervals and harmonic minor songs:
"El cóndor pasa," p. 46
"Sometimes I Feel Like a Motherless Child," p. 241

1 INTRODUCE

1c Share with students the information in Across the Curriculum below. Tell students that the song *"Lo yisa"* is a Hebrew song of peace. Use the Pronunciation Practice track **CD 7-26** and the Pronunciation Guide on Resource Book p. A-12 to teach the Hebrew words.

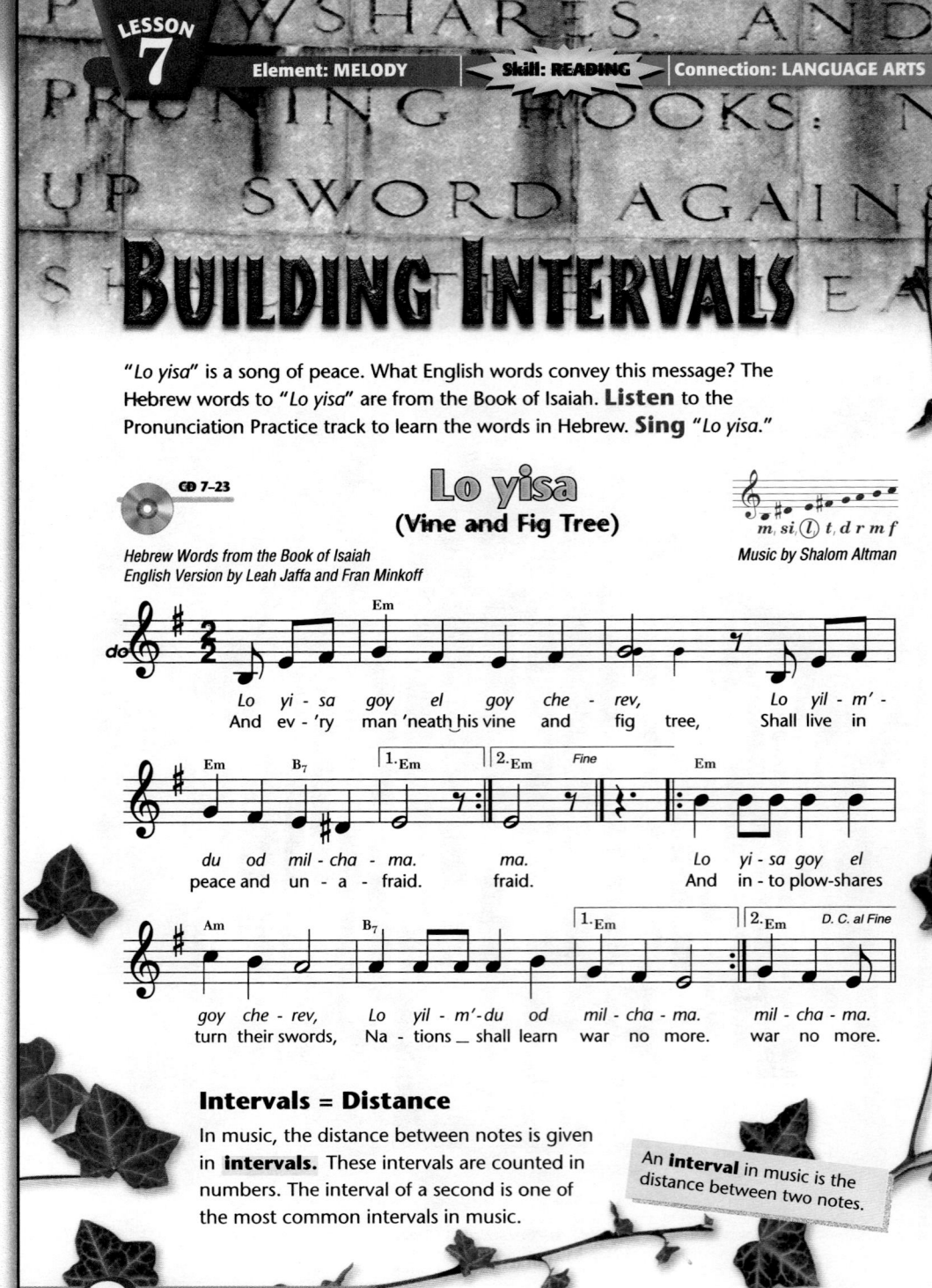

BUILDING INTERVALS

"Lo yisa" is a song of peace. What English words convey this message? The Hebrew words to *"Lo yisa"* are from the Book of Isaiah. **Listen** to the Pronunciation Practice track to learn the words in Hebrew. **Sing** *"Lo yisa."*

CD 7-23

Lo yisa
(Vine and Fig Tree)

Hebrew Words from the Book of Isaiah
English Version by Leah Jaffa and Fran Minkoff

Music by Shalom Altman

Lo yi-sa goy el goy che-rev,
And ev-'ry man 'neath his vine and fig tree,
Lo yil-m'-du od mil-cha-ma. ma.
peace and un-a-fraid. fraid.
Lo yi-sa goy el
And in-to plow-shares
goy che-rev, Lo yil-m'-du od mil-cha-ma.
turn their swords, Na-tions __ shall learn war no more.
mil-cha-ma.
war no more.

Intervals = Distance

In music, the distance between notes is given in **intervals.** These intervals are counted in numbers. The interval of a second is one of the most common intervals in music.

An **interval** in music is the distance between two notes.

130 Reading Sequence 15

Footnotes

ACROSS THE CURRICULUM

▶ **Language Arts** Share the book *The Day the Earth Was Silent* by Michael McGuffee (Inquiring Voices, 1996) and invite students to talk about children changing their world for the better.

Guide students in a discussion of the meaning of the lyrics of *"Lo yisa."* Point out key words such as *peace, unafraid, into plow-shares turn their swords,* and *learn war no more.* Ask students how they would like to see the world change for the better.

BUILDING SKILLS THROUGH MUSIC

▶ **Writing** Discuss the lyrics from *"Lo yisa."* Share Across the Curriculum above. Ask students to write a brief paragraph describing how they would like to see the world change for the better.

TEACHER TO TEACHER

▶ **Interval Charts** Visual feedback may assist students with inner hearing, as they learn to identify, listen to, and sing intervals and scales.

Reinforcement Have eight students create a "living" interval chart by lining up and spacing themselves in an "interval chart" line. Have them sing a major and minor scale with each student singing one note of the scale.

On Target Using a large interval chart on the board, have students sing a major or minor scale using hand signs and pitch syllables.

Challenge As you point to intervals on a large interval chart, have students echo (sing) those intervals.

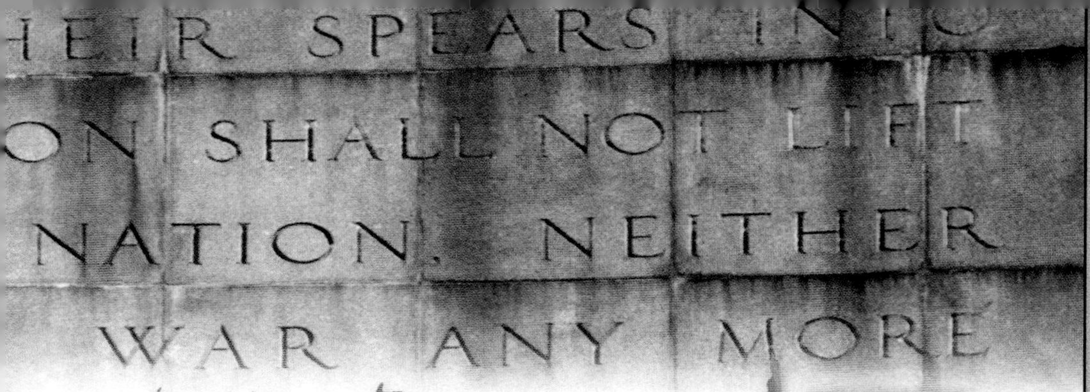

A Major Interval Chart—Seconds

All notes on neighboring lines and spaces of the staff are seconds. Some of these intervals are major seconds and some are minor seconds.

This interval chart shows the intervals of a second in a major scale. Make a list of the intervals. With the help of your teacher, **identify** and bracket the major and minor seconds.

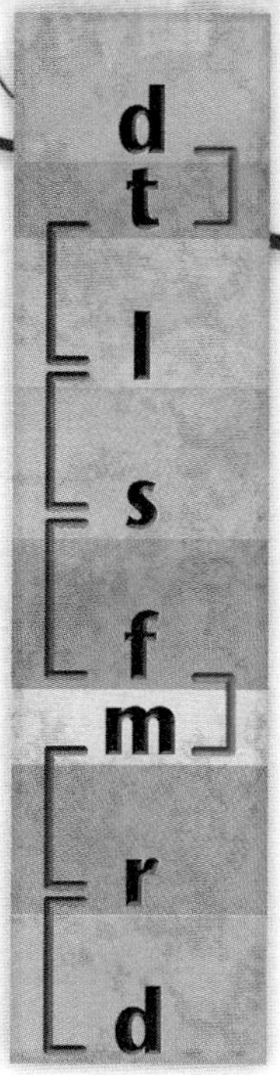

Analyze a Song

Analyze the notation of "Lo yisa" and **identify** the intervals in the song. Which interval is the most common?

Using pitch syllables, **sing** the E harmonic-minor scale. The note D♯ is sung as *si*. The pitch syllables *si-la* are used in the harmonic-minor scale.

Building Scales One Step at a Time

You can use mallet instruments to hear how major and minor seconds sound. Use C as *do*. **Play** up the scale (C-D-E-F-G-A-B-C) and **listen** to the major and minor seconds. Match the sound to your list of intervals.

Now use F as *do*. **Play** up the scale as before. On what pitch does the interval sound incorrect? Fix this by exchanging the B bar for a B-flat bar. **Play** the scale again. Does it sound correct this time?

Which pitches will you need if you use G as *do*?

2 DEVELOP

Listening

5e Play the recording of "Lo yisa" **CD 7-23** and have students read the notation as they listen, then sight-sing along with the recording. Have them identify that the song is in a minor key. (E harmonic-minor)

Analyzing

6c Write the pitch set for "Lo yisa" on the board (above the song notation in the Teacher's Edition, p. 130). Lead students in comparing the key signature of the song to the pitch set. Have them identify that G is *do*, that the tonic, low *la,* is E, and that the accidental, D♯, is a sharped *so*.

SAY When a sharped *so* is used in a minor scale, it is called *si*; when *si* is used in a minor scale, it is a harmonic-minor scale.

Singing

Have students read and sing "Lo yisa," using pitch syllables.

Analyzing

6a Have students understand that the distances between pitches are called intervals. Ask them to identify the major and minor seconds in "Lo yisa." Then identify the other intervals in the song (thirds and fourths).

6b Lead students to the interval chart on p. 131. Tell them that this chart is for a major, not minor, scale. Have students identify the major seconds and minor seconds in the major scale. Invite students to create an interval chart for a harmonic-minor scale starting on E-*la.* and bracket the major and minor intervals in the harmonic-minor scale. Students may also wish to perform the mallet activity on p. 131.

3 CLOSE

Skill: READING   ASSESSMENT

Performance/Observation Observe students' ability to accurately read and sing the notation of "Lo yisa" and identify the major and minor seconds.

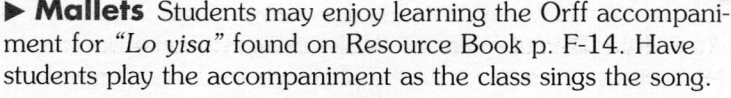

SKILLS REINFORCEMENT

▶ **Mallets** Students may enjoy learning the Orff accompaniment for "Lo yisa" found on Resource Book p. F-14. Have students play the accompaniment as the class sings the song.

▶ **Reading** For practice working with intervals in major and minor scales, have students use Reading Music Worksheet D-18 in the Resource Book.

Invite students to sing a countermelody to "Lo yisa" in Reading Sequence 15 on p. 495, or Resource Book p. E-16.

▶ **Singing** Students will enjoy singing the A and B sections of "Lo yisa" as a canon. Group 2 enters with the three-note pick-up as Group 1 is singing the second ending of the A section.

TECHNOLOGY/MEDIA LINK

5d **Sequencing Software** Divide the class into small groups and have them record the melody for "Lo yisa," using sequencing software. Then have them create two more tracks and use the sequencer's copy and paste functions to create a three-part round. Encourage students to experiment with different timbres for each track and to explore the loop function. Ask students to find "clashing" harmonic intervals (dissonance) in their rounds and to identify these intervals.

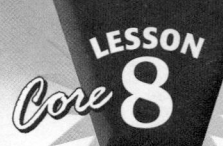

Core LESSON 8

LESSON AT A GLANCE

Element Focus	**MELODY** Melodic sequences	
Skill Objective	**READING** Read melodic sequences	
Connection Activity	**MATHEMATICS** Examine a mathematical sequence in a word problem	

MATERIALS
- "Alleluia"   **CD 7-30**
- **Recording Routine:** Intro (4 m.); vocal; interlude (4 m.); vocal (round); vocal (round)
- **Music Reading Practice, Sequence 16**   **CD 7-32**
- *Canon No. 110 in G* (excerpt)   **CD 7-35**
- **Resource Book** pp. C-2, D-19, E-17
- mallet instruments

VOCABULARY

whole step   half step   melodic sequence

◆ ◆ ◆ ◆ **National Standards** ◆ ◆ ◆ ◆

1d Sing music written in three parts
2a Play instruments accurately in small ensembles
5a Read half, quarter, and eighth notes in alla breve time
6c Understand and use basic principles of intervals in music analysis
8b Identify ways music relates to math

MORE MUSIC CHOICES

For more practice in singing melodic sequence:
"Strike Up the Band," p. 135
"Hava nagila," p. 153

1 INTRODUCE

8b **SAY** In music, a sequence is a melody repeated at an interval above or below itself. Sequences occur in math, too.

Lead a discussion of how sequences occur in math and in daily life. See Across the Curriculum, p. 133.

Moving Motives

A motive can be repeated at different pitches to create a **melodic sequence.** Melodic sequences can move upward (ascending) or downward (descending).

> A **melodic sequence** is the repetition of a melodic pattern usually at different stepwise pitch levels.

Here is a descending melodic sequence. Notice that the first pitch of each motive descends—*so-fa-mi.*

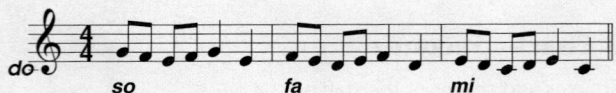

Here is an ascending melodic sequence. Notice that the first note of each motive ascends—*so, la, ti.*

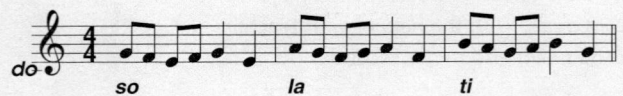

Spotting Sequences

Analyze the melody of "Alleluia," a three-part canon by Mozart. In which phrases can you **identify** a melodic sequence? What is the starting pitch of each motive in the sequence?

Sometimes composers change the rhythm of the repeated motives. **Identify** the motives in "Alleluia" that have rhythmic changes.

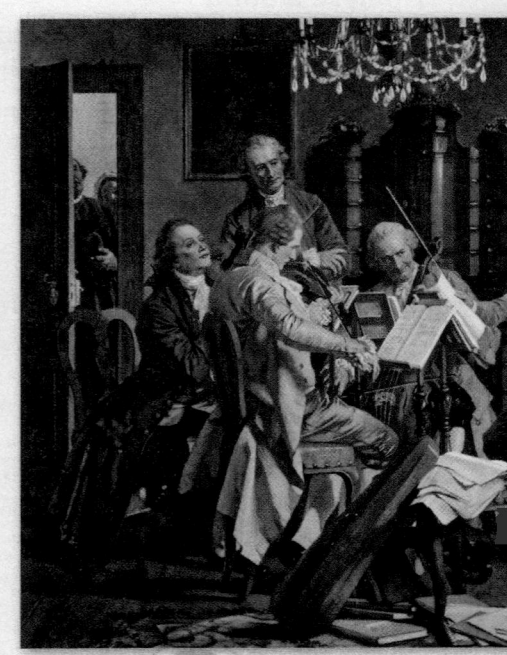

Arts Connection

Engraving of Franz Joseph Haydn conducting and playing in a string quartet ▶

132 🎵 Reading Sequence 16

Footnotes

SPOTLIGHT ON

▶ **The Composer** Encourage students to find out all they can about the composer Franz Joseph Haydn (1732–1809). For more about Haydn and other composers and musicians, invite students to read and listen further in *Story of the Orchestra: A Child's Introduction to the Instruments, the Music and the Musicians* by Robert T. Levine and Meredith Hamilton (Black Dog & Leventhal, 2000).

BUILDING SKILLS THROUGH MUSIC

▶ **Reading** Tell students that Mozart and Haydn, the two composers whose music appeared in this lesson, lived during the same time period. Have them read about each composer, then develop a comparison chart, using Resource Book p. C-2, to show ways in which their lives were alike and different.

SKILLS REINFORCEMENT

▶ **Notating** Have students use standard symbols to notate pitches of the B♭ major diatonic scale, using Resource Book p. D-19. Invite students to circle the pitch set of "Alleluia" in the scale and sing the notes of the pitch set in ascending and descending patterns, using pitch syllables.

8b Help students create one-measure melodic sequences by using addition and subtraction to transpose intervals up or down (+2 = transpose up a major second). Have students adjust the notes to stay in the diatonic scale.

2a Invite students to play their sequences from Resource Book, p. D-19, in canon, on mallet instruments. Voice 2 starts on m. 3.

▶ **Reading** See p. 495, or Resource Book p. E-17, for additional reading practice.

Sing "Alleluia." As you sing, conduct in $\frac{4}{4}$, then in $\frac{2}{2}$.

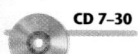

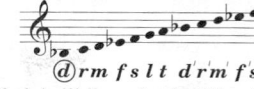

Alleluia

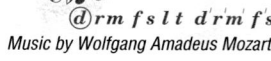

d rm f s l t d'r'm'f s'

Music by Wolfgang Amadeus Mozart

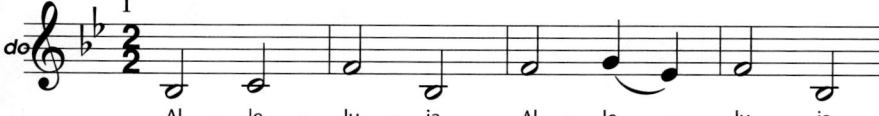

Al – le – lu – ia, Al – le – lu – ia.

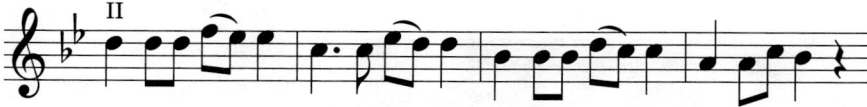

Sing al-le-lu – ia, al-le-lu – ia, sing al-le-lu – ia, al-le-lu–ia.

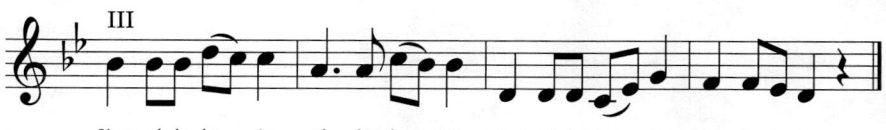

Sing al-le-lu – ia, al-le-lu – ia, sing al-le-lu – ia, al-le-lu–ia.

Listening Sequences

Listen to this canon by Haydn. Can you **identify** a melodic sequence?

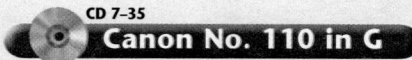

CD 7–35

Canon No. 110 in G

by Franz Joseph Haydn

This Haydn canon is a four-part canon.

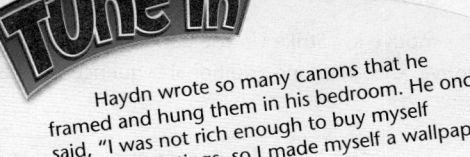

Haydn wrote so many canons that he framed and hung them in his bedroom. He once said, "I was not rich enough to buy myself beautiful paintings, so I made myself a wallpaper that not everybody can have."

Unit 4 **133**

2 DEVELOP

Singing

Have students read p. 132. Ask them to sing both sequences on p. 132 with the pitch syllable on the first note and a neutral syllable on the remaining notes of each measure, noting the descent or ascent of the first pitch in each motive.

Reading

Help students to find the motive that is in m. 5 of "Alleluia" and find the descending sequence in mm. 6, 7, and 8.

ASK Is the rhythm of the motive the same in each repetition? (No, it changes in measures 6 and 8.)

Does the third line have the same sequence? (No, the third line has a two-measure sequence that starts a third lower than line 2.)

Play the recording of "Alleluia" **CD 7-30** and help students independently sing each phrase in unison and with accurate intonation. Then sing the song as a three-part round, demonstrating basic performance techniques. Then, have them read and conduct in $\frac{4}{4}$ then $\frac{2}{2}$.

Listening

Play the recording of *Canon No. 110 in G* **CD 7-35**. Explain that the motive has two heavy beats, and that each voice part is four beats long. Help students to identify the melodic sequence and the four voices.

3 CLOSE

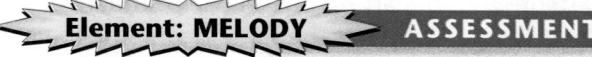

Element: MELODY   ASSESSMENT

Performance/Observation Direct students to Reading Sequence 16 on p. 495. Ask them to read and sing the countermelody using pitch syllables and hand signs. Observe students' ability to read and sing the countermelody accurately.

ACROSS THE CURRICULUM

► **Math** A mathematical series can be created with a word problem: Four members of a family had a three-week vacation. On vacation they all gained 2 pounds by week two and another 1 pound by the end of the third week. Here is a chart of their weights before (original melody), the weights for the second week, and at the end of the trip. Take the last digits of each of these rows of numbers and you will have a melody made of a major triad and two higher repetitions, forming a sequence. Notate them in C major.

	Father	Mark	Carla	Mother	*Melody*
Start	151	113	105	121	*1, 3, 5, 1*
Wk. 2	153	115	107	123	*3, 5, 7, 3*
End	154	116	108	124	*4, 6, 8, 4*

CHARACTER EDUCATION

► **Cooperation** Tell students that singing a round requires cooperation, discipline, and commitment. Have them create a list of activities that require cooperation (playing a team sport, building a house). Ask them: Why is cooperation important? What is required for successful cooperation? (not always having your own way, finding compromises) Discuss the benefits of working more cooperatively at home and at school.

TECHNOLOGY/MEDIA LINK

Notation Software Students may use notation software to notate and play back the sequences in canon they composed in the Skills Reinforcement on p. 132.

LESSON AT A GLANCE

Element Focus — **MELODY** Sequences

Skill Objective — **SINGING** Sing a song that employs sequences

Connection Activity — **RELATED ARTS** Compare sequences in visual art to sequences in music

MATERIALS

- "Strike Up the Band"   **CD 7-36**
  Recording Routine: Intro (4 m.); vocal; interlude (8 m.); vocal; coda
- **Resource Book** pp. B-13, I-13
- melody bells or other melody instruments
- paper, colored pencils or pens

VOCABULARY

motive   sequence   enharmonic tones

◆◆◆◆ National Standards ◆◆◆◆

1a Sing accurately in small ensembles
2a Play instruments alone accurately
4c Compose, using electronic media
6c Understand and use basic principles of intervals in music analysis
8a Show how different arts portray the same idea in unique ways

MORE MUSIC CHOICES

For more practice finding sequences:
"Goin' to Boston," p. 433
"Take Time in Life," p. 292

1 INTRODUCE

8a Draw attention to the art on p. 134. Help students discover that the artist repeats the same geometric figure but changes its color slightly on each repetition. Students can see that repetitions give form to art, as they do to music. See Across the Curriculum below for more on visual sequences.

SEQUENCE-IT

In music, as you have learned, ideas can repeat at a higher or lower pitch. This repetition is called a "sequence."

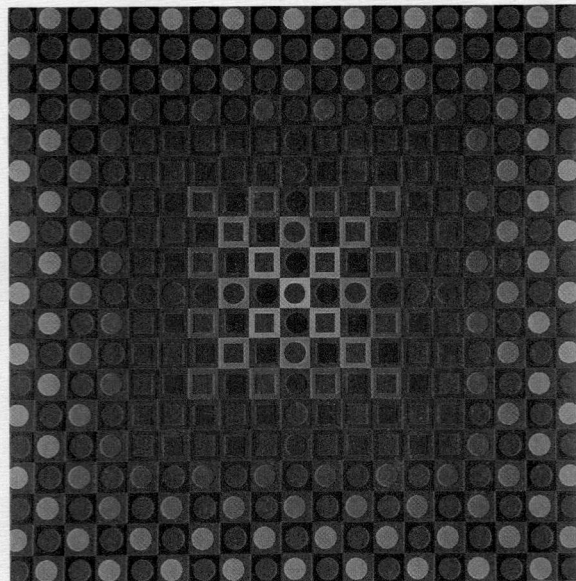

Look at the melodic ideas, or motives, in "Strike Up the Band." The main motive is shaded purple. The secondary motive is shaded orange. **Sing** "Strike Up the Band" to discover how George Gershwin used motives and sequences to build this song.

Arts Connection

◄ The form of this painting, *Alom* by Victor Vasarely (1908–1997), is composed of repeated patterns that are positioned at different levels and angles.

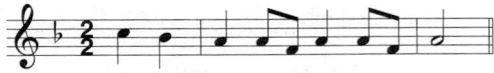
Show What You Know!

Find this motive in "Strike Up the Band" and **identify** the sequences based on this motive. **Create** one additional sequence for this motive.

(134)

Footnotes

SPOTLIGHT ON

▶ **Title Song** "Strike Up the Band" is the title song from a musical comedy originally produced on Broadway in 1930. This antiwar satire boasts one of George and Ira Gershwin's best scores, featuring such great hits as "I've Got a Crush on You," "The Man I Love," "Soon," and the classic title song. The book, by legendary playwright George S. Kaufman, concerns an imaginary war between the United States and Switzerland over the issue of tariffs on chocolate.

BUILDING SKILLS THROUGH MUSIC

▶ **Writing** Tell students that repetition in poetry or prose is similar to sequences in music. Ask students to write a poem about a parade in which they use a phrase (or slight variations on the phrase) repeatedly throughout the poem.

ACROSS THE CURRICULUM

▶ **Visual Arts** Victor Vasarely (1908–1997) was born in Pecs, Hungary, and moved to Paris in 1930 to launch his career. During the 1950s and 1960s, Vasarely became the leader of the op art movement, which studied the effects of form, line, and color on perception and implemented optical illusions in artwork. The artists also sought to create a form of modern art that was democratic, or easily comprehended by anyone, regardless of his or her knowledge of fine art.

8a Students will also enjoy viewing the work of the Dutch artist M. C. Escher (1898–1972) in *M. C. Escher: 29 Master Prints* by Maurits Cornelis Escher (Harry N. Abrams, 1983). This book contains detailed black and white lithographs, many with imitative and sequential design.

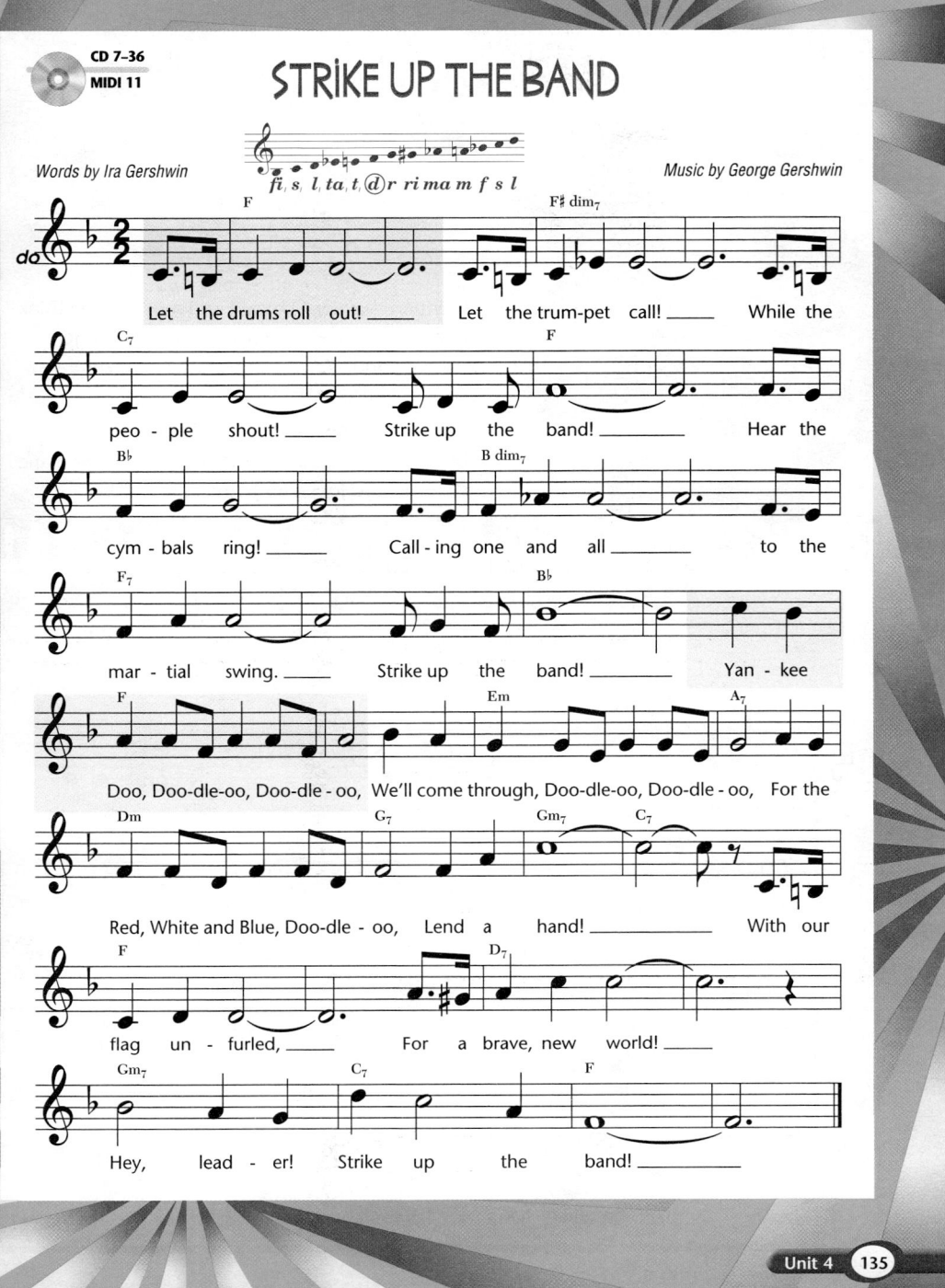

STRIKE UP THE BAND

Words by Ira Gershwin   Music by George Gershwin

Let the drums roll out! _____ Let the trum-pet call! _____ While the

peo - ple shout! _____ Strike up the band! _____ Hear the

cym - bals ring! _____ Call - ing one and all _____ to the

mar - tial swing. _____ Strike up the band! _____ Yan - kee

Doo, Doo-dle-oo, Doo-dle - oo, We'll come through, Doo-dle-oo, Doo-dle - oo, For the

Red, White and Blue, Doo-dle - oo, Lend a hand! _____ With our

flag un - furled, _____ For a brave, new world! _____

Hey, lead - er! Strike up the band!

Unit 4 135

2 DEVELOP

Singing

Invite students to

1a
- Sing "Strike Up the Band" **CD 7-36.**
- Play the main motive (shaded blue), then its first sequence of repetitions (mm. 3–7) on a melody instrument.

You may wish to share with students the information on George Gershwin from p. 251.

Analyzing

Explain that a sequence can be an exact repetition of the original idea on a different pitch level, or it can vary slightly. Invite students to play the secondary motive (p. 134) on a melody instrument, then find this motive (mm. 17–18) and its sequence (mm. 19–23). Have students sing mm. 1–8, and then mm. 9–16.

6c
ASK What is the relationship between these two longer phrases (mm. 1–8, mm. 9–16)? (The second phrase is a repetition of the first, but on a higher level; they form a sequence.)

Moving

Invite students to create hand movements (suggest arcs) that model the melodic sequences they hear. Play the recording of "Strike Up the Band" **CD 7-36** as the students perform their movements.

3 CLOSE

Element: MELODY   ASSESSMENT

Performance/Observation Have students sing "Strike Up the Band" **CD 7-36**, moving their hands in arcs to show phrases and raising and lowering arc levels to show ascending and descending sequences. Observe each type of motion for accuracy. For additional assessment, ask students to perform the Show What You Know activity on p. 134, or Resource Book p. B-13.

SKILLS REINFORCEMENT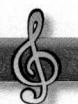

2a
▶ **Recorder** The part below can be played on soprano recorder with mm. 9–16 of "Strike Up the Band." The entire recorder countermelody can be found on Resouce Book p. I-13. Before students play, show them how to finger G♯ on their soprano recorders. Explain that G♯ and A♭ are enharmonic tones. Explain to students that they will play the fingering for G♯ each time they see an A♭.

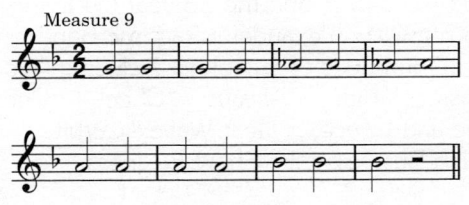

TECHNOLOGY/MEDIA LINK

4c
MIDI/Sequencing Software Add an electronic accompaniment to the MIDI song file for "Strike Up the Band." Divide the class into small groups. Encourage students to explore the percussion bank on the classroom MIDI keyboard(s). Students may improvise percussion solos to be played during the long notes of "Strike Up the Band." Have some students play this electronic percussion part while the rest of the class sings the song.

LESSON AT A GLANCE

Element Focus **TIMBRE** Band instrumentation

Skill Objective **LISTENING** Listen for the differences between a big band and a concert band

Connection Activity **GENRE** Understand the role and history of different kinds of bands

MATERIALS

- "Alexander's Ragtime Band"   **CD 8-1**
  Recording Routine: Intro (4 m.); vocal; vocal; coda
- "March" from *Suite No. 2 in F,* Op. 28b   **CD 8-3**
- *Fanfare for Freedom*   **CD 8-4**

VOCABULARY

concert band	motive	woodwinds
brass	percussion	half step

◆ ◆ ◆ ◆ National Standards ◆ ◆ ◆ ◆

1d Sing music written in two parts
5a Read dotted notes in duple meter
6b Listen and analyze uses of timbre in music from diverse genres
8b Identify ways music relates to math
9a Describe characteristics of music genres from a variety of cultures

MORE MUSIC CHOICES

For more experience with brass timbres:

Variations on "The Carnival of Venice," p. 161
Galliard battaglia, p. 362
Marche militaire, Op. 51, No. 1, p. 17

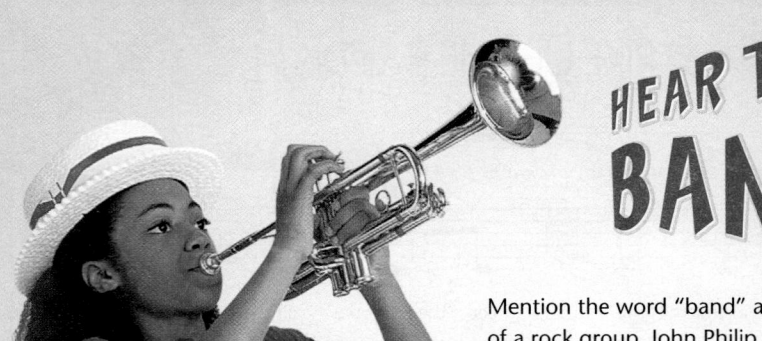

HEAR THE BAND!

Mention the word "band" and most people think of a rock group, John Philip Sousa, or a large parade band. But there are many different types of bands around the world.

Sing "Alexander's Ragtime Band" by Irving Berlin. Berlin was influenced by the ragtime piano style of Scott Joplin and others.

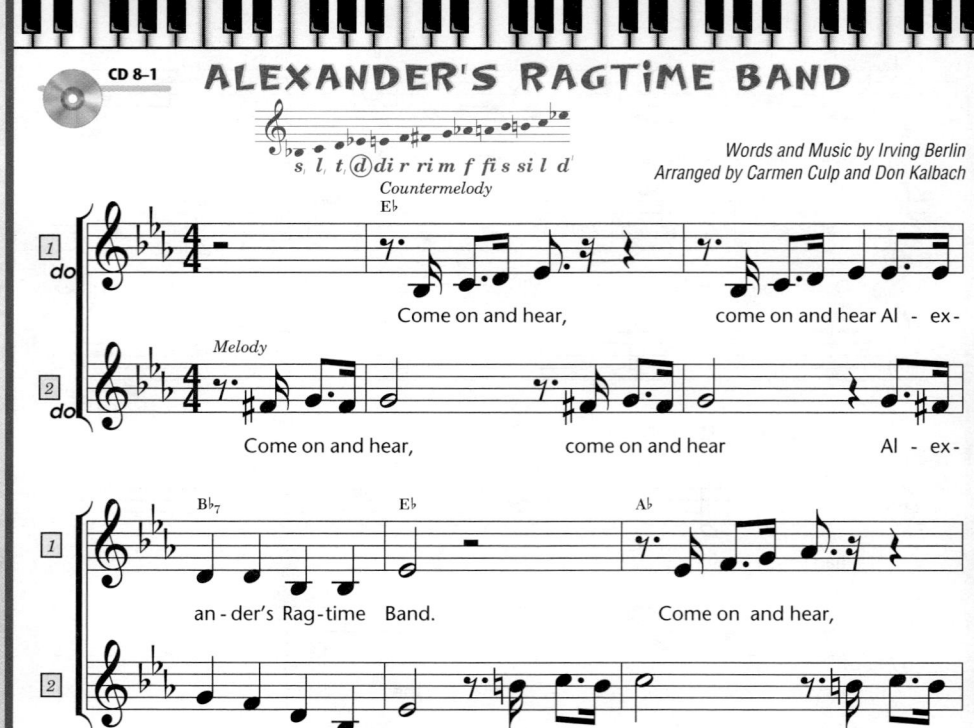

CD 8-1   **ALEXANDER'S RAGTIME BAND**

Words and Music by Irving Berlin
Arranged by Carmen Culp and Don Kalbach

136

Footnotes

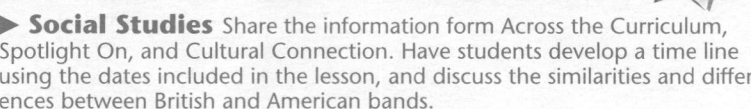

SKILLS REINFORCEMENT

6b ▶ **Listening** Play half steps and whole steps on a keyboard, and ask students to distinguish between them. Divide the class into pairs of students. Give each pair a note on a staff and ask them to write a half step above or below the given note. Encourage students to think of familiar melodies that contain important half-step motives, such as the theme from the movie *Jaws* and the theme from *Overture to Candide* on p. 218, m. 3.

BUILDING SKILLS THROUGH MUSIC

▶ **Social Studies** Share the information form Across the Curriculum, Spotlight On, and Cultural Connection. Have students develop a time line using the dates included in the lesson, and discuss the similarities and differences between British and American bands.

ACROSS THE CURRICULUM

▶ **Social Studies** Share with students these interesting historical events from the year 1911.

In 1911, Roald Amundsen became the first human to reach the South Pole; the Manchu dynasty was about to fall in China; the deserted Inca city of Machu Picchu was rediscovered in Peru; Stravinsky premiered his ballet *Pétrouchka;* and Marie Curie received the Nobel Prize in chemistry. In 1911, Gustav Holst wrote his *Suite No 2 in F,* and the 23-year-old Irving Berlin had his first smash hit with "Alexander's Ragtime Band." Irving Berlin went on to write hundreds of hit songs, including "God Bless America," "Easter Parade," "Always," "Cheek to Cheek," "Let's Face the Music and Dance," "Heat Wave," "White Christmas," and "There's No Business Like Show Business."

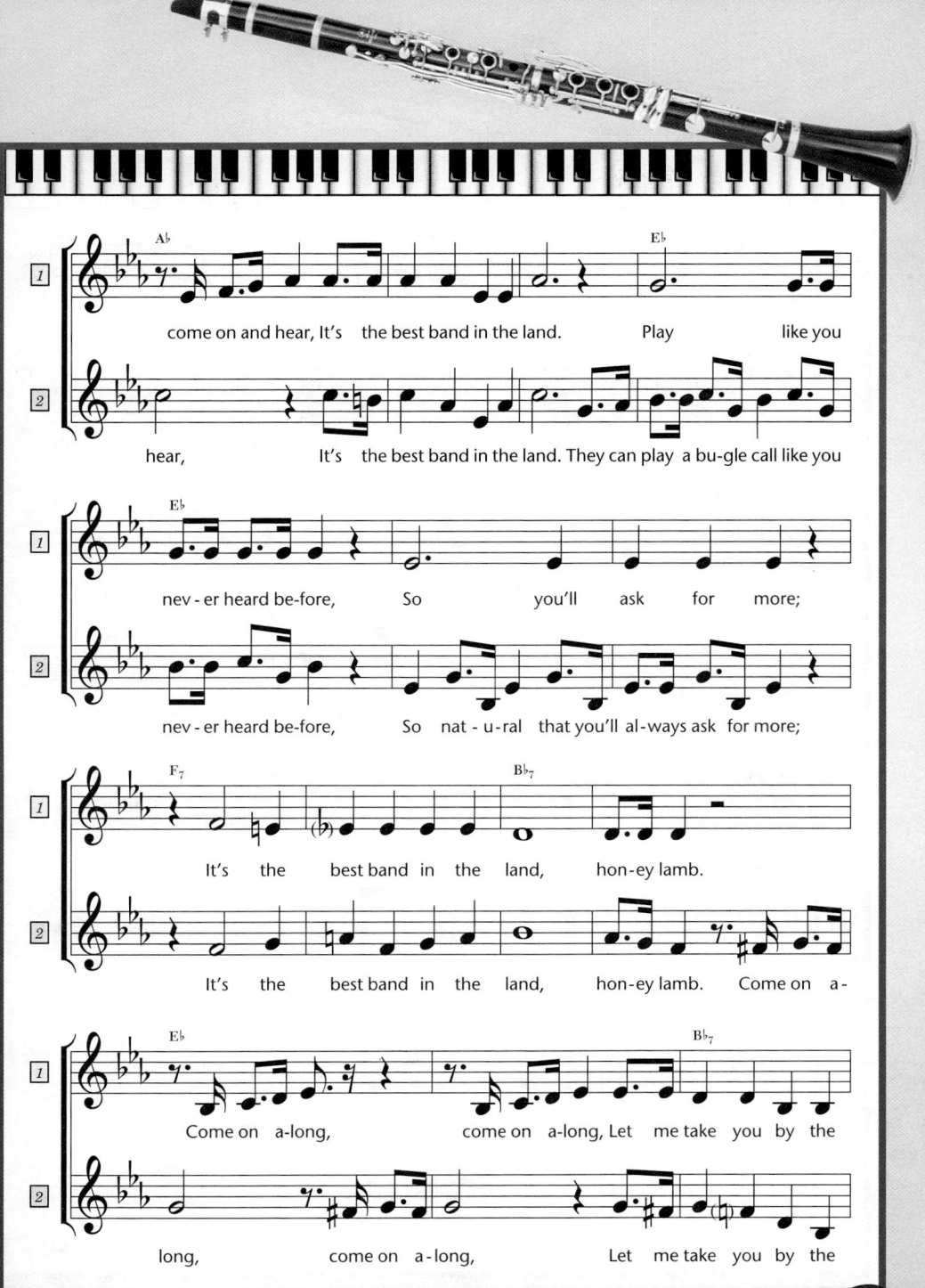

1 INTRODUCE

Ask students to try to remember the first time they heard a band playing live. Was it at a parade? Was it at a sports event? Was it at a concert?

2 DEVELOP

Reading

Share with students some information about the historical setting for Irving Berlin's "Alexander's Ragtime Band." See Across the Curriculum on p. 136.

Play the recording of "Alexander's Ragtime Band" **CD 8-1** and invite students to

5a
- Follow the melody (bottom staff) in their books.
- Identify the rhythmic motive that is used throughout the song (*Come on and hear*).

ASK **How many times is the rhythmic motive used in both parts?** (22)

Singing

Divide the class into two groups and guide students to

- Alternate saying the rhythmic motive, using *ta-dah ta-dah*.

1d
- Sing the first set of four *Come on and hear* motives, and realize that the melody is singing a half-step pattern while the countermelody is singing a pattern from *so* up the scale to *do*.
- Sing the second set of *Come on and hear* motives (mm. 5–7), and learn that the pattern is the same but sung a fourth higher.

ASK **Where in the song do the exact alternations come back?** (mm. 17–24)

What is different about the beginning and the last set of alternations (last four measures of the piece)? (The last melody is a third higher than at the beginning.)

continued on page 138

SPOTLIGHT ON

9a ▶ **The Concert Band** The modern concert band evolved from American military bands and their English counterparts. In the period following the Civil War (1861–1865) up to World War II (1939–1945), concert bands such as the John Philip Sousa Band (1892–1932) established the basic instrumentation and the basis for literature for the nonmilitary concert band. Once the concert band became well established in schools, colleges, and towns, its future was ensured. After World War II the wind ensemble movement under the leadership of Frederick Fennell further refined the concert band movement. Besides Gustav Holst and Morton Gould, major composers who have written for the concert band include Vaughan Williams, Paul Hindemith, Aaron Copland, Vincent Persichetti, William Schuman, and Igor Stravinsky.

CULTURAL CONNECTION

9a ▶ **The British Brass Band** Besides the military band and the concert band, another kind of non-jazz band is the British brass band. The history of this kind of brass ensemble dates back to the early nineteenth century and England's Industrial Revolution. Large companies involved in coal mining or manufacturing sponsored bands as a way of providing alternative leisure-time options. The two bands with the longest traditions are the Bessies O' the Barn Brass Band and the Black Dyke Mills Brass Band. By 1860 there were over 750 brass bands in England.

Today there are over 5,000 brass bands in England, and many are more than 100 years old. A typical brass band contains B♭ and E♭ cornets, flügelhorns, tenor horns, baritone horns, trombones, euphoniums, B♭ and E♭ basses, and percussion.

Where does the melody sound like a bugle call?
(mm. 12 and 13)

1d Invite all students to sing the entire melody (bottom line) with the recording **CD 8-1.** Next, ask them to sing the countermelody along with the recording. Then, divide the class into two groups and have them sing both parts with the recording.

Listening

ASK How many of you play band instruments?

Invite students to individually demonstrate their instruments in class and describe the characteristic timbre of the instrument to the class. Discuss the concert band and its history using information in Spotlight On, p. 137.

Ask students to write these section letters for the form of *Suite No. 2 in F:* ABCAB

Invite students to

- Listen to *Suite No. 2 in F* **CD 8-3.**

6b - Use music terms to describe the timbre and character of the music and musical instruments they hear in each section. (A: vigorous and accented brass opening followed by woodwinds; B: legato [smooth] section; C: minor section featuring woodwinds)

- Read about composer Gustav Holst in the Music Maker on p. 139.

- Use standard terminology to describe the differences in timbre found in band music compared to other music ensembles. (Concert bands are comprised of wind and percussion instruments, and have no string instruments.)

Help students to

- Listen to *Fanfare for Freedom* **CD 8-4.**

- Listen again and call out instrument families they hear for you to write on the board. (brass, percussion, woodwinds)

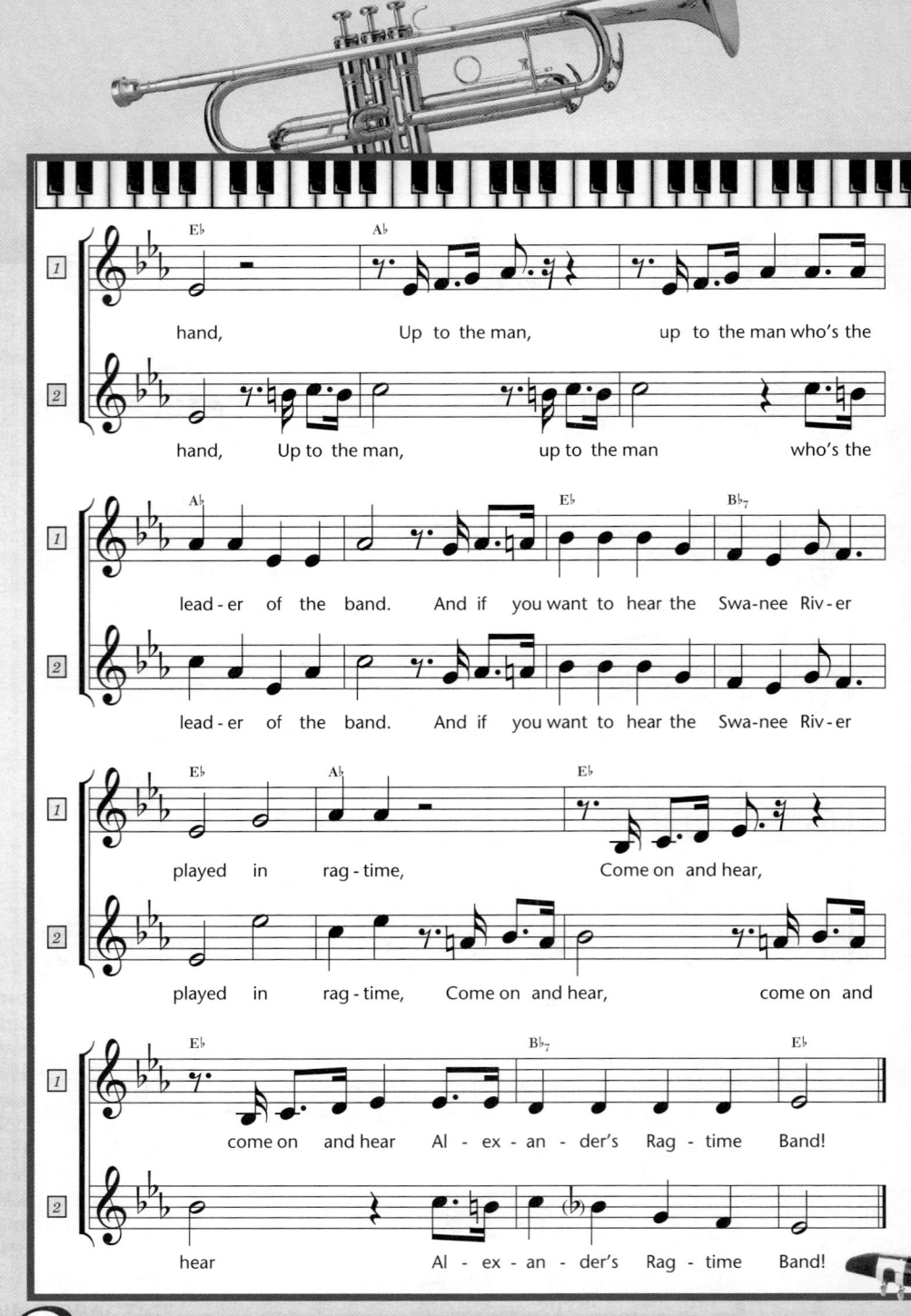

Footnotes

SPOTLIGHT ON

▶ **The Composer** Morton Gould (1913–1996) was one of America's most prominent composers and conductors. His honors include the Kennedy Center Honor (1994), the Pulitzer Prize in Music (1995), a Grammy Award (1965), and election as president of the American Society of Composers, Authors, and Publishers (1986–1994). Gould started composing at age six and as a youngster gave recitals all over New York City. Gould promoted serious concert band music through his compositions for that genre, though his best-known works are for orchestra. He also composed for Broadway shows (*Billion Dollar Baby*, 1945), ballet (*Fall River Legend*, 1947), film (*Windjammer*, 1958), and a TV movie (*Holocaust*, 1978). Music education was an important cause for Morton Gould. He taught composition and conducted student ensembles.

ACROSS THE CURRICULUM

8b ▶ **Math** A bugle is a soprano brass instrument that looks like a trumpet but has a larger, conical bore. The valveless bugle can produce only the second through sixth notes in the series of tones called the harmonic series. The harmonic series is mathematically derived. A B♭ bugle can play only the bracketed notes in this complete B♭ harmonic series.

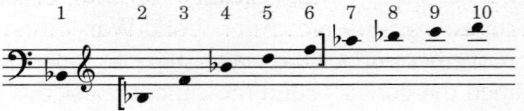

Ask students if the intervals get larger or smaller as the series goes up. (smaller)

The Concert Band

The concert, or symphonic, band is found in just about every school and university in America. This ensemble plays music of many different genres—from classical to pop to patriotic.

The concert band is made up of woodwinds, brass, and percussion. (See the Sound Bank for information on specific band instruments.)

Listen to this piece from the British concert band literature.

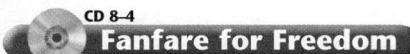

CD 8–3
Suite No. 2 in F

**Movement 1, "March"
by Gustav Holst**

Holst based this suite on English country tunes.

Listen to another selection for concert band and **identify** the families of instruments mentioned above.

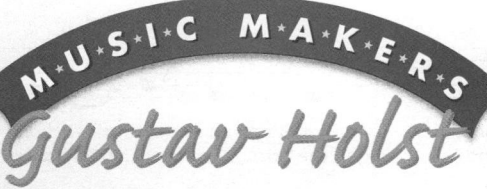

CD 8–4
Fanfare for Freedom

by Morton Gould

American composer Morton Gould (1913–1996) wrote this patriotic fanfare in 1971.

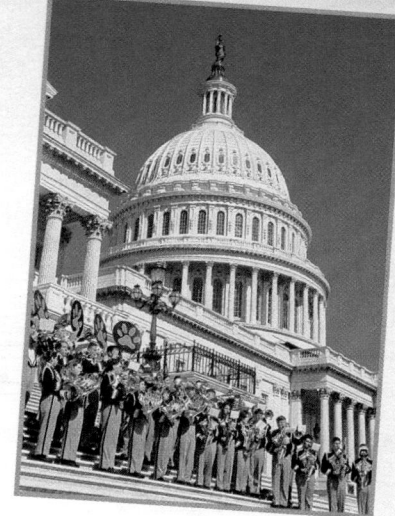

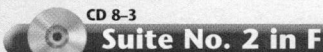
M·U·S·I·C M·A·K·E·R·S
Gustav Holst

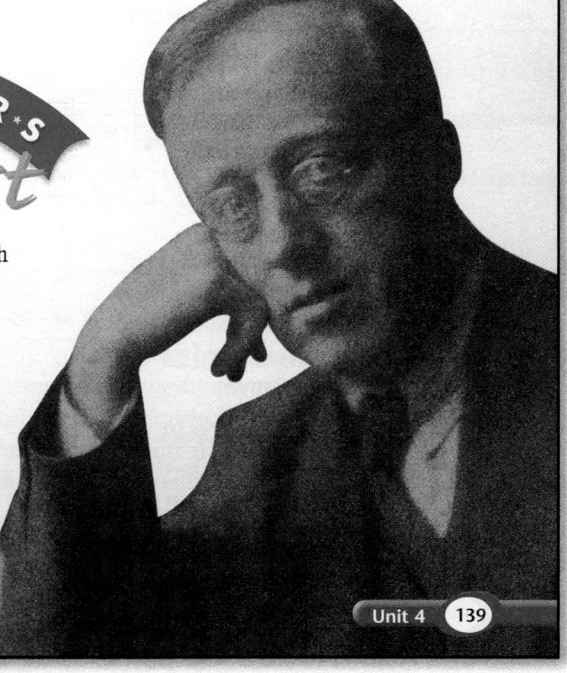

Gustav Holst (1874–1934) was an English composer and well-known teacher and educator. His most famous work is *The Planets*, a suite for orchestra. His two "military" suites are among the best and most important works for concert band. Holst loved English folk songs of the sixteenth and seventeenth centuries. He was also influenced by the music and folklore of India and the Far East.

Unit 4 139

- Listen and determine if Gould used the families of instruments together most of the time or in alternation. (in alternation)

- Learn more about the composer, Morton Gould, in Spotlight On, p. 138.

3 CLOSE

Analyzing

Tell students that there are other types of bands, in addition to concert bands and military bands. Marching bands are found in many high schools and colleges. They generally have percussion, brass, and woodwinds in their ensemble. Some university marching bands only use brass and percussion instruments. A different type of marching band is the drum-and-bugle-corp style band. These bands have a very powerful sound with only brass and percussion instruments. Drum-and-bugle-corp bands have unique brass instruments and a unique style of marching. The British brass band is similar to these bands, utilizing only brass and percussion. Share with students the information in Cultural Connection, p. 137, on British brass bands.

Skill: LISTENING   ASSESSMENT

Music Journal Writing Have students listen to the instrumental tracks of "Alexander's Ragtime Band" **CD 8-1**, *Suite No. 2 in F* **CD 8-3**, and *Fanfare for Freedom* **CD 8-4**. Encourage students to write a paragraph about the use of instrumental timbre in each listening selection. They should

- Refer to all three families of instruments used in the selections: brass, percussion, and woodwinds.

- Compare and contrast use of instrumental timbre in the selections; they may wish to write about which use of timbre they find most effective.

- Add this page of writing to their portfolios.

TEACHER TO TEACHER

6b ▶ **Listening** Create a listening assignment for this lesson's examples of jazz big band ("Alexander's Ragtime Band" performance track), and concert band (*Suite No. 2 in F* and *Fanfare for Freedom*). Offer students (on the board or on individual papers) a list of musical terms to which they may refer during their listening assignment, for example, tempo, meter, dynamics, harmony, form, style, instrumentation.

While listening to each example, students may list the names of the instruments they hear, and then use musical terms to describe the music they are hearing (for example, fast tempo, tight harmony, improvisation, repeated sections). Ask students to share aloud their ideas about each selection. Play the selection again. Use students' musical descriptions to create a large, descriptive class list for each genre.

SCHOOL TO HOME CONNECTION

▶ **Interviews** Invite students to ask older relatives about band concerts in parks—a great American institution. Students may ask: "What kind of music did the bands play?" "What is your favorite band piece?" Students may discuss their findings.

TECHNOLOGY/MEDIA LINK

Electronic Keyboard Invite students to locate sounds for band instruments on their MIDI keyboards. (Trumpet, trombone, tuba, flute, clarinet, and so on.) Ask students to create an accompaniment part for their chosen instrument by improvising as the class sings the song with the recording. Suggest that the countermelody (top line) be performed as an accompaniment.

LESSON AT A GLANCE

Element Focus	**TEXTURE/HARMONY** Chordal accompaniment
Skill Objective	**PLAYING** Play an accompaniment in reggae style
Connection Activity	**CULTURE** Recognize that popular culture today is influenced by cultures from all over the world

MATERIALS

- "Give a Little Love"   **CD 8-5**

  Recording Routine: Intro (4 m.); refrain 1; v. 1; refrain 1; v. 2; refrain 2; bridge; refrain 2; coda

- *Reggae Is Now*   **CD 8-7**

- high and low drums, keyboard, guitar, shakers, bass instrument

VOCABULARY

reggae   accompaniment   call-and-response form

◆ ◆ ◆ ◆ National Standards ◆ ◆ ◆ ◆

1c Sing music from diverse cultures
2a Play instruments accurately in small ensembles
2c Perform instrumental music from diverse cultures
3a Improvise simple harmonic accompaniments
6b Listen and analyze uses of texture in music from diverse cultures
7b Students use specific criteria for evaluating performances, and offer constructive suggestions for improvement

MORE MUSIC CHOICES

For more practice with D and A₇ chords:

"Adiós, amigos," p. 57

"Down in the Valley," p. 375

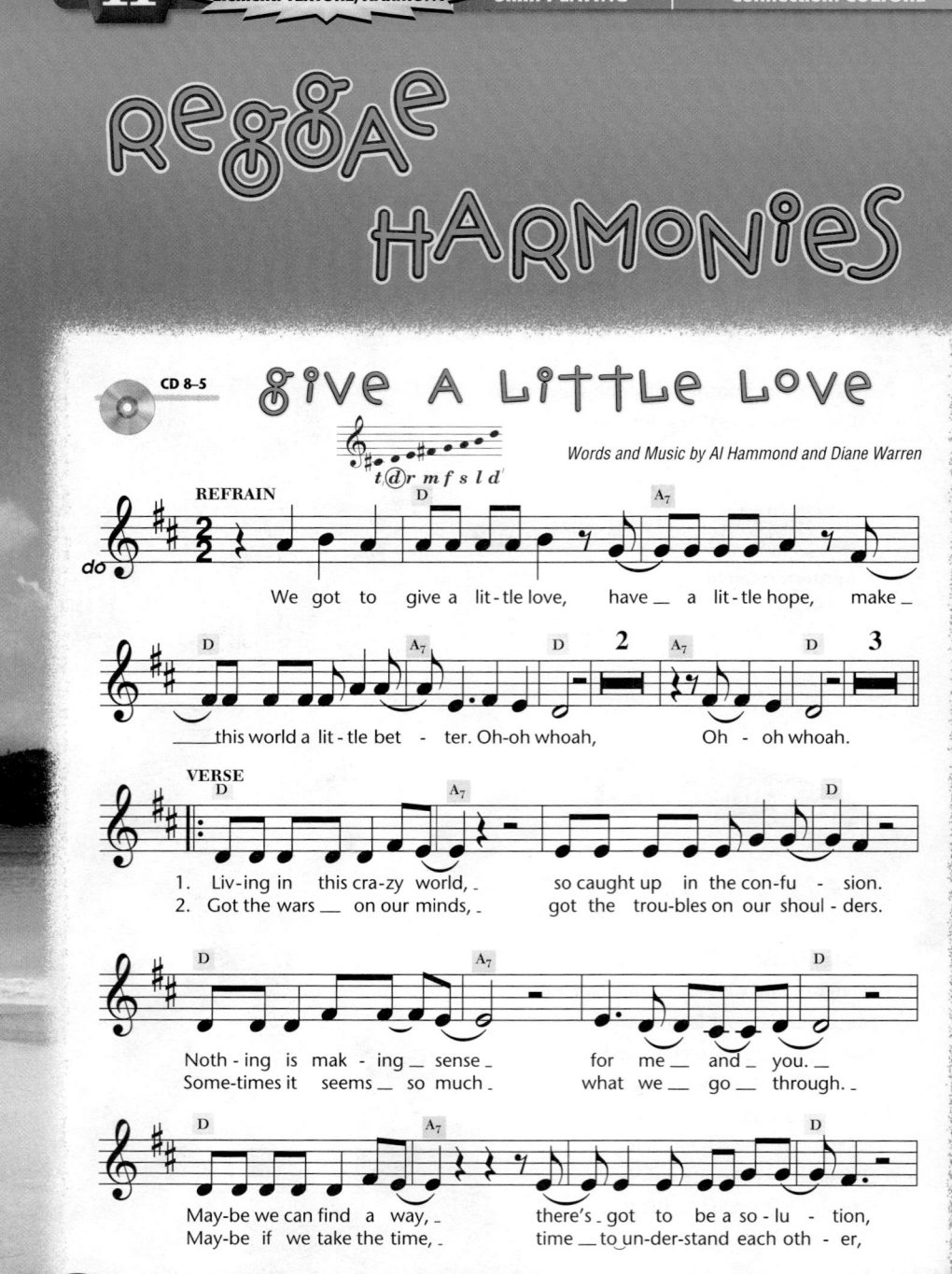

Reggae Harmonies

Give a Little Love

Words and Music by Al Hammond and Diane Warren

Footnotes

MEETING INDIVIDUAL NEEDS

▶ **Syncopated Lyrics** These activities may assist students.

Reinforcement English Language Learners may clearly speak the lyrics in a regular rhythm on the beat.

On Target Students may read the lyrics at a slow tempo, and in a straight rhythm, then read the lyrics in rhythm.

Challenge Students may read syncopated lyrics and rhythms simultaneously—tap a steady beat with one hand, and the syncopated rhythm with the other as they sing.

BUILDING SKILLS THROUGH MUSIC

▶ **Language** Have students read the web-based article about the music of Jamaica in Technology/Media Link on p. 143. Then have them write an outline of the information presented.

SKILLS REINFORCEMENT

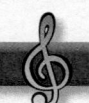

▶ **Recorder** Students can play this reggae accompaniment on alto recorders during the verses of "Give a Little Love." For an ensemble experience, have some students play the recorder while others play D and A₇ chords (as indicated in the music) on guitar or keyboard while the class sings verse 1. Have students demonstrate small-ensemble performance techniques in this informal concert by using appropriate volume, balance, and blend to obtain a good sound.

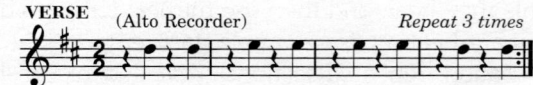

Reggae Is Pop

Reggae is a popular music style that was born in Jamaica. It is a blend of African American music, rock, and traditional African Jamaican music. This modern reggae song uses mostly two chords.

Sing "Give a Little Love."
Listen to the harmonies and the rhythm as you sing.

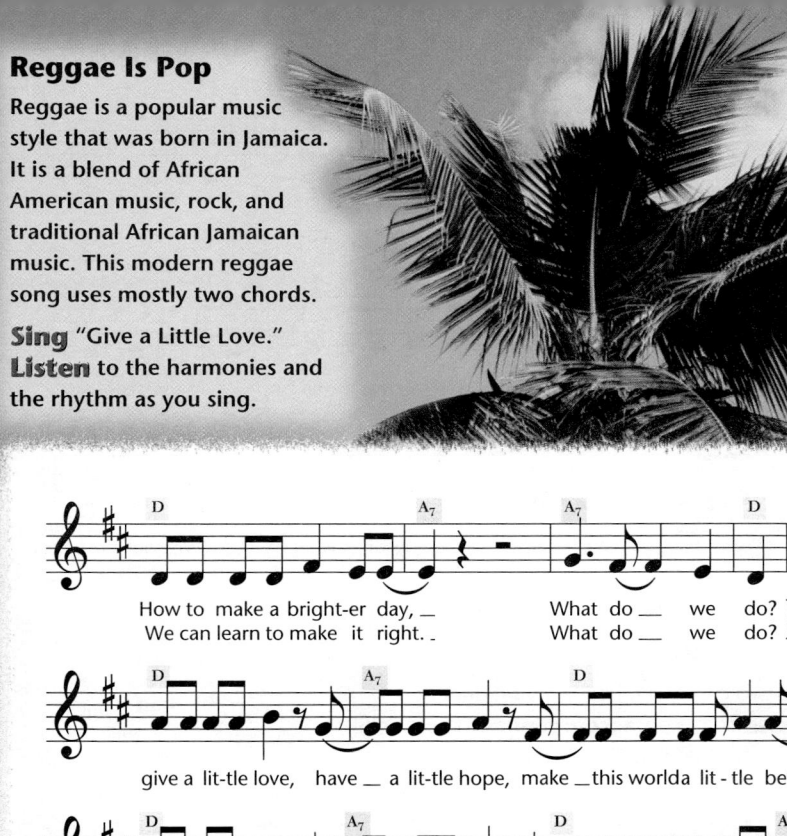

REFRAIN

How to make a bright-er day, _ What do _ we do?
We can learn to make it right. _ What do _ we do? } We got to

give a lit-tle love, have _ a lit-tle hope, make _ this worlda lit-tle bet - ter.

Try a lit-tle more, hard - er than be-fore, let's do what we can do to-geth - er. Oh _

whoah - oh, _____ We can ev-en make it bet - ter, yeah. _

1.
(last time repeat refrain ad lib)
Oh whoah, _ la, la, la, On-ly if we try. ___ ___ We got to

2. D   Bm   Em
___ If ev-'ry-bod-y took some-bod-y by the hand, _

Unit 4 **141**

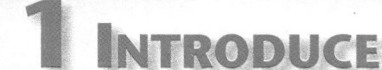

1 INTRODUCE

Engage students in a short discussion about how our music and popular culture is influenced by cultures from all over the world. Explain that reggae is a style of music originally from Jamaica. Share information on reggae's predecessor, the Jamaican *ska,* in Cultural Connections, p. 143. Invite students to discover information on the history of Jamaica in Across the Curriculum below.

2 DEVELOP

Listening

Help students to

- Listen to "Give a Little Love" **CD 8-5** as they follow the music.
- Discover the repeats and first and second endings in the music, as well as directions to go back to the refrain at certain places. Ask students to identify the musical form from the notation. (verse refrain)

Singing

Invite students to perform independently and demonstrate fundamental skills. Have them

- Sing the song with the recording **CD 8-5**.
- Tap, clap, or play the heavy beat on a drum as they sing the song again.

Analyzing

ASK How many heavy beats did you hear in each measure? (two)

How many different chords are used in this song? (four: D, A₇, Bm, and Em)

Which chords are used most frequently? (D and A₇)

continued on page 142

SPOTLIGHT ON

▶ **Harmony** Demonstrate to students that all of the notes in a major scale can be found in these chords: I, IV, and V. Write these chords in D major on the board. Divide the class into small groups and distribute at least one melody instrument and one chording instrument to each group. Ask each group to create a short melody in D major in duple meter, using from four to eight notes. Then invite students to assign appropriate chords to accompany each note. Point out that for some melody notes, more than one chord could work. In these cases they will have to try both chords and decide which one they prefer. When all groups have finished, have them perform their harmonized melodies for the class.

ACROSS THE CURRICULUM

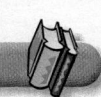

▶ **Social Studies** Invite students to find Jamaica on a map. It is about 500 miles south of Florida. The indigenous group, the Arawak Nation, were nearly destroyed when Christopher Columbus landed in 1494 and claimed the island for Spain. But Spain did not care to settle or develop the island because of a lack of gold. The Arawak people were forced to work as slaves for the Spaniards; enslaved Africans were also brought to Jamaica to work. These Africans became the new people of Jamaica, along with some immigrants from Europe and Asia including Syria. In 1670, Britain invaded and gained control, and Jamaica remained a British colony until 1962, when it gained independence. The people of Jamaica have a history of trying to make this world *a little bit better* despite outside oppression.

Playing

Invite students to

- Look at the chord diagrams for the A₇ and D chords on keyboard and on guitar.

- Practice each chord on either keyboard or guitar until they are comfortable switching from chord to chord. Tell students to use the color shading to help determine when to switch chords.

 • Perform an accompaniment for "Give a Little Love" **CD 8-5** by playing the A₇ and D chords as they occur in the song.

- Perform the accompaniment again as the rest of the class sings the song.

Invite students to learn the clap, guitar chord, shaker, and bass patterns at the top of p. 143 for the refrain.

ASK How many times will you play each chord in a measure? (twice, because there are two beats in each measure)

Can these two chords be played throughout the entire song? (No, they can't be played during the Em and Bm measures at the bottom of p. 141 and top of p. 142.) Some students can lightly tap the guitar body during these measures.

Help students to

- Perform this accompaniment on the refrain as they sing the song with the Stereo Performance track **CD 8-6.**

- Sing the song and perform the A₇ and D chords on verses and the rhythm complex from p. 143 on the refrain.

You may wish to substitute resonator bells or hand chimes for keyboard and bass if necessary.

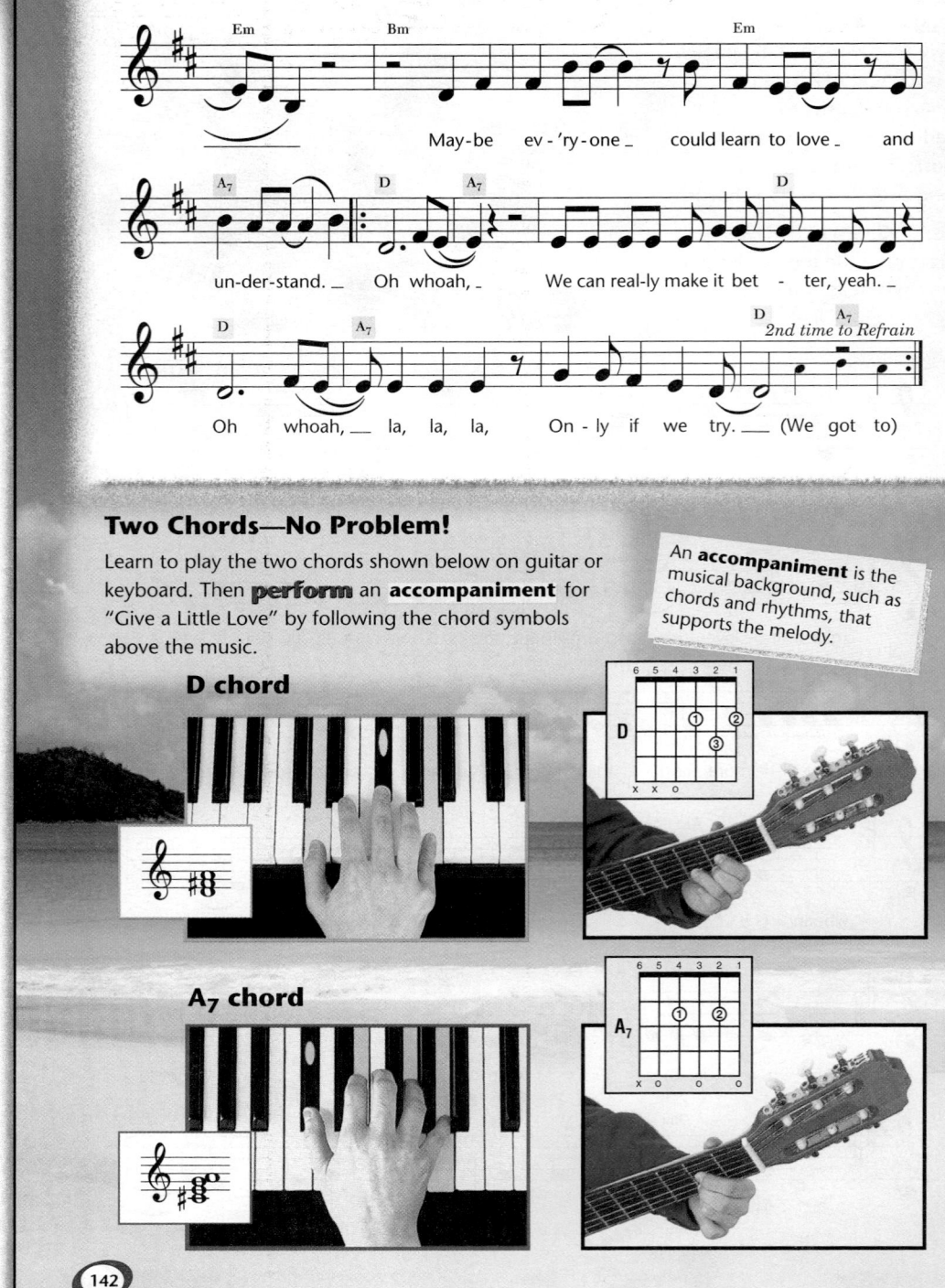

Two Chords—No Problem!

Learn to play the two chords shown below on guitar or keyboard. Then **perform** an **accompaniment** for "Give a Little Love" by following the chord symbols above the music.

An **accompaniment** is the musical background, such as chords and rhythms, that supports the melody.

D chord

A₇ chord

Footnotes

SKILLS REINFORCEMENT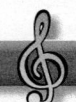

▶ **Improvising** After listening to and singing the reggae song "Give a Little Love," have students improvise a drum part for the song. Provide a high and a low drum for this activity. Invite a volunteer to improvise a two-measure drum part and play it as the class sings "Give a Little Love." Encourage the volunteer to keep the drum part going throughout the whole song. Have students constructively critique the improvised pattern. Repeat the activity with as many volunteers as possible, then discuss which patterns worked best and why.

▶ **Singing** Invite students to sing songs from other diverse cultures that are in verse refrain form: *"Eres tú"* on p. 473, *"Riendo el río corre"* on p. 263, and "Skye Boat Song" on p. 372.

CHARACTER EDUCATION

▶ **Kindness and Social Responsibility** Discuss with students the message of "Give a Little Love." Encourage students to consider what they could do to "make this world a little better." Ask them how they would describe the message of this song to their classmates. How would they demonstrate this message to them? (be caring, be courteous, offer help when someone needs it) Have students consider specific behaviors they might demonstrate at home (cleaning their room, being kind to their siblings and parents, doing chores without being asked) and at school (keeping the school grounds clean, acting respectfully toward teachers and classmates, helping others, following rules) that would make their world a better place. Discuss how students might make a positive difference in their community (volunteer at an animal shelter, pick up litter, show kindness to others).

Reggae Rhythm Box

Perform this reggae-style rhythm complex when you sing the refrain.

(Beats)	1		2		1		2	
Clap		X		X		X		X
Guitar Chords		D		D		A₇		A₇
Shakers	X	X	X	X	X	X	X	X	X	X	X	X	X	X	X	X
Bass	D		D		A		A	

Listen to Ziggy Marley's performance of *Reggae Is Now*.

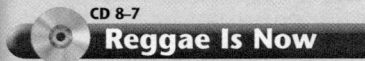

CD 8–7
Reggae Is Now

by Ziggy Marley
performed by Ziggy Marley and the Melody Makers
Ziggy Marley's performance of *Reggae Is Now* features
reggae-style rhythms and call-and-response form.

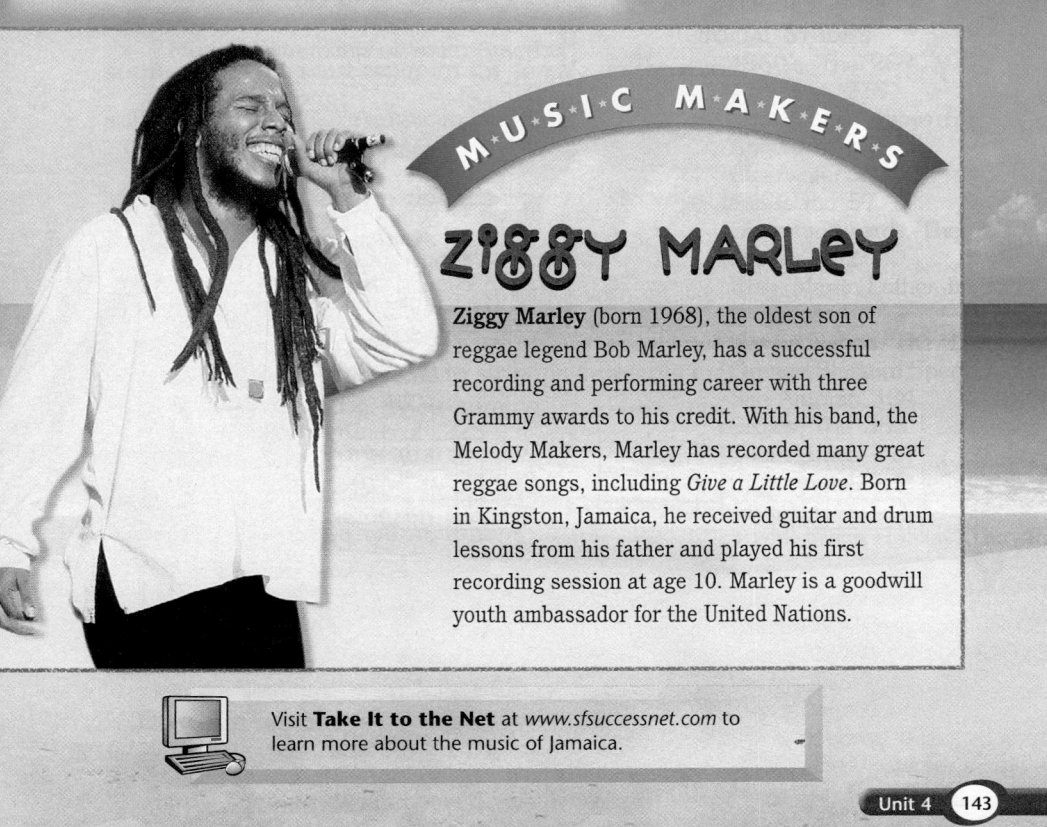

M·U·S·I·C M·A·K·E·R·S

ZIGGY MARLEY

Ziggy Marley (born 1968), the oldest son of
reggae legend Bob Marley, has a successful
recording and performing career with three
Grammy awards to his credit. With his band, the
Melody Makers, Marley has recorded many great
reggae songs, including *Give a Little Love*. Born
in Kingston, Jamaica, he received guitar and drum
lessons from his father and played his first
recording session at age 10. Marley is a goodwill
youth ambassador for the United Nations.

Visit **Take It to the Net** at *www.sfsuccessnet.com* to
learn more about the music of Jamaica.

Listening

6b Invite students to

- Listen to *Reggae Is Now* **CD 8-7** focusing on the change in texture that is the result of Ziggy Marley's use of call-and-response form (call is solo voice, response is in homophonic close harmony).
- Read about the highly successful Jamaican reggae artist Ziggy Marley.

For additional activities, invite students to play the recorder pattern in Skills Reinforcement, p. 140. Then invite students to explore improvising reggae patterns in Skills Reinforcement, p. 142. Finally, guide students to see how chords are related to harmony in Spotlight On, p. 141.

3 CLOSE

Element: TEXTURE/HARMONY — ASSESSMENT

7b **Performance/Peer Critique** Divide the class into groups of four. Have two students in each group perform the chord and rhythm complex accompaniments while the other two students sing "Give a Little Love" with the Stereo Performance track **CD 8-6**. Invite singers to evaluate the accompanists' ability to perform in a reggae style. Have students offer constructive comments on how they might improve, then have students switch roles and repeat.

Invite the whole class to sing the song in unison without the recording and without any accompaniment. Ask students to comment on what happens to the texture when the harmony and other accompaniment elements are gone.

CULTURAL CONNECTION

▶ **Jamaican *Ska*** A dance style popular in the mid-1960s, *ska* was a predecessor of the reggae style in Jamaica. It grew out of an urban tradition that was influenced by the rhythm and blues style of artists in the United States, like Fats Domino. People in Jamaica listened to radio broadcasts of rhythm and blues music from New Orleans in the 1950s. Soon musicians in Jamaica were imitating this style with offbeat rhythms played in a fast tempo. Artists known for their *ska* style include Minnie Small and the Skatalites. By the mid-1960s, this *ska* style slowed down a bit into another called "rock steady." Reggae developed from the rock-steady style and quickly became popular not just in Jamaica but all over the world.

TECHNOLOGY/MEDIA LINK

CD-ROM After students have learned to sing "Give a Little Love," help them take turns entering the song's chord progression into the *Band-in-a-Box* program (have each student enter a measure or two). Have students sing the song with several different accompaniment styles. Ask students which styles seem most appropriate for this song.

Web Site Go to *www.sfsuccessnet.com* to learn more about the music of Jamaica.

LESSON AT A GLANCE

Element Focus   **TEXTURE/HARMONY** Homophonic texture

Skill Objective   **PLAYING** Accompany a song on the guitar, Autoharp, or piano using the F, B♭, and C_7 chords

Connection Activity   **SOCIAL STUDIES** Explore the history of cowboy culture in the West

MATERIALS

- "El payo"   **CD 8-8**
- "The Cowpoke"   **CD 8-9**

  Recording Routine: Intro (4 m.); v. 1; interlude (4 m.); v. 2; coda
- **Pronunciation Practice/Translation** p. 527
- keyboard, guitars with capo at third fret
- **Resource Book** pp. A-12, F-16, I-14

VOCABULARY

root position   inversion

♦ ♦ ♦ ♦ National Standards ♦ ♦ ♦ ♦

1c Sing music from diverse cultures
2a Play instruments accurately in small ensembles
5c Identify standard notation symbols for pitch
6c Understand and use basic principles of chords in music analysis
8b Identify ways music relates to social studies

MORE MUSIC CHOICES

For more practice using the F, B♭, and C_7 chords:

"Las mañanitas," p. 481

"Red River Valley," p. 11

1 INTRODUCE

Discuss with students the fact that the life of the cowboy is full of hard work and loneliness. For more information on cowboy culture, have students read *Cowboy: An Album* by Linda Granfield (Ticknor and Fields, 1994).

Guitar Textures

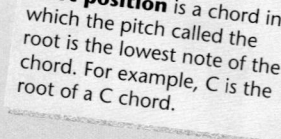

Vaqueros and cowboys roamed the western plains from Mexico to Canada from the 1860s to the 1880s, driving cattle from one place to another. They played simple chords on their guitars and sang to entertain themselves.

Sing *"El payo."* **Listen** to the simple harmonies as you sing. How many different chords are used?

Cowboy Chords

"El payo" is harmonized with three chords: I (F), IV (B♭), and V_7 (C_7). These chords are built on the first, fourth, and fifth degrees of the F scale.

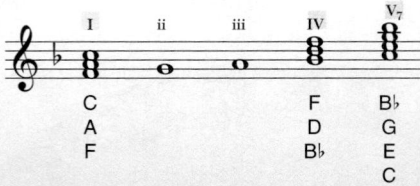

The I, IV, and V_7 chords appear above in **root position.** To **perform** *"El payo"* on the guitar, place a capo on fret 3 and play the chords D (I), G (IV), and A_7 (V_7).

> **Root position** is a chord in which the pitch called the root is the lowest note of the chord. For example, C is the root of a C chord.

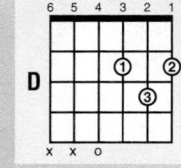
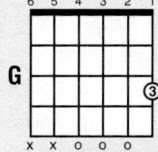
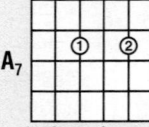

Footnotes

SKILLS REINFORCEMENT

▶ **Mallets** Students may enjoy learning to play the Orff accompaniment on Resource Book p. F-16 for *"El payo."* Have some students play the accompaniment while the class sings the song.

▶ **Recorder** Have some students practice and play the soprano recorder part on Resource Book p. I-14. Students may play the part as an accompaniment for *"El payo."*

BUILDING SKILLS THROUGH MUSIC

▶ **Math** Have students create a chart showing the chords that are built on each note of the F major scale. For each scale tone, have them tabulate in how many chords the scale tone is played.

SKILLS REINFORCEMENT

▶ **Guitar** Challenge your students to accompany *"El payo"* on guitar, using one of the following rhythms. (Arrows indicate the direction of the strum.)

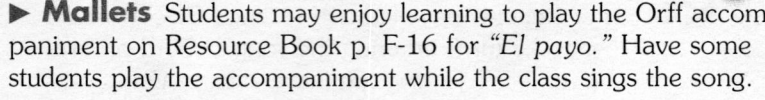

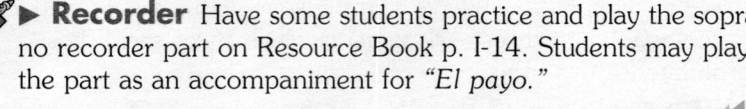

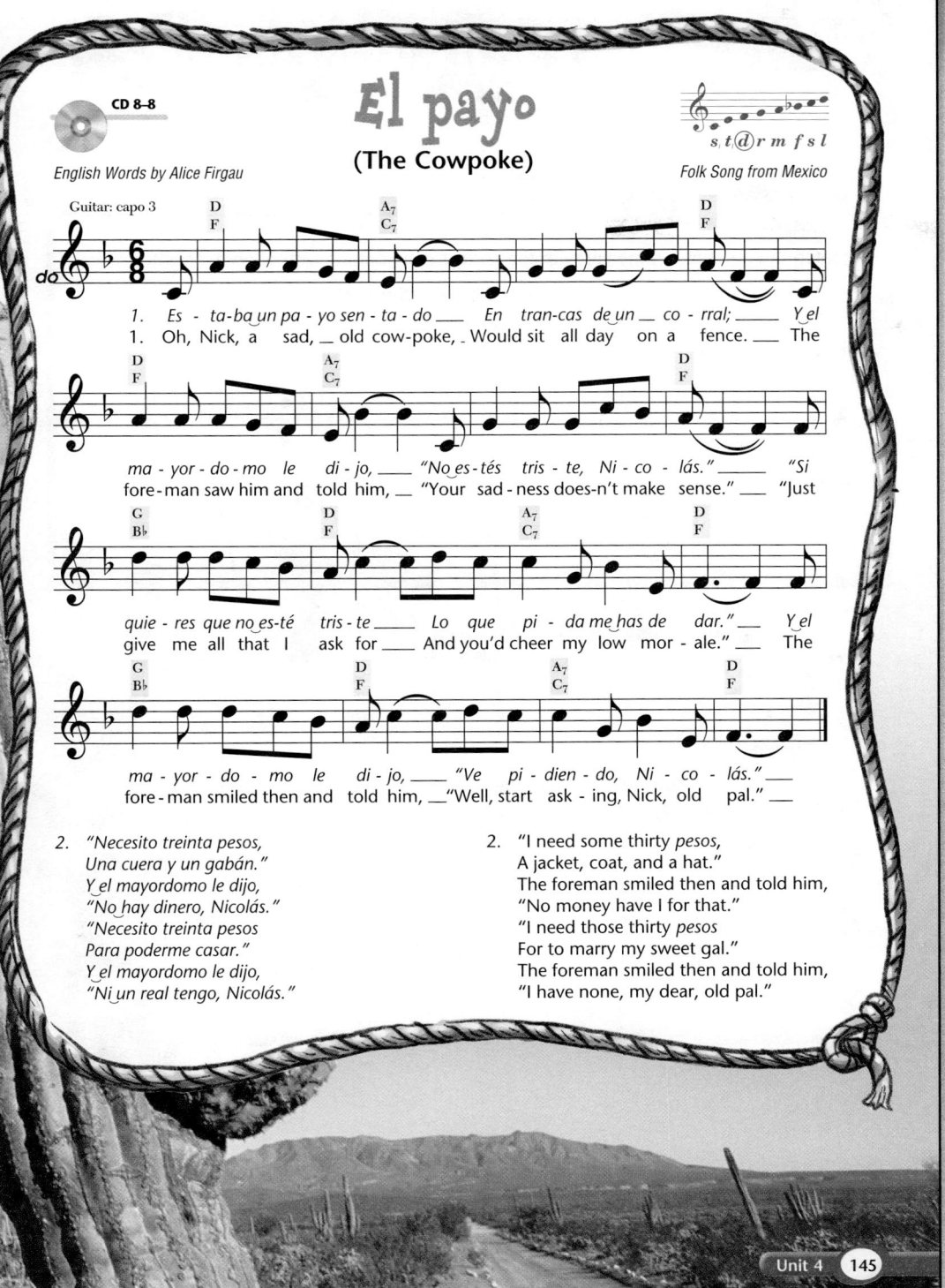

CD 8-8

El payo
(The Cowpoke)

English Words by Alice Firgau

Folk Song from Mexico

s, t, d, r, m, f, s, l

Guitar: capo 3

1. Es - ta - ba_un pa - yo sen - ta - do ___ En tran - cas de_un ___ co - rral; ___ Y el
1. Oh, Nick, a sad, ___ old cow - poke, ___ Would sit all day on a fence. ___ The

ma - yor - do - mo le di - jo, ___ "No_es - tés tris - te, Ni - co - lás." ___ "Si
fore - man saw him and told him, ___ "Your sad - ness does - n't make sense." ___ "Just

quie - res que no_es - té tris - te ___ Lo que pi - da me_has de dar." ___ Y el
give me all that I ask for ___ And you'd cheer my low mor - ale." ___ The

ma - yor - do - mo le di - jo, ___ "Ve pi - dien - do, Ni - co - lás." ___
fore - man smiled then and told him, ___ "Well, start ask - ing, Nick, old pal." ___

2. "Necesito treinta pesos,
Una cuera y un gabán."
Y_el mayordomo le dijo,
"No_hay dinero, Nicolás."
"Necesito treinta pesos
Para poderme casar."
Y_el mayordomo le dijo,
"Ni_un real tengo, Nicolás."

2. "I need some thirty *pesos,*
A jacket, coat, and a hat."
The foreman smiled then and told him,
"No money have I for that."
"I need those thirty *pesos*
For to marry my sweet gal."
The foreman smiled then and told him,
"I have none, my dear, old pal."

Unit 4 **145**

2 DEVELOP

Singing

Invite students to listen to *"El payo"* CD 8-8.

ASK Did you feel six or two heavy beats per measure? (two)

Help students to

- Sing the song with the recording.
- Learn to sing the song in Spanish, using the Pronunciation Practice Guide on Resource Book p. A-12, and the Pronunciation Practice track **CD 8-11.**
- Sing the song, "The Cowpoke," in English **CD 8-9.**

Playing

Encourage students to

- Learn to play the F, B♭, and C₇ chords on keyboard, or D, G, and A₇ on guitar, with a capo at the third fret.
- Read the chord changes for *"El payo"* as they play two chords per measure.

- Sing and accompany the song with *"El payo"* **CD 8-8** and recognize the texture as homophonic.

Help students discover that

- Chords can be built on each degree of the scale.
- The chord takes its name from the degree of the scale on which it is built.

3 CLOSE

Skill: PLAYING **ASSESSMENT**

Performance/Observation Ask pairs of students to play a chord accompaniment to *"El payo"* on guitar or Autoharp, as the class sings the song in Spanish **CD 8-8.** Observe and assess their performance.

TEACHER TO TEACHER

▶ **Resonator Bells and Hand Chimes** Resonator bells or hand chimes may be substituted for or used with keyboards or guitars in this lesson. If using bells and chimes, assign a different student or group of students to play each note of a chord. Have students each play their bell on the appropriate chord. Divide the class into three groups.

Group 1: bells F (F and B♭ chord) and E (C chord)

Group 2: bells A (F chord) and B♭ (B♭ chord)

Group 3: bells C (F chord and C chord) and D (B♭ chord)

Invite students to sing chord tones on a neutral syllable while playing the bells. Then sing the chords as a vocal accompaniment. Finally, substitute the song's lyrics for the neutral syllable. They will be singing in homophonic style.

SCHOOL TO HOME CONNECTION

▶ **Interview and Report** Students will have learned from p. 144 that cowboys must often travel to do their work. Encourage students to interview an adult relative or friend who travels extensively for work. They may wish to report to the class on how that person copes with commuting to work or with trips away from family and friends.

TECHNOLOGY/MEDIA LINK

Web Site Go to *www.sfsuccessnet.com* to learn more about Mexican music. Ask students to describe the style of *mariachi* songs and the instruments used in *mariachi* bands.

WHAT DO YOU KNOW?

> **MATERIALS**
> • **Resource Book** p. B-14

Have students review the definitions and examples of meter on pp. 118–120 and 204–205. Then, have students answer the questions on p. 146, matching the correct definition or symbol to the notation from Resource Book, p. B-14. Have students read and answer the questions and check their answers with a partner.

WHAT DO YOU HEAR?

> **MATERIALS**
> • *What Do You Hear? 4A*   **CD 8-12 to CD 8-15**
> • *What Do You Hear? 4B*   **CD 8-16 to CD 8-19**
> • **Resource Book** pp. B-14, B-15

Review the lessons, listenings, and definitions of fugue (p. 128), round (p. 122), and canon (p. 124) with the class. Remind them that a song that tells a story, often with multiple verses, is called a ballad, or verse form. Have students listen to the selections on p. 146 *(What Do You Hear? 4A)* and ask students to identify the form that best describes the listening selection, using Resource Book p. B-14.

Review the lessons on timbre on pp. 136–139 and band ensembles. Remind students of the differences between a Dixieland band, a concert band, and a polka band. Ask students to listen to the selections on p. 147 *(What Do You Hear? 4B)* and identify the correct ensemble to the listening selection from Resource Book p. B-15.

What Do You Know?

Match the notation on the left with the correct definition or symbol on the right.

Notation	Definition/Symbol
1. 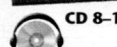	**a.** C
2. $\frac{4}{4}$	**b.** simple meter
3. $\frac{2}{2}$	**c.** compound meter
4.	**d.** ¢

What Do You Hear? 4A

CD 8–12

Form

Listen to the following selections. Identify the term in the right column that best describes the form of the selection.

Selection	Form
1. "Dance for the Nations"	**a.** verse form (ballad form)
2. *Canon for Violin and Cello*	**b.** fugue
3. "Barb'ry Allen"	**c.** round
4. "Little" Organ Fugue in G Minor	**d.** canon

146

Footnotes

ANSWER KEY

▶ **What Do You Know?**

1. b. simple meter
2. a. C
3. d. ¢
4. c. compound meter

▶ **What Do You Hear? 4A**

1. c. round
2. d. canon
3. a. verse form (ballad form)
4. b. fugue

▶ **What Do You Hear? 4B**

1. b. concert band
2. b. concert band
3. a. big band
4. c. polka band

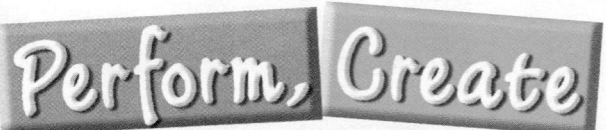

Perform, Create

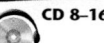

What Do You Hear? 4B

CD 8–16

Timbre

Listen to the timbre of these selections and match each with the correct musical ensemble.

Selection
1. *Suite No. 2 in F*
2. *The Stars and Stripes Forever*
3. *"Alexander's Ragtime Band"*
4. *Kerenski*

Musical Ensemble
a. big band
b. concert band
c. polka band

What You Can Do

Sing with Expression

As a class, sing "Swanee," page 118, with the recording. Follow the notation and conduct a two-beat pattern. Then sing the song without the recording at a slow tempo and again at a fast tempo. Point to the correct Italian terms below for "slow" and "fast."

• *moderato* • *adagio* • *prestissimo* • *allegro*

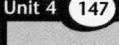

Sing Sequences

Sing the melody of "Alleluia," page 133. Perform small steady-beat movements as you sing. Point to the melodic sequence in the second line of the music. Is this sequence ascending or descending?

Play Chords

Play the D and A chords on guitar or keyboard. Sing "Give a Little Love," page 140, with the recording. Add harmony by playing the accompaniment part on guitar or keyboard with the recording. Play the chords accurately and in time with the song.

Unit 4 147

WHAT YOU CAN DO

MATERIALS	
• "Swanee," p. 118	**CD 7-3**
• "Alleluia," p. 123	**CD 7-30**
• "Give a Little Love," p. 140	**CD 8-5**
• **Resource Book** pp. B-15, J-7	
• guitar, keyboard	

Sing with Expression

Review with students the definitions and lesson on tempo markings on p. 114. Tell students that they will sing the song "Swanee" with different tempos. Ask students to sing with the recording **CD 7-3** while they conduct. Ask students to point to the correct Italian term for *slow (adagio)* and *fast (allegro).* Assess students on their ability to perform the tempo changes indicated on p. 147.

Sing Sequences

Review melodic sequences on pp. 132–133. Invite students to sing "Alleluia" **CD 7-30** on p. 133 as they perform steady-beat movements. Have students point out and identify the melodic sequences in the piece. Ask them if the sequence in the second line is ascending or descending. (descending)

Play Chords

Review with students the chords for guitar and keyboard to "Give a Little Love" on pp. 140–143. Have students practice the A_7 and D chords on their choice of instrument. Ask students to play a guitar or keyboard accompaniment to "Give a Little Love" **CD 8-5** with the recording.

Crossword Puzzle

Invite students to fill out a crossword puzzle worksheet found on Resource Book p. J-7. The vocabulary used in this puzzle is a review of Units 1 through 4.

▶ **What You Can Do**

Sing with Expression

slow = *adagio*

fast = *allegro*

Sing Sequences

The melodic sequence in the second line of *"Alleluia"* is descending.

TECHNOLOGY/MEDIA LINK

▶ **Rubrics**

Visit *www.sfsuccessnet.com* for rubrics to assess students' achievement in music skills.

Lesson	Elements	Skills	
LESSON 1 **CORE** **Speed Up/Slow Down** pp. 152–155 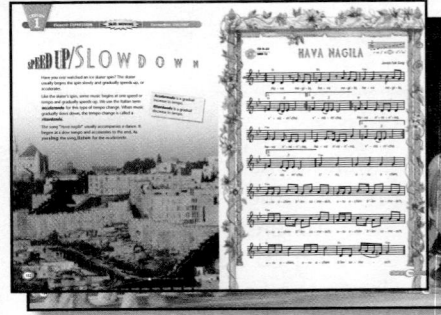	**Element: Expression** **Concept:** Tempo **Focus:** Changing tempos **Secondary Element** Form: aabbcc **National Standards** 1c 1e 2c 4c 5c 5d 6a	**Skill: Moving** **Objective:** Perform a folk dance that includes an *accelerando* **Secondary Skills** • **Listening** Listen for changes in tempo and for *accelerando;* listen for *ritardando* • **Singing** Sing in tempo and with an *accelerando;* sing Hebrew lyrics	**SKILLS REINFORCEMENT** • **Recorder** Play a melody on recorder • **Creating** Create a percussion composition that incorporates changing tempos
LESSON 2 **CORE** **Syncopated Rhythms** pp. 156–157 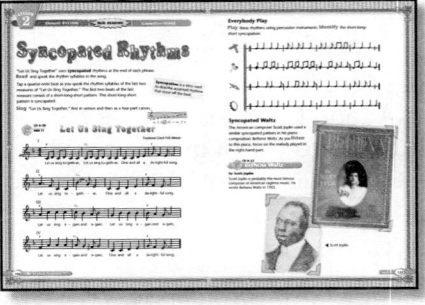 Reading Sequence 17, p. 496	**Element: Rhythm** **Concept:** Pattern **Focus:** Syncopation **Secondary Element** Form: canon **National Standards** 5a 6c 9a	**Skill: Reading** **Objective:** Read from notation that includes syncopation **Secondary Skills** • **Reading** Locate "short-long-short" rhythms in a score • **Singing** Sing parts of a song with pitch syllables, then lyrics • **Listening** Compare syncopated patterns	**SKILLS REINFORCEMENT** • **Recorder** Practice a downward leap and learn a countermelody on recorder • **Listening** Compare syncopated patterns; perform an ostinato with a recording
LESSON 3 **Double the Speed** pp. 158–159 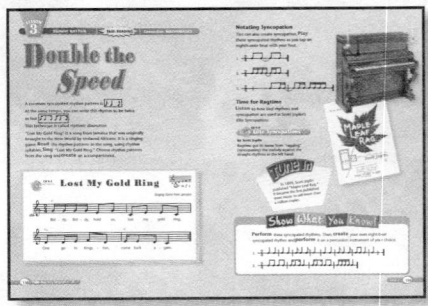 Reading Sequence 18, p. 496	**Element: Rhythm** **Concept:** Pattern **Focus:** Syncopation **Secondary Element** Tonality: tonal center **National Standards** 1c 5a 5c 6b	**Skill: Reading** **Objective:** Read from notation that includes syncopation **Secondary Skills** • **Singing** Sing a song with pitch syllables, then lyrics • **Listening** Listen to a selection for syncopation • **Creating** Create an accompaniment from the rhythms in a song	**SKILLS REINFORCEMENT** • **Playing** Play an Orff accompaniment to a song

Connections

Music and Other Literature

Connection: Culture

Activity: Explore Jewish culture with the *hora*

ACROSS THE CURRICULUM   **Social Studies** Read a book on Israel

SPOTLIGHT ON
The Hora Facts about this Israeli dance
The Conductor Facts on Zubin Mehta

CULTURAL CONNECTION   **Jewish Americans** Jewish migration to America

MOVEMENT   **Pattern Dance** Learn the *hora*

BUILDING SKILLS THROUGH MUSIC   **Language** Determine the purpose of an author

Song *"Hava nagila"*

Listening Selection "The Great Gate of Kiev" from *Pictures at an Exhibition*

M·U·S·I·C M·A·K·E·R·S
Zubin Mehta

More Music Choices
"At the Same Time," p. 115
"Don't Cry for Me, Argentina," p. 74

ASSESSMENT

Performance/Self Assessment Perform pattern dance movements that include an *accelerando* while singing

TECHNOLOGY/MEDIA LINK

Sequencing Software Manipulate the tempo of song

Connection: Genre

Activity: Explore the role of ragtime in the history of jazz

SPOTLIGHT ON   **Ragtime** Facts about ragtime

BUILDING SKILLS THROUGH MUSIC   **Social Studies** Create a timeline

Song "Let Us Sing Together"

Listening Selection
Bethena Waltz

More Music Choices
"Give My Regards to Broadway," p. 39
"Ain't Gonna Let Nobody Turn Me 'Round," p. 85
"Hava nagila," p. 153

ASSESSMENT

Performance/Observation Read and sing a song with syncopation; read and play a percussion ensemble piece with syncopation

TECHNOLOGY/MEDIA LINK

MIDI/Sequencing Software Use vocal tracks to help learn the parts of a song

---

Connection: Mathematics

Activity: Explain how rhythmic duration can be changed by a factor of 2

TEACHER TO TEACHER   **String Game** Play a game to reinforce steady beat

ACROSS THE CURRICULUM
Social Studies Research Jamaica
Mathematics Create a rhythm pattern

BUILDING SKILLS THROUGH MUSIC   **Reading** Discuss a history article

Song "Lost My Gold Ring"

Listening Selection
Elite Syncopations

More Music Choices
"A Brand New Day," p. 7
"The Rhythm is Gonna Get You," p. 348

ASSESSMENT

Performance/Observation Read and play a percussion part with syncopation

TECHNOLOGY/MEDIA LINK

Video Library View a steel drum ensemble in *Steel Drums*

Lesson	Elements	Skills	
LESSON 4 **CORE** **Theme and Variations** pp. 160–161 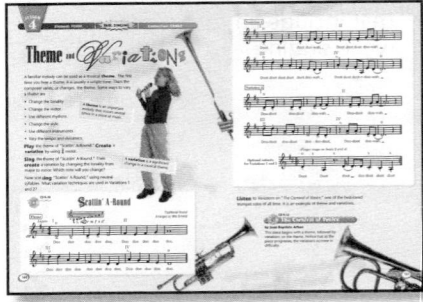	**Element: Form** **Concept:** Form **Focus:** Theme and variations **Secondary Element** Expression: legato and staccato **National Standards** 1a 1d 4c 6a 6c	**Skill: Singing** **Objective:** Sing a theme and variations **Secondary Skills** • **Listening** Listen to and identify variations within a theme-and-variation form	**SKILLS REINFORCEMENT** • **Guitar** Play a guitar accompaniment using two chords
LESSON 5 **American Variations** pp. 162–163 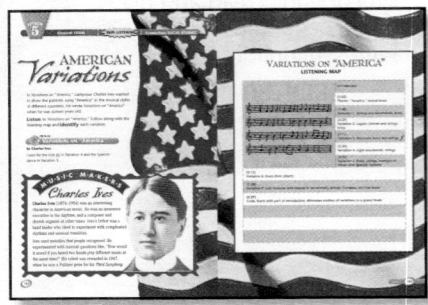	**Element: Form** **Concept:** Form **Focus:** Theme and variations **Secondary Element** Melody: ornamentation **National Standards** 1a 4c 6a 6b 8b	**Skill: Listening** **Objective:** Follow theme-and-variation form on a listening map **Secondary Skills** • **Singing** Sing a well-known theme from a theme and variations • **Listening** Listen to a theme and variations and discuss the cultures and styles that are represented	**SKILLS REINFORCEMENT** • **Creating** Create variations on a familiar theme and discuss how themes are varied
LESSON 6 **Melodic Distances** pp. 164–165 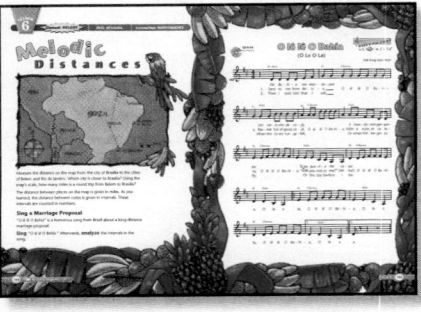 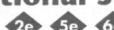 Reading Sequence 19, p. 497	**Element: Melody** **Concept:** Pitch and direction **Focus:** Half and Whole Steps **Secondary Element** Form: solo-chorus antiphonal response **National Standards** 1b 2e 5e 6a	**Skill: Reading** **Objective:** Identify half and whole steps when reading a song from notation **Secondary Skills** • **Analyzing** Identify pitch movement of different voice parts in a song • **Reading** Identify all intervals in a major scale using a tone ladder • **Singing** Sing various intervals using pitch syllables	**SKILLS REINFORCEMENT** • **Playing** Play rhythmic ostinatos as an accompaniment • **Mallets** Play an Orff accompaniment • **Reading** Read intervals in major and minor scales using a worksheet

Connections

Music and Other Literature

Connection: Genre
Activity: Identify theme-and-variation form in two different genres

TEACHER TO TEACHER
Singing in Tune Singing major thirds in tune
Singing Legato and Staccato Focus on *legato* and *staccato* articulations
Breathing Develop longer breath control

CULTURAL CONNECTION **Scat Singers** Background on scat singing and Louis Armstrong

BUILDING SKILLS THROUGH MUSIC **Writing** Describe variations

Song "Scattin' A-Round"

Listening Selection
Variations on "The Carnival Venice" (excerpt)

More Music Choices
"Let Us Sing Together," p. 156
"Lost My Gold Ring," p. 158
"Gloria, Gloria," p. 459

ASSESSMENT

Performance/Observation
Sing a song while showing theme and variation using body percussion

TECHNOLOGY/MEDIA LINK
CD-ROM Use *Band-in-a-Box* to create background accompaniments disabilities play

---

Connection: Social Studies
Activity: Explore immigration and our multicultural society as presented in a musical work

ACROSS THE CURRICULUM **Social Studies** Read a book on immigration to the United States

SPOTLIGHT ON **"America"** Facts on the origin of the song "America"

CHARACTER EDUCATION **Character Traits** Discuss the character traits valued by a free society

BUILDING SKILLS THROUGH MUSIC **Writing** Elaborate on text

Song *Variations on "America"*

Listening Map
Variations on "America"
M·U·S·I·C M·A·K·E·R·S
Charles Ives

More Music Choices
"Scattin' A-Round," p. 160
Variations on "The Carnival of Venice," p. 161

ASSESSMENT

Observation Listen to variations of a song and point them out on a listening map

TECHNOLOGY/MEDIA LINK
Transparency Follow a listening map of a theme and variations

---

Connection: Mathematics
Activity: Compare measurements of distance and measurement in music

TEACHER TO TEACHER **Listening** Teach students to listen to and identify intervals of a second and fourth

CULTURAL CONNECTION **Bahía, Brazil** Facts on this culturally diverse Brazilian state

BUILDING SKILLS THROUGH MUSIC **Math Obj. 4/Math** Convert miles to kilometers

Songs
"O lê lê O Bahía"
"O Le O La"

More Music Choices
"Vive l'amour," p. 176
"Everybody Loves Saturday Night," p. 296

ASSESSMENT

Performance/Observation
Use pitch syllables and hand signs to read and sing a song

TECHNOLOGY/MEDIA LINK
CD-ROM Use a CD-ROM for more practice with intervals

Lesson	Elements	Skills	

LESSON 7

CORE
Distance = Intervals
pp. 166–167

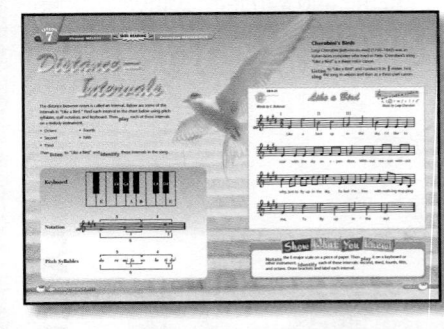

Reading Sequence 20, p. 497

Element: Melody
Concept: Intervals
Focus: Melodic intervals

Secondary Element
Form: canon

National Standards
4c 5a 5b 5c 5d

Skill: Reading
Objective: Read, identify, and sing intervals

Secondary Skills
• **Reading** Identify major, minor, and perfect intervals
• **Singing** Sing a song with pitch syllables and hand signs, then with the lyrics, then as a three-part canon

SKILLS REINFORCEMENT
• **Reading** Use a card game to improve skills with intervals

---

LESSON 8

Rows of Tones
pp. 168–169

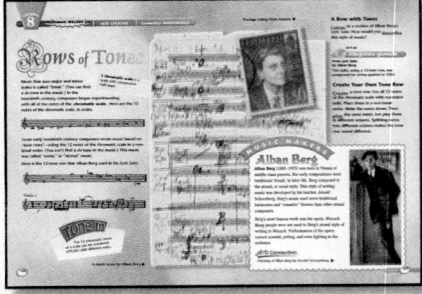

Element: Melody
Concept: Pattern
Focus: 12-tone melodies

Secondary Element
Timbre: string quartet

National Standards
4c 6a 6b 8b

Skill: Creating
Objective: Create and notate 12-tone row and its retrograde

Secondary Skills
• **Playing** Play a chromatic scale and a tone row
• **Listening** Listen to a contemporary music selection that uses a tone row
• **Creating** Create a 12-tone melody

SKILLS REINFORCEMENT
• **Creating** Create a six-note tone row and experiment with inversions and retrogrades

---

LESSON 9

CORE
Different Cultures and Timbres
pp. 170–171

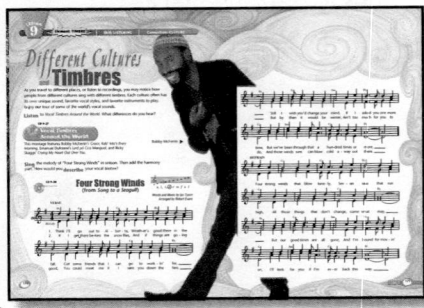

Element: Timbre
Concept: Vocal
Focus: Vocal timbres

Secondary Element
Texture/Harmony: two-part harmony in thirds and sixths

National Standards
1d 4b 6b 7a

Skill: Listening
Objective: Describe vocal timbres common to different cultures

Secondary Skills
• **Singing** Sing a song in two-part harmony using pitch syllables
• **Playing** Play an accompaniment on guitar using G, C, and D₇ chords

SKILLS REINFORCEMENT
• **Vocal Development** Help students to sing in sixths
• **Recorder** Learn a harmony part for a song
• **Guitar** Learn to an accompaniment in groups

Connections

Music and Other Literature

Connection: Mathematics

Activity: Measure the distance between intervals by naming the interval

ACROSS THE CURRICULUM ▶ **Language Arts** Discuss birds as symbols of freedom; read a book about this imagery

MEETING INDIVIDUAL NEEDS ▶ **Including Everyone** Create tone rows to practice working with intervals

BUILDING SKILLS THROUGH MUSIC ▶ **Language** Identify the mood of lyrics

---

Song "Like a Bird"

More Music Choices
"Bury Me Not on the Lone Prairie," p. 19
"Down in the Valley," p. 375
"My Dear Companion," p. 23

ASSESSMENT

Performance/Observation
Read, sing, and identify melodic intervals

TECHNOLOGY/MEDIA LINK

Notation Software
Create and transpose a melody

Connection: Mathematics

Activity: Discuss the applications of mathematics in the composition of serial music

SPOTLIGHT ON ▶ **The Composer** Facts on Arnold Schoenberg

ACROSS THE CURRICULUM ▶ **Math** Discuss permutations of a 12-tone row

BUILDING SKILLS THROUGH MUSIC ▶ **Language** Speculate about the reception of a composer in his day

---

Listening Selection
"Allegretto giovale" from *Lyric Suite*
M·U·S·I·C M·A·K·E·R·S
Alban Berg

More Music Choices
"Finale" from *Serenade for Strings in C,* Op. 48, p. 363
"Summer" from *Concerto No. 2,* p. 102

ASSESSMENT

Written Assessment
Create and notate a six-tone row and write its retrograde

TECHNOLOGY/MEDIA LINK

Notation Software
Notate a six-tone row and experiment with inversions and retrogrades

---

Connection: Culture

Activity: Discuss the ways in which preferences for the arts, food, and customs may vary among cultures

CULTURAL CONNECTION ▶ **Comparing Cultural Preferences** Insights on cultural preferences

ACROSS THE CURRICULUM ▶ **Language Arts** Share a book with poems about the wind

BUILDING SKILLS THROUGH MUSIC ▶ **Writing** Write a paragraph about vocal styles

---

Song "Four Strong Winds" from *Song to a Seagull*

Listening Selection
Vocal Timbres Around the World (montage)

Poem "The Wind"

More Music Choices
"Vive l'amour," p. 176
"Run! Run! Hide!" p. 340

ASSESSMENT

Music Journal Writing
Listen to vocal timbres and write descriptions of them

TECHNOLOGY/MEDIA LINK

Notation Software
Create an arrangement of a song

Lesson	Elements	Skills

LESSON 10

CORE

Spanish Textures

pp. 172–175

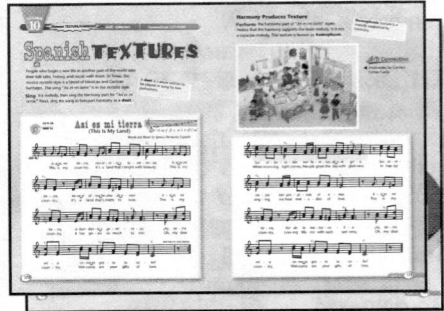

Element: Texture/Harmony

Concept: Harmony and texture

Focus: Harmony in thirds, homophonic texture

Secondary Element
Form: aaba

National Standards
1a 1c 1d 2a 3a 6b 9b

Skill: Singing

Objective: Sing two songs with harmony in thirds

Secondary Skills
- **Singing** Sing a song in two parts
- **Analyzing** Analyze the harmony, intervals of parallel thirds, and homophonic texture in a Hispanic song
- **Playing** Create an accompaniment for a Hispanic song
- **Improvising** Create an improvisation to accompany a Hispanic song

SKILLS REINFORCEMENT
- **Playing** Learn a rhythmic ostinato to accompany a song
- **Keyboard** Play a rhythmic ostinato accompaniment to a song
- **Percussion** Perform a two-measure ostinato as an accompaniment

---

LESSON 11

Steps to Harmony

pp. 176–179

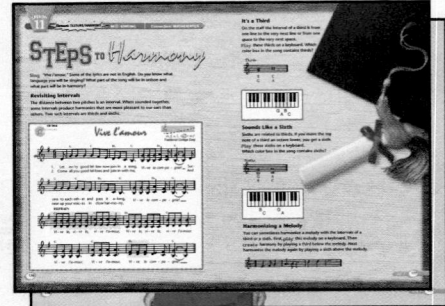
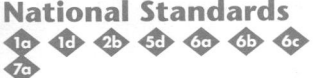

Element: Texture/Harmony

Concept: Harmony

Focus: Intervals

Secondary Element
Texture: homophonic

National Standards
1a 1d 2b 5d 6a 6b 6c 7a

Skill: Singing

Objective: Sing a two-part song in thirds and sixths

Secondary Skills
- **Analyzing** Analyze intervals of a sixth in a song
- **Singing** Sing a song in two part harmony with a recording
- **Playing** Play a melody on bells or keyboard, then harmonize the melody using sixths

SKILLS REINFORCEMENT
- **Guitar** Play a three-chord accompaniment using the G, C, and D$_7$ chords on guitar
- **Vocal Development** Discuss vibrato and good breath support while singing

---

LESSON 12

Calypso Textures

pp. 180–183

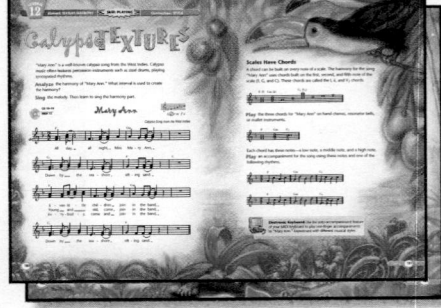

Element: Texture/Harmony

Concept: Chordal accompaniment

Focus: Chordal accompaniment

Secondary Element
Rhythm: rhythm patterns

National Standards
1d 2b 2c 4c

Skill: Playing

Objective: Play a chordal accompaniment while singing a song

Secondary Skills
- **Singing** Sing a song in calypso style
- **Analyzing** Analyze chords used in a song
- **Playing** Perform an accompaniment on bells or chimes
- **Moving** Perform movements to song in calypso style

SKILLS REINFORCEMENT
- **Vocal Development** Techniques for singing in thirds
- **Recorder** Play a recorder duet that accompanies a song

Connections

Connection: Culture

Activity: Discover folk traditions of Latin American, and their influence on American music

CULTURAL CONNECTION
Música Norteña Discuss this Mexican and German stylistic blend
Music of Puerto Rico Background on Puerto Rican tradition in music

ACROSS THE CURRICULUM
Language Arts Read a book about the pioneer spirit
Social Studies Learn about Puerto Rico

TEACHER TO TEACHER **Degrees of Bodily Movement** Tell students that learning to dance is a gradual process

MOVEMENT **Nonlocomotor Movement** Associate movements with different chords in a song

BUILDING SKILLS THROUGH MUSIC **Social Studies** Research communities of mixed cultures

Connection: Mathematics

Activity: Use counting to find intervals of a sixth and a third

CULTURAL CONNECTION **French Culture** Facts on French culture

TEACHER TO TEACHER
Changing Voices Assist boys with changing voices
Singing Harmony Sing parallel sixths with success
Listening Learn to listen to music without notation or listening map

AUDIENCE ETIQUETTE **Audience Etiquette and Participation** Contrast etiquette for a performance of a college song at a public place and an opera or pop concert

SPOTLIGHT ON **Requiems** Background on *Pie Jesu* and the requiem mass

BUILDING SKILLS THROUGH MUSIC **Language** Identify the purpose of a writing

Connection: Style

Activity: Discuss calypso style and its origins in the West Indies

TEACHER TO TEACHER
Percussion Instruments Use professional instruments
Playing Chords Have student groups play chords on resonator bells
Modeling an Instrumental Part Demonstrate how to hold and play a an instrument to make it easier for students to learn

CULTURAL CONNECTION **Foods of the Caribbean** Facts on island foods

ACROSS THE CURRICULUM **Language Arts** Share a collection of poems from Jamaica

BUILDING SKILLS THROUGH MUSIC **Language** Make inferences and support conclusions through textual evidence

Music and Other Literature

Songs
"*Así es mi tierra*" ("This Is My Land")
"*Habemos llegado*" ("We Have Arrived")

More Music Choices
"*Las mañanitas,*" p. 481
"Abraham, Martin, and John," p. 466

Song "*Vive l'amour*"

Listening Selections
"Pie Jesu" from *Requiem*
"Pie Jesu" from *Requiem* (Church) (excerpt)
Listening Map
Pie Jesu
M·U·S·I·C M·A·K·E·R·S
   Charlotte Church

More Music Choices
"Four Strong Winds," p. 170
"Abraham, Martin, and John," p. 466
"*Fais do do,*" p. 403

Song "Mary Ann"

More Music Choices
"Evening Chaconne," p. 202
"Give a Little Love," p. 140
"Water Come a Me Eye," p. 300
"By the Waters of Babylon," p. 311

ASSESSMENT
Performance/Observation
Sing a song in two parts and indicate when singing parallel thirds

TECHNOLOGY/MEDIA LINK
CD-ROM Explore Latin American styles using *Band-in-a-Box*
Electronic Keyboard Explore styles using the auto-accompaniment function

---

ASSESSMENT
Performance/Observation
Sing a song with harmony in thirds and sixths in tune

TECHNOLOGY/MEDIA LINK
Notation Software Harmonize a melody using thirds and sixths
Web Site Find out more about Andrew Lloyd Webber
Transparency Display listening map for *Pie Jesu*

ASSESSMENT
Performance/Observation
Perform chordal accompaniment to a song

TECHNOLOGY/MEDIA LINK
Web Site Explore the music and instruments of the Caribbean
MIDI/Sequencing Software Create mallet and percussion textures
Electronic Keyboard Play a Caribbean-style accompaniment using auto-accompaniment

INTRODUCING THE UNIT

Discovering New Musical Horizons is important in the development of music appreciation by students. Exposure to new and exciting styles (scat singing, calypso), cultures (Puerto Rican, Israeli, Czech), and musical eras (60s folk-rock, 12-tone modernism) will open the door to a wider world of music. Unit highlights are listed in the footnotes and a brief overview of the skills assessed in this unit can be found on p. 149. Students will enjoy discovering new musical horizons.

UNIT PROJECT

Discuss with students how musical styles combine with other styles to create new styles. Tell students to follow the process below in analyzing how new styles are created.

- Begin with a simple song like *"Frère Jacques."*

  ASK What would it take to perform this song in styles such as classical, rock, jazz, or country? (appropriate instruments, appropriate vocal timbre, stylistic performance techniques on notes, such as bends, glissando, trills, and so on, and modified rhythms)
- Challenge students to take this song (or another) and perform it in a new style.
- Analyze Lesson 4, which treats the song "Row, Row, Row Your Boat" as a set of jazz variations.
- Ask students to find examples of songs that artists or groups have set in a new style. Jazz is a style that often transforms songs originally created in other styles. Have them bring recordings to class to share with others.

  Have students look for songs with many different recordings. Recording web sites offer a quick reference service for finding multiple recordings.
- Have students share their findings with the class.

Play a Song for Me

The 1960s was a decade of social and political change, and popular music experienced a transformation of its own. As the Beatles and other British groups stormed the U.S., America answered with poet/songwriter Bob Dylan and groups like the Byrds.

Listen to this recording of the Byrds singing Dylan's *Mr. Tambourine Man.*

Then turn the page and **sing** your own rendition of the song.

CD 8–20
Mr. Tambourine Man

by Bob Dylan
as performed by the Byrds
The Byrds' unique folk-rock style features distinctive harmonies and a 12-string Rickenbacker guitar sound.

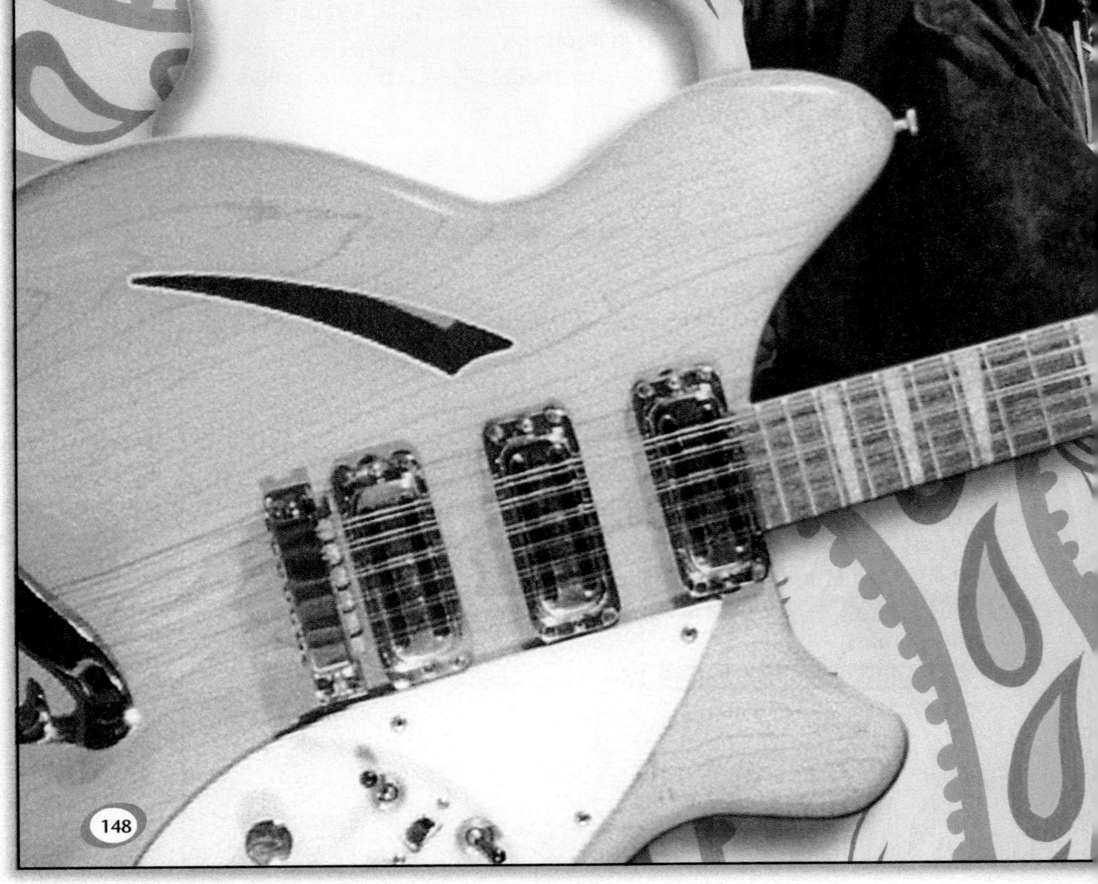

148

ACROSS THE CURRICULUM

Unit Highlights The following interdisciplinary activities in this unit are related to the music elements presented in the lessons and are intended to enhance student learning. For a more detailed topical description, see the Unit at a Glance on pp. 147a–147h.

▶ **LANGUAGE ARTS**

- Discuss birds as symbols of freedom (p. 166)
- Read a poem about the wind (p. 170)
- Read a book about the pioneer spirit (p. 172)
- Share poems from Jamaica (p. 182)

▶ **MATH**

- Create a diminution of a rhythm and determine the mathematical factor by which the apparent tempo changed (p. 159)
- Learn about the number of permutations of a 12-tone row (p. 169)

▶ **SOCIAL STUDIES**

- Share a book with information on Israel (p. 152)
- Locate Jamaica on a map and research its history (p. 159)
- Dramatize scenes in a book about immigration to America (p. 162)
- Learn facts about Puerto Rico (p. 172)

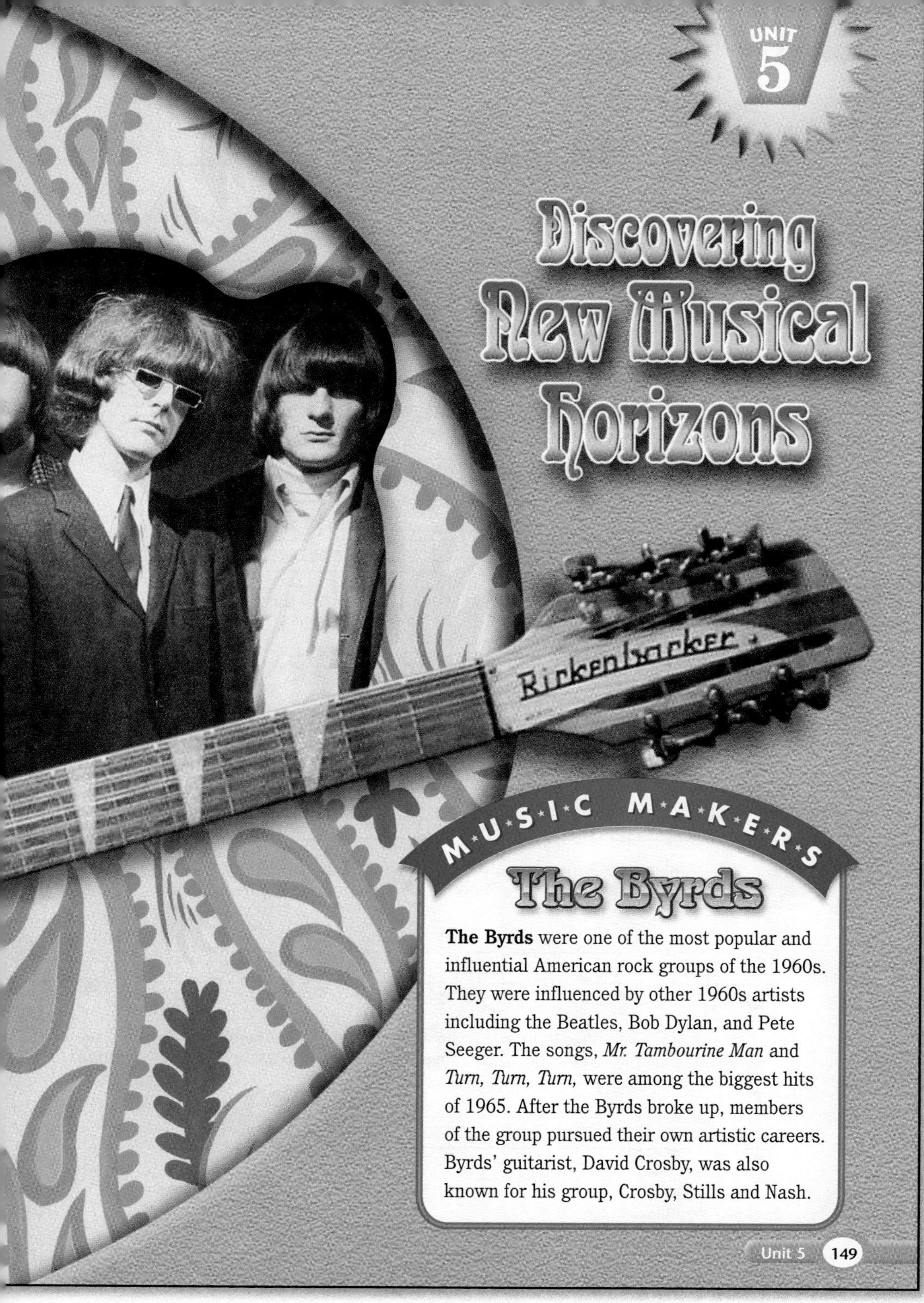

UNIT 5

Discovering New Musical Horizons

M·U·S·I·C M·A·K·E·R·S
The Byrds

The Byrds were one of the most popular and influential American rock groups of the 1960s. They were influenced by other 1960s artists including the Beatles, Bob Dylan, and Pete Seeger. The songs, *Mr. Tambourine Man* and *Turn, Turn, Turn,* were among the biggest hits of 1965. After the Byrds broke up, members of the group pursued their own artistic careers. Byrds' guitarist, David Crosby, was also known for his group, Crosby, Stills and Nash.

Unit 5 149

MUSIC SKILLS
ASSESSED IN THIS UNIT

Reading Music: Rhythm

- Read and perform syncopated rhythms in a percussion ensemble (p. 157)
- Read and perform the syncopated rhythms in "Lost My Gold Ring" (p. 159)

Reading Music: Pitch

- Read and sing whole steps and half steps using pitch syllables (p. 165)
- Read, sing, and identify the intervals in the E-major scale (p. 167)

Performing Music: Singing

- Sing the variations of the song "Scattin' A-Round" (p. 161)
- Sing a melody and harmony part in homophonic texture (p. 175)
- SIng a song in two parts with intervals of thirds and sixths (p. 179)

Performing Music: Playing

- Play a rhythm accompaniment as they sing a calypso song (p. 183)

Listening to Music

- Listen to and identify the variations in *Variations on "America"* (p. 163)
- Listen to *Vocal Timbres Around the World* and describe the vocal timbres (p. 171)

Moving to Music

- Perform movements to the *hora* (p. 155)

Creating Music

- Create a tone row, notate it and write its retrograde (p. 169)

CULTURAL CONNECTION

Unit Highlights The musical literature in this unit provides many opportunities for students to explore a variety of world cultures. A more detailed description of the resources and activities listed below can be found in the Unit at a Glance on pp. 147a–147h.

▶ CARIBBEAN

- Learn about the music of Puerto Rico (p. 175)
- Learn about and discuss the foods of the Caribbean (p. 181)

▶ SOUTH AMERICA

- Discover information about Bahía, Brazil (p. 164)

▶ UNITED STATES

- Learn about the Jewish migration to the United States (p. 153)
- Discover facts about Louis Armstrong and scat singing (p. 161)
- Learn and compare cultural preferences from cultures around the world (p. 170)
- Find the roots of the *música norteña* style (p. 172)

OPENING ACTIVITIES

MATERIALS

- "Mr. Tambourine Man" **CD 8-21**

  Recording Routine: Intro (9 m.); vocal; coda

- *Mr. Tambourine Man* **CD 8-20**

- guitars, Autoharps, keyboards, drums, tambourines, or other percussion

Listening

Have students read the Music Makers feature on The Byrds. Discuss the term *folk-rock* as an example of a hybrid combination of folk and rock. Listen to the recording of Mr. Tambourine Man **CD 8–20** by The Byrds.

ASK What aspects of the recording contribute to the "rock" part of the style? (electric guitars, drum set)

Reading

Ask students to look for the following in the music:

- Lyrics. Bob Dylan is as much a poet as a songwriter and performer. Discuss with students the meaning of the lyrics of the verse.
- Key signature and *do* (C major; *do* = C).

  ASK Why does the song sound incomplete at the bottom of the page? (ends on the dominant chord and the note D)

  ASK How does the *D.C. al Fine* to the refrain give the song a more satisfying ending? (ends on the tonic note and chord)

- Syncopations. Ask students to find measures with off-beat syncopations in them.

Singing

Ask students to listen to the song "Mr. Tambourine Man" **CD 8–21.** Then, have them sing the song with the recording.

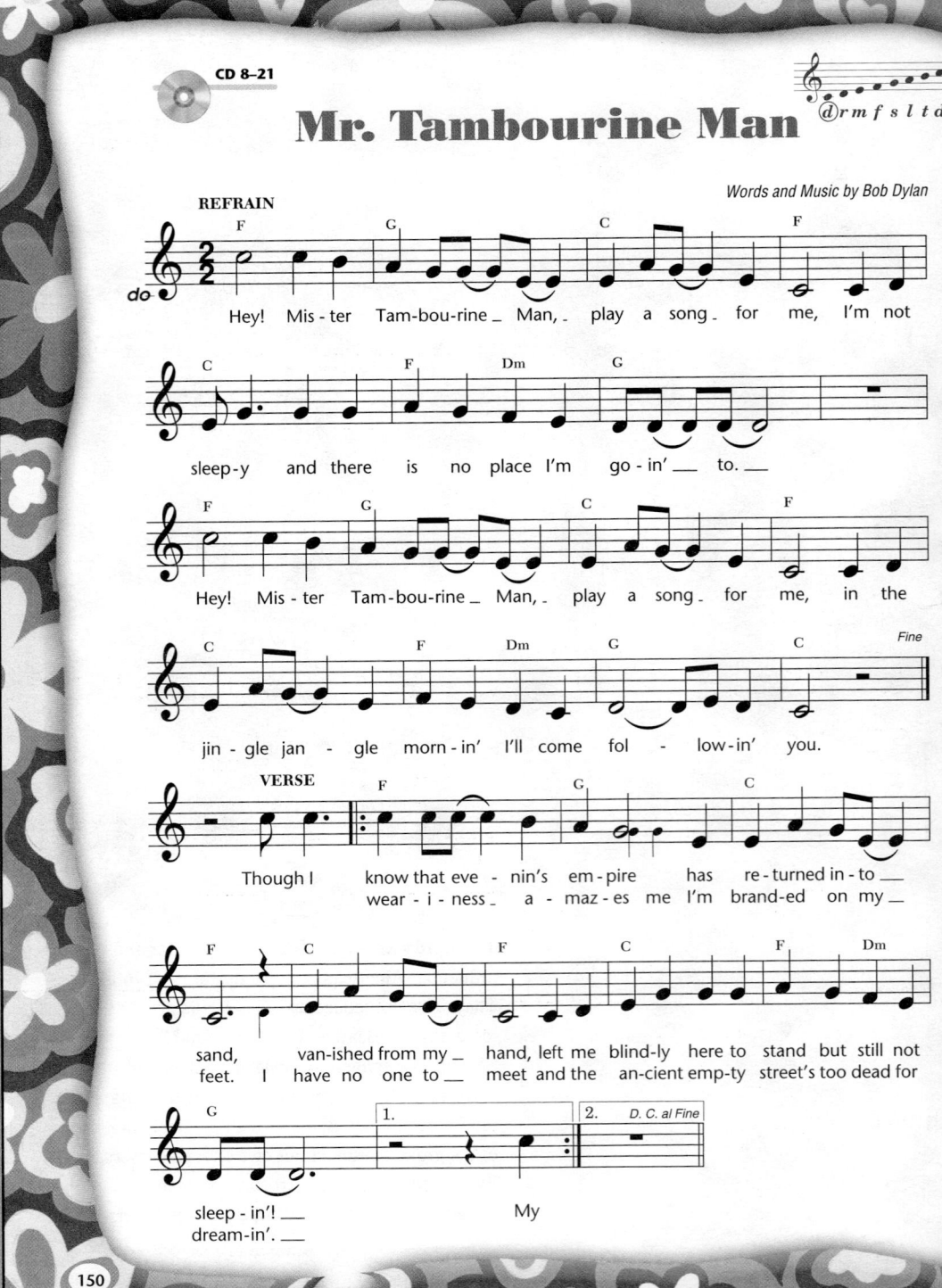

Mr. Tambourine Man

Words and Music by Bob Dylan

150

(ASSESSMENT banner)

Unit Highlights This unit includes a variety of strategies and methods, described below, to track students' progress and assess their understanding of lesson objectives. Reproducible masters for Show What You Know! and Review, Assess, Perform, Create can be found in the Resource Book.

▶ **FORMAL ASSESSMENTS**

The following assessments, using written language, cognitive, and performance skills, help teachers and students conceptualize the learning that is taking place.

- **Show What You Know!** Element-specific assessments, on the student page, for Rhythm (p. 159) and Melody (p. 167)
- **Review, Assess, Perform, Create** This end-of-unit activity (pp. 184–185) can be used for review and to assess students' learning of the core lessons in this unit.

▶ **INFORMAL ASSESSMENTS**

At the close of each Teacher's Edition lesson in this unit, one of the following types of assessments is used to evaluate the learning of the key element focus or skill objective.

- Music Journal Writing (p. 171)
- Observation (p. 163)
- Performance/Observation (pp. 157, 159, 161, 165, 167, 175, 179, 183)
- Performance/Self Assessment (p. 155)
- Written Assessment (p. 169)

▶ **RUBRICS**

Visit *www.sfsuccessnet.com* for rubrics to assess students' achievement in music skills.

Tune In

Bob Dylan had mega-hits of his own in the 1960s. His song *Like a Rolling Stone* (1965) is a classic of the folk-rock genre.

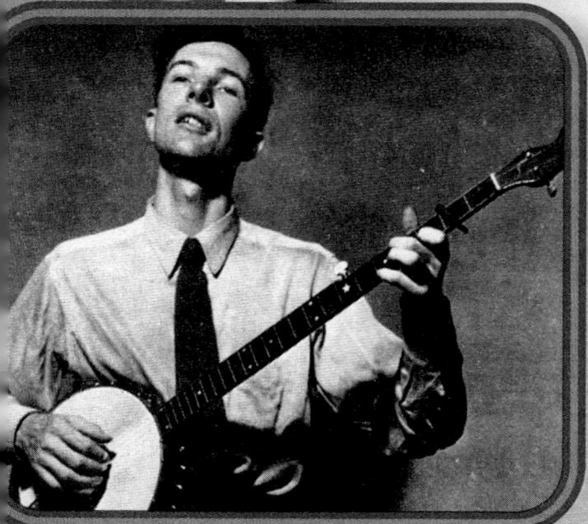

▲ Pete Seeger

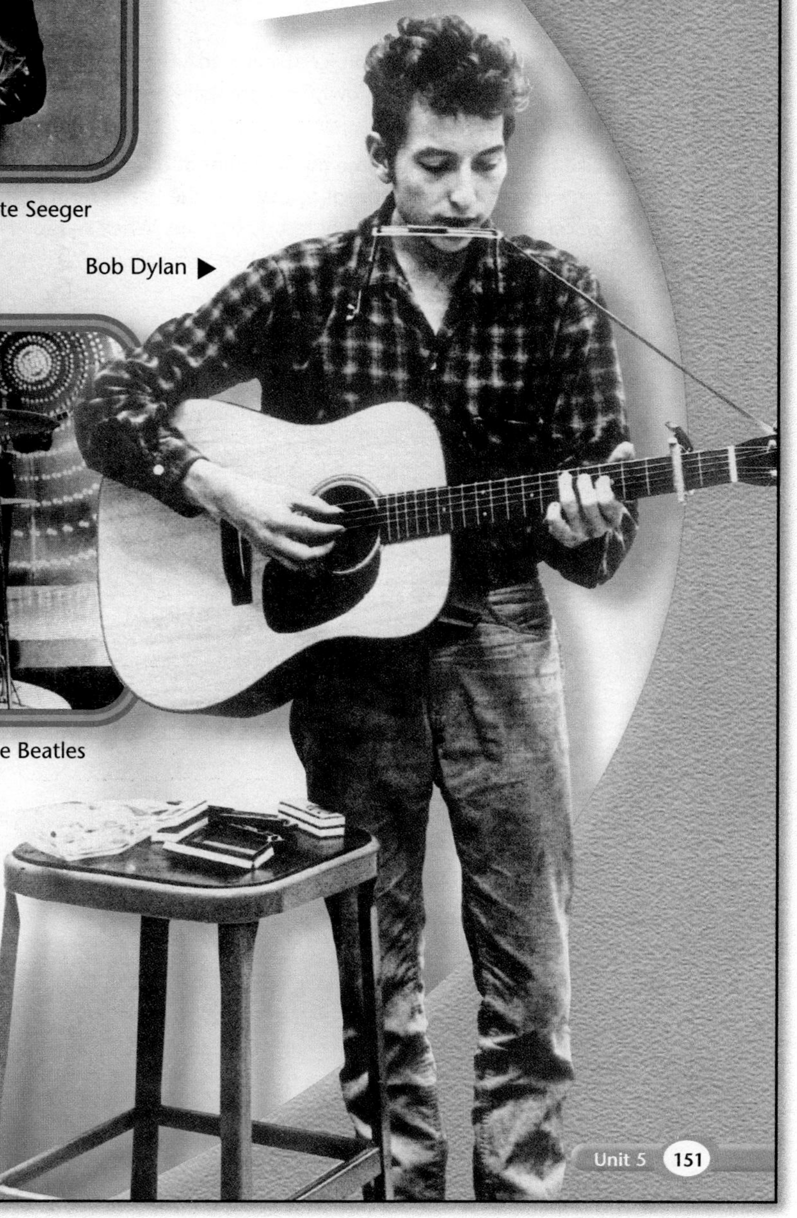

Bob Dylan ▶

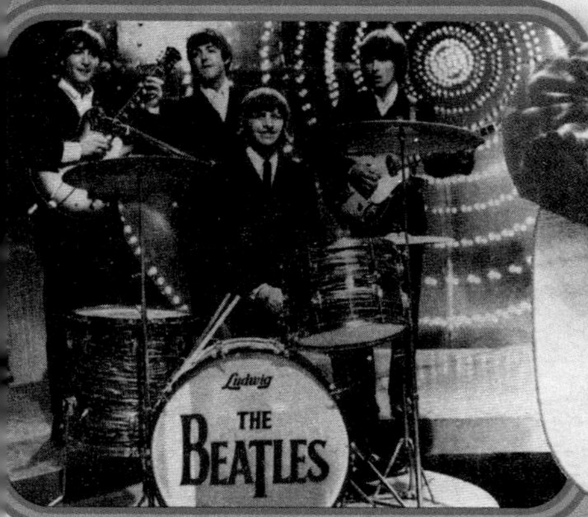

▲ The Beatles

When they know the melody to the refrain, have them sing the melody with very straight, unsyncopated rhythms.

ASK How do the syncopations bring the song to life? (They give the song a syncopated style common to pop or rock.)

Playing

Invite students to play the chords to this song on guitar, Autoharp, or keyboard.

Guitars may find it easier to play with a capo at fret 5, using the following chord substitutes:

Printed Chords		Capo Chords
C	=	G
F	=	C
G	=	D
Dm	=	Am

Add drums, tambourine, or other percussion to fill out the accompaniment.

INNOVATIVE TEACHER SUPPORT FOR THIS UNIT

- **MAKING MUSIC DVD, Grade 6** contains video segments that support lessons, including signing and movement.
- **MAKING MUSIC with Movement and Dance** provides more opportunities for large group activities in music or physical education classes.
- **MAKING MUSIC with Technology** provides lesson plans for many technology applications; includes MIDI files.
- **¡A cantar!** features recorded songs and lessons from around the Spanish-speaking world; includes strategies for bilingual classes and for English-speaking teachers working with Spanish-speaking students.
- **Bridges to Asia** features recorded songs and lessons from Asian and Pacific region cultures.
- **www.sfsuccessnet.com** provides an online lesson planner to conveniently create lesson plans at school or at home. Includes rubrics for assessment, lesson modifications to meet the needs of all students, performance musicals based on program content, and more.

Unit 5　151

TECHNOLOGY/MEDIA LINK

Unit Highlights The following components are used in this unit to reinforce and expand students' understanding of music elements and related themes.

▶ **CD-ROM**
- Use *Band-in-a-Box* to create an accompaniment (p. 161)
- Use *Alfred's Essentials of Music Theory* to practice intervals (p. 165)
- Use *Band-in-a-Box* to explore Latin musical styles (p. 175)

▶ **ELECTRONIC KEYBOARD**
- Use auto-accompaniments (p. 175 and p. 183)

▶ **MIDI/SEQUENCING SOFTWARE**
- Use a MIDI song file to learn the vocal parts to a song (p. 157)
- Create a percussion accompaniment for a MIDI file (p. 183)

▶ **NOTATION SOFTWARE**
- Create a melody (p. 167) and a tone row (p. 169)
- Use notation software to create an arrangement (p. 171)
- Notate a melody and harmonize it in thirds and sixths (p. 179)

▶ **SEQUENCING SOFTWARE**
- Enter a song melody and experiment with tempo (p. 155)

▶ **TRANSPARENCY**
- Display the listening maps (p. 163 and p. 179)

▶ **VIDEO LIBRARY**
- Show the video *Steel Drums* (p. 159)

▶ **WEB SITE**
- Learn more information about Andrew Lloyd Webber (p. 179)
- Explore the music and instruments of the Caribbean (p. 183)

LESSON AT A GLANCE

Element Focus   **EXPRESSION** Changing tempos

Skill Objective   **MOVING** Perform a folk dance that includes an *accelerando*

Connection Activity   **CULTURE** Explore Jewish culture with the *hora*

MATERIALS

- *"Hava nagila"*   **CD 8-23**

  Recording Routine: Intro (2 m.); vocal; interlude (2 m.); vocal
- **Pronunciation Practice/Translation** p. 520
- *"The Great Gate of Kiev"* from *Pictures at an Exhibition*   **CD 8-27**
- **Dance Directions** for *"Hava nagila"* p. 557
- **Resource Book** pp. A-14, I-15

VOCABULARY

accelerando   *ritardando*

> ◆ ◆ ◆ ◆ **National Standards** ◆ ◆ ◆ ◆
>
> **1c** Sing music from diverse cultures
> **1e** In groups, sing moderately easy pieces with expression
> **2c** Perform instrumental music from diverse cultures
> **4c** Compose, using traditional sound sources
> **5c** Define standard notation symbols for tempo and dynamics
> **5d** Use standard notation to record musical ideas
> **6a** Listen and describe events in music, using appropriate terms

MORE MUSIC CHOICES

For more practice with changing tempos:

"At the Same Time," p. 115

"Don't Cry for Me, Argentina," p. 74

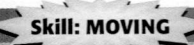

sPEED UP/SLOW DOWN

Have you ever watched an ice skater spin? The skater usually begins the spin slowly and gradually speeds up, or accelerates.

Like the skater's spin, some music begins at one speed or tempo and gradually speeds up. We use the Italian term **accelerando** for this type of tempo change. When music gradually slows down, the tempo change is called a **ritardando**.

The song "Hava nagila" usually accompanies a dance. It begins at a slow tempo and accelerates to the end. As you **sing** the song, **listen** for the *accelerando*.

> **Accelerando** is a gradual increase in tempo.
>
> **Ritardando** is a gradual decrease in tempo.

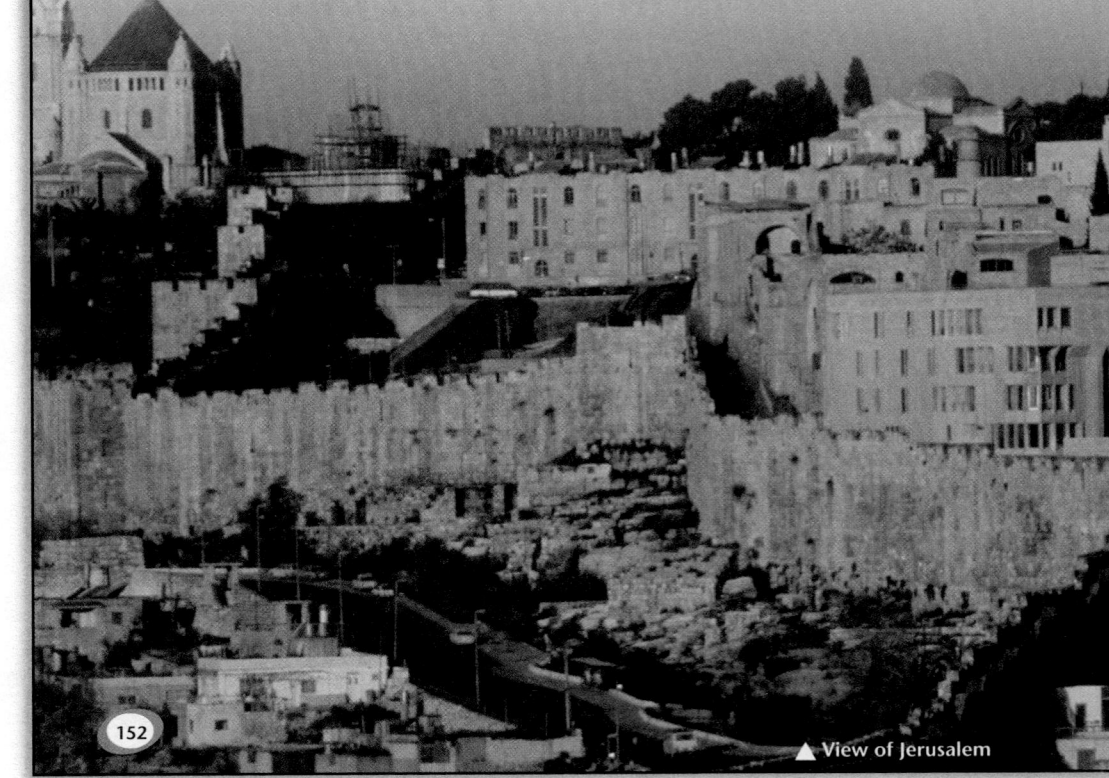

▲ View of Jerusalem

152

Footnotes

ACROSS THE CURRICULUM

▶ **Social Studies** Share the book *Israel* by Jose Patterson (Raintree/Steck Vaughn, 1997). Assign groups of students to each of the categories discussed in the book. (landscape, climate, natural resources, population, industry, laws) Have each group give an oral presentation, with visuals, on the aspect of Israel it has selected.

BUILDING SKILLS THROUGH MUSIC

▶ **Language** After reading the Music Maker on Zubin Mehta on p. 155, ask students to determine the author's purpose. Is it to entertain, to persuade, to inform, or to express? Have them show what in the writing led to their answer.

SKILLS REINFORCEMENT

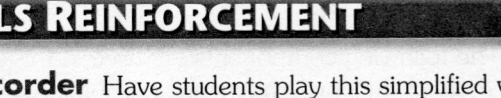

▶ **Recorder** Have students play this simplified version of the last section of the melody for *"Hava nagila"* (beginning m. 11).

2c This melody will give students additional practice playing B♭ on the soprano recorder. Have them practice the melody slowly, and then play it with the recording **CD 8-23**. For a recorder challenge using *"Hava nagila,"* see Resource Book p. I-15.

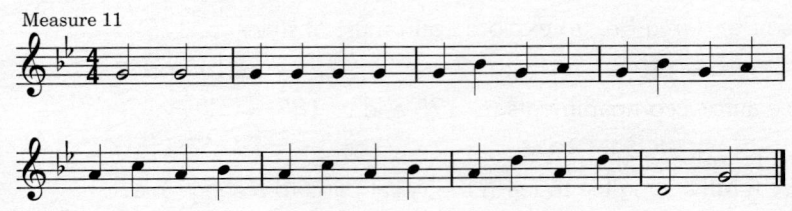

Measure 11

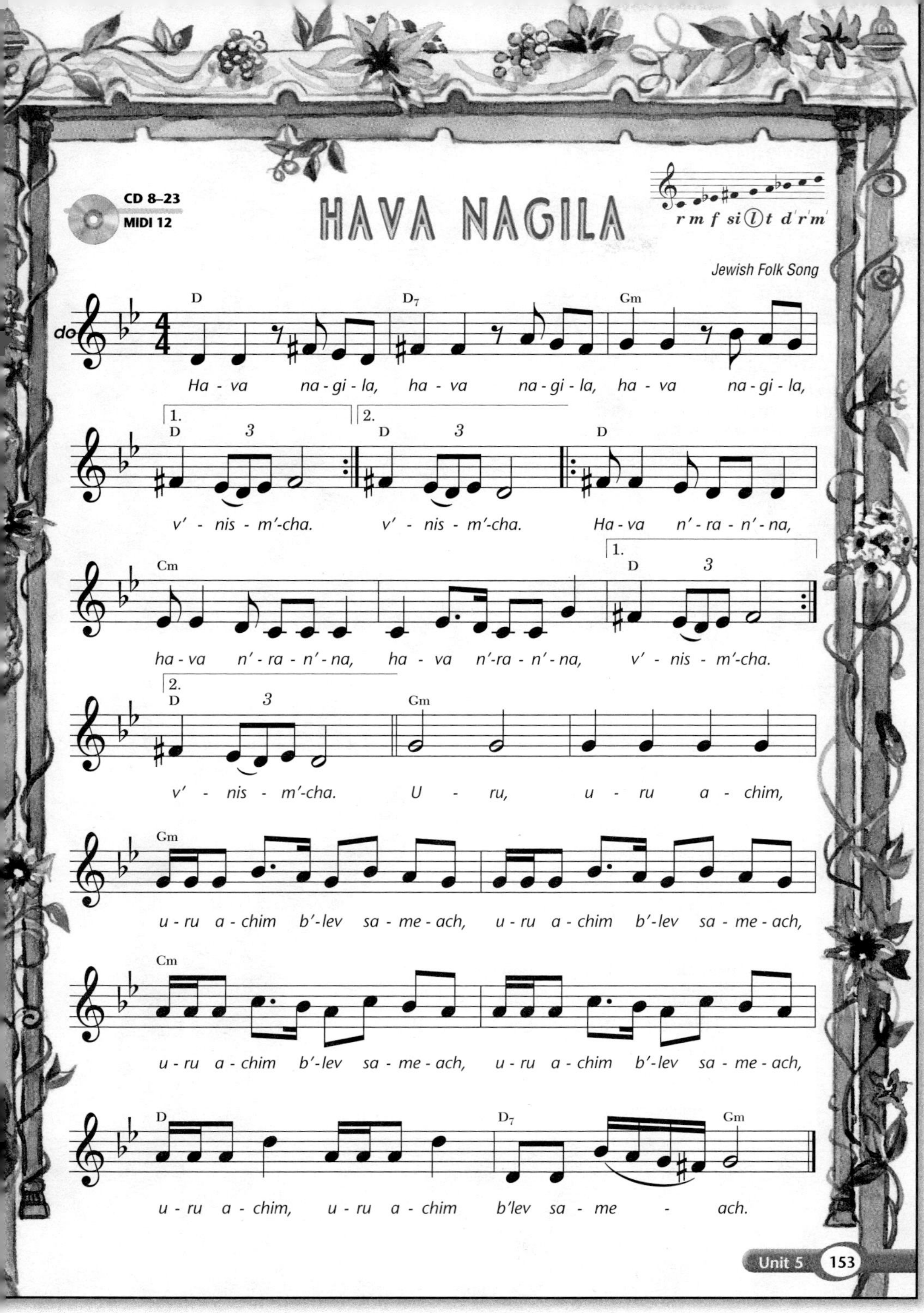

HAVA NAGILA

CD 8–23
MIDI 12

r m f si ⓛ t d′ r′ m′

Jewish Folk Song

Ha - va na - gi - la, ha - va na - gi - la, ha - va na - gi - la,

v' - nis - m'-cha. v' - nis - m'-cha. Ha - va n' - ra - n' - na,

ha - va n' - ra - n' - na, ha - va n' - ra - n' - na, v' - nis - m' - cha.

v' - nis - m'-cha. U - ru, u - ru a - chim,

u - ru a - chim b'-lev sa - me - ach, u - ru a - chim b'-lev sa - me - ach,

u - ru a - chim b'-lev sa - me - ach, u - ru a - chim b'-lev sa - me - ach,

u - ru a - chim, u - ru a - chim b'lev sa - me - ach.

Unit 5 153

---

1 INTRODUCE

Invite students to imagine going for a ride on a bicycle, in a car, or on a train. Help students recognize that they would

- Begin slowly, and gradually increase in speed.
- Ride at a constant speed for a period of time.
- After a period of time, gradually slow down to a full stop.

ASK What is the musical term that indicates speed? *(tempo)*

2 DEVELOP

Listening

6a Encourage students to lightly tap the steady beat as they listen to *"Hava nagila"* **CD 8-23.**

ASK Did the tempo remain steady throughout? (No, it became faster.)

Did the tempo change suddenly or gradually? (gradually)

5c SAY The musical term for "gradually getting faster" is *accelerando.*

ASK When did the *accelerando* begin? (after the interlude, at the beginning of the last section)

Singing

1c Encourage students to learn the Hebrew text for *"Hava nagila."* Have students

- Use Resource Book p. A-14 and look at the phonetics guide as they listen to the Pronunciation Practice **CD 8-25.**
- Sing the Hebrew phrases, modeling the speaker.
- Sing *"Hava nagila"* **CD 8–23,** performing expressively, from notation, a varied repertoire of music representing styles from diverse cultures.

continued on page 154

SPOTLIGHT ON

▶ **The *Hora*** The *hora* is one of many European circle dances that began in ancient times and is still performed today. *Hora* means "circle," which is the formation for the dance. Imported to Israel from the Balkans, the Israeli hora has neither social importance nor specific festive significance. Instead, it is an expression of happiness and is performed on many occasions. The dance is usually performed to the well-known song *"Hava nagila."* It is frequently danced at weddings, *bar* and *bat mitzvahs,* and festive occasions associated with religious holidays. *Bar mitzvahs* (for boys) and *bat mitzvahs* (for girls) are the ceremonies that mark the passage of young teenagers of the Jewish faith into adulthood.

CULTURAL CONNECTION

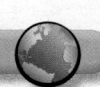

▶ **Jewish Americans** Many Jewish people in America can trace their ancestors to Russia, Eastern Europe, Germany, Western Europe, and Israel. Jewish migration to the United States has been continuous since the first group of 23 Jews arrived in New York (then New Amsterdam) in 1654. Successive migrations brought Spanish-speaking Jews (Sephardim) and Jews from the German-speaking areas of central Europe and Poland (Ashkenazim). Some twenty-first century Jewish Americans still speak the languages of their ancestors, including Hebrew, Yiddish, *Ladino,* Russian, Arabic, German, Hungarian, and Spanish. Despite their cultural diversity, Jewish Americans are united by their common faith and traditions.

Remind students that when performing *"Hava nagila,"* they should maintain a steady tempo until the last measure of line 2, when a very gradual *accelerando* begins and continues until the end. After the interlude, the song begins at the original tempo and accelerates the same way.

When interpretting how to perform an *accelerando,* remind students not to speed up too quickly or too much, or the song won't stay together.

Moving

Explain that *"Hava nagila"* is a popular song in Israel and with Jewish people all over the world. It is performed at many celebrations, including weddings, *bar mitzvahs,* and *bat mitzvahs.*

Share the information on Jewish American culture with students in Cultural Connection, p. 153.

Share with students the background information on the *hora* in Spotlight On, p. 153. More detailed information on performing the *hora* can be found in the Dance Directions on p. 557.

SAY The *hora* is danced in a closed circle with your hands holding your neighbors' hands at your side. The dance begins by moving to the left.

Encourage students to learn the dance steps for the *hora* by using the Dance Practice **CD 8-26** and following the directions on p. 155. This practice track is performed at a slower tempo to assist students in learning the dance steps.

After students know the movements, have them prepare for the last section of the dance by gradually increasing the speed of the steps.

Invite students to dance the *hora* using the song *"Hava nagila"* and the Dance Performance **CD 8-23.** Have students sing the song as they dance.

An Exhibition of Tempo

The job of the conductor is to lead a group of musicians in playing a piece of music. The conductor gives the music expression by telling the musicians how to play. One of the most famous conductors in the world is Zubin Mehta. He conducts the Israel Philharmonic Orchestra and makes guest appearances with many other orchestras around the world.

Listen to Zubin Mehta conduct an excerpt from Russian composer Mussorgsky's *The Great Gate of Kiev.* How does Mehta use tempo changes, such as *ritardandos,* to make the music more expressive?

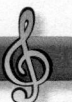
CD 8–27
The Great Gate of Kiev

**from *Pictures at an Exhibition*
by Modest Mussorgsky
as performed by Zubin Mehta and
the New York Philharmonic**
This selection features both tempo and meter changes.

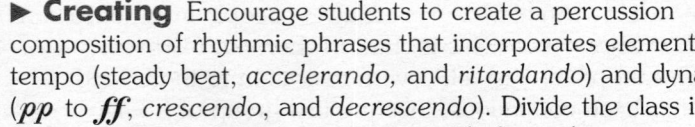

Zubin Mehta (born 1936) is known for his grandiose and intense conducting style. He is a world-class conductor. Born in the city of Mumbai (formerly Bombay), India, Mehta initially wanted to become a doctor; however, his father, who co-founded the Bombay Symphony Orchestra, encouraged his son to pursue music. At the age of eighteen, Mehta went to the famous Academy of Music in Vienna, Austria. Mehta has been the musical director in Montreal, Los Angeles, New York City, and Florence, Italy. Presently, he serves as the permanent Music Director for the Israel Philharmonic Orchestra.

154

Footnotes

SKILLS REINFORCEMENT

4c
5c
▶ **Creating** Encourage students to create a percussion composition of rhythmic phrases that incorporates elements of tempo (steady beat, *accelerando,* and *ritardando*) and dynamics (*pp* to *ff*, *crescendo,* and *decrescendo*). Divide the class into four groups. Have groups create an eight-beat phrase to use as an ostinato, using nonpitched instruments or body percussion. (Remind students to include both sound and silence.) Each group should perform their composition for the class.

MOVEMENT

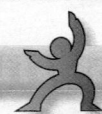

▶ **Pattern Dance** *"Hava nagila"* is a favorite song to which one can dance the *hora.* Learn more about the *hora* and its close relationship to the Arabic *debke* in the Dance Directions section on p. 557.

Perform these optional movements when the music accelerates.

Step 3: Jump on both feet.
Step 4: Kick right while hopping on left.
Step 5: Jump on both feet.
Step 6: Kick right while hopping on right.

Israeli Dance

"Hava nagila" is a favorite song for dancing the *hora*. The movements to *"Hava nagila"* can be performed at different tempos.

Perform the movements below. The traditional *hora* is danced moving to the left. The music begins slowly and gradually becomes faster.

1. Step Left

2. Step Right (in front or in back of Left)

3. Step Left

4. Lift Right

5. Step Right

6. Lift Left

▼ The *hora* is danced in a circle and uses steps and lifts. Dancers feel the energy increase as the music and dancing get faster and faster.

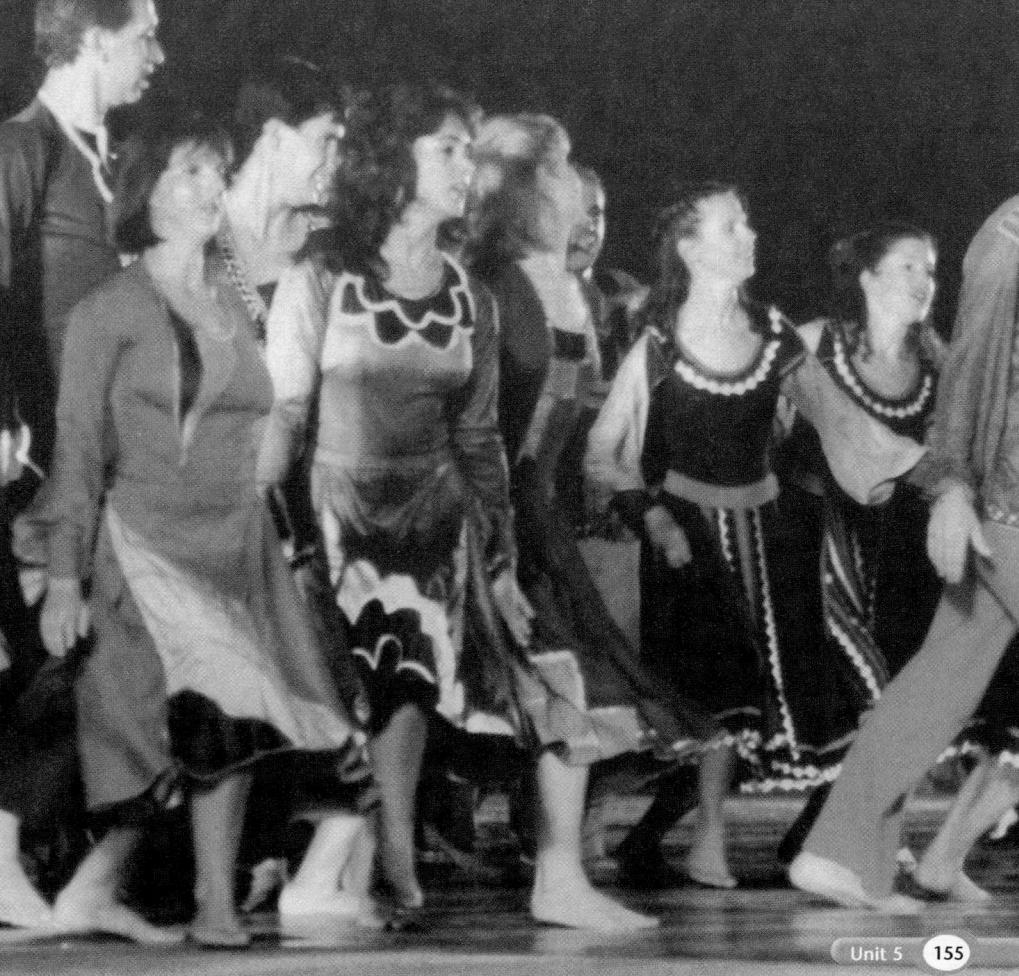

Unit 5 **155**

Listening

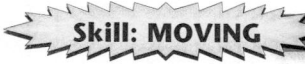 Ask students to listen to *The Great Gate of Kiev* **CD 8-27**. It is the final section of a larger piece entitled *Pictures at an Exhibition,* by Russian composer Modest Mussorgsky.

ASK In a piece with a large group of players, such as an orchestra, which person controls the tempo and decides at what rate the group should perform an *accelerando* or *ritardando?* (the conductor)

Introduce students to Zubin Mehta by sharing Spotlight On below. Then, guide them to hear the *ritardando* in Mehta's performance of *The Great Gate of Kiev.*

SAY As you listen to the selection again, conduct in meter in 4, and conduct following the tempo changes.

Encourage students to read the information about the role of the conductor in achieving expression and the Music Makers profile of Zubin Mehta. Invite students to discuss a career or vocation as a conductor.

3 CLOSE

Skill: MOVING   ASSESSMENT

Performance/Self-Assessment Have students perform the *hora* with *"Hava nagila"* **CD 8–23** as they sing the song. Ask students to identify criteria for evaluating their performance for both singing and movement (such as the following), and self-assess their performance.

- Did they perform the movement patterns correctly and remember the sequence of steps throughout the song?

- Did they maintain the steps through the *accelerando?*

- Were they able to sing with an expression of energetic spirit as they performed the movements?

SPOTLIGHT ON

▶ **The Conductor** Maestro Zubin Mehta and the Israeli Philharmonic have been partners in making music since 1968, when Mehta was made director of the Israeli Philharmonic. In 1981, Mehta's appointment as music director was extended for life. He has won many prestigous awards, including the Order of the Lotus from India and an honorary doctorate degree from Tel Aviv University.

Zubin Mehta is also an international conductor, serving as director of other major orchestras—New York, Montreal, Los Angeles, and recently, the Bavarian State Opera. Mehta is recognized for his interpretations of both romantic symphonic literature and opera.

TECHNOLOGY/MEDIA LINK

Sequencing Software Have students enter the melody for *"Hava nagila,"* then experiment with the tempo of the song, using *accelerando* and *ritardando.* Remind students that *"Hava nagila"* is usually performed while people are dancing, so abrupt starts and stops are not appropriate. Play some of the results for the class and discuss which versions are more successful, and why.

LESSON AT A GLANCE

Element Focus	**RHYTHM** Syncopation	
Skill Objective	**READING** Read from notation that includes syncopation	
Connection Activity	**GENRE** Explore the role of ragtime in the history of jazz	

MATERIALS

- "Let Us Sing Together" — **CD 8-28**
  Recording Routine: Intro (4 m.); vocal (unison); interlude (4 m.); vocal (4-part canon); coda
- *Music Reading Practice,* Sequence 17 — **CD 8-30**
- *Bethena Waltz* (excerpt) — **CD 8-33**
- **Resource Book** p. D-20, E-18
- rhythm sticks, wood block, drum

VOCABULARY

syncopation   ostinato   ragtime

◆ ◆ ◆ ◆   National Standards   ◆ ◆ ◆ ◆

5a Read half notes, quarter notes, eighth notes, and dotted notes in duple meter

6c Understand and use basic principles of rhythm in music analysis

9a Describe characteristics of music genres from a variety of cultures

MORE MUSIC CHOICES

For more practice singing songs with syncopated rhythms:

"Give My Regards to Broadway," p. 39

"Ain't Gonna Let Nobody Turn Me 'Round," p. 85

"Hava nagila," p. 153

1 INTRODUCE

Explore with students how ragtime bridged minstrel tunes and jazz, by sharing Spotlight On below.

Syncopated Rhythms

"Let Us Sing Together" uses **syncopated** rhythms at the end of each phrase. **Read** and speak the rhythm syllables in the song.

Tap a quarter-note beat as you speak the rhythm syllables of the last two measures of "Let Us Sing Together." The first two beats of the last measure consist of a short-long-short pattern. This short-long-short pattern is syncopated.

> **Syncopation** is a term to describe accented rh that occur off the beat.

Sing "Let Us Sing Together," first in unison and then as a four-part canon.

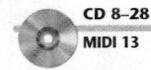
s, l, t (d) di r m f s

CD 8–28
MIDI 13

Let Us Sing Together

Traditional Czech Folk Melody

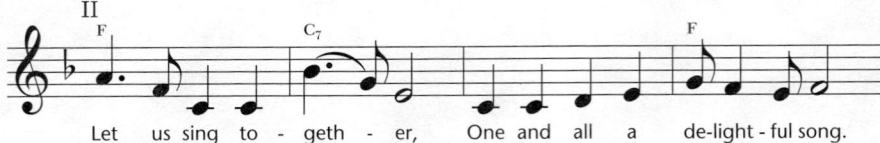
Let us sing to-geth-er,   Let us sing to-geth-er,   One and all a   de-light-ful song.

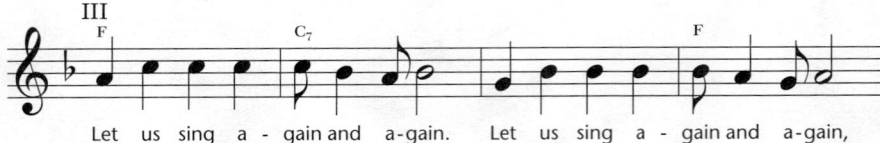
Let   us sing to - geth - er,   One and all a   de-light - ful song.

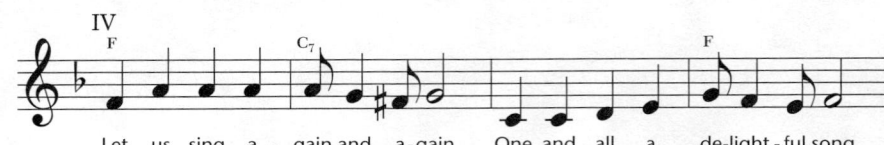
Let   us sing a - gain and a-gain.   Let   us sing a - gain and a-gain,

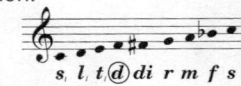
Let   us sing a - gain and a-gain,   One and all a   de-light - ful song.

Footnotes

SKILLS REINFORCEMENT

▶ **Recorder** Invite students to review the fingering for the downward leap from F to middle C on soprano recorder. When they are ready, have students play this accompaniment with "Let Us Sing Together."

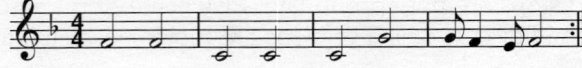

BUILDING SKILLS THROUGH MUSIC

▶ **Social Studies** Have students use the information presented in the Spotlight On, p. 156, to create a time line of the events and musical styles from ragtime through jazz.

SPOTLIGHT ON

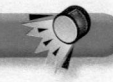

9a ▶ **Ragtime** Arising from camp meetings and minstrel tunes such as "Turkey in the Straw," an exciting new musical form was developed by Missouri pianists during the 1890s. Often played by people who could not read notation, the music had syncopated rhythms and dissonant, contrapuntal effects. When this nameless new form was played at the 1893 Chicago World's Fair, visitors were thrilled by its jubilant sound. (Scott Joplin attended the fair.) By 1897, probably because of its "ragged rhythms," the style was dubbed "ragtime." Around the 1910s, a virtuosic form of ragtime was developed in New York's Harlem. It was called "stride." This style had an expanded rhythmic language, a wider range, a "stride bass," and faster tempos. Stride was the forerunner of jazz; and by the 1920s, many ragtime musicians, such as Jelly Roll Morton, simply called themselves jazz musicians.

Everybody Play

Play these rhythms using percussion instruments. **Identify** the short-long-short syncopation.

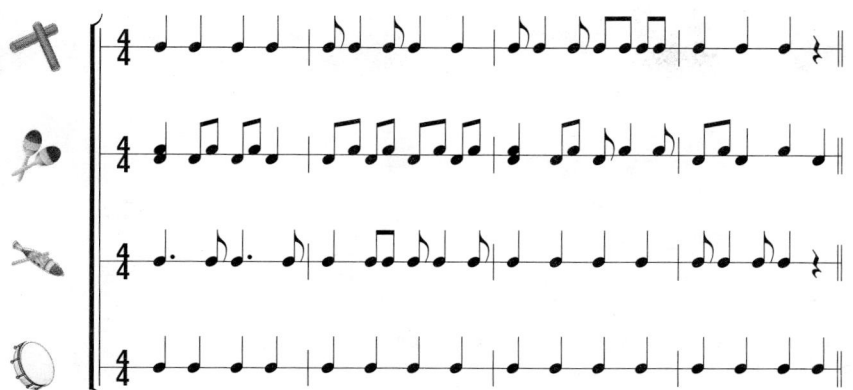

Syncopated Waltz

The American composer Scott Joplin used a similar syncopated pattern in his piano composition *Bethena Waltz*. As you **listen** to this piece, focus on the melody played in the right-hand part.

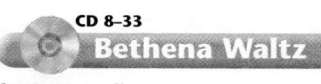

CD 8–33
Bethena Waltz

by Scott Joplin

Scott Joplin is probably the most famous composer of American ragtime music. He wrote *Bethena Waltz* in 1905.

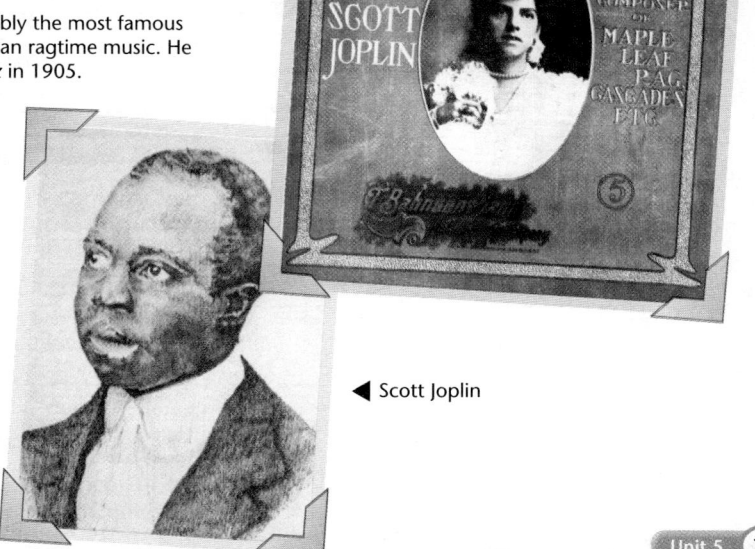

 Scott Joplin

---

2 DEVELOP

Reading

5a Direct students' attention to the notation of "Let Us Sing Together." Ask them to find a "short-long-short" rhythm pattern *(ti-ta-ti)* in the song, and to identify the measure numbers in which it appears. (mm. 4, 8, 10, 12, 14, 16)

ASK Which parts have the same rhythm? (III, IV)

Have students tap a quarter-note beat and say the rhythm syllables. For additional reading practice, see p. 496, or Resource Book, p. E-18.

Singing

Play the recording of "Let Us Sing Together" **CD 8-28.** Ask students to independently sing each of the parts, using pitch syllables, singing the syncopated rhythms accurately and demonstrating fundamental skills.

Listening

6c Guide students to realize that syncopation is found in many musical styles from canons to ragtime. Play the recording of *Bethena Waltz* **CD 8-33** and have students compare with "Let Us Sing Together." See Skills Reinforcement below for the comparison. Ask students to describe the musical characteristics of the ragtime style. (syncopated rhythms, piano is a favorite instrument, melody with left-hand boom-chick accompaniment)

3 CLOSE

Skill: READING   ASSESSMENT

Performance/Observation Organize the class into four groups. Have students sing "Let Us Sing Together" in four parts while following the notation. Then have students demonstrate fundamental skills by reading and playing the percussion ensemble on p. 157 with accurate rhythm, first with body percussion and then with percussion instruments. Observe students' ability to play the syncopated rhythms accurately.

SKILLS REINFORCEMENT

6c ► Listening Have students listen to and compare the syncopated patterns in *Bethena Waltz* and "Let Us Sing Together." Point out that, although they are in different meters and diverse styles, both pieces use the same pattern.

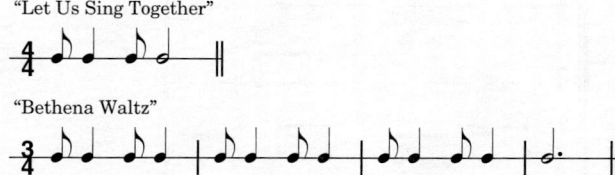

As students listen to *Bethena Waltz* again, have them perform a three-beat ostinato (pat-clap-clap). Explain that this composition is a concert waltz and contains some *rubato*.

TECHNOLOGY/MEDIA LINK

MIDI/Sequencing Software Using the MIDI song file for "Let Us Sing Together," display the melody tracks in notation view. Mute all tracks except one and play the file for students to learn that vocal part. Repeat with other vocal tracks. Play and display all vocal tracks to support class singing in parts.

LESSON AT A GLANCE

Element Focus   **RHYTHM** Syncopation and diminution

Skill Objective   **READING** Read from notation that includes syncopation

Connection Activity   **MATHEMATICS** Explore how rhythmic duration can be changed by a factor of 2

MATERIALS

- "Lost My Gold Ring"   **CD 9-1**
  Recording Routine: Intro (4 m.); vocal; interlude (4 m.); vocal; coda
- **Music Reading Practice, Sequence 18**   **CD 9-3**
- *Elite Syncopations*   **CD 9-9**
- **Resource Book** p. E-19, F-18
- string with a ring on it (tied to form a large circle)
- claves, cowbell, maracas, bongos

VOCABULARY

syncopation   diminution

◆ ◆ ◆ National Standards ◆ ◆ ◆

1c Sing music from diverse cultures
5a Read quarter notes, eighth notes, and sixteenth notes in duple meter
5c Identify standard notation symbols for rhythm
6b Listen and analyze uses of rhyhm in music from diverse genres

MORE MUSIC CHOICES

For more practice with tied rhythms that create syncopation:
"A Brand New Day," p. 7
"The Rhythm is Gonna Get You," p. 348

1 INTRODUCE

Share with students the rhythm exercise in Across the Curriculum (Math), p. 159, to explore how they can divide by two to achieve diminution.

Double the Speed

A common syncopated rhythm pattern is ♪♩♪.

At the same tempo, you can write this rhythm to be twice as fast.

This technique is called *rhythmic diminution*.

"Lost My Gold Ring" is a song from Jamaica that was originally brought to the New World by enslaved Africans. It is a singing game. **Read** the rhythm patterns in the song, using rhythm syllables. **Sing** "Lost My Gold Ring." Choose rhythm patterns from the song and **create** an accompaniment.

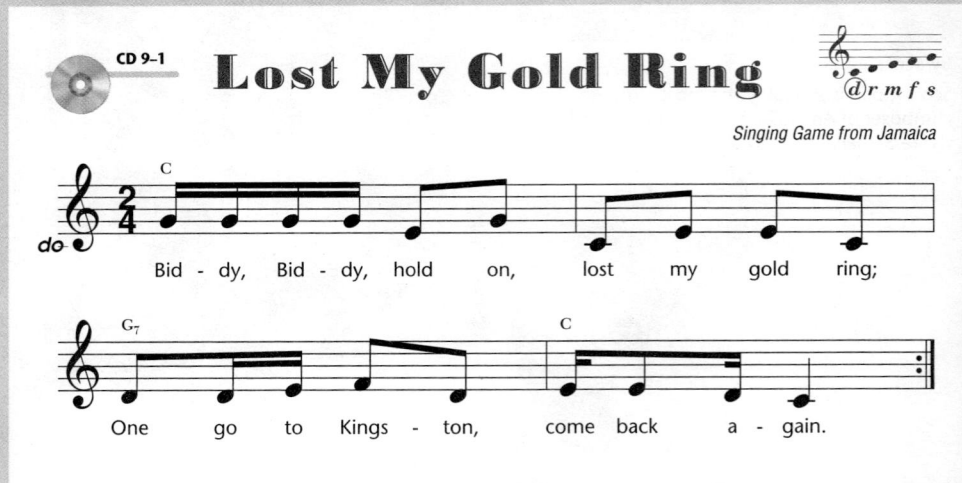

CD 9–1
Lost My Gold Ring

Singing Game from Jamaica

Bid - dy, Bid - dy, hold on, lost my gold ring;

One go to Kings - ton, come back a - gain.

Footnotes

TEACHER TO TEACHER

▶ **String Game** To play this game with "Lost My Gold Ring," students form a circle and hold a circular string with both hands closed around the string, onto which a ring has been placed. One player is in the center of the ring, with eyes closed to start. While singing the song three times, players move their hands on the beat, as they secretly pass the ring. At the conclusion, the center player guesses where the ring is.

BUILDING SKILLS THROUGH MUSIC

▶ **Reading** Have students visit *www.sfsuccessnet.com* and read the history section of the article on Jamaican Music and Musicians. Have them discuss the information found in the article.

SKILLS REINFORCEMENT

▶ **Playing** Have students perform this percussion ensemble with "Lost My Gold Ring;" then, have them play the Orff accompaniment on Resource Book p. F-18.

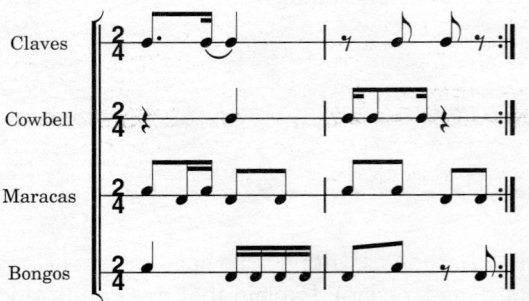

Claves
Cowbell
Maracas
Bongos

Notating Syncopation

Ties can also create syncopation. **Play** these syncopated rhythms as you tap an eighth-note beat with your foot.

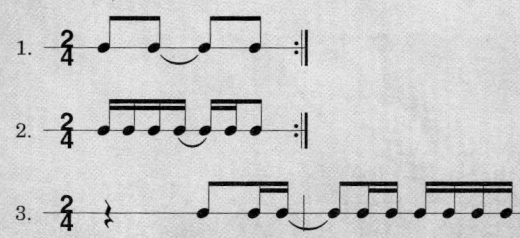

1.
2.
3.

Time for Ragtime

Listen to how tied rhythms and syncopation are used in Scott Joplin's *Elite Syncopations.*

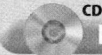

Elite Syncopations

by Scott Joplin

Ragtime got its name from "ragging" (syncopating) the melody against the straight rhythms in the left hand.

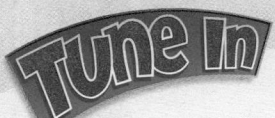

In 1899, Scott Joplin published "Maple Leaf Rag." It became the first published sheet music to sell more than a million copies.

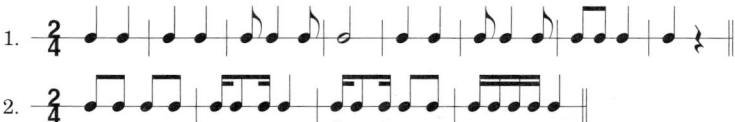

Perform these syncopated rhythms. Then, **create** your own eight-beat syncopated rhythm and **perform** it on a percussion instrument of your choice.

1.
2.

2 DEVELOP

Singing

5a Refer students to the text and rhythm patterns on p. 158 that illustrate syncopation and diminution.

Ask students to look at the notation for "Lost My Gold Ring" **CD 9-1.** Have them

- Tap the beat and say the rhythm syllables.
5c
- Identify the key signature and tonic (C-*do*).
1c
- Sight-read the song, using pitch syllables and then lyrics.

As an optional activity, teach the class the singing game in Teacher to Teacher on p. 158.

Reading

5a Tell students that another way syncopation is created is through the use of tied rhythms. Provide a steady beat and have students tap their feet on an eighth-note beat as they clap each rhythm pattern at the top of p. 159.

For additional reading practice, see p. 496, or Resource Book p. E-19.

Listening

6b Tell students that Scott Joplin also used syncopation to create characteristic ragtime rhythms. As an example, play Joplin's *Elite Syncopations* **CD 9-9.**

Creating

Invite students to choose rhythms from "Lost My Gold Ring" and create an accompaniment from those rhythms.

3 CLOSE

Skill: READING   **ASSESSMENT**

Performance/Observation Ask students to read the rhythms in Skills Reinforcement on p. 158. Have them perform the accompaniment on percussion instruments as the class sings "Lost My Gold Ring." Ask students to identify the syncopated patterns in the song and accompaniment. Assess students' abilities to read and identify the syncopation.

ACROSS THE CURRICULUM

▶ **Social Studies** Invite students to find Jamaica on a map of the Caribbean. Ask them to research the country's history and geography, then share with the class what they have learned.

▶ **Math** Encourage students to work in small groups to create a rhythm pattern. Ask students to notate the rhythm. Then ask them to make the rhythm two times faster by changing the note values. Ask them to identify this technique. (diminution) Then assist students to use a metronome to determine the tempo of each pattern (original and diminution) and to write the tempo down. Ask students by what factor is the tempo changed? (a factor of 2; the faster tempo of the diminution should be approximately 2 times faster than the original tempo)

CHARACTER EDUCATION

▶ **Honesty** To help students understand honesty, ask what they would do if they found a gold ring. How would they define honesty? Why is honesty an important character trait to possess? What are the benefits of being honest? Why is it difficult to always be honest? What are some behaviors that demonstrate dishonesty (lying, cheating)? How would they feel if they discovered someone had been dishonest with them?

TECHNOLOGY/MEDIA LINK

Video Library Show the video *Steel Drums* to present a performance by a Caribbean steel drum ensemble.

LESSON AT A GLANCE

Element Focus **FORM** Theme and variations

Skill Objective **SINGING** Sing a theme and variations

Connection Activity **GENRE** Identify theme-and-variation form in two different genres

MATERIALS

- "Scattin' A-Round" **CD 9-10**

  Recording Routine: Intro (4 m.); theme: unison, 4-part round 1 time; interlude (7 m.); var. 1: unison, 4-part round 1 time; interlude (8 m.); ostinato 2 times; var. 2: unison, 4-part round 1 time; coda

- *Variations on "The Carnival of Venice"* (excerpt) **CD 9-12**

- selected mallet instruments, keyboard

VOCABULARY

theme   variation   scat singing

◆ ◆ ◆ ◆ National Standards ◆ ◆ ◆ ◆

1a Sing accurately with good breath control
1d Sing music written in two and in three parts
4c Arrange using electronic media
6a Listen and describe events in music using appropriate terms
6c Understand and use basic principles of tonality in music analysis

MORE MUSIC CHOICES

For more rounds or canons:
"Let Us Sing Together," p. 156
"Lost My Gold Ring," p. 158
"Gloria, Gloria," p. 459

1 INTRODUCE

Explain to students that every snowflake has a unique pattern of crystals. But the theme is still "snowflake." In music the theme-and-variation form is similar. A composer begins with a basic tune (theme) and changes it (variations).

Theme and Variations

A familiar melody can be used as a musical **theme.** The first time you hear a theme, it is usually a simple tune. Then the composer varies, or changes, the theme. Some ways to vary a theme are

- Change the tonality.
- Change the meter.
- Use different rhythms.
- Change the style.
- Use different instruments.
- Vary the tempo and dynamics.

> A **theme** is an important melody that occurs several times in a piece of music.

Play the theme of "Scattin' A-Round." **Create** a **variation** by using $\frac{3}{4}$ meter.

Sing the theme of "Scattin' A-Round." Then **create** a variation by changing the tonality from major to minor. Which note will you change?

Now scat **sing** "Scattin' A-Round," using neutral syllables. What variation techniques are used in Variations 1 and 2?

> A **variation** is a significant change in a musical theme.

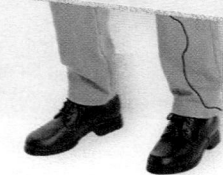

CD 9–10

Scattin' A-Round

*Traditional Round
Arranged by Will Schmid*

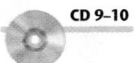
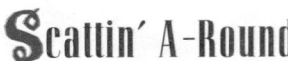
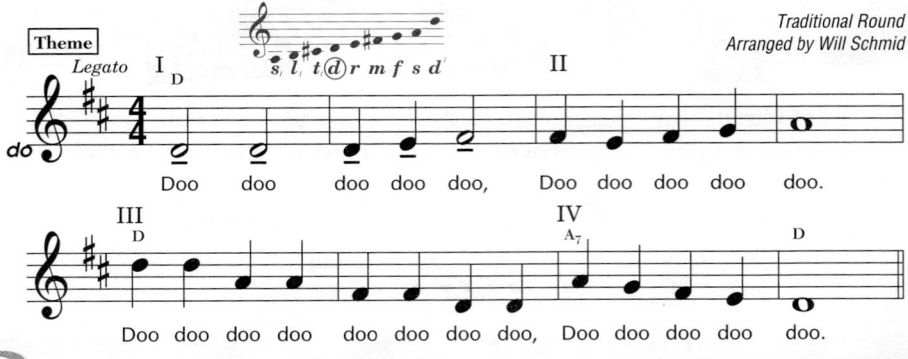

Doo   doo   doo doo doo,   Doo doo doo doo   doo.

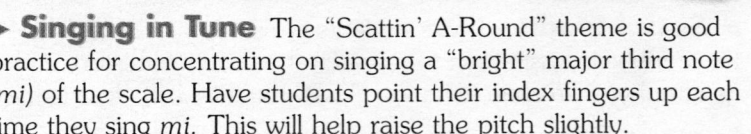

Doo doo doo doo   doo doo doo doo,   Doo doo doo doo   doo.

Footnotes

SKILLS REINFORCEMENT

▶ **Guitar** Adding guitar accompaniment to "Scattin' A-Round" can make the song even more fun while being performed numerous times. A simple down strum with the thumb of the right hand is appropriate, two strums per measure. Draw attention to the common fingerings or hand positions as students move from chord to chord. In this case, when forming the D chord, the first and second fingers keep their basic position, moving up one string when moving to A₇.

BUILDING SKILLS THROUGH MUSIC

▶ **Writing** After listening to *Variations on "The Carnival of Venice"* and writing brief descriptions of select variations, have students organize and expand upon those descriptions to create a more complete description of the variations in this piece of music.

TEACHER TO TEACHER

▶ **Singing in Tune** The "Scattin' A-Round" theme is good practice for concentrating on singing a "bright" major third note *(mi)* of the scale. Have students point their index fingers up each time they sing *mi*. This will help raise the pitch slightly.

▶ **Singing *Legato* and *Staccato*** To teach *legato*, tie knots on a string at regular intervals and run the string between your thumb and finger, creating an unbroken line with bumps at the beginning of each note. Ask students to identify the *legato* and *staccato* articulations in the song notation, and accurately interpret them as they sing the song.

1a ▶ **Breathing** Challenge students to sing "Scattin' A-Round" in only one or two breaths while they sing it as a round.

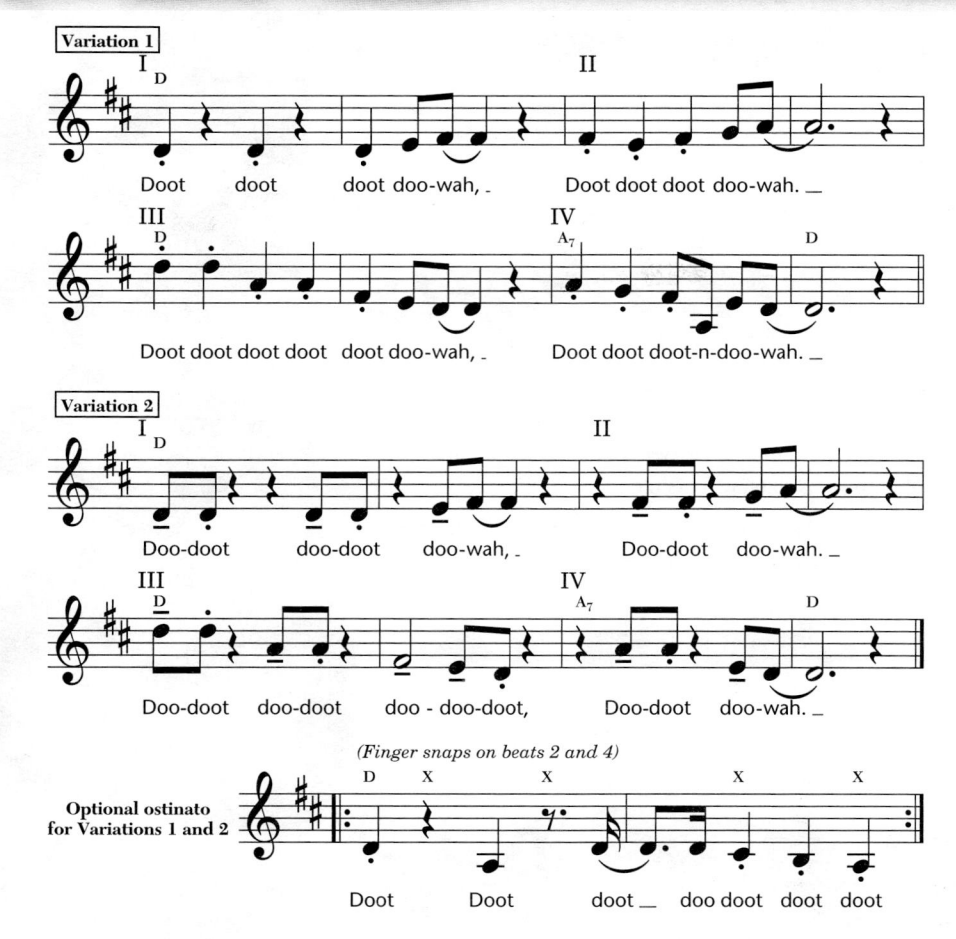

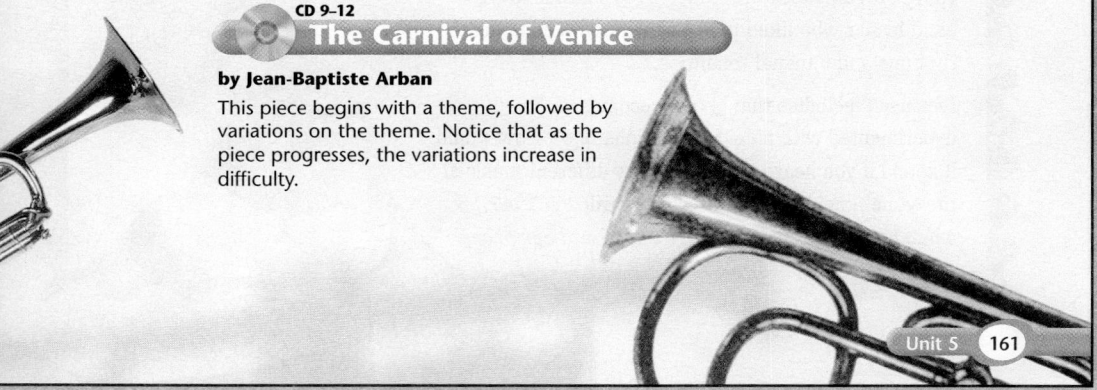

Listen to *Variations on "The Carnival of Venice,"* one of the best-loved trumpet solos of all time. It is an example of theme and variations.

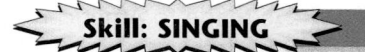

CD 9–12
The Carnival of Venice

by Jean-Baptiste Arban
This piece begins with a theme, followed by variations on the theme. Notice that as the piece progresses, the variations increase in difficulty.

2 DEVELOP

Singing

1d Invite students to read the text on p. 160. Have students discuss the ways a composer can vary a theme. Have them follow the notation of "Scattin' A-Round" **CD 9-10**, p. 160, as they sing the song in unison and then as a round.

Have students listen to "Scattin' A-Round," Variation 1 **CD 9-10** and then sing along.

Invite a group of students to sing the ostinato. Have students listen and sing it along with "Scattin' A-Round," Variation 2 **CD 9-10.**

Playing

Have students play the theme of "Scattin' A-Round" on keyboard or mallet instruments. Have them create a variation on the theme by changing the tonality from major to minor.

6c **ASK What note needs to be changed to turn this theme from major to minor?** (F♯ becomes F.)

Listening

6a Invite students to listen to *Variations on "The Carnival of Venice"* **CD 9-12.** Guide students to write brief descriptions of select variations, using music terms to explain the musical performance, and share their descriptions. Ask them also to contrast the use of theme-and-variation form in these two genres.

3 CLOSE

Skill: SINGING   **ASSESSMENT**

Performance/Observation Divide the class into two groups. Assign variation 1 and variation 2, one to each group. Have one group snap fingers during their variation, and the other clap offbeats during their variation. Observe for accuracy as students sing "Scattin' A-Round" **CD 9-10** with assigned body percussion.

CULTURAL CONNECTION

▶ **Scat Singers** Louis Armstrong (1898–1971), who was an internationally known jazz trumpeter, also popularized a style of singing that was more like an instrumental jazz solo than a vocal solo. This style, called scat singing, uses the human voice like a wind or brass instrument to sing jazz variations on a basic melody, with nonsense syllables. Students can hear Armstrong's scat singing in the recording *Hotter Than That* **CD 4-25** on p. 65. Louis Armstrong and Ella Fitzgerald (1918–1996) were two of the best-known scat singers.

Although authentic scat singing is an African American creation, the Irish also have a fascinating tradition of singing variations on fiddle tunes, using syllables.

TECHNOLOGY/MEDIA LINK

4c **CD-ROM** Use *Band-in-a-Box* to provide motivating background accompaniments for students as they perform "Scattin' A-Round." Have students

- Enter the song's chord progression into the computer. (Have each student type in a measure or two.)
- Experiment with the song accompaniment by selecting different musical styles.
- Sing the song with these accompaniments in various styles.
- Discuss with students the styles that seem best for the song and also those which do not work well.

Challenge students to improvise their own variations on the song with *Band-in-a-Box* accompaniment.

LESSON AT A GLANCE

Element Focus **FORM** Theme and variations

Skill Objective **LISTENING** Follow theme-and-variation form on a listening map

Connection Activity **SOCIAL STUDIES** Explore immigration and our multicultural society in America

MATERIALS
- "America" .... **CD 23-1**
- *Variations on "America"* .... **CD 9-13**

VOCABULARY
theme   variations

◆ ◆ ◆ ◆ National Standards ◆ ◆ ◆ ◆
1a Sing accurately in large ensembles
4c Arrange using non-traditional sound sources
6a Listen and describe events in music using appropriate terms
6b Listen and analyze uses of form in music from diverse genres
8b Identify ways music relates to social studies

MORE MUSIC CHOICES
Other examples of theme and variations:
"Scattin' A-Round," p. 160
Variations on "The Carnival of Venice," p. 161

1 INTRODUCE

8b Invite student volunteers to share stories of their families' immigration to the United States. See Across the Curriculum below for a book suggestion on immigration. Encourage students to recognize the many contributions that immigrants have made to American culture. Tell students that during this lesson they will listen to a composition by twentieth-century composer Charles Ives. The composition is *Variations on "America."*

AMERICAN Variations

In *Variations on "America,"* composer Charles Ives wanted to show the patriotic song "America" in the musical styles of different countries. He wrote *Variations on "America"* when he was sixteen years old.

Listen to *Variations on "America."* Follow along with the listening map and **identify** each variation.

CD 9-13
Variations on "America"

by Charles Ives

Listen for the Irish jig in Variation 4 and the Spanish dance in Variation 5.

M·U·S·I·C M·A·K·E·R·S
Charles Ives

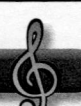

Charles Ives (1874–1954) was an interesting character in American music. He was an insurance executive in the daytime, and a composer and church organist at other times. Ives's father was a band leader who liked to experiment with complicated rhythms and unusual tonalities.

Ives used melodies that people recognized. He experimented with musical questions like, "How would it sound if you heard two bands play different music at the same time?" His talent was rewarded in 1947, when he won a Pulitzer prize for his *Third Symphony.*

162

Footnotes

ACROSS THE CURRICULUM

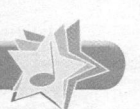

▶ **Social Studies** Read aloud the book *Coming to America: The Story of Immigration* by Betsy Maestro (Scholastic, 1996). Invite students to discuss the experiences of immigrants arriving in the United States. Then, have groups of students create dramatic scenes portraying vignettes from the book. Share additional facts about immigration as students perform.

BUILDING SKILLS THROUGH MUSIC

▶ **Writing** Using information from the listening map and the lesson, have students list the phrases and words that describe one of the variations in *Variations on "America."* Have them rewrite the information into a paragraph using complete sentences.

SKILLS REINFORCEMENT

4c ▶ **Creating** Charles Ives was a maverick composer because he tried things that were completely unconventional in his time, with very interesting, often beautiful results. Ask students to consider some unconventional approaches to creating their own variations on a familiar theme, using their imaginations to design new, yet workable, ideas. Help them make lists of their ideas and share them in class. Discussion should focus on *what* is being varied, *how* it is being varied, and *why.* This process will help the students understand the importance of planning in the creative process. It will also increase their motivation for realizing these ideas in sound in a subsequent lesson.

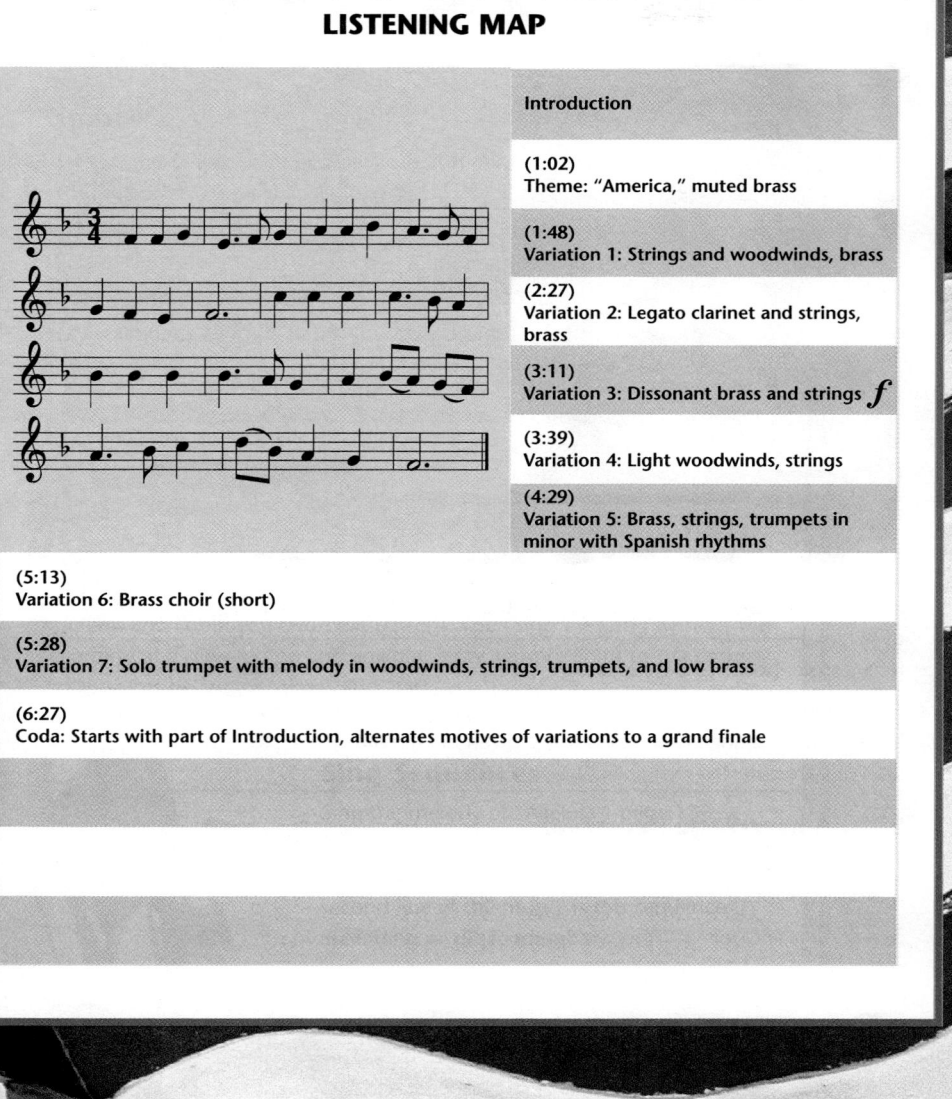

VARIATIONS ON "AMERICA"
LISTENING MAP

Introduction

(1:02)
Theme: "America," muted brass

(1:48)
Variation 1: Strings and woodwinds, brass

(2:27)
Variation 2: Legato clarinet and strings, brass

(3:11)
Variation 3: Dissonant brass and strings *f*

(3:39)
Variation 4: Light woodwinds, strings

(4:29)
Variation 5: Brass, strings, trumpets in minor with Spanish rhythms

(5:13)
Variation 6: Brass choir (short)

(5:28)
Variation 7: Solo trumpet with melody in woodwinds, strings, trumpets, and low brass

(6:27)
Coda: Starts with part of Introduction, alternates motives of variations to a grand finale

Unit 5 **163**

2 DEVELOP

Singing

1a Invite students to sing one verse of "America" **CD 23-1** with the recording. Have students follow the music on p. 484.

Share with students the background information on the history of "America" in Spotlight On below.

Listening

Have students read the information about Charles Ives on p. 162.

SAY During most of his life, Charles Ives's music was not appreciated. Finally, at age 73, he was awarded the Pulitzer Prize for his *Third Symphony*.

For an example of Ives's musical experiments, ask students to imagine themselves walking in a shopping mall. Tell them that they hear different musical styles coming from several stores and many conversations at the same time. Tell them that this "sound montage" is one concept that Ives experimented with in his music. When Ives was young, his father sometimes played in one key and had Charles sing in another key.

6a Have students study the listening map to prepare for the differences in the variations. Have them listen to **6b** the recording of *Variations on "America"* **CD 9-13** while following the listening map. Encourage students to use standard terminology to discuss the musical styles, cultures, and performances. See Technology/Media Link below for using the transparency.

3 CLOSE

Skill: LISTENING   ASSESSMENT

Observation Have students listen to *Variations on "America"* **CD 9-13** and point to the appropriate variations on the listening map. Observe students' ability to accurately identify the variations on the listening map.

SPOTLIGHT ON

▶ **"America"** "My Country! 'tis of Thee" was first sung on July 4, 1831, in the Park Street Church, Boston. The Rev. Samuel Francis Smith, a Baptist clergyman, wrote the words. He set his new words to the melody "Heil, Dir im Siegerkranz," which he found in a German hymnal, unaware that it was also the tune for the British anthem, "God Save the King/Queen."

CHARACTER EDUCATION

▶ **Character Traits** Discuss the character traits valued by a free society (honesty, hard work, compassion, respect for ethnic diversity, patriotism). Ask students to select a character trait, define it, and show how they might use it in their lives. Ask them how they might show this trait in their lives, as they get older.

SCHOOL TO HOME CONNECTION

▶ **American Immigration** Encourage students to discuss their family history with immediate family and other relatives. Students may be surprised to learn that most American families have ancestors who immigrated to America. Ask students to make a chart of immigration patterns for the families represented in their class.

TECHNOLOGY/MEDIA LINK

Transparency Display the listening map transparency for *Variations on "America."* Invite students to trace the progress of the song with a finger on the map in their books as you trace on the overhead projection.

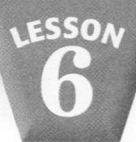

LESSON AT A GLANCE

Element Focus	**MELODY** Half and whole steps
Skill Objective	**READING** Identify half and whole steps when reading a song from notation
Connection Activity	**MATHEMATICS** Compare measurements of distance and measurement in music

MATERIALS
- "O lê lê O Bahía"   **CD 9-14**
- "O Le O La"   **CD 9-15**

  Recording Routine: Intro (7 m.); vocal; interlude (4 m.); vocal; coda
- **Music Reading Practice, Sequence 19**   **CD 9-18**
- **Pronunciation Practice/Translation** p. 528
- **Resource Book** pp. A-15, D-22, E-20
- mallet instruments

VOCABULARY

interval   ostinato   dissonance

◆ ◆ ◆ ◆ National Standards ◆ ◆ ◆ ◆
1b Sing easy pieces with technical accuracy
2e In instrumental ensembles, perform moderately easy pieces with technical accuracy
5e In performance classes, sightread easy music accurately
6a Listen and describe events in music using appropriate terms

MORE MUSIC CHOICES

For more practice in reading half and whole steps in major:
"Vive l'amour," p. 176
"Everybody Love Saturday Night," p. 296

1 INTRODUCE

Share with students the information on Bahía, Brazil in Cultural Connection below. Have students measure the distances between cities on p. 164. Tell students that the distances between pitches are called intervals that are measured by counting steps between them.

Melodic Distances

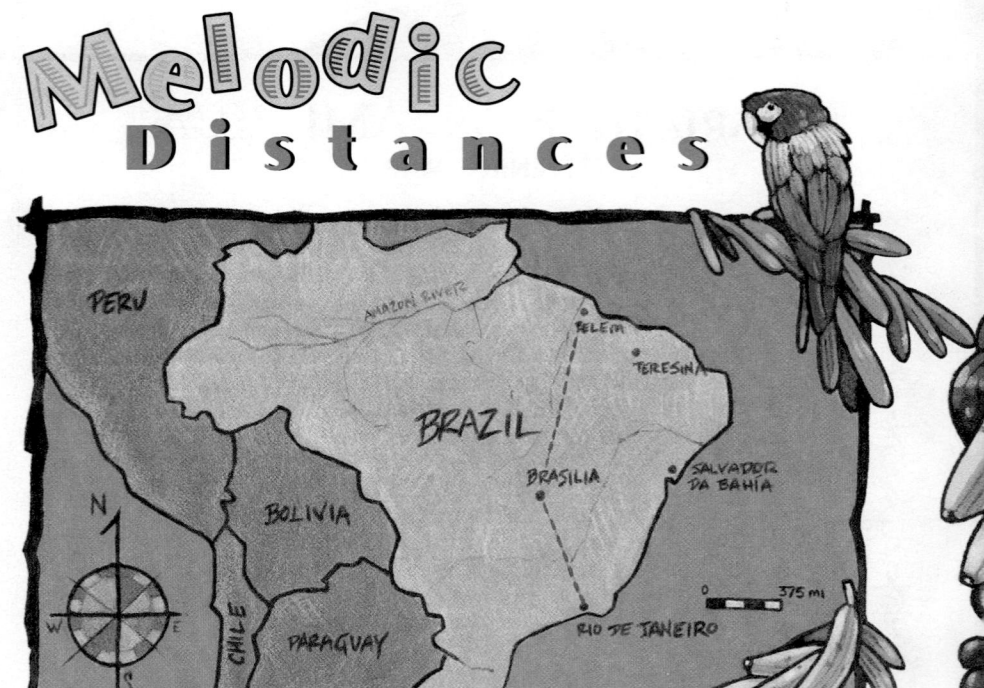

Measure the distance on the map from the city of Brasilia to the cities of Belem and Rio de Janeiro. Which city is closer to Brasilia? Using the map's scale, how many miles is a round trip from Belem to Brasilia?

The distance between places on the map is given in miles. As you learned, the distance between notes is given in intervals. These intervals are counted in numbers.

Sing a Marriage Proposal

"O lê lê O Bahía" is a humorous song from Brazil about a long-distance marriage proposal.

Sing "O lê lê O Bahía." Afterwards, **analyze** the intervals in the song.

164   Reading Sequence 19

Footnotes

TEACHER TO TEACHER

6a ▶ **Listening** The intervals sung in the "O lê lê O Bahía" chorus are seconds (*do–re*; *re–mi*; *mi–fa*) and a fourth (*so–do¹*). To help students learn these intervals, tell them that you are going to play one of the intervals on the piano. Have students listen carefully and tell you whether the interval you played was a second or a fourth. Repeat until this is secure, then add some of the intervals of a third used in the solo part (*fa–la*; *mi–do*; *ti₁–so₁*; *so–mi*; *do–la₁*; *re–ti₁*), and have students differentiate between seconds, thirds, and fourths.

BUILDING SKILLS THROUGH MUSIC

▶ **Math** Using a map of Brazil, have students answer the questions about distance found on p. 164 and convert those measurements from miles to kilometers.

CULTURAL CONNECTION

▶ **Bahía, Brazil** Bahía, which means "bay," is a state in the central-eastern coastal region of Brazil. Salvador, a port city, is the capital of Bahía. The blending of indigenous Indian, Portuguese, black African, Spanish, and black Brazilian peoples in Brazil has created a wide variety of folk song and dance genres.

"O lê lê O Bahía" is an amusing folk song about unrequited love. Another kind of folk song popular throughout Brazil is the *aboio*. *Aboios* are sung while herding cattle and, like "O lê lê O Bahía," they are in call-and-response form.

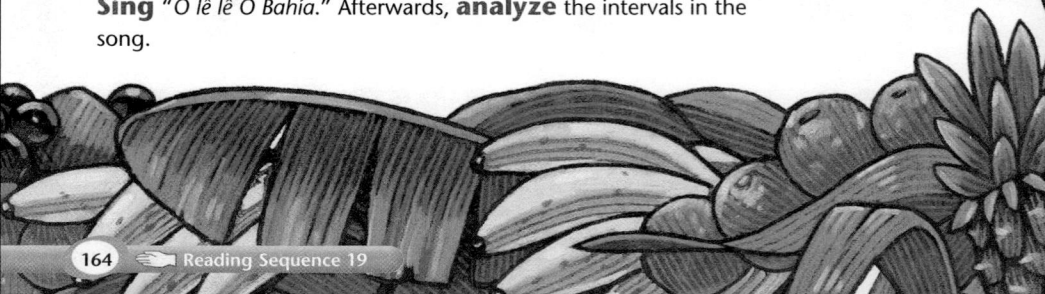

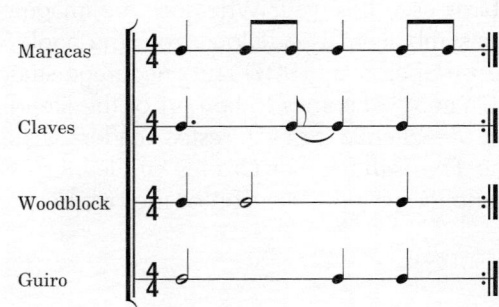

O lê lê O Bahía

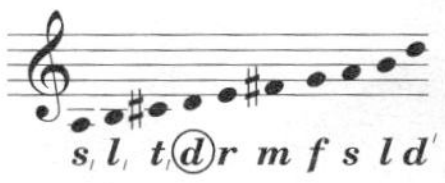

(O Le O La)

CD 9–14

Folk Song from Brazil

D Solo / G Chorus

Da Ba-hí-a me man-da-ram
1. Sent to me from Ba-hí - a, ____ O lê lê O Ba-hí -
2. Then I told him that I will, ____

G Solo / D Chorus / Solo

Um ces-ti-nho de ca-já, *E man-da-ram per-gun-*
a, Bas-ket full of good ca-já, O lê lê O Ba-hí - a, With a note, et ce-te -
When the riv-ers run up-hill, Or when fish be-gin to

A₇ Chorus / Solo / D Chorus

tar *Se eu que-ri-a me ca-sar.*
ra, O lê lê O Ba-hí - a, "Will you mar-ry me?" (Ah - ha!) O lê lê O Ba-hí -
fly, Or the day be-fore I die.

D Solo / A₇ Chorus / Solo

a, O le o la, O lê lê O Ba-hí - a, O le o

D Chorus / 1. Solo / 2.

la, O lê lê O Ba-hí - a, O le o a.

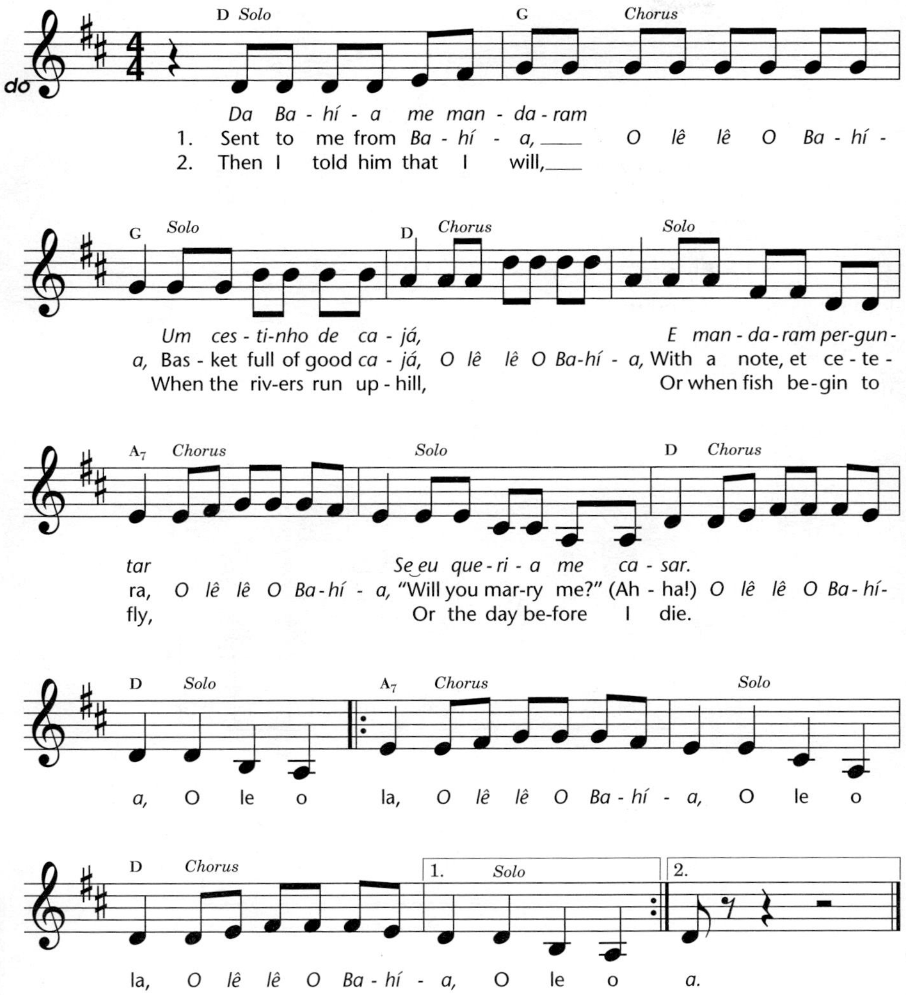

Unit 5 **165**

---

2 DEVELOP

Analyzing

6a Play *"O lê lê O Bahía"* **CD 9-14** and ask students what they notice about the solo and chorus parts (they alternate), and identify pitch movement by steps (choruses 3, 4, 5, 6), skips (chorus 2) and repeated pitch (chorus 1).

Singing

1b Have students sight-sing the choruses of *"O lê lê O Bahía"* **CD 9-14** as you sing the solos. Use the Pronunciation Practice **CD 9–17** to teach the Portuguese lyrics.

Reading

Draw a vertical tone ladder from *do* to *do¹* on the board. Help students read and identify all the intervals created from *do*.

Use Resource Book p. D-22 to help students see that intervals are measured from all of the pitches in a scale. Sing the seconds and help students identify that the seconds are not all the same size.

For additional reading practice, see Resource Book p. E-20, or p. 497.

Singing

Help students read and sing the seconds, thirds, and fourths in *"O lê lê O Bahía"* using pitch syllables. Use Resource Book p. D-22 to have students identify the major and minor seconds in the C-*do;* G-*do,* and D-*do* scale.

3 CLOSE

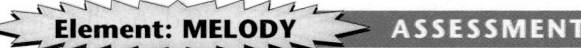

Element: MELODY ASSESSMENT

5e **Performance/Observation** Have students use pitch syllables to read and sing *"O lê lê O Bahía."*
2e Observe their ability to accurately read and sing whole steps and half steps, using pitch syllables.

SKILLS REINFORCEMENT

2e ▶ **Playing** Have students play these rhythmic ostinatos as an accompaniment for *"O lê lê O Bahía."*

Maracas

Claves

Woodblock

Guiro

TECHNOLOGY/MEDIA LINK

CD-ROM Invite students to use the CD-ROM, *Alfred's Essentials of Music Theory,* Volumes 1 and 2, for more practice with intervals.

LESSON AT A GLANCE

Element Focus **MELODY** Melodic intervals

Skill Objective **READING** Read, identify, and sing intervals

Connection Activity **MATHEMATICS** Measure the distance between pitches by naming the interval

MATERIALS

- "Like a Bird" **CD 9-21**

  Recording Routine: Intro (4 m.); vocal (unison); interlude (4 m.); vocal (3-part canon); coda

- Music Reading Practice, Sequence 20 **CD 9-23**
- Resource Book pp. B-16, D-23, E-21

VOCABULARY

interval   major   minor   perfect   octave

◆ ◆ ◆ ◆ National Standards ◆ ◆ ◆ ◆

4c Compose, using electronic media

5a Read half notes, quarter notes, and eighth notes in alla breve time

5b Sightread melodies in treble clef

5c Identify standard notation symbols for pitch

5d Use standard notation to record musical ideas

MORE MUSIC CHOICES

For more practice with identifying intervals in songs:

"Bury Me Not on the Lone Prairie," p. 19

"Down in the Valley," p. 375

"My Dear Companion," p. 23

1 INTRODUCE

Remind students that they can use easy math to find interval distances: simply count half steps to find the distance just like they count miles to find the distance between two cities. Seconds with one half step equal the distance of a minor second; seconds with two half steps equal the distance of a major second.

Distance = Intervals

The distance between notes is called an interval. Below are some of the intervals in "Like a Bird." Find each interval in the chart below using pitch syllables, staff notation, and keyboard. Then **play** each of these intervals on a melody instrument.

- Octave
- Second
- Third
- Fourth
- Fifth

Then **listen** to "Like a Bird" and **identify** these intervals in the song.

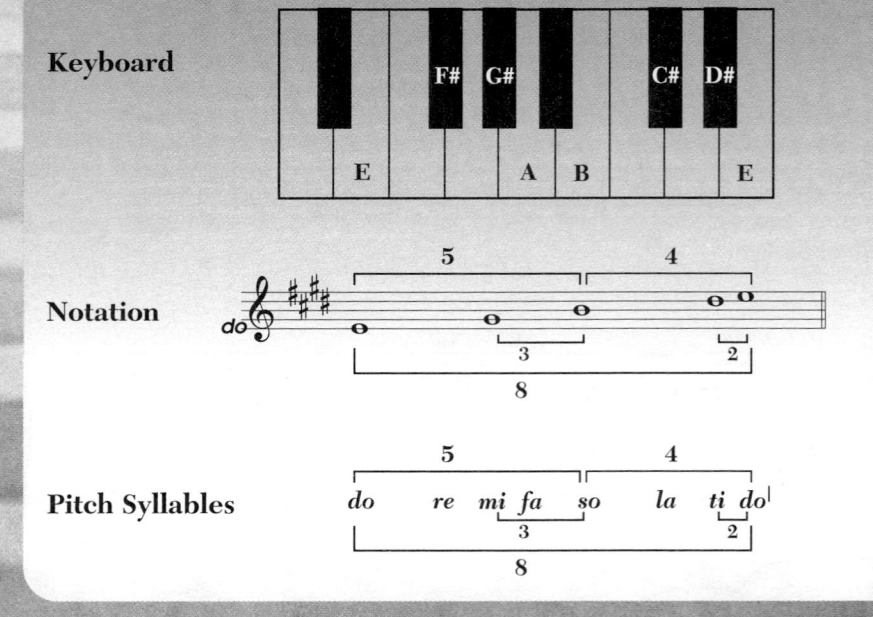

Footnotes

SKILLS REINFORCEMENT

▶ **Reading** Invite students to sing and play the Mystery Interval game. Prepare five cards showing the intervals specified in this lesson on the staff in E-*do*. Use one interval per card. Draw only the note heads. Divide the class into two teams. In turn, team members draw a card, sing the pitch and interval name, and then play it on a tone bell set or a keyboard. Allow students to create new games using other scales, pitch sets, or intervals.

BUILDING SKILLS THROUGH MUSIC

▶ **Language** Ask students to identify the mood the lyricist projects through the lyrics. Have them identify specific words or phrases that contribute to that mood.

ACROSS THE CURRICULUM

▶ **Language Arts** Invite students into a conversation about the use of birds to symbolize freedom. Where else have they seen or heard birds used this way? Why does the image of a bird lend itself to this symbolism? Read aloud from the book *Sadako* by Eleanor Coerr (Paper Star, 1997) and encourage students to consider how this imagery comes to be part of the life of a young girl dying of leukemia. For interested readers, suggest *Sadako and the Thousand Paper Cranes* by Eleanor Coerr (Puffin, 1999), the longer novel version of the picture book above.

Cherubini's Birds

Luigi Cherubini [keh-roo-BEE-nee] (1760–1842) was an Italian-born composer who lived in Paris. Cherubini's song "Like a Bird" is a three-voice canon.

Listen to "Like a Bird" and conduct it in $\frac{2}{2}$ meter. First **sing** the song in unison and then as a three-part canon.

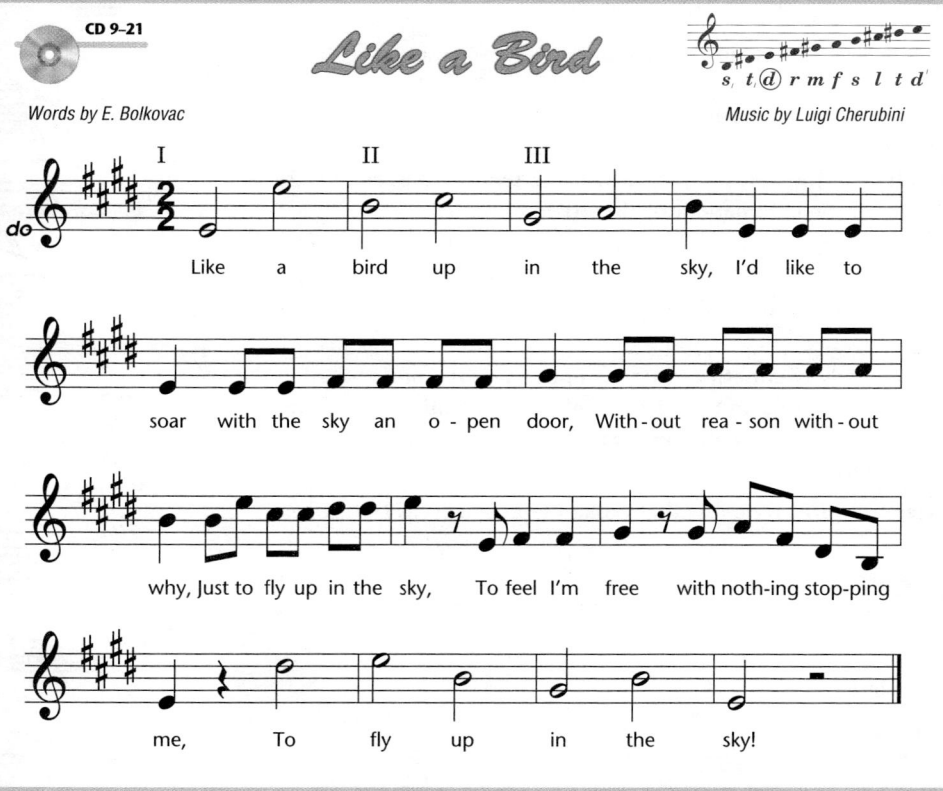

CD 9-21

Like a Bird

Words by E. Bolkovac

Music by Luigi Cherubini

Like a bird up in the sky, I'd like to soar with the sky an o-pen door, With-out rea-son with-out why, Just to fly up in the sky, To feel I'm free with noth-ing stop-ping me, To fly up in the sky!

Show What You Know!

Notate the E-major scale on a piece of paper. Then **play** it on a keyboard or other instrument. **Identify** each of these intervals: second, third, fourth, fifth, and octave. Draw brackets and label each interval.

2 DEVELOP

Reading

Explain to students that seconds, thirds, sixths, and sevenths can be measured as major or minor. Unisons, fourths, fifths, and octaves are called perfect. Their measurement is always the same: the distance of a perfect fifth always measures seven half steps.

5b Have students sing letter names as they touch each key on the keyboard on p. 166, then sing the pitches notated, using pitch syllables. Have students read and identify each interval on the chart on p. 166. Use the Reading Music Worksheet on Resource Book p. D-23 to give students extra practice identifying intervals.

Encourage students to play each interval on a melody instrument.

For additional music reading practice, invite students to sing a countermelody to "Like a Bird" on p. 497, or Resource Book p. E-21.

Singing

5a Invite students to listen to "Like a Bird" **CD 9-21** while conducting in $\frac{2}{2}$. Have them sing the song with pitch syllables and hand signs, then with the lyrics, and finally as a three-part canon, when they are ready.

3 CLOSE

Skill: READING   ASSESSMENT

Performance/Observation Have students complete the Show What You Know activity on Resource Book p. B-16 (E-major scale).

5c Write the intervals in E–*do* from the lesson on the board. Have students individually sing the pitch names and identify one interval by name. Assess each student's ability to read, sing, and identify the interval.

MEETING INDIVIDUAL NEEDS

5d ► Including Everyone To reinforce practice with intervals, encourage students to create major scale "tone rows."

Reinforcement Students needing assistance may be placed with a supportive peer. One student can record choices and write the row for his or her partner, who chooses notes for the row by pointing to different notes in a major scale.

On Target Students should work independently to create their tone rows. They may choose their notes by their letter names, or by playing them on the keyboard. Have students analyze the intervals in their rows.

Challenge Have students create tone rows based on major and minor scales, or modes. Have them label the intervals in their rows.

TECHNOLOGY/MEDIA LINK

Notation Software Encourage students to use notation software to create and notate a melody. Have students create melodic phrases and combine them into a melody. Then, have them count half steps to find the intervals from note to note in that melody, and transpose the melody a chosen interval up or down from the original. Have students play their melodies and transpositions for the class.

LESSON AT A GLANCE

Element Focus **MELODY** Twelve-tone melodies

Skill Objective **CREATING** Create and notate a 12-tone row and its retrograde

Connection Activity **MATHEMATICS** Discuss the applications of mathematics in composition of serial music

MATERIALS
- "Allegretto gioviale" from *Lyric Suite*   **CD 9-26**
- **Resource Book** p. J-14
- keyboard(s), resonator bells, music manuscript paper

VOCABULARY
12-tone row   chromatic scale

◆ ◆ ◆ ◆ National Standards ◆ ◆ ◆ ◆
4c Compose, using traditional sound sources
6a Listen and describe events in music using appropriate terms
6b Listen and analyze uses of pitch in music from diverse genres
8b Identify ways music relates to math

MORE MUSIC CHOICES
Other listening pieces with string instruments:
"Finale" from *Serenade for Strings in C,* Op. 48, p. 363
"Summer" from *Concerto in No. 2,* p. 102

1 INTRODUCE

SAY In a tonal piece, we usually know where the tonal center is.

Play the Berg tone row on this page.

ASK Can you sing *do?* (no)

SAY There is no feeling of *do* in 12-tone music. Read about Alban Berg and his 12-tone music in the Music Makers feature on p. 169.

Rows of Tones

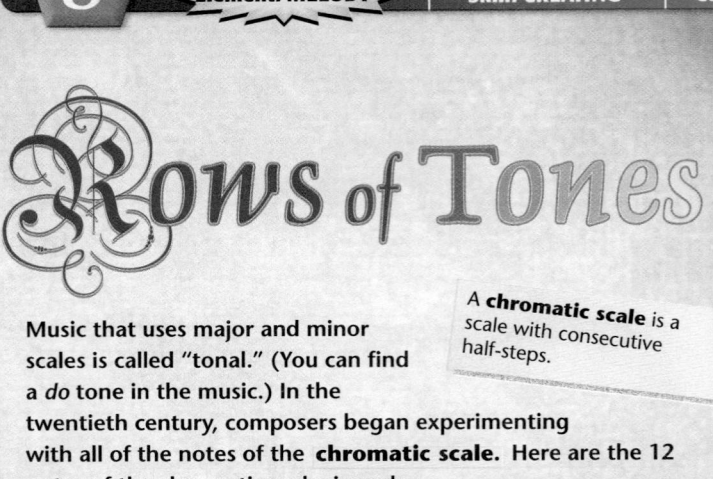

Music that uses major and minor scales is called "tonal." (You can find a *do* tone in the music.) In the twentieth century, composers began experimenting with all of the notes of the **chromatic scale.** Here are the 12 notes of the chromatic scale, in order.

> A **chromatic scale** is a scale with consecutive half-steps.

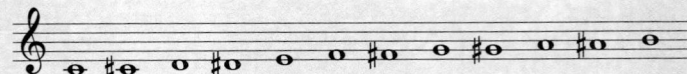

Some early twentieth-century composers wrote music based on "tone rows"—using the 12 notes of the chromatic scale in a non-tonal order. (You can't find a *do* tone in the music.) This music was called "serial," or "atonal" music.

Here is the 12-tone row that Alban Berg used in his *Lyric Suite.*

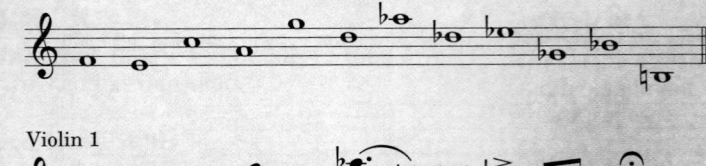

Violin 1

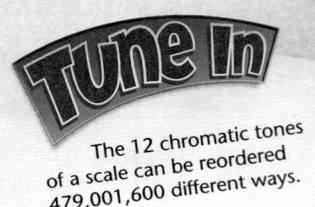

Tune In

The 12 chromatic tones of a scale can be reordered 479,001,600 different ways.

A music score by Alban Berg ▶

Footnotes

SPOTLIGHT ON

▶ **The Composer** Viennese composer Arnold Schoenberg (1874–1951) introduced the method of composition based on a tone row (series of 12 tones), called *serialism.* (He also painted the portrait of Berg on p. 169.) His most important pupils were Alban Berg, Anton Webern, and John Cage. Schoenberg taught at the Prussian Academy of Arts, U.S.C., and at U.C.L.A. A special building at the University of Southern California is dedicated to housing his works, his library, and other materials.

BUILDING SKILLS THROUGH MUSIC

▶ **Language** Have students read the Music Maker on Alban Berg, p. 169, and answer these questions: Did audiences, during his life, seem to enjoy his use of an atonal style of writing? What information supports that view?

SKILLS REINFORCEMENT

▶ **Creating** Students can modify their tone rows by arranging the pitches in reverse order (retrograde) or writing the intervals upside down, as in a mirror (inversion), starting from the first note. Here are examples of an original six-tone row, the retrograde, and the inversion.

Original Row

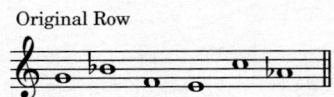

Retrograde

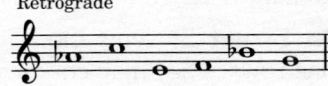

Inversion

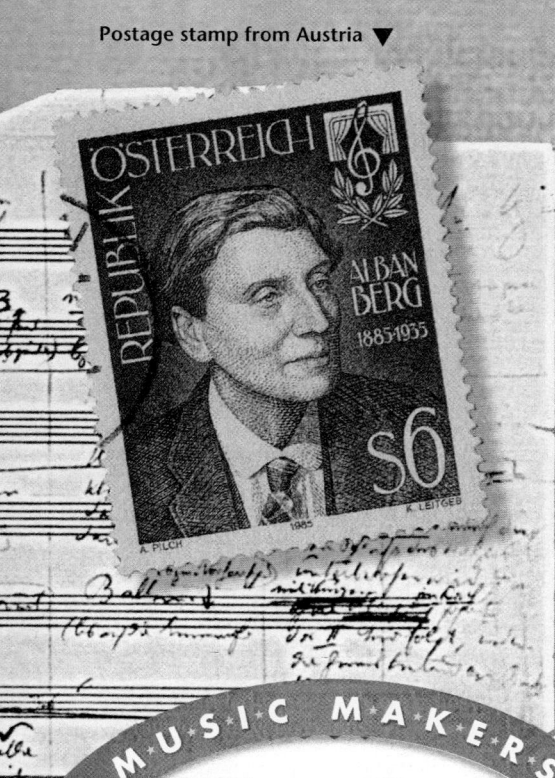

Postage stamp from Austria ▼

A Row with Tones

Listen to a section of Alban Berg's *Lyric Suite*. How would you **describe** this style of music?

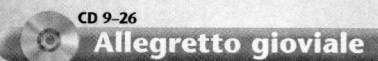

CD 9–26
Allegretto gioviale

from *Lyric Suite*
by Alban Berg
This suite, using a 12-tone row, was composed for string quartet in 1926.

Create Your Own Tone Row

Create a tone row. Use all 12 notes of the chromatic scale with resonator bells. Place them in a non-tonal order. Write the notes down. Then **play** the same notes, but play them in different octaves. Splitting notes into different octaves makes the tone row sound different.

MUSIC MAKERS

Alban Berg

Alban Berg (1885–1935) was born in Vienna of middle class parents. His early compositions were traditional (tonal). In later life, Berg composed in the atonal, or serial style. This style of writing music was developed by his teacher, Arnold Schoenberg. Berg's music used more traditional harmonies and "romantic" themes than other atonal composers.

Berg's most famous work was his opera, *Wozzeck*. Many people were not used to Berg's atonal style of writing in *Wozzeck*. Performances of the opera caused scandal, yelling, and even fighting in the audience.

Arts Connection

Painting of Alban Berg by Arnold Schoenberg ▶

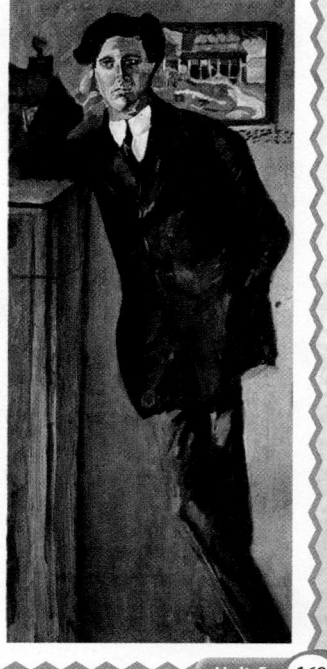

Unit 5 **169**

2 DEVELOP

Playing

6a Have students listen and follow on p. 168 as you play the chromatic scale. Have them listen and watch the notation as you play Berg's 12-tone row. Invite volunteers to play the scale and tone row.

8b Discuss with students the fact that there are mathematically many possible melodies in 12-tone composition. See Across the Curriculum below.

Listening

6b Have students follow the notation, p. 168, as you play the first violin theme from Berg's *Lyric Suite* on keyboard.

Play the excerpt from *Lyric Suite* **CD 9-26** for students and invite them to share their reactions.

Creating

4c Invite students to be 12-tone composers. Have them arrange 12 resonator bells in a non-tonal order, and experiment with octaves and rhythms to create a 12-tone melody. Ask students to notate their melody.

Share with students the Skills Reinforcement information, p. 168, on how composers can manipulate a tone row with inversion and retrograde. Ask students to arrange melodic phrases by writing a retrograde of their melody on manuscript paper. See Resource Book p. J-14 for manuscript paper.

3 CLOSE

Element: MELODY **ASSESSMENT**

Written Assessment Have students create and notate another tone row on manuscript paper, then write its retrograde.

ACROSS THE CURRICULUM

8b ▶ **Math** The chances of two composers using the same 12-tone row are very small, because there are many possible combinations of 12 pitches. You can use math to find the maximum number of ways that groups of pitches or numbers can be combined. The numbers 1 2 3 can be combined six different ways. That is, the number 3 has six permutations: 1 2 3, 1 3 2, 2 1 3, 2 3 1, 3 1 2, 3 2 1.

To find the number of permutations for a number, multiply the number by the permutation of the number just below it. Permutation of 3 is 6 (3 × perm. of 2, which is 2); permutation of 4 is 24 (4 × perm. of 3, which is 6); permutation of 5 is 120 (5 × perm. of 4, which is 24). So, the permutation of 12 is 479,001,600 (12 × perm. of 11, which is 39,916,800). That is a lot of possible melodies!

TECHNOLOGY/MEDIA LINK

Notation Software Using notation software, have students

- Create and enter a 6-note tone row into the software.
- Create a retrograde of the row and, if possible, an inversion.
- Make a classroom poster of the tone rows from students. (Print in different sizes and colors.)

LESSON AT A GLANCE

Element Focus — **TIMBRE** Vocal timbres

Skill Objective **LISTENING** Describe vocal timbres common to different cultures

Connection Activity **CULTURE** Discuss the ways in which preferences for the arts, food, and customs may vary among cultures

MATERIALS

- "Four Strong Winds"   **CD 9-28**
  Recording Routine: Intro (4 m.); v. 1; interlude (4 m.); v. 2; coda
- *Vocal Timbres Around the World*   **CD 9-27**
- "The Wind" (poem)
- **Resource Book** p. I-16
- guitar

VOCABULARY

timbre

◆ ◆ ◆ National Standards ◆ ◆ ◆ ◆

1d Sing music written in two parts
4b Arrange pieces for voices and instruments
6b Listen and analyze uses of timbre in music from diverse cultures
7a Students evaluate the music they hear

MORE MUSIC CHOICES

Other songs in two parts:
"Vive l'amour," p. 176
"Run! Run! Hide!" p. 340

1 INTRODUCE

Have a few students close their eyes. Select four students to say, "Every voice has a different timbre." Ask the students with eyes closed to identify speakers by voice.

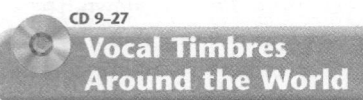

Different Cultures and Timbres

As you travel to different places, or listen to recordings, you may notice how people from different cultures sing with different timbres. Each culture often has its own unique sound, favorite vocal styles, and favorite instruments to play. Enjoy our tour of some of the world's vocal sounds.

Listen to *Vocal Timbres Around the World.* What differences do you hear?

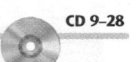

CD 9-27
Vocal Timbres Around the World

Bobby McFerrin ▶

This montage features Bobby McFerrin's *Grace*, Keb' Mo's *Every Morning*, Emanual Dufrasne's *Leró pá Cico Mangual*, and Ricky Skaggs' *Crying My Heart Out Over You.*

Sing the melody of "Four Strong Winds" in unison. Then add the harmony part. How would you **describe** your vocal timbre?

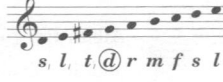

CD 9–28 **Four Strong Winds**
(from *Song to a Seagull*)

Words and Music by Ian Tyson
Arranged by Robert Evans

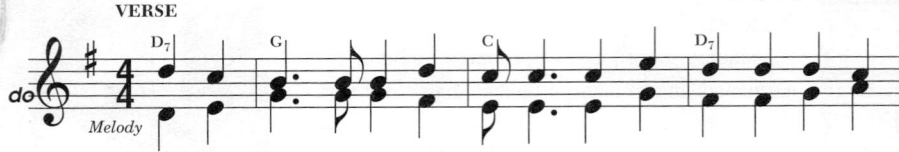

1. Think I'll go out to Al-ber-ta, Weath-er's good there in the
2. If I get there be-fore the snow flies, And if things are go-ing

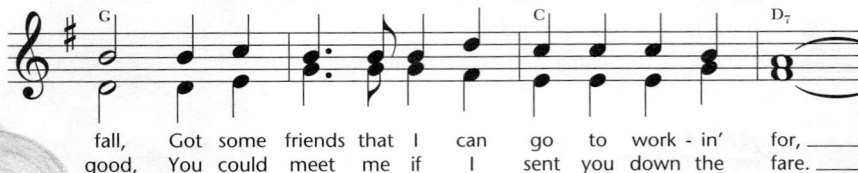

fall, Got some friends that I can go to work-in' for, _____
good, You could meet me if I sent you down the fare. _____

Footnotes

CULTURAL CONNECTION

▶ **Comparing Cultural Preferences** Just as people of different cultures may prefer different vocal timbres and styles, people all over the world have a wide variety of preferences for food, art, architecture, and so on. Invite students to choose one of the areas of preference listed above, then ask a person who is from a country different from their own about the preferences he or she has in the area. Students may report their findings to the class.

BUILDING SKILLS THROUGH MUSIC

▶ **Writing** Have students use their music journal writing assessment activity to write a paragraph discussing their preferences about one of the vocal styles heard. They should include the descriptive adjectives they selected to describe it, and express their preferences and opinions on the listening.

ACROSS THE CURRICULUM

▶ **Language Arts** Share the book *Make Things Fly: Poems About the Wind* edited by Dorothy Kennedy (Margaret McElderry, 1998). Students may also enjoy "The Wind" by James Reeves (*Random House Book of Poetry for Children* by Jack Prelutsky, 1983).

The Wind

I can get through a doorway without any key,
And strip the leaves from the great oak tree.
I can drive storm-clouds and shake tall towers,
Or steal through a garden and not wake the flowers.
Seas I can move and ships I can sink;
I can carry a house-top or the scent of a pink.
When I am angry I can rave and riot;
And when I am spent, I lie quiet as quiet.

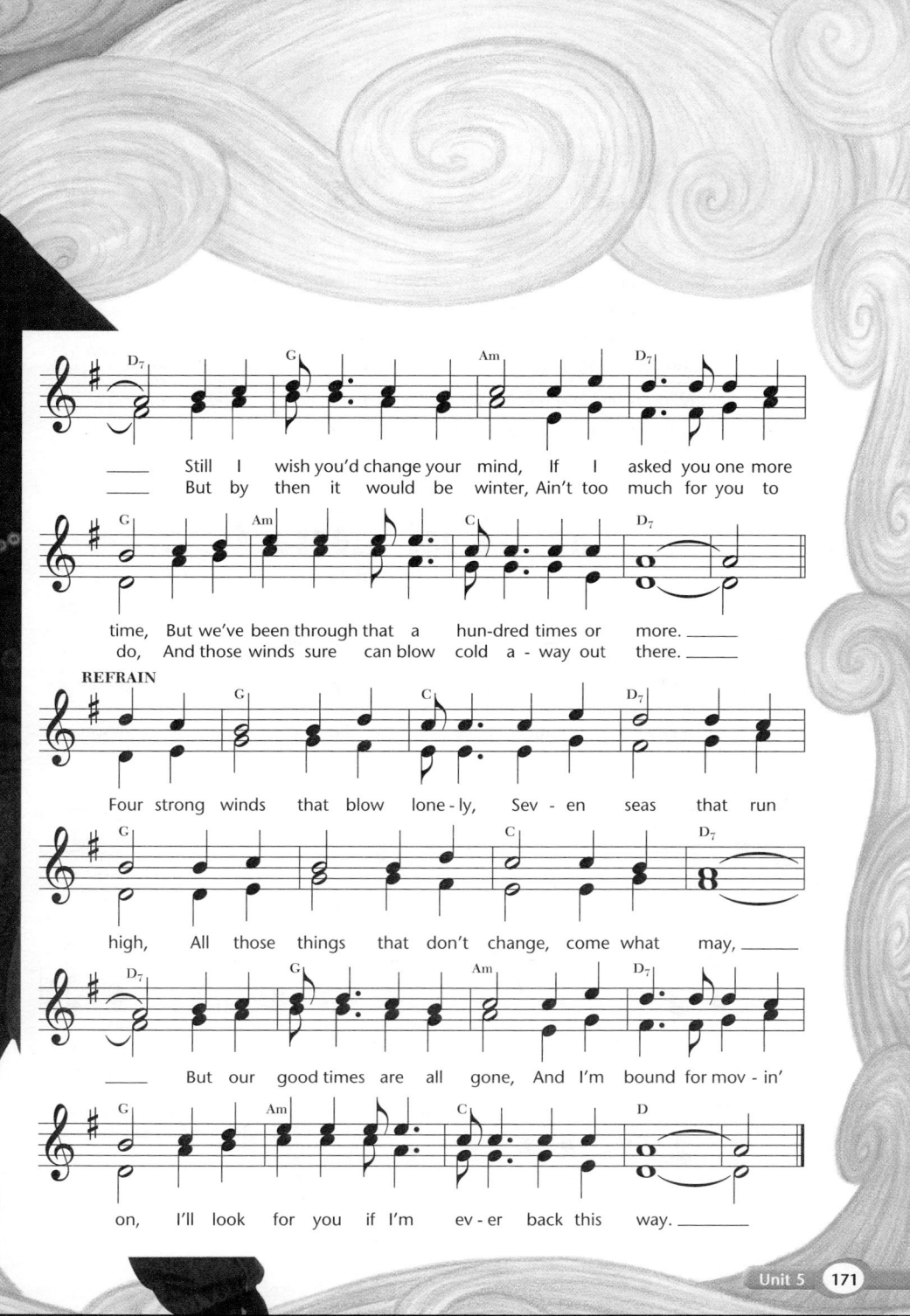

Still I wish you'd change your mind, If I asked you one more
But by then it would be winter, Ain't too much for you to

time, But we've been through that a hun-dred times or more. _____
do, And those winds sure can blow cold a - way out there. _____

REFRAIN

Four strong winds that blow lone-ly, Sev - en seas that run

high, All those things that don't change, come what may, _____

But our good times are all gone, And I'm bound for mov - in'

on, I'll look for you if I'm ev - er back this way. _____

2 DEVELOP

Listening

SAY Each person has a unique vocal timbre. Cultural groups can have a unique style of vocal timbre as well.

6b Select a familiar song. Have students individually sing it several times, demonstrating a different characteristic vocal timbre each time. Discuss the timbres and related cultural factors. See Cultural Connection, p. 170. Play *Vocal Timbres Around the World* **CD 9-27** asking students to describe each aurally-presented music example representing diverse cultures.

Singing

Have students echo sing the melody of "Four Strong Winds" **CD 9-28** as you model it, with pitch syllables.

Divide the class into two groups, one singing the melody, the other, harmony. Then, have students sing the song with soloists or small groups on the verse and the whole class on the refrain.

Playing

"Four Strong Winds" has only three chords—G, C, and D_7. Invite students to accompany the song on guitar. (See Skills Reinforcement below for a recorder counter-melody.)

3 CLOSE

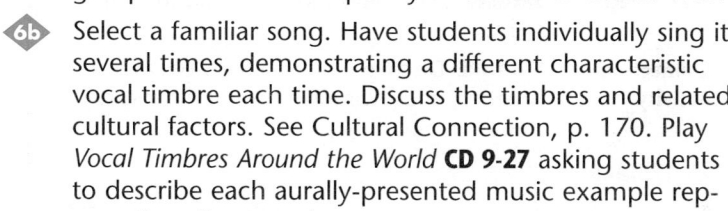
Element: TIMBRE   **ASSESSMENT**

7a **Music Journal Writing** Have students listen to *Vocal Timbres Around the World* **CD 9-27** and write three adjectives in their music journals, using standard terminology to describe the vocal timbre in each example. Then, students may write about their preferences with regard to the examples of vocal timbre.

SKILLS REINFORCEMENT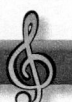

1d ▶ **Vocal Development** To help students sing in sixths, practice singing scales and simple folk songs or phrases in sixths. Model the harmony part first while students sing the melody.

Use *Hot Cross Buns* in G major for singing sixths below the melody. The harmony part is in a good range for cambiata voices.

▶ **Recorder** You may wish to have some students learn and play the recorder part on Resource Book p. I-16 as additional harmony for "Four Strong Winds."

▶ **Guitar** Beginning guitar students may be more successful playing G, C, and D_7 chords if the class is divided into three groups. Have each group play the same, single chord each time it occurs in the song.

TECHNOLOGY/MEDIA LINK

4b **Notation Software** Have students use notation software to create their own arrangement of "Four Strong Winds." Invite students to set up two staves in treble clef and one staff in bass clef.

Have students select the key of G and notate the melody and harmony parts of the song on the treble staves. Ask them to create an accompaniment on the bass staff, using the chord roots found in the song notation and selecting their own rhythm patterns. Invite students to experiment with the playback timbre of the song.

LESSON AT A GLANCE

Element Focus **TEXTURE/HARMONY** Harmony in thirds, homophonic texture

Skill Objective **SINGING** Sing two songs with harmony in thirds

Connection Activity **CULTURE** Discover folk traditions of Latin America, and their influence on American music

MATERIALS

- "Así es mi tierra" **CD 9-30**
- "This Is My Land" **CD 9-31**

    Recording Routine: Intro (4 m.); vocal; coda

- **Pronunciation Practice/Translation** p. 529
- "Habemos llegado" **CD 10-1**
- "We Have Arrived" **CD 10-2**

    Recording Routine Intro (8 m.); v. 1; interlude (4 m.); v. 2; instrumental (16 m.); v. 1; coda

- **Pronunciation Practice/Translation** p. 530
- **Dance Directions** for "Así es mi tierra" p. 557
- **Resource Book** pp. A-16, A-17, H-16
- keyboard, mallet instruments, guitar, conga drums, maracas, *guiro*, claves, and cowbell

VOCABULARY

duet   interval   thirds   homophonic

música norteña   chords   *tremolo*

◆ ◆ ◆ ◆ National Standards ◆ ◆ ◆ ◆

1a Sing accurately with good breath control
1d Sing music written in two parts
2a Play instruments accurately alone and in small ensembles
3a Improvise simple harmonic accompaniments
6b Listen and analyze uses of harmony and texture in music from diverse cultures
9b Describe characteristics of music styles from a variety of cultures

MORE MUSIC CHOICES

For more practice singing thirds:

"Las mañanitas," p. 481

"Abraham, Martin, and John," p. 466

Spanish TEXTURES

People who begin a new life in another part of the world take their folk tales, history, and music with them. In Texas, the *música norteña* style is a blend of Mexican and German heritages. The song "Así es mi tierra" is in the *norteña* style.

> A **duet** is a piece written to be played or sung by two performers.

Sing the melody, then sing the harmony part for "Así es mi tierra." Next, sing the song in two-part harmony as a **duet**.

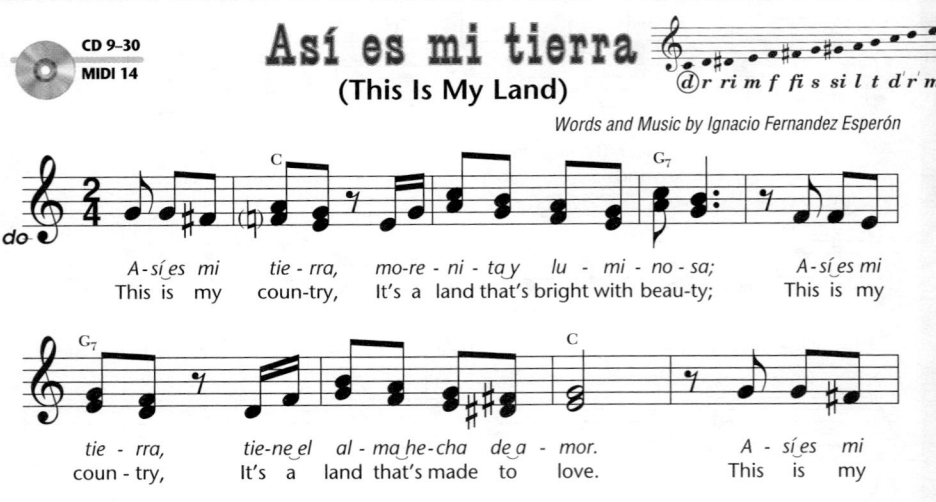

CD 9–30
MIDI 14

Así es mi tierra
(This Is My Land)

Words and Music by Ignacio Fernandez Esperón

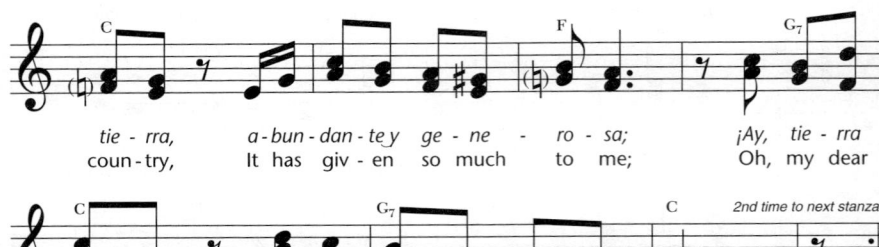

A-sí es mi   tie - rra,   mo-re-ni - ta y   lu - mi - no - sa;   A-sí es mi
This is my   coun-try,   It's a   land that's bright with beau-ty;   This is my

tie - rra,   tie-ne el   al - ma he-cha   de a - mor.   A - sí es   mi
coun - try,   It's a   land that's made to   love.   This is   my

tie - rra,   a-bun-dan-te y   ge - ne -   ro - sa;   ¡Ay, tie - rra
coun - try,   It has giv - en   so much   to me;   Oh, my dear

mí -   a   co-mo es   gra - to   tu   ca - lor!   2nd time to next stanza
coun - try,   Wel-come are   your   gifts   of   love.

172

Footnotes

CULTURAL CONNECTION

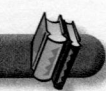

▶ *Música Norteña* "Así es mi tierra" is a good example of *música norteña*. It began in Texas as a blend of the Mexican American Latino style of music (harmony in thirds) with the German American polka tradition. Today, the style is well known in Mexican American communities far beyond Texas.

BUILDING SKILLS THROUGH MUSIC

▶ **Social Studies** Have students do independent research to identify communities where there is a blend of German and Mexican heritage (Texas) or the blend of two cultures in their communities.

ACROSS THE CURRICULUM

▶ **Language Arts** Read aloud the book *I Have Heard of a Land* by Joyce Carol Thomas (HarperCollins, 1998). It is a tribute to the pioneer spirit necessary to tame a new land. Invite students to consider the importance of their homes and to list things they would need to begin a new life in another country.

▶ **Social Studies** Invite students to learn about Puerto Rico. In 1917, Puerto Rico became an official territory of the United States. Its people were granted American citizenship and open passage to the mainland. In 1952, Puerto Rico became a commonwealth of the United States with its own constitution. Today, Puerto Ricans are deciding the issue of statehood. About 3.8 million people live in Puerto Rico, and more than two million Puerto Ricans live in the mainland United States.

Harmony Produces Texture

Perform the harmony part of *"Así es mi tierra"* again. Notice that the harmony supports the main melody. It is not a separate melody. This texture is known as **homophonic**.

Homophonic texture is a melody supported by harmony.

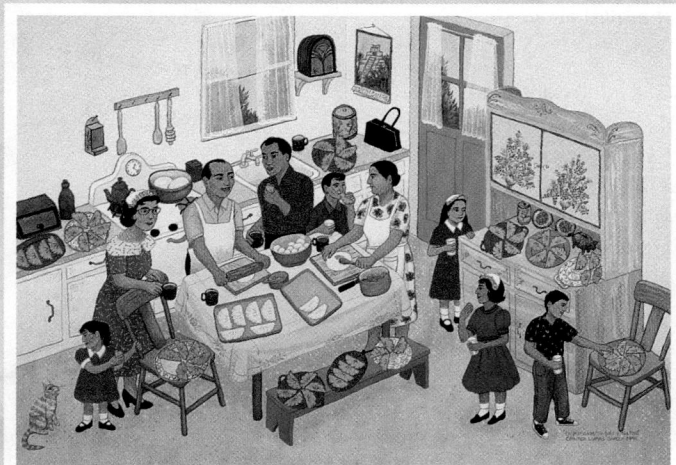

Arts Connection

◄ *Empanadas* by Carmen Lomas Garza

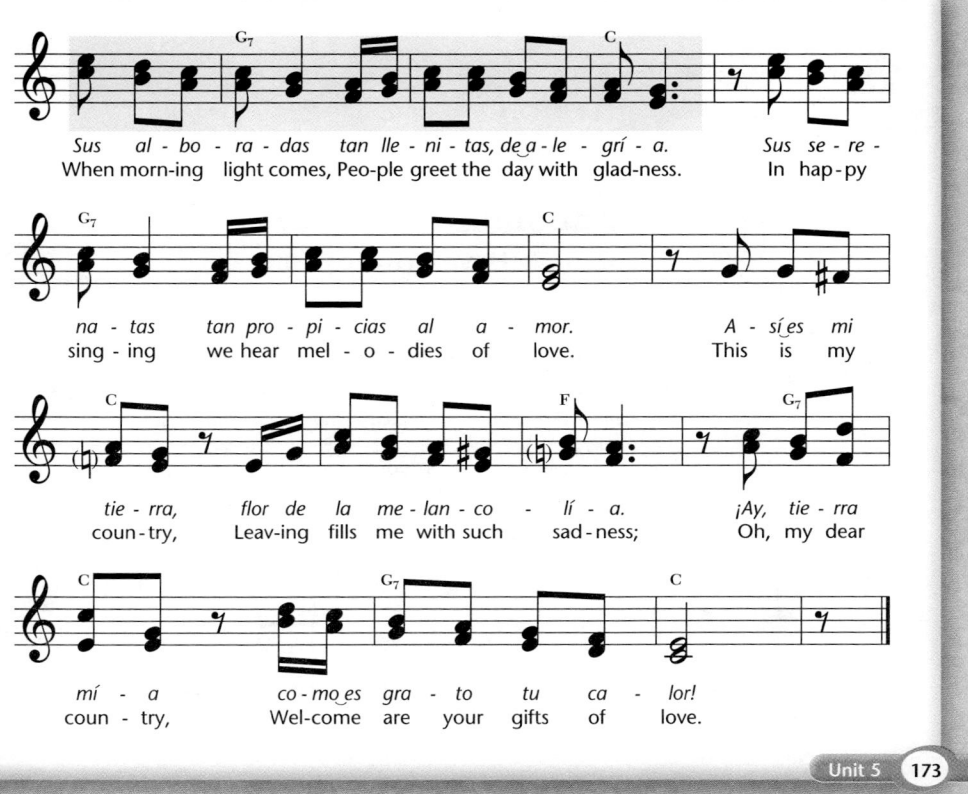

Sus al - bo - ra - das tan lle - ni - tas, de_a - le - grí - a.
When morn-ing light comes, Peo-ple greet the day with glad-ness.
Sus se - re -
In hap-py

na - tas tan pro - pi - cias al a - mor.
sing - ing we hear mel - o - dies of love.
A - sí_es mi
This is my

tie - rra, flor de la me - lan - co - lí - a.
coun - try, Leav-ing fills me with such sad-ness;
¡Ay, tie - rra
Oh, my dear

mí - a co - mo_es gra - to tu ca - lor!
coun - try, Wel-come are your gifts of love.

Unit 5　173

1 INTRODUCE

Tell students that Latin America includes Mexico, the Caribbean, and Central and South America. Have them find these areas on a map. Lead them to discover that Latin American music is popular in the United States and that Latin style sometimes blends with other cultural styles *(música norteña)*. Share the information in Cultural Connection on p. 172.

2 DEVELOP

Singing

1c **1d** Encourage the students to use the Pronunciation Practice **CD 9-33** to learn the Spanish text of *"Así es mi tierra."* Have students independently sing the melody **CD 9-33**, then sing the harmony **CD 9-34**. Then have them sing the song **CD 9-30** in two parts with accurate intonation, demonstrating fundamental skills.

Analyzing

Have students sing just the harmony part for *"Así es mi tierra"* without the recording, then the top line.

1a **ASK Did the harmony part stand alone well as a melody?** (no)

6b Help students understand that the two parts have the same rhythm and words, but different pitches that are close together. Explain that melody supported by harmony is known as homophonic texture.

Moving

Invite students to learn the patterned dance routine for *"Así es mi tierra,"* in the Dance Directions on p. 557. Use the Dance Practice **CD 9-36** to teach the routine; then, use the Dance Performance **CD 9-35** when students are ready to perform the dance.

Students may wish to create a movement pattern for *"Así es mi tierra."* Ask them to vary their movements according to phrases, or melody vs. melody with harmony.

continued on page 174

SKILLS REINFORCEMENT

▶ **Playing** Have students play the following ostinato on rhythm instruments as an accompaniment for *"Así es mi tierra."*

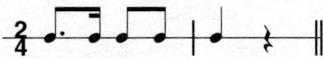

 ▶ **Keyboard** For a complete keyboard accompaniment for *"Así es mi tierra"* that uses the rhythm ostinato above, see Resource Book p. H-16.

TEACHER TO TEACHER

▶ **Degrees of Bodily Movement** Guide students to become more confident in using movement to express what they hear in the music.

Reinforcement Students who lack confidence in dancing may begin with smaller gestures, or even movement in place, such as subtle swaying with *"Habemos llegado"* **CD 10-1.**

On Target Have students perform a nonlocomotor movement (see Movement, p. 174) as a next step to dancing. Add other movement activities, such as steps and formations.

Challenge Invite students to model movements you create and to improvise their own movements. Modeling movement can be a means of both challenging advance students and encouraging hesitant students.

Listening

Ask students to listen to *"Habemos llegado"* **CD 10-1.** Guide them to describe the cultural and musical characteristics of the song. (Spanish language, guitars, *cuatros,* harmony in thirds)

Analyzing

Direct students to the song notation for *"Habemos llegado."* Have them

- Analyze and describe the melody and the interval of the harmony (a third below the melody).
- Understand that the melody and harmony have the same rhythm and words, but they have different pitches that are close together (harmony).

Tell students that melody supported by harmony is known as homophonic texture.

Guide students to analyze the chord changes (i, iv, V) in the song and understand that a root-note with two thirds (or third and fifth) stacked above it is called a chord.

Singing

Invite students to use Pronunciation Practice **CD 10-4** and **CD 10-5** to learn the Spanish lyrics to *"Habemos llegado."* Then, have students independently

- Sight-sing the melody on a neutral syllable.
- Sing the melody while listening for chord changes, indicating whether the chord is i, iv, or V.
- Sing just the harmony part, a third lower than the melody with the recording.
- Sing the song in two parts as a duet.

Playing

Help students review the chord changes in *"Habemos llegado"* **CD 10-1.** As they listen, have them indicate with one, four, or five fingers the tonic (i), subdominant (iv), and dominant (V$_7$) chords.

Invite students to create an accompaniment to *"Habemos llegado"* on guitar or keyboard. Have students

Caribbean Harmonies

Homophonic texture, using harmony in thirds, is also a part of the music of Caribbean and other Latin cultures. Singers often create harmony by singing intervals of a third above or below a melody.

Listen to *"Habemos llegado,"* a folk song from Puerto Rico. As you listen, indicate where the homophonic texture and harmony in thirds occur. Use the Pronunciation Practice track to learn the Spanish words, melody, and harmony parts. When you are ready, **sing** *"Habemos llegado."*

From Harmony to Chords

Caribbean singers are often accompanied by guitars or *cuatros.* These chord instruments play chords based on the harmony of a song.

Analyze the three chords in *"Habemos llegado."* **Sing** the root of each chord and then **play** it on keyboard.

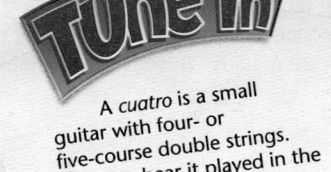

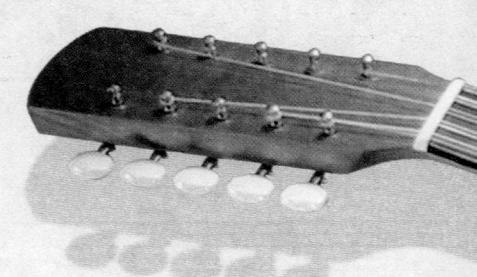

A *cuatro* is a small guitar with four- or five-course double strings. You may hear it played in the music of South America, Mexico, and the Caribbean.

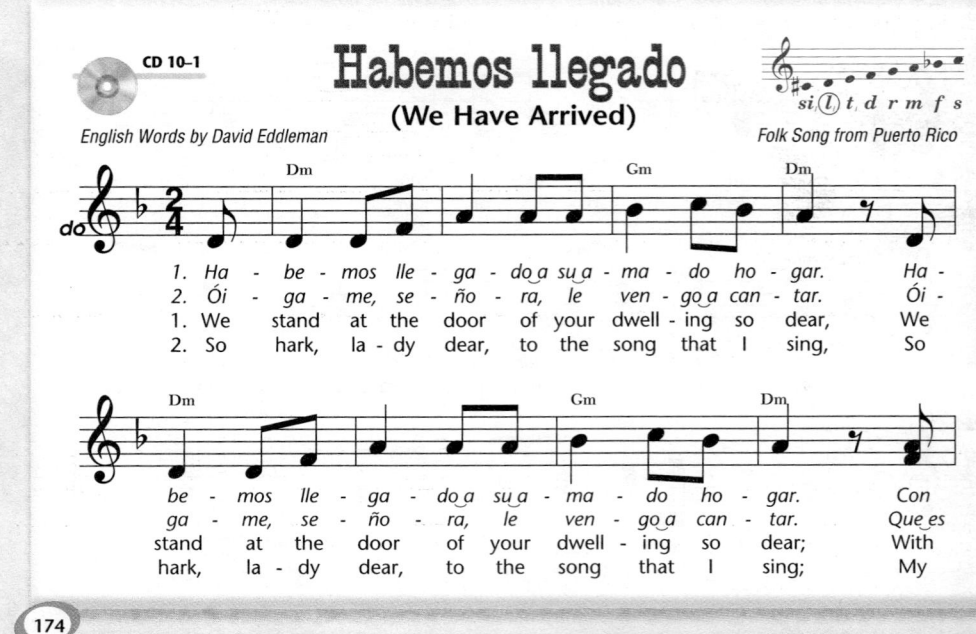

Habemos llegado
(We Have Arrived)

CD 10–1

English Words by David Eddleman

Folk Song from Puerto Rico

1. Ha - be - mos lle - ga - do a su a - ma - do ho - gar. Ha -
2. Ói - ga - me, se - ño - ra, le ven - go a can - tar. Ói -
1. We stand at the door of your dwell - ing so dear, We
2. So hark, la - dy dear, to the song that I sing, So

be - mos lle - ga - do a su a - ma - do ho - gar. Con
ga - me, se - ño - ra, le ven - go a can - tar. Que es
stand at the door of your dwell - ing so dear; With
hark, la - dy dear, to the song that I sing; My

174

Footnotes

MOVEMENT

▶ **Nonlocomotor Movement** Ask students to follow the chord progression to *"Habemos llegando"* **CD 10-1.** as they listen to the recording. Tell students they will use their entire body to face in the direction associated with a given chord. On I, face forward/front, turn right for the IV chords, and turn left for the V chords. Have students perform the movements as you play the recording again.

SKILLS REINFORCEMENT

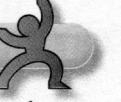 ▶ **Percussion** Ask students to perform this two-measure ostinato as an accompaniment to *"Habemos llegado."*

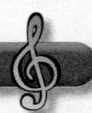

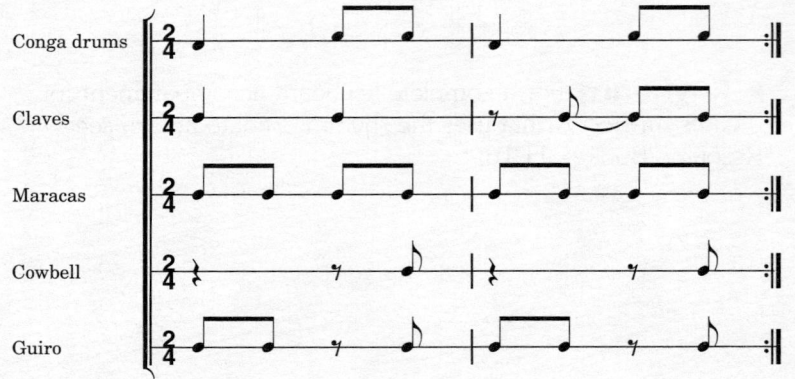

Conga drums

Claves

Maracas

Cowbell

Guiro

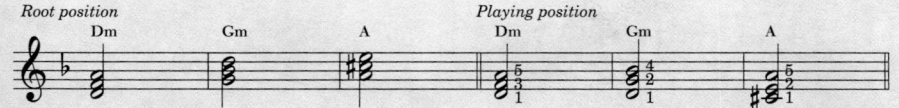

Root position   Playing position

Play the chords for *"Habemos llegado"* on keyboard, or bells. Experiment with creating rhythms that may accompany the song.

Keyboard chords for Habemos llegado

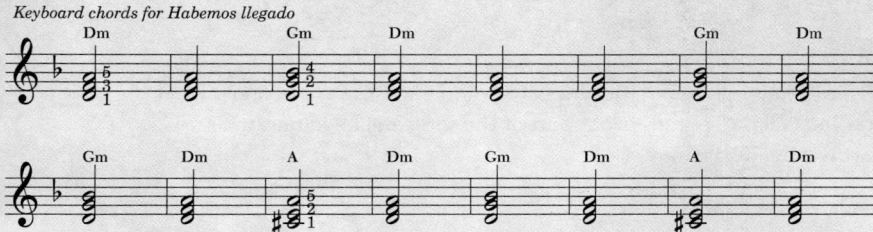

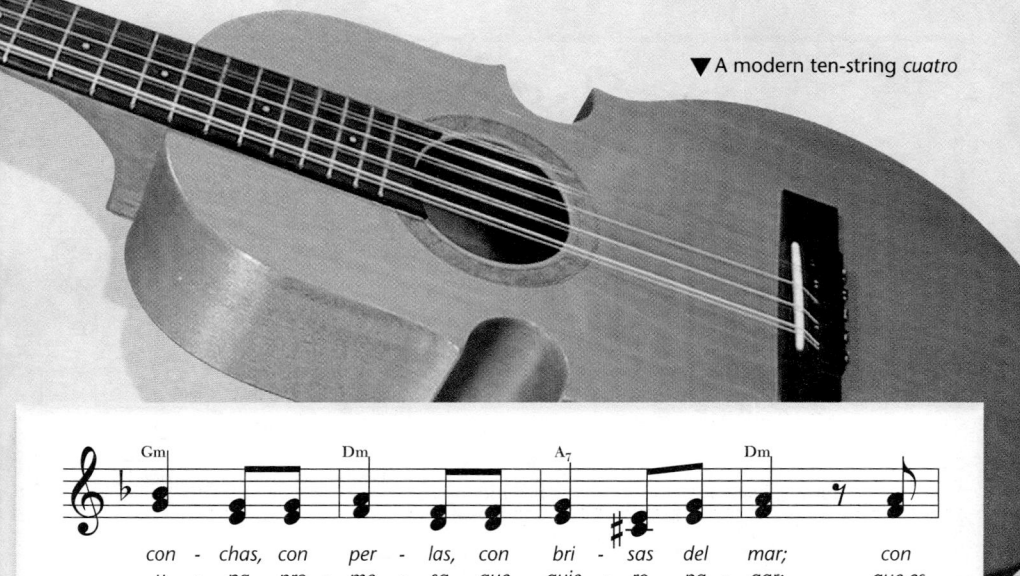

▼ A modern ten-string *cuatro*

con - chas, con per - las, con bri - sas del mar;   con
u - na pro - me - sa que quie - ro pa - gar;   que es
shells and with pearls and with sea breez - es near,   With
prom - ise to keep is the song that I bring,   My

con - chas, con per - las, con bri - sas del mar.
u - na pro - me - sa que quie - ro pa - gar.
shells and with pearls and with sea breez - es near.
prom - ise to keep is the song that I bring.

Unit 5   **175**

2a
- Play the Dm, Gm, and A₇ chords for *"Habemos llegado,"* on keyboard or guitar. (See p. 175, and pp. 508–509.)
- On keyboard, play the chords in root position (p. 175). Have them analyze the letter-names of the chord tones and locate them in the Dm scale.
- On keyboard, learn to play chords in "playing position" (p. 175) so that their hands remain more stationary rather than move about the keyboard.
- Play the chord progression for *"Habemos llegado."*

When ready, divide the class into groups. Invite each group to perform their chord accompaniment to *"Habemos llegado"* as the class sings the song in harmony.

Improvising

3a   Invite students to create an improvisation to accompany *"Habemos llegado."* Have students

- Play the chords for *"Habemos llegado"* on mallet instruments (Alto 1, Alto 2). Tell students, Alto 1 can play the root and third while Alto 2 can play the root and fifth. To sustain the sound of the pitches on wooden xylophones, play in a *tremolo* manner.
- Play the chords on guitar with a rhythm strum.
- Use Puerto Rican percussion instruments (conga drums, claves, cowbell, maracas, and *guiro*) to improvise a rhythm accompaniment.

3 CLOSE

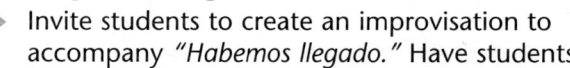

Element: TEXTURE/HARMONY —ASSESSMENT

Performance/Observation Divide the class into groups of four. Have two students in each group sing the melody of *"Así es mi tierra"* and the other two sing only the harmony part without the recording. Switch parts. Repeat with other groups until you have assessed everyone's ability to sing in homophonic texture.

CULTURAL CONNECTION

▶ **Music of Puerto Rico** Students may be interested in learning about the music of Puerto Rico. Puerto Rico is home to frequent music-making activity, especially during holidays. The Puerto Rican communities in the United States carry on this tradition of song, dance, and lively instrumental music. At Christmas, *aguinaldos* permeate the homes of Puerto Ricans. Like carols, they are learned "by heart" at an early age. While the melodies of *aguinaldos* may settle into minor keys, the communal harmonies and brisk tempos communicate the joys of the season.

TECHNOLOGY/MEDIA LINK

CD-ROM Invite students to use *Band-in-a-Box* to explore the musical styles of Mexico, *música norteña,* Puerto Rico, the islands of the Caribbean, and other Latin American countries. Ask students to enter the chord progression for *"Así es mi tierra"* and *"Habemos llegado"* into the software. Invite them to explore various Latin styles of music using this chord progression. Remind students to change the tempo if the musical style requires a different tempo.

Electronic Keyboard Have students use the auto-accompaniment feature of a keyboard to play one-finger accompaniments in Mexican, *música norteña,* Puerto Rican, Caribbean, and other Latin American musical styles.

LESSON AT A GLANCE

Element Focus   **TEXTURE/HARMONY** Harmony in thirds and sixths

Skill Objective   **SINGING** Sing a two-part song in thirds and sixths

Connection Activity   **MATHEMATICS** Use counting to find intervals of a sixth and a third

MATERIALS

- "Vive l'amour"   **CD 10-6**
  Recording Routine: Intro (8 m.), v. 1, refrain, v. 2, refrain, coda
- "Pie Jesu" from *Requiem*   **CD 10-8**
- "Pie Jesu" from *Requiem* (Church) (excerpt)   **CD 10-9**
- **Resource Book** p. J-8
- keyboard or resonator bells, guitar, Autoharp

VOCABULARY

third   sixth   soprano   duet
monophonic   homophonic   polyphonic

◆ ◆ ◆ ◆ National Standards ◆ ◆ ◆ ◆

1a Sing accurately with good breath control
1d Sing music written in two parts
2b Perform easy instrumental pieces with technical accuracy
5d Use standard notation to record musical ideas
6a Listen and describe events in music using appropriate terms
6b Listen and analyze uses of harmony and texture in music from diverse genres
6c Understand and use basic principles of intervals in music analysis
7a Create standards for evaluating performances

MORE MUSIC CHOICES

For more practice singing in thirds and sixths:
"Four Strong Winds," p. 170
"Abraham, Martin, and John," p. 466
"Fais do do," p. 403

STEPS TO Harmony

Sing *"Vive l'amour."* Some of the lyrics are not in English. Do you know what language you will be singing? What part of the song will be in unison and what part will be in harmony?

Revisiting Intervals

The distance between two pitches is an interval. When sounded together, some intervals produce harmonies that are more pleasant to our ears than others. Two such intervals are thirds and sixths.

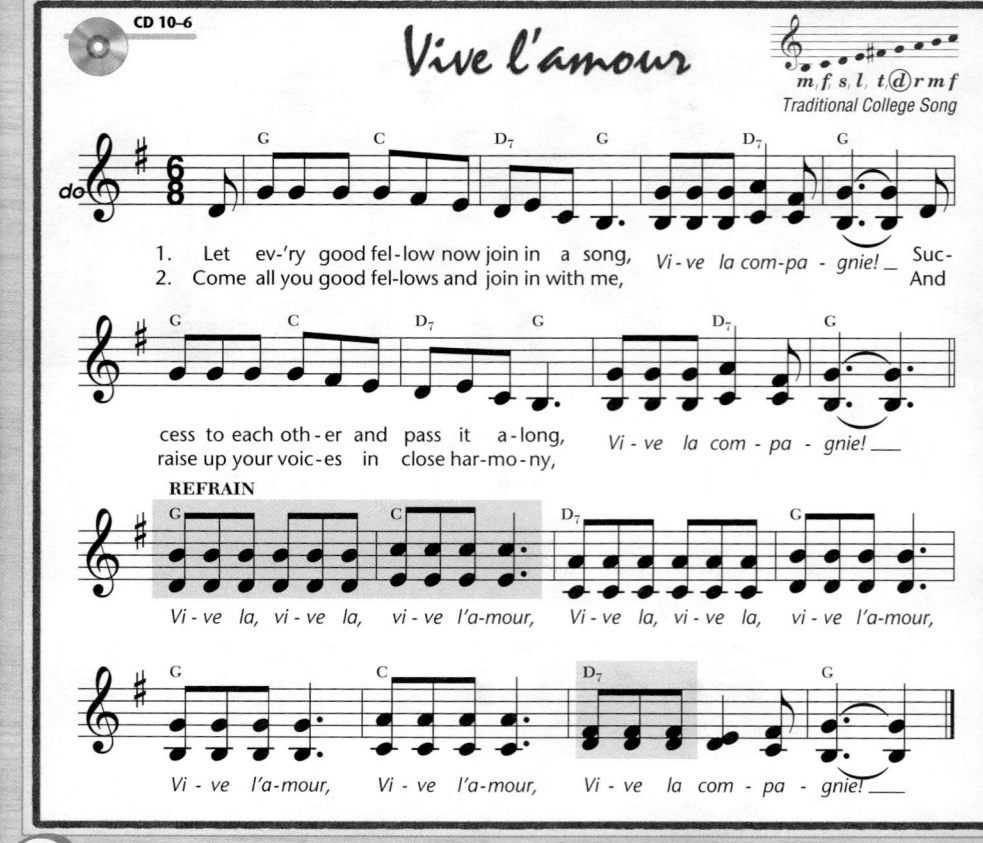

Footnotes

CULTURAL CONNECTION

▶ **French Culture** French culture is renowned for its art, food, wine, architecture, literature, and fashion, among many other things. Travelers to Paris, the capital of France, enjoy the architecture of Notre Dame de Paris and the art of Le Louvre. Students may enjoy researching France and its culture.

BUILDING SKILLS THROUGH MUSIC

▶ **Language** Have students read the Music Maker on Charlotte Church on p. 178, then identify the author's purpose in writing this.

SKILLS REINFORCEMENT

▶ **Guitar** *"Vive l'amour"* is a three-chord song (G, C, and D₇) that can be accompanied with guitar.

2b First have students accompany the refrain. Ask students to practice a G, C, D₇, G progression before they accompany the verse. They will strum each chord four times before changing, then two times, and finally only one time. The open G tuning on guitar on p. 358 may make the accompaniment easier to play. Allow students to review all chords on p. 360 and students can use a G (partial) chord in place of the full G chord.

Remind students that the challenge of playing guitar is a combination of memorizing fingerings, placing the fingers, and changing chords in time to music. Playing and coordination will improve with practice and time.

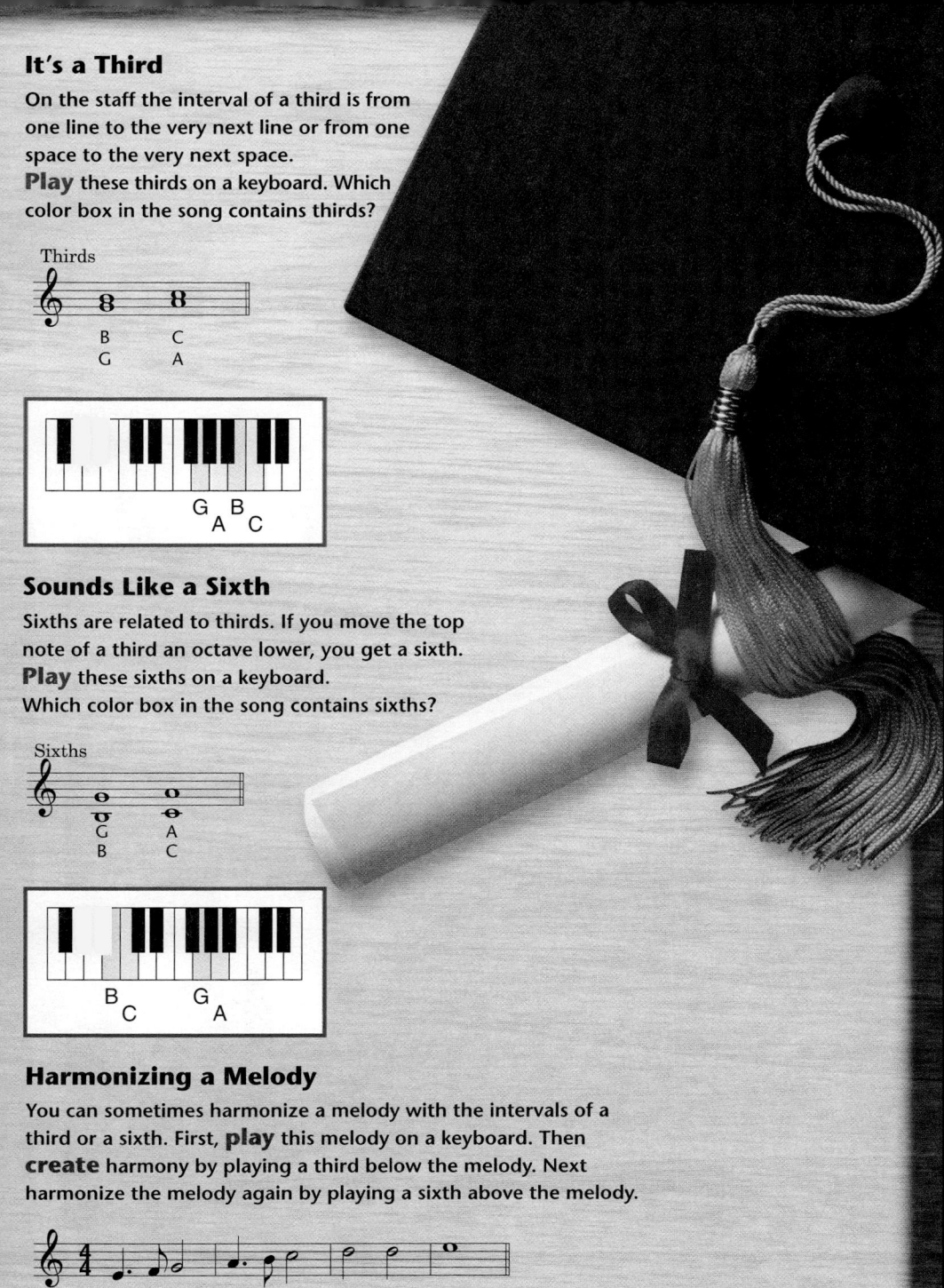

It's a Third

On the staff the interval of a third is from one line to the very next line or from one space to the very next space.

Play these thirds on a keyboard. Which color box in the song contains thirds?

Sounds Like a Sixth

Sixths are related to thirds. If you move the top note of a third an octave lower, you get a sixth.
Play these sixths on a keyboard.
Which color box in the song contains sixths?

Harmonizing a Melody

You can sometimes harmonize a melody with the intervals of a third or a sixth. First, **play** this melody on a keyboard. Then **create** harmony by playing a third below the melody. Next harmonize the melody again by playing a sixth above the melody.

Unit 5   **177**

1 INTRODUCE

Ask students to identify songs they have sung on camping trips, scouting events, church outings, field trips, or other social events. Explain that *"Vive l'amour"* is a "social event" song that has been sung for generations by college groups. Tell students that in this lesson, they will sing and listen to music that has harmony in thirds and sixths.

2 DEVELOP

Analyzing

Explain to students that they can find an interval by starting on the bottom note (counting it as 1) and counting up the scale steps to the top note. The number of the top note is the number of the interval.

6c Help students to

6b
- Discover that the harmony of *"Vive l'amour"* is mostly sixths (thirds are used in the penultimate measure).

- Find that *"Vive l'amour"* uses two languages and two textures in the vocal line: French = homophonic texture, English = unison singing.

- Review the sound of sixths and of thirds before singing them, playing them as shown on p. 177 on keyboard or resonator bells.

Additional activities with intervals can be found in Resource Book p. J-8.

TEACHER TO TEACHER

1d ▶ **Changing Voices** Boys with changing voices are often capable of singing only a limited range of pitches. The harmony part for *"Vive l'amour"* uses only four pitches (B, C, D, and E) and provides a comfortable range for boys whose voices are changing.

▶ **Singing Harmony** Singing parallel sixths is difficult for many young singers. To help students achieve success singing *"Vive l'amour"* in two parts, limit initial experiences to singing only the verse in harmony. Help harmony singers notice that the last unison pitch (B) of the verse is also the first pitch of the harmony part. Have students sing the first phrase in unison, then hold the first two-part chord. Sing the refrain in harmony only after students can sing the verse in two parts.

AUDIENCE ETIQUETTE

▶ **Audience Etiquette and Participation** Ask students if they have ever sung as a group in a public setting (a restaurant, a birthday party, a wedding). *Vive l'amour* is a traditional college song that may have been sung by students in public places such as restaurants. Guide students to understand that when singing as a group in public places, there are rules to follow. For example, ask if it is all right to sing in that location. Be considerate of other people in the area, and, perhaps, don't sing too loudly. Being considerate and courteous is a good general guideline to follow at all times.

Contrast this with proper audience etiquette at a performance of Charlotte Church either at an opera or in one of her pop concerts.

Lesson 11 Continued

Singing

1d Invite students to sing the melody of *"Vive l'amour"* **CD 10-6.** Select a small group of students to sing the harmony part. Have students sing the song in two parts with the recording.

Playing

Invite students to independently perform the melody on p. 177 on keyboard or bells and harmonize it using thirds. Then, encourage them to harmonize the melody, using sixths. Have students perform with accurate rhythm, demonstrating performance techniques.

Listening

Engage students in a discussion of the requiem as a musical genre that comes from a religious setting. See Spotlight On below.

Draw students' attention to the listening map for *Pie Jesu* [PEE-ay-YAY-soo]. Tell students that candles represent one beat. The large candle shows the downbeat.

ASK **Which lines are played only by instruments?** (the first and fourth lines)

    Will any part of the music repeat? (Yes, lines 2 and 3 will repeat.)

6a Encourage students to tap or point to each candle (beat) as they listen to *Pie Jesu* **CD 10-8.** Note that the rhythm of the introduction is mostly eighth notes.

ASK **How many voices did you hear?** (two, a female soprano and a boy soprano)

    Did the voices sing in unison or harmony? (They each sing alone, then sing in harmony.)

Encourage students to listen to the recording again and to identify which line is mostly in thirds. (the third line)

6b **ASK** **Is this music mostly monophonic, polyphonic, or homophonic in texture?** (homophonic)

    Which are the two sections with no voices? (introduction and interlude)

Harmonies of Angels

Pie Jesu is a duet sung by a woman soprano and a boy soprano. Part of this duet is sung in thirds.

Follow the listening map on page 179. As you **listen** to the music, identify the sections where you hear thirds in the melody.

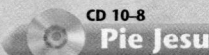
CD 10-8
Pie Jesu

**from *Requiem*
by Andrew Lloyd Webber**

Now **listen** to a solo performance.

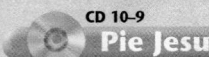
CD 10-9
Pie Jesu

**from *Requiem*
by Andrew Lloyd Webber
as performed by Charlotte Church**

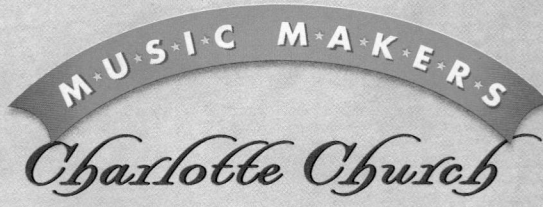

MUSIC MAKERS

Charlotte Church

Charlotte Church (born 1986) is one of today's biggest young superstars. Church's international career began at age 11 when she performed *Pie Jesu* on a British television show. Her debut album, *Voice of an Angel*, has sold over two million records.

Church has expanded her singing repertoire from that of opera to a variety of musical styles that include Broadway musicals, Gaelic songs, and popular music. By age 16, her achievements included four albums with international sales of over 10 million records, a platinum record in the United States, and performances to sellout crowds.

Church has performed for many famous people including President Clinton, Prince Charles, and the Queen of England.

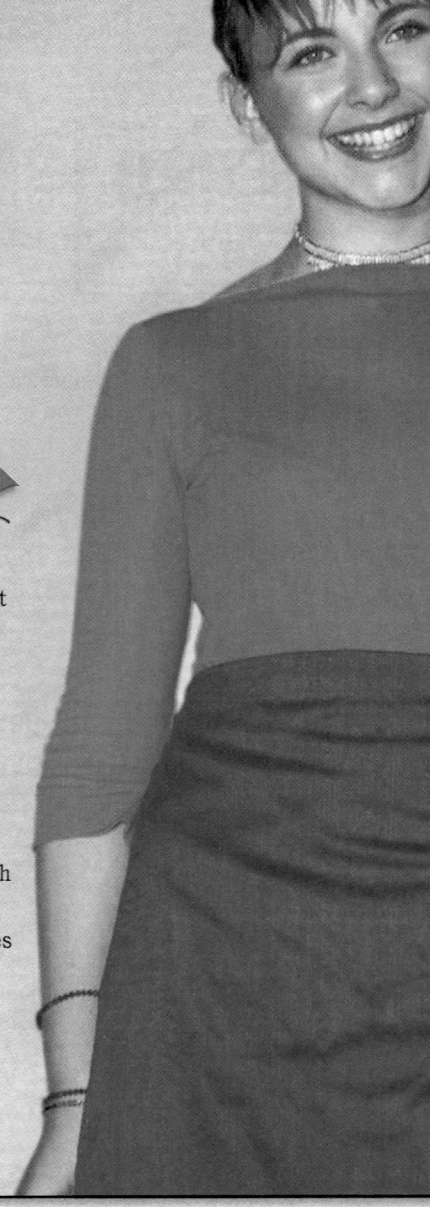

178

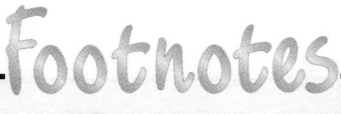

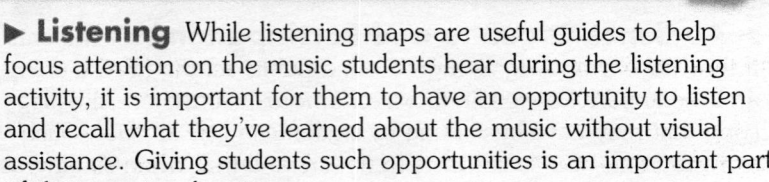 **TEACHER TO TEACHER**

▶ **Listening** While listening maps are useful guides to help focus attention on the music students hear during the listening activity, it is important for them to have an opportunity to listen and recall what they've learned about the music without visual assistance. Giving students such opportunities is an important part of their music education.

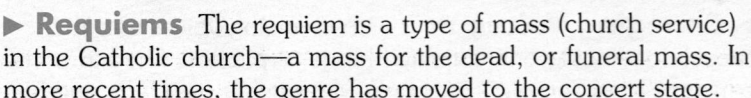 **SPOTLIGHT ON**

▶ **Requiems** The requiem is a type of mass (church service) in the Catholic church—a mass for the dead, or funeral mass. In more recent times, the genre has moved to the concert stage.

Pie Jesu is an important part of the requiem. Your students might enjoy hearing the *Pie Jesu* from the requiem by French composer Gabriel Fauré. Performed by a soprano soloist, the text of Fauré's *Pie Jesu* is identical to that of the *Pie Jesu* written by Webber because it uses the requiem mass text, and all musical settings of the requiem mass will have very nearly the same text, usually in Latin.

Mapping Harmony

Follow the listening map for *Pie Jesu*. Where are the singers singing in thirds? Where are they singing in sixths?

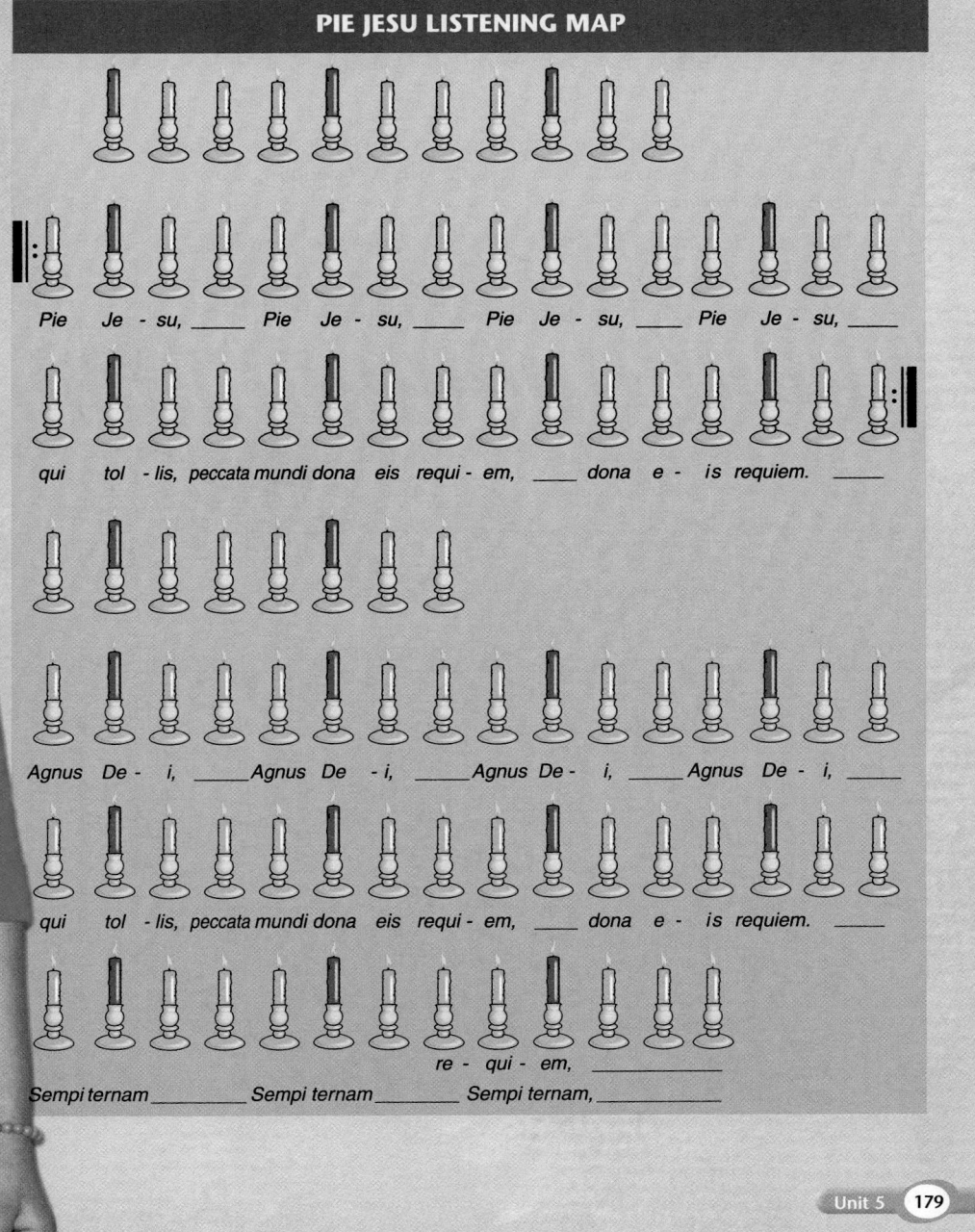

PIE JESU LISTENING MAP

Pie   Je - su, _____   Pie   Je - su, _____   Pie   Je - su, _____   Pie   Je - su, _____

qui   tol - lis, peccata mundi dona eis requi - em, ____ dona e - is requiem. _____

Agnus De - i, _____Agnus De - i, _____Agnus De - i, _____Agnus De - i, _____

qui   tol - lis, peccata mundi dona eis requi - em, ____ dona e - is requiem. _____

re - qui - em, _____
Sempiternam _____ Sempiternam _____ Sempiternam, _____

Have students read the Music Makers on Charlotte Church. Then, ask them to listen to *Pie Jesu* once more, with Charlotte Church singing **CD 10-9**.

7a Invite students to evaluate the quality of the music, and musical performance, in both listening selections for *Pie Jesu* as if they were writing a concert review for a newspaper. Have students first identify the criteria for evaluating the performance before they begin writing. Their review and criteria may include

- Was the music well written? Was the melody pleasing?
- Did the expression of the music match its purpose? (soft and melancholy; purpose—music for a requiem)
- Was the singing accurate in intonation and rhythm?
- Did the singers phrase the melody appropriately? (Yes; long, legato phrases.)
- Was the vocal timbre and quality of the singers pleasing? Did the pair of singers blend well?
- How was Charlotte Church's performance and singing technique? (Performance: great performance. Technique: beautiful vocal quality and timbre, able to sing in a high range, good control of voice, good breath control and phrasing, sings in tune.)

Have students write their review (evaluations and impressions) in their music journals.

3 CLOSE

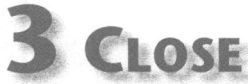

Element: TEXTURE/HARMONY   ASSESSMENT

Performance/Observation Have students sing *"Vive l'amour"* in two parts. Observe and assess their ability to sing the intervals of thirds and sixths in tune.

SKILLS REINFORCEMENT

1a ▶ **Vocal Development** Vibrato is a slight fluctuation in pitch that sounds like a single pitch. In singing, vibrato is the result of developing a good vocal technique. Students who support and sustain the breath will naturally sing with a vibrato. A natural vibrato will have a resonant and rich tone.

Too much vibrato can sound like out-of-tune singing and is the result of poor breath management. Students who sing with too much vibrato typically are forcing the vibration with their throat rather than sustaining the vibration through breath management. This type of singing should not be encouraged. Practice breath support and control exercises if this problem occurs.

TECHNOLOGY/MEDIA LINK

5d **Notation Software** Have students use notation software to harmonize a melody with thirds and sixths. Have pairs harmonize their melody by copying the melody to a "new" staff, and raising and lowering the notes, compared to the melody, by a third or sixth.

Web Site Encourage students to visit *www.sfsuccessnet.com* to find out more about Andrew Lloyd Webber and his music.

Transparency Display the listening map transparency for *Pie Jesu*. Invite students to trace the progress of the selection with a finger on the map in their books as you trace on the overhead projection.

LESSON AT A GLANCE

Element Focus TEXTURE/HARMONY Chordal accompaniment

Skill Objective PLAYING Play a chordal accompaniment while singing a song

Connection Activity STYLE Discuss calypso style and its origins in the West Indies

MATERIALS

- "Mary Ann" CD 10-10

  Recording Routine: Intro (4 m.); v. 1; interlude (4 m.); v. 2; interlude (4 m.); v. 3; coda
- **Dance Directions** for "Mary Ann" p. 559
- **Resource Book** p. I-17
- hand chimes or resonator bells, glockenspiel, alto metallophone, bass xylophone, maracas, claves, bongo drums, conga drums, world map

VOCABULARY

calypso harmony chords

◆ ◆ ◆ ◆ National Standards ◆ ◆ ◆ ◆

1d Sing music written in two parts
2b Perform easy instrumental pieces with technical accuracy
2c Perform instrumental music from diverse cultures
4c Compose, using electronic media

MORE MUSIC CHOICES

Another song with mallet accompaniment:
"Evening Chaconne," p. 202
Other songs from the Caribbean:
"Give a Little Love," p. 140
"Water Come a Me Eye," p. 300
"By the Waters of Babylon," p. 311

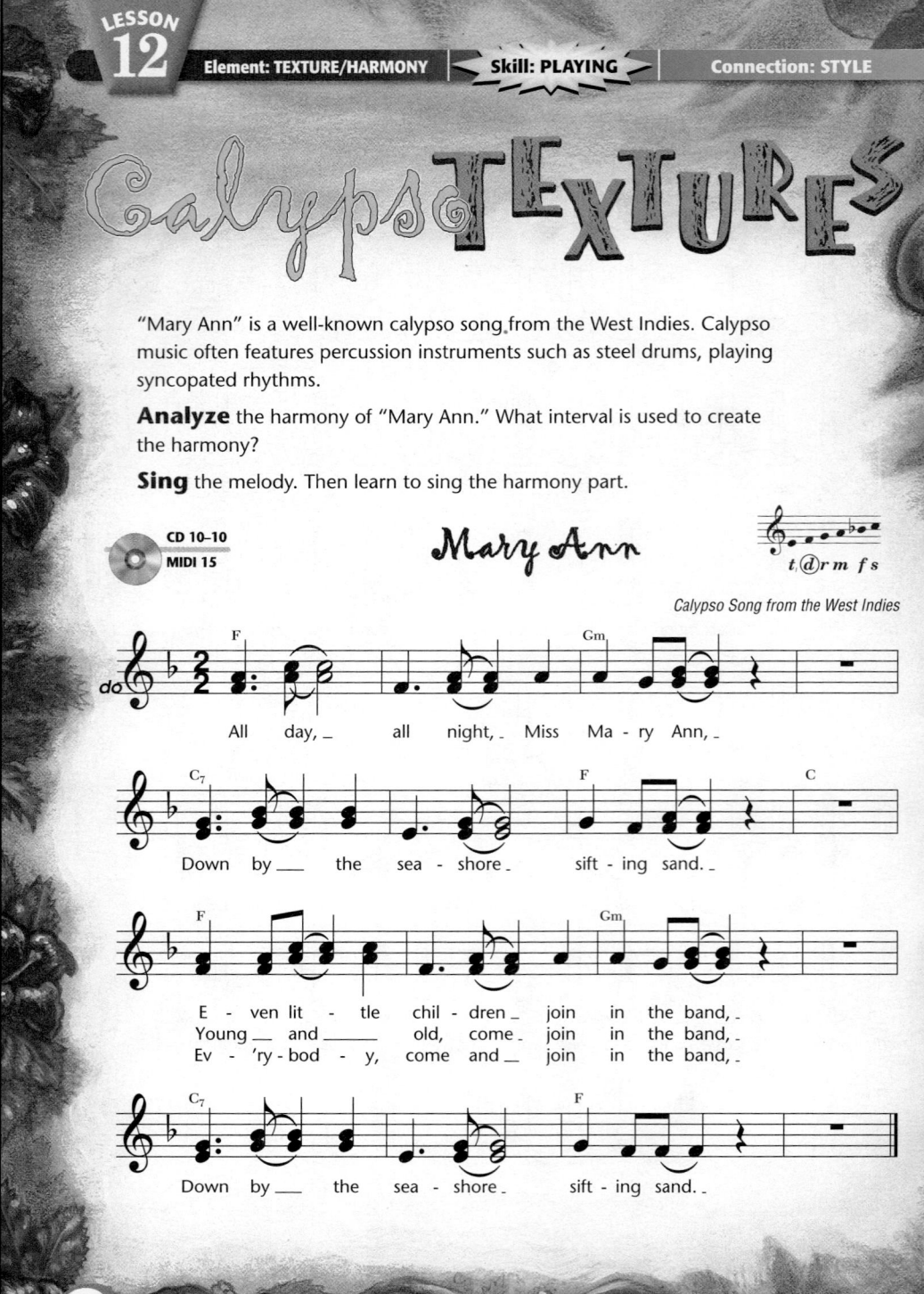

Calypso TEXTURES

"Mary Ann" is a well-known calypso song from the West Indies. Calypso music often features percussion instruments such as steel drums, playing syncopated rhythms.

Analyze the harmony of "Mary Ann." What interval is used to create the harmony?

Sing the melody. Then learn to sing the harmony part.

CD 10-10
MIDI 15

Mary Ann

Calypso Song from the West Indies

All day, __ all night, __ Miss Ma-ry Ann, __

Down by __ the sea - shore __ sift - ing sand. __

E - ven lit - tle chil - dren __ join in the band, __
Young __ and _____ old, come __ join in the band, __
Ev - 'ry-bod - y, come and __ join in the band, __

Down by __ the sea - shore __ sift - ing sand. __

180

Footnotes

TEACHER TO TEACHER

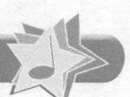

▶ **Percussion Instruments** Professional percussion instruments should be used whenever possible because they produce the best sound. Too frequently, inexpensive imitations look and sound like toys. Upper-elementary and middle-school students recognize the difference and will more readily participate when they know they are playing "real" instruments.

BUILDING SKILLS THROUGH MUSIC

▶ **Language** Have students read the article on Caribbean Music and Musicians on the *www.sfsuccessnet.com* web site. Ask them to identify which islands are the likely source of the song "Mary Ann" and support their answer with text references.

SPOTLIGHT ON

▶ **The West Indies** The West Indies is a large group of islands that stretches more than 2,000 miles from south of Florida to the northern coast of Venezuela. The islands separate the Caribbean Sea from the Atlantic Ocean. The best-known islands in this group are Cuba, Jamaica, Haiti, the Dominican Republic, Puerto Rico, Trinidad, and Tobago. On some islands, English is the official language, but French or Spanish is the official language on others.

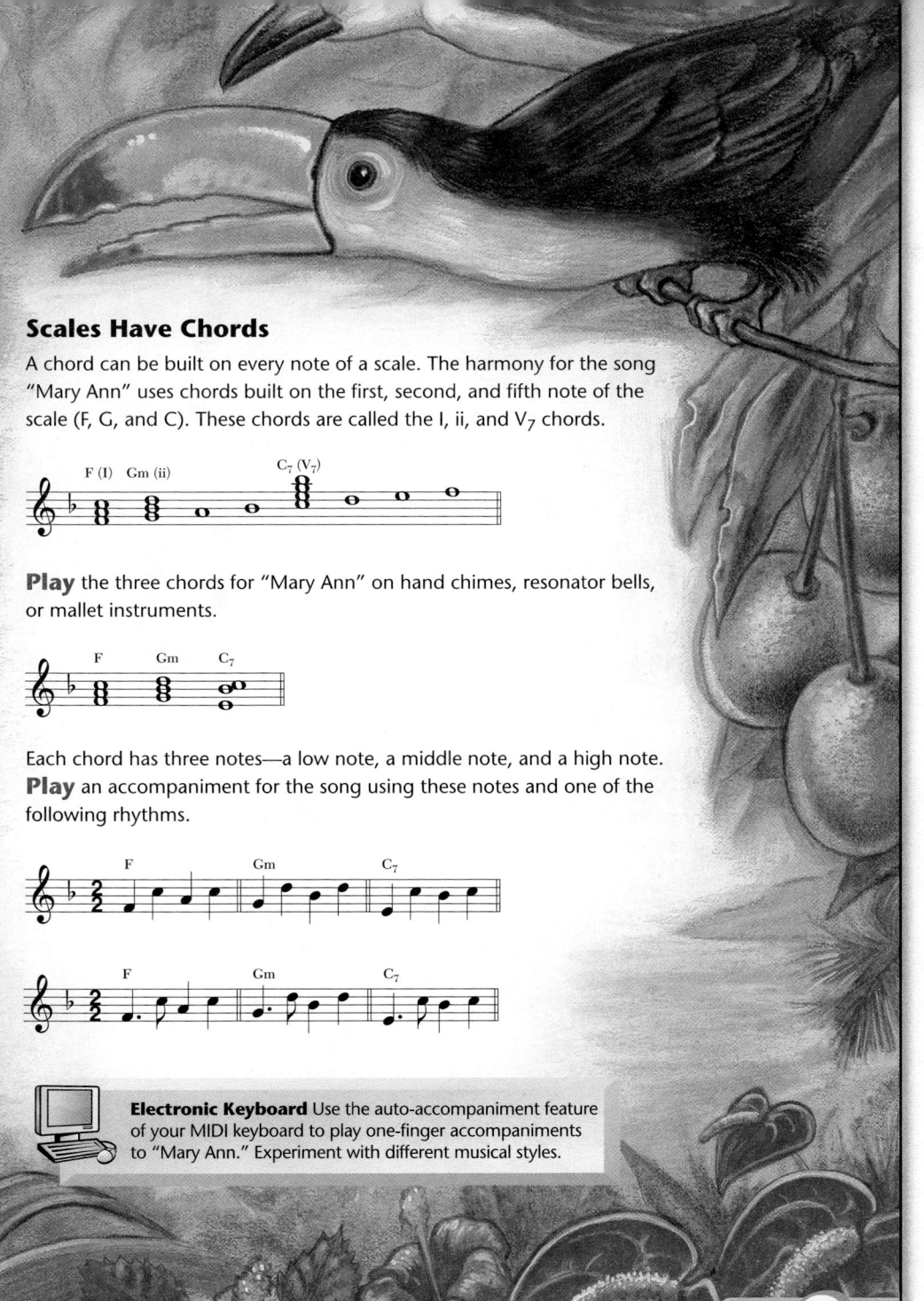

Scales Have Chords

A chord can be built on every note of a scale. The harmony for the song "Mary Ann" uses chords built on the first, second, and fifth note of the scale (F, G, and C). These chords are called the I, ii, and V₇ chords.

Play the three chords for "Mary Ann" on hand chimes, resonator bells, or mallet instruments.

Each chord has three notes—a low note, a middle note, and a high note. **Play** an accompaniment for the song using these notes and one of the following rhythms.

Electronic Keyboard Use the auto-accompaniment feature of your MIDI keyboard to play one-finger accompaniments to "Mary Ann." Experiment with different musical styles.

Unit 5   181

1 INTRODUCE

Using a world map, help students locate the Caribbean Sea, Trinidad, and the West Indies. Share Spotlight On, p. 180, with students.

Explain that calypso is a style of music that originated in this area. Calypso songs are usually improvised, and the words are often based on a current topic or satirize a current topic. "Mary Ann" is a popular calypso song.

2 DEVELOP

Singing

Invite students to sing "Mary Ann" with the recording **CD 10-10**.

ASK Is the song in unison or in harmony? (harmony)

What interval is used to harmonize the song? (the third)

Invite a group of students to sing the harmony part with the recording. Then, have students sing the song in two parts with the recording.

Analyzing

Encourage students to read the information about chords on p. 181. Help students discover that "Mary Ann" is harmonized using three chords: F, Gm, and C₇. The chords are built on the first, second, and fifth notes of the F-major scale.

continued on page 182

SKILLS REINFORCEMENT

▶ **Vocal Development** Singing in thirds is difficult for many young singers. Those challenged by the interval might find it easier to sing the harmony part for "Mary Ann" after they discover that in mm. 2, 3, 6, 7, 10, 11, and 14 they create harmony by repeating the previous pitch. Other students might achieve success singing harmony only in mm. 3, 7, and 11 initially, then adding the remaining measures listed above, and finally adding mm. 1, 5, 9, and 13.

CULTURAL CONNECTION

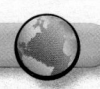

▶ **Foods of the Caribbean** The 7,000 islands of the Caribbean are known for their abundance of fruits, such as mangoes, bananas, passion fruit, and coconuts. Staple foods of the region include callaloo (leafy greens), Scotch Bonnet chile peppers (very hot), and land crabs. The national dish of one Caribbean island, Jamaica, is *akee* and saltfish. It is made with dried salted cod and cooked *akee*, a fruit that is poisonous if eaten raw. Jerk is a famous barbeque sauce of the region. Its fiery flavor is made by combining over twenty ingredients, including hot chiles, garlic, onions, allspice, and ginger. Expect fresh fruit and hot dishes if you intend to eat on a Caribbean island.

Unit 5 *Discovering New Musical Horizons*   **181**

Lesson 12 Continued

Playing

2c Distribute the appropriate hand chimes or resonator bells to students to play all three chords. Provide an opportunity for students to practice playing the chords.

Have students accompany "Mary Ann" on hand chimes or resonator bells, playing the appropriate chord on the first beat of each measure while the rest of the class sings the song with **CD 10-10.**

ASK What texture did we create by singing the song in harmony and adding the chords? (homophonic texture)

Challenge students to perform the accompaniment for "Mary Ann" with one of the rhythm arrangements on p. 181.

When students are comfortable with the bell or chime accompaniment, add the percussion accompaniment for "Mary Ann" on this page.

When the bell or chime and percussion parts are played successfully, add the mallet instrument accompaniment for "Mary Ann" on p. 183.

Guide students to perform independently, with accurate intonation, and demonstrate basic performance techniques.

For a recorder countermelody for "Mary Ann," have some students learn the recorder part in the Skills Reinforcement on p. 183.

Mellow Movements

People in the West Indies like to move to music. Sometimes they follow specific patterns or steps.

Learn this basic calypso step with your partner. **Perform** the calypso step to the music of "Mary Ann." Move in a relaxed manner. When you are ready, **improvise** and **create** your own calypso steps.

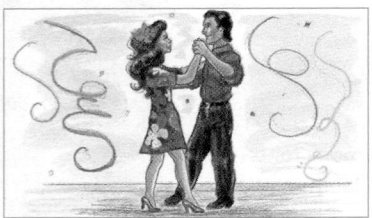

▲ Count 1: Step right foot in front of left, with a small twist

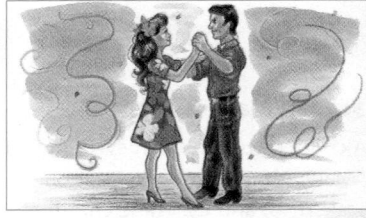

▲ Count 2: Step left foot in place

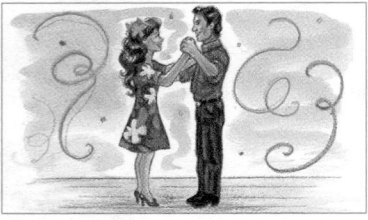

▲ Count 3: Step right foot next to left foot

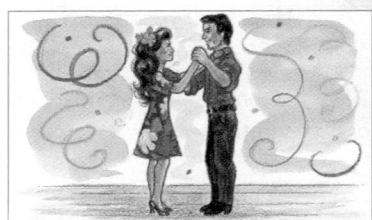

▲ Count 4: Step left foot in place

Mellow Percussion

Calypso rhythms can be played on mallet and percussion instruments. Learn these percussion parts. When you are ready, **play** the percussion accompaniment with "Mary Ann."

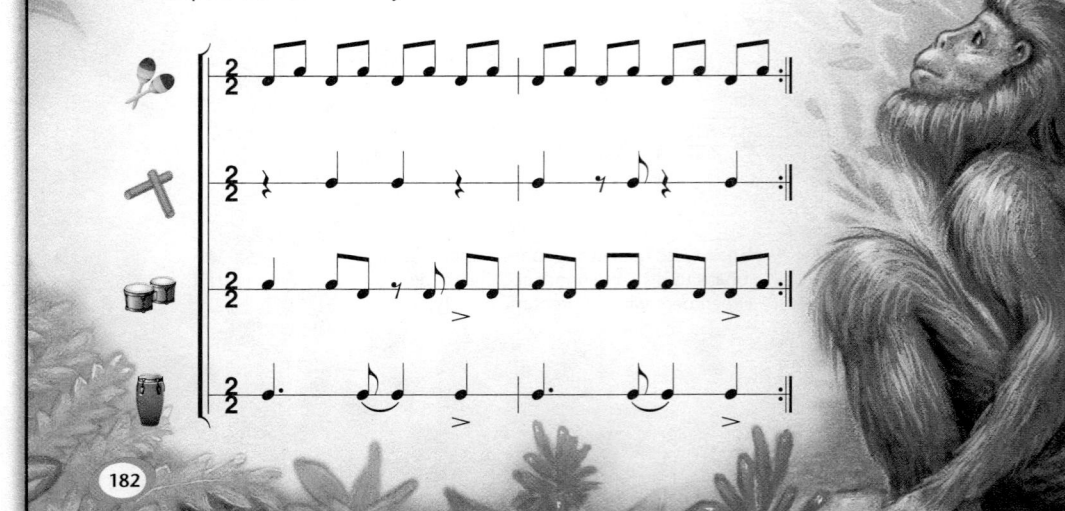

Footnotes

TEACHER TO TEACHER

▶ **Playing Chords** Students may find it easier to play chords on resonator bells and hand chimes if they are invited to stand as a chord group, that is, F-chord bells stand together, G-minor-chord bells stand together, and C₇-chord bells stand together. This will make it much easier for students to perform the accompaniments suggested in the lesson.

▶ **Modeling an Instrumental Part** Modeling saves valuable instruction time when teaching students how to hold an instrument properly and how to play a rhythm.

Play the rhythm on the instrument and demonstrate how to hold it before handing the instrument to the student. Allow the student an opportunity to practice the rhythm on the instrument before adding the rhythm to the song.

ACROSS THE CURRICULUM

▶ **Language Arts** Share a collection of poems from Jamaica in the book *Under the Breadfruit Tree: Island Poems* by Monica Gunning (Boyds Mills, 1998). Invite groups of students to select a poem and create an illustration and performance for it. These poem performances can be used for a school-wide presentation or in presentations for younger students.

A Calypso Ensemble

This orchestration adds mallet instruments to accompany "Mary Ann." Learn the orchestration and when you are ready, **perform** both ensembles to accompany the song.

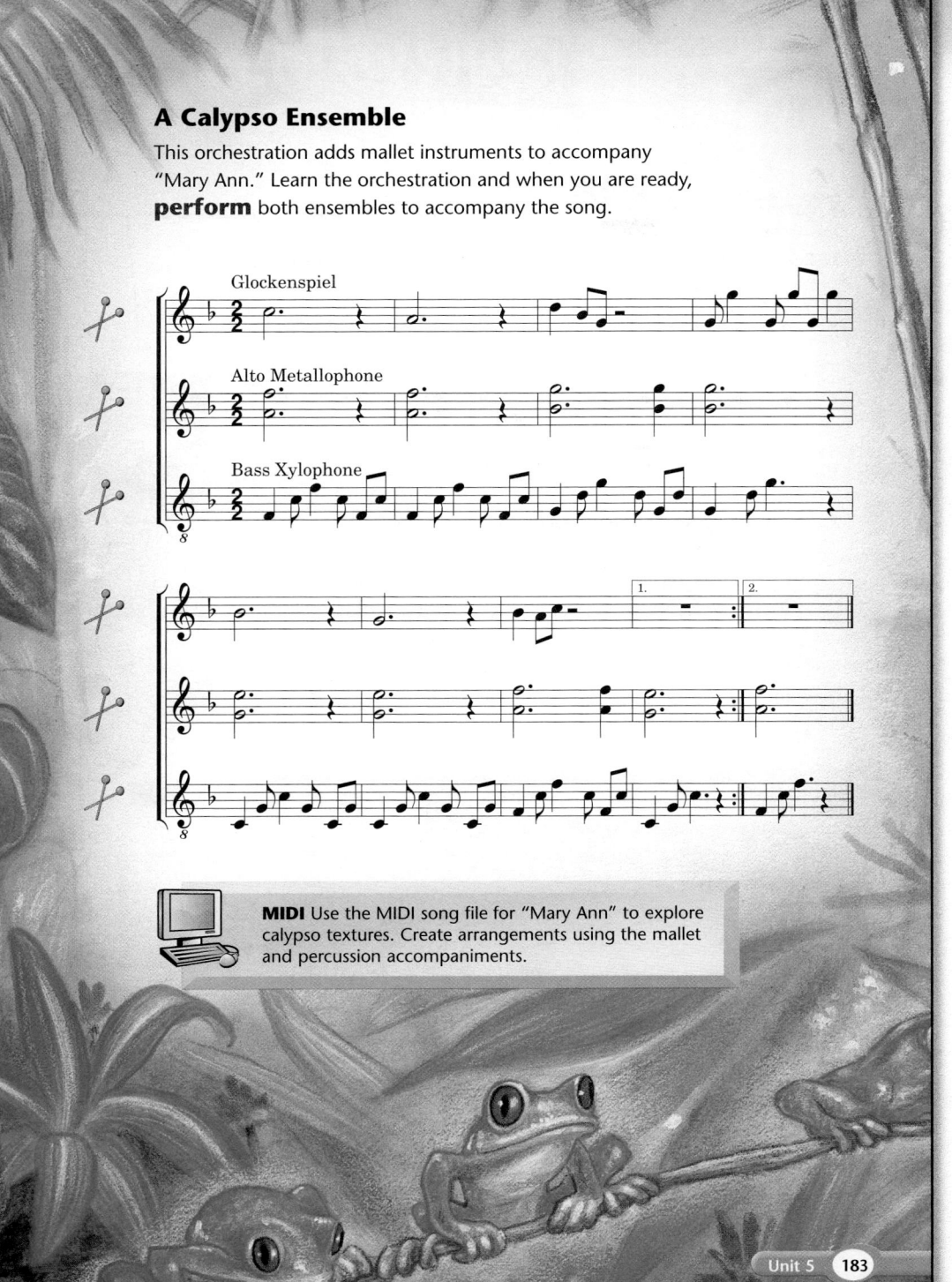

 MIDI Use the MIDI song file for "Mary Ann" to explore calypso textures. Create arrangements using the mallet and percussion accompaniments.

Moving

Encourage students to try the movement ideas for "Mary Ann" on p. 182. Then, invite them to improvise movements for the song, using their own ideas. Refer to Dance Directions, p. 559, for background information and a dance routine for "Mary Ann." Have them practice with Dance Practice **CD 10-12.** When students are comfortable with the routine, have them perform it with Dance Performance **CD 10-10.**

3 CLOSE

Skill: PLAYING   **ASSESSMENT**

Performance/Observation Invite students to sing "Mary Ann" **CD 10-10** while playing the accompaniment rhythms on p. 181 by softly tapping the palm of a hand. Then, divide the class into groups that will play together to form chordal accompaniments, and have students play the accompaniments with the recording. Watch to see if students change their note of the chord at the right time to be with each other and with the recording.

SKILLS REINFORCEMENT

▶ **Recorder** Review the fingering for B♭ on the soprano recorder. To help students play the rhythm of this accompaniment, relate it to the rhythm of the melody of "Mary Ann." They are both the same. For an alto recorder accompaniment, *see* Resource Book p. I-17.

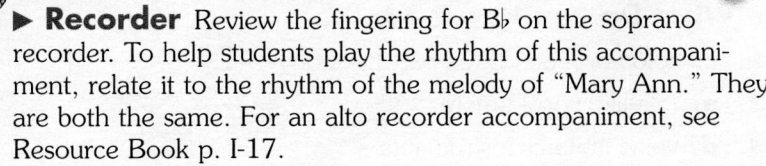

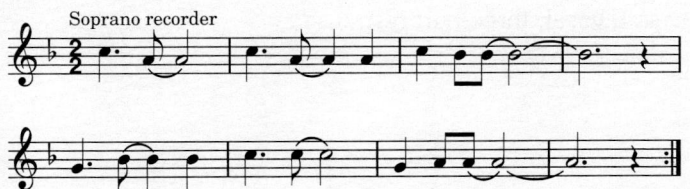

TECHNOLOGY/MEDIA LINK

Web Site Invite students to visit *www.sfsuccessnet.com* to explore the music and instruments of the Caribbean.

MIDI/Sequencing Software Invite students to use the MIDI file for "Mary Ann" to create mallet and percussion textures and accompaniments.

Electronic Keyboard Allow students to play a Caribbean-style accompaniment using the auto-accompaniment feature of a MIDI keyboard.

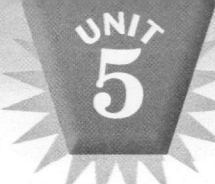

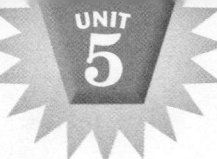
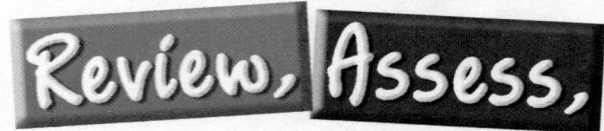

WHAT DO YOU KNOW?

> **MATERIALS**
> • **Resource Book** p. B-17

Review with students the concepts of syncopation and intervals as necessary. Then, have them complete the worksheet on Resource Book p. B-17.

WHAT DO YOU HEAR? 5A

> **MATERIALS**
> • *What Do You Hear? 5A*   **CD 10-13 to 10-16**
> • **Resource Book** p. B-18

Review the montage *Vocal Timbres Around the World* **CD 9-27**. Help students describe what they hear. Then, play the music again *(What Do You Hear? 5A)* **CD 10-13 to 10-16** and have students identify and match each selection with the most appropriate description in the list provided, using the worksheet on Resource Book p. B-18.

Point out that the students should listen for characteristics that determine the style of the music.

What Do You Know?

1. Read the rhythms below. Identify the rhythms that contain syncopation.

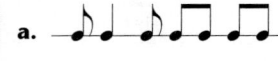 a.   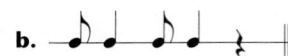 b.

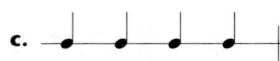 c.   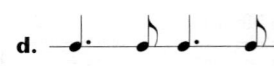 d.

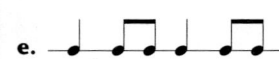 e.   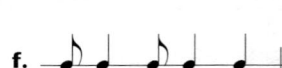 f.

2. Select the correct name for each musical interval.

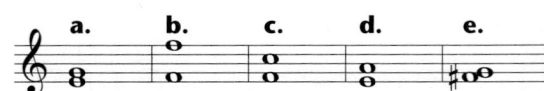

- octave
- fourth
- second
- fifth
- third

What Do You Hear? 5A

 CD 10–13

Timbre

Listen to *Vocal Timbres Around the World*, page 170. Match the most appropriate description to each musical style.

Musical Style	**Description**
1. country-western	**a.** folksy and rough vocal timbre, blues progression, guitar accompaniment
2. folk blues	**b.** solo vocal answered by three-part response, drum accompaniment
3. vocal imitation	**c.** solo vocal with vocal inflections, three-part harmony in refrain, country sound
4. African call and response	**d.** voice imitates instruments

(184)

Footnotes

ANSWER KEY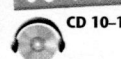

▶ What Do You Know?

1 The rhythms that contain syncopation are **a, b,** and **f.**

2. a. third
    b. octave
    c. fifth
    d. fourth
    e. second

▶ What Do You Hear? 5A

1. c. solo vocal and three-part harmony

2. a. folk-like vocal timbre

3. d. voice imitates instruments

4. b. solo vocal, three-part response

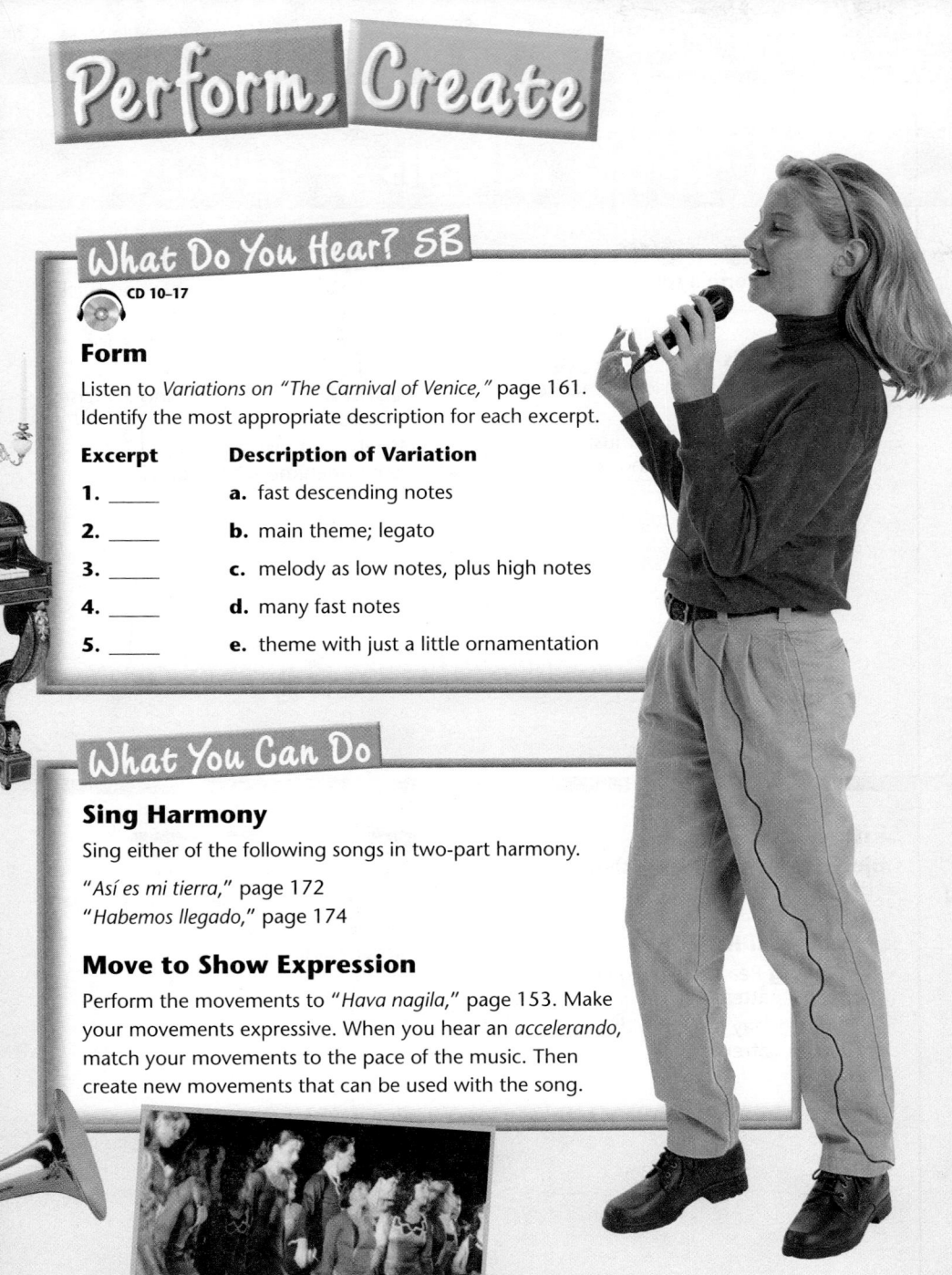

Perform, Create

What Do You Hear? 5B

CD 10–17

Form

Listen to *Variations on "The Carnival of Venice,"* page 161. Identify the most appropriate description for each excerpt.

Excerpt	Description of Variation
1. _____	**a.** fast descending notes
2. _____	**b.** main theme; legato
3. _____	**c.** melody as low notes, plus high notes
4. _____	**d.** many fast notes
5. _____	**e.** theme with just a little ornamentation

What You Can Do

Sing Harmony

Sing either of the following songs in two-part harmony.

"Así es mi tierra," page 172
"Habemos llegado," page 174

Move to Show Expression

Perform the movements to *"Hava nagila,"* page 153. Make your movements expressive. When you hear an *accelerando,* match your movements to the pace of the music. Then create new movements that can be used with the song.

Unit 5 **185**

WHAT DO YOU HEAR? 5B

MATERIALS
- *What Do You Hear? 5B* **CD 10-17 to 10-21**
- **Resource Book** p. B-18

Review the idea of variation with students. Then, have them listen to *Variations on "The Carnival of Venice"* (*What Do You Hear? 5B*) **CD 10-17 to 10-21** and determine which description best matches each variation, using the worksheet on Resource Book p. B-18. If necessary, pause the recording after each variation.

WHAT YOU CAN DO

MATERIALS
- *"Así es mi tierra,"* p. 172 **CD 9-30**
- *"Habemos llegado,"* p. 174 **CD 10-1**
- **Resource Book** p. B-19

Sing Harmony

Ask students to review and sing *"Así es mi tierra"* on p. 172 and *"Habemos llegado"* on p. 174, paying attention to singing in two-part harmony. When students are ready, have them choose a song and sing it as a class in harmony.

Move to Show Expression

Review with students the movements to the *hora,* following the directions on p. 154 of the Teacher Edition. Complete dance directions can be found in the Dance Directions on p. 557. Then, ask students to perform the movements to *"Hava nagila,"* p. 153.

Remind students to dance with expression and to match the pace of the *accelerando.* When ready, ask the class to dance the *hora* with the song. Then, ask students to create new movements that can be performed with the song.

► **What Do You Hear? 5B**

1. **e.** theme with just a little ornamentation
2. **a.** fast descending notes
3. **d.** many fast notes
4. **c.** melody as low notes, plus high notes
5. **b.** main theme; *legato*

TECHNOLOGY/MEDIA LINK

► Rubrics

Visit *www.sfsuccessnet.com* for rubrics to assess students' achievement in music skills.

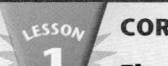

Lesson	Elements	Skills

LESSON 1 · CORE
Flowing Tempos

pp. 190–193

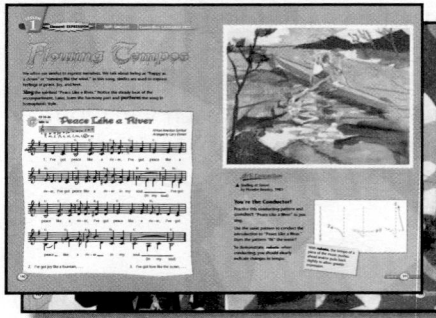

Element: Expression
Concept: Tempo
Focus: Tempo *rubato*

Secondary Element
Rhythm: beat

National Standards
1c　4c　6b　8b　9a

Skill: Singing
Objective: Perform a spiritual using *rubato*

Secondary Skills
- **Singing** Sing an African American spiritual
- **Moving** Conduct and musical examples that use both *rubato* and a steady beat
- **Listening** Identify *rubato*

SKILLS REINFORCEMENT
- **Listening** Recognize thin and thick texture
- **Signing** Learn sign language for a song
- **Vocal Development** Sing exercises in *rubato*
- **Keyboard** Play a keyboard accompaniment to a song

LESSON 2
Adjust the Accents

pp. 194–195

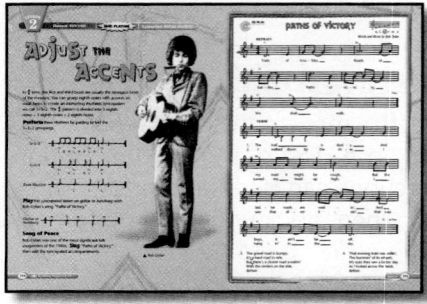

Reading Sequence 21, p. 498

Element: Rhythm
Concept: Pattern
Focus: Eighth notes grouped in 3+3+2

Secondary Element
Genre: ballad

National Standards
2a　5a　6b　8b

Skill: Reading
Objective: Play 3+3+2 eighth-note rhythm patterns

Secondary Skills
- **Reading** Read and echo clap 3+3+2 rhythm patterns
- **Playing** Play a song with various rhythm patterns

SKILLS REINFORCEMENT
- **Keyboard** Play a keyboard accompaniment using three chords
- **Mallets** Learn an Orff accompaniment

LESSON 3 · CORE
Meters Move

pp. 196–197

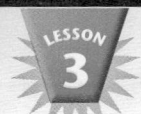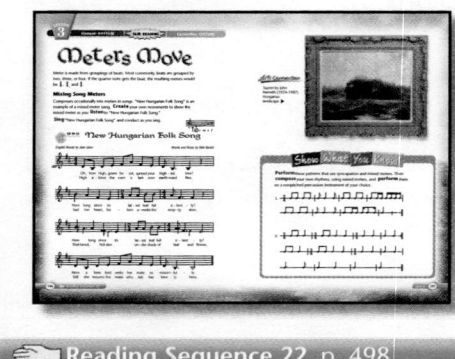

Reading Sequence 22, p. 498

Element: Rhythm
Concept: Meter
Focus: Mixed meter

Secondary Element
Tonality: tonal center

National Standards
1c　2a　4c　5a　7b　8b

Skill: Playing
Objective: Read rhythm patterns that use syncopation and mixed meter

Secondary Skills
- **Moving** Create movements for mixed meter
- **Singing** Sing a song with pitch syllables, then lyrics
- **Composing** Compose a pentatonic melody

SKILLS REINFORCEMENT
- **Playing** Play a rhythm pattern on percussion instruments

Connections	**Music and Other Literature**	
Connection: Language Arts **Activity:** Discover that similes can be effectively used in song lyrics **MEETING INDIVIDUAL NEEDS** **English Language Learners** Match photos to words **SPOTLIGHT ON** **The Conductor's Baton** Facts about batons **The Composer** Facts on Johann Strauss, Jr. **CULTURAL CONNECTION** **African American Spirituals** Background on African American spirituals **ACROSS THE CURRICULUM** **Social Studies** Facts about the Danube River **BUILDING SKILLS THROUGH MUSIC** **Language** Interpret lyrics	**Song** "Peace Like a River" **Listening Selections** "Minuet" from *Orchestral Suite No. 2 in B Minor* *The Blue Danube* **Poem** "Autumn" **More Music Choices** *Glory, Glory Hallelujah,* p. 54 *Swing Low, Sweet Chariot,* p. 234	**ASSESSMENT** **Performance/Peer Critique** Sing a spiritual in *rubato* style **TECHNOLOGY/MEDIA LINK** **Notation Software** Create an arrangement of a song
Connection: Social Studies **Activity:** Discuss the political significance of social unrest in the 1960s **ACROSS THE CURRICULUM** **Social Studies** Read a book on conflict and peace **MEETING INDIVIDUAL NEEDS** **Including Everyone** Suggestions for helping students to learn rhythms **SCHOOL TO HOME CONNECTION** **The 1960s** Discuss the 1960s with friends and relatives **BUILDING SKILLS THROUGH MUSIC** **Language** Write a fictitious conversation based on research	**Song** "Paths of Victory" **More Music Choices** "*Má Teodora,*" p. 301 *El Salón México,* p. 199	**ASSESSMENT** **Performance/Observation** Have students read and play rhythm patterns **TECHNOLOGY/MEDIA LINK** **Web Site** Explore information on Bob Dylan
Connection: Culture **Activity:** Explore the geographic and social origins of a composed song **SPOTLIGHT ON** **The Composer** Facts on Béla Bartók **CULTURAL CONNECTION** **Folk Music of Hungary** Facts about Hungarian folk music **BUILDING SKILLS THROUGH MUSIC** **Language** Discuss the tradition of folk songs	**Song** "New Hungarian Folk Song" **More Music Choices** "Love in Any Language," p. 476 "One Moment in Time," p. 352	**ASSESSMENT** **Performance/Peer Critique** Perform rhythm patterns that use syncopation and mixed meter **TECHNOLOGY/MEDIA LINK** **Sequencing Software** Explore graphic editing features, looping tracks, and adding percussion **Web Site** Research Béla Bartók and the music of Hungary

Lesson	Elements	Skills

LESSON 4
Adjust the Meters

pp. 198–199

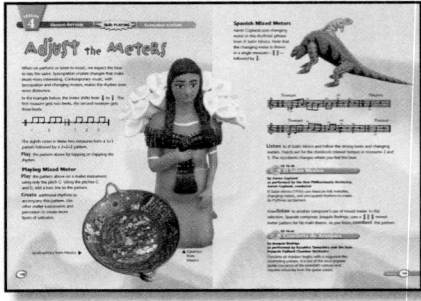

Element: Rhythm
Concept: Meter
Focus: $\frac{6}{8}$ and $\frac{3}{4}$ meter

Secondary Element
Expression: accents

National Standards
2a 2c 4c 6b 6c

Skill: Playing
Objective: Play rhythm ostinatos in $\frac{6}{8}$ and $\frac{3}{4}$ meter

Secondary Skills
- **Playing** Play syncopated rhythms with changing meters
- **Creating** Create a bass line for the rhythm patterns
- **Listening** Listen to and conduct music with mixed meters

SKILLS REINFORCEMENT
- **Guitar** Play a guitar accompaniment in *mariachi* style

LESSON 5
CORE
Through-Composed Songs

pp. 200–201

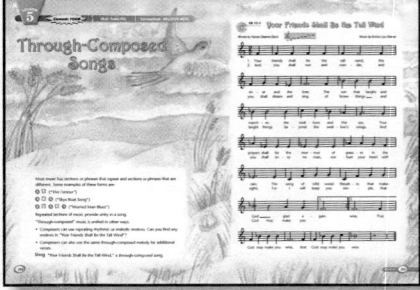
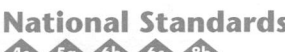

Element: Form
Concept: Sectional forms
Focus: Through-composed form

Secondary Element
Melody: accidentals

National Standards
4c 5a 6b 6c 8b

Skill: Singing
Objective: Sing a song in through-composed form

Secondary Skills
- **Listening** Listen to a through-composed song
- **Singing** Sing a through-composed song and discuss it's characteristics

SKILLS REINFORCEMENT
- **Listening** Listen to selected songs and identify the form

---

LESSON 6
An Evening Dance

pp. 202–203

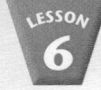
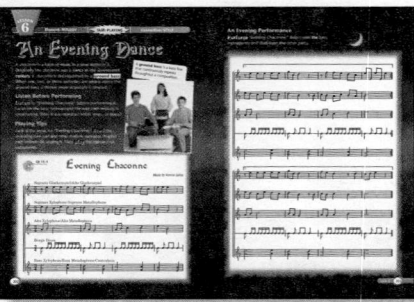
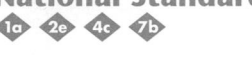

Element: Melody
Concept: Pattern
Focus: Melodic ostinatos

Secondary Element
Texture/Harmony: texture

National Standards
1a 2e 4c 7b

Skill: Playing
Objective: Play a chaconne with melodic ostinatos and ground bass
Secondary Skills
- **Listening** Listen to a song and pay attention to the bass part
- **Singing** Echo-sing, then sing and play parts in the air with a recording
- **Analyzing** Discuss melodic ostinatos and melodic patterns

SKILLS REINFORCEMENT
- **Mallets** Play mallet and percussion parts

Connections

Music and Other Literature

Connection: Culture

Activity: Explore cultural influences on a composition by an American composer

SPOTLIGHT ON **The Composer** Facts on composer Aaron Copland

CULTURAL CONNECTION
Mexican Influences Cultural information on a Mexican musical style
Spanish Influence Facts about Joaquín Rodrigo and his influence

BUILDING SKILLS THROUGH MUSIC **Language** Complete a Venn diagram comparing two compositions

Listening Selection *El Salón México* (excerpt)

More Music Choices
"New Hungarian Folk Song," p. 196
"Paths of Victory," p. 195

ASSESSMENT

Performance/Observation
Perform rhythm patterns that use syncopation and mixed meter

TECHNOLOGY/MEDIA LINK
Web Site Research the music of Aaron Copeland

Connection: Related Arts

Activity: Discuss ways in which nature is portrayed in music and the visual arts

MEETING INDIVIDUAL NEEDS **Including Everyone** Express appreciation of peers

BUILDING SKILLS THROUGH MUSIC **Writing** Write to describe and compare through-compositions

Song "Your Friends Shall Be the Tall Wind"

More Music Choices
"Four Strong Winds," p. 170
"*Riendo el río corre*," p. 263

ASSESSMENT

Music Journal Writing
Sing a song and identify its form

TECHNOLOGY/MEDIA LINK
Notation Software
Create a through-composed piece

Connection: Style

Activity: Participate in an ensemble arrangement for mallet instruments and drum

SPOTLIGHT ON **Orff Instruments** Facts about Carl Orff and his instruments

AUDIENCE ETIQUETTE **Preparing to Attend a Performance** Tips on preparing students for a live performance

BUILDING SKILLS THROUGH MUSIC **Reading** Read indicative text and choose a tempo based on it

Song "Evening Chaconne"

More Music Choices
"Mary Ann," p. 180

ASSESSMENT

Performance/Peer Critique Play melodies with ostinatos on percussion instruments

TECHNOLOGY/MEDIA LINK
Notation Software
Compose an Orff arrangement

Lesson	Elements	Skills	
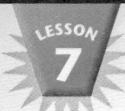 **LESSON 7** **CORE** **Lumberjack Intervals** pp. 204–205 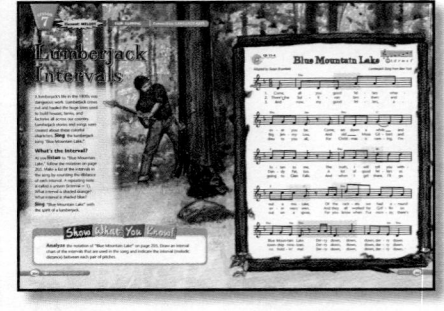 👉 Reading Sequence 23, p. 499	**Element: Melody** **Concept:** Intervals **Focus:** Intervals of fourths and fifths **Secondary Element** Melody: minor scales **National Standards** 5b 6b 6c	**Skill: Reading** **Objective:** Read a song containing fourths and fifths **Secondary Skills** • **Reading** Review the intervals founds in a major scale • **Listening** Listen to a song in a minor key and discuss the intervals found in a minor scale • **Singing** Sing a song in a compound meter	**SKILLS REINFORCEMENT** • **Reading** Understand the variations of the minor scale • **Recorder** Learn an alto and soprano recorder duet accompaniment
LESSON 8 **'Round a Melody** pp. 206–207 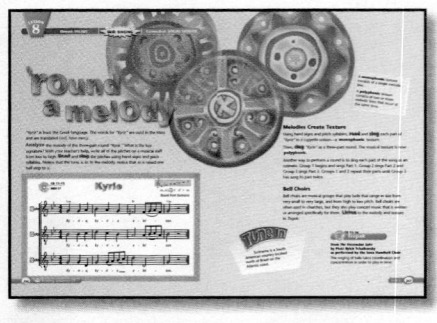 👉 Reading Sequence 24, p. 499	**Element: Melody** **Concept:** Texture **Focus:** Rounds and Canons **Secondary Element** Form: canon **National Standards** 1c 1d 2b 6b	**Skill: Singing** **Objective:** Sing a canon in minor **Secondary Skills** • **Analyzing** Examine three distinct parts of a melody • **Singing** Sight-sing using pitch syllables and hand signs and sing in a three-part round	**SKILLS REINFORCEMENT** • **Keyboard** Play a trio arrangement of a three-part round • **Hand Bells** Play an accompaniment
LESSON 9 **Take a Chance** pp. 208–209 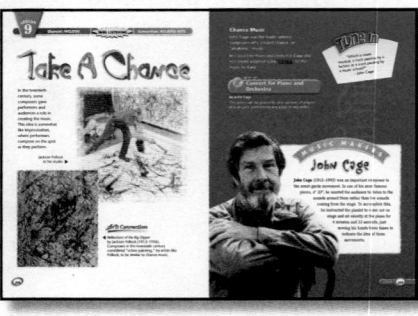	**Element: Melody** **Concept:** Atonality **Focus:** Chance (aleatory) music **Secondary Element** Timbre: instrumental **National Standards** 4a 4b 4c 6a 6b 8a	**Skill: Listening** **Objective:** Listen to and describe an example of aleatory **Secondary Skills** • **Creating** Create a graphic composition with a text • **Listening** Listen to a piece of aleatoric music and discuss melody, timbre, and pitch choice	**SKILLS REINFORCEMENT** • **Creating** Plan and perform an aleatory composition for five radios

Connections

Music and Other Literature

Connection: Language Arts

Activity: Discuss the lyrics and story of a lumberjack song from the Adirondack Mountains

ACROSS THE CURRICULUM **Language Arts** Write lyrics based on a theme related to a song

SPOTLIGHT ON **Contra Dance** Facts on the contra dance

SCHOOL TO HOME CONNECTION **Getting Back to Nature** Have students commune with nature

BUILDING SKILLS THROUGH MUSIC **Math** Use math to help understand meter

Song "Blue Mountain Lake"

More Music Choices
"Skye Boat Song," p. 372
"Your Friends Shall Be the Tall Wind," p. 201

ASSESSMENT

Performance/Observation
Have students use pitch syllables to sing a song; observe their ability to sing fourths and fifths

TECHNOLOGY/MEDIA LINK

Notation Software
Create and notate a two-measure ostinato

Connection: Social Studies

Activity: Link a round with information about its country of origin

SPOTLIGHT ON **The Text** Backround on the Latin text *Kyrie eleison*

ACROSS THE CURRICULUM **Social Studies** Facts about the country Suriname

BUILDING SKILLS THROUGH MUSIC **Social Studies** Learn about Suriname

Song *"Kyrie"*

Listening Selection
"Trepak" from *The Nutcracker Suite*

More Music Choices
"Hey, Ho! Nobody Home," p. 28
"Dance for the Nations," p. 122

ASSESSMENT

Performance/Observation
Perform a song as a three part round in polyphonic texture

TECHNOLOGY/MEDIA LINK

MIDI/Sequencing Software Use software to help learn a round with parts separately, then together

---

Connection: Related Arts

Activity: Discuss ways in which unplanned, or "chance," events can be incorporated into musical composition and the visual arts

ACROSS THE CURRICULUM **Language Arts** Read a book about John Cage

SPOTLIGHT ON
The Composer Facts about John Cage
The Artist Facts about Jackson Pollock

CHARACTER EDUCATION **Audience Behavior** Encourage respect when listening to all types of music

BUILDING SKILLS THROUGH MUSIC **Science** Observe and write down ambient sounds

Listening Selection Concert for Piano and Orchestra (excerpt)

More Music Choices
Ionisation, p. 357
"Allegretto giovale" from Lyric Suite, p. 169

ASSESSMENT

Music Journal Writing
Listen to an aleatoric piece and have students write how pitch, timbre, texture, and dynamics are used

TECHNOLOGY/MEDIA LINK

Multimedia Have students create a multimedia concert

Lesson	Elements	Skills

LESSON 10

CORE

Choir Sounds

pp. 210–211

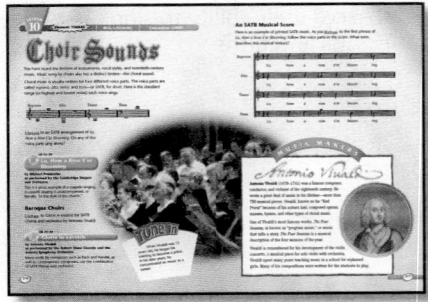

Element: Timbre
Concept: Vocal
Focus: SATB choir

Secondary Element
Melody: tonality

National Standards
5a 6b 9b

Skill: Listening
Objective: Describe selected examples of choral singing

Secondary Skills
- **Listening** Introduce the vocal ranges of the different voice parts with a piano; compare timbre in two different pieces
- **Reading** Study a choral score and take note of the different clefs

SKILLS REINFORCEMENT
- **Listening** Listen to several choral recordings and identify what voice parts or singing

---

LESSON 11

African Choir Sounds

pp. 212–215

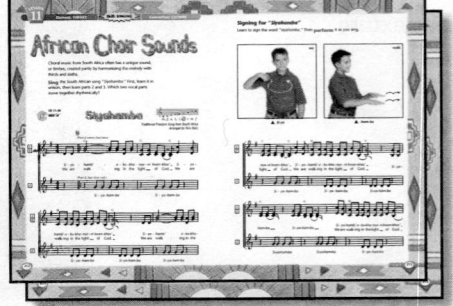

Element: Timbre
Concept: Vocal
Focus: South African choral timbre

Secondary Element
Rhythm: pattern

National Standards
1c 1d 4c 5c 7b 8b

Skill: Singing
Objective: Perform a South African song in three-part harmony

Secondary Skills
- **Reading** Follow the road map for the notation of a song; listen to and follow the notation
- **Singing** Sing a Zulu song while following the score
- **Playing** Play a drum ensemble as the class sings the song
- **Moving** Perform creative movements to a Zulu song

SKILLS REINFORCEMENT
- **Mallets** Play an Orff accompaniment to a song
- **Vocal Development** Assign vocal parts and ranges
- **Playing** Perform a highlife drum ensemble with a song
- **Signing** Learn the sign language for a song

LESSON 12

CORE

Bernstein's Textures

pp. 216–219

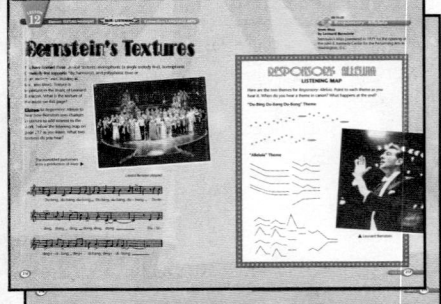

Element: Texture/Harmony
Concept: Texture
Focus: Polyphonic and homophonic textures

Secondary Element
Rhythm: syncopation

National Standards
1c 6a 6b 8a 8b

Skill: Listening
Objective: Discern polyphonic and homophonic textures in a listening selection

Secondary Skills
- **Singing** Sing a selection that sounds like bells
- **Listening** Listen for the usage of homophonic and polyphonic textures in a piece
- **Moving** Use movements to reinforce different textures in a piece of music

SKILLS REINFORCEMENT
- **Singing** Sing or listen to other examples of scat singing; sing a song that uses a canon

Connections

Music and Other Literature

Connection: Genre

Activity: Explore the historical and social setting of choral singing

SPOTLIGHT ON
The Composer Facts about Michael Praetorius
Choral Music Background on choral music

ACROSS THE CURRICULUM Language Arts Facts about Latin lyrics in church music

SCHOOL TO HOME CONNECTION SATB Encourage students to ask friends and family if they have ever sung in a choir

BUILDING SKILLS THROUGH MUSIC Language Describe music

Listening Selections
Lo, How a Rose E'er Blooming (excerpt)
Gloria in excelsis

M·U·S·I·C M·A·K·E·R·S
Antonio Vivaldi

More Music Choices
Give Us Hope, p. 337
Stopping by Woods on a Snowy Evening, p. 40
"Vem kan segla?" p. 417

ASSESSMENT

Music Journal Writing Listen to and describe timbre and other performance aspects of selected recordings of choral performances

TECHNOLOGY/MEDIA LINK
Notation Software Input a choral score and play it back

Connection: Culture

Activity: Explore the social and cultural setting of a Zulu freedom song

CULTURAL CONNECTION The Zulu Facts about the Zulu nation

ACROSS THE CURRICULUM
Social Studies Facts about South Africa
Language Arts Read a poem with the same mood as the song

MOVEMENT Creative Movement Perform a dance to a song

BUILDING SKILLS THROUGH MUSIC Language Chronologically document steps required for a performance

Songs *"Siyahamba"* (Zulu and English)

Poem "Roads Go Ever Ever On"

More Music Choices
"Ise oluwa," p. 230
"Take Time in Life," p. 292

ASSESSMENT

Performance/Peer Critique Perform a South African song in three-part harmony with movement, signing, and drumming

TECHNOLOGY/MEDIA LINK
MIDI/Sequencing Software Experiment with graphic editing features; create vocal and instrumental parts

---

Connection: Language Arts

Activity: Identify the literary source of a contemporary opera

ACROSS THE CURRICULUM
Social Studies Read a book about Leonard Bernstein
Language Arts Facts about Voltaire's *Candide*

SPOTLIGHT ON The Composer Facts on Leonard Bernstein

CULTURAL CONNECTION Bernstein's Mass Background on the work

CHARACTER EDUCATION Life Textures Relate textures in music to everyday life

BUILDING SKILLS THROUGH MUSIC Language List given information

Listening Selections
"Responsary: Alleluia" from *Mass Overture to Candide*
Overture to Candide
Overture to Candide (excerpt)

More Music Choices
"Little" Organ Fugue in G Minor (organ), p. 129
"Little" Organ Fugue in G Minor (brass), p. 129
"Scattin' A-Round," p. 160

ASSESSMENT

Observation/Music Journal Writing Identify polyphonic and homophonic texture in a listening selection; write about texture in music journals

TECHNOLOGY/MEDIA LINK
Transparency Follow a listening map and point the way as students follow along and listen
Web Site Research Leonard Bernstein

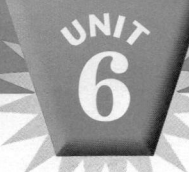

INTRODUCING THE UNIT

Unit 6, *Making Music Our Own*, offers students a view of the wide world of musical styles. Whether it is Native American drumming, Bob Dylan's folk guitar rhythms, the music of John Cage, or the rounds of Suriname, students will learn that the music they listen to in the United States has been influenced by the music, culture, and styles from around the world, and from other eras. A brief overview of the skills assessed in this unit can be found on p. 187. Unit highlights and are listed in the footnotes.

UNIT PROJECT

Invite students to read about Native American drumming on p. 186, then listen to *Dineh Round Dance* **CD 8-15.**

ASK What beats are stressed in the music? (first beat)

ASK Which instruments stand out? (wood flute) **Which instruments are in the background?** (mallets, claves)

Listen again to identify the appearance of each instrument listed on p. 186.

Read the biography of Valerie Dee Naranjo on p. 186 to learn more about the performer.

Focus student attention on the picture on p. 187. Explain that the performers are probably singing as they drum.

ASK How are the performers arranged? (In a circle around a large drum.)

Discuss other performance practices used by drummers.

* A single person at a trap set.
* Several people switching from one instrument to another in a symphony orchestra.
* A large group of people playing many different drums (conga, bongos, etc.)
* A line of drummers in a marching band.

New Native American Drumming

Native American music has a rich tradition of drumming. Contemporary Native Americans are creating new versions of traditional music.

Listen to this contemporary rendition of *Dinéh Round Dance* performed on Native American instruments. Then listen to an interview with the performer.

 CD 10–22
Dinéh Round Dance

**Traditional Navajo Dance
as performed by Valerie Dee Naranjo**

A marimba, hoe blade, alto log drum, water sounds, claves, and *kechua* flute are the instruments that accompany the voice in this piece.

CD 10–23
**Interview with
Valerie Dee Naranjo**

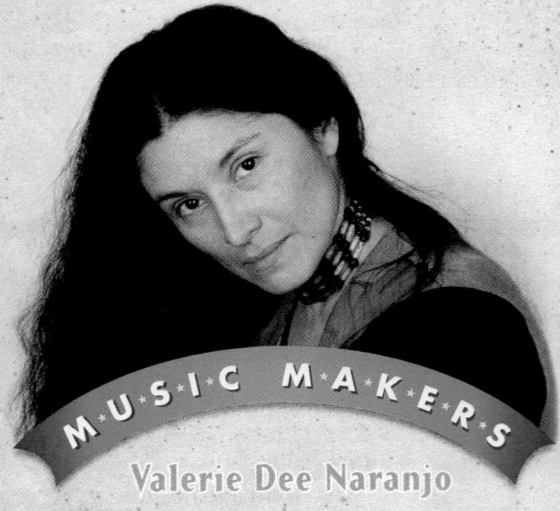

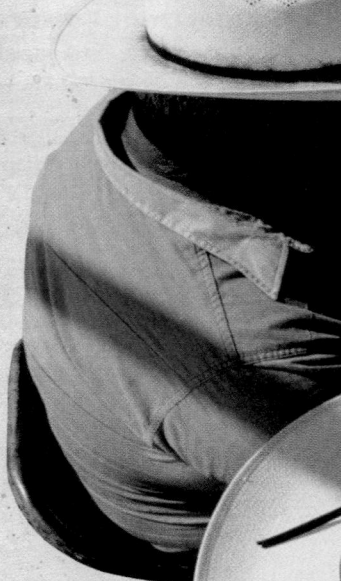

MUSIC MAKERS
Valerie Dee Naranjo

Valerie Dee Naranjo is a performer, singer, and educator proficient in the music and drumming styles of Native American and African cultures. She began singing with her family at an early age in the Southwest and in Mexico. She learned to play Native American musical instruments.

Naranjo has performed with Philip Glass, David Byrne, Selena, and Tori Amos. She has played in Broadway's *The Lion King* and in NBC's *Saturday Night Live Band.*

186

ACROSS THE CURRICULUM

Unit Highlights The following interdisciplinary activities in this unit are related to the music elements presented in the lessons and are intended to enhance student learning. For a more detailed topical description, see the Unit at a Glance on pp. 185a–185h.

▶ **LANGUAGE ARTS**

* Discuss how the lyrics of a song are illustrated by melodic contour (p. 201)
* Write lyrics based on a lumberjack theme (p. 204)
* Share the writings of composer John Cage (p. 208)
* Learn about the influence of Latin on Romance languages (p. 211)
* Read the J. R. R. Tolkien poem, "Roads Go Ever Ever On" (p. 214)
* Discover information on Voltaire's *Candide* (p. 218)

▶ **SOCIAL STUDIES**

* Learn facts about the Danube River (p. 192)
* Learn about the facts and history of Suriname (p. 206)
* Learn about South Africa's resources, geography, and wildlife (p. 213)
* Read a book on Leonard Bernstein (p. 216)

▶ **VISUAL ARTS**

* Discuss how nature is portrayed in art (p. 201)

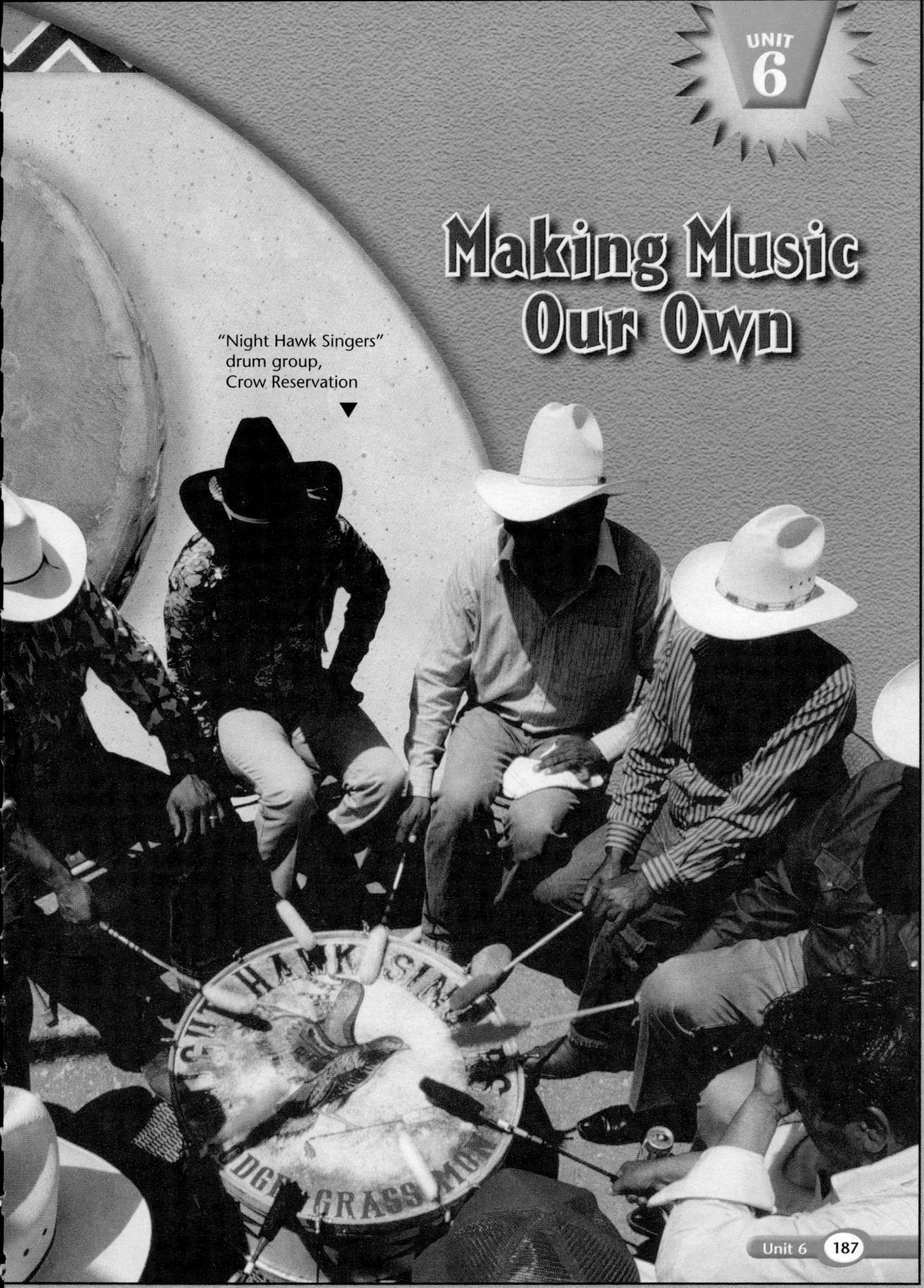

UNIT 6

Making Music Our Own

"Night Hawk Singers"
drum group,
Crow Reservation
▼

MUSIC SKILLS
ASSESSED IN THIS UNIT

Reading Music: Rhythm

- Read and perform syncopated rhythm patterns (p. 195)
- Read and perform syncopated and mixed-meter rhythms (p. 197)

Reading Music: Pitch

- Read and sing a song with fourths and fifths (p. 205)
- Read and sing a three-part round (p. 207)

Performing Music: Singing

- Sing a song expressively, with *rubato* (p. 193)
- Sing and identify the form of a through-composed song (p. 201)
- Sing and evaluate the performance of "Siyahamba" (p. 215)

Performing Music: Playing

- Pat a mixed-meter ostinato (p. 199)
- Perform an Orff arrangement titled "Evening Chaconne" (p. 203)

Listening to Music

- Listen to and describe the musical elements in a John Cage piece (p. 209)
- Listen to and describe the voicing and timbre of choral selections (p. 211)
- Listen to and identify the musical texture of a Bernstein piece (p. 219)

Unit 6 187

CULTURAL CONNECTION

Unit Highlights The musical literature in this unit provides many opportunities for students to explore a variety of world cultures. A more detailed description of the resources and activities listed below can be found in the Unit at a Glance on pp. 185a–185h.

▶ AFRICAN/AFRICAN AMERICAN

- Learn about the history and roots of African American spirituals (p. 191)
- Learn about the Zulu nation in South Africa (p. 212)

▶ EUROPEAN

- Discover facts about the folk music of Hungary (p. 197)

▶ MEXICAN; SPANISH

- Learn about Mexican *mariachi* music (p. 199)
- Discover the influence of mixed-meters in the music of Joaquín Rodgrio (p. 199)

▶ UNITED STATES

- Learn about Leonard Bernstein's *Mass* (p. 217)

OPENING ACTIVITIES

MATERIALS

• "Go, My Son"	**CD 10–24**

Recording Routine: Intro (7 m. spoken); v. 1; v. 2; coda

• *Dinéh Round Dance*	**CD 10–22**
• Interview with Valerie Dee Naranjo	**CD 10–23**
• keyboards	

Listening

Clap the rhythm of the first four measures of "Go, My Son" for students. Help them discover that mm. 1-2 is the same as mm. 3-4. Invite all students to clap this rhythm.

Clap the rhythm of mm. 5-8.

ASK Is this the same or different rhythm? (The first two measures are the same; the second two measures are different.)

Repeat this activity for p. 189, working four measures at a time.

Help students discover that each eighth measure phrase ends with dotted half and whole notes, the only long notes in the piece.

Singing

Invite students to sing "Go, My Son" **CD 10–22** with the recording. Encourage them to use good breath support for the long phrases. Have students practice holding notes for their full value.

Reading

Invite students to read the rhythm of "Go, My Son" aloud, using rhythm syllables. Remind them to read the stems going up, as the stems going down are only for one verse. Tell students, the song has many patterns, which can be used to learn the song.

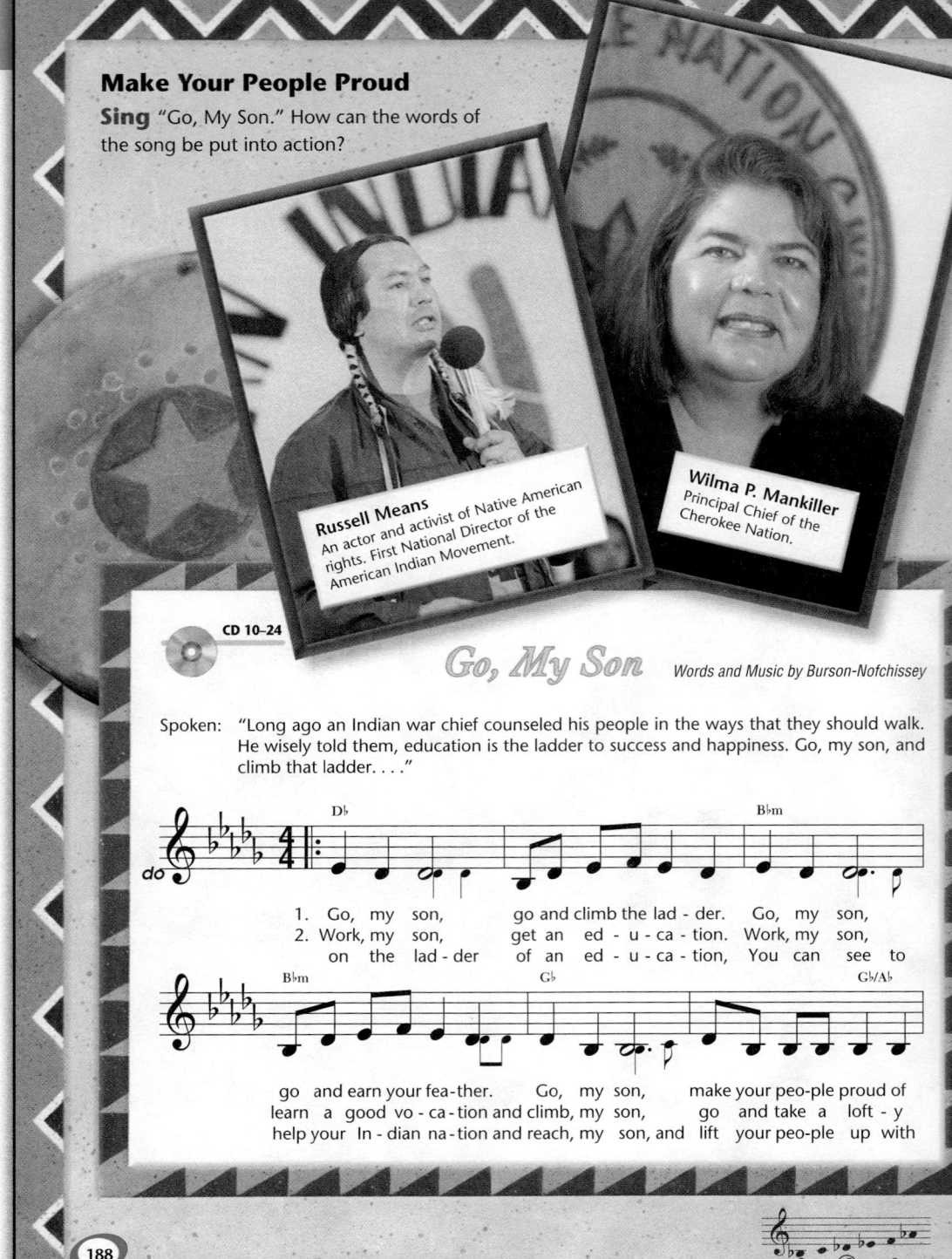

Make Your People Proud

Sing "Go, My Son." How can the words of the song be put into action?

Russell Means
An actor and activist of Native American rights. First National Director of the American Indian Movement.

Wilma P. Mankiller
Principal Chief of the Cherokee Nation.

CD 10–24

Go, My Son
Words and Music by Burson-Nofchissey

Spoken: "Long ago an Indian war chief counseled his people in the ways that they should walk. He wisely told them, education is the ladder to success and happiness. Go, my son, and climb that ladder...."

1. Go, my son, go and climb the lad - der. Go, my son,
2. Work, my son, get an ed - u - ca - tion. Work, my son, on the lad - der of an ed - u - ca - tion, You can see to

go and earn your fea - ther. Go, my son, make your peo - ple proud of
learn a good vo - ca - tion and climb, my son, go and take a loft - y
help your In - dian na - tion and reach, my son, and lift your peo - ple up with

188

ASSESSMENT

Unit Highlights This unit includes a variety of strategies and methods, described below, to track students' progress and assess their understanding of lesson objectives. Reproducible masters for Show What You Know! and Review, Assess, Perform, Create can be found in the Resource Book.

▶ **FORMAL ASSESSMENTS**

The following assessments, using written language, cognitive, and performance skills, help teachers and students conceptualize the learning that is taking place.

- **Show What You Know!** Element-specific assessments, on the student page, for Rhythm (p. 197) and Melody (p. 204)
- **Review, Assess, Perform, Create** This end-of-unit activity (pp. 220–221) can be used for review and to assess students' learning of the core lessons in this unit.

▶ **INFORMAL ASSESSMENTS**

At the close of each Teacher's Edition lesson in this unit, one of the following types of assessments is used to evaluate the learning of the key element focus or skill objective.

- Music Journal Writing (pp. 209, 211)
- Observation/Music Journal Writing (p. 219)
- Performance/Observation (pp. 195, 199, 205, 207)
- Performance/Music Journal Writing (p. 201)
- Performance/Peer Critique (pp. 193, 197, 203, 215)

▶ **RUBRICS**

Visit *www.sfsuccessnet.com* for rubrics to assess students' achievement in music skills.

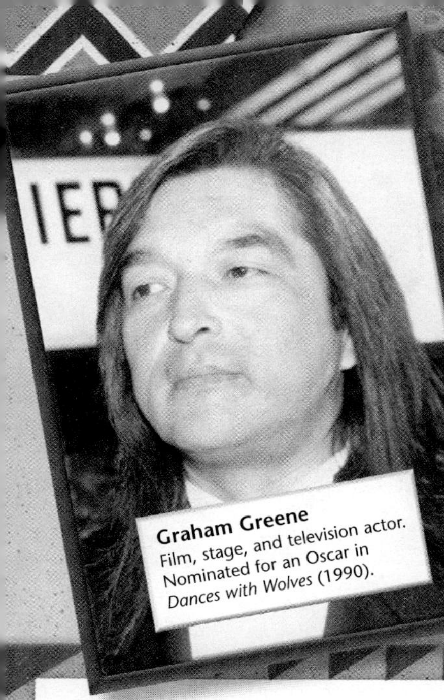

Graham Greene
Film, stage, and television actor. Nominated for an Oscar in *Dances with Wolves* (1990).

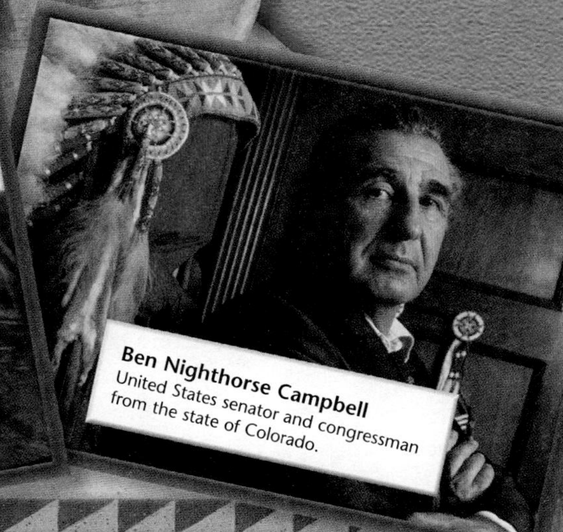

Ben Nighthorse Campbell
United States senator and congressman from the state of Colorado.

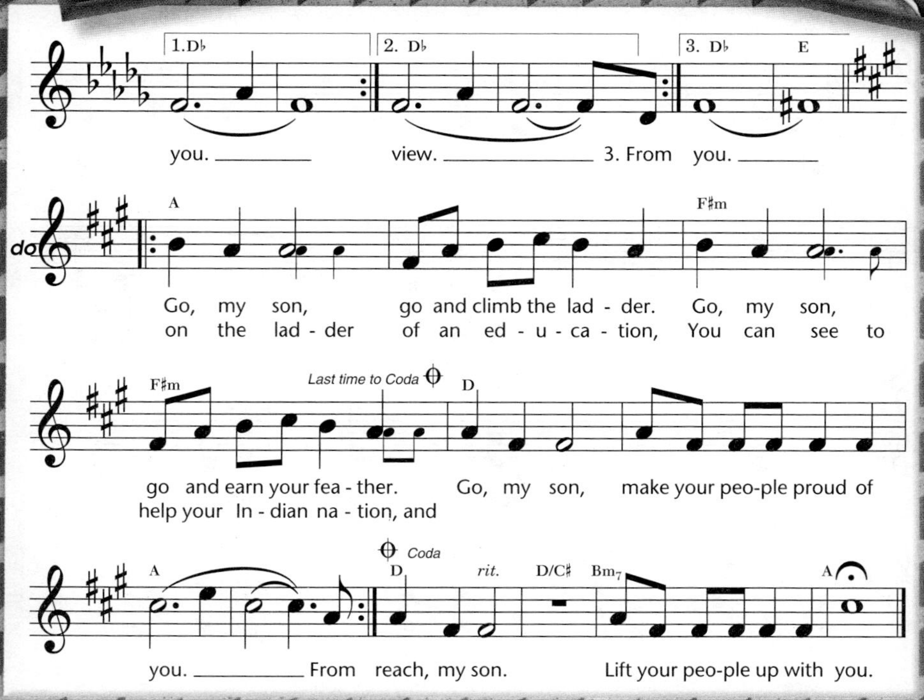

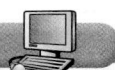

Moving

Invite students to play a passing game. Have students sit knee to knee in a circle on the floor, a pair of sticks in front of each person. Then, have students perform these movements with the song.

Beat

1 Pick up your own.

2 Pass to the right (leave them on the floor).

3 Pick up your own.

4 Pass to the right (leave them on the floor).

5 Pick up your own.

6 Tap sticks together.

7 Tap floor.

8 Tap sticks together.

Improvising

Guide students to see that "Go, My Son" uses a pentatonic scale. Invite them to improvise a melody on the black keys of the piano. Have other students play a steady beat on drums.

INNOVATIVE TEACHER SUPPORT FOR THIS UNIT

- **MAKING MUSIC DVD, Grade 6** contains video segments that support lessons, including signing and movement.
- **MAKING MUSIC with Movement and Dance** provides more opportunities for large group activities in music or physical education classes.
- **MAKING MUSIC with Technology** provides lesson plans for many technology applications; includes MIDI files.
- *¡A cantar!* features recorded songs and lessons from around the Spanish-speaking world; includes strategies for bilingual classes and for English-speaking teachers working with Spanish-speaking students.
- **Bridges to Asia** features recorded songs and lessons from Asian and Pacific region cultures.
- *www.sfsuccessnet.com* provides an online lesson planner to conveniently create lesson plans at school or at home. Includes rubrics for assessment, lesson modifications to meet the needs of all students, performance musicals based on program content, and more.

Go, my son, go and climb the lad-der. Go, my son,
on the lad-der of an ed-u-ca-tion, You can see to

go and earn your fea-ther. Go, my son, make your peo-ple proud of
help your In-dian na-tion, and

you. From reach, my son. Lift your peo-ple up with you.

Unit 6 189

TECHNOLOGY/MEDIA LINK

Unit Highlights The following components are used in this unit to reinforce and expand students' understanding of music elements and related themes.

▶ **MIDI/SEQUENCING SOFTWARE**

- Record the melody of a round and create a round (p. 207)
- Use a MIDI file to isolate and learn vocal parts (p. 215)

▶ **MULTIMEDIA**

- Create an avant-garde multimedia concert (p. 209)

▶ **NOTATION SOFTWARE**

- Use notation software to create an arrangement of a song (p. 193)
- Create a through-composed composition (p. 201)
- Give students a handout on how to compose an Orff arrangement, using notation software (p. 203)

- Use notation software to create a two-measure ostinato (p. 205)
- Notate and play back a SATB choral score (p. 211)

▶ **SEQUENCING SOFTWARE**

- Record an original mixed-meter composition (p. 197)

▶ **TRANSPARENCY**

- Display the listening map transparencies for *Responsory: Alleluia* and *Overture to Candide* (p. 219)

▶ **WEB SITE**

- Find out more information on Bob Dylan (p. 195)
- Learn more about Béla Bartok and the music of Hungary (p. 197)
- Look up information on Aaron Copland (p. 199)
- Learn more about Leonard Bernstein and his music (p. 219)

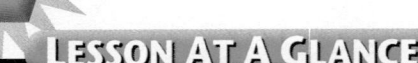

LESSON AT A GLANCE

Element Focus	**EXPRESSION** Tempo *rubato*
Skill Objective	**SINGING** Perform a spiritual using *rubato*
Connection Activity	**LANGUAGE ARTS** Discover that similes can be effectively used in song lyrics

MATERIALS

- "Peace Like a River"   **CD 10-26**
  Recording Routine: Intro (free tempo, then 4 m.); v. 1; v. 2; interlude (4 m.); v. 3
- "Minuet" from *Orchestral Suite No. 2 in B Minor* (excerpt)   **CD 10-28**
- *The Blue Danube* (excerpt)   **CD 10-29**
- "Autumn" (poem)
  Resource Book pp. G-11, H-18
- conductor's baton

VOCABULARY

rubato   conducting   introduction

◆ ◆ ◆ ◆ National Standards ◆ ◆ ◆ ◆

1c Sing music from diverse genres, with appropriate expression
4c Arrange, using electronic media
6b Listen and analyze uses of rhythm, timbre, and texture in music from diverse genres
8b Identify ways music relates to language arts
9a Describe characteristics of music genres from a variety of cultures

MORE MUSIC CHOICES

For more experience with *rubato*:
Glory, Glory, Hallelujah, p. 54
Swing Low, Sweet Chariot, p. 234

Flowing Tempos

We often use similes to express ourselves. We talk about being as "happy as a clown" or "running like the wind." In this song, similes are used to express feelings of peace, joy, and love.

Sing the spiritual "Peace Like a River." Notice the steady beat of the accompaniment. Later, learn the harmony part and **perform** the song in homophonic style.

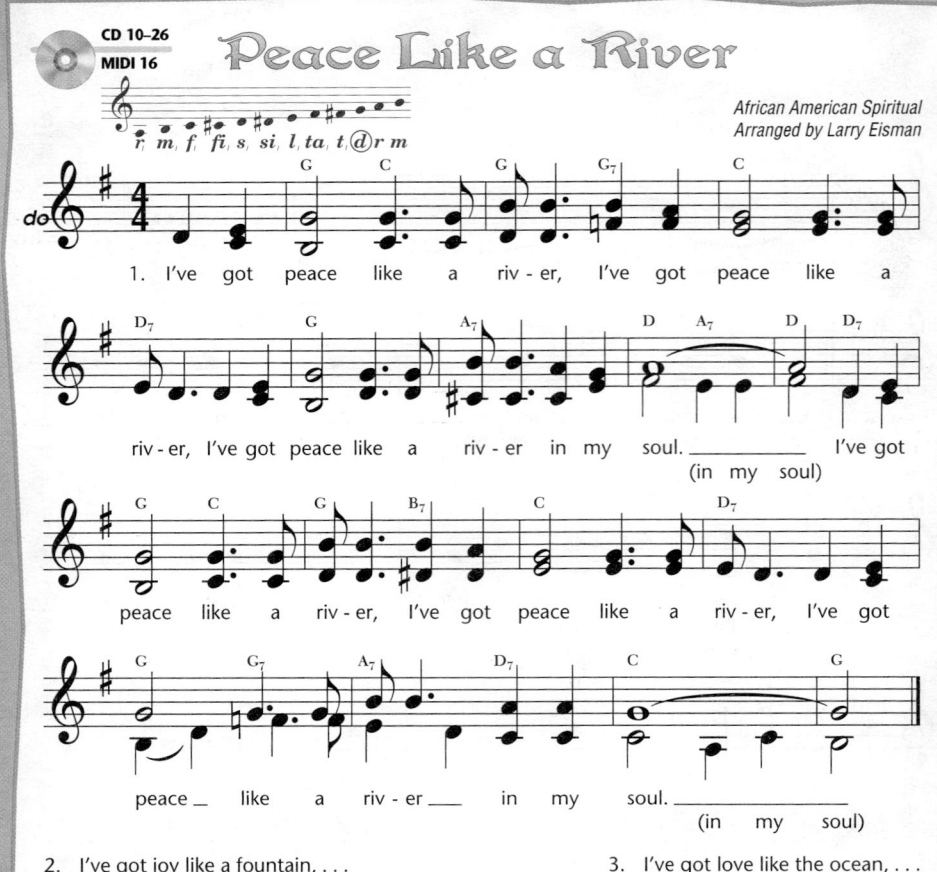

Peace Like a River

CD 10–26   MIDI 16

African American Spiritual
Arranged by Larry Eisman

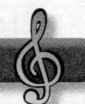

1. I've got peace like a riv-er, I've got peace like a riv-er, I've got peace like a riv-er in my soul. (in my soul) I've got

peace like a riv-er, I've got peace like a riv-er, I've got

peace _ like a riv-er _ in my soul. (in my soul)

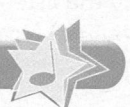 2. I've got joy like a fountain, . . .   3. I've got love like the ocean, . . .

190

Footnotes

MEETING INDIVIDUAL NEEDS

▶ **English Language Learners** Using various photos of rivers, fountains, and the ocean, ask students to select among these photos for the correct picture to match the word as they sing "Peace Like a River." Add distracter items to ensure that students really do understand the words.

BUILDING SKILLS THROUGH MUSIC

▶ **Language** Have students read the lyrics to "Peace Like a River." By using *river, fountain,* and *ocean* as similes for *peace, joy,* and *love,* the writer was adding meaning to those words. Ask students to describe their interpretation of those meanings. Working in small groups, have the students write a poem about peace.

SKILLS REINFORCEMENT

6b ▶ **Listening** Help students recognize thin and thick texture in the recording of "Peace Like a River." Point out that the texture is thin at first (only a solo flute) and becomes thicker as voices and instruments are added. Explain that the texture of this piece can be described as "chordal," or *homophonic.*

Several different styles can be observed in the recorded performance of "Peace Like a River." The introduction of the song is played by solo flute. Verse 1 features a gentle vocal solo, accompanied by piano and cello. Verse 2 adds vocal harmony, accompanied by strings, piano, and harp. Verse 3 employs a gospel style in both the voices and the accompaniment.

▶ **Signing** Invite students to learn sign language for "Peace Like a River" on Resource Book p. H-18.

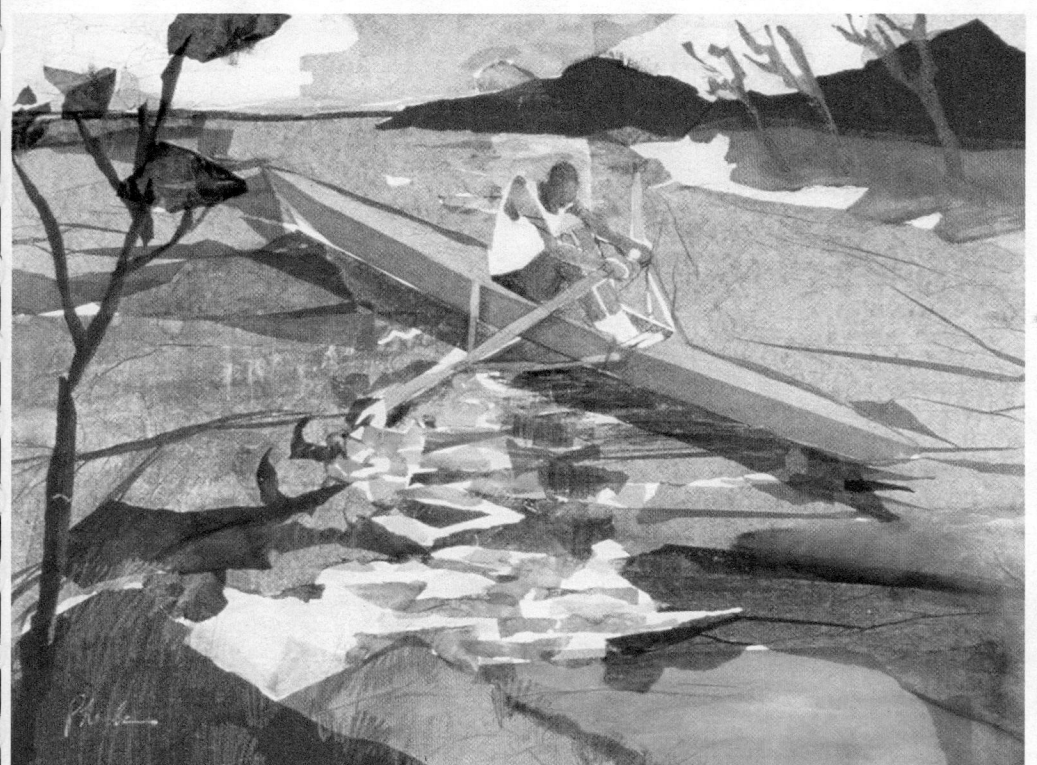

1 **INTRODUCE**

1 **INTRODUCE**

Engage students in a short discussion of similes and invite them to share similes they have heard or to create new ones. (For example: *sly as a fox, gentle as a lamb, happy as a lark, lonely as a cloud.*)

Ask students to read the poem "Autumn," on p. 193, and identify the similes in the text.

8b Challenge students to examine the text of the song "Peace Like a River" to find similes. *(peace like a river, joy like a fountain, love like the ocean)*

2 **DEVELOP**

Singing

Invite students to sing "Peace Like a River" **CD 10-26.** Select a few students to sing the harmony part with the recording. Then have students sing the song in two parts with the recording.

Moving

1c Invite students to conduct "Peace Like a River" in meter in 4. Have students

- Perform expressively, from the notation, this song from American culture.
- Practice the conducting pattern $\frac{4}{4}$ on p. 191.
- Conduct "Peace Like a River" while singing it without the recording.
- Conduct and sing the song with the recording.

Help students discover that it is difficult to conduct the introduction because the beat is not steady. Explain that the flute plays *rubato* during the introduction. Introduce students to the definition of *rubato* on p. 191.

SAY Although the underlying beat stays the same, *rubato* "plays" with the beat, pushing it ahead or pulling it back slightly to allow greater expression.

Arts Connection

▲ *Sculling at Sunset*
by Phoebe Beasley, 1983

You're the Conductor!

Practice this conducting pattern and **conduct** "Peace Like a River" as you sing.

Use the same pattern to conduct the introduction to "Peace Like a River." Does the pattern "fit" the music?

To demonstrate **rubato** when conducting, you should clearly indicate changes in tempo.

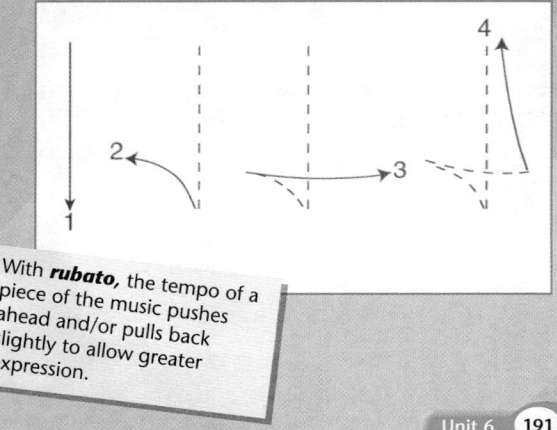

With **rubato,** the tempo of a piece of the music pushes ahead and/or pulls back slightly to allow greater expression.

 Unit 6 **191**

continued on page 192

SPOTLIGHT ON

▶ **The Conductor's Baton** Students might enjoy knowing more about the baton used by conductors of instrumental and large choral groups. The baton is a delicate "instrument" that is light and perfectly balanced. It assumed its present form only after hundreds of years of experimentation. A skilled conductor uses the baton to communicate with the performers.

To hold a baton properly, the conductor places the stick in the right hand between the tip of the thumb and the side of the index finger. The heel, or ball, of the baton rests in the palm of the hand, between the center of the palm and the base of the thumb. The tip of the baton should point forward, and the time-beating pattern should be very clear at the end of the stick.

CULTURAL CONNECTION

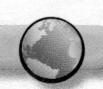

9a ▶ **African American Spirituals** The African American spiritual can be traced back to the call-and-response singing styles of sub-Saharan Africa. When Africans came to the New World, they continued this practice in work songs, leisure songs, and spirituals. Most spirituals display a strong rhythmic feel (even slow, lyrical examples such as "Peace Like a River" use syncopation) and the influence of the European harmonies sung by white colonial settlers.

Spirituals represent one aspect of African American slaves' musical response to their condition. The religious content and syncopated rhythms helped to make the hard work more bearable. Spirituals were also the first genuine African American music to be popularized after the Civil War by African American college choirs such as the Fisk Jubilee Singers.

Lesson 1 Continued

Allow students to

- Examine a conductor's baton.
- Practice holding it correctly. (See Spotlight On below.)
- Practice conducting meter in 4 with it.

Playing

Invite students to learn a keyboard part for "Peace Like a River" in Skills Reinforcement on p. 193.

Moving

Invite students to learn signs for "Peace Like a River" on Resource Book p. G-11.

Listening

6b Invite students to

- Observe and practice the conducting pattern for meter in 3 ($\frac{3}{4}$) on p. 192.
- Conduct the pattern as they listen to Bach's *Minuet* **CD 10-28.**

Help students discover that the beat in this selection is very steady, making it easy to conduct the pattern.

Invite students to conduct meter in 3 as they listen to *The Blue Danube* **CD 10-29.**

ASK Did the tempo remain steady throughout? (No; *rubato* was used.)

Guide students to understand that *The Blue Danube* is a challenging selection to conduct. The introduction is conducted in 3 but will be interrupted by *rubato* passages, pauses, and an *accelerando*. Once the main theme arrives (approximately 1:37), it begins with a *rubato* pickup followed by the main theme in a fast 3. Guide students to learn that a fast meter in 3 can be conducted in meter in 1. Have students imitate your conducting in both a fast meter in 3 and meter in 1.

Invite students to listen again to *The Blue Danube* **CD 10-29** and conduct the main theme, using their choice of meter in 1, or meter in 3.

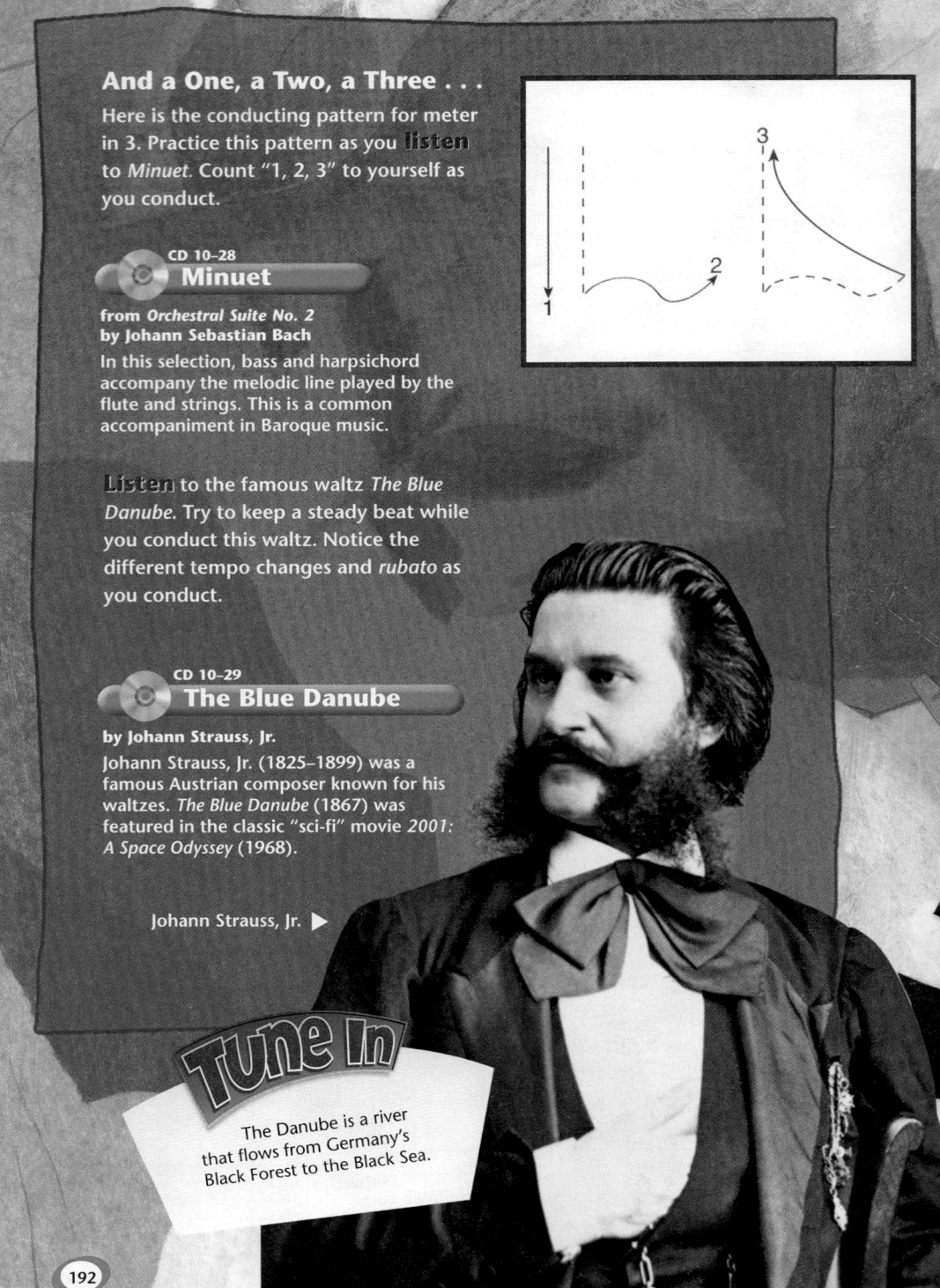

And a One, a Two, a Three . . .

Here is the conducting pattern for meter in 3. Practice this pattern as you **listen** to *Minuet*. Count "1, 2, 3" to yourself as you conduct.

CD 10–28
Minuet

from *Orchestral Suite No. 2* by Johann Sebastian Bach

In this selection, bass and harpsichord accompany the melodic line played by the flute and strings. This is a common accompaniment in Baroque music.

Listen to the famous waltz *The Blue Danube*. Try to keep a steady beat while you conduct this waltz. Notice the different tempo changes and *rubato* as you conduct.

CD 10–29
The Blue Danube

by Johann Strauss, Jr.
Johann Strauss, Jr. (1825–1899) was a famous Austrian composer known for his waltzes. *The Blue Danube* (1867) was featured in the classic "sci-fi" movie *2001: A Space Odyssey* (1968).

Johann Strauss, Jr. ▶

Tune In

The Danube is a river that flows from Germany's Black Forest to the Black Sea.

192

Footnotes

SPOTLIGHT ON

▶ **The Composer** Johann Strauss II (1825–1899) was told by his father, a prominent composer and violinist, to go into banking instead of music. Music must have been in Strauss's genes, though, because at age six he was already composing music. His mother saw the child's talent and arranged for him to secretly take violin lessons with the leader of his father's orchestra. Eventually, the younger Strauss formed his own orchestra, hiring his composer brothers as conductors and violinists. When his father died, the younger Strauss combined orchestras and inherited his father's title, the Waltz King. Johann, in fact, perfected the Viennese waltz with his gifts for melody, interesting harmonies, and unique orchestrations. He also wrote polkas, quadrilles, and stage works such as *Die Fledermaus*. He died a wealthy man, celebrated in both Europe and America.

ACROSS THE CURRICULUM

▶ **Social Studies** The Danube River, the subject of one of Strauss's best-known waltzes, is the only major river in Europe that flows from west to east. It begins in the Black Forest region and empties into the Black Sea. The Danube Valley in Austria, between Linz and Vienna, is especially renowned for its scenery. In Strauss's time, the river became an important link between industrial Germany and the agrarian Balkans. Today the Danube, like many other rivers, is suffering the results of pollution. Various organizations are, however, determined to make it beautiful once again.

Invite students to locate the Danube on a map of Europe and trace its course from west to east.

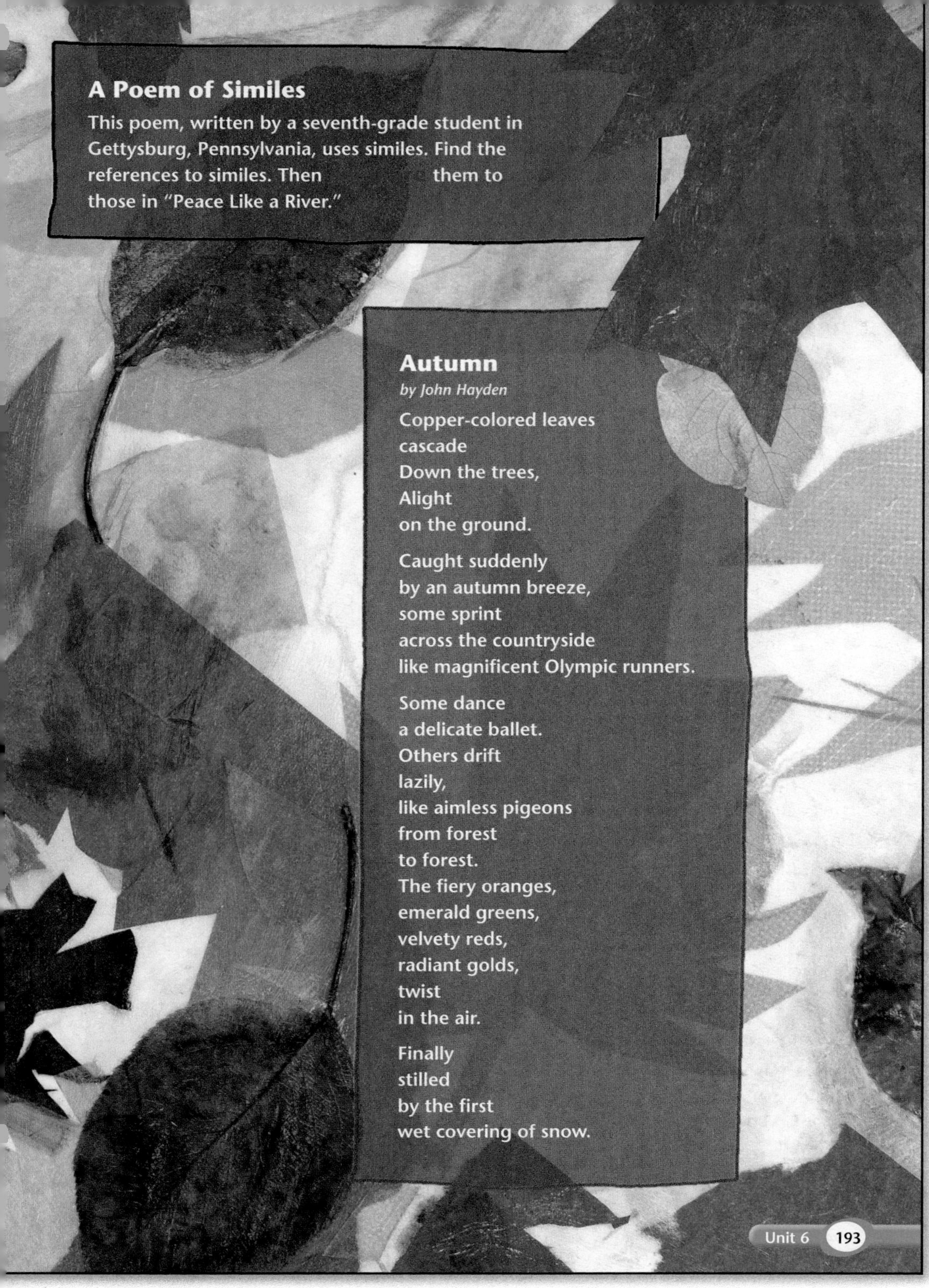

A Poem of Similes

This poem, written by a seventh-grade student in Gettysburg, Pennsylvania, uses similes. Find the references to similes. Then   them to those in "Peace Like a River."

Autumn
by John Hayden

Copper-colored leaves
cascade
Down the trees,
Alight
on the ground.

Caught suddenly
by an autumn breeze,
some sprint
across the countryside
like magnificent Olympic runners.

Some dance
a delicate ballet.
Others drift
lazily,
like aimless pigeons
from forest
to forest.
The fiery oranges,
emerald greens,
velvety reds,
radiant golds,
twist
in the air.

Finally
stilled
by the first
wet covering of snow.

Unit 6   **193**

3 CLOSE

Element: EXPRESSION   **ASSESSMENT**

1c   **Performance/Peer Critique** Organize the class into three groups. Assign each group to sing a different verse of "Peace Like a River," without the recording, incorporating *rubato* in the performance to heighten expression of the lyrics. Invite each group to choose a conductor.

Provide an opportunity for the groups to sing their verse for the rest of the class. Invite the listeners to critique each performance and determine how well each group interpreted and used *rubato* to add to the expression of the lyrics in their performance.

SKILLS REINFORCEMENT

1c ▶ **Vocal Development** *Rubato*, the slight slowing down of certain notes or phrases in a song, is used in certain styles of music to increase expression. As an additional experience with rubato, have students try the following exercise: On a treble staff, in $\frac{4}{4}$ time, write two measures of eighth notes on first-space F. Under each note, write alternately *doo* and *deh*. Ask students to sing the exercise in strict rhythm to a metronome marking of 60 (quarter note). Then ask students to sing the exercise following your *rubato* conducting. Return to the original tempo after the *rubato*.

 ▶ **Keyboard** Students may learn and play the tenor and bass keyboard part on Resource Book p. H-18 with "Peace Like a River."

TECHNOLOGY/MEDIA LINK

4c **Notation Software** Use notation software to create an arrangement of "Peace Like a River." Have students

- Set three staff lines (for the melody, harmony, and one bass clef staff). Use standard symbols to notate the meter. $\frac{4}{4}$
- Choose the key of G (one sharp), then notate the treble staves of "Peace Like a River" by selecting the desired rhythmic value and clicking on the staff to notate the pitch.
- Create a bass part on the bass staff using chord roots with student-selected rhythms.
- Challenge students to sight-read the bass part written in the bass clef.
- Select a playback timbre for each of the song's staves.

LESSON AT A GLANCE

Element Focus	**RHYTHM** Eighth notes grouped in 3+3+2
Skill Objective	**PLAYING** Play 3+3+2 eighth-note rhythm patterns
Connection Activity	**SOCIAL STUDIES** Discuss the political significance of social unrest in the 1960s

MATERIALS
- "Paths of Victory"   **CD 10-30**
  Recording Routine: Intro (8 m.); refrain; v. 1; refrain; v. 2; refrain; interlude (8 m.); v. 3; refrain; v. 4; refrain; coda
- **Music Reading Practice, Sequence 21**   **CD 10-32**
- **Resource Book** pp. E-22, F-19, H-19
- guitar, Autoharps, drums, mallet instruments, claves

VOCABULARY
syncopation

◆ ◆ ◆ ◆ **National Standards** ◆ ◆ ◆ ◆

2a Play instruments accurately alone
5a Read quarter and eighth note syncopated rhythm patterns
6b Listen and analyze uses of rhythm in music from diverse genres
8b Identify ways music relates to social studies

MORE MUSIC CHOICES
For more songs and listenings with 3+3+2:
"Má Teodora," p. 301
El Salón México, p. 199

1 INTRODUCE

8b Lead a discussion about the social issues in the United States in the 1960s and that folk music, poetry, and movies from that time often centered on peace. Have students read and listen to the lyrics for Bob Dylan's "Paths of Victory" **CD 10-30.** Guide them to identify the theme of hope. Invite students to sing the song.

ADJUST THE ACCENTS

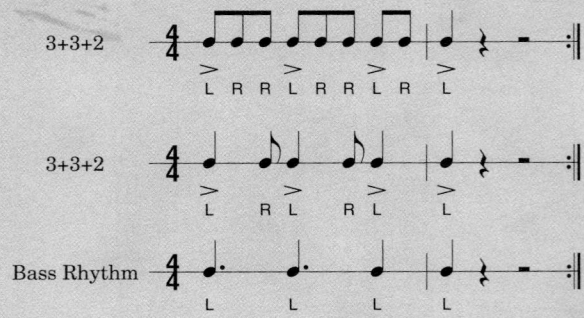

In ⁴₄ time, the first and third beats are usually the strongest beats of the measure. You can group eighth notes with accents on weak beats to create an interesting rhythmic syncopation we call 3+3+2. The ⁴₄ pattern is divided into 3 eighth notes + 3 eighth notes + 2 eighth notes.

Perform these rhythms by patting to feel the 3+3+2 groupings.

3+3+2
L R R L R R L R   L

3+3+2
L R L R L   L

Bass Rhythm
L L L L

Play this syncopated strum on guitar or Autoharp with Bob Dylan's song "Paths of Victory."

Guitar or Autoharp

Song of Peace
Bob Dylan was one of the most significant folk songwriters of the 1960s. **Sing** "Paths of Victory," then add the syncopated accompaniments.

▲ Bob Dylan

Footnotes

ACROSS THE CURRICULUM

▶ **Social Studies** Read aloud the book *War and Peace* by Toni Goffe (Childs Play, 1991), which discusses the causes of conflict and the difficulty of achieving peace. Invite students to write in their journals about peace. Using the prompt in the book about individual responsibility, ask students to consider what they are willing to do for peace.

BUILDING SKILLS THROUGH MUSIC

▶ **Language** After learning about the 1960's in School to Home Connection, have students create a conversation between two sixth graders in the 1960s. Ask them to write in present tense. Ask for volunteers to share their dialogues.

SKILLS REINFORCEMENT

▶ **Keyboard** Students will enjoy learning the close-position chords on the keyboard with "Paths of Victory." The three chords from the song are notated on Resource Book p. H-19, along with a keyboard accompaniment. Select a student to play the accompaniment as the class sings the song.

▶ **Mallets** Invite students to learn the Orff accompaniment for "Paths of Victory," found on p. F-19 in the Resource Book. Mallet players may wish to join the keyboard and guitar players for a full accompaniment as the class sings the song.

▶ **Reading** For more music reading practice, see p. 498 or Resource Book p. E-22.

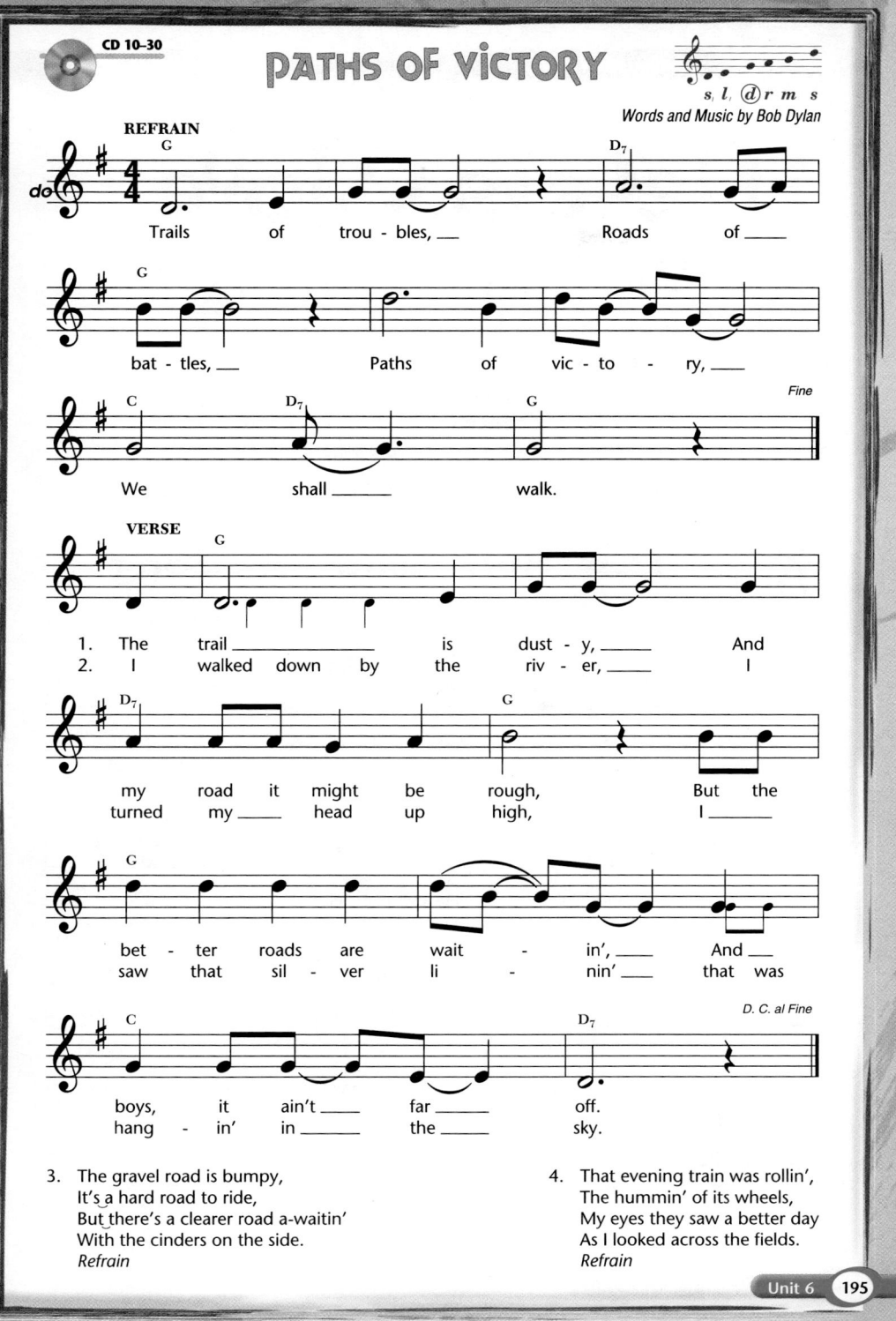

PATHS OF VICTORY

s, l, (d) r m s

Words and Music by Bob Dylan

REFRAIN

Trails of trou-bles, ___ Roads of

bat-tles, ___ Paths of vic-to-ry, ___

Fine

We shall _____ walk.

VERSE

1. The trail _____ is dust-y, _____ And
2. I walked down by the riv-er, _____ I

my road it might be rough, But the
turned my ___ head up high, I _____

bet-ter roads are wait-in', ___ And ___
saw that sil-ver li-nin' ___ that was

D. C. al Fine

boys, it ain't ___ far off.
hang-in' in the ___ sky.

3. The gravel road is bumpy,
   It's a hard road to ride,
   But there's a clearer road a-waitin'
   With the cinders on the side.
   Refrain

4. That evening train was rollin',
   The hummin' of its wheels,
   My eyes they saw a better day
   As I looked across the fields.
   Refrain

Unit 6 **195**

2 DEVELOP

Playing

6b Write one measure of paired eighth notes in $\frac{4}{4}$ meter on the board, with accents on the first eighth note of beats 1 and 3. Have one group of students pat the beat as another group claps the rhythm. Have them switch parts. Ask students to repeat this activity at a *piano* dynamic, as you play the first 3+3+2 rhythm (p. 194) on claves. Help students discover that their rhythm is straight, and yours is syncopated.

Reading

5a Have students read about changing accents on p. 194. As they read each rhythm ostinato, have them pat the accented rhythms and clap the unaccented rhythms, suspending their hands in the air during the rests.

Playing

2a Play "Paths of Victory" **CD 10-30** and have students perform each pattern, switching to subsequent patterns with each new verse. On verse 4, let students choose which pattern they will read and perform.

Ask students to read the syncopated rhythm on p. 194 and strum it on an "air guitar," then on a real guitar or Autoharp. Review the G (partial), D_7, and C chords for guitar on pp. 508–509. Using Skills Reinforcement on p. 194, encourage students to learn the mallet accompaniment on Resource Book, p. F-19.

3 CLOSE

Skill: PLAYING   **ASSESSMENT**

5a **Performance/Observation** Ask students to read and perform the syncopated rhythm patterns on p. 194. Then, have them perform the syncopated rhythm strum on p. 194 on "air guitar" as they sing "Paths of Victory." Observe students' ability to accurately perform the syncopated rhythms.

MEETING INDIVIDUAL NEEDS

▶ **Including Everyone** Students can learn to focus as they clap and tap syncopated rhythms.

Reinforcement For students having difficulty, consider beginning with less complex patterns, limiting the time working with one pattern, or using an aural model for patterns.

On Target If students lose focus as they watch notated patterns for long periods or the tasks become more complex, have students take a break or simplify tasks.

Challenge Invite students to play the syncopated strum on guitar as a chord accompaniment to "Paths of Victory." Further challenge students to sing the song as they play their syncopated guitar accompaniment.

SCHOOL TO HOME CONNECTION

8b ▶ **The 1960s** Ask students to discuss the 1960s with older relatives and friends. Students may wish to include topics such as the war in Vietnam, the draft, the antiwar movement, and music that was a product of that movement. Lighter topics for discussion may include clothes, hairstyles, movies, rock concerts, and poetry.

TECHNOLOGY/MEDIA LINK

Web Site Invite students to visit *www.sfsuccessnet.com* for more information on Bob Dylan.

LESSON AT A GLANCE

Element Focus	**RHYTHM** Mixed meter
Skill Objective	**READING** Read rhythm patterns that use syncopation and mixed meter
Connection Activity	**CULTURE** Explore the geographic and social origins of a composed song

MATERIALS
- "New Hungarian Folk Song" **CD 10-35**
  Recording Routine: Intro (2 m.); v. 1; interlude (3 m.); v. 2; coda
- **Music Reading Practice, Sequence 22** **CD 10-37**
- **Resource Book** pp. B-20, D-25, E-23
- nonpitched percussion instruments (rhythm sticks, claves, drums), mallet instruments

VOCABULARY
mixed meter

> ◆ ◆ ◆ ◆ **National Standards** ◆ ◆ ◆ ◆
> **1c** Sing music from diverse cultures
> **2a** Play instruments accurately alone and in small ensembles
> **4c** Compose using traditional sound sources and electronic media
> **5a** Read half, quarter, eighth, and dotted notes in duple meter
> **7b** Students use specific criteria for evaluating their own performances and compositions
> **8b** Identify ways music relates to social studies

MORE MUSIC CHOICES
For more practice with mixed meter:
"Love in Any Language," p. 476
"One Moment in Time," p. 352

1 INTRODUCE

Share the information in Cultural Connection, p. 197, with students to explore the geographical and social origins of "New Hungarian Folk Song."

Meters Move

Meter is made from groupings of beats. Most commonly, beats are grouped by two, three, or four. If the quarter note gets the beat, the resulting meters would be $\frac{2}{4}$, $\frac{3}{4}$, and $\frac{4}{4}$.

Mixing Song Meters
Composers occasionally mix meters in songs. "New Hungarian Folk Song" is an example of a mixed meter song. **Create** your own movements to show the mixed meter as you **listen** to "New Hungarian Folk Song."

Sing "New Hungarian Folk Song" and conduct as you sing.

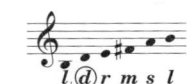

CD 10-35 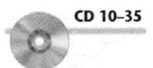 **New Hungarian Folk Song**

English Words by Jean Sinor *Words and Music by Béla Bartók*

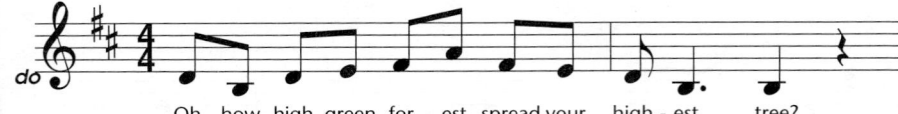

Oh, how high, green for - est, spread your high - est tree?
High a - bove the corn a lark now earth-ward flies.

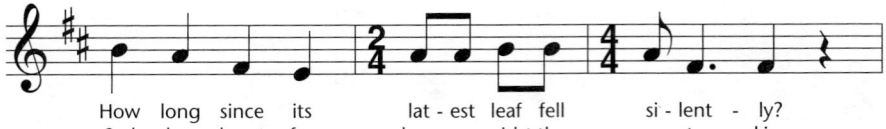

How long since its lat - est leaf fell si - lent - ly?
Sad her heart, for - lorn a - midst the emp - ty skies.

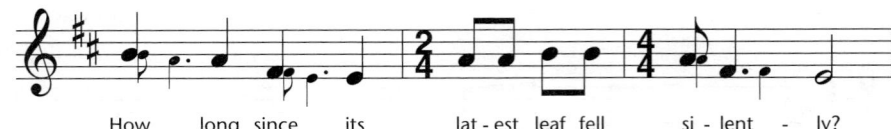

How long since its lat - est leaf fell si - lent - ly?
Shel-tered, hid-den un - der shade of leaf and flower,

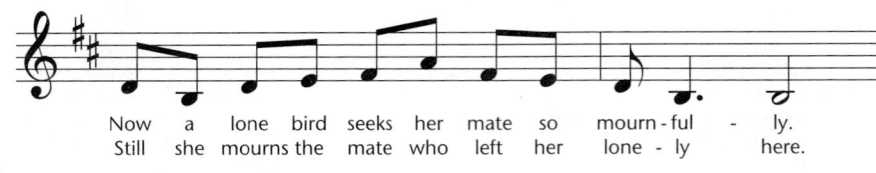

Now a lone bird seeks her mate so mourn - ful - ly.
Still she mourns the mate who left her lone - ly here.

Footnotes

SPOTLIGHT ON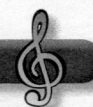

▶ **The Composer** Béla Bartók (1881–1945), one of Hungary's greatest composers, was a shy child with many illnesses. He did, however, always enjoy music. At age 9, he composed his first pieces, including *The Course of the Danube*. He eventually attended the Academy of Music in Budapest on the advice of Ernst von Dohnányi. Bartók developed a unique style of composition, fusing folklike musical elements with art music techniques.

BUILDING SKILLS THROUGH MUSIC

▶ **Language** Share the information from Cultural Connection on p. 197 with students. Lead students in a discussion of comparing Hungary's oral tradition of passing down folk songs to that of America's similar tradition. Create a list of American folk songs that may have been passed down orally (Stephen Foster songs, African American spirituals, cowboy songs).

SKILLS REINFORCEMENT

5a **2a** ▶ **Playing** The rhythm below is from *Mikrokosmos No. 137.* Have students pat the downbeat of each measure and fingertip clap the remaining beats, while saying the rhythm syllables. Then divide the class in half. Have Group 1 use a foot stomp to perform the beat as Group 2 plays the rhythm on nonpitched percussion instruments.

Play 4 times

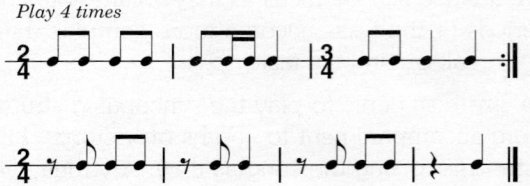

▶ **Reading** For more music reading practice, see p. 498 or Resource Book p. E-23, and Resource Book p. D-25.

Arts Connection

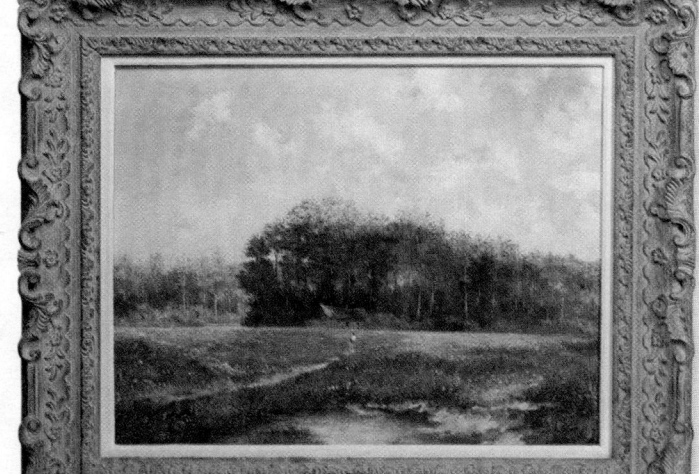

Sopron by John Nemeth (1924–1987). Hungarian landscape ▶

Show What You Know!

Perform these patterns that use syncopation and mixed meters. Then **compose** your own rhythms, using mixed meters, and **perform** them on a nonpitched percussion instrument of your choice.

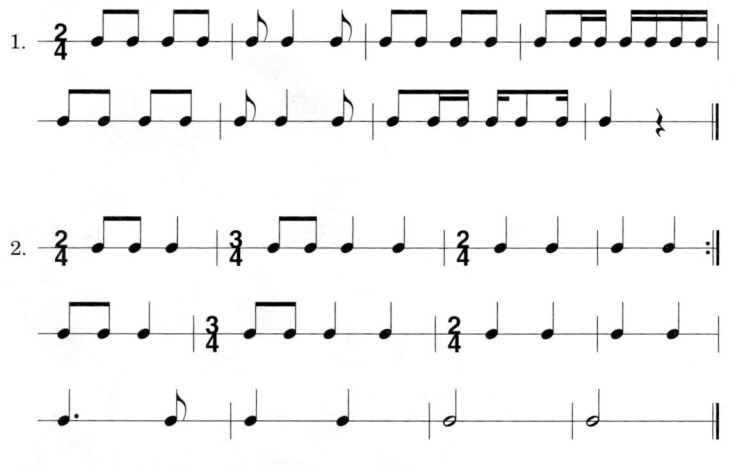

Unit 6 ⟨197⟩

2 DEVELOP

Reading

5a Direct students to the song notation of "New Hungarian Folk Song" **CD 10-35.** Have students pat the downbeat of each measure and fingertip clap the remaining beats. Then, provide an audible steady beat as they read and say the rhythm syllables silently. Ask students to listen again and conduct in mixed meter as they read the song notation.

Moving

Have students work in small groups to create movements for meter in 4 and meter in 2. Have each group perform their movements with the recording **CD 10-35.**

Singing

Direct students to the song notation. Have them

- Tap the beat as they read and sing pitch syllables.
- Read the text and determine what season is implied (summer) and what emotions are evoked (sadness, loneliness).
1c • Sing the song with the lyrics.

Composing

4c Have students create melodic phrases in *do*-pentatonic, using the pitch set and mixed-meter rhythms of "New Hungarian Folk Song."

3 CLOSE

Skill: READING   **ASSESSMENT**

7b **Performance/Peer Critique** Have students read the rhythms on Resource Book p. B-20. Have them read and perform the syncopated and mixed meter rhythms on rhythm sticks or claves as another group plays the beat on drums. Ask students to evaluate the quality of their peers' musical performances and ability to read syncopated rhythms and mixed meters.

CULTURAL CONNECTION

8b ▶ **Folk Music of Hungary** Around 1903, when nationalistic feelings were sweeping Europe, Béla Bartók and his friend Zoltán Kodály became determined to collect the folk songs of the Hungarian people. They traveled widely, asking peasants to record their voices on a wax cylinder. Kodály and Bartók recorded, collected, and analyzed peasant songs throughout their lives. Bartók's mature style incorporated many of the folk elements he learned, such as modal and pentatonic scales, exotic rhythms, and polytonality. In addition to his numerous orchestral and chamber works, Bartók published nearly 2,000 folk tunes, drawn mainly from Hungary and Romania. ("New Hungarian Folk Song" is from *Mikrokosmos*, a six-volume set of progressive piano pieces composed between the years 1926 and 1939.)

TECHNOLOGY/MEDIA LINK

4c **Sequencing Software** Encourage students to use sequencing software to arrange their rhythmic and melodic phrases. Have them

- Record their original mixed-meter compositions.
- Explore graphic editing features to alter their compositions.
- Experiment with combining and looping tracks.
- Choose a variety of percussion instruments from the GM Instrument List.

Web Site Go to *www.sfsuccessnet.com* to learn more about Béla Bartók and the music of Hungary.

LESSON AT A GLANCE

Element Focus RHYTHM $\frac{6}{8}$ and $\frac{3}{4}$ meter

Skill Objective PLAYING Play rhythm ostinatos in $\frac{6}{8}$ and $\frac{3}{4}$ meter

Connection Activity CULTURE Explore the cultural influences on a composition by an American composer

MATERIALS
- *El Salón México* (excerpt) **CD 10-40**
- *Concierto de Aranjuez* (excerpt) **CD 10-41**
- **Resource Book** p. C-8
- mallet instruments, nonpitched percussion

VOCABULARY

changing meter syncopation ostinato

◆ ◆ ◆ ◆ National Standards ◆ ◆ ◆ ◆
2a Play instruments accurately alone and in small ensembles
2c Perform instrumental music from diverse cultures
4c Compose, using traditional sound sources
6b Listen and analyze uses of rhythm in music from diverse cultures
6c Understand and use basic principles of meter in music analysis

MORE MUSIC CHOICES
Other music with changing meters or 3+3+2:
"New Hungarian Folk Song," p. 196
"Paths of Victory" (guitar strum), p. 195

1 INTRODUCE

Tell students that American composer Aaron Copland's symphonic work *El Salón México* is one of the most famous works that uses mixed meter. Mixed meter is an important element of style in twentieth-century music. Mixed meter rhythms are also found in *mariachi* music—a Mexican style that influenced the composition of Copland.

Share the Cultural Connection on p. 199 with students.

Adjust the Meters

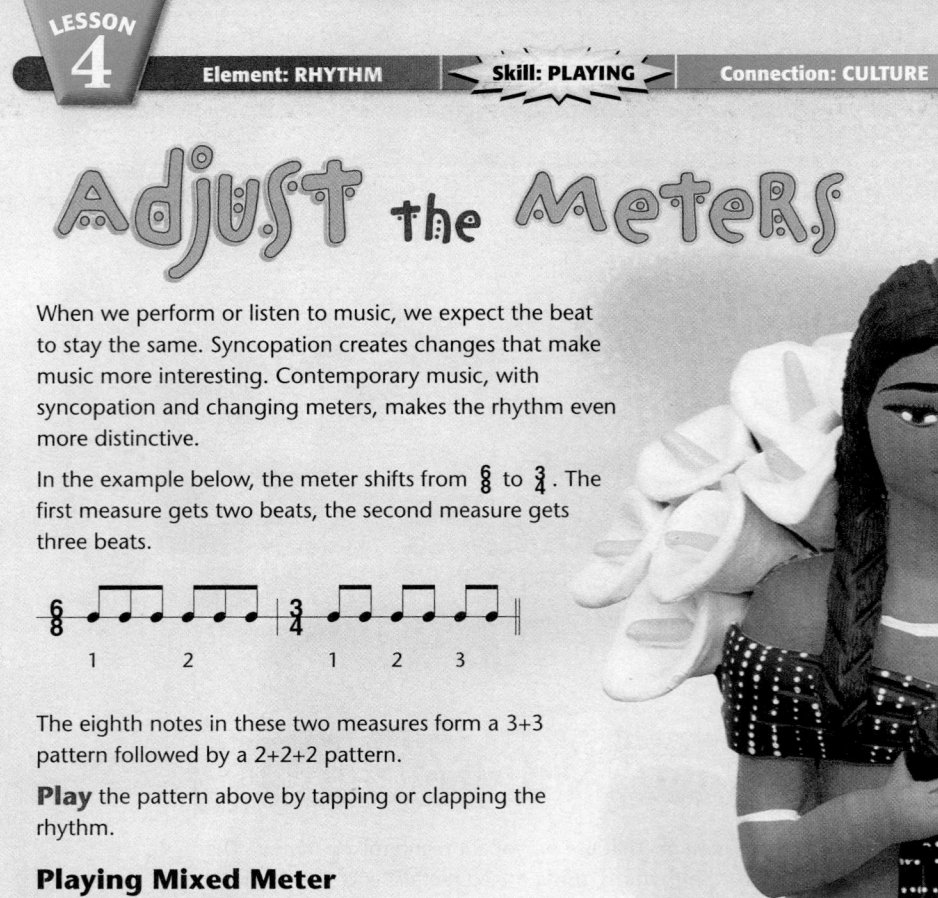

When we perform or listen to music, we expect the beat to stay the same. Syncopation creates changes that make music more interesting. Contemporary music, with syncopation and changing meters, makes the rhythm even more distinctive.

In the example below, the meter shifts from $\frac{6}{8}$ to $\frac{3}{4}$. The first measure gets two beats, the second measure gets three beats.

The eighth notes in these two measures form a 3+3 pattern followed by a 2+2+2 pattern.

Play the pattern above by tapping or clapping the rhythm.

Playing Mixed Meter

Play the pattern above on a mallet instrument, using only the pitch G. Using the pitches G and D, add a bass line to the pattern.

Create additional rhythms to accompany this pattern. Use other mallet instruments and percussion to create more layers of ostinatos.

Iguala pottery from Mexico ▶

▲ Ceramic from Mexico

198

Footnotes

SPOTLIGHT ON

▶ **The Composer** Aaron Copland (1900–1990) decided to become a composer at age 15. As a child, he learned piano from his older sister and took a correspondence course in harmony. By 1921, he went to Paris to study with the famous teacher Nadia Boulanger. Copland composed in many styles, but he is best known for his style of using simple harmonies and melodies. Copland is recognized as one of America's foremost composers.

BUILDING SKILLS THROUGH MUSIC

▶ **Language** Have students read about and listen to *El Salón México* by Aaron Copland and *Concierto de Aranjuez* by Spanish composer Joaquín Rodrigo. Have students complete a Venn diagram on Resource Book p. C-8 comparing the two compositions.

SKILLS REINFORCEMENT

▶ **Guitar** Encourage students to practice combining rhythms in Mexican *mariachi* style by patting a guitar rhythm with the left hand (labeled "Strong Hand" below) and a typical *guitarrón* rhythm with the right hand (labeled "Weak Hand" below). Tell students that they are patting $\frac{3}{4}$ with the right hand and $\frac{6}{8}$ with the left hand. Transfer the rhythms to chosen chords and notes on guitar and bass for a taste of *mariachi* style.

Strong Hand: $\frac{3}{4}$
Weak Hand: $\frac{6}{8}$

Both strong weak strong Both strong weak strong

Spanish Mixed Meters

Aaron Copland uses changing meter in this rhythmic phrase from *El Salón México*. Note that the changing meter is shown in a single measure—§ ¾ — followed by ⅜.

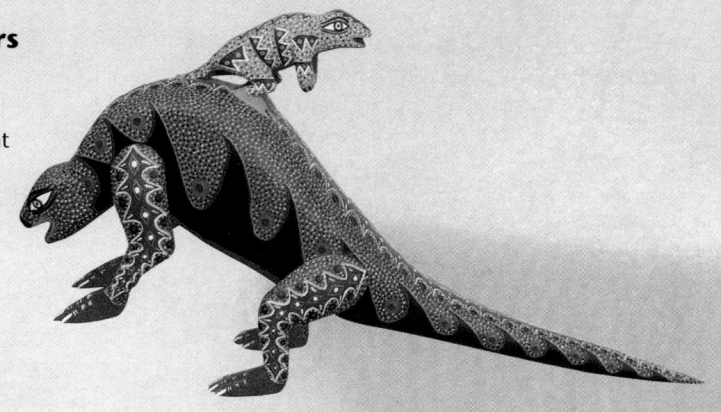

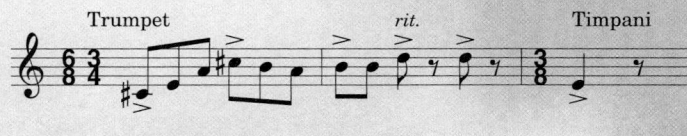

Trumpet   *rit.*   Timpani

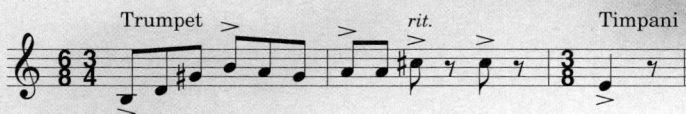

Trumpet   *rit.*   Timpani

Listen to *El Salón México* and follow the strong beats and changing meters. Watch out for the *ritardando* (slower tempo) in measures 2 and 5. The *ritardando* changes where you feel the beat.

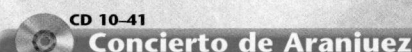

CD 10–40
El Salón México

by Aaron Copland
as performed by the New Philharmonia Orchestra, Aaron Copland, conductor

El Salón México (1936) uses Mexican folk melodies, changing meters, and syncopated rhythms to create its rhythmic excitement.

Now **listen** to another composer's use of mixed meter. In this selection, Spanish composer, Joaquín Rodrigo, uses a § ¾ § mixed-meter pattern for his main theme. As you listen, **conduct** this pattern.

CD 10–41
Concierto de Aranjuez

by Joaquín Rodrigo
as performed by Kazuhito Yamashita and the Jean-François Paillard Chamber Orchestra

Concierto de Aranjuez begins with a *rasgueado*-like strumming pattern. It is one of the most popular guitar concertos of the twentieth century and requires virtuosity from the guitar soloist.

Unit 6   **199**

---

2 DEVELOP

Playing

2c Have students read p. 198 and then follow the rhythm pattern as you clap it. Ask students to count the rhythm pattern aloud as you play it and then pat the pattern on their thighs, using the left hand for strong beats and the right hand for weak beats. See Skills Reinforcement on p. 198.

Creating

4c Encourage students to create a bass line for the pattern, using the pitches G and D on mallet instruments. Invite
2a volunteers to share their bass lines with the class.

Listening

6b Have students read and discuss the information on p. 199 about Aaron Copland's changing meter theme in *El Salón México* **CD 10-40** and then follow the theme as you play it on a keyboard. Demonstrate the conducting patterns for a § measure. Ask volunteers to conduct as you play the theme.

6c Have students listen to the excerpt from *El Salón México* **CD 10-40** and raise their hands when they hear the theme. Point out that in the recording there is a *ritardando* starting in measure 2 that adds a brief pause after each accented note in measures 2, 3, 5, and 6.

Invite students to listen to *Concierto de Aranjuez*, **CD 10-41.** Guide them to identify the § ¾ § mixed meter pattern as they listen. See Cultural Connection below.

3 CLOSE

Skill: PLAYING   ASSESSMENT

Performance/Observation Have students pat the ostinato on p. 198 as you play the theme on p. 199 on a keyboard. Observe students' ability to accurately perform the meter shift.

CULTURAL CONNECTION

▶ **Mexican Influences** *Mariachi* music is central to Mexican culture and represents a blend of indigenous and Spanish influences. The practice of combining meters, known as the *son* style, is the unifying feature of *mariachi* music all over Mexico. *Mariachi* has always been tied to dancing. Performers learn the music by ear and stroll about as they play and sing.

▶ **Spanish Influences** Joaquín Rodrigo (1901–1999) is recognized as one of Spain's foremost composers. Blind from the age of three, he became an accomplished pianist, violinist, and composer. His most famous piece, *Concierto de Aranjuez*, shows the influence of classical guitar and flamenco from his Spanish homeland. Spanish music is rich in mixed meters. The § ¾ alternating meter on, p. 198, is known as *flamenco compras*.

TECHNOLOGY/MEDIA LINK

Web Site Encourage students to visit *www.sfsuccessnet.com* for more information on composer Aaron Copland.

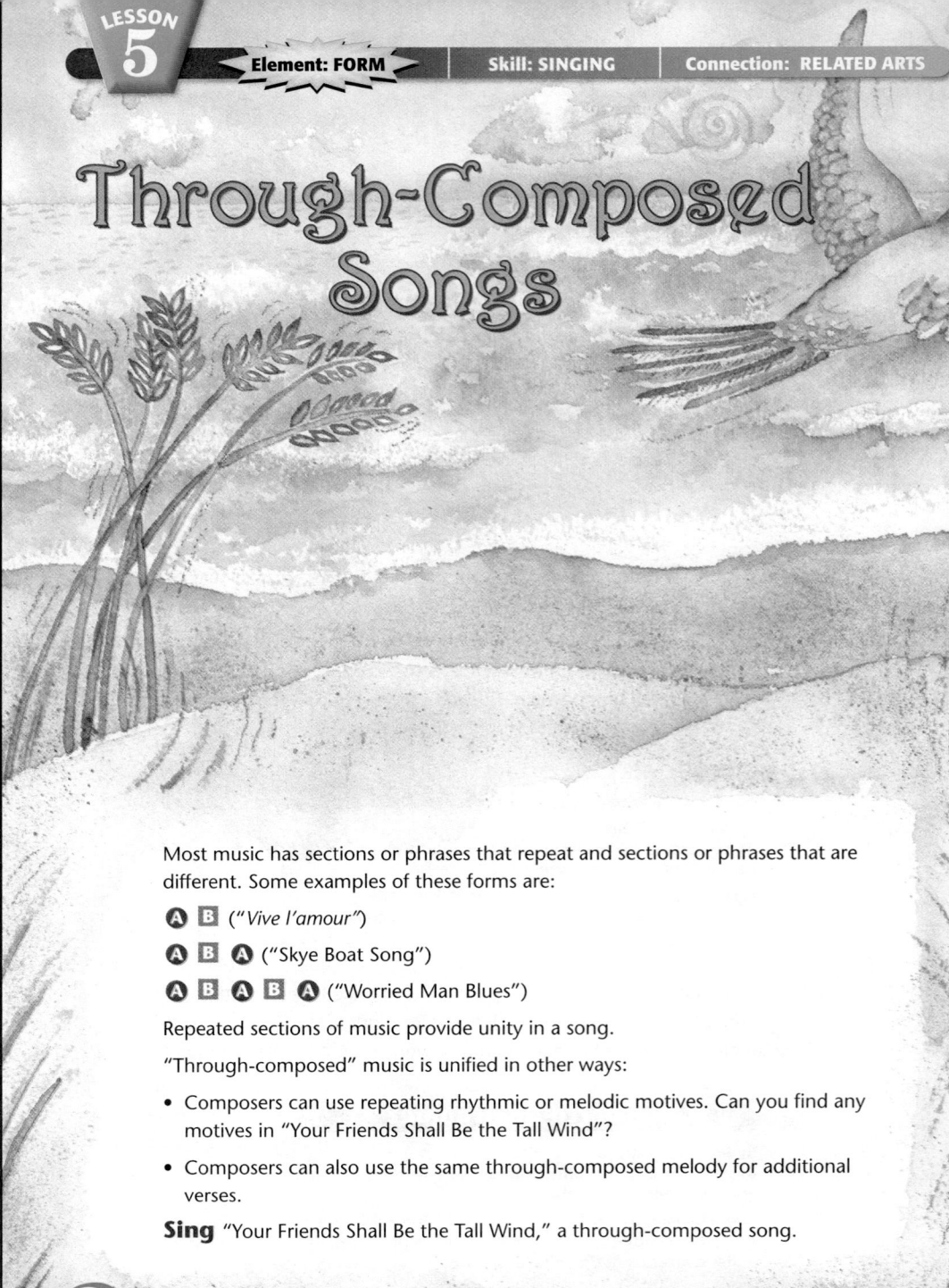

Through-Composed Songs

Element Focus	**FORM** Through-composed form
Skill Objective	**SINGING** Sing a song in through-composed form
Connection Activity	**RELATED ARTS** Discuss ways in which nature is portrayed in music and the visual arts

MATERIALS

• "Your Friends Shall Be the Tall Wind"   **CD 11-1**

Recording Routine: Intro (4 m.); v. 1; interlude (4 m.); v. 2; coda

VOCABULARY

through-composed

◆ ◆ ◆ ◆ **National Standards** ◆ ◆ ◆ ◆

4c Compose, using electronic media
5a Read quarter, half, and dotted notes in duple meter
6b Listen and analyze uses of pitch, rhythm, and form in music from diverse genres
6c Understand and use basic principles of rhythm in music analysis
8b Identify ways music relates to language arts and visual arts

MORE MUSIC CHOICES

For more songs with nature themes:
"Four Strong Winds," p. 170
"*Riendo el río corre,*" p. 263

1 INTRODUCE

8b Invite students to share descriptions of some of their favorite places in nature and to tell why those places hold special memories. Ask students to think of songs or instrumental pieces that might describe the beauty of their favorite natural places. See Across the Curriculum (Visual Arts) on p. 201.

Most music has sections or phrases that repeat and sections or phrases that are different. Some examples of these forms are:

A **B** ("Vive l'amour")

A **B** **A** ("Skye Boat Song")

A **B** **A** **B** **A** ("Worried Man Blues")

Repeated sections of music provide unity in a song.

"Through-composed" music is unified in other ways:

• Composers can use repeating rhythmic or melodic motives. Can you find any motives in "Your Friends Shall Be the Tall Wind"?

• Composers can also use the same through-composed melody for additional verses.

Sing "Your Friends Shall Be the Tall Wind," a through-composed song.

200

Footnotes

MEETING INDIVIDUAL NEEDS

▶ **Including Everyone** Because students with disabilities are often socially isolated, you might talk with the class about friendship and belonging. It might help to use an appreciation circle in which students share something they like about someone else in the circle. Make sure that each student has been appreciated by someone!

BUILDING SKILLS THROUGH MUSIC

▶ **Writing** Ask students to write a description of the ways through-composed songs differ from songs with sectional forms (such as AB or ABA), or phrase forms (such as aaba or aabb). Have them include reasons why they think the composer of "Your Friends Shall Be the Tall Wind" chose to write in through-composed style.

SKILLS REINFORCEMENT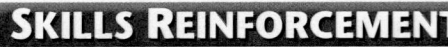

6b ▶ **Listening** Refer to the following list of songs when administering the assessment activity (form) under Close.

AB:	"Green, Green Grass of Home," p. 248 "Jambalaya," p. 244
ABA:	"Free at Last," p. 468 "Paths of Victory," p. 195
aabb:	"*El cóndor pasa,*" p. 46 "Greensleeves," p. 49
aaba:	"Blue Skies," p. 88 "Strike Up the Band," p. 135
Through-composed:	"*Bắt kim thang,*" p. 13 "I Walk the Unfrequented Road," p. 79

Your Friends Shall Be the Tall Wind

Words by Fannie Stearns Davis

Music by Emma Lou Diemer

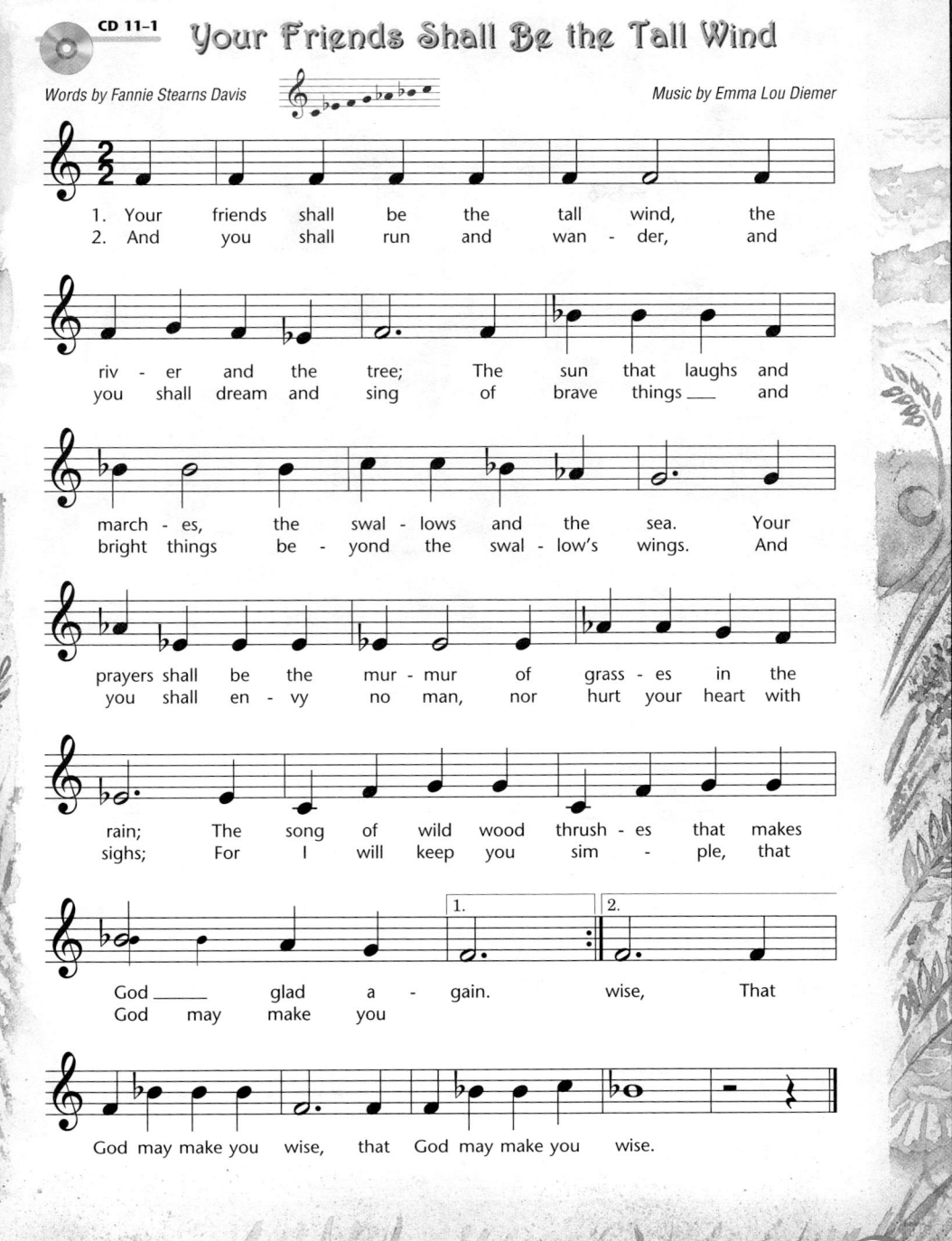

1. Your friends shall be the tall wind, the
2. And you shall run and wan - der, and

riv - er and the tree; The sun that laughs and
you shall dream and sing of brave things ____ and

march - es, the swal - lows and the sea. Your
bright things be - yond the swal - low's wings. And

prayers shall be the mur - mur of grass - es in the
you shall en - vy no man, nor hurt your heart with

rain; The song of wild wood thrush - es that makes
sighs; For I will keep you sim - ple, that

1. God ____ glad a - gain.
2. God may make you

wise, That

God may make you wise, that God may make you wise.

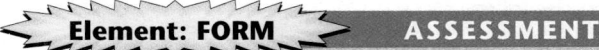

2 DEVELOP

Listening

Have students read the review information on p. 200 about song forms and through-composed songs and then listen to "Your Friends Shall Be the Tall Wind" **CD 11-1.**

6c **SAY** This song is through-composed, which means that no part of the melody repeats throughout the verse.

Guide students to identify rhythmic repetition in through-composed forms, and compare it to identifying rhythmic repetition in repeating forms, such as aaba. (more difficult).

5a **ASK** Is there rhythmic repetition that gives the song unity? (Yes. The first three phrases have the same rhythm.)

Singing

Tell students that they can sight-read simple music in treble clef in various meters, including mixed meters, using the same sight-reading skills they have already developed. Then, invite them to sight-sing "Your Friends Shall Be the Tall Wind" **CD 11–1.**

Ask students to discuss how the melodic contour illustrates the natural elements in the lyrics. See Across the Curriculum below.

3 CLOSE

Element: FORM   **ASSESSMENT**

Performance/Music Journal Writing Have students sing "Your Friends Shall Be the Tall Wind" **CD 11-1** and identify its form (through-composed) in their journals.

Write "Section" (AB, ABA) and "Phrase" (aabb, aaba) on the board. For extra credit, have students listen to selected songs as listed in Skills Reinforcement, p. 200. Ask students to identify the music forms presented aurally and write the form of each song or listening selection in their journals.

ACROSS THE CURRICULUM

8b ▶ **Language Arts** Invite students to discuss how the words of "Your Friends Shall Be the Tall Wind" are illustrated by the melodic contour. (The first line is like a *straight blowing wind* in v. 1, and *run and wander* in a straight line in v. 2; second line begins with undulating stepwise motion showing *river*, v. 1; followed by disjunct intervals of *sun that laughs and marches*, v. 1, and *brave things and bright things*, v. 2; the rest of the melody is soothing and calm, illustrating the rest of the words.)

▶ **Visual Arts** The background art for this lesson is an illustration of a natural scene. Ask students to find items of nature they see in the art. Lead a discussion about the way nature is portrayed in the art on pp. 41, 66, and 198 (ceramic bowl).

TECHNOLOGY/MEDIA LINK

4c **Notation Software** After discussing through-composed form with students, challenge them to create their own through-composed pieces, using their notation software. Have students

- Create their own lyrics, using the same rhythm found in "Your Friends Shall Be the Tall Wind." (It may be helpful to suggest topics to begin with, such as "school lunch" or "homework.")

- Use notes of the E-minor-pentatonic scale (E-G-A-B-D) to create and notate their melodies. (Remind students that they may repeat notes, as in "Your Friends Shall Be the Tall Wind.")

- Print a hard copy of their work to post in the hallway outside the music room.

LESSON 6

LESSON AT A GLANCE

Element Focus **MELODY** Melodic ostinatos

Skill Objective **PLAYING** Play a *chaconne* with melodic ostinatos and ground bass

Connection Activity **STYLE** Participate in an ensemble arrangement for mallet instruments and drum

MATERIALS
- "Evening Chaconne" **CD 11-3**
  Recording Routine: Instruments enter successively —bongos; bass, alto, soprano xylophones; glockenspiel; all instruments (1x) to 2nd ending
- bass, alto, and soprano xylophones or metallophones; soprano glockenspiel; bongos

VOCABULARY

ground bass   *chaconne*   ostinato   texture

◆ ◆ ◆ ◆ National Standards ◆ ◆ ◆ ◆

1a Sing accurately in small ensembles

2e In instrumental ensembles, perform moderately easy pieces with technical accuracy

4c Compose, using electronic media

7b Students use specific criteria for evaluating-performances, and offer constructive suggestions for improvement

MORE MUSIC CHOICES

For more experience with mallet instruments: "Mary Ann," p. 180

1 INTRODUCE

SAY A *chaconne* is a type of music in a slow meter in 3. The distinguishing characteristic of a *chaconne* is a melodic pattern in the bass part (called a *ground bass*) that repeats. One, two, or even three melodies are added above the ground bass to create a thicker texture.

An Evening Dance

A *chaconne* is a form of music in a slow meter in 3. Originally the *chaconne* was a dance in the seventeenth century. A *chaconne* is distinguished by a **ground bass.** When one, two, or three melodies are added above the ground bass, a thicker musical texture is created.

> A **ground bass** is a bass line that continuously repeats throughout a composition.

Listen Before Performing

Listen to "Evening Chaconne" before performing it. Focus on the bass ostinato and the way each melody is constructed. Does it use repeated notes, steps, or leaps?

Playing Tips

Look at the music for "Evening Chaconne." **Read** the repeating bass part and other melodic ostinatos. Practice each ostinato by singing it. Then **play** the ostinatos on instruments.

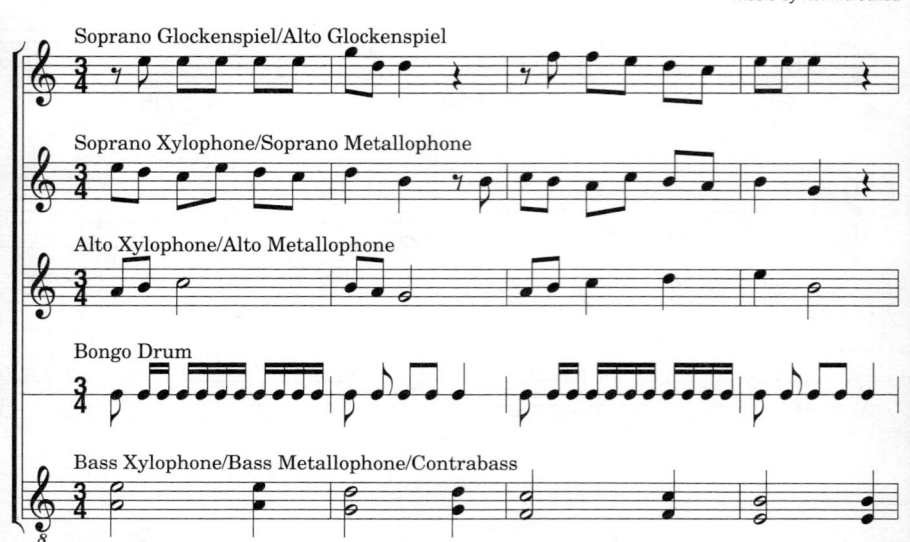

CD 11–3

Evening Chaconne

Music by Konnie Saliba

Soprano Glockenspiel/Alto Glockenspiel

Soprano Xylophone/Soprano Metallophone

Alto Xylophone/Alto Metallophone

Bongo Drum

Bass Xylophone/Bass Metallophone/Contrabass

202

Footnotes

SKILLS REINFORCEMENT

▶ **Mallets** The recording routine of "Evening Chaconne" is as follows. Each instrument part enters individually beginning with the bongos and then proceeding from low to high parts. Each instrument plays to the 1st ending and repeats until all instruments are playing. All instruments play one final time proceeding to the 2nd ending. Encourage the contrabass player to play the root of each chord, not the open fifth.

BUILDING SKILLS THROUGH MUSIC

▶ **Reading** Have students read the text information describing the *chaconne* on p. 202. Then, ask students to determine an appropriate tempo for the performance of this piece.

SPOTLIGHT ON

▶ **Orff Instruments** When Carl Orff (1895–1982) first worked with students of gymnastics and dance in the 1920s at the Güntherschule in Munich, Germany, only nonpitched percussion instruments such as gongs, rattles, and drums were used. At the suggestion of musicologist Curt Sachs, Orff chose the recorder as a melody instrument.

Orff's direct prototype for adding barred percussion to the ensemble was an African xylophone, a "Kaffir piano." He took the xylophone to instrument builder and friend Karl Maendler to tune it to the Western scale. This first alto xylophone was followed by sopranos, then metallophones and glockenspiels in these ranges; the bass instruments came last. The Orff instrumentarium integrates sounds of Asia, Africa, and Europe.

An Evening Performance

Perform "Evening Chaconne." Begin with the bass instruments and then layer the other parts.

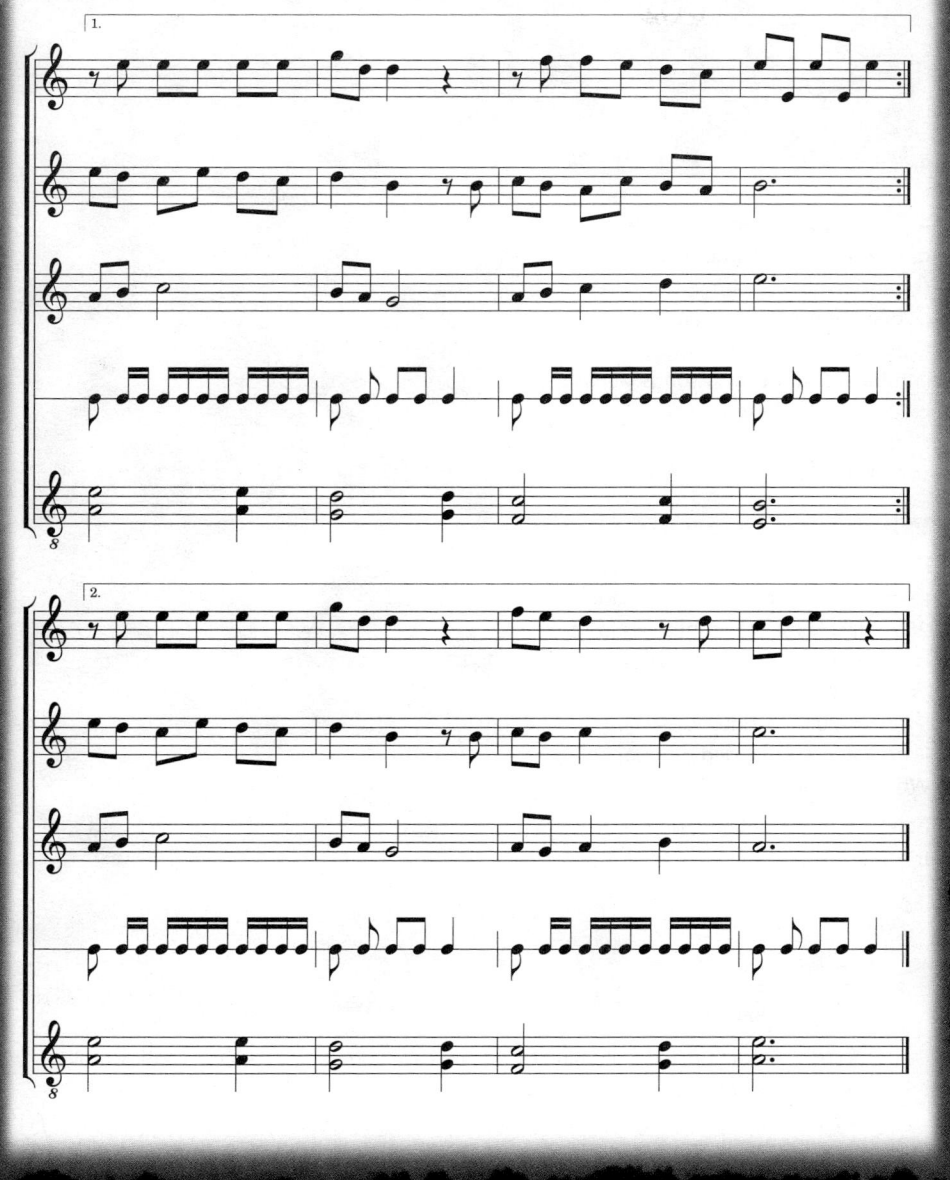

2 DEVELOP

Listening

Have students listen to "Evening Chaconne" **CD 11-3**, paying special attention to the bass part.

ASK How many descending pitches do you hear in the bass pattern? (four)

Singing

1a Invite students to

- Echo sing, in a comfortable register, each pitched part of "Evening Chaconne" as you model it, using numbers, pitch syllables, or note letter names.
- Play each part in the air while singing it with the recording.

Playing

Ask students to learn the percussion parts to "Evening Chaconne." Have them practice each part separately. Then have them perform the piece with the recording **CD 11-3**, following the routine in Skills Reinforcement, p. 202.

Analyzing

Analyze the melodic lines in "Evening Chaconne" for melodic movement, sequences, and ostinato patterns. Ask students to identify two-measure melodic patterns that are prominent in the parts.

3 CLOSE

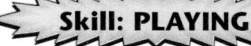
Skill: PLAYING   **ASSESSMENT**

7b **Performance/Peer Critique** Separate the class into groups. Each group will perform "Evening Chaconne" following the routine in Skills Reinforcement on p. 202. Have listeners evaluate each performance with regard to rhythmic accuracy and correct pitches.

AUDIENCE ETIQUETTE

▶ **Preparing to Attend a Performance** Students may be interested in attending a live concert performance of instrumental or vocal music. Students will be more attentive as informed listeners when they are prepared for what they will see and hear. To prepare, have students

- Research the performers and composers. Include facts about the composers' lives, time period, and culture.
- Listen to recordings of the music they will hear. Engage students in the music through movement, listening maps, written responses, or singing and playing of themes or rhythms.
- Read information about the music, plots, or story lines.
- Prepare interview questions for musicians who visit the school or classroom, or write a letter to musicians they have heard.

TECHNOLOGY/MEDIA LINK

4c **Notation Software** Prepare a handout for students, containing the following points, on how to compose an Orff arrangement using notation software.

- Set up a score with four mallet-instrument staves and two percussion staves.
- Select a meter signature and create a total of four measures, with a repeat sign at the end.
- Use the following pitches: C, D, E, G, and A.
- Compose a 1-measure bass line and repeat it in each measure.
- Compose another part and listen to both parts. Change as needed.
- Continue until all staves are full.

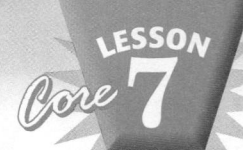

LESSON AT A GLANCE

Element Focus **MELODY** Intervals of fourths and fifths

Skill Objective **READING** Read a song containing intervals of fourths and fifths

Connection Activity **LANGUAGE ARTS** Discuss the lyrics of a song from the Adirondack Mountains

MATERIALS

• "Blue Mountain Lake" CD 11-4
  Recording Routine: Intro (4 m.); v. 1; interlude (4 m.); v. 2; interlude (4 m.); v. 3; coda
• **Music Reading Practice, Sequence 23** CD 11-6
• *Four Potatoes Medley* CD 11-9
• **Dance Directions** for *Four Potatoes Medley* p. 560
• hand drums
• **Resource Book** pp. D-26, E-24, I-18

VOCABULARY

interval fourth fifth compound meter

◆ ◆ ◆ ◆ National Standards ◆ ◆ ◆ ◆

5b Sightread melodies in treble clef
6b Listen and analyze uses of rhythm in music from diverse cultures
6c Understand and use basic principles of intervals in music analysis

MORE MUSIC CHOICES

For more songs with fourths and fifths:
"Your Friends Shall Be the Tall Wind," p. 201
"Skye Boat Song," p. 372

1 INTRODUCE

SAY "Blue Mountain Lake" is a ballad, or song that tells a story, about life as a lumberjack. Discuss with students the lyrics and story of "Blue Mountain Lake."

ASK What other songs do you know that tell a story? ("Barb'ry Allen," p. 44; "Harrison Town," p. 97)

Lumberjack Intervals

A lumberjack's life in the 1800s was dangerous work. Lumberjack crews cut and hauled the huge trees used to build houses, farms, and factories all across our country. Lumberjack stories and songs were created about these colorful characters. **Sing** the lumberjack song "Blue Mountain Lake."

What's the Interval?

As you **listen** to "Blue Mountain Lake," follow the notation on page 205. Make a list of the intervals in the song by counting the distance of each interval. A repeating note is called a unison (interval = 1). What interval is shaded orange? What interval is shaded blue?

Sing "Blue Mountain Lake" with the spirit of a lumberjack.

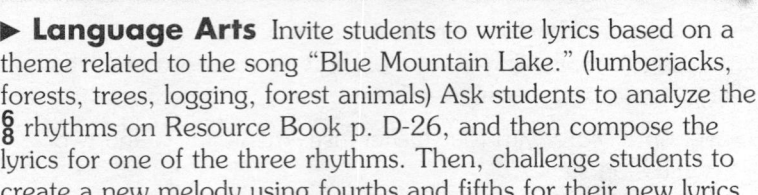

Show What You Know!

Analyze the notation of "Blue Mountain Lake" on page 205. Draw an interval chart of the intervals that are used in the song and indicate the interval (melodic distance) between each pair of pitches.

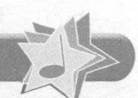 204 Reading Sequence 23

Footnotes

ACROSS THE CURRICULUM

▶ **Language Arts** Invite students to write lyrics based on a theme related to the song "Blue Mountain Lake." (lumberjacks, forests, trees, logging, forest animals) Ask students to analyze the $\frac{6}{8}$ rhythms on Resource Book p. D-26, and then compose the lyrics for one of the three rhythms. Then, challenge students to create a new melody using fourths and fifths for their new lyrics.

BUILDING SKILLS THROUGH MUSIC

▶ **Math** Remind students that $\frac{6}{8}$ compound meter has three subdivisions per main beat. Ask students to create an equation to calculate how many main beats would occur when 36 subdivisions are present. ($36 \div 3 = 12$)

SKILLS REINFORCEMENT

6c ▶ **Reading** Guide students to understand that the minor scale tone ladder in the Resource Book is harmonic minor and that if they construct a tone ladder in D-harmonic minor, some of the notes will be different from the song. (There is no C♯, just a C♮; also the note B♭ is missing in the song.) Note that the key of "Blue Mountain Lake" could be categorized as D-natural minor, or D-mixolydian mode.

For more music reading practice, see p. 499, or Resource Book pp. D-26 and E-24.

▶ **Recorder** Have some students learn the soprano and alto recorder duet acccompaniment in the Resource Book on **2a** p. I-18 for "Blue Mountain Lake." When students are comfortable, they may play the duet as the class sings the songs.

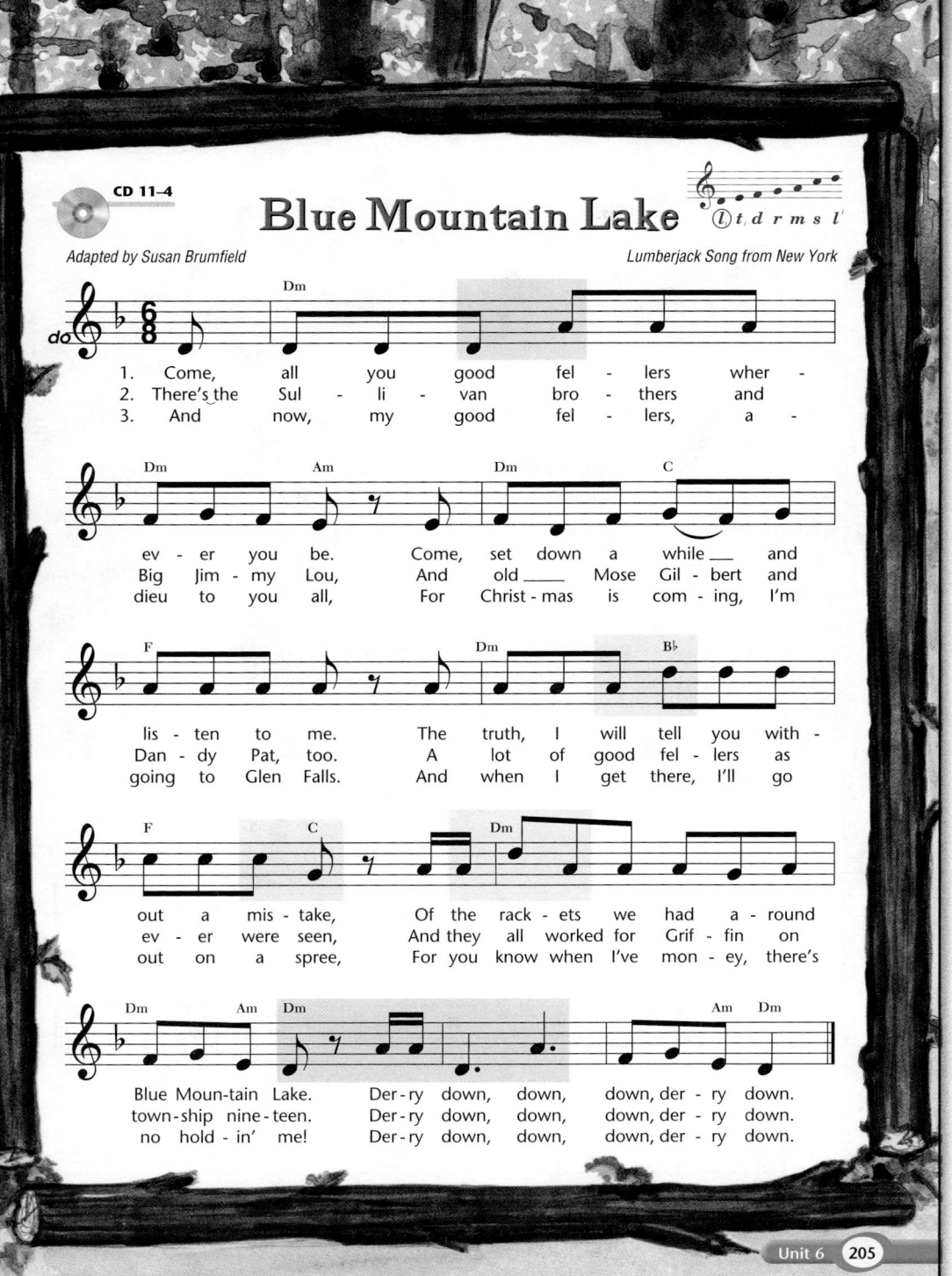

CD 11–4

Blue Mountain Lake

Adapted by Susan Brumfield

Lumberjack Song from New York

1. Come, all you good fel - lers wher -
2. There's the Sul - li - van bro - thers and
3. And now, my good fel - lers, a -

ev - er you be. Come, set down a while ___ and
Big Jim - my Lou, And old ___ Mose Gil - bert and
dieu to you all, For Christ - mas is com - ing, I'm

lis - ten to me. The truth, I will tell you with -
Dan - dy Pat, too. A lot of good fel - lers as
going to Glen Falls. And when I get there, I'll go

out a mis - take, Of the rack - ets we had a - round
ev - er were seen, And they all worked for Grif - fin on
out on a spree, For you know when I've mon - ey, there's

Blue Moun-tain Lake. Der-ry down, down, down, der - ry down.
town-ship nine-teen. Der-ry down, down, down, der - ry down.
no hold - in' me! Der-ry down, down, down, der - ry down.

Unit 6 **205**

2 DEVELOP

Reading

6c Remind students that distances between pitches are measured in intervals. Draw a vertical tone ladder from *do* to *do¹* on the board and review the intervals in a major scale.

Listening

Play "Blue Mountain Lake" **CD 11-4** and have students identify that the song is in minor. Ask what pitch syllables are needed to construct a tone ladder in minor? (*la₁* to *la*)

Draw a vertical tone ladder on the board and help students identify seconds, thirds, fourths, and fifths when *la* is the tonic. Use Resource Book p. D-26 to have students independently identify and perform these intervals with accurate intonation, demonstrating fundamental skills.

Singing

6b Direct students to the notation of "Blue Mountain Lake" and explain that in quick-tempo ⁶⁄₈ songs, the six eighth-note beats are often felt as two dotted-quarter beats per measure. Remind students that ⁶⁄₈ meter is called compound meter. Have students sight-sing "Blue Mountain Lake."

Reading

6c Have students read the notation of "Blue Mountain Lake" and identify the intervals of fourths and fifths. (Fourths: m. 5–*mi-la*; m. 6–*so-re*; m. 6–7–*mi-la* and *la-mi*); (Fifths: m. 1–*la₁-mi*; m. 8–9–*la₁-mi* and *mi-la₁*).

3 CLOSE

Element: MELODY   ASSESSMENT

5b **Performance/Observation** Have students use pitch syllables to read and sing "Blue Mountain Lake." Observe students' ability to accurately read and sing the intervals of fourths (*mi-la* and *so-re*) and fifths (*la₁-mi*).

SPOTLIGHT ON

▶ **Contra dance** Found in New England, the contra dance is a modified English country dance. It was probably brought over from England with early settlers in Colonial times, but it is still enjoyed today. The word *contra* describes the two lines of dancers facing or opposing each other (from the French *contre*). Sometimes known as barn dancing, this is a dance that the lumberjack in "Blue Mountain Lake" may have danced when he went into town for the Christmas festivities (verse 3).

This particular dance, found in the Dance Directions on p. 561, is called the "Pam and Pat Reel," named after two Ohio music teachers. Invite students to perform a contra dance to the selection *Four Potatoes Medley* **CD 11-9**.

SCHOOL TO HOME CONNECTION

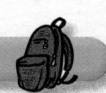

▶ **Getting Back to Nature** Ask students if there is a forest, a large park, or any other place near their homes where they can go for a walk in the woods or commune with nature. Have students select a favorite natural spot, visit it with family or friends, and write about their experiences in their journals.

TECHNOLOGY/MEDIA LINK

Notation Software Have students use notation software to create and notate a two-measure ostinato for "Blue Mountain Lake." Have students select ⁶⁄₈ meter. Encourage them to use intervals of fourths and fifths in their ostinato. Students may play their ostinatos as the class sings the song.

LESSON 8

LESSON AT A GLANCE

Element Focus	**MELODY** Rounds and canons
Skill Objective	✦ **SINGING** Sing a canon in minor
Connection Activity	**SOCIAL STUDIES** Link a round with information about its country of origin

MATERIALS

- "Kyrie"   **CD 11-11**
  Recording Routine: Intro (4 m.); vocal; instrumental; vocal
- **Music Reading Practice, Sequence 24**   **CD 11-13**
- "Trepak" from *The Nutcracker Suite*   **CD 11-16**
- **Resource Book** p. D-27, E-25, H-21
- hand bells or chimes, resonator bells, keyboard

VOCABULARY

round   canon   monophonic/polyphonic texture

✦ ✦ ✦ ✦ National Standards ✦ ✦ ✦ ✦

- **1c** Sing music from diverse genres
- **1d** Sing music written in three parts
- **2b** Perform easy instrumental pieces with technical accuracy
- **6b** Analyze uses of pitch and texture in music from diverse cultures

MORE MUSIC CHOICES

For more practice in singing rounds and canons:
"Hey, Ho! Nobody Home," p. 28
"Dance for the Nations," p. 122

1 INTRODUCE

Share with students background information on the South American country of Suriname from Across the Curriculum below. Explain that the class will be singing a round from this country.

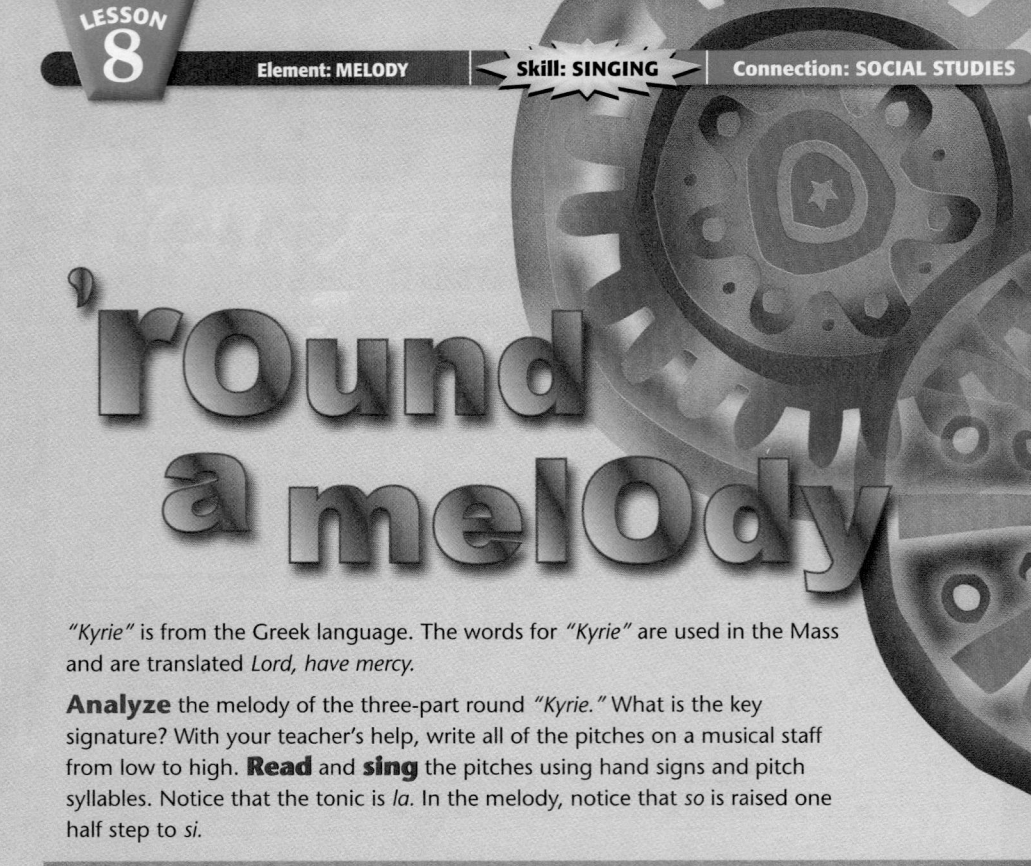

'round a melody

"Kyrie" is from the Greek language. The words for "Kyrie" are used in the Mass and are translated *Lord, have mercy.*

Analyze the melody of the three-part round "Kyrie." What is the key signature? With your teacher's help, write all of the pitches on a musical staff from low to high. **Read** and **sing** the pitches using hand signs and pitch syllables. Notice that the tonic is *la.* In the melody, notice that *so* is raised one half step to *si.*

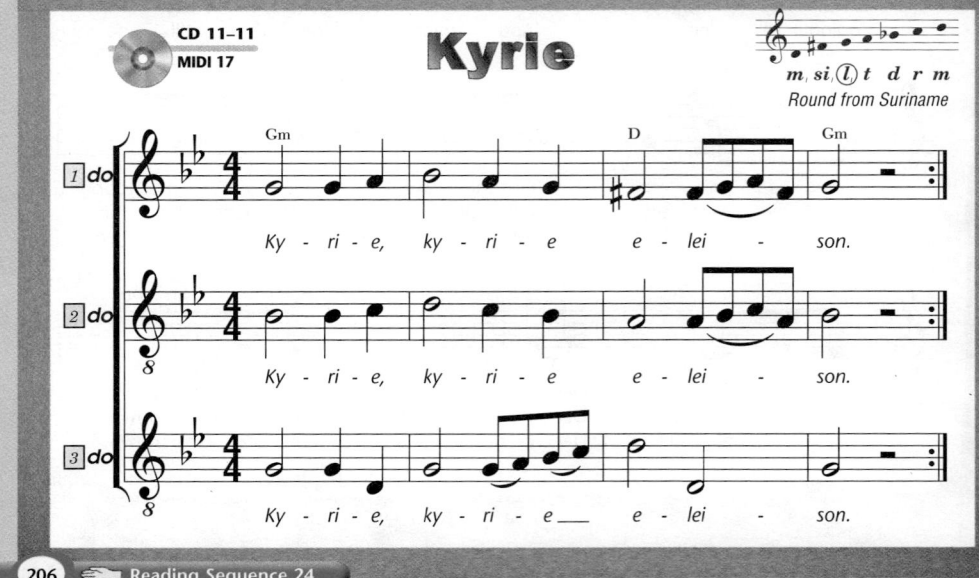

CD 11-11   MIDI 17

Kyrie

Round from Suriname

Ky - ri - e, ky - ri - e   e - lei - son.

206   Reading Sequence 24

Footnotes

SPOTLIGHT ON

▶ **The Text** *Kyrie eleison* ("Lord, have mercy") has been used in response to a litany since the fourth or fifth century. Its use in the Ordinary of the Roman Mass was established by St. Gregory the Great, who was pope from 590 to 604.

BUILDING SKILLS THROUGH MUSIC

▶ **Social Studies** Have students locate Suriname on a world map or globe. Have students locate the Netherlands and England on the map. Share the information on Suriname from Across the Curriculum. Lead students in a discussion about how Suriname achieved independence.

ACROSS THE CURRICULUM

▶ **Social Studies** Located on the northern coast of South America between Guyana and French Guiana, Suriname is about the size of the state of Georgia. Because more than 80 percent of the country is covered by the Amazon rain forest, 95 percent of its population lives along the coast. Dutch is the official language of Suriname, but other languages, including Sranan tongo, a local Creole language, are widely spoken.

Originally part of the coastal area called Guiana, Suriname changed ownership between the Dutch and the British many times. Finally in 1667, after signing the Treaty of Breda, the British traded the area with the Dutch for what is now New York City. Suriname gained independence from the Netherlands in 1975. Its main source of income is derived from export of bauxite (the principle ore of aluminum), gold, rice, and bananas.

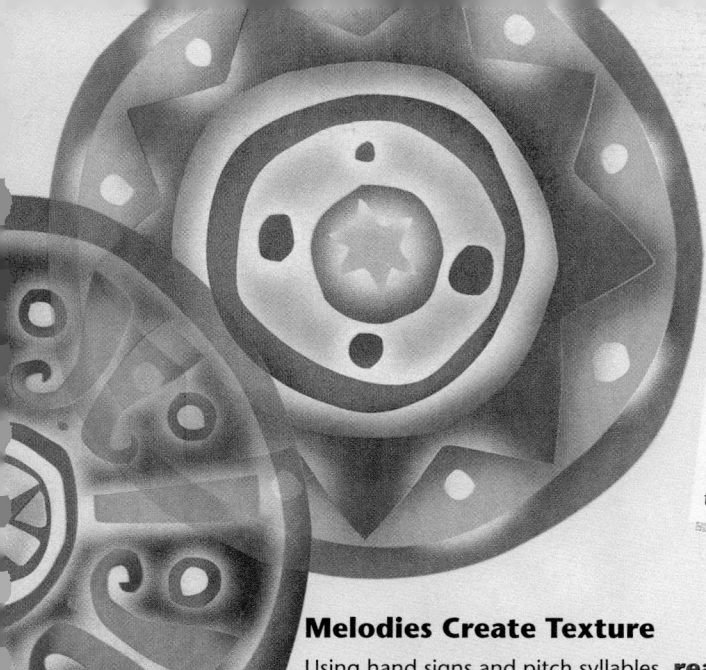

> A **monophonic** texture consists of a single melodic line.

> A **polyphonic** texture consists of two or more melodic lines that occur at the same time.

Melodies Create Texture

Using hand signs and pitch syllables, **read** and **sing** each part of *"Kyrie"* in *a cappella* unison—a **monophonic** texture.

Then, **sing** *"Kyrie"* as a three-part round. The musical texture is now **polyphonic.**

Another way to perform a round is to sing each part of the song as an ostinato. Group 1 begins and sings Part 1. Group 2 sings Part 2 and Group 3 sings Part 3. Groups 1 and 2 repeat their parts until Group 3 has sung its part twice.

Bell Choirs

Bell choirs are musical groups that play bells that range in size from very small to very large, and from high to low pitch. Bell choirs are often used in churches, but they also play concert music that is written or arranged specifically for them. **Listen** to the melody and texture in *Trepak.*

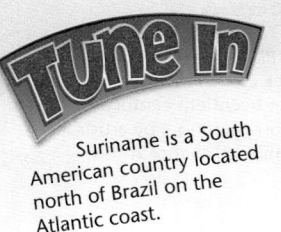
Tune In

Suriname is a South American country located north of Brazil on the Atlantic coast.

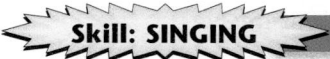
CD 11–16
Trepak

from *The Nutcracker Suite* by Piotr Ilyich Tchaikovsky as performed by the Sona Handbell Choir

The ringing of bells takes coordination and concentration in order to play in time.

Unit 6 **207**

---

2 DEVELOP

Analyzing

6b Direct students to *"Kyrie"* on p. 206. Help them to discover that the song has three parts. Write the pitch-set of the song on a staff, from lowest to highest on the board. Have students identify that *la* is the tonic, the key signature is G-*la,* and the melody contains a raised *so,* or *si.*

Invite students to examine each of the three parts of the melody. Have them determine which part sounds major (Part 2); which part contains the interval of an octave (Part 3); and which part contains the interval of a fourth (Part 3).

Singing

1c Have students sight-read each part, using pitch syllables and hand signs. Have them switch parts. Invite students to sing the entire song in unison.

6b Tell students that when they sing the song in *a cappella* unison, they are creating a monophonic texture—a single melody, without accompaniment. Have students sing *"Kyrie"* as a three-part round in polyphonic texture.

Invite students to perform the round (as three repeated ostinatos), as suggested on p. 206.

Listening

Invite students to listen to the bell choir in *Trepak* **CD 11-16,** then perform a bell choir accompaniment to *"Kyrie"* found in Skills Reinforcement below.

3 CLOSE

Skill: SINGING — ASSESSMENT

1d **Performance/Observation** Have students sing *"Kyrie"* in unison using pitch syllables and hand signs. Then, have them sing *"Kyrie"* as a three-part round. Observe students' ability to accurately sing a round in three parts.

SKILLS REINFORCEMENT

2b
▶ **Keyboard** Students can experience all three parts of *"Kyrie"* at once by playing the trio arrangement of the song for keyboard found on Resource Book p. H-21.

▶ **Hand Bells** Invite students to sight-read this pattern on hand bells or hand chimes as an accompaniment to *"Kyrie."* Assign one student to play the G bell and another student to play the D bell.

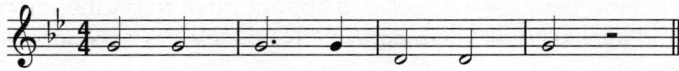

▶ **Reading** See Resource Book p. E-25, or p. 499, for additional music reading practice.

TECHNOLOGY/MEDIA LINK

MIDI/Sequencing Software Have students use the classroom computer, keyboard, and MIDI sequencing software to help them learn the round *"Kyrie."* Have students record the round's melody, first on track 1. Then, have them use the copy and paste functions to input the round on two more tracks. Remind students to start the second voice in m. 5, and the third voice in m. 9. Then, have students

- Use the loop function to keep each voice repeating.
- Listen to all the MIDI tracks together while following the notation in the book.
- Sing with one of the MIDI tracks.
- Sing with all the MIDI tracks together.

LESSON AT A GLANCE

Element Focus   **MELODY** Chance (aleatory) music

Skill Objective   **LISTENING** Listen to and describe an example of chance music

Connection Activity   **RELATED ARTS** Discuss ways in which unplanned, or "chance," events can be incorporated into musical composition and the visual arts

MATERIALS

- *Concert for Piano and Orchestra* (excerpt)   **CD 11-17**
- **Resource Book** p. J-9

VOCABULARY

chance (aleatory) music   prepared piano

◆ ◆ ◆ ◆ National Standards ◆ ◆ ◆ ◆

4b Arrange pieces for instruments
4c Compose, using non-traditional sound sources
6a Listen and describe events in music using appropriate terms
6b Listen and analyze uses of texture in music from diverse genres
8a Show how different arts portray the same idea in unique ways

MORE MUSIC CHOICES

For more experience with contemporary music:

Ionisation, p. 357

"Allegretto gioviale" from *Lyric Suite,* p. 169

1 INTRODUCE

Organize the class into groups of three. Have each group find a familiar song in their books. Have the groups begin singing their songs at the same time, changing dynamics and rhythms freely.

Explain to students that they have performed an example of chance (aleatory) music. Tell them that the term *aleatory* comes from the Latin word *alea,* which means "die" (as in "one of a pair of dice," which is used in games of chance).

Take A Chance

In the twentieth century, some composers gave performers and audiences a role in creating the music. This idea is somewhat like improvisation, where performers compose on the spot as they perform.

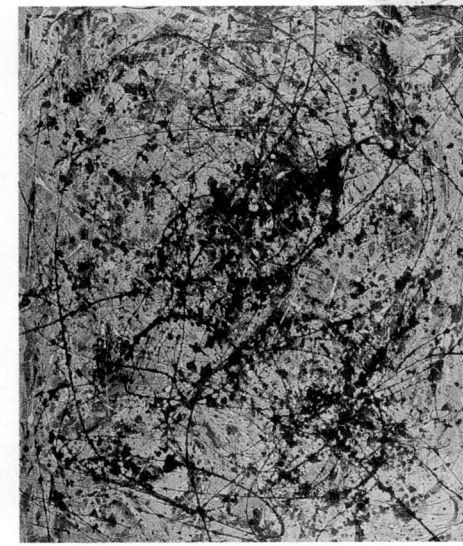

Jackson Pollock in his studio ▶

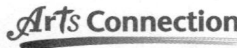

Arts Connection

◀ *Reflections of the Big Dipper* by Jackson Pollock (1912–1956). Composers in the twentieth century considered "action painting," by artists like Pollock, to be similar to chance music.

 208

Footnotes

ACROSS THE CURRICULUM

▶ **Language Arts** John Cage considered himself to be not only a composer, but also a philosopher, visual artist, and poet. Interested readers may read more about the other sides of Cage in *John Cage: Composed in America* edited by Marjorie Perloff and Charles Junkerman (University of Chicago, 1994).

BUILDING SKILLS THROUGH MUSIC

▶ **Science** Have students read the information in Music Makers. Lead them in a discussion of what the audience might have heard during the performance of *4'33"*. Give students a sheet of paper, ask the class to get silent, then ask them to observe and write down what they hear during the next 4 minutes and 33 seconds.

SKILLS REINFORCEMENT

4c ▶ **Creating** The following is an additional classroom activity for creating chance music.

- Assemble four or five portable radios at different points around the classroom. Then, choose a volunteer to be the "operator/performer" for each radio.

- Tell the class that the volunteers will be performing the composition "Piece for Five Aleatory Radios." Ask each radio operator/performer to select a spot at random on the radio band (dial) without listening to it. Then, select a conductor.

- The operators may change stations at any time. The conductor will conduct the volume of each radio, cut off and bring in the radios, and end the piece as he or she wishes.

Chance Music

John Cage was the leader among composers who created chance, or "aleatoric," music.

In *Concert for Piano and Orchestra*, Cage did not create a typical score. **Listen** to this music by Cage.

CD 11-17

Concert for Piano and Orchestra

by John Cage

This piece can be played by any number of players and singers, performing any page in any order.

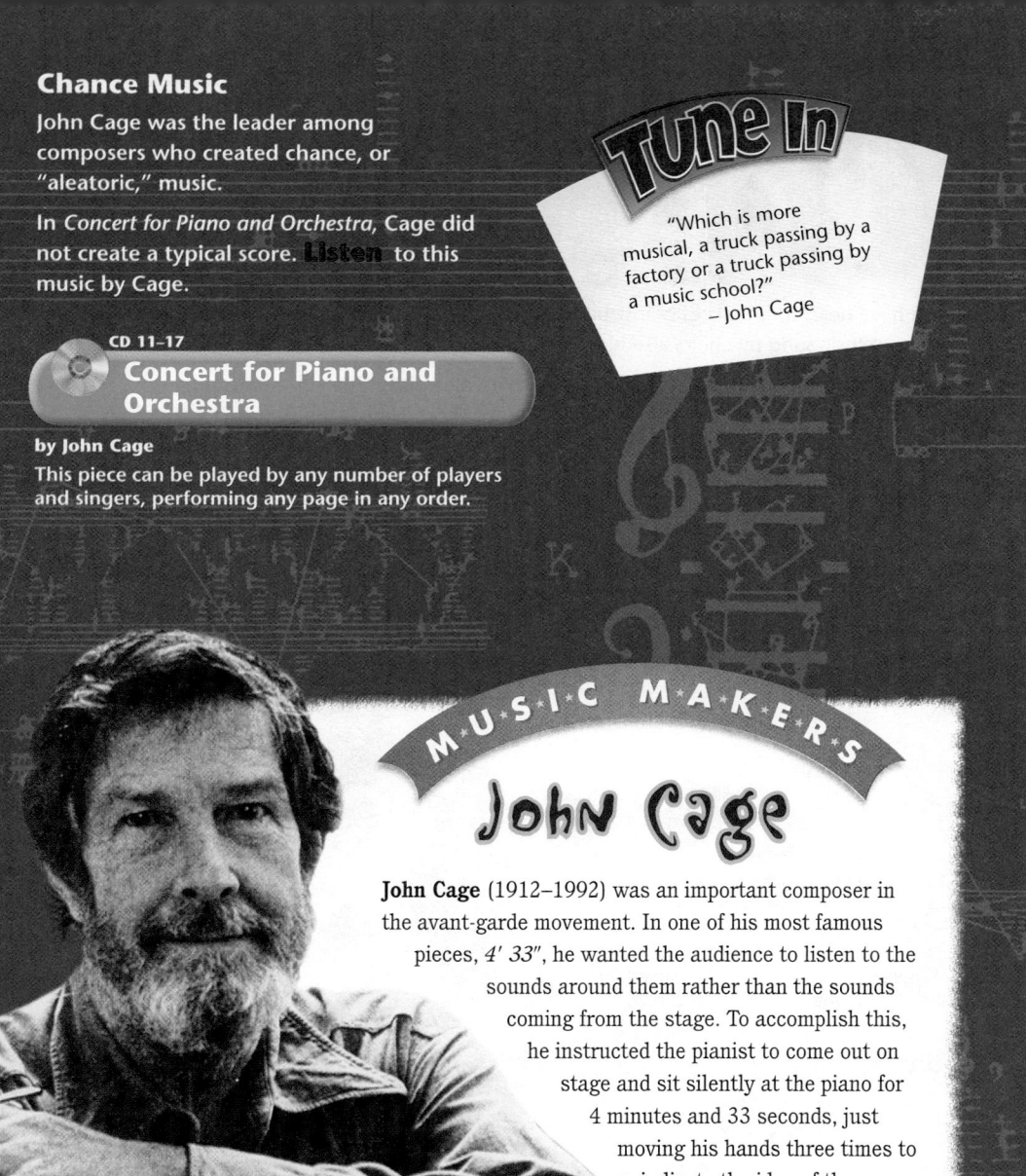

Tune In

"Which is more musical, a truck passing by a factory or a truck passing by a music school?"
– John Cage

M·U·S·I·C M·A·K·E·R·S

John Cage

John Cage (1912–1992) was an important composer in the avant-garde movement. In one of his most famous pieces, *4' 33"*, he wanted the audience to listen to the sounds around them rather than the sounds coming from the stage. To accomplish this, he instructed the pianist to come out on stage and sit silently at the piano for 4 minutes and 33 seconds, just moving his hands three times to indicate the idea of three movements.

2 DEVELOP

Listening

6a Invite students to read about John Cage and Jackson Pollock on pp. 208–209 and in Spotlight On below. Play Cage's *Concert for Piano and Orchestra* **CD 11-17.** Point out that the players determine what they play. Ask students to listen to the melodic ideas in the music and discuss their pitch and timbre. Tell students that Cage often asks musicians to play instruments in unusual ways, such as bowing on the violin's tailpiece, or playing a "prepared" piano.

Then, have students view the art on p. 208 and discuss how "chance" is part of Pollock's creation.

Creating

4c Guide students in creating their own graphic composi-
8a tions. Using a poem or original lyrics, have students write the words in a way that indicates the following elements.

Dynamics: size of letters—large = loud, small = soft.

Pitch: place words high or low.

Rhythm: close together = fast, far apart = slow.

Texture: thick = dense grouping, thin = sparse grouping.

Separate the class into small groups and have them prepare and perform the pieces for the class.

An additional activity for creating a chance music composition can be found on Resource Book p. J-9.

3 CLOSE

Skill: LISTENING   **ASSESSMENT**

6b **Music Journal Writing** Have students listen as you play the recording of *Concert for Piano and Orchestra* **CD 11-17.** Ask students to describe in their journals how pitch, timbre, texture, and dynamics are used.

SPOTLIGHT ON

▶ **The Composer** American composer John Cage (1912–1992) studied with composers Henry Cowell and Arnold Schoenberg. Cage developed the "prepared piano," a piano that is modified to produce new and interesting timbres. He wrote music for dance companies and was interested in indeterminate techniques, as well as in Zen, which treasures "nonintention."

▶ **The Artist** Jackson Pollock (1912–1956) Abstract expressionist painter Jackson Pollock wanted his work to be an expression of his unconscious moods, so he made his paintings with no points of emphasis or defined parts. He put his canvases on the floor and poured or dripped paint, often mixed with sand or broken glass, on them. The application of paint in this manner adds an aleatoric element to the painting.

CHARACTER EDUCATION

▶ **Audience Behavior** Encourage students to listen to all music respectfully. Have them list good audience etiquette for listening. Ask them why they should exhibit respect and proper concert etiquette as an informed listener during varied live performances? Why do people choose not to act appropriately when listening? As the class listens to music that is different from what they typically listen to, have students rate the audience etiquette of the class, and discuss their behavior.

TECHNOLOGY/MEDIA LINK

4b **Multimedia** Invite students to create a multimedia concert, using improvisation, chance music, "prepared" and "found" sounds, abstract art and slides, and modern dance.

LESSON AT A GLANCE

Element Focus **TIMBRE** SATB choir

Skill Objective **LISTENING** Describe selected examples of choral singing

Connection Activity **GENRE** Explore the social and historical setting of choral singing

MATERIALS
- *Lo, How a Rose E'er Blooming* (excerpt) **CD 11-18**
- *Gloria in excelsis* **CD 11-19**
- keyboard

VOCABULARY
a cappella SATB (soprano, alto, tenor, bass)

◆ ◆ ◆ ◆ National Standards ◆ ◆ ◆ ◆
5a Read half notes and quarter notes in duple meter
6b Listen and analyze uses of timbre in music from diverse genres
9b Classify high-quality musical works by genre

MORE MUSIC CHOICES
For more experience with choral music timbre:

Give Us Hope, p. 337

"Stopping by Woods on a Snowy Evening" from *Frostiana*, p. 40

"*Vem kan segla?*" p. 417

1 INTRODUCE

Invite students to share their experiences singing in a choir. Then, ask them to share their experiences listening to choirs whose singers were high school age or older. (Students may be interested in hearing *Give Us Hope* **CD 17–8**, demonstrating the rich vocal timbre and three-part harmony (SSA) of the Young People's Choir of NYC—New York City. See More Music Choices.) Share the information about choral music in Spotlight On below.

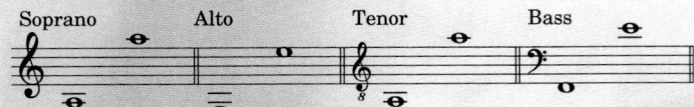
Choir Sounds

You have heard the timbres of instruments, vocal styles, and twentieth-century music. Music sung by choirs also has a distinct timbre—the choral sound.

Choral music is usually written for four different voice parts. The voice parts are called *soprano, alto, tenor,* and *bass*—or SATB, for short. Here is the standard range (or highest and lowest notes) each voice sings:

Soprano   Alto   Tenor   Bass

Listen to an SATB arrangement of *Lo, How a Rose E'er Blooming.* Do any of the voice parts sing alone?

CD 11-18
Lo, How a Rose E'er Blooming

by Michael Praetorius as performed by the Cambridge Singers and Orchestra

This is a good example of *a cappella* singing. *A cappella* singing is unaccompanied, or literally, "in the style of the church."

Baroque Choirs

Listen to *Gloria in excelsis* for SATB chorus and orchestra by Antonio Vivaldi.

CD 11-19
Gloria in excelsis

by Antonio Vivaldi as performed by the Robert Shaw Chorale and the Atlanta Symphony Orchestra

Many works by composers such as Bach and Handel, as well as contemporary composers, use the combination of SATB chorus with orchestra.

Tune In

When Vivaldi was 15 years old, he began his training to become a priest. In his later years, he concentrated on music as a career.

210

Footnotes

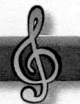
SKILLS REINFORCEMENT

6b ▶ Listening Explain to students that composers often write choral music for voicings (different voice parts) other than SATB. Tell them that these combinations might include: SA, SSA (treble choirs); TB, TTBB (men's choirs); and SAB, double choirs, and antiphonal choirs (mixed choirs).

Select several recordings of choral music. Have students listen to the performances and identify what voice parts they hear.

BUILDING SKILLS THROUGH MUSIC

▶ Language After reading the Music Maker on Antonio Vivaldi, have students describe the types of choral music and instrumental music that he wrote.

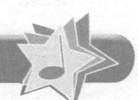
SPOTLIGHT ON

▶ The Composer German composer Michael Praetorius (1571–1621), who was an organist, composer, and musicologist, is famous for his 1619 text *Syntagma musicum.* It tells about the performance practice and theory of the day.

▶ Choral Music The genre of choral music in Western European culture was dominated by church music for many years. Christian churches were, along with the royal courts, the biggest employers of musicians in the days of Praetorius and Vivaldi. Over the past few hundred years, however, choral singing has become a way of sharing music in a social way. Many cities have choral societies full of talented singers who perform major works from all periods of music history.

An SATB Musical Score

Here is an example of printed SATB music. As you **listen** to the first phrase of *Lo, How a Rose E'er Blooming*, follow the voice parts in the score. What term describes this musical texture?

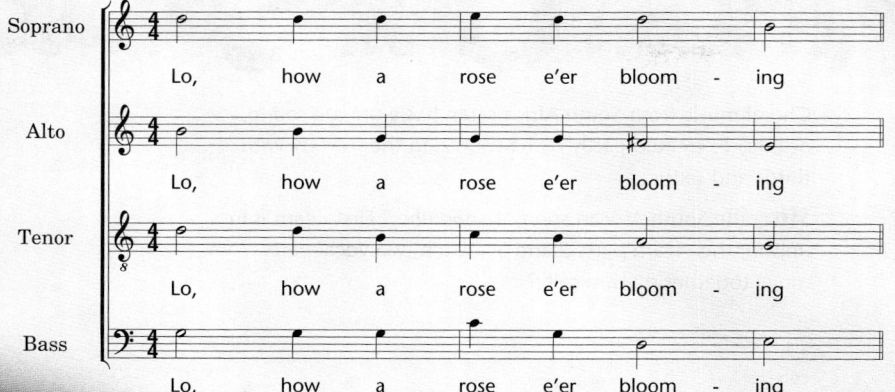

Soprano
Lo, how a rose e'er bloom - ing

Alto
Lo, how a rose e'er bloom - ing

Tenor
Lo, how a rose e'er bloom - ing

Bass
Lo, how a rose e'er bloom - ing

MUSIC MAKERS

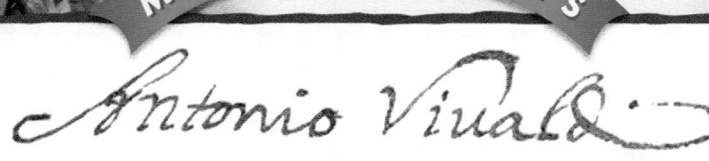

Antonio Vivaldi (1678–1741) was a famous composer, conductor, and violinist of the eighteenth century. He wrote a great deal of music in his lifetime—more than 750 musical pieces. Vivaldi, known as the "Red Priest" because of his auburn hair, composed operas, masses, hymns, and other types of choral music.

One of Vivaldi's most famous works, *The Four Seasons,* is known as "program music," or music that tells a story. *The Four Seasons* is a musical description of the four seasons of the year.

Vivaldi is remembered for his development of the violin concerto, a musical piece for solo violin with orchestra. Vivaldi spent many years teaching music in a school for orphaned girls. Many of his compositions were written for the students to play.

2 DEVELOP

Listening

9b Have students read the information on p. 210 about choral voice parts. Then, describe the soprano, alto, tenor, and bass in an SATB choir. On the keyboard, play the professional vocal ranges indicated on p. 210. Have students sing scales within the voice part ranges, as they are able. Then, introduce the term *a cappella* as unaccompanied choral singing. Have students listen to *Lo, How a Rose E'er Blooming* **CD 11-18** (SATB choir).

Reading

5a Have students sight-read the individual parts, in clefs other than treble in various meters, pointing out that the tenor part, written in the "treble 8vb" clef, is sung an octave lower than written. Play *Lo, How a Rose E'er Blooming* again **CD 11-18**.

Listening

Have students listen to Vivaldi's *Gloria in excelsis* **CD 11-19** for SATB choir and orchestra.

6b **ASK** What differences in timbre do you hear between *Lo, How a Rose E'er Blooming* and *Gloria in excelsis?* (The orchestral accompaniment in *Gloria in excelsis;* the distinct choral parts in *Lo, How a Rose E'er Blooming.*)

3 CLOSE

Element: TIMBRE   **ASSESSMENT**

Music Journal Writing Play the recordings from "More Music Choices," p. 210, and have students write a brief description of the performance, focusing on voicing (SATB) and timbre (*a cappella* or accompanied), using correct standard terminology.

ACROSS THE CURRICULUM

▶ **Language Arts** Latin, the language used in Vivaldi's *Gloria in excelsis,* was the universal language of the Catholic Church during the time of Vivaldi and Praetorius. Latin also served as the basis for many modern languages including French, Italian, Spanish, Portuguese, Catalán, Provençal, Romanian, and Rhaeto-Romanic (from Switzerland and the Tyrol). Because Latin was spoken by the Romans, who conquered and influenced many European cultures, Latin-based languages are often called Romance languages.

Have students look up the Latin roots of some common musical words, such as *chorus, music, auditorium, a cappella, instrument, soprano, alto,* and *tenor.*

SCHOOL TO HOME CONNECTION

▶ **SATB** Invite students to ask friends and relatives at home if they ever sang in an SATB choir. If so, students may ask them which voice part they sang, and if there were any particular challenges involved in singing that part. The discussion could also include particular choral pieces of interest to the singer.

TECHNOLOGY/MEDIA LINK

Notation Software Invite students to enter the score on p. 211 into a notation program, setting up four staves, including the "treble 8vb" and bass clefs. Then, have them select vocal MIDI timbres and play back their notation. Remind students that the tenor part sounds one octave lower.

LESSON AT A GLANCE

Element Focus **TIMBRE** South African choral timbre

Skill Objective **SINGING** Perform a South African song in three-part harmony

Connection Activity **CULTURE** Explore the social and cultural setting of a Zulu freedom song

MATERIALS

- "Siyahamba" (Zulu)   **CD 11-20**
- "Siyahamba" (English)   **CD 11-21**
  Recording Routine: Intro (6 m.); vocal; coda
- **Pronunciation Practice/Translation** p. 531
- "Roads Go Ever Ever On" (poem)
- **Resource Book** pp. A-18, F-21, G-13
- *tubanos* (or conga-type drums) in high, medium, and/or low pitches; two cowbells; rattles; talking drums (optional)

VOCABULARY

choral music   close harmony
intervals of thirds and sixths

◆ ◆ ◆ ◆ National Standards ◆ ◆ ◆ ◆

1c Sing music from diverse cultures
1d Sing music written in three parts
4c Arrange, using electronic media
5c Identify standard notation symbols for pitch, rhythm, and articulation
7b Students use specific criteria for evaluating their own performances
8b Identify ways music relates to social studies

MORE MUSIC CHOICES

For more African songs:
"Ise oluwa," p. 230
"Take Time in Life," p. 292

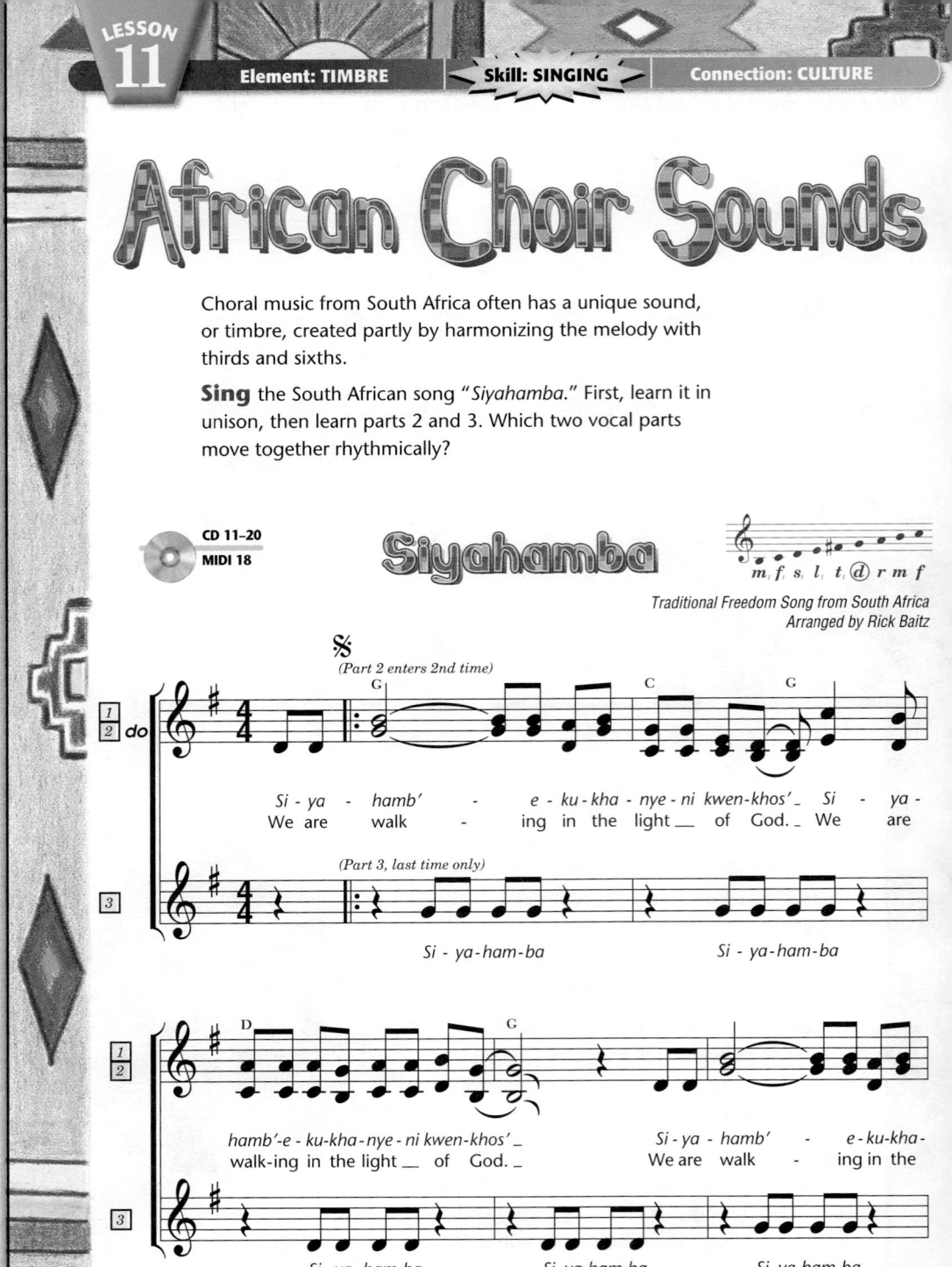

African Choir Sounds

Choral music from South Africa often has a unique sound, or timbre, created partly by harmonizing the melody with thirds and sixths.

Sing the South African song "Siyahamba." First, learn it in unison, then learn parts 2 and 3. Which two vocal parts move together rhythmically?

 CD 11–20
MIDI 18

Siyahamba

Traditional Freedom Song from South Africa
Arranged by Rick Baitz

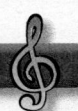

(Part 2 enters 2nd time)

Si - ya - hamb' — e - ku - kha - nye - ni kwen-khos' _ Si - ya -
We are walk - ing in the light __ of God. _ We are

(Part 3, last time only)

Si - ya - ham - ba   Si - ya - ham - ba

hamb'-e - ku - kha - nye - ni kwen-khos' _ Si - ya - hamb' — e - ku - kha -
walk-ing in the light __ of God. _ We are walk - ing in the

Si - ya - ham - ba   Si - ya - ham - ba   Si - ya - ham - ba

212

Footnotes

SKILLS REINFORCEMENT

▶ **Mallets** Encourage students to learn the Orff accompaniment for "Siyahamba" on Resource Book p. F-21. Have students play the Orff accompaniment and others play the percussion ensemble parts in Skills Reinforcement, p. 214. Have students add dynamic symbols to their copies of the notation and follow the dynamics while performing.

BUILDING SKILLS THROUGH MUSIC

▶ **Language** After learning this piece, ask students to write a chronology of the steps the class followed in learning all the parts. They should include the order in which parts were learned as well as how and when they were combined to create the whole performance.

CULTURAL CONNECTION

▶ **The Zulu** Historically, *Zulu* refers to the clan of Shaka, who created the powerful Zulu nation of South Africa during the early nineteenth century. By the end of the century, however, the Zulu had lost much of their land and wealth through warfare with European settlers. The more than 9 million Zulu people alive today speak Zulu, a Bantu language.

Other African culture groups in South Africa, in addition to the Zulu, include the Xhosa, Swazi, Ndebele, Sotho, Venda, Tsonga, San, and Khoikhoi.

Signing for "Siyahamba"

Learn to sign the word "siyahamba." Then **perform** it as you sing.

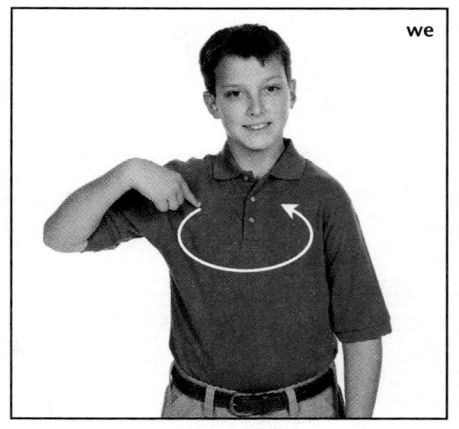

we

▲ *Si-ya*

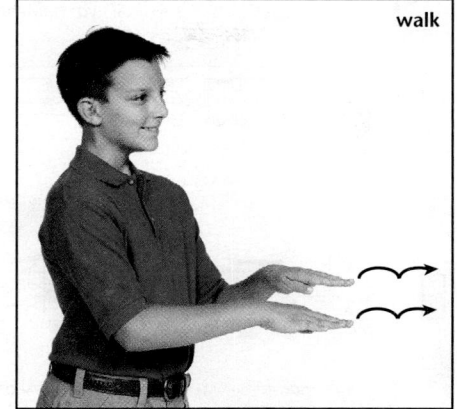

walk

▲ *-ham-ba*

*nye-ni kwen-khos'_ Si - ya - hamb'-e - ku-kha-nye-ni kwen-khos'_*
light _ of God. _ We are walk-ing in the light _ of God. _

Si - ya -

Si - ya-ham-ba   Si - ya-ham-ba   Si-ya-ham-ba

*ham-ba___   Si-ya-ham-ba___   Si - ya-hamb'- e - ku-kha-nye - ni kwen-khos'_*
We are walk-ing in the light _ of God. _

Si-ya-ham-ba   Si-ya-ham-ba   Si - ya-ham-ba

continued on page 214

1 INTRODUCE

8b Ask students to share what they know about the civil rights struggles of African Americans. Share with students the information that South Africans lived under a system known as *apartheid* where persons were required to live in segregated areas and were subject to discrimination. After years of struggle, apartheid finally came to an end. *"Siyahamba"* was the battle cry of the antiapartheid movement.

Also share with students the information on South Africa found in Across the Curriculum below.

2 DEVELOP

Reading

Have students

- Read the information about African choral music on p. 212.
- Follow the road map for the notation of *"Siyahamba"* by looking for musical road signs, such as repeat signs, *D.S. al Coda,* first and second endings, *Last time to Coda* marking, and *Coda.* (Students should be guided by you during this step.)
- Listen to *"Siyahamba"* **CD 11-21,** sung in English, while following the score with their fingers.

Singing

Have students

- Use the Pronunciation Practice track to echo speak the Zulu words of *"Siyahamba"* **CD 11-23.**
- Listen to *"Siyahamba"* **CD 11-20** sung in Zulu while again following the score with their fingers.

1c
- Sing the melody in Zulu with the recording.

Invite students to learn more about Zulu history and culture. See Cultural Connection on p. 212.

SKILLS REINFORCEMENT

▶ **Vocal Development** Voice range and quality determine what voice part a person should sing. The four vocal categories and their standard professional singing ranges are as follows.

- **Soprano** (range: A3–A5) is a female voice with a light, pure vocal quality that has a fuller tone in the upper range.
- **Alto** (range: F3–E5) is a female voice with a heavier, or darker, quality than the soprano voice. The alto voice has a fuller tone in the lower range.
- **Tenor** (range: A2–A4) is a male voice with a light, lyrical vocal quality that has a fuller tone in the upper range.
- **Bass** (range: F2–E4) is a male voice with a rich, resonant vocal quality and a deeper, fuller tone in the lower range.

ACROSS THE CURRICULUM

▶ **Social Studies** South Africa is a country of diverse climate, landscapes, and natural resources. The climate varies from humid sub-tropical to temperate. It also varies from dry desert to snow-covered mountain passes. Less than 1 percent of South Africa is forested. Its terrain includes coastal lowlands, high plateaus, the Great Escarpment, the Kalahari Desert, and the spectacular Drakensberg Mountains. The high plateaus, known as the *high veld,* contain most of South Africa's impressive mineral wealth.

South Africa also enjoys a diverse wildlife population, which includes rhinoceroses, elephants, giraffes, zebras, antelopes, an amazing variety of birds, and many species of snakes. Its Kruger National Park is a famous wildlife refuge.

Playing

You may wish to invite some students to play Drum Ensemble 3 from p. 295 and the mallet accompaniment, as the rest of the class sings the song. See Skills Reinforcement below and on p. 212 for these playing activities.

Singing

The Pronunciation Practice/Translation information on p. 520 and the Pronunciation Practice tracks **CD 11-23** (melody) and **CD 11-24** (harmony) will assist students in learning the Zulu lyrics, pronunciation, and harmony parts.

SAY In *"Siyahamba,"* there is a melody, called Part 1, and two additional vocal parts. Look at Parts 2 and 3 carefully.

 ASK What differences do you see between Parts 2 and 3 in the A section of the song, from the beginning to the first ending on p. 214? (Part 2 follows the rhythm of the melody and is mostly in thirds and sixths below the melody. Part 3 is more of a rhythmic "response" to the "call" of the lyrics in Parts 1 and 2. There are only two different pitches sung in Part 3.)

Have students

- Echo sing each phrase of Part 2 as you model it.
- Read and sing Part 3 as you model it, saying aloud "4–1" on the rests to reinforce counting skills.

Divide the class into three groups and assign a different part to each group. See Skills Reinforcement on p. 213 for tips on assigning parts. Have students

- Sing section A in Zulu and in three-part harmony with the recording **CD 11-20.**
- Sight-sing Part 1 of section B (from the second ending of the second system on p. 214).
- Echo sing Part 2 of section B as the teacher models it.

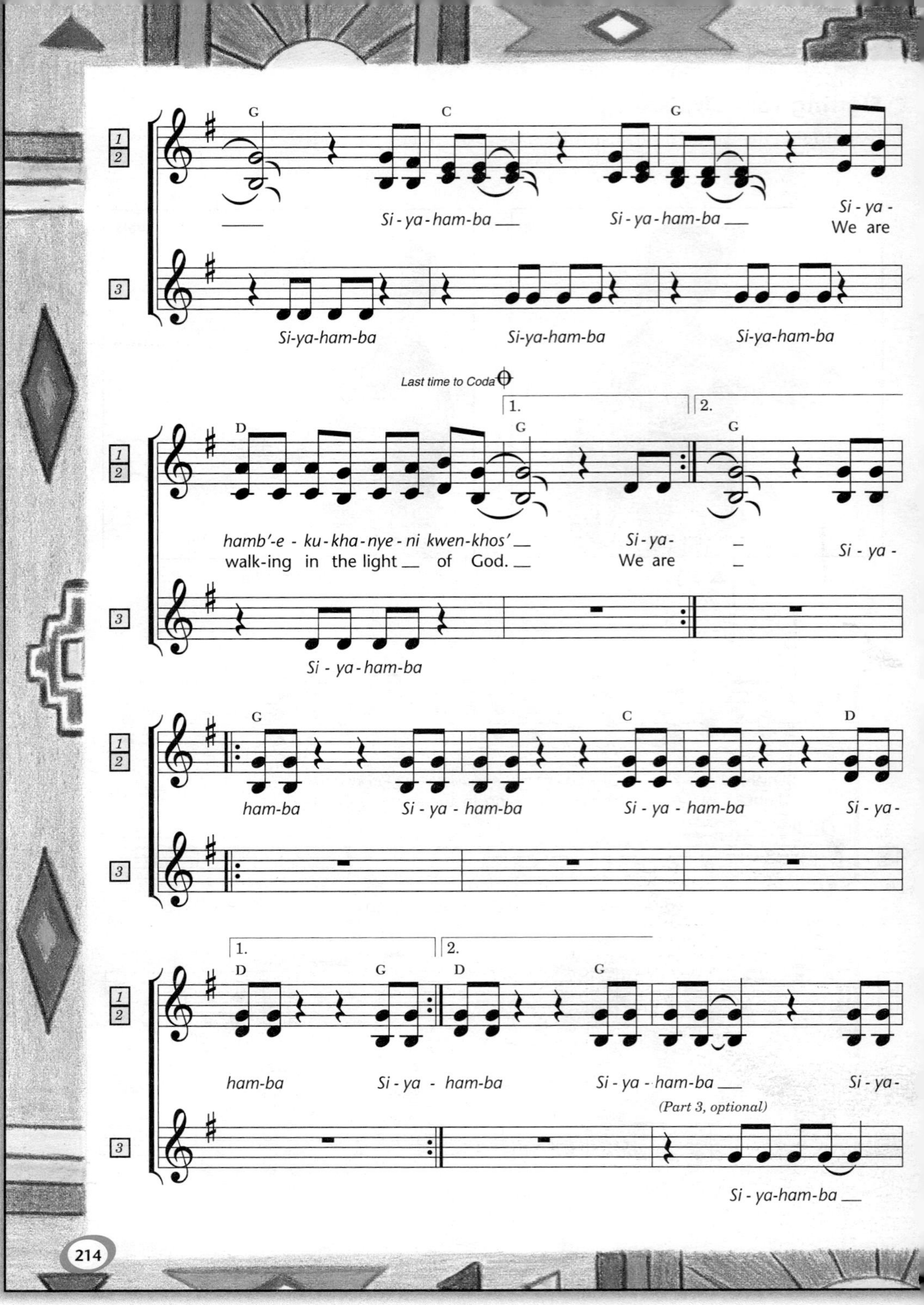

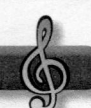

214

Footnotes

ACROSS THE CURRICULUM

▶ **Language Arts** The following excerpt from this poem by J. R. R. Tolkien shares with *"Siyahamba"* a strong sense of determination.

Roads Go Ever Ever On
from *The Hobbit* by J.R.R. Tolkien

Roads go ever ever on
Over rock and under tree
By caves where never sun has shone
By streams that never find the sea.
Over snow by winter sown
And through the merry flowers of June
Over grass and over stone
And under mountains in the moon.

SKILLS REINFORCEMENT

▶ **Playing** Refer students to p. 295 (Drum Ensemble 3) for a form of highlife drumming that can be performed with *"Siyahamba."* The drum ensemble should be played in a tempo at which the half-note beat matches the speed of the quarter-note beat of *"Siyahamba."*

Then, have students practice entering on the first ending, on this page. On the syllable *ya*, the rattles and the medium drum enter; the *shekere* and bell enter on the first beat of the following measure. Consider having the talking drum or other "master" drummer play a solo over the singing and accompaniment during the B section, which begins on p. 214.

 ▶ **Signing** Encourage students to learn the sign language for *"Siyahamba,"* found on Resource Book p. G-13.

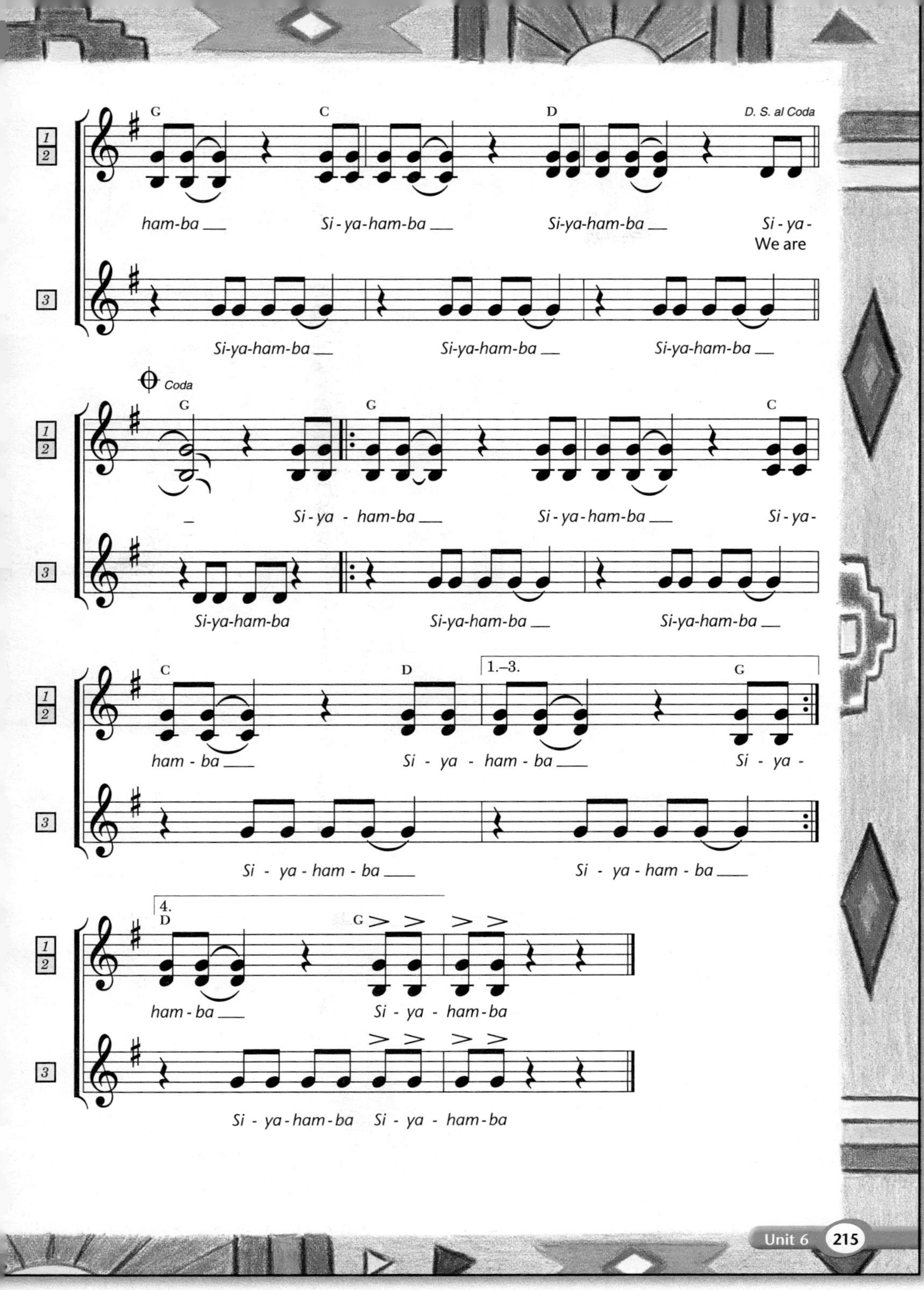

The sheet music for "Siyahamba" with lyrics: ham-ba, Si-ya-ham-ba, Si-ya-ham-ba, Si-ya- / We are. Si-ya-ham-ba (repeated), Coda, Si-ya-ham-ba, ham-ba, Si-ya-ham-ba, Si-ya-, etc.

ASK How many different pitches do you sing in Part 2, and what are those pitches? (three: B, C, and D)

Have students echo clap and sight-sing Part 3 of section B as you model it. Then, separate students into three groups, assign a part to each group, and have groups sing *"Siyahamba"* **CD 11-20, 11-21** in Zulu or English in three-part harmony with the recording.

Moving

Share with students that in west coast, central, and southern Africa, music and dance are integrally tied together. Encourage students to perform these easy steps to *"Siyahamba"* found in Movement below.

Guide students in

- Learning the signs for *Siyahamba* on p. 213.
- Incorporating the signs into their performance of the song.

3 CLOSE

Skill: SINGING   **ASSESSMENT**

1c **Performance/Peer Critique** Arrange for students to perform "Siyahamba" for an audience of fellow students, teachers, families, or community members. Remind students to demonstrate appropriate ensemble performance techniques and etiquette during the concert. Have students

- Sing *"Siyahamba"* in Zulu **CD 11-20** and English **CD 11-21**, in three-part harmony from memory, with movement, signing, and drumming. Perform expressively and from memory.
- Teach the audience to sing Part 3 in section B. Then, sing the song once more with audience participation.

7b In follow-up discussions, have students conduct a group evaluation of the effectiveness of the live concert performance, with suggestions on how specific elements might be improved.

MOVEMENT

▶ **Creative Movement** Encourage students to perform the following movements with *"Siyahamba."*

Section A: Hold hands with neighbors; alternate gliding.

(Beats)	1	2	3	4	1	2	3	4
	Glide–L		Glide–R		Glide–L		Glide–R	

Section B: Hold hands in a "W"; alternate a double glide.

(Beats)	1	2	3	4	1	2	3	4
	Glide–L		Glide–L		Glide–R		Glide–R	

Coda: Hold hands in a "W"; glide to the left and raise right leg. Glide to the right and raise left leg.

(Beats)	1	2	3	4	1	2	3	4
	Glide–L		Lift–R		Glide–R		Lift–L	

TECHNOLOGY/MEDIA LINK

4c **MIDI/Sequencing Software** Using the MIDI song file for *"Siyahamba,"* have students

- Select the software program's graphic editor and isolate each of the vocal parts.
- Experiment with various graphic editing features, such as changing pitches and assigning different timbres.
- Create additional vocal and instrumental parts.

LESSON AT A GLANCE

Element Focus   **TEXTURE/HARMONY** Polyphonic and homophonic textures

Skill Objective   **LISTENING** Discern polyphonic and homophonic textures in a listening selection

Connection Activity   **LANGUAGE ARTS** Identify the literary source of a contemporary opera

MATERIALS

- "Responsory: Alleluia" from *Mass*   **CD 11-25**
- *Overture to Candide*   **CD 11-26**
- *Overture to Candide* (excerpt)   **CD 11-27**
- sheets of paper (two per student)—half with the letter *P* (for polyphonic) printed on them, and the other half with the letter *H* (for homophonic)

VOCABULARY

monophonic   homophonic   polyphonic

texture   canon

◆ ◆ ◆ ◆ National Standards ◆ ◆ ◆ ◆

1c Sing music from diverse genres
6a Listen and describe events in music using appropriate terms
6b Listen and analyze uses of texture in music from diverse genres
8a Show how different arts portray the same idea in unique ways
8b Identify ways music relates to social studies and language arts

MORE MUSIC CHOICES

For more practice with polyphonic texture:
"Little" Organ Fugue in G Minor (organ), p. 129
"Little" Organ Fugue in G Minor (brass), p. 129
"Scattin' A-Round," p. 160

Bernstein's Textures

You have learned three musical textures: monophonic (a single melody line), homophonic (a melody line supported by harmony), and polyphonic (two or more melody lines, moving at the same time). Texture is important in the music of Leonard Bernstein. What is the texture of the music on this page?

Listen to *Responsory: Alleluia* to hear how Bernstein uses changes in texture to add interest to the work. Follow the listening map on page 217 as you listen. What two textures do you hear?

The assembled performers from a production of *Mass* ▶

Leonard Bernstein (Adapted)

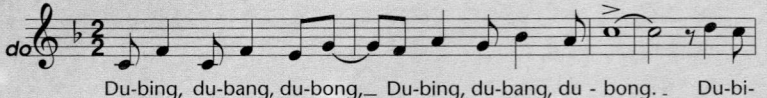

Du-bing, du-bang, du-bong,_ Du-bing, du-bang, du - bong. _ Du-bi-

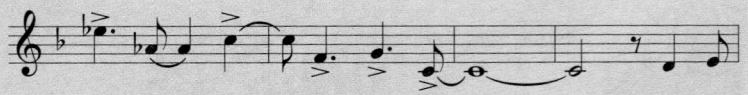

ding, dong, _ ding, _ dong, ding, dong. _____ Du - bi -

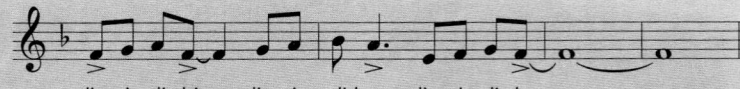

ding-i - di - bing, _ ding-i - di-bang, ding-i - di - bong. _____

216

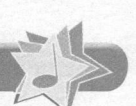

Footnotes

ACROSS THE CURRICULUM

▶ **Social Studies** Read aloud from the book *Leonard Bernstein* by Mike Venezia (Children's Press, 1998) to help students get to know this legendary musician.

BUILDING SKILLS THROUGH MUSIC

▶ **Language** Share the information about Leonard Bernstein throughout the lesson. Ask students to read about and then list the different careers in which Bernstein excelled and give examples of his accomplishments in each.

SPOTLIGHT ON

▶ **The Composer** Conductor, composer, pianist, lecturer, television personality, and author Leonard Bernstein (1918–1990) had good teachers. He learned the basics of music with Walter Piston, conducting with Fritz Reiner, and orchestration with Randall Thompson. After his studies at Harvard and the Curtis Institute, he studied at Tanglewood with Serge Koussevitzky. Bernstein made his debut as assistant conductor in 1943 with the New York Philharmonic, when he substituted for Bruno Walter—with no rehearsal. He composed music for stage productions such as *Candide* and *West Side Story*. Among his many other works are three symphonies, ballets (*Fancy Free, On the Town*), film music (*On the Waterfront*), and a setting of passages from the book of Psalms (*Chichester Psalms*).

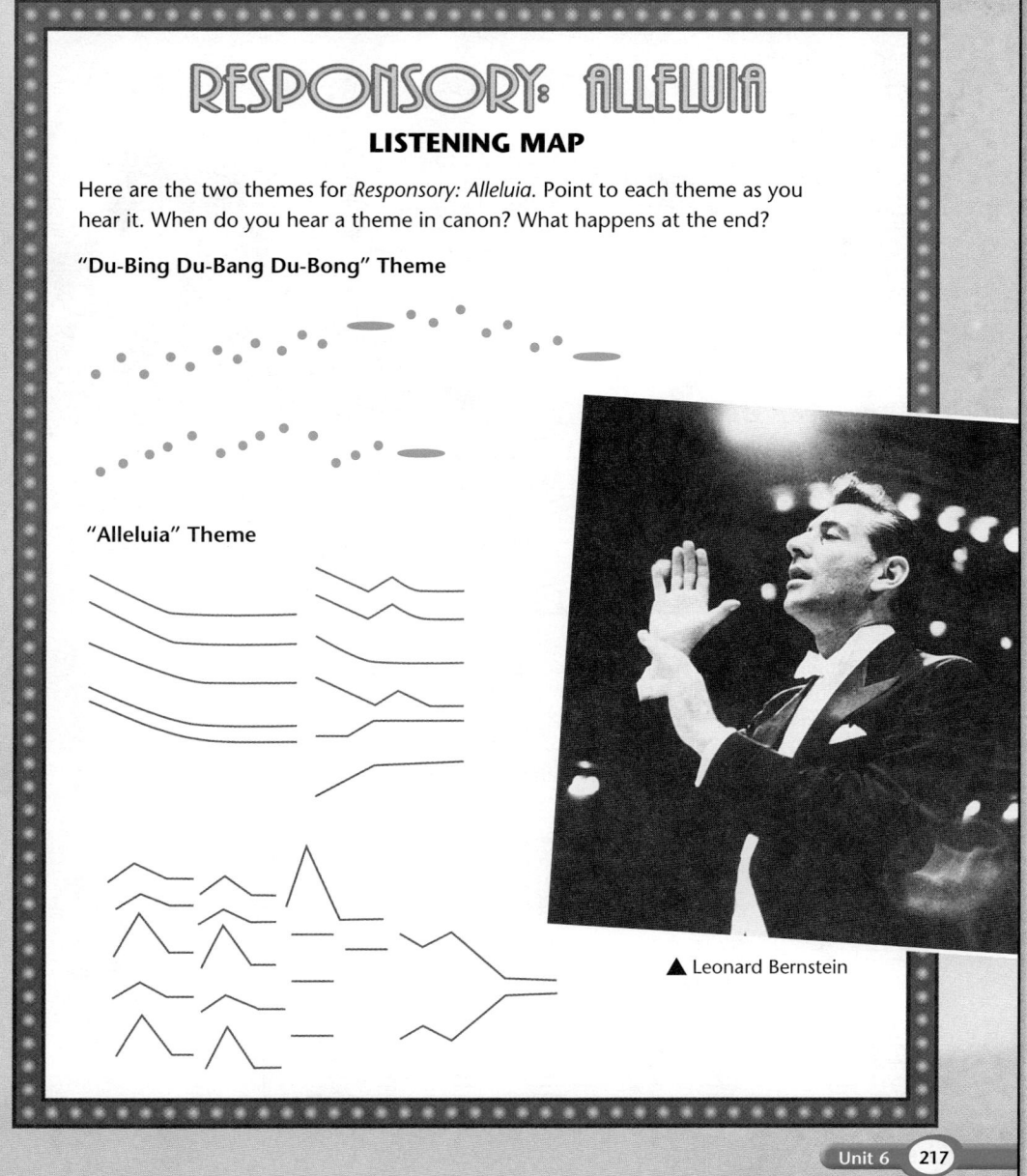

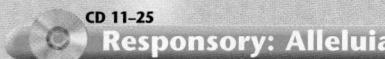

CD 11–25

Responsory: Alleluia

from *Mass*
by Leonard Bernstein

Bernstein's *Mass* premiered in 1971 for the opening of the John F. Kennedy Center for the Performing Arts in Washington, D.C.

RESPONSORY: ALLELUIA

LISTENING MAP

Here are the two themes for *Responsory: Alleluia.* Point to each theme as you hear it. When do you hear a theme in canon? What happens at the end?

"Du-Bing Du-Bang Du-Bong" Theme

"Alleluia" Theme

▲ Leonard Bernstein

Unit 6 **217**

1 INTRODUCE

Invite students to read the material on p. 216 of the student text. Review with them the definitions of monophonic, homophonic, and polyphonic. Tell students they will learn to identify these textures when listening to the music of Leonard Bernstein.

2 DEVELOP

Singing

1c Invite students to individually sing the excerpt from *Responsory: Alleluia* **CD 11-25** with the recording.

ASK What instrument were you imitating with your voice? (bells)

Inform students that this excerpt is part of a larger work, called *Mass,* written by American composer and conductor Leonard Bernstein. Have students describe how composing can be an avocation or a vocation. See Spotlight On, p. 216, and Cultural Connection below.

Listening

6a Ask students to describe the instrument they hear as they listen to *Responsory: Alleluia* (bells) **CD 11-25.**

ASK Did the voices imitate this instrument throughout the music? (No; they also sang the word *Alleluia.*)

Explain that this piece uses both polyphonic and homophonic textures.

(Note: The first section—*Du-bing, du-bang, du-bong*—is monophonic, then polyphonic when the theme is sung in canon; the second section—*Alleluia*—is homophonic; the third section returns to the first theme and is polyphonic since it is all done in canon.)

Direct students' attention to the listening map on p. 217. Ask students to follow the graphic representation of each theme as they listen to *Responsory: Alleluia.* See Technology/Media Link, p. 219, for suggestions on using the listening map transparency.

continued on page 218

CULTURAL CONNECTION

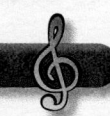

8b ▶ **Bernstein's *Mass*** Leonard Bernstein believed that one of the biggest problems facing the twentieth century was a crisis of faith. He felt that if people could be made to feel, they could call on their spiritual life to help them with their everyday lives. Bernstein got his chance when he was commissioned by Jacqueline Kennedy to write *Mass* in honor of the slain President. In this "theatre piece for singers, players, and dancers," Bernstein brought in a cast of nearly 40 people, a full orchestra, a street band, pop singers, tape recordings, the Alvin Ailey Dance Company, two choirs, and others.

Mass opened at the Kennedy Center in Washington, D.C., on September 8, 1971. Despite initial lukewarm reviews, *Mass* was eventually recognized as one of the great works of our time.

SKILLS REINFORCEMENT

1c ▶ **Singing** The style of singing used in Leonard Bernstein's *Responsory: Alleluia* is similar to jazz scat singing. Give students the opportunity to sing or listen to the following scat songs: "Just a Snap-Happy Blues" on p. 388 and "Scattin' A-Round" on p. 160.

CHARACTER EDUCATION

▶ **Life Textures** Different situations in life act as "life textures." Discuss how a person acts independently (monophonic/taking a test); with others, supporting them (homophonic/a surgical team in an operation); and with others, each having his/her own responsibility (polyphonic/the many people who manufacture a car).

Listening

Share with students information on Voltaire's *Candide* from Across the Curriculum below, explaining that this literary work served as the basis and inspiration for an opera by Bernstein.

Introduce *Overture to Candide* by informing students that this Bernstein selection, too, uses both homophonic and polyphonic textures. Then, play the complete recording **CD 11-26** and have students listen to the variety of Bernstein's themes and textures.

Direct students' attention to the listening map on p. 219. Explain that the three large sections shown on the map represent how Bernstein uses one theme, p. 218, in a variety of textures.

6b Play the excerpt **CD 11-27** as students follow the listening map. See Technology/Media Link, p. 219, for suggestions on using the listening map transparency.

ASK How does this theme differ from one section to the next? (It is performed using different textures and timbres.)

Point out that

- In section A, the theme is performed using light, homophonic texture.
- In section B, the theme is performed using light, polyphonic texture.
- In section C, the theme is performed using thicker, more prominent polyphonic texture.

Moving

8a Encourage students to use the Movement activity, p. 219, to illustrate and reinforce the different textures of the excerpted theme in *Overture to Candide*.

Bernstein as Conductor

Leonard Bernstein was first known as a conductor. He had a brilliant career with the New York Philharmonic Orchestra and the New York City Center Orchestra. He was a guest conductor for many international orchestras.

Bernstein as Teacher

Bernstein was a gifted teacher of both adults and children. His *Philharmonic Concerts for Young People* appeared on television in 1958 and continued for 15 years.

A Textured Overture

The *Overture to Candide* is another example of Bernstein's use of melody and texture. **Listen** to *Overture to Candide* and its melodic themes.

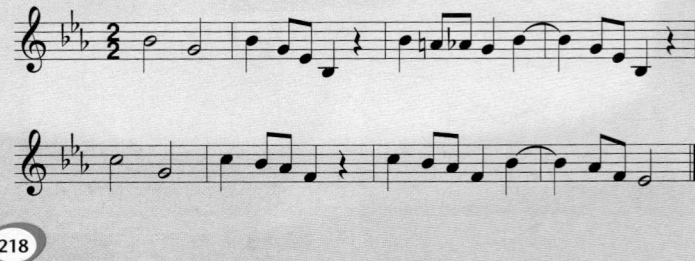
CD 11–26
Overture to Candide

by Leonard Bernstein
Bernstein uses many short themes and motives that include a brass fanfare, a lively comic melody, and a beautiful *legato* theme played by strings.

Now **listen** to an excerpt from the same piece, in which Bernstein uses a section of the melody below as a canon. Follow this theme on the listening map. Describe the musical textures you hear.

218

Footnotes

SKILLS REINFORCEMENT

1c ▶ **Singing** Students often find the task of singing and listening to rounds, canons, countermelodies, and polyphonic textures challenging. Singing and listening to separate moving parts requires "independent singing." Here are some techniques from other parts of the book to develop this skill.

Reinforcement Have students use Skills Reinforcement on p. 124 to sing a warm-up scale in a two-part canon.

On Target Use Meeting Individual Needs on p. 104 for an activity on developing independence in singing countermelodies, using "Going upon the Mountain."

Challenge Have students sing rounds and canons as ostinatos, as found on p. 206 of the student text, using *"Kyrie."* Then, challenge students to sing it as a standard canon.

ACROSS THE CURRICULUM

8b ▶ **Language Arts** *Candide* (1759) is a story written by the French writer and philosopher François Voltaire (1694–1778). The story satirizes eighteenth-century life and thought, especially class distinction, war, optimism, and the reliance on Providence. In the story, Candide's teacher, Pangloss, accepts with equanimity such suffering as earthquakes, shipwrecks, the Spanish Inquisition, and crime. He does this by saying over and over, "All is for the best in this best of all possible worlds." At first, Candide accepts this philosophy and uses it to get through many perils. Ultimately, though, he sees that the philosophy is unrealistic. Candide decides that the world is bizarre and that he should just "cultivate his own garden."

Bernstein's *Candide*

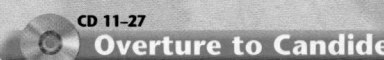

CD 11–27
Overture to Candide

by Leonard Bernstein

Bernstein wrote the *Overture to Candide* in 1956. The second voice of the canon enters when the first voice starts the second measure.

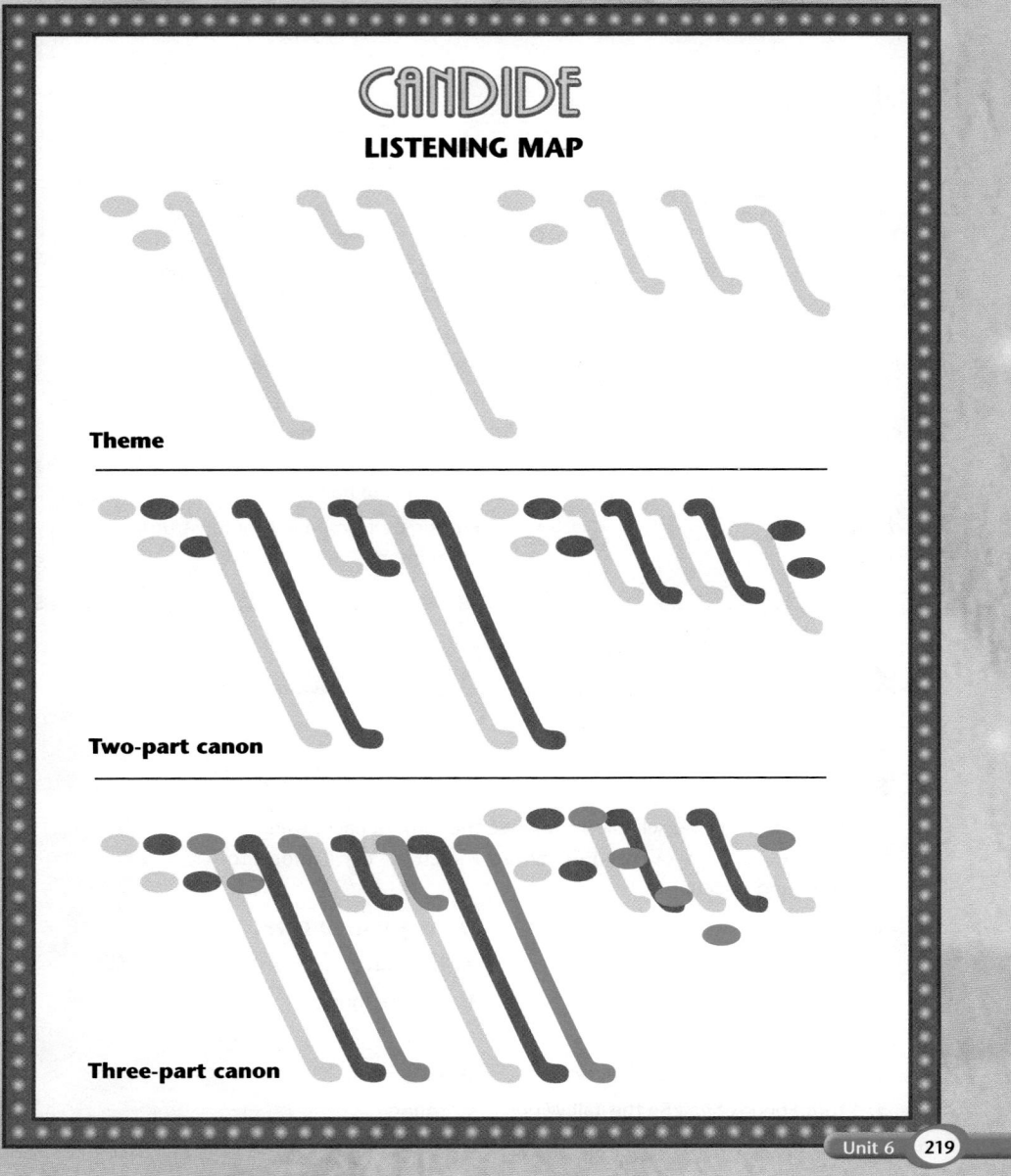

CANDIDE

LISTENING MAP

Theme

Two-part canon

Three-part canon

Unit 6 219

3 CLOSE

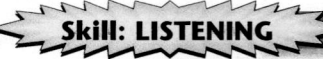

Skill: LISTENING   ASSESSMENT

6b **Observation/Music Journal Writing** Distribute sheets of paper, prepared as described under Materials. Instruct students to raise the *P* when they hear polyphonic texture and the *H* when they hear homophonic texture as they listen to *Responsory: Alleluia* **CD 11-25.** Play the recording again to allow students to confirm or correct their responses.

Have students write in their music journals their own summary descriptions of homophonic and polyphonic textures.

MOVEMENT

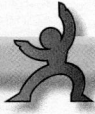

8a ▶ **Creative Movement** Encourage students to illustrate the different textures of the listening map theme in *Overture to Candide.* Have students work in groups of three (partner A, B, and C). Point out that each statement of the theme is made up of two eight-beat phrases. For each of their assigned phrases, have the groups move as follows.

- A: Make a movement that twists from low to high.
- B: Make a movement from high to low.
- C: Make a movement while traveling around A and B; change direction for the second phrase.

Begin with the A's scattered in the space, doing their movement for two phrases. They are joined by their B partners for the next two phrases, then the C's for the last two phrases.

TECHNOLOGY/MEDIA LINK

6b **Transparency** Display the listening map transparencies for *Responsory: Alleluia* and *Overture to Candide* as you play the recordings. Point to each section of each piece on the first listening to help students follow along. On subsequent listenings, invite a student to point to the sections as you play the recording.

Web Site Go to *www.sfsuccessnet.com* to learn more about Leonard Bernstein and his music.

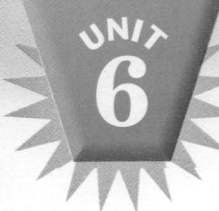
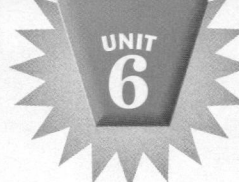
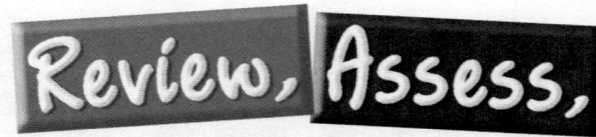
WHAT DO YOU KNOW?

MATERIALS
• **Resource Book** p. B-21

Review with students the intervals on pp. 204 and 205. Ask students to identify intervals on a music staff. Have them look at the notation on p. 220 and select the correct name for each interval, using the worksheet on Resource Book p. B-21. Students may use a keyboard visual to do this.

WHAT DO YOU HEAR? 6A

MATERIALS
• *What Do You Hear? 6A*   **CD 11-28 to 11-32**
• **Resource Book** p. B-22

Review with students the forms, or style of composing, for the songs and listenings on p. 220. Review rounds, through-composed music, chance music, AB form, and ABA form. When ready, play each selection *(What Do You Hear? 6A)* **CD 11-28 to 11-32**. Ask students to work in pairs and select the description that best fits each listening, using the worksheet on Resource Book p. B-22.

What Do You Know?

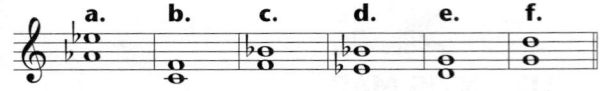

1. Identify the intervals of a fourth and fifth.

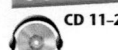

2. Match each term with its definition.

Term	Definition
a. through-composed	• a change in tempo in which the music pushes ahead and/or pulls back slightly to allow greater expression
b. *a capella*	• a musical piece in which the musical sections do not repeat
c. *rubato*	• a musical texture in which two or more melodic parts occur at the same time, creating layers of harmony
d. polyphonic	• vocal music performed without instrumental accompaniment

What Do You Hear? 6A

CD 11-28

Form

Listen to the following selections. Analyze the form of each, using letter names for the sections in the music. Match the correct form to each listening selection.

Selection	Description of Form
1. "Skye Boat Song"	**a.** through-composed
2. "Kyrie"	**b.** chance music
3. *"Vive l'amour"*	**c.** ABA
4. Concert for Piano and Orchestra	**d.** AB
5. "Your Friends Shall Be the Tall Wind"	**e.** round

220

Footnotes

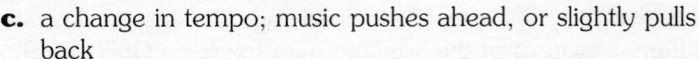

ANSWER KEY

▶ What Do You Know?

1. a. fifth
  b. fourth
  c. fourth
  d. fifth
  e. fourth
  f. fifth

2. a. musical piece in which sections do not repeat
  b. vocal music performed without instrumental accompaniment

  c. a change in tempo; music pushes ahead, or slightly pulls back
  d. musical texture in which two or more melodic parts occur at the same time

▶ What Do You Hear? 6A

1. c. ABA form
2. e. round
3. d. AB form
4. b. chance music
5. a. through-composed

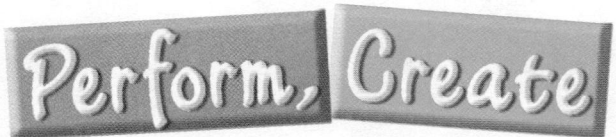

Perform, Create

What Do You Hear? 6B

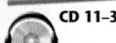 CD 11-33

Timbre

Listen to the following choral selections. Point to the description of the timbre that best describes each listening selection.

Selection	Description of Timbre
1. *Gloria in excelsis*	**a.** African chorus
2. *Lo, How a Rose E'er Blooming*	**b.** chorus and orchestra
3. "*Siyahamba*"	**c.** *a cappella* chorus
4. "America, the Beautiful"	

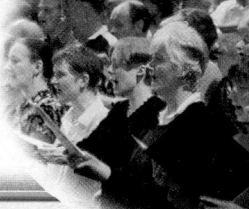

What You Can Do

Analyzing Texture

Review the use of texture in your choice of *Responsory: Alleluia* on page 217, or *Overture to Candide* on page 218. You may wish to listen to the recording you choose. Then, describe the texture of your selection using the words *homophonic* or *polyphonic*.

Play Syncopated Rhythms

Play the rhythm parts on page 197, following the notation. First perform the rhythms using body percussion and then again using percussion instruments.

Perform with Expression

Select a song from this unit. Decide where to use *rubato* in the song. Perform the song with the class, using *rubato* to add expression to the music. Discuss the effect of *rubato* on the character of the song.

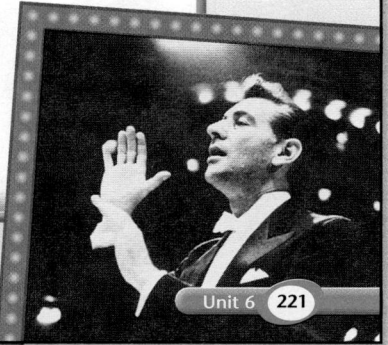

WHAT DO YOU HEAR? 6B

> **MATERIALS**
> - *What Do You Hear? 6B*   **CD 11-33 to 11-36**
> - **Resource Book** p. B-22

Review timbre in choral ensembles. Then, play the selections listed above (*What Do You Hear? 6B*) **CD 11-33 to 11-36**. Have students work with a partner to decide which type of group was performing each selection and record their answers on the worksheet on Resource Book p. B-22.

WHAT YOU CAN DO

> **MATERIALS**
> - *Responsory: Alleluia,* p. 217   **CD 11-25**
> - *Overture to Candide,* p. 218   **CD 11-26**
> - **Resource Book** pp. B-23, J-10

Sing Different Textures

Review the use of texture in your choice of *Responsory: Alleluia,* p. 217, or *Overture to Candide,* p. 218. Then, describe the texture of your selection. Write your description in your music journal.

Play Syncopated Rhythms

Review syncopation with the class. Then, invite students to perform the percussion parts on p. 197, first using body percussion and then with percussion instruments.

Perform with Expression

Review performing in various meters. Then, select a song or a listening selection from this unit and invite students to perform it, using *rubato* and expressing the feeling.

▶ What Do You Hear? 6B

1. b. chorus and orchestra
2. c. *a cappella* chorus
3. a. African chorus
4. b. chorus and orchestra

▶ What You Can Do

Analyzing Texture

Responsory: Alleluia = polyphonic

Overture to Candide = homophonic, polyphonic

Perform with Expression

Rubato, the slight push and pull of tempo, allows music to be more expressive and free-flowing.

TECHNOLOGY/MEDIA LINK

▶ Rubrics

Visit *www.sfsuccessnet.com* for rubrics to assess students' achievement in music skills.

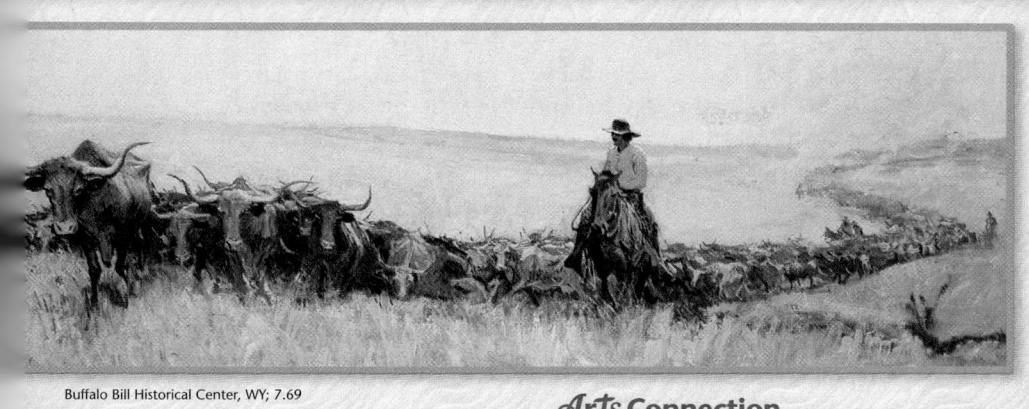

Buffalo Bill Historical Center, WY; 7.69

Arts Connection

▲ *Trail Herd to Abilene* (1923) by W. H. D. Koerner (1878–1938) depicts a cattle drive.

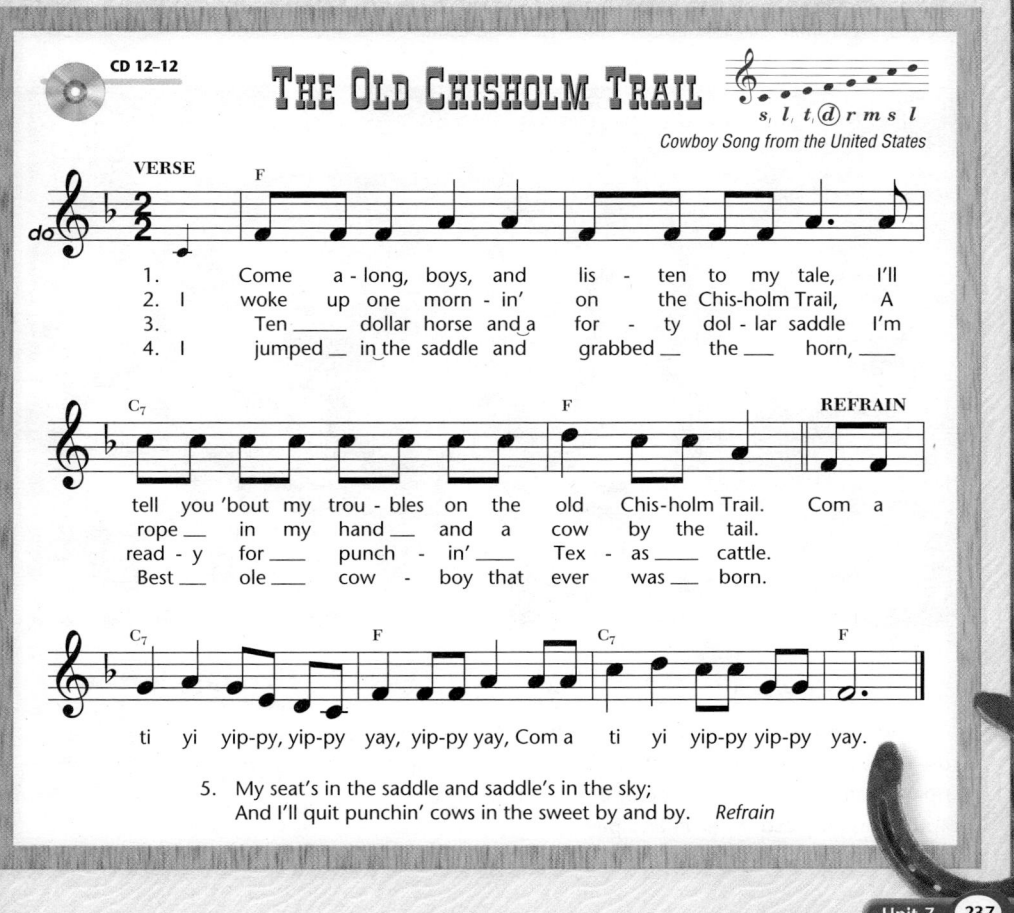

CD 12–12

THE OLD CHISHOLM TRAIL

s, l, t, (d) r m s l

Cowboy Song from the United States

VERSE

1. Come a-long, boys, and lis-ten to my tale, I'll
2. I woke up one morn-in' on the Chis-holm Trail, A
3. Ten ____ dollar horse and a for-ty dol-lar saddle I'm
4. I jumped __ in the saddle and grabbed __ the __ horn, ____

REFRAIN

tell you 'bout my trou-bles on the old Chis-holm Trail. Com a
rope __ in my hand __ and a cow by the tail.
read-y for __ punch-in' __ Tex-as __ cattle.
Best __ ole __ cow - boy that ever was __ born.

ti yi yip-py, yip-py yay, yip-py yay, Com a ti yi yip-py yip-py yay.

5. My seat's in the saddle and saddle's in the sky;
And I'll quit punchin' cows in the sweet by and by. *Refrain*

1 INTRODUCE

ASK From what you have seen in movies, how might you describe the life of a cowboy on a cattle drive? (Accept a variety of answers, such as herding cattle down a trail; eating by the campfire at night)

8b Invite the class to imagine soldiers coming home to Texas after the Civil War (1865), seeing nearly five million cows running wild. All they had to do was round them up, brand them, and drive them north to be fattened up and shipped to cities in the East.

Tell students that in this lesson they will learn about the life of a cowboy on cattle trails after the Civil War.

2 DEVELOP

Analyzing

Invite students to identify and locate the Chisholm Trail on p. 236 of the student text. Then, using a more detailed map of Texas and Kansas, have students

8b
- Study the map of the Chisholm Trail leading from San Antonio, Texas up to Abilene, Kansas where they could connect with the railroad to ship the cows to Kansas City and other points north and east.

- Identify and count the number of rivers that must be crossed.

- Read the paragraph on Cowboy Life on p. 236.

ASK What do you think life was like as a young cowboy of 19 to 22 years of age? (hard work, long days, poor pay of a dollar a day, dusty trail rides, fording rivers with nests of snakes, cattle stampedes, and so on)

SAY Let's listen to Charlie Daniels's recording of *The Old Chisholm Trail*; then we will sing the song. We can add to the list of things about cowboy life after we listen.

Listening

Have students listen to *The Old Chisholm Trail*
CD 12–11.

continued on page 238

6b ► **Cowboy Instruments** Students may be interested in learning more about the instruments that cowboys played. Have students describe the timbre of each instrument.

- **Banjo** An African American creation, the banjo became popular in America around 1830–1840 and was featured in minstrel shows.

- **Guitar** C. F. Martin, the first American guitar manufacturer, established his company in New York in 1833.

- **Harmonica** Matthias Hohner, German clockmaker, sent harmonicas to America in 1865, where they quickly became popular.

- **Fiddle** The fiddle is just another word for violin, an orchestral instrument first made in Italy between 1520 and 1550.

6b ► **Listening** Invite students to listen to country music selections and identify the guitar-like instruments that often play melodies that "slide around." Ask students how they may describe the timbre of steel-string guitars. (electric, steel, sharp, clean, nasal, notes have slides or *glissandos*) Two types of steel-string guitars are:

- **Acoustic slide guitars** The Dobro and National Steel are two acoustic slide guitars. These guitars are often played with a metal cylinder. They may be played flat on the lap or in regular guitar position. Many of these guitars feature a metal "pie-plate looking" resonator over the sound hole.

- **Pedal steel guitars** These electric guitars are played sitting down with the guitar on a stand, and look like a fingerboard on legs. They produce a sustained sound that has become a signature sound of mainline country music.

6b **ASK** **What timbres are used to set the mood during the opening narrative?** (harmonica, wind, crickets, bird calls, herding sounds)

What instruments/voices do you hear in the Charlie Daniels's recording? (fiddle, steel-string guitar, drum set, harmonica, pedal steel guitar, back-up vocals)

Singing

Share with students the information in Across the Curriculum on p. 236. Then continue the discussion of cowboy life on the cattle trail through Texas, Oklahoma, and Kansas.

1c Invite students to sing "The Old Chisholm Trail" **CD 12–12** with the recording.

Playing

2d Ask students to identify the key of "The Old Chisholm Trail" on p. 237 (F major). Use Skills Reinforcement on p. 239 to help students understand the use of a capo to simplify playing chords. When ready, have students

- Write "F major" and the chords "F and C_7."
- Write "D major" and the chords "D and A_7"on the next line.
- Review the guitar fingerings for D and A_7 on pp. 508–509 of the student text.

2a
- Play a simple two-chord accompaniment to "The Old Chisholm Trail" on Autoharp, guitar (capo 3 and play D and A_7 to sound F and C_7), or keyboard.

Listening

Have students read the paragraph on A Cowboy Dance on p. 238 and discuss the instruments used by cowboys both in the ranch bunkhouse and on the trail. (See Spotlight On, p. 237.)

ASK **Why do you think cowboys valued someone who could sing, play an instrument, or tell a story?** (There were no radios, TVs, phonographs, or interactive games and other forms of entertainment.)

A Cowboy Dance

After all their hard work, cowboys were happy to have a break. They enjoyed music, dancing, stories, or poetry. Instruments such as the guitar, harmonica, concertina, banjo, mandolin, and fiddle were popular. Those instruments were also easy to carry on the trail. A man who could tell a good story was a valued companion in the cowboy bunkhouse or the lumberjack shanty.

Listen to Michael Martin Murphy perform his version of *Cowboys' Christmas Ball*. Notice how Murphy and the band end the recording with a number of dance tunes including *Good King Wenceslas*, *Under the Double Eagle*, *Redwing*, and *Oh, Them Golden Slippers*. What instruments do you hear in the band?

 CD 12–14
Cowboys' Christmas Ball

**Traditional Cowboy Song
as performed by Michael Martin Murphy**

Larry Chittenden, a New York writer turned cowboy poet, wrote the poem *Cowboys' Christmas Ball* after attending a cowboy Christmas dance in the 1880s.

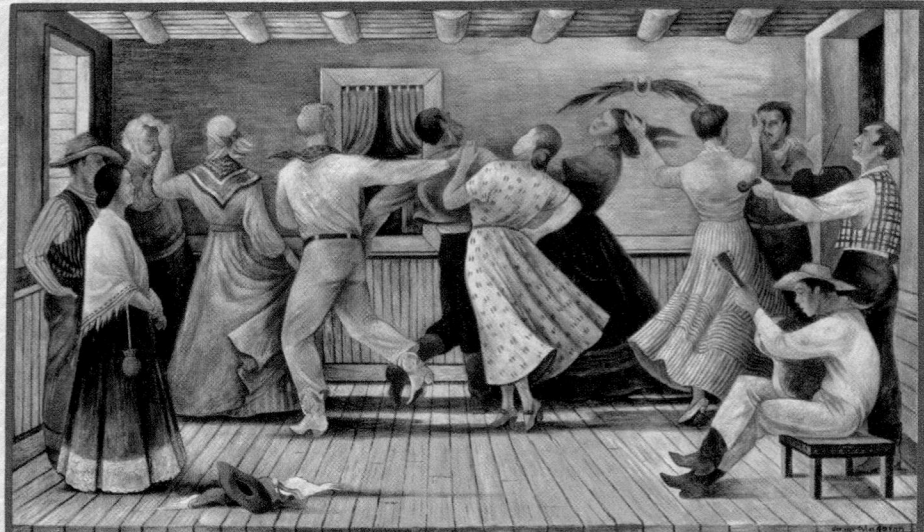

Dancing Cowboys

Around Christmas time, cowboys were invited down to the main ranch house for a festive dinner and dance. If no women were present, some of the men put on aprons and danced the woman's part. **Sing** "Cowboys' Christmas Ball," which describes the dance.

 Arts Connection

▲ *Cowboy Dance*, or *Fiesta de Vaqueros*, by Jenne Magafan (1915–1952) shows a festive cowboy dance.

238

Footnotes

ACROSS THE CURRICULUM

8a ▶ **Visual Arts** Allow students to discover that young western artists such as Frederic Remington (1861–1909) and Charles Russell (1864–1926) heeded the call "go west, young man" in search of adventure and a new start. They captured the spirit of the cowboy era in their art.

Remington, from Ogdensburg, NY, was well known for his drawings and bronze sculptures of horses. The epitaph on his gravestone is "He knew horses." His drawings, sculptures, and paintings of cowboys and other western scenes can be found in museums all over the United States.

Russell, from St. Louis, was best known for his action paintings of cowboys and western life. His paintings are featured in a museum dedicated to his work in Great Falls, Montana.

238

SPOTLIGHT ON

8b ▶ **Lawrence "Larry" Chittenden** Students may be interested in learning about poet-rancher Larry Chittenden **8a** (1862–1934). He wrote *Cowboys' Christmas Ball* about a dance he attended in Anson, Texas in 1890. Most of his poems were published in an 1893 book, *Ranch Verses*.

The first and last verses of his poem "Texas Types—The Cowboy" are:

He wears a big hat and big spurs and all that,
* And leggins of fancy fringed leather;*
He takes pride in his boots and the pistol he shoots
* And he's happy in all kinds of weather.*

Hence I say unto you, give the cowboy his due,
* And be kinder, my friends, to his folly;*
For he's generous and brave, though he may not behave
* Like your dudes, who are so melancholy.*

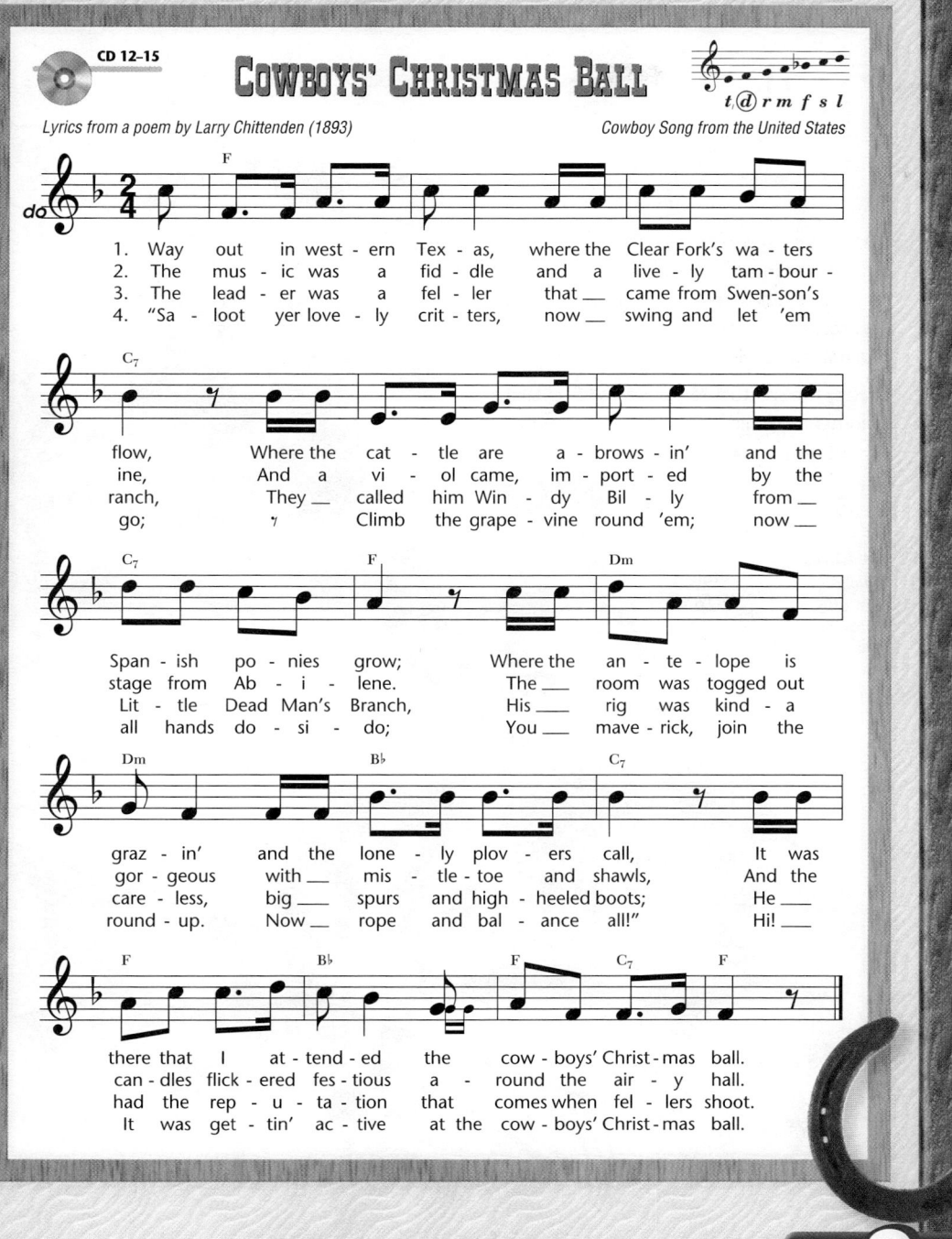

CD 12-15

COWBOYS' CHRISTMAS BALL

Lyrics from a poem by Larry Chittenden (1893)

Cowboy Song from the United States

1. Way out in west-ern Tex-as, where the Clear Fork's wa-ters
2. The mus-ic was a fid-dle and a live-ly tam-bour-
3. The lead-er was a fel-ler that __ came from Swen-son's
4. "Sa-loot yer love-ly crit-ters, now __ swing and let 'em

flow, Where the cat-tle are a-brows-in' and the
ine, And a vi-ol came, im-port-ed by the
ranch, They __ called him Win-dy Bil-ly from __
go; Climb the grape-vine round 'em; now __

Span-ish po-nies grow; Where the an-te-lope is
stage from Ab-i-lene. The __ room was togged out
Lit-tle Dead Man's Branch, His __ rig was kind-a
all hands do-si-do; You __ mave-rick, join the

graz-in' and the lone-ly plov-ers call, It was
gor-geous with __ mis-tle-toe and shawls, And the
care-less, big __ spurs and high-heeled boots; He __
round-up. Now __ rope and bal-ance all!" Hi! __

there that I at-tend-ed the cow-boys' Christ-mas ball.
can-dles flick-ered fes-tious a-round the air-y hall.
had the rep-u-ta-tion that comes when fel-lers shoot.
It was get-tin' ac-tive at the cow-boys' Christ-mas ball.

Unit 7 **239**

Guide students to

8a
- Discuss the importance of dancing as a diversion as Americans moved westward. Tell them the fiddle was the instrument of choice for dances.
- Listen to *Cowboys' Christmas Ball* **CD 12-14** performed by Michael Martin Murphy. Ask students to notice the background music ("I Heard the Bells On Christmas Day") behind Bruce Kiskadden's poem recited by Waddie Mitchell.

ASK What instruments or voices do you hear in the Michael Murphy recording? (fiddle, accordion, steel-string guitar, drum set, harmonica, string bass)

Have students listen to the dance tunes played at the end of the recording. *(Good King Wenceslas; Under the Double Eagle; Redwing; Oh, Them Golden Slippers)* Have students signal when they think each new piece is beginning.

Singing

1c Invite students to sing "Cowboys' Christmas Ball" **CD 12-14** with the recording.

Ask students to describe some of the stylistic techniques that make instruments sound like dance or cowboy music (for example, violin playing the "dee dig-ga, dee dig-ga" rhythm played by fiddlers; the "boom-chick" or bass-strum on guitar).

3 CLOSE

Skill: LISTENING   ASSESSMENT

Observation Invite students to bring to class recordings of the instruments featured in this lesson. (harmonica, fiddle, accordion, steel-string guitar)

Using these recordings, or the recordings in this lesson, play several selections and have students identify the instruments and timbres they hear on the recording. Observe students' abilities to correctly identify the instruments and their timbres.

SKILLS REINFORCEMENT

2d ▶ **Using a Guitar Capo** Playing guitar in a key such as F major is difficult. Using a capo allows a player to sound in F major while playing in an easier key such as D.

Remind students that each fret space on guitar represents a half step. To determine what key is best and where the capo should be placed, have students follow these steps (using B♭ major for example):

- Move downward in pitch from the original key (B♭) until you reach one of the easy guitar playing keys (C, D, G, A, or Am).
- Count the number of half-steps from the original key (B♭) to the new playing key (G or A) and place the capo in that fret space (G = capo 3; A = capo 1). The capo raises the pitch of the playing key to the original key. Capo 3 means to place the capo on fret 3. Play in the easier key.

TECHNOLOGY/MEDIA LINK

▶ **Electronic Keyboard** Invite students to find and explore MIDI keyboard sounds that can be used in an arrangement of a cowboy song. Have students make a list of the instruments or sounds and their locations for later use in arranging songs with sequencing software.

Guide students to experiment with an electric steel-guitar sound. Ask them how they might use a MIDI keyboard to create "slides" that are part of its sound. Have students

- Use the Pitch Bend control on most MIDI keyboards to create a bend or slide on the pitch.
- Set the Pitch Bend to a minus (−) position, then play the note while slowly moving the control to its normal position.

LESSON AT A GLANCE

Element Focus — EXPRESSION Blues style

Skill Objective — CREATING Create new verses for a blues song

Connection Activity — STYLE Discover how the blues gave voice to the African American experience in the twentieth century

MATERIALS

- "Sometimes I Feel Like a Motherless Child" **CD 12–17**
  Recording Routine: Intro (4 m.); v. 1; v. 2; v. 1; coda
- "Sun Gonna Shine" **CD 12–19**
  Recording Routine: Intro (4 m.); v. 1; v. 2; v. 3; v. 4; v. 5; coda
- "Key to the Highway" **CD 12–22**
  Recording Routine: Intro (4 m.); v. 1; v. 2; instrumental; v. 3; coda
- *Key to the Highway* **CD 12–21**
- **Resource Book** pp. G-14, H-22, H-23, I-20
- guitars, keyboards, Autoharp (optional), recorders

VOCABULARY

country blues   classic blues   urban blues

◆ ◆ ◆ ◆ National Standards ◆ ◆ ◆ ◆

1b Sing easy pieces with expression
1d Sing music written in two parts
2a Play instruments accurately alone
2d Perform simple accompaniments by ear
4a Compose short pieces, demonstrating unity and variety through music
6b Listen and analyze uses of form in music from diverse genres
9a Describe characteristics of music genres from a variety of cultures

MORE MUSIC CHOICES

For more practice with blues form and style:
"Birthday," p. 90
"Rock and Roll Is Here to Stay," p. 36
"Worried Man Blues," p. 371

The Blues Feeling

The **blues** is sometimes described as a feeling, such as "I'm feeling down and out. My baby has just left me." Feelings of loneliness or sadness were also expressed in earlier African American musical styles, such as spirituals and work songs.

Sing the spiritual "Sometimes I Feel Like a Motherless Child." Then **create** your own verses about how you feel.

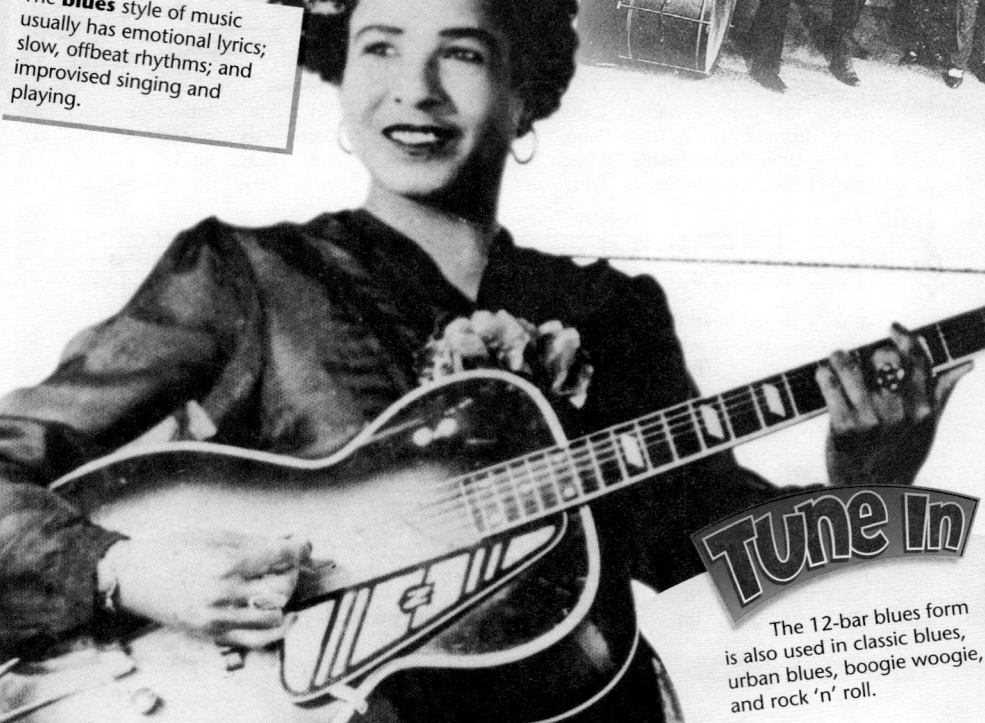

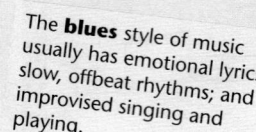
The **blues** style of music usually has emotional lyrics; slow, offbeat rhythms; and improvised singing and playing.

Tune In
The 12-bar blues form is also used in classic blues, urban blues, boogie woogie, and rock 'n' roll.

240

Footnotes

ACROSS THE CURRICULUM

9a ▶ **Social Studies** In the early part of the twentieth century many African Americans in the South moved north to find better-paying jobs in large city factories. The country blues style also traveled north and eventually turned into both the classic blues and the urban blues styles. See Spotlight On, pp. 241 and 242. Blues lyrics reflected the poor living conditions in the cities. Encourage students to explore this subject in more detail.

BUILDING SKILLS THROUGH MUSIC

▶ **Social Studies** Share the information from Across the Curriculum above, and from Spotlight On, pp. 241 and 242, with students. Ask them to select Country Blues, Classic Blues, or Urban Blues to complete a concept map of the style they select.

CULTURAL CONNECTION

▶ **Switching Cultures** Explain to students that jazz (including blues) is a cultural performance style as much as a category of music. Invite students to select a favorite song from a culture that is not jazz oriented. Students could select "Harrison Town," p. 97. Discuss with students what musical changes they could make to convert the song from a folk song from the Ozarks to a jazzy song. (Swing straight eighth-note rhythms, add syncopation, sing downbeats slightly ahead of the beat, create and use scat syllables, add a jazzy accompaniment, and so on)

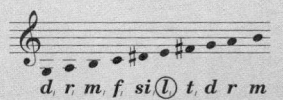

d, r, m, f, si ① t, d r m

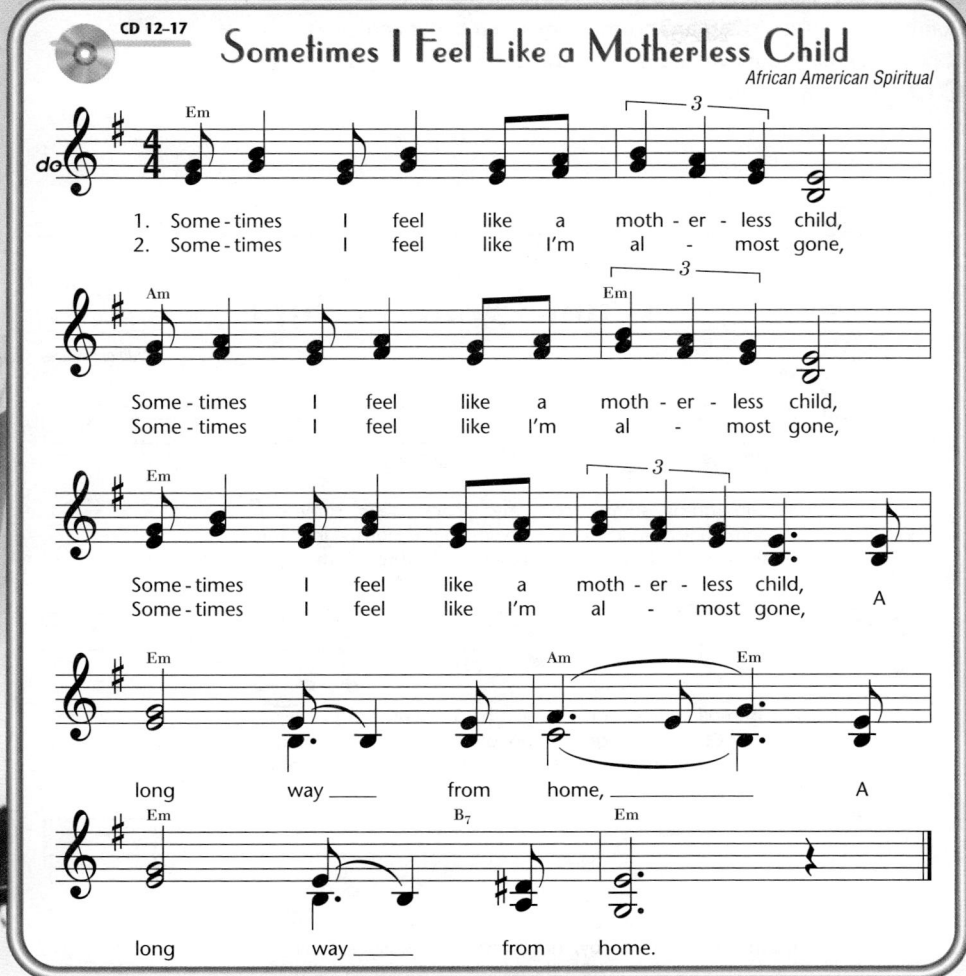

CD 12–17

Sometimes I Feel Like a Motherless Child
African American Spiritual

do

1. Some - times I feel like a moth - er - less child,
2. Some - times I feel like I'm al - most gone,

Some - times I feel like a moth - er - less child,
Some - times I feel like I'm al - most gone,

Some - times I feel like a moth - er - less child,
Some - times I feel like I'm al - most gone,

long way _____ from home, _____

long way _____ from home.

The 12-Bar Blues

Early country blues recorded in the 1920s was simply one singer
accompanied by a guitar. Many country blues artists used a form called
12-bar blues (12 measures long), which had three phrases in an
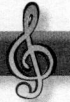 lyric structure. "Sun Gonna Shine," on the next page, is a
good example of this traditional blues form.

◀ Memphis Minnie (left) and Ma Rainey (top right, with her
band) were among blues' most important female artists.

Unit 7 **241**

1 INTRODUCE

Ask students if they are familiar with the term "feeling
blue." Let students know that singing can help express
the blues and that a whole style of music developed
just for this reason. Help students discover how blues
gave voice to African American experience in the twentieth century. Share the information in Across the
Curriculum and Cultural Connection, p. 240, and
Spotlight On, below and on p. 242.

2 DEVELOP

Singing

SAY Some spirituals were precursors to the blues
style. "Sometimes I Feel Like a Motherless Child" is
such a spiritual.

1b Have students listen to "Sometimes I Feel Like a
Motherless Child" **CD 12–17** as they follow the music.
After listening, ask students to describe the style of the
music. Students may then sing the melody (top part)
with the recording or with other forms of accompaniment, such as guitar or keyboard.

ASK This song is a spiritual; what makes it seem like
a blues song? (the feelings it expresses)

How does the soloist on the recording express
the blues feeling of the song? (by "stretching" the
tempo and rhythms to emphasize the words; by "sliding" from one note to the next)

1d Have students sing the harmony (lower part) with the
recording of the song, then divide the class into two
groups and sing the entire song with both parts.

Creating

Encourage students to create new verses for
"Sometimes I Feel Like a Motherless Child." Point out
that they only need to think of a short phrase to follow
Sometimes I feel like _____.

continued on page 242

SKILLS REINFORCEMENT

2a ▶ **Keyboard** Have students play the following broken chords
to accompany "Sometimes I Feel Like a Motherless Child" on
keyboard. See Resource Book p. H-22 for a complete accompaniment.

Em   Am   B(7)

Students may wish to play the tritone blues accompaniment for
"Sun Gonna Shine," on Resource Book p. H-23.

▶ **Recorder** Students may enjoy playing the stylized recorder
part for "Sun Gonna Shine," on Resource Book p. I-20.

SPOTLIGHT ON

9a ▶ **Country Blues** The earliest blues recorded in the 1920s
and 1930s was country blues, which featured an African
American male singer with acoustic steel-string guitar. This style,
from the Mississippi Delta and Texas, was represented by artists
Robert Johnson, Charley Patton, Son House, Blind Lemon
Jefferson, Eubie Blake, Huddie Ledbetter (Leadbelly), Mississippi
John Hurt, and Lightnin' Hopkins.

▶ **Classic Blues** The sophisticated classic blues style of the
1920s and 1930s, from Memphis, Kansas City, Chicago, and
New York, featured a female soloist with a small Dixieland jazz
band or piano. Some who sang classic blues were Bessie Smith,
Ma Rainey, Mamie Smith, Ethel Waters, and Alberta Hunter.
Later singers of classic blues were Billie Holiday, Ella Fitzgerald,
and Sarah Vaughn.

Moving

Encourage students to create movements that reflect the music and words of "Sometimes I Feel Like a Motherless Child" and to learn the signing found on Resource Book p. G-14.

Analyzing

Have students

6b

- Sing verse 1 of "Sun Gonna Shine" **CD 12–19** with the recording or other accompaniment, such as guitar or keyboard.
- Examine the typical aab 12-bar blues rhyme scheme used in this song.
- Discuss the use of 12-bar blues in this song and in various other types of blues. See Spotlight On, p. 241 and below.

Singing

Have students sing all the verses of "Sun Gonna Shine."

Have them sing it again with the traveling-step routine on selected verses, as described in Movement below.

Creating

Encourage students to create new verses for "Sun Gonna Shine," based on the aab rhyme scheme. See Skills Reinforcement, p. 243.

Reading

Have students

- Sing verse 1 of "Key to the Highway" **CD 12–22** several times as they follow the music.
- Sing the entire song.

ASK If "Sun Gonna Shine" is a 12-bar blues, how many bars are in "Key to the Highway"? (Eight. Point out that the partial measures at the beginning and end count as only one whole measure.)

ASK What is the rhyme scheme? (two phrases with a rhyming word at the end, or "couplets")

Let the Sunshine In

No matter how blue you may feel, you know that the sun will come out and shine again. It's a good feeling. **Sing** "Sun Gonna Shine." Then **play** an accompaniment on guitar and **create** some of your own blues verses using the 12-bar blues lyric structure.

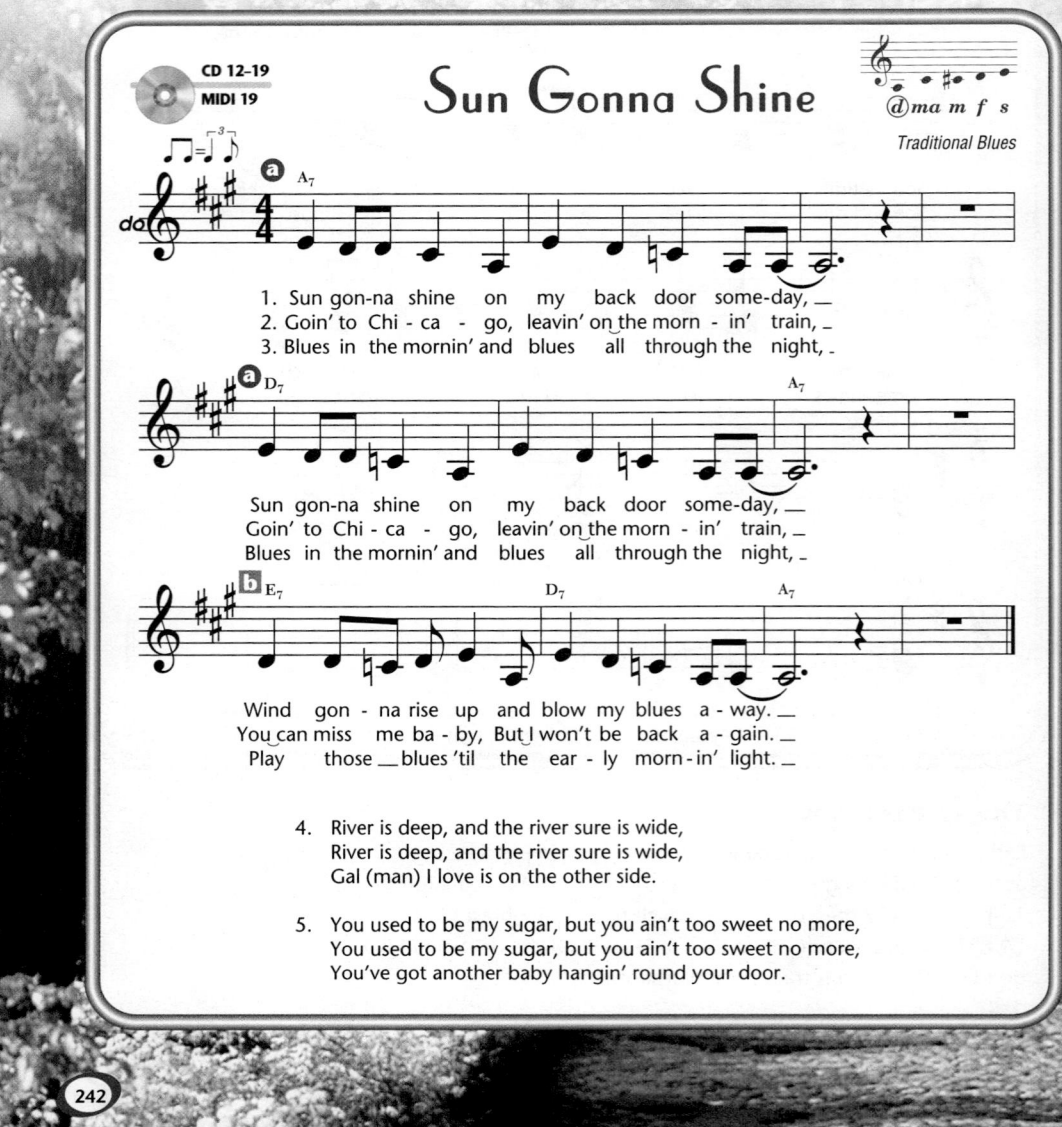

Sun Gonna Shine

Traditional Blues

1. Sun gon-na shine on my back door some-day, __
2. Goin' to Chi-ca-go, leavin' on the morn-in' train, __
3. Blues in the mornin' and blues all through the night, .

Sun gon-na shine on my back door some-day, __
Goin' to Chi-ca-go, leavin' on the morn-in' train, __
Blues in the mornin' and blues all through the night, _

Wind gon-na rise up and blow my blues a-way. __
You can miss me ba-by, But I won't be back a-gain. __
Play those __ blues 'til the ear-ly morn-in' light. __

4. River is deep, and the river sure is wide,
   River is deep, and the river sure is wide,
   Gal (man) I love is on the other side.

5. You used to be my sugar, but you ain't too sweet no more,
   You used to be my sugar, but you ain't too sweet no more,
   You've got another baby hangin' round your door.

242

Footnotes

SPOTLIGHT ON

▶ **Urban Blues** A 1930s to 1950s style, urban blues (also known as rhythm and blues or R&B) features a vocalist and a small band with instruments such as electric guitar, harmonica, piano, string bass (electric bass by the 1950s), drum set, and sometimes saxophones and trumpets. The hotbeds of this style were Chicago, New York, Memphis, and Kansas City.

The leading urban blues guitarists were Muddy Waters, Howlin' Wolf, Jimmy Reed, Elmore James, Bo Diddley, Willie Dixon, T-Bone Walker, Lowell Fulson, John Lee Hooker, Brownie McGhee, Big Bill Broonzy, and Gatemouth Brown. Harmonica (blues harp) players included Little Walter, Sonny Boy Williamson, and Sonny Terry. Urban blues laid the groundwork for 1950s rock 'n' roll.

MOVEMENT

▶ **Patterned Dance** Invite students to perform a 12-bar-blues movement routine with "Sun Gonna Shine." Tell them that in the blues style, a traveling step involves a loose-limbed, subtle movement. They should use a slow step-bend, keeping the feet close to the ground in a shuffle. Improvised movements during the instrumental riffs can be small pivots, swivels, and syncopated steps.

Mm. 1–4: Travel to stage right. Improvise in place during riff.

Mm. 5–8: Travel to stage left. Improvise in place during riff.

Mm. 9–12: Travel diagonally downstage. Improvise back to place during riff.

Keyed to the Blues

Sing "Key to the Highway," an urban blues popularized by Big Bill Broonzy. Is this song a 12-bar blues? To **play** along on guitar, place your guitar capo on fret 1 to play in E, or on fret 3 to play in D.

Key to the Highway

by Big Bill Broonzy and Charles Segar
as performed by Big Bill Broonzy
Broonzy's music reflects the gospel style of his Southern roots. Between 1928 and his death in 1958, he made more than 300 recordings.

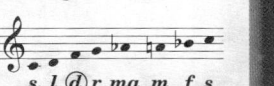

s, l, (d) r ma m f s

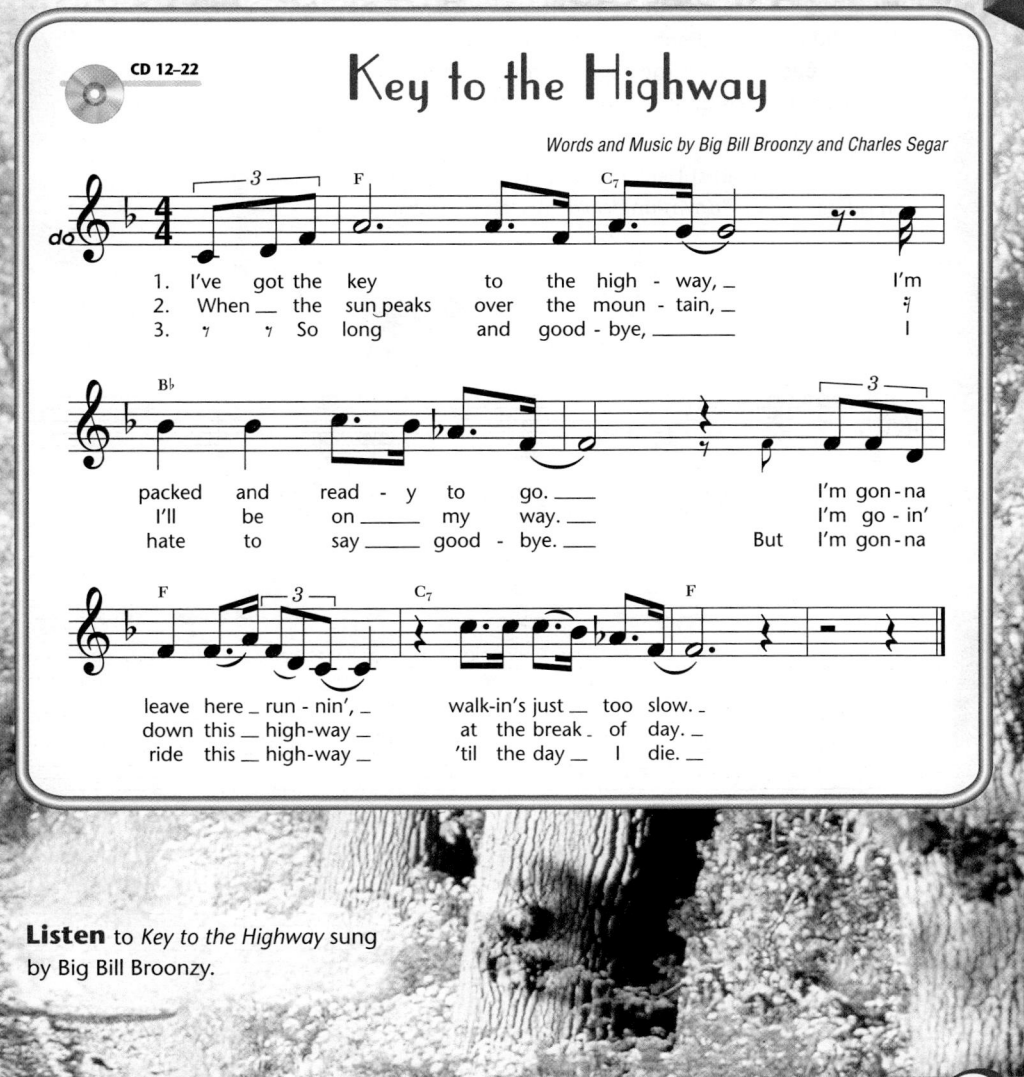

CD 12–22

Key to the Highway

Words and Music by Big Bill Broonzy and Charles Segar

1. I've got the key to the high - way, __ I'm
2. When __ the sun peaks over the moun - tain, __
3. So long and good - bye, ___

packed and read - y to go. ___ I'm gon-na
I'll be on __ my way. __ I'm go - in'
hate to say __ good - bye. ___ But I'm gon-na

leave here __ run - nin', walk-in's just __ too slow. _
down this __ high-way __ at the break _ of day. _
ride this __ high-way __ 'til the day I die. _

Listen to *Key to the Highway* sung by Big Bill Broonzy.

Unit 7 **243**

Exploring America's Music

Listening

Have students listen to the Big Bill Broonzy version of *Key to the Highway* **CD 12–21**.

ASK How does it differ from the printed version of the song? (Broonzy sings the melody differently on each verse; some words are different.)

What instrument is used to play the solo at the beginning and in the middle of the recording? (harmonica; also called the blues harp)

Playing

Using guitar, keyboard, Autoharp, or other instruments that play chords, students can easily accompany the three songs in this lesson. See Skills Reinforcement on p. 241, and below.

Have students

- Play a broken-chord accompaniment on keyboard, using the designated harmonies for "Sometimes I Feel Like a Motherless Child."

- Play a rhythm-and-blues strum accompaniment on guitar for "Key to the Highway."

- Play a tritone blues accompaniment on keyboard for "Sun Gonna Shine."

3 CLOSE

Element: EXPRESSION ASSESSMENT

Self-Assessment/Music Journal Writing Have students assess their own responses to blues expression as they

- Write their own verses to "Sometimes I Feel Like a Motherless Child" and "Sun Gonna Shine" in a music journal.

- Write a short piece about a time in their life when they had the blues.

ASK How did you feel when you had the blues? How did you "chase the blues away"?

SKILLS REINFORCEMENT

▶ **Creating** To help students create 12-bar blues lyrics, suggest sample first lines and have students make a list of possible rhyming words; then create a rhyming second line. For example (underlined words indicate beat 1 of a measure):

1. I got the <u>blues</u> at night, and <u>they</u> don't leave till <u>day.</u> *(repeat)*

2. I <u>woke</u> up this mornin', the <u>blues</u> all in my <u>head</u> *(repeat)*

Point out that the typical blues line ends on the first beat of bar 3, to allow for the entrance of the instrumental solo.

▶ **Guitar** "Key to the Highway" is most authentically played with the rhythm-and-blues strum on guitar. Use an electric guitar, if possible

▶ **Signing** Invite students to perform the signing to "Sometimes I Feel Like a Motherless Child" on Resource Book p. G-14.

TECHNOLOGY/MEDIA LINK

CD-ROM Set up a 12-bar-blues background on *Band-in-a-Box* for students to improvise over. Use resonator bells, recorders, or keyboards. To set up keyboard for *Band-in-a-Box*, first invite students to select a blues style. Then ask them to enter chords (one chord per measure) for a 12-bar blues in the key of E.

E_7 / / / | E_7 / / / | E_7 / / / | E_7 / / / |
A_7 / / / | A_7 / / / | E_7 / / / | E_7 / / / |
B_7 / / / | A_7 / / / | E_7 / / / | E_7 / / / ‖

Encourage students to improvise breaks over the choruses.

LESSON AT A GLANCE

Element Focus **RHYTHM** Quarter-note/eighth-note pattern

Skill Objective **MOVING** Move to the Cajun two-step

Connection Activity **GENRE** Explore elements of country and western music from Appalachia and the southwestern United States

MATERIALS

- "Jambalaya" **CD 13–1**

  Recording Routine: Intro (8 m.); v. 1; refrain; interlude (4 m.); v. 2; refrain; interlude (8 m.); v. 1; refrain; coda

- "You Are My Sunshine" **CD 13–4**

  Recording Routine: Intro (4 m.); refrain; refrain; verse; refrain; interlude (2 m.); refrain

- "Green, Green Grass of Home" **CD 13–7**

  Recording Routine: Intro (4 m.); v. 1; refrain; vocal interlude (4 m.); v. 2; refrain; vocal coda

- *Jambalaya* **CD 13–3**
- *You Are My Sunshine* **CD 13–6**
- *Don't Look Down* **CD 13–9**
- **Resource Book** pp. F-24, G-16, I-21
- guitars, washboard, triangle, keyboard, Autoharp

VOCABULARY

country and western   Cajun

◆ ◆ ◆ ◆ National Standards ◆ ◆ ◆ ◆

1c Sing music from diverse genres

5a Read quarter notes and eighth notes in alla breve time

6b Listen and analyze uses of timbre in music from diverse genres

8b Identify ways music relates to social studies

9a Describe characteristics of music genres from a variety of cultures

MORE MUSIC CHOICES

For practice with other songs in country style:

"Bury Me Not on the Lone Prairie," p. 19

"Down in the Valley," p. 375

"Red River Valley," p. 11

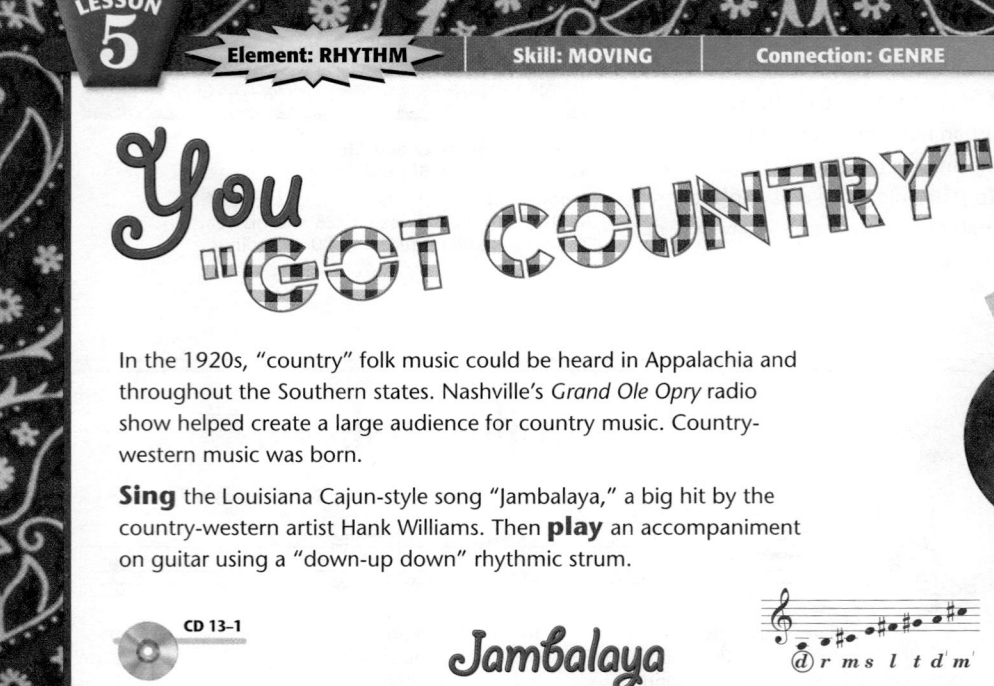

You "Got Country"

In the 1920s, "country" folk music could be heard in Appalachia and throughout the Southern states. Nashville's *Grand Ole Opry* radio show helped create a large audience for country music. Country-western music was born.

Sing the Louisiana Cajun-style song "Jambalaya," a big hit by the country-western artist Hank Williams. Then **play** an accompaniment on guitar using a "down-up down" rhythmic strum.

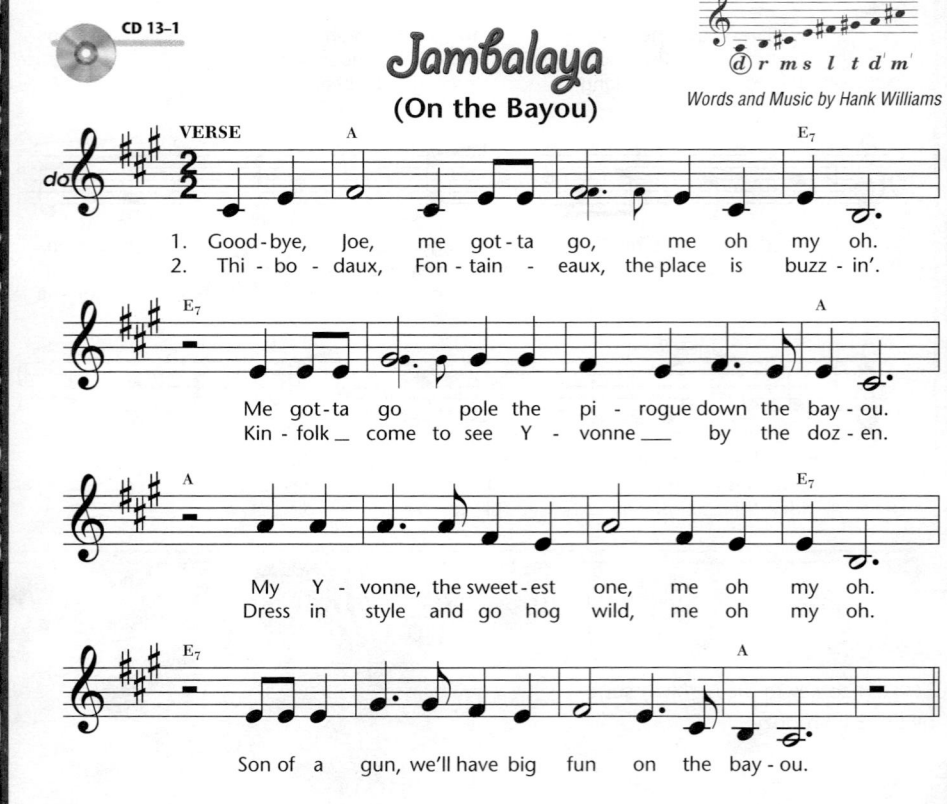

CD 13–1

Jambalaya
(On the Bayou)

Words and Music by Hank Williams

1. Good-bye, Joe, me got-ta go, me oh my oh.
2. Thi-bo-daux, Fon-tain-eaux, the place is buzz-in'.

Me got-ta go pole the pi-rogue down the bay-ou.
Kin-folk come to see Y-vonne by the doz-en.

My Y-vonne, the sweet-est one, me oh my oh.
Dress in style and go hog wild, me oh my oh.

Son of a gun, we'll have big fun on the bay-ou.

244

Footnotes

ACROSS THE CURRICULUM

8b ▶ **Social Studies** Country music got much of its sentimentality directly from nineteenth-century popular songs by Stephen Foster, Henry Work, James Bland, and others. The most common nostalgic themes found in country ballads today are mom and dad, the old home place, down South, trains, cowboys, religion, love gone wrong, and getting out of prison. Like blues, country and western music of the 1920s to 1940s mirrored the gradual shift of people from the farm to the city.

BUILDING SKILLS THROUGH MUSIC

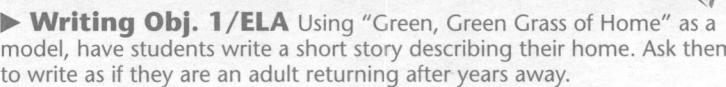

▶ **Writing Obj. 1/ELA** Using "Green, Green Grass of Home" as a model, have students write a short story describing their home. Ask them to write as if they are an adult returning after years away.

SPOTLIGHT ON

▶ **Country and Western** Country and western was the perfect name for a musical style that represented two different regions and musical traditions. The chart below outlines the two main branches of country and western music.

	Eastern	**Western**
Region	Appalachia	Texas
Capital	Nashville	Austin
Example	Carter Family	Jimmie Rodgers
Venue	Grand Ole Opry	Austin City Limits

Listen to this Cajun recording of *Jambalaya*, which features the accordion and the fiddle.

CD 13–3
Jambalaya
by Hank Williams
as performed by Jo-El Sonnier
This performance of *Jambalaya* is sung entirely in Cajun dialect.

Tune In

References in the lyrics of "Jambalaya" that may be unfamiliar include:

bayou—An area of shallow, slow-moving water
pirogue—A dugout canoe, usually fashioned from a single log
gumbo—A thick soup, made with okra

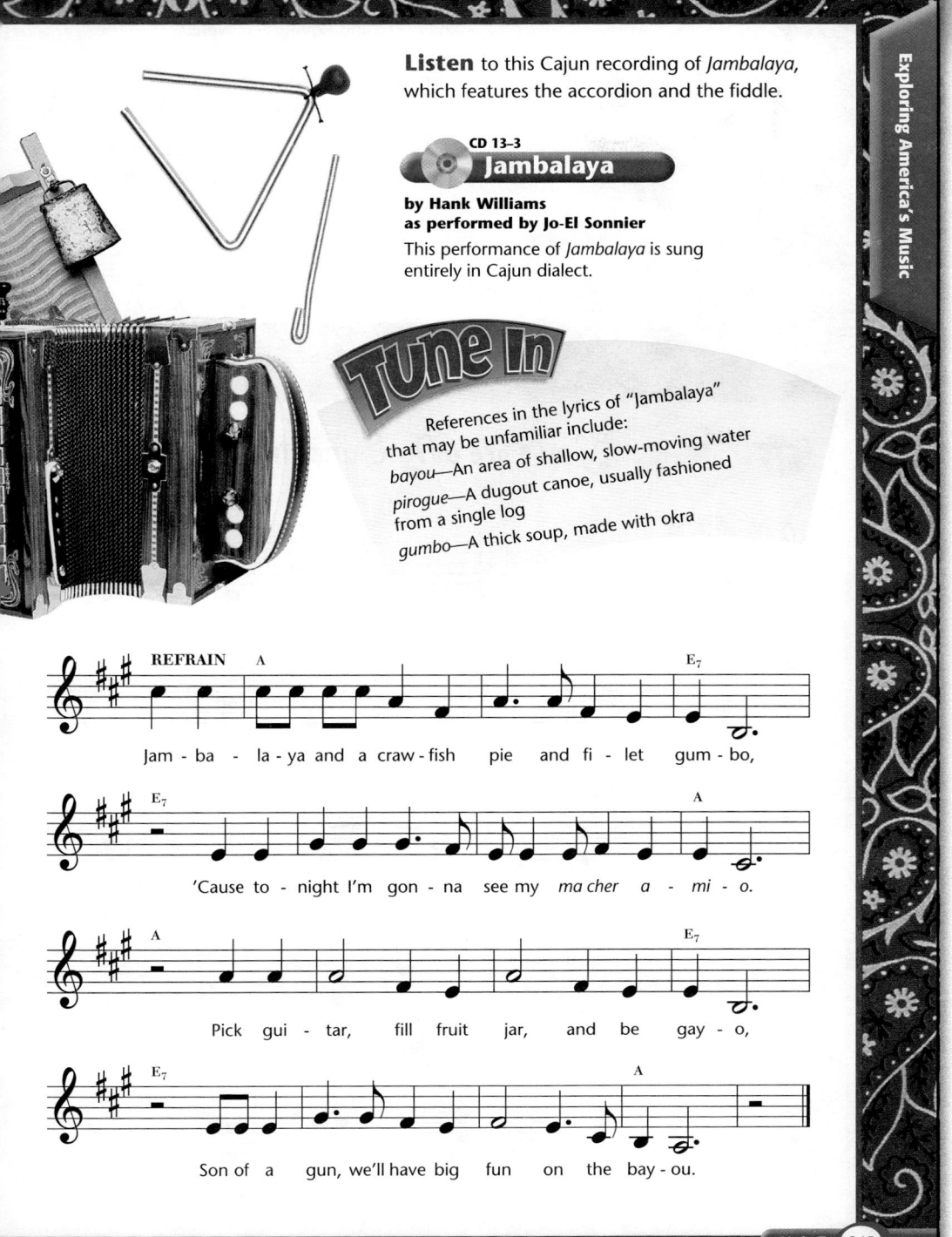

REFRAIN

Jam - ba - la - ya and a craw-fish pie and fi - let gum - bo,

'Cause to - night I'm gon - na see my *ma cher a - mi* - o.

Pick gui - tar, fill fruit jar, and be gay - o,

Son of a gun, we'll have big fun on the bay - ou.

Unit 7 **245**

1 INTRODUCE

As *down-home* as baseball, hot dogs, or apple pie, country music represents a tradition that comes from the European American settlers of the United States. This lesson features some highlights of this tradition. Discuss with students country singers, musicians, and songs with which they may be familiar. Share the information in Spotlight On and Across the Curriculum on p. 244 with students to help them explore elements of country and western music from Appalachia and the southwestern United States.

2 DEVELOP

Singing

1c Have students

- Listen to "Jambalaya" **CD 13–1**.
- Sing "Jambalaya" with the recording or other accompaniment, such as guitar or keyboard.

5a **ASK What is the basic underlying rhythm of this Cajun-style song, as heard in the accompaniment?**
(♩ ♫) (This is also the basic rhythm of highlife music from West Africa. See Unit 8: Lesson 5, p. 294.)
See Cultural Connection below for a glossary of terms used in "Jambalaya."

Playing

Have students

- Learn the A and E₇ chords on guitar, keyboard, or Autoharp to accompany "Jambalaya" **CD 13–1**.
- Add washboard and triangle to the accompaniment by playing the rhythm pattern above, or new patterns based on this rhythm. See Spotlight On, p. 246.

continued on page 246

CULTURAL CONNECTION

▶ **Glossary for "Jambalaya"**

jambalaya:	A spicy dish with sausage, chicken, tomatoes, and onions over rice
pirogue:	A shallow Cajun canoe
bayou:	A creek or small river
crawfish pie:	A Cajun dish made with crawfish (crayfish)
gumbo:	A thick, robust soup
ma cher amio:	My sweetheart
Thibodaux, Fontaineaux:	Cajun family names

MEETING INDIVIDUAL NEEDS

▶ **Learning Foreign Terms** Some of the concepts and words in "Jambalaya" may be foreign to many students. Have students use these techniques to learn the words and concepts.

Reinforcement For English language learners, use *realia*—real objects—or pictures to illustrate the various ideas in this song. For example, bring in a crawfish or a picture of one.

On Target Ask students to engage in a study of other words in the song, such as *bayou, gumbo,* and *pirogue.* Have students write descriptions of each term and illustrate them with pictures.

Challenge Students may wish to explore the origin of foreign words to add to their understanding of the terms.

Have all students share their findings with the class.

Lesson 5 Continued

Listening

 Have students listen to the Cajun recording of *Jambalaya* **CD 13–3** by accordion player Jo-El Sonnier and his band.

ASK Besides the accordion, what other instruments play solos in this piece? (violin and pedal steel guitar)

What differences do you hear in the two recordings of "Jambalaya"? (vocal timbres, language, instrumentation, verse/refrain routine)

See Cultural Connection, p. 247, for information about Cajun culture and history.

Invite students to listen to a recording of the accordion in the Sound Bank, starting on p. 512.

Moving

Encourage students to perform a Cajun two-step with *Jambalaya* **CD 13–3.**

Formation: Partners stand face to face. One partner travels forward and the other travels backward. Couples travel around the room in a large circle.

Verse
- Partner moving forward starts with right foot, partner moving backward starts with left foot.
- Step-together-step-touch on forward diagonal, using small steps.
- Alternate step-together-step-touch, moving right, then left.

Refrain   One partner turns under the arm of the other partner, using the same step-together-step-touch footwork, either in-place or moving.

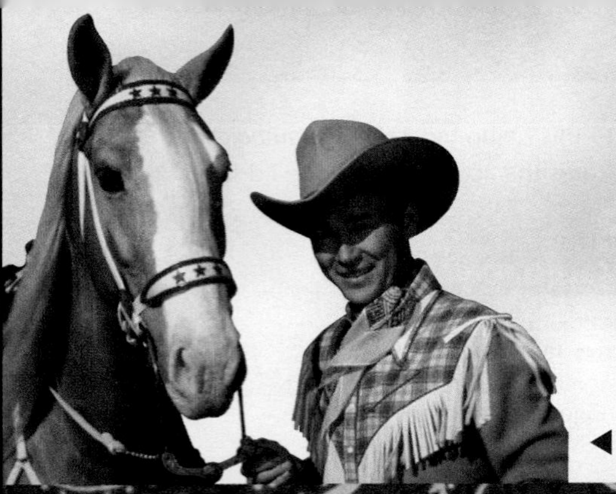

Happy Trails!

Gene Autry and Roy Rogers were two of the biggest singing cowboy movie stars of the twentieth century. They helped create the "western" part of country-western music.

Sing one of Gene Autry's all-time biggest hits, "You Are My Sunshine." Then **play** an accompaniment on guitar using a "down down-up" rhythmic strum.

◄ Roy Rogers and Trigger

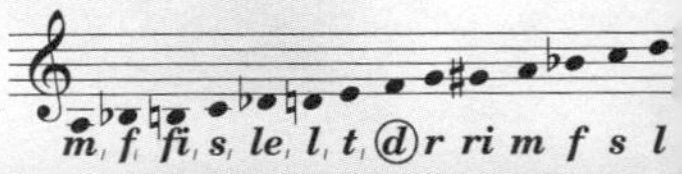

CD 13–4

You Are My Sunshine

Words and Music by Jimmie Davis and Charles Mitchell

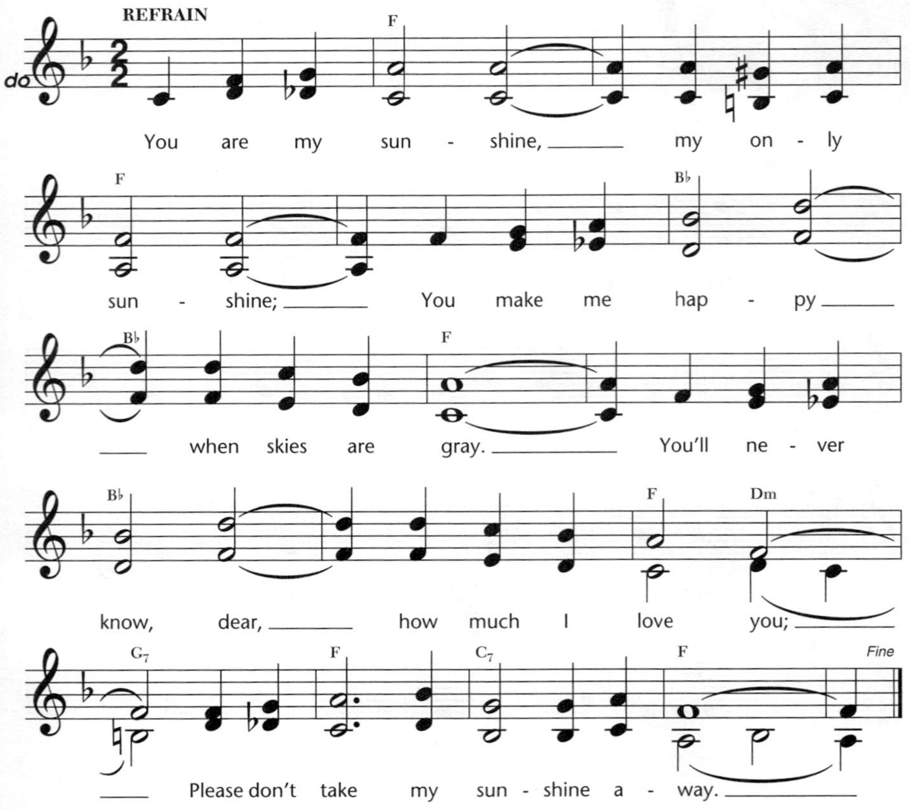

REFRAIN

You are my sun - shine, _____ my on - ly sun - shine; _____ You make me hap - py _____ when skies are gray. _____ You'll ne - ver know, dear, _____ how much I love you; _____ Please don't take my sun - shine a - way. _____

246

Footnotes

SPOTLIGHT ON

▶ **The Songwriter** Hank Williams (1923–1953) was one of country and western music's greatest songwriters and performers. In his short life he wrote hundreds of songs, including "Jambalaya," "I'm So Lonesome I Could Die," and "Hey, Good Lookin'." As a young boy in Georgiana, Alabama, Williams learned a lot from black street musician Rufus Payne.

▶ **Nontraditional Instruments** Students can use a washboard and a triangle to accompany "Jambalaya." The washboard can be played with spoons, metal thimbles on fingers, or gloves with bottle caps fastened to the finger pads.

SKILLS REINFORCEMENT

▶ **Signing** Refer to Resource Book p. G-16 for the sign language for "You Are My Sunshine."

▶ **Mallets** See Resource Book p. F-24 for an Orff arrangement of "You Are My Sunshine."

Country Sunshine

Listen for the "western swing" style of playing in this performance by Autry.

CD 13–6
You Are My Sunshine

by Jimmie Davis and Charles Mitchell
as performed by Gene Autry

Jimmie Davis, the composer of "You Are My Sunshine," served two terms as governor of Louisiana.

Gene Autry ▶

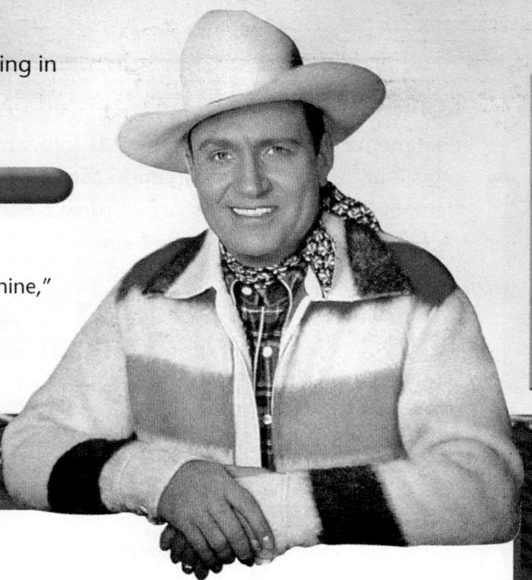

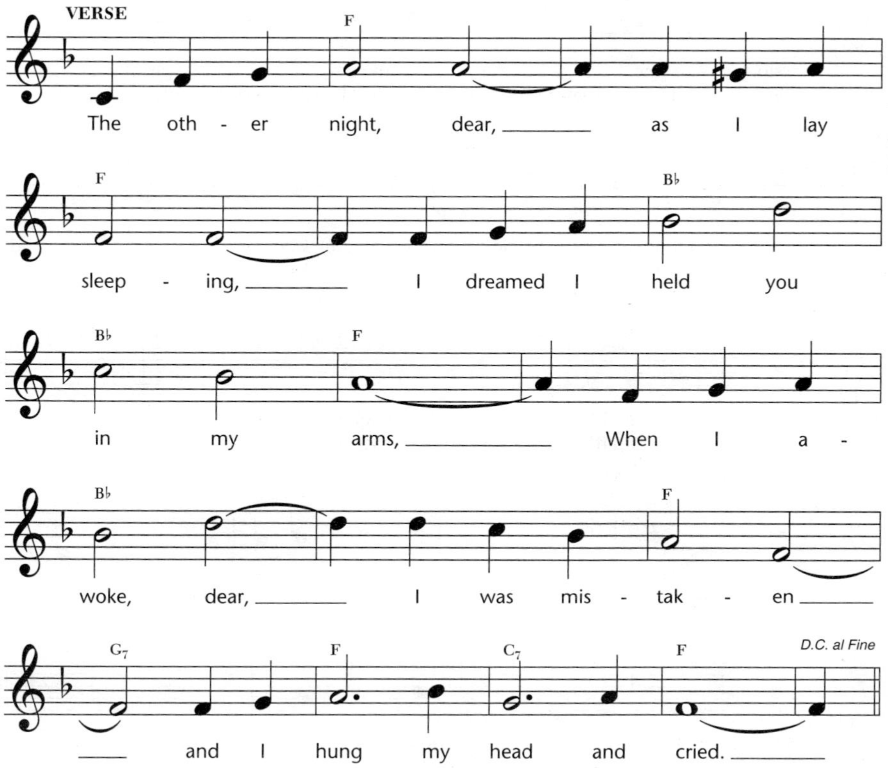

VERSE

F

The oth - er night, dear, _____ as I lay

F
B♭

sleep - ing, _____ I dreamed I held you

B♭
F

in my arms, _____ When I a -

B♭
F

woke, dear, _____ I was mis - tak - en _____

G₇
F
C₇
F
D.C. al Fine

_____ and I hung my head and cried. _____

Unit 7 **247**

Singing

Have students

- Listen to *You Are My Sunshine* **CD 13–6.**
- Discuss the importance of movie cowboys in the development of country music. (Relate the popularity of movie cowboys to the popularity of western wear, such as cowboy boots and hats.)

- Sing "You Are My Sunshine" with **CD 13–4** or other accompaniment, such as guitar, Autoharp, or keyboard.
- Discover that "You are My Sunshine" is one of many songs that are part of American heritage. Ask students to name other songs that are classic American songs.

Playing

Have students learn the F, B♭, Dm, G₇, and C₇ chords on guitar, keyboard, or Autoharp to accompany "You Are My Sunshine" **CD 13–4.** Students may need practice time for this activity.

The Dm chord on guitar is difficult to perform at this tempo. Ask students to locate the Dm chord in the song notation (p. 246, line 4). Tell them they may play the F chord as a substitute for the Dm chord, making it easier to perform.

Listening

Invite students to listen to Gene Autry's recording of *You Are My Sunshine* **CD 13–6.** Point out some of Autry's other hits that students may be familiar with, such as "Rudolph, the Red-Nosed Reindeer" or "Here Comes Peter Cottontail."

9a **ASK** Does Gene Autry sing the melody exactly as notated on pp. 246–247? (No; the opening pickup notes are different.)

ACROSS THE CURRICULUM

▶ **Science** There are more than 300 species of crayfish in North America, mainly in Kentucky and in the Mississippi Basin area of Louisiana. Crayfish, also called "crawfish" or "crawdads," are related to the lobster. Most live in freshwater streams that have a decent food supply, including plants, snails, tadpoles, fish, fungi, and bacteria. Crayfish are not, however, above dining on carrion should the opportunity float their way.

Encourage interested students to learn more about the important role of crayfish in traditional New Orleans cooking.

CULTURAL CONNECTION

8b ▶ **Cajuns of Lousiana** *"Laissez les bons temps roulez!"* [lay-zay leh boh(n) toh(n) roo-lay] "Let the good times roll!" This motto comes from the fun-loving Cajun people of Louisiana. The word *Cajun* comes from "Acadian." The Acadians, exiled from New Acadia (Nova Scotia) in 1765, were the ancestors of today's Louisiana Cajuns. More than 10,000 Acadians migrated, mostly to Louisiana, where they continued to speak French. Many settled along the bayous and swamps of southern Louisiana and lived as hunters, trappers, fishers, farmers, and boat builders. Favorite spicy Cajun dishes include jambalaya, gumbo, turtle sauce piquante, andouille sausage, and crawfish pie. Traditional Cajun musical instruments include the fiddle, accordion, triangle, and, recently added, drums and guitars.

Singing

Ask students to think about a place where they used to live.

ASK Have you ever gone back to that place after being away for a long time? What did it feel like?

Invite students to

- Sing "Green, Green Grass of Home" **CD 13–7** with the recording or other accompaniment, such as guitar or keyboard.
- Sing the song again, this time joining in on the vocal interlude and coda (last phrase of the refrain as it repeats).
- Discuss what makes this song sentimental.

Relate the discussion topic above to the sentimentality of nineteenth-century popular songs, such as those of Stephen Foster. See Across the Curriculum on p. 244.

Listening

Have students listen to the recording of *Don't Look Down* **CD 13–9** performed by Sweethearts of the Rodeo.

 ASK What makes this recording sound different from the older styles of country music you have heard? (In its rhythm and overall performance style, the performance on the recording contains strong elements of contemporary pop music.)

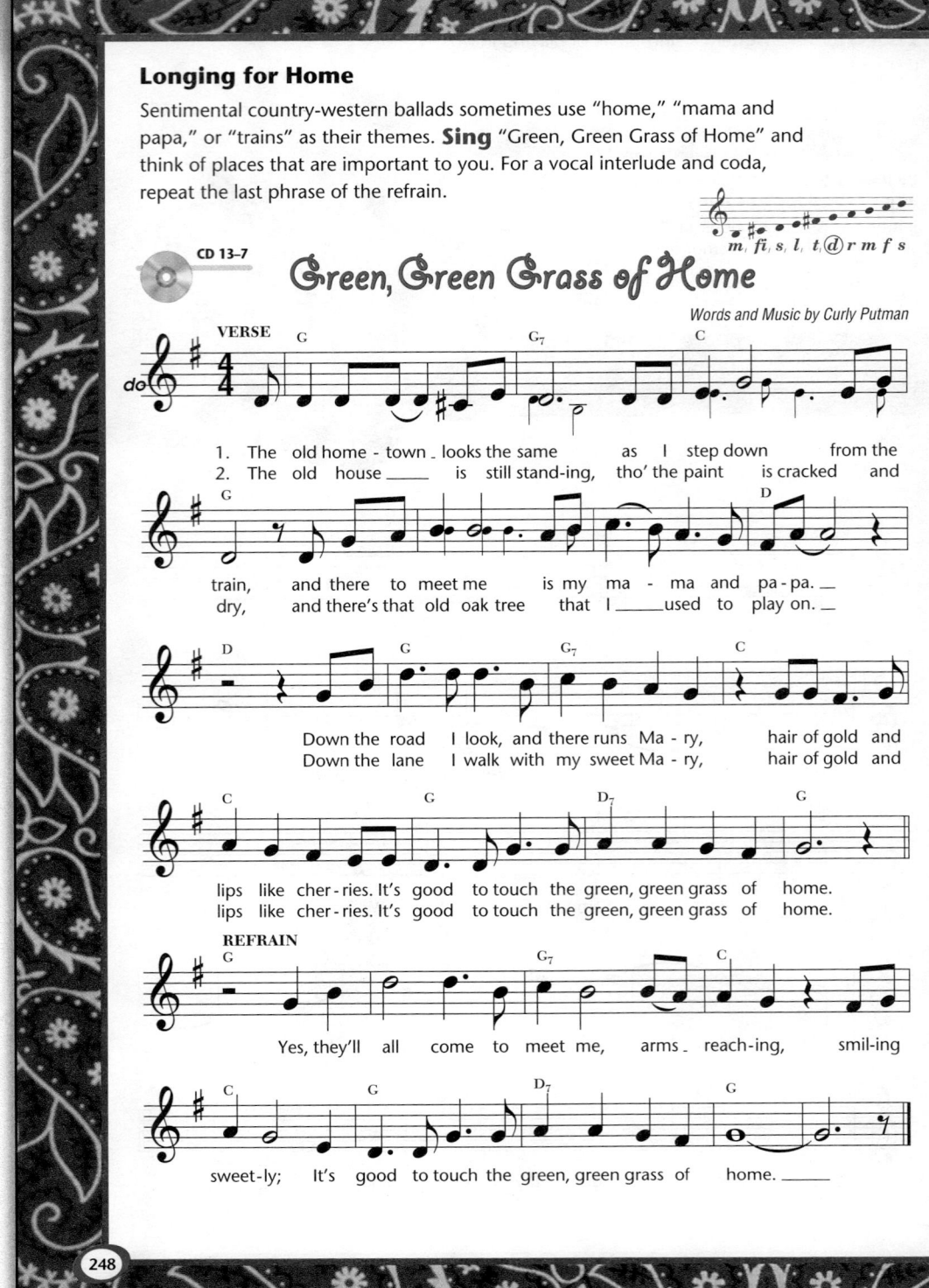

Longing for Home

Sentimental country-western ballads sometimes use "home," "mama and papa," or "trains" as their themes. **Sing** "Green, Green Grass of Home" and think of places that are important to you. For a vocal interlude and coda, repeat the last phrase of the refrain.

CD 13–7

Green, Green Grass of Home

Words and Music by Curly Putman

VERSE

1. The old home-town looks the same as I step down from the train, and there to meet me is my ma-ma and pa-pa.
2. The old house is still stand-ing, tho' the paint is cracked and dry, and there's that old oak tree that I used to play on.

Down the road I look, and there runs Ma-ry, hair of gold and lips like cher-ries. It's good to touch the green, green grass of home.

Down the lane I walk with my sweet Ma-ry, hair of gold and lips like cher-ries. It's good to touch the green, green grass of home.

REFRAIN

Yes, they'll all come to meet me, arms reach-ing, smil-ing sweet-ly; It's good to touch the green, green grass of home.

248

Footnotes

SKILLS REINFORCEMENT

▶ **Recorder** Students can play the following harmonic accompaniment on soprano recorder with "Jambalaya." Before playing, students should review the fingering for G♯.

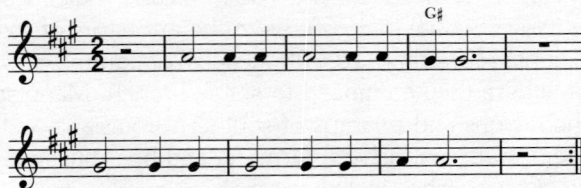

For a recorder ensemble accompaniment for "Green, Green Grass of Home," see Resource Book p. I-21.

SPOTLIGHT ON

▶ **Guitars** To truly understand country music, one must know about important innovations in guitar design and construction. Two models, the Martin Dreadnought steel-string guitar and the Fender solid-body electric guitar, have had an enormous impact on the development of various styles of country music. The Dreadnought, first made by Martin in 1916, is a large, flat-top acoustic guitar. The flat-top design was used mostly by blues, country, and folk performers, while the arch-top was favored by dance bands and jazz musicians. In 1948, Leo Fender developed the world's first commercially produced solid-body electric guitar, the Broadcaster (renamed the Telecaster in 1950).

Country Stars

Listen to the two-part harmony vocals in *Don't Look Down*.

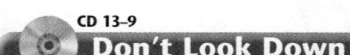
CD 13–9
Don't Look Down

**by Wendy Waldman and Steve Buckingham
as performed by Sweethearts of the Rodeo**

From their hit album in 1988, *Don't Look Down* features the Sweethearts' close vocal harmony and country sound.

Country Dancing

Country music and dance go together like ham and eggs. Country and western dancing is very popular, and many people take country dancing lessons.

Two well-known dances in country music are line dancing and the "two-step." Learn the two-step and **perform** it to "Jambalaya," on page 244.

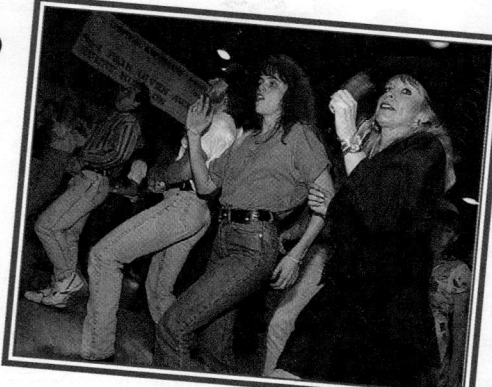
▲ Country line dancing

MUSIC MAKERS

Sweethearts of the Rodeo

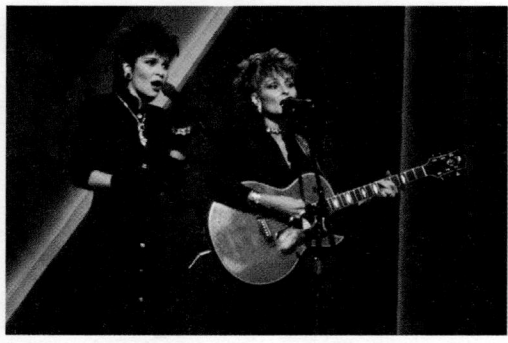
▲ Sisters Janice and Kristine Oliver of Sweethearts of the Rodeo

Sweethearts of the Rodeo are another in the long line of sister or brother duets in country music dating back to the 1930s. Janice and Kristine Oliver grew up in southern California. After Janice taught herself how to play guitar, she and Kristine started to sing harmony together. The Sweethearts of the Rodeo took their name from the Byrds' 1968 recording by the same name. They cut their debut album in 1986 and have recorded several other albums.

Unit 7 **249**

---

3 CLOSE

Element: RHYTHM — **ASSESSMENT**

Performance/Observation Assess how well students have mastered the basic Cajun rhythms in "Jambalaya" as you

- Listen to them play the rhythm of the melody on the washboard (or other nonpitched percussion instrument) with **CD 13–1**.

- Watch them do the Cajun two-step with the recording.

- Observe whether they can play guitar in rhythm with the chords of the song.

MEETING INDIVIDUAL NEEDS

▶ **Including Everyone** Students enjoy singing and playing energetic, happy songs such as those in this lesson. Give all students frequent opportunities to sing, play, and memorize these and other songs and accompaniments.

Some students spend much of their time after school alone. When they can play or sing songs by memory, they will have an activity that will make time by themselves joyous instead of lonely.

Memorization of the words is not entirely necessary, since playing and humming can bring pleasure, too.

TECHNOLOGY/MEDIA LINK

Video Library Show students the video, *Pam Tillis* featuring country singer Pam Tillis in performance.

Unit 7 *Exploring America's Music* **249**

LESSON AT A GLANCE

Element Focus	**EXPRESSION** Solo improvisation
Skill Objective	**LISTENING** Listen to and evaluate individual examples of jazz improvisation
Connection Activity	**GENRE** Understand jazz as an expression of an era, as well as a musical style

MATERIALS
- "Summertime" **CD 13–10**
  Recording Routine: Intro (free tempo); vocal; coda
- *Summertime* **CD 13–12**
- guitars, xylophones, recorders, keyboards, or resonator bells

VOCABULARY
chord root   jazz standard

◆ ◆ ◆ ◆ **National Standards** ◆ ◆ ◆ ◆

1c Sing music from diverse genres
2c Perform instrumental music from diverse genres
3b Improvise melodic variations on given melodies
3c Improvise melodies with consistent style, meter, and tonality, accompanied by a given rhythmic background
8a Show how different arts portray the same scene in unique ways
9b Classify high-quality musical works by genre

MORE MUSIC CHOICES
For more experience with jazz songs:
"Hit Me with a Hot Note and Watch Me Bounce," p. 112
"I Got Rhythm," p. 101
"Scattin' A-Round," p. 160

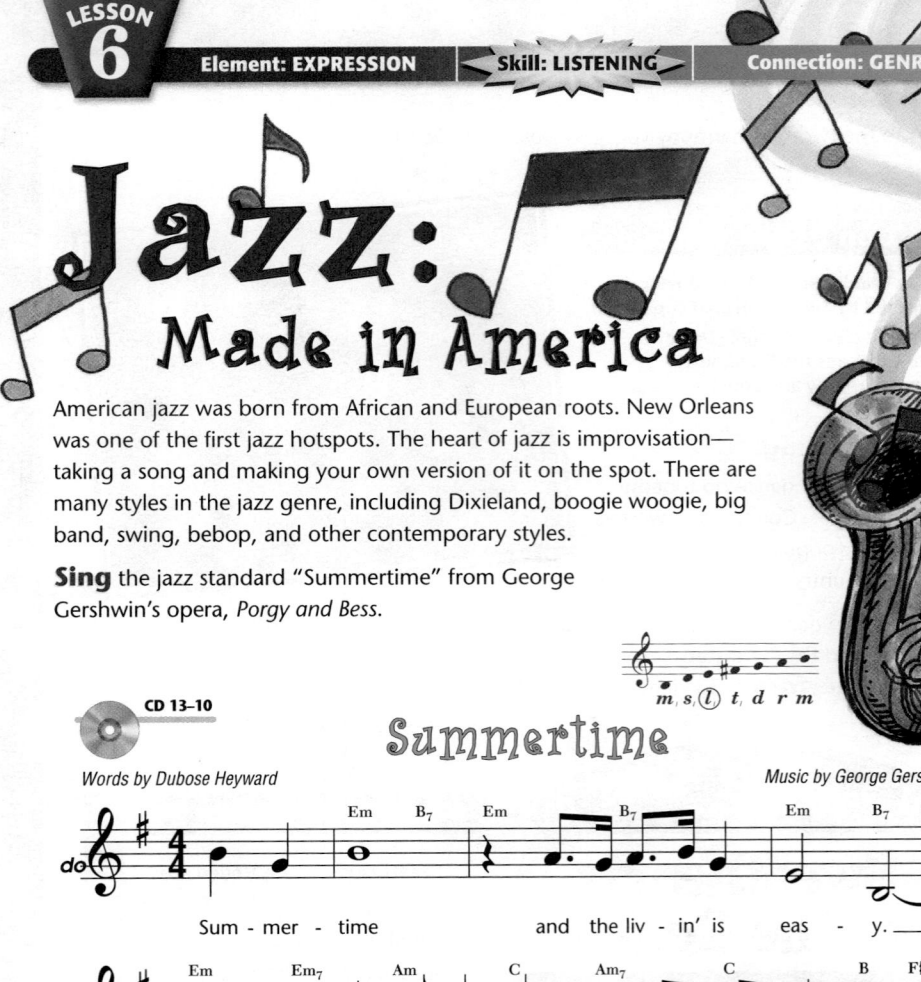

Jazz: Made in America

American jazz was born from African and European roots. New Orleans was one of the first jazz hotspots. The heart of jazz is improvisation—taking a song and making your own version of it on the spot. There are many styles in the jazz genre, including Dixieland, boogie woogie, big band, swing, bebop, and other contemporary styles.

Sing the jazz standard "Summertime" from George Gershwin's opera, *Porgy and Bess*.

CD 13–10

Summertime

Words by Dubose Heyward

Music by George Gershwin

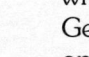

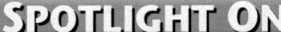

Sum - mer - time   and the liv - in' is eas - y. ___

Fish are jump - in' ___   and the cot - ton is high. ___

___ Oh, your dad - dy's rich ___   and your ma is good - look - in'.

So hush, lit - tle ba - by, don't ___ you cry. ___

(250)

Footnotes

MOVEMENT

8a ► **Creative Movement** In "Summertime," Gershwin uses certain musical elements (slow tempo, legato quality) to suggest a place—the steamy American South in summer. Ask students to imagine they are in a hot, humid place. Then communicate the idea of summertime heat without words. Consider posture, type and speed of movements (smooth or sharp, fast or slow), and other heat-related movements (fanning, wiping sweat from forehead) to create movement to accompany "Summertime."

BUILDING SKILLS THROUGH MUSIC

► **Language** The lyrics of the last half of "Summertime" on p. 251 uses the flight of a bird as a metaphor for the future. Ask students to discuss what the writer means with this metaphor.

SPOTLIGHT ON

► **The Opera** George Gershwin's opera *Porgy and Bess* was based on a novel called *Porgy*, published by DuBose Heyward in 1925. In 1934, Gershwin and his brother, Ira, spent the summer writing *Porgy and Bess*. George Gershwin wrote the music. Ira Gershwin and DuBose Heyward wrote lyrics and dialogue. The opera is about a disabled man named Porgy and his love for a difficult woman named Bess. The rest of the plot concerns the other people of the fictional Catfish Row. Although *Porgy and Bess* was first performed in New York in 1935, it only became popular in the 1940s, after Gershwin's death. Today, it is a well-known and well-loved American opera. The song "Summertime" is a lullaby, sung early in the opera.

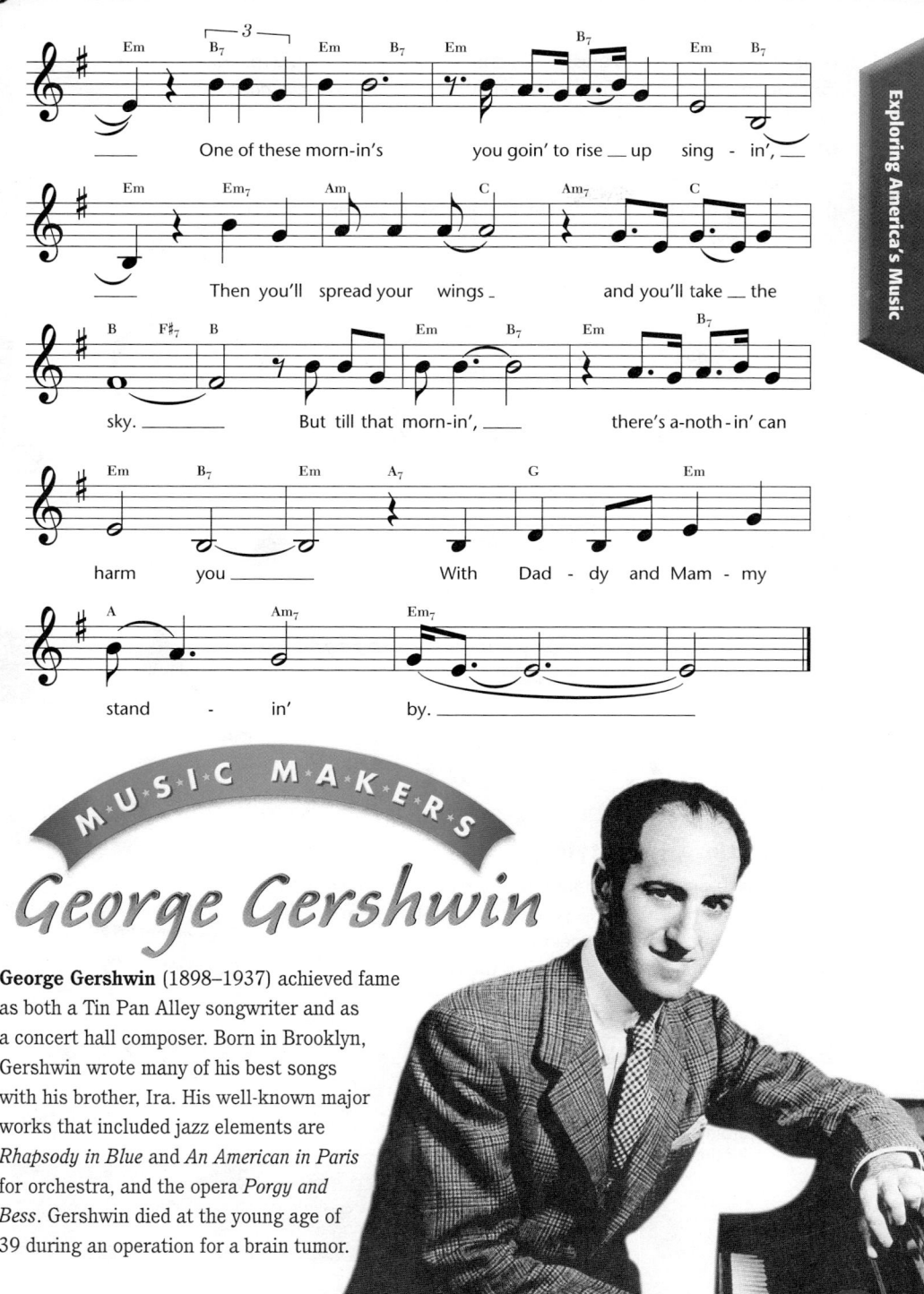

One of these morn-in's   you goin' to rise __ up   sing - in',__

Then you'll spread your   wings _   and you'll take __ the

sky. _____   But till that morn-in', ____   there's a-noth-in' can

harm   you _____   With   Dad - dy and Mam - my

stand - in'   by. _____

M·U·S·I·C · M·A·K·E·R·S

George Gershwin

George Gershwin (1898–1937) achieved fame as both a Tin Pan Alley songwriter and as a concert hall composer. Born in Brooklyn, Gershwin wrote many of his best songs with his brother, Ira. His well-known major works that included jazz elements are *Rhapsody in Blue* and *An American in Paris* for orchestra, and the opera *Porgy and Bess*. Gershwin died at the young age of 39 during an operation for a brain tumor.

Unit 7   **251**

1 INTRODUCE

Discuss with students the meaning of the word *improvise* and lead them into a discussion of musical improvisation—making up a solo on the spot, based on the chords of a piece, rather than reading a written melody.

Point out that improvisation is the essence of jazz—a musical genre made in America. In this lesson, students will have the opportunity to improvise in the same basic way as the jazz greats.

Help students begin to understand jazz as an expression of an age as well as a musical style. Use the information and activities in Across the Curriculum below, and in Spotlight On, p. 252, to start a discussion of the jazz era and some of its greatest musicians.

2 DEVELOP

Singing

SAY **Listen for the feelings that the words and music of this song express.** (laid back, slowed down, relaxed)

Have students

- Listen to "Summertime" **CD 13–10** as they follow the music on pp. 250–251.

- Sing the song with the recording or other accompaniment, such as guitar or keyboard.

continued on page 252

ACROSS THE CURRICULUM

▶ **Language Arts** Encourage students to

- Read more about the lives and careers of great jazz musicians, including Louis Armstrong, Count Basie, Duke Ellington, Ella Fitzgerald, Billie Holiday, and Charlie Parker, in biographies from the reading series *Black Americans of Achievement* (Chelsea House, 1988).

- Create a bulletin board with pictures of great jazz artists of both past and present. Ask students to write short biographies of selected jazz artists to display on the bulletin board or to add to their music journals.

MEETING INDIVIDUAL NEEDS

▶ **English Language Learners** Because "Summertime" is so rich in visual images, it would be easy to teach its words by a game of charades. Before students sing the song, write some of its key words on pieces of paper (*mama, daddy, wings, good-lookin', cotton, fish, jumpin' high*, and so on). Divide the class into two teams. Have a student from one team pick a word to act out, and have the student's own team guess what it is. When the word is guessed, that team gets a point. There would, of course, be a time limit (45 seconds, for example) for each word to be guessed.

After the word has been correctly guessed, it would be helpful to show students a picture of the word to solidify the concept. Then sing the song.

9b Discuss with students the information on p. 250 and the Music Makers feature on Gershwin, and how jazz influenced George Gershwin's music.

Playing

Have students

2c • Use guitars, xylophones, recorders, keyboards, or resonator bells to play the E-minor pentatonic scale, including D below the staff. (This will be used for improvising on "Summertime" and on the 12-bar blues progression. Students need to have these notes "under their fingers" before improvising. If xylophones are used, remove all bars not in the E-minor pentatonic scale.)

• Review the definition of *chord root;* then play the chord roots (whole and half notes) of "Summertime," as notated on p. 252. (The black noteheads are for improvisation.)

• Answer you in a series of interesting one-measure rhythms on E. Stress the use of syncopation to give the rhythms a "jazzy" sound.

• Answer you or another student in improvising a series of two-measure phrases based on the notes E, G, and D. For example:

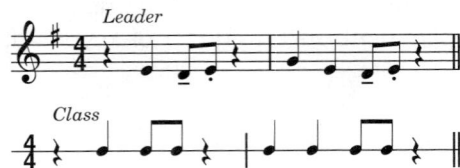

3b • Answer you or another student in improvising a series of two-measure phrases based on pentatonic pitches, as desired.

Help students understand that the D♯ in the B₇ chord is not a mistake but is a "blues" note.

Play an Improvisation

Learn how to **improvise** using the chords below. Most of the melody for "Summertime" uses notes in the blues minor pentatonic (*la, do, re, mi, so*). You will use these notes (E, G, A, B, and D) to improvise.

Play along on a keyboard. Each slash is worth one beat and tells you to keep playing the same notes. If you play the whole note, you are playing the "root" of the chord. Add the extra notes when you are ready and improvise new rhythms.

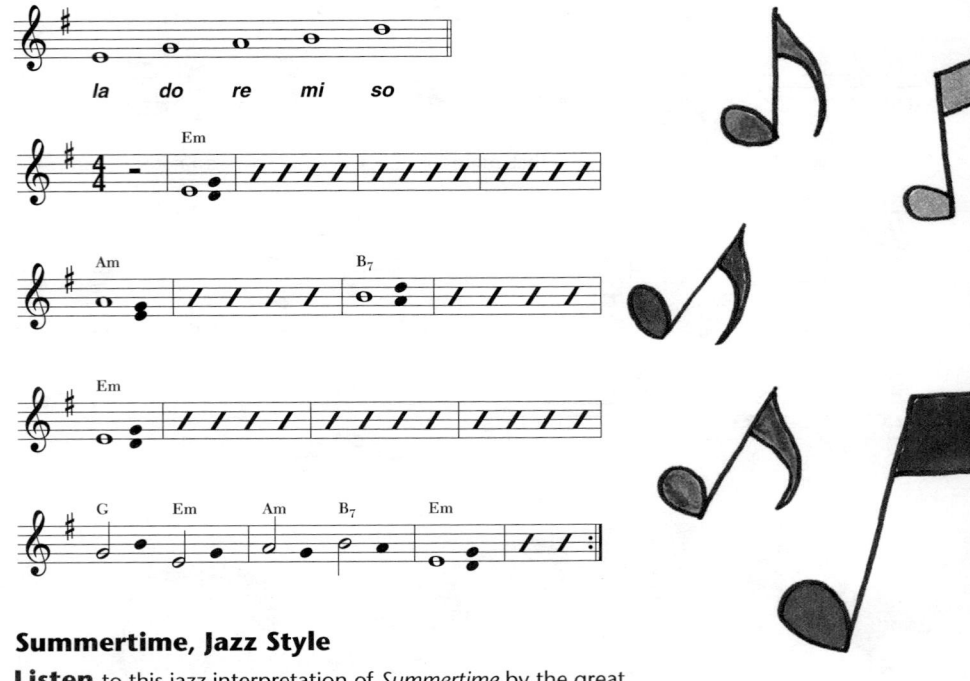

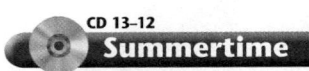

Summertime, Jazz Style

Listen to this jazz interpretation of *Summertime* by the great trumpet player Miles Davis as you follow the listening map on page 253. You will hear the melody played first, followed by improvisations based on the tune and the chords.

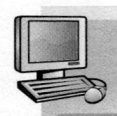

CD 13–12
Summertime

by George Gershwin
as performed by Miles Davis

On this recording, Davis uses a Harmon mute to color the sound of the trumpet.

CD-ROM Make your own jazz arrangement and explore improvisation using *Band-in-a-Box.*

Footnotes

▶ **The Performer** Miles Davis (1926–1991) was a twentieth-century jazz trumpet great. He started playing trumpet at age 13 in East St. Louis, Illinois. Davis played in his high school band, then went to New York to study music at Juilliard. He didn't stay at the traditional music school long, though, because his calling was jazz. (Traditional schools now do have jazz as an important part of the curriculum.) Davis became a mainstay of bebop, cool jazz, and fusion. These were jazz styles of the 1950s to 1970s, after the big-band swing era. Davis played with all of the jazz greats of his time, including Charlie Parker, Thelonious Monk, John Coltrane, and Dizzy Gillespie. Some of his landmark albums include *Kind of Blue* and *The Birth of the Cool.*

3c ▶ **Improvising** When students begin improvising, they often want to play a great many notes. Suggest that they follow B. B. King, who believes that "less is more."

Some helpful tips

• Motives (or licks) rule! If you get a good idea, play it again.

• Syncopations star! Play interesting rhythms.

• Hang around home! Weave your solos around chord roots.

• Put windows in your music! Leave some breathing space.

• There is safety in numbers! Having all students improvise their solos at the same time provides a sense of comfort that is *essential* to "no-fault" improvisation.

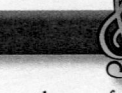

Summertime
LISTENING MAP

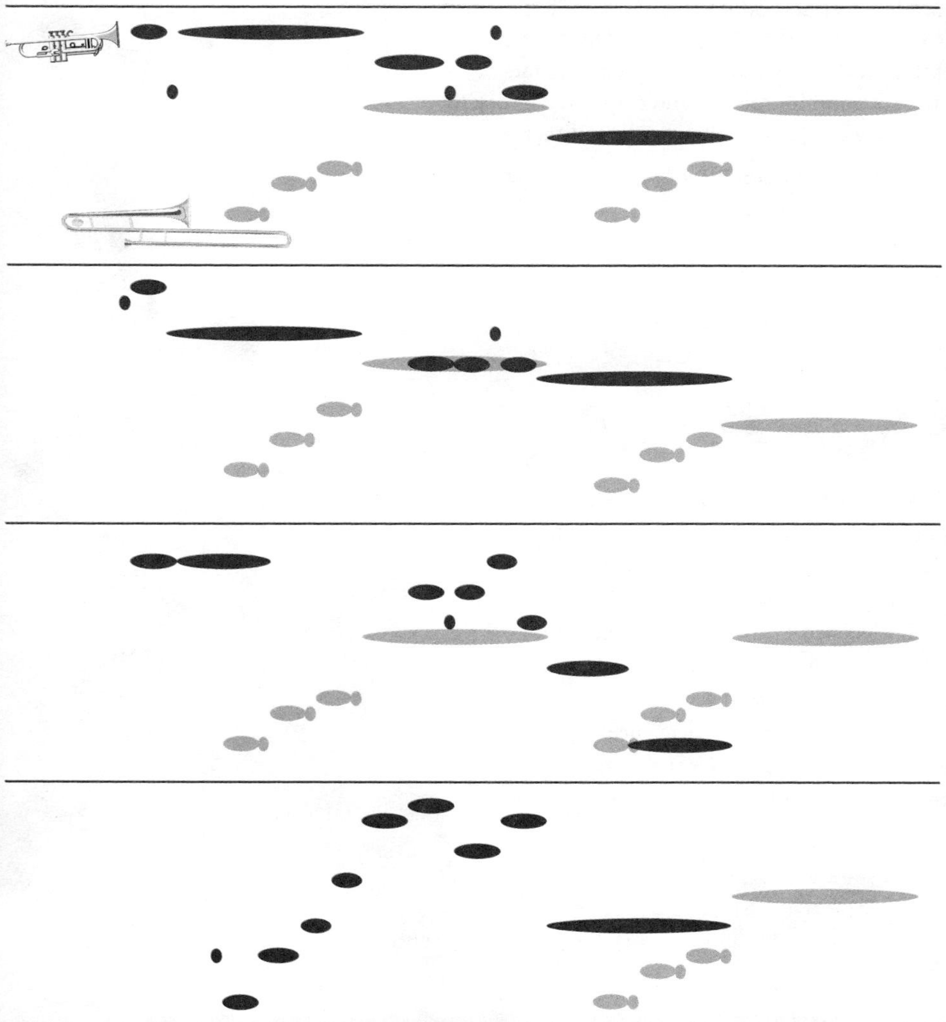

- Simultaneously improvise with the recording of "Summertime" **CD 13–10.**
- Record their improvisations.

See Skills Reinforcement on p. 252 and Teacher to Teacher below for tips on managing classroom improvisation activities.

Listening

Have a student, teacher, or parent who plays trumpet demonstrate various kinds of mutes and how the mutes change the timbre of the trumpet.

Have students listen to Miles Davis's recording of *Summertime* **CD 13–12.** Share with students the biographical information on Miles Davis in Spotlight On, p. 252.

ASK How closely does Miles Davis follow the original melody? (Not very closely. He is improvising mostly on the chord structure of the piece, rather than on the melody.)

Have students listen to Miles Davis's recording again while following the listening map on p. 253. The listening map illustrates the first time through the melody, up to 0:34. See Technology/Media Link below for use of the listening map transparency.

3 CLOSE

Skill: LISTENING   **ASSESSMENT**

Performance/Self-Assessment Play for students the recordings of their "Summertime" improvisations. Ask them to listen and assess themselves on a 5 (high) to 1 (low) scale, using the following statements.

- I could keep my place in the music while improvising. (5 4 3 2 1)
- I felt comfortable playing different E-minor pentatonic notes. (5 4 3 2 1)
- I used interesting rhythms. (5 4 3 2 1)

TEACHER TO TEACHER

▶ **Classroom Management** One effective classroom management technique is to establish and provide clear guidelines so that students will know how they are expected to act and what to expect if they don't follow proper procedures.

Another method is to make a social contract; that is, involve the class in the decision-making process when setting the class rules. Reduce student-recommended rules to a few positively stated broad-spectrum rules, such as "Be on time."

The students will learn more, and the teacher will be more relaxed, if good management techniques are used.

TECHNOLOGY/MEDIA LINK

CD-ROM Invite students to improvise over the chords for "Summertime," as played by *Band-in-a-Box.* Students may use resonator bells, recorder, or keyboard instruments.

Set up the computer and keyboard for *Band-in-a-Box.* Ask students to enter the chords for "Summertime" (pp. 250–251).

Ask students to select a style that best fits this song.

Invite students (as a group, then individually) to improvise, using the notes of the E-minor pentatonic scale (E-G-A-B-D) during the breaks between the lyrics.

Transparency Display the listening map transparency for *Summertime* as you play the recording. On first listening, point to musical events as they occur in the recording.

LESSON AT A GLANCE

Element Focus	**RHYTHM** Rock 'n' roll shuffle and even rock rhythms
Skill Objective	**PLAYING** Perform examples of rock 'n' roll shuffle and even rock patterns
Connection Activity	**CULTURE** Explore British and American pop culture of the 1950s and 1960s

MATERIALS

- "Don't Be Cruel" — CD 13–13
  Recording Routine: Intro (4 m.); vocal; coda
- "Downtown" — CD 13–18
  Recording Routine: Intro (4 m.); v. 1; interlude (3 m.); v. 2; coda
- *That'll Be the Day* — CD 13–15
- *Let's Twist Again* — CD 13–16
- *Penny Lane* — CD 13–17
- *Interview with Petula Clark* — CD 13–20
- guitars or keyboard, drumsticks (or pencils)
- **Resource Book** p. H-24

VOCABULARY

backup vocals   fill   shuffle   rhythm and blues (R&B)

◆ ◆ ◆ ◆ National Standards ◆ ◆ ◆ ◆

2a Play instruments accurately with good stick technique

3c Improvise melodies with consistent style, meter, and tonality, accompanied by a given rhythmic background

4c Compose, using electronic media

6a Listen and describe events in music using appropriate terms

8b Identify ways music relates to social studies

9a Describe characteristics of music genres from a variety of cultures

MORE MUSIC CHOICES

For more experience with rock songs:

"Birthday," p. 90

"Rock and Roll Is Here to Stay," p. 36

"Surfin' U.S.A." p. 260

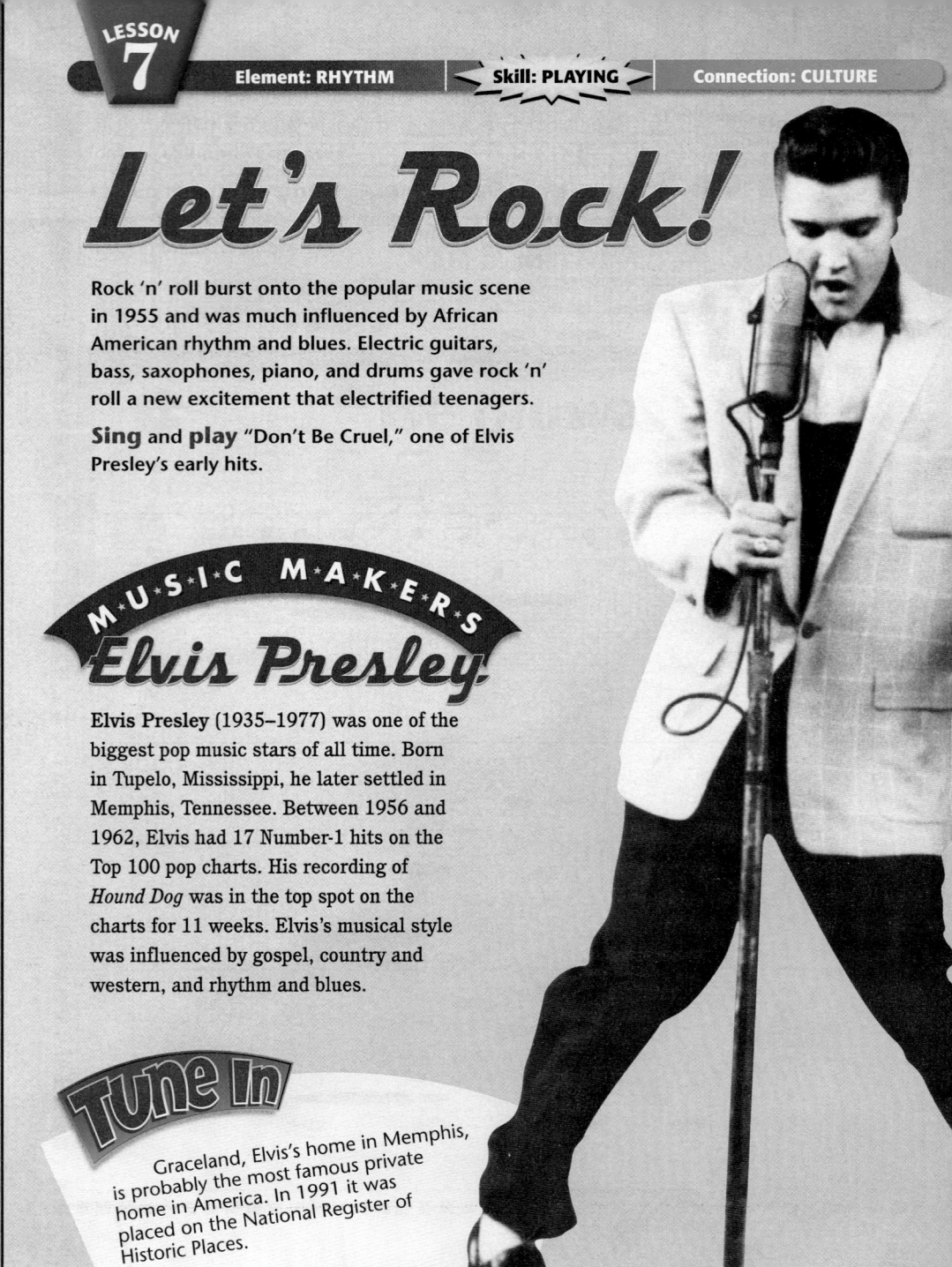

Let's Rock!

Rock 'n' roll burst onto the popular music scene in 1955 and was much influenced by African American rhythm and blues. Electric guitars, bass, saxophones, piano, and drums gave rock 'n' roll a new excitement that electrified teenagers.

Sing and **play** "Don't Be Cruel," one of Elvis Presley's early hits.

MUSIC MAKERS
Elvis Presley

Elvis Presley (1935–1977) was one of the biggest pop music stars of all time. Born in Tupelo, Mississippi, he later settled in Memphis, Tennessee. Between 1956 and 1962, Elvis had 17 Number-1 hits on the Top 100 pop charts. His recording of *Hound Dog* was in the top spot on the charts for 11 weeks. Elvis's musical style was influenced by gospel, country and western, and rhythm and blues.

Tune In

Graceland, Elvis's home in Memphis, is probably the most famous private home in America. In 1991 it was placed on the National Register of Historic Places.

Footnotes

ACROSS THE CURRICULUM

▶ **Language Arts** Students can meet "The King" through the book *Shake Rag: From the Life of Elvis Presley* by Amy Littlesugar (Putnam, 1998). This book documents Presley's early life and musical influences.

Interested readers can also check out *Elvis Presley: The King* by Katherine Krohn (Lerner, 1993).

BUILDING SKILLS THROUGH MUSIC

▶ **Social Studies** Have students create a chart in which all the music in the lesson is categorized as (a) using shuffle rhythms, or (b) using even rock rhythms.

SPOTLIGHT ON

▶ **The Entertainer** Born in Tupelo, Mississippi, Elvis Presley (1935–1977) is called the King of Rock 'n' Roll because of his amazing number of hits. He holds the Number 1 spot on the Billboard Top 500 Artists list, with 9,576 points (far ahead of the second-place Beatles, at 5,330 points). Elvis had 149 chart hits, and his *Heartbreak Hotel* was the first record to top the pop, R&B, and country and western charts at the same time. From 1956 on, he created a lasting image through his unique vocal stylings, gyrations, TV appearances, and movies.

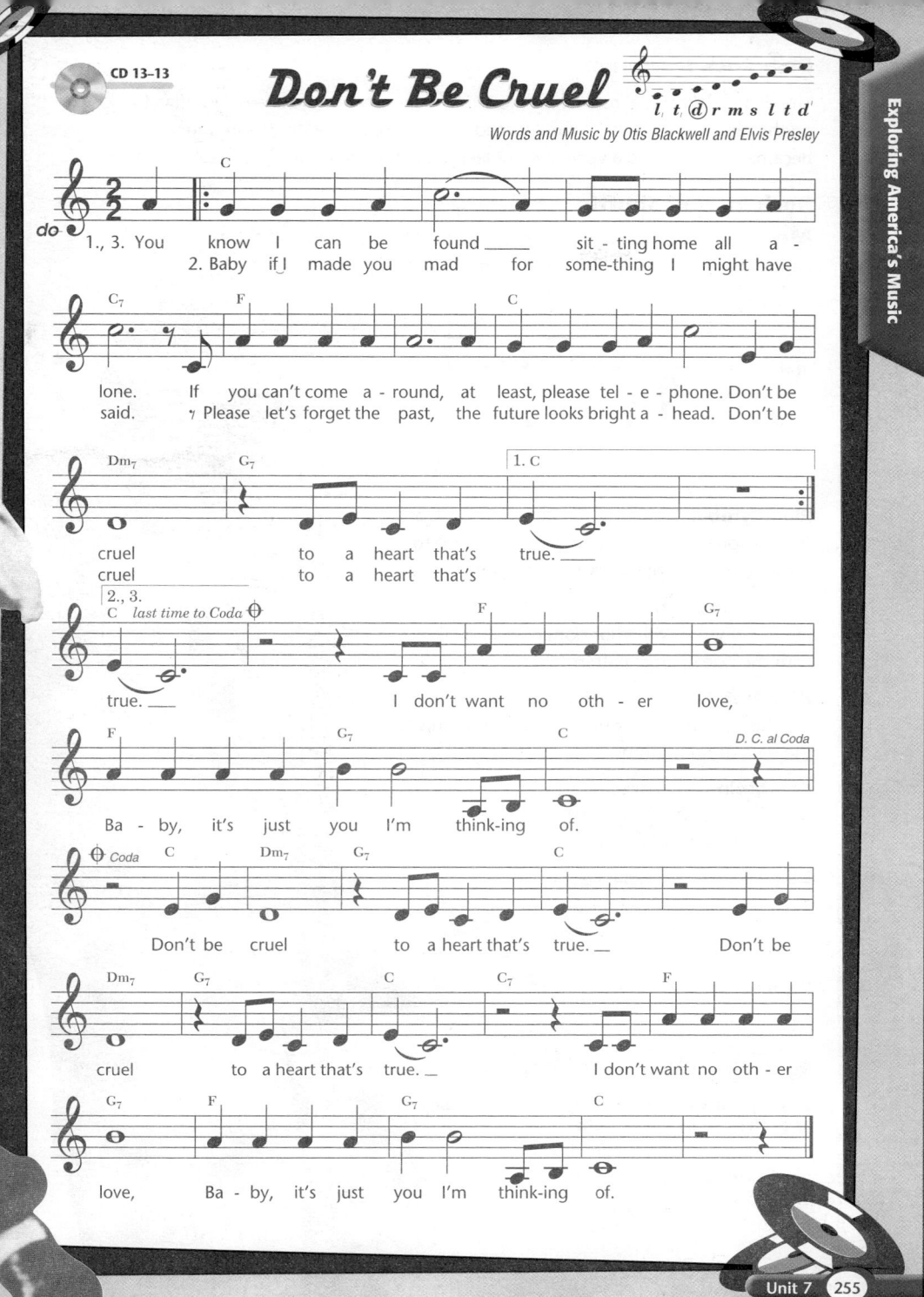

Don't Be Cruel

CD 13-13

Words and Music by Otis Blackwell and Elvis Presley

1., 3. You know I can be found ___ sit - ting home all a -
2. Baby if I made you mad for some-thing I might have

lone. If you can't come a - round, at least, please tel - e - phone. Don't be
said. Please let's forget the past, the future looks bright a - head. Don't be

cruel to a heart that's true. ___
cruel to a heart that's

true. ___ I don't want no oth - er love,

Ba - by, it's just you I'm think - ing of.

Don't be cruel to a heart that's true. ___ Don't be

cruel to a heart that's true. ___ I don't want no oth - er

love, Ba - by, it's just you I'm think - ing of.

Unit 7 **255**

1 INTRODUCE

8b Briefly discuss with students the history of early rock 'n' roll as described on this page. Rock 'n' roll combined both African American and European American musical styles. It transcended racial barriers and became wildly popular in the mid-1950s, with artists like Bill Haley and the Comets ("Rock Around the Clock"), Chuck Berry ("Maybelline"), and Elvis Presley ("Hound Dog"). The popularity of rock reflected the growing influence of teenagers in American culture. It also showed the influence of the media (records, radio, television, and movies) on teenagers' tastes.

Tell students that they will explore American (pp. 254–256) and British (pp. 257–259) rock 'n' roll styles. Share with students the information in Cultural Connection below and on p. 258, and Across the Curriculum, p. 258, to start a discussion of American and British pop culture in the 1950s and 1960s.

2 DEVELOP

Singing

9a Introduce "Don't Be Cruel" by emphasizing that rock 'n' roll combined elements of African American rhythm and blues with European American country and western styles.

Have students listen to "Don't Be Cruel" **CD 13–13** and then sing along with the recording or other accompaniment, such as guitar or keyboard.

ASK What is the role of the backup vocals in the recording of "Don't Be Cruel"? (They fill in spaces where the melody holds a long note.)

What rock 'n' roll instruments (in addition to backup vocals) are used for fills? (electric guitar, piano, saxophone, drums)

Discuss with students the musical term *fill*. (added music that fills the spaces on long notes or rests in the music)

continued on page 256

CULTURAL CONNECTION

8b ▶ **Teen Idols** In each era it seems that the public becomes enthralled with some musical star or group. In the 1950s it was Elvis Presley who made the girls swoon. He had a tremendous influence on the music, dance, and popular culture of the time. The Beatles were adored in the 1960s, their "long" hairstyles and fashions widely imitated. Their music reflected a time of unrest, protests, drug experimentation, and antiwar sentiment. Ask students to discuss current popular groups or individual performers. Discuss the influence these artists have on society through their musical messages, innovative performance styles, and dress and appearance.

SKILLS REINFORCEMENT

▶ **Keyboard** Students may accompany "Don't Be Cruel" by playing these chords on beats 2 and 3 of each measure. The full accompaniment is on Resource Book p. H-24.

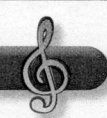

Playing

2a Give each student a drumstick or a wooden pencil that can be used as a drumstick. Tell students they will learn to play two different drum set patterns: the rock 'n' roll shuffle and the even rock rhythm.

To teach the rock 'n' roll shuffle, have students

- Play the ride cymbal part on the desktop with a pencil or stick while saying the sound with their voices (*tcsh—dit di-tcsh—dit di*).

- Play the bass drum part with the dominant foot (keeping the heel down), making the low sound (*doom- doom- doom- doom*) with their voices. Then add the ride cymbal to the bass drum part.

- Play the high hat part with the other foot (keep the heel down) while saying the sound (*[rest]-chick-[rest]- chick*). Put the bass drum and high hat together by starting with the bass drum and adding the high hat; then add the ride cymbal.

Divide the class into three groups. Have each group say and play one of the parts. Then, put the three parts together.

Listening

6a Have students listen to *That'll Be the Day* **CD 13–15** by Buddy Holly and the Crickets. Discuss the fact that the Beatles copied their instrumentation from Buddy Holly's band. Point out the similarity between the groups' names (Crickets and Beatles).

ASK **What is the instrumentation on this recording?** (two guitars, bass, and drums)

Invite students to listen to the recording of drums in the Sound Bank, starting on p. 512.

Playing

2a Invite students to play the shuffle rhythm parts with *That'll Be the Day* **CD 13–15**.

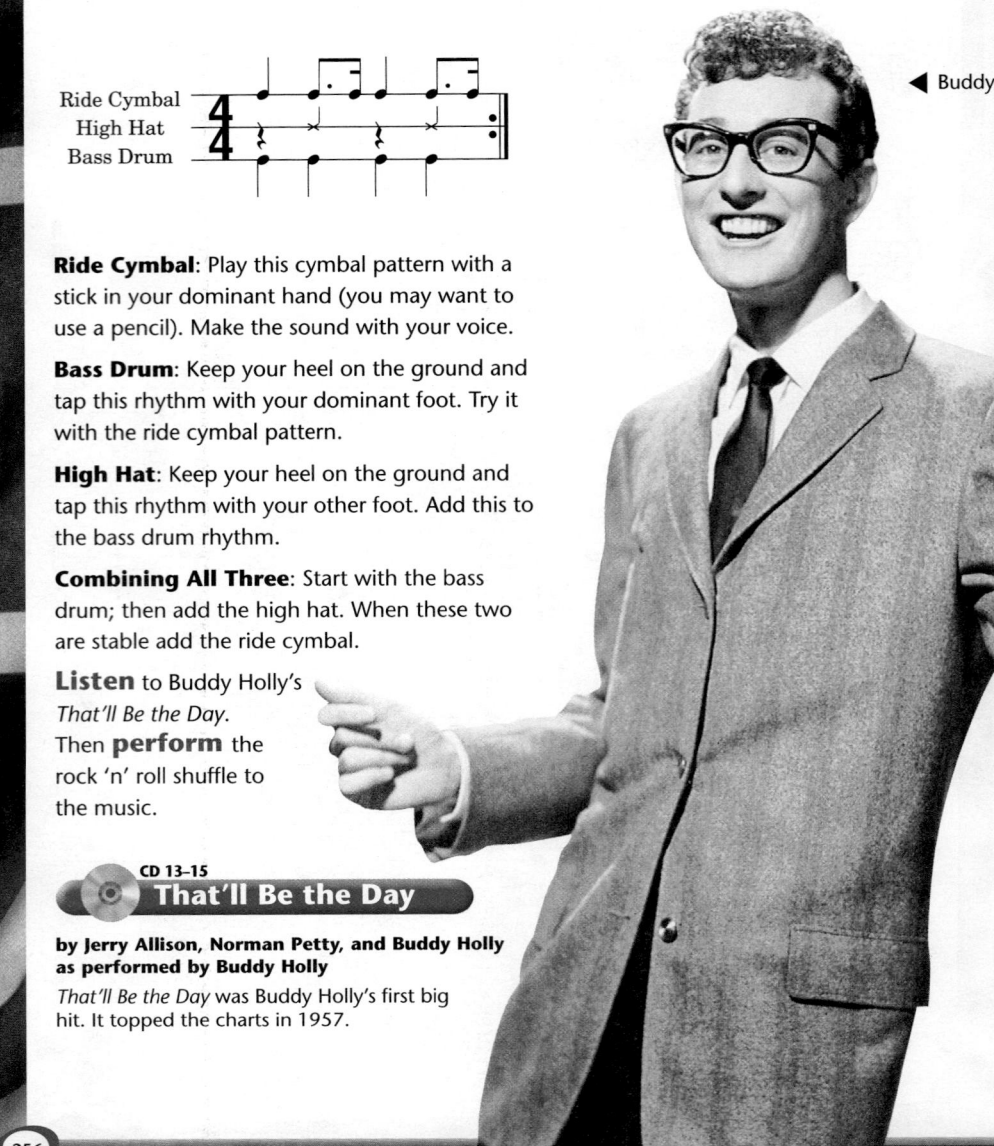

Be a Rock Drummer

The rhythm of rock 'n' roll during the 1950s was based on the uneven shuffle of rhythm and blues. As rock 'n' roll turned into rock of the 1960s, the rhythms became even and had a very different feel. What rhythm creates the "shuffle" feel?

Rock 'n' Roll Shuffle

Move as though you are playing a shuffle on the "air" drum set using your hands and feet. Then **play** the rhythms below on percussion instruments.

Ride Cymbal
High Hat
Bass Drum

Ride Cymbal: Play this cymbal pattern with a stick in your dominant hand (you may want to use a pencil). Make the sound with your voice.

Bass Drum: Keep your heel on the ground and tap this rhythm with your dominant foot. Try it with the ride cymbal pattern.

High Hat: Keep your heel on the ground and tap this rhythm with your other foot. Add this to the bass drum rhythm.

Combining All Three: Start with the bass drum; then add the high hat. When these two are stable add the ride cymbal.

Listen to Buddy Holly's *That'll Be the Day*. Then **perform** the rock 'n' roll shuffle to the music.

◀ Buddy

 CD 13–15
That'll Be the Day

by Jerry Allison, Norman Petty, and Buddy Holly as performed by Buddy Holly

That'll Be the Day was Buddy Holly's first big hit. It topped the charts in 1957.

256

Footnotes

MEETING INDIVIDUAL NEEDS

▶ **Classroom Management** Boys and girls both like to play drums, but boys, in particular, will respond to music in a more positive way if they can be active participants. Drums give boys a much-needed outlet for their physical enthusiasm. Since many boys are lost to music during the middle school years, having a drum set in your room could make quite a difference. Jeanne Julseth-Heinrich, a well-known Wisconsin middle school choral and general music teacher, was famous for recruiting as many boys as girls into her choirs. Her secret? A red drum set right inside the door of her room!

SPOTLIGHT ON

▶ **The Performers** The Beatles were the most important rock group of the 1960s. The members of the "Fab Four" from Liverpool were guitarists John Lennon and George Harrison, bass player Paul McCartney, and drummer Ringo Starr. The Beatles were influenced by American rock 'n' roll artists Chuck Berry, Elvis Presley, Little Richard, and the Everly Brothers, and copied their instrumentation from Buddy Holly and the Crickets. The Beatles came to the United States in 1964, and "Beatlemania" was born. With most of their songs written by Lennon and McCartney, they had an incredible series of hit records throughout the 1960s. In 1970 they disbanded to pursue solo careers.

Even Rock Rhythm

To change the shuffle beat to an even rock rhythm, substitute straight eighth notes for the ride cymbal. **Play** these patterns on percussion instruments.

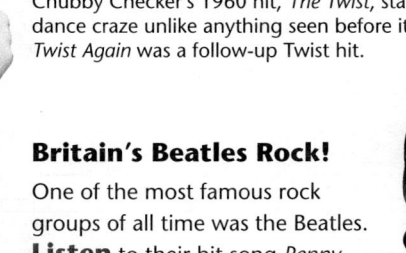

Chubby Checker helped to firmly establish the rock revolution in the 1960s with hits such as *The Twist* and *Let's Twist Again*. These hits are a good example of even rock rhythms.

Listen to *Let's Twist Again*. Then **perform** even rock rhythms with the music.

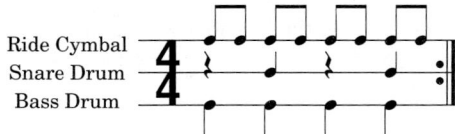
CD 13–16
Let's Twist Again

by David Appell and Kal Mann as performed by Chubby Checker

Chubby Checker's 1960 hit, *The Twist*, started a new dance craze unlike anything seen before it. *Let's Twist Again* was a follow-up Twist hit.

Britain's Beatles Rock!

One of the most famous rock groups of all time was the Beatles. **Listen** to their hit song *Penny Lane*.

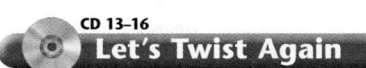
CD 13–17
Penny Lane

by John Lennon and Paul McCartney

Penny Lane was written about a local bus stop in Liverpool, England, near where Beatles Lennon and McCartney grew up.

The Beatles ▶

Exploring America's Music (side tab)

Listening

Have students

- Listen to *Penny Lane* **CD 13–17**.
- Discuss the fact that, in this song, John Lennon and Paul McCartney of the Beatles used Baroque-style fanfares.

ASK What orchestral instrument is featured in *Penny Lane?* (piccolo trumpet)

Playing

2a Invite students to play the shuffle rhythm parts with *Penny Lane* **CD 13–17**.

To help students learn the even rock rhythm, have them play the ride cymbal part on the desktop with a pencil or stick, while saying the sound with the voice (*ding-ding ding-ding ding-ding ding-ding*). Emphasize the difference between the two ride cymbal parts. Mention the quote from Earl Palmer, Little Richard's drummer, about how the straight eighth-note style began. See Skills Reinforcement below.

Have students

- Play the bass drum part with their dominant foot, making the low sound (*doom-doom-doom-doom*) with their voices. Add the ride cymbal to the bass drum part.
- Play the snare drum part with the other hand, saying it (*[rest]-tack-[rest]-tack*) as they play. Put the bass drum and snare drum together, starting with the bass drum; then add the ride cymbal.

ASK In the shuffle rhythm, what instrument plays only on beats 2 and 4? (high hat)

Divide the class into three groups. Have each group say and play one of the parts. Then put the three parts together.

If possible, provide a simple drum set for students to try. A student who plays drums might be able to bring a set from home.

continued on page 258

ACROSS THE CURRICULUM

▶ **Language Arts** For more information on the Beatles, refer students to *The Beatles* by Mike Venezia (Children's Press, 1997).

8b ▶ **Related Arts** The British invasion began officially in 1964 with the arrival of the Beatles but included other British groups like Gerry and the Pacemakers, the Kinks, the Who, and the Rolling Stones. Topping the American charts, their sound was based on the traditions of American rock 'n' roll, blues, and R&B, with role models that included Elvis, Little Richard, Chuck Berry, and Buddy Holly.

The pattern of many of the British artists was to first record American blues and R&B songs. Later they played their own songs, which retained the influences of the African American music. Their new music was largely hard-driving and uninhibited.

SKILLS REINFORCEMENT

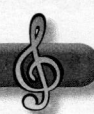

▶ **Playing** Share this background material with students before they play the even rock rhythm pattern above.

Earl Palmer, former drummer for rock 'n' roll legend Little Richard, said in a *New York Times* interview (April 25, 1999) that in 1956, Little Richard forced him to play straight eighth-note rock to "match Richard's right hand [on the piano] *Ding-ding-ding-ding* . . . Most everything I had done before was a shuffle or slow triplets . . ., but Little Richard moved from a shuffle to that straight eighth-note feeling." Palmer also credits guitarist Chuck Berry as pioneering the straight-eighth sound.

Listening

Have students listen to *Let's Twist Again* **CD 13–16** performed by Chubby Checker.

6a **ASK** **How is this song similar in style to other songs by British rock groups, such as the Beatles?** (catchy tune, basic chords, use of guitars and drums)

Playing

2a Have students play the even rock rhythm with *Let's Twist Again* **CD 13–16.**

Moving

Ask students to invent one set of dance steps for the rock 'n' roll shuffle, and another set for the even rock rhythm.

Singing

8b Introduce "Downtown" as you

9a • Discuss the influence that British rock had on the United States. See Cultural Connection below.

• Invite students to read about Petula Clark on p. 259 and listen to the recorded interview **CD 13–20.**

ASK **Does this song have shuffle rhythms or even rock rhythms?** (even rock rhythms)

Does "Downtown" use backup vocals? (yes)

Have students listen to "Downtown" **CD 13–18,** then sing along with the recording or other accompaniment, such as guitar or keyboard.

Playing

2a Invite students to perform the even rock rhythm parts with the recording of "Downtown" **CD 13–18.**

The British Are Here

Starting in 1964 with the Beatles' first tour, British groups began to dominate the rock scene. In addition to the Beatles, British performers included the Dave Clark Five, the Rolling Stones, and Petula Clark. "Downtown" was one of Petula Clark's biggest international hits.

Listen to and then **sing** "Downtown." Does the song have shuffle rhythms or even rhythms?

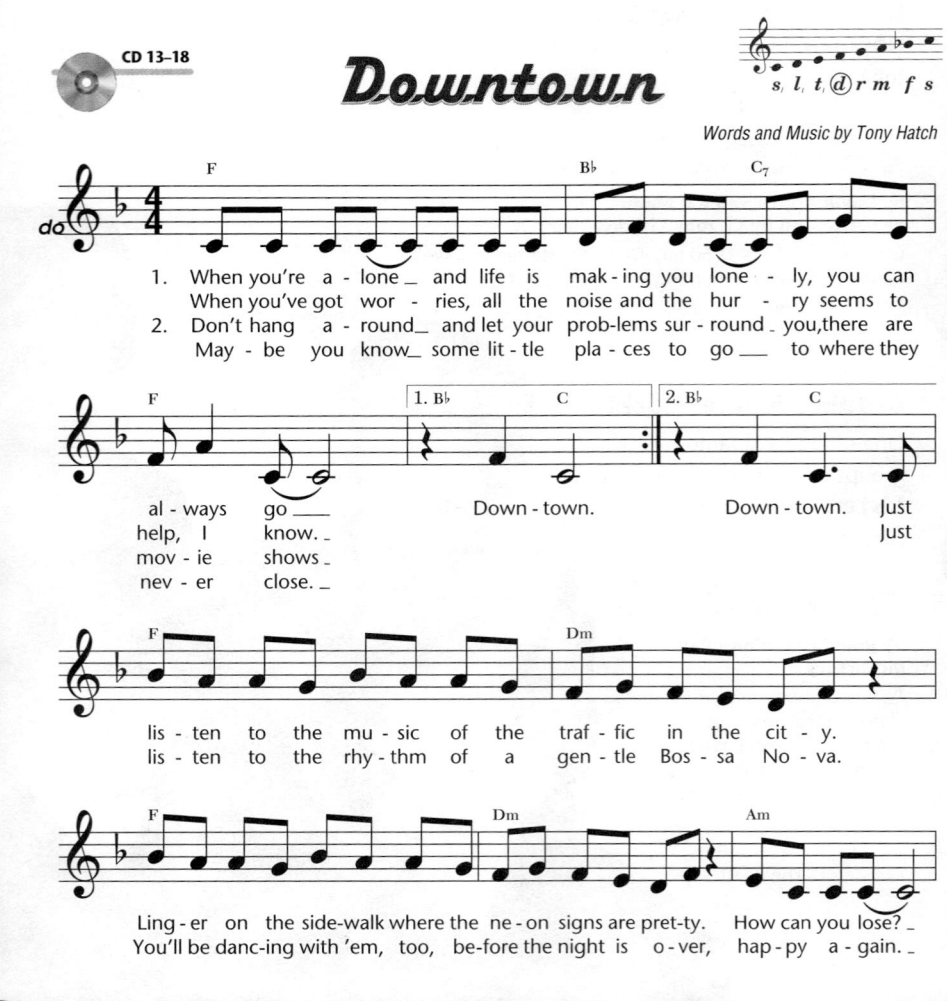

CD 13–18

Downtown

Words and Music by Tony Hatch

1. When you're a-lone _ and life is mak-ing you lone-ly, you can
   When you've got wor-ries, all the noise and the hur-ry seems to
2. Don't hang a-round _ and let your prob-lems sur-round _ you, there are
   May-be you know _ some lit-tle pla-ces to go _ to where they

al-ways go _ Down-town. Down-town. Just
help, I know. _ Just
mov-ie shows _
nev-er close. _

lis-ten to the mu-sic of the traf-fic in the cit-y.
lis-ten to the rhy-thm of a gen-tle Bos-sa No-va.

Ling-er on the side-walk where the ne-on signs are pret-ty. How can you lose? _
You'll be danc-ing with 'em, too, be-fore the night is o-ver, hap-py a-gain. _

258

Footnotes

CULTURAL CONNECTION

9a ▶ **A Friendly Invasion** American blues and rock 'n' roll played a huge part in the development of the British rock scene of the 1950s and 1960s. African American blues artists toured extensively in Britain, influencing the sound and content of groups such as the Rolling Stones, the Beatles, and Cream. After the British groups had absorbed and put their own stamp on the American sound, they brought it back to the United States in what was called the British invasion. Then, American groups absorbed ideas from the British groups. So rock has really been a cooperative effort between American, British, and now, worldwide cultures.

SPOTLIGHT ON

▶ **The Performer** A true rock pioneer, Buddy Holly (1936–1959) made two guitars, bass, and drums the standard rock performance ensemble. It was the young Elvis Presley who inspired Holly to try rock 'n' roll. Although his rock career lasted only two years (he died in a plane crash while on tour), Holly produced a string of influential hits, including "That'll Be the Day," "Peggy Sue," and "Oh, Boy!"

▶ **The Performer** Chubby Checker (born Ernest Evans in 1941) became famous with his hit song "The Twist" and his follow-up hit "Let's Twist Again." Checker started the "Twist," the dance phenomenon that changed how people moved—alone and separate from their partner.

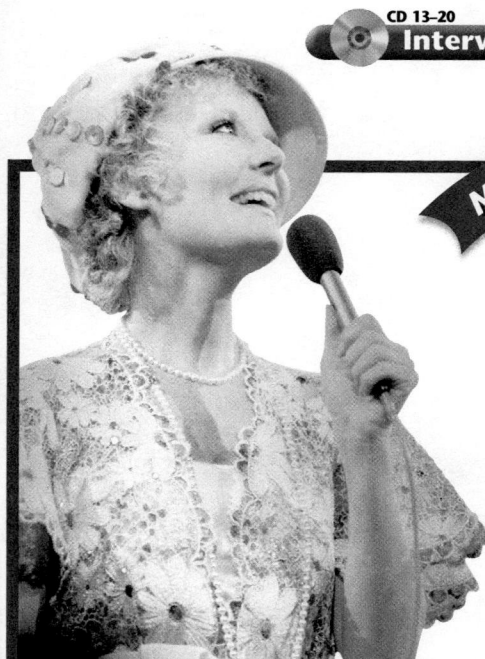

CD 13–20
Interview with Petula Clark

MUSIC MAKERS

Petula Clark

Petula Clark (born 1933) was a star in England at age eight. She sang for British troops in World War II and even starred in a comic strip! Her movie career has spanned almost 30 films. In 1965 she received her first Grammy Award for her recording of "Downtown." Clark has appeared on Broadway and London's West End in *Blood Brothers, The Sound of Music,* and *Sunset Boulevard.*

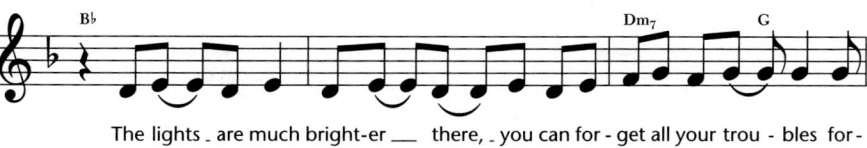

The lights _ are much bright-er ___ there, _ you can for - get all your trou - bles for-

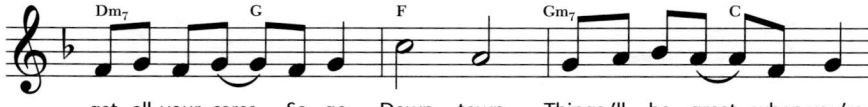

get all your cares. _ So go Down - town. Things-'ll be great _ when you're

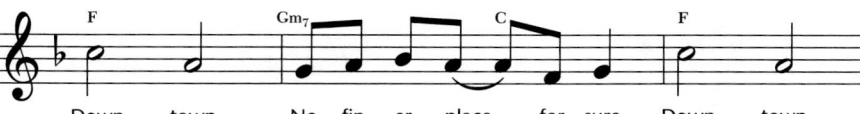

Down - town. No fin - er place _ for sure, Down - town.

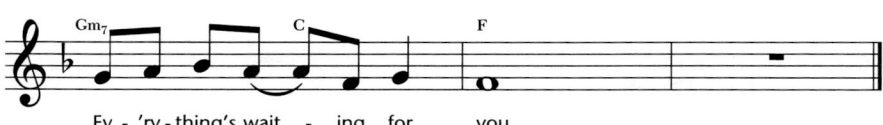

Ev - 'ry - thing's wait - ing for you. ____

Unit 7 **259**

Creating

Invite students to explore rock styles using *Band-in-a-Box*. Write the styles listed in Technology/Media Link below on the board. Ask students to

- Create a four-measure introduction to the song using the C chord for three measures and the G chord on the final measure.
- Enter the chords for "Don't Be Cruel," found in Skills Reinforcement on p. 255, after the introduction. Guide students to understand that the style determines the meter. Have them enter the chords in meter in 4 (the default meter), although the song is in meter in 2.
- Change the style of the arrangement by selecting the style from the menu or style button.
- Play the new arrangement and determine if the style uses shuffle rhythm patterns or even rhythm patterns.

3 CLOSE

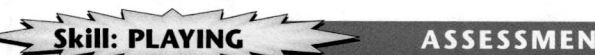

Skill: PLAYING   **ASSESSMENT**

Performance/Self-Assessment Have students work in groups of three to practice the drum set patterns. Ask them to help each other; then have each student rate his or her own drumming ability, using the following rubric.

5 I accurately play all three parts at once; the playing is totally steady.

4 I play all three parts at once; the playing is fairly steady.

3 I play all three parts at once but sometimes have trouble.

2 I can play two parts at once but am working on adding the third.

1 I can play each part separately but have difficulty combining parts.

Instead of using numbers for the rubric, students may enjoy making up their own labels. They might use rock 'n' roll names that they create (5 = Awesome).

AUDIENCE ETIQUETTE

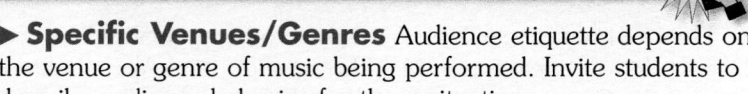

▶ **Specific Venues/Genres** Audience etiquette depends on the venue or genre of music being performed. Invite students to describe audience behavior for these situations.

- A rock concert held outdoors. (It is appropriate to move, dance, clap, and sing along with the music.)
- A chorus, band, or orchestra concert in an auditorium. (Quiet and stillness are best. Applaud only at the end of pieces.)
- A jazz concert. (Audiences tend to nod or tap feet to the music. It's okay to applaud after a solo, even if the piece is not over.)
- An opera performance. (It is appropriate to call out "Bravo" or "Brava" after a singer has sung an exceptional rendition of an aria.)

SCHOOL TO HOME CONNECTION

▶ **Rock in the '50s and '60s** Ask students to talk to adult friends and relatives about their favorite rock 'n' roll artists and the pros and cons of a career as a rock 'n' roll star.

TECHNOLOGY/MEDIA LINK

3c
4c

CD-ROM Students may use the following styles in *Band-in-a-Box* to create new arrangements of "Don't Be Cruel."

- Light Rock and Shuffle Rock
- Blues Even and Blues Shuffle
- Chuck Berry Style (Chuk_B_1.Sty)

Element: MELODY | Skill: SINGING | Connection: GENRE

The Surfin' Sound

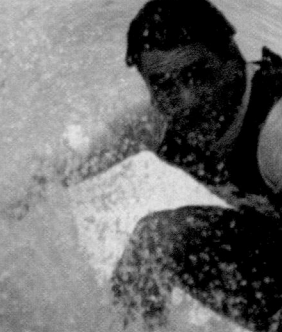

LESSON AT A GLANCE

Element Focus **MELODY** Flatted-seventh blues note

Skill Objective **SINGING** Sing a "surf rock" hit song with a flatted-seventh blues note

Connection Activity **GENRE** Explore the history and stylistic elements of surf rock

MATERIALS
- "Surfin' U.S.A." **CD 13–21**
  Recording Routine: Intro (4 m.); v. 1; v. 2; coda
- *Surfin' Safari* **CD 13–23**

VOCABULARY
surf rock   flatted-seventh blues note

◆ ◆ ◆ ◆ **National Standards** ◆ ◆ ◆ ◆

1c Sing music from diverse genres
2d Perform simple accompaniments by ear
4c Arranging, using electronic media
6a Listen and describe events in music using appropriate terms
6b Listen and analyze uses of pitch in music from diverse genres
8b Identify ways music relates to social studies

MORE MUSIC CHOICES
For more experience with rock songs:
"Birthday," p. 90
"Rock and Roll Is Here to Stay," p. 36

Not all rock music in the early 1960s was sung with a British accent. From Southern California, groups like Jan and Dean, the Surfaris, and the Beach Boys helped produce "surf rock," a new sound that was uniquely American.

The main elements of surf rock are high vocal harmony, carefree lyrics (mostly about beach parties and hot rods), Chuck Berry-like guitar riffs, and a strong drumbeat.

Sing "Surfin' U. S. A.," one of the Beach Boys' biggest hits.

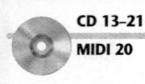
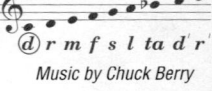

1 INTRODUCE

8b Part of the distinctive sound of surf rock came from the high falsetto vocals. The other part came from such surf guitarists as Dick Dale, who created an exciting new sound. Share the information in Spotlight On below and Cultural Connection, p. 261, to help students explore the history and stylistic elements of surf rock.

CD 13–21
MIDI 20

Surfin' U.S.A.

Words by Brian Wilson
Music by Chuck Berry

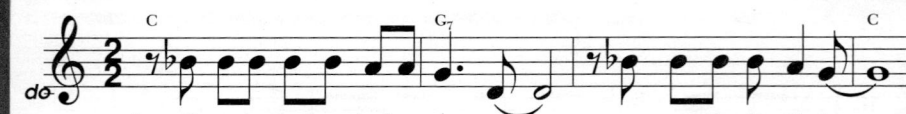
1. If ev-'ry-bod - y had an o - cean ___ a - cross the U. S. A., ___
2. We'll all be plan-nin' out a route _____ we're gon - na take real soon. ___

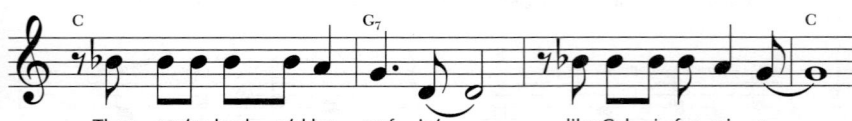
Then ev-'ry-bod - y'd be surf - in' ___ like Cal - i - for - ni - a. ___
We're wax-in' down ___ our surf - boards, ___ we can't ___ wait for June. ___

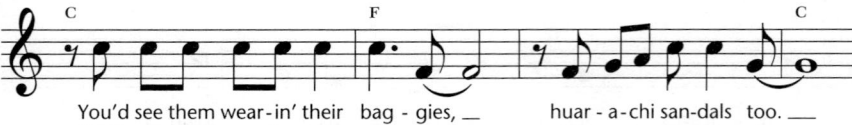
You'd see them wear-in' their bag - gies, ___ huar - a-chi san-dals too. ___
We'll all be gone for the sum - mer, ___ we're on sa - fa - ri ___ to stay. ___

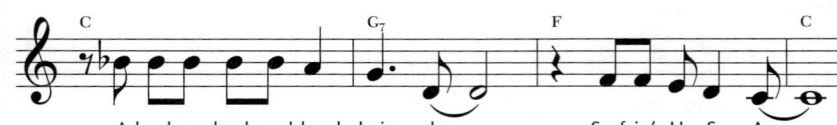
A bush-y, bush - y blond hair - do. ___ Surf-in' U. S. A. ___
7 Tell the teach-er we're surf - in', ___ Surf-in' U. S. A. ___

260

Footnotes

SKILLS REINFORCEMENT

2d ▶ **Singing** Play the recording of "Surfin' U.S.A." and ask students to focus on the backup vocal parts. Give students an opportunity to improvise their own vocal backup, based on the recorded routine.

▶ **Playing** Ask students to improvise a chord progression based on the I and flatted-seventh (♭VII) degrees of the G major scale. (G and F chords)

BUILDING SKILLS THROUGH MUSIC

▶ **Writing** Lead students in a discussion of surfing as a sport. Have them write a brief paragraph about their favorite sport. Ask them to include their reason for selecting the sport.

SPOTLIGHT ON

▶ **The Performers** In 1961 three brothers, Brian, Carl, and Dennis Wilson, their cousin Mike Love, and friend Alan Jardin formed the Beach Boys in a suburb of Los Angeles. Their songs celebrated California, the sport of surfing, Californians' love of hot-rod racing, and high schoolers' school spirit. Brian Wilson, the group's leader, was responsible for writing most of their songs, as well as arranging and recording. He created thick, close harmonies and intricate vocals and accompaniments. In addition to "Surfin' U.S.A.," the group's big hits include "California Girls," "Little Deuce Coupe," and "Be True to Your School," among many others. The group was inducted into the Rock and Roll Hall of Fame in 1989.

Surf's Up

In addition to the Beach Boys, Jan and Dean were also known for their surf music. **Listen** to the duo's 1962 hit, *Surfin' Safari*.

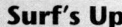
CD 13–23
Surfin' Safari

by Mike Love and Brian Wilson
as performed by Jan and Dean

Love and Wilson were members of the Beach Boys. Until their record companies objected, Jan and Dean and the Beach Boys often appeared on each others' recordings.

◀ The Beach Boys ▶

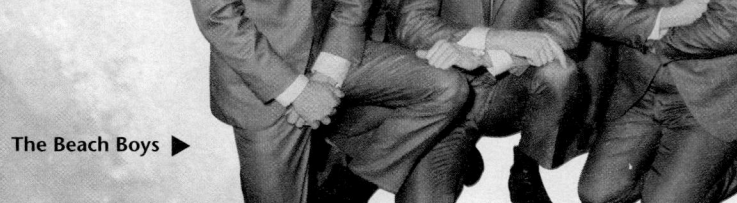

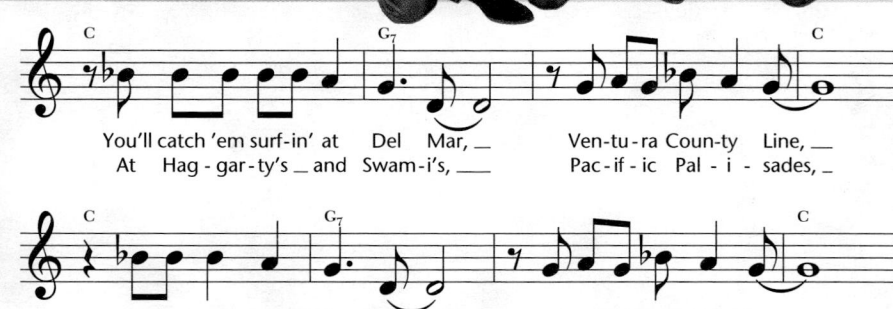

You'll catch 'em surf-in' at Del Mar, ___ Ven-tu-ra Coun-ty Line, ___
At Hag-gar-ty's __ and Swam-i's, ___ Pac-if-ic Pal-i-sades, ___

San-ta Cruz and Tress-els, ___ Aus-tra-lia's Nar-a-bine.
San O-no-fre and Sun-set, ___ Re-don-do Beach, L. A. ___

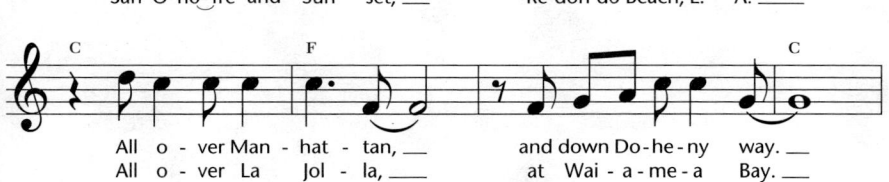

All o-ver Man-hat-tan, ___ and down Do-he-ny way. ___
All o-ver La Jol-la, ___ at Wai-a-me-a Bay. ___

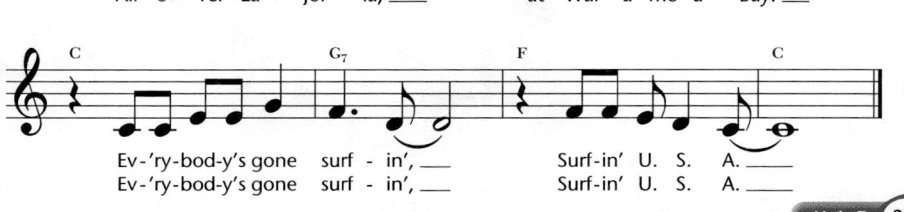

Ev-'ry-bod-y's gone surf-in', ___ Surf-in' U. S. A. ___
Ev-'ry-bod-y's gone surf-in', ___ Surf-in' U. S. A. ___

Unit 7 261

2 DEVELOP

Reading

6b Have students listen to "Surfin' U.S.A." **CD 13–21** while following the notation.

ASK In "Surfin' U.S.A.," which melody note does not belong in the C-major scale? (B♭)

Which note of the scale is represented by this altered pitch, and how is it changed? (The seventh note, *ti*, is lowered by a half step to *ta*.)

Tell students that the flatted-seventh of a scale is common in rock music. This is often called a "blues" note.

Singing

Ask students to

- Sing the notes of the C scale with a flatted-seventh.

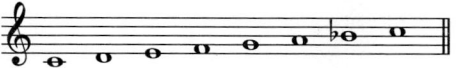

1c
- Sing "Surfin' U.S.A." with the recording or keyboard accompaniment.

Listening

6a Have students listen to *Surfin' Safari* **CD 13–23** and compare the stylistic elements of the song to "Surfin' U.S.A." Ask students to describe the vocal style and performance of both songs.

3 CLOSE

Element: MELODY   ASSESSMENT

Performance/Observation Have students listen to, sing, and identify pairs of scales in which one is major and the other contains a flatted-seventh.

Then have them sing "Surfin' U.S.A.," a surf rock song with a flatted-seventh blues note. Observe students' ability to sing the lowered seventh of this scale. Invite students to evaluate and discuss their performance.

CULTURAL CONNECTION

8b ▶ **The Surf Scene** Surf music, which started as a California phenomenon, embraced a new postwar generation that had both affluence and the leisure time to play. The ability of the young male to spend a summer getting a tan, riding a wave, partying forever, and driving his car was venerated in surf music. Hollywood jumped into the water, too, by creating beach movies to go along with the trend. The tidal wave of surf music eventually covered America.

TECHNOLOGY/MEDIA LINK

4c **MIDI/Sequencing Software** Using the MIDI song file for "Surfin' U.S.A.," have students

- Change the melody from a flatted-seventh to major and describe the effect.

- Transpose the song into other keys and identify the pitch names of the new scale.

LESSON AT A GLANCE

Element Focus	**RHYTHM** Latin rhythm patterns
Skill Objective	**LISTENING** Listen for specific rhythm patterns in Latin pop music
Connection Activity	**SOCIAL STUDIES** Relate elements of Latin American music to cultural traditions from the Caribbean and Mexico

MATERIALS

- *"Riendo el río corre"*   **CD 13–24**
- *"Run, Run, River"*   **CD 13–25**

  Recording Routine: Intro (4 m.); refrain; v. 1; interlude (4 m.); refrain; v. 2; refrain; coda
- **Pronunciation Practice/Translation** p. 532
- *Ayer*   **CD 14–1**
- *Si tú no estás* (excerpt)   **CD 14–2**
- available Latin percussion instruments, guitars
- **Resource Book** p. A-20

VOCABULARY

salsa	Tejano	conjunto	cha-cha
rumba	tango	samba	

◆◆◆◆ National Standards ◆◆◆◆

1c Sing music from diverse cultures
2c Perform instrumental music from diverse cultures
4c Arrange, using electronic media
5a Read syncopation in duple meter
6a Listen and describe events in music using appropriate terms
8b Identify ways music relates to social studies and science
9a Describe characteristics of music styles from a variety of cultures

---

MORE MUSIC CHOICES

For more experience with Latin rhythms:

"El payo," p. 145

"Má Teodora," p. 301

"Magnolia," p. 16

"O lê lê O Bahía," p. 165

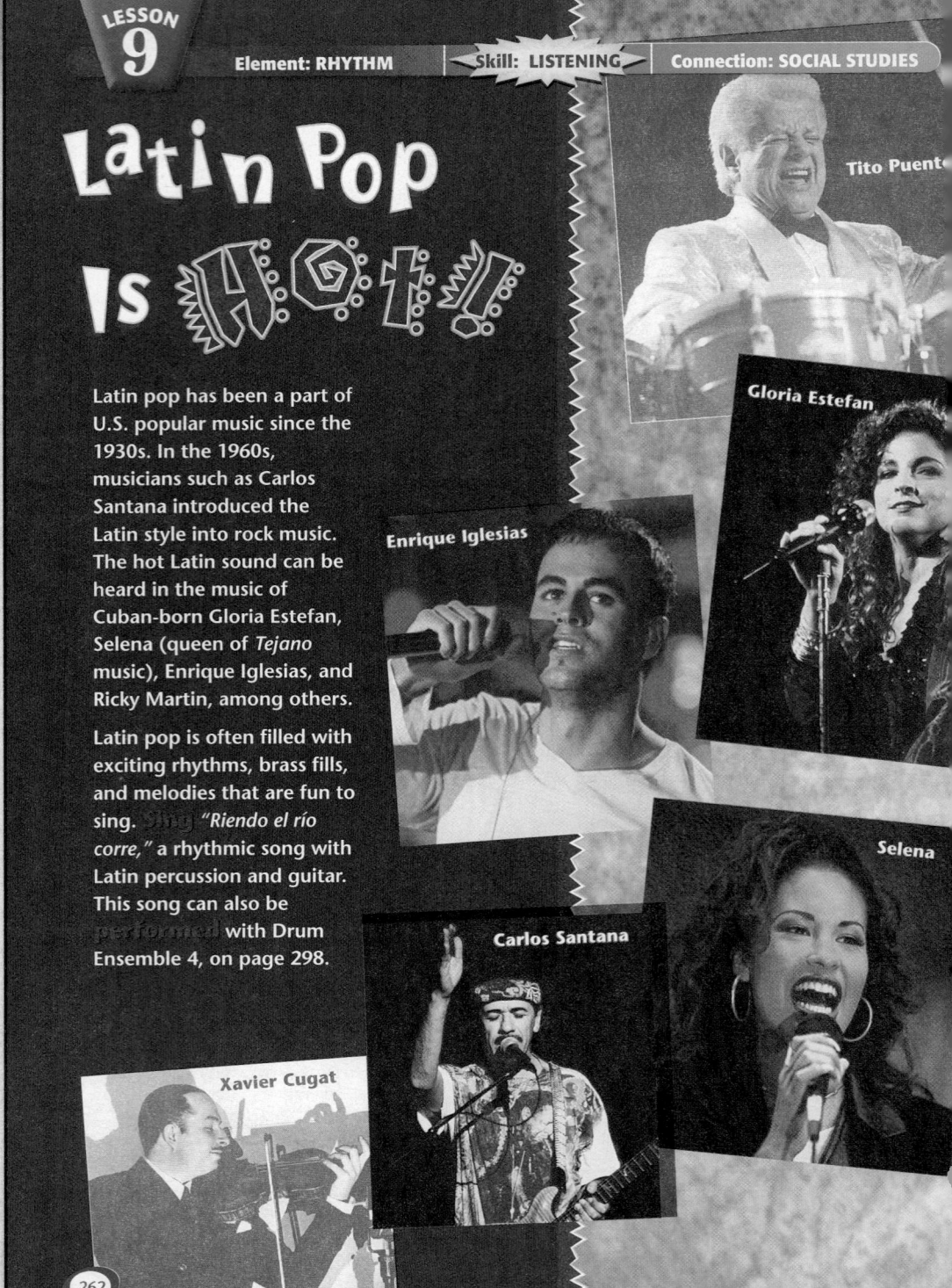

Latin Pop Is HOT!

Tito Puente

Gloria Estefan

Enrique Iglesias

Selena

Carlos Santana

Xavier Cugat

Latin pop has been a part of U.S. popular music since the 1930s. In the 1960s, musicians such as Carlos Santana introduced the Latin style into rock music. The hot Latin sound can be heard in the music of Cuban-born Gloria Estefan, Selena (queen of *Tejano* music), Enrique Iglesias, and Ricky Martin, among others.

Latin pop is often filled with exciting rhythms, brass fills, and melodies that are fun to sing. **Sing** *"Riendo el río corre,"* a rhythmic song with Latin percussion and guitar. This song can also be **performed** with Drum Ensemble 4, on page 298.

262

Footnotes

CULTURAL CONNECTION

8b ▶ **Tejano** *Tejano* music is the music of the Tejanos of South Texas and the Norteños of northern Mexico. Its roots are in the sacred and secular songs of Mexico. Tejano music is the sounds of the *mariachis* and the *bandas* from Sinaloa. It embraces the urban orchestras, the rural string bands, the *bolero* singers, and the gutsy, rural *ranchero* stars. It includes accordion players, fiddlers, and falsetto singers. It is truly reflective of the soul of the people.

BUILDING SKILLS THROUGH MUSIC

▶ **Language** Have students read about Tish Hinojosa in Music Makers and ask them to restate the information in outline form.

SPOTLIGHT ON

▶ **Latin Music Legends** Known as the Mambo King, Tito Puente (1923–2000) started learning to be a percussionist at age ten. By the 1940s, he and his band were famous for their exciting Latin music. His song *"Oye como va"* became a crossover hit for Carlos Santana in the 1970s.

Carlos Santana (born 1947) is known for his blending of rock riffs, blues, and Afro-Latin rhythms set off by his melodic and sustained guitar style. Highlights of his long career include 30 million albums sold and a history-making performance at Woodstock.

Selena (1971–1995) had 12 Top-40 singles on the Billboard charts and won a Grammy Award. Her tragic death in 1995 drew even more attention to *Tejano* music, inspiring candlelight vigils, a movie, and a musical about the life of the queen of *Tejano* music.

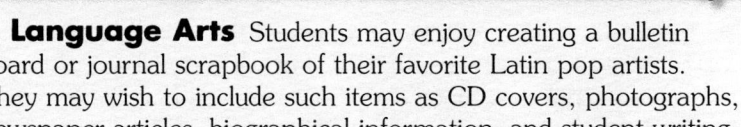

Riendo el río corre
(Run, Run, River)

English Words by Sue Ellen LaBelle
Words and Music by Tish Hinojosa

CD 13–24

REFRAIN

Co - rre, co - rre, __ co - rre el rí - o, __ Ri - en - do el rí - o __
Run, run, riv - er, __ Run, run, riv - er, __ With laugh-ter runs __ the __

co - rre. __ Co - rre, co - rre, __ co - rre el rí - o, __ Ri -
riv - er. __ Run, run, riv - er, __ Run, run, riv - er, __ With

Last time to Coda

VERSE

en - do el rí - o __ co - rre. __
laugh-ter runs __ the __ riv - er. __

1. Cuén - ta - me __ de __ las
2. Sa - bes tú __ de __ la
1. Tell a - bout __ the __ high __
2. Tell a - bout __ the __ great __

__ mon - ta - ñas __ de tu em - pe - zar,
__ dis - tan - cia que pien - sas al - can - zar,
__ moun - tains where your jour - ney be - gan,
__ dis - tance you've gone to reach __ the __ sea,

Cuén - ta - me ____ de ____ pie - dra y pe - na ____
Co - mo sue - ño ____ de ____ la lu - na que
Tell a - bout __ the __ pla - ces ____ you
Whis - p'rings of ____ your __ tra - vels _____ seem

D.C. al Coda ⊕ *Coda*

que lle - vas __ al __ mar. __ en - do el rí - o __ co - rre. __
me das para __ so - ñar. __ laugh-ter runs __ the __ riv - er. __
passed a - long __ the __ way. __
like a dream __ to __ me. __

Unit 7 **263**

---

1 INTRODUCE

9a Begin a discussion by asking students if they are familiar with any Latin music, singers, or singing groups. Mention that the popularity of Latin-based pop music has grown along with the Hispanic population of the United States. Music from different Hispanic cultures has slightly different flavors, depending on the history of the specific culture. "*Riendo el río corre*" is a mix of Texan and Mexican elements. *Ayer* uses Cuban and *salsa* styles.

Share the information in Cultural Connection, pp. 262, 264, and 270; and Spotlight On, pp. 262 and 267 to help students relate elements of American Latin pop music to cultural traditions from the Caribbean and Mexico.

2 DEVELOP

Singing

8b Share with students the information on *Tejano* music, in Cultural Connection on p. 262.

ASK Which of the Latin percussion instruments shown on p. 264 do you hear in this recording? (All are present in the recording.)

Then, have students listen to "*Riendo el río corre*" **CD 13–24** while following the notation.

continued on page 264

ACROSS THE CURRICULUM

▶ **Language Arts** Students may enjoy creating a bulletin board or journal scrapbook of their favorite Latin pop artists. They may wish to include such items as CD covers, photographs, newspaper articles, biographical information, and student writing.

The following books provide interesting information and photos for student Latin pop projects and displays.

Ricky Martin: Livin' La Vida Loca by Letisha Marrero (Harper Entertainment, 1999)

Selena: The Queen of Tejano by Jill C. Wheeler (ABDO, 1995)

Gloria Estefan by Sue Boulais (Mitchell Lane Publications, 1999)

SKILLS REINFORCEMENT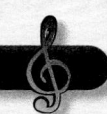

▶ **Guitar** "*Riendo el río corre*" is in the key of D minor, which makes it easy to sing but fairly difficult to play on guitar. Placing a capo on the fifth fret will help. In this way, the barred chords are eliminated. For every Dm chord, students can now play Am; for Gm, play Dm; for A and A_7, play E and E_7. Placing the capo on the fifth fret will also make the guitar sound like a *requinto*, a folk instrument characteristic of much Latin folk music. Have students play a relaxed down strum, using their thumb, which will place the attention where it belongs—on the melody and words.

▶ **Playing** Drum Ensemble 4, p. 298, may also be used to accompany both "*Riendo el río corre*," p. 263, and *Ayer* on p. 266.

Lesson 9 Continued

Have students read about Tish Hinojosa in the Music Makers feature on p. 264. Explain to students that *conjunto* style is a combination of Mexican and European folk styles, and it originated in southern Texas in the 1930s.

Have students

- Use the Pronunciation Practice **CD 13–27** to learn the Spanish lyrics for "*Riendo el río corre*." Refer also to the Pronunciation Practice Guide on Resource Book p. A-20.

1c
- Sing "*Riendo el río corre*" **CD 13–24** with the recording, or with keyboard or guitar accompaniment.

Playing

Teach students the guitar chords for "*Riendo el río corre*." See Skills Reinforcement, p. 263, for more information on capo placement and chords.

2c Encourage students to perform a Latin percussion ensemble accompaniment to "*Riendo el río corre* " **CD 13–24**. See Skills Reinforcement, p. 263.

Moving

Using "*Riendo el río corre*" **CD 13–24**, ask students to perform the following rhythm warmup. See Movement on p. 265.

- Keep the rhythm with just one body part.
- Put the rhythm in the shoulders. (Challenge students to move only their shoulders, not the whole body.)
- Put the rhythm in the elbows, head, back, hands, or knees.

Encourage students to create their own dance steps to "*Riendo el río corre*."

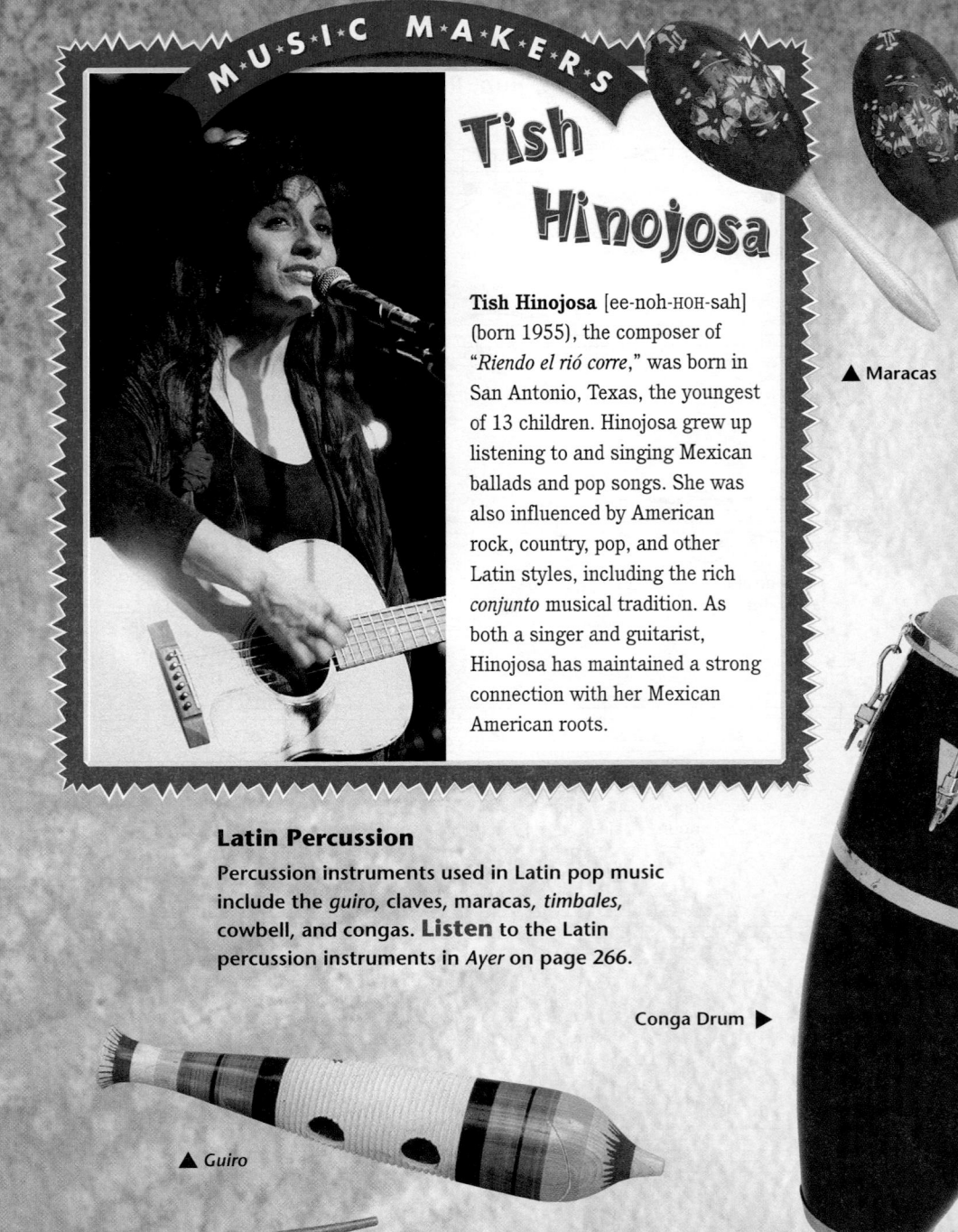

MUSIC MAKERS

Tish Hinojosa

▲ Maracas

Tish Hinojosa [ee-noh-HOH-sah] (born 1955), the composer of "*Riendo el rió corre*," was born in San Antonio, Texas, the youngest of 13 children. Hinojosa grew up listening to and singing Mexican ballads and pop songs. She was also influenced by American rock, country, pop, and other Latin styles, including the rich *conjunto* musical tradition. As both a singer and guitarist, Hinojosa has maintained a strong connection with her Mexican American roots.

Latin Percussion

Percussion instruments used in Latin pop music include the *guiro*, claves, maracas, *timbales*, cowbell, and congas. **Listen** to the Latin percussion instruments in *Ayer* on page 266.

Conga Drum ▶

▲ *Guiro*

264

Footnotes

CULTURAL CONNECTION

8b ▶ **Music of the Caribbean** Caribbean musical styles grew from an interesting mixture of European and West African cultural and musical roots. The main contributions of each are

West Coast African Music
- Drums, bells, and rattles
- Call-and-response form, dance music
- Syncopation, layered rhythms, and polyrhythms (3 against 2)

European Music
- Guitars, keyboards, basses, brass, and woodwinds
- Ballads (songs that tell stories), dance music
- Tonal melodies (major and minor scales)

ACROSS THE CURRICULUM

 ▶ **Science** Rivers collectively represent the world's water resources to humans because they carry virtually all the water available for our use. Since early times, people have been dependent on the rivers and the fertile soils that developed in their floodplains. For example, the Sumerians depended on the Tigris and the Euphrates; the early Egyptians on the Nile; the Chinese on the Huang ("Yellow"); and the Harappans (in the land that is now Pakistan) on the Indus.

The significance of a river is measured by its flow. The Amazon, the world's largest river, has a flow rate that is five times that of the second largest river, the Congo. Discuss with students the powerful imagery and inspiration that rivers lend to the music and literature of cultures around the world. See Skills Reinforcement on p. 265.

264

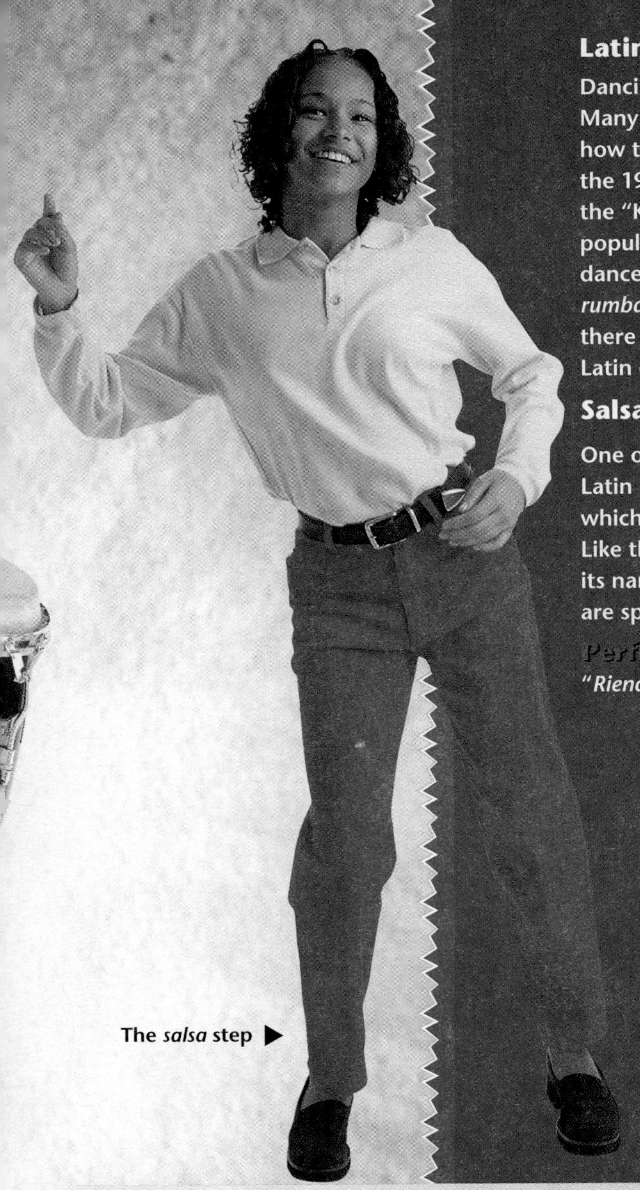

Latin Moves

Dancing to Latin music is hot! Many people take lessons to learn how to dance to Latin music. In the 1930s Xavier Cugat, known as the "King of the Rumba," helped popularize many Latin American dances such as the *cha-cha, rumba, tango,* and *samba.* Today, there are many modern styles of Latin dance.

Salsa Step

One of the most popular styles of Latin music and dance is *salsa,* which comes from Puerto Rico. Like the Spanish sauce that shares its name, *salsa's* rhythm and style are spicy.

Perform the *salsa* step to "Riendo el río corre."

The *salsa* step ▶

CD-ROM Use *Band-in-a-Box* to create your own Latin pop song.

Unit 7 **265**

Listening

Play the recording of *Ayer* **CD 14–1.**

 ASK **What Latin music term would best describe the style of each of the two sections that make up this music?** (first section: Cuban style; second section: *salsa*)

What musical elements help create the Cuban and salsa styles? (Latin percussion, prominent horn section, singable melody, syncopated eighth-note rhythm patterns, *salsa* section with more percussion, a slightly faster tempo, and vocal harmonies)

Students can hear another recording of the conga drum in the Sound Bank, starting on p. 512.

Creating

 Invite students to create a Latin pop song or dance arrangement, using *Band-in-a-Box.* (See Technology/Media Link on p. 267.) Guide students to

- Select a style from the Latin styles in *Band-in-a-Box.*
- Determine a key for their song. (For example, D minor.)
- Write the basic chords of that key on paper. (For example, the i, iv and V_7 chords in D minor are Dm, Gm, and A_7.)
- Enter a chord progression into *Band-in-a-Box* using those chords and build the chords into a song.
- Play the song and evaluate if the chord progression and style work well together.
- Experiment with different Latin styles and chord progressions.

Invite students to play their songs for the class. Have students create movements to accompany the songs or dance arrangements.

continued on page 266

SKILLS REINFORCEMENT

▶ **Listening** For centuries, composers have found inspiration in the literal and metaphorical attributes of rivers. The following list is just a small sampling. Invite students to share with the class recordings of these or other theme-related works of their choosing.

- *The Moldau* (Bedřich Smetana)
- *The Beautiful Blue Danube* (Johann Strauss)
- *Mississippi Suite* (Ferde Grofé)
- *The River* (Virgil Thomson)
- *The River* (Duke Ellington)
- *The River of Dreams* (Billy Joel)
- *River Run* (Philip Glass)

MOVEMENT

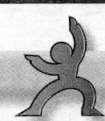

▶ **Nonlocomotor Movement** Encouraging students to move can be made easier by giving a very specific movement task. Focusing the directions very specifically for students this age helps to create a nonthreatening, doable task.

For a warmup exercise, work with students to create a pattern of moving for 8 or 16 counts with shoulders, elbows, knees, and back. These kinds of exercises are valuable for use in small spaces and can even be done seated in chairs or on risers.

Moving

Encourage students to learn a basic *salsa* dance step to perform with the *salsa* section of *Ayer* **CD 14–1.** See Movement below.

Playing

5a

Have students use a pencil or rhythm sticks to

- Play the rhythm for the conga drum part on this page.
- Play the rhythm for the *timbale* drum part.

Ask for volunteers to play the parts with the *salsa* section of *Ayer* **CD 14–1** on a conga drum and *timbales* if these instruments are available. See also Skills Reinforcement on p. 263.

Latin Sounds

Latin music is sometimes influenced by a combination of musical styles. Two important styles found in Latin music are those of *salsa* and Cuban music.

Salsa, a well-known Latin sound, is a style that emerged in the 1940s. *Salsa* is energetic and vibrant. It uses syncopated bass rhythms, horn sections, and expanded percussion.

Cuban music's distinct sound features continuous eighth-note rhythms, percussion textures, guitar, vocal harmonies, and brass punctuation.

Listen to Gloria Estefan's performance of *Ayer.* It shows Cuban and *salsa* musical influences.

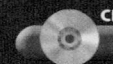

CD 14–1
Ayer

by Juanito R. Marquez
as performed by Gloria Estefan

Ayer (Yesterday) begins in the style of Cuban music. After the *accelerando,* the song takes on a *salsa* style.

Learn and **play** the rhythms below on the conga and *timbale* drums. When you are ready, perform them with the recording.

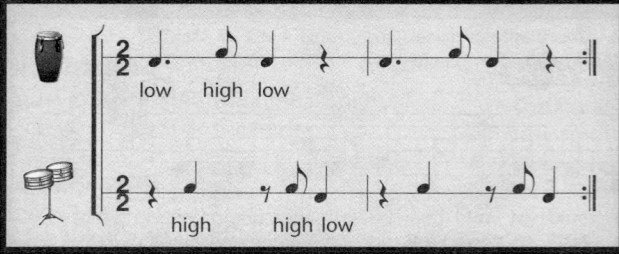

low   high low

high   high low

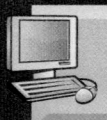

Take It to the Net Visit *www.sfsuccessnet.com* to discover more about Latin music.

266

Footnotes

CULTURAL CONNECTION

8b ▶ *Salsa* Salsa (meaning "sauce") is considered a Puerto Rican style of dance. Its introduction to the United States, however, was mainly through the influx of Cubans to Florida in the 1960s. A recording company executive who liked a 1968 album title, *Llegó la salsa,* named the genre. This lively music features a prominent horn and percussion section and has a driving rhythm that makes you want to dance. (See Movement on this page.) Latin dances that preceded *salsa* include the *cha-cha,* tango, *rumba,* and *mambo.*

MOVEMENT

▶ **Patterned Dance** *Salsa* style is similar to that of many other Latin dances. The upper body stays relatively still while most of the movement is done with the lower body. Knees are bent, and the feet make small, flat footsteps. The hips move subtly side to side, following the action of the feet.

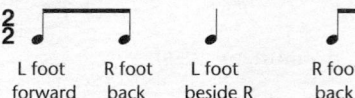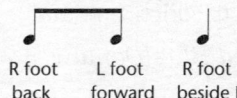

L foot forward | R foot back | L foot beside R | R foot back | L foot forward | R foot beside L

Venezuela's Treasures

Venezuela is a country of mountains, forests, vast plains, mighty rivers, Caribbean beaches, and vibrant cities. It is a land rich in natural resources and rich in its musical heritage.

Among Venezuela's musical treasures is singer and songwriter Franco de Vita. He is internationally known for his music and vocal recordings. De Vita often writes in a contemporary pop style that combines pop and Latin musical elements.

Listen to de Vita's hit ballad, *Si tú no estás* (If You're Not Here). Which musical elements give the song its Latin character?

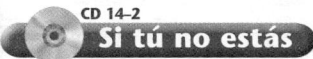

CD 14–2
Si tú no estás

written and performed by Franco de Vita

The Latin flavor of *Si tú no estás* comes from its blend of guitar, exciting rhythms, and a brass section.

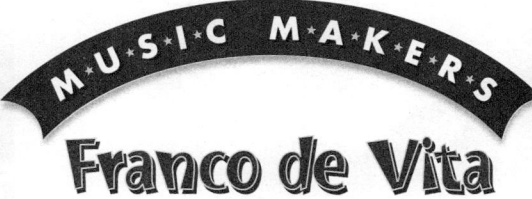

Franco de Vita

Franco de Vita (born 1954 in Caracas, Venezuela) spent his childhood in Italy but returned to Venezuela as a teenager. He began musical training after high school and studied formally at the Music Conservatory. De Vita first achieved success as a singer and songwriter in the 1980s. His albums have sold millions of copies throughout the world.

Franco de Vita achieved international fame when he wrote Ricky Martin's first single, *Vuelve* (Come Back). De Vita is also known for his songs and lyrics on social issues. His ballad *Lluvia* (Rain), was written about floods that took many lives in Venezuela. The *cuatro* and *tonado* rhythms in *Lluvia* are traditional in Venezuelan music (see page 332).

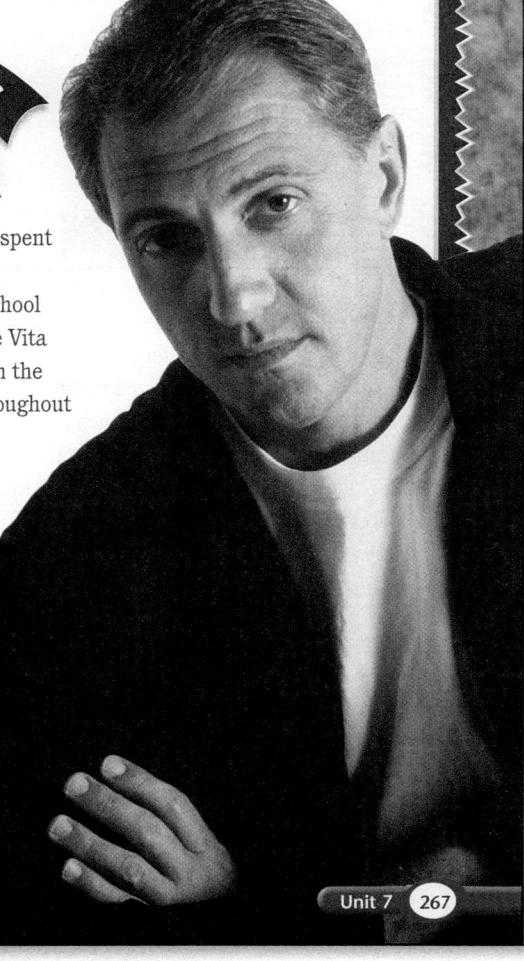

Unit 7 **267**

Listening

ASK Which Latin musical elements do you hear in *Si tú no estás?* (brass section featured, Latin rhythms, and use of guitar)

Invite students to listen as you play *Si tú no estás* **CD 14–2.**

Invite students to read the Music Makers feature on Venezuelan songwriter/performer Franco de Vita.

3 CLOSE

Skill: LISTENING   **ASSESSMENT**

6a **Music Journal Writing** Play short samples of musical selections from this lesson. Ask students to listen and

- Write down what they have learned about each selection. (selection title, performer, style, instrumentation)
- Identify a sample Latin rhythm and write it in their journals.

SPOTLIGHT ON

▶ **Traditional Venezuelan Music** The use of flute, harps, and mandolin is central to the traditional music of Venezuela. The mandolin was brought to Venezuela in the mid-nineteenth century. Interested students may listen to groups such as *Más Allá de Venezuela, El Tramao, El Trancao,* and *Arisca* (includes solo mandolin) for a taste of traditional Venezuelan music.

Some artists in Venezuela are fusing elements of urban pop from Europe and North America with traditional music to form their own world-music styles. Groups students may wish to sample include *El Agridulce* and *El Paito.* For other Venezuelan artists, students may visit the international section of their local record store.

SCHOOL TO HOME CONNECTION

▶ **Latin Influence** Ask students to listen to the types of Latin styles or performing artists their family and friends like. Students can also make note of other locations in their neighborhood where they hear Latin music played. Ask students to share their discoveries.

TECHNOLOGY/MEDIA LINK

4c

CD-ROM Students may use *Band-in-a-Box* to create their own Latin songs or dance arrangements. Other students may play rhythm instruments along with the arrangements.

Web Site Visit *www.sfsuccessnet.com* to learn more about Latin pop performers.

LESSON AT A GLANCE

Element Focus **RHYTHM** World beat

Skill Objective **LISTENING** Listen for specific stylistic features in world beat

Connection Activity **SOCIAL STUDIES** Relate some styles of music from around the world to their culture of origin

MATERIALS

- *The Same* (excerpt)   **CD 14–3**
- *Hindewhu* (whistle) *solo*   **CD 14–4**
- *Watermelon Man* (excerpt)   **CD 14–5**
- *Watchers of the Canyon*   **CD 14–6**
- *Colours of the World*   **CD 14–7**
- *Brolga* (excerpt)   **CD 14–8**
- available nonpitched percussion instruments

VOCABULARY

world beat   fusion

Afropop   hip-hop   *didgeridoo*

◆ ◆ ◆ ◆ National Standards ◆ ◆ ◆ ◆

6a Listen and describe events in music using appropriate terms
6b Listen and analyze uses of rhythm/pitch/timbre in music from diverse cultures
8b Identify ways music relates to social studies
9a Describe characteristics of music styles from a variety of cultures
9c Compare, in several cultures, functions music serves

MORE MUSIC CHOICES

For more experience with world beat music:

Evening Samba, p. 297

Gidden riddum, p. 299

"Give a Little Love," p. 140

WORLD MUSIC

"World beat" is a musical style created by the merger of American pop styles and vocal and instrumental elements from Africa, Latin America, Australia, and other parts of the world.

Listen to *The Same*, a good example of "world beat" music. The rhythm patterns, which are influenced by African and Caribbean drumming, are accompanied by pop harmonies and instruments.

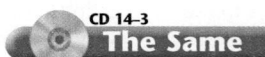

CD 14–3
The Same

by Youssou N'Dour and Habib Faye as performed by Youssou N'Dour

The lyrics of *The Same* tell how much of the world's music is "the same."

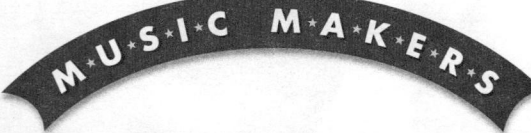
M·U·S·I·C M·A·K·E·R·S

YOUSSOU N'DOUR

Youssou N'Dour (born 1959) was born in Dakar, Senegal. As a child, he learned to sing from his mother, a *griot* (storyteller). N'Dour performs and tours with artists around the world and has collaborated with musicians such as Peter Gabriel and Paul Simon. He wrote the music for the World Cup Soccer anthem and his album *Eyes Open* received a Grammy nomination. N'Dour performs and writes music in a world music style.

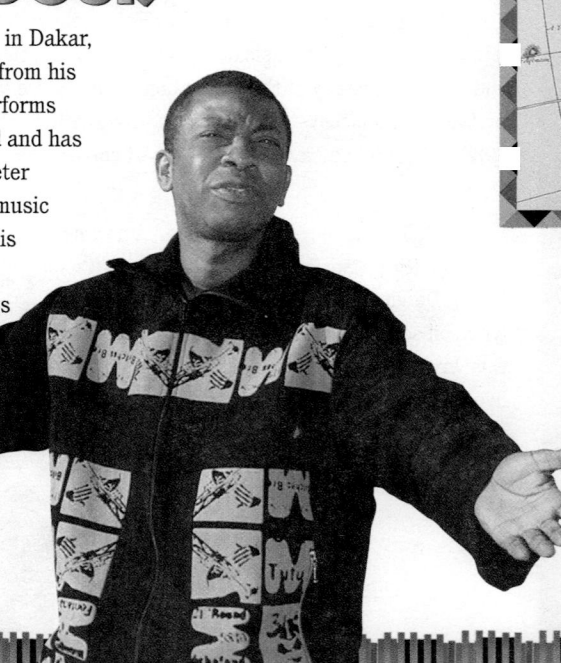

Footnotes

SPOTLIGHT ON

▶ **World Beat Music Around the World** Youssou N'Dour is one of many artists who write and perform some of their music in world beat style. Other artists include Paul Simon, Peter Gabriel, Zap Mama, and Ladysmith Black Mambazo.

BUILDING SKILLS THROUGH MUSIC

▶ **Writing** Have students write a brief paragraph describing how changes in transportation and communication have affected the influence that music from other countries has on American music (from the early 1900s to today). Ask students to volunteer to share their paragraphs.

ACROSS THE CURRICULUM

 ▶ **Related Arts** Students may enjoy designing a world beat bulletin board. Start with style categories, including Afropop, hip-hop, funk, jazz, *a cappella, salsa,* and folk. Students may post a world map, photos, CD covers, and names of current world beat artists, including the ones featured in this lesson. Use yarn or string to connect the style categories to the appropriate artists, countries, and so on.

For more on the influence of world beat, refer students to *The Roots of Rhythm,* a video series narrated by Harry Belafonte. It includes background information on Afro-Cuban music, *salsa,* and other world beat styles.

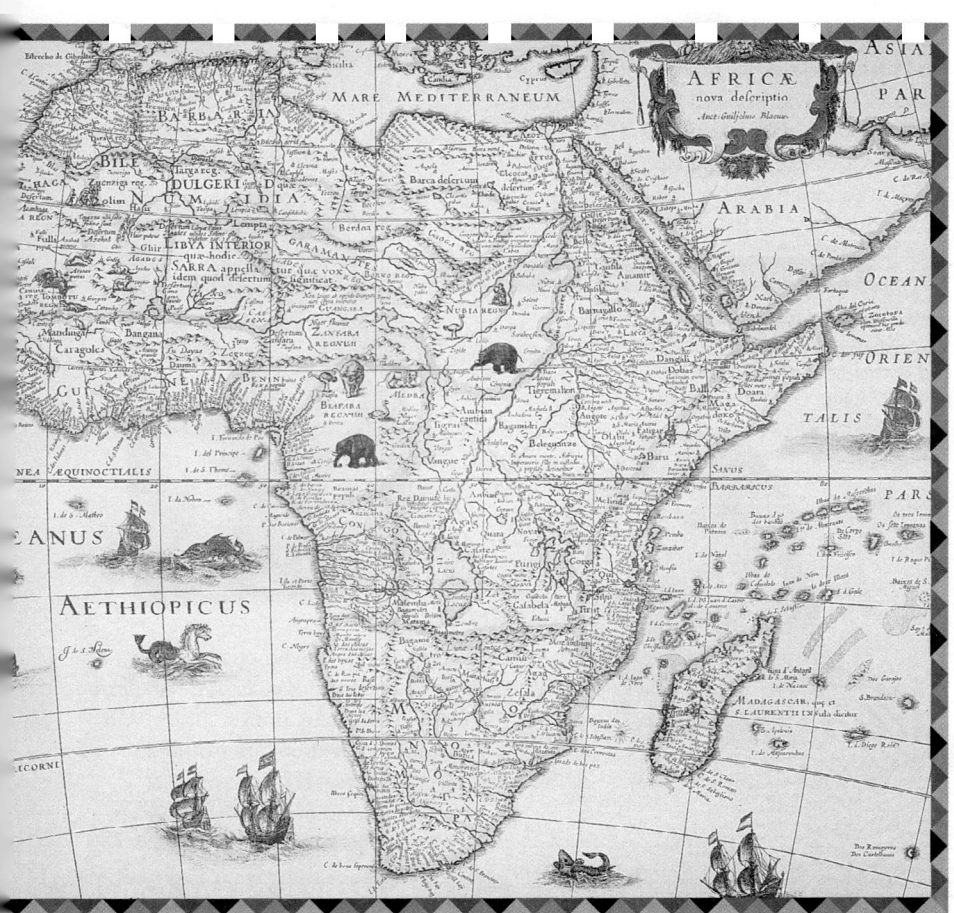

Go to the Source

African and aboriginal music are a source of ideas and inspiration to musicians, such as Herbie Hancock. **Listen** to a recording of the Ba-Benzélé pygmies.

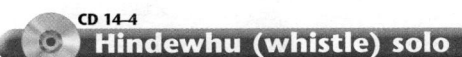

CD 14–4

Hindewhu (whistle) solo

Traditional pygmy voice and whistle solo by the Ba-Benzélé pygmies

This delightful combination of whistle and voice can give you ideas about how to experiment with your own voice.

1 INTRODUCE

Ask students about different kinds of food or art that they like from different cultures. Discuss how cultures share ideas.

Mention that the growth of worldwide communication networks, such as the Internet, has helped people all over the world share elements of culture, including styles of music. This lesson guides students to relate styles of music to their culture of origin. Be sure to include the information in Spotlight On, pp. 268 and 270; Across the Curriculum, p. 268; and Cultural Connection, p. 270 and below, in your discussion.

Today, influences on new music can come from any-where on Earth. This lesson is also all about world beat—cultures sharing music across the world.

2 DEVELOP

Listening

Have students

8b

- Read and discuss the background of Senegal-born vocalist Youssou N'Dour, on p. 268.

6a

- Listen to *The Same* CD **14–3**. Ask students to focus on the Afro-Caribbean drumming, the jazz har-monies, and the message of the song's lyrics.

6b

Playing

World beat rhythm patterns are prominent in D'Nour's *The Same*. Encourage students to

- Choose a nonpitched percussion instrument and improvise world beat patterns similar to what they hear in the recording.

- Layer additional rhythm patterns to create a world beat style.

- Adapt rhythm patterns from the other world drumming cultures and listening selections found in this lesson.

continued on page 270

CULTURAL CONNECTION

▶ **Ba-Benzélé Pygmies** The pygmies of the southwestern Central African Republic are nomadic hunter-gatherers, who hunt, fish, and collect wild plants in the forest for food. Most Pygmy communities have fewer than 50 people. Average height for adult pygmies is about 4 feet 4 inches. Pygmy religious beliefs are centered on the forest. Pygmy musicians make the unique sound heard in the *Hindewhu* recording by alternately singing and blowing notes on a panpipe made from the hollow stems of papaya leaves. Another piece of music inspired by *Hindewhu* is *Walking Song* by Kevin Volans (Chandos; Netherlands Wind Ensemble).

SKILLS REINFORCEMENT

6b ▶ **Listening** The students might enjoy the challenge of a Drop-the-Needle game, using the six examples presented in this lesson. Allow students to become thoroughly familiar with the selections. Suggest that they learn to recognize the music, the style, the artists, and the country of origin of each piece. Then, when students come to class, play a few phrases of several of the pieces. (A selection may be repeated if a different part is used.) Ask students to write and describe information about the musical characteristics and cultural traits of each listening example they hear.

Listening

Encourage students to read p. 269 and

- Discuss the Ba-Benzélé Pygmies of the Central African Republic and their musical style. See Cultural Connection, p. 269, for more information on the Pygmies.

- Listen to *Hindewhu (whistle) solo* **CD 14–4.**

ASK How would you describe this effect of combining yodeling and whistling? (Accept all valid responses.)

Have students read the information on Herbie Hancock on p. 270 and

- Discuss Herbie Hancock's role (U.S.A.) as a leading figure in the fusion style that brought world music into the context of jazz.

- Listen for the solo at the beginning of *Watermelon Man* **CD 14–5.**

ASK How is this similar to the sound of the Ba-Benzélé Pygmies' *Hindewhu*? (In creating *Watermelon Man*, Hancock was inspired by *Hindewhu*.)

Play *Watermelon Man* again and ask students to

- Listen for how the music builds in layers. (Point out that this is a very important trait of African music.)

- Listen for the B section (saxophone solo) that sounds more like mainstream jazz, and the return of the A section in a more African style.

Play *Watchers of the Canyon* **CD 14–6,** written and performed by the group Burning Sky. Explain to students that the two flute players are from the Diné Nation and the White River Ute Nation of Native Americans.

ASK What cultural musical style elements do you hear? (folk guitar, Native American flute, African American syncopation, modern jazz harmonies)

Pygmy Inspired Music

Listen to a classic jazz recording by Herbie Hancock that was inspired by the Ba-Benzélé pygmy vocal style on page 269. Hancock used this African inspiration to help create a new jazz style called fusion.

Burning Sky ▼

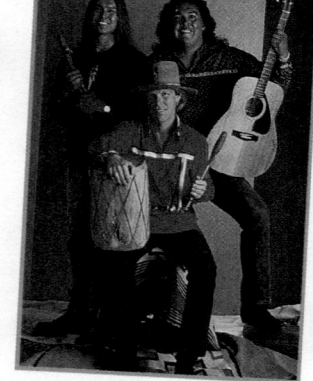

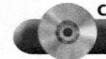
CD 14–5
Watermelon Man

written and performed by Herbie Hancock

Hancock uses a pygmy theme at the beginning and end of the piece. He builds typical African layered patterns that go with the theme.

Herbie Hancock
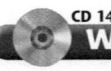

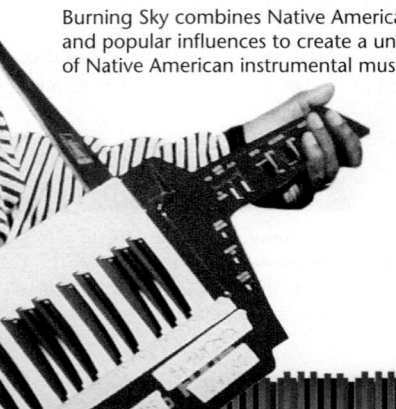

Sky Sounds

Listen to the Native American group Burning Sky perform *Watchers of the Canyon*. The guitar, bass, flute, drums, rattles, and the African *djembe* drum are featured in this selection. **Identify** the musical instruments that sound Native American.

CD 14–6
Watchers of the Canyon

written and performed by Burning Sky

Burning Sky combines Native American, African, and popular influences to create a unique sound of Native American instrumental music.

270

Footnotes

CULTURAL CONNECTION

▶ **Aborigines of Australia** Before Europeans arrived in Australia, there were about 750,000 Aborigines. Their present population is estimated at about 125,000. There were originally about 500 different tribal groups. Each had its own language or dialect and region of the continent. Although Aborigines were mostly nomadic hunter-gatherers, they traded goods and shared religious ceremonies with neighboring tribes. Much like the native peoples of North America, Australian Aborigines' religious beliefs connect them closely with nature and all other living things. Aborigines have elaborate musical, ceremonial, and artistic traditions.

SPOTLIGHT ON

▶ **The Performer** Called the Mariah Carey of the East, CoCo Lee has sold over 6 million albums worldwide. She attends the University of California, Irvine, with a double major in biochemistry and bioscience. Born in Hong Kong in 1975, CoCo Lee was raised in San Francisco and entered singing contests, following her sisters' leads. While vacationing in Hong Kong, she entered a contest, just for fun—and won! Her unique style earned her a recording contract.

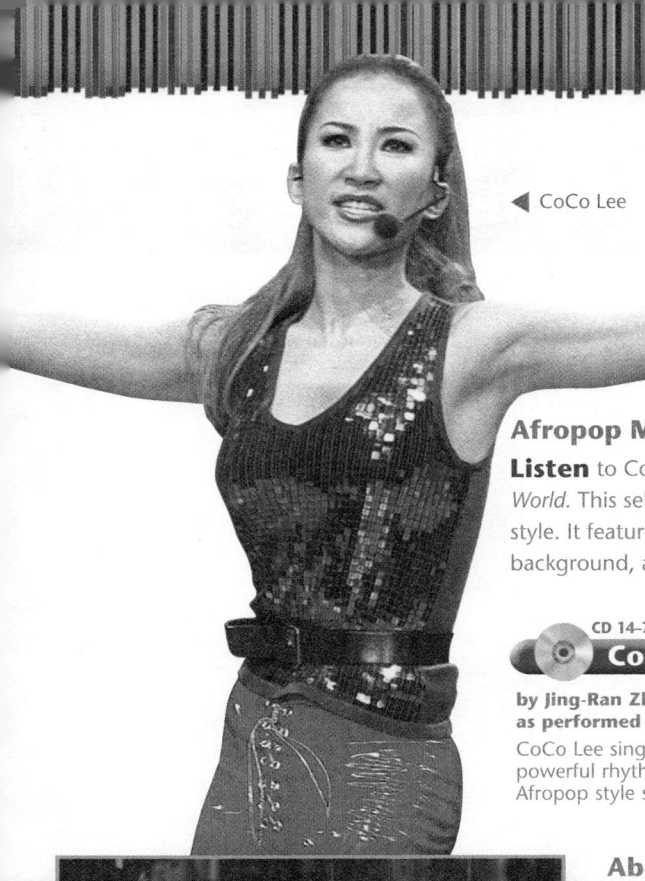

◄ CoCo Lee

Afropop Meets Rap

Listen to CoCo Lee perform *Colours of the World*. This selection is in a typical world beat style. It features Afropop, hip-hop, DJ background, and an emcee rap.

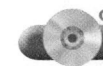
CD 14–7
Colours of the World

by Jing-Ran Zhu and Qui-Hong Her as performed by CoCo Lee

CoCo Lee sings with a big pop sound over a powerful rhythmic background. This sample of Afropop style shows a world music influence.

Aboriginal Sounds

Listen to the bird sounds in *Brolga*. The piece begins with a recording of the Aborigines on Elcho Island, north of Australia. The sound imitates the Brolga bird, crying as it beats its wings on the water of the sacred water hole.

▲ Aborigine playing a *didgeridoo*

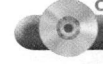
CD 14–8
Brolga

by Graham Wiggins, Mark Revell, and Ian Campbell as performed by Dr. Didg and Outback

Brolga uses traditional Australian Aboriginal instruments, including *didgeridoos* and clapping sticks.

Tune In

The *didgeridoo* is a long hollow tube played with the breath and vibrating lips in a fashion much like the tuba. Players use circular breathing (blowing out of the mouth while breathing in from the nose) to sustain long drone tones.

Listening

Invite students to read about CoCo Lee and

9a
- Discuss the influences of Afropop and hip-hop (rap) on Chinese American singer CoCo Lee.

6b
- Listen for this basic "*doom chik-a doom chik-a*" Afropop beat in *Colours of the World* **CD 14–7.**

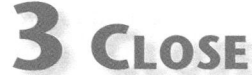

- Listen for the hip-hop/rap section in the middle of the selection, Middle Eastern flavors, and African American vocal stylings.

Invite students to read about Aboriginal sounds and

- Discuss how the Australian *didgeridoo* is played.

8b
- Discuss the Australian Aborigines. See Cultural Connection, p. 270.

Invite students to listen to a recording of the *didgeridoo* in the Sound Bank, beginning on p. 512.

Play *Brolga* **CD 14–8** and ask students to

- Listen for Aboriginal music at the beginning of this selection: voices, sticks, and the didgeridoo.

6a
- Listen for entrances of Western instruments layered with the Aboriginal music and how the new music takes over.

- Listen for a featured solo instrument (melodica).

- Listen for how the piece ends.

3 CLOSE

Skill: LISTENING   ASSESSMENT

6b
Music Journal Writing Play all of the recordings from this lesson (*The Same* **CD 14–3**, *Hindewhu (whistle) solo* **CD 14–4**, *Watchers of the Canyon* **CD 14–6**, *Watermelon Man* **CD 14–5**, *Colours of the World* **CD 14–7**, and *Brolga* **CD 14–8**) For each selection, have students write a description of the different musical influences, especially with regard to rhythm, from various parts of the world.

TEACHER TO TEACHER

8b ▶ **Make a *Didgeridoo*** The Aboriginal *didgeridoo* of northern Australia is a thin tree hollowed out naturally by termites. For classroom use, you can make a fine *didgeridoo* out of a length of $1\frac{1}{2}$" PVC pipe about 5 feet long. Students can experiment with the unique sound it makes. Tell students it is played in the same way as a brass instrument, by buzzing the lips. Most *didgeridoo* players practice circular breathing—simultaneously breathing in through the nose while blowing out through the mouth—thus enabling them to produce a long tone without interruption. It is also possible to sing and play the *didgeridoo* at the same time, but that might take a bit of practice on your class-made instrument!

TECHNOLOGY/MEDIA LINK

CD-ROM Divide the class into groups of three. Using the computer as a learning center, ask students to create and record their own composition using *Band-in-a-Box*. Have students

- Create a new file and enter chords for the composition. (Students can use I, IV, V as a starting point.)

- Explore several different musical styles (African.sty, Caribean.sty, Eurobea3.sty, and LtnBrazl.sty) from the program's style menu, then choose a style for their piece.

- Set an appropriate tempo for their style.

- Play their compositions for the class.

Lesson	Elements	Skills

LESSON 1

Drums Around the World

pp. 276–279

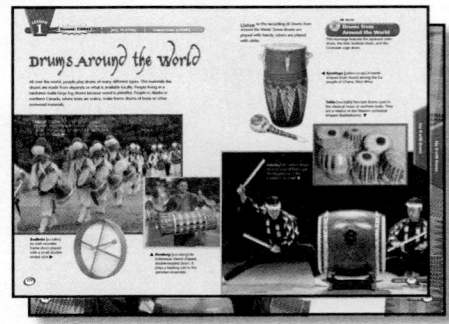

Element: Timbre
Concept: Instrumental
Focus: Drums from around the world

Secondary Element
Rhythm: pattern

National Standards
2a 2c 3b 6b 7a 8b 9c

Skill: Playing
Objective: Perform echo and question-and-answer drumming patterns

Secondary Skills
- **Listening** Listen to a variety of drums from across the world
- **Playing** Play "open" and "bass" tones on conga drum
- **Creating** Create two-beat question-and-answer drum patterns

SKILLS REINFORCEMENT
- **Playing** Play a steady beat on drums

LESSON 2

Musical Teamwork

pp. 280–283

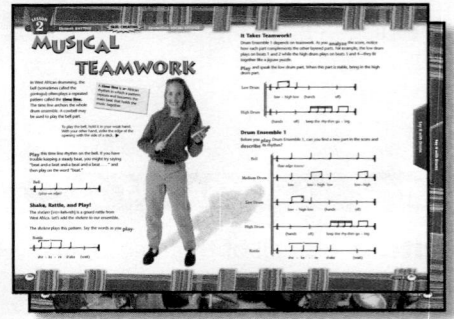

Element: Rhythm
Concept: Pattern
Focus: West African layered rhythms

Secondary Element
Timbre: instrumental

National Standards
2a 2c 4a 5a 6b 8b 9a

Skill: Creating
Objective: Create a drum piece to be performed by a classroom drum ensemble

Secondary Skills
- **Playing** Practice playing a cowbell and shekere; perform in an African drum ensemble
- **Singing** Sing a song with drum ensemble
- **Listening** Listen to and recognize the influence of African percussion

SKILLS REINFORCEMENT
- **Keyboard** Play a keyboard accompaniment
- **Listening/Playing** Have a drum ensemble play along with various styles of recordings

---

LESSON 3

Native American Drumming

pp. 284–287

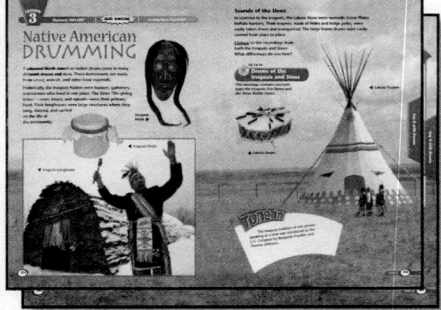

Element: Melody
Concept: Pitch and direction
Focus: Native American melody using vocables

Secondary Element
Timbre: vocal

National Standards
1c 2c 6b 8b 9a 9c

Skill: Singing
Objective: Sing a Native American song while performing a simple round dance

Secondary Skills
- **Listening** Listen to and discuss Native American drummings; listen to and discuss a Navajo selection
- **Singing** Sing a Native American song with vocables
- **Moving** Perform a circle dance with song

SKILLS REINFORCEMENT
- **Playing** Sight read a drum pattern with mixed meter

Connections

Music and Other Literature

Connection: Science

Activity: Discuss the science of local drum construction

ACROSS THE CURRICULUM
Science Read about how drums are made
Language Arts Read a book about Japanese drum history

CHARACTER EDUCATION **Respect** Promote respect by means of cooperation and teamwork

CULTURAL CONNECTION **Natural Resources** Local materials influence instruments

TEACHER TO TEACHER **Management Tips** Keeping everyone involved in drumming

MEETING INDIVIDUAL NEEDS **Including Everyone** Motivate students with question-and-answer drumming

SCHOOL TO HOME CONNECTION **Interactive Bulletin Board** Find more information about drums and drummers from around the world

BUILDING SKILLS THROUGH MUSIC **Science** Discuss the location of rainforests

---

Listening Selection *Drums from Around the World*

More Music Choices
"*Bát kim thang*," p. 13
"*O lê lê O Bahí a*," p. 165
"*Siyahamba*," p. 212
"*Wai bamba*," p. 26

ASSESSMENT

Performance/Peer Critique Perform question-and-answer drumming with proper technique

TECHNOLOGY/MEDIA LINK
Web Site Information on African drumming

Connection: Social Studies

Activity: Examine how teamwork is developed by performing in a drum ensemble

MEETING INDIVIDUAL NEEDS **Visual/Motor Coordination** Assisting students with drumming

CULTURAL CONNECTION **Liberia** Facts on Liberia

ACROSS THE CURRICULUM
Social Studies Discuss social relevance of question-and-answer drumming
Language Arts/Drama Read a Liberian story and dramatize

TEACHER TO TEACHER
Teaching Tips: Drum Ensemble 1 Tips on ensemble drumming
Management Tip Teamwork in drumming

AUDIENCE ETIQUETTE **Rehearsal Etiquette for Performers** Points on rehearsal etiquette

SCHOOL TO HOME CONNECTION **Drumming Clinic** Teach friends and family

BUILDING SKILLS THROUGH MUSIC **Writing** Describe teamwork

Song "*Nana Kru*"

Listening Selection *Lost River*

More Music Choices
"Lost My Gold Ring," p. 158
"New Hungarian Folk Song," p. 196

ASSESSMENT

Performance/Peer Critique Create and perform a drum ensemble; assess the performance

TECHNOLOGY/MEDIA LINK
Electronic Keyboard Use West African percussion sounds as accompaniment

---

Connection: Culture

Activity: Examine diverse Native American cultures

CULTURAL CONNECTION
A Way of Life Importance of the Iroquois Longhouse
The Navajo A Navajo creation story

ACROSS THE CURRICULUM
Social Studies Facts on the Iroquois
Language Arts Read books about the Navajo

SPOTLIGHT ON **The Great Sioux Nation** History of the Sioux

MOVEMENT **Patterned Dance** Learn the circle dance

BUILDING SKILLS THROUGH MUSIC **Social Studies** Learn about Native American tribes

---

Song "Yo-shi nai"

Listening Selections
Drums of the Iroquois and Sioux
Jo'ashila
M·U·S·I·C M·A·K·E·R·S
Marilyn Hood

More Music Choices
"Go My Son," p. 188
Round Dance (excerpt), p. 445

ASSESSMENT

Performance/Peer Critique Sing a song in small groups and have them assess their performances

TECHNOLOGY/MEDIA LINK
Web Site Information on Native American music and instruments

Lesson	Elements	Skills

LESSON 4

Rhythms from West Africa

pp. 288–293

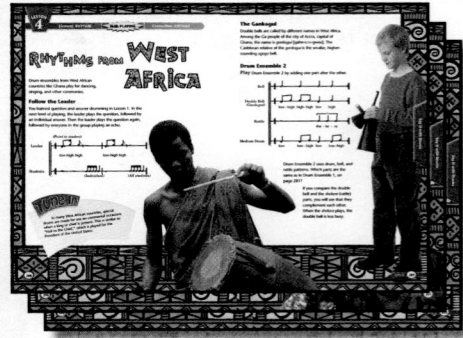

Element: Rhythm
Concept: Pattern
Focus: West African rhythm patterns

Secondary Element
Harmony: thirds and sixths

National Standards
1c 2b 2c 4a 5a 6b 9c

Skill: Playing
Objective: Perform as part of a drum ensemble

Secondary Skills
- **Playing** Perform question-and-answer drumming patterns; play a West African drum ensemble; play a gankogui (double bell)
- **Notating** Notate each instrument part of a drum ensemble
- **Singing** Sing two African songs with rhythm accompaniment
- **Listening** Listen to and discuss a Ghanaian master drummer
- **Creating** Create a drum ensemble in highlife style

SKILLS REINFORCEMENT
- **Notating** Notate each part of a drum ensemble
- **Mallets** Play an accompaniment
- **Creating** Create a time line rhythm pattern on a gankogui
- **Recorder** Play harmony parts on soprano and alto recorder

---

LESSON 5

A Taste of the Highlife

pp. 294–297

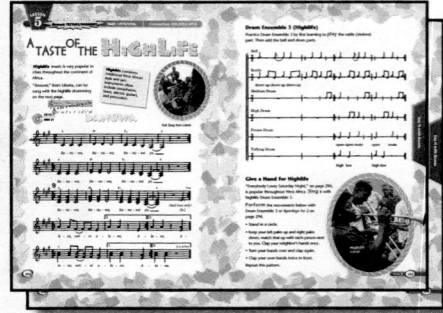

Element: Texture/Harmony
Concept: Texture
Focus: Thick texture

Secondary Element
Rhythm: syncopation

National Standards
1c 1d 2c 4c 5c 6b 9c

Skill: Listening
Objective: Listen to a percussion ensemble piece while following a listening map

Secondary Skills
- **Singing** Sing a Liberian song in harmony; sing a highlife song
- **Playing** Play a drum piece in highlife style
- **Listening** Listen to a master drummer
- **Moving** Perform hand-clapping movements to a highlife song

SKILLS REINFORCEMENT
- **Notating** Notate triads
- **Reading** Read a highlife rhythm
- **Recorder** Play an accompaniment on soprano recorder
- **Keyboard** Play a finger exercise
- **Mallets** Play an accompaniment in highlife style
- **Signing** Learn signing to a highlife song

LESSON 6

Caribbean Connections

pp. 298–301

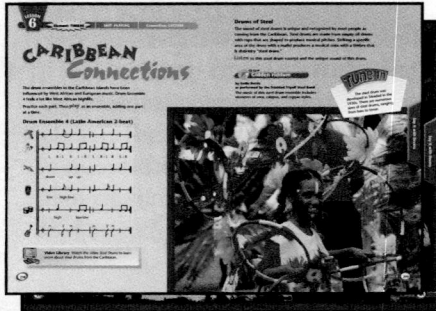

Element: Timbre
Concept: Instrumental
Focus: Caribbean percussion instruments

Secondary Element
Harmony: thirds and sixths

National Standards
1c 1d 2b 2c 2d 4c

Skill: Playing
Objective: Perform in a Latin drum ensemble

Secondary Skills
- **Listening** Listen to a steel drum
- **Playing** Learn to play the claves, maracas, guiro and bongos
- **Singing** Sing songs with a call and response in harmony

SKILLS REINFORCEMENT
- **Singing** Sing harmony in thirds and sixths
- **Mallets** Play an accompaniment
- **Guitar** Play an accompaniment
- **Recorder** Play an accompaniment on the soprano and alto recorder

Connections

Music and Other Literature

Connection: Culture

Activity: Examine the role of the master drummer in West African culture

ACROSS THE CURRICULUM
Social Studies Share a geography book on Ghana
Language Arts Share a book set in Liberia

CULTURAL CONNECTION Ghana Facts on Ghana

MEETING INDIVIDUAL NEEDS **Including Everyone** Alternate drumming techniques

SPOTLIGHT ON
Master Drummer Master drummers in Ghana
The Performer Information on the drummer, Sowah Mensah

CHARACTER EDUCATION **Taking Time for Yourself**

TEACHER TO TEACHER **Management Tips** Listening skills

MOVEMENT Patterned Dance Learn a dance to an African song

BUILDING SKILLS THROUGH MUSIC **Social Studies** Discuss careers in music

Song *Kelo aba w'ye*

Listening Selection *Obokete* (excerpt)
M•U•S•I•C M•A•K•E•R•S
Sowah Mensah

More Music Choices
Ionisation, p. 357
Kebjar teruna, p. 385

ASSESSMENT

Performance/Peer Critique Play a drum ensemble and assess using provided criteria

TECHNOLOGY/MEDIA LINK
Web Site Research African percussion instruments

Connection: Related Arts

Activity: Discuss the folk art of African *kente* cloth

MEETING INDIVIDUAL NEEDS **Including Everyone** Hand clapping activities

SPOTLIGHT ON **Highlife** Facts on this influential African musical style

CULTURAL CONNECTION *Kente* Cloth from Ghana Facts on this African cloth

MOVEMENT Patterned Dance Learn a highlife dance

BUILDING SKILLS THROUGH MUSIC **Social Studies** Learn about relevant African locations

Songs
"*Banuwa*"
"Everybody Loves Saturday Night"

Listening Selections
Kpanlogo for 2 (excerpt)
Evening Samba
Listening Map *Evening Samba*

More Music Choices
"Siyahamba," p. 212
"Wai bamba," p. 26

ASSESSMENT

Music Journal Writing Listen to a recording and describe texture changes in student journal

TECHNOLOGY/MEDIA LINK
Sequencing Software Create African drum tracks
Transparency Display the listening map transparency for *Evening Samba*

Connection: Culture

Activity: Discuss Caribbean geography and culture

CULTURAL CONNECTION
Calypso Style Facts on the calypso musical style
Two Caribbean Nations Trinidad and Tobago; Cuba

ACROSS THE CURRICULUM **Language Arts** Discuss famous individuals from Cuba

MEETING INDIVIDUAL NEEDS **Learning Idioms** Discuss idioms to understand lyrics

SPOTLIGHT ON "*Má Teodora*" Background on the song

CHARACTER EDUCATION **Sensitivity** Discuss the benefits of crying

BUILDING SKILLS THROUGH MUSIC **Language** Discuss the meaning of lyrics

Songs
"Water Come a Me Eye"
"*Má Teodora*"

Listening Selection
Gidden riddum (excerpt)

More Music Choices
"Give a Little Love," p. 140
"Lost My Gold Ring," p. 158

ASSESSMENT

Portfolio Create and share a list of Caribbean music sounds

TECHNOLOGY/MEDIA LINK
CD-ROM Use *Band-in-a-Box* to create a Caribbean accompaniment
Video Library Show the video *Steel Drums*

Lesson	Elements	Skills

LESSON 7
Asian Drums
pp. 302–303

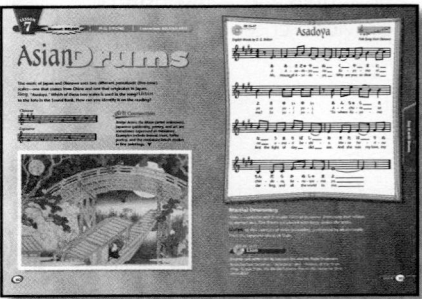

Element: Melody
Concept: Tonality
Focus: Pentatonic scales

Secondary Element
Rhythm: beat

National Standards
1c 3b 8a 9a 9c

Skill: Singing
Objective: Sing a folk song in Japanese

Secondary Skills
• **Singing** Sing a song in English and Japanese with vocables
• **Listening** Listen to and discuss taiko drumming

SKILLS REINFORCEMENT
• **Mallets** Play an accompaniment

LESSON 8
Indian Rhythms
pp. 304–305

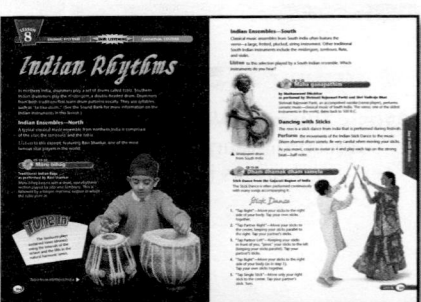

Element: Rhythm
Concept: Pattern
Focus: Indian drum improvisation within a *tala*

Secondary Element
Timbre: instrumental

National Standards
2c 6a 6b 9a

Skill: Listening
Objective: Listen to and echo the rhythms played by North Indian tabla drummers

Secondary Skills
• **Listening** Listen to and discuss Indian drumming ensembles
• **Movement** Learn the movements to the Indian stick dance

SKILLS REINFORCEMENT
• **Playing** Play and echo tabla drum rhythm patterns

LESSON 9
Shades of the Middle East
pp. 306–309

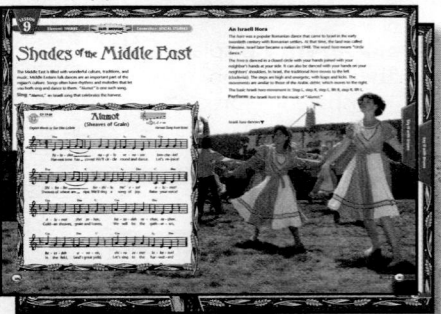

Element: Timbre
Concept: Instrumental
Focus: Percussion from the Middle East

Secondary Element
Expression: tempo

National Standards
1c 2c 5a 8b 9a

Skill: Moving
Objective: Sing and move to two Middle Eastern celebration songs

Secondary Skills
• **Singing** Sing an Israeli harvest song in Hebrew; sing a Palestinian folk song
• **Movement** Introduce the *hora* and *debke* dances to students
• **Playing** Play a *dombak* to accompany the *debke*

SKILLS REINFORCEMENT
• **Creating** Create embellished rhythms with recording

LESSON 10
African Influences
pp. 310–311

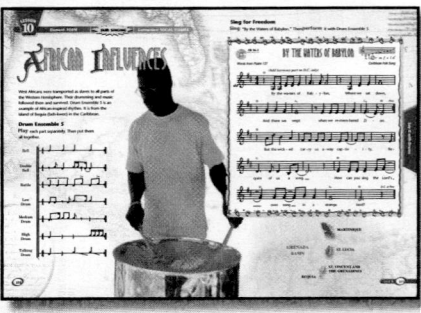

Element: Form
Concept: Form
Focus: aabaa phrase form; ABA section form

Secondary Element
Expression: dynamics

National Standards
1c 2c 7b 8b

Skill: Singing
Objective: Sing a Caribbean folk song

Secondary Skills
• **Playing** Play a drum ensemble accompaniment
• **Singing** Sing in two-part harmony

SKILLS REINFORCEMENT
• **Playing** Teach a low drum part

Connections	Music and Other Literature	

Connection: Related Arts
Activity: Discuss minimalism in Japanese fine arts

CULTURAL CONNECTION **Japanese Fine Arts** Information on fine arts in Japan

SPOTLIGHT ON
Taiko Facts on Japanese taiko drumming
Asadoya Learn about the song

BUILDING SKILLS THROUGH MUSIC **Language** Learn about Kodo Drummers

Song "Asadoya"

Listening Selection *Lion* (excerpt)

More Music Choices
"*Bát kim thang*," p. 13

ASSESSMENT

Performance/Observation Improvise a pentatonic melody for provided lyrics

TECHNOLOGY/MEDIA LINK
MIDI/Sequencing Software Create MIDI drum tracks in *taiko* style

Connection: Culture
Activity: Examine Indian culture and dance

ACROSS THE CURRICULUM **Social Studies** Read a book on Indian culture

MOVEMENT **Patterned Dance** Perform the traditional Indian stick dance

BUILDING SKILLS THROUGH MUSIC **Social Studies** Research and discuss North and South India

Listening Selections
Máru-bihág (excerpt)
Maha ganapathin (excerpt)
Dham dhamak dham samelu (excerpt)

More Music Choices
"*La mariposa*," p. 58

ASSESSMENT

Written Assessment Listen to a selection and identify the function of each instrument

TECHNOLOGY/MEDIA LINK
Web Site Information on the music and instruments of India
Video Library Watch video Instrumental Ensemble

Connection: Social Studies
Activity: Examine the geography and history of the Middle East

CULTURAL CONNECTION **Israel** Facts about Israel and its people

ACROSS THE CURRICULUM **Social Studies** Discuss the history of Palestine

SPOTLIGHT ON
The Hora Share facts on this Israeli dance
The Debke Share facts on this Arabic dance

MOVEMENT **Patterned Dance** Learn the steps to the hora and the debke

BUILDING SKILLS THROUGH MUSIC **Dance** Compare and contrast dance types

Songs
"Alumot" ("Sheaves of Grain")
"Al yadee"

Listening Selection *Yemeni baglamis telli basina* (excerpt)

More Music Choices
"Hava nagila," p. 153
"Shalom aleichem," p. 409

ASSESSMENT

Performance/Observation Perform two Middle Eastern songs with traditional dance movements and compare the two

TECHNOLOGY/MEDIA LINK
Web Site Information on Middle Eastern music

Connection: Social Studies
Activity: Discuss the influence of West African music on the music of the Caribbean

ACROSS THE CURRICULUM **Social Studies** Read about the Caribbean

SPOTLIGHT ON **Bequia** Discuss facts on the Grenadine Islands

BUILDING SKILLS THROUGH MUSIC **Social Studies** Research islands of the Carribean

Song "By the Waters of Babylon"

More Music Choices
"Give a Little Love," p. 140
"Water Come a Me Eye," p. 300

ASSESSMENT

Performance/Self-Assessment Create a classroom performance of a song that reinforces the form of the song

TECHNOLOGY/MEDIA LINK
Sequencing Software Use digital recording to record ensemble performances

INTRODUCING THE UNIT

Today's world music is influenced by drumming from around the world. Drums are an important part of many musical styles. From African, Native American, Asian, and Indian drumming to contemporary Afropop, drumming is prominent in our music. In this unit, students will *Say it with Drums* from a variety of cultures and musical styles.

UNIT PROJECT

As students learn to play together in ensembles, they will naturally want to share the joy with others.

Tell students that in this unit they will put together an *informance* (A performance focused on sharing what students have learned) that involves the audience.

Have students

- Learn some of the ensembles and related songs.
- Decide which pieces are ready to share with others and prepare them for presentation. This should include issues such as how to start, stop, when to sing, or perhaps whether individuals are going to take solos. Question-and-answer drumming can also be shared.
- Decide whether they wish to showcase any of their own student ensembles.
- Discuss whether they think the informance should include short selections of recordings of drumming from around the world.
- Consider whether they wish to teach any members of the audience how to play one of the easy ensembles.
- Develop visual material showing what they have learned from drumming together in ensembles. Concepts could include teamwork, focusing, listening, respect, unity, taking turns, and cooperation.

Welcome to World Drumming

There is an explosion of interest in "world drumming"—the drumming styles and music from around the world.

Listen to *Welcome to Our World* by Lebo M. This song combines choral and rhythmic styles of the African continent with contemporary pop style.

CD 14–9
Welcome to Our World
written and performed by Lebo M.

The lyrics of this song are in Zulu, Sethoso, Wolof, and English and are intended to "honor the people of the entire world."

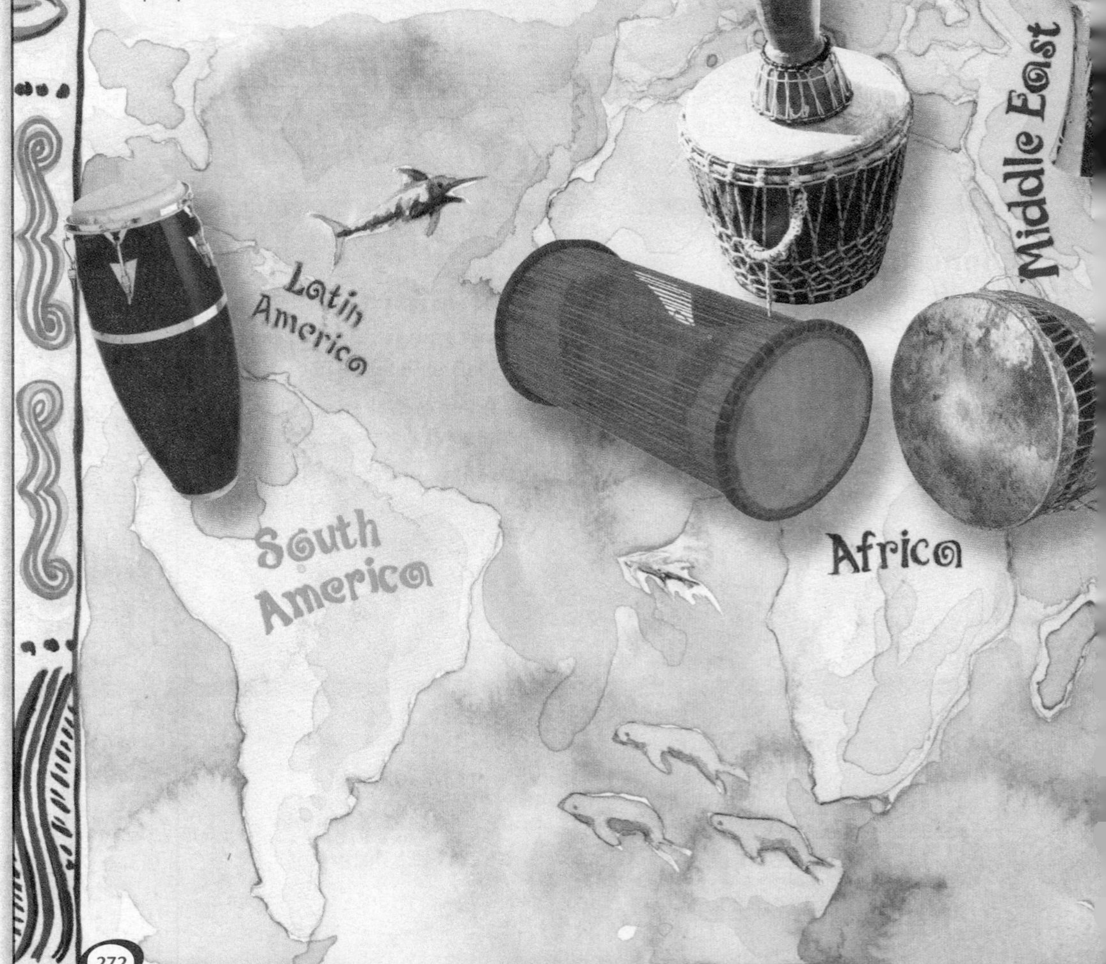

272

ACROSS THE CURRICULUM

Unit Highlights The following interdisciplinary activities in this unit are related to the music elements presented in the lessons and are intended to enhance student learning. For a more detailed topical description, see the Unit at a Glance on pp. 271a–271f.

▶ **ART/DRAMA**

- Read a Liberian story and dramatize it (p. 283)

▶ **LANGUAGE ARTS**

- Read a book about Japanese drum history (p. 278)
- Read a Liberian story and dramatize it (p. 283)
- Read books about the Navajo (p. 286)
- Discuss famous individuals from the Caribbean (p. 298)

▶ **LITERATURE**

- Share a book set in Liberia (p. 291)

▶ **SOCIAL STUDIES**

- Discuss social relevance of question-and-answer drumming (p. 281)
- Learn facts about the Iroquois people (p. 284)
- Share a geography book on Ghana (p. 288)
- Read a book on Indian culture (p. 304)
- Learn about the history of Palestine (p. 306)
- Read about the Caribbean (p. 310)

▶ **SCIENCE**

- Discuss how drums are made (p. 276)

272

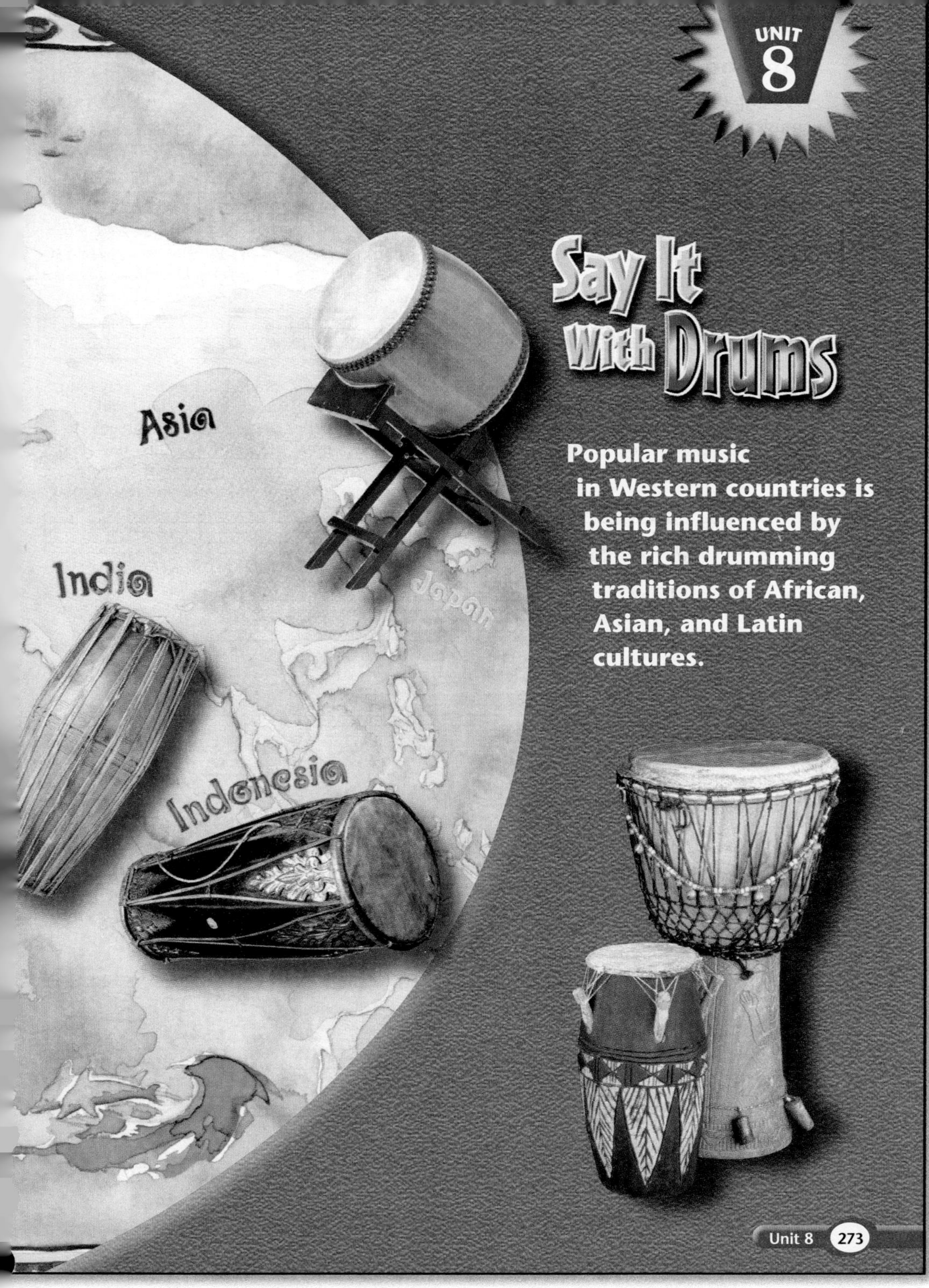

Say It with Drums

UNIT 8

Popular music in Western countries is being influenced by the rich drumming traditions of African, Asian, and Latin cultures.

Asia

India

Japan

Indonesia

Unit 8 273

MUSIC SKILLS ASSESSED IN THIS UNIT

Reading Music: Rhythm

- Practice two-beat echo and question-and-answer drumming (p. 279)
- Play a time line rhythm (p. 280)
- Play a drum ensemble (pp. 281, 289, 295, 298, 310)

Reading Music: Pitch

- Improvise a new melody for a phrase, based on a pentatonic scale (p. 303)

Performing Music: Singing

- Sing "Yo-shi-nai" and assess the performance (p. 287)
- Organize the class into different groups for a performance of "By the Waters of Babylon" (p. 311)

Performing Music: Playing

- Play Drum Ensemble 2 (p. 293)

Creating Music

- Create drum ensemble pieces (p. 283)
- Create a list of sounds that characterize Caribbean music (p. 301)
- Improvise a new melody for a phrase, based on a pentatonic scale (p. 303)

Listening to Music

- Follow a listening map for *Evening Samba* and indicate changes in texture (p. 297)
- Listen to *Maha ganapathim* and write a brief description of the instruments' functions (p. 305)

Moving to Music

- Sing and dance to "*Alumot*" and "*Al yadee*" (p. 309)

CULTURAL CONNECTION

Unit Highlights The musical literature in this unit provides many opportunities for students to explore a variety of world cultures. A more detailed description of the resources and activities listed below can be found in the Unit at a Glance on pp. 271a–271f.

▶ AFRICAN/AFRICAN AMERICAN

- Find out how local materials influence instruments in West Africa and many other regions (p. 277)
- Learn facts about Liberia (p. 280)
- Discover facts about Ghana (p. 288)
- Learn about *kente*, a cloth from Ghana (p. 295)

▶ ASIAN; AUSTRALIAN

- Gather more information about on Japanese fine arts (p. 302)

▶ CARIBBEAN

- Explore the history and style of calypso music (p. 298)
- Discuss the Caribbean nations of Trinidad and Tobago, and Cuba (p. 300)

▶ MIDDLE EASTERN

- Learn more information on Israel and its people (p. 306)

▶ NATIVE AMERICAN

- Learn about the importance of the Iroquois Longhouse (p. 284)
- Find out about the Navajo creation story (p. 286)

OPENING ACTIVITIES

MATERIALS

- "It's Time," p. 274   CD 14–10

  Recording Routine:
  Intro (6 m.); v.1; refrain; interlude (4 m.); v.2;
  refrain; coda

- percussion instruments

Listening

Have students listen to the recording of "It's Time" **CD 14–10** as they follow along in their books. Ask them to identify its regional influence. (Africa—call-and-response singing)

Reading

Ask students to look for the following features in the music:

- The road signs. (D.C., repeats)
- The rhythmic motive in m. 1 that is used in other parts of the song. (mm. 5, 7, 9)
- Melodic phrases or motives that use pitches D and A. (mm. 6, 8, 10, and *Let's celebrate.*)

Playing

Teach students the percussion parts first using body percussion or voices; then using real instruments.

After students have learned some of the drumming patterns presented in this unit, have them play drums and other classroom instruments along with *Welcome to Our World* **CD 14–9** and the Stereo Performance track of "It's Time" **CD 14–11.**

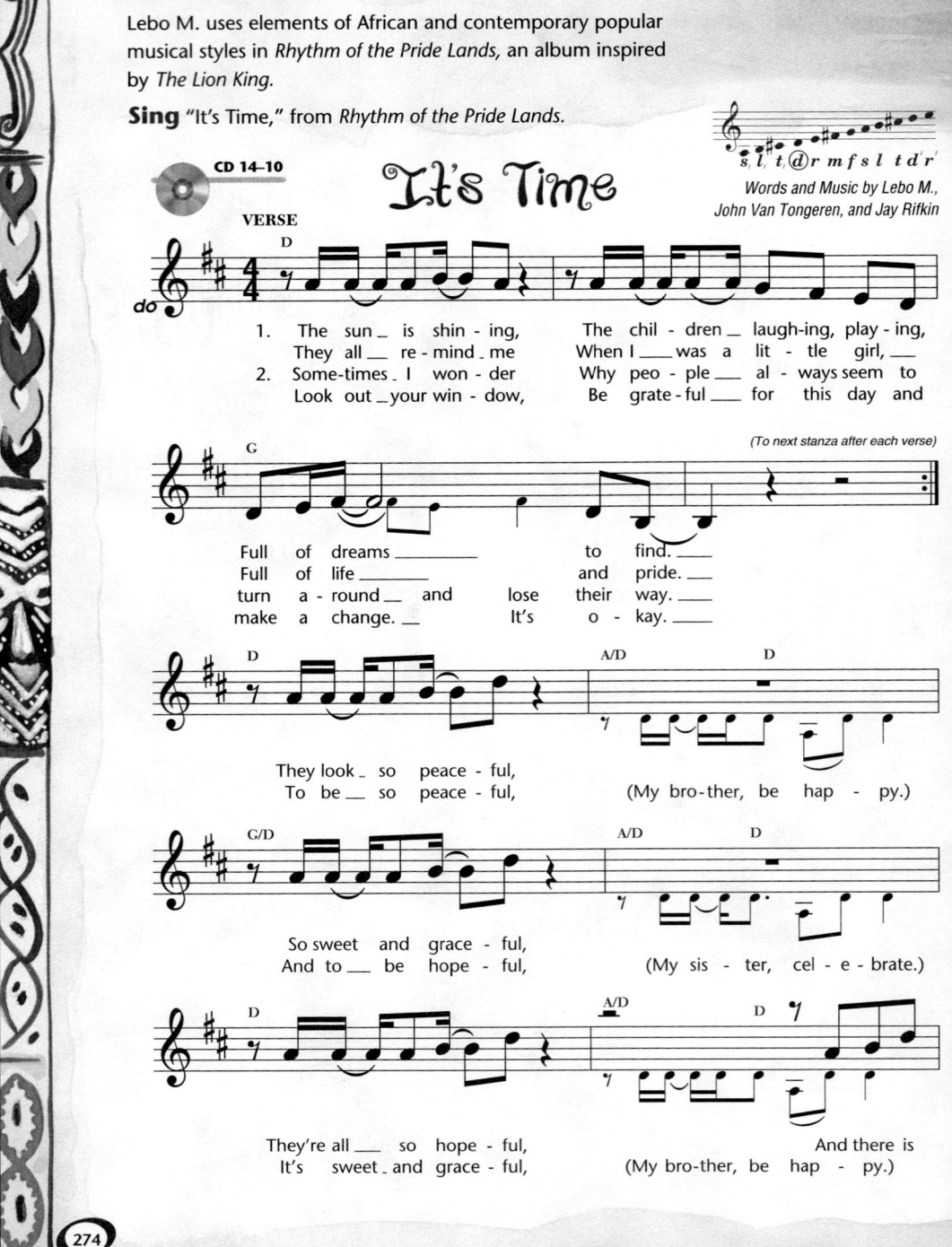

Life and Pride

Lebo M. uses elements of African and contemporary popular musical styles in *Rhythm of the Pride Lands,* an album inspired by *The Lion King.*

Sing "It's Time," from *Rhythm of the Pride Lands.*

274

Unit Highlights The lessons in this unit were chosen and developed to support the theme *Say It with Drums.* Each lesson, as always, presents a clear element focus, a skill objective, and an end-of-lesson assessment. The overall sequence of lessons, however, is organized according to this theme, rather than concept or skill development. In this context, formal assessment strategies, such as those presented in Units 1–6, are no longer applicable.

▶ **INFORMAL ASSESSMENTS**

At the close of each Teacher's Edition lesson in this unit, one of the following types of assessments is used to evaluate the learning of the key element focus or skill objective.

- Music Journal Writing (p. 297)
- Performance/Observation (pp. 303, 309)
- Performance/Peer Critique (pp. 279, 283. 287, 293)
- Performance/Self-Assessment (p. 311)
- Portfolio (p. 301)
- Written Assessment (p. 305)

▶ **RUBRICS**

Visit *www.sfsuccessnet.com* for rubrics to assess students' achievement in music skills.

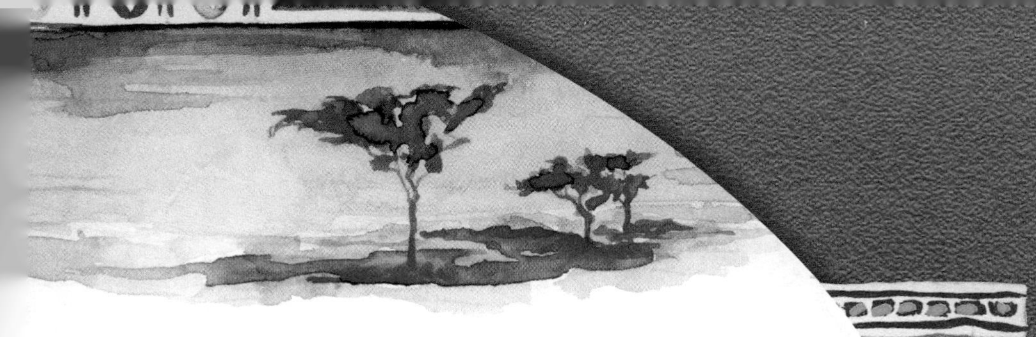

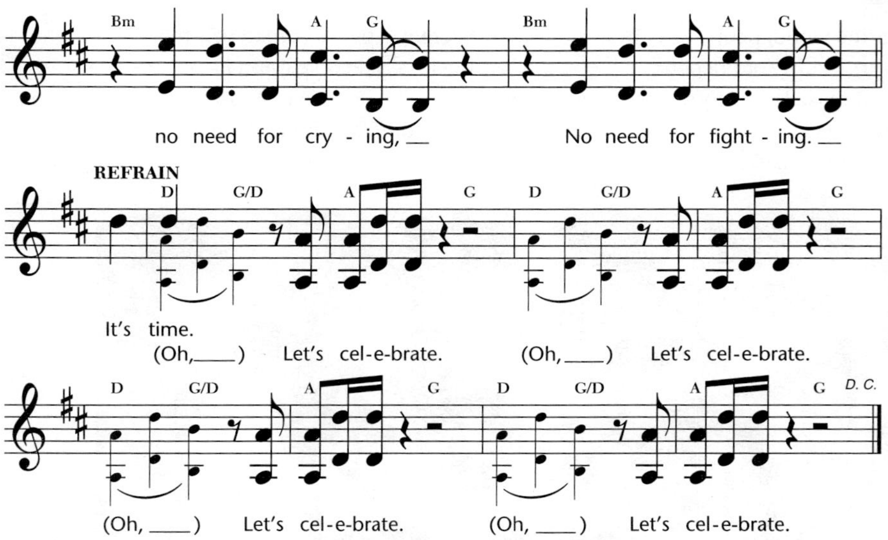

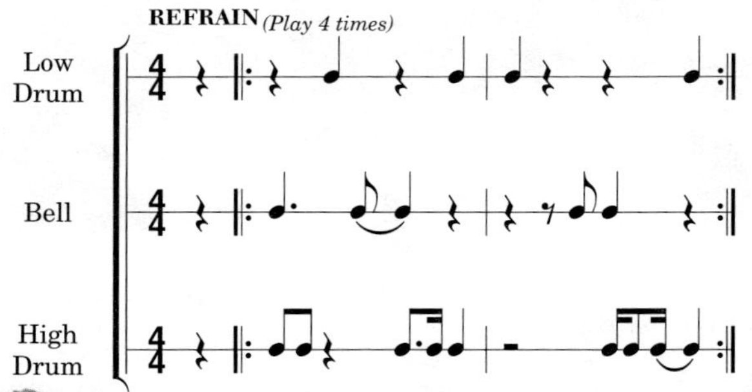

Singing

Focus on learning the song by singing along with the recording. If sections are too high for some singers, have them sing an octave lower as suggested in the Refrain.

Have students learn and echo the sixteenth-note syncopated rhythms.

When ready, select a small group to sing the small notes; the rest of the class sings the song. Point out that the groups are singing in a call-and-response style, frequently found in African music.

Moving

Invite students to make up their own movements or dances to sections of the song.

Creating

Have students create other percussion parts that can be played along with the recording.

INNOVATIVE TEACHER SUPPORT FOR THIS UNIT

- **MAKING MUSIC DVD, Grade 6** contains video segments that support lessons, including signing and movement.
- **MAKING MUSIC with Movement and Dance** provides more opportunities for large group activities in music or physical education classes.
- **MAKING MUSIC with Technology** provides lesson plans for many technology applications; includes MIDI files.
- **¡A cantar!** features recorded songs and lessons from around the Spanish-speaking world; includes strategies for bilingual classes and for English-speaking teachers working with Spanish-speaking students.
- **Bridges to Asia** features recorded songs and lessons from Asian and Pacific region cultures.
- **www.sfsuccessnet.com** provides an online lesson planner to conveniently create lesson plans at school or at home. Includes rubrics for assessment, lesson modifications to meet the needs of all students, performance musicals based on program content, and more.

---

no need for cry-ing, ___ No need for fight-ing. ___

REFRAIN

It's time.
(Oh, ___) Let's cel-e-brate. (Oh, ___) Let's cel-e-brate.

(Oh, ___) Let's cel-e-brate. (Oh, ___) Let's cel-e-brate.

A Rhythm Celebration

Learn to **play** one of the percussion parts below. Then perform it with the refrain of "It's Time."

REFRAIN *(Play 4 times)*

Low Drum

Bell

High Drum

Unit 8 275

TECHNOLOGY/MEDIA LINK

Unit Highlights The following components are used in this unit to reinforce and expand students' understanding of music elements and related themes.

▶ **CD-ROM**

- Use *Band-in-a-Box* to create a Caribbean accompaniment (p. 301)

▶ **ELECTRONIC KEYBOARD**

- Use West African percussion sounds to accompany two selections (p. 283)

▶ **MIDI/SEQUENCING SOFTWARE**

- Create African drum tracks (p. 297)
- Create MIDI drum tracks in *taiko* style (p. 303)
- Use digital recording equipment to record performances (p. 311)

▶ **TRANSPARENCY**

- Display the listening map transparency for *Evening Samba* (p. 297)

▶ **VIDEO LIBRARY/DVD**

- Show the video *Steel Drums* (p. 301)
- Watch a video featuring an Indian ensemble (p. 305)

▶ **WEB SITE**

- Gather more information on African drumming (p. 279)
- Find out more information on Native American music and instruments (p. 287)
- Research African percussion instruments (p. 293)
- Look up information on the music and instruments of India (p. 305)
- Study Middle Eastern music (p. 309)

LESSON AT A GLANCE

Element Focus — **TIMBRE** Drums from around the world

Skill Objective **PLAYING** Perform echo and question-and-answer drumming patterns

Connection Activity **SCIENCE** Discuss the science of local drum construction

MATERIALS
- *Drums from Around the World* CD 14–12
- **Resource Book** p. J-11
- *tubanos* (conga-type drums)
- world map

VOCABULARY

bodhrán	dholak	kendang	kpanlogo
tabla	odaiko	question-and-answer drumming	

◆ ◆ ◆ National Standards ◆ ◆ ◆

2a Play instruments accurately in large ensembles
2c Perform instrumental music from diverse cultures
3b Improvise rhythmic variations on given melodies
6b Listen and analyze uses of rhythm in music from diverse genres
7a Students evaluate the music they perform
8b Identify ways music relates to science
9c Compare, in several cultures, conditions under which music is performed

MORE MUSIC CHOICES

For more practice with percussion timbre:
"*Bắt kim thang*" p. 13
"*O lê lê O Bahía,*" p. 165
"*Siyahamba,*" p. 212
"*Wai bamba,*" p. 26

Drums Around the World

All over the world, people play drums of many different types. The materials the drums are made from depends on what is available locally. People living in a rainforest make large log drums because wood is plentiful. People in Alaska or northern Canada, where trees are scarce, make frame drums of bone or other nonwood materials.

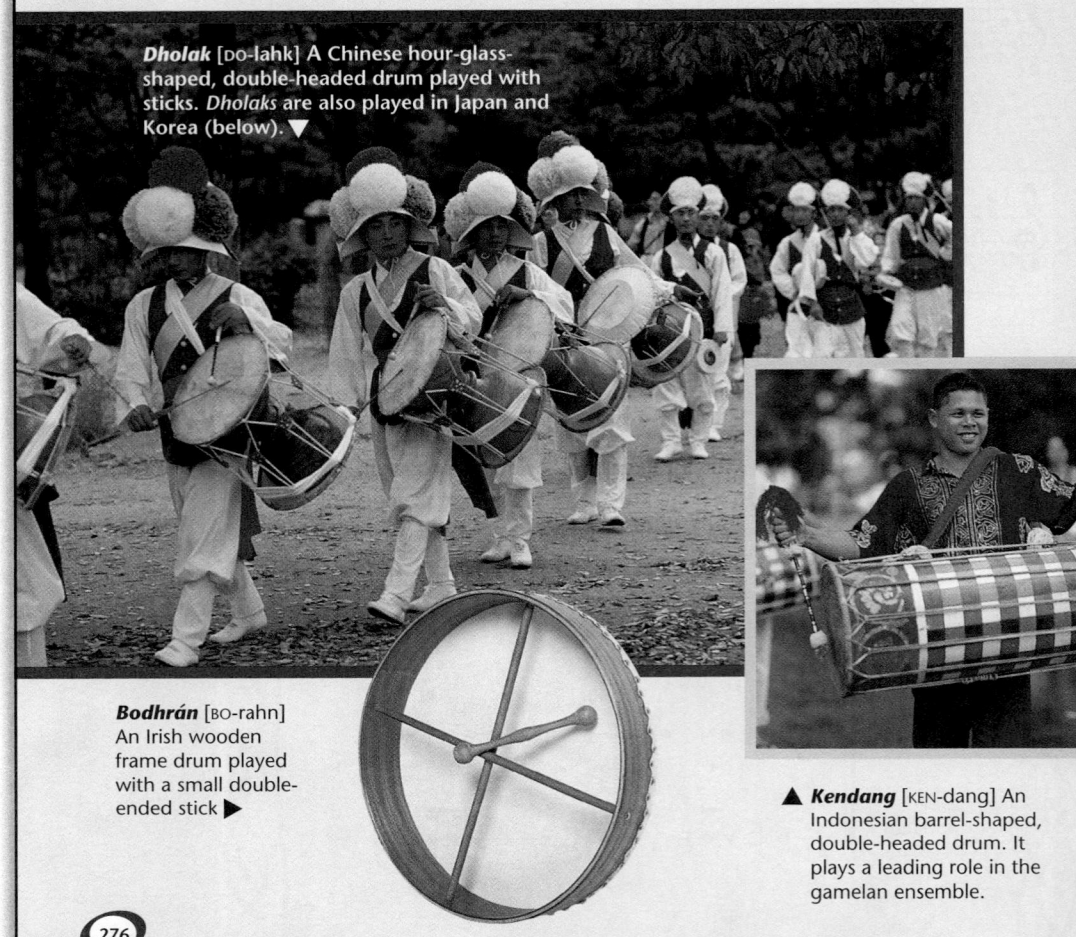

Dholak [DO-lahk] A Chinese hour-glass-shaped, double-headed drum played with sticks. *Dholaks* are also played in Japan and Korea (below). ▼

Bodhrán [BO-rahn] An Irish wooden frame drum played with a small double-ended stick ▶

▲ *Kendang* [KEN-dang] An Indonesian barrel-shaped, double-headed drum. It plays a leading role in the gamelan ensemble.

Footnotes

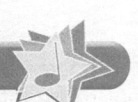

SKILLS REINFORCEMENT

2a ▶ **Playing** Keeping a steady beat while drumming may be a challenge for the class. To strengthen students' feeling for the steady beat, have them play a simple, continuous beat as they wait for their turn to play an individual echo or an answer to the drummed question.

BUILDING SKILLS THROUGH MUSIC

▶ **Science** Rain forests exist only in Central America, South America, India, Africa, Southeast Asia, and Australia (see Across the Curriculum, p. 276). Have students locate rain forests on the globe. Ask them why they think that there are rain forests in those areas of the world and not in North America. (The rain forests are all located near the equator.)

ACROSS THE CURRICULUM

8b ▶ **Science** Ask students what they think would happen if increasing numbers of wooden drums were made from rain forest trees. (depletion of the world's rain forests) Share with students that drums are now manufactured from recycled wood particles in place of wood from trees. These wood particles are made into a heavy form of wood-fiber paper, which is rolled and glued in layers to produce drums like the *tubano* (a conga-type drum). Once the basic tube for the drum is formed, it is dipped in resin to give the drum the acoustic properties of regular wooden drums. The outsides of these drums are then covered in tropical design fabrics. The drumheads are made of a form of nylon that looks and plays like natural leather drumheads.

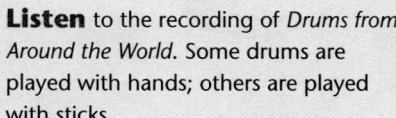

CD 14–12

Listen to the recording of *Drums from Around the World*. Some drums are played with hands; others are played with sticks.

Drums from Around the World

This montage features the Japanese *taiko* drum, the Irish *bodhrán* drum, and the Ghanaian *sogo* drum.

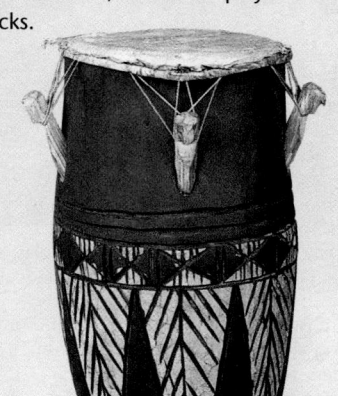

◄ *Kpanlogo* [pahn-LOH-go] A barrel-shaped drum found among the Ga people of Ghana, West Africa

Tabla [TAH-blah] Principal drums used in the classical music of northern India. They are a relative of the Western orchestral timpani (kettledrums). ▼

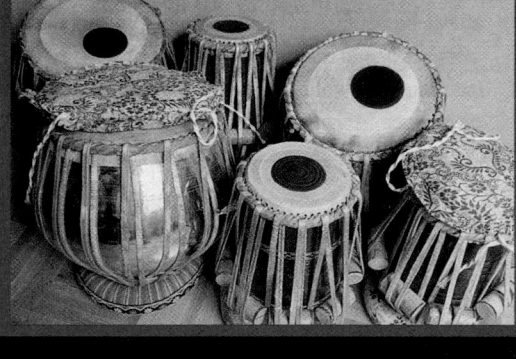

Odaiko [oh-DIE-ko] drum One of several Japanese drums played in the tradition of *taiko* ▼

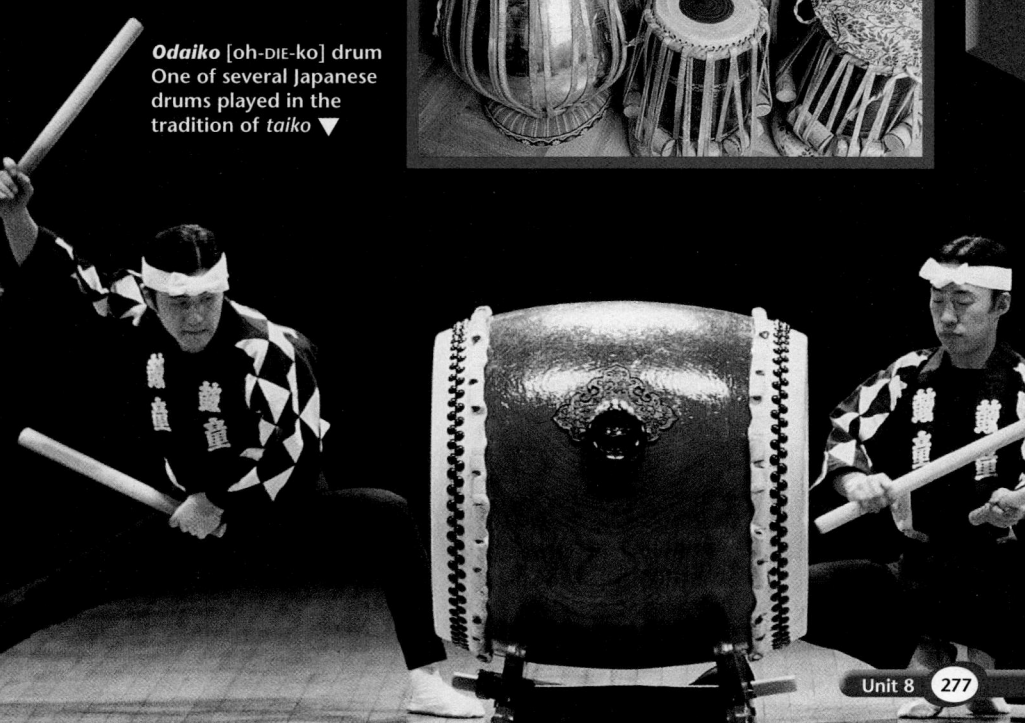

Say It with Drums

Unit 8 **277**

1 INTRODUCE

Share with students that drumming is practiced throughout the world and that people make drums out of whatever is locally available. Ask students to explain why drumming is universally important. (Basic drumming is easy to learn. It is music for dancing; it is tied to ritual and celebration.) Share with students information from Across the Curriculum, p. 276, and Cultural Connection below.

2 DEVELOP

Listening

ASK In the following selection featuring drums, what differences do you hear between the drums? (Some drums are high and others very low. Some excerpts have all the drums playing together; others involve layers of many drums playing different patterns.)

6b Have students listen to *Drums from Around the World* **CD 14–12.** Additional recordings of the *bodhrán, kendang, tabla, kpangolo,* and *odaiko* drum can be heard in the Sound Bank, beginning on p. 512.

Playing

Before passing out instruments, prepare students by sharing the information in Teacher to Teacher, p. 278.

2c Have students sit in a circle or semicircle with their drums. To keep all students involved, encourage those without drums to play the drum patterns on their thighs. See Teacher to Teacher, p. 278, for suggestions on ensuring student involvement.

To teach students to play the open tone (called "high"), have them

- Use all of their fingers (from palm to tip) to strike the drumhead.
- Bounce their hands off the drumhead to avoid a muffled sound.
- Alternate hands as they drum.

continued on page 278

CHARACTER EDUCATION

▶ **Respect** A goal of this unit is to promote an attitude of respect among students by means of cooperation and teamwork.

Have students show respect for the musical instruments by

- Moving them carefully from place to place.
- Keeping the drumheads free of other objects.
- Striking them only with hands or the appropriate stick.

Encourage students to demonstrate respect for one another by

- Recognizing one another's efforts.
- Working as a group to accomplish the drumming goal.

CULTURAL CONNECTION

9c ▶ **Natural Resources** Available natural resources often dictate the types of drums a culture creates. People who live in the rain forests of West Africa have abundant access to the trees from which they make drums. Many of these drums have large wooden barrel-like shells, either carved out of a whole log or constructed from staves. The *kpanlogo,* pictured above, is from the Ga tribe of Ghana, West Africa. Native peoples of Alaska and northern Canada, who live in climates where trees are scarce, make frame drums that do not require wood. A frame drum has a large skin head stretched across a hoop made of bone or other hard substances. The large skin head still produces a deep tone, even though it does not have a wooden resonator.

To teach students to play the bass tone (called "low"), have them

- Place their hands in the middle of the drumhead, as shown.
- Keep their hands relaxed.
- Bounce their hands off the drumhead as if they were dribbling a basketball.

2a Using the example on p. 278, teach students echo playing. Expand to a two-beat pattern and ask them to play expressively and echo the pattern, from memory, on their drums. Then, have them

- Speak and play a two-beat question and two-beat answer, as shown on p. 279.
- Maintain the two-beat pattern in a strict tempo.

In the question-and-answer drumming activities on p. 279, select a student to be the leader. Remind students that the leader provides the question to which an answer is required. As the leader speaks or plays the question rhythm pattern, he/she points to a student. In this manner, the leader selects who will respond to the question. The student who is pointed to responds by singing or playing the answer rhythm pattern. Modify the activity by allowing the leader to select a small group, or the entire class, when pointing.

Creating

3b When students are comfortable with the question-and-answer format, ask individuals to drum their own two-beat answers to each two-beat question drummed by you.

2c Observe students' playing position and ability as each student responds to the leader's drum question. In providing general feedback about playing position, remind students to

- Use all their fingers on the drumhead to play the high tone.
- Alternate hands.

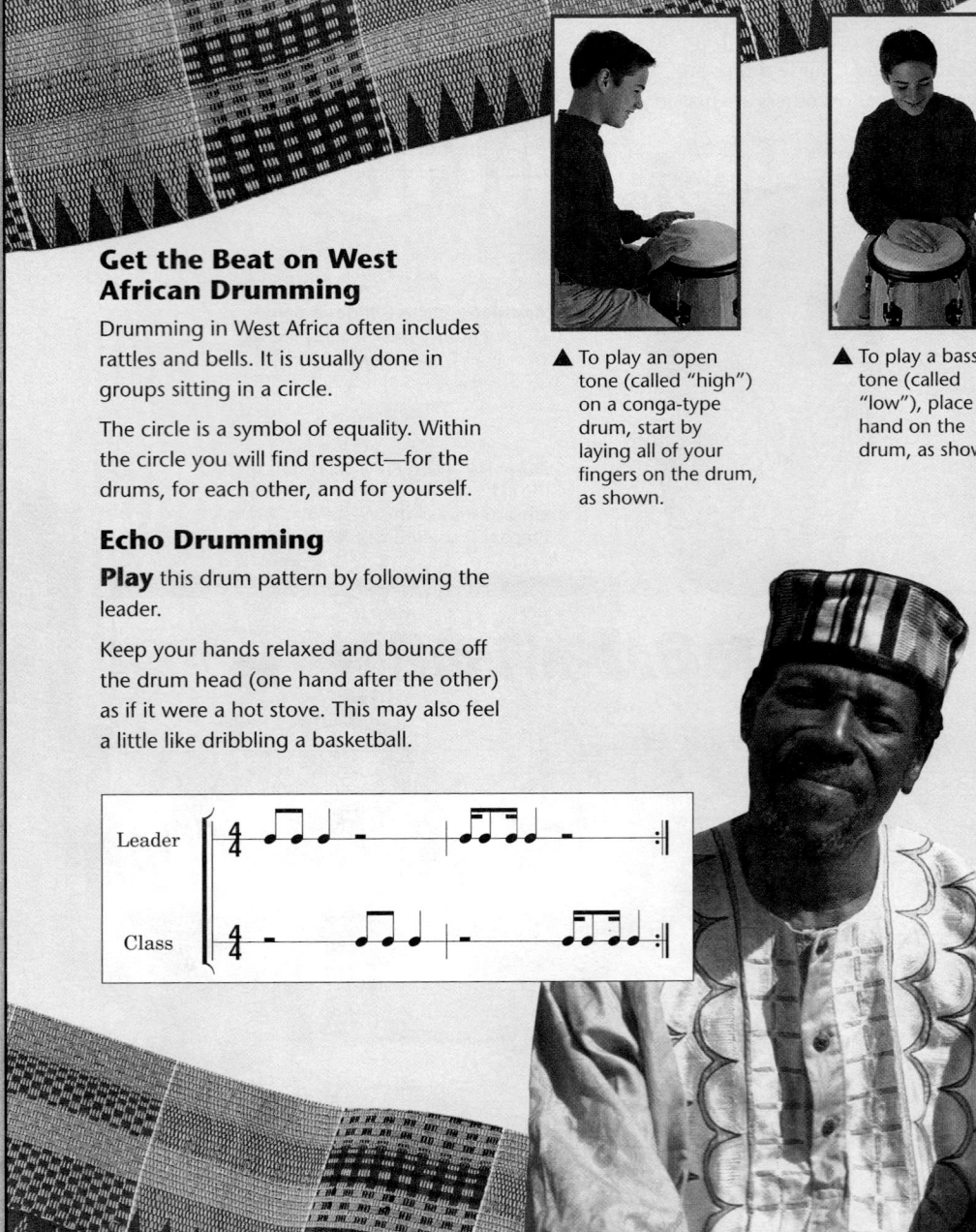

Get the Beat on West African Drumming

Drumming in West Africa often includes rattles and bells. It is usually done in groups sitting in a circle.

The circle is a symbol of equality. Within the circle you will find respect—for the drums, for each other, and for yourself.

▲ To play an open tone (called "high") on a conga-type drum, start by laying all of your fingers on the drum, as shown.

▲ To play a bass tone (called "low"), place your hand on the drum, as shown.

Echo Drumming

Play this drum pattern by following the leader.

Keep your hands relaxed and bounce off the drum head (one hand after the other) as if it were a hot stove. This may also feel a little like dribbling a basketball.

278

Footnotes

ACROSS THE CURRICULUM

▶ **Language Arts** Read aloud and dramatize *Drums of Noto Hanto* by J. Alison James (Dorling Kindersley, 1999). The book commemorates the yearly celebration of a 400-year-old event in which Japanese villagers defended themselves from a fleet of invading *samurai* with bells, drums, and frightening masks made of bark and seaweed. The text of the book is full of percussive language and action that captures the power and intensity of Japanese drumming. The students could present a performance of this legend, complete with sounds from real percussion instruments, to a group of younger students.

TEACHER TO TEACHER

2a ▶ **Management Tips** To keep students involved in drumming, provide as many drums or drum substitutes as possible (cardboard boxes, round oatmeal boxes, empty plastic water bottles, desktops, and so on). Encourage two or three students to share a drum by taking turns playing on the drumhead. Students who do not have immediate access to a drum or drum substitute can play the drumming patterns on their thighs.

Whenever possible, arrange drummers in a circle. If your room does not permit students to sit in a circle, try to create a semicircle or another shape that allows students to establish eye contact necessary for question-and-answer drumming.

Question and Answer

Start this activity by speaking the questions and answers.

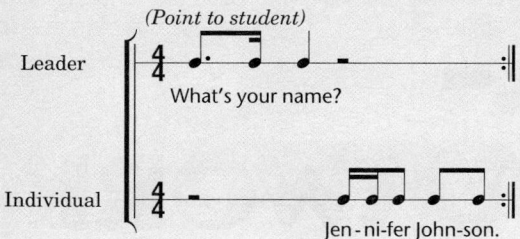

Leader

(Point to student)

What's your name?

Individual

Jen - ni-fer John-son.

Now, speak and **play** the question and answer on your drum.

Try a different question, first by speaking, then by both speaking and playing the drum. When playing, bounce off the middle of the drum with the whole hand relaxed.

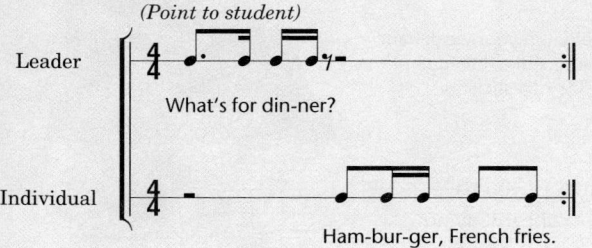

Leader

(Point to student)

What's for din-ner?

Individual

Ham-bur-ger, French fries.

When you are ready, try **question-and-answer drumming** with drums only. As the leader plays the same question over and over, answer with any two-beat pattern.

> **Question-and-answer drumming** is an African style of playing rhythms. A leader plays a phrase, which is answered by other phrases from the group.

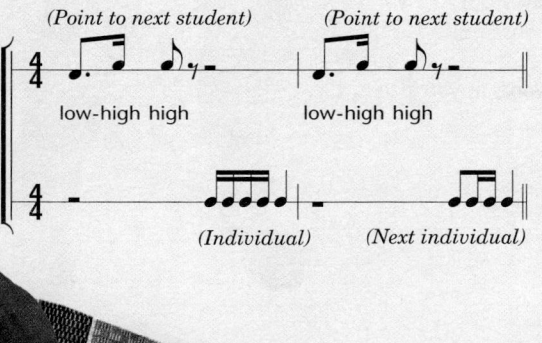

(Point to next student)

low-high high

(Individual)

(Point to next student)

low-high high

(Next individual)

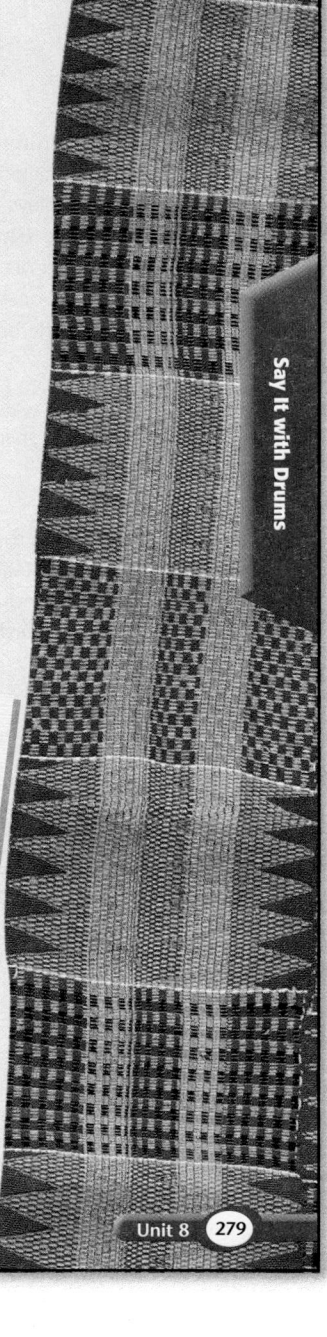

Say It with Drums

Unit 8 **279**

- Bounce their hands off the drumhead.
- Play high and low tones.

Invite students who are interested in drumming to read a Japanese story about drums in Across the Curriculum on p. 278.

For additional activities on question-and-answering drumming, see Activity Master 10, Musical Questions and Answers, on Resource Book p. J-11.

3 CLOSE

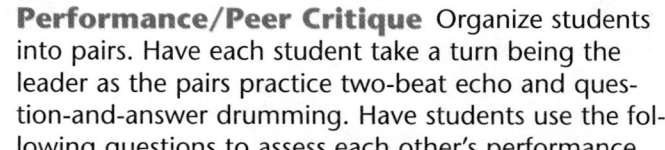

Element: TIMBRE   **ASSESSMENT**

7a **Performance/Peer Critique** Organize students into pairs. Have each student take a turn being the leader as the pairs practice two-beat echo and question-and-answer drumming. Have students use the following questions to assess each other's performance.

- Does the timbre of the bass (low) tone sound low?
- Does the timbre of the open (high) tone sound high?
- Can you hear the difference in timbre between the low and high tones?
- Do your partner's hands bounce off the drumhead correctly, which helps in producing a good sound?
- On the open (high) tone, does your partner use all his or her fingers on the drumhead?

MEETING INDIVIDUAL NEEDS

▶ **Including Everyone** Question-and-answer drumming and echo drumming provide activities that reinforce interaction.

Reinforcement Pair students who may not easily initiate interacting with peers with a student who has demonstrated patience, kindness, and enthusiasm.

On Target Have students work with partners to practice open and bass tones and technique. Tell them to look directly at each other as they "communicate." Partners maintain eye contact as they alternate listening and performing patterns.

Challenge Invite students to practice this skill with partners and small groups where eye contact is used to indicate which member is to respond. Ask the group to create and perform more difficult question-and-answer patterns for the class.

SCHOOL TO HOME CONNECTION

▶ **Interactive Bulletin Board** Invite students to enlist friends and family members to help them find more information and illustrations about drums and drummers from cultures around the world. As students bring their information to class, provide a world map to which students can attach inserts of their creations or discoveries.

TECHNOLOGY/MEDIA LINK

Web Site Go to *www.sfsuccessnet.com* to learn more about African drumming.

LESSON AT A GLANCE

Element Focus   **RHYTHM** West African layered rhythms

Skill Objective   **CREATING** Create a drum piece to be performed by a classroom drum ensemble

Connection Activity   **SOCIAL STUDIES** Examine how teamwork is developed by performing in a drum ensemble

MATERIALS

- *"Nana Kru"*   CD 14–13
  Recording Routine: Intro (12 m.); vocal; interlude (4 m.); vocal; coda
- *Lost River*   CD 14–15
- **Resource Book** p. H-26
- *tubanos* (conga-type drums) in high, medium, and low pitches; cowbells; *shekeres* (or other rattles); keyboard

VOCABULARY

time line   cowbell   *shekere*

complementary rhythm

◆ ◆ ◆ ◆ National Standards ◆ ◆ ◆ ◆

2a Play instruments accurately in small ensembles
2c Perform instrumental music from diverse cultures
4a Compose short pieces, demonstrating balance through music
5a Read quarter, eighth, sixteenth, and dotted notes in duple meter
6b Listen and analyze uses of rhythm and timbre in music from diverse cultures
8b Identify ways music relates to social studies
9a Describe characteristics of music styles from a variety of cultures

MORE MUSIC CHOICES

For more practice with drumming patterns:
"Lost My Gold Ring," p. 158
"New Hungarian Folk Song, " p. 196

MUSICAL TEAMWORK

In West African drumming, the bell (sometimes called the *gankogui*) often plays a repeated pattern called the **time line.** The time line anchors the whole drum ensemble. A cowbell may be used to play the bell part.

> A **time line** is an African rhythm in which a pattern repeats and becomes the main beat that holds the music together.

To play the bell, hold it in your weak hand. With your other hand, strike the edge of the opening with the side of a stick. ▶

Play this time line rhythm on the bell. If you have trouble keeping a steady beat, you might try saying "beat and-a beat and-a beat and-a beat . . ." and then play on the word "beat."

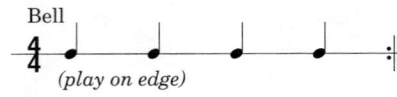

Bell
(play on edge)

Shake, Rattle, and Play!

The *shekere* [SHEH-keh-reh] is a gourd rattle from West Africa. Let's add the *shekere* to our ensemble.

The *shekere* plays this pattern. Say the words as you **play**.

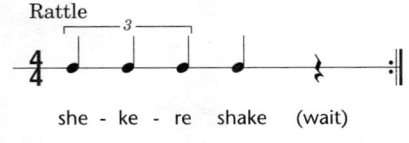

Rattle

she - ke - re   shake   (wait)

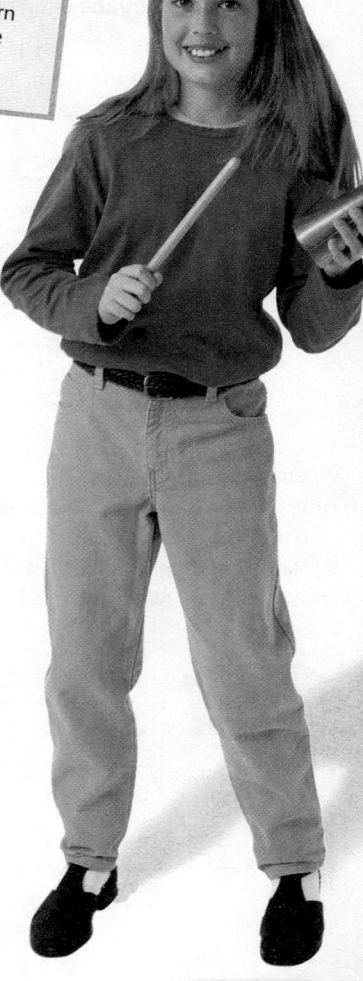

Footnotes

MEETING INDIVIDUAL NEEDS

▶ **Visual/Motor Coordination** When you ask students to create their own drum ensemble, you may want to ensure that the student with a disability is in a group with peers who have provided assistance in the past. These other sixth graders will have ideas about how the student with a disability can participate in the drum ensemble.

BUILDING SKILLS THROUGH MUSIC

▶ **Writing** Share the information from Across the Curriculum, p. 281. Ask students to write a description of the teamwork that was involved as the class learned to play Drum Ensemble 1.

CULTURAL CONNECTION

▶ **Liberia** Independent since 1847, Liberia is the only nation in black Africa that was never under colonial rule. It was partly settled by freed American slaves during the 19th century. The capital city, Monrovia, was named for U.S. President James Monroe. Liberia's landscape varies from sandy beaches to plains to hills in the north. The climate is hot and humid with an average temperature of 80°F. Liberia's major natural resources include timber and minerals (iron, diamonds, gold). Principal tribes include the *Kpelle, Bassa, Gio, Kru, Grebo, Mano, Krahn, Mandingo,* and *Loma*. During the 1990s, Liberia suffered greatly from the effects of civil war.

It Takes Teamwork!

Drum Ensemble 1 depends on teamwork. As you **analyze** the score, notice how each part complements the other layered parts. For example, the low drum plays on beats 1 and 2 while the high drum plays on beats 3 and 4—they fit together like a jigsaw puzzle.

Play and speak the low drum part. When this part is stable, bring in the high drum part.

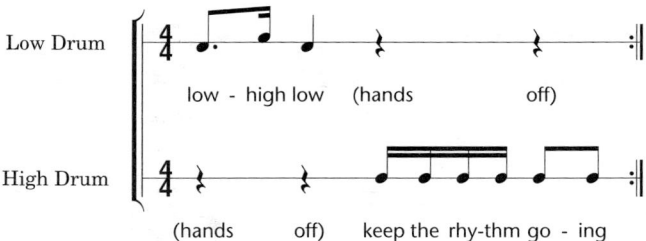

Drum Ensemble 1

Before you **play** Drum Ensemble 1, can you find a new part in the score and **describe** its rhythm?

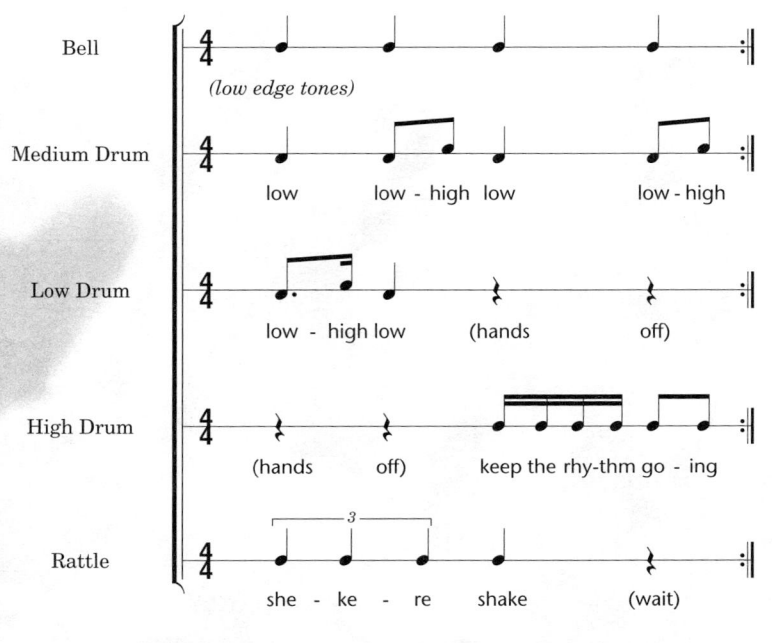

1 INTRODUCE

9a Share with students that West African drumming is based on layered complementary bell, rattle, and drum parts. All members of a drumming ensemble must work together as a team. Share information on African drumming from Across the Curriculum below.

2 DEVELOP

Playing

Direct students' attention to the hand positions for playing a cowbell, as shown on p. 280. Have students

- Observe closely as you demonstrate the hand positions.
- Listen for the many different tones the bell makes.

ASK What causes the cowbell to make different tones? (the position in which the bell is held; where on the bell the player strikes)

2a Direct students to

- Take turns playing the bell.
- Help one another to hold the bell and stick correctly.

Share with students the importance of the time line, which is played by the bell.

6b ASK Why is the time line considered the "anchor" of the drum ensemble? (It provides the steady beat.)

9a Why does the time line often start an African drum ensemble piece? (Hearing the time line tells the other players the rhythm and tempo they need to follow.)

Invite students to clap, say, and then play the time line rhythm (the bell part) of Drum Ensemble 1.

For additional playing activities, see Skills Reinforcement on p. 282.

continued on page 282

ACROSS THE CURRICULUM

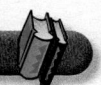

8b ▶ Social Studies Share with students that the complementary layered patterns inherent in most African and Caribbean drumming are a form of social interaction much like having a conversation. Ask students to list the characteristics of a good conversation. (Each person listens to the others, each responds in a timely manner without interrupting others, no one person does most of the talking.) Remind students that conversations and drumming require teamwork, one of the most important life skills taught in school.

TEACHER TO TEACHER

2a ▶ Teaching Tips: Drum Ensemble 1 Teach the class to play their drumming parts, saying the appropriate phrases. (On the phrase *hands off,* a gesture is made to the side.) Let low drum players establish their part, using both bass and open tones. Add high drums to the ensemble. Remind high drum players to use open tones. Next, teach the medium drum part, having students use their dominant hand to play steady bass tones in the middle of the drumhead while saying *low, low, low, low.* Have them add the other hand on the high (open) tones as they say *low, low, high: low, low, high.*

▶ Management Tip Teamwork in the drumming circle requires everyone to work together. Remove uncooperative students from the drumming circle until they modify their behavior so they can return to the circle.

Lesson 2 Continued

Share with students that many cultures make and use rattles as musical instruments. Some rattles have seeds or beads inside them to make sound. The *shekere's* beads are on the outside of the rattle.

Have students

- Observe as you play the *shekere* by hitting it against either the hand or the thigh.
- Play the *shekere* (rattle) part from Drum Ensemble 1, saying "*she-ke-re* shake" as they play.
- Avoid shaking the rattle when you are not playing rhythms so that only the correct rhythms are heard.

To prepare students to perform Drum Ensemble 1, on p. 281, invite them to echo drum your simple patterns; then drum examples of question-and-answer patterns. See Teacher to Teacher, p. 281. Next, have students

- Play the low drum part, then the high part.
- Choose the low or high drum part and play in a whole-class two-part ensemble.
- Play the medium drum part.
- Choose one of the three drum parts and play in a whole-class three-part ensemble.

- Combine all five parts, bringing them in according to score order. (Never add a new part until the ensemble is stable.)

- Perform Drum Ensemble 1 with the recording of "*Nana Kru*" **CD 14–13.** (Note: The recorded introduction includes an additional part, shown below, for double bell, or *gankogui*. This part follows the entrance of the high drum.)

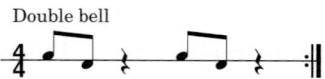

Play and Sing

Drum ensembles in West African countries such as Ghana, Sierra Leone, Ivory Coast, and Liberia are often combined with singing and dancing.

Sing "*Nana Kru*" while some members of the class **play** Drum Ensemble 1. Then, choose a rhythm part and play and sing at the same time. Which parts are the easiest to play while you sing?

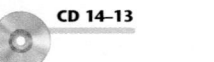
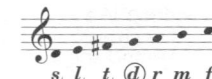

NANA KRU

Traditional Song from the Kou Tribe of Liberia (Adapted)

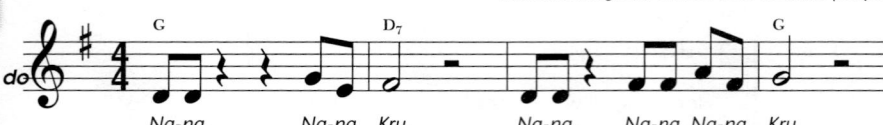

Na-na,   Na-na Kru,   Na-na,   Na-na, Na-na Kru,

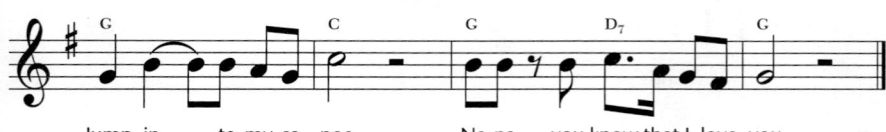

Jump in - to my ca - noe,   Na-na,   you know that I love you.

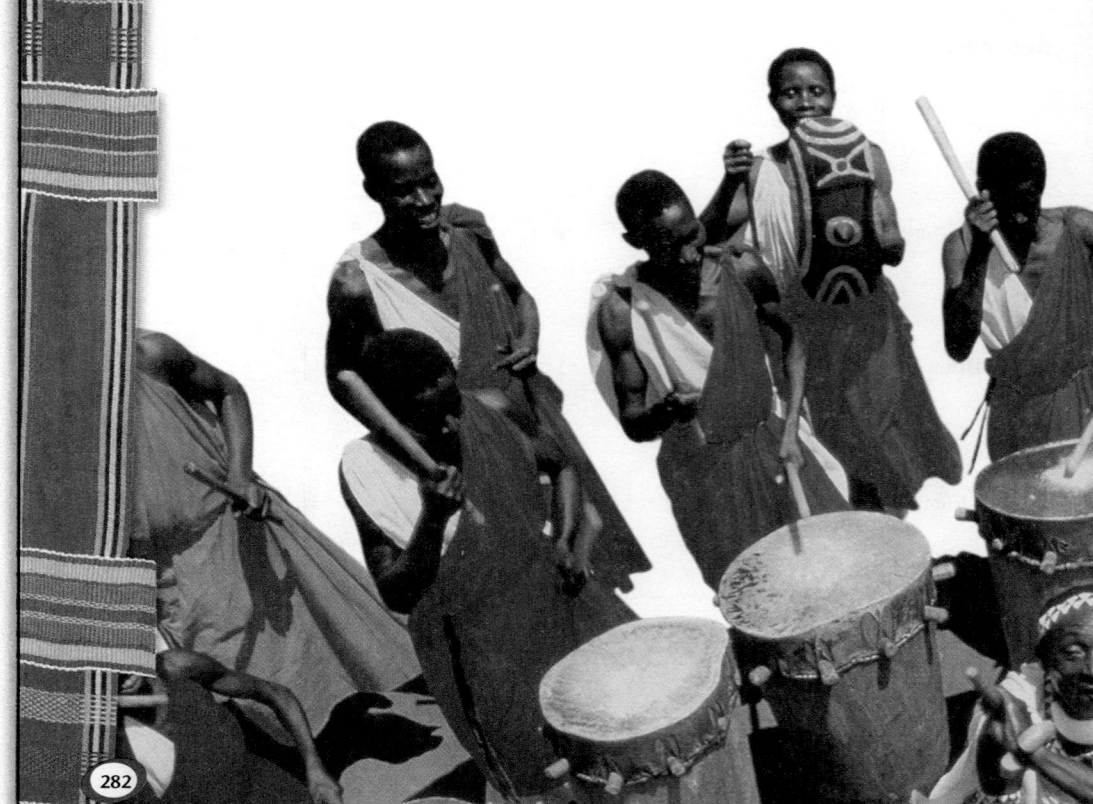

282

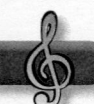

Footnotes

AUDIENCE ETIQUETTE

▶ **Rehearsal Etiquette for Performers** Productive rehearsals prepare musicians for the best performance possible. Each ensemble member is responsible for participating attentively. Help students develop a set of "rehearsal etiquette" guidelines, such as

- Be on time and listen to all instructions.
- Converse with friends only after the rehearsal is finished.
- Come prepared for rehearsal with a pencil and your music.
- Listen to others in your section and to other sections.
- Be aware of your own space, and respect the space of others.
- Say "thank you" to the leaders of the group at the end of rehearsal.

SKILLS REINFORCEMENT

▶ **Keyboard** Encourage students to play a keyboard accompaniment to "*Nana Kru*," based on the rhythm of the double bell part, found on Resource Book p. H-26.

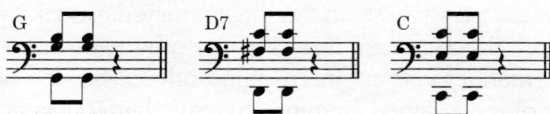

▶ **Listening/Playing** One of the fun ways to enhance students' experience with Drum Ensemble 1 is to have students find recordings that work well with the feel of the ensemble, then bring the recordings to class and play along with them. Drum Ensemble 1 works well with many styles of music, including rock, pop, Latin, and hip-hop. (Always preview a recording before using it in class.)

A Beat of Your Own

To **create** your own drum piece, you will need four or five fellow musicians to play the following instruments.

- bell
- rattle
- two or three drums of different pitches

The bell starts by playing a time line. Then each of the other instruments makes up a part that is complementary. Add one part at a time, coming in only when the other parts are stable.

Listen to *Lost River*, performed by Mickey Hart of the Grateful Dead, along with percussionists and vocalists from all over this planet.

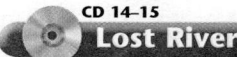

CD 14–15
Lost River

created and performed by Mickey Hart and the musicians of Planet Drum

Lost River uses the following instruments: *djembe, dundun,* drum set, *duggi tarang,* conch shell, cymbals, shakers, wood blocks, floor tom, metal percussion, and voices.

Describe the ways in which *Lost River* sounds like rock music. How has African and other world percussion become part of rock?

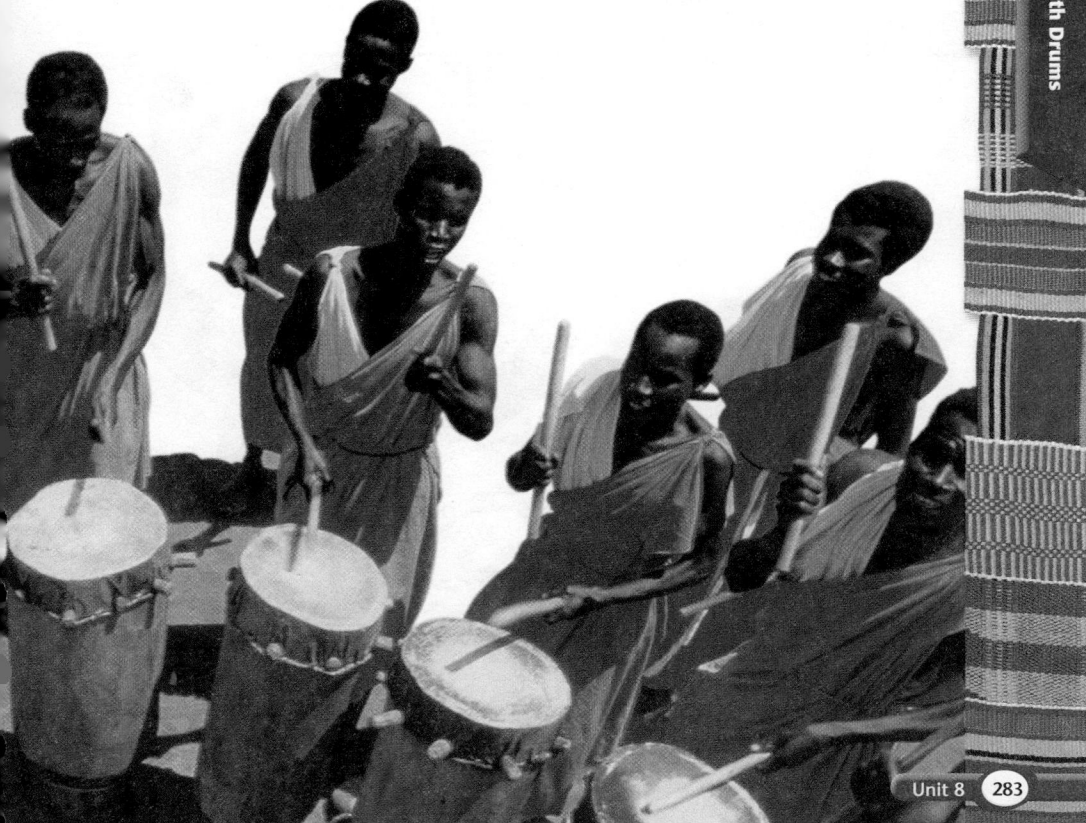

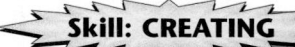

Say It with Drums

Unit 8 283

Singing

Invite students interested in Africa to share with the class an African story in Across the Curriculum below, and facts on Liberia, from Cultural Connection on p. 280.

Share with students the importance West African cultures place on combining singing, movement, and drumming. Organize the class into singers, drummers, and dancers. Have students

- Listen to *"Nana Kru"* **CD 14–13.**
- Sing *"Nana Kru"* with Drum Ensemble 1.
- Create a movement pattern to accompany the performance.

Listening

Have students listen to *Lost River* **CD 14–15.**

6b ASK In what ways does *Lost River* sound like rock music? (It uses drums and other percussion to create a strong beat and repetitive patterns, important elements in both rock and world drumming.)

9a SAY The music of Africa is an important ingredient in rock music. Rock developed from the musical style called *rhythm and blues*—an African American style that is rich in African musical characteristics such as syncopation and polyrhythms.

3 CLOSE

Skill: CREATING   ASSESSMENT

4a Performance/Peer Critique Organize the class into groups of four or five. Have students follow the guidelines on p. 283 to create their own drum ensemble pieces. Allow students to assess each group's drum pieces using the following criteria.

- Do the drum parts work well together?
- Is the tempo steady and stable?
- Is the performance exciting?

ACROSS THE CURRICULUM

▶ **Language Arts/Drama** Read aloud *Koi and the Kola Nuts: A Tale from Liberia* by Verna Aardema (Atheneum, 1999), a charming and beautifully illustrated authentic tale of a young Liberian boy and his quest to become the leader of his people. This tale could be dramatized for younger children and used in performances of music from West Africa.

SCHOOL TO HOME CONNECTION

▶ **Drumming Clinic** At a parent/teacher conference or open school night, have students teach their parents and others to play Drum Ensemble 1. Ask students to explain how ensemble drumming promotes good teamwork, positive social interaction, and good listening and playing coordination.

TECHNOLOGY/MEDIA LINK

4a Electronic Keyboard Have students use West African percussion sounds on the MIDI keyboard to accompany Drum Ensemble 1 on p. 281 and *"Nana Kru"* on p. 282.

LESSON AT A GLANCE

Element Focus **MELODY** Native American melody using vocables

Skill Objective **SINGING** Sing a Native American song while performing a simple round dance

Connection Activity **CULTURE** Examine diverse Native American cultures

MATERIALS

- *Drums of the Iroquois and Sioux*   CD 14–16
- "Yo-shi nai"   CD 14–17

  Recording Routine: Intro (6 m.); vocal (two times); interlude (6 m.); vocal (two times)

- *Jo'ashila*   CD 14–19

VOCABULARY

vocables   circle dance   accents

◆ ◆ ◆ ◆ National Standards ◆ ◆ ◆ ◆

1c Sing music from diverse cultures

2c Perform instrumental music from diverse cultures

6b Listen and analyze uses of timbre and rhythm in music from diverse cultures

8b Identify ways music relates to social studies

9a Describe characteristics of music styles from a variety of cultures

9c Compare, in several cultures, conditions under which music is performed

MORE MUSIC CHOICES

For more experience with Native American music:

"Go, My Son," p. 188

Round Dance (excerpt), p. 445

Native American DRUMMING

Traditional North American Indian drums come in many different shapes and sizes. These instruments are made from wood, animals, and other local materials.

Historically, the Iroquois Nation were hunters, gatherers, and farmers who lived in one place. The three "life-giving sisters"—corn, beans, and squash—were their primary food. Their longhouses were large structures where they sang, danced, and carried on the life of the community.

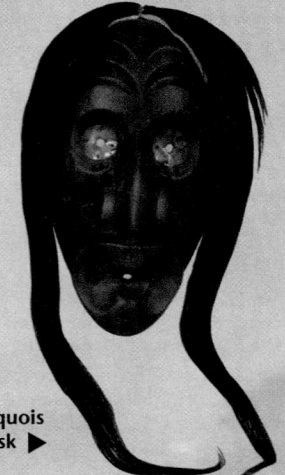

Iroquois Mask ▶

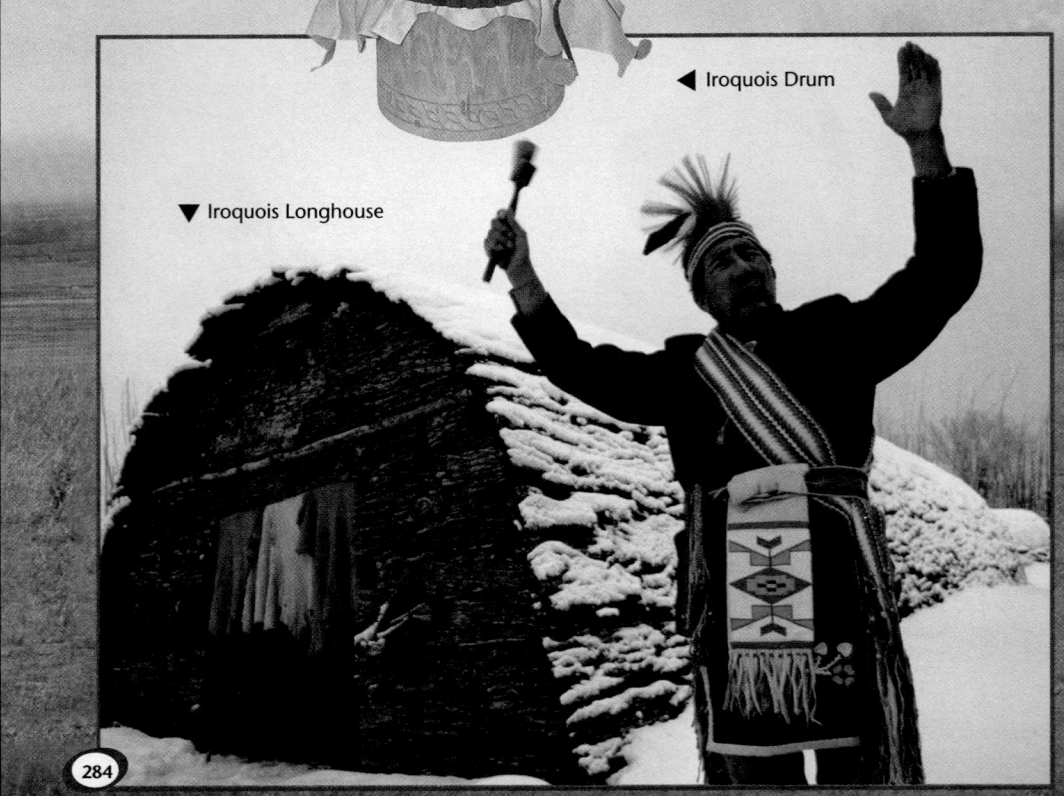

◀ Iroquois Drum

▼ Iroquois Longhouse

284

Footnotes

CULTURAL CONNECTION

8b ▶ **A Way of Life** The Iroquois Longhouse is a way of life in which many nations live peacefully under a common law confederation. The traditional "longhouse," 50 to 100 feet in length and covered with bark, contained as many as 20 families and was protected by a stockade. Outside were extensive cornfields, orchards, and fields of squash, beans, and tobacco. At social dances, musicians played the water drum or horn rattle; dancers moved to the "stomp," "fish," and "side-step shuffle."

BUILDING SKILLS THROUGH MUSIC

▶ **Social Studies** Have students identify at least three facts they read about the Iroquois Nation, the Lakota Sioux, and the Navajo. Ask them to use these facts to compare and contrast the three tribal groups.

ACROSS THE CURRICULUM

▶ **Social Studies** Share with students that the *Haudenosaunee* (the Iroquois) was the first league of nations in this land. Six nations, including the Seneca, Onondaga, and Mohawk, make up the Iroquois. The nations coexist under the oldest continually operating form of government. The league was established about 1570 through the effort of Hiawatha (River Maker), probably of the Mohawk tribe. The Iroquois form of government is based on the clan. The women's council from each tribe, chosen from the mothers of the tribe, makes decisions in all matters of public importance, including the nomination of members of the chief's council.

Sounds of the Sioux

In contrast to the Iroquois, the Lakota Sioux were nomadic Great Plains buffalo hunters. Their teepees, made of hides and lodge poles, were easily taken down and transported. The large frame drums were easily carried from place to place.

Listen to the recordings from both the Iroquois and Sioux. What differences do you hear?

CD 14–16

Drums of the Iroquois and Sioux

This montage contains excerpts from the Iroquois *Fish Dance* and the Sioux *Rabbit Dance*.

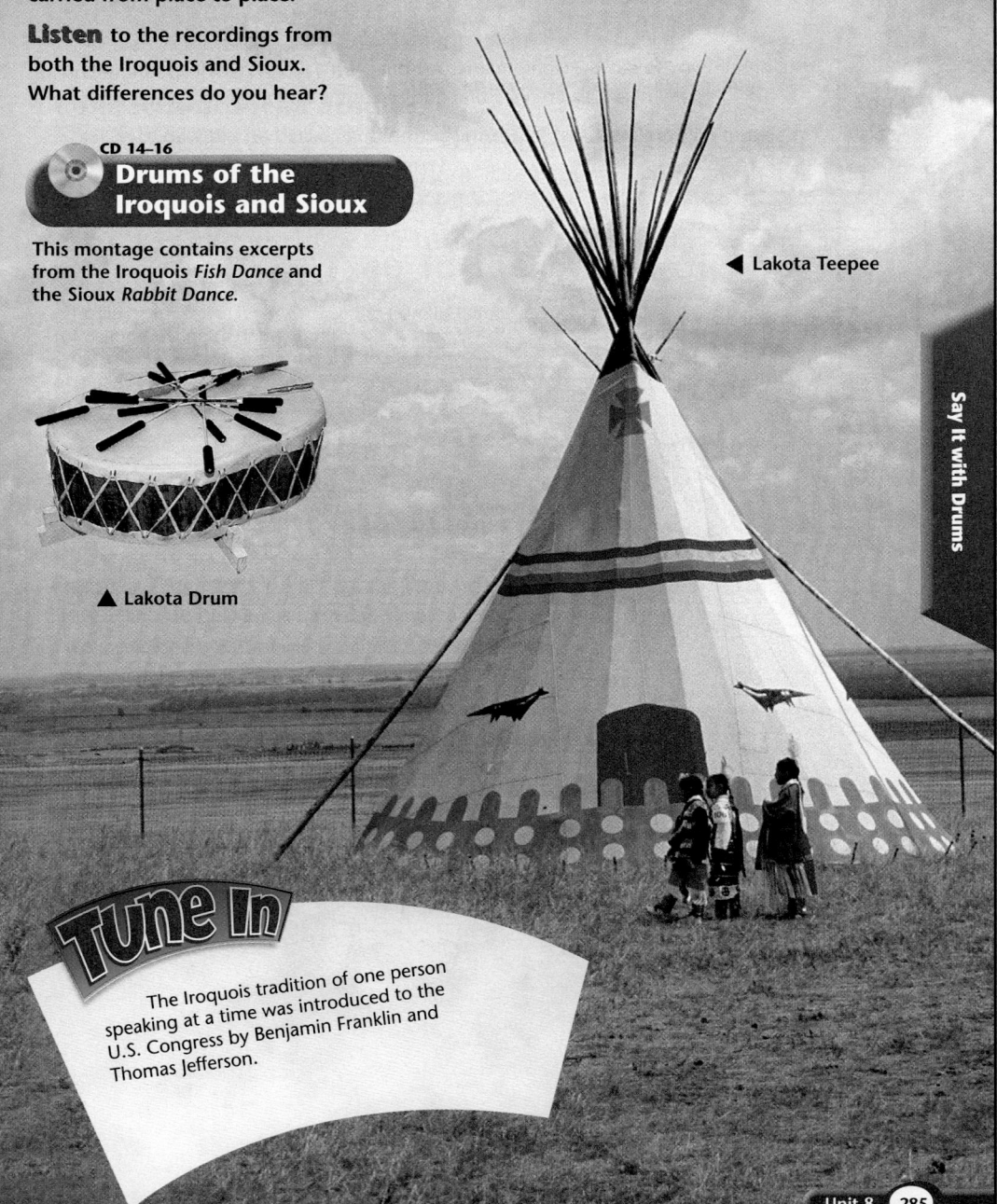

▶ Lakota Teepee

▲ Lakota Drum

Say It with Drums

Tune In

The Iroquois tradition of one person speaking at a time was introduced to the U.S. Congress by Benjamin Franklin and Thomas Jefferson.

Unit 8 285

1 INTRODUCE

9c Ask students to list ways that African cultures use drums. (for communication, in celebration, in their spiritual life, in music-making)

Share with students that North American Indians also view drums as a very important part of their music and spiritual life. In fact, the drum is seen as the heartbeat of the people. Ask students to list factors that might affect the types of drums used by different Native American tribes. (available natural resources, lifestyle, cultural traditions)

2 DEVELOP

8b Ask students to read about the Iroquois Nation, on p. 284. Then share the information in Across the Curriculum, p. 284. Point out the photo of the Iroquois longhouse and share with students the information in Cultural Connection, p. 284, about the longhouse way of life. Then discuss with students the photos and information about the Lakota Sioux, in Spotlight On below. Have the class make a list of the similarities and differences between the two cultures.

Listening

Invite students to listen to *Drums of the Iroquois and Sioux* **CD 14–16.**

SAY Because you now know something about the culture of the Iroquois people of upstate New York and the Lakota Sioux from the Great Plains, you probably have some expectations about the sounds of their drums.

6b **ASK** **What kinds of drums do you expect to hear?** (Answers will vary, but students should indicate that the Iroquois drum will be high-pitched and the larger Lakota Sioux drum will have a lower sound.)

continued on page 286

SPOTLIGHT ON

▶ **The Great Sioux Nation** The seven original bands of the Great Sioux Nation, in an alliance called the Seven Council Fires, dominated the northern Plains, an area including most of the Dakotas, northern Nebraska, eastern Wyoming, and southeastern Montana. The Lakota followed the buffalo as their principal source of food, constructing teepees of buffalo skins stretched over long poles, which could be moved quickly to stay near the buffalo. Large frame drums were used as an easily transportable form of musical accompaniment along with rattles for singing and dancing. The Great Sioux Nation was gradually forced onto reservations after many major battles with the U.S. Army.

SKILLS REINFORCEMENT

6b
2c ▶ **Playing** *Jo'ashila,* **CD 14–19** uses a combination of three different meters, as shown below. Have students follow the metric arrangement as they listen, and then sight-read the steady beat rhythm pattern below on drums with the recording.

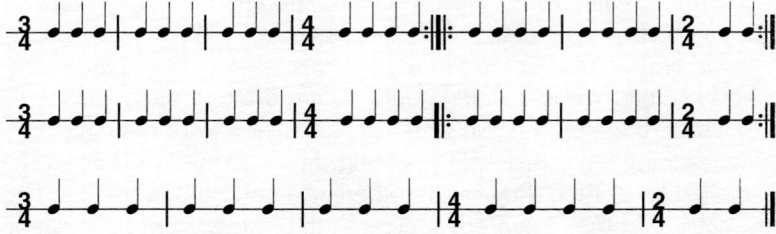

9a **ASK** What differences do you hear in the sounds of the singing? (The Lakota Sioux example has a higher-pitched sound with descending lines; the Iroquois example has a more relaxed tone quality sung in a range consistently lower than that of the Lakota.)

Singing

Ask students to read the information at the top of p. 286. Share with students that *"Yo-shi nai"* includes words and vocables, which are syllables without a specific, literal meaning.

Have students

1c
- Listen to *"Yo-shi nai"* **CD 14–17** while following the music.
- Sing the song with the recording.
- Perform the song from memory so it can be sung while doing the circle dance.

Moving

SAY The circle shape is an important part of Native American culture and spiritual life.

Share with students a quotation of Black Elk, a member of the Oglala Lakota Sioux: "You have noticed that everything an Indian does is in a circle, and that is because the Power of the World always works in circles, and everything tries to be round.... Even the seasons form a great circle in their changing, and always come back again to where they were."

Teach students the circle dance to accompany *"Yo-shi nai."* See Movement, p. 287.

Listening

Have students

- Read about Marilyn Hood, on p. 287.
- **6b 9a** Listen to *Jo'ashila* **CD 14–19** and compare the sounds of the vocal and percussion parts with those of *"Yo-shi nai"* **CD 14–17**.

Navajo Celebration

The Navajo were originally nomadic hunters. They later settled in the Southwest and became sheepherders and farmers, somewhat like their neighbors, the Pueblos.

"Yo-shi nai" is a circle dance song that means "come and dance." It is a public part of the Navajo Enemy Way, a ceremony honoring the return of Navajo warriors. **Sing** *"Yo-shi nai."* Which part of the melody repeats?

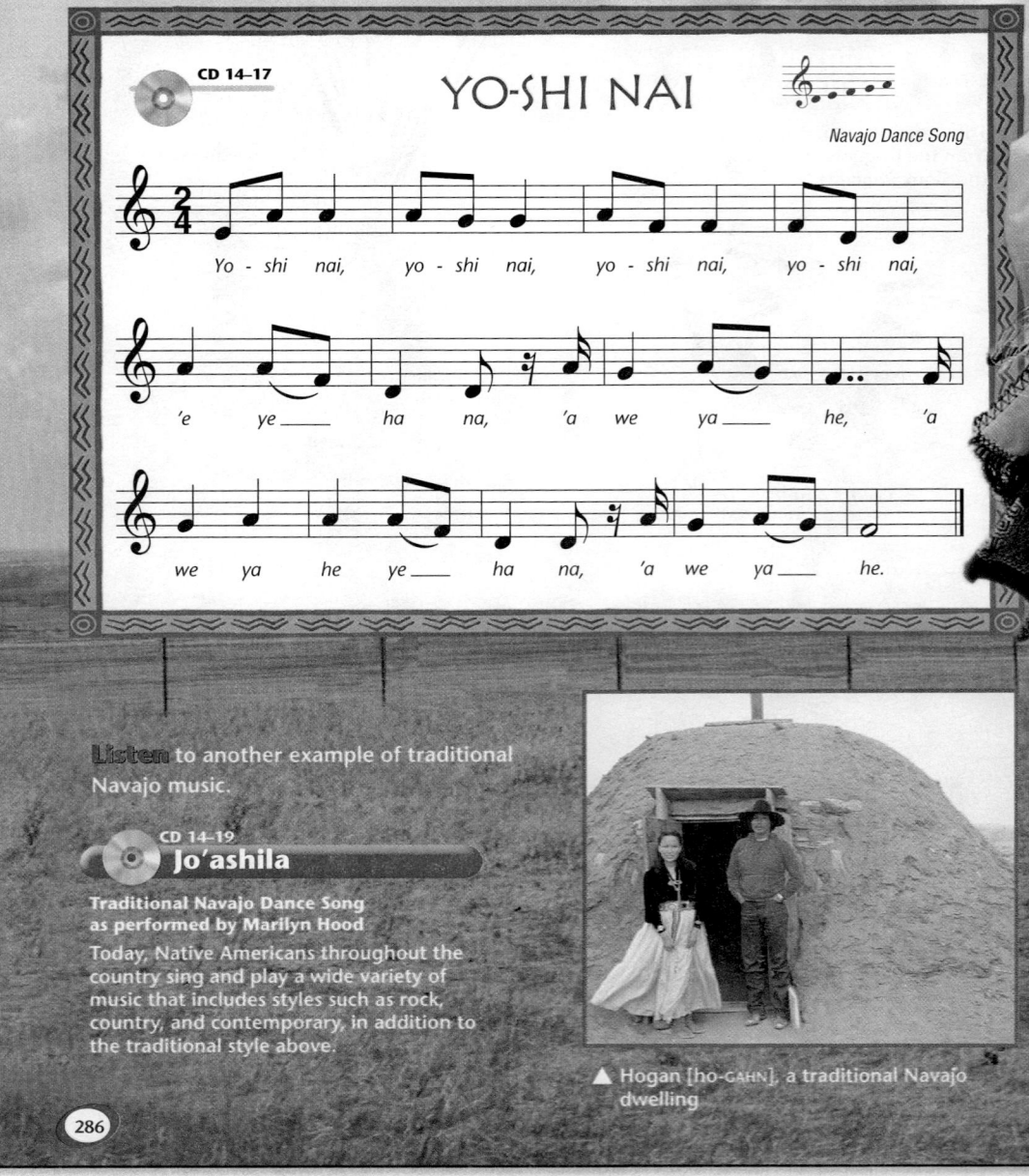

CD 14–17

YO-SHI NAI
Navajo Dance Song

Yo - shi nai, yo - shi nai, yo - shi nai, yo - shi nai,

'e ye ___ ha na, 'a we ya ___ he, 'a

we ya he ye ___ ha na, 'a we ya ___ he.

Listen to another example of traditional Navajo music.

 CD 14–19
Jo'ashila

Traditional Navajo Dance Song as performed by Marilyn Hood

Today, Native Americans throughout the country sing and play a wide variety of music that includes styles such as rock, country, and contemporary, in addition to the traditional style above.

▲ Hogan [ho-GAHN], a traditional Navajo dwelling

286

Footnotes

CULTURAL CONNECTION

▶ **The Navajo** Students might enjoy hearing a traditional Navajo creation story.

Only the Creator knows where the beginning is. The Creator had a thought that created Light in the East. Then the thought went South to create Water, West to create Air, and North to create Pollen from emptiness. This Pollen became Earth. Light, air, water, and earth became the four elements—all of the natural world is interconnected and equal. When the four elements mixed together, the Holy People were created. They were responsible for teaching what is right and wrong. Holy people were given the original laws; then they created the earth and human beings. The Creator and the Holy People created the natural world and put it into *hozjo* (harmony, balance, and peace).

ACROSS THE CURRICULUM

▶ **Language Arts** Read aloud excerpts from *The Girl Who Chased Away Sorrow: The Diary of Sarah Nita, a Navajo Girl, New Mexico, 1864* by Ann Warren Turner (Scholastic, 1999). This book describes the journey of a 13-year-old Navajo Indian girl on the Long Walk in 1863–1864.

For more about the Navajo, recommend the Newbery honor book *Sing Down the Moon* by Scott O'Dell (Yearling Books, 1992).

Explore Navajo art with students. One useful resource is *Enduring Traditions: Art of the Navajo* by Lois Essary Jacka (Northland, 1994).

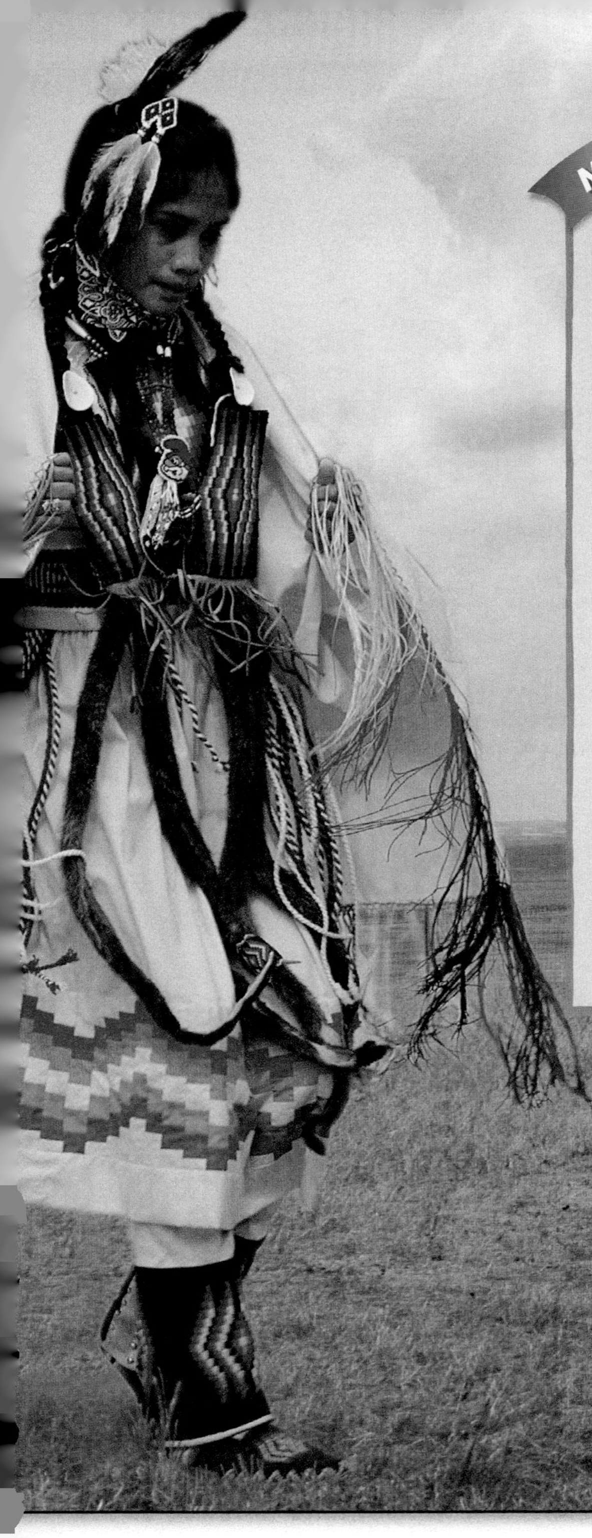

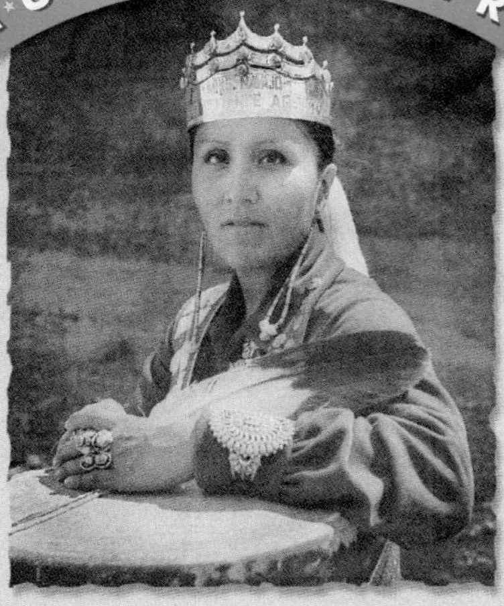

Marilyn Hood

Marilyn Hood, a Navajo singer, dancer, and painter, was born in Arizona and now lives in a traditional hogan outside Gallup, New Mexico. Hood lives with her four children, teaching them the traditional songs she learned as a child. She feels deeply that the old ways should be honored.

Join the Dance!

The traditional circle dance, called the "round" dance, can be performed to *"Yo-shi nai."* It is performed "sunwise" (clockwise, to the left), moving to the left with a sideways movement.

◀ Young Navajo dancer

Invite students to read about a Navajo story and art, in Across the Curriculum on p. 286. Share with students the Navajo creation story, in Cultural Connection on p. 286.

Playing

Copy the notation from Skills Reinforcement on p. 285 onto the board. Ask students to read and follow the notation as they listen to *Jo'ashila* **CD 14–19** again. Ask students if they were surprised to learn that the notation is in mixed meter.

Invite students to perform the beat on a drum with the recording **CD 14–19.** Tell students that all beats should be performed without accents.

3 CLOSE

Analyzing

In a class discussion, review with students the information in this lesson about the culture and music of the Iroquois, Lakota Sioux, and Navajo.

Skill: SINGING   **ASSESSMENT**

Performance/Peer Critique Assign students to two groups. Have each group sing *"Yo-shi nai"* **CD 14–17.** Ask students in each group to assess the other group's singing using the following criteria.

- Clarity of sound (vocables and words)
- Good melodic and rhythmic execution
- Correct performance of accents

Afterward, allow students to offer positive suggestions for improvement.

MOVEMENT

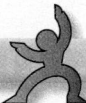

▶ **Patterned Dance** The traditional circle dance, also called the "round" dance, is performed "sunwise" (clockwise, to the left).

Formation: Students form a circle with arms interlocked. (If space is limited, form two concentric circles.)

- Side-step to the left to the beat: left–together, left–together.
- Dance with erect posture.
- Bend the knees when stepping to the left. (This move will make the circle dip slightly.)

When students are comfortable with the dance, encourage them to sing *"Yo-shi nai"* as they dance.

TECHNOLOGY/MEDIA LINK

Web Site Go to *www.sfsuccessnet.com* to learn more about Native American music and instruments.

LESSON AT A GLANCE

Element Focus	**RHYTHM** West African rhythm patterns	
Skill Objective	**PLAYING** Perform as part of a drum ensemble	
Connection Activity	**CULTURE** Examine the role of the master drummer in West African culture	

MATERIALS

- *"Kelo aba w'ye"* — **CD 14–20**
  Recording Routine: Intro (8 m.); vocal (two times)
- *"Take Time in Life"* — **CD 14–22**
  Recording Routine: Intro (8 m.); vocal; interlude (4 m.); vocal; coda
- *Obokete* (excerpt) — **CD 14–21**
- **Resource Book** p. F-26
- *tubanos* (conga-type drums) in medium or low pitches, cowbells, *gankoguis* (or double bells), *shekeres* (or other rattles), soprano or alto recorders
- map of Africa

VOCABULARY

drum ensemble	gankogui (double bell)	shekere
time line	complementary patterns	

◆ ◆ ◆ ◆ National Standards ◆ ◆ ◆ ◆

1c Sing music from diverse cultures
2b Perform easy instrumental pieces with technical accuracy
2c Perform instrumental music from diverse cultures
4a Compose short pieces, demonstrating balance through music
5a Read quarter notes and eighth notes in duple meter
6b Listen and analyze uses of rhythm and timbre in music from diverse cultures
9c Compare, in several cultures, the roles of musicians

MORE MUSIC CHOICES

For more experience with percussion ensembles:
Ionisation, p. 357
Kebjar teruna (Balinese gamelan), p. 385

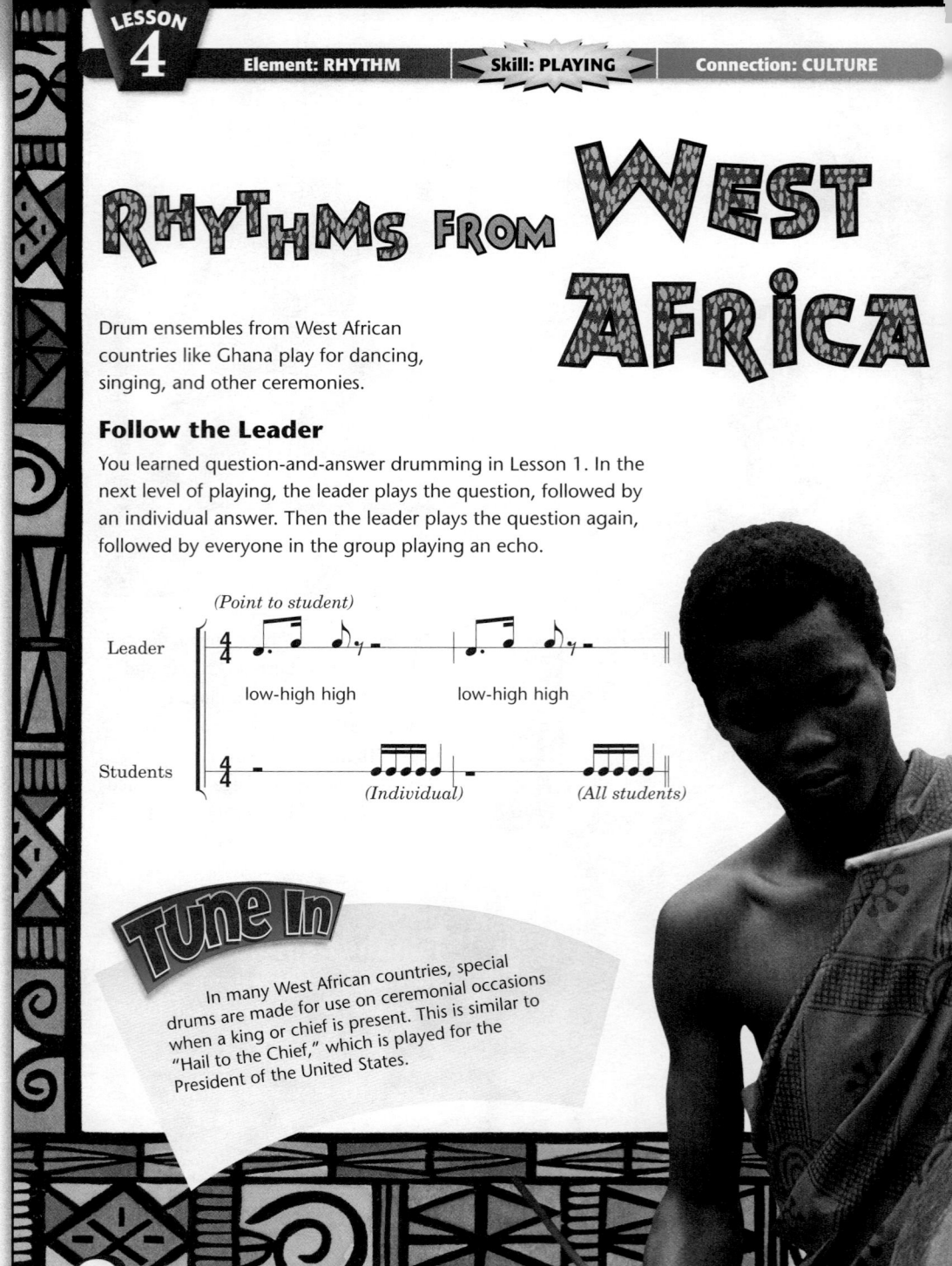

RHYTHMS FROM WEST AFRICA

Drum ensembles from West African countries like Ghana play for dancing, singing, and other ceremonies.

Follow the Leader

You learned question-and-answer drumming in Lesson 1. In the next level of playing, the leader plays the question, followed by an individual answer. Then the leader plays the question again, followed by everyone in the group playing an echo.

(Point to student)
Leader
low-high high   low-high high

Students
(Individual)   (All students)

Tune In

In many West African countries, special drums are made for use on ceremonial occasions when a king or chief is present. This is similar to "Hail to the Chief," which is played for the President of the United States.

288

Footnotes

ACROSS THE CURRICULUM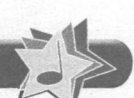

▶ **Social Studies** The Gold Coast, now known as Ghana, intrigues many students. In the visual geography book *Ghana in Pictures* by Lydia Verona Zemba (Lerner Publications, 1988), students learn about the history, geography, government, economy, culture, and people of this African country.

BUILDING SKILLS THROUGH MUSIC

▶ **Social Studies** Ask students to identify the four musical vocations in which Sowah Mensah participates. Lead students in a discussion of each career (composer, arranger, ethnomusicologist, performer). Ask them to name other people in those careers. Discuss each career's place in American society.

CULTURAL CONNECTION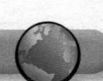

▶ **Ghana** Formerly a British colony, Ghana was the first black African colony to receive independence, on March 6, 1957. The capital city of Accra is located on the southern coast. Much of Ghana is lowlands, with a sandy beach coast, plains, and saltwater lagoons. One third of the country is a forested area that produces cacao, Ghana's most important export, used in making chocolate, and timber. The climate is tropical, with humid air in the southern rain forests and hot, dry air in the northern grassy savannas. The Volta River system dominates the country. The major tribes (among 75 ethnic groups) include the *Akan*, *Ewe*, and *Ga*. English is the official language taught in the schools.

The Gankogui

Double bells are called by different names in West Africa. Among the Ga people of the city of Accra, capital of Ghana, the name is *gankogui* [gahn-KOH-gwee]. The Caribbean relative of the *gankogui* is the smaller, higher-sounding *agogo* bell.

Drum Ensemble 2

Play Drum Ensemble 2 by adding one part after the other.

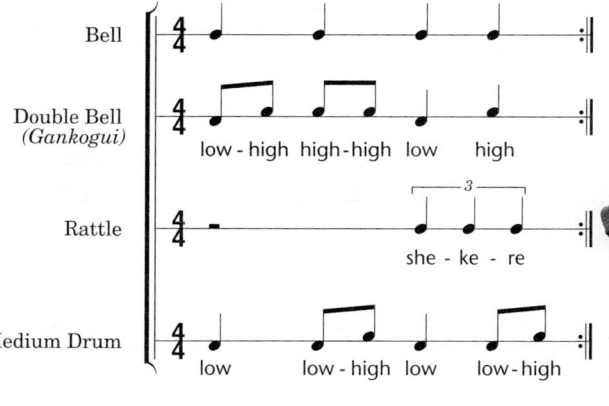

Bell

Double Bell (*Gankogui*) — low - high high - high low   high

Rattle — she - ke - re

Medium Drum — low   low - high low   low - high

Drum Ensemble 2 uses drum, bell, and rattle patterns. Which parts are the same as in Drum Ensemble 1, on page 281?

If you compare the double bell and the *shekere* (rattle) parts, you will see that they complement each other. When the *shekere* plays, the double bell is less busy.

Say It with Drums

1 INTRODUCE

Ask students to recall the most important quality of a good drum ensemble performance. (teamwork) Then have them list the two musical forms that are often combined with drum ensemble playing. (singing and dancing) Drum several short rhythm patterns and encourage students to echo the patterns on their desktops.

2 DEVELOP

Have students

- Read the information about drum ensembles in Ghana.
- Locate Ghana on a map of Africa.

Share with students the information on Ghana found in Cultural Connection and Across the Curriculum on p. 288.

Playing

In this question-and-answer drumming session, have students

- Sit in a circle with their drums.
- Echo drum your drummed patterns. (The patterns should include high [open] and low [bass] tones. Refer to Lesson 1 for examples.)
- Create drum "answers" to your (or student leader's) drummed "questions." (Refer to Lesson 1.)
- Read the information on p. 288 about question-and-answer drumming with echo.
- Play question-and-answer drumming with echo as a group. (Moving around the drumming circle, allow each student to take a turn drumming an "answer" that all students then echo.)

continued on page 290

SKILLS REINFORCEMENT

 ▶ **Notating** Ask students to use standard symbols to notate the meter and rhythm of Drum Ensemble 2 onto staff paper. Have them leave the *shekere* part until last. Suggest that students count the parts out loud as they notate. As they notate the *shekere* part, guide students to understand the quarter-note triplet rhythm in the part.

 ▶ **Mallets** Invite students to play an accompaniment to "Take Time in Life" on mallets, found on Resource Book p. F-26. Consider using parts of this arrangement as an introduction or interlude in a live concert performance of this song.

MEETING INDIVIDUAL NEEDS

▶ **Including Everyone** For students with difficulties playing the various drum parts, try some of these techniques.

- Seat the student next to a strong player on the same part.
- Have the student play a simplified version of the part, leaving out some tones. For example, he or she may play the medium drum part with a bass tone on each beat with the strong hand, or play the *gankogui* part as straight quarter notes: low–high–low–high.
- Have another student lightly tap the rhythm of the part on the student's shoulder corresponding to the hand being used.

Distribute among students the instruments needed to play Drum Ensemble 2. (If necessary, have students use drum substitutes for the medium drum and body percussion for the bell [cowbell] and double bell [gankogui]. The medium drum part can also be played on the low drum.)

Review with students the definition and function of a time line. (A repeated rhythm pattern that becomes the main beat and anchors the drum ensemble.) Before students refer to the notation on p. 289, have them

- Echo your playing of the *gankogui* part, saying the words *low-high, high-high, low, high.*
- Play the *shekere* (rattle) part, saying *she-ke-re,* while the *gankoguis* continue playing.
- Echo your playing of the medium drum part.
- Play the drum, *gankogui,* and *shekere* parts together.
- Echo your playing of the bell (cowbell) part.
2c
- Combine all four parts. The parts should enter the piece in the order in which they're listed in the score.

Additional activities on creating time lines can be found in Skills Reinforcement below.

Notating

5a
When students know Drum Ensemble 2 well, ask them to notate the various parts using Skills Reinforcement on p. 289. Then have them perform the ensemble from their notation or the notation on p. 289.

A Fishing Song

The words of the song "*Kelo aba w'ye,*" from the Ga people of Ghana, mean "bring us fish to eat." When you have learned to **sing** it, **perform** it with Drum Ensemble 2.

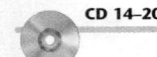 CD 14–20

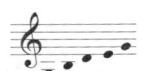

KELO ABA W'YE

Traditional Song from Ghana

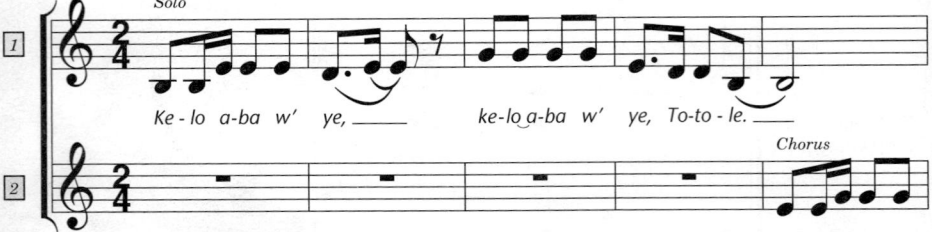

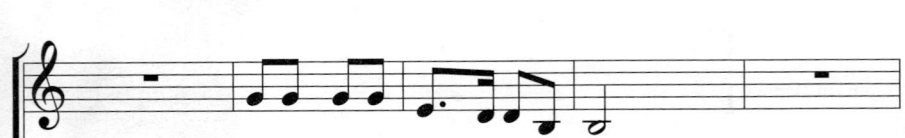

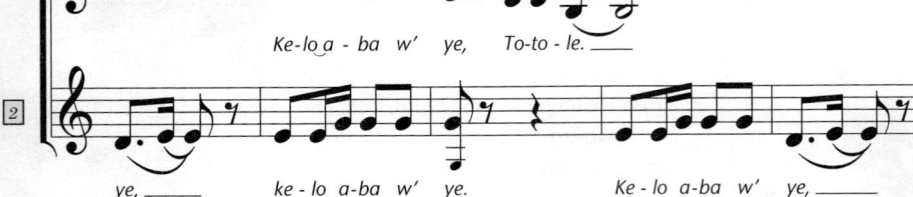

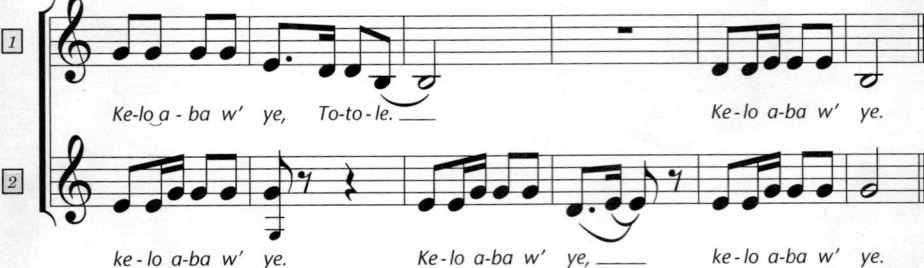

290

Footnotes

SKILLS REINFORCEMENT

4a ▶ **Creating** As an extension to the concept of a time line, invite students to use the *gankogui* (a dual-pitched, two-pronged African bell) to play a time line common to Ghanaian music and create their own layered rhythm patterns. Provide shakers and drums of different pitches to round out the drumming ensemble. As a guideline for exploration, remind students that there are three universally observed principles for achieving a variety of drumming sounds: 1) use open strokes; 2) play bass tones in the middle of the drum; 3) alternate hands to play varied patterns. Keep track among your playing groups of how each group negotiates these principles in its performance.

SPOTLIGHT ON

9c ▶ **Master Drummer** A master drummer plays the following musical roles: teaches and leads the drum ensemble, plays solos over the ensemble, works with the lead dancer(s) to move from one piece to the next, leads singing, plays drum signals to signal the start and stop of different pieces or sections of music, often plays other instruments such as flute or xylophone, and composes new songs and ensembles. Traditional master drummers in Ghana learn by working as apprentices for other master drummers.

Listen to the Pros

Listen to *Obokete*, traditional royal music from Ghana.

Focus on these features.

- the time line played by the bells (Does it stay the same throughout?)
- different drum parts (How many different drum parts do you hear?)
- the interaction of the drum parts

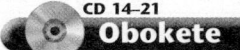
CD 14–21
Obokete

**traditional royal music from Ghana
as performed by Sowah Mensah**

This recording illustrates drum ensembles, which are an important part of West African culture.

M·U·S·I·C   M·A·K·E·R·S

Sowah Mensah

Sowah Mensah is a composer, arranger, ethnomusicologist, and a master drummer from Ghana. He is on the music faculty both of Macalester College and the University of St. Thomas in St. Paul, Minnesota. His compositions have been performed by the Minnesota Orchestra. Mensah enjoys performing throughout North and South America and conducting workshops throughout the United States.

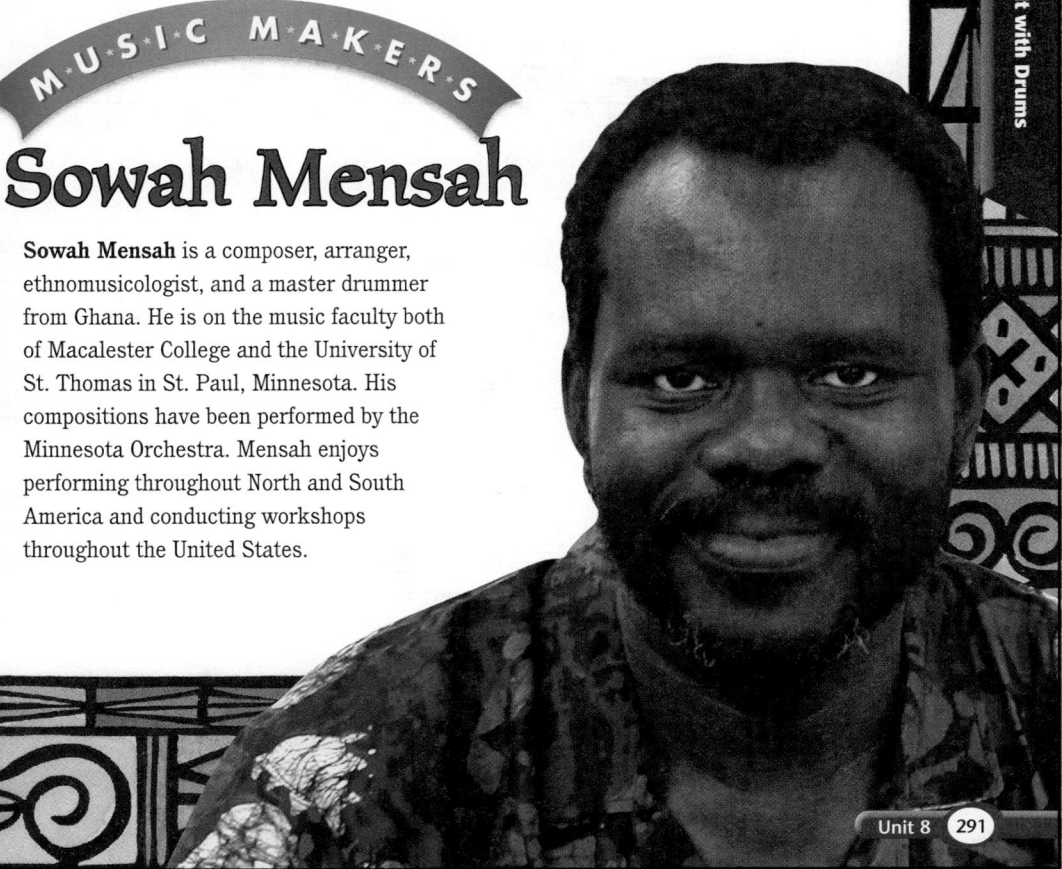

Say It with Drums

Singing

Invite students to

- Read the information about *"Kelo aba w'ye"* on p. 290.
- Listen to *"Kelo aba w'ye"* **CD 14–20,** then sing the solo part.

When students are comfortable singing the song, divide the class into two groups; have one group sing while the other group claps the *shekere* rhythm from Drum Ensemble 2.

Have students listen to *"Kelo aba w'ye"* **CD 14–20,** then echo your singing of the chorus part.

 When students are comfortable with both parts, separate the class into three groups. Have one group begin singing the solo part of *"Kelo aba w'ye"* while a second group claps the *shekere* rhythm from Drum Ensemble 2. Then, have the third group join in, singing the choral response.

 Select eight students to play Drum Ensemble 2 as an accompaniment to the class's two-part singing of *"Kelo aba w'ye."*

Listening

Share with students the information in Spotlight On, p. 290 about the role of a master drummer in Ghana.

Have students

- Read about the musical elements to listen for in *Obokete*.
- Listen to *Obokete* **CD 14–21.**
- Discuss the elements of the piece, using the list of features as a discussion guide. For answers to the questions on p. 291, refer to Teacher to Teacher below.
- Read about master drummer Sowah Mensah.
- Listen to the sound of the *gankogui* in the Sound Bank recordings, beginning on p. 512.

continued on page 292

ACROSS THE CURRICULUM

▶ **Language Arts** Refer interested readers to *Beyond the Mango Tree* by Amy Bronwen Zemser (Greenwillow, 1998). This is an enchanting story of an American girl who moves with her family to Liberia and is unhappy until she makes a new friend and understands another world.

CHARACTER EDUCATION

▶ **Taking Time for Yourself** Help students understand the importance of taking time for themselves (spend time with family and friends, exercise, play a sport) What are the benefits of taking time for yourself? (makes life more enjoyable, helps balance work and play, gives you time to enjoy activities and people, and allows you to enjoy the beauty of nature)

TEACHER TO TEACHER

▶ **Management Tips** The following questions and answers may prove helpful in guiding students' listening to *Obokete*.

- Does the time line stay the same throughout the piece? (No, the tone changes; it begins with a low bell, then a high bell, then low, then high.)
- Is there a *shekere* part? (No, there are no rattles used in the piece.)
- How many different drum parts do you hear? (Initially, there are two—low and high. Next, three are heard—low, medium, and high. Finally, there are many different parts.)
- How do the drum parts interact? (There is alternation of drums and call-and-response drumming.)

Singing

Guide students in recalling that they learned to sing a West African song, "Nana Kru," in an earlier lesson. (Lesson 2)

ASK From what country does "Nana Kru" come? (Liberia)

If time permits, have students sing "Nana Kru" on p. 282.

Invite students to

- Listen to the recording of "Take Time in Life" **CD 14–22.**
- Sing the chorus when it occurs on the recording.

When students are comfortable with the chorus, select several students to clap the *shekere* rhythm from Drum Ensemble 2 while the others sing the chorus of "Take Time in Life."

6b ASK How are the rhythms of the chorus and the *shekere* complementary? (When the chorus is busy rhythmically in beats 1 and 2, the *shekere* is silent; when the *shekere* plays, the chorus is less busy.)

Have students

- Sing the solo parts and the chorus of "Take Time in Life" **CD 14–22** with the recording.
- Sing the harmony parts in the chorus.

2b When students feel comfortable with the song, select six to eight students to play Drum Ensemble 2 while the class sings the song.

Invite students who have an interest in Liberia to read a story from Across the Curriculum on p. 291.

Moving

Teach students the patterned dance in Movement below. Have students perform the movements as they sing "Take Time in Life."

Enjoy a Little Harmony

Sing "Take Time in Life," from Liberia. It can also be **performed** with Drum Ensemble 2.

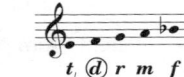

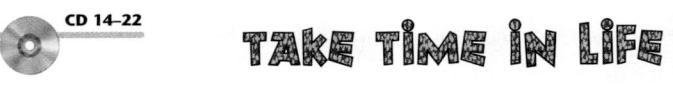

CD 14–22

Folk Song from Liberia

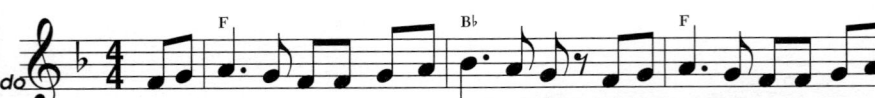

I was pass-ing by, My broth-er called to me, And he said to me you bet-ter sis - ter she

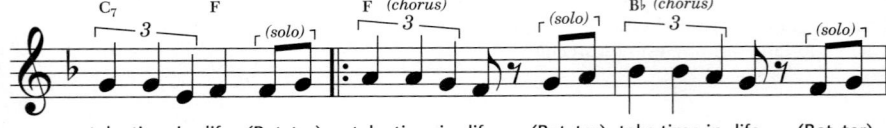

take time in life. (Bet-ter) take time in life, (Bet-ter) take time in life, (Bet-ter)

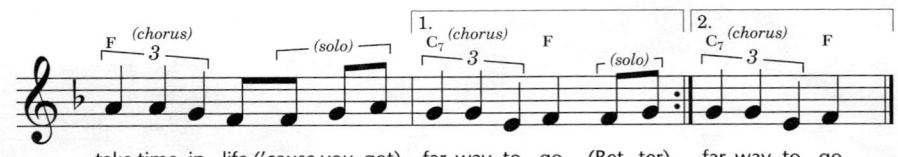

take time in life ('cause you got) far way to go. (Bet-ter) far way to go.

For variety, **perform** the chorus parts of "Take Time in Life" in harmony.

Chorus (with harmony parts 2 and 3)

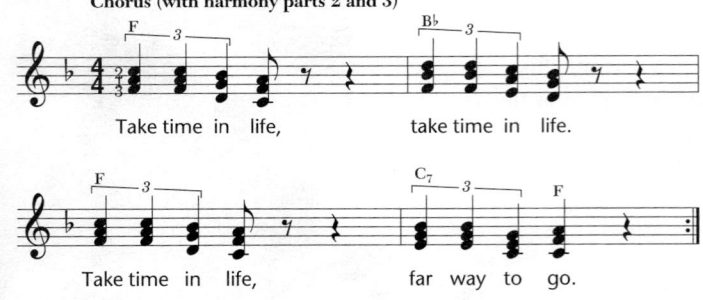

Take time in life, take time in life.

Take time in life, far way to go.

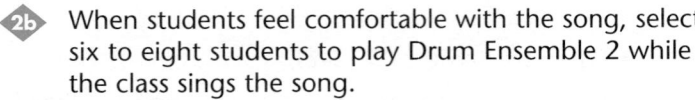

292

Footnotes

MOVEMENT

► **Patterned Dance** Students will enjoy performing this movement with "Take Time in Life."

Formation: Students stand in a circle (or two semicircles).

- To a count of four, step left-together, right-together.
- Clap on the right-foot step on beat 3.
- While moving, sing the chorus of "Take Time in Life."

SPOTLIGHT ON

► **The Performer** A contemporary master drummer, Sowah Mensah is proficient in computer music technology and composes for traditional instruments and symphony orchestra. He records his own CDs, and composes and plays African gospel music with piano and other instruments. Besides teaching world music drumming at summer workshops, this master drummer performs with a wide variety of chamber music, popular music, and Latin music ensembles.

Play Those Patterns

Show that you understand how African drum ensembles use complementary layered patterns by forming small ensembles of four players (two bells, two drums, one rattle); then **create** and **play** your own rhythms, using the following routine.

- The first bell player starts with a time line. The *gankogui* player enters with a short pattern that repeats many times.
- The rattle player then adds a complementary pattern that fits with the bell.
- The drummers then add complementary parts.
- **Play** your ensemble for the class or record it.
- If time permits, switch instruments and **create** another ensemble.

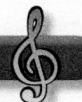

Say It with Drums

Unit 8 **293**

Creating

 Separate the class into groups of four or five students with these instruments in each group: one *gankogui* (double bell), one *shekere* (rattle), two or three drums of different pitches.

Ask each group to create a drum ensemble piece in which

- The bell plays a simple repeated pattern.
- The rattle plays a complementary pattern.
- One by one the drums enter with their complementary patterns.

To add recorders to the ensemble, see Skills Reinforcement below.

3 CLOSE

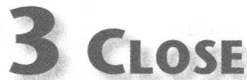
Skill: PLAYING   **ASSESSMENT**

Performance/Peer Critique Organize the class into four groups. Provide each group with the percussion instruments to play Drum Ensemble 2, p. 289. As a class, play Drum Ensemble 2. Then have each group perform Drum Ensemble 2.

Each group should assess the other groups' performances using the following criteria

- Does each part enter correctly?
- Does each part play its rhythm correctly?
- Does the group maintain a steady tempo?
- Does the group have a nice balance? (Each part is the same volume and can be heard.)

SKILLS REINFORCEMENT

▶ Recorder Students can play the harmony parts for "Take Time in Life," using soprano and alto recorders. Have them play the lower part on the alto recorder and the upper parts on soprano recorders.

Soprano recorder players will need to review the fingering for B♭ before playing their parts. Remind students of the half-step rule.

- Think of the fingering for the note that is a half step higher than the note with the accidental.
- To learn B♭, students should first finger B on the recorder; then skip a hole and cover the next two holes.

TECHNOLOGY/MEDIA LINK

Web Site Have students choose one African percussion instrument and research it at *www.sfsuccessnet.com*. Have students discuss what they learned about each instrument.

LESSON AT A GLANCE

Element Focus   **TEXTURE/HARMONY** Thick texture

Skill Objective   **LISTENING** Listen to a percussion ensemble piece while following a listening map

Connection Activity   **RELATED ARTS** Discuss the folk art of African *kente* cloth

MATERIALS

- *"Banuwa"*   CD 15–1

  Recording Routine: Intro (32 m.); vocal; interlude (16 m.); vocal; coda

- **Pronunciation Practice/Translation** p. 533

- "Everybody Loves Saturday Night"   CD 15–4

  Recording Routine: Intro (32 m.); vocal; interlude (8 m.); vocal; coda

- *Kpanlogo for 2* (excerpt)   CD 15–6

- **Dance Directions** for *Kpanlogo for 2* (highlife) p. 561

- *Evening Samba*   CD 15–8

- **Resource Book** pp. A-22, F-28, G-20, H-27

- *tubanos* (conga-type drums) in high, medium, and low pitches; cowbells; rattles; soprano recorders; guitars

VOCABULARY

highlife music

◆ ◆ ◆ ◆ **National Standards** ◆ ◆ ◆ ◆

1c Sing music from diverse cultures
1d Sing music written in three parts
2c Perform instrumental music from diverse cultures
4c Arrange, using electronic media
5c Identify standard notation symbols for pitch
6b Listen and analyze uses of harmony and timbre in music from diverse cultures
9c Compare, in several cultures, functions music serves

MORE MUSIC CHOICES

For more practice with texture in thirds and sixths:
"Siyahamba," p. 212
"Wai bamba," p. 26

A TASTE OF THE HIGHLIFE

Highlife music is very popular in cities throughout the continent of Africa.

"Banuwa," from Liberia, can be sung with the highlife drumming on the next page.

CD 15–1
MIDI 21

Highlife combines traditional West African style and jazz. Instruments often include saxophones, brass, electric guitars, and percussion.

BANUWA

Folk Song from Liberia

Ba - nu - wa, ba - nu - wa, ba - nu - wa yo.

Ba - nu - wa, ba - nu - wa, ba - nu - wa yo.

Ba - nu - wa, ba - nu - wa, ba - nu - wa yo. *(2nd time only) (A-)*   *Fine*

la - no, neh - ni a - la - no. A - la - no. A -

la - no, neh - ni a - la - no. A - la - no.   *D.S. al Fine*

294

Footnotes

MEETING INDIVIDUAL NEEDS

▶ **Including Everyone** When preparing students for the movement activity on p. 295 that accompanies "Everybody Loves Saturday Night," arrange chairs in a circle so that students can sit rather than stand to do the hand clapping. You may also want to create picture prompts of the hand-clapping activity so that students with disabilities can practice with these prompts a few times.

BUILDING SKILLS THROUGH MUSIC

▶ **Social Studies** Share the information from Spotlight On, p. 294, and Cultural Connection, p. 295. Have students locate Africa on the map. Focus their attention on the places in Africa included in the lesson.

SPOTLIGHT ON

9c ▶ **Highlife** A major influence on pop styles throughout the world, highlife music originated in Ghana and Sierra Leone and has become one of Africa's most popular forms of contemporary music. Highlife is a fusion of Ghanaian dance rhythms and melodies and Western influences. Early forms of highlife included dance bands, village brass bands, and rural guitar bands. Musicians used "found" instruments, such as old and discarded European brass, winds, and drums in these early bands.

In 1948, E. T. (Sowah) Mensah and his band incorporated West African melodies and rhythms into the music. By the 1980s, highlife experienced a major revival in Ghana and other parts of the world. One of the forms of highlife in Ghana is *kpanlogo*. Today, highlife has absorbed Western electric instruments and elements of Afro-Caribbean reggae.

Drum Ensemble 3 (Highlife)

Practice Drum Ensemble 3 by first learning to **play** the rattle (shekere) part. Then add the bell and drum parts.

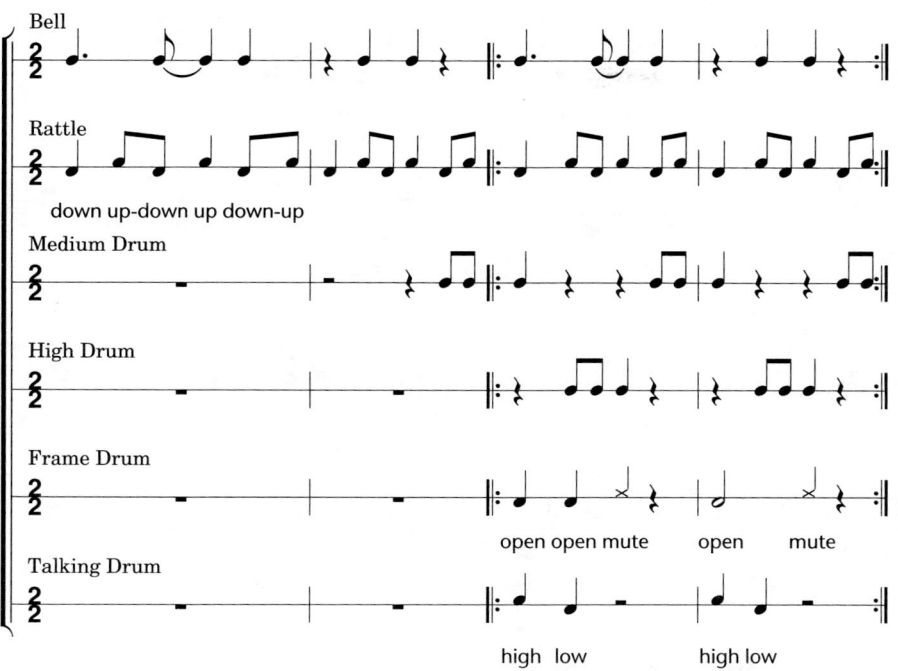

Bell

Rattle

down up-down up down-up

Medium Drum

High Drum

Frame Drum

open open mute   open   mute

Talking Drum

high low   high low

Say It with Drums

Give a Hand for Highlife

"Everybody Loves Saturday Night," on page 296, is popular throughout West Africa. **Sing** it with highlife Drum Ensemble 3.

Perform the movements below with Drum Ensemble 3 or *Kpanlogo for 2* on page 296.

- Stand in a circle.
- Keep your left palm up and right palm down; match that up with each person next to you. Clap your neighbor's hands once.
- Turn your hands over and clap again.
- Clap your own hands twice in front.

Repeat this pattern.

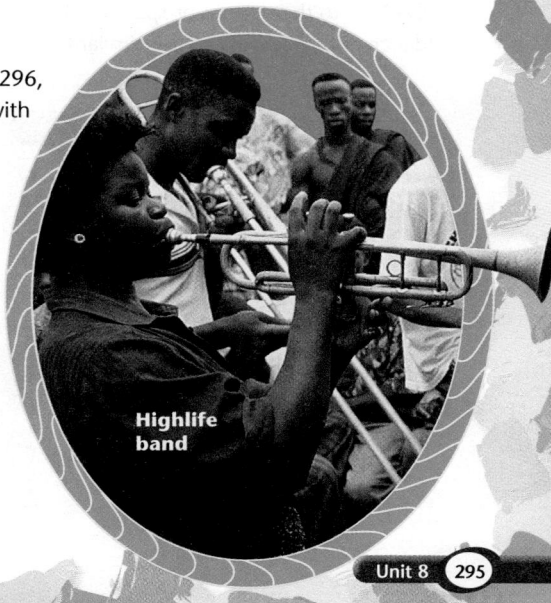

Highlife band

Unit 8 **295**

1 INTRODUCE

Share with students information on African arts and culture, in Spotlight On, p. 294, and in Cultural Connection below. Lead students in a discussion of the rich tradition of African music and folk art.

Tell students they will learn about layers and textures in African highlife music.

2 DEVELOP

Singing

1c Share with students that the words of the Liberian song *"Banuwa,"* p. 294, mean "Don't cry, pretty little girl."

Invite students to listen to the recording of *"Banuwa"* **CD 15–1**, then use the Pronunciation Practice Guide on Resource Book p. A-22 and the Pronunciation Practice **CD 15–3** to sing the song.

When students can sing the melody, have them

- Sing the melody with the recording to practice holding a melody while hearing the harmony.
- Echo sing part 2 (a third above the melody).
- Echo sing part 3 (the remaining note in the triad).

Analyzing

Share with students that an A-major triad is constructed of a root (A), a third (C♯), and a fifth (E).

5c **ASK** On which note of the triad does the melody of *"Banuwa"* start? (third)

> **On which note does part 2 start?** (fifth)
>
> **On which note does part 3 start?** (root)

Singing

1d Have students echo sing the melody for the verse of *"Banuwa,"* and then echo-sing the verse's harmony. Assign parts to students and invite them to sing a harmonized *"Banuwa"* with the recording **CD 15–1**.

continued on page 296

SKILLS REINFORCEMENT

5c ▶ **Notating** Guide students in discovering the primary triads and chord symbols used in *"Banuwa"*: A (I), D (IV), and E (V). Assist students in notating these triads and symbols. If guitars are available, teach students to play the A, D, and E (or E₇) chords. Use the guitar accompaniment in a class performance of *"Banuwa."*

▶ **Reading** Invite students to read the following rhythm. Then add the hand-clapping highlife movements, on p. 295, to *"Banuwa."*

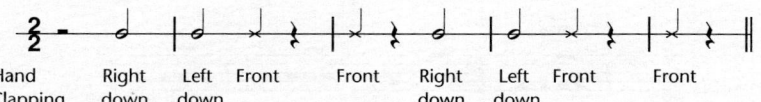

| Hand Clapping | Right down | Left down | Front | | Front | Right down | Left down | Front | | Front |

CULTURAL CONNECTION

▶ *Kente Cloth from Ghana* Share with students that *kente* cloth, made by the Asante people of Ghana and the Ewe people of Ghana and Togo, is the best known of all African textiles. The practice of weaving this cloth in strips began in the former Gold Coast of West Africa as festive dress for special occasions. *Kente* comes from the word *kenten*, which means "basket." The Asante people also refer to *kente* as *nwentoma*, or "woven cloth." Today *kente* cloth is used for a wide variety of decorative coverings of various objects, including drums.

Playing

Invite students to listen to the Stereo Performance track of *"Banuwa"* **CD 15–1** as they follow Drum Ensemble 3 on p. 295. (Note: The recording includes a double bell part that follows the entrance of the bell.)

Double bell

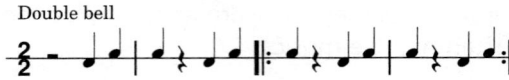

2c Have students observe as you play the rattle part. Then ask students to play the rattles while saying the rhythm syllables.

SAY This pattern is the basis of the highlife rhythm.

Have students

- Clap the bell part as you play the bell.
- Move on the beat to a pattern of right-together, left-together, while saying the bell pattern.
- Play the bell part on the cowbell.

Invite students to play the rattle and bell parts together. Ask students without instruments to clap the bell part.

Have students

- Play the high drum part while saying rhythm syllables in a high voice.
- Play the medium drum part while saying rhythm syllables in a lower voice.

For additional activites, have students create a guitar accompaniment and hand-clapping movements to *"Banuwa."* See Skills Reinforcement on p. 295.

Singing

1c Have students listen to "Everybody Loves Saturday Night" **CD 15–4.** Then, sing the song with the recording.

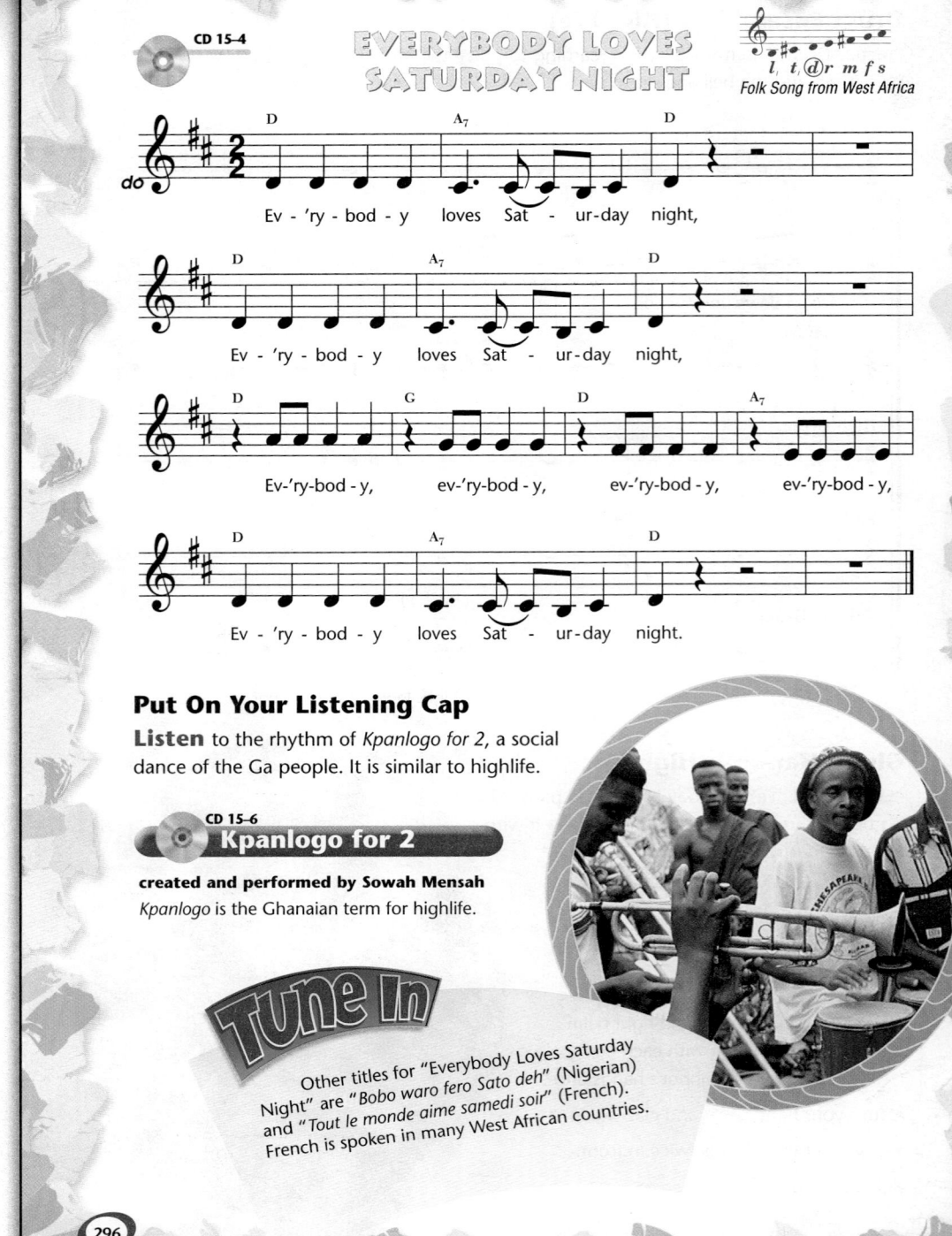

EVERYBODY LOVES SATURDAY NIGHT

Folk Song from West Africa

l, t, @r m f s

Ev - 'ry - bod - y loves Sat - ur - day night,

Ev - 'ry - bod - y loves Sat - ur - day night,

Ev - 'ry - bod - y, ev - 'ry - bod - y, ev - 'ry - bod - y, ev - 'ry - bod - y,

Ev - 'ry - bod - y loves Sat - ur - day night.

Put On Your Listening Cap

Listen to the rhythm of *Kpanlogo for 2*, a social dance of the Ga people. It is similar to highlife.

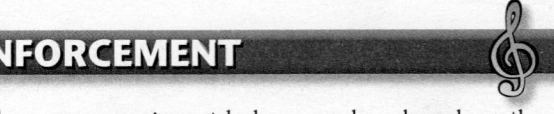

Kpanlogo for 2

created and performed by Sowah Mensah
Kpanlogo is the Ghanaian term for highlife.

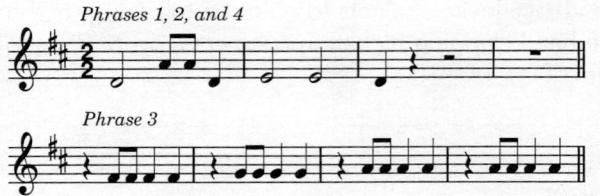

Other titles for "Everybody Loves Saturday Night" are "Bobo waro fero Sato deh" (Nigerian) and "Tout le monde aime samedi soir" (French). French is spoken in many West African countries.

296

Footnotes

MOVEMENT

▶ **Patterned Dance** Students will enjoy learning to move to highlife. First have students perform the highlife hand-clapping rhythm and movement activity in Skills Reinforcement on p. 295. Then share with students the background information and pattern dance movements for highlife in Dance Directions, p. 561. Students will perform the highlife dance to *Kpanlogo for 2* **CD 15–6.**

SKILLS REINFORCEMENT

▶ **Recorder** The accompaniment below can be played on the soprano recorder with "Everybody Loves Saturday

2c Night." Have students compare the rhythm of the recorder part with the rhythm of the song melody. Ask students, "In which phrase is the rhythm the same but the melody different?" (phrase 3)

Phrases 1, 2, and 4

Phrase 3

Everybody Loves a *Samba*

Listen to *Evening Samba* as you follow the listening map. Notice how similar this South American *samba* is to the African highlife style.

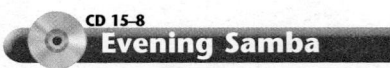
CD 15–8
Evening Samba

created and performed by Mickey Hart and the musicians of Planet Drum

Many of the world's greatest drummers joined together to make this recording. Performers include Airto Moreira, Babatunde Olatunji, Sikiru Adepoju, Zakir Hussain, and T. H. Vinayakram.

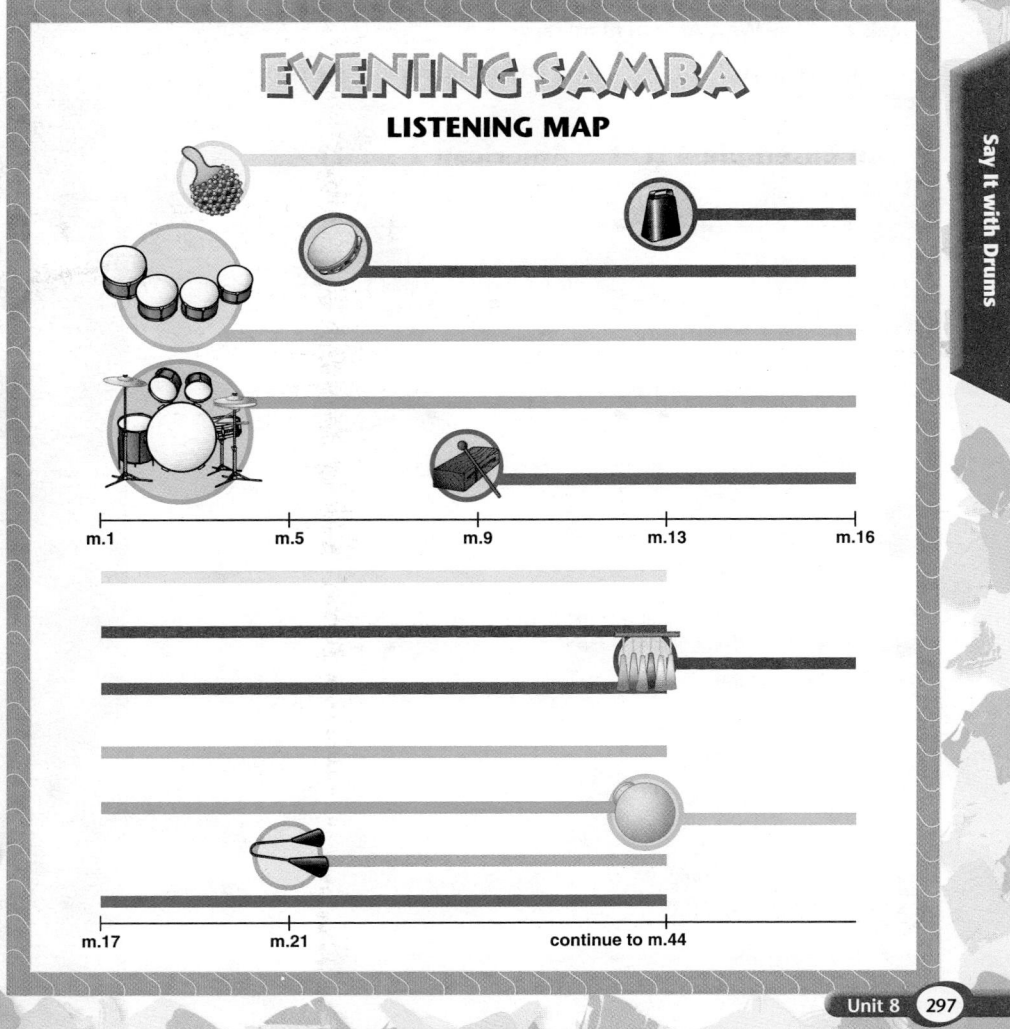

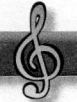

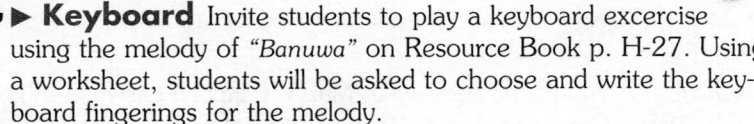

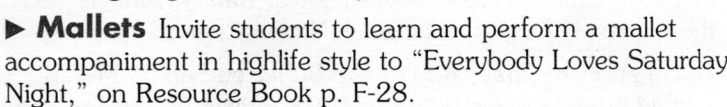

Unit 8   297

Moving

Invite students to perform the hand-clapping movements, on p. 295, with either "Everybody Loves Saturday Night," *Kpanlogo for 2,* or Drum Ensemble 3. See Movement below and Dance Directions, p. 561, for more movement activities.

Students may also wish to learn and perform the signing to "Everybody Loves Saturday Night." See Skills Reinforcement on p. 297.

Listening

9c Share with students that the Ga people of Ghana enjoy a social dance called *kpanlogo*. Invite them to listen to *Kpanlogo for 2*, as performed by Sowah Mensah.

Playing

2c Have students perform a highlife piece as follows.

- Play Drum Ensemble 3, beginning with one instrument then adding the others in turn.
- Sing *"Banuwa"* **CD 15–1** with vocal harmony and instruments.
- Play Drum Ensemble 3 as an interlude.
- Sing "Everybody Loves Saturday Night" **CD 15–4** with Drum Ensemble 3.

Invite students to play a recorder countermelody with "Everybody Loves Saturday Night." See Skills Reinforcement on p. 296.

3 CLOSE

Element: TEXTURE/HARMONY   ASSESSMENT

6b   Music Journal Writing Play *Evening Samba* **CD 15–8** as students follow the listening map on p. 297. Have students listen to the piece and indicate the distinct texture changes as they occur. Then have them describe, by writing in their music journals, the changes of texture in terms of rhythm patterns and instrumental timbres.

See Technology/Media Link below for tips on using the listening map transparency.

SKILLS REINFORCEMENT

▶ **Keyboard** Invite students to play a keyboard excercise using the melody of "*Banuwa*" on Resource Book p. H-27. Using a worksheet, students will be asked to choose and write the keyboard fingerings for the melody.

▶ **Mallets** Invite students to learn and perform a mallet accompaniment in highlife style to "Everybody Loves Saturday Night," on Resource Book p. F-28.

▶ **Signing** Students may be interested in learning and performing the signing to "Everybody Loves Saturday Night" on Resource Book p. G–20.

TECHNOLOGY/MEDIA LINK

4c   Sequencing Software Prepare the computer to be used as a learning center. In small groups, students will create a multiple-track recording using MIDI drum sounds. After they learn the drum ensemble for "*Banuwa*," have students

- Set keyboard for percussion sounds and explore those sounds that most closely emulate those of the "*Banuwa*" drum ensemble.
- Perform and record several tracks of rhythms using various percussion sounds.

Transparency Display the listening map transparency for *Evening Samba* as you play the recording. You may wish to point to each section of the piece on the first listening to help students follow along.

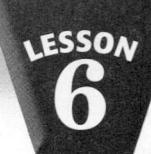

LESSON AT A GLANCE

Element Focus — **TIMBRE** Caribbean percussion instruments

Skill Objective **PLAYING** Perform in a Latin drum ensemble

Connection Activity **CULTURE** Discuss geography and cultures of the Caribbean

MATERIALS

- "Water Come a Me Eye" **CD 15–10**

  Recording Routine: Intro (12 m.); v. 1; refrain; interlude (8 m.); v. 2; refrain; coda
- *"Má Teodora"* **CD 15–12**
- *"Má Teodora"* (English) **CD 15–13**

  Recording Routine: Intro (12 m.); vocal; interlude (8 m.); vocal; coda
- **Pronunciation Practice/Translation** p. 533
- *Gidden riddum* (excerpt) **CD 15–9**
- **Resource Book** pp. A-23, F-29, I-22
- *tubanos* (conga-type drums) in medium or low pitches; two pairs of claves; two pairs of maracas; two *guiros,* bongos or *timbales;* guitars (optional); soprano and alto recorders
- map of Caribbean

VOCABULARY

claves	maracas	*guiro*	bongos
timbales	steel drums	calypso	

◆ ◆ ◆ ◆ National Standards ◆ ◆ ◆ ◆

1c Sing music from diverse cultures
1d Sing music written in two parts
2b Perform easy instrumental pieces with technical accuracy
2c Perform instrumental music from diverse genres
2d Perform simple accompaniments by ear
4c Arrange, using electronic media

MORE MUSIC CHOICES

For more practice with Caribbean songs:
"Give a Little Love," p. 140
"Lost My Gold Ring," p. 158

CARIBBEAN Connections

The drum ensembles in the Caribbean islands have been influenced by West African and European music. Drum Ensemble 4 feels a lot like West African highlife.

Practice each part. Then **play** as an ensemble, adding one part at a time.

Drum Ensemble 4 (Latin American 2-beat)

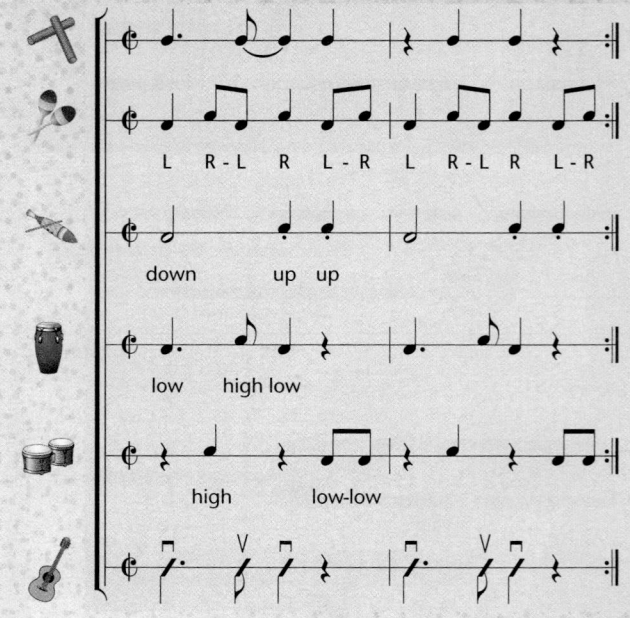

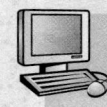

Video Library Watch the video *Steel Drums* to learn more about steel drums from the Caribbean.

Footnotes

CULTURAL CONNECTION

▶ **Calypso Style** The essential music of Trinidad and Tobago is calypso. This style grew out of the nineteenth-century celebration of Carnaval (like Mardi Gras) and is part satire, news, commentary, and defiance. The style features exaggerated, distorted, and accented speech, with a syncopated counter rhythm. The singer either creates an original tune or uses a known melody to get across a political or satirical point. *Soca,* a more recent style, is a combination of calypso and soul music.

BUILDING SKILLS THROUGH MUSIC

▶ **Language** Ask students the meaning of the title "Water Come a Me Eye." Ask them what in the text and their personal experience supports their answer.

ACROSS THE CURRICULUM

▶ **Language Arts** Invite students to discuss famous people from the island of Cuba.

- *Rafael Palmeiro* by Barbara J. Marvis (Mitchell Lane, 1997). In 1987, Chicago Cubs baseball player Rafael Palmeiro had the highest batting average of all National League rookies.
- *Alicia Alonso: First Lady of the Ballet* by Sandra Martin Arnold (Walker & Co. Library, 1993). Alicia Alonso became a prima ballerina, dancing in North and South America, Europe, and Asia, even though detached retinas in both eyes left her virtually blind in her early twenties.

Drums of Steel

The sound of steel drums is unique and recognized by most people as coming from the Caribbean. Steel drums are made from empty oil drums with tops that are shaped to produce musical pitches. Striking a specific area of the drum with a mallet produces a musical note with a timbre that is distinctly "steel drum."

Listen to this steel drum excerpt and the unique sound of this drum.

CD 15–9
 Gidden riddum

by Emile Borde
as performed by the Trinidad Tripoli Steel Band
The music of this steel drum ensemble includes elements of soca, calypso, and reggae styles.

Tune In

The steel drum was developed in Trinidad in the 1930s. There are numerous sizes of steel drums, ranging from bass to tenor.

Say It with Drums

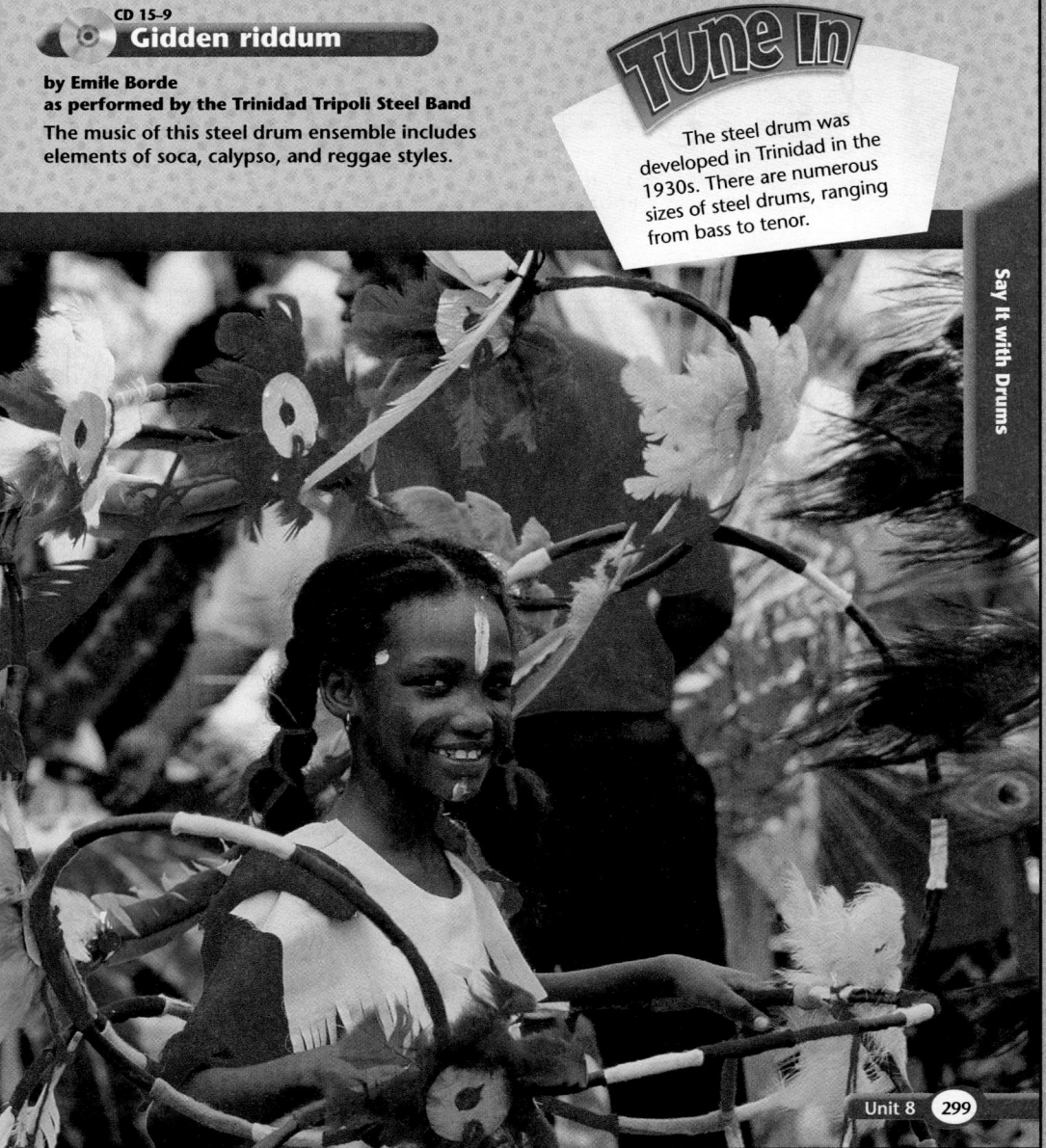

Unit 8 **299**

1 INTRODUCE

Play a short excerpt from Drum Ensemble 4 **CD 15–10** (the recorded introduction of "Water Come a Me Eye"). Share with students that music of the Caribbean influenced the music of West Africa and of highlife.

2 DEVELOP

Listening

Have students use a map of the Caribbean to locate the islands of Trinidad, Tobago, and Cuba. Share the information in Cultural Connection, pp. 298 and 300. Refer students with an interest in Cuba to books in Across the Curriculum on p. 298. Then play the steel drum piece *Gidden riddum* **CD 15–9**.

Let students listen to more examples of steel drums in the Sound Bank, starting on p. 512.

Playing

2b To teach students to play the claves, ask them to

- Hold the claves with one clave cradled loosely in their weak hand and the other clave held in their strong hand.
- Play the clave pattern for Drum Ensemble 4, saying *bup, boo, bup, rest, bup, bup, rest.*

ASK When have you heard and played this rhythm before? (the bell part in Drum Ensemble 3)

Invite students to play the claves and say the pattern. Students without claves should clap and say the pattern.

To teach students to play the maracas, invite them to

- Play with one in each hand; the wrists held rather stiffly.
- Play the maracas part for Drum Ensemble 4, saying *cha chick-a cha chick-a.* (Students without maracas should play imaginary ones.)

continued on page 300

SKILLS REINFORCEMENT

1d ▶ **Singing** "Water Come a Me Eye" and *"Má Teodora"* provide the opportunities for students to practice singing harmony in thirds and sixths.

- Have students determine that the harmony of "Water Come a Me Eye" is parallel to the melody, except for the final note in the refrain.
- Divide the class, with more students on melody than harmony.

"Má Teodora" has a single response that begins at the interval of a sixth, with the last note of the call being the first of the harmony part.

▶ **Mallets** Invite students to perform a mallet accompaniment to "Water Come a Me Eye," on Resource Book, p. F-29.

MEETING INDIVIDUAL NEEDS

▶ **Learning Idioms** Students often find the use of idioms to be confusing. Use the song "Water Come a Me Eye" to reinforce the learning of idioms.

Reinforcement For English language learners, idioms (phrases with a different meaning from the words themselves) are difficult to understand. Ask foreign language students to share with the class a culturally appropriate idiom.

On Target Once the class understands the idiom *water come a me eye* (crying), invite students to create a list of other idioms. (Baseball: *out of the park* = homerun)

Challenge Invite students to create a brand new idiom that no one has ever heard. Stimulate their imagination by suggesting a topic (basketball) and an activity (a dunk). Possible answer = *flying point slammer.*

Unit 8 *Say It with Drums* **299**

ASK When have you heard and played this rhythm?
(the rattle part in Drum Ensemble 3)

2b To teach students to play the *guiro,* ask them to

- Hold the *guiro* in the weak hand with fingers in the holes; with stick in strong hand, scrape downward once (away from the body), then scrape upward (toward the body) twice in *staccato* fashion.

- Play the *guiro* while saying *drrrrrr dut dut* to prepare for Drum Ensemble 4.

To prepare students for playing the bongos on page 298, have them use body percussion. Invite them to

- Pat the steady beat (half note in cut time) on the side of their thigh with their weak hand.

- Pat the off-beats on the side of their other thigh with their strong hand. (The rhythm is as follows: "weak-strong-weak-strong/strong.")

- Transfer their playing to the bongos or *timbales* on page 298. (Have them pat the side of the drum on the steady beat.)

2c To teach students to play Drum Ensemble 4, have them

- Play and say the parts for claves, maracas, *guiro,* and bongos or *timbales.*

- Play and say *low-high/low* on the low conga *(tubano)* part.

- Play the guitar strum (down-up-down) to the same rhythm as the conga. See Skills Reinforcement below. (This part is optional.)

Combine the parts, adding each new part (when the ensemble is stable) according to score order.

Singing

Have students

- Echo sing the response melody of "Water Come a Me Eye."

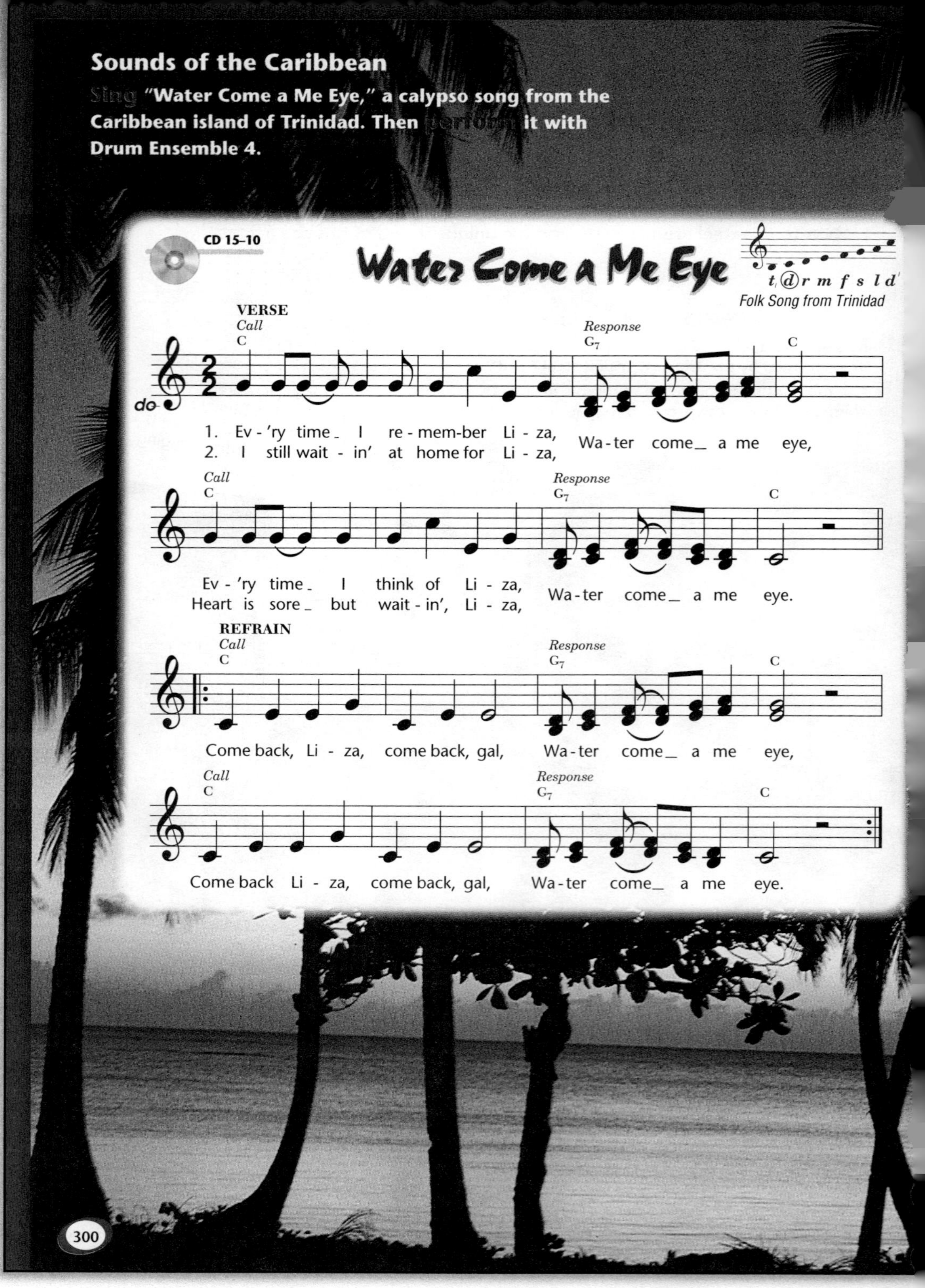

Sounds of the Caribbean

Sing "Water Come a Me Eye," a calypso song from the Caribbean island of Trinidad. Then perform it with Drum Ensemble 4.

CD 15–10

Water Come a Me Eye

t, @ r m f s l d'

Folk Song from Trinidad

VERSE

Call

Response

1. Ev-'ry time I re-mem-ber Li-za, Wa-ter come a me eye,
2. I still wait-in' at home for Li-za, Wa-ter come a me eye.

Ev-'ry time I think of Li-za, Wa-ter come a me eye,
Heart is sore but wait-in', Li-za, Wa-ter come a me eye.

REFRAIN

Call *Response*

Come back, Li-za, come back, gal, Wa-ter come a me eye,

Come back Li-za, come back, gal, Wa-ter come a me eye.

300

 Footnotes

CULTURAL CONNECTION

▶ **Two Caribbean Nations** The independent nation and member of the Commonwealth of Nations made up of the two islands of Trinidad and Tobago is famous for steel bands, calypso, and Carnaval. The capital city is Port of Spain. Explored by Christopher Columbus in 1498, the islands have been under the influence of five different cultures: Spanish, British, Carib Indian, Dutch, and French.

Cuba, at 750 miles long and 125 miles wide, is the largest island in the Greater Antilles. A Spanish colony until 1898, its capital is Havana. Cuba's official language is Spanish. Although sugar is the major export crop, potatoes, rice, sweet potatoes, eggs, tobacco, and citrus are produced and exported.

SKILLS REINFORCEMENT

▶ **Guitar** Invite students to use the guitar strum below to accompany "Water Come a Me Eye." If students have difficulty **2d** with this strum, have them play half-note down-strums on the beat.

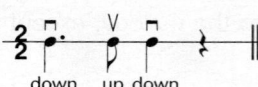

down   up down

▶ **Recorder** Invite students to play a soprano and alto recorder accompaniment to "Water Come a Me Eye," on Resource Book p. I-22.

Sing "Má Teodora." In the song, *chopping up the firewood* refers to dancing.

Play Drum Ensemble 4 to accompany "Má Teodora."

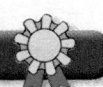

Má Teodora

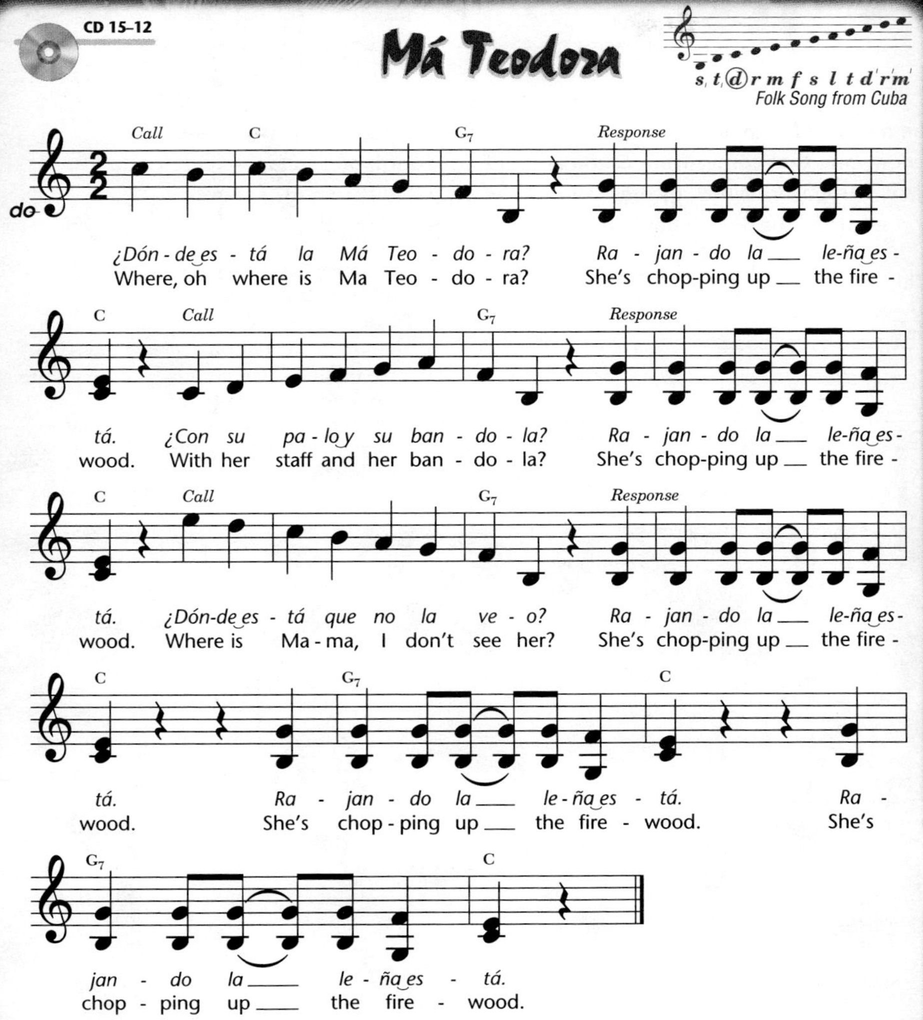

s, t, (d) r m f s l t d' r m'
Folk Song from Cuba

CD 15–12

Call C G₇ *Response*

¿Dón - de es - tá la Má Teo - do - ra? Ra - jan - do la __ le - ña es -
Where, oh where is Ma Teo - do - ra? She's chop-ping up __ the fire -

C *Call* G₇ *Response*

tá. ¿Con su pa - lo y su ban - do - la? Ra - jan - do la __ le - ña es -
wood. With her staff and her ban - do - la? She's chop-ping up __ the fire -

C *Call* G₇ *Response*

tá. ¿Dón - de es - tá que no la ve - o? Ra - jan - do la __ le - ña es -
wood. Where is Ma - ma, I don't see her? She's chop-ping up __ the fire -

C G₇ C

tá. Ra - jan - do la __ le - ña es - tá. Ra -
wood. She's chop - ping up __ the fire - wood. She's

G₇ C

jan - do la __ le - ña es - tá.
chop - ping up __ the fire - wood.

- Sing the responses with the recording **CD 15–10**.
- Echo sing the response harmony, using Skills Reinforcement, p. 299.

1d Divide the class and have half sing the response melody and half sing the harmony with the recording. Then have them sing the calls with the recording.

Share with students the information about Teodora Gines in Spotlight On below. Then, play the recording of "Má Teodora" in English **CD 15–13**. (Remind students that *chopping up the firewood* means "dancing up a storm.")

Explain to students that the rhythm of the response is a typical Latin American pattern of grouping eighth notes:

1 – 2 – 3   **1** – 2 – 3   **1** – 2

Clap and say this rhythm with students.

1c Use the Pronunciation Practice Guide on Resource Book p. A-23, and the Pronunciation Practice **CD 15–15** and **CD 15–16** to help students learn to sing "Má Teodora" in Spanish. Then, have them sing the song in Spanish with the recording **CD 15–12**.

2c Select ten students to play Drum Ensemble 4 as an accompaniment to either "Water Come a Me Eye" **CD 15–10** or "Má Teodora" **CD 15–12**. Begin with the instruments and then bring in the song.

3 CLOSE

Element: TIMBRE   ASSESSMENT

Portfolio Organize students into groups of three or four. Have each group create a list of five sounds that characterize Caribbean music to add to a class portfolio. Allow the groups to share their lists with the class. (instruments from Drum Ensemble 4, Spanish language, steel drums, call and response, 3 + 3 + 2 rhythms)

SPOTLIGHT ON

▶ *Má Teodora* Teodora Gines, of African descent, was born into slavery. Because she and her sister, Michaela, showed great musical gifts, they were freed to enter the service of the Cathedral at Santiago de Cuba as musicians. Gines is credited with being the mother of modern Cuban folkloric music.

CHARACTER EDUCATION

▶ **Sensitivity** Tell students the phrase *water come a me eye* refers to crying. Ask them: What are the benefits of crying? (stress reliever, allows us to express emotions) What are some ways other than crying to deal with your emotions? (take a walk, play music, write about your feelings) Have them share their feelings about crying with the class.

TECHNOLOGY/MEDIA LINK

4c **CD-ROM** Have students use *Band-in-a-Box* to build a Caribbean accompaniment for "Water Come a Me Eye" or "Má Teodora." Have students

- Enter the song settings—key, length, chorus, intro.
- Enter the chord changes in the measures.
- Select a Caribbean style from the style menu.
- Click play to hear the accompaniment. Invite some students to perform rhythm patterns in the accompaniment.

Video Library Show the video *Steel Drums* to have students learn more about steel drums. Invite students to discuss this unique instrument.

LESSON AT A GLANCE

Element Focus MELODY Pentatonic scales

Skill Objective SINGING Sing a folk song in Japanese

Connection Activity RELATED ARTS Discuss minimalism in Japanese fine arts

MATERIALS
- *"Asadoya"* (Japanese) — CD 15–17
- *"Asadoya"* (English) — CD 15–18
  Recording Routine: Intro (2 m.); vocal; coda
- *Pronunciation Practice/Translation* p. 534
- *Lion* (excerpt) — CD 15–21
- *Resource Book* pp. A-24, F-31
- keyboard or mallet instruments

VOCABULARY
pentatonic   *taiko* drumming

◆ ◆ ◆ ◆ **National Standards** ◆ ◆ ◆ ◆
- **1c** Sing music from diverse cultures
- **3b** Improvise melodic variations on given melodies
- **8a** Show how different arts portray the same idea in unique ways
- **9a** Describe characteristics of music genres from a variety of cultures
- **9c** Compare, in several cultures, functions music serves

MORE MUSIC CHOICES
For more practice with Asian music:
"Bắt kim thang" p. 13

1 INTRODUCE

8a
9c
Explain to students that the many people who live on the small islands of Japan and Okinawa have little personal space. As a result, they have learned to "make much from little," particularly in their arts. Share with students information, in Cultural Connection below, about Japanese fine arts.

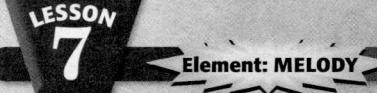

Asian Drums

The music of Japan and Okinawa uses two different pentatonic (five-tone) scales—one that comes from China and one that originates in Japan. **Sing** *"Asadoya."* Which of these two scales is used in the song? **Listen** to the *koto* in the Sound Bank. How can you identify it on the recording?

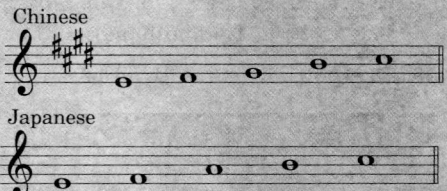

Chinese

Japanese

Arts Connection

Bridge Across the Moon (artist unknown). Japanese gardening, poetry, and art are sometimes expressed in miniature. Examples include bonsai trees, haiku poetry, and the miniature brush strokes in fine paintings. ▼

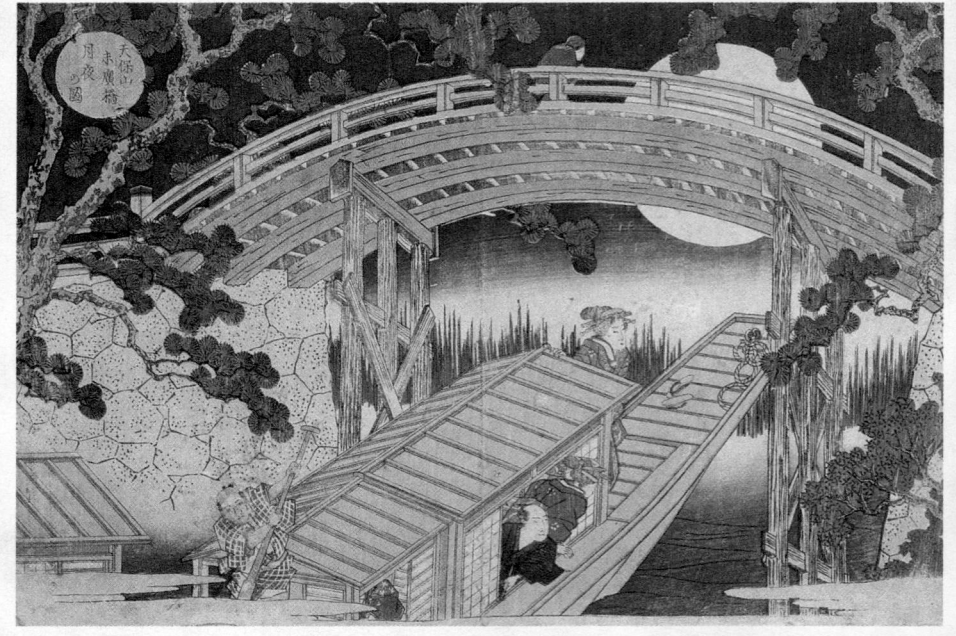

302

Footnotes

SKILLS REINFORCEMENT

 ▶ **Mallets** Pentatonic songs such as *"Asadoya"* lend themselves to performance on mallet instruments. However, *"Asadoya's"* key of E-pentatonic is not an appropriate key for mallets. For an F-pentatonic ostinato accompaniment to *"Asadoya,"* see Resource Book p. F-31. Students may sing along in F-pentatonic as others play on mallet instruments.

BUILDING SKILLS THROUGH MUSIC

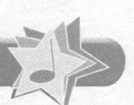

▶ **Language** After listening to Lion and reading the information about *taiko* drumming, ask students to write their answer to the question: Why did the performers choose the name "Kodo Drummers" for their ensemble?

CULTURAL CONNECTION

8a ▶ **Japanese Fine Arts** The Japanese concept of "making much from little" is a strong influence on the culture's fine arts. *Bonsai* [BAHN-si], a 2,000-year-old Asian horticultural art, literally means "tree-in-a-pot." A tree planted in a small pot is not a bonsai until it has been pruned, shaped, and trained into the desired shape, harmony, proportion, and scale. *Sumi-e,* Japanese brush paintings with ink, show nature in tiny well-crafted scenes. *Haiku* [hi-koo] is Japanese poetry written vertically in one line or, in English, three lines that paint a simple scene. Haiku usually has at least two images, but no more than three, that paint a scene.

CD 15–17

Asadoya

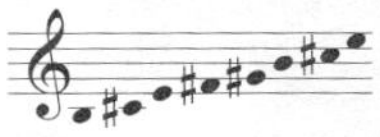

English Words by D. G. Britton

Folk Song from Okinawa

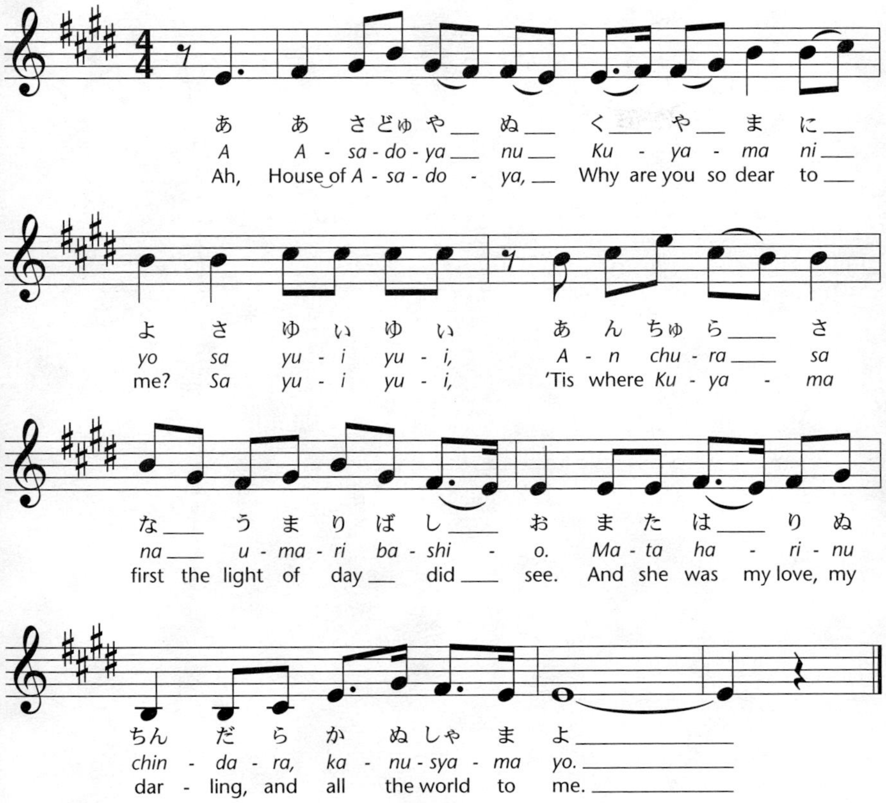

あ　あ　さどゅや＿　ぬ＿　く＿や＿ま　に＿
A　　A - sa-do-ya＿　nu＿　Ku - ya - ma　ni＿
Ah,　House of A - sa - do - ya,＿　Why are you so dear　to＿

よ　さ　ゆ　い　ゆ　い　　あ　ん　ちゅ　ら＿＿　さ
yo　sa　yu - i　yu - i,　A - n　chu - ra＿＿　sa
me?　Sa　yu - i　yu - i,　'Tis where Ku - ya - ma

な＿　う - ま　り　ば　し＿　お　ま　た　は＿　り　ぬ
na＿　u - ma - ri　ba - shi＿ - o.　Ma - ta　ha - ri - nu
first the light of　day＿　did＿　see.　And she was　my love, my

ちん　だ　ら，　か　ぬ　しゃ　ま　よ＿＿＿＿＿＿
chin - da - ra,　ka - nu - sya - ma　yo.＿＿＿＿＿
dar - ling, and　all　the world　to　me.＿＿＿＿＿

Say It with Drums

Martial Drumming

Taiko is a popular and dramatic form of Japanese drumming that relates to martial arts. The drums are played with large dowel-like sticks.

Listen to this example of *taiko* drumming, performed by an ensemble from the Japanese island of Sado.

CD 15–21
Lion

created and performed by Leonard Eto and the Kodo Drummers

Kodo has two meanings: "heartbeat" and "children of the drum." Why, do you think, did the performers choose this name for their ensemble?

Unit 8 **303**

2 DEVELOP

Singing

Invite students to read aloud the English lyrics of *"Asadoya."* Explain that *Sa yui yui* are vocables—syllables without any specific meaning that produce good singing sounds.

Have students

- Sing *"Asadoya"* **CD 15–18** in English with the recording.
- Learn the Japanese lyrics by singing with the Pronunciation Practice **CD 15–20.** (Resource Book p. A-24)

- Follow the notation on p. 302 while listening to the two forms of pentatonic scales—Japanese and Chinese—as you play them on a keyboard.

ASK **Which of the two scales is used in** *"Asadoya"?* (Chinese)

Playing

Invite students to play the mallet accompaniment to *"Asadoya,"* on Resource Book p. F-31.

Listening

Point out to students that Japanese music can also be very exciting, as in *taiko* drumming. Ask students to listen to *Lion* **CD 15–21**, a recording of *taiko* drumming. See Spotlight On below for facts on *taiko*.

3 CLOSE

Element: MELODY **ASSESSMENT**

Performance/Observation Divide the class into three groups and assign each group one phrase of lyrics from *"Asadoya."* Have students in each group

- Improvise a new melody for their phrase, based on the first pentatonic scale shown on p. 302. (Transpose to *F*-pentatonic if students are to use Orff instruments.)
- Sing and play the phrases in the proper order.

SPOTLIGHT ON

▶ *Taiko* Modern Japanese *taiko*, performed as an ensemble *(kumi-daiko)*, was created in 1951 by Daihachi Oguchi. Oguchi, a jazz drummer, found an old piece of *taiko* music and arranged it for a *taiko* drum ensemble of various-sized drums, including the high-pitched *shime-daiko* (which plays the backing rhythm), the large barrel-shaped *odaiko* (which plays a simple rhythm that grounds the pulse), a variety of smaller barrel-shaped *nagado-daiko* (which play riffs that push the music along), and the metallic *tetsu-zutsu* (a bell-like instrument made of three pieces of pipe). *Taiko* today is performed by ensembles all over the world.

▶ *Asadoya* In *"Asadoya,"* *Kuyama* is the name of a girl the singer once loved. *House of Asadoya* refers to Kuyama's family and ancestors.

TECHNOLOGY/MEDIA LINK

MIDI/Sequencing Software Have students work in small groups to create a multiple-track recording using MIDI drum sounds. After listening to recordings of *taiko* drum ensembles, have students

- Explore percussion sounds that most closely emulate *taiko* drums. (See Spotlight On for drum descriptions.)
- Improvise and record several tracks of rhythms using various percussion sounds.

LESSON AT A GLANCE

Element Focus **RHYTHM** Indian drum improvisation within a *tala*

Skill Objective **LISTENING** Listen to and echo the rhythms played by North Indian *tabla* drummers

Connection Activity **CULTURE** Examine Indian culture and dance

MATERIALS
- *Máru-bihág* (excerpt)   **CD 15–22**
- *Maha ganapathim* (excerpt)   **CD 15–23**
- *Dham dhamak dham samelu* (excerpt)   **CD 15–24**
- **Dance Directions** for *Dham dhamak dham samelu* p. 562
- sticks, drums

VOCABULARY
tabla   mridangam   sitar   tamboura   tala   veena

◆ ◆ ◆ ◆ National Standards ◆ ◆ ◆ ◆
2c Perform instrumental music from diverse cultures
6a Listen and describe events in music using appropriate terms
6b Listen and analyze uses of rhythm in music from diverse cultures
9a Describe characteristics of music styles from a variety of cultures

MORE MUSIC CHOICES
For more practice with eighth- and sixteenth-note rhythms: "La mariposa," p. 58

1 INTRODUCE

9a **SAY** North and South India have different musical and cultural traditions. *Hindustani* music of northern India features two drums called *tabla* [tah-blah]; *Carnatic* music of southern India uses a two-headed barrel-shaped drum called a *mridangam* [mree-dahn-gahm]. Indian dance is also associated with a geographic region.

Indian Rhythms

In northern India, drummers play a set of drums called *tabla*. Southern Indian drummers play the *mridangam*, a double-headed drum. Drummers from both traditions first learn drum patterns vocally. They use syllables, such as "ta-tika-doom." (See the Sound Bank for more information on the Indian instruments in this lesson.)

Indian Ensembles—North

A typical classical music ensemble from northern India is comprised of the *sitar*, the *tamboura*, and the *tabla*.

Listen to this excerpt, featuring Ravi Shankar, one of the most famous sitar players in the world.

CD 15–22
Máru-bihág

Traditional Indian Raga as performed by Ravi Shankar

Máru-bihág begins with a short, non-rhythmic section played by *sitar* and *tamboura*. This is followed by a longer, rhythmic section in which the *tabla* joins in.

Tune In

The *tamboura* plays sustained tones (drones) using the intervals of the octave and the fifth in the natural harmonic series.

Tabla from northern India ▶

304

Footnotes

ACROSS THE CURRICULUM

▶ **Social Studies** For more information about India's fascinating people, arts, and culture, refer students to *India: The People* by Bobbie Kalman (Crabtree, 1989) and *Gandhi, Peaceful Warrior* by Rae Bains (Troll, 1996), a moving account of the life of India's famous leader of nonviolent social reform, Mahatma Gandhi. Suggest to students that they compare the philosophy and social activism of Gandhi and Dr. Martin Luther King, Jr.

BUILDING SKILLS THROUGH MUSIC

▶ **Social Studies** Have students locate India on a world map. Have them discuss what they know about North and South India. Suggest to students that they research India and share in class what they learn.

SKILLS REINFORCEMENT

2c ▶ **Playing** Echo the following *tabla* rhythm. Then, play the pattern on a drum. On *toon*, play the low drum.

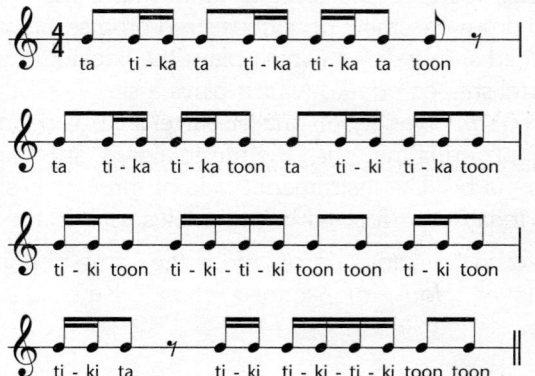

ta   ti - ka ta   ti - ka ti - ka ta   toon

ta   ti - ka   ti - ka toon   ta   ti - ki   ti - ka toon

ti - ki toon   ti - ki - ti - ki toon toon   ti - ki toon

ti - ki ta   ti - ki   ti - ki - ti - ki toon toon

Indian Ensembles—South

Classical music ensembles from South India often feature the *veena*—a large, fretted, plucked, string instrument. Other traditional South Indian instruments include the *mridangam, tamboura,* flute, and violin.

Listen to this selection played by a South Indian ensemble. Which instruments do you hear?

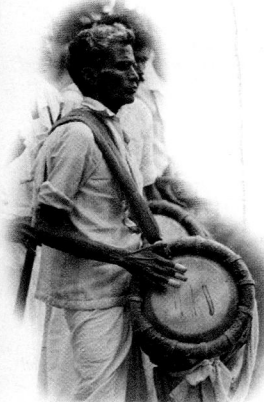

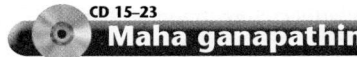
CD 15–23
Maha ganapathim

by Muthuswami Dikshitar
as performed by Shrimati Rejeswari Pariti and Shri Vadiraja Bhat

Shrimati Rajeswari Pariti, an accomplished *vainika* (*veena* player), performs *carnatic* music—classical music of South India. The *veena,* one of the oldest instruments in the world, dates back to 500 B.C.

Dancing with Sticks

The *raas* is a stick dance from India that is performed during festivals.

Perform the movements of the Indian Stick Dance to the music *Dham dhamak dham samelu.* Be very careful when moving your sticks.

As you move, count in meter in 4 and play each tap on the strong beat—half note.

▲ *Mridangam* drum from South India

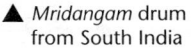
CD 15–24
Dham dhamak dham samelu

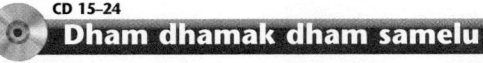
Stick Dance from the Gujarati Region of India
The Stick Dance is often performed continuously with many songs accompanying it.

Stick Dance

1. "Tap Right"—Move your sticks to the right side of your body. Tap your own sticks together.

2. "Tap Partner Right"—Move your sticks to the center, keeping your sticks parallel to the right. Tap your partner's sticks.

3. "Tap Partner Left"—Keeping your sticks in front of you, "pivot" your sticks to the left (keeping your sticks parallel). Tap your partner's sticks.

4. "Tap Right"—Move your sticks to the right side of your body (as in step 1). Tap your own sticks together.

5. "Tap Single Stick"—Move only your right stick to the center. Tap your partner's stick. Turn.

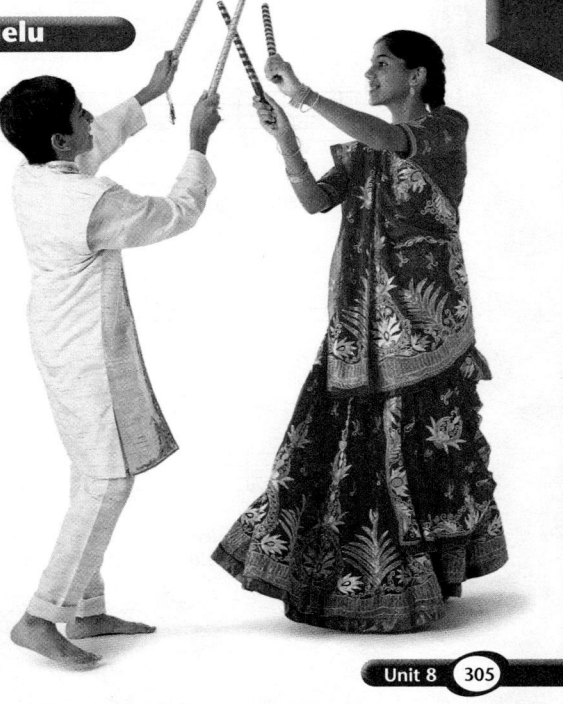

Say It with Drums

Unit 8 **305**

2 DEVELOP

Listening

Share with students that drummers from North and South India improvise rhythms within a cycle of beats, called *tala.* A *tala* may be from 3 to 128 beats, but most do not exceed 20 beats. Write the *Jhaptal* on the board and point out how the beats are grouped. Invite students to slowly count and tap the *tala* in rhythm.

1 2 3 4 5 6 7 8 9 10

6b Have students listen to *Máru-bihág* **CD 15–22** and count the *Jhaptal* along with Ravi Shankar.

Invite students to play the *tabla* rhythm in Skills Reinforcement on p. 304.

Play the recording of *Maha ganapathim* **CD 15–23** as an example of a South Indian ensemble featuring the *veena* and *mridangam.*

Have students listen to the *tamboura* and *mridangam* in the Sound Bank, starting on p. 512.

Moving

Invite students to learn the movements of the Indian stick dance as shown on p. 305. Share background information on the stick dance from Movement below. Then, perform the dance *Dham dhamak dham samelu* **CD 15–24** with the recording.

3 CLOSE

Skill: LISTENING   **ASSESSMENT**

6a **Written Assessment** Have students listen to *Maha ganapathim.* Ask students to write on paper a brief description of the function of the *veena* and the *mridangam* in the South India ensemble. (The *veena* plays the melody and drone harmony. The *mridangam* provides the rhythmic accompaniment.)

MOVEMENT

▶ **Patterned Dance** The Indian Stick Dance (also called *Raas, Ras,* or *Raj*) is a traditional folk dance of Gujarati, India, celebrated during the festival of *Raas Garaba.* Sticks are painted with colors or wrapped with shiny laces. Dancers wear colorful clothing—girls wear *saris, chania-chori* and jewelry; boys wear *habbha, durta* and *lehnga.* Dance instructions on the stick dance can be found in Dance Directions on p. 562.

Dham dhamak dham samelu is a folk dance that is sung and danced when villagers make flour from grain. Villagers pound the grain with a *samelu,* a painted wooden pole 5 to 6 feet tall. The grain is placed in a *khayna,* a concrete hole in the ground. Villagers sing and dance while making the flour. The sound and rhythm of the pounding of the grains is *dham dhamak dham dham dham.*

TECHNOLOGY/MEDIA LINK

Web Site Go to *www.sfsuccessnet.com* to learn more about the music and instruments of India.

Video Library See the video *Instrumental Ensemble from India* for a segment featuring improvisations by musicians from India.

LESSON AT A GLANCE

Element Focus | **TIMBRE** Percussion from the Middle East

Skill Objective | **MOVING** Sing and move to two Middle Eastern celebration songs

Connection Activity | **SOCIAL STUDIES** Examine the geography and history of the Middle East

MATERIALS

- "Alumot" (excerpt) — **CD 15–26**
- "Sheaves of Grain" — **CD 15–27**
  Recording Routine: Intro (4 m.); vocal; interlude (4 m.); vocal; coda
- **Pronunciation Practice/Translation** p. 535
- "Al yadee" — **CD 15–32**
  Recording Routine: Intro (4 m.); v. 1; instrumental (12 m.); v. 2; coda
- Yemeni baglamis telli basina (excerpt) — **CD 15–36**
- **Dance Directions** for "Alumot" and "Al yadee" p. 563
- dombak (or other available drums), videotape recorder (optional), world map
- **Resource Book** p. A-25

VOCABULARY

dombak   debke   hora

◆ ◆ ◆ National Standards ◆ ◆ ◆ ◆

1c Sing music from diverse cultures
2c Perform instrumental music from diverse cultures
5a Read quarter, eighth, sixteenth and dotted notes in duple meter
8b Identify ways music relates to social studies
9a Describe characteristics of music styles from a variety of cultures

MORE MUSIC CHOICES

For more practice with music of the Middle East:
"Hava nagila," p. 153
"Shalom aleichem," p. 409

Shades of the Middle East

The Middle East is filled with wonderful culture, traditions, and music. Middle Eastern folk dances are an important part of the region's culture. Songs often have rhythms and melodies that let you both sing and dance to them. "Alumot" is one such song.

Sing "Alumot," an Israeli song that celebrates the harvest.

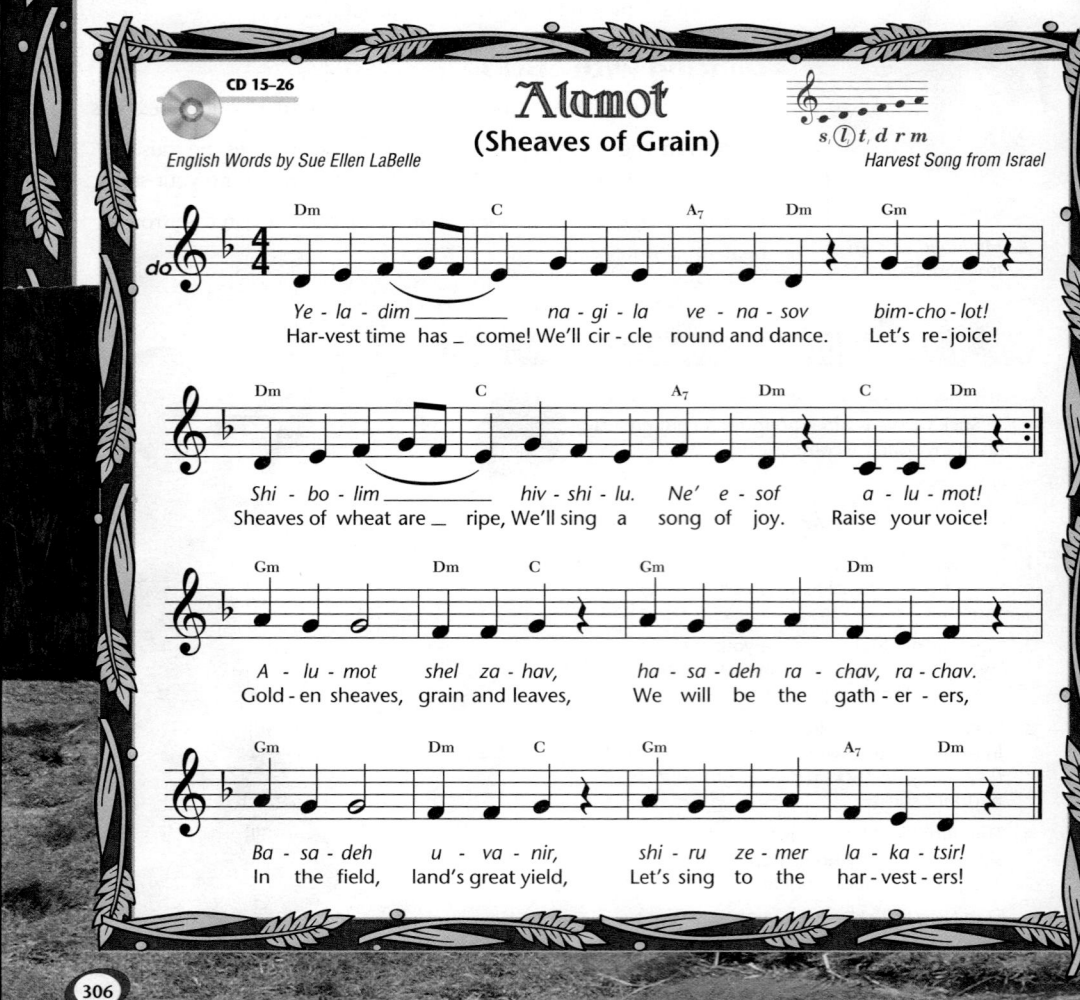

CD 15–26

Alumot
(Sheaves of Grain)

English Words by Sue Ellen LaBelle

Harvest Song from Israel

s (l) t, d r m

Ye - la - dim _____ na - gi - la ve - na - sov bim - cho - lot!
Har - vest time has _ come! We'll cir - cle round and dance. Let's re - joice!

Shi - bo - lim _____ hiv - shi - lu. Ne' e - sof a - lu - mot!
Sheaves of wheat are _ ripe, We'll sing a song of joy. Raise your voice!

A - lu - mot shel za - hav, ha - sa - deh ra - chav, ra - chav.
Gold - en sheaves, grain and leaves, We will be the gath - er - ers,

Ba - sa - deh u - va - nir, shi - ru ze - mer la - ka - tsir!
In the field, land's great yield, Let's sing to the har - vest - ers!

306

Footnotes

CULTURAL CONNECTION

▶ **Israel** Israel is situated in an area considered to be holy land for Christians, Jews, and Muslims. The Jewish state of Israel was established on May 14, 1948, on British-controlled land called Palestine. The official languages of Israel are Hebrew and Arabic, although English is also common. About 83% of its people are Jewish, coming from different national backgrounds all over the globe, while about 17% are Arab. The three largest cities are Jerusalem, Tel Aviv–Jaffa, and Haifa.

BUILDING SKILLS THROUGH MUSIC

▶ **Dance** Have students read about the hora and the debke. Then, ask students to identify the most prominent differences between the two dances.

ACROSS THE CURRICULUM

▶ **Social Studies** Palestine, originally the home of ancient Israel and Judah, is located today in the modern states of Israel and Jordan. Since A.D. 70, Palestine has been controlled by the Romans and Byzantines, the Islamic Caliphate, European crusaders, Egyptians, Turks, and the British.

Write on the board the Arabic and Hebrew words for "peace," shown below. Then discuss the similarities between the two words. Ask students to suggest reasons for the similarities. (Both languages share similar roots.)

SHALOM (Hebrew)

SALAAM (Arabic)

An Israeli Hora

The *hora* was a popular Romanian dance that came to Israel in the early twentieth century with Romanian settlers. At that time, the land was called Palestine. Israel later became a nation in 1948. The word *hora* means "circle dance."

The *hora* is danced in a closed circle with your hands joined with your neighbors' hands at your side. It can also be danced with your hands on your neighbors' shoulders. In Israel, the traditional *hora* moves to the left (clockwise). The steps are high and energetic, with leaps and kicks. The movements are similar to those of the Arabic *debke*, which moves to the right.

The basic Israeli *hora* movement is: Step L, step R, step L, lift R, step R, lift L.

Perform the Israeli *hora* to the music of "*Alumot.*"

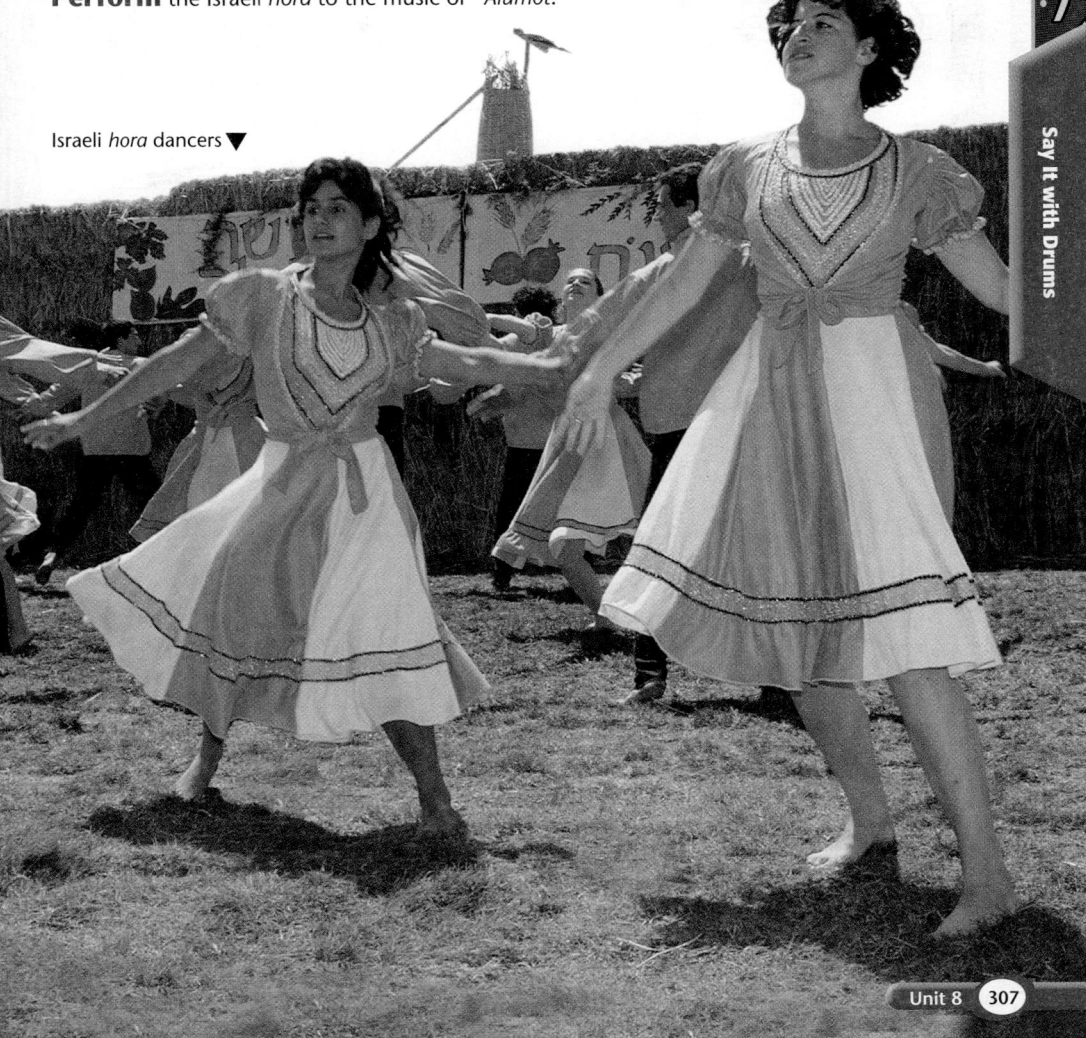
Israeli *hora* dancers ▼

Say it with Drums

Unit 8 **307**

1 INTRODUCE

Guide students in locating the Middle East (also known as western Asia) on a world map. Ask them to locate Israel on the same map. Share with students the information found in Cultural Connection and Across the Curriculum, p. 306. Then ask students to think of similarities the two cultures might share. (livelihood, dress, music, dance, food)

2 DEVELOP

Singing

8b Share with students that the song "*Alumot,*" p. 306, is an Israeli song that celebrates a plentiful wheat harvest.

Have students

1c
- Learn the song's Hebrew words, using the Pronunciation Practice **CD 15–29** and the Pronunciation Practice Guide on Resource Book p. A-25.
- Sing the song with the recording **CD 15–26**, and then in English with **CD 15–27**.
- Memorize the song so that they can sing it while performing the *hora.*

Moving

Using the information on p. 307 and in Spotlight On below, introduce students to the *hora,* a traditional circle dance. Then guide students in learning the dance, using the directions in Movement below.

Gradually increase the tempo at which the steps are performed until an appropriate tempo for singing "*Alumot*" is achieved. Then have students

- Join hands in the circle.
- Dance the *hora* while singing "*Alumot.*"

Singing

Share with students that the song "*Al yadee,*" p. 308, is a Palestinian dance song. It accompanies the *debke,* a Palestinian line dance.

continued on page 308

SPOTLIGHT ON

8b ▶ **The *Hora*** The word *hora* means "circle dance." The Israeli *hora* was originally done in closed circles with each dancer's hands joined with neighbors' hands, and arms either held down at sides (V position) or on neighbors' shoulders (T position). In Israel, the traditional *hora* moves to the left, although modern *horas* can move in any direction. The steps are high and joyous, with leaps and kicks.

The *hora* is remarkably similar to the Arabic *debke* dance. Guide students to realize that cultures that live together and share common geography and history often have common traits in their art, folk art, and music.

MOVEMENT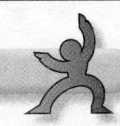

▶ **Patterned Dance** Teach students to dance the *hora.* Tell students to say the steps (in caps) on each beat. Repeat all steps moving to the left.

Formation: Students form a circle, facing inward, with hands at their sides.

- Step LEFT
- Cross RIGHT
- Step LEFT
- Right KICK
- Step RIGHT
- Left KICK

Unit 8 *Say It with Drums* **307**

5a Have students

- Listen to the recording of the song **CD 15–32** while following the music.
- Read aloud in rhythm the song's lyrics.

9a **ASK** **What similarities do you find between** *"Alumot"* **and** *"Al yadee"?* (Both songs have a strong, steady beat that makes dancing to them easier; both talk about nature; both are in minor keys.)

Then, have students

1c
- Sing *"Al yadee"* with the recording.
- Memorize the song.

Playing

Ask students to read the information about the *dombak.* Share with them that the body of the *dombak* may be ceramic or metal (usually silver or aluminum).

Invite students to listen to a recording of the *dombak* in the Sound Bank, p. 514.

ASK **Why do you think the** *dombak* **is capable of such clear low and high tones?** (Because of the goblet shape, with a deep resonator under the middle of the drum and a shallow resonator under the edges.)

How is the *dombak* **different from the West African drums we've studied?** (It is made from ceramic or metal, not from wood; it is goblet-shaped rather than cylindrical or round.)

Share with students that when *dombak* players are learning new rhythm patterns, they use syllables for different sounds in much the same way as *tabla* players from northern India do. (See Lesson 8.)

- *Dom* = A bass sound made by striking the center of the drum
- *Bak* (or *tak*) = A high sound made by striking near the rim

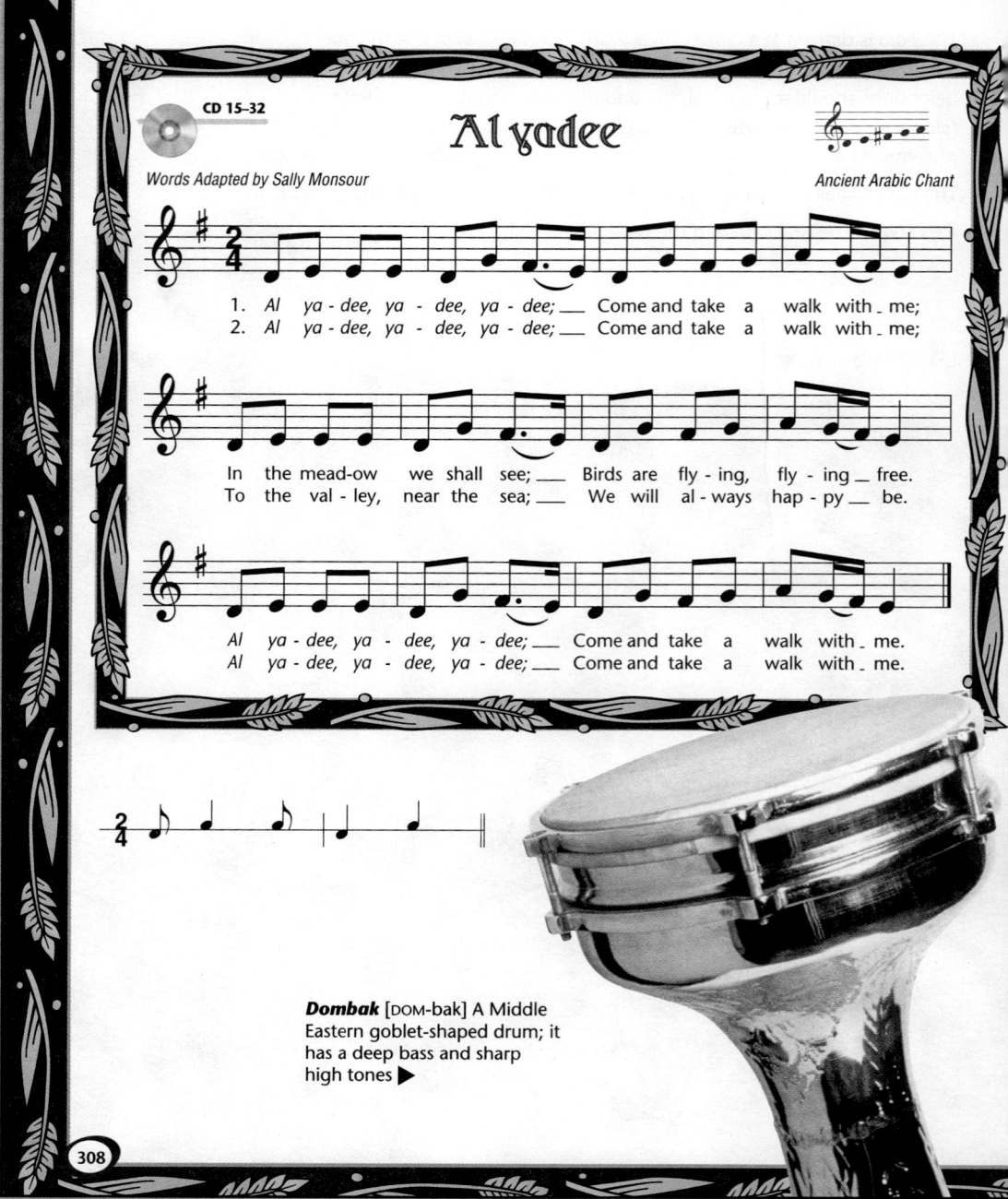

A Palestinian Debke Dance

Sing *"Al yadee,"* a Palestinian dance song (*debke*). Afterwards, learn and **play** the *dombak* rhythm below while you sing the song.

Al yadee

Words Adapted by Sally Monsour

Ancient Arabic Chant

1. Al ya - dee, ya - dee, ya - dee; ___ Come and take a walk with _ me;
2. Al ya - dee, ya - dee, ya - dee; ___ Come and take a walk with _ me;

In the mead - ow we shall see; ___ Birds are fly - ing, fly - ing _ free.
To the val - ley, near the sea; ___ We will al - ways hap - py _ be.

Al ya - dee, ya - dee, ya - dee; ___ Come and take a walk with _ me.
Al ya - dee, ya - dee, ya - dee; ___ Come and take a walk with _ me.

Dombak [DOM-bak] A Middle Eastern goblet-shaped drum; it has a deep bass and sharp high tones ▶

308

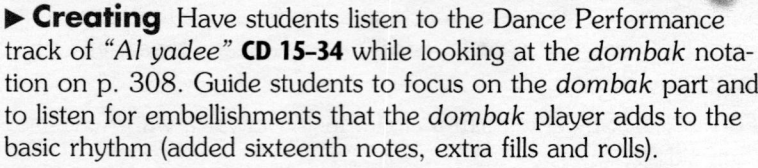

SKILLS REINFORCEMENT

▶ **Creating** Have students listen to the Dance Performance track of *"Al yadee"* **CD 15–34** while looking at the *dombak* notation on p. 308. Guide students to focus on the *dombak* part and to listen for embellishments that the *dombak* player adds to the basic rhythm (added sixteenth notes, extra fills and rolls).

Ask students to play and create new embellished rhythms based on the *dombak* rhythm pattern as they play along with the recording.

SPOTLIGHT ON

8b ▶ **The** *Debke* Share with students that the *debke,* sometimes called *debky,* is one of the most common dances of Palestinians and Arabic people who live in Lebanon, Jordan, and Syria. Traditional *debkes* are often done in short lines. Hands are generally joined down at the side, with dancers moving shoulder to shoulder in a tight formation to the right (counterclockwise). The step pattern is similar to that of the Israeli *hora,* but *debke* steps are more up-and-down, sharp and powerful, with stamps and strong knee movements.

Debke Movement

The *debke* (sometimes called *debky*) is one of the most common dances of the Arabic people who live in Lebanon, Jordan, and Syria and of the Palestinian people. *Debke* means "line dance," and traditional *debke* are often done in short lines. Although similar to the Israeli *hora,* the *debke* steps are sharp and powerful and have more up and down stamps and knee movements.

The basic Arabic *debke* is performed moving to the right, hands down at your sides and joined with neighbors' hands. The steps are: Step R, step L, step R, stamp L, step L, stamp R.

The same dance pattern can be found in eastern European and Asian countries. In Bulgaria, it is called *horo;* in Hungary, *kor;* in Serbia and Croatia, *kolo;* in Macedonia, *oro;* and in Greece, *choros.*

Arab *debke* dancers ▼

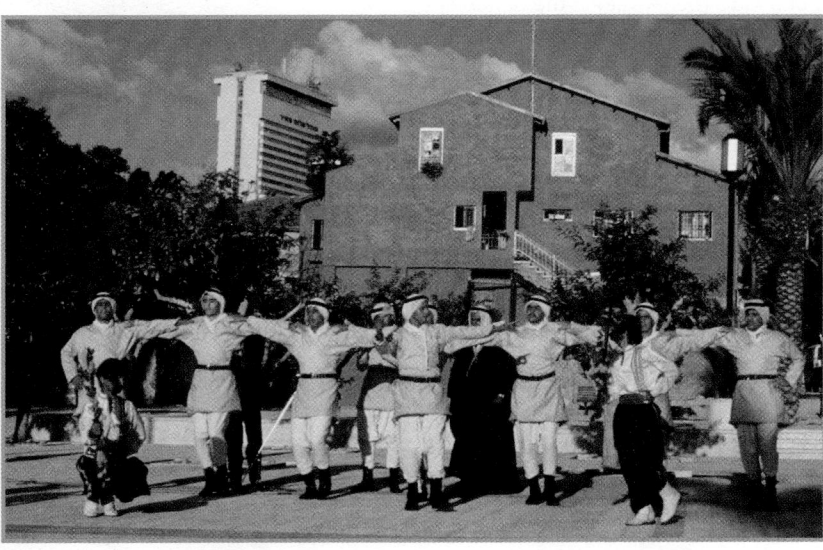

Listen to this recording of a *dombak* being played with a violin, tambourine, and a Turkish instrument called the *oud* (similar to a lute).

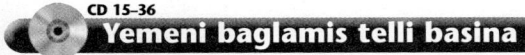

CD 15–36
Yemeni baglamis telli basina

**Traditional Turkish Dance
as performed by Farabi**
The *dombak* has a rich bass tone ("dom") when played in the middle of the drumhead, and a high, sharp tone ("bak") when played near the edge of the drumhead.

Have students

5a
• Play the *dombak* rhythm on p. 308, commonly known as *baladi,* by patting their left thigh with their left hand for *dom* and patting their right thigh with their right hand for *bak.*

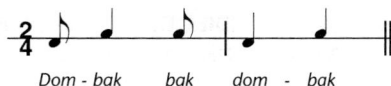

Dom - bak   bak   dom - bak

2c
• Play a *dombak,* if one is available, or another drum substitute, while singing *"Al yadee"* **CD 15-32.**

Moving

Using the information on p. 309 and in Spotlight On, p. 308, introduce students to the *debke.* Then invite them to learn the dance. Have students dance the *debke* while singing *"Al yadee."*

When students are comfortable singing and dancing, select three or four students to play the *dombak* rhythm, either on drums or with body percussion, while the rest of the class sings and dances.

Listening

Have students listen to *Yemeni baglamis telli basina,* a Turkish dance performed by Farabi.

3 CLOSE

Skill: MOVING   **ASSESSMENT**

1c **Performance/Observation** Separate students into four groups. Have half of the groups sing and dance to *"Alumot"* **CD 15-26** and the other half sing and dance to *"Al yadee"* **CD 15-32.**

Have some students perform the *dombak* rhythm on p. 308 with *"Al yadee."* Ask students

• How does the *dombak's* sound (timbre) and rhythm affect the dance?

Observe students' ability to perform the movements and to play both of the *dombak's* timbres accurately.

MOVEMENT

▶ **Patterned Dance** The basic steps to the Arabic *debke* are similar to the *hora* but begin in a counterclockwise direction. Moving to the right: Step R, step L, step R, stamp L, step L, stamp R. As already mentioned the steps are more energetic and have sharp stamps characteristic of the dance.

For more cultural information and a summary of the *debke* and the *hora,* see Spotlight On on pp. 307 and 308.

For Dance Directions for both the *debke* and *hora,* see p. 563.

TECHNOLOGY/MEDIA LINK

Web Site Go to *www.sfsuccessnet.com* to explore Middle Eastern music.

LESSON AT A GLANCE

Element Focus **FORM** aaba phrase form; ABA section form

Skill Objective **SINGING** Sing a Caribbean folk song

Connection Activity **SOCIAL STUDIES** Discuss the influence of West African music on music of the Caribbean

MATERIALS

- "By the Waters of Babylon" **CD 16–1**
  Recording Routine: Intro (8 m.); vocal; interlude (8 m.); vocal
- *tubanos* (conga-type drums) in low, medium, and high pitches; cowbells with sticks; double bells; rattles; talking drums (optional)

VOCABULARY

time line

◆ ◆ ◆ ◆ National Standards ◆ ◆ ◆ ◆

1c Sing music from diverse cultures
2c Perform instrumental music from diverse cultures
7b Students use specific criteria for evaluating their own performance
8b Identify ways music relates to social studies

MORE MUSIC CHOICES

For more practice singing Caribbean songs:
"Give a Little Love," p. 140
"Water Come a Me Eye," p. 300

1 INTRODUCE

8b Share with students that when West African people were enslaved and brought to the New World, they longed for their homes and freedom. In spite of many difficulties, they kept their culture alive through their language, music, and folk stories.

Students interested in the Caribbean may read the books listed in Across the Curriculum below.

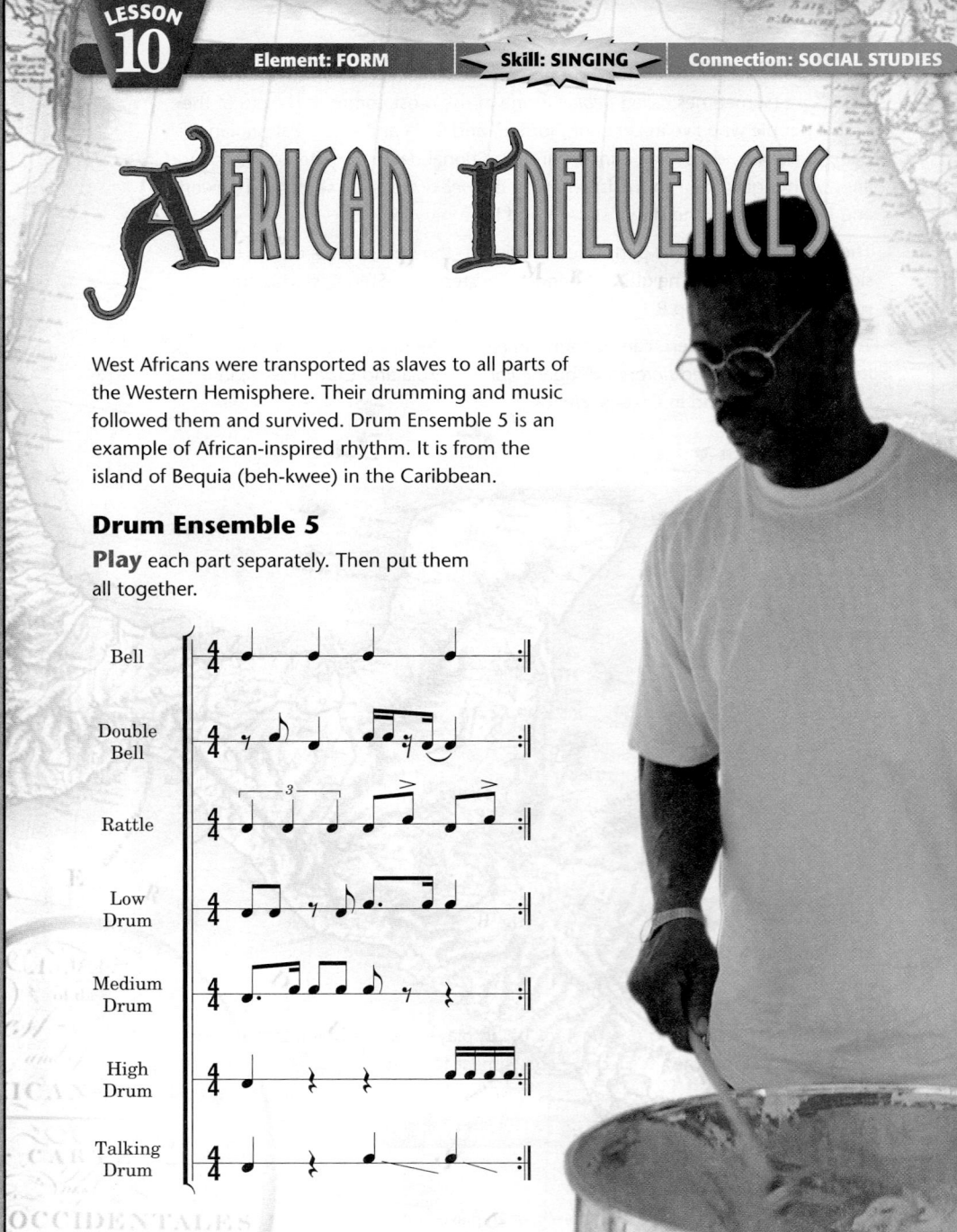

AFRICAN INFLUENCES

West Africans were transported as slaves to all parts of the Western Hemisphere. Their drumming and music followed them and survived. Drum Ensemble 5 is an example of African-inspired rhythm. It is from the island of Bequia (beh-kwee) in the Caribbean.

Drum Ensemble 5

Play each part separately. Then put them all together.

310

Footnotes

ACROSS THE CURRICULUM

▶ **Social Studies** Introduce students to life in each country or region of the Caribbean with *The Caribbean* by Linda Illsley (Raintree/Steck Vaughn, 1999).

For information on Babylon and its people, refer students to *Mysteries of Lost Civilizations* by Anne Millard (Copper Beech Books, 1996).

BUILDING SKILLS THROUGH MUSIC

▶ **Social Studies** Building on the information from Spotlight On, p. 311, have students research other islands in the Caribbean to determine the origins of other countries that had an influence on the islands.

SKILLS REINFORCEMENT

2c ▶ **Playing** Here is a way of teaching the low drum part in Drum Ensemble 5 in progressively easy to more difficult steps.

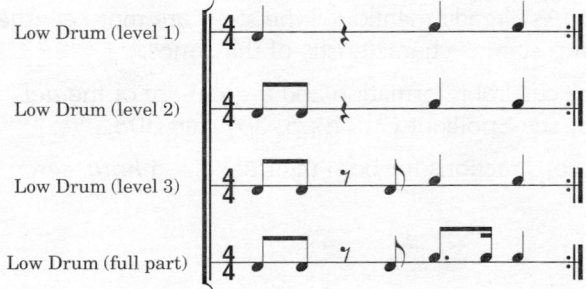

Sing "By the Waters of Babylon." Then **perform** it with Drum Ensemble 5.

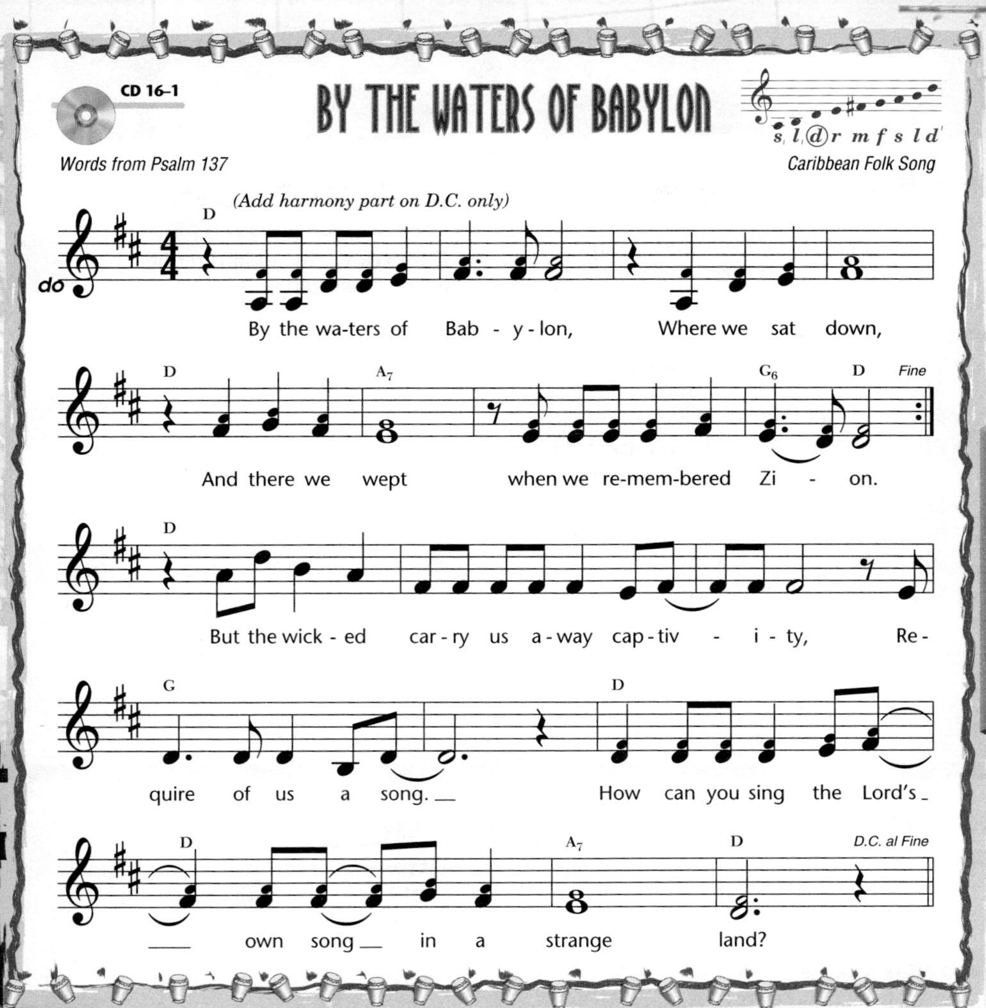

CD 16–1

BY THE WATERS OF BABYLON

s, l, @ r m f s l d'

Words from Psalm 137

Caribbean Folk Song

(Add harmony part on D.C. only)

do

By the wa-ters of Bab - y - lon, Where we sat down,

And there we wept when we re-mem-bered Zi - on.

But the wick - ed car-ry us a-way cap-tiv - i - ty, Re-

quire of us a song. ___ How can you sing the Lord's ___

___ own song ___ in a strange land?

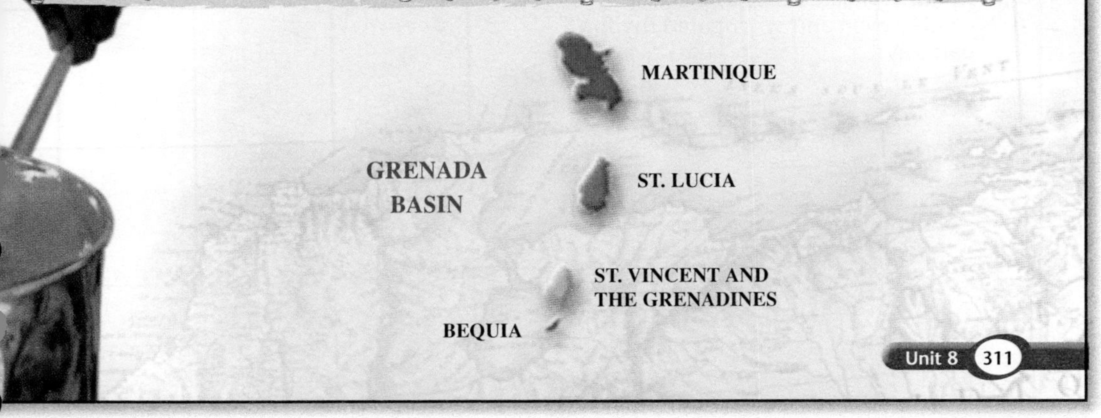

MARTINIQUE

GRENADA
BASIN

ST. LUCIA

ST. VINCENT AND
THE GRENADINES

BEQUIA

Unit 8 **311**

2 DEVELOP

Playing

Position students in a drumming circle and distribute the instruments needed to play Drum Ensemble 5 on p. 310. Use drum substitutes when necessary.

2c Teach the drum ensemble patterns in this order: low, medium, and high drums; talking drum; rattle; bell (the time line). Then have students play the patterns in score order. (Drum Ensemble 5 can be heard as the recorded introduction to "By the Waters of Babylon" **CD 16–1.**)

Use the rhythm patterns in Skills Reinforcement on p. 310 to assist students in learning the low drum part.

Singing

1c Have students first listen to and then sing the melody of "By the Waters of Babylon" **CD 16–1.** Next, teach them the harmony. Point out to students that the song's phrases make up two main sections (A and B). Ask students to identify the section form (ABA) and describe the similarities and differences between the two sections.

3 CLOSE

Skill: SINGING   **ASSESSMENT**

7b **Performance/Self-Assessment** For a classroom performance of "By the Waters of Babylon," organize the class into the following groups: drum ensemble, melody singers, harmony singers, soloists.

Ask students to suggest ways the performance can reinforce the aabaa (ABA) form of the song. (Change dynamics, vary the combination of instruments, have a soloist perform the B section.)

Have students evaluate their singing on the basis of technical accuracy and use of expression.

Say It with Drums

SPOTLIGHT ON

▶ **Bequia** Some of the less familiar Caribbean islands are the Grenadines, about 600 small islands that stretch from St. Vincent in the north to Grenada [gre-NAY-dah] in the south. Bequia, the home of Drum Ensemble 5, is one of the Grenadines. Grenada is a mountainous, heavily wooded country with a tropical climate and a beautiful harbor. Christopher Columbus was the first European to discover Grenada (in 1498). The chief export crops are nutmeg, cocoa, and bananas. About 95% of the population of Grenada is of African descent.

TECHNOLOGY/MEDIA LINK

Sequencing Software Use a digital audio program to record students' ensemble performance of "By the Waters of Babylon." On separate tracks, record the class

- Playing Drum Ensemble 5.
- Singing the melody.
- Singing the harmony part.

7b Use the mixer function to balance the parts. Then post the final mix as a WAV file to the class Web site. Ask students to describe the strong points and weaker points of the recorded performance.

Lesson	Elements	Skills

LESSON 1

A Melody for a King

pp. 316–319

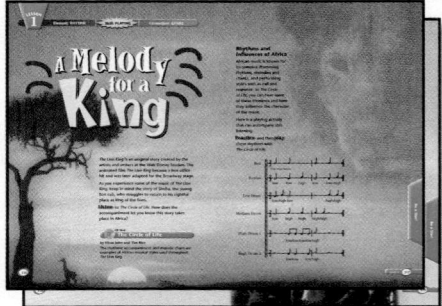
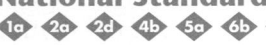

Element: Rhythm
Concept: Pattern
Focus: African rhythm patterns

Secondary Element
Form: question and answer

National Standards
1a 2a 2d 4b 5a 6b 9c

Skill: Playing
Objective: Perform African rhythm patterns in a drum ensemble along with a listening selection and song

Secondary Skills
- **Listening** Listen to and discuss African-inspired effects in music; listen to call and response
- **Playing** Play African drum ensemble rhythms and play an accompaniment
- **Signing** Learn and perform the signs for a traditional African American song
- **Creating** Create, perform, and record a production number

SKILLS REINFORCEMENT
- **Creating** Create a puppet show
- **Recorder** Play an alto recorder accompaniment

LESSON 2

The Best of Dancin' Feet

pp. 320–321

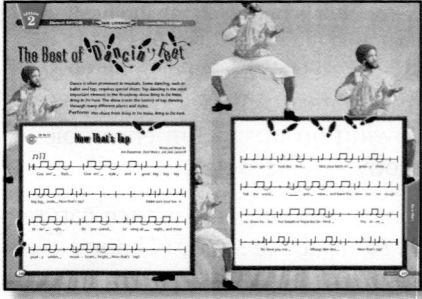

Element: Rhythm
Concept: Pattern
Focus: Syncopated rhythm patterns

Secondary Element
Form: aaba

National Standards
1c 5a 6b

Skill: Listening
Objective: Listen to a Broadway tap dance routine containing syncopated rhythms

Secondary Skills
- **Reading** Read a speech piece and identify even and syncopated rhythm patterns

SKILLS REINFORCEMENT
- **Listening** Listen to and tap a steady beat to a highly syncopated tap dance

---

LESSON 3

Dance—a Body Language

pp. 322–325

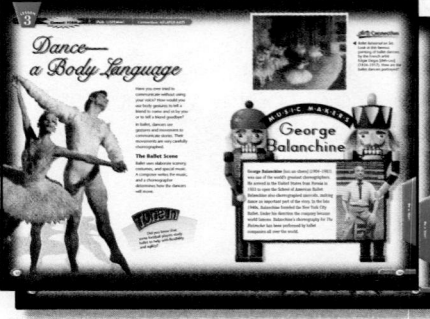

Element: Form
Concept: Form
Focus: ABA

Secondary Element
Timbre: instrumentation of themes

National Standards
6b 7a 8b 9c

Skill: Listening
Objective: Identify and trace the sequence of themes in a listening selection

Secondary Skills
- **Analyzing** Analyze and describe ballet as an art form; follow a listening map and analyze its melodic roadmap
- **Listening** Listen to and discuss a ballet
- **Moving** Improvise movements to a waltz

SKILLS REINFORCEMENT
- **Listening** Listen to and read about the harp in ballet; analyze the form of a ballet selection

Connections

Connection: Genre
Activity: Discuss the genre of stage musicals

MEETING INDIVIDUAL NEEDS **English Language Learners** Help students understand idioms in songs

SPOTLIGHT ON
The Lion King **Story** Facts on *The Lion King*
Musical Theater Information on Broadway and music

ACROSS THE CURRICULUM **Related Arts** Discuss the art of animation
Drama Read a book about *The Lion King*

CHARACTER EDUCATION **Compassion** Define the qualities of compassion and discuss how to promote them

AUDIENCE ETIQUETTE
Performance Behavior Perform a traditional African American song with proper etiquette
Audience Behavior Exhibit concert etiquette as an actively involved listener during live performances

BUILDING SKILLS THROUGH MUSIC **Social Studies** Write a paragraphs about ambitions

Connection: Culture
Activity: Explore African American cultural experience as expressed in dance

SPOTLIGHT ON **Tap Dancing** Facts on tap dance style

CULTURAL CONNECTION *Bring In Da Noise, Bring In Da Funk* Facts on this musical

SCHOOL TO HOME CONNECTION **Tap Dance Demonstration** Invite students and their families to a tap dance demonstration

BUILDING SKILLS THROUGH MUSIC **Reading** Discuss how tap dance has changed over time

Connection: Related Arts
Activity: Discuss ballet as another art form that takes place on both stage and screen

MEETING INDIVIDUAL NEEDS **Nonvocal Communication** Discuss alternative ways of communication

ACROSS THE CURRICULUM **Dance** Read about ballet training

CULTURAL CONNECTION **Nutcrackers** Facts on eighteenth-century nutcrackers

SPOTLIGHT ON **The Artist** Facts on the artist Edgar Degas
The Nutcracker **Ballet** Facts on *The Nutcracker* ballet

BUILDING SKILLS THROUGH MUSIC **Theater** Organize *The Nutcracker* on paper

Music and Other Literature

Song "There Is Love Somewhere"

Listening Selections
The Circle of Life
It's Time
Interview with David "Dakota" Sanchez
M·U·S·I·C M·A·K·E·R·S
   David "Dakota" Sanchez

More Music Choices
"Banuwa," p. 294
"Nana Kru," p. 282

Song "Now That's Tap"

Listening Selection *Now That's Tap*

More Music Choices
"Hit Me with a Hot Note and Watch Me Bounce," p. 112
"At the Same Time," p. 115

Listening Selections *Waltz of the Flowers*
Listening Map: *Waltz of the Flowers*
M·U·S·I·C M·A·K·E·R·S
   George Balanchine
   Piotr Illych Tchaikovsky

More Music Choices
"Blue Skies" (AABA), p. 88
"El condor pasa" (AABB), p. 46
Jesu, Joy of Man's Desiring (AABA), p. 87

ASSESSMENT

Performance/Observation
Perform African drum ensemble rhythms with a listening selection

TECHNOLOGY/MEDIA LINK
Sequencing Software
Create a rhythmic phrase or ostinato for a traditional African American song

---

ASSESSMENT

Music Journal Writing
Describe the effects of syncopation on music

TECHNOLOGY/MEDIA LINK
Sequence Software
Create and record a live tap dance

ASSESSMENT

Music Journal Writing
Listen to a selection and write a form map of musical themes and instruments

TECHNOLOGY/MEDIA LINK
Transparency Listening map for *Waltz of the Flowers*

Lesson	Elements	Skills

Dance, Irish Style

pp. 326–327

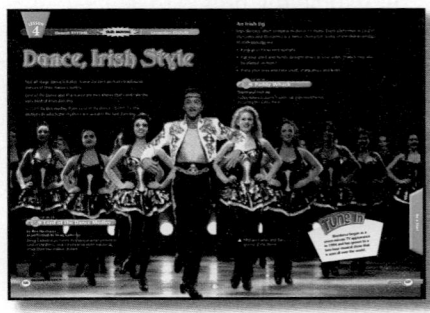

Element: Rhythm
Concept: Pattern
Focus: Dance rhythm patterns

Secondary Element
Expression: dynamics and tempo in dance performance

National Standards
6a 6b 7b

Skill: Moving
Objective: Perform an Irish jig

Secondary Skills
• **Listening** Listen to Irish music featuring dance

SKILLS REINFORCEMENT
• **Patterned Dance** Perform an Irish jig

"Stomp" Rhythms

pp. 328–329

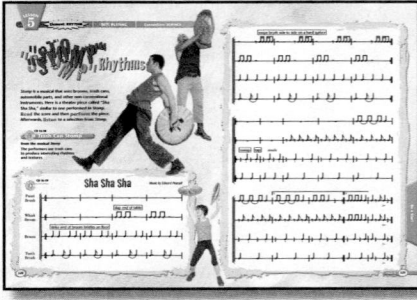
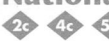

Element: Rhythm
Concept: Pattern
Focus: *Stomp* rhythm patterns

Secondary Element
Timbre: instruments made of junk

National Standards
2c 4c 5a

Skill: Playing
Objective: Read and perform a rhythm piece in the style of the Broadway show *Stomp*

Secondary Skills
• **Listening** Listen to music featuring junk instruments
• **Reading** Read notation, meter, articulation, and rhythm patterns
• **Playing** Play a rhythmic score using brooms as instruments
• **Creating** Compose and perform a short work using junk instruments
• **Moving** Create movements to a rhythmic score

SKILLS REINFORCEMENT
• **Playing** Gain proficiency in playing various kinds of brooms

---

Good Listening By Design

pp. 330–331

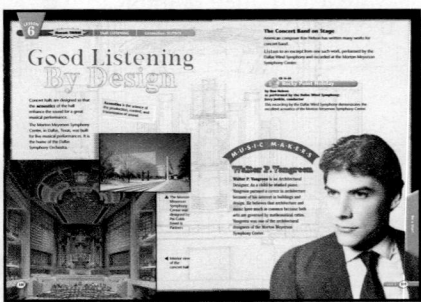

Element: Timbre
Concept: Instrumental
Focus: Wind and percussion instruments

Secondary Element
Expression: expressive musical elements in music for winds and percussion

National Standards
6b 8b 9b

Skill: Listening
Objective: Identify groups of wind and percussion instruments aurally

Secondary Skills
• **Listening** Listen to and describe the instruments in a piece for wind band

SKILLS REINFORCEMENT
• **Listening** Review wind and percussion instruments using the sound bank

Connections | Music and Other Literature

Connection: Culture
Activity: Explore Irish culture and dance

CULTURAL CONNECTION Irish Culture The Irish jig, folk dances, and songs

SPOTLIGHT ON Irish Instruments Facts on Irish instruments

BUILDING SKILLS THROUGH MUSIC Social Studies Discuss Irish culture

Listening Selections
Lord of the Dance Medley (excerpt)
Paddy Whack

More Music Choices
Kerenski, p. 78
Sellenger's Round, p. 44

ASSESSMENT

Performance/Peer Critique Perform an Irish jig

TECHNOLOGY/MEDIA LINK

Multimedia Create a multimedia presentation on the Irish jig
Digital Video Record and edit performances
Digital Still Photography Create a slideshow

Connection: Science
Activity: Recognize that almost any objects can serve as a sound source

SPOTLIGHT ON Stomp Facts on the *Stomp* stage production

CULTURAL CONNECTION Different Cultural Timbres Facts on cultures creating instruments from junk

BUILDING SKILLS THROUGH MUSIC Writing Write a short story

Song "Sha Sha Sha"

Listening Selection *Trash Can Stomp*

More Music Choices
"Bury Me Not on the Lone Prairie," p. 19
"Red River Valley," p. 11

ASSESSMENT

Performance/Observation Perform a rhythm piece with percussion or junk instruments

TECHNOLOGY/MEDIA LINK

Sequencing Software Create a rhythm composition using "found sounds"

Connection: Science
Activity: Explore the science of acoustics

ACROSS THE CURRICULUM Science Discuss acoustics and concert halls

SPOTLIGHT ON
The Composer Facts on composer Ron Nelson
Rocky Point Holiday Discusses the orchestration of this composition

BUILDING SKILLS THROUGH MUSIC Science Experiment with room acoustics

Listening Selection *Rocky Point Holiday*
M·U·S·I·C M·A·K·E·R·S
Walter P. Vangreen

More Music Choices
Farandole, p. 68
Symphony No. 5, Movement 1 (excerpt), p. 98
Wedding Day at Troldhaugen, Op. 65, No. 6, p. 9

ASSESSMENT

Music Journal Writing Listen to and write about timbre in a piece for winds and percussion

TECHNOLOGY/MEDIA LINK

Sequencing Software Add reverb to rhythm track

Lesson	Elements	Skills	

LESSON 7 — Latin Style!
pp. 332–335

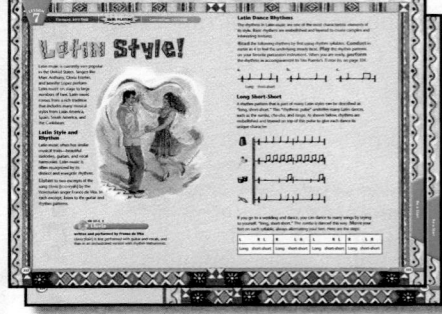

Element: Rhythm
Concept: Pattern
Focus: Latin rhythm patters

Secondary Element
Timbre: Latin percussion instruments

National Standards
2c 4c 5a 6a 6b 7b 8b 9a

Skill: Playing
Objective: Perform a Latin rhythm accompaniment

Secondary Skills
- **Listening** Listen to the rhythmic elements in Venezuelan, Cuban, and Latin pop ballad styles
- **Reading** Read Latin dance rhythm patterns
- **Playing** Perform a rhythm pattern to a recording
- **Moving** Perform "long, short-short" movements for the cha-cha and rumba dance movements

SKILLS REINFORCEMENT
- **Playing** Play a syncopated Latin rhythm on percussion; play a percussion accompaniment to a Latin ballad

LESSON 8 — Choirs on Stage
pp. 336–337

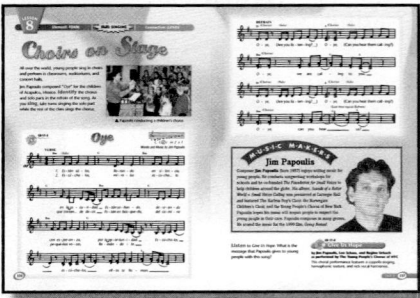

Element: Form
Concept: Architecture
Focus: Verse-refrain form

Secondary Element
Texture

National Standards
1a 2a 6a 6b 7b

Skill: Singing
Objective: Sing a song in verse-refrain form with solo-chorus response

Secondary Skills
- **Analyzing** Analyze the form and texture of a song
- **Listening** Discuss the use of solo and chorus response
- **Playing** Create a rhythm accompaniment using nonpitched percussion

SKILLS REINFORCEMENT
- **Singing** Tips for learning two-part harmonies in a song

LESSON 9 — Sing a Special Arrangement
pp. 338–343

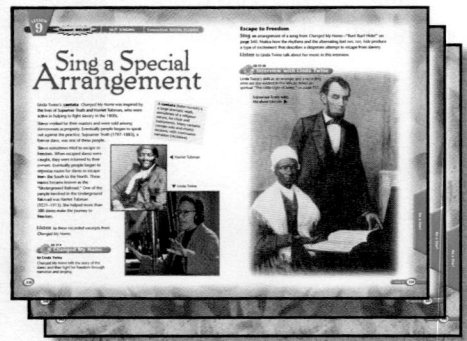

Element: Melody
Concept: Pattern
Focus: Melodic motive

Secondary Element
Rhythm: eighth note patterns and syncopation

National Standards
1c 1d 1e 5a 5c 6a 8b 9c

Skill: Singing
Objective: Sing an arrangement of a song containing melodic motives

Secondary Skills
- **Analyzing** Analyze and discuss a cantata; discuss themes of freedom and the Underground Railroad
- **Listening** Listen to a special cantata arrangement
- **Playing** Learn and play the rhythms to a spiritual
- **Singing** Sing an African American selection from a cantata
- **Performing** Present a dramatic performance of a cantata

SKILLS REINFORCEMENT
- **Creating** Create and perform a cantata with a story line, characters, and songs
- **Recorder** Play the vocal parts of a cantata on the recorder for support

Connections

Music and Other Literature

Connection: Culture
Activity: Explore Latin culture through dance

CULTURAL CONNECTION
Origins of Cha-Cha Facts on the cha-cha
Rumba Facts on the rumba
Origins of Salsa Facts on salsa music

SPOTLIGHT ON
The Composer Facts on Franco de Vita
The Composer Facts on Tito Puente

SCHOOL TO HOME CONNECTION Latin Influence Discuss Latin music with friends and family

BUILDING SKILLS THROUGH MUSIC Social Studies Document origins of musical styles

Listening Selections
Lluvia
Ti mon bo (excerpt)
You Sang to Me
M•U•S•I•C M•A•K•E•R•S
Marc Anthony

More Music Choices
Mi tierra, p. 365
Si tú no estás (excerpt), p. 267

ASSESSMENT

Performance/Self-Assessment Perform a Latin percussion score

TECHNOLOGY/MEDIA LINK
Web Site Information on Latin dance styles

Connection: Genre
Activity: Discuss choral music for young people's choice

ACROSS THE CURRICULUM Social Studies Discuss Acapulco, Mexico
SPOTLIGHT ON Young People's Chorus of New York City Discuss this famous choir

BUILDING SKILLS THROUGH MUSIC Language Organize information in an outline

Song *"Oye"*

Listening Selection *Give Us Hope*
M•U•S•I•C M•A•K•E•R•S
Jim Papoulis

More Music Choices
"Free at Last," p. 468
"Water Come a me Eye," p. 300

ASSESSMENT

Performance/Peer Critique Sing a song with solo and chorus parts

TECHNOLOGY/MEDIA LINK
Sequencing Software Create a percussion accompaniment for a children's song

---

Connection: Social Studies
Activity: Explore the Underground Railroad, Sojourner Truth, Harriet Tubman

CULTURAL CONNECTION
Secret Code Secret codes in spirituals sung by slaves
A Divided Country Discuss abolition and the Civil War
Songs of the Civil War Discuss famous songs of this period

SPOTLIGHT ON
The Cantata Facts on the cantata *Changed My Name*
Sojourner Truth Facts on Sojourner Truth and her fight against slavery
Harriet Tubman Facts on Harriet Tubman

ACROSS THE CURRICULUM Social Studies Women's rights and slavery; Lincoln and the Emancipation Proclamation
MOVEMENT Creative Movement Portray emotions
AUDIENCE ETIQUETTE Educating the Audience Proper etiquette
CHARACTER EDUCATION Courage Explore courage and other emotions that might conflict with it
BUILDING SKILLS THROUGH MUSIC Social Studies Identify individuals in the fight against slavery

Song "Run! Run! Hide!"

Listening Selections
Changed My Name
Interview with Linda Twine

More Music Choices
"Ain't Gonna Let Nobody Turn Me 'Round," p. 85
"Free At Last," p. 468
"The Gospel Train," p. 398
"I Wish I Knew How It Would Feel to Be Free," p. 470

ASSESSMENT

Music Journal Writing Sing an arrangement of a cantata and write answers to relevant questions

TECHNOLOGY/MEDIA LINK
Sequencing Software Use digital audio software to record a cantata

Lesson	Elements	Skills	
LESSON 10 **Music in the Movies** pp. 344–347 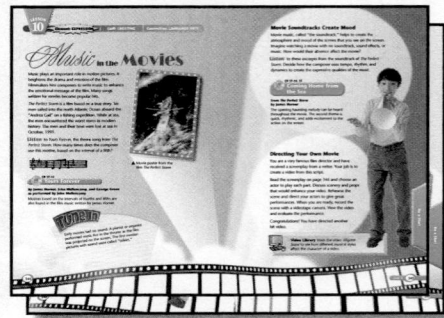	**Element: Expression** **Concept:** Tempo **Focus:** Combining musical elements for dramatic effect **Secondary Element** Melody: melodic motives **National Standards** 5a 6a 6c 7b 9a 9c	**Skill: Creating** **Objective:** Create a film scene and choose music to help express drama in the scene **Secondary Skills** • **Listening** Listen to melodic motives from a movie theme; listen to melodic motives and musical expression in two contrasting film episodes • **Creating** Create, rehearse and record a film scene, then choose a soundtrack that best fits their performance	**SKILLS REINFORCEMENT** • **Creating** Create a film using techniques used in the film-making industry • **Listening** Play a "Guess That Movie Soundtrack" listening game
LESSON 11 **Music Videos** pp. 348–349 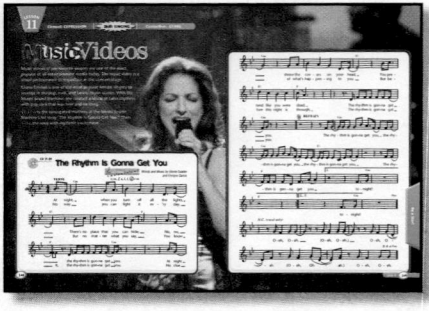	**Element: Expression** **Concept:** Articulation **Focus:** Expressive elements in Latin music **Secondary Element** Rhythm: syncopated and dotted-rhythm patterns **National Standards** 1c 2c 6b	**Skill: Singing** **Objective:** Perform a Latin pop song with expression **Secondary Skills** • **Listening** Listen to a pop song in Latin style • **Singing** Sing a Latin pop song with a recording • **Creating** Create a rhythmic accompaniment and video to a Latin pop song	**SKILLS REINFORCEMENT** • **Creating** Create and play Latin, layered, percussion patterns for a pop song; create a music video for the song

Connections

Music and Other Literature

Connection: Language Arts

Activity: Explore the written and the spoken word as used in screenplays

SPOTLIGHT ON

Music and Film Encourage students to research more about film composers

The Composer Facts on film composer James Horner

The Performer Facts on rock star John Mellencamp

Movie Soundtracks Background on recording soundtracks

ACROSS THE CURRICULUM

Science Discuss facts about the storm from the film *The Perfect Storm*

Social Studies Discuss careers in filmmaking

BUILDING SKILLS THROUGH MUSIC **Theater** Write a plan for a music score.

Listening Selections
Yours Forever
Coming Home from the Sea I, II (excerpt)
One Fine Day
Jungle Beat
Illusions

More Music Choices
"A Brand New Day," p. 7
"Don't Cry for Me, Argentina," p. 74

ASSESSMENT

Music Journal Writing View students' film scenes and critique their production

TECHNOLOGY/MEDIA LINK

Multimedia Create a movie using a DV camcorder and digital editing software

---

Connection: Genre

Activity: Discuss music videos and Latin pop

CULTURAL CONNECTION **Latin Pop** Encourage students to learn about pop performer Gloria Estefan

SPOTLIGHT ON **Music Videos** History of music videos

SCHOOL TO HOME CONNECTION **Music Videos from Home** Ask family and friends to find music videos that use a song's lyrics to dictate the images

BUILDING SKILLS THROUGH MUSIC **Math** Create a timeline

Song "The Rhythm Is Gonna Get You"

More Music Choices
"Má Teodora," p. 301

ASSESSMENT

Performance/Observation Perform a Latin pop song with expression using a Latin layered rhythm accompaniment

TECHNOLOGY/MEDIA LINK

CD-ROM Use *Band-in-a-Box* to create a Latin accompaniment

INTRODUCING THE UNIT

At some time and place in their lives, everyone deserves a chance to be a star!

Unit 9 gives students a glance at many different aspects of music and dance performance and opportunities to "meet" stars of performance and performance-related fields.

If students have dreams of becoming a star, this is a great place to start learning what it takes.

UNIT PROJECT

Help your students create their own songs using teamwork. Organize the class so each student is assigned a creative role (composer or lyricist). Then, have them work in pairs, one composer and one lyricist in each team.

Have each pair

- Compose a sixteen-measure song.
- Use a xylophone or keyboard to work out their melodies.
- Offer suggestions for presentation of the song. (Costumes, movements, props, and so on.)

Focus student attention on the pictures and text on pages 312–313. Invite them to read about, and then listen to the interview with Jeanine Tesori and Brian Crawley **CD 16-3.**

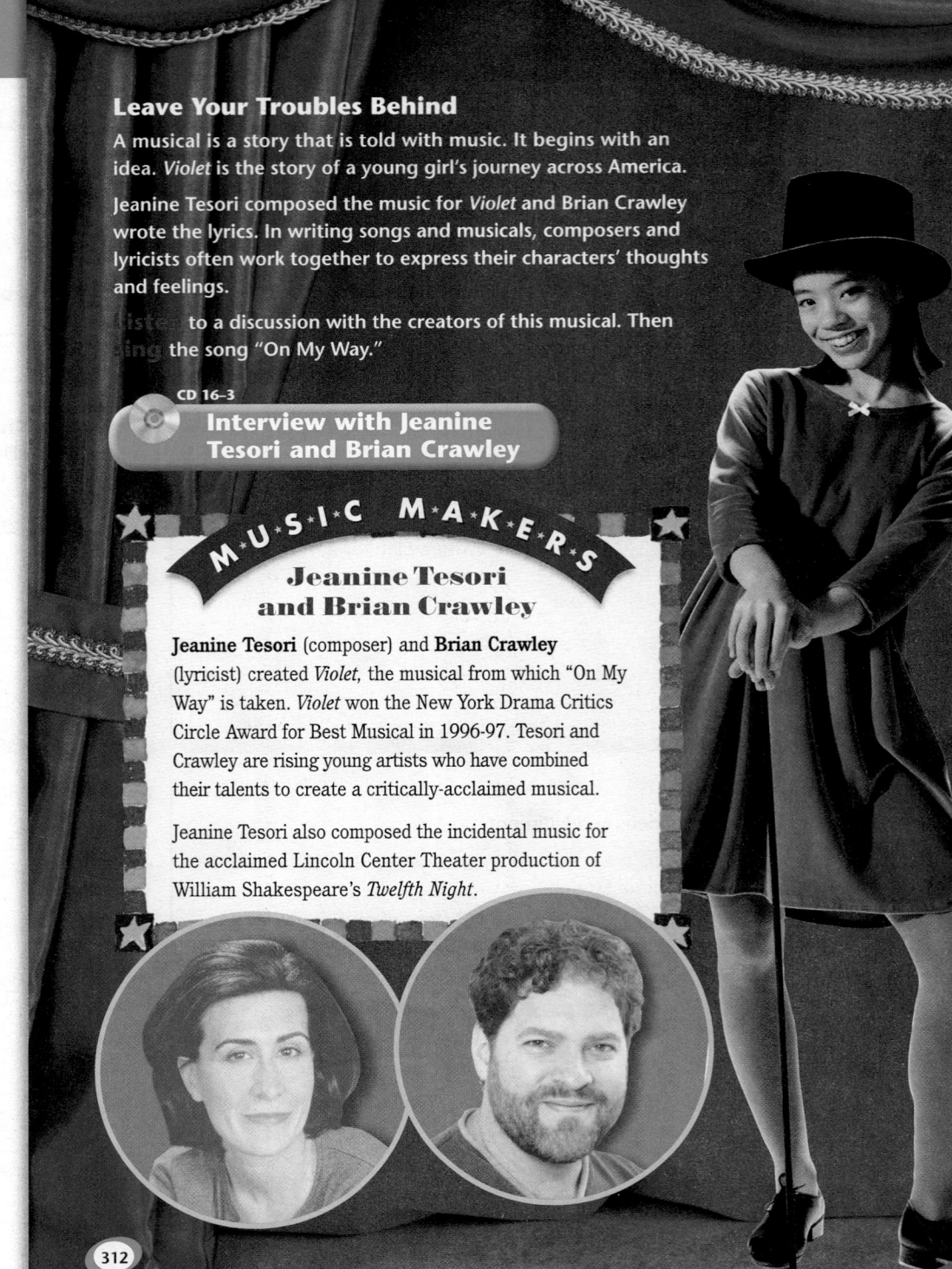

Leave Your Troubles Behind

A musical is a story that is told with music. It begins with an idea. *Violet* is the story of a young girl's journey across America.

Jeanine Tesori composed the music for *Violet* and Brian Crawley wrote the lyrics. In writing songs and musicals, composers and lyricists often work together to express their characters' thoughts and feelings.

Listen to a discussion with the creators of this musical. Then sing the song "On My Way."

CD 16-3

Interview with Jeanine Tesori and Brian Crawley

MUSIC MAKERS

Jeanine Tesori and Brian Crawley

Jeanine Tesori (composer) and **Brian Crawley** (lyricist) created *Violet*, the musical from which "On My Way" is taken. *Violet* won the New York Drama Critics Circle Award for Best Musical in 1996-97. Tesori and Crawley are rising young artists who have combined their talents to create a critically-acclaimed musical.

Jeanine Tesori also composed the incidental music for the acclaimed Lincoln Center Theater production of William Shakespeare's *Twelfth Night*.

312

ACROSS THE CURRICULUM

Unit Highlights The following interdisciplinary activities in this unit are related to the music elements presented in the lessons and are intended to enhance student learning. For a more detailed topical description, including related arts activities, see the Unit at a Glance, pp. 311a–311h.

▶ **ART/RELATED ARTS**

- Learn how animated films are created and produced (p. 317)
- Learn more about the training and experiences of ballet dancers (p. 322)

▶ **SCIENCE**

- Study the physics of sound and the design of concert halls (p. 330)
- Learn about storms (p. 344)

▶ **SOCIAL STUDIES**

- Learn about some of the features of Acapulco, on Mexico's Pacific coast (p. 336)
- Read about the Underground Railroad, Harriet Tubman, and Sojourner Truth (p. 339)
- Learn about the Emancipation Proclamation and slavery (p. 340)
- Investigate career possibilities in filmmaking (p. 347)

▶ **DRAMA**

- Read about and see photographs of a Broadway show (p. 318)

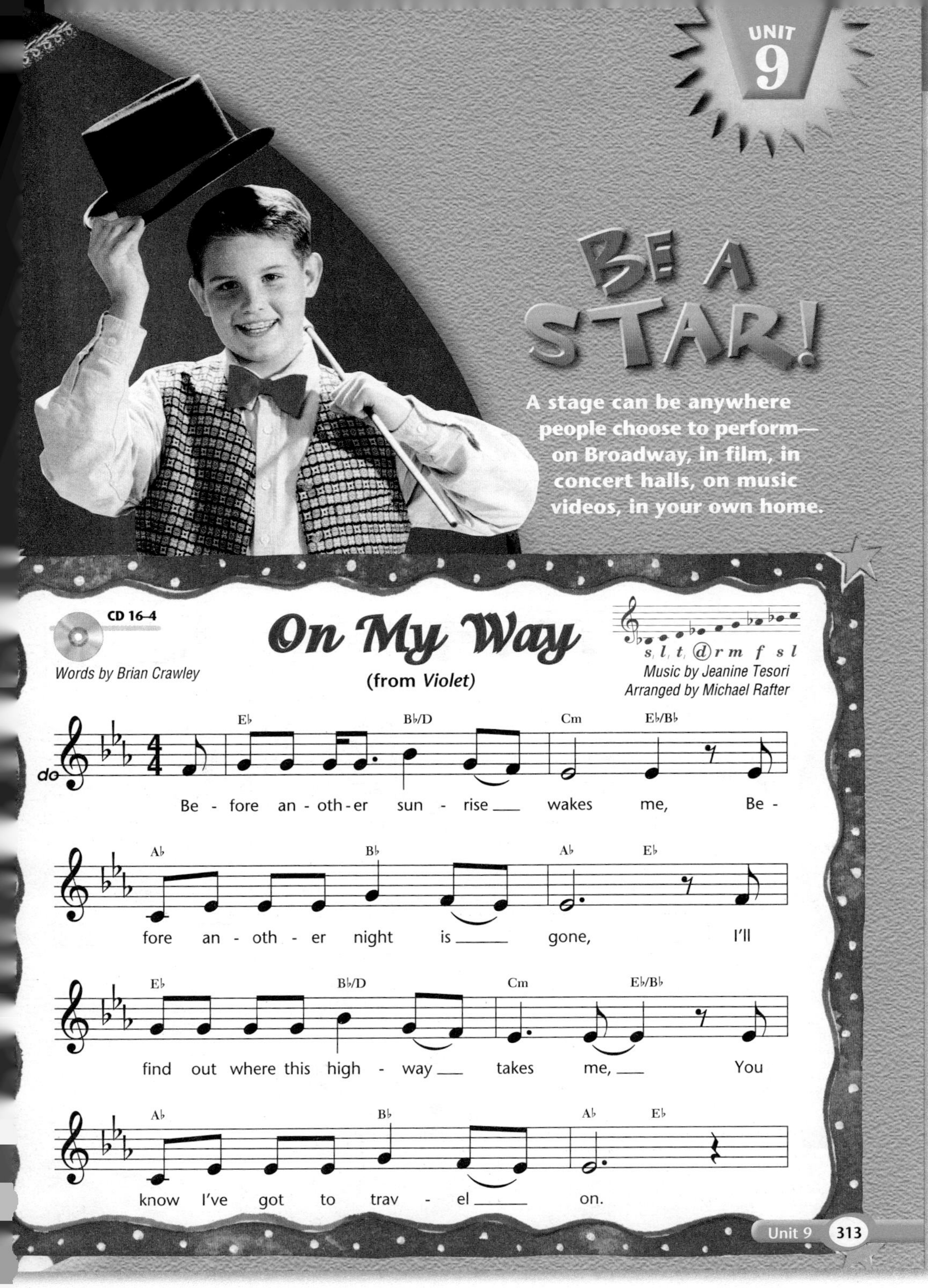

MUSIC SKILLS ASSESSED IN THIS UNIT

Reading Music: Rhythm

- Play drums as an accompaniment to singing (p. 319)

Performing Music: Singing

- Discuss and critique performance of solo parts in a song (p. 337)
- Sing a song, and write the answers to specific questions (p. 343)
- Sing a syncopated song (p. 349)

Performing Music: Playing

- Perform a rhythm piece with the recording of a song (p. 329)
- Discuss and critique the performance of a percussion ensemble as a song accompaniment (p. 335)

Performing Music: Dancing

- Perform and critique dancing, using observation (p. 327)

Creating Music

- Create a videotape, and critique its production (p. 347)
- Create a rhythm accompaniment for a song (p. 349)

Listening to Music

- Listen to and describe the effects of syncopation (p. 321)
- Listen to determine the form, specific instruments, and reaction to a piece of music (p. 325)
- Listen to music and write descriptions of the instrumental combinations (p. 331)

BE A STAR!

A stage can be anywhere people choose to perform— on Broadway, in film, in concert halls, on music videos, in your own home.

CD 16–4

On My Way

(from *Violet*)

Words by Brian Crawley

s, l, t, @ r m f s l

Music by Jeanine Tesori
Arranged by Michael Rafter

Be - fore an - oth - er sun - rise ___ wakes me, Be -
fore an - oth - er night is ___ gone, I'll
find out where this high - way ___ takes me, You
know I've got to trav - el ___ on.

Unit 9 **313**

CULTURAL CONNECTION

Unit Highlights The musical literature in this unit provides many opportunities for students to explore aspects of performing and performance-related fields. A more detailed description of the resources and activities listed below can be found in the Unit at a Glance on pp. 311a–311h.

▶ **AFRICAN/AFRICAN AMERICAN**

- "There Is Love Somewhere" (p. 318)
- *Rocky Point Holiday* (p. 331): A work by an American composer
- "Run! Run! Hide!" (p. 340): From a cantata by an African American composer

▶ **AMERICAN REGIONAL**

- "Now, That's Tap" (p. 320): Selection from a Broadway show
- "Sha Sha Sha" (p. 328): Selection from a Broadway show

- "The Rhythm Is Gonna Get You" (p. 348)
- *Yours Forever* (p. 344): From the soundtrack of a popular movie

▶ **LATIN AMERICAN**

- *Lluvia* (p. 332): Written by a Venezuelan composer
- "Oye" (p. 336): Composed for the children of Acapulco, Mexico
- *You Sang to Me* (p. 355): A contemporary Latin ballad

▶ **EUROPEAN**

- *Waltz of the Flowers* from "The Nutcracker" (p. 325): A ballet by Tchaikovsky
- *Paddy Whack* (p. 327): A traditional Irish jig

OPENING ACTIVITIES

MATERIALS

- Interview with Jeanine Tesori and
  Brian Crawley   **CD 16-3**
- "On My Way"   **CD 16-4**

  Recording Routine:
  Intro (4 m.); vocal; coda
- **Dance Directions** for "On My Way," p. 554

Listening

Invite your students to listen to "On My Way" without looking at the music. Play the I, IV, and V chords used in the first section of the song (E♭, A♭, B♭).

SAY These chords are used in the first part of the song, but later on they are replaced by other chords. Raise your hand when you hear this happen.

Have students discuss

- Where the change (modulation) occurred.
- How the melody changed. (longer notes, higher key)
- How the sections before and after the modulation were similar or different.

Singing

Have the students sing the song "On My Way" in unison, then in two parts.

Point out: the lower harmony part uses only six notes.

Practice the harmony part separately, two measures at a time, to give students a chance to find patterns.

Encourage students to add the harmony part during this lesson and whenever the class revisits the song.

Reading

Help students find and clap the dotted rhythms in "On My Way." Break the song into segments so your students can find similar and different rhythms more easily.

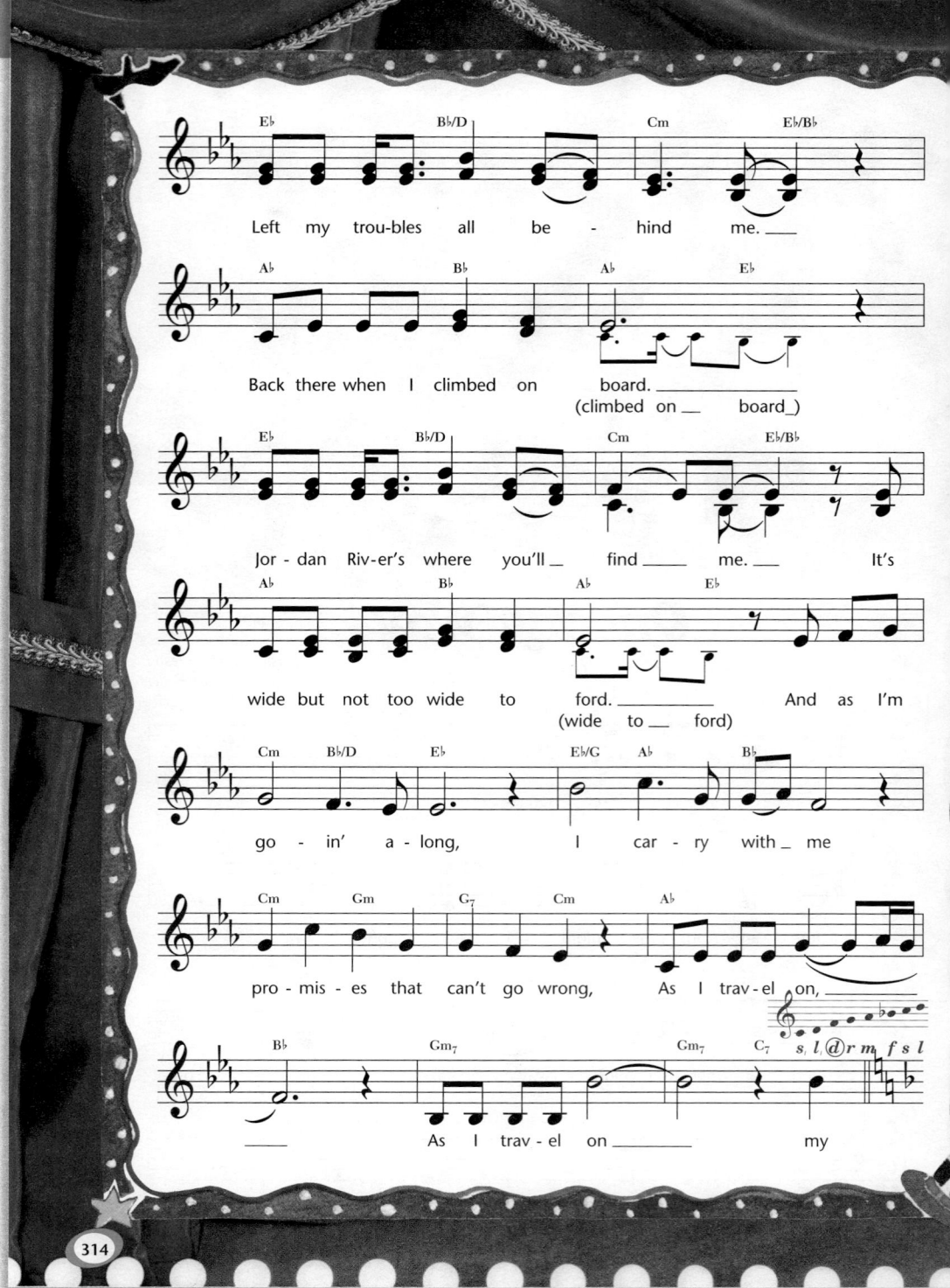

314

ASSESSMENT

Unit Highlights The lessons in this unit were chosen and developed to support the theme "Be a Star!" Each lesson, as always, presents a clear element focus, a skill objective, and an end-of-lesson assessment. The overall sequence of lessons, however, is organized according to this theme, rather than concept or skill development. In this context, formal assessment strategies, such as those presented in Units 1-6, are no longer applicable.

▶ **INFORMAL ASSESSMENTS**

At the close of each Teacher's Edition lesson in this unit, one of the following types of assessments is used to evaluate the learning of the key element focus or skill objective.

- Music Journal Writing (pp. 321, 325, 331, 343, 347)
- Performance/Observation (pp. 319, 329, 349)
- Performance/Peer Critique (pp. 327, 337)
- Performance/Self-Assessment (p. 335)

▶ **RUBRICS**

Visit *www.sfsuccessnet.com* for rubrics to assess students' achievement in music skills.

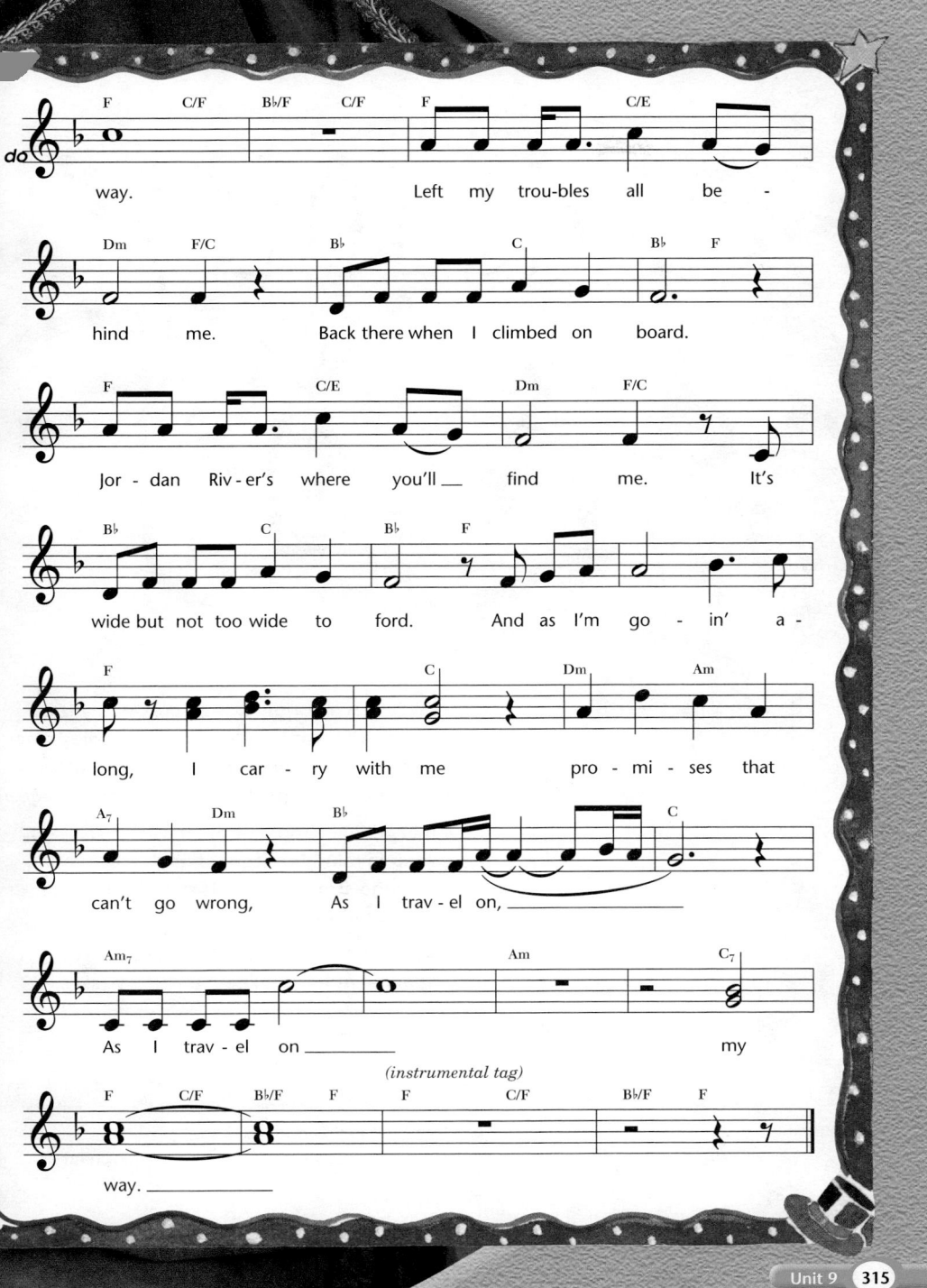

Remind students that
- A dot at the end of a note lengthens its value by 50%.
- Rhythms that are joined together take up one beat (for example, two eighth notes).
- The long note may appear at the beginning or at the end of a pair of rhythms.

Moving

Your students may create their own motions for "On My Way," or they may follow the Dance Directions on p. 563.

Improvising

"On My Way" describes someone leaving a troubled past.

Invite your students to create their own stories that would include "On My Way." Divide the class into at least three groups.

Group A: Writes a story that *begins* with "On My Way."

Group B: Writes a story with "On My Way" at its *midpoint*.

Group C: Writes a story that *ends* with "On My Way."

INNOVATIVE TEACHER SUPPORT FOR THIS UNIT

- **MAKING MUSIC DVD, Grade 6** contains video segments that support lessons, including signing and movement.
- **MAKING MUSIC with Movement and Dance** provides more opportunities for large group activities in music or physical education classes.
- **MAKING MUSIC with Technology** provides lesson plans for many technology applications; includes MIDI files.
- *¡A cantar!* features recorded songs and lessons from around the Spanish-speaking world; includes strategies for bilingual classes and for English-speaking teachers working with Spanish-speaking students.
- **Bridges to Asia** features recorded songs and lessons from Asian and Pacific region cultures.
- *www.sfsuccessnet.com* provides an online lesson planner to conveniently create lesson plans at school or at home. Includes rubrics for assessment, lesson modifications to meet the needs of all students, performance musicals based on program content, and more.

TECHNOLOGY/MEDIA LINK

Unit Highlights The following components are used in this unit to reinforce and expand students' understanding of performance and recording music and related themes.

▶ **CD–ROM**
- Generate Latin accompaniments for a song (p. 349)

▶ **DIGITAL VIDEO**
- Create and edit a video (p. 327)

▶ **DIGITAL STILL PHOTOGRAPHY**
- Plan a storyboard of pictures (p. 327)

▶ **MIDI/SEQUENCING SOFTWARE**
- Create an ostinato for a song (p. 319)
- Create and record a live "tap dance" performance (p. 321)
- Create a composition using "found sounds" (p. 329)

- Add reverb to a track, using *Micro Logic AV* (p. 331)
- Create a percussion accompaniment for a song (p. 337)
- Self-evaluate a singing performance of a song (p. 343)

▶ **MULTIMEDIA**
- Create a multimedia presentation for the Irish jig (p. 327)
- Create and edit a movie (p. 347)

▶ **TRANSPARENCY**
- Display a listening map transparency while playing a recording (p. 325)

▶ **WEB SITE**
- Visit *www.sfsuccessnet.com* to learn more about Latin dance styles (p. 335)

LESSON AT A GLANCE

Element Focus **RHYTHM** African rhythm patterns

Skill Objective **PLAYING** Perform African rhythm patterns in a drum ensemble with a listening selection and song

Connection Activity **GENRE** Discuss the genre of stage musicals

MATERIALS

- "There Is Love Somewhere" **CD 16-7**
  Recording Routine: Intro (14 m.); v. 1; v. 2; instrumental (16 m.); v. 3; v. 4; coda
- *The Circle of Life* **CD 16-6**
- *It's Time* **CD 16-9**
- *Interview with David "Dakota" Sanchez* **CD 16-10**
- **Resource Book** p. G-21, I-24
- cowbell (bell); rattles; low, medium, and high drums
- materials for making puppets or animation production

VOCABULARY

Broadway musical   rhythm patterns

◆ ◆ ◆ ◆ National Standards ◆ ◆ ◆ ◆

1a Sing accurately in small ensembles
2a Play instruments accurately in small ensembles
2d Perform simple accompaniments by ear
4b Arrange pieces for voices and instruments
5a Read quarter, eighth, and sixteenth notes in duple meter
6b Listen and analyze uses of rhythm, timbre, and form in music from diverse genres
9c Compare, in several cultures, the roles of musicians

MORE MUSIC CHOICES

For more practice with percussion ensembles:
"*Banuwa,*" p. 294
"*Nana Kru,*" p. 282

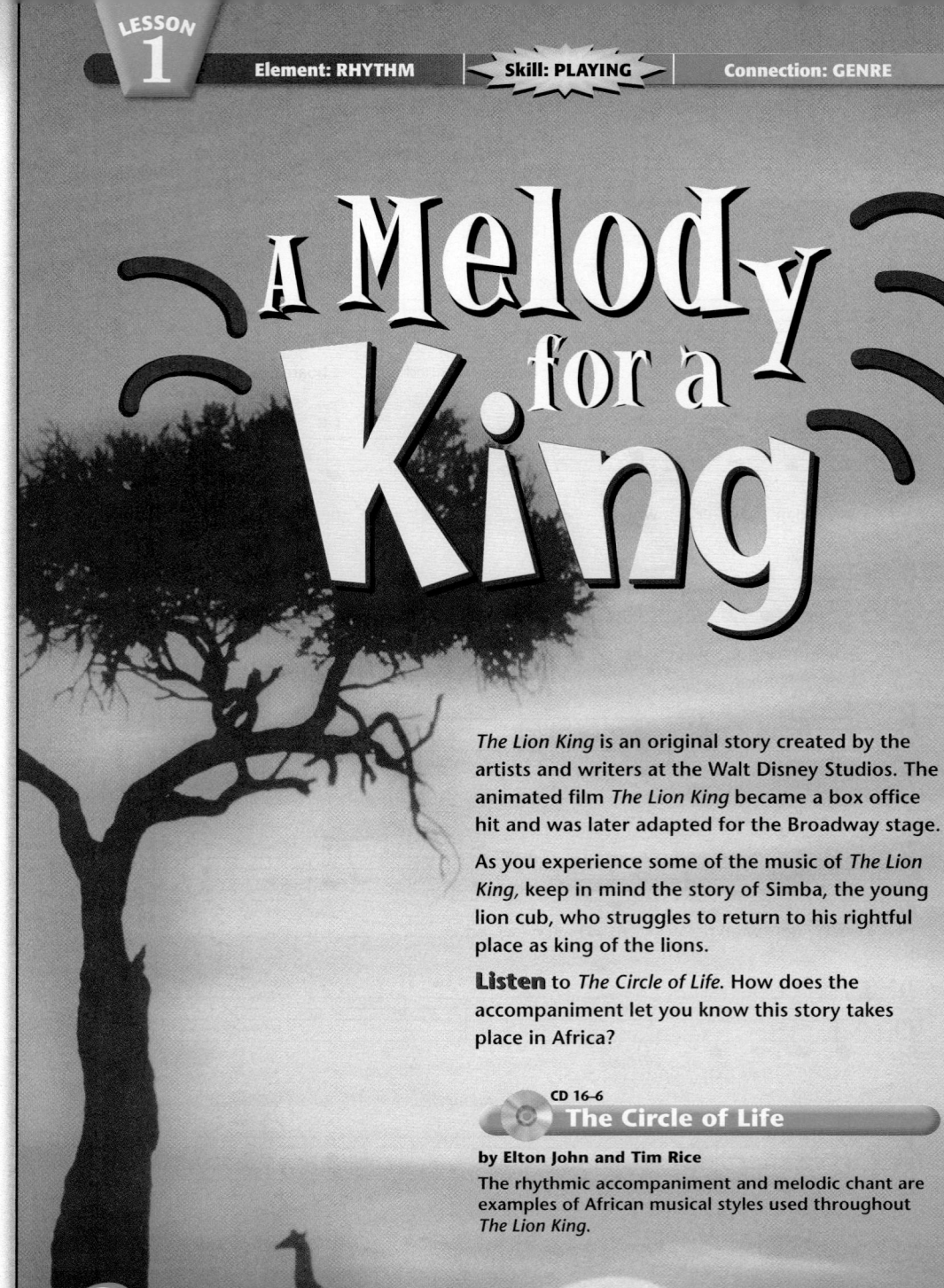

A Melody for a King

The Lion King is an original story created by the artists and writers at the Walt Disney Studios. The animated film *The Lion King* became a box office hit and was later adapted for the Broadway stage.

As you experience some of the music of *The Lion King,* keep in mind the story of Simba, the young lion cub, who struggles to return to his rightful place as king of the lions.

Listen to *The Circle of Life.* How does the accompaniment let you know this story takes place in Africa?

CD 16–6
The Circle of Life
by Elton John and Tim Rice
The rhythmic accompaniment and melodic chant are examples of African musical styles used throughout *The Lion King.*

316

Footnotes

MEETING INDIVIDUAL NEEDS

▶ **English Language Learners** Idioms are often confusing for students who are not fluent in English. *The Circle of Life* provides an opportunity for you to talk about idioms and how they are used in song texts. Discuss what *circle of life* might mean. Ask students if hearing the whole song helps them to understand the meaning of the phrase. Have students list other idioms they have heard and whose meanings are confusing.

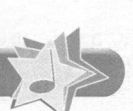
BUILDING SKILLS THROUGH MUSIC

▶ **Social Studies** Have students read the Music Maker on David "Dakota" Sanchez, p. 319. Have them write a brief paragraph about their ambition in life.

SPOTLIGHT ON

▶ *The Lion King* **Story** When Simba, a young lion prince, is born in Africa, his uncle Scar becomes second in line for the throne. Unhappy that he will not become king when Simba's father, King Mafasa, dies, Scar plots with the hyenas to kill both Prince Simba and King Mafasa, thus making himself king. After King Mafasa is killed, Scar convinces Simba that his father's death was Simba's fault. Feeling guilty and ashamed, Prince Simba flees the kingdom. After years in exile, Prince Simba is persuaded to return home to overthrow his uncle and claim the kingdom as his own.

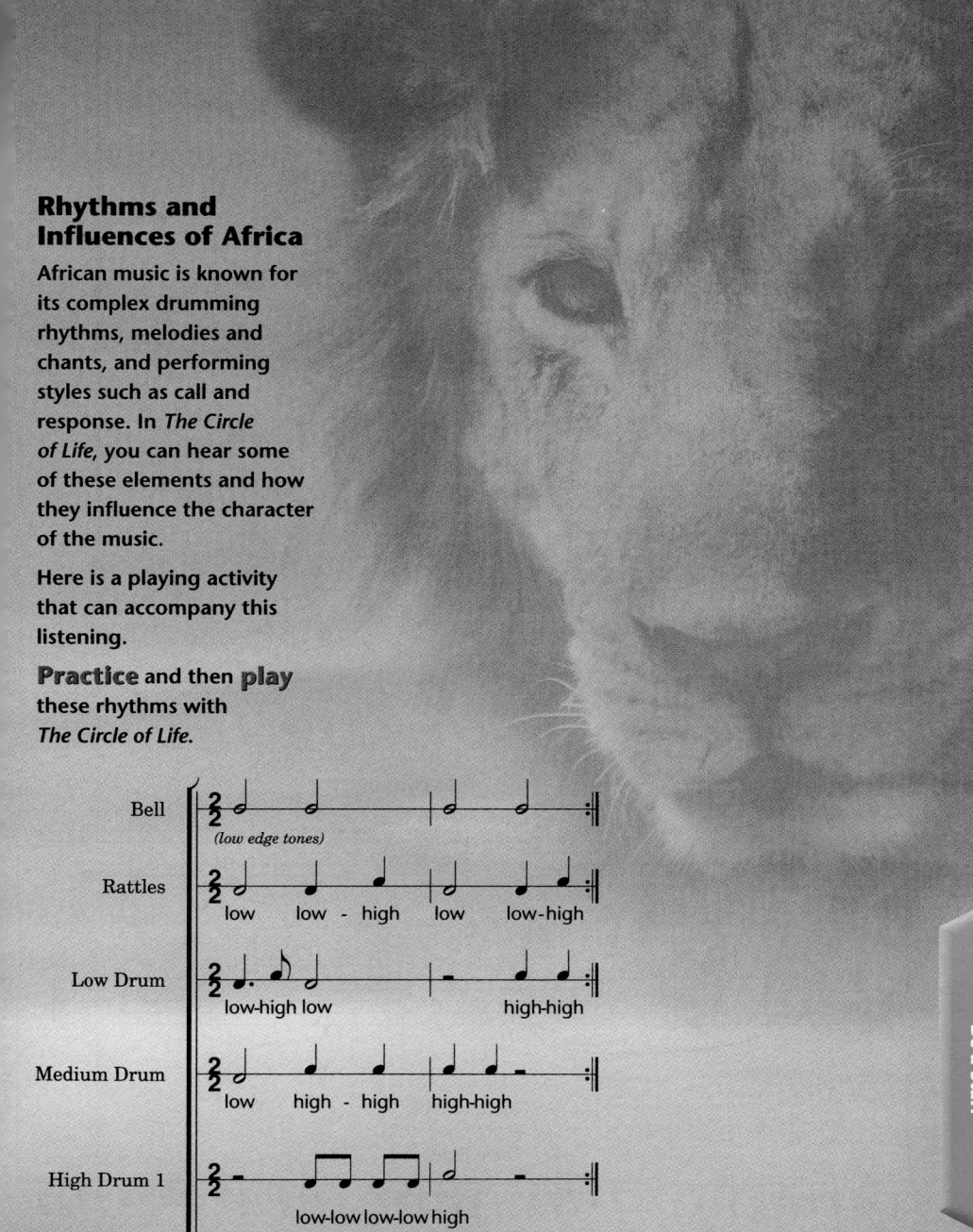

Rhythms and Influences of Africa

African music is known for its complex drumming rhythms, melodies and chants, and performing styles such as call and response. In *The Circle of Life*, you can hear some of these elements and how they influence the character of the music.

Here is a playing activity that can accompany this listening.

Practice and then **play** these rhythms with *The Circle of Life*.

Bell
(low edge tones)

Rattles
low · low - high · low · low-high

Low Drum
low-high low · high-high

Medium Drum
low · high - high · high-high

High Drum 1
low-low low-low high

High Drum 2
low-low · low high

Be a Star!

Unit 9 **317**

1 INTRODUCE

Invite students to

- Create a list of various musical productions that take place on a stage or on screen.
- Share with the class the titles of their favorite animated films.
- Read about *The Lion King*, on p. 316.

Tell students that music is often related to other fine arts on stage and screen. Inform them that

- Musicals are theatrical productions with musical numbers and dialogue based on a story.
- Musicals can be presented either on a stage or through film.
- *The Lion King* is a musical that was first an animated film and later became a Broadway musical.

Share with the class the story of *The Lion King* in Spotlight On, p. 316 and background on the genre of musicals in Spotlight On, p. 318.

2 DEVELOP

Listening

 Invite students to listen to *The Circle of Life* CD **16-6**. Then discuss the African-inspired effects in the music (the rhythmic accompaniment and melodic chant).

Tell students that

- Songs are an important part of musical theater. They are used to set a scene, express a character's emotions, or reflect on something that has happened in the story.
- *The Circle of Life* is both the first and the last song in *The Lion King*.

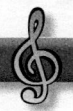 Encourage a small group of students to improvise an ostinato on a rhythm instrument with the recording of *The Circle of Life* CD **16-6**.

continued on page 318

ACROSS THE CURRICULUM

▶ **Related Arts** Traditional animated films are hand-drawn, frame by frame, on a piece of celluloid ("cell") that measures 12″ × 10″. It takes approximately 1,500 cells to produce one minute of film. Every motion is created from a series of drawings, each one slightly different from the one preceding and the one following. The animated drawings (more than 1 million of which were used for *The Lion King*) are scanned into a computer system, colored online, and put onto film. After frames are drawn, they are photographed in sequence, one frame at a time, using a special camera. The voices of the characters are usually recorded before the animators or artists begin the drawings. This allows the animators to perfectly match the movement of characters with sounds.

SKILLS REINFORCEMENT

▶ **Creating** Encourage students to create a puppet show to accompany *The Circle of Life*. Make puppets easily by drawing the face of a character on one side of a paper bag, and animate it with a hand inside the bag. Puppets can also be made out of socks, with faces on the toe. Using a table, puppeteers could hide underneath and manipulate puppets on the tabletop "stage." Remind puppeteers to allow puppets to make eye contact with the audience and to keep puppets moving while talking or singing, as movement draws the audience's attention to their characters.

 ▶ **Recorder** Have students learn the alto recorder parts for *The Circle of Life* on Resource Book, p. I-24.

Playing

Prepare students to independently perform the rhythm ensemble on p. 317 with accurate rhythm, demonstrating appropriate large ensemble performance techniques suitable for a formal concert. Invite them to echo drum each pattern with the teacher or a student leader. Then, have students

- Play the low drum part, followed by the two high drum parts.
- Choose the low or high drum parts and play in a whole-class three-part ensemble.
- Play the medium drum part.
- Choose one of the four drum parts and play in a whole-class four-part ensemble.

- Combine all six parts, bringing them in according to score order. (Never add a new part until the ensemble is stable.)
- Perform the drum ensemble with *The Circle of Life* **CD 16-6**, demonstrating ensemble performance techniques appropriate for a formal concert.

Singing

Have students read about African musical heritage on p. 318. Invite them to sing "There Is Love Somewhere" **CD 16-7** with the recording.

Playing

Have students play the rhythms on p. 317 and perform it as accompaniment to "There Is Love Somewhere."

Signing

Invite students to learn the signs for "There Is Love Somewhere" on Resource Book p. G-21. Ask students to write a thematic narration for one verse of the song and to look up the signs for their narration in *The American Sign Language Dictionary* or *The Joy of Signing*. Then, invite students to perform the signing and the narration on the instrumental section, with the Stereo Performance track **CD 16-8**.

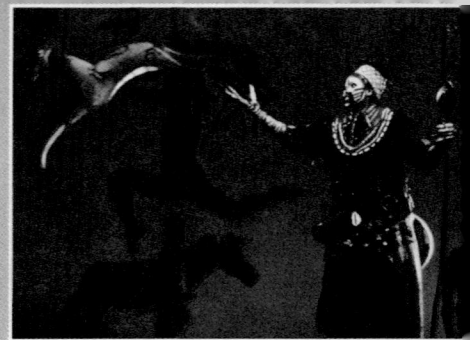

The African Heritage

When Africans came to America, they brought their musical traditions, songs, and rhythms with them. Thus, the heritage of the music of the African people can be found in African American music as well.

Sing this traditional African American song. As you sing, conduct a two-beat pattern and **listen** to the African-style rhythms that accompany "There Is Love Somewhere."

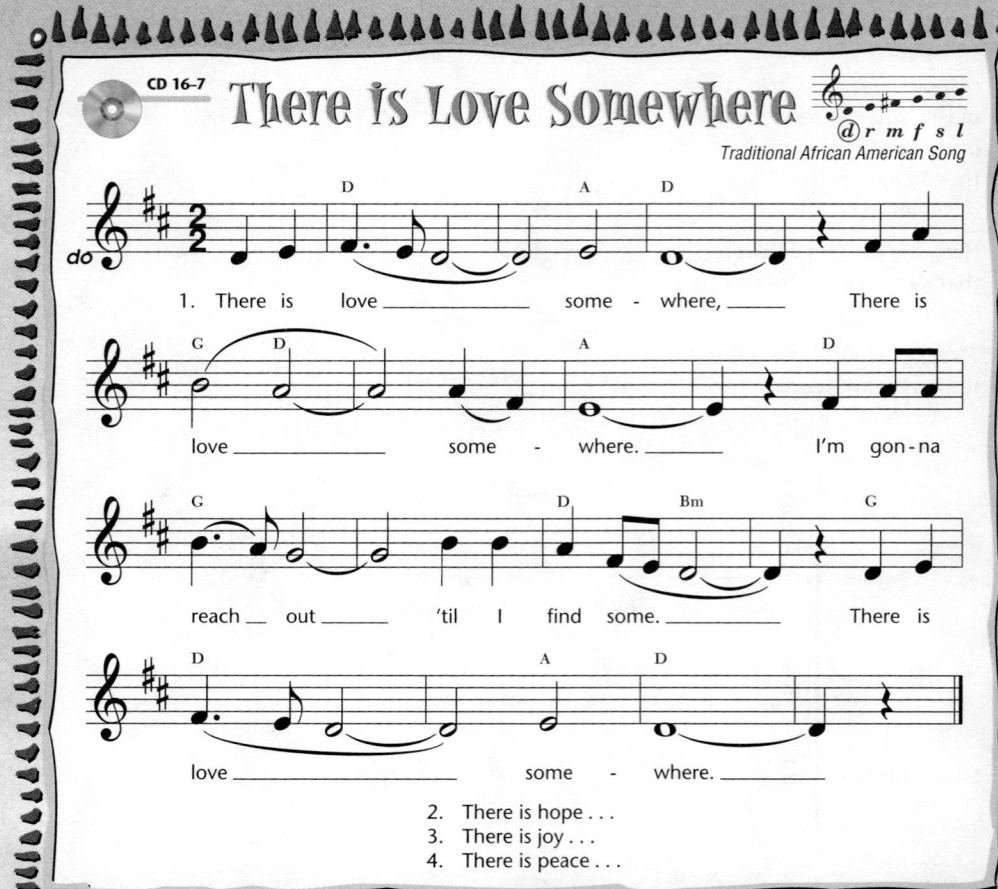

CD 16-7

There Is Love Somewhere
Traditional African American Song

d r m f s l

do

1. There is love _____ some - where, _____ There is
love _____ some - where. _____ I'm gon-na
reach __ out _____ 'til I find some. _____ There is
love _____ some - where. _____

2. There is hope . . .
3. There is joy . . .
4. There is peace . . .

Play the rhythms on page 317. Determine if these rhythms will work with "There Is Love Somewhere." **Analyze** the lyrics and choose which rhythms you will play for each verse. When you are ready, **perform** your accompaniment as the class sings.

318

Footnotes

SPOTLIGHT ON

▶ **Musical Theater** Also known as musical comedy, the genre of musical theater is a popular form of entertainment developed in the United States and England during the twentieth century. These productions tell a story, with songs and dances integrated, contributing to plot and character development. Productions in New York City and London, centers of musical theater, are usually of the highest caliber and display elaborate costumes and scenery. The best and most expensive productions eventually appear on Broadway, in New York City, where most of the city's theaters were once located. In more recent years, "Broadway" refers to an area adjacent to this famous street.

ACROSS THE CURRICULUM

▶ **Drama** For more about *The Lion King*, read *Disney Presents the Lion King: With Photographs from the Broadway Musical, Winner of the 1998 Tony Award* by Joan Marcus (Disney, 1998).

CHARACTER EDUCATION

▶ **Compassion** "There Is Love Somewhere" expresses a longing for love, hope, joy, and peace. How would you define these qualities, and how can we promote and demonstrate them? Why is it important for people to experience these qualities? How does possessing them and demonstrating them to others make you feel?

Pride Land Rhythms

Performer, singer, and songwriter Lebo M. recorded the album *Rhythm of the Pride Lands,* which contains songs inspired by the music of *The Lion King.*

Listen to *It's Time,* as performed by Lebo M. and an African chorus. The call and response between Lebo M.'s solo and the chorus is just one of many African musical elements.

 CD 16-9

It's Time

from *Rhythm of the Pride Lands* by Lebo M., John Van Tongeren, and Jay Rifkin as performed by Lebo M. and chorus

The positive message of *It's Time* is emphasized by the joyful lyrics and singing of the African chorus.

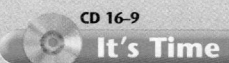

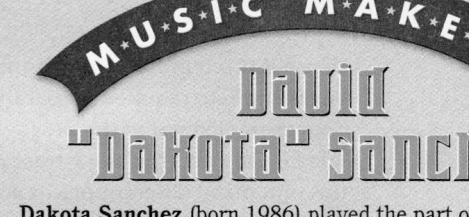

M·U·S·I·C M·A·K·E·R·S
David "Dakota" Sanchez

Dakota Sanchez (born 1986) played the part of Young Simba in the Broadway production of *The Lion King.* He made his Broadway debut in this musical when he was in seventh grade. Sanchez loves to sing. While in elementary school, the future Broadway performer sang in the school chorus and for school assemblies and celebrations. Sanchez currently attends the Professional Performing Arts School in New York City. He lives in New York with his mother and father and his siblings, Raquel and Nicolas. In his free time, he loves to read science fiction. His ambition is to be a scientist.

Listen to Dakota Sanchez talk about his musical career and his experience with *The Lion King.*

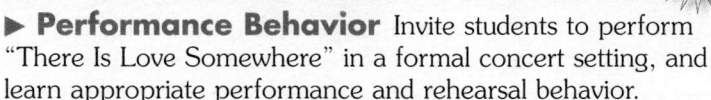 CD 16–10

Interview with David "Dakota" Sanchez

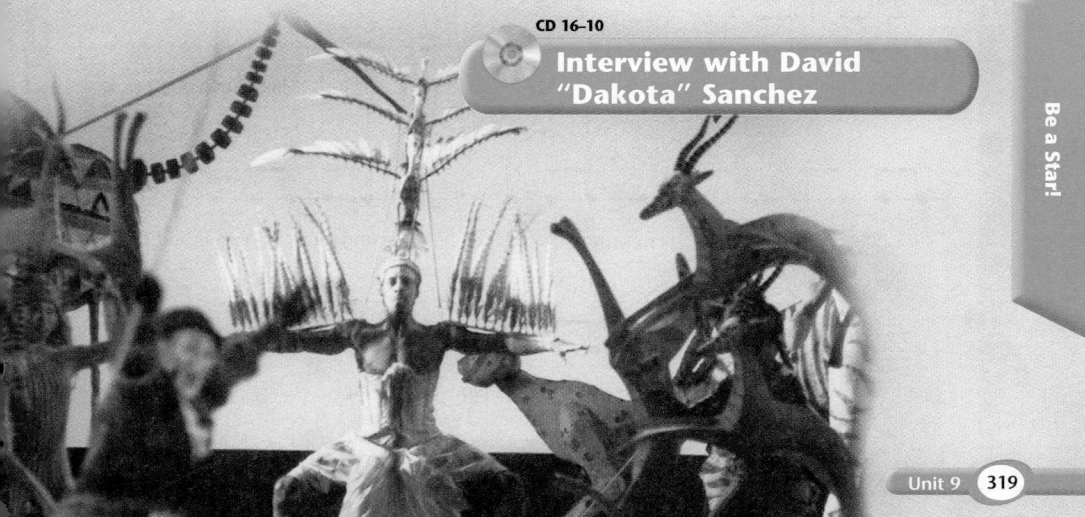

Be a Star!

Unit 9 **319**

Listening

6b Invite students to read the background material on p. 319 on Lebo M. and the inspiration for the album *Rhythm of the Pride Lands.*

Help students to

- Listen to *It's Time* **CD 16-9** and identify the chorus as an African chorus.
- Identify call-and-response form.
- Discuss any other musical elements that contribute to the spirit of the song. (African-style flute, rhythmic ostinato)

9c Encourage students to read the Music Makers feature on David "Dakota" Sanchez and listen to the recorded interview **CD 16-10** with this young artist.

Creating

Divide the class into small groups. Invite students to plan and perform a production number. Have students

- Choose a song that tells a story and decide on characters and actions needed to tell the story.
- Design and make puppets for an animated film presentation. See Skills Reinforcement on p. 317.
- Perform and videotape the puppet show, or save the animated production on film.

3 CLOSE

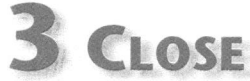 **Skill: PLAYING** 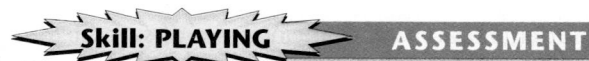 **ASSESSMENT**

2a **Performance/Observation** Divide the class into small groups. Ask each group to perform the rhythms on p. 317 as the class sings "There Is Love Somewhere." Tell them to choose a different drumming pattern for each verse. Observe and evaluate each performance for basic performance techniques such as independence, rhythmic accuracy, and style. Ask students to discuss and evaluate the quality and effectiveness of the music and of their performances.

AUDIENCE ETIQUETTE

▶ **Performance Behavior** Invite students to perform "There Is Love Somewhere" in a formal concert setting, and learn appropriate performance and rehearsal behavior.

▶ **Audience Behavior** Invite students to exhibit concert etiquette as an actively involved listener during live performances.

- Arrive on time for the performance and stay with your group. No eating or drinking in the theater.
- Use soft, "inside" voices while waiting for the performance to begin. Stay seated during the performance.
- Concentrate on listening and watching. Give the performers your attention and applaud at the conclusion.
- Write thank-you cards to show your appreciation for the performance. Tell your family about your experience.

TECHNOLOGY/MEDIA LINK

4b **Sequencing Software** Using sequencing software, have students create a rhythm phrase, or ostinato, for "There Is Love Somewhere." Have students

- Find and list the appropriate MIDI sounds (percussion or pitched) with its General MIDI number.
- Set the correct tempo to match the song.
- Set the number of measures for the ostinato or phrase.
- Create a MIDI track for each instrument.
- Play the phrase ostinato as the class sings the song.

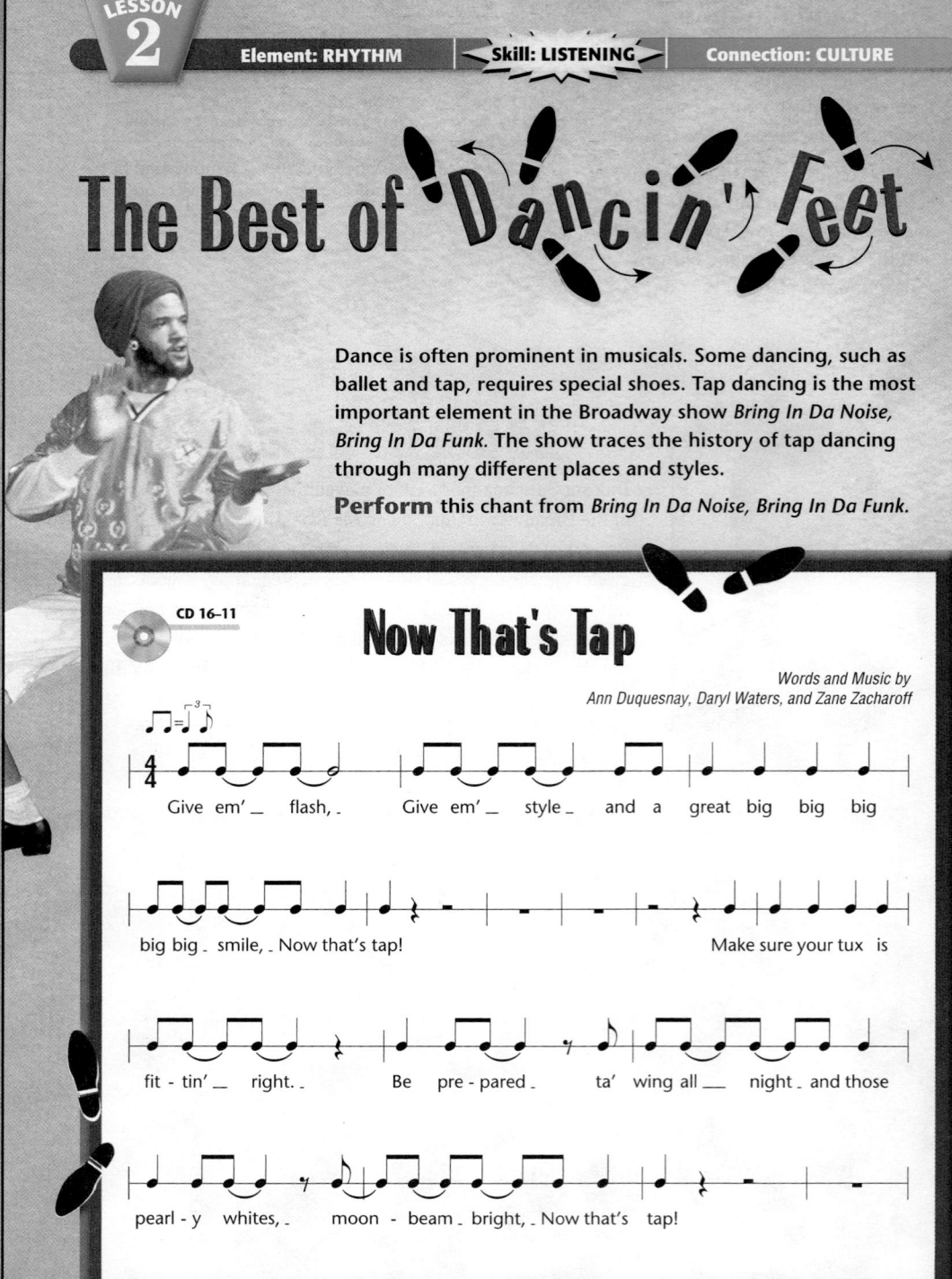

LESSON AT A GLANCE

Element Focus   **RHYTHM** Syncopated rhythm patterns

Skill Objective   **LISTENING** Listen to a Broadway tap dance routine containing syncopated rhythms

Connection Activity   **CULTURE** Explore African American cultural experience as expressed in dance

MATERIALS

- "Now That's Tap"   **CD 16-11**

    Recording Routine: Intro (4 m.); vocal; coda

VOCABULARY

tap dancing   syncopated patterns/even patterns

◆ ◆ ◆ ◆ **National Standards** ◆ ◆ ◆ ◆

1c Sing music from diverse genres
5a Read eighth and quarter notes and rests in duple meter
6b Listen and analyze uses of rhythm and timbre in music from diverse genres

MORE MUSIC CHOICES

For more practice with syncopation:
"Hit Me with a Hot Note and Watch Me Bounce," p. 112
"At the Same Time," p. 115

1 INTRODUCE

Inform students that in tap dancing, one of several types of dance performed on stage, the dancers tap out rhythm with their feet. Share with students the information on tap dance in Spotlight On below, and Cultural Connection, p. 321, to help them explore African American cultural experience as expressed in dance.

The Best of "Dancin' Feet"

Dance is often prominent in musicals. Some dancing, such as ballet and tap, requires special shoes. Tap dancing is the most important element in the Broadway show *Bring In Da Noise, Bring In Da Funk*. The show traces the history of tap dancing through many different places and styles.

Perform this chant from *Bring In Da Noise, Bring In Da Funk*.

CD 16-11

Now That's Tap

Words and Music by Ann Duquesnay, Daryl Waters, and Zane Zacharoff

Give em' flash, Give em' style and a great big big big

big big smile, Now that's tap! Make sure your tux is

fit-tin' right. Be pre-pared ta' wing all night and those

pearl-y whites, moon-beam bright, Now that's tap!

320

Footnotes

SKILLS REINFORCEMENT

▶ **Listening** Invite students to tap the steady beat with a toe as they listen to "Now That's Tap" **CD 16-11.** This may be a challenge, since there is much syncopation. On a second listening, have them locate the spots in the recording where they hear rhythms that could be made by dancers' feet. Students may wish to tap an original rhythm when they reach these passages on a subsequent listening.

BUILDING SKILLS THROUGH MUSIC

▶ **Reading** Share the information on tap dancing from Spotlight On. Have students read the information on p. 320, learn the chant *Now That's Tap* and answer this question: Has tap dancing always been the same or has it changed over time? They should use information in the text to support their answer.

SPOTLIGHT ON

▶ **Tap Dancing** Tap dancing originated in the United States before 1800. The dance form evolved from a combination of African drumming and European clog and step dancing. Tapping first appeared on street corners, where people tried to perform better than other street-corner dancers. Tapping became popularized when vaudeville's Bill "Bojangles" Robinson and John Bubbles refined the steps. Later, films featuring Fred Astaire, Eleanore Powell, and the Nicholas Brothers helped to establish tap dancing as an art form. Today, the world-famous Rockettes of Radio City Music Hall in New York City always include tap-dancing routines in their performances.

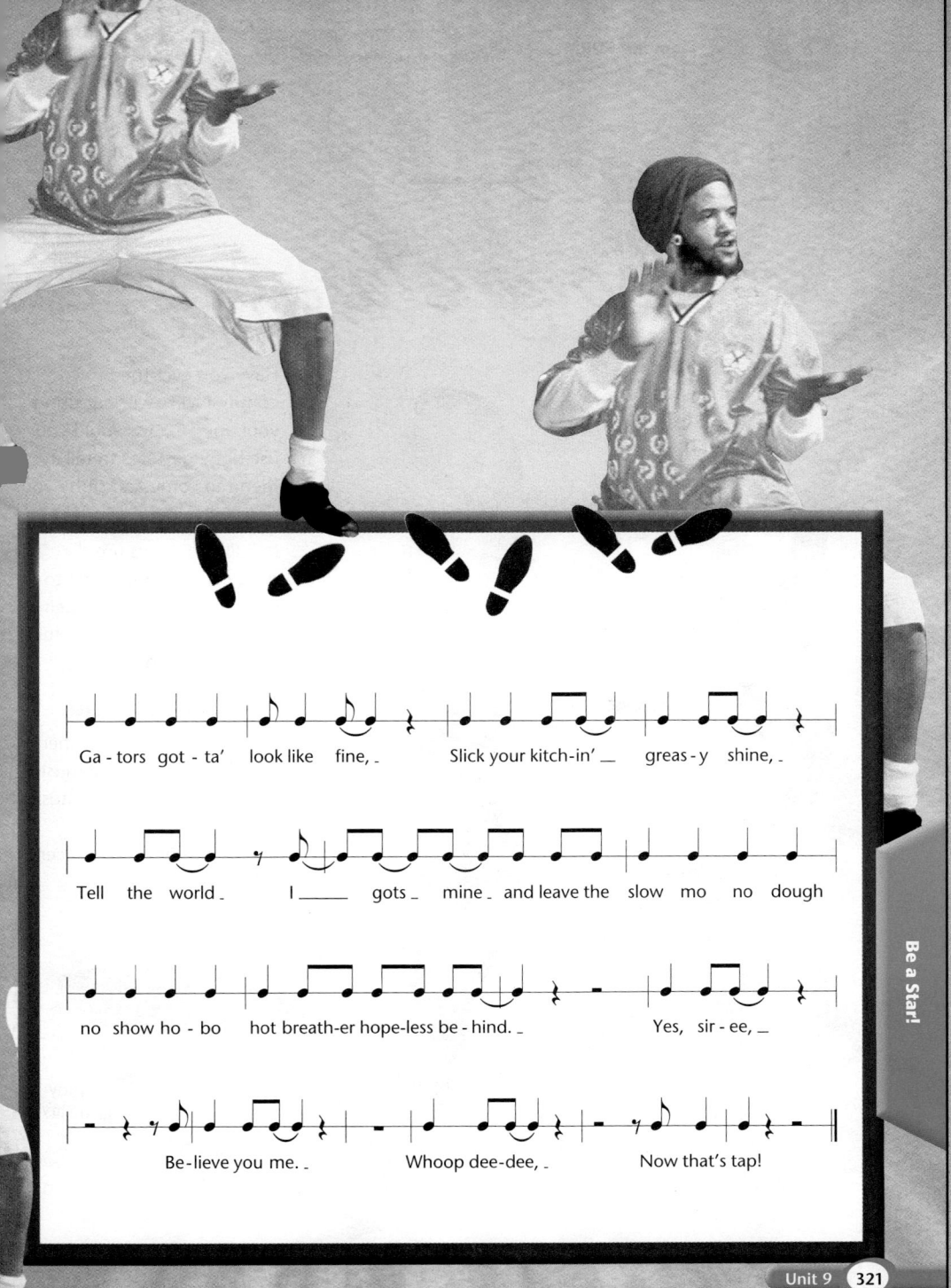

Ga - tors got - ta' look like fine, _ Slick your kitch-in' __ greas - y shine, _

Tell the world _ I ____ gots _ mine _ and leave the slow mo no dough

no show ho - bo hot breath-er hope-less be - hind. _ Yes, sir - ee, __

Be - lieve you me. _ Whoop dee-dee, _ Now that's tap!

Be a Star!

2 DEVELOP

Reading

Have students

5a • Sight-read the speech piece "Now That's Tap" **CD 16-11** while listening to the recording.

1c • Perform the chant with the recording.

6b Ask students to identify in the score those measures that contain even rhythm patterns (3 and 9, for example) and those that contain syncopated patterns (1, 2, and 4, for example).

Listening

SAY Tap dancing requires special shoes with taps, metal plates attached to toe and heel that allow the dancer's feet to sound like a percussion instrument.

Inform students that there are three terms familiar to all tap dancers: *stealing steps,* where one dancer copies another dancer's steps, and *challenges* or *trading fours,* where one dancer tries to top, or outdo, another dancer's steps to four measures (16 beats).

Invite students to listen to "Now That's Tap" **CD 16-11.**

Have students improvise their own movement routines. See Skills Reinforcement, p. 320.

3 CLOSE

Skill: LISTENING   ASSESSMENT

6b **Music Journal Writing** Have students

• Listen once again to "Now That's Tap" **CD 16-11.**

• Describe in their music journals the effects of syncopation and the sound of dancing feet in the performance.

CULTURAL CONNECTION

▶ **Bring In Da Noise, Bring In Da Funk** This contemporary musical tells of the African American experience through music, dance, and song. The selection *Now That's Tap* contains lyrics that proclaim to the listener that this dancer is leaving thoughts of money trouble and a hard life behind. Premiering in November 1995, in New York City, the musical is based on African American musical styles from the past century, including blues, jazz, R&B (rhythm and blues), hip-hop, and street drumming. The show's choreographer and main dancer, Savion Glover, received much acclaim for his unique tap dancing style. The show won four Tony awards in 1996: Best Director, musical (George C. Wolfe); Best Choreography (Glover); Best Featured Actress, musical (Ann Duquesnay); and Best Lighting Design, musical (Jules Fisher and Peggy Eisenhauer).

SCHOOL TO HOME CONNECTION

▶ **Tap Dance Demonstration** Students and their families may enjoy participating in a tap dance demonstration. Invite a local tap artist or group to come to your school and perform for students. Ask the artist(s) to teach students and family members a few basic tap steps. Local tap artists can be located by calling dance schools and organizations in your community.

TECHNOLOGY/MEDIA LINK

Sequencing Software Invite students to create and then record a live "tap dance" performance of "Now That's Tap," using the digital audio recording feature of their sequencing software.

LESSON AT A GLANCE

Element Focus **FORM** ABA

Skill Objective **LISTENING** Identify and track the sequence of themes in a listening selection

Connection Activity **RELATED ARTS** Discuss ballet as another art form that takes place on both stage and screen

MATERIALS

• "Waltz of the Flowers" from *The Nutcracker* **CD 16-13**

VOCABULARY

ballet	choreographer	form
melodic contour	dynamics	timbre

◆ ◆ ◆ ◆ National Standards ◆ ◆ ◆ ◆

6b Listen and analyze uses of timbre and form in music from diverse genres

7a Students evaluate the music they hear

8b Identify ways music relates to language arts and other school subjects

9c Compare, in several cultures, functions music serves and the roles of musicians

MORE MUSIC CHOICES

For more experience with form:

"Blue Skies" (AABA), p. 88

"El condor pasa" (AABB), p. 46

Jesu, Joy of Man's Desiring (AABA), p. 87

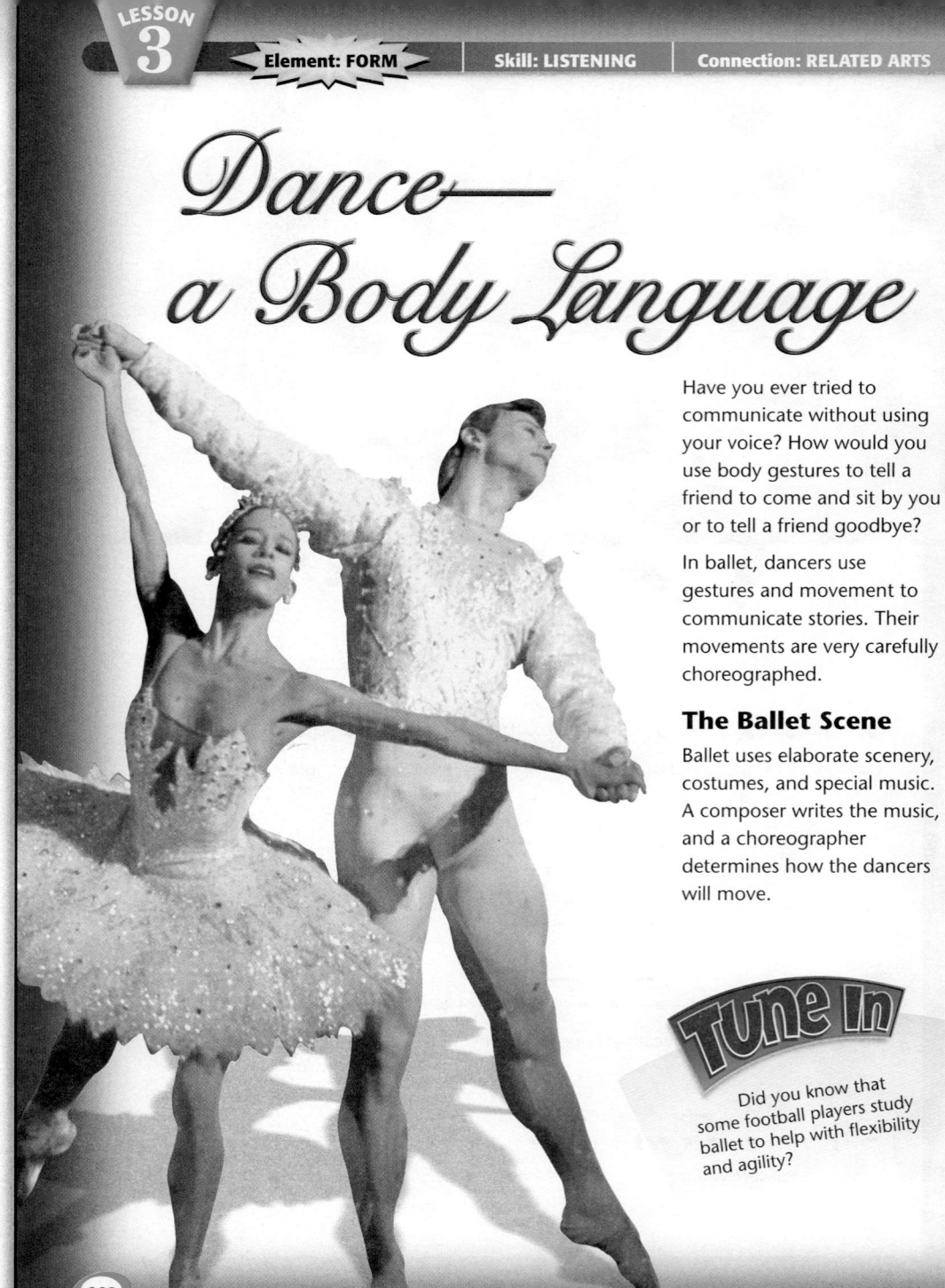

Dance—
a Body Language

Have you ever tried to communicate without using your voice? How would you use body gestures to tell a friend to come and sit by you or to tell a friend goodbye?

In ballet, dancers use gestures and movement to communicate stories. Their movements are very carefully choreographed.

The Ballet Scene

Ballet uses elaborate scenery, costumes, and special music. A composer writes the music, and a choreographer determines how the dancers will move.

Did you know that some football players study ballet to help with flexibility and agility?

322

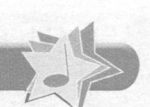Footnotes

MEETING INDIVIDUAL NEEDS

▶ **Nonvocal Communication** You may want to make students aware of the fact that not everyone communicates with their voice. For example, some people use sign language. Others use speech synthesizers. *The Boy Who Ate Words* by Thierry Dedieu (Harry Abrams, 1997) is an inspiring story of a boy who stops talking and learns the language of nature instead of words. Inspire sensitivity to the fact that not everyone can speak.

BUILDING SKILLS THROUGH MUSIC

▶ **Theater** Have students read the description of the story of *The Nutcracker* on p. 324. Ask them to organize the story into three acts, and list the characters that would appear in each act.

ACROSS THE CURRICULUM

▶ **Dance** Invite students to read about the first public school in America to train professional ballet dancers in *Kids Dance: The Students of Ballet Tech* by Jim Varriale (Penguin Putnam, 1999). The school program, founded by dancer/choreographer Eliot Feld, introduces hundreds of students to ballet each year while they continue their regular academic courses. The book focuses on the experiences of the students—how they audition, the hours of discipline and practice involved, rehearsals, and final performances. Excellent, exciting photographs of racially diverse students dancing, as well as the words of students themselves, make this fine book an appealing introduction to the world of ballet.

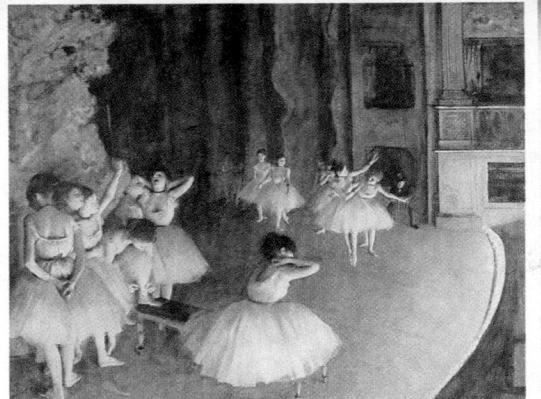

Arts **Connection**

◄ *Ballet Rehearsal on Set.*
Look at this famous
painting of ballet dancers
by the French artist
Edgar Degas [deh-GAH]
(1834–1917). How are the
ballet dancers portrayed?

M·U·S·I·C M·A·K·E·R·S

George Balanchine

George Balanchine [BAL-an-sheen] (1904–1983)
was one of the world's greatest choreographers.
He arrived in the United States from Russia in
1933 to open the School of American Ballet.
Balanchine also choreographed musicals, making
dance an important part of the story. In the late
1940s, Balanchine founded the New York City
Ballet. Under his direction the company became
world famous. Balanchine's choreography for *The
Nutcracker* has been performed by ballet
companies all over the world.

Be a Star!

Unit 9 **323**

1 INTRODUCE

Engage students in a discussion of nonverbal communication.

**ASK How can body gestures be used to make a
statement, ask a question, or communicate an idea?**
(waving goodbye, telling someone to move from one
place to another, shrugging your shoulders, showing if
you're cold or if you're hot, and so on)

2 DEVELOP

Analyzing

Have students read the information on p. 322 on ballet
as an art form and guide students to see how other
arts, such as ballet, are related to music.

Inform students that

- Ballet is a form of nonverbal communication that
takes place on stage and screen.
- Ballet tells a story through dance, music, movement, and gestures.
- Each dancer's movements are carefully planned, or
choreographed.

8b Ask students to focus on the painting by Degas.

**ASK How would you describe the movement por-
trayed in this ballet scene?** (graceful, flowing)

**What type of music might be accompanying
the solo dancer?** (Accept a variety of reasonable
responses.)

9c Invite students to read about George Balanchine.

**ASK Why would dancers and choreographers have
to understand music?** (Their movements have to be
synchronized with the music.)

continued on page 324

SPOTLIGHT ON

▶ **The Artist** Painter and sculptor Hilaire Germain Edgar
Degas (1834–1917) was born into a wealthy Parisian banking
family. Although he studied under the classicist painter J. A. D.
Ingres, and was a friend of Impressionists Manet and Van Gogh,
he developed a style all his own. Unlike the classicists, he composed pictures on odd visual angles, often cropping his subjects
at the edges. Unlike the Impressionists, though, he was not at all
interested in natural light. He preferred painting indoors. He also
preferred painting theatrical subjects rather than nature scenes.

Degas was a sharp observer who tried to grasp the moment. For
example, he painted a dancer scratching her back and a discarded dress still keeping some of the shape of the wearer. He did
not flatter people. He painted them as he saw them. This may
be why he was not viewed as a great artist until after his death.

SKILLS REINFORCEMENT

6b ▶ **Listening** Although the harp is an orchestral instrument,
many composers do not include it in their compositions.
Tchaikovsky, however, gave the harp a significant role in *The
Nutcracker*, especially in the introduction. Have students listen to
the introduction and identify the harp, a member of the string
family. Share with students that the harp has been around for
more than 2,500 years. The Western symphonic version has 47
strings, which are plucked with the fingers. The C and F strings
are in different colors, usually red and blue, to help the harpist
identify them. The harpist uses the pedals at the base of the
instrument to raise or lower pitches of the strings by a half step.

For more practice listening for harp timbre within an orchestra,
invite students to listen to *Wedding Day at Troldhaugen*
CD 1-5.

Listening

Ask students to

- Read the story of *The Nutcracker,* on p. 324.

- Read about Piotr Ilyich Tchaikovsky in the Music Makers feature on p. 324.

Direct students' attention to the listening map on p. 325 and the title of this selection from *The Nutcracker* ballet.

ASK In what meter do you expect this selection to be? (Waltzes are usually in meter in 3.)

What types of movement would you expect to be used with this piece? (light, airy, delicate, and so on)

Play the first one or two minutes of *Waltz of the Flowers* **CD 16-14;** then engage students in a follow-up discussion of the questions above.

In the context of the listening, ask students to describe why aurally-presented music of diverse periods is important to their listening experience. (Music from other historical periods provides an insight into their culture, musical style, entertainment, and history of the period.) Ask them to describe some of their musical insights in the context of *Waltz of the Flowers.* (The orchestra was important to performing music; the waltz was a popular dance and musical form; the ballet was a popular form of entertainment.)

Moving

As students listen to a longer portion of *Waltz of the Flowers,* encourage them to improvise appropriate arm and upper body movements that reflect the style of the music.

Analyzing

Direct students' attention to the listening map on p. 325.

ASK How many different melodies are used in this selection? (four)

A Holiday Ballet

The Nutcracker is one of the most popular ballets of all time.

The story begins when Marie, a young girl, receives a nutcracker carved in the shape of a little man. When her brother and his friends break it playing roughly, Marie becomes upset. Later that night Marie dreams that the nutcracker comes to life as a gallant soldier. The soldier goes to battle with the king of a gang of mice. When the Mouse King dies, the nutcracker becomes a prince. The prince escorts Marie on a wonderful journey. Eventually they go to a dance where many kinds of sweets, toys, and even flowers dance in their honor.

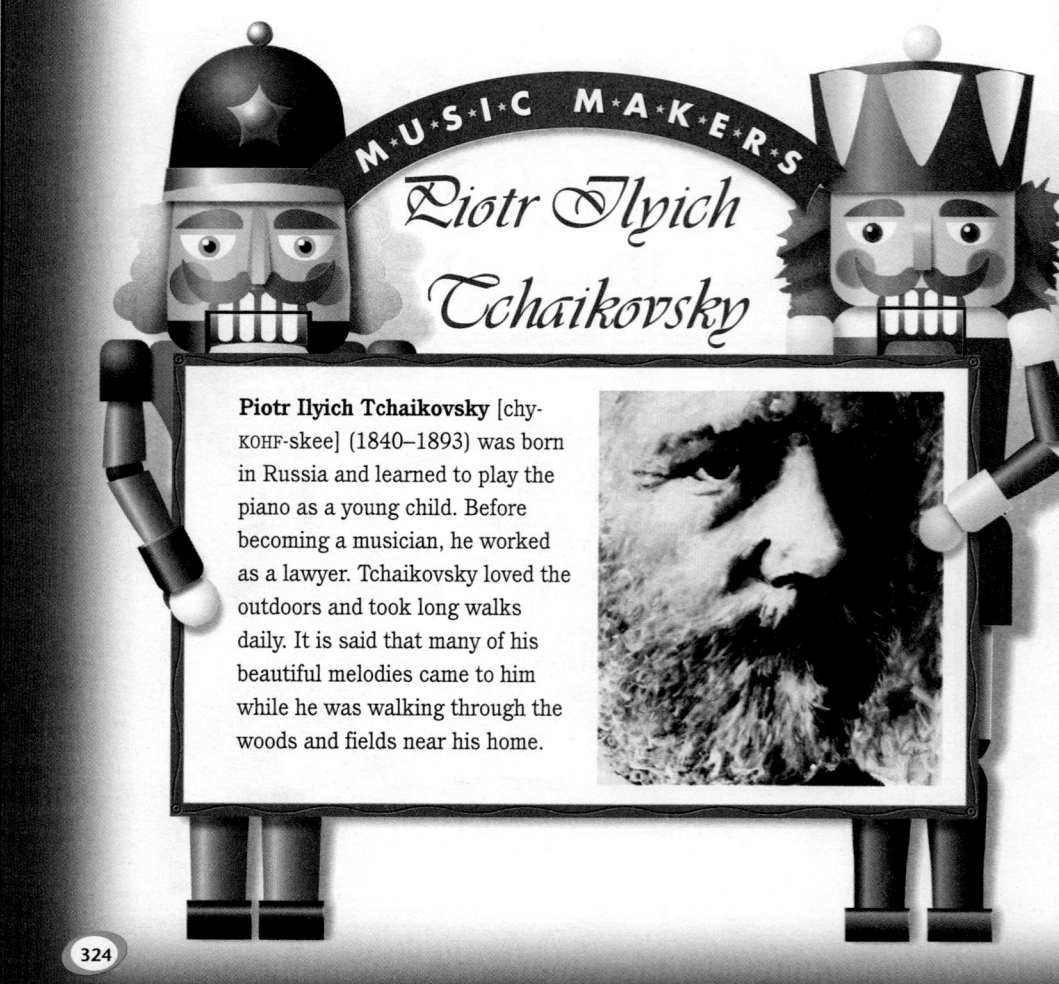

Piotr Ilyich Tchaikovsky [chy-KOHF-skee] (1840–1893) was born in Russia and learned to play the piano as a young child. Before becoming a musician, he worked as a lawyer. Tchaikovsky loved the outdoors and took long walks daily. It is said that many of his beautiful melodies came to him while he was walking through the woods and fields near his home.

324

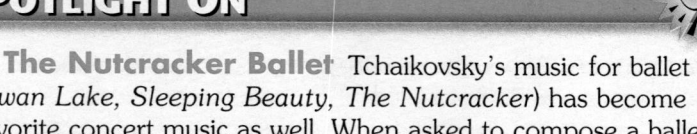

SPOTLIGHT ON

▶ **The Nutcracker Ballet** Tchaikovsky's music for ballet (*Swan Lake, Sleeping Beauty, The Nutcracker*) has become favorite concert music as well. When asked to compose a ballet for the Russian Imperial Theater, Tchaikovsky chose E. T. A. Hoffman's Christmas tale, *The Nutcracker and the Mouse King,* as the story line for the ballet. Hoffman's original story, considered to be too mean, had to be revised by Alexander Dumas.

CULTURAL CONNECTION

▶ **Nutcrackers** Prized gifts in the mid-eighteenth century, when Tchaikovsky wrote *The Nutcracker,* nutcrackers were useful tools that took on the form of a human figure. They were usually made of wood and had large heads with large mouths into which a nut was placed. The shell was cracked by closing the nutcracker's mouth with a lever on the back of the figure. Nutcrackers were given as keepsakes to bring good luck and to protect one's home. Their popularity soared after the premiere in 1892 of Tchaikovsky's ballet.

A Nutcracker Map

Look at the listening map as you **listen** to "Waltz of the Flowers" from *The Nutcracker*. Follow the map and determine the form as you listen.

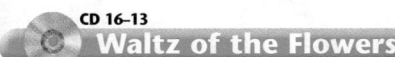

CD 16–13
Waltz of the Flowers

from *The Nutcracker*
by Piotr Ilyich Tchaikovsky

The Nutcracker is very popular at holiday time, due to its setting and colorful characters.

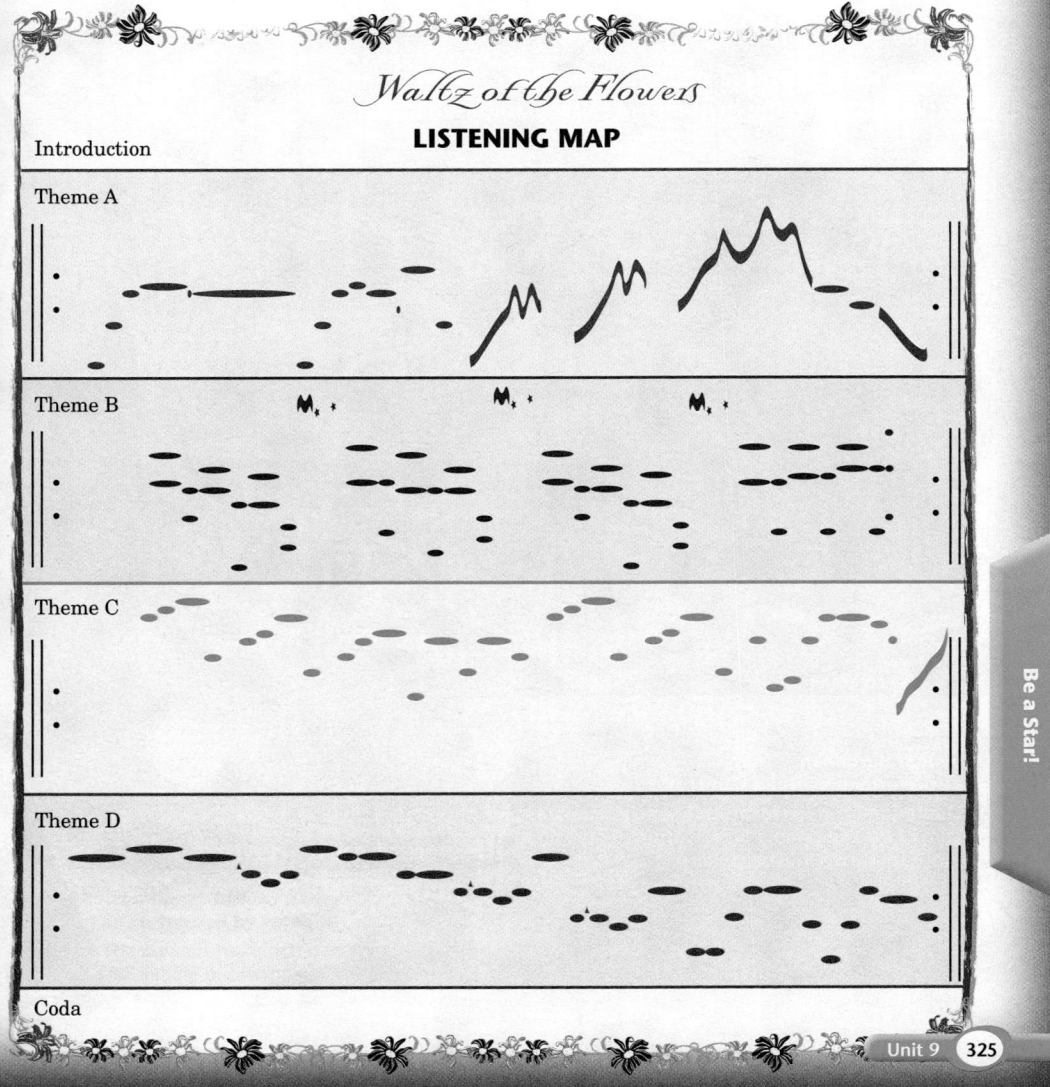

Waltz of the Flowers
LISTENING MAP

Introduction

Theme A

Theme B

Theme C

Theme D

Coda

Be a Star!

Unit 9 **325**

Play the entire recording of *Waltz of the Flowers* as students follow the listening map. See Technology/Media Link, p. 325, for tips on using the transparency.

ASK Were the four melodies always presented in the same, consecutive order? (no)

How are the four melodies different from one another? (For their responses, encourage students to focus on such elements as melodic contour, dynamics, and timbre.)

3 CLOSE

Element: FORM | **ASSESSMENT**

Music Journal Writing As you play *Waltz of the Flowers* **CD 16-13**, encourage students to follow the listening map once again. Ask students to identify music forms presented aurally. Have them

• Determine the form of the piece by mapping out the sequence of themes A, B, C, and D. See Skills Reinforcement below.

• Identify, where possible, specific instruments heard playing each theme.

• Write their analysis of and reaction to the music, evaluating the effectiveness of the music.

Invite students to share and discuss their responses with the class.

SKILLS REINFORCEMENT

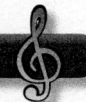
▶ **Listening** Not counting sections that immediately repeat, the form of *Waltz of the Flowers* may be outlined as follows.

(Introduction) ABAB CDC ABAB (Coda)

In a larger sense, the form may be considered ABA.

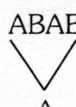　　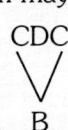　　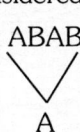

ABAB　　CDC　　ABAB

A　　B　　A

TECHNOLOGY/MEDIA LINK

Transparency Display the listening map transparency for *Waltz of the Flowers* as you play the recording. Point to each theme as it is played to help students follow along. On subsequent listenings, invite individual students to point to the sections as you play the recording.

LESSON AT A GLANCE

Element Focus   **RHYTHM** Dance rhythm patterns

Skill Objective   **MOVING** Perform an Irish jig

Connection Activity   **CULTURE** Explore Irish culture and dance

MATERIALS
* *Lord of the Dance Medley* (excerpt)   **CD 16-14**
* *Paddy Whack*   **CD 16-15**
* **Dance Directions** for *Paddy Whack* p. 564

VOCABULARY

choreography   tempo   dynamics

crescendo   *accelerando*

◆ ◆ ◆ ◆ National Standards ◆ ◆ ◆ ◆

6a Listen and describe events in music using appropriate terms

6b Listen and analyze uses of rhythm and timbre in music from diverse cultures

7b Students use specific criteria for evaluating performances, and offer constructive suggestions for improvement

MORE MUSIC CHOICES

For more experience with European folk dance:

Kerenski, p. 78

Sellenger's Round, p. 44

1 INTRODUCE

Explain to students that people everywhere in the world have their own folk songs, folk stories, and folk dances and that they have been passed on from one generation to the next. Share with students information in Cultural Connection, below, about Irish culture, and dance and Irish instruments, in Spotlight On below.

Dance, Irish Style

Not all stage dance is ballet. Some dancers perform traditional dances of their native country.

Lord of the Dance and *Riverdance* are two shows that celebrate the very best of Irish dancing.

Listen to this medley from *Lord of the Dance.* Identify the sections in which the rhythms are suitable for fast dancing.

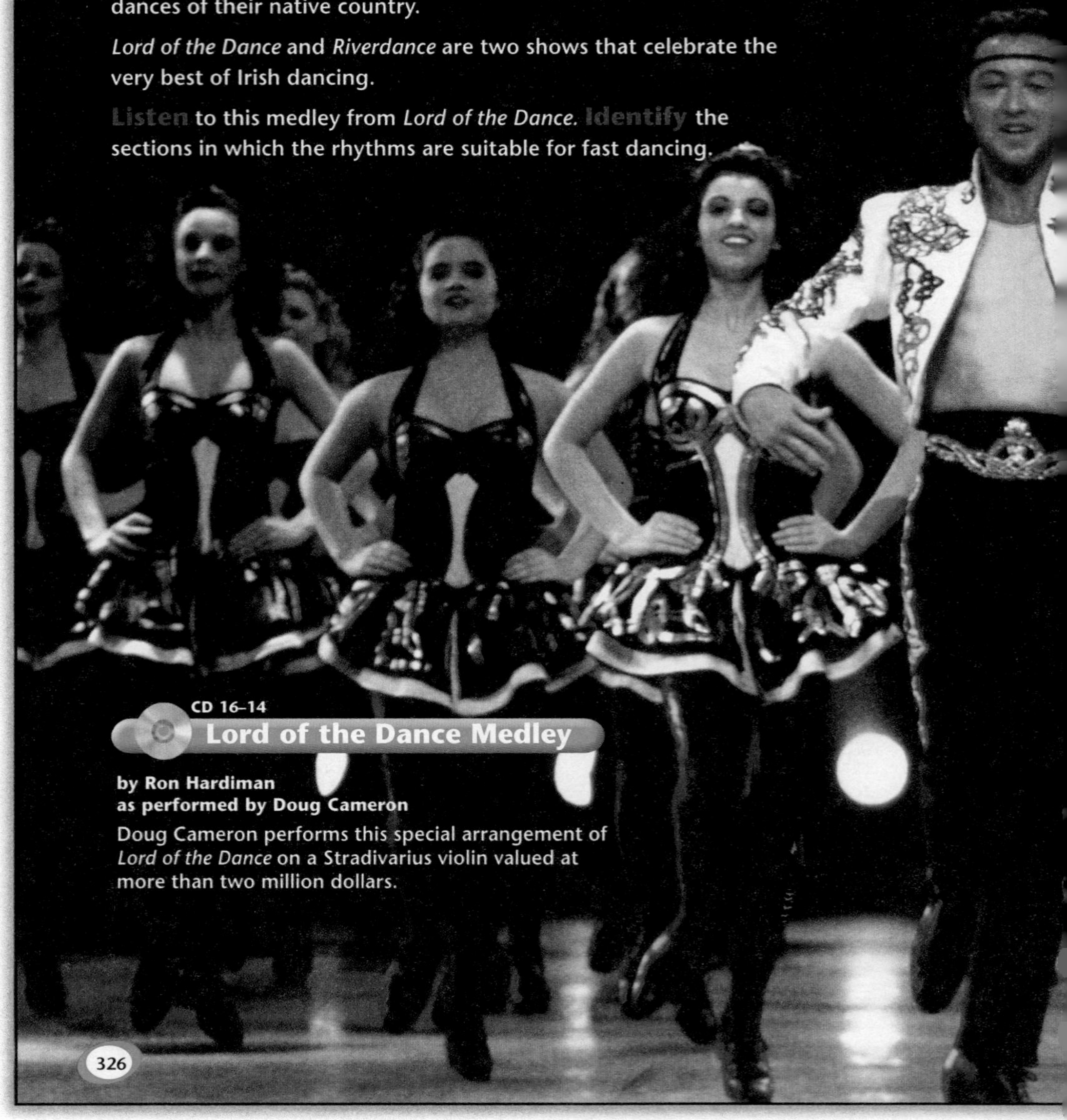

CD 16–14
Lord of the Dance Medley

by Ron Hardiman
as performed by Doug Cameron

Doug Cameron performs this special arrangement of *Lord of the Dance* on a Stradivarius violin valued at more than two million dollars.

Footnotes

CULTURAL CONNECTION

▶ **Irish Culture** Native Irish melodies have been popular since their re-emergence in the 1800s. Folk songs and dances such as the jig are a huge part of Irish culture. Jigging competitions are popular in Irish communities; judges sit under the stage to listen for the speed and accuracy of the dancer's tap.

BUILDING SKILLS THROUGH MUSIC
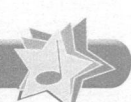

▶ **Social Studies** Share the information on Irish Culture in Cultural Connection. Discuss the practice of jigging competitions. Discuss the terms listed in Assessment on p. 327. Have students work in small groups. Guide them to develop a rubric to critique their peers' dance performance.

SPOTLIGHT ON

▶ **Irish Instruments** The following Irish instruments are featured in *Lord of the Dance Medley.*

* *Celtic flute* and *whistles*
* *Uilleann pipes* (sometimes called union pipes): Irish bag-pipes. An indoor instrument with a sweet tone, it is still very popular in Ireland today.
* *Bodhrán:* An 18" one-sided drum made of goatskin stretched over a circular wooden frame; played with a "tipper," or beater.

An Irish Jig

Irish dancers often compete in dance contests. Every performer in *Lord of the Dance* and *Riverdance* is a dance champion. Some of the characteristics of Irish dancing are:

- Keep your torso very upright.
- Put your arms and hands straight down at your sides. (Hands may also be placed on hips.)
- Point your toes and take small, sharp steps and kicks.

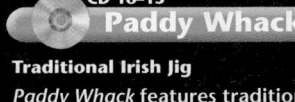

CD 16–15
Paddy Whack

Traditional Irish Jig

Paddy Whack features traditional Irish instruments, including the Celtic harp.

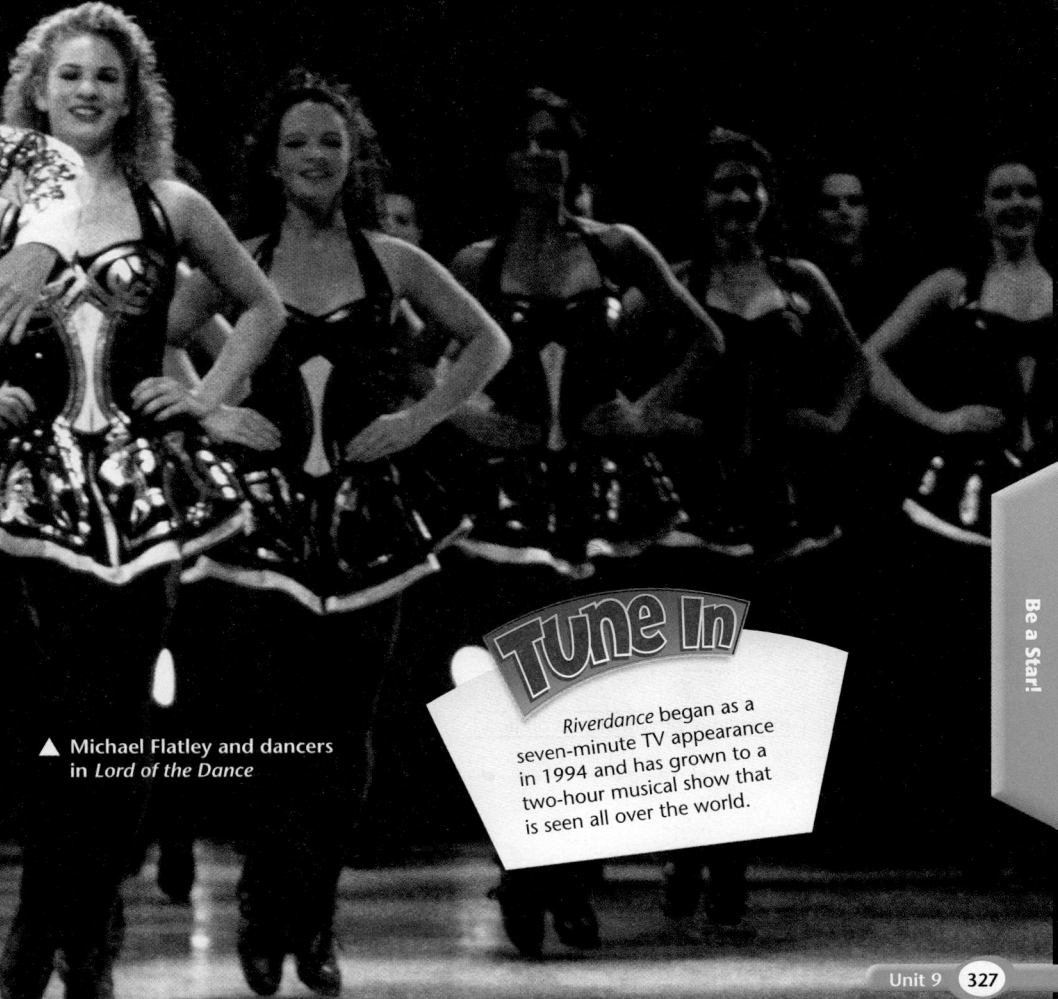

Riverdance began as a seven-minute TV appearance in 1994 and has grown to a two-hour musical show that is seen all over the world.

▲ Michael Flatley and dancers in *Lord of the Dance*

Be a Star!

Unit 9　**327**

---

2 DEVELOP

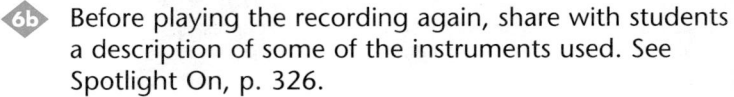

Listening

6a Write the following terms on the board: *steady beat, loud percussion, slow tempo, fast tempo, accelerando.*

6b Then, invite students to listen for each of these features in *Lord of the Dance Medley* **CD 16-14.** Approximate timings are as follows:

- Steady beat—0:57
- Loud percussion—1:36
- Slow tempo—2:22
- Steady beat—2:57
- Fast tempo—3:42
- *Accelerando*—4:02 and 4:50

6b Before playing the recording again, share with students a description of some of the instruments used. See Spotlight On, p. 326.

Moving

Help students

- Learn an Irish jig (see Movement below).
- Follow the Dance Practice **CD 16-16** and refer to Dance Directions, p. 564, to learn the steps.
- Perform the dance with *Paddy Whack* **CD 16-15.**

3 CLOSE

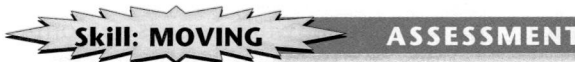

Skill: MOVING　　ASSESSMENT

7b **Performance/Peer Critique** Divide the class into two groups. Encourage each group to develop criteria and critique the other group's dance performance and give constructive suggestions, observing ensemble, artistry, and synchronization of movement to the rhythm of the music.

MOVEMENT

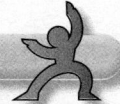

▶ **Patterned Dance** Help students learn and perform these practice movements for an Irish jig, a traditional folk dance with quick $\frac{6}{8}$ rhythms. See the complete Dance Directions on p. 564.

Formation:　All dancers stand facing the same direction.

Part A

Meas. 1:　Standing on L foot, touch R toe in front.

Meas. 2:　Hop on L foot as R foot kicks out and up.

Meas. 3–4:　Take four quick steps in place and hold for two counts (R-L-R-L hold).

Part B

Meas. 1–4:　Slide to R (side-close) three times, side-touch. Repeat, sliding to left.

TECHNOLOGY/MEDIA LINK

Multimedia Invite small groups of students to create a multimedia presentation that demonstrates how to dance the Irish jig (see Movement).

Digital Video Have students write a script, rehearse dancers, and videotape the movements. Use a DV camcorder, computer, and software to edit the video. Students can add titles, transitions, music, narration, and digital photographs to their video ("post production"), then play their videos for the class.

Digital Still Photography Have students plan a storyboard. Using a digital still camera, have them photograph the dancers' movements. Have students download the photographs into a computer, organize their photos into a slide show, add music, and then present their slide show to the class.

Unit 9　*Be a Star!*　**327**

| Element: RHYTHM | Skill: PLAYING | Connection: SCIENCE |

LESSON AT A GLANCE

Element Focus	**RHYTHM** *Stomp* rhythm patterns
Skill Objective	**PLAYING** Read and perform a rhythm piece in the style of the Broadway show *Stomp*
Connection Activity	**SCIENCE** Recognize that almost any object can serve as a sound source

MATERIALS
- *Trash Can Stomp*   **CD 16-17**
- "Sha Sha Sha"   **CD 16-18**
- several of each of the following: paint brushes, whisk brooms, straight brooms, and push brooms

VOCABULARY
noise   music   accent   *staccato*

◆◆◆◆ National Standards ◆◆◆◆
2c Perform instrumental music from diverse genres
4c Compose, using non-traditional sound sources
5a Read quarter, eighth, half, and dotted notes and rests in duple meter

MORE MUSIC CHOICES
For more practice reading and playing rhythms:
"Bury Me Not on the Lone Prairie," p. 19
"Red River Valley," p. 11

1 INTRODUCE

SAY Music is organized sound, while noise is random or unorganized sound. Anything you can blow across or through, or that vibrates when you hit it, scrape it, tap it, pluck it, or drag it can be an instrument.

Share Spotlight On, below, and Cultural Connection, p. 329, with students for more sound source ideas.

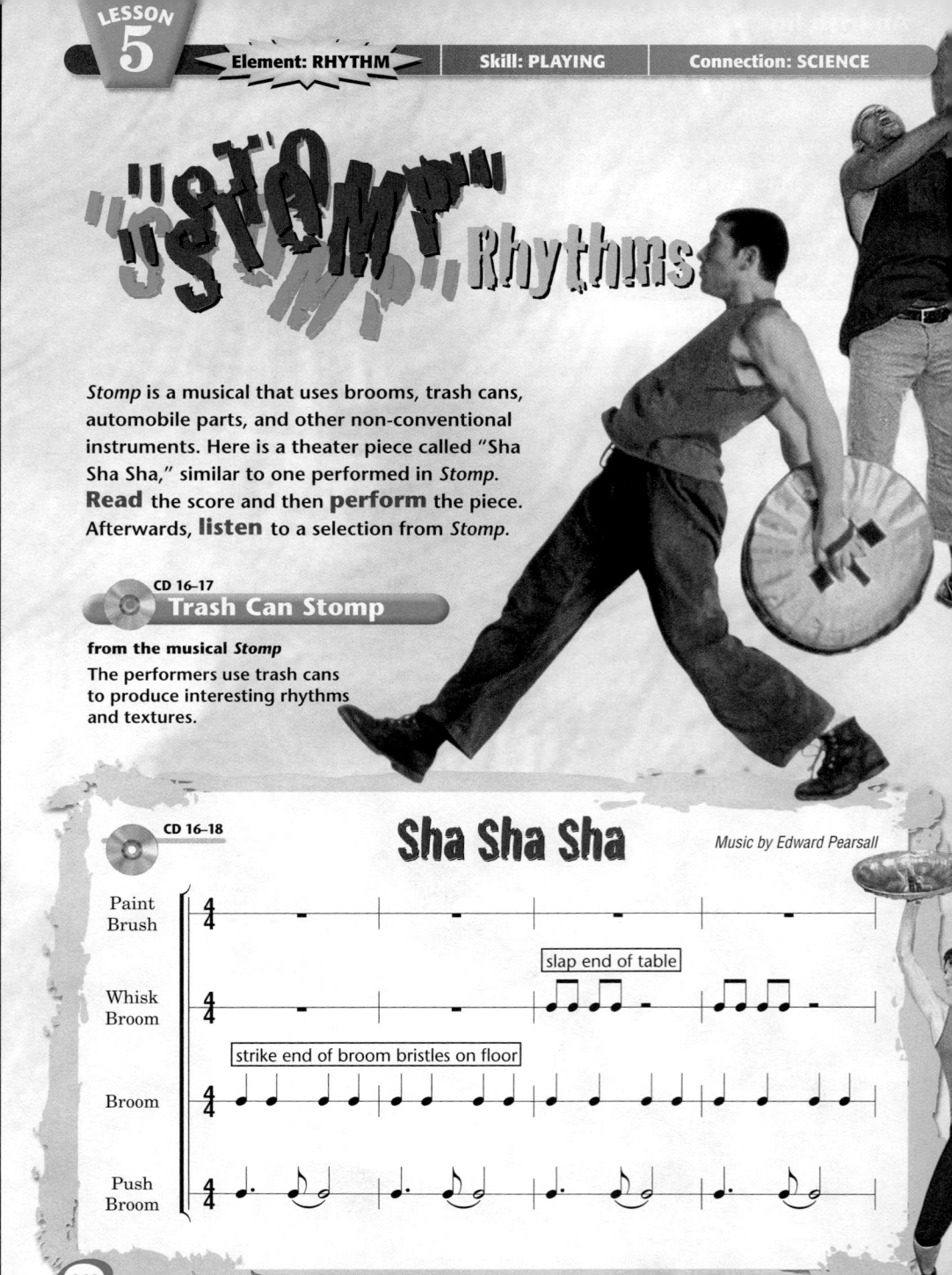

"STOMP" Rhythms

Stomp is a musical that uses brooms, trash cans, automobile parts, and other non-conventional instruments. Here is a theater piece called "Sha Sha Sha," similar to one performed in *Stomp*. **Read** the score and then **perform** the piece. Afterwards, **listen** to a selection from *Stomp*.

CD 16–17
Trash Can Stomp

from the musical *Stomp*
The performers use trash cans to produce interesting rhythms and textures.

CD 16–18

Sha Sha Sha
Music by Edward Pearsall

Paint Brush

Whisk Broom — slap end of table

Broom — strike end of broom bristles on floor

Push Broom

328

Footnotes

SPOTLIGHT ON

▶ **Stomp** This theater show of rhythm and movement has no dialogue, no story, and no melody. *Stomp* is totally rhythmical. The show finds beauty and music in the mundane. Junk, trash cans, corrugated metal sheets, pieces of scrap metal, brooms, and other objects are transformed into instruments. Eight musicians perform and move about the stage. The show opens with a piece entitled "Brooms," which is similar to "Sha Sha Sha."

BUILDING SKILLS THROUGH MUSIC

▶ **Writing** Have students write a very short story of a child discovering all the possible musical sounds that can be created with the objects found in one location (such as a kitchen, garage, barn, junk yard, arcade, or restaurant). Ask students to describe the objects, the sounds, and the process of discovering them.

SKILLS REINFORCEMENT

▶ **Playing** The following tips will help students as they perform "Sha Sha Sha."

Reinforcement Students with difficulty in motor coordination may perform the rhythms with mouth or other sounds.

On Target Tell the push broom performers to listen to the broom part to be sure they are brushing the second note with the tie at the right time.

Challenge Invite students to discover new instruments that may be used in this work (PVC piping, light pencil-tapping on plastic soda bottles). Then, have them improvise new complementary rhythm patterns as an accompaniment for "Sha Sha Sha."

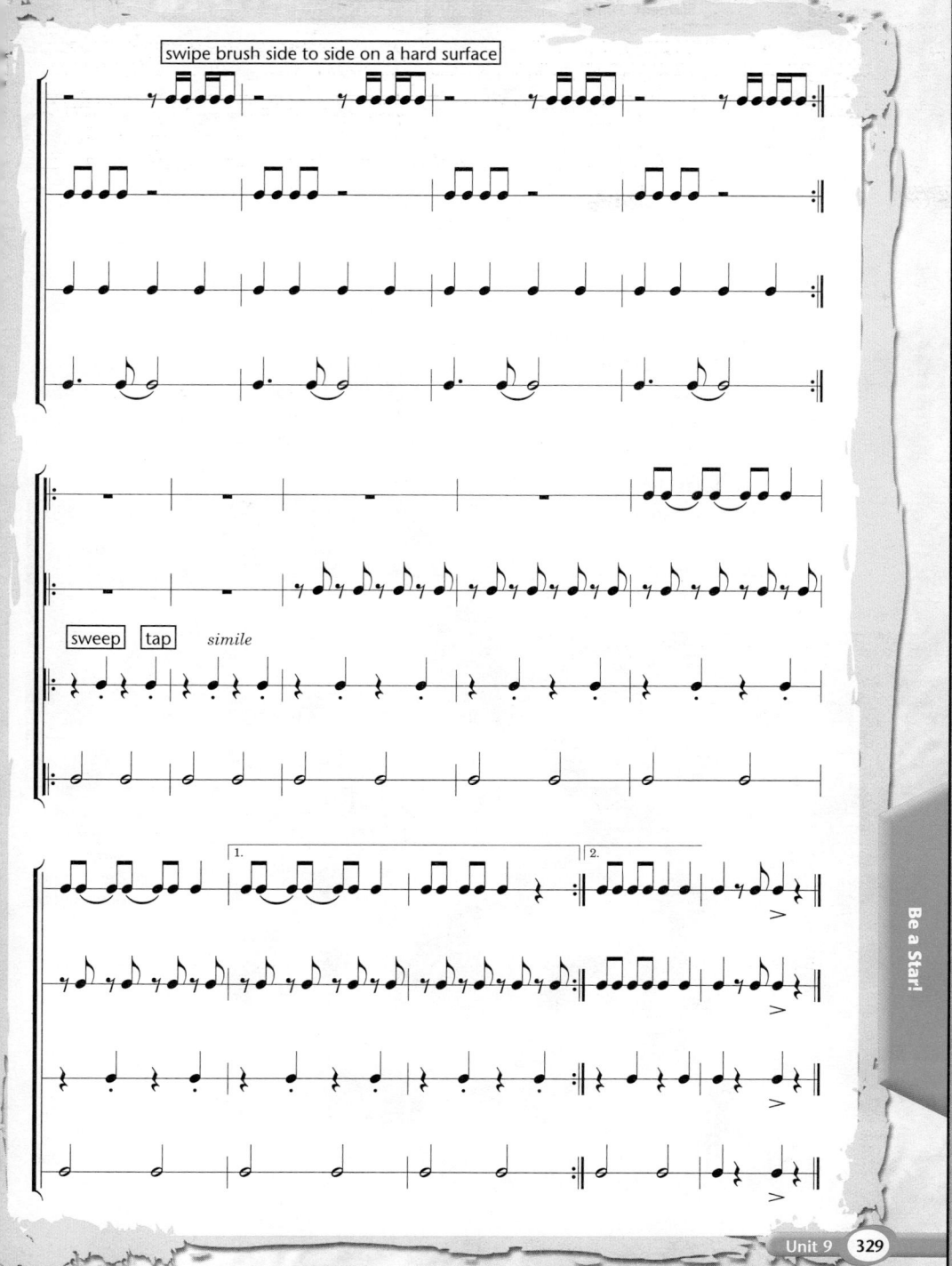

swipe brush side to side on a hard surface

sweep | tap | simile

Unit 9 **329**

2 DEVELOP

Listening

Invite students to read about the musical *Stomp,* on p. 328, and then listen to a selection from the show, *Trash Can Stomp* **CD 16-18.**

Reading

Direct students' attention to "Sha Sha Sha" and help them identify and discuss the meter, repeat marks, first and second endings, accent marks, and staccato marks.

5a Invite students to sight-read simple music in other clefs (percussion) in various meters, tapping each rhythm with the recording **CD 16-19.**

Playing

Divide the class into four groups and assign a "Sha Sha Sha" rhythm part to each group.

2c Distribute brooms and brushes to each group of students and invite them to experiment with the "instruments." Then, have students perform the piece.

Creating

4c Invite students to compose and perform an original, short composition, using all four sound sources. See Technology/Media Link below for additional activities.

Moving

Inform students that the musicians in *Stomp* move when they perform. Encourage students to plan movements for their performance of "Sha Sha Sha."

3 CLOSE

Element: RHYTHM   **ASSESSMENT**

Performance/Observation Divide the class into groups and encourage each group to perform the rhythm piece with "Sha Sha Sha" **CD 16-19.** Evaluate each group's performance for rhythmic accuracy.

CULTURAL CONNECTION

▶ **Different Cultures, Different Timbres** *Stomp* was not the first group of musicians to transform functional, everyday objects into instruments. Various cultures throughout the world have made musical instruments from gourds, hollow logs, and other materials some would consider less than artistic. As studied in Unit 8, abandoned steel oil drums are made into tuned musical instruments in Trinidad and Tobago. Blue Man Group, another innovative performing group, uses PVC plumbing pipe of different lengths and sizes, as well as many other interesting nonmusical items, to create a unique musical experience.

TECHNOLOGY/MEDIA LINK

4c **Sequencing Software** Invite students to create a rhythm composition (a four-measure ostinato), using "found sounds" in the classroom. Students will use the digital audio feature of their sequencing software to record their compositions. Have students

- Find four sound sources in the classroom. (foot tapping, tapping pencils, body percussion sounds, other object sounds)
- Create and notate four rhythm parts. Assign each part to a student who will perform it as an ostinato.
- Record each rhythm part onto an armed track of the sequencing software. Create a "mix" of the four tracks.
- Play back their composition for the class. Save their composition as an MP3, or audio CD, for their student portfolio.

Unit 9 *Be a Star!* **329**

LESSON AT A GLANCE

Element Focus   **TIMBRE** Wind and percussion instruments

Skill Objective   **LISTENING** Identify groups of wind and percussion instruments aurally

Connection Activity   **SCIENCE** Explore the science of acoustics

MATERIALS
- *Rocky Point Holiday*   **CD 16-20**
- instrument posters or name cards

VOCABULARY

acoustics   brass   percussion   woodwinds

◆ ◆ ◆ ◆ **National Standards** ◆ ◆ ◆ ◆

6b Listen and analyze uses of timbre in music from diverse genres
8b Identify ways music relates to science
9b Classify high-quality musical works by historical period and composer

MORE MUSIC CHOICES

For more practice with orchestral timbre:
"Farandole" from *L'Arlésienne Suite No. 2,* p. 68
Symphony No. 5, Movement 1 (excerpt), p. 98
Wedding Day at Troldhaugen, Op. 65, No. 6, p. 9

1 INTRODUCE

ASK **Where do you go to listen to music?** (Accept a variety of responses.)

Have any of you ever attended a performance in a concert hall?

SAY Concert halls are auditoriums specifically designed for listening to music.

Share with students the information on acoustics in Across the Curriculum below, and about appropriate audience etiquette at concerts, listed throughout the Teacher Edition.

Good Listening By Design

Concert halls are designed so that the **acoustics** of the hall enhance the sound for a great musical performance.

Acoustics is the science of the production, control, and transmission of sound.

The Morton Meyerson Symphony Center, in Dallas, Texas, was built for live musical performances. It is the home of the Dallas Symphony Orchestra.

▲ The Morton Meyerson Symphony Center was designed by Pei Cobb Freed & Partners

◄ Interior view of the concert hall

330

Footnotes

SKILLS REINFORCEMENT

► **Listening** Before listening to *Rocky Point Holiday,* encourage students to review wind and percussion instruments of the orchestra using the Sound Bank with pictures of instruments on p. 512 and the recordings of orchestral instruments beginning on **CD 23-11.**

BUILDING SKILLS THROUGH MUSIC

► **Science** Have students select a sound that can be repeated, then select three locations of different size in your school (for example, the gym, music room, office). In each location they should repeat the sound, write down their observations about the sound (loudness, echo, how far it carries, and so on), and write descriptions of the locations, identifying things that might affect the acoustical properties.

ACROSS THE CURRICULUM

8b ► **Science** Inform students that concert halls are designed by architects who understand how materials used in the construction of the hall will affect the sound. If too much sound is absorbed by carpeting, or sound-absorbing tiles on the walls or ceiling, the room will be "dead." If the room is too "live," the sound will bounce off the hard surfaces and produce too much echo.

For more about the physics of sound, encourage students to try the experiments in *Music (Science Encounters)* by Julian Rowe (Heineman, 1997).

For more information about the facility featured in this lesson, refer students to *The Meyerson Symphony Center: Building a Dream* by Laurie Shulman (Univ. of North Texas Press, 2000).

The Concert Band on Stage

American composer Ron Nelson has written many works for concert band.

Listen to an excerpt from one such work, performed by the Dallas Wind Symphony and recorded at the Morton Meyerson Symphony Center.

CD 16–19
Rocky Point Holiday

by Ron Nelson
as performed by the Dallas Wind Symphony;
Jerry Junkin, conductor

This recording by the Dallas Wind Symphony demonstrates the excellent acoustics of the Morton Meyerson Symphony Center.

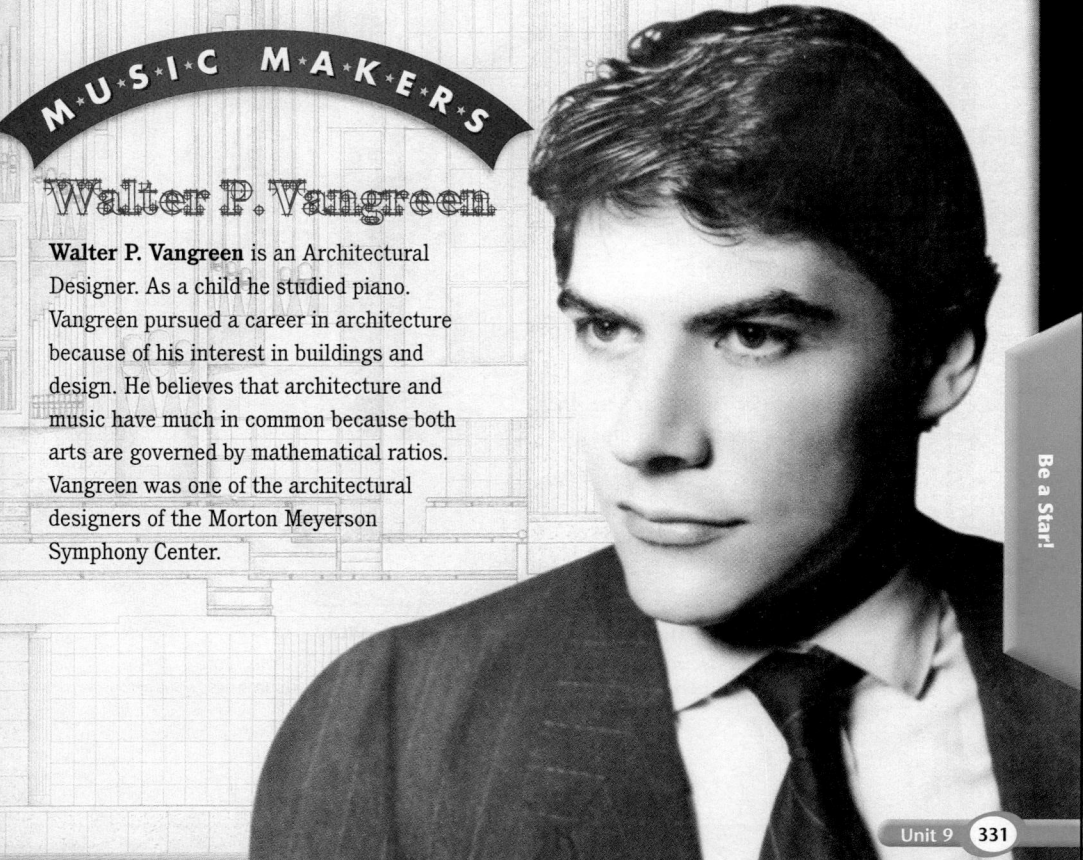

M·U·S·I·C M·A·K·E·R·S

Walter P. Vangreen

Walter P. Vangreen is an Architectural Designer. As a child he studied piano. Vangreen pursued a career in architecture because of his interest in buildings and design. He believes that architecture and music have much in common because both arts are governed by mathematical ratios. Vangreen was one of the architectural designers of the Morton Meyerson Symphony Center.

Be a Star!

Unit 9 **331**

---

2 DEVELOP

Listening

Ask students to read the information on p. 330 and the Music Makers feature on this page. Discuss details students find in the photo of Morton Meyerson Symphony Center on p. 330.

8b Inform students that the architectural designer must carefully engineer the acoustics of a concert hall to allow the audience to hear both a solo instrument and a symphony orchestra equally well.

9b Students may be interested in learning about a career as a composer. Share information on the contemporary American composer Ron Nelson (see Spotlight On below). Ask students to describe the music vocation or avocation of a composer.

Before playing *Rocky Point Holiday* **CD 16-19,** explain that the title refers to a seaside resort in Rhode Island. Then, divide the class into four groups: high brass, low brass, woodwinds, percussion. Distribute appropriate posters or name cards of specific instruments to students in each group (see Spotlight On below).

6b As they listen to the recording, ask students to raise their posters only when they hear an instrument or instruments from their assigned group. Families of instruments play together at times.

See Skills Reinforcement, p. 330, for a preliminary listening practice.

3 CLOSE

Element: TIMBRE   **ASSESSMENT**

Music Journal Writing On subsequent listening experiences with *Rocky Point Holiday* **CD 16-19,** have students write detailed descriptions of the instrumental combinations. As an aid, play the music in smaller segments.

SPOTLIGHT ON

9b ▶ **The Composer** Ron Nelson, born in 1929 in Joliet, Illinois, wrote his first composition at age six. His work includes 90 choral works, two operas, a mass, a cantata, an oratorio, music for films and television, and more than 40 instrumental works.

▶ **Rocky Point Holiday** The piece is scored for the following wind and percussion instruments.

- High Brass: trumpets, French horns
- Low Brass: trombones, baritone, tuba
- Woodwinds: piccolo, flutes, oboes, English horn, clarinets, bassoons, saxophones
- Percussion: timpani, snare drum, bass drum, glockenspiel, xylophone, marimba, vibraphone, celesta, triangle, cymbals

TECHNOLOGY/MEDIA LINK

Sequencing Software Remind students that a concert hall sounds good because of its acoustics. Tell students that music on CDs, in movies, and on television is recorded and mixed by a "recording engineer." One element of controlling space in recorded music is reverberation, or reverb. Using *Micro Logic AV,* challenge students to add reverb to a track. Have students

- Record a MIDI rhythm part onto Track 10.
- Go to the Mixer window and locate MIDI Track 10.
- Add reverb to MIDI Track 10, if possible.
- Play back Track 10 from the Transport bar and listen to the effect reverb has on the sound.

LESSON AT A GLANCE

Element Focus	**RHYTHM** Latin rhythm patterns	
Skill Objective	**PLAYING** Perform a Latin rhythm accompaniment	
Connection Activity	**CULTURE** Explore Latin culture through dance	

MATERIALS
- *Lluvia* (guitar and vocals) (excerpt)   **CD 17-1**
- *Lluvia* (rhythm instruments)   **CD 17-2**
- *(Chi Chi Chi) Cha Cha Cha* (excerpt)   **CD 17-3**
- *You Sang to Me*   **CD 17-4**
- selected Latin rhythm instruments (claves, congas, *guiro*, bongos, cowbell, maracas, woodblock)

VOCABULARY
rhythm pattern   *rumba*   cha-cha
Latin ballad   syncopation

◆ ◆ ◆ ◆ National Standards ◆ ◆ ◆ ◆
2c Perform instrumental music from diverse cultures
4c Arrange, using electronic media
5a Read half, quarter, and eighth notes in duple meter
6a Listen and describe events in music using appropriate terms
6b Listen and analyze uses of rhythm and timbre in music from diverse cultures
7b Students use specific criteria for evaluating performances, and offer constructive suggestions for improvement
8b Identify ways music relates to social studies
9a Describe characteristics of music styles from a variety of cultures

MORE MUSIC CHOICES
For more experience with Latin music:
Mi tierra, p. 365
Si tú no estás (excerpt), p. 267

Latin Style!

Latin music is currently very popular in the United States. Singers like Marc Anthony, Gloria Estefan, and Jennifer Lopez perform Latin music on stage to large numbers of fans. Latin music comes from a rich tradition that includes many musical styles from Latin America, Spain, South America, and the Caribbean.

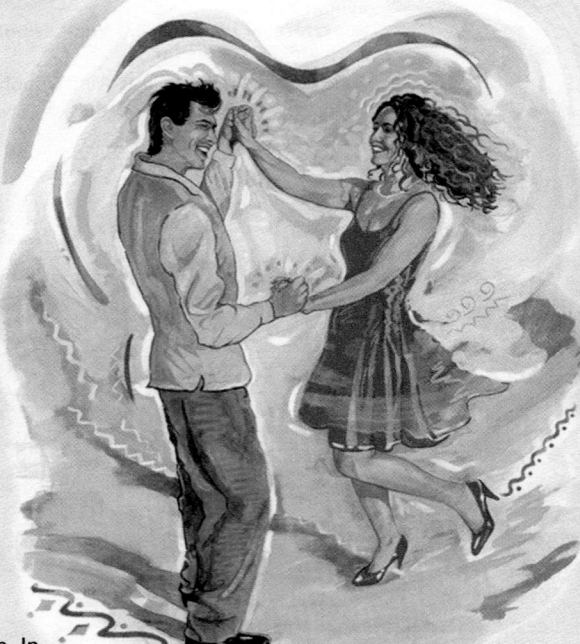

Latin Style and Rhythm

Latin music often has similar musical traits—beautiful melodies, guitars, and vocal harmonies. Latin music is often recognized by its distinct and energetic rhythms.

Listen to two excerpts of the song *Lluvia* [YOO-vyah] by the Venezuelan singer Franco de Vita. In each excerpt, listen to the guitar and rhythm patterns.

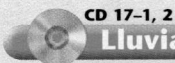

CD 17–1, 2
Lluvia
written and performed by Franco de Vita
Lluvia (Rain) is first performed with guitar and vocals, and then in an orchestrated version with rhythm instruments.

332

Footnotes

CULTURAL CONNECTION

8b ▶ **Origins of *Cha-Cha*** The *cha-cha* gets its name from a seedpod-producing plant of the same name that was used as a shaker by Haitian voodoo bands.

In 1953 the Cuban orchestra America developed the modern *cha-cha* by playing a *mambo* slowly enough to allow some hip movements. These hip movements became the small triple step that characterizes the dance. By 1959, the *cha-cha* became wildly popular in the United States and remains a popular Latin dance.

BUILDING SKILLS THROUGH MUSIC

▶ **Social Studies** Have students document the origins of the musical styles in this unit *(cha-cha, rumba, mambo, salsa)* and trace the movement of those influences using maps or globes.

SPOTLIGHT ON

▶ **The Composer** Of Italian descent, Franco de Vita was born in Caracas, Venezuela, in the mid-1950s. At age 3 he went to Italy but returned to Venezuela when he was 13. After high school, he studied at the music conservatory in Caracas, where he decided to dedicate his life to music.

From the start, de Vita's albums were extremely successful. His second album contained "Solo importas tú," a song that became the theme song of a soap opera. His latest album, *Nada es igual,* contains the hit song *Lluvia.*

Franco de Vita's music has many faces. It is personal and introspective, romantic, and socially conscious. It is traditional, festive, tropical, and, above all, it is Latin.

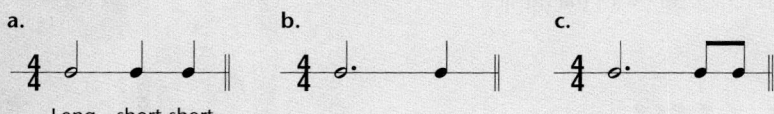

Latin Dance Rhythms

The rhythms in Latin music are one of the most characteristic elements of its style. Basic rhythms are embellished and layered to create complex and interesting textures.

Read the following rhythms by first using rhythm syllables. **Conduct** in meter in 4 to feel the underlying steady beat. **Play** the rhythm patterns on your favorite percussion instrument. When you are ready, **perform** the rhythms as accompaniment to Tito Puente's *Ti mon bo*, on page 334.

a.   b.   c.

Long   short-short

Long Short-Short

A rhythm pattern that is part of many Latin styles can be described as "long, short-short." This "rhythmic pulse" underlies many Latin dances, such as the *rumba*, *cha-cha*, and *tango*. As shown below, rhythms are embellished and layered on top of this pulse to give each dance its unique character.

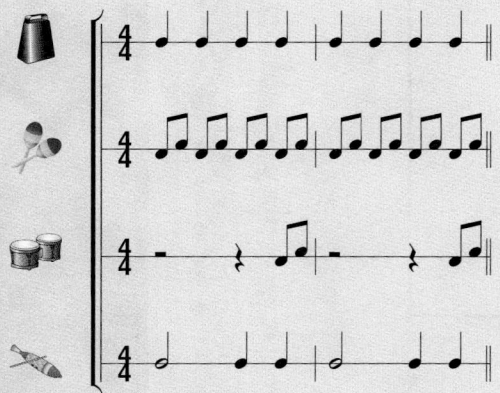

If you go to a wedding and dance, you can dance to many songs by saying to yourself, "long, short-short." The *rumba* is danced this way. **Move** your feet on each syllable, always alternating your feet. Here are the steps:

L	R L	R	L R	L	R L	R	L R
Long	short-short	Long	short-short	Long	short-short	Long	short-short

Unit 9   **333**

---

1 INTRODUCE

Select a volunteer to read the introductory paragraph on p. 332. Invite students to name additional Latin performers, past and present.

2 DEVELOP

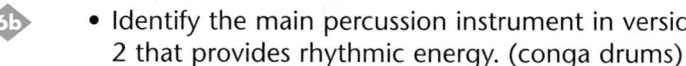

Listening

Play both versions of *Lluvia* **CD 17-1, CD 17-2**. See Spotlight On, p. 332, for information on the performer. Have students

6a
- Describe and compare, in general terms, the two arrangements.
- Lightly pat the rhythm pattern played by guitar in version 1. (Point out that, even without the presence of percussion instruments, rhythmic energy is provided by the guitar.)

6b
- Identify the main percussion instrument in version 2 that provides rhythmic energy. (conga drums)

Point out that, in version 2, rhythmic energy is also provided by the layering of different rhythm patterns.

Reading

5a Have students refer to the three rhythm patterns labeled a., b., c. at the top of p. 333 and

- Pat and count each pattern.
- Count each pattern while conducting meter in 4.
- Play each rhythm on a selected percussion instrument.

continued on page 334

CULTURAL CONNECTION

8b ▶ *Rumba* Often called the "dance of romance," the *rumba* started as an energetic African folk dance. About a hundred years ago, it migrated to Cuba. Becoming progressively slower, it has often been called a *son* by Cubans. In the hot climate of Cuba, people danced during the chorus and fanned themselves during the verses.

In the early twentieth century, the *rumba* traveled to the United States and other parts of the world with Cuban immigrants. The American *rumba* has very smooth steps. It is characterized by a "Cuban motion," a hip movement in which weight is transferred from foot to foot. This dance was established in the United States by Xavier Cugat and his orchestra.

SKILLS REINFORCEMENT

2c ▶ **Playing** Encourage students to add syncopated patterns to the percussion ensemble on this page.

Reinforcement Invite students to play a non-syncopated steady beat pattern (time line). Then, gradually introduce syncopated rhythms into the pattern.

On Target Invite students to play the following pattern.

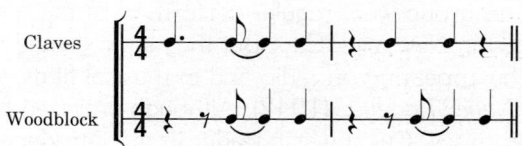

Challenge Invite students to improvise syncopated patterns.

Unit 9   *Be a Star!*   **333**

Playing

Play the recording of *(Chi Chi Chi) Cha Cha Cha* **CD 17-3** and ask students to focus on the rhythmic feel of the music. Then have students

- Choose one of the three rhythm patterns from the previous activity.

2c
- Perform their rhythm patterns with the recording.

Moving

9a Introduce students to the "long, short-short" rhythm pattern on p. 333, which is typical of many Latin styles of music and dance. Ask students to

- Pat the rhythm as an ostinato at a moderate tempo.
- Perform the *rumba* step pattern, as shown at the bottom of p. 333.

Following the same procedure, introduce students to the *cha-cha* rhythm and movement activity on this page.

8b Share background information with students on Latin culture as revealed through dance. (For the *cha-cha*, see Cultural Connection, p. 332; for the *rumba*, see Cultural Connection, p. 333; and for *salsa*, see Cultural Connection, p. 335.)

Playing

2c Help a group of students learn each of the patterns in the Latin rhythm score on p. 333. Have the group accompany the *rumba* and *cha-cha* movement activities.

Creating

Encourage students to create rhythmic phrases of their own to accompany Latin songs from the book, beginning with *"Mi tierra"* and *"Si tú no estás."* They should follow the example of the patterns in the Latin rhythm score on p. 333 and evaluate each other's decisions, offering suggestions for improvement if necessary.

A Popular Latin Dance

Many people dance socially. The *cha-cha* is a favorite type of Latin social dance. The *cha-cha* rhythm is a variation of the "long, short-short" rhythm. **Play** the *cha-cha* rhythm pattern below as you say "1-2, cha-cha-cha." Then **perform** the *cha-cha* movements to *(Chi Chi Chi) Cha Cha Cha*. When you are ready, **perform** the rhythm accompaniment on page 333 with the music.

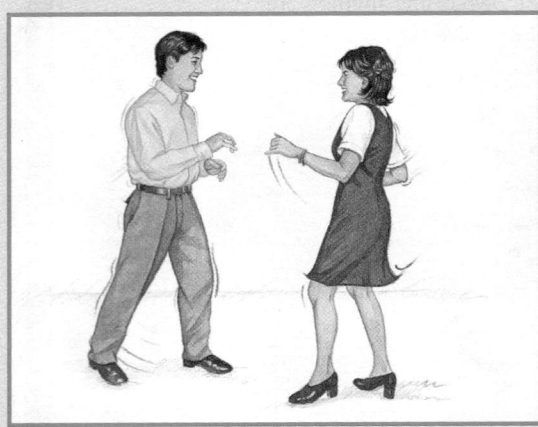

Cha-cha

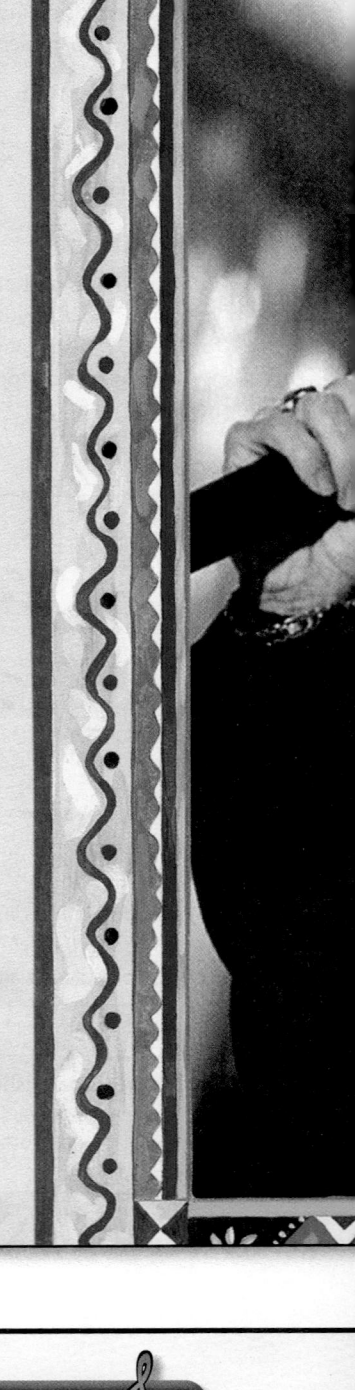

▲ Left-two, cha-cha-cha
Right-two, cha-cha-cha

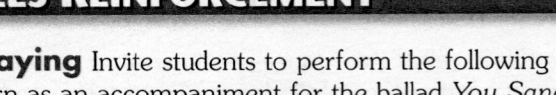

CD 17–3
(Chi Chi Chi) Cha Cha Cha

**by Marco Rizo and Kevin Morgan
as performed by Xavier Cugat and His Orchestra**

Xavier Cugat, known as "King of the Rumba," brought Spanish and Latin American dance rhythms to the United States. What dance rhythms can you identify in this piece?

334

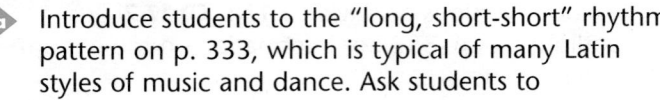

Footnotes

SPOTLIGHT ON

▶ **The Performer** Latin bandleader Xavier Cugat (1900–1990) was born in Spain (his full name was Francisco de Asis Javier Cugat Mingall de Bru y Deulofeo) and grew up in Cuba, where he trained as a classical violinist. His fame as a master of Latin dance music began in 1915 with the tango craze. By the 1930s, his band was known for its flaming red jackets and entertaining mix of novelty numbers and popular dance tunes. Cugat and his group were regular performers at the new Waldorf Astoria Hotel in New York City. But they soon gained nationwide popularity by appearing on radio and in musical films, such as *You Were Never Lovelier* (1942). Although criticized for his stylistic compromises, Cugat was a leader in the introduction of Latin music into America's mainstream musical culture.

SKILLS REINFORCEMENT

2c ▶ **Playing** Invite students to perform the following rhythm pattern as an accompaniment for the ballad *You Sang to Me* **CD 17-4.** Students may also wish to improvise their own rhythmic accompaniment to go with the selection.

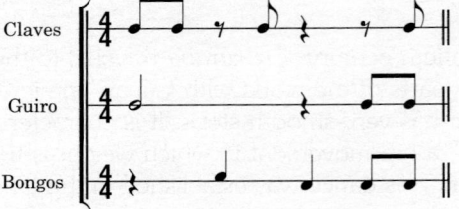

Claves

Guiro

Bongos

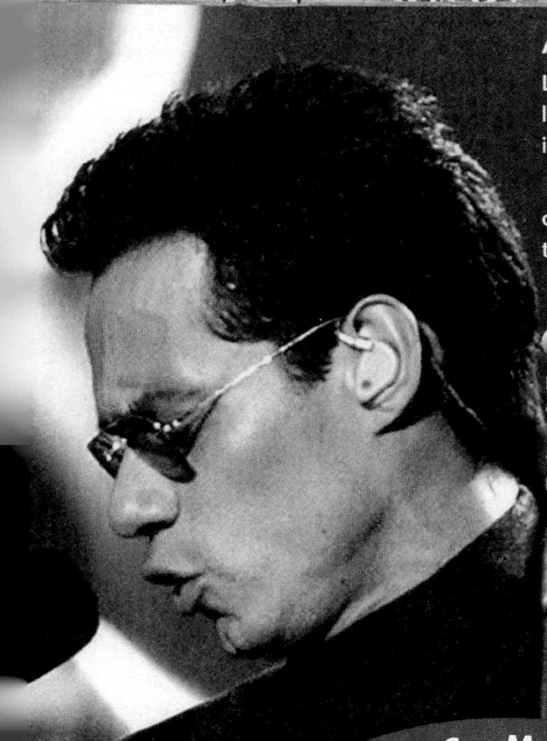

A Latin Ballad

Latin music also includes ballads and love songs in traditional Latin style and in new contemporary pop styles.

Listen to *You Sang to Me*, a contemporary Latin ballad, and notice the syncopation of the melody.

CD 17–4

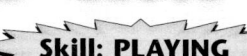
You Sang to Me

by Marc Anthony and Mark C. Rooney as performed by Sophia Salguero

You Sang to Me tells of love and emotions that are common themes in many Latin ballads and pop songs.

M·U·S·I·C M·A·K·E·R·S
Marc Anthony

Marc Anthony (born 1968) is one of today's biggest Latin pop stars. He first learned about music from his father, a Latino musician and composer, who encouraged Marc and his seven older brothers to sing and perform. When Anthony was a teenager, he began his career by writing club and dance music. A producer heard Marc's singing and invited him to make an entire album of Latino music. The album, *When the Night Is Over*, featured the work of several famous salsa musicians and marked the beginning of Anthony's interest in Latin and salsa music.

Anthony has performed with Latin salsa stars, including Tito Puente and Ruben Blades. Today, Anthony composes and performs in both the Latin salsa and contemporary pop styles.

Be a Star!

Unit 9 **335**

Listening

Discuss the information on Latin ballads. Have students read about pop star Marc Anthony in the Music Makers feature.

6b For an example of a contemporary Latin ballad, play the recording of *You Sang to Me* **CD 17-4.**

SAY Even though it is in a more relaxed style, this selection also uses rhythmic layering and syncopation to create a sense of energy and movement.

Ask volunteers to illustrate this point by patting or singing a portion of this melody in an even rhythm; that is, without syncopation.

Invite students to learn a rhythmic ostinato for three instruments that they can play as accompaniment for *You Sang to Me*. See Skills Reinforcement, p. 334.

3 CLOSE

Skill: PLAYING   ASSESSMENT

Performance/Self-Assessment Divide the class into groups of four students each, one for each instrument in the percussion ensemble on p. 333. Review the percussion ensemble score on p. 333 with students.

2c
7b When ready, have each group perform its part with the recording of *(Chi Chi Chi) Cha Cha Cha* **CD 17-3.** In follow-up discussion, ask each group to critique its own performance, using the following criteria, and offer suggestions for improvement.

- Rhythmic accuracy of individual percussion parts
- Coordination of ensemble playing
- Proper, stable tempo

Tell students that the class, at a school assembly or informal concert, could perform the percussion ensemble piece. Guide students to learn and demonstrate small–ensemble performance techniques during formal concerts.

CULTURAL CONNECTION

8b ▶ **Origins of *Salsa*** An ancestor of much of today's Latin pop styles is *salsa*. *Salsa* is a mixture of Caribbean rhythms with African and Latin influences. New York and Florida were the destinations of many Caribbean immigrants, mainly from Puerto Rico and Cuba. Longing for their Caribbean roots, they continued to make Afro-Caribbean music but adapted it to the metropolitan lifestyle. They mixed sounds from their homelands with North American jazz. Authentic *salsa* is spontaneous and intricate, and the dancing is lively. It can be quite slow or very fast, and the rhythm can change within the same song. During the 1970s, thanks to many outstanding performers from Cuba, Venezuela, Puerto Rico, and Panama, *salsa* spread throughout the entire world, becoming extremely popular among people from all walks of life.

SCHOOL TO HOME CONNECTION

▶ **Latin Influence** Ask students to listen to the types of Latin styles or performing artists their families and friends like. Students can also make note of locations in their neighborhood where they may hear Latin music played. Ask students to share their discoveries.

TECHNOLOGY/MEDIA LINK

4c **Web Site** Students may visit *www.sfsuccessnet.com* to learn more about Latin dance styles.

Unit 9 *Be a Star!* **335**

LESSON AT A GLANCE

Element Focus   **FORM** Verse-refrain form

Skill Objective   **SINGING** Sing a song in verse-refrain form with solo-chorus response

Connection Activity   **GENRE** Discuss choral music for young people's choirs

MATERIALS

- *"Oye"*   **CD 17-5**

  Recording Routine: Intro (5 m.); v. 1; refrain; interlude (8 m.); v. 2; refrain; refrain (in E); coda

- *Give Us Hope*   **CD 17-8**

- nonpitched percussion instruments

VOCABULARY

a cappella   homophonic texture   solo   chorus

◆ ◆ ◆ ◆ National Standards ◆ ◆ ◆ ◆

1a Sing accurately alone and in small ensembles
2a Play instruments accurately in small ensembles
6a Listen and describe events in music using appropriate terms
6b Listen and analyze uses of rhythm, timbre, and form in music from diverse genres
7b Students use specific criteria for evaluating their own performances.

MORE MUSIC CHOICES

For more practice with verse-refrain form and solo-chorus response:

"Free at Last," p. 468
"Water Come a Me Eye," p. 300

1 INTRODUCE

Ask students to list on the board the choirs in which they have sung and the places they have performed.

Tell students that in this lesson they will sing a song by Jim Papoulis, who writes music for young people.

Choirs on Stage

All over the world, young people sing in choirs and perform in classrooms, auditoriums, and concert halls.

Jim Papoulis composed "Oye" for the children of Acapulco, Mexico. **Identify** the chorus and solo parts in the refrain of the song. As you **sing**, take turns singing the solo part while the rest of the class sings the chorus.

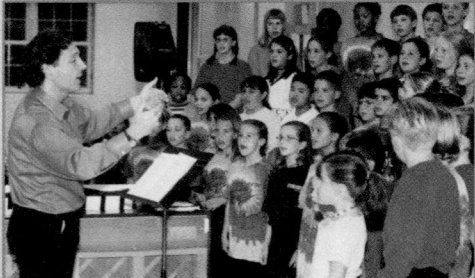

▲ Papoulis conducting a children's chorus

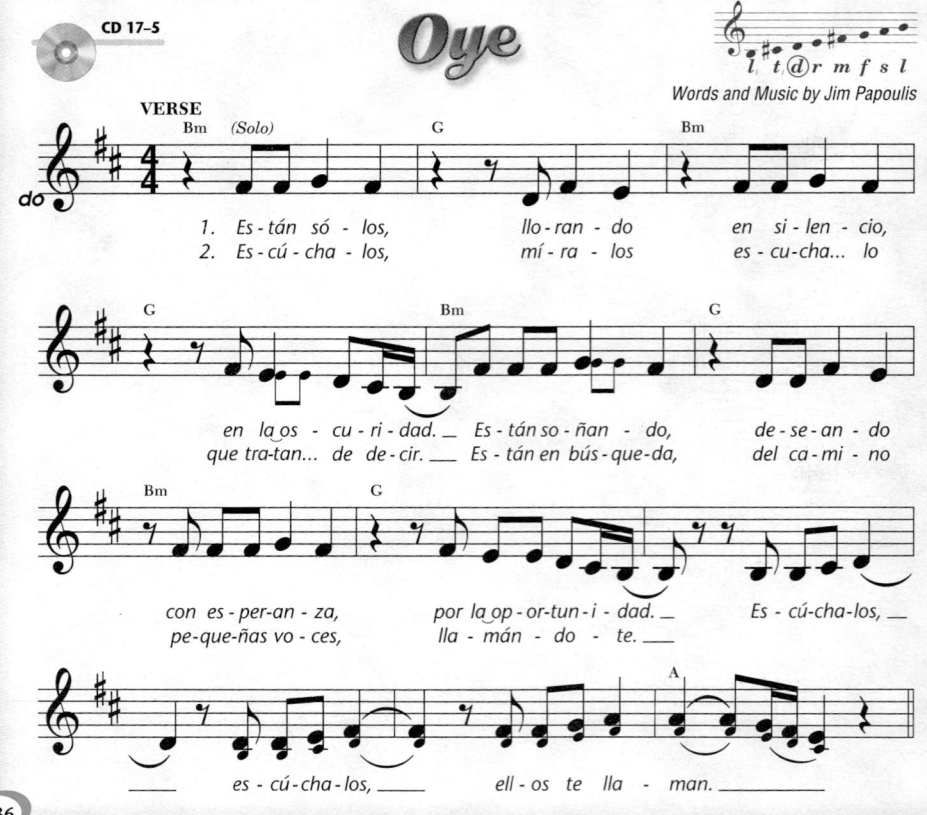

CD 17–5

Oye

Words and Music by Jim Papoulis

VERSE

1. Es-tán só-los,   llo-ran-do   en si-len-cio,
2. Es-cú-cha-los,   mí-ra-los   es-cu-cha... lo

en la os-cu-ri-dad. _ Es-tán so-ñan-do,   de-se-an-do
que tra-tan... de de-cir. ___ Es-tán en bús-que-da,   del ca-mi-no

con es-per-an-za,   por la op-or-tun-i-dad. _ Es-cú-cha-los, ___
pe-que-ñas vo-ces,   lla-mán-do-te. ___

___ es-cú-cha-los, _____   ell-os te lla-man. _____

336

Footnotes

ACROSS THE CURRICULUM

▶ **Social Studies** Acapulco, Mexico, is a beautiful city on Mexico's Pacific coast. It has long been a vacation headquarters for movie stars and tourists, with posh hotels and white-sand beaches. One of the city's most famous attractions is its cliff divers, or *le quebrada*. These athletes dive 136 feet into the Pacific Ocean from the top of rocky cliffs. They land in water that is just under ten feet deep, equal to the deep end of some swimming pools.

BUILDING SKILLS THROUGH MUSIC

▶ **Language** Share the information from Spotlight On. After reading the Music Maker on Jim Papoulis, p. 337, have students organize the information into outline form.

SPOTLIGHT ON

▶ **Young People's Chorus of New York City**
Members of this outstanding ensemble represent 150 different schools from every part of New York City. Students in this choir are between the ages of 12 and 17 years old. They must be willing to perform 30–40 times a year. They perform at top venues, including Carnegie Hall, and on television broadcasts in the United States and Mexico. The choir also performs on tours of Europe during summer vacation. The choir sings all types of music including pop, gospel, opera, folk, and other musical styles. Music education is an important part of each student's training while in the choir.

Director Francisco J. Nunez is an award-winning composer, conductor, and pianist.

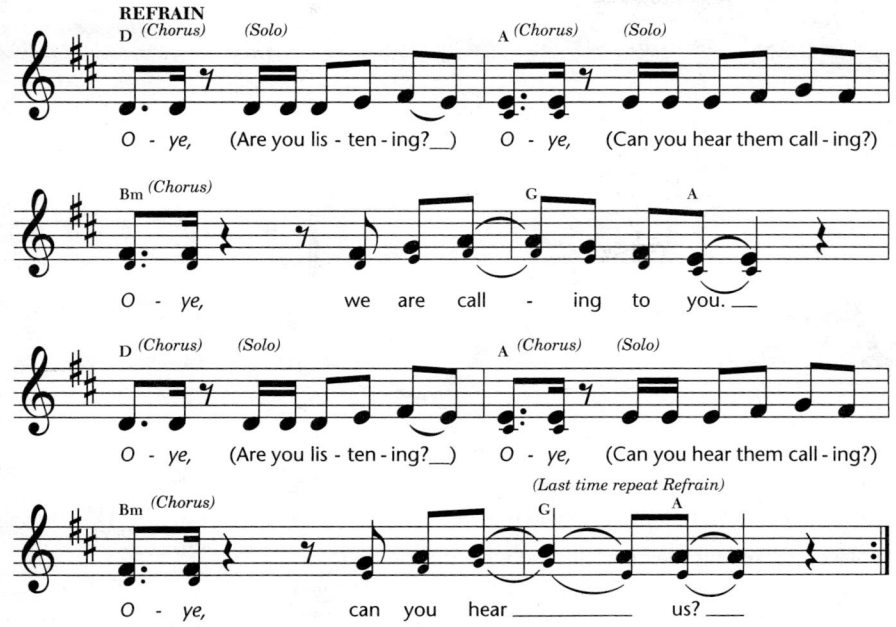

REFRAIN

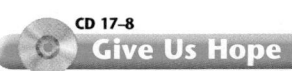

M·U·S·I·C M·A·K·E·R·S

Jim Papoulis

Composer **Jim Papoulis** (born 1957) enjoys writing music for young people. He conducts songwriting workshops for schools and he co-founded *The Foundation for Small Voices* to help children around the globe. His album, *Sounds of a Better World = Small Voices Calling* was premiered at Carnegie Hall and featured The Harlem Boy's Choir, the Norwegian Children's Choir, and the Young People's Chorus of New York. Papoulis hopes his music will inspire people to respect the young people in their care. Papoulis composes in many genres. He scored the music for the 1999 film, *Going Nomad*.

Listen to *Give Us Hope*. What is the message that Papoulis gives to young people with this song?

CD 17–8

Give Us Hope

by Jim Papoulis, Leo Schass, and Regine Urbach as performed by The Young People's Chorus of NYC

This choral performance features *a cappella* singing, homophonic texture, and rich vocal harmonies.

Unit 9 **337**

2 DEVELOP

Analyzing

6b Invite students to look at the song notation for *"Oye,"* on pp. 336–337. Ask them to analyze the form of the song (verse-refrain or AB form) and its texture (mostly monophonic in verse, homophonic in refrain).

Listening

Have students listen to the recording of *"Oye"* **CD 17-5.** Discuss the use of solo and chorus response.

Playing

2a Invite students to create a rhythm accompaniment using nonpitched percussion instruments for *"Oye."*

Singing

1a Invite the class to sing *"Oye,"* adding the percussion accompaniment as the class sings.

Listening

6a Invite students to listen to "Give Us Hope" **CD 17-8.**

Ask students to identify and describe the texture. (homophonic). Ask students what term means "unaccompanied singing" (a cappella).

3 CLOSE

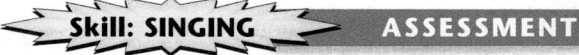

Skill: SINGING | **ASSESSMENT**

1a **Performance/Peer Critique** Ask students to sing
7b the solo parts in the verse and refrain as the class sings the song, paying attention to the verse-refrain form. Ask students to critique their performance, and if they accurately followed the form and solo-chorus responses.

SKILLS REINFORCEMENT

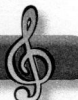

1a ▶ **Singing** Students may be able to better learn the two-part singing in *"Oye"* with mental guideposts found in the music. For example, where is a note coming from or going to? Guide students to sing in two parts using these tips.

- p. 336, bottom line—Low part repeats previous measure; both parts move up the scale.
- p. 337—Lines 1 and 3 are exactly the same.
- p. 337—Line 2 uses the same notes as the last 2 measures on p. 336.

TECHNOLOGY/MEDIA LINK

Sequencing Software Have students create a percussion accompaniment for *"Oye"* using sequencing software. Remind them that the song was written for children in Acapulco, Mexico, and they need to select appropriate Latin rhythm instruments (MIDI sounds) to give the accompaniment an authentic feel. Have students

- Map the correct number of measures for each section.
- Set the correct tempo for the accompaniment.
- Establish a MIDI track for each instrument.
- Create and then record each instrumental track.
- Play their accompaniment as the class sings the song.

LESSON AT A GLANCE

Element Focus — **MELODY** Melodic motive

Skill Objective — **SINGING** Sing an arrangement of a song containing melodic motives

Connection Activity — **SOCIAL STUDIES** Explore the Underground Railroad and the lives of Sojourner Truth and Harriet Tubman

MATERIALS

- "Run! Run! Hide!"   **CD 17-11**
  Recording Routine: Intro (4 m.); vocal
- *Changed My Name*   **CD 17-9**
- *Interview with Linda Twine*   **CD 17-10**
- pencils and paper

VOCABULARY

cantata	narration	triad	motive
crescendo	dynamics	accent	*staccato*

◆ ◆ ◆ ◆ National Standards ◆ ◆ ◆ ◆

1c Sing music from diverse genres
1d Sing music written in three parts
1e In groups, sing moderately easy pieces with expression
5a Read eighth notes, quarter notes, half notes, and rests in duple meter
5c Identify standard notation symbols for pitch and dynamics
6a Listen and describe events in music using appropriate terms
8b Identify ways music relates to social studies
9c Compare, in several cultures, functions music serves

MORE MUSIC CHOICES

For more experience with African American freedom songs:
"Ain't Gonna Let Nobody Turn Me 'Round," p. 85
"Free at Last," p. 468
"The Gospel Train," p. 398
"I Wish I Knew How It Would Feel to Be Free," p. 470

Sing a Special Arrangement

Linda Twine's **cantata** *Changed My Name* was inspired by the lives of Sojourner Truth and Harriet Tubman, who were active in helping to fight slavery in the 1800s.

Slaves worked for their masters and were sold among slaveowners as property. Eventually people began to speak out against this practice. Sojourner Truth (1797–1883), a former slave, was one of these people.

Slaves sometimes tried to escape to freedom. When escaped slaves were caught, they were returned to their owners. Eventually people began to organize routes for slaves to escape from the South to the North. These routes became known as the "Underground Railroad." One of the people involved in the Underground Railroad was Harriet Tubman (1821–1913). She helped more than 300 slaves make the journey to freedom.

A **cantata** (kahn-TAH-tuh) is a large dramatic work, sometimes of a religious nature, for choir and instruments. Many cantatas contain solo and chorus sections, with continuous narration (recitative).

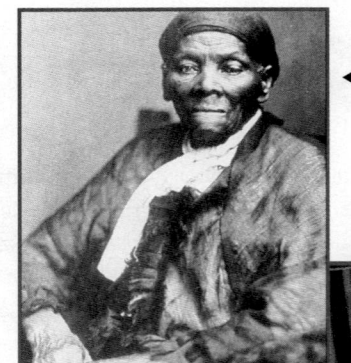
◀ Harriet Tubman

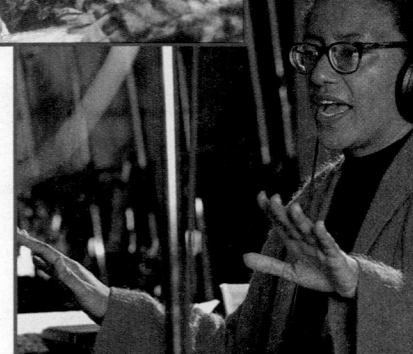
▼ Linda Twine

Listen to these recorded excerpts from *Changed My Name.*

 CD 17–9
Changed My Name

by Linda Twine
Changed My Name tells the story of the slaves and their fight for freedom through narration and singing.

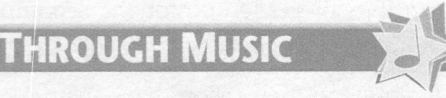 Footnotes

CULTURAL CONNECTION

9c ▶ **Secret Code** Because slaves were prohibited from congregating in groups and prohibited from talking to each other, they communicated by singing spirituals. The slave masters thought the slaves were singing about the Christian belief in a better life after death. Through the casual singing of these "religious" songs, slaves would pass on vital messages about escape plans and timing of the "run for freedom." One such song was "'Tis the Old Ship of Zion."

BUILDING SKILLS THROUGH MUSIC

▶ **Social Studies** Using facts from the lesson, have students identify and discuss the significance of Sojourner Truth and Harriet Tubman in the fight against slavery in the 1800s.

SPOTLIGHT ON

▶ **The Cantata** *Changed My Name,* by Linda Twine, is a cantata about Sojourner Truth and Harriet Tubman and how they helped enslaved people escape to freedom. Before the Civil War, slaves were the property of their masters. They were bought and sold at auctions. Many slaves were sold for the first time when they were children. Some never saw their families again. It was not uncommon for a slave to be sold five or more times during a lifetime. The slave's name changed after each sale.

The title of the cantata was taken from "I Told Jesus It Would Be Alright if He Changed My Name," a spiritual that, as expressed by Linda Twine, "suggests we can reshape our thinking, behavior and circumstance if we commit ourselves to do so. What we think affects how we act. How we act affects the treatment of our fellow man."

Escape to Freedom

Sing an arrangement of a song from *Changed My Name*—"Run! Run! Hide!" on page 340. Notice how the rhythms and the alternating text *run, run, hide* produce a type of excitement that describes a desperate attempt to escape from slavery.

Listen to Linda Twine talk about her music in this interview.

CD 17–10
Interview with Linda Twine

Linda Twine's skills as an arranger and a recording artist are also evident in the African American spiritual "This Little Light of Mine," on page 232.

Sojourner Truth with Abraham Lincoln ▶

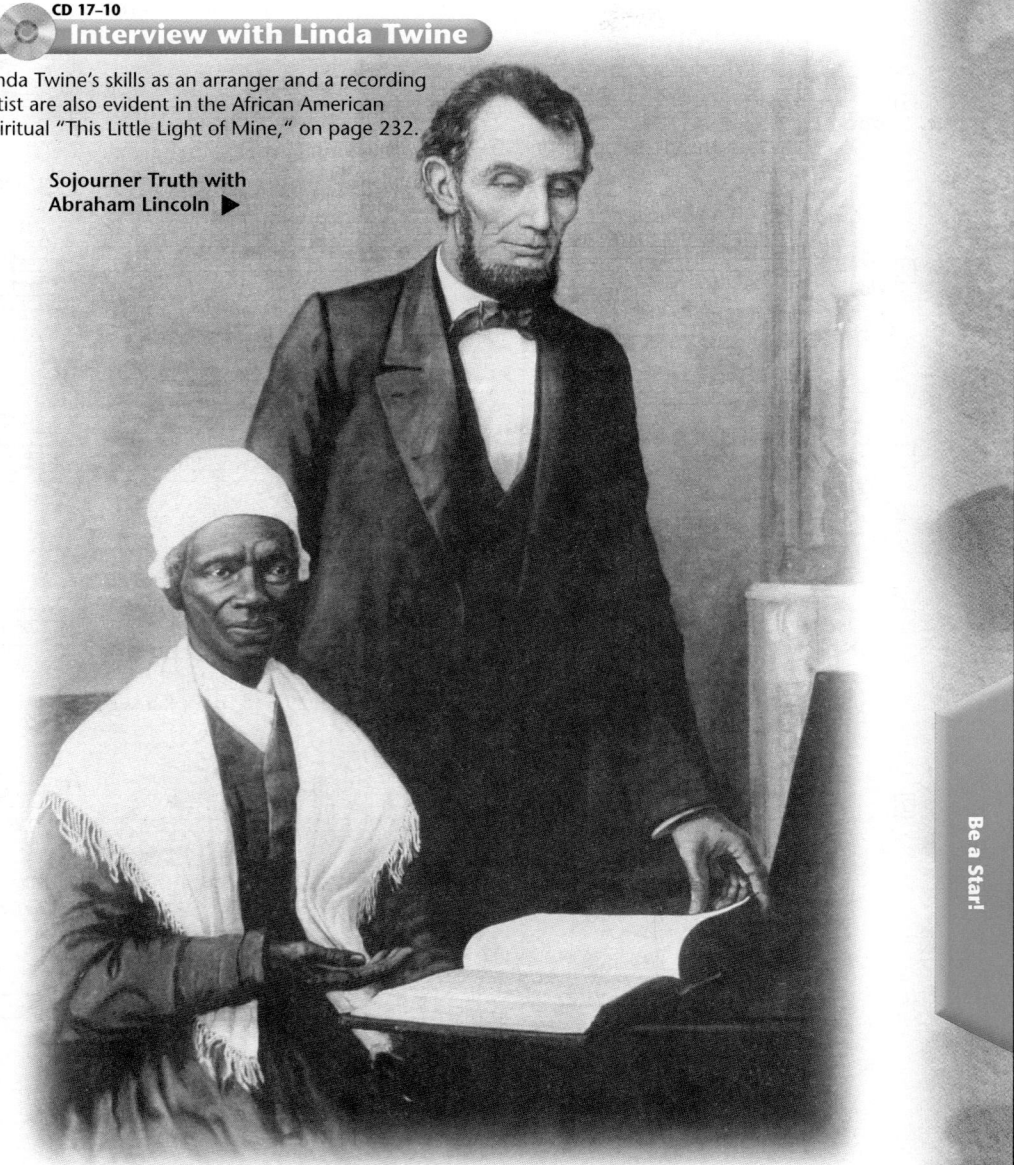

Be a Star!

Unit 9 **339**

1 INTRODUCE

Inform students that cantatas are

- Dramas that are sung by soloists, small groups of singers, and choirs.
- Performed on stage but without costumes and without acting.
- Based on either sacred or secular subject matter.

2 DEVELOP

Analyzing

8b Invite students to read the information on p. 338 about cantatas and about *Changed My Name,* a cantata inspired by spirituals and the lives of Sojourner Truth and Harriet Tubman.

Share with students information about Sojourner Truth, a former slave, and her mission against slavery, on p. 338. See also Spotlight On, p. 340.

9c Share with students information on the Underground Railroad and the use of spirituals with a hidden meaning to communicate coded information in Cultural Connection on p. 338.

Discuss the information on p. 338 about Harriet Tubman, especially her importance to the Underground Railroad. See also Spotlight On, p. 342.

ASK What is the special significance of the picture on p. 339? (Sojourner Truth's message was heard by many important people, including Abraham Lincoln, who was also against slavery. He was the person who could make the most difference on this issue. He is standing behind her in a supportive way in the picture.)

continued on page 340

SKILLS REINFORCEMENT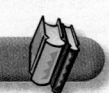

▶ **Creating** Students might enjoy organizing familiar material around a chosen theme to create their own cantata. Invite students to

- Select several songs from this book that share a common theme.
- Decide the order in which the songs should be performed.
- Write a narration to tie the songs together.
- Determine which songs should be performed by a soloist, which by a small group, and which by a chorus.
- Perform the cantata for their parents and friends.

ACROSS THE CURRICULUM

▶ **Social Studies** Encourage students to read the following books for more information about the Underground Railroad, Harriet Tubman, Sojourner Truth, the fight for the end of slavery, and the establishment of rights for women.

Harriet Tubman: Conductor on the Underground Railroad by Ann Petry (Harper Trophy, 1995) presents the story of the woman who helped hundreds of slaves escape to freedom.

Sojourner Truth (Black Americans of Achievement) by Peter Krass (Chelsea House, 1988) is about the life of an illiterate former slave who went on to become one of the most outspoken and articulate advocates for the abolition of slavery and establishment of women's rights.

Lesson 9 Continued

Listening

8b Invite students to listen to a condensed version of *Changed My Name* **CD 17-9.**

6a Help students discover that

- The songs are connected by a narration.
- The narrators represent Harriet Tubman and Sojourner Truth.
- Many of the songs are spirituals.

Invite students to listen to "Run! Run! Hide!" **CD 17-11** as they follow the music.

ASK **Why are the people running?** (They want to escape slavery, to get to freedom.)

Why are they hiding? (They don't want to be discovered and returned to their owner or sold to another slave master.)

What effect do the rhythms of the parts have? (They build energy and excitement and a feeling of urgency.)

Invite students to listen to and discuss the recorded interview with composer Linda Twine **CD 17-10.**

Playing

Tell students they can use this song to learn the skill of sight-reading simple music in treble clef and various meters. Divide the class into two groups.

Invite the first group to lightly clap the rhythms of Part 1 and the second group to lightly clap the rhythms of Part 2 as they listen to "Run! Run! Hide!"

5a Select some students to form a third group for Part 3, which enters at the top of p. 342 and ends on the first measure of p. 343.

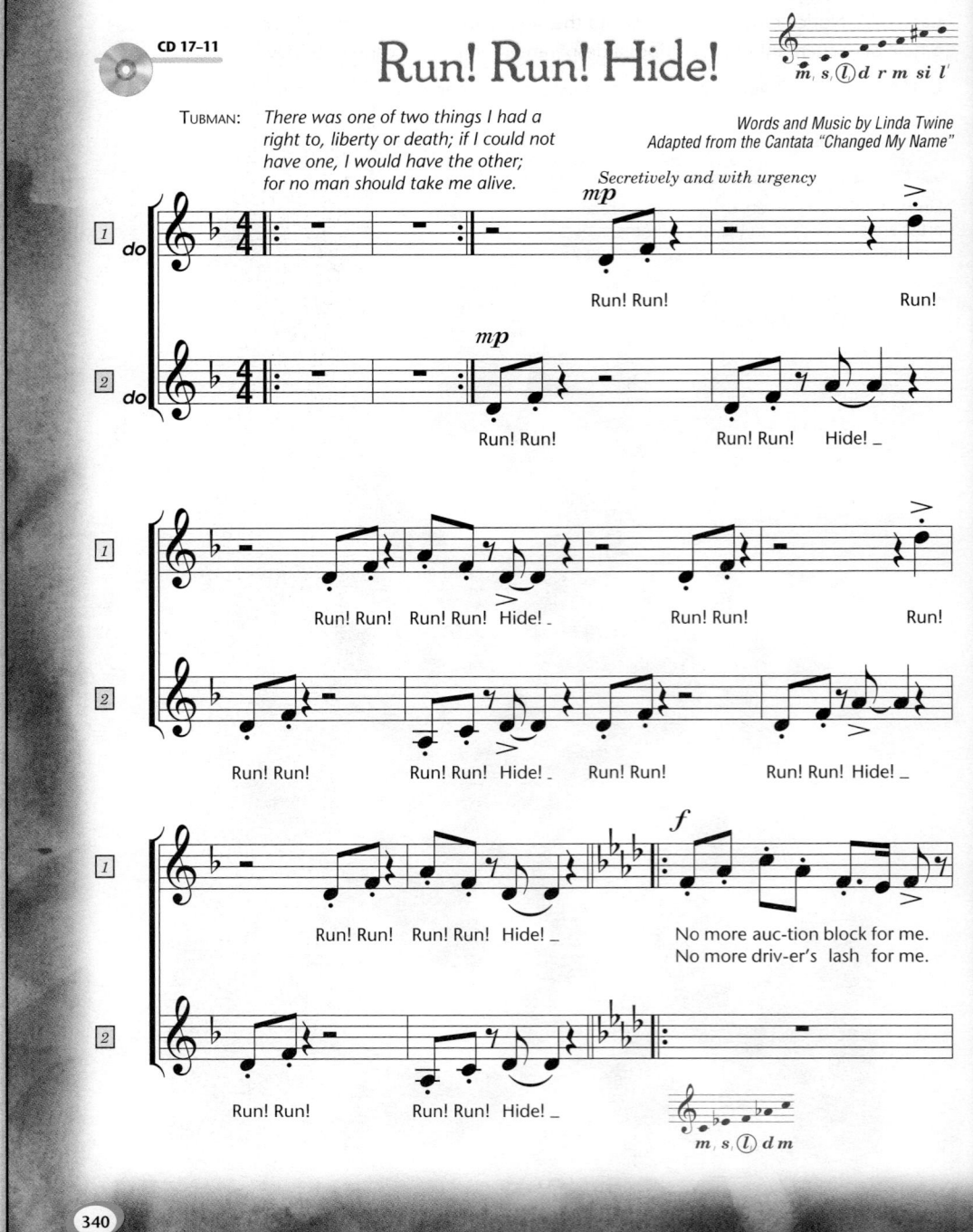

Footnotes

SPOTLIGHT ON

▶ **Sojourner Truth** A former slave, Sojourner Truth (1797–1883) believed no one should live in slavery. She became a preacher after she was released from slavery. She changed her name from Isabella to Sojourner Truth after gaining her freedom. Sojourner Truth worked tirelessly to end slavery and helped many slaves escape to freedom. She was an eloquent and witty speaker and one of the first black women to give speeches on women's rights.

ACROSS THE CURRICULUM

▶ **Social Studies** On September 22, 1862, President Lincoln stated in his famous Emancipation Proclamation that as of January 1, 1863, all slaves in the *territories in rebellion* against the North would be free. The Proclamation freed no slaves in the North or in the border states that were aligned with the North. It also did not free slaves in southern areas that were controlled by the North. It did, however, make clear that slavery was the issue for which the Civil War was fought.

Lincoln came to his position slowly. Originally a white supremacist, he viewed the war only as a means to preserving the Union. As the war continued, however, he became more aware of the plight of the slaves and more sympathetic to the abolition of slavery. The slaves were actually freed on December 18, 1865, with the passage of the Thirteenth Amendment to the Constitution.

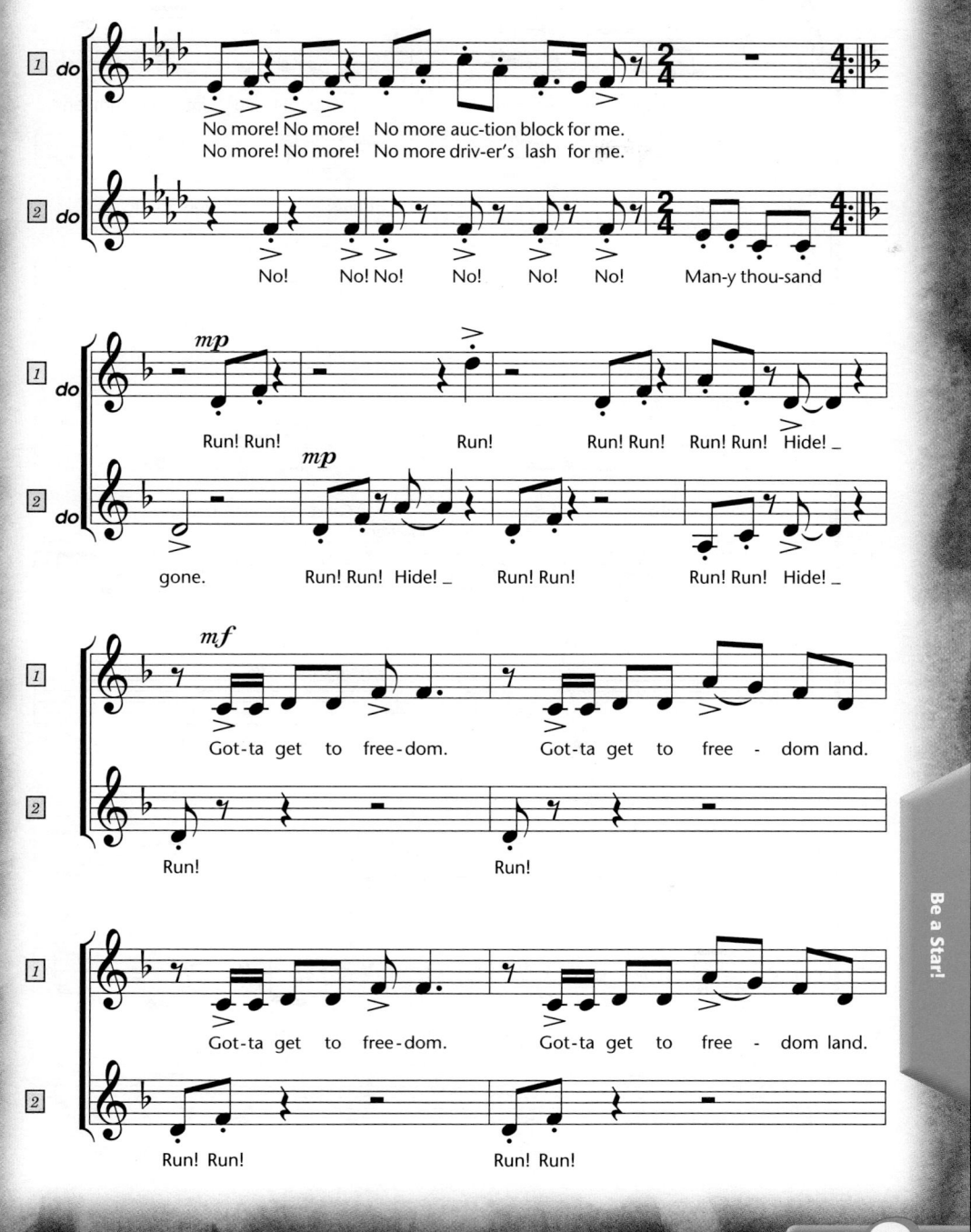

continued on page 342

Pose the following questions to each group, asking them to evaluate the quality of their music performances.

ASK Where in the song did you have difficulties? (Answers may include knowing when to come in, counting rests, following the repeat from p. 341 back to p. 340, and observing the meter change.)

What do you think would help you with this problem? (Answers may include counting the rhythm, watching the rests, clapping the song slower, placing a finger to mark the return for the repeat sign, and so on.)

Have students stay in their assembled groups and clap the rhythms with the recording again.

Singing

1c Invite students to sing their assigned part quietly with the recording of "Run! Run! Hide!" **CD 17-11**, using crisp **1d** diction.

Tell students that their goal, when performing a varied repertoire of music representing styles from diverse cultures, including American, is to perform expressively, from notation. Help students decide that

- The song should be performed energetically.
- The dynamic contrasts emphasize the change in mood of the text from furtive and anxious (quiet), to defiant (loud), to goal-oriented (medium growing to very loud at the end). Remind students that they need to identify music symbols referring to dynamics and to interpret them appropriately when performing.
- The alternating rhythm between the two parts adds energy and excitement.
- Good diction helps make the song move.
- Some notes are staccato; some are accented, or emphasized. Ask students to identify music symbols referring to articulation and to interpret them appropriately when performing.

Unit 9 **341**

CULTURAL CONNECTION

▶ **A Divided Country** The mid-nineteenth century economic culture of the American South, which was based on slave labor, caused whites in the southern states to fear abolition. Some white Southerners whose livelihood depended on slave labor feared their culture and lifestyle would change with abolition. When many antislavery states joined the Union, the South seceded, and civil war was declared.

During the Civil War there was also tension in muticultural New York City. Race riots came about because some members of various cultural groups in New York resented the fact that African Americans, like everyone else, were paid a good sum of money by the government to fight as soldiers in the Union Army. These African American soldiers had two motivations to fight: freedom from slavery and income.

MOVEMENT

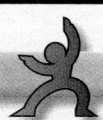

▶ **Creative Movement** When slaves ran away from their owners, they might have shown very different emotions. Some may have been bravely anticipating their life to come. Some may have been terrified. Others may have been wary, or reluctant to leave the only life they knew.

Divide the class into groups. Play the recording of "Run! Run! Hide!" **CD 17-11**. Have students portray, through movement, a particular emotion as they "run" to a "safe" location in the room. Ask them to use their whole bodies to dramatize how they feel when they finally reach "freedom." Bear in mind that this activity is not a game, but a serious portrayal of emotions.

Unit 9 *Be a Star!* **341**

Lesson 9 Continued

ASK In what key does the song start? (D minor)

How do you spell the D-minor triad? (D-F-A)

5c Ask students to identify where, in the first line of the song, the D-minor triad is spelled out. (the last measure in Part 2)

Point out to students that the minor triad is the main melodic motive throughout the song.

Performing

1e To prepare students to present a dramatic performance of "Run! Run! Hide!" **CD 17-11.**

- Choose volunteers to speak the dialogue of Harriet Tubman.

- Encourage students to observe the dynamics found in the song, as well as the gradual crescendo in the middle of p. 342.

- Remind students to use articulation and dynamics to express the urgency and intensity of the setting when they perform the song.

Audience Etiquette

As students prepare for a formal concert performance, they will be interested in learning proper etiquette for how to act and perform during rehearsals (see p. 282) and during a concert (see pp. 319, 46, and 259).

Share this information with students and guide them to discover appropriate behavior.

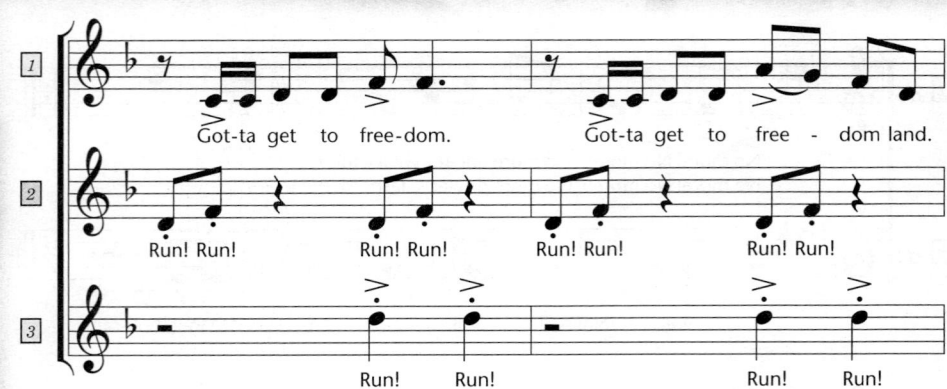

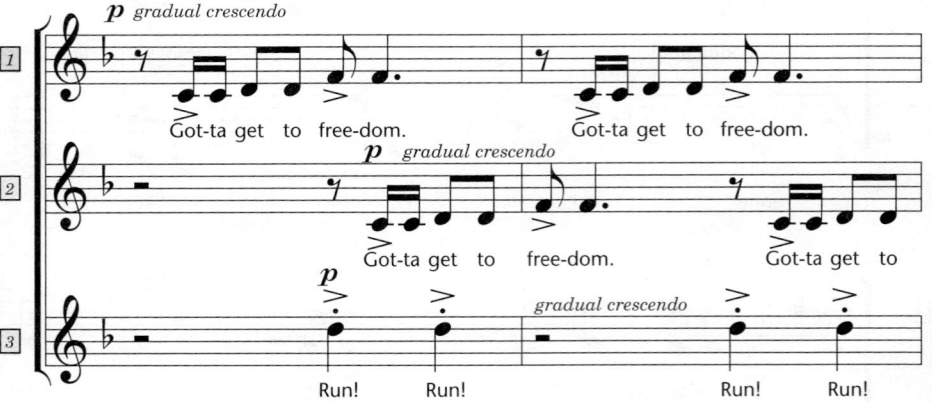

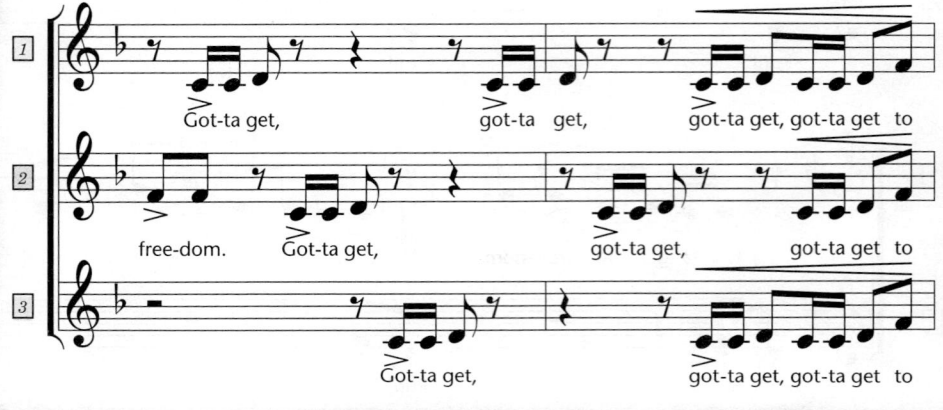

342

Footnotes

SPOTLIGHT ON

▶ **Harriet Tubman** This amazing woman was called the Moses of her people because she helped so many slaves flee from the hardship of slavery. A former slave, Harriet Tubman (1821–1913) made 19 dangerous journeys to the "promised land" (the North and Canada), helping more than 300 slaves reach freedom. Tubman was affectionately known as "The General" because of her organizational and tactical abilities.

AUDIENCE ETIQUETTE

▶ **Educating the Audience** Students will be anxious to learn proper etiquette for themselves as performers, and for their peers and family as the audience. See Audience Etiquette in the side column above for tips on how to develop these skills.

SKILLS REINFORCEMENT

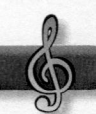

▶ **Recorder** Students can play the parts of "Run! Run! Hide!" on their recorders to support the singing of the song. (They just change the low A, which is out of range, to a middle C. Have students rest during the top system of p. 341.) This song will help students practice staccato and accented articulation, as well as the lower and upper ranges of the instrument.

Because sixteenth notes may be too difficult for students to articulate, students may wish to use an eighth note to replace each sixteenth-note pair in any of the three parts.

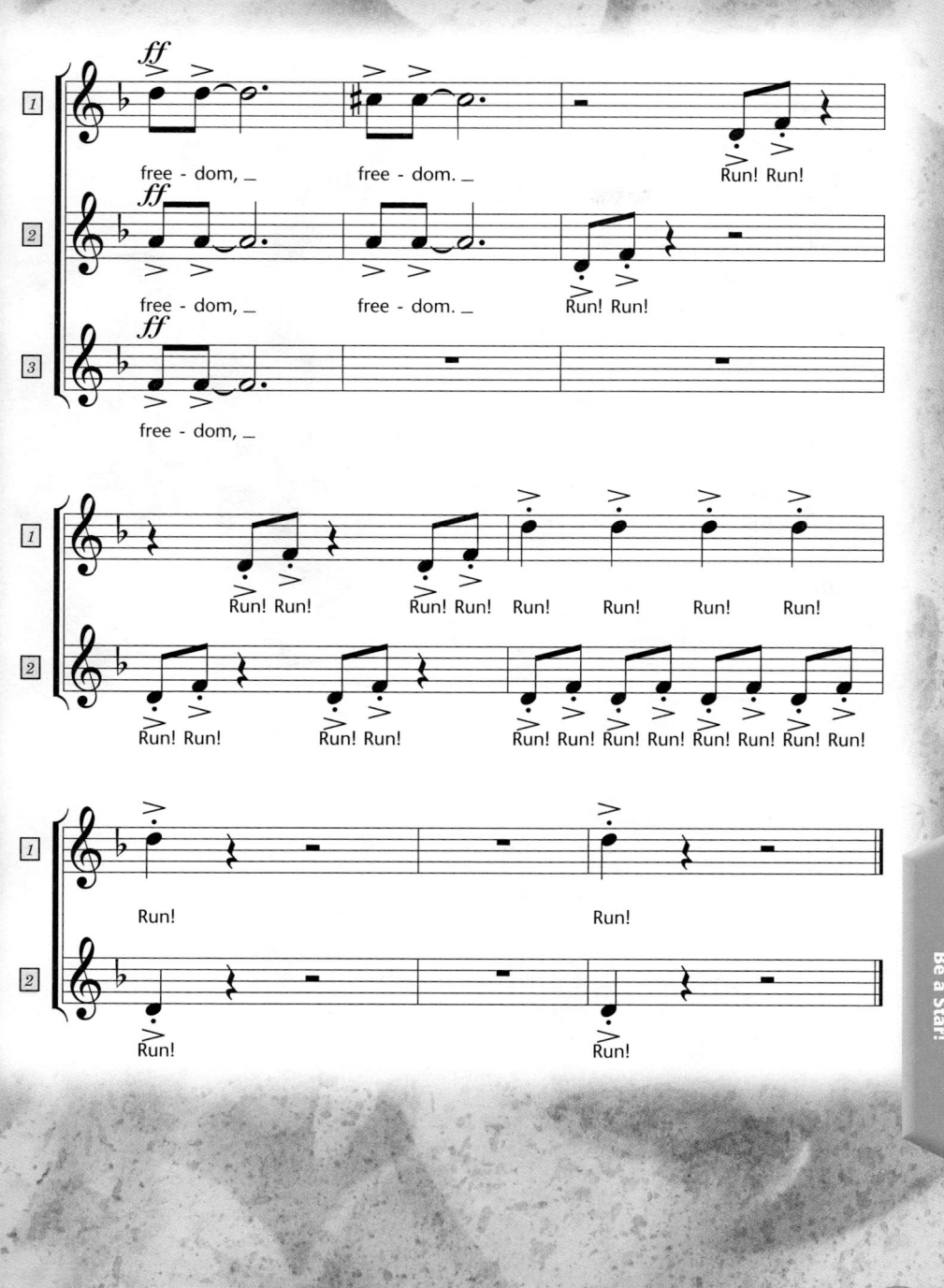

The performance of this dramatic piece within the context of a larger formal concert (such as Black History Month) sets the stage for developing a set of guidelines for the audience (friends, peers, and parents) that they can use as well when attending concerts. The following "audience etiquette" guidelines can be printed in the school newspaper or in the concert program. Encourage students to develop guidelines in the spirit of providing the best performance opportunity for themselves and other student musicians. Suggestions to the audience may include

- Be punctual for the concert.
- Turn all pagers, cell phones, and other electronic equipment to the silent mode.
- No flash photography while students are performing.
- If video cameras are allowed, do not place them in the aisles or between seats. Do not bock the view of other audience members.
- Hold applause until the end of a selection.
- Do not bring food or drinks to the concert.

3 CLOSE

Element: MELODY ASSESSMENT

Music Journal Writing Have students sing "Run! Run! Hide!" Then have them write the answers to the following questions in their journals. Students may refer to their books to answer the questions.

- What is the name of the minor triad in "Run! Run! Hide!" that serves as the main melodic motive? (D minor)
- How is this triad spelled? (D-F-A)
- On what word do all three parts sing the complete triad at the same time? (*freedom;* measure 1 on this page)

CULTURAL CONNECTION

▶ **Songs of the Civil War** There were many songs sung by soldiers on both sides in the Civil War. "Battle Hymn of the Republic," written by Julia Ward Howe, was sung by the Union soldiers. The Confederate soldiers sang "When Johnny Comes Marching Home" as they traveled.

CHARACTER EDUCATION

▶ **Courage** What characteristics might be possessed by a person who is escaping from slavery and a person who is helping slaves seek freedom (courage, commitment to freedom, knowledge of what is right and wrong)? Explore the conflicting emotions felt by slaves (excitement about freedom, apprehension, reluctance to leave, fear, bravery). Allow students to discuss situations in which they have felt conflicting emotions.

SCHOOL TO HOME CONNECTION

▶ **Causes** Ask students to find out the names of people who fight for important rights and causes in today's world. What are some of the organizations that advocate and fight for civil rights, world hunger, children's rights, animal rights, protection of the environment, and other important causes? Have students ask their families and friends about causes that are important to them.

TECHNOLOGY/MEDIA LINK

Sequencing Software Use a digital audio program to record students singing "Run! Run! Hide!" Play the track for students' self-evaluation.

LESSON AT A GLANCE

Element Focus — **EXPRESSION** Combining musical elements for dramatic effect

Skill Objective — **CREATING** Create a film scene and choose music to help express the drama in the scene

Connection Activity — **LANGUAGE ARTS** Explore the written and the spoken word as used in screenplays

MATERIALS

• *Yours Forever*	CD 17-13
• *Coming Home from the Sea I* (excerpt)	CD 17-14
• *Coming Home from the Sea II* (excerpt)	CD 17-15
• *One Fine Day*	CD 17-16
• *Jungle Beat*	CD 17-17
• *Illusions*	CD 17-18

• keyboard or other melodic instrument

• music journals, VCR and monitor, videotape and video-taping equipment, DV camcorder and computer video editing software (optional)

VOCABULARY

motive	soundtrack	screenplay
expressive qualities	score	

◆ ◆ ◆ ◆ National Standards ◆ ◆ ◆ ◆

5a Read eighth notes, sixteenth notes, half notes in duple meter

6a Listen and describe events in music using appropriate terms

6c Understand and use basic principles of intervals in music analysis

7b Students use specific criteria for evaluating their own performances

9a Describe characteristics of music genres from a variety of cultures

9c Compare, in several cultures, functions music serves

MORE MUSIC CHOICES

For more experience with music from the movies:

"A Brand New Day," p. 7

"Don't Cry for Me, Argentina," p. 74

Music in the Movies

Music plays an important role in motion pictures. It heightens the drama and emotion of the film. Filmmakers hire composers to write music to enhance the emotional message of the film. Many songs written for movies become popular hits.

The Perfect Storm is a film based on a true story. Six men sailed into the north Atlantic Ocean aboard the "Andrea Gail" on a fishing expedition. While at sea, the men encountered the worst storm in modern history. The men and their boat were lost at sea in October, 1991.

Listen to *Yours Forever*, the theme song from *The Perfect Storm*. How many times does the composer use this motive, based on the interval of a fifth?

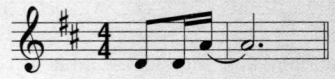

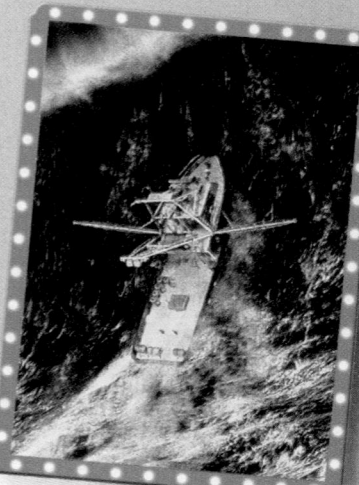

▲ Movie poster from the film *The Perfect Storm*

CD 17–13
Yours Forever

by James Horner, John Mellencamp, and George Green as performed by John Mellencamp

Motives based on the intervals of fourths and fifths are also found in the film music written by James Horner.

Tune In

Early movies had no sound. A pianist or organist performed music live in the theater as the film was projected on the screen. The first motion pictures with sound were called "talkies."

Footnotes

SPOTLIGHT ON

▶ **Music and Film** Encourage interested students to research the focus of this lesson in more depth and report to the class. Possible report topics include film composers (such as Max Steiner, Alfred Newman, Miklós Rózsa, Bernard Herrmann, John Williams, Rachel Portman, John Barry, Nino Rota, Elmer Bernstein, and Danny Elfman) and classical composers who wrote for film (such as Aaron Copland, Leonard Bernstein, Sergei Prokofiev, and Virgil Thomson).

BUILDING SKILLS THROUGH MUSIC

▶ **Theater** Ask students to write a plan for music they would compose for *The Perfect Storm,* visualizing a scene when the storm is just beginning. They should include the instruments they would use and some description of the expressive elements of their music.

ACROSS THE CURRICULUM

▶ **Science** In October 1991, the *Andrea Gail,* a fishing vessel, and a six-man crew set sail from Gloucester, Massachusetts, for the fishing grounds of the North Atlantic Ocean. After catching a large quantity of fish, the men headed home, encountering winds of 120 miles per hour, with waves as high as a ten-story building. Neither the men nor their ship survived this "storm of the century." The movie *The Perfect Storm* depicts their struggle.

Discuss with students ways to locate information on the biggest storms of the past 100 years. Create a list of possible resources to research (for example, Internet, weather books, local TV weather reporters, university science departments) and encourage students to learn about storm formation, measurement, tracking, and property and other damage.

Movie Soundtracks Create Mood

Movie music, called "the soundtrack," helps to create the atmosphere and mood of the scenes that you see on the screen. Imagine watching a movie with no soundtrack, sound effects, or music. How would their absence affect the movie?

Listen to these excerpts from the soundtrack of *The Perfect Storm*. Decide how the composer uses tempo, rhythm, and dynamics to create the expressive qualities of the music.

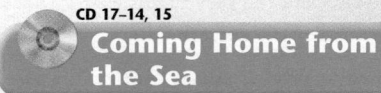

CD 17–14, 15

Coming Home from the Sea

from *The Perfect Storm*
by James Horner

The opening haunting melody can be heard throughout the movie. The second theme is quick, rhythmic, and adds excitement to the action on the screen.

Directing Your Own Movie

Imagine that you are a very famous film director and have received a screenplay from a writer. Your job is to create a video from this script.

Read the screenplay on page 346 and choose an actor to play each part. Discuss scenery and props that would enhance your video. Rehearse the scene and direct your actors to give great performances. When you are ready, record the scene with a videotape camera. View the video and evaluate the performance.

Congratulations! You have directed another hit video.

Video Library Watch the video *Alligator Scene* to see how different musical styles affect the character of a video.

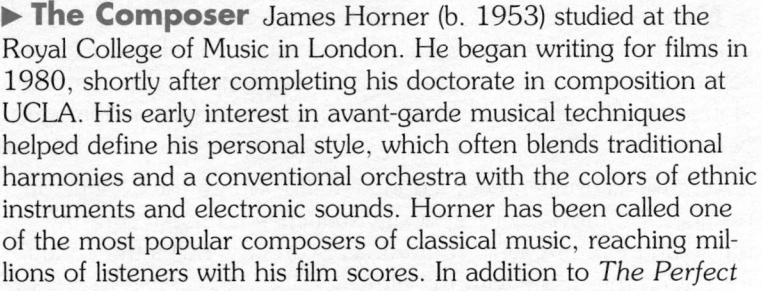

Be a Star!

Unit 9 **345**

---

1 INTRODUCE

Encourage students to read about film music and about *The Perfect Storm*, on p. 344. See also Across the Curriculum, p. 344, and Spotlight On, p. 346.

2 DEVELOP

Listening

6c Play the recording of *Yours Forever* **CD 17-13**. Help students discover that the opening three notes of the song are repeated many times throughout the selection.

ASK What do we call these three notes? (a motive)

5a Play the motive on a keyboard or other melody instrument, pointing out that it is based on the interval of a fifth. Invite keyboard players in class to demonstrate this motive in different keys and octaves as students refer to the notation on p. 344.

Play *Yours Forever* again and have students raise their hands and sing each time they hear the motive.

Invite students to listen to *Coming Home from the Sea, I and II*, **CD 17-14, 17-15**, more soundtrack excerpts from *The Perfect Storm*. Have them raise their hands when the mood of the music changes.

6a **ASK How did the composer change the mood?** (The tempo became faster and the dynamics became louder.)

Did the change in dynamics and tempo add more or less suspense or excitement? (more)

Was the music similar to, or different from, the theme song? (It was similar to the song.)

6a Play the recording again and ask students to raise their hands each time they hear material from the theme song.

For information on the composer, James Horner, see Spotlight On below.

continued on page 346

SPOTLIGHT ON

▶ **The Composer** James Horner (b. 1953) studied at the Royal College of Music in London. He began writing for films in 1980, shortly after completing his doctorate in composition at UCLA. His early interest in avant-garde musical techniques helped define his personal style, which often blends traditional harmonies and a conventional orchestra with the colors of ethnic instruments and electronic sounds. Horner has been called one of the most popular composers of classical music, reaching millions of listeners with his film scores. In addition to *The Perfect Storm*, his scores include *An American Tale*, *Glory*, *Braveheart*, *Titanic*, and *How the Grinch Stole Christmas*.

▶ **The Performer** See pp. 2–5 ("Your Life Is Now") for information on songwriter and performer John Mellencamp.

SKILLS REINFORCEMENT

▶ **Creating** As your students prepare to create their own film, suggest that they employ a technique commonly used in film-making. Share with them that movies consist of many different scenes. Filmmakers usually shoot, or film, these scenes one at a time. However, they do not start at the beginning of the story and continue to the end. Instead, they shoot all the scenes that happen in a given location at one time, before they move on to the next location. Later the filmmaker uses a process called editing to put the scenes in the required sequence to tell the story. After the filmmaker completes the editing, the composer scores the soundtrack. (See Spotlight On, p. 346.)

Creating

Explain to students that the written and spoken words used in screenplays drive all of the other elements in a movie: scenery and props, characters, costumes, mood, action, sound effects, and music to name a few.

Invite students to make a video of the screenplay scenario on pp. 346–347. After students read the screenplay carefully, have them answer these questions.

- Who will be the actors and what part will each actor play?

- Who will be the director and tell the actors what to do and when?

- Who will design and create the background?

- Who will be responsible for special sound effects if sound effects are needed?

- Who will decide what props are needed (green stones and other objects) and be responsible for collecting or making them?

- Who will be the camera person to videotape the scene?

Allow students to plan the scene and rehearse it a few times, then videotape their performance.

 After students are satisfied with their videotape, have them listen to the three different soundtracks composed to accompany their film **CD 17-16, CD 17-17, CD 17-18.** Lead a discussion of the musical and dramatic qualities of each soundtrack, evaluating the effectiveness of the music.

Ask students to decide which soundtrack best fits their performance. See Skills Reinforcement, p. 345, and Spotlight On below for more ideas and information on shooting scenes and how a soundtrack is made.

Screenplay

Beach Scene: A group of students are at a beach playing tug-of-war. One of the students calls attention to a shining stone, and the game stops. Everyone examines the stone. Soon more stones are found, one after another. The students decide to follow the trail created by the stones, which leads to a great cavern with a beautiful pool of water at the bottom. The students look away for a moment; but when they look back, there is a pirate ship in the pool. They whisper in awe. Again they look away for a moment. When they look back, the pirate ship has vanished! Did they really see it? They believe they did, and they make a pact to keep it a secret!

Dialogue: GROUPS OF STUDENTS ARE PLAYING TUG-OF-WAR WHEN SUDDENLY THE GAME HALTS.

Student 1: Hey, you guys! Look at this!
Several students: What? Where?
Student 1: Look at that shiny thing on the ground.

EVERYONE DROPS THE ROPE AND RUNS TO SEE THE DISCOVERY

Student 2: That's the brightest green stone I've ever seen!
Student 3: Look! There's another one!

SOON EVERYONE IS FINDING THESE BRILLIANT STONES

Student 4: It's a trail! Let's follow it!
All students: Maybe it leads to a buried treasure!

EXCITEDLY, THEY ALL HEAD OFF TO FOLLOW THE TRAIL.

Student 5: Whoa! Watch out—it's a cavern!
Student 6: Look way down there! It's a huge pool of water!

THEY LOOK AWAY AND MURMUR AMONG THEMSELVES

Student 8: (LOOKING BACK AT THE CAVERN) It's a pirate ship! A real pirate ship!
Student 9: Hey, isn't that the captain?
Student 10: Captain Hook!
Student 11: Aren't ships supposed to be really huge? This thing is puny!
Student 12: You're right! That's a really small ship!

346

Footnotes

SKILLS REINFORCEMENT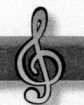

▶ **Listening** To illustrate how closely soundtracks are associated with the movies for which they were created, play the game Guess That Movie Soundtrack. Organize students into two or more teams. Have volunteers bring movie soundtracks from home or use your own. Blocking students' views of the recording, let teams collect points by identifying the associated movie from hearing excerpts played.

SPOTLIGHT ON

▶ **Movie Soundtracks** After a movie is edited, the composer writes music for the film. Although the music, or film score, has several purposes, its main functions are to heighten the emotional impact of the film and to fill empty spaces where no dialogue occurs.

The music is usually recorded in a studio, where the conductor watches the movie, with special visual cues, to make sure the music and film are synchronized. This process helps the conductor match the music with the film.

THE GROUP LOOKS AWAY FOR A MOMENT TO DISCUSS.

Student 13: Hey, you guys! It's *gone!*

THE GROUP MOANS IN DISAPPOINTMENT

Student 14: OK, we cracked! It just wasn't there! We didn't really see it.

Student 1: No, it was there! I know we saw it!

Student 15: Yeah, that's cool! We all know we saw it!

Student 16: Nobody is going to believe us, though.

Student 1: So we don't tell anyone—deal? This stays with us!

THE STUDENTS CHATTER AMONG THEMSELVES AGAIN, AND THEY AGREE TO KEEP THIS A SECRET.

Adding Music to Your Movie

Your movie has been filmed and has spoken dialogue. To add more drama to the film, you need to add a musical score to the film. Here are three different orchestral soundtracks to accompany your film. **Listen** to each soundtrack and decide which one best fits your film.

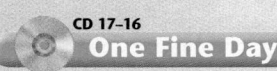
CD 17–16
One Fine Day

by Edward Pearsall

This orchestral arrangement features string and woodwind melody lines over strings.

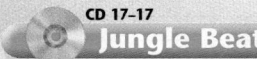
CD 17–17
Jungle Beat

by Edward Pearsall

A jungle-like rhythm is the backdrop for unusual chords and mysterious melodic figures.

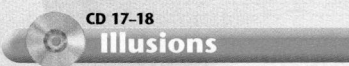
CD 17–18
Illusions

by Edward Pearsall

This string orchestra piece has a melodic **A** section and a rhythmic **B** section.

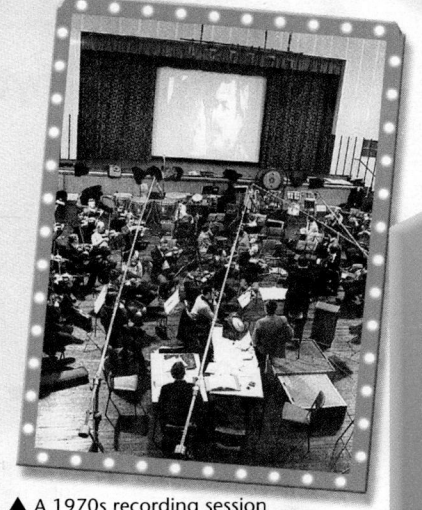

▲ A 1970s recording session for a Bernard Herrmann film score

Be a Star!

---

3 CLOSE

7b **Music Journal Writing** Encourage students to

- View their production while listening to the chosen soundtrack.

- Write a critique of their production (including a discussion of the musical elements of the chosen soundtrack that enhance expression of the action in the production), to be added to their music journals.

ACROSS THE CURRICULUM

9c ▶ **Social Studies** Students might like to know about some of the career possibilities in filmmaking. Some of these careers require sensitivity to sound and to music, skills that are gained through music study.

People have filmmaking careers as actors, producers, directors, composers, stunt people, sound engineers, designers, camera operators, wardrobe people, makeup artists, and special effects experts.

TECHNOLOGY/MEDIA LINK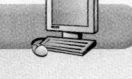

Multimedia Invite students to create their own movie by using a DV camcorder and a video editing program. Have students

- Write a scene, choose actors, and rehearse them.

- Shoot the video using a DV camcorder, and then download the "shoot" in short "clips" to your movie editing software.

- Using the software, edit the video clips into one scene for the movie. Add titles, transitions (just a couple), and narration.

- Challenge students to create a music soundtrack for the scene using sequencing software. Then, import the audio file into the movie. Play it for the class.

LESSON AT A GLANCE

Element Focus **EXPRESSION** Expressive elements in Latin music

Skill Objective **SINGING** Perform a Latin pop song with expression

Connection Activity **GENRE** Discuss music videos and Latin pop

MATERIALS

- "The Rhythm Is Gonna Get You" **CD 17-19**
  Recording Routine: Intro (6 m.); v. 1; refrain; v. 2; refrain; coda
- video camera, blank videotape, VCR, monitor
- cowbell, conga drums, bongo drums, maracas

VOCABULARY

lyrics   syncopation   *salsa*   Latin pop

◆ ◆ ◆ National Standards ◆ ◆ ◆

1c Sing music from diverse genres
2c Perform instrumental music from diverse genres
6b Listen and analyze uses of rhythm in music from diverse genres

MORE MUSIC CHOICES

For more practice playing rhythm accompaniments: "*Má Teodora*," p. 301

1 INTRODUCE

Explain to students that music videos became popular in the 1980s with the appearance of MTV. Many popular artists, including Gloria Estefan, make music videos when they release a new CD.

Have students read the information about Gloria Estefan, Latin pop music, and music videos. Share with students information on Latin pop music in Cultural Connection below, and information on music videos in Spotlight On, p. 349.

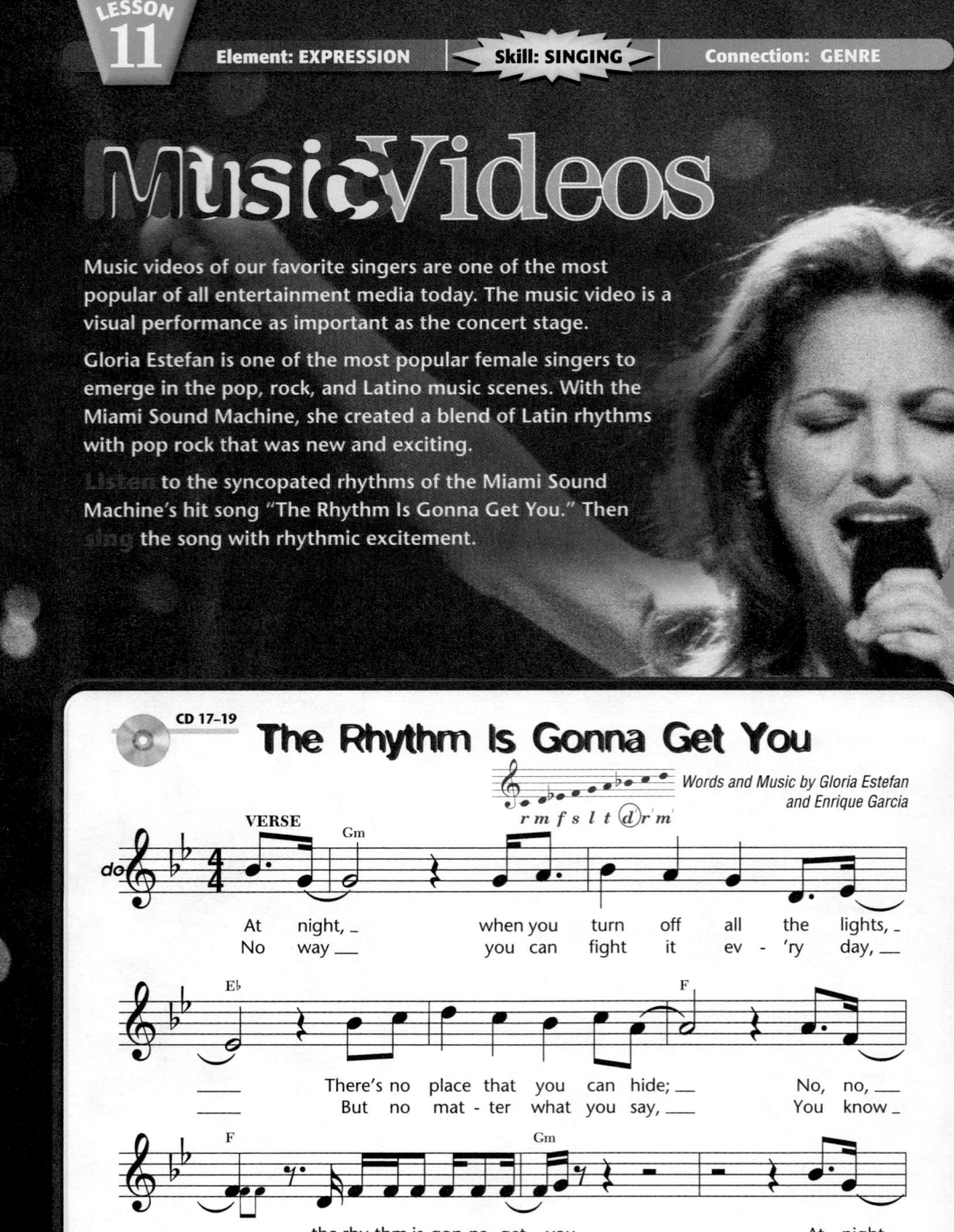

Music Videos

Music videos of our favorite singers are one of the most popular of all entertainment media today. The music video is a visual performance as important as the concert stage.

Gloria Estefan is one of the most popular female singers to emerge in the pop, rock, and Latino music scenes. With the Miami Sound Machine, she created a blend of Latin rhythms with pop rock that was new and exciting.

Listen to the syncopated rhythms of the Miami Sound Machine's hit song "The Rhythm Is Gonna Get You." Then **sing** the song with rhythmic excitement.

CD 17–19
The Rhythm Is Gonna Get You

Words and Music by Gloria Estefan and Enrique Garcia

VERSE

At night, _ when you turn off all the lights, _
No way __ you can fight it ev - 'ry day, __

There's no place that you can hide; _ No, no, __
But no mat - ter what you say, ___ You know _

____ the rhy-thm is gon-na get _you. At night _
____ it, the rhy-thm is gon-na get _you. No clue __

348

Footnotes

CULTURAL CONNECTION

▶ **Latin Pop** Encourage students to learn more about Latin pop music and the life, artistry, and influence of Gloria Estefan, a sensational Latin performer and songwriter, by reading *Gloria Estefan* (A&E Biography) by Michael Benson (Lerner, 2000).

BUILDING SKILLS THROUGH MUSIC

▶ **Math** Share the information from Spotlight On. Have students create a time line that could be used in planning a music video for this song that incorporates the timing of each scene that would be included. Students will need to make decisions regarding number of scenes and placement of scene changes within the song.

SKILLS REINFORCEMENT

2c ▶ **Creating** Invite students to create a layered rhythm accompaniment for "The Rhythm Is Gonna Get You" **CD 17-19** that will use expressive Latin rhythm elements they have learned in this unit. Students may choose Latin instruments and notate a rhythm for each instrument. Have students perform the accompaniment with the song.

▶ **Creating** Students can create a music video for "The Rhythm Is Gonna Get You." Determine students responsible for the screenplay, singing, dancing, acting, videotaping, props, and set. Expression of the lyrics should drive decision making. Rehearse the scene to synchronize all activities with the recording. A student may then videotape the action while the singers perform with the recording.

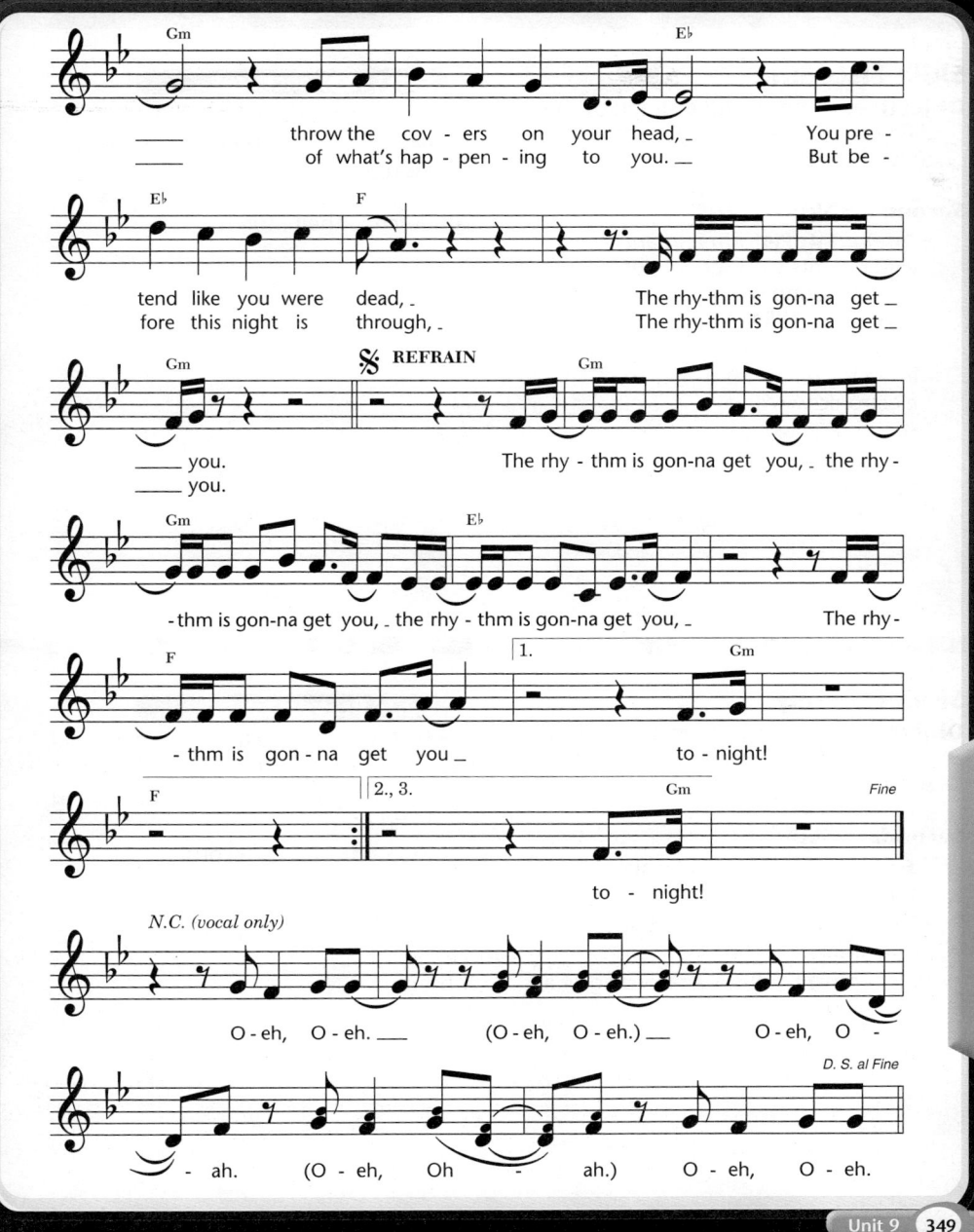

(lyrics under the music)

throw the cov-ers on your head, / of what's hap-pen-ing to you. — You pre- / tend like you were dead, — / fore this night is through, —

The rhy-thm is gon-na get — / The rhy-thm is gon-na get —

REFRAIN

— you. The rhy-thm is gon-na get you, — the rhy- / — you.

-thm is gon-na get you, — the rhy - thm is gon-na get you, — The rhy-

- thm is gon-na get you — to - night!

(2., 3.) to - night!

N.C. (vocal only) O - eh, O - eh. — (O - eh, O - eh.) — O - eh, O -

- ah. (O - eh, Oh - ah.) O - eh, O - eh.

Be a Star!

Unit 9 **349**

2 DEVELOP

Listening

Invite students to listen to "The Rhythm Is Gonna Get You" **CD 17-19.**

6b **ASK** **What category of popular music best describes this song?** (*salsa* or Latin pop)

Is the rhythm mostly even, or mostly syncopated? (syncopated)

What rhythm instruments are used in this *salsa* music? (bongos, congas, claves, maracas, cowbells)

Singing

1c Invite students to sing "The Rhythm Is Gonna Get You" **CD 17-19** with the recording. After students know the song, encourage a small group to sing the verses, and the entire class to sing the refrain.

Creating

2c Have students create and perform an accompaniment to "The Rhythm Is Gonna Get You." See Skills Reinforcement, p. 348.

Invite students to make a music video of their own performance of "The Rhythm Is Gonna Get You," using ideas in Skills Reinforcement, p. 348.

Stress the importance of expressing the song lyrics in every decision students make.

3 CLOSE

Skill: SINGING **ASSESSMENT**

Performance/Observation Have students sing "The Rhythm Is Gonna Get You" with their rhythm accompaniment. Observe their use of expressive Latin rhythm elements in their performance, such as singing accented syncopations and bringing out the uniqueness of each layer in the rhythm accompaniment.

SPOTLIGHT ON

▶ **Music Videos** A combination of popular music with visual images, music videos were initially used to promote recordings. *Don't Go Breaking My Heart,* an early Elton John music video, showed the artists singing in the studio.

After Music Television (MTV) began in 1981, short films were created to accompany a song. Toni Basil's *Mickey* used choreography, and Michael Jackson's *Beat It* told a story. Music videos now either show the performer in concert, tell a story (which may or may not relate to the lyrics), or have abstract visuals or dreamlike images.

Creators rely heavily on the use of computers to distort and manipulate the images. The digital video disc (DVD) format allows the video and music to appear on the same disc.

SCHOOL TO HOME CONNECTION

▶ **Music Videos from Home** Encourage students to ask their families and friends to help them find suitable music videos in their private collections that use a song's lyrics to dictate the visual images. Some students may be allowed to bring the videos to class. Note: Preview videos for suitability before showing them in class.

TECHNOLOGY/MEDIA LINK

CD-ROM Have students type the chord progression of "The Rhythm Is Gonna Get You" into *Band-in-a-Box.* Have students use the progression to generate Latin accompaniments for the percussion instruments and singers.

Lesson	Elements	Skills	
LESSON 1 — **Vibration: the Basis of Sound** pp. 354–357 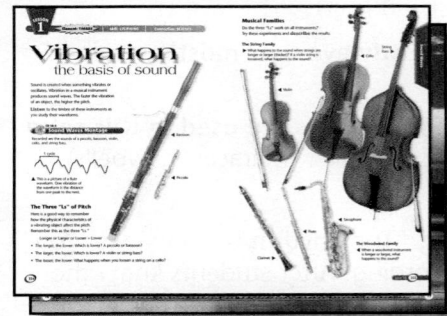	**Element: Timbre** **Concept:** Environmental, instrumental **Focus:** Instrumental timbre and sound families, sound vibration, and waveforms **Secondary Element** Form: free form (*Ionisation*) **National Standards** 6a 6b 8b	**Skill: Listening** **Objective:** Listen to and distinguish the different timbres of instruments within musical families **Secondary Skills** • **Analyzing** Perform and analyze experiments with sound vibrations; analyze sound vibration using the Three "Ls" of Pitch • **Listening** Listen to sound waves; listen to sound timbres in an electronic work	**SKILLS REINFORCEMENT** • **Playing** Play a drumroll to demonstrate a vibrating drumhead • **Listening** Listen to various instruments in the Sound Bank and describe the timbres
LESSON 2 — **Jug Band Sounds** pp. 358–361 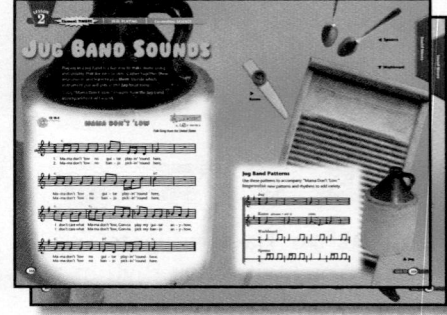	**Element: Timbre** **Concept:** Instrumental **Focus:** Instruments in a jug band **Secondary Element** Rhythm: eighth- and sixteenth-note rhythm patterns **National Standards** 1a 2a 2c 3b 6b 8b	**Skill: Playing** **Objective:** Play jug band instruments as accompaniment to an American folk song **Secondary Skills** • **Singing** Sing an Appalachian folk song • **Playing** Play various jug band instruments • **Listening** Listen to a recording of a jug band	**SKILLS REINFORCEMENT** • **Guitar** Play a guitar accompaniment tuning a guitar to open G • **Creating** Create new verses to a jug band song • **Recorder** Play a recorder accompaniment
LESSON 3 — **Types of Vibrations** pp. 362–367 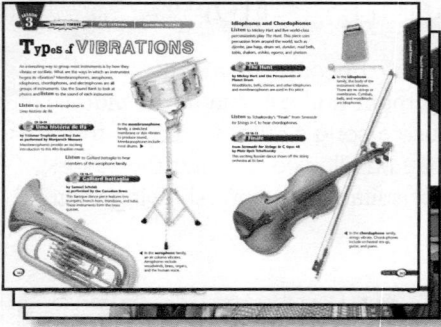	**Element: Timbre** **Concept:** Instrumental **Focus:** Instrument families and timbre **Secondary Element** Melody: melodic sequence **National Standards** 2a 2c 6b 8b	**Skill: Listening** **Objective:** Listen to and identify instrument timbres **Secondary Skills** • **Listening** Listen to groups of instruments organized by the way their sounds are produced • **Singing** Sing a song in English then Spanish • **Playing** Experiment with mambo rhythms to a Cuban song	**SKILLS REINFORCEMENT** • **Recorder** Play a countermelody on alto recorder; play an accompaniment on soprano recorder • **Playing** Play Latin or Cuban rhythms using auto-accompaniment on a MIDI keyboard • **Creating** Create Latin rhythms using MIDI sequencing software • **Keyboard** Explore broken chord accompaniments

Connections

Music and Other Literature

Connection: Science

Activity: Discuss the science of timbre, sound vibration, and sound waves

ACROSS THE CURRICULUM **Science** Discuss how sound waves are produced; read books on acoustics

TEACHER TO TEACHER
Do Vibrations Exist? Perform an experiment to prove vibrations exist
Waveform: The Rope Trick Perform a rope experiment that displays a waveform

SPOTLIGHT ON
Oscilloscope Waveforms Use an oscilloscope to view waveforms
Vibrations and Sand Perform an experiment that proves sound vibrates

BUILDING SKILLS THROUGH MUSIC **Language** Compare and contrast characteristics of compositions

Listening Selections
Sound Waves Montage
Ionisation
Listening Map: *Ionisation*

More Music Choices
Symphony No. 5 in C Minor, "Movement 1" (orchestra, excerpt), p. 98
Uma história de Ifá (percussion), p. 362
Think (excerpt) (electronic), p. 367

ASSESSMENT

Written/Oral Assessment
Listen to a variety of instruments and describe them

TECHNOLOGY/MEDIA LINK
Electronic Keyboard Experiment with electronic timbres
Transparency *Ionisation*

Connection: Science

Activity: Examine how jug band instruments produce sound through playing

TEACHER TO TEACHER **Safety Tips** Tips on playing a jug in a class

MOVEMENT **Patterned Dance** learn an Appalachian dance
Signing Perform a signing interpretation

SPOTLIGHT ON
Making a Gutbucket (Washtub Bass) How to make and play a gutbucket
Making Musical Spoons How to make musical spoons
Playing the Spoons How to play the spoons

SCHOOL TO HOME CONNECTION **Home "Found Sounds"** Have students teach others how to play rhythms on instruments at home

BUILDING SKILLS THROUGH MUSIC **Math** Use ratios

Song "Mama Don't Low"

Listening Selections *Jug Band Music*

More Music Choices
"Jambalaya," p. 244
"Paths of Victory," p. 195

ASSESSMENT

Performance/Observation
Play a game where instruments are identified by timbre

TECHNOLOGY/MEDIA LINK
Web Site Information on jug and skiffle bands

Connection: Science

Activity: Discuss how instrument families create sound

CULTURAL CONNECTION
Afro-Brazilian Music Facts on this style of music
How to Make a Diddley Bow Instructions on making a zither

ACROSS THE CURRICULUM
Science Share history on the instrument family classifications; perform an experiment using a "straw" reed
Language Arts/Social Studies Migrant working families

SPOTLIGHT ON
Instrument Sound Groups Facts on different instrument family groups
The Performer Facts on rock star Gloria Estefan

CHARACTER EDUCATION **Perseverance** Migrant workers
TEACHER TO TEACHER **Careers in Music** Related fields
SCHOOL TO HOME CONNECTION **Homemade Instruments** Have students create various types of instruments
BUILDING SKILLS THROUGH MUSIC **Reading** Organize facts

Listening Selections
Uma história de Ifá
Galliard battaglia
The Hunt
"Finale" from *Serenade for Strings in C,* Op. 48 (excerpt)
"Corta la caña"("Head for the Canefields")
Mi tierra
Wild Bull (excerpt)
Think (excerpt)
M·U·S·I·C M·A·K·E·R·S
Morton Subotnick

More Music Choices
"Everybody Loves Saturday Night," p. 296
"By the Waters of Babylon," p. 311

ASSESSMENT

Observation Play a listening game to categorize instruments by timbre and instrument family

TECHNOLOGY/MEDIA LINK
Web Site Information on instruments and how they produce sound

---

Lesson	Elements	Skills

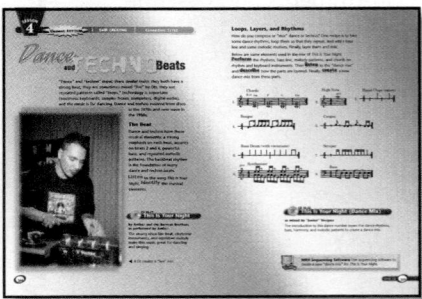

LESSON 4

Dance and Techno Beats

pp. 368–369

Element: Rhythm
Concept: Beats
Focus: Backbeat/dance beat/techno beat

Secondary Element
Syncopation

National Standards
2a 5a 6b 7b

Skill: Creating
Objective: Create a dance mix for a listening selection

Secondary Skills
- **Listening** Listen to a song and discuss the different dance beats that are heard
- **Playing** Play African drumming rhythms
- **Creating** Create a dance beat

SKILLS REINFORCEMENT
- **Playing** Play African drumming patterns

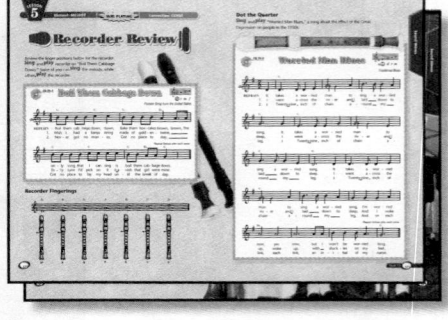
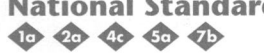

LESSON 5

Recorder Review

pp. 370–373

Element: Melody
Concept: Pitch and direction
Focus: Folk melodies

Secondary Element
Rhythm: 6/8 meter

National Standards
1a 2a 4c 5a 7b

Skill: Playing
Objective: Play folk melodies from three different cultures on the recorder

Secondary Skills
- **Singing** Sing a folk song
- **Playing** Review recorder fingering and play a folk song
- **Reading** Read dotted quarter-note rhythms
- **Performing** Perform a folk song on mallets and recorder

SKILLS REINFORCEMENT
- **Mallets** Create a mallet accompaniment using chord notes; learn an Orff accompaniment to a folk song
- **Recorder** Play an ostinato on alto recorder; play alto and soprano recorder parts to two folk songs
- **Keyboard** Play a broken-chord accompaniment to a folk song

---

LESSON 6

Playing Guitar and Autoharp

pp. 374–377

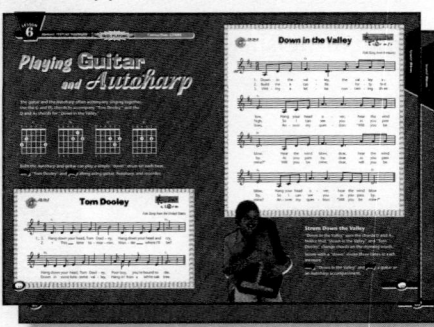

Element: Texture/Harmony
Concept: Harmony
Focus: Chords

Secondary Element
Rhythm: 6/8 meter

National Standards
1a 2a 2b 5a 6b 8b

Skill: Playing
Objective: Play Autoharp and guitar chords for three folk songs

Secondary Skills
- **Singing** Sing three folk songs from diverse cultures; sing a folk song in Spanish
- **Playing** Learn the chords for and accompany folk songs

SKILLS REINFORCEMENT
- **Recorder** Play a countermelody on recorder
- **Mallets** Play an Orff arrangement to a folk song

Connections

Connection: Style
Activity: Explore dance and techno styles

ACROSS THE CURRICULUM **Language Arts** Develop body percussion to accompany rhyming verse

SPOTLIGHT ON **Techno Historical Benchmarks** Explores the development of techno music

SCHOOL TO HOME CONNECTION **Radio** Listen to and critique radio stations that play dance music

BUILDING SKILLS THROUGH MUSIC **Writing** Describe a dance mix

Connection: Genre
Activity: Examine the recorder as a solo and accompaniment instrument

TEACHER TO TEACHER
Reading Skeleton Melodies Melodic outlines
Recorder Teaching Sequence Method for teaching recorder

SCHOOL TO HOME CONNECTION **Home Performance** Have students play the recorder for their families

BUILDING SKILLS THROUGH MUSIC **Language** Recognize meaning behind lyrics

Connection: Genre
Activity: Examine guitar and Autoharp folk song accompaniments and harmony

SPOTLIGHT ON
The Guitar Historical background on the guitar
Guitars Facts on types of guitars
Guitar Manufacturers Facts on two makers of guitars

ACROSS THE CURRICULUM
Language Arts/Drama Write a story about Tom Dooley's life
Social Studies/Language Arts Share books on South America and Chile

TEACHER TO TEACHER **Guitar Management Tips** Tips on playing guitars in class

MEETING INDIVIDUAL NEEDS **Including Everyone** Assist students with guitar playing

BUILDING SKILLS THROUGH MUSIC **Language** Use lyrics to write a story

Music and Other Literature

Listening Selections
This Is Your Night (excerpt)
This Is Your Night (Dance Mix) (excerpt)

More Music Choices
Drum Ensemble 1, p. 281
Drum Ensemble 2, p. 289

Songs
"Boil Them Cabbage Down"
"Worried Man Blues"
"Skye Boat Song"

More Music Choices
"Four Strong Winds," p. 170
"Nana Kru," p. 282

Songs
"Tom Dooley"
"Down in the Valley"
"Cuando pa' Chile mee voy" ("Leavin' for Chile")

More Music Choices
"Everybody Loves Saturday Night," p. 296
"Water Come a Me Eye," p. 300
"Jambalaya," p. 244

ASSESSMENT

Performance/Peer Critique Play students' dance mixes and have peers offer suggestions

TECHNOLOGY/MEDIA LINK
Sequencing Software Create a dance mix with rhythm patterns, melody and bass

ASSESSMENT

Performance/Peer Critique Play a song on recorder and have a peer critique

TECHNOLOGY/MEDIA LINK
Notation Software Create folk song accompaniments
Web Site Information on the recorder

ASSESSMENT

Performance/Self-Assessment Play chord accompaniments on guitar and Autoharp

TECHNOLOGY/MEDIA LINK
CD-ROM Play guitar and Autoharp with Band-in-a-Box arrangements

Lesson	Elements	Skills

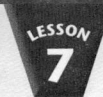

LESSON 7
The Life of a Sound

pp. 378–381

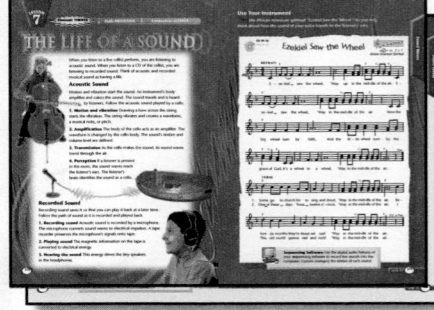

Element: Timbre
Concept: Environmental
Focus: Acoustic stages of sound and timbre

Secondary Element Form: verse-refrain form

National Standards
1d 2a 2c 2d 4c 5a 6b
8b

Skill: Analyzing
Objective: Analyze the four steps in the life of a sound and how sound is produced by instruments

Secondary Skills
- **Analyzing** Analyze science experiments on sound
- **Singing** Sing an American spiritual in two-part harmony
- **Playing** Perform accompaniments to an American spiritual

SKILLS REINFORCEMENT
- **Keyboard** Play two-handed accompaniment to a spiritual; play a full accompaniment to a spiritual in the Resource Book
- **Playing** Play an accompaniment on an Orff instrument; Learn how to play a Boomwhacker®

LESSON 8
Nature's Instruments

pp. 382–383

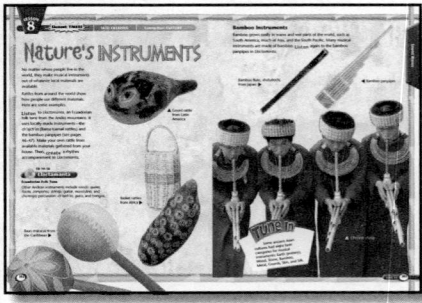

Element: Timbre
Concept: Instrumental
Focus: Instruments made from locally available materials

Secondary Element
Rhythm: Andean rhythm patterns

National Standards
4c 6b 7c 8b

Skill: Creating
Objective: Make a homemade rattle and create a rattle composition

Secondary Skills
- **Listening** Listen to bamboo and other instruments from the Andes
- **Creating** Create rattles and create compositions using them

SKILLS REINFORCEMENT
- **Listening** Listen to timbres and rhythms of Andean instruments

---

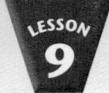

LESSON 9
Gamelan Orchestras

pp. 384–385

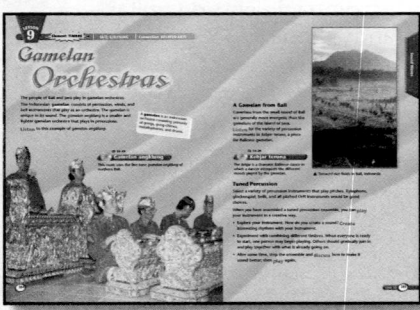

Element: Timbre
Concept: Instrumental
Focus: Gamelan timbres

Secondary Element
Rhythm: improvising rhythm patterns with tuned percussion instruments

National Standards
4c 6b 9a

Skill: Listening
Objective: Listen to gamelan timbres

Secondary Skills
- **Creating** Create a tuned percussion piece that illustrates timbre
- **Playing** Play in a tuned percussion ensemble

Connections

Music and Other Literature

Connection: Science

Activity: Write about the principles of musical sound and recording

TEACHER TO TEACHER **Science Fair** Demonstrate acoustic projects at fairs

ACROSS THE CURRICULUM **Science** Discuss digital recording in music

SPOTLIGHT ON
Science of Music Facts on sounds and instruments
Early Recording Techniques Facts on the first audio recordings

BUILDING SKILLS THROUGH MUSIC **Science** Collect data on sound decay

Song "Ezekiel Saw the Wheel"

More Music Choices
Lesson 1, pp. 354–357 (science and acoustics)

ASSESSMENT

Music journal Writing
Analyze the "Life of a Sound" for each instrument family

TECHNOLOGY/MEDIA LINK
Sequencing Software
Experiment with digital audio recording

Connection: Culture

Activity: Discuss how instruments are made from locally available materials in different cultures

CULTURAL CONNECTION **Bamboo Instruments** Share books on bamboo instruments

ACROSS THE CURRICULUM **Social Studies** Create a bulletin board displaying cultural and regional instruments

BUILDING SKILLS THROUGH MUSIC **Writing** Create a fictitious locale and an indigenous instrument

Listening Selections *Llactamanta*

More Music Choices
"El cóndor pasa," p. 46
Gamelan angklung, p. 384
Drums of the Iroquois and Sioux, p. 285

ASSESSMENT

Performance/Peer Critique Critique original rhythm compositions played on homemade rattles

TECHNOLOGY/MEDIA LINK
CD-ROM Use *Making More Music* to create and notate rattle rhythms

---

Connection: Related Arts

Activity: Discuss Balinese dance

ACROSS THE CURRICULUM **Social Studies** Circumnavigate a world globe to find Bali

SPOTLIGHT ON **Balinese Dance** Facts on Balinese dance

CULTURAL CONNECTION **Musical Onomatopoeia** Discuss instruments named for their sounds

CHARACTER EDUCATION **Creativity** Discuss the elements of creativity

BUILDING SKILLS THROUGH MUSIC **Language** Create an orchestration

Listening Selections
Gamelan angklung (excerpt)
Kebjar teruna (excerpt)

More Music Choices
Hindewhu (whistle) solo, p. 269
"Yo-shi nai," p. 286
"Banuwa," p. 294

ASSESSMENT

Music Journal Writing
Listen to a gamelan selection and write about the timbres in the gamelan

TECHNOLOGY/MEDIA LINK
Sequencing Software
Use digital audio recording to create a collage of sounds

INTRODUCING THE UNIT

The unit "Sound Waves" brings together the fields of music, science, and mathematics to help students explore how sound and instruments work. Students can go beyond the simpler categories for instruments to a more sophisticated understanding of acoustics.

UNIT PROJECT

Put together a Sound Sampler Showcase presentation that demonstrates acoustics and how instruments work.

Have students

- Sing and play "Mama Don't 'Low" (p. 358) with jug band as an opening song.
- Demonstrate the various forms of sound vibration or oscillation (p. 354). Illustrate the Three "Ls" of Pitch (p. 354). Use the Waveform: The Rope Trick (Teacher to Teacher, p. 356) with members of the audience.
- Play brief sections of the recordings found on p. 357.
- Show how the recorder, guitar, and Autoharp work, and sing and play songs from Lessons 5 and 6 of this unit.
- Demonstrate "The Life of a Sound" as illustrated in Lesson 7.
- Do "Sound Wizard" demonstrations of the Hose-a-phone (p. 381) and Whacky Music (p. 381).
- Show examples of gourd and bamboo instruments and play them, if possible. Students may wish to collect and show other utensils made from either of these natural resources.

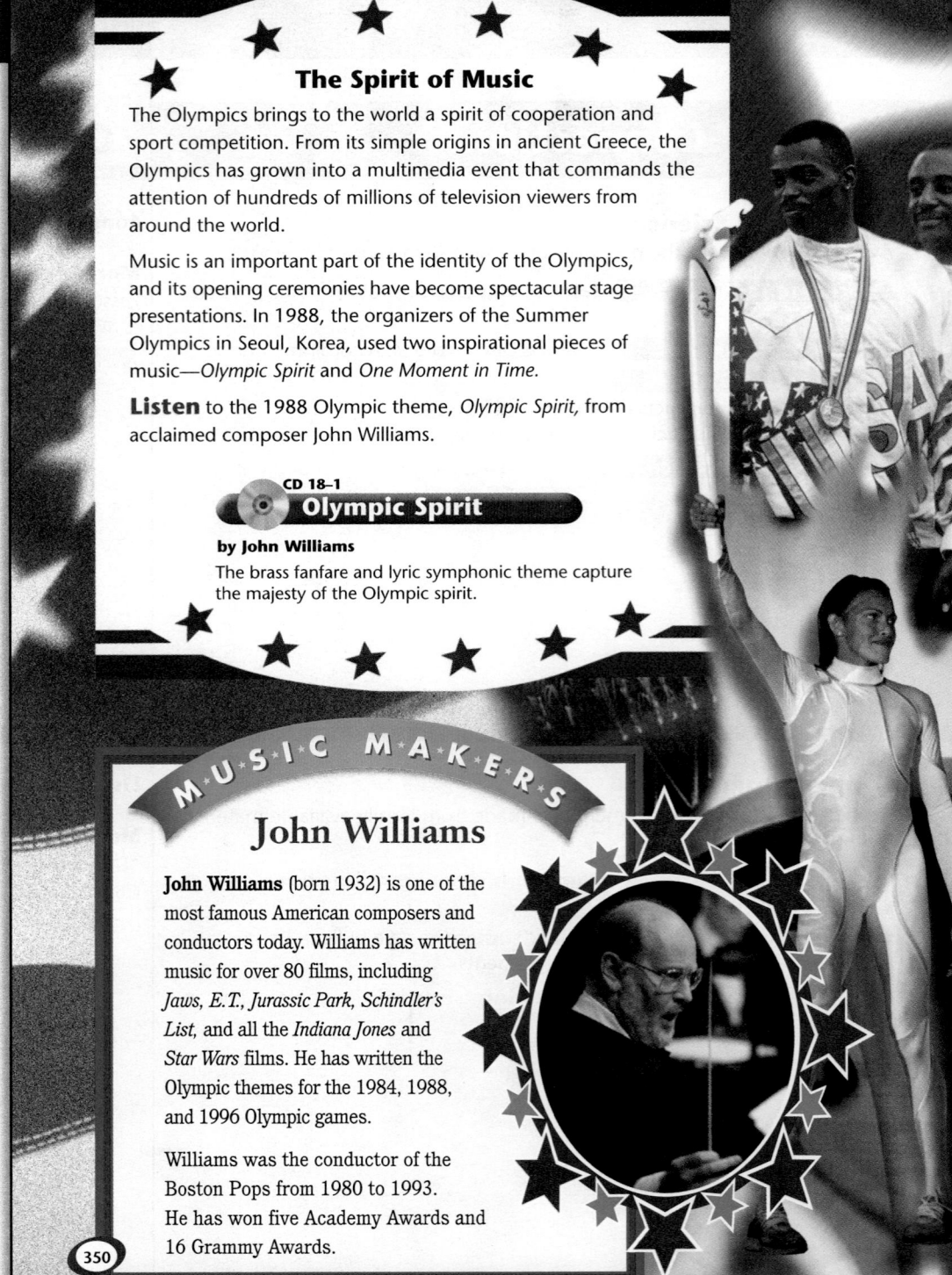

The Spirit of Music

The Olympics brings to the world a spirit of cooperation and sport competition. From its simple origins in ancient Greece, the Olympics has grown into a multimedia event that commands the attention of hundreds of millions of television viewers from around the world.

Music is an important part of the identity of the Olympics, and its opening ceremonies have become spectacular stage presentations. In 1988, the organizers of the Summer Olympics in Seoul, Korea, used two inspirational pieces of music—*Olympic Spirit* and *One Moment in Time.*

Listen to the 1988 Olympic theme, *Olympic Spirit,* from acclaimed composer John Williams.

CD 18–1
Olympic Spirit
by John Williams
The brass fanfare and lyric symphonic theme capture the majesty of the Olympic spirit.

MUSIC MAKERS

John Williams

John Williams (born 1932) is one of the most famous American composers and conductors today. Williams has written music for over 80 films, including *Jaws, E.T., Jurassic Park, Schindler's List,* and all the *Indiana Jones* and *Star Wars* films. He has written the Olympic themes for the 1984, 1988, and 1996 Olympic games.

Williams was the conductor of the Boston Pops from 1980 to 1993. He has won five Academy Awards and 16 Grammy Awards.

350

ACROSS THE CURRICULUM

Unit Highlights The following interdisciplinary activities in this unit are related to the music elements presented in the lessons and are intended to enhance student learning. For a more detailed topical description, including related arts activities, see the Unit at a Glance, pp. 349a–349f.

▶ **LANGUAGE ARTS**

- Develop individual body percussion, movement, and vocal sound backbeats (p. 368)
- Write an imaginary story about a person's life (p. 375)

▶ **SOCIAL STUDIES**

- Read about a family whose members make their living working the fields (p. 364)
- Read stories with folk tales, descriptions of the Andes, and South American geography and customs (p. 376)

- Create a bulletin board to display instruments from different cultures and geographic regions around the world (p. 383)
- Examine destinations on a globe of the world (p. 384)

▶ **SCIENCE**

- Learn about how sounds are created and recognized (p. 354)
- Examine waveforms and other acoustic principles (p. 356)
- Become aware of a classification system of organizing music instruments (p. 362)
- Conduct an experiment to create a double reed from a soda straw (p. 367)
- Learn about recording techniques and how they have changed over the years (p. 378)

UNIT 10

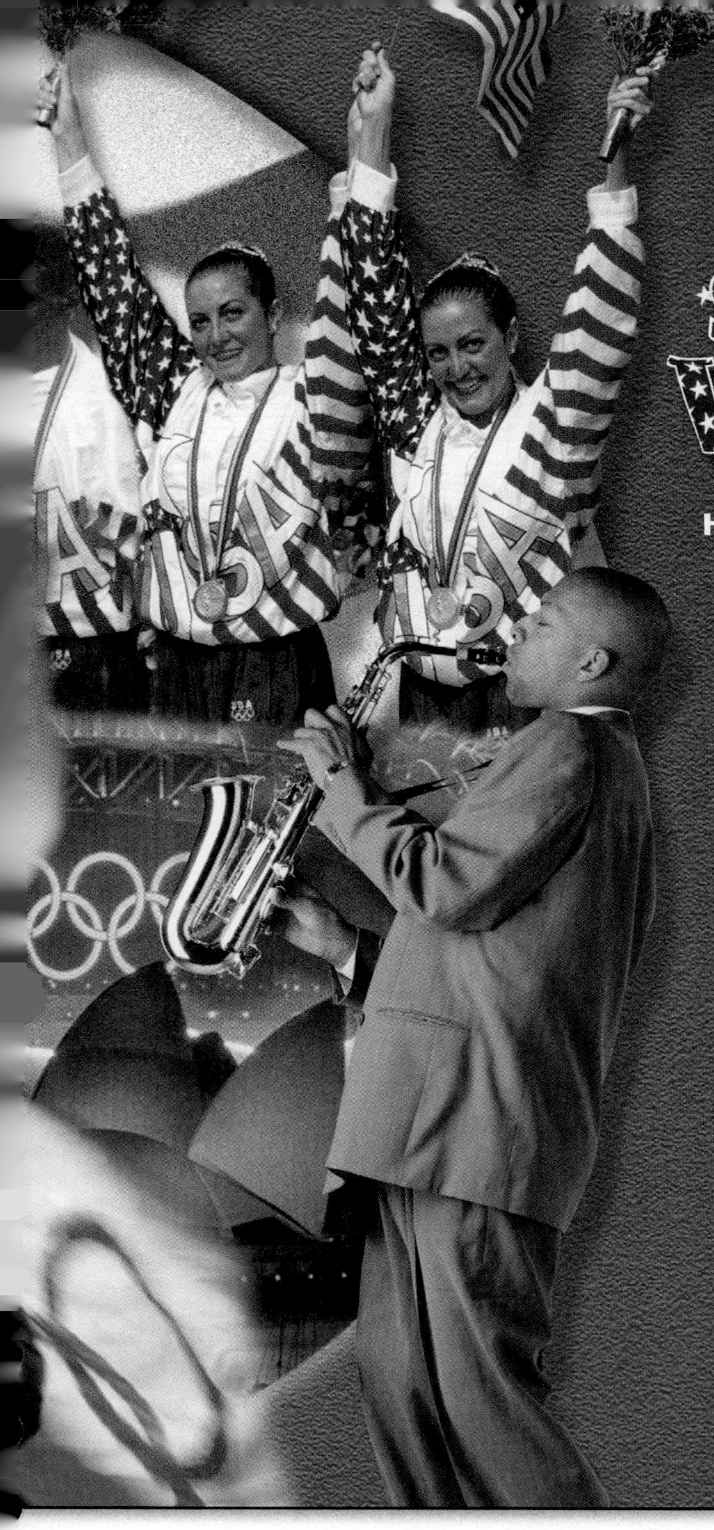

Sound Waves

How is sound produced, and how does it travel? In this unit, you will explore the worlds of sound, science, and music.

MUSIC SKILLS ASSESSED IN THIS UNIT

Reading Music: Rhythm

- Play a folk melody using the correct rhythms (p. 373)

Reading Music: Pitch

- Use the correct pitches when playing a folk melody (p. 373)

Performing Music: Singing

- Sing a folk song while accompanying it on Autoharp or guitar (p. 377)

Performing Music: Playing

- Play jug band instruments (p. 361)
- Perform an accompaniment on Autoharp or guitar (p. 377)

Creating Music

- Create a dance mix (p. 369)
- Create a composition using homemade rattles (p. 383)

Listening to Music

- Write the pitch and timbre of instruments (p. 357)
- Identify instruments by timbre (p. 361)
- Identify instruments by family (p. 367)
- Listen to and describe timbres heard in a gamelan (p. 385)

CULTURAL CONNECTION

Unit Highlights The musical literature in this unit provides many opportunities for students to explore a aspects of performing and recording music. A more detailed description of the resources and activities listed below can be found in the Unit at a Glance on pp. 349a–349f.

SOUTH AMERICAN

- *"Cuando pa' Chile me voy"* (p. 376)

AFRICAN/AFRICAN AMERICAN

- "Ezekiel Saw the Wheel" (p. 379)

AFRO-BRAZILIAN MUSIC

- Learn about the origins and characteristics of Afro-Brazilian music (p. 362)

AMERICAN REGIONAL

- How to Make a Diddley Bow (p. 364)
- "Mama Don't 'Low" (p. 358); "Boil Them Cabbage Down" (p. 370); "Worried Man Blues" (p. 371); "Tom Dooley" (p. 374); "Down in the Valley" (p. 375)

ASIAN; AUSTRALIAN

- Bamboo Instruments: Read about a boy who learns to play a bamboo flute (p. 382)
- Musical Onomatopoeia: Become aware of how instruments are named after the sound they make (p. 385)

CARIBBEAN/PUERTO RICO

- *"Corta la caña"* (p. 364)

EUROPEAN

- "Skye Boat Song" (p. 372)

OPENING ACTIVITIES

MATERIALS

- *Olympic Spirit*   **CD 18–1**
- "One Moment in Time"   **CD 18–2**

    Recording Routine:
    Intro (5 m.); vocal; coda

- music writing journals

Listening

Have students listen to the recording of *Olympic Spirit* **CD 18–1,** and identify the instrument family they hear in this fanfare (brass). Ask students why brass instruments are often used in fanfares (powerful sound). Tell students that John Williams, featured on p. 350, is an important film composer of today.

Reading

Ask students to look for the following things in the notation of "One Moment in Time:"

- First and second endings.
- Repeat signs.
- Key changes.

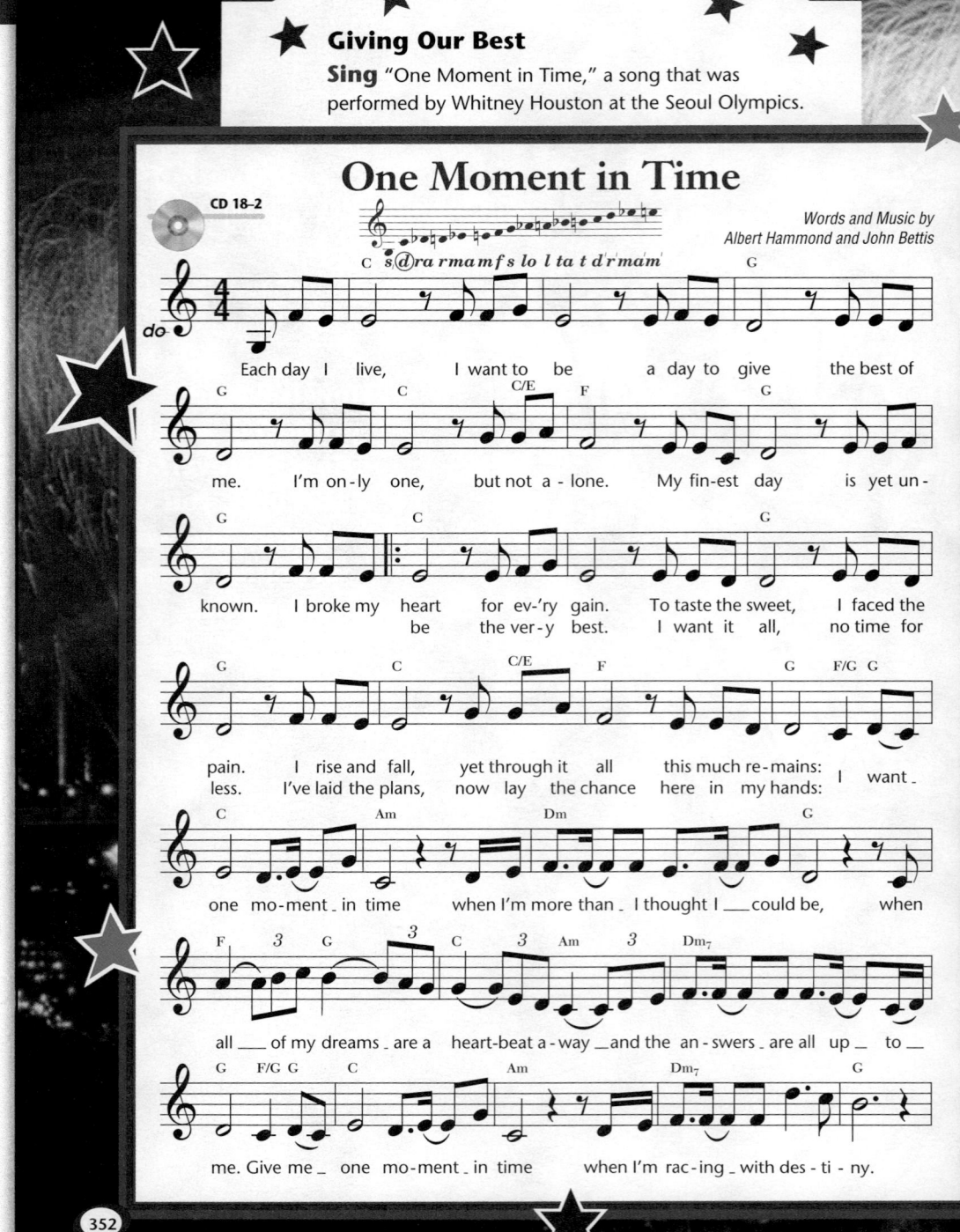

Giving Our Best

Sing "One Moment in Time," a song that was performed by Whitney Houston at the Seoul Olympics.

ASSESSMENT

Unit Highlights The lessons in this unit were chosen and developed to support the theme "Sound Waves." Each lesson, as always, presents a clear element focus, a skill objective, and an end-of-lesson assessment. The overall sequence of lessons, however, is organized according to this theme, rather than concept or skill development. In this context, formal assessment strategies, such as those presented in Units 1–6, are no longer applicable.

▶ **INFORMAL ASSESSMENTS**

At the close of each Teacher's Edition lesson in this unit, one of the following types of assessments is used to evaluate the learning of the key element focus or skill objective.

- Music Journal Writing (pp. 381, 385)
- Performance/Observation (p. 361)
- Performance/Peer Critique (pp. 369, 373, 383)
- Performance/Self-Assessment (p. 377)
- Written/Oral Assessment (p. 357)
- Observation (p. 367)

▶ **RUBRICS**

Visit *www.sfsuccessnet.com* for rubrics to assess students' achievement in music skills.

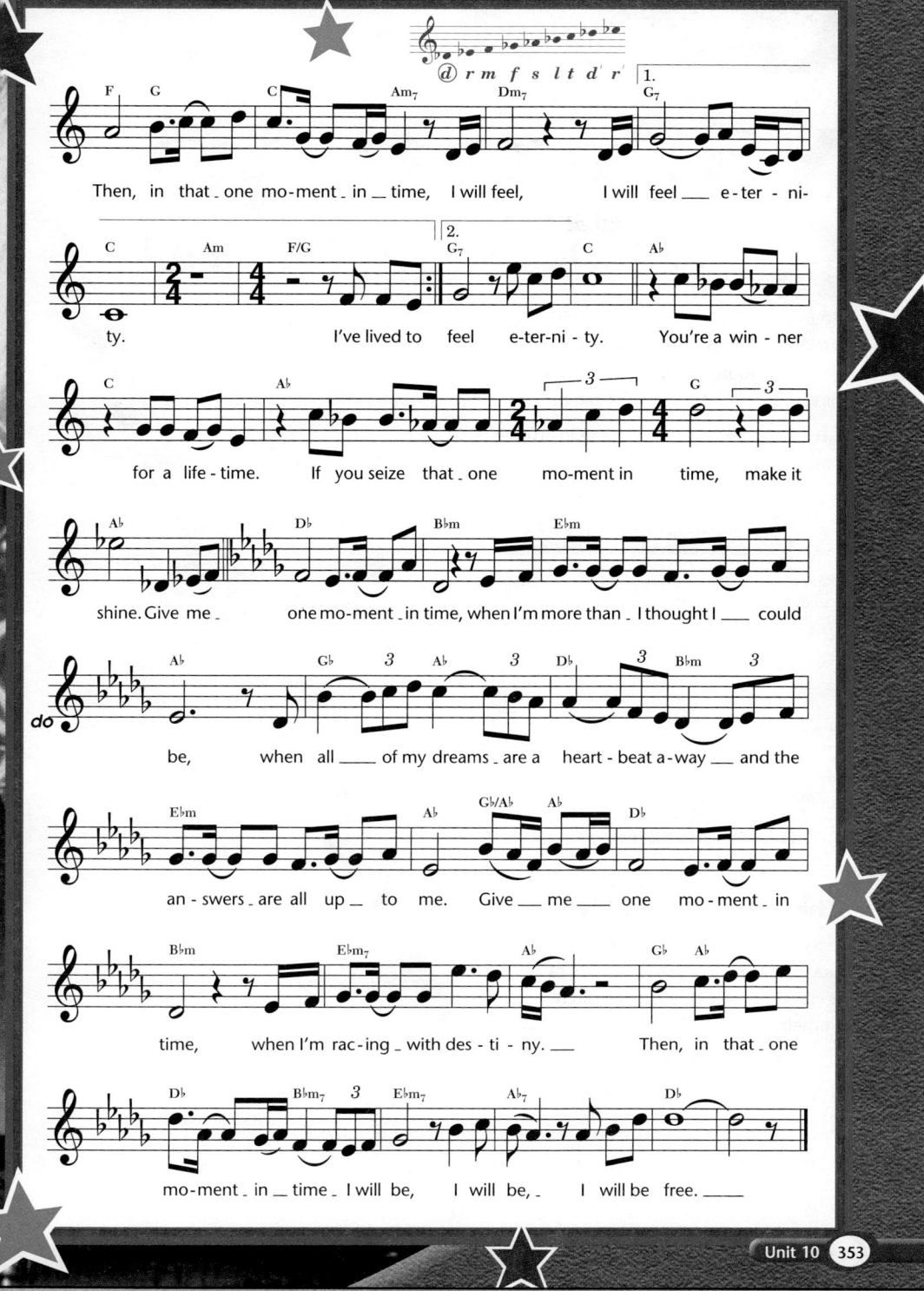

Then, in that one mo-ment in time, I will feel, I will feel ___ e-ter-ni-ty. I've lived to feel e-ter-ni-ty. You're a win-ner for a life-time. If you seize that one mo-ment in time, make it shine. Give me ___ one mo-ment in time, when I'm more than I thought I ___ could be, when all ___ of my dreams are a heart-beat a-way ___ and the an-swers are all up ___ to me. Give ___ me one mo-ment in time, when I'm rac-ing with des-ti-ny. ___ Then, in that one mo-ment in time ___ I will be, I will be, ___ I will be free. ___

Singing

Have students listen to the recording of "One Moment in Time" and follow the roadmap of the song.

ASK How did you feel when the key was raised from C to D♭ on the second page? (Accept a variety of answers.)

Discuss how this has become a common technique used in pop and country music.

Sing the song along with the recording.

Analyzing

Discuss with students the message of the lyrics to "One Moment in Time." Here are some examples of phrases from the lyrics.

- "More than I thought I could be."
- "To taste the sweet, I faced the pain."
- "I've laid the plans, now lay the choice here in my hands."
- "In that one moment in time, I will be free."

Have students write some personal goals in their journals.

INNOVATIVE TEACHER SUPPORT FOR THIS UNIT

- **MAKING MUSIC DVD, Grade 6** contains video segments that support lessons, including signing and movement.
- **MAKING MUSIC with Movement and Dance** provides more opportunities for large group activities in music or physical education classes.
- **MAKING MUSIC with Technology** provides lesson plans for many technology applications; includes MIDI files.
- **¡A cantar!** features recorded songs and lessons from around the Spanish-speaking world; includes strategies for bilingual classes and for English-speaking teachers working with Spanish-speaking students.
- **Bridges to Asia** features recorded songs and lessons from Asian and Pacific region cultures.
- **www.sfsuccessnet.com** provides an online lesson planner to conveniently create lesson plans at school or at home. Includes rubrics for assessment, lesson modifications to meet the needs of all students, performance musicals based on program content, and more.

TECHNOLOGY/MEDIA LINK

Unit Highlights

▶ **CD-ROM**

- Play and record guitar and Autoharp accompaniments (p. 377)
- Create and notate selected percussion or rattle rhythms (p. 383)

▶ **ELECTRONIC KEYBOARD**

- Explore how sounds can be created and modified on an electronic keyboard (p. 357)

▶ **MIDI/SEQUENCING SOFTWARE**

- Create a dance mix (p. 369)
- Record using the audio features of a sequencing program (p. 381)
- Create a collage of tuned percussion sounds (p. 385)

▶ **NOTATION SOFTWARE**

- Create accompaniments for folk songs (p. 373)

▶ **TRANSPARENCY**

- Assist students in hearing and identifying prominent percussion instruments in the music (p. 357)

▶ **WEB SITE**

- Visit *www.sfsuccessnet.com* to learn more about jug and skiffle bands (p. 361)
- Learn more about how instruments produce sound (p. 367)
- Visit *www.sfsuccessnet.com* to learn more about the recorder and its history (p. 373)

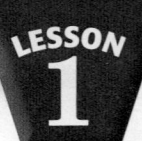

LESSON 1

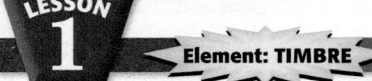

LESSON AT A GLANCE

Element Focus — **TIMBRE** Instrumental timbre and sound families, sound vibration, and waveforms

Skill Objective — **LISTENING** Listen to and distinguish the different timbres of instruments within musical families

Connection Activity — **SCIENCE** Discuss the science of timbre, sound vibration, and sound waves

MATERIALS
- *Sound Waves Montage* — CD 18–4
- *Ionisation* — CD 18–5
- **Resource Book** pp. C-8, J-12
- snare drum, drumsticks, drums (varying sizes), dimes, guitar, recorder, band or string instruments (played by students), oscilloscope (if available), fine sand, clothesline rope (15')

VOCABULARY
vibration   waveform   cycle   oscillation

◆ ◆ ◆ ◆ National Standards ◆ ◆ ◆ ◆
6a Listen and describe events in music using appropriate terms
6b Listen and analyze uses of timbre in music from diverse cultures
8b Identify ways music relates to science

MORE MUSIC CHOICES
For more listening selections that demonstrate timbre:
Symphony No. 5 in C Minor, "Movement 1" (orchestra, excerpt), p. 98
Uma história de Ifá (percussion), p. 362
Think (excerpt) (electronic), p. 367

LESSON 1

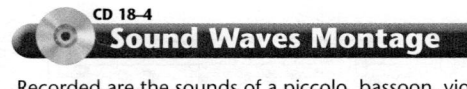

Vibration
the basis of sound

Sound is created when something vibrates or oscillates. Vibration in a musical instrument produces sound waves. The faster the vibration of an object, the higher the pitch.

Listen to the timbre of these instruments as you study their waveforms.

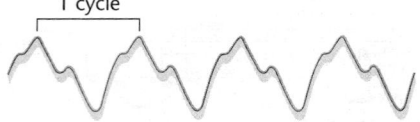
CD 18–4 Sound Waves Montage

Recorded are the sounds of a piccolo, bassoon, violin, cello, and string bass.

1 cycle

▲ This is a picture of a flute waveform. One vibration of the waveform is the distance from one peak to the next.

◄ Bassoon

◄ Piccolo

The Three "Ls" of Pitch
Here is a good way to remember how the physical characteristics of a vibrating object affect the pitch. Remember this as the three "Ls."

Longer or Larger or Looser = Lower

- The *longer,* the lower: Which is lower? A piccolo or bassoon?
- The *larger,* the lower: Which is lower? A violin or string bass?
- The *looser,* the lower: What happens when you loosen a string on a cello?

(354)

Footnotes

ACROSS THE CURRICULUM

8b ▶ **Science** Share with students how sounds are created and recognized. First, a musical instrument vibrates, or oscillates, and creates a waveform. Then, the waveform produces sound waves in the air (changes in air pressure). Next, the sound waves cause our eardrums (tympanic membranes) to vibrate in the same pattern as that of the instrument being played. The brain translates the eardrum vibrations, and we recognize the instrument.

BUILDING SKILLS THROUGH MUSIC

▶ **Language** Have students listen to *Ionisation.* Have them list the characteristics of the composition. Have the students listen to *Symphony No. 5 in C minor* listed in Lesson at a Glance: More Musical Choices, and list the characteristics. Have them complete a Venn Diagram (Resource Book p. C-8) comparing and contrasting the compositions.

TEACHER TO TEACHER

▶ **Do Vibrations Exist?** Review with students that the sound or timbre of an instrument is determined by its vibration and waveform. Ask students how they can prove vibrations exist. (Feeling vibrations as you sing musical notes is one proof.) Have students perform an easy experiment to prove that vibrations exist.

Experiment: Ask students to put a dime in the middle of a drumhead; then hit the drumhead in a different spot and watch the dime jump from the vibration of the drumhead. Ask students how this proves that vibrations create sound. (Hitting the drumhead starts the vibration. The bouncing of the dime on the drumhead demonstrates that the drumhead is vibrating. Sound is heard when the drum is struck.)

Musical Families

Do the three "Ls" work on all instruments?
Try these experiments and **describe** the results.

The String Family

▶ What happens to the sound when strings are longer or larger (thicker)? If a violin string is loosened, what happens to the sound?

◀ Violin

String Bass ▶

◀ Cello

◀ Saxophone

◀ Flute

Clarinet ▶

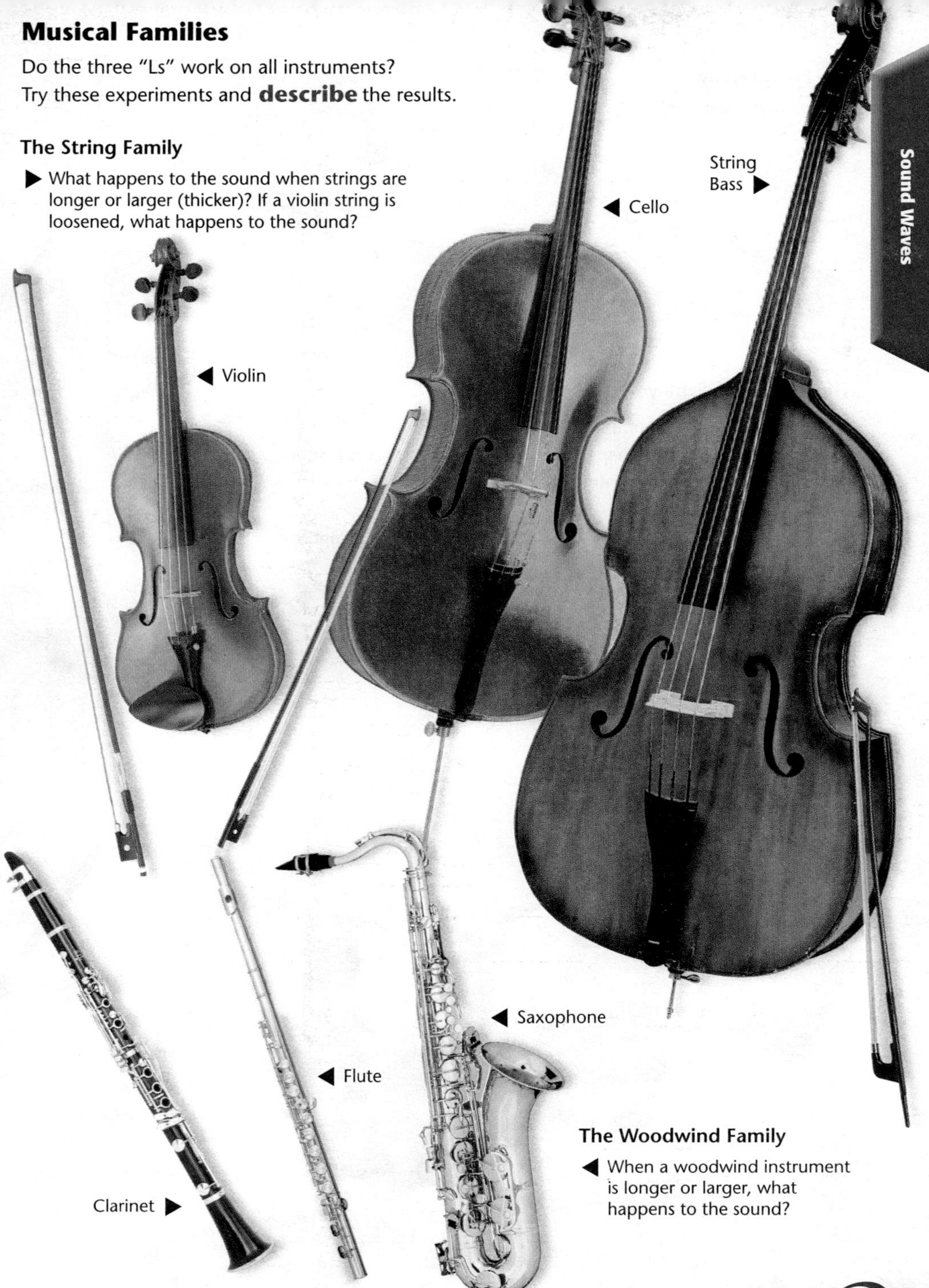

The Woodwind Family

◀ When a woodwind instrument is longer or larger, what happens to the sound?

Unit 10 355

---

1 INTRODUCE

Invite students to lightly place two fingers on their throat (larynx). Then, have them hum a low pitch. Ask them what occurs as they hum. (a vibration in their larynx) Share with students that all sound begins with vibration (oscillation). See Across the Curriculum on p. 354.

2 DEVELOP

Analyzing

8b Discuss with students the information in Teacher to Teacher and Across the Curriculum on p. 354. Divide the class into groups and give each group a drum and a dime. Have students

- Perform the experiment to demonstrate that vibrations do exist.
- Read the information about waveforms on p. 354.
- Use an oscilloscope if available to demonstrate waveforms for other instruments using Spotlight On below.

Listening

6a Invite students to listen to *Sound Waves Montage* **CD 18–4.** Have students identify the instruments and describe the characteristics of each instrument's timbre. (A bassoon sounds buzzy; it has a low sound.)

Ask students to read The Three "Ls" of Pitch on p. 354. Have students

- Echo the three "Ls" of pitch.
- Order the instruments in *Sound Waves Montage* by size and the three "Ls" of pitch (piccolo—smallest, highest pitch; violin—small, high pitch; bassoon—large, low pitch; cello—larger, lower pitch; string bass—largest, lowest pitch).

See Teacher to Teacher on p. 354 for a discussion of and an experiment with sound vibrations.

continued on page 356

SKILLS REINFORCEMENT

▶ **Playing** If a student plays drums, ask him or her to demonstrate how a beginning drumroll is played on a snare drum.

- Using the dominant hand, hold the drumstick in a relaxed manner and let the drumstick naturally bounce on the drumhead. (The drumstick should bounce a number of times before coming to a rest.) Do the same with the alternate hand.
- Continue alternating hands (L-R-L-R), gradually increasing tempo. (If the hands are relaxed and the drumsticks are bouncing naturally, the sound will be perceived as a drumroll.)
- For the advanced student, in a true drum roll, each stick hits the drum just twice, rather than continuing to bounce. To make all the sounds evenly spaced and of equal volume takes much practice.

SPOTLIGHT ON

▶ **Oscilloscope Waveforms** If an oscilloscope is available, use it to show students the waveforms of different musical instruments. Share with them that the waveform for each instrument is determined by a complex series of overtones. This distinctive mixture of overtones produces a waveform that determines an instrument's timbre.

▶ **Vibrations and Sand** If they are available, use a bass drum or timpani for this experiment. Have students

- Put fine sand on the drumhead, then gently strike the edge of the drumhead with a mallet.
- Watch as the vibrations of the head create radial patterns in the sand.

Lesson 1 Continued

Invite students to look at the instruments pictured on pp. 355–356 and read the caption for each picture. If possible, have students who play instruments demonstrate them in class.

SAY Using the principles of the three "Ls" of pitch, classify and compare the instruments shown on pp. 355–356. (Larger instruments are lower in pitch.) See Resource Book p. J-12 for a worksheet on the three "Ls" of pitch.

String Family

ASK How do the length and thickness of the strings on violin and cello affect their pitch? (The cello will have a lower pitch than the violin because the cello's strings are longer and larger [thicker] than the violin's.)

Demonstrate the principle of "the looser, the lower," using a guitar. Play each string, loosening or tightening the string each time it is plucked.

ASK What happens to the sound of a string when it is loosened? (The pitch goes down.)

Woodwind Family

Have students compare the pitches of the woodwind instruments shown on p. 355, based on the length and diameter of the pipe. (A tenor saxophone is longer and has a thicker pipe, and therefore has a lower pitch than a flute, which is shorter and has a higher pitch.)

Share with students that the holes in woodwind instruments allow a player to change the length of the vibrating air column in an instrument's pipe.

ASK In order to play a high note on a woodwind instrument, should there be a short or long air column? (short)

Brass Family

ASK Which of the brass instruments pictured on p. 356 will have the highest sound, based on the three "Ls" of pitch? (The trumpet; it is the shortest instrument, and the diameter of its pipes is the smallest.)

Music's Heavy Hitters

The Brass Family

► Compare the sound of brass instruments that are longer and larger.

◄ Trumpet

◄ Trombone

▲ French Horn

The Percussion Family

Compare the sound of a larger drumhead to that of a smaller drumhead. What happens to pitch when the pedal on a timpani loosens or tightens the drumhead?

◄ Conga

▼ Xylophone

Timpani ►

The Electronic Instrument Family

If the sound is electronic and not acoustic, do the three "Ls" apply?

◄ Synthesizer

356

Footnotes

ACROSS THE CURRICULUM

8b ► **Science** Use an illustrated science or acoustics book to show waveforms and other acoustic principles. Ask students to find the waveforms for the following waves and compare them to a representative instrument: sine wave (flute) **CD 23–25**, square wave (clarinet) **CD 23–17**, sawtooth wave (cello) **CD 23–16**, and noise (drums) **CD 23–23**. Then, ask students to draw these waveforms and listen to audio samples from the Sound Bank, pp. 512–519.

Ask students why some sounds are pitches (repeating waveform) and others are nonpitched (random, noise, nonrepeating).

TEACHER TO TEACHER

► **Waveform: The Rope Trick** This experiment illustrates a waveform without an oscilloscope. Have two students take opposite ends of a 15-foot clothesline rope.

- One student holds one rope end steady while the other student moves the opposite end up and down, counting "one thousand, two thousand . . ." at the bottom of each up and down motion. (This movement makes one simple loop, illustrating one vibration, or waveform, per second.)

- Repeat the up and down motion at double the speed by doing two strokes per second. (This faster movement will cause the rope to make a figure-8 pattern with two loops.)

- Ask all students to draw the rope waveform and compare it with the flute waveform shown on p. 354.

Electric Percussion

Edgar Varèse (1885–1965) created a unique contemporary musical work with his percussion piece *Ionisation*. This famous work stands as a classic example of twentieth-century *avant-garde* music. In *avant-garde* music, composers often use sound itself as the main element in music.

Listen to *Ionisation* and follow the listening map.

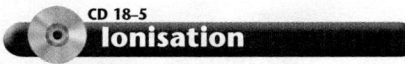

CD 18–5
Ionisation

by Edgar Varèse

Ionisation uses more than 40 percussion instruments to create a variety of musical sounds and events.

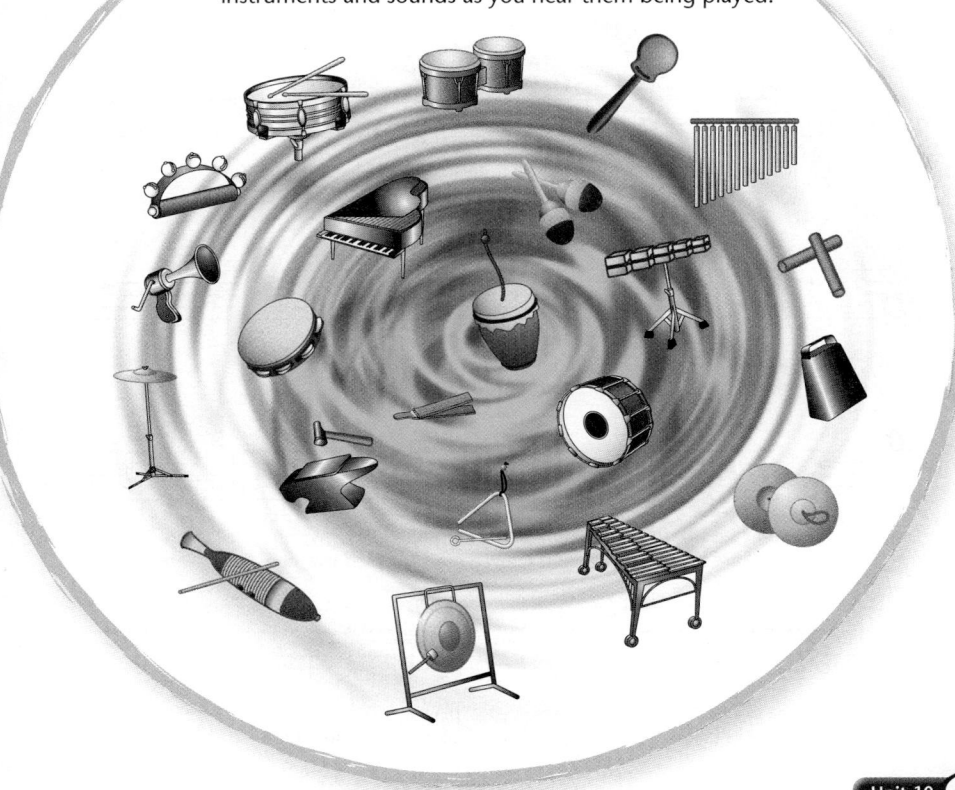

IONISATION

LISTENING MAP

Listen to *Ionisation* and **identify** each of the instruments and sounds as you hear them being played.

Describe how the valves on a trumpet affect the air column and pitch.

Percussion Family

Invite students to look at the xylophone on p. 356.

ASK How does the length of a xylophone bar affect its pitch? (Longer=lower; shorter=higher.)

Using drums of varying sizes, students should experiment to confirm the principle, the larger (the drumhead), the lower the pitch. Demonstrate vibration as suggested in Skills Reinforcement on p. 355.

Share with students that the three "Ls" of pitch do not apply to synthesizers or other electronic instruments, where sound is produced through oscillation of electrical current, or digital sampling.

Listening

6b Invite students to listen to Edgard Varèse's *Ionisation* **CD 18–5** for percussion instruments. Have students

- Describe this example of twentieth-century music.
- Identify the instruments in the recording as they follow the listening map on p. 357.
- On a separate piece of paper, draw a time line and indicate the most prominent instruments as they occur on the recording.

For tips on using the listening map transparency see Technology/Media Link below.

3 CLOSE

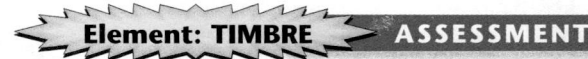

Element: TIMBRE ▸ **ASSESSMENT**

6a **Written/Oral Assessment** Have students

- Listen to instruments from the Sound Bank, pp. 354–357, or in Skills Reinforcement below.
- Use standard terminology in explaining musical instruments or voices and describe, orally or in writing, the pitch (three "Ls" of pitch) and timbre of each instrument.

SKILLS REINFORCEMENT

▶ **Listening** Have students listen to the musical families of instruments and analyze the differences in timbres between the families. Then listen to examples from the Sound Bank, pp. 512–519, as they view the instruments on pp. 355–357.

violin	**CD 23–48**	clarinet	**CD 23–17**
cello	**CD 23–16**	flute	**CD 23–25**
string bass	**CD 23–40**	saxophone	**CD 23–36**
trumpet	**CD 23–46**	bassoon	**CD 23–14**
trombone	**CD 23–45**	conga	**CD 23–18**
French horn	**CD 23–26**	timpani	**CD 23–44**
synthesizer	**CD 23–41**	xylophone	**CD 23–49**

TECHNOLOGY/MEDIA LINK

Electronic Keyboard Explain to students that modern electronic keyboards produce realistic timbres that sound almost identical to those of real instruments. Many also let you manipulate, edit, and create new timbres. Have students explore how sounds can be created and modified on an electronic keyboard.

Transparency Use the *Ionisation* listening map transparency to assist students in hearing and identifying prominent percussion instruments in the music. As students listen, point to the instruments on the projected map. The instrument in the center is a "lion's roar" and is played by pulling a rope through a drum head.

LESSON AT A GLANCE

Element Focus — **TIMBRE** Instruments in a jug band

Skill Objective — **PLAYING** Play jug band instruments as accompaniment to an American folk song

Connection Activity — **SCIENCE** Examine how jug band instruments produce sound through playing

MATERIALS

- "Mama Don't 'Low"   **CD 18–6**
  Recording Routine: Intro (4 m.); v. 1; v. 2; interlude (16 m.); v. 1; v. 2; coda
- *Jug Band Music*   **CD 18–9**
- **Dance Directions** for "Mama Don't 'Low" p. 565
- **Resource Book** pp. G-23, I-25
- guitar, Autoharp, one or more glass gallon jugs, plastic liter (1, 2, 3) soda bottles, metal or wooden washboard, kazoos, metal thimbles (or teaspoons), metal tablespoons, tape, gutbucket supplies

VOCABULARY

gutbucket	washboard	spoons
kazoo	*glissando*	

◆ ◆ ◆ ◆ National Standards ◆ ◆ ◆ ◆

1a Sing accurately in large ensembles
2a Play instruments accurately in small ensembles
2c Perform instrumental music from diverse genres
3b Improvise melodic embellishments on given melodies
6b Listen and analyze uses of timbre in music from diverse genres
8b Identify ways music relates to science

MORE MUSIC CHOICES

For more songs to play with a jug band:

"Jambalaya," p. 244

"Paths of Victory," p. 195

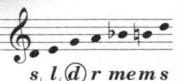

JUG BAND SOUNDS

Playing in a jug band is a fun way to make music using instruments that are easy to play. Gather together these instruments and learn to play them. Decide which instrument you will play in this jug band song.

Sing "Mama Don't 'Low." Imagine how the jug band accompaniment will sound.

CD 18–6

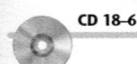

MAMA DON'T 'LOW

s, l (d) r mems

Folk Song from the United States

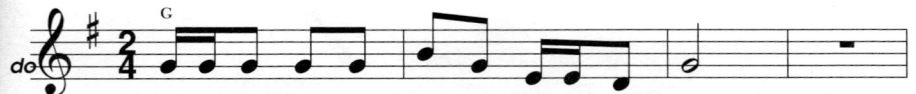

1. Ma-ma don't 'low no gui-tar play-in' 'round here,
2. Ma-ma don't 'low no ban-jo pick-in' 'round here,

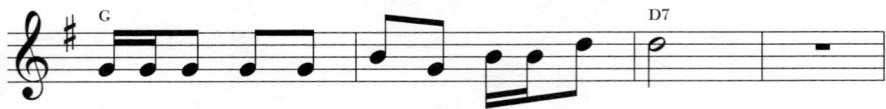

Ma-ma don't 'low no gui-tar play-in' 'round here,
Ma-ma don't 'low no ban-jo pick-in' 'round here,

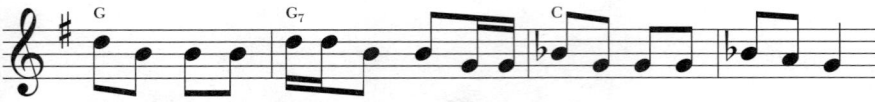

I don't care what Ma-ma don't 'low, Gon-na play my gui-tar an-y-how,
I don't care what Ma-ma don't 'low, Gon-na pick my ban-jo an-y-how,

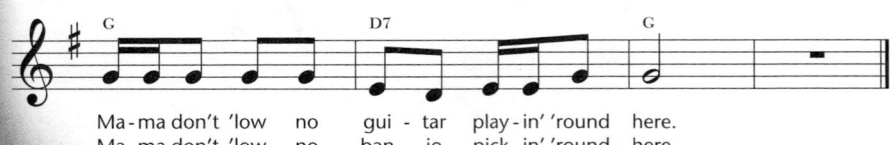

Ma-ma don't 'low no gui-tar play-in' 'round here.
Ma-ma don't 'low no ban-jo pick-in' 'round here.

(358)

Footnotes

TEACHER TO TEACHER

▶ **Safety Tips** For health reasons, students should not pass a jug from one to another unless there is an antiseptic available to spray and wipe the jug mouth after each use. If preferred, students could bring one-, two-, and three-liter plastic soda bottles. These are easier to collect, so more would be available in class. A small piece of masking tape will work well for students to label their bottles and their kazoos. Remind students that they should not use someone else's items.

BUILDING SKILLS THROUGH MUSIC

▶ **Math** Ask students to use ratios to report the results of the game activity in the Assessment. They could show the ratio of each team's correct answers compared to total questions asked or the ratio of how often each instrument was identified correctly or incorrectly.

SKILLS REINFORCEMENT

▶ **Guitar** Use the following chart to tune the guitar to open G for the "Mama Don't 'Low" activity in Skills Reinforcement on p. 361.

Tuning the Guitar to Open G						
String	1	2	3	4	5	6
Standard tuning	E	A	D	G	B	E
Adjustment	down 1	down 1	none	none	none	down 1
Open-G tuning	D	G	D	G	B	D

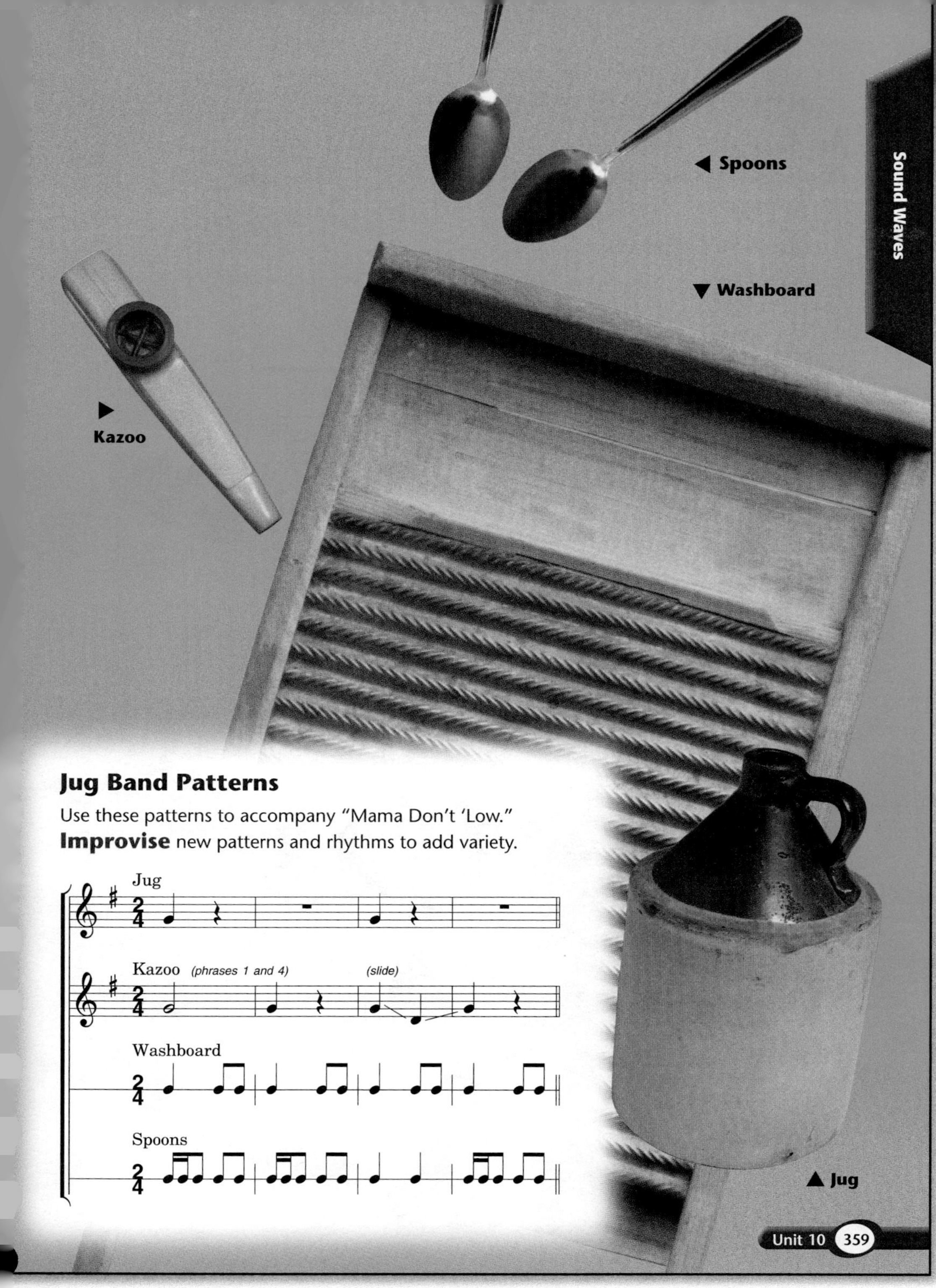

◀ Spoons

▼ Washboard

▶ Kazoo

Jug Band Patterns

Use these patterns to accompany "Mama Don't 'Low."
Improvise new patterns and rhythms to add variety.

▲ Jug

1 INTRODUCE

Invite students to share their experiences making musical instruments from kitchen articles such as pots, spoons, or graters. Share with students that people throughout history have used a variety of unlikely articles to create music. Tell them that in this lesson they will play some creative instruments as part of a jug band.

2 DEVELOP

Singing

Have students

- Sight-read, in rhythm, the words to "Mama Don't 'Low" in treble clef and duple meter.
- Listen to the recording **CD 18–6.**
- Echo sing each phrase of the song.

ASK If the instruments in a jug band were to play solos during "Mama Don't 'Low," in what measures should they play? (4, 8, and 16)

Have students sing "Mama Don't 'Low" with the recording, saying the words *solo, solo, solo* on each beat after the word *here* each time it occurs.

Playing

The Jug Students will use plastic soda bottles in the class jug band. To produce the "jug sound," follow these steps.

- Place the opening of the jug against the lower lip; keep the bottle against the body so it is vertical.
- Jut out the lower lip a little while pursing the lips. Don't pull your lips back tight against your teeth.
- Blow *across* the opening, not into it. Blow at the rim farthest from you.
- Experiment a little to get the best sound.

Have the students play their plastic soda bottles as an accompaniment to "Mama Don't 'Low." See Teacher to Teacher, p. 358, for safety tips.

continued on page 360

SKILLS REINFORCEMENT

▶ **Creating** After they have learned the song "Mama Don't 'Low," students should

- Gather together various jug band instruments.
- Discuss how this song has been used for generations to teach improvisation.
- Improvise an entire "verse" of the song after their instrument is called out during the previous verse.
- Expand upon standard jug band instruments to include "corpophones" (body percussion) and "found sounds" (natural sources such as tabletops, pencils) that can be used in their improvising.

SPOTLIGHT ON

▶ **Making a Gutbucket (Washtub Bass)** Using a large metal washtub turned upside down, drill or punch a small hole in the middle of the washtub. Add a washer on each side of the hole, insert an eyebolt (eye sticking up), and put a nut underneath to hold it securely. Take an old broom handle about 4–5 feet long and cut a V-shaped notch in the flat end so that it rests securely on the edge of the overturned washtub. Screw a small eye screw into the handle's rounded end and attach a clothesline rope between the end and the eyebolt.

To play a gutbucket bass, the player puts one foot on the tub to hold it in place, then uses the broom handle to tighten or loosen the string, which produces musical notes when plucked.

Washboard Ask students to watch as you place three to five metal thimbles on the fingers of your dominant hand and hold a metal washboard against your chest. (If metal thimbles are not available, use a teaspoon.) Have students

- Listen to the washboard part on p. 359.

- Take turns playing the washboard rhythm.

- Make interesting rhythms, using a combination of fingers and strumming motions. (Practice "air" washboard when it is someone else's turn.)

If a washboard is not available, a guiro can be used.

Kazoo If possible, have enough kazoos available so that every student can play his or her own. Tell students that a kazoo sounds best when the player sings, instead of blows, into it. Have students sing the kazoo part on p. 359, then practice the part.

 Students can improvise solos to be played during the vocally quiet parts of "Mama Don't 'Low." Suggest that kazoo solos start on the pitch sung on *here* and use pitches that just preceded it. For example, in measures 3–4, the solo would begin on G and also include E and D; in measures 7–8, the solo would begin on D and also use B.

Have students play their solos, including glissandos, as the class sings the song with the recording **CD 18–6.**

Spoons Have students practice the spoons rhythm on p. 359, patting their thighs. Demonstrate how to correctly play the spoons in Spotlight On below. For "Mama Don't 'Low," strike the spoons on every eighth note while singing. To play the sixteenth notes, hold the nondominant hand 6 inches above the thigh and alternate striking thigh and raised hand. Continue practicing the spoons part until students are confident.

Jug Band Guitar

The song "Mama Don't 'Low" has three basic guitar chords, shown below. **Play** a basic $\frac{2}{4}$ pattern with one strum on each beat.

Autoharp

Learn the G, D_7 and C chords on the Autoharp as part of the jug band accompaniment.

Gutbucket (Washtub Bass)

Making a gutbucket is a project for the adventurous. If you can't make one, you can play the "air" gutbucket. (The technique is the same as the "air" guitar.)

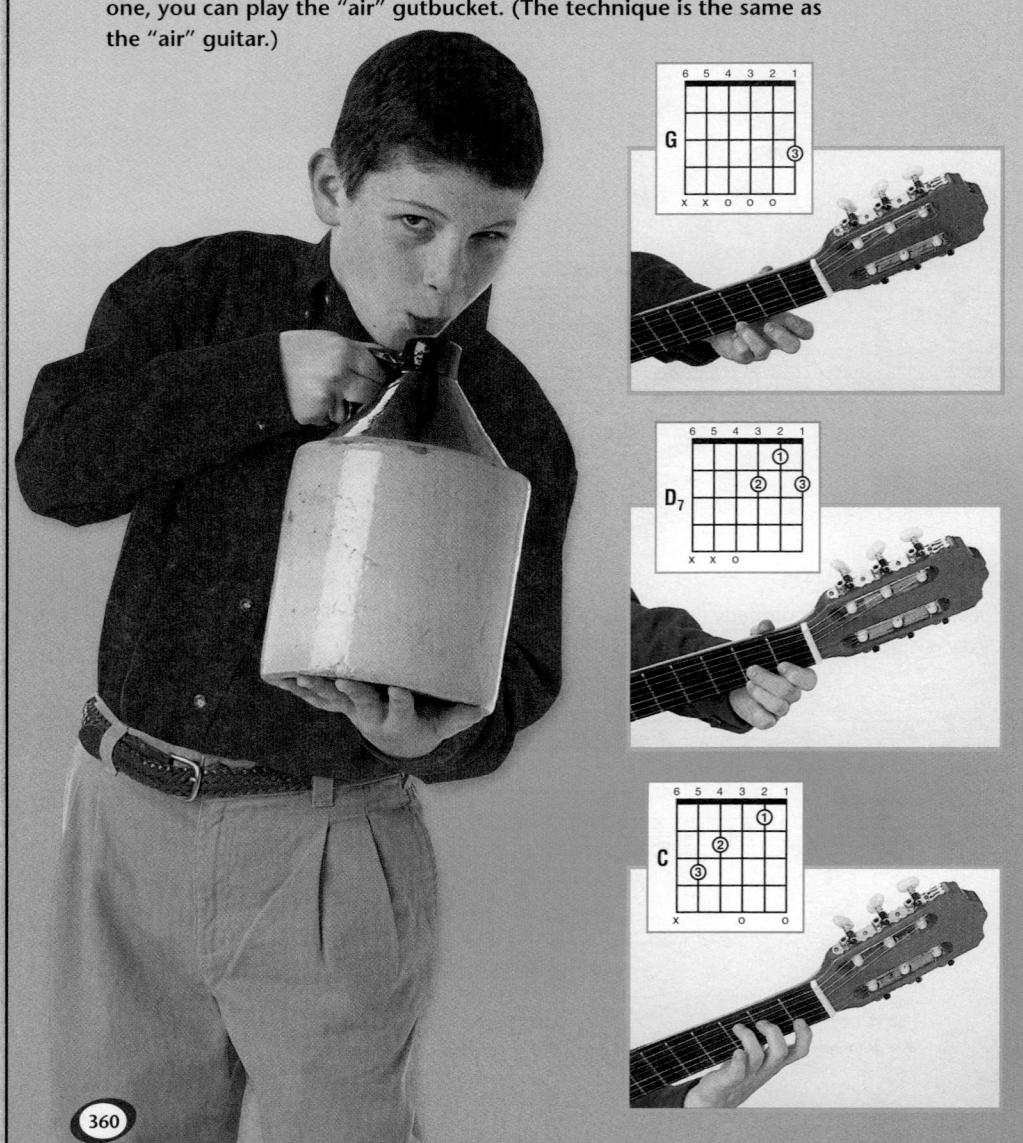

Footnotes

MOVEMENT

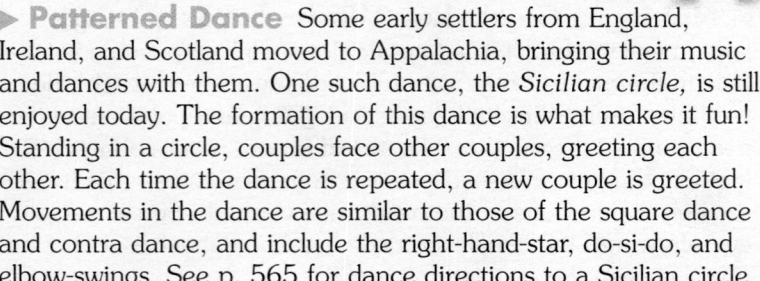

▶ **Patterned Dance** Some early settlers from England, Ireland, and Scotland moved to Appalachia, bringing their music and dances with them. One such dance, the *Sicilian circle,* is still enjoyed today. The formation of this dance is what makes it fun! Standing in a circle, couples face other couples, greeting each other. Each time the dance is repeated, a new couple is greeted. Movements in the dance are similar to those of the square dance and contra dance, and include the right-hand-star, do-si-do, and elbow-swings. See p. 565 for dance directions to a Sicilian circle for "Mama Don't 'Low."

 ▶ **Signing** Invite students to perform a signing interpretation to "Mama Don't 'Low." Refer to Resource Book, p. G–23.

SPOTLIGHT ON

▶ **Making Musical Spoons** Have students look at the picture of the spoons on p. 359. Demonstrate the creation of a spoons instrument by turning two metal tablespoons back-to-back and wrapping 1-inch duct tape several times around the ends of the spoon handles. Be sure to leave enough room between the handles to insert an index finger. Bend the spoons until the rounded parts almost touch.

▶ **Playing the Spoons** Demonstrate to students how to play the spoons. Insert the index finger between the handles about 2 inches up (or tape a small piece of wood between the handles). Then strike the spoon ends against the top of the thigh so that they click and spring back to the open position. Play rhythms between the thigh and the other hand.

Ready, Set, Play!

Your jug band is now ready.

Play a jug band accompaniment as you **sing** "Mama Don't 'Low." When you are ready, you can add some solos to the accompaniment as well.

Now that you have played in a jug band, **listen** to a professional jug band.

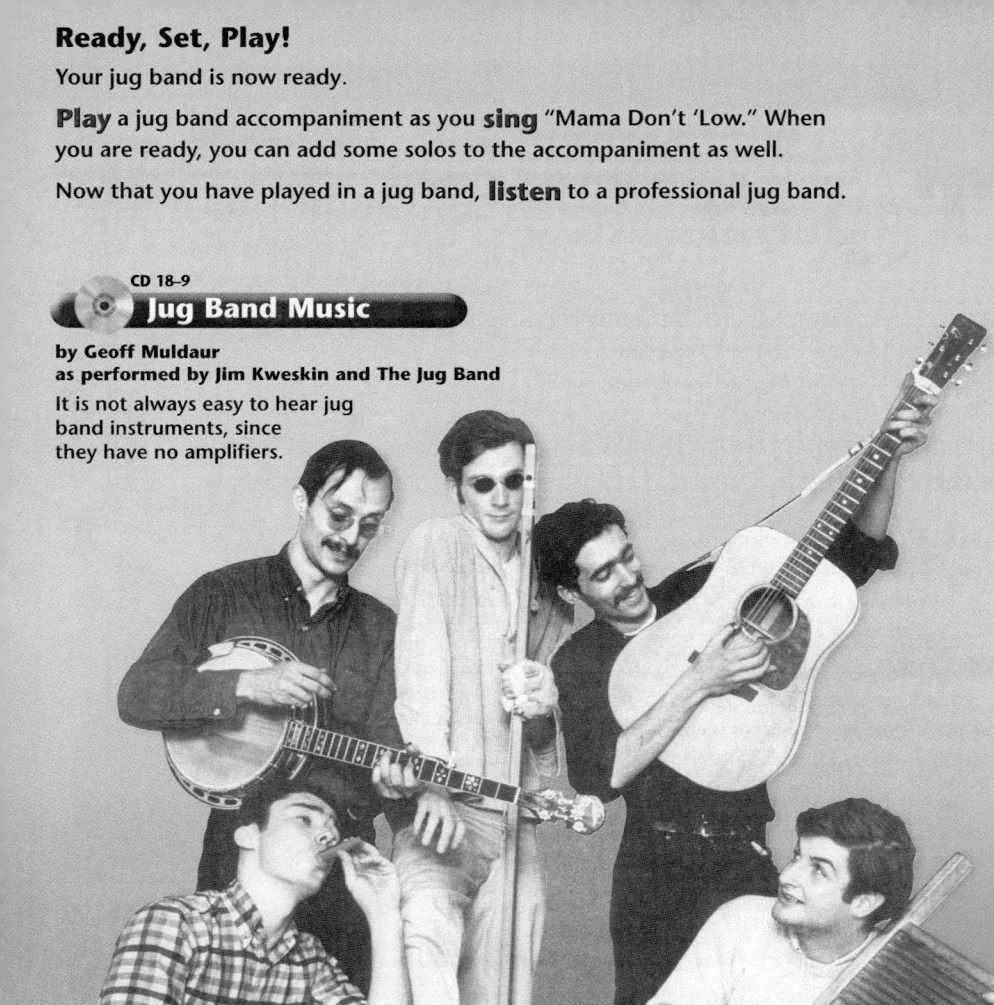

CD 18–9
Jug Band Music

by Geoff Muldaur
as performed by Jim Kweskin and The Jug Band

It is not always easy to hear jug band instruments, since they have no amplifiers.

Unit 10 **361**

Gutbucket (Washtub Bass) To make a gutbucket, see Spotlight On, p. 359. To play the gutbucket, put one foot on the far edge of the washtub to steady it. Tighten and loosen the rope or string to change pitch by pulling back on the handle as you pluck the "string."

Guitar and Autoharp Have students practice the chords on p. 360 (G, C, and D₇), on guitar and Autoharp. See Skills Reinforcement below and on p. 358 for guitar playing activities using open G tuning.

2a **Jug Band** Select six or more students to play in the jug band. Band instruments can include guitar, Autoharp, gutbucket, jug, soft washboards, soft spoons, and kazoos. Have students sing "Mama Don't 'Low" accompanied by the jug band. Have the jug band members play solos at the end of each verse. Allow all students to play in the band.

Listening

6b Have students listen to and identify the instruments in *Jug Band Music* by Geoff Muldaur, as performed by Jim Kweskin and The Jug Band **CD 18–9.**

3 CLOSE

Element: TIMBRE   ASSESSMENT

6b **Performance/Observation** Have students play Name That Instrument, in which they identify an instrument by its timbre. Divide the class into groups.

- Arrange the jug band instruments in a hidden area of the classroom.
- Play one of the jug band instruments and allow the first group 15 seconds to identify the instrument. If the group is successful, award it one point. If the group cannot successfully identify the instrument, ask the next group to identify it.
- Continue playing with each jug band instrument.

SKILLS REINFORCEMENT

2c ▶ **Guitar** On most guitars, the fifth and seventh frets are marked with a dot. When the guitar is tuned to open G, these frets can be used to play the C and D chords. The player can hold the guitar across the lap or on a desk or table. Hold a pen or pencil in the left hand and use it like a slider (as a slide-guitar player would) to produce the C and D chords to accompany "Mama Don't 'Low."

Slide-guitar players also use a device called a *bottleneck*, which is just what you would expect—the neck of a long bottle, cut off, sanded to remove rough edges, and slipped over the finger.

▶ **Recorder** Have students play the soprano recorder countermelody in Resource Book, p. I-25, to "Mama Don't 'Low."

SCHOOL TO HOME CONNECTION

▶ **Home "Found Sounds"** Encourage students to teach family and friends to play short rhythmic patterns on instruments found or created at home. Students could copy the words to "Mama Don't 'Low" and teach the melody or choose another familiar song. If possible, have students record the music-making session to share with the music class.

TECHNOLOGY/MEDIA LINK

Web Site Have students visit *www.sfsuccessnet.com* to learn more about jug and skiffle bands. Ask students to write a paragraph about the kinds of instruments in the bands and the kinds of music the bands play.

LESSON AT A GLANCE

Element Focus — **TIMBRE** Instrument families and timbre

Skill Objective — **LISTENING** Listen to and identify instrument timbres

Connection Activity — **SCIENCE** Discuss how instrument families create sound

MATERIALS

- *Uma história de Ifá* — CD 18–10
- *Galliard battaglia* — CD 18–11
- *The Hunt* — CD 18–12
- "Finale" from *Serenade for Strings in C,* Op. 48 (excerpt) — CD 18–13
- "Corta la caña" — CD 18–14
- "Head for the Canefields" — CD 18–15
  Recording Routine: Intro (8 m.); vocal; instrumental; vocal; coda
- **Pronunciation Practice/Translation** p. 536
- *Mi tierra* — CD 18–18
- *Wild Bull* (excerpt) — CD 18–19
- *Think* (excerpt) — CD 18–20
- **Resource Book** pp. A-27, C-6, I-26, I-27
- drums, recorders, guitars, wood block, kazoo, waxed paper, combs, soft drink bottles, PVC pipe, tone bells

VOCABULARY

membranophone	aerophone
chordophone	idiophone electrophone

◆ ◆ ◆ ◆ **National Standards** ◆ ◆ ◆ ◆

2a Play instruments accurately alone and in small ensembles
2c Perform instrumental music from diverse cultures
6b Listen and analyze uses of timbre in music from diverse genres
8b Identify ways music relates to science

MORE MUSIC CHOICES

For more songs with membranophones:
"Everybody Loves Saturday Night," p. 296
"By the Waters of Babylon," p. 311

Types of VIBRATIONS

An interesting way to group most instruments is by how they vibrate or oscillate. What are the ways in which an instrument begins its vibration? Membranophones, aerophones, idiophones, chordophones, and electrophones are all groups of instruments. Use the Sound Bank to look at photos and **listen** to the sound of each instrument.

Listen to the membranophones in *Uma história de Ifá.*

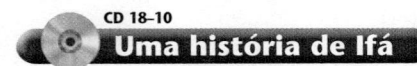
CD 18–10
Uma história de Ifá

by Ytthmar Tropicália and Rey Zulu as performed by Margareth Menezes
Membranophones provide an exciting introduction to this Afro-Brazilian music.

In the **membranophone** family, a stretched membrane or skin vibrates to produce sound. Membranophones include most drums. ▶

Listen to *Galliard battaglia* to hear members of the aerophone family.

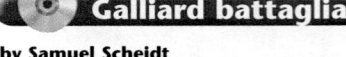
CD 18–11
Galliard battaglia

by Samuel Scheidt as performed by the Canadian Brass
This Baroque dance piece features two trumpets, French horn, trombone, and tuba. These instruments form the brass quintet.

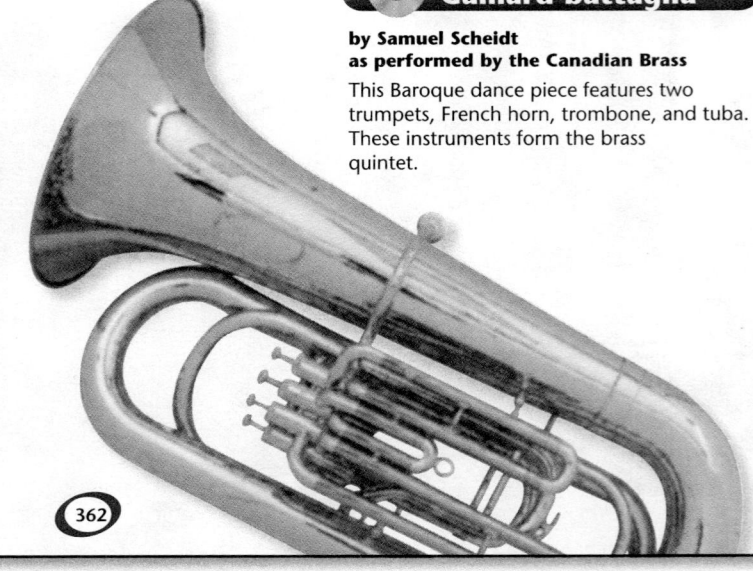

◀ In the **aerophone** family, an air column vibrates. Aerophones include woodwinds, brass, organs, and the human voice.

Footnotes

CULTURAL CONNECTION

▶ **Afro-Brazilian Music** This exciting music comes from Bahía, located in northeastern Brazil. It contains many African elements. The music is blended with native Brazilian music, making a vibrant sound. Afro-Brazilian music is characterized by the *agogo* rhythm, which is often tapped on a two-horned cowbell of the same name. It is also pounded on "deaf drums," which are the loud, low drums heard in *"Uma história de Ifá."*

BUILDING SKILLS THROUGH MUSIC

▶ **Reading** Using Resource Book p. C-6 (Semantic Map), have students organize the facts they read and learn about the classification system of organizing musical instruments in Across the Curriculum and Spotlight On. Divide the class into small groups. Give them teacher-made cards with each system name (idiophones, membranophones, etc.). Using index cards, have them classify classroom folk and orchestral instruments.

ACROSS THE CURRICULUM

8b ▶ **Science** Musicologists Sachs and Von Hornbostel came up with a classification system of organizing musical instruments by how they vibrated and produced sound. This classification assigned the following system names to the instrument families: idiophones, membranophones, chordophones, aerophones, and electrophones. The new system helps ethnomusicologists organize their study of world instruments and museums organize their collections of instruments. Previous classification of instruments was difficult: the percussion family was large and unorganized; instruments like the piano belonged to more than one family (strings, percussion). The Sachs and Von Hornbostel system solved these problems. The study of musical instruments and their classification is called *organology.*

Idiophones and Chordophones

Listen to Mickey Hart and five world-class percussionists play *The Hunt*. This piece uses percussion from around the world, such as *djembe*, jaw harp, drum set, *dundun*, *naal* bells, *tabla*, shakers, *ashiko*, *ngoma*, and *ghatam*.

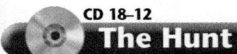

CD 18–12
The Hunt

by Mickey Hart and the Percussionists of Planet Drum

Woodblocks, bells, chimes, and other idiophones and membranophones are used in this piece.

Listen to Tchaikovsky's "Finale" from *Serenade for Strings in C* to hear chordophones.

CD 18–13
Finale

from *Serenade for Strings in C*, Opus 48 by Piotr Ilych Tchaikovsky

This exciting Russian dance shows off the string orchestra at its best.

▲ In the **idiophone** family, the body of the instrument vibrates. There are no strings or membranes. Cymbals, bells, and woodblocks are idiophones.

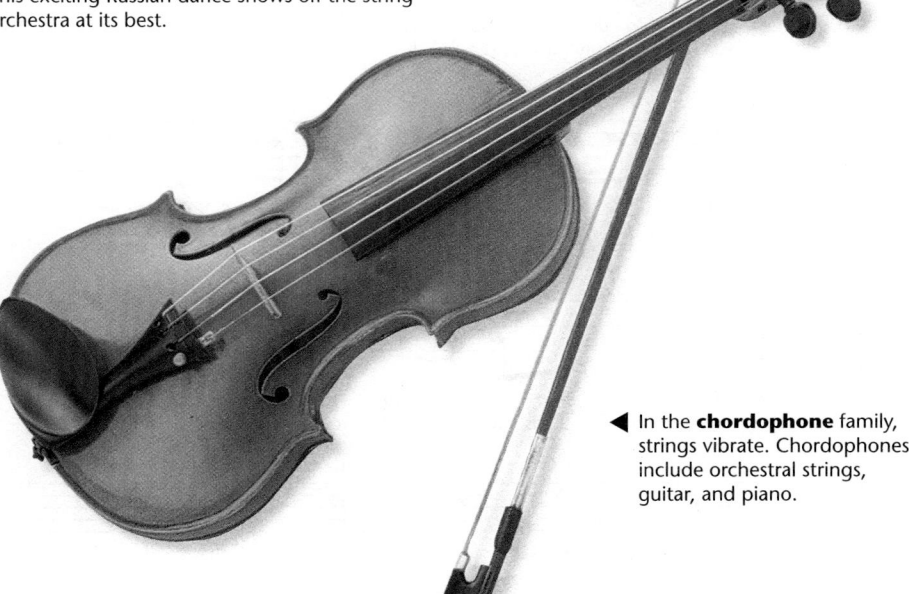

◄ In the **chordophone** family, strings vibrate. Chordophones include orchestral strings, guitar, and piano.

Unit 10 **363**

Sound Waves

---

1 INTRODUCE

Ask students to name the families of musical instruments. (Answers will include woodwinds, brass, strings, percussion.) Ask them to name the piano's family. (chordophone; percussion/strings is traditional classification) Share with students information on the classification of instruments in Across the Curriculum on p. 362 and Spotlight On below.

2 DEVELOP

Listening

8b
6b
Membranophones Ask students to describe a *membrane*. (Guide them to understand that a membrane is a thin, soft, pliable sheet of material.) Then share with students that *-phone* is an English suffix that comes from the Greek word for "sound."

SAY Remember that a musical instrument's sound is produced by vibration.

ASK How does an instrument in the membranophone family produce sound? (by the vibration of a stretched membrane or skin)

What instruments are called membranophones? (most drums)

Have students play several drums and observe the vibrations of the drum skins.

Open a kazoo and show students the membrane. Then, distribute a comb to each student. (If there are not enough combs for all, the teacher can demonstrate the activity.) Have students

- Put waxed paper around a comb and sing into it as they would into a kazoo.

- Choose a partner and observe the waxed paper as their partner plays the "comb kazoo."

continued on page 364

SPOTLIGHT ON

▶ **Instrument Sound Groups**

Membranophones—Struck, rattled, friction drums; the membrane is vibrated by a stick or cord (*cuica,* lion's roar), and singing membranes, such as those of kazoos.

Idiophones—Struck, such as castanets, claves, xylophones, guiros, and friction idiophones (sandpaper blocks).

Chordophones—Zithers, such as Autoharps and kotos; lutes, such as violins, guitars, and mandolins; harps.

Aerophones—Harmonica, flutes, reed pipes, trumpets, trombone, and *didgeridoo*.

Electrophones—Synthesizers and MIDI controllers for keyboards, microphones, and strings; electronic enhancement on guitars and electric basses.

SKILLS REINFORCEMENT

▶ **Recorder** Students can play a countermelody to "*Corta la caña*" on the alto recorder. See Resource Book p. I–26 for the accompaniment and a review of the alto fingerings for C, D, F, and G.

Students can also play an accompaniment to "*Corta la caña*" on the soprano recorder. See Resource Book p. I–27 for this accompaniment and a review of the soprano fingerings for D, G, and A.

Unit 10 *Sound Waves* **363**

Invite students to listen to the membranophones in *Uma história de Ifá* **CD 18–10.** Share information on Afro-Brazilian music from Cultural Connection on p. 362.

Another example of the snare drum sound can be found in the Sound Bank, beginning on p. 512.

Listening

 Aerophones Invite students to explain how an aerophone creates sound. (the vibration of an air column) Challenge students to list members of the aerophone family without consulting the textbook. (woodwinds, brass, organs, human voice) Then, have students read p. 362 to check their lists. Based on the number of aerophones in the classroom, invite volunteers to

- Blow across a soft-drink bottle to simulate playing a flute.
- Play a recorder to demonstrate how most woodwinds produce sound.
- Make the "raspberry" sound (see Lesson 2, p. 359) while blowing into a PVC pipe to demonstrate how brass instruments produce sound.
- Listen to the aerophones in *Galliard battaglia* **CD 18–11.**

Visit the Sound Bank, beginning on p. 512, to hear another example of the tuba.

Chordophones Share with students that the Latin word *chorda* means "string." Challenge students to list instruments that can be classified as chordophones. (the orchestral string family, piano families, guitar)

Invite volunteers to play the guitar as the class observes the vibrating guitar strings.

Have students listen to the chordophones in *Finale* **CD 18–13.**

SAY You know that in order to produce sound, an instrument has to vibrate.

ASK **What part of an idiophone vibrates?** (The body of the instrument vibrates.)

A Working Song

Sing "*Corta la caña*," a Puerto Rican song that uses an interesting mixture of idiophones, membranophones, and chordophones in its accompaniment.
Identify which instruments are used.

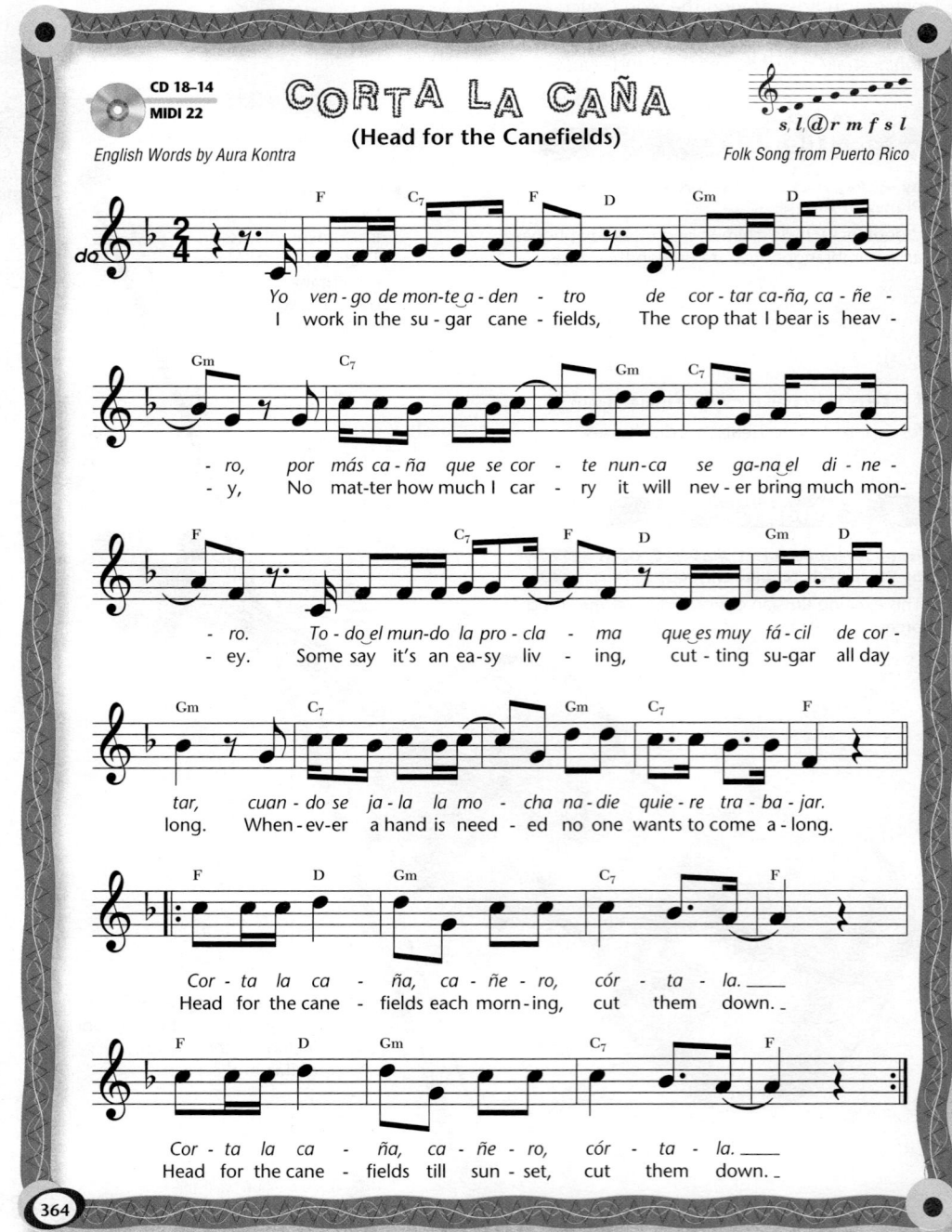

364

Footnotes

CULTURAL CONNECTION

▶ **How to Make a Diddley Bow** In the southern United States, a form of simple zither, called the diddley bow, is actually a string stretched across the side of a barn. We will substitute a long plank for the barn. Partially insert an eye screw into each end of the plank about three inches from the end, attach the ends of a wire firmly to each screw, and slide a small spice jar under each end of the wire near each screw to form bridges for the string. Tighten the screws until the wire sounds a clear pitch; change pitch by using a third spice jar as a "bottleneck," moving it up and down. Either bow or pluck with a pick. For more amplification and resonance, place the diddley bow on a hollow wooden box or tabletop.

ACROSS THE CURRICULUM

▶ **Language Arts/Social Studies** Share with students *A Migrant Family* by Larry Dane Brimner (Lerner Publications, 1992), which is a thoughtful portrayal of the life of a family whose members make their living working the fields.

CHARACTER EDUCATION

▶ **Perseverance** Discuss the scenario of typical migrant workers. What characteristics might they develop as a result of their life experiences (hard-work ethic, appreciation for money, industriousness, following through with commitments, responsibility, willingness to work hard in exchange for a reward, value of community and family)? What life experiences have shaped your character and beliefs?

Latin Rhythms

Gloria Estefan is one of the premiere performers of Latin music. **Listen** to *Mi tierra* (My Homeland). It is a song about missing the Cuban homeland. **Listen** for the pattern that the *conga* plays.

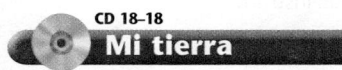

CD 18–18
Mi tierra

by Estefano
as performed by Gloria Estefan

Mi tierra has the quick tempo, continuous eighth-note rhythms, *conga* rhythms, and brass punctuation characteristic of Latin music.

Conga Rhythms

The *conga* drum is important in Latin music. *Congas* are most often played in pairs (low-high). They provide the rhythmic basis of Puerto Rican and Cuban music. Sometimes these rhythms are similar to *mambo* rhythms.

Learn and **play** the following rhythms in the *mambo* style. When you are ready, **play** along with *Mi tierra*. Later, **create** and **improvise** new *mambo* rhythms on your favorite instrument.

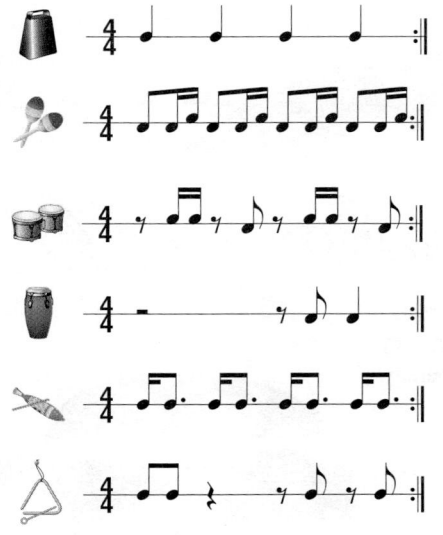

Gloria Estefan ▼

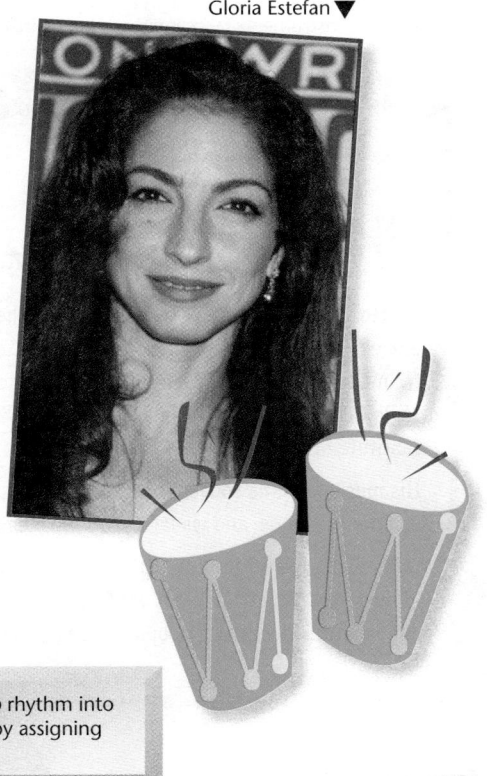

Sequencing Software Input the *mambo* rhythm into the sequencing software. Explore timbre by assigning different instruments to the rhythm.

Unit 10 **365**

Have students

- Play the woodblocks, cymbals, and other wood and metal objects available in the classroom.
- Listen to the idiophones in *The Hunt* **CD 18–12** and make a list of them.
- Find and play various metal and wood objects from home.

Singing

Have students

- Listen for idiophones, membranophones, and chordophones in *"Corta la caña"* **CD 18–14.**
- Find the challenging rhythm patterns in the song, including the sixteenth-eighth-sixteenth note patterns and dotted rests.
- Echo speak each phrase in English as you model it.
- Sing the English version of *"Corta la caña"* several times with the recording **CD 18–15.**

ASK How are the melodies in phrases 1 and 2 similar? (Phrase 2 is a sequence of phrase 1; it is the same melody one step higher than phrase 1.)

Have students

- Use the Pronunciation Practice Guide on p. 536, Resource Book p. A-27, and the Pronunciation Practice **CD 18–17** to teach students the Spanish lyrics of *"Corta la caña."*
- Sing *"Corta la caña"* in Spanish with the recording **CD 18–14.**
- Play two recorder accompaniments to *"Corta la caña"* on Resource Book pp. I-26 and I-27.

Listening

6b Separate the class into three groups: the aerophones, the membranophones, and the chordophones. Tell the groups that they will hear *Mi tierra,* a Cuban song.

Have the groups listen to *Mi tierra* **CD 18–18** and raise their hands when they hear instruments from their group's family in the accompaniment.

continued on page 366

SPOTLIGHT ON

▶ **The Performer** Gloria Estefan is one of the most successful Latin American singers today. Her music is widely recognized as being a blend of Cuban and American popular styles. Her album *Mi tierra* ("My Homeland") is all Spanish (with English translation) and offers a variety of contemporary pop and rock music in the Latin style.

Gloria Estefan supports music education in a variety of ways, including allowing her music to be used in classroom publications. She is a special person in addition to being a major pop star of this generation.

Invite students to discuss the music and message of *Mi tierra.* Students may wish to sing Estefan's "The Rhythm Is Gonna Get You," on p. 348.

SKILLS REINFORCEMENT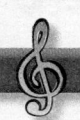

▶ **Playing** Encourage students to use a MIDI keyboard that has auto-accompaniment as they explore and play Cuban or Latin rhythms that are similar in style to those of *Mi tierra.* Have them play auto-accompaniment rhythms and one-finger chord accompaniments in meter in 4. Let them explore different chord patterns and changing tempos.

▶ **Creating** Ask advanced students to create a Latin rhythm dance beat, using a MIDI keyboard and sequencing software. They should begin by creating a basic rhythm for a Latin percussion instrument. Have them add new rhythms, one by one, until the layered patterns are a solid dance beat in Latin style.

Listening

ASK In *Mi tierra,* which instrument families can be heard most clearly? (chordophones—bass, guitar, keyboard; aerophones—brass; membranophones—drums)

Playing

Ask students to look at the mambo rhythm for *Mi tierra.* Have students learn the parts by using rhythm syllables. Have the groups

- Listen to *Mi tierra* **CD 18–18.**
- Play their percussion instruments with the recording.
- Experiment with Latin rhythms, as suggested in Skills Reinforcement on p. 365.

Listening

Electrophones Share with students that electrophones, like the other instrument families, produce sound through vibration. But, unlike the other families, electrophones use an oscillating (or vibrating) current transmitted through speakers to produce a sound. If possible, demonstrate the sound of an electronic keyboard or electric guitar. Have students

- Listen to *Wild Bull* **CD 18–19,** an electronic music composition by Morton Subotnick.
- Discuss how composers create electronic music.
- Read about the composer.

Dance and Techno Music Share with students the example of dance and techno music. Have students listen to *Think* **CD 18–20** by Paul Robb and Information Society.

ASK What sound source do you hear? (synthesizer)

How do you create a dance beat? (Create a basic rhythm for one instrument; layer new rhythms for other instruments on top of each other; and build to a powerful dance beat.)

Electrophones

Electrophones are electronic instruments. Instead of acoustic vibrations, sound is created by an oscillating current. When these waveforms are transmitted through speakers, we hear musical sound.

The electrophone family includes most contemporary electronic instruments such as synthesizers, drum machines, and samplers.

Electronic Music From a Pioneer

"Electronic music" is a genre of music composition that was prominent in the 1970s and 1980s. Composers began to write electronic music because electronic instruments were manufactured by Robert Moog, Donald Buchla, and Arp Instruments. Morton Subotnick is an important composer in electronic music.

Listen to *Wild Bull,* an electronic music composition by Subotnick. What musical timbres do you hear? Discuss how composers created electronic music.

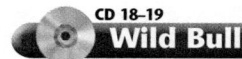

CD 18–19
Wild Bull

by Morton Subotnick
These electronic sounds were created by early electronic instruments (some with no keyboard).

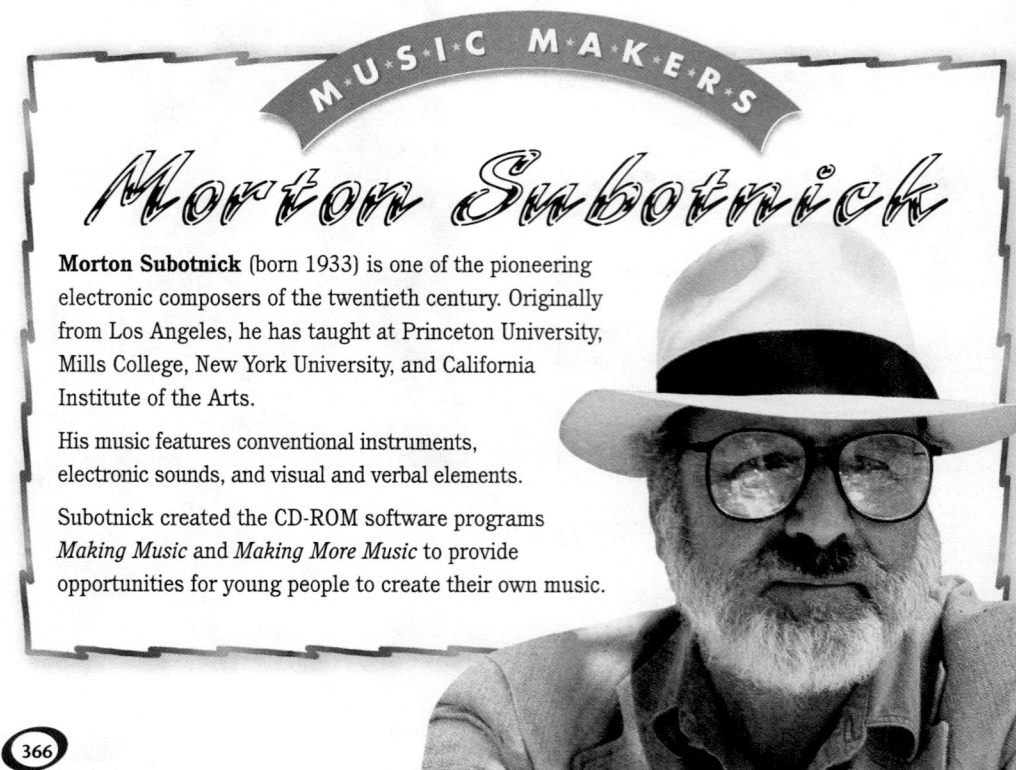

M·U·S·I·C M·A·K·E·R·S

Morton Subotnick

Morton Subotnick (born 1933) is one of the pioneering electronic composers of the twentieth century. Originally from Los Angeles, he has taught at Princeton University, Mills College, New York University, and California Institute of the Arts.

His music features conventional instruments, electronic sounds, and visual and verbal elements.

Subotnick created the CD-ROM software programs *Making Music* and *Making More Music* to provide opportunities for young people to create their own music.

366

Footnotes

SKILLS REINFORCEMENT

▶ **Keyboard** The traditional piano keyboard is a chordophone (it has strings that vibrate). The piano is a wonderful accompaniment instrument. Ask students to explore how accompaniments can be created for songs by using broken chords.

Begin by selecting a song with simple chords and notating the chord names as a chord progression (similar to a lead sheet). Then, write the notes for each chord (use simple triads). Finally, improvise a rhythm pattern that fits the song, using the broken notes of each chord. Remind students that this process is similar to how keyboard players perform in bands.

TEACHER TO TEACHER

▶ **Careers in Music** Share with students some of the scholarly, scientific, and technical music careers that are related to instruments. Have students describe the music-related vocations and avocations in their music journals.

Instrument Maker—An artisan who makes musical instruments by hand.

Musicologist—A person who studies music history.

Acoustician—A person who studies the science of acoustics. This knowledge is used in the design of instruments.

Recording Engineer—A person who studies and practices the science and art of recording music.

New Electronics

Electronic instruments developed from their early beginnings to today's sophisticated synthesizers, keyboards, computers, samplers, and digital music systems. Today, much of the world's pop and commercial music is created using electronics.

Techno and dance music is sometimes created, or mixed, by DJs using electronic equipment. It can also be created in a traditional recording studio using synthesizers and other electronic keyboards. The result is the same—exciting pop electronic music.

Dance and Techno Music

Dance and techno music is a worldwide phenomenon. Singers, musicians, DJs, and producers in countries all over the planet are producing music that has a great beat and is fun to dance to.

Listen to *Think*, an example of techno and dance music. The music is performed by the group Information Society. **Identify** the electronic sounds as they occur in the music.

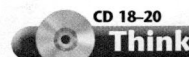
CD 18–20
Think

by Paul Robb
as performed by Information Society

The steady dance beat, electronic rhythms, and melodic "hooks" are characteristic of dance and techno music.

A recording engineer creating a "mix" in a Nashville recording studio ▼

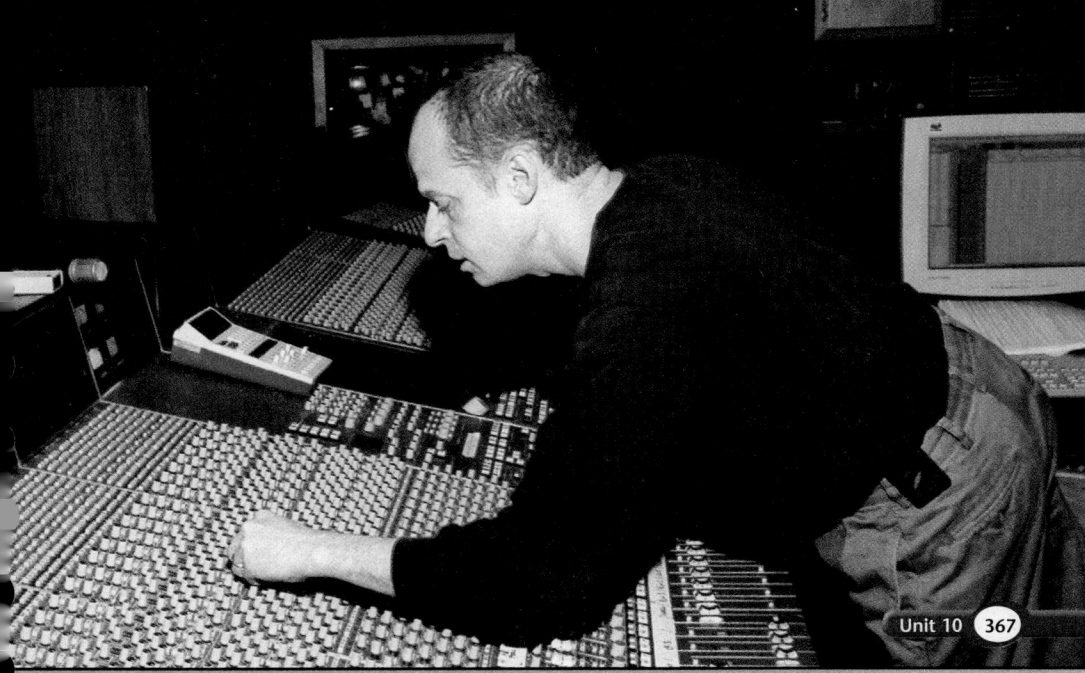

Sound Waves

Ask students to identify (and play) the melodic hook that repeats in the song. Relate to students that keyboards are important in this music. See Skills Reinforcement on p. 366.

3 CLOSE

Element: TIMBRE | **ASSESSMENT**

Observation Organize the class into groups of five or six and tell students that their groups will be playing Name That Family, in which they will identify an instrument by its timbre. Have students listen as you play an instrument sound from the Sound Bank (see list below). Allow the first group 15 seconds to

- Identify the instrument. (5 points)
- Decide what vibrates on the instrument. (10 points)
- Identify the family or families (idiophone, membranophone, chordophone, aerophone, or electrophone) to which the instrument belongs. (20 points)

Continue with an example of these instruments:

snare drum—membranophone **CD 23–38;**

trombone—aerophone **CD 23–45;**

violin—chordophone **CD 23–48;** and

synthesizer—electrophone **CD 23–41.**

ACROSS THE CURRICULUM

▶ **Science** (Note: This experiment requires very careful handling of sharp items.) Remind students that oboes, bassoons, and English horns require the vibrations of a double reed to produce sound. For a class project, make a soda-straw double reed, pinching one end of the straw so it has creases on each side of the pinched end. Use scissors to cut ¼" down the crease on each side of the straw. Have a volunteer attempt to play the straw. Place the "double reed" far enough into the mouth so that the lips are not touching the reed, breathe very deeply, and blow hard. The resulting sound is rather like a duck's call. Have students demonstrate the three "Ls" of pitch by snipping off pieces of the straw's open end to hear the pitch rise.

SCHOOL TO HOME CONNECTION

▶ **Homemade Instruments** Invite students to create and bring to class their homemade versions of idiophones, membranophones, chordophones, and aerophones. Separate the class into the four instrument sound groups. Encourage students to name their instruments and demonstrate range and variety of sounds. Create a class composition, using these instruments.

TECHNOLOGY/MEDIA LINK

Web Site Have students go to *www.sfsuccessnet.com* for information on instruments and how they produce sound.

LESSON AT A GLANCE

Element Focus   **RHYTHM** Backbeat/dance beat/techno beat

Skill Objective   **CREATING** Create a dance mix for a listening selection

Connection Activity   **STYLE** Explore dance and techno styles

MATERIALS
- *This Is Your Night* (excerpt)   **CD 18–21**
- *This Is Your Night* (Dance Mix) (excerpt)   **CD 18–22**
- **Resource Book** pp. J-13, J-14
- bell, low drum, medium drum, high drums, rattles, snare, bongos, congas, bass drum, scraper, synthesizer, bass

VOCABULARY

dance   techno   disco   new wave

◆ ◆ ◆ ◆ **National Standards** ◆ ◆ ◆ ◆

2a Play instruments accurately in small ensembles
5a Read whole notes, quarter notes, eighth notes, sixteenth notes, and dotted rhythms in duple meter
6b Listen and analyze uses of rhythm in music from diverse cultures
7b Students use specific criteria for evaluating their own compositions

MORE MUSIC CHOICES

For more African drumming examples playable with *This Is Your Night*:

Drum Ensemble 1, p. 281

Drum Ensemble 2, p. 289

1 INTRODUCE

SAY Have you ever watched a disc jockey (DJ) work—using turntables to mix rhythms from several sources? In this lesson we will apply the backbeat idea to dance and techno music and explore these two styles.

Dance and TECHNO Beats

"Dance" and "techno" music share similar traits: they both have a strong beat, they are sometimes mixed "live" by DJs, they use repeated patterns called "loops," technology is important (electronic keyboards, sampler boxes, computers, digital audio), and the music is for dancing. Dance and techno evolved from disco in the 1970s and new wave in the 1980s.

The Beat

Dance and techno have these musical elements: a strong emphasis on each beat, accents on beats 2 and 4, powerful bass, and repeated melodic patterns. The backbeat rhythm is the foundation of many dance and techno beats.

Listen to the song *This Is Your Night*. **Identify** the musical elements.

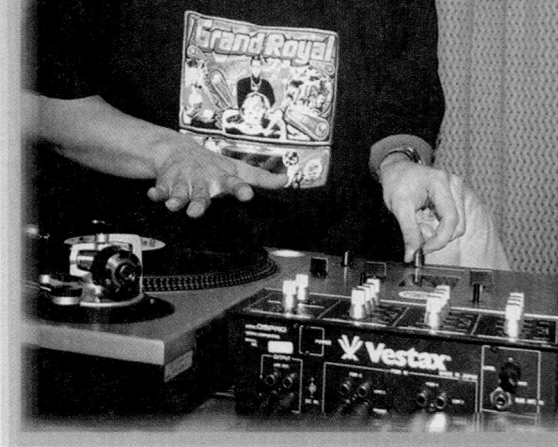

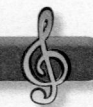 **CD 18–21**
This Is Your Night

by Amber and the Berman Brothers as performed by Amber

The strong disco-like beat, electronic instruments, and repetitive melody make this music great for dancing and singing.

◀ A DJ creates a "live" mix.

Footnotes

ACROSS THE CURRICULUM

▶ **Language Arts** When your students have mastered the concept of backbeat, encourage them to develop their own body percussion, movement, and vocal sound backbeats to be performed with original humorous rhyming poetry, limericks, or other rhyming verse.

BUILDING SKILLS THROUGH MUSIC

▶ **Writing** Have students write a description of their dance mix, including what elements they chose, what order they used them in, and a self-evaluation of its effectiveness.

SKILLS REINFORCEMENT

▶ **Playing** Add these African drumming rhythms to the recording of *This Is Your Night* (Dance Mix) **CD 18–22**.

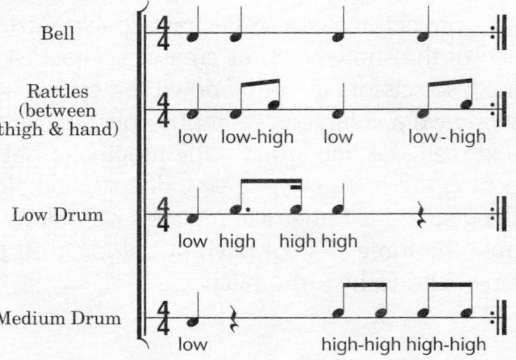

Loops, Layers, and Rhythms

How do you compose or "mix" dance or techno? One recipe is to take some dance rhythms, loop them so that they repeat, and add a bass line and some melodic motives. Finally, layer them and mix.

Below are some elements used in the mix of *This Is Your Night*. **Perform** the rhythms, bass line, melody patterns, and chords on rhythm and keyboard instruments. Then **listen** to the "dance mix" and **describe** how the parts are layered. Finally, **create** a new dance mix from these parts.

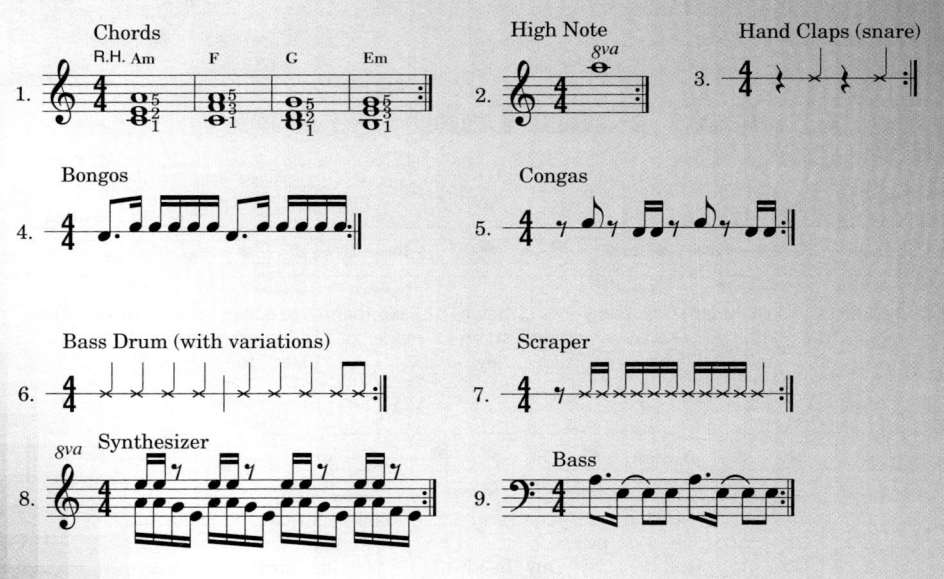

Chords

Bongos

Bass Drum (with variations)

Synthesizer

High Note

Congas

Scraper

Hand Claps (snare)

Bass

CD 18–22
This Is Your Night (Dance Mix)

as mixed by "Junior" Vasquez

The introduction to this dance number layers the dance rhythms, bass, harmony, and melodic patterns to create a dance mix.

MIDI Sequencing Software Use sequencing software to create a new "dance mix" for *This Is Your Night*.

Unit 10 **369**

2 DEVELOP

Moving

Invite students to listen and move to the recording of *This Is Your Night* **CD 18–21**, using small steps, left–together–right–together. Then, add a soft clap pattern on beat 2 and a subdivided clap (♪ ♪) on beat 4.

Listening

Ask students to listen again to the recording of *This Is Your Night* **CD 18–21** and identify and discuss each dance style element they hear. (strong disco beat, electronic instruments, repeated melody)

Playing

Ask students to play the African drumming rhythms (see Skills Reinforcement, p. 368) along with *This Is Your Night* **CD 18–21**.

Creating

Help students to

- Play the chords, rhythms, bass line, and melody patterns on p. 369.

- Listen again to the selection **CD 18–21** and discuss how the parts are layered in this techno version.

- Create a dance mix of their own, arranging the rhythmic and melodic phrases on p. 369. See Resource Book pp. J–13 and J–14, and Technology/Media Link below.

See Spotlight On below for a history of techno.

3 CLOSE

Element: RHYTHM — **ASSESSMENT**

Performance/Peer Critique Have students play their new dance mix for the class. After each performance, have classmates critique the dance mix with regard to danceability, new use of elements, and use of backbeat.

SPOTLIGHT ON

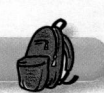

▶ **Techno Historical Benchmarks** You may wish to have students make time lines.

1920   Leon Theremin invents the Theremin, an early synthesizer.

1960   Robert Moog introduces the first analog synthesizer.

1970   Kraftwerk, the first electronic band, arrives.

1970s   Soul, disco, punk established; new wave begins.

1980s   House music/DJs; noise; ambient styles.

1987   Techno arrives. Later techno variations include global house nation, neo-techno, ambient wave, breakbeat, and trance.

SCHOOL TO HOME CONNECTION

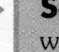

▶ **Radio** Ask students to listen to radio stations at home to evaluate the quality of the music, and determine which plays the best dance music. Students may take notes on dance elements of songs from each station and report their findings to the class.

TECHNOLOGY/MEDIA LINK

Sequencing Software Students may use sequencing software to create a dance mix, composing patterns for rhythm, bass, and melody lines.

LESSON AT A GLANCE

Element Focus   **MELODY** Folk melodies

Skill Objectives   **PLAYING** Play folk melodies from three different cultures on the recorder

Connection Activity   **GENRE** Examine the recorder as a solo and an accompaniment instrument

MATERIALS

- "Boil Them Cabbage Down"   **CD 19–1**

  Recording Routine: Intro (2 m.); refrain; v. 1; refrain; interlude (4 m.); refrain; v. 2; refrain; coda

- "Worried Man Blues"   **CD 19–3**

  Recording Routine: Intro (8 m.); refrain; v. 1; refrain; interlude (8 m.); v. 2; refrain; coda

- "Skye Boat Song"   **CD 19–5**

  Recording Routine: Intro (8 m.); refrain; v. 1; refrain; v. 2; refrain; coda

- **Resource Book** pp. F-32, I-28

- recorders for all students

VOCABULARY

aerophone   skeleton melody

◆ ◆ ◆ National Standards ◆ ◆ ◆ ◆

1a Sing accurately in large ensembles

2a Play instruments accurately alone and in large ensembles

4c Compose, using electronic media

5a Read dotted notes in duple and triple meter

7b Students use specific criteria for evaluating performances, and offer constructive suggestions for improvement

MORE MUSIC CHOICES

For more songs that are easy to play on recorder:

"Four Strong Winds," p. 170

"Nana Kru," p. 282

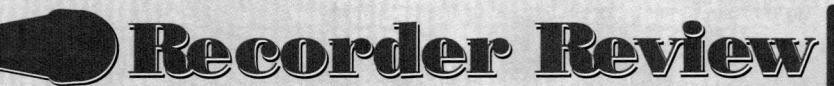
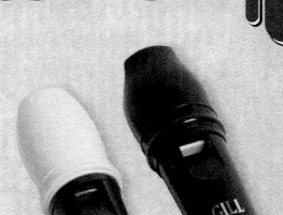

Recorder Review

Review the finger positions below for the recorder. **Sing** and **play** recorder on "Boil Them Cabbage Down." Some of you can **sing** the melody, while others **play** the recorder.

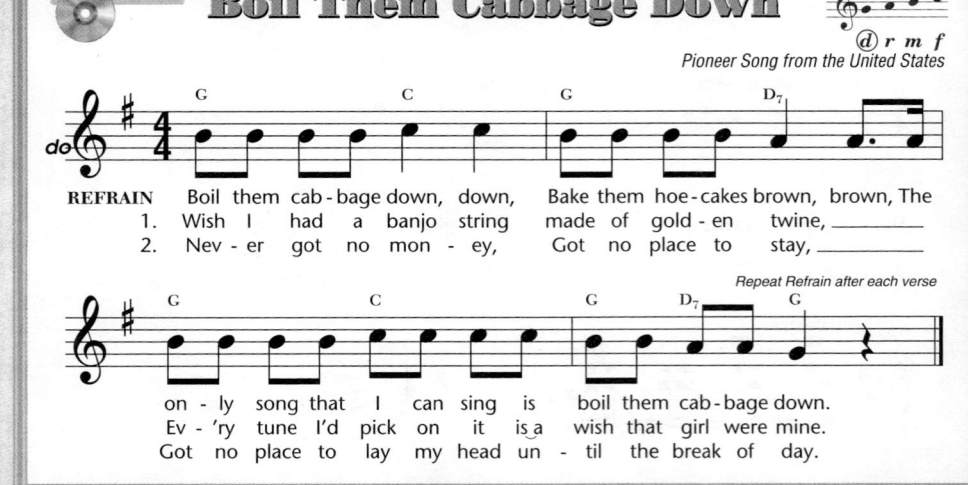

CD 19–1 Boil Them Cabbage Down

Pioneer Song from the United States

REFRAIN: Boil them cab-bage down, down, Bake them hoe-cakes brown, brown, The
1. Wish I had a banjo string made of gold-en twine, _____
2. Nev-er got no mon-ey, Got no place to stay, _____

Repeat Refrain after each verse

on-ly song that I can sing is boil them cab-bage down.
Ev-'ry tune I'd pick on it is a wish that girl were mine.
Got no place to lay my head un-til the break of day.

Recorder Fingerings

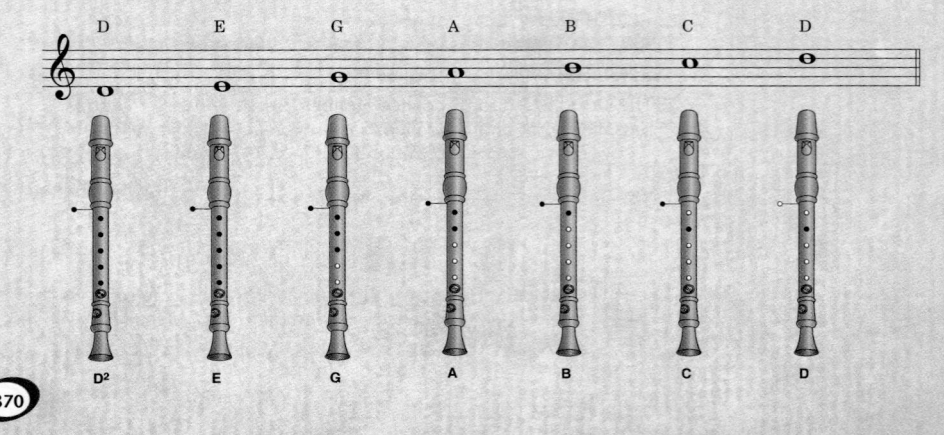

D   E   G   A   B   C   D

D²   E   G   A   B   C   D

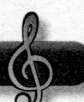

Footnotes

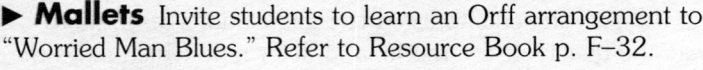 ▶ **Mallets** Invite students to learn an Orff arrangement to "Worried Man Blues." Refer to Resource Book p. F–32.

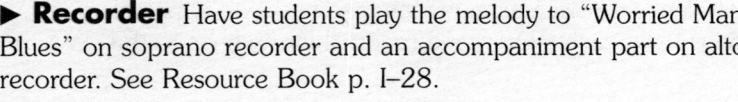 ▶ **Recorder** Have students play the melody to "Worried Man Blues" on soprano recorder and an accompaniment part on alto recorder. See Resource Book p. I–28.

BUILDING SKILLS THROUGH MUSIC

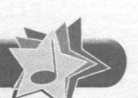

▶ **Language** After learning "Skye Boat Song," ask students to identify the setting, and what they believe to be the plot of the lyrics. Ask them to support their answers with text evidence.

SKILLS REINFORCEMENT

 ▶ **Recorder** Encourage students to play the alto recorder. To assist students in the transition, relate the alto recorder fingering to that of the soprano recorder.

2a

- C on the alto is the same as G on the soprano.
- D on the alto is the same as A on the soprano.

Have students play the ostinato below on alto recorder as an accompaniment to "Boil Them Cabbage Down."

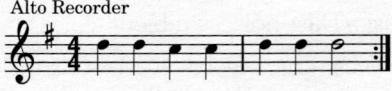

Alto Recorder

Visit the Sound Bank, beginning on p. 512, to hear the recorder.

Dot the Quarter

Sing and **play** "Worried Man Blues," a song about the effect of the Great Depression on people in the 1930s.

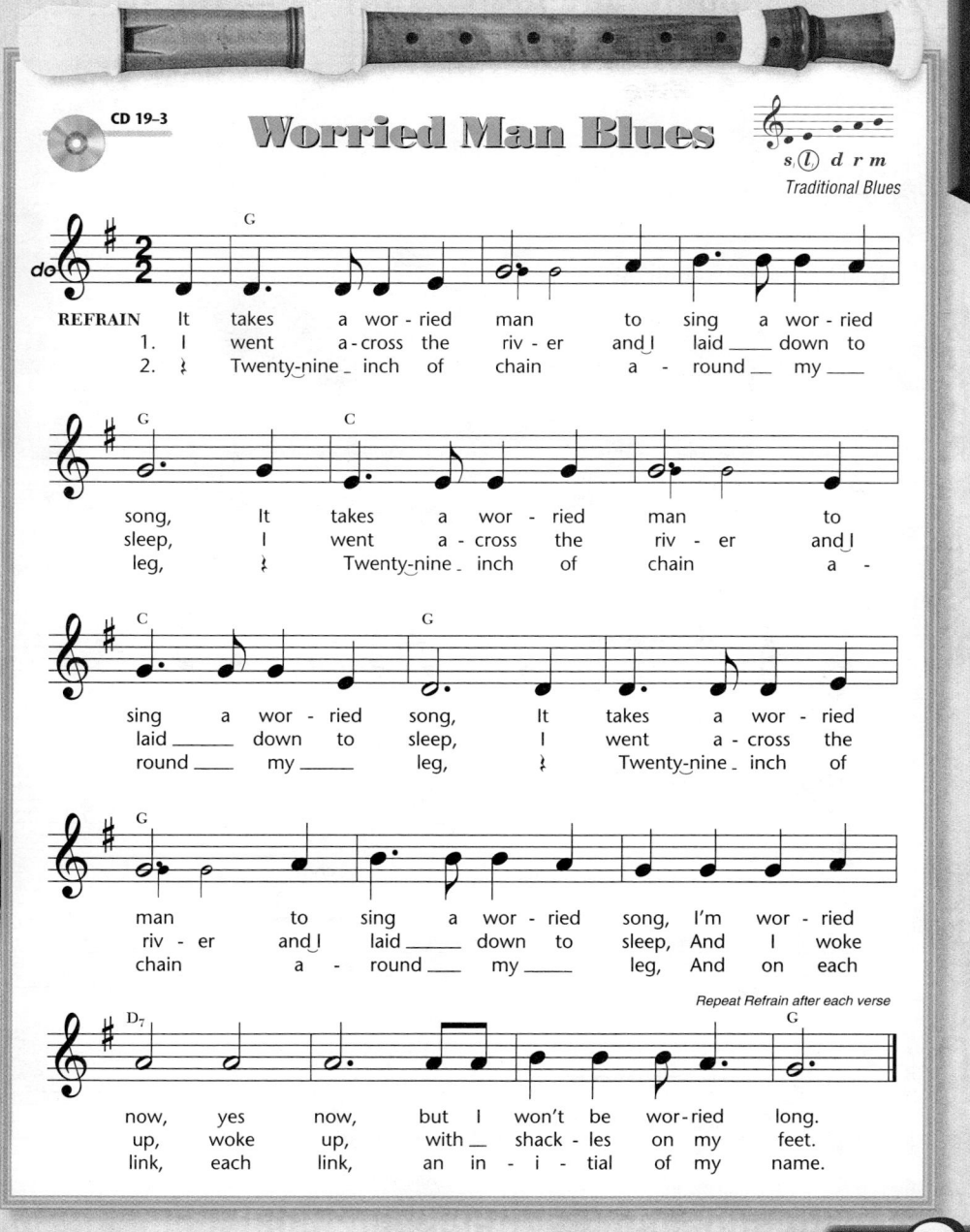

Worried Man Blues

CD 19–3

s, l d r m

Traditional Blues

REFRAIN   It   takes   a   wor-ried   man   to   sing   a   wor-ried
1. I   went   a-cross   the   riv-er   and I   laid ___ down   to
2. ₹ Twenty-nine _ inch   of   chain   a - round ___ my ___

song,   It   takes   a   wor-ried   man   to
sleep,   I   went   a-cross   the   riv-er   and I
leg,   ₹   Twenty-nine _ inch   of   chain   a -

sing   a   wor-ried   song,   It   takes   a   wor-ried
laid ___ down   to   sleep,   I   went   a-cross   the
round ___ my ___   leg,   ₹   Twenty-nine _ inch   of

man   to   sing   a   wor-ried   song,   I'm   wor-ried
riv-er   and I   laid ___ down   to   sleep,   And   I   woke
chain   a -   round ___ my ___   leg,   And   on   each

Repeat Refrain after each verse

now,   yes   now,   but I   won't   be   wor-ried   long.
up,   woke   up,   with ___ shack-les   on   my   feet.
link,   each   link,   an   in-i-tial   of   my   name.

Unit 10 371

---

1 INTRODUCE

Invite students to share their experiences playing the recorder and other wind instruments.

ASK To which sound group does the recorder belong? (aerophones)

See Lesson 3, p. 362, for more on instrumental sound groups.

2 DEVELOP

Singing

Have students

* Sight-read, in rhythm, the words of "Boil Them Cabbage Down" on p. 370.
* Listen to the recording of the song **CD 19–1**.
* Sing with the recording.

1a

Playing

To prepare for playing the recorder, invite students to

* Look at the recorder fingering chart on p. 370. Then, demonstrate the proper way to hold a recorder.
* Follow your example for fingering and blowing technique for playing C, B, A, and G, as shown on the chart on p. 370. Repeat fingering for notes frequently.

2a **Recorder Teaching Sequence:** Teach students to play "Boil Them Cabbage Down," p. 370, on recorder. Have students follow these basic steps for playing the songs in this lesson and others, using the Recorder Teaching Sequence in Teacher to Teacher below. Students may find it helpful to sing the part with rhythm syllables and pitch names before using recorders.

(See Resource Book p. I-1 for the complete Resource Book list of activities on playing the recorder.)

continued on page 372

TEACHER TO TEACHER

▶ **Recorder Teaching Sequence** Use this basic sequence to teach recorder parts for any song. Have students

* Practice playing notes used in the song. (the warm up)
* Whisper the rhythms of the song, using the syllable *daah*, in order to practice tonguing and articulation.
* Rest recorder on chin, and finger the notes of the song while listening to the recording.
* Play the melody of the song on recorders with the CD accompaniment. (Remind students to blow and play gently and whisper *daah* into the recorder as they play each note.)
* Sing the song with CD accompaniment and play the recorder during the song's instrumental interludes.

SKILLS REINFORCEMENT

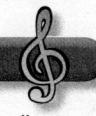

▶ **Keyboard** Perform with "Boil Them Cabbage Down."

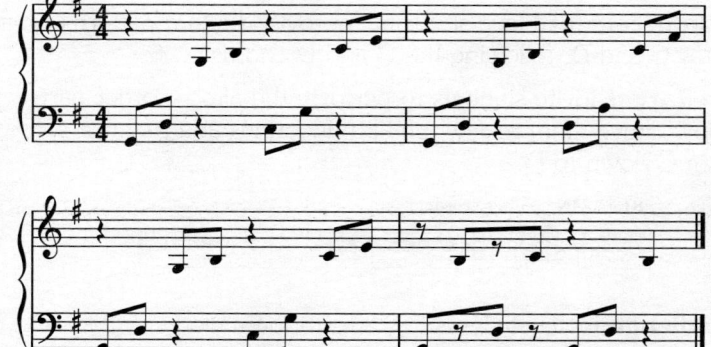

Lesson 5 Continued

Have students

- Practice playing notes used in this song. (C, B, A, and G)
- Rest recorder on chin, and finger the notes of the song while listening to the recording.
- Play the melody of the song on recorders with the Stereo Performance **CD 19–2.** (Remind students to play gently and whisper *daah* into the recorder as they play each note.)
- Sing "Boil Them Cabbage Down" with the Stereo Performance track and play the recorder during the song's instrumental interludes.

Invite students to learn to play the alto recorder part in Skills Reinforcement on p. 370. Students can also play a broken-chord accompaniment on keyboard, as shown in Skills Reinforcement on p. 371.

Reading

 Challenge students to find the dotted quarter notes in "Worried Man Blues," on p. 371. (mm. 1, 3, 5, 7, 9, 11, and 15) Have students echo the rhythm with you. Then, listen to and sing "Worried Man Blues" **CD 19–3.**

Performing

ASK What notes are in the melody of "Worried Man Blues"? (D, E, G, A, B)

Using Teacher to Teacher on p. 373, have students

- Learn the melody of "Worried Man Blues" on recorder.
- Sing "Worried Man Blues" **CD 19–3** with the recording and play the recorder during the instrumental interludes.
- Learn the mallet and recorder accompaniments on Resource Book pp. F-32 and I-28.

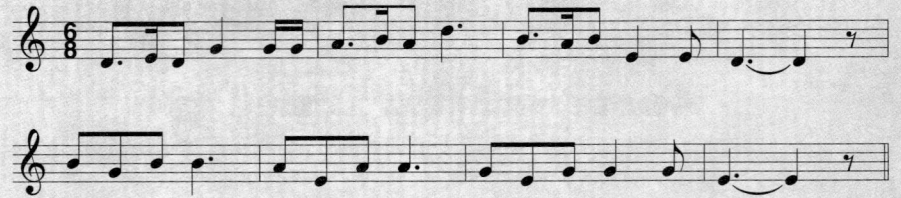

Time for 6/8

Play this warm-up for "Skye Boat Song." Pay careful attention to the rhythms in 6/8 meter.

Sing and **play** the Scottish "Skye Boat Song."

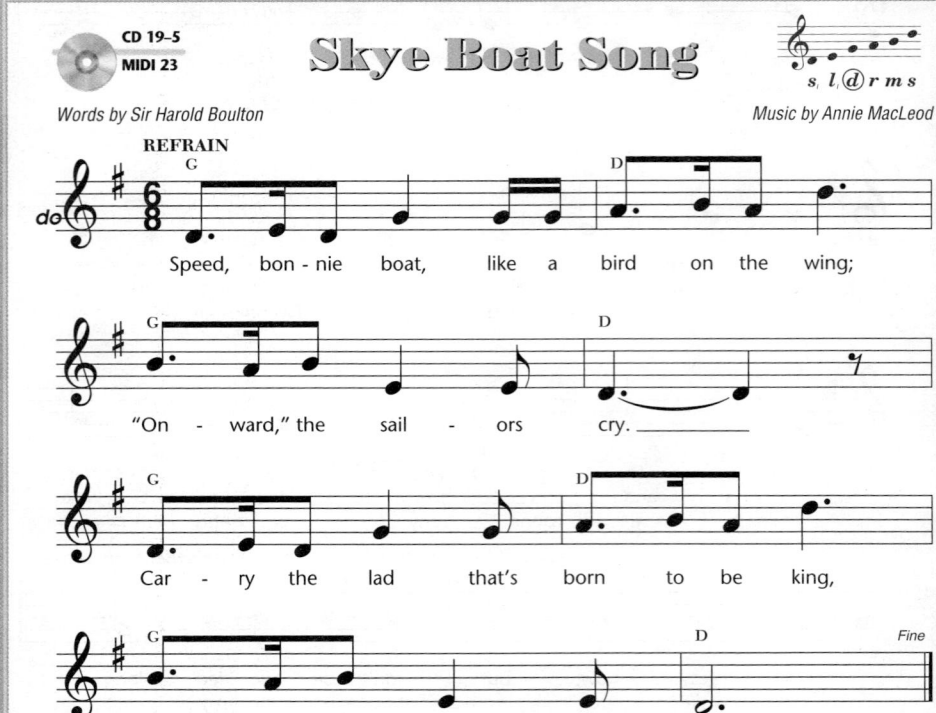

Words by Sir Harold Boulton

Music by Annie MacLeod

REFRAIN

Speed, bon-nie boat, like a bird on the wing;

"On - ward," the sail - ors cry. _____

Car - ry the lad that's born to be king,

O - ver the sea to Skye.

372

Footnotes

SKILLS REINFORCEMENT

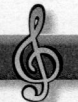 ► **Recorder** Invite students to perform a recorder accompaniment to the refrain of "Skye Boat Song."

Reinforcement Have students improvise rhythm patterns on the notes G and D, following the G and D chords.

On Target Invite students to perform the alto recorder part below. Have them review the alto fingerings and practice the leap from G down to D.

REFRAIN (Alto Recorder)

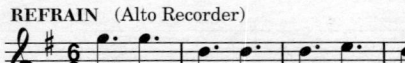

Challenge Invite students to perform the melody of "Skye Boat Song" on soprano recorder. Challenge them to improvise new countermelodies, following the G and D chords.

SKILLS REINFORCEMENT

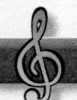 ► **Mallets** A xylophone is an idiophone that plays pitches. Share with students that you can often create accompaniments for songs by using the root and fifth of the chords. Write the chords of a song and notate the root and fifth of each chord. Then, create rhythm ostinatos, using the chord notes, to accompany the song.

Use the mallet part below to accompany the recorder on "Skye Boat Song." Use two mallets and play dotted quarter notes, using the following pitches for each chord.

G   = G and D

D   = D and A

Em = E and B

Am = A and E

372

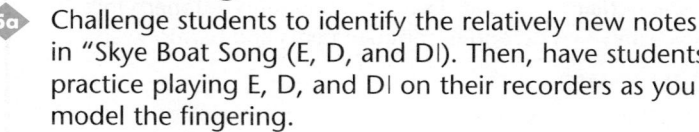

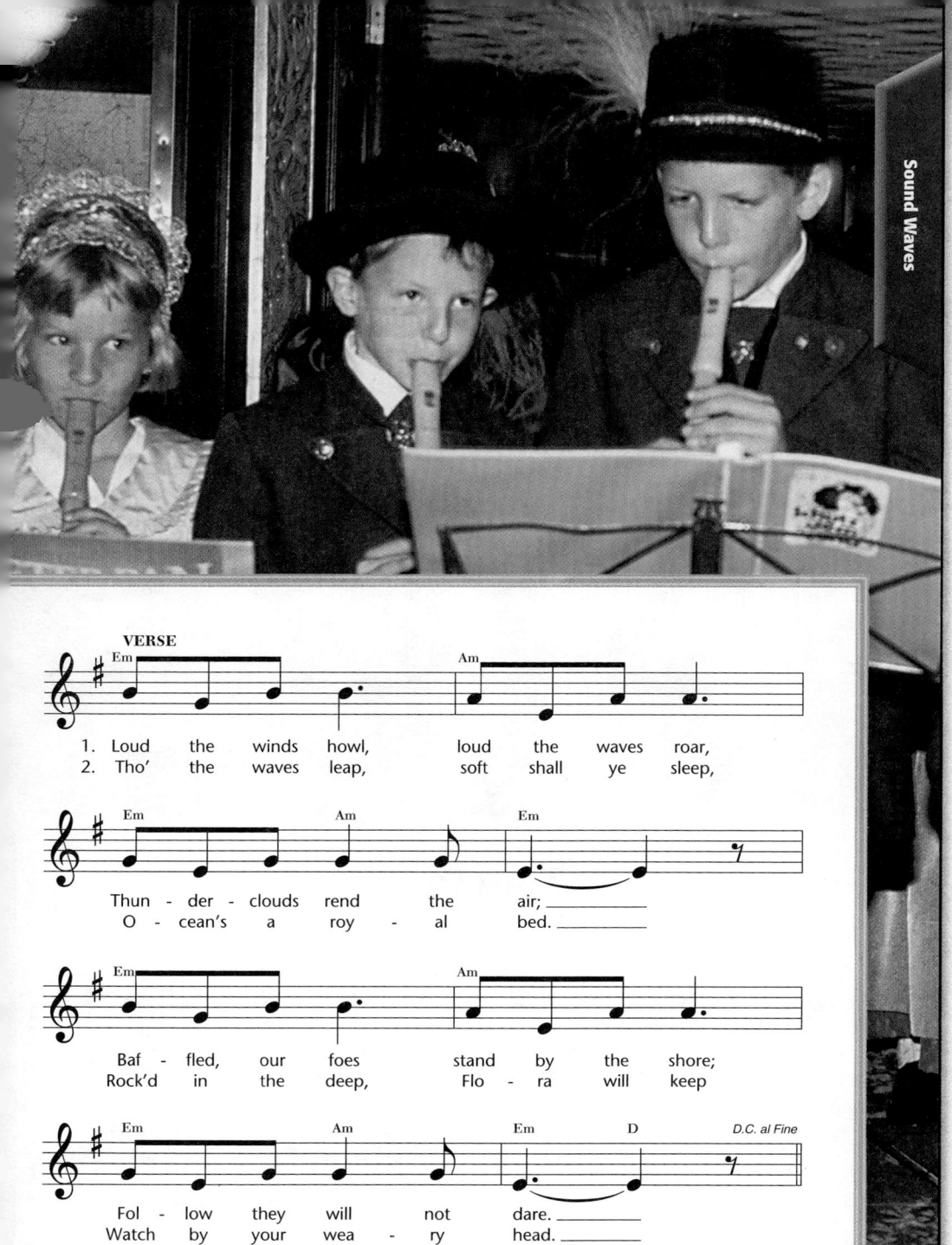

VERSE

1. Loud the winds howl, loud the waves roar,
2. Tho' the waves leap, soft shall ye sleep,

Thun - der - clouds rend the air; _____
O - cean's a roy - al bed. _____

Baf - fled, our foes stand by the shore;
Rock'd in the deep, Flo - ra will keep

Fol - low they will not dare. _____
Watch by your wea - ry head. _____

D.C. al Fine

Unit 10 373

Singing

Have students

- Echo clap the rhythm of each line of "Skye Boat Song" as you model it.
- **1a** • Listen to and sing "Skye Boat Song" **CD 19–5.**

Performing

5a Challenge students to identify the relatively new notes in "Skye Boat Song (E, D, and D♭). Then, have students practice playing E, D, and D♭ on their recorders as you model the fingering.

Have students play the warm-up at the top of p. 372 several times.

Share with students the skeleton melody of "Skye Boat Song" in Teacher to Teacher below.

Invite students to play "Skye Boat Song" on the alto recorder and on mallets. See Skills Reinforcement, p. 372.

2a Have students

- Finger and play the skeleton melody and melody to "Skye Boat Song."
- Sing "Skye Boat Song" **CD 19–5** with the recording and play the recorder during the instrumental interludes.

3 CLOSE

Skill: PLAYING   **ASSESSMENT**

7b **Performance/Peer Critique** Organize students into pairs. Have each student perform one of the three folk melodies in this lesson, using the following questions to assess the partner's performance.

- Did your partner play the correct notes?
- Did your partner maintain the rhythm?
- Did your partner whisper *daah* on every note? (If each note is heard clearly and distinctly, your partner is articulating, or tonguing, *daah* on each note.)

TEACHER TO TEACHER

▶ **Reading Skeleton Melodies** As students learn to read music, help them look for patterns, such as the skeleton melody ("bare bones" or most basic notes) of a piece. Encourage students to find the long-note skeleton melodies below.

- "Boil Them Cabbage Down"

    B C B A B C B A G

- "Worried Man Blues"

    D G B G E G G D

    D G B G A A B G

- "Skye Boat Song"

    D G A D♭ B E D 𝄽   Repeat line

    B B A A G G E 𝄽   Repeat line

SCHOOL TO HOME CONNECTION

▶ **Home Performance** Students can demonstrate playing the recorder for their families and friends.

TECHNOLOGY/MEDIA LINK

4c **Notation Software** Have students create accompaniments for folk songs, using notation software. Have them notate a melody, a bass part of quarter-note roots and fifths, and sixteenth-note arpeggios on separate staves.

Web Site Invite students to visit *www.sfsuccessnet.com* to learn more about the recorder and its history.

LESSON AT A GLANCE

Element Focus	**TEXTURE/HARMONY** Chords	
Skill Objective	**PLAYING** Play Autoharp or guitar chords for three folk songs	
Connection Activity	**GENRE** Examine guitar and Autoharp folk song accompaniments and harmony	

MATERIALS

- "Tom Dooley"   **CD 19–7**

  Recording Routine: Intro (4 m.); v. 1; interlude (4 m.); v. 2; instrumental; v. 3; coda

- "Down in the Valley"   **CD 19–9**

  Recording Routine: Intro (8 m.); v. 1; interlude (6 m.); v. 2; instrumental; v. 3; coda

- *"Cuando pa' Chile me voy"*   **CD 19–11**
- "Leavin' for Chile"   **CD 19–12**

  Recording Routine: Intro (15 m.); v. 1; refrain; interlude (15 m.); v. 2; refrain

- **Pronunciation Practice/Translation** p. 537
- **Resource Book** pp. A-28, F-34
- guitars, Autoharps, recorders

VOCABULARY

aerophone   chordophone

◆ ◆ ◆ ◆ National Standards ◆ ◆ ◆ ◆

1a Sing accurately in large ensembles
2a Play instruments accurately alone and in small ensembles
2b Perform easy instrumental pieces expressively
5a Read dotted notes in $\frac{6}{8}$ meter
6b Listen and analyze uses of harmony and texture in music from diverse genres
8b Identify ways music relates to other school subjects

MORE MUSIC CHOICES

For more easy-to-play guitar and Autoharp songs:

"Everybody Loves Saturday Night," p. 296

"Water Come a Me Eye," p. 300

"Jambalaya," p. 244

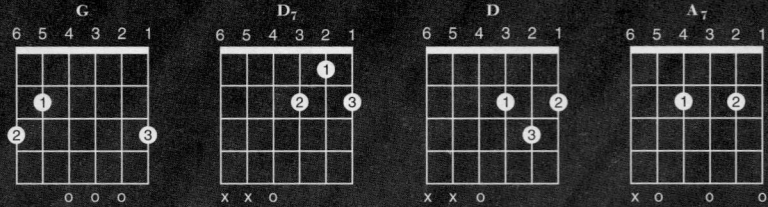

Playing Guitar and Autoharp

The guitar and the Autoharp often accompany singing together. Use the G and D$_7$ chords to accompany "Tom Dooley," and the D and A$_7$ chords for "Down in the Valley."

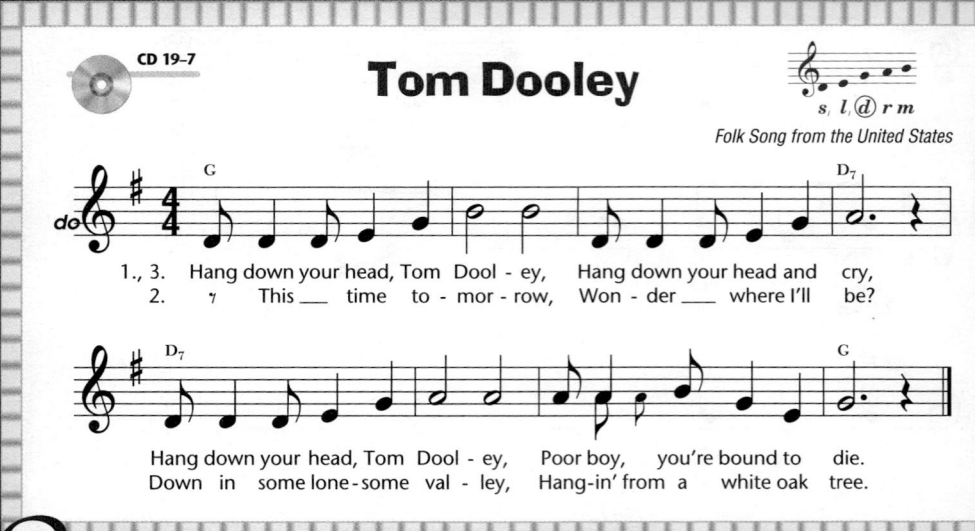

Both the Autoharp and guitar can play a simple "down" strum on each beat. Sing "Tom Dooley" and play along using guitar, Autoharp, and recorder.

CD 19–7

Tom Dooley

s, l, (d) r m

Folk Song from the United States

1., 3.   Hang down your head, Tom Dool - ey,   Hang down your head and   cry,
2.   This __ time to - mor - row,   Won - der __ where I'll   be?

Hang down your head, Tom Dool - ey,   Poor boy,   you're bound to   die.
Down in some lone - some val - ley,   Hang - in' from a   white oak   tree.

Footnotes

▶ **The Guitar** The students may enjoy learning more about the guitar. Prototypes of the guitar date back to the fourth century and were likely introduced into Spain by Arabs. The modern guitar from Spain exists in a whole family of sizes. Guitars generally fall into these categories: nylon-stringed classic guitars; steel-stringed guitars; solid-body electric guitars with steel strings; and acoustic electric guitars.

BUILDING SKILLS THROUGH MUSIC

▶ **Language** Ask students how the author of the lyrics for "Tom Dooley" uses point of view to involve them in the story. Note that the two verses are written from differing points of view.

SKILLS REINFORCEMENT

▶ **Recorder** Throughout the year, it is a good idea to review recorder fingerings. After reviewing the notes below, have students play this accompaniment to "Tom Dooley" on the soprano recorder. Invite advanced students to play the song melody of "Tom Dooley."

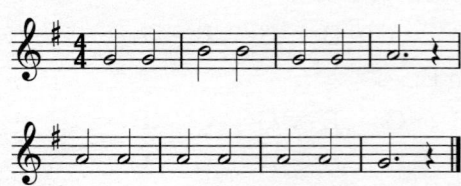

▶ **Mallets** For an Orff accompaniment to "Tom Dooley," refer to Resource Book p. F-34.

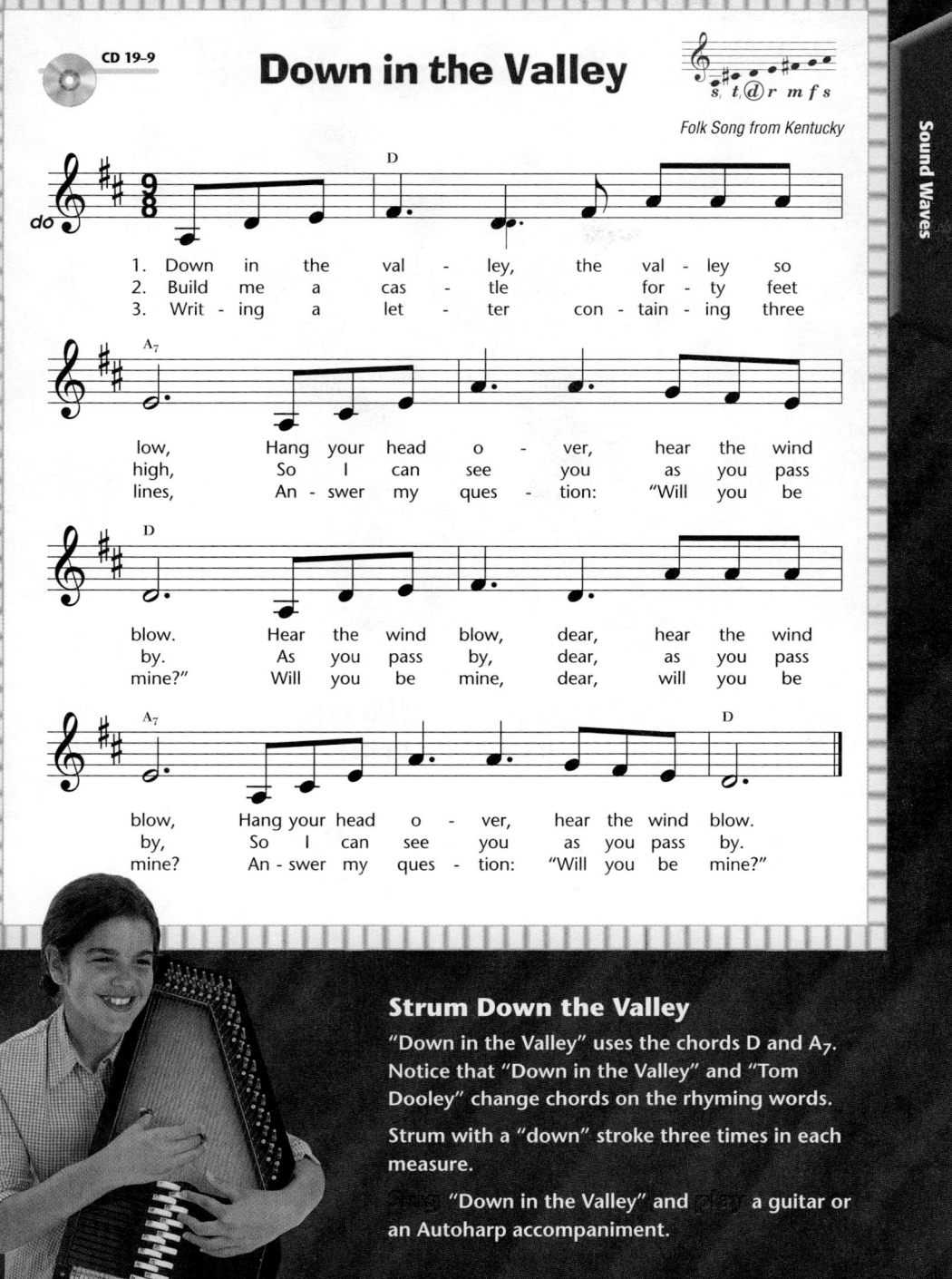

Down in the Valley

Folk Song from Kentucky

do

1. Down   in   the   val - ley,   the   val - ley   so
2. Build   me   a   cas - tle   for - ty   feet
3. Writ - ing   a   let - ter   con - tain - ing   three

low,   Hang   your   head   o - ver,   hear   the   wind
high,   So   I   can   see   you   as   you   pass
lines,   An - swer   my   ques - tion: "Will   you   be

blow.   Hear   the   wind   blow,   dear,   hear   the   wind
by.   As   you   pass   by,   dear,   as   you   pass
mine?"   Will   you   be   mine,   dear,   will   you   be

blow,   Hang   your   head   o - ver,   hear   the   wind   blow.
by,   So   I   can   see   you   as   you   pass   by.
mine?   An - swer   my   ques - tion: "Will   you   be   mine?"

Strum Down the Valley

"Down in the Valley" uses the chords D and A₇. Notice that "Down in the Valley" and "Tom Dooley" change chords on the rhyming words.

Strum with a "down" stroke three times in each measure.

Sing "Down in the Valley" and play a guitar or an Autoharp accompaniment.

Unit 10 375

---

1 INTRODUCE

8b Share with students that many cultures use string instruments to accompany folk songs. Guitar, Autoharp, and fiddle are some of the instruments. Tell students that they will accompany folk songs from Chile and the United States with guitar and Autoharp.

Students may be interested in information on the guitar found in Spotlight On, p. 377. Tips on teaching the guitar may be found in Meeting Individual Needs on p. 376 and in Teacher to Teacher below.

2 DEVELOP

Singing

1a Share with students that "Tom Dooley" is a folk song about a man who is about to be hanged. Have students

- Echo clap the song's rhythm.
- Say the lyrics in rhythm.
- Listen to the recording **CD 19–7**.
- Sing the song with the recording.

Playing

2a Separate students into pairs. Distribute the tuned guitars and Autoharps. Have students observe as you model the playing of the G and D₇ chords on guitar, as illustrated on p. 374.

Have students practice playing the G and D₇ chords.

Check that students are playing with arched fingers and with one finger on each string. After students play guitar, have them

- Observe as you demonstrate playing the Autoharp by holding the instrument up to the chest and using the left-hand fingers to play the G and D₇ chord bars while strumming with a thumb pick (or flat pick) in the right hand.

continued on page 376

ACROSS THE CURRICULUM

8b ▶ **Language Arts** Invite students to write an imaginary story about Tom Dooley's life. Ask them to explain how he ended up in the terrible situation described in the song. Have volunteers read their stories to the class. If time permits, have the class select a favorite story and create a minidrama. In the drama, include an opportunity for the class to sing "Tom Dooley" with guitar, Autoharp, and recorder accompaniment.

TEACHER TO TEACHER

▶ **Guitar Management Tips** To make class guitar playing a pleasant and organized experience, consider the following.

- When students are not playing their guitars, have them turn the instruments over in their laps so that the strings are muffled against their thighs.
- Make it clear to students that they should not turn the guitars' tuners.
- When students are to sing and strum simultaneously, have them begin by strumming for one or two measures before they start singing.
- Ask students to play more softly than they sing when they are accompanying themselves.

Lesson 6 Continued

1a
- Sing "Tom Dooley" while observing your Autoharp accompaniment.

ASK What is an easy way to remember where the chords change in "Tom Dooley?" (on the rhyme at the end of each line)

2b Have student pairs

- Practice playing the G and D₇ chords on the Autoharp.
- Strum on each beat (or on each half note) with the Stereo Performance track of "Tom Dooley" **CD 19–8.**
- Sing and strum the chords, on either guitar or Autoharp, with the recording.

Invite some students to play "Tom Dooley" on the recorder in Skills Reinforcement, p. 374, and on mallets, as suggested on Resource Book p. F-34. Ask the accompanists to play during the instrumental interludes as the class sings with the recording **CD 19–8.**

Singing

1a Share with students that "Down in the Valley" is another American folk song, but its mood is different. Ask students to decide the mood. Have students listen to the recording of "Down in the Valley" **CD 19–7.** Then, have them sing with the recording, taking note of the chord markings above each line of music.

Playing

ASK When do the chords change in "Down in the Valley"? (at measures 1, 2, 4, 6, and 8)

Distribute guitars to each student pair. Have pairs sing and strum the chords to accompany "Down in the Valley" without the recording.

Then invite students to play Autoharps and guitars while singing "Down in the Valley" with the recording. (The song's range is not suited to playing recorder.)

Chord Challenge

Review the G and D₇ chords on page 374. Then practice the three chords below. The guitar should play a simple "down" strum on the first beat of each measure in *"Cuando pa' Chile me voy."*

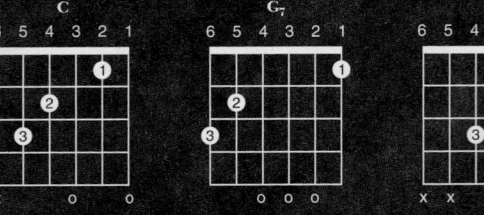

If you are playing Autoharp, find the chords ahead of time. Leave your left-hand fingers on the chord bars even when you are not pressing them. Autoharps should strum on the first beat of each measure, also.

Sing and play guitar and Autoharp on *"Cuando pa ' Chile me voy."*

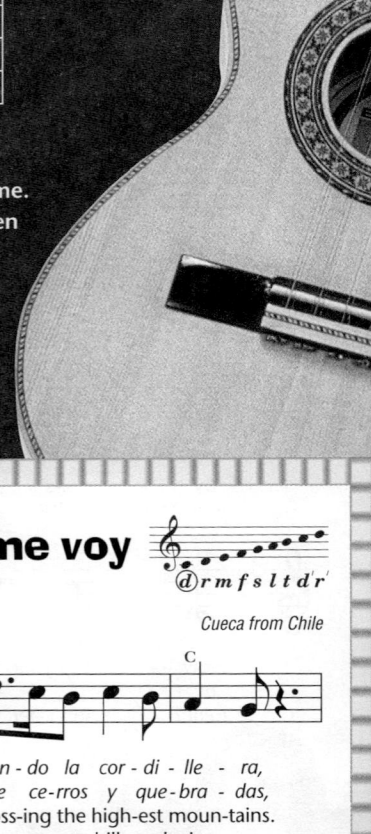

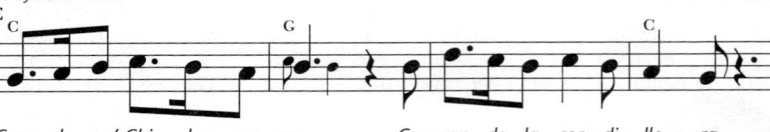

CD 19–11

Cuando pa' Chile me voy
(Leavin' for Chile)

English Words by Aura Kontra

Cueca from Chile

VERSE

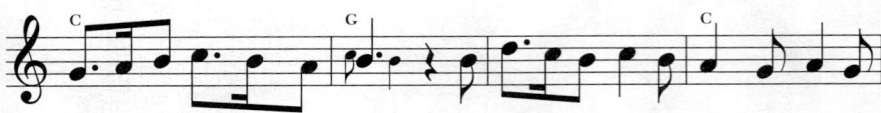

1. Cuan-do pa' Chi - le   me voy,   Cru-zan-do la cor-di - lle - ra,
   Y cuan-do vuel - vo   de Chi - le,   En - tre ce-rros y que-bra - das,
1. Leav - in' for Chi - le   a - gain,   I'm cross-ing the high-est moun-tains.
   And when I come home from Chi - le,   I cross o - ver hills and riv - ers.

Cuan-do pa' Chi - le   me voy,   Cru-zan-do la cor-di - lle - ra, La-te el
Y cuan-do vuel - vo   de Chi - le,   En - tre ce-rros y que-bra - das, La-te el
Leav - in' for Chi - le   a - gain,   I'm cross-ing the high-est moun-tains. And my
And when I come home from Chi - le,   I cross o - ver hills and riv - ers. And my

Footnotes

☺ MEETING INDIVIDUAL NEEDS

▶ **Including Everyone** Use the following strategies to help students who are struggling to play the guitar.

Reinforcement Pair students who are having difficulty with guitar with a partner who is an accomplished player. Ask students to model correct playing techniques at a slow tempo.

On Target These tips may help students improve.
- Make sure that the guitar is the right size for them.
- Use partial chords for G, G₇, C, or F.
- Strum less frequently (such as the first beat of each measure).
- Play only some of the chords.

Challenge Invite advanced students to improvise new strumming patterns, without slowing the tempo.

📖 ACROSS THE CURRICULUM

8b ▶ **Language Arts** As students learn *"Cuando pa' Chile me voy,"* share the folk tale *Mariana and the Merchild: A Folk Tale from Chile* by Caroline Pitcher (Eerdmans, 2000) about a child who lives at the seashore.

▶ **Social Studies** Introduce students to Chile's geography by sharing *This Place Is High: The Andes Mountains of South America* by Vicki Cobb (Walker & Co., 1993). This book describes the Andes and the animals and people who live there.

Learn more about South American geography and customs in the book *Argentina, Chile, Paraguay, Uruguay* by Anna Selby (Raintree/Steck Vaughn, 1999).

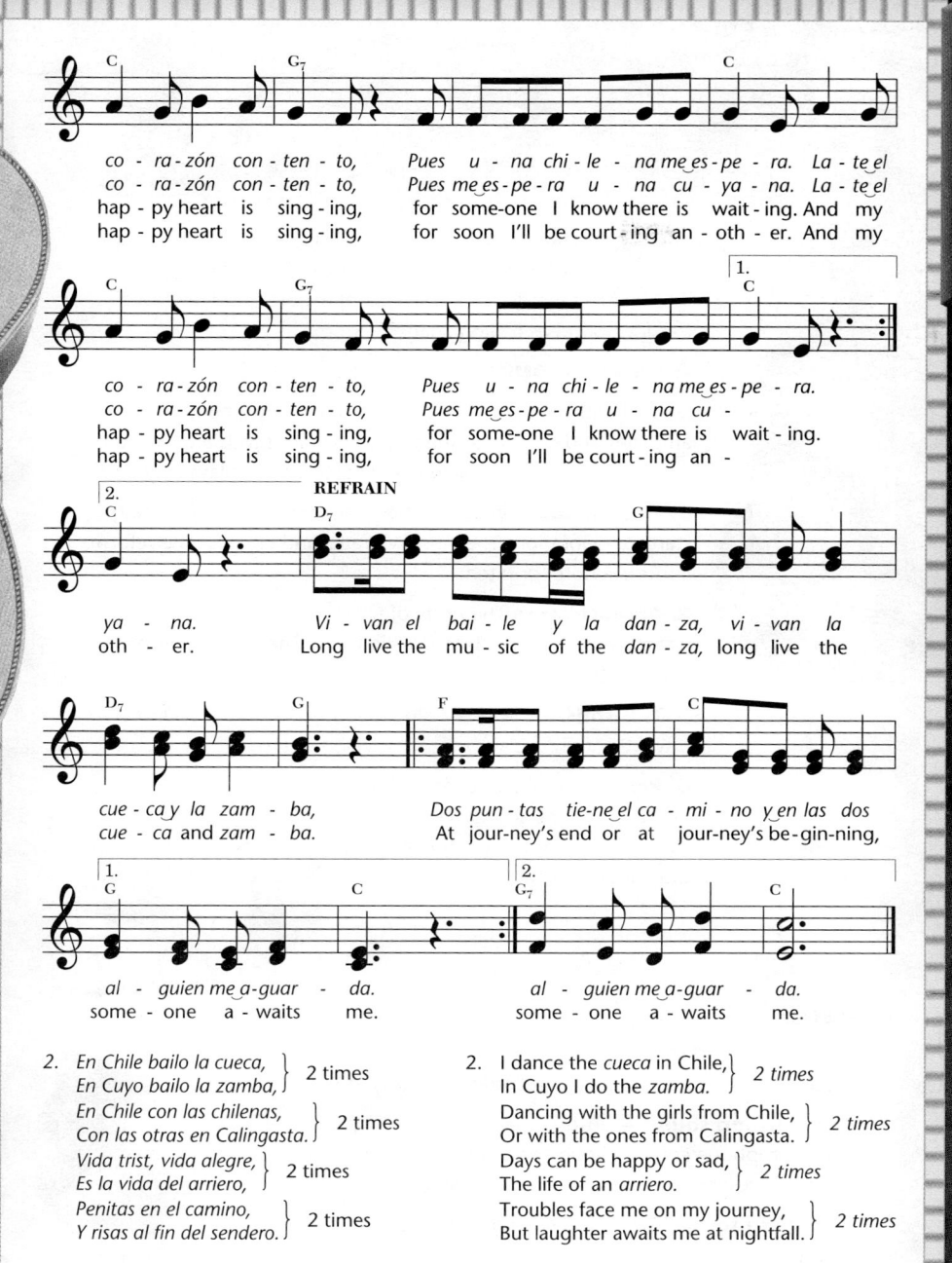

 co - ra - zón con - ten - to, / Pues u - na chi - le - na me_es - pe - ra. La - te_el
co - ra - zón con - ten - to, / Pues me_es - pe - ra u - na cu - ya - na. La - te_el
hap - py heart is sing - ing, / for some - one I know there is wait - ing. And my
hap - py heart is sing - ing, / for soon I'll be court - ing an - oth - er. And my

 co - ra - zón con - ten - to, / Pues u - na chi - le - na me_es - pe - ra.
co - ra - zón con - ten - to, / Pues me_es - pe - ra u - na cu -
hap - py heart is sing - ing, / for some - one I know there is wait - ing.
hap - py heart is sing - ing, / for soon I'll be court - ing an -

REFRAIN

ya - na. / Vi - van el bai - le y la dan - za, vi - van la
oth - er. / Long live the mu - sic of the dan - za, long live the

cue - ca y la zam - ba, / Dos pun - tas tie - ne_el ca - mi - no y_en las dos
cue - ca and zam - ba. / At jour - ney's end or at jour - ney's be - gin - ning,

al - guien me_a - guar - da. / al - guien me_a - guar - da.
some - one a - waits me. / some - one a - waits me.

2. En Chile bailo la cueca, } 2 times
En Cuyo bailo la zamba, }

En Chile con las chilenas, } 2 times
Con las otras en Calingasta. }

Vida trist, vida alegre, } 2 times
Es la vida del arriero, }

Penitas en el camino, } 2 times
Y risas al fin del sendero. }

Refrain

2. I dance the *cueca* in Chile, } 2 times
In Cuyo I do the *zamba*. }

Dancing with the girls from Chile, } 2 times
Or with the ones from Calingasta. }

Days can be happy or sad, } 2 times
The life of an *arriero*. }

Troubles face me on my journey, } 2 times
But laughter awaits me at nightfall. }

Refrain

Unit 10 **377**

Singing

5a To teach *"Cuando pa' Chile me voy,"* have students

- Listen to the recording **CD 19–11** and clap the refrain rhythm each time it occurs.
- Sing the song in English with the recording **CD 19–12.**
- Use the Pronunciation Practice Guide on p. 537 and Resource Book p. A-28 to learn the Spanish lyrics to *"Cuando pa' Chile me voy."* (Refer also to Pronunciation Practice **CD 19–14** and **CD 19–15.**)
- Sing the song in Spanish with the recording **CD 19–11.**

Playing

6b Invite students to study the guitar chord charts on p. 376 for chords C, G₇, and F. Demonstrate the guitar chord options for G₇ (playing a one-finger chord on string 1, fret 1) and for F (bar across fret 1 and playing strings 1 and 2 only). Using guitar and Autoharp, student pairs will

- Practice strumming and changing the C, G, G₇, D₇, and F chords on each dotted quarter-note beat while singing *"Cuando pa' Chile me voy."*
- Perform the song without the recording.

3 CLOSE

Skill: PLAYING   ASSESSMENT

2b **Performance/Self-Assessment** Separate students into pairs. Have each student perform an accompaniment to "Down in the Valley" or *"Cuando pa' Chile me voy"* on Autoharp or guitar. Then, have each student assess his or her own performance, using these criteria.

- Can you play the chords?
- Did you change chords in time?
- Can you sing and play chords at the same time?

SPOTLIGHT ON

▶ **Guitars** As students learn to play guitar chords, share that the chords they learn can be used in other guitar styles, such as rock 'n' roll. Ask students to discuss the differences between playing folk guitar and rock guitar. (Answers may include amplified vs. acoustic sound; nylon vs. steel strings; finger picking vs. flatpick; and strumming styles.)

Hear more examples of the guitar sound by visiting the Sound Bank, beginning on p. 512.

▶ **Guitar Manufacturers** Students may be interested in seeing styles of guitars used in rock music today. Explore guitar Web sites, such as Fender and Martin. Consider bringing in a pop guitar magazine to show students new styles of guitars.

TECHNOLOGY/MEDIA LINK

CD-ROM As students learn to play guitar and Autoharp accompaniments to the songs in this lesson, have them take turns entering accompaniments into *Band-in-a-Box*. Playing and singing along with these accompaniments can provide for a more motivating musical experience.

LESSON AT A GLANCE

Element Focus **TIMBRE** Acoustic stages of sound and timbre

Skill Objective **ANALYZING** Analyze the four steps in the life of a sound and how sound is produced by instruments

Connection Activity **SCIENCE** Write about the scientific principles of musical sound and recording

MATERIALS

- "Ezekiel Saw the Wheel" **CD 19–16**
  Recording Routine: Intro (4 m.); refrain; v. 1; refrain; v. 2; refrain
- Boomwhackers®, bass xylophone, bass metallophone, alto glockenspiel, tambourine, triangle, trumpet mouthpiece, 6-to-8-foot rubber hose, small funnel
- **Resource Book** p. H-28

VOCABULARY

amplification	transmission	perception
acoustic	digital	analog	*tremolo*

◆ ◆ ◆ ◆ National Standards ◆ ◆ ◆ ◆

1d Sing music written in two parts
2a Play instruments accurately alone and in small ensembles
2c Perform instrumental music from diverse genres
2d Perform simple melodies by ear
4c Arrange, using electronic media
5a Read eighth, quarter, half, whole, and dotted notes in duple meter
6b Listen and analyze uses of timbre in music from diverse cultures
8b Identify ways music relates to science

MORE MUSIC CHOICES

For information on the science of acoustics and vibration:
See Lesson 1, pp. 354–357

THE LIFE OF A SOUND

When you listen to a live cellist perform, you are listening to acoustic sound. When you listen to a CD of the cellist, you are listening to recorded sound. Think of acoustic and recorded musical sound as having a life.

Acoustic Sound

Motion and vibration start the sound. An instrument's body amplifies and colors the sound. The sound travels and is heard by listeners. Follow the acoustic sound played by a cello.

1. Motion and vibration Drawing a bow across the string starts the vibration. The string vibrates and creates a waveform, a musical note, or pitch.

2. Amplification The body of the cello acts as an amplifier. The waveform is changed by the cello body. The sound's timbre and volume level are defined.

3. Transmission As the cello makes the sound, its sound waves travel through the air.

4. Perception If a listener is present in the room, the sound waves reach the listener's ears. The listener's brain identifies the sound as a cello.

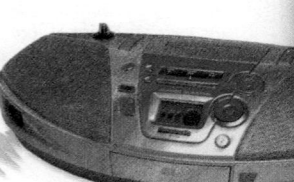

Recorded Sound

Recording sound saves it so that you can play it back at a later time. Follow the path of sound as it is recorded and played back.

1. Recording sound Acoustic sound is recorded by a microphone. The microphone converts sound waves to electrical impulses. A tape recorder preserves the microphone's signals onto tape.

2. Playing sound The magnetic information on the tape is converted to electrical energy.

3. Hearing the sound This energy drives the tiny speakers in the headphones.

Footnotes

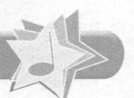

TEACHER TO TEACHER

8b ▶ **Science Fair** Science fairs are a great way to excite students about creative projects. The science of music is a wonderful way to incorporate music and sound into these projects. Encourage students to create science projects or homemade instruments that demonstrate the science of sound. Students may wish to consult with their school science teachers. Invite students to enter their projects (or instruments) in a school science fair.

BUILDING SKILLS THROUGH MUSIC

▶ **Science** Have students collect data on the rate of decay for instrument sounds using various percussion and/or string instruments available in the classroom. For each, students should document the source of the vibration, the material that vibrates, and the length of time in seconds that the sound lasts.

ACROSS THE CURRICULUM

8b ▶ **Science** The recording of music and sound is undergoing a revolution. Sound recording was traditionally known as *analog*, or the recording of live, acoustic signals onto magnetic tape. Today, sound recording is often in the digital domain. Sound information is stored as digital information, as 0s and 1s. Digital tape recorders (DATs) store their information on digital tape; recordable CDs (CD-R, CD-RW) and DVDs (DVD-R, DVD-RW) store their information on compact discs; computers, digital audio workstations, and digital audio equipment store sound on computer hard drives or other media. Ask students about the advantages of digital recording (higher fidelity, no loss of quality when copying, ability to manipulate sound digitally).

Sing the African American spiritual "Ezekiel Saw the Wheel." As you sing, think about how the sound of your voice travels to the listeners' ears.

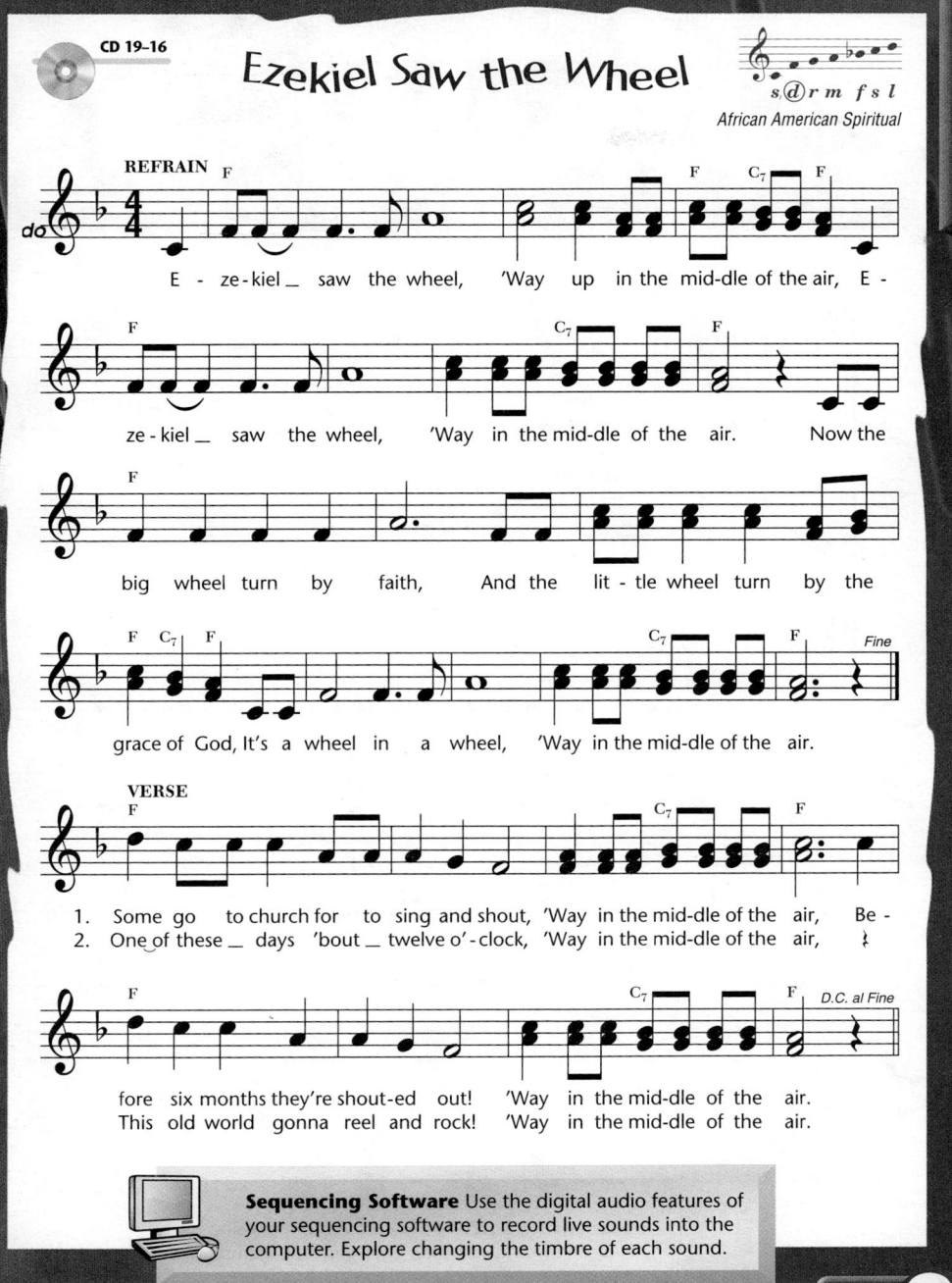

Ezekiel Saw the Wheel

CD 19–16

African American Spiritual

REFRAIN

E - ze-kiel __ saw the wheel, 'Way up in the mid-dle of the air, E -
ze-kiel __ saw the wheel, 'Way in the mid-dle of the air. Now the
big wheel turn by faith, And the lit-tle wheel turn by the
grace of God, It's a wheel in a wheel, 'Way in the mid-dle of the air.

VERSE

1. Some go to church for to sing and shout, 'Way in the mid-dle of the air, Be -
2. One of these __ days 'bout __ twelve o'-clock, 'Way in the mid-dle of the air,

fore six months they're shout-ed out! 'Way in the mid-dle of the air.
This old world gonna reel and rock! 'Way in the mid-dle of the air.

Sequencing Software Use the digital audio features of your sequencing software to record live sounds into the computer. Explore changing the timbre of each sound.

Unit 10 **379**

1 INTRODUCE

8b Ask students to recall what it is that determines the timbre of a guitar or a recorder. (the instrument's vibration or waveform) Then, ask them to explain what starts the vibration in a guitar or recorder. (guitar: fingers strumming or picking the strings; recorder: air flowing over a sharp edge, called a *fipple*) Share with students that a sound can be thought of as having a life.

2 DEVELOP

Analyzing

8b Invite students to read Acoustic Sound on p. 378.

ASK To what instrument sound family does the cello belong? (chordophones)

Other than bowing, what other ways are there of starting the vibration on a chordophone? (plucking or picking: orchestral string family, guitar, harpsichord; strumming: guitar; hammering: piano, dulcimer)

Remind students that the physical characteristics of an instrument will affect its pitch (see Lesson 1, pp. 354–357). Have students read Amplification, p. 378.

ASK What forms of amplification do chordophones have? (a piano's soundboard; the hollow body of an orchestral string instrument—violin, viola, cello, bass; a dulcimer's hollow box; a sitar's attached gourd; a solid-body electric guitar's amplifier or speaker)

Guide students in discovering how a sound begins, vibrates, and is amplified in other sound families. See Spotlight On below.

8b Have students read Recorded Sound, on p. 378 and discuss the life of a recorded sound.

See Spotlight On, p. 380, and share with students the fact that the process of recording has changed greatly since Edison first invented the phonograph, in 1878.

continued on page 380

SPOTLIGHT ON

8b ▶ **Science of Music** Use this chart to help students understand the science of music.

Instrument	Motion	Vibration	Amplification
Clarinet and Sax	single reed	air column	body and bell
Brass family	vibrating lips	air column	bell
Violin family	bow, pluck	strings	hollow body
Piano	hammer	strings	sound board
Xylophone	hit w/mallet	wooden bars	tubes
Most drums	hit	membrane	drum shell

SKILLS REINFORCEMENT

▶ **Keyboard** Students may enjoy learning a two-handed accompaniment to "Ezekiel Saw the Wheel." The "boom-chick" **2a** accompaniment below is based on two patterns.

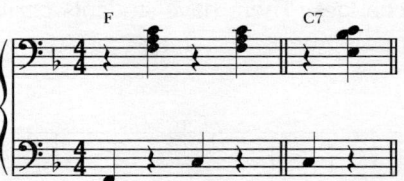

Students may wish to learn and play a full accompaniment to "Ezekiel Saw the Wheel." See Resource Book, p. H–28, for the full two-handed accompaniment.

Lesson 7 Continued

Singing

Have students listen to "Ezekiel Saw the Wheel"
CD 19–16 and follow the music on p. 379.

ASK This African American spiritual uses an alternation between a soloist and chorus. What is that style called? (call and response)

Have students

- Listen to the recording and sight-sing the refrain melody with the recording.

5a
- Echo-clap the refrain of "Ezekiel Saw the Wheel" as you model it.

- Echo-sing the refrain melody (the lower notes of the two-part harmony).

- Echo-sing the higher notes of the refrain's two-part harmony as you model it.

1d Divide the class into two groups. Ask one group to sing the refrain melody and the other group to sing the harmony. Invite volunteers to sing the verses. Have students

- Sing "Ezekiel Saw the Wheel" with the recording. (Have soloists sing the call and the rest of the class sing the harmonized response.)

- Think about how they produce the notes as they sing.

6b **ASK** Why do people sound different when they sing? (because they have a different timbre)

How are voices different from one another? (higher and lower pitch; lighter, heavier, nasal-sounding, and throaty timbre)

Playing

Invite students to read Percussive Sounds on p. 380. Ask students to identify each instrument part. Then, have students

- Identify the names of the notes that will be played on the bass part.

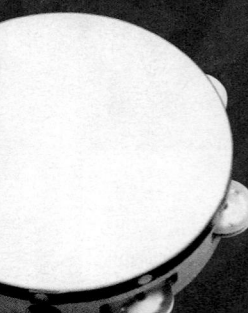

Percussive Sounds

Percussion instruments make many different sounds. A mallet striking a wooden xylophone and a mallet striking a metal glockenspiel produce different sounds. A tambourine makes its sound using both a membrane and metallic jingles. The solid body of a triangle produces its distinctive sound.

Play this accompaniment to "Ezekiel Saw the Wheel." As you play, think about how each instrument produces its sound.

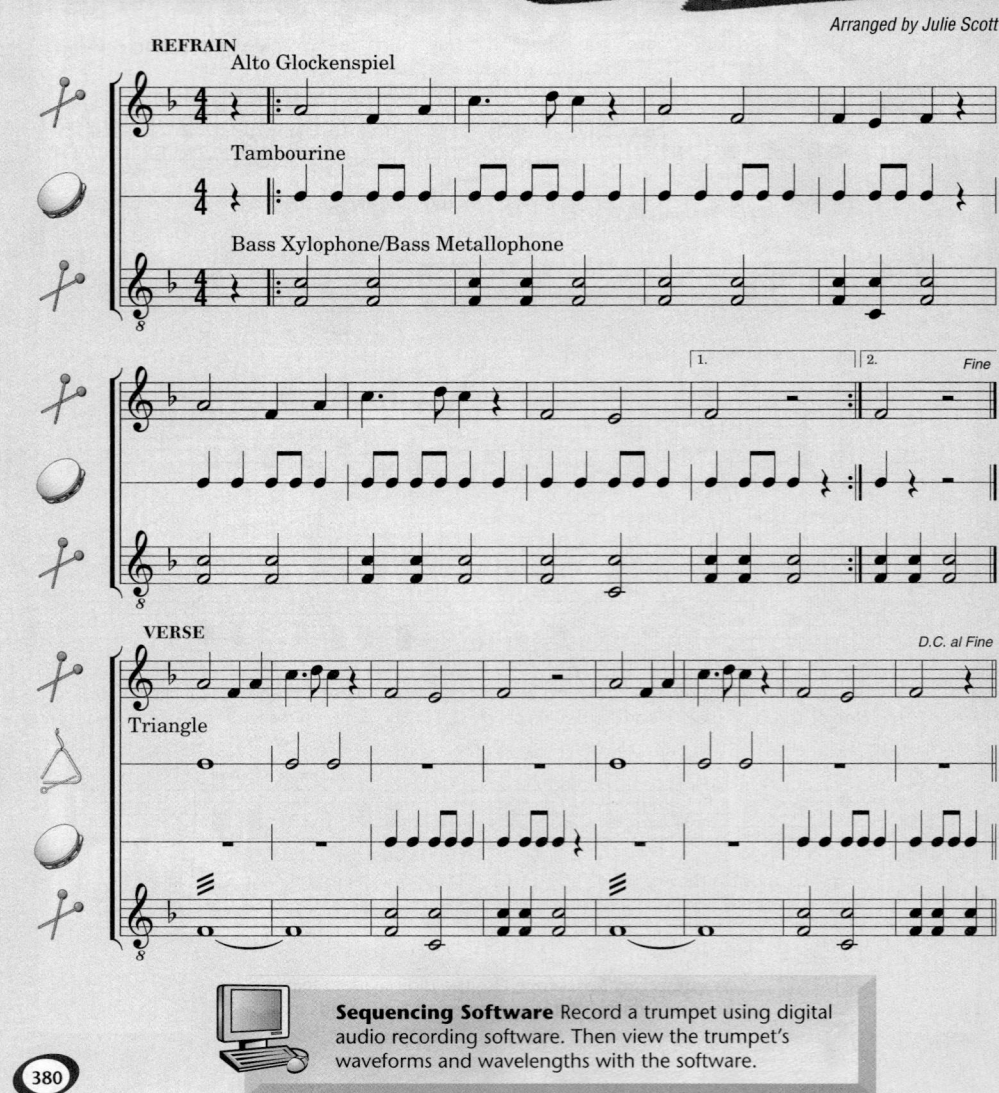

Arranged by Julie Scott

Sequencing Software Record a trumpet using digital audio recording software. Then view the trumpet's waveforms and wavelengths with the software.

380

Footnotes

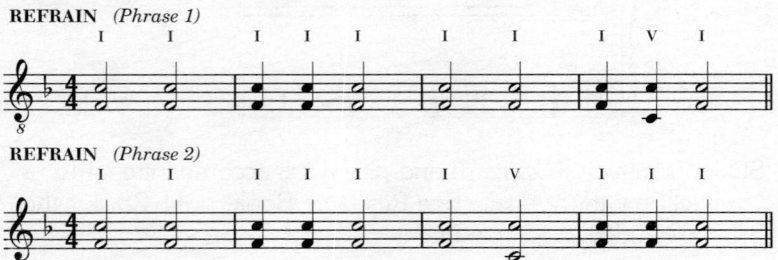

SKILLS REINFORCEMENT

2a
2d
▶ **Playing** Have students listen for chord changes, using the bass part for the refrain of "Ezekiel Saw the Wheel." Have them perform these patterns on Orff instruments as they listen to the "I" and "V" chord changes. Then, have students perform the accompaniment on p. 380.

REFRAIN *(Phrase 1)*

REFRAIN *(Phrase 2)*

SPOTLIGHT ON

▶ **Early Recording Techniques** Until 1925, sound recordings were made with large megaphones, which collected the sound and transferred the mechanical energy directly to cylinders or disks. Interestingly, the key to the development of modern phonographs, the vacuum tube amplifier created by Lee de Forest, was actually invented in 1912. By 1925, de Forest's invention led to the development of amplified recording and playback systems at Bell Telephone Laboratories, and the first electrical recordings using the microphone came out shortly thereafter. This new technology paved the way for the development of sound films (1927), better radio transmissions, and higher-quality phonograph recordings and reproductions.

Whacky Music

Plastic tubes like Boomwhackers® are fun to play. You can use them to make background patterns that go with songs. They come in different lengths to make a range of pitches. They illustrate one of the Three "Ls" of Pitch described on page 354—The Longer, The Lower.

Describe the timbre of a Boomwhacker® or other tuned tube.

Play each of these rhythms by hitting the tube(s). Start with the first rhythm and then add each pattern until all of the parts are playing together. When you are ready, **perform** "The Whacky Wheel" with the recording of "Ezekiel Saw the Wheel" on page 379.

Sound Waves

The Whacky Wheel Ensemble

Music by Will Schmid

1st Boomer

Bass Boomer (optional)

2nd Boomer

3rd Boomer

4th Boomer

Tune In

On the Caribbean Island of Trinidad, musicians play "Bamboo Tamboo" using different lengths of bamboo tubes hit on the ground to create a variety of rhythm patterns.

Create Your Own Hose-a-phone

To do this experiment, you will need a trumpet mouthpiece, a six- to eight- foot length of rubber hose that just fits over the mouthpiece end, and a small funnel that will also fit into the hose.

Demonstrate the three parts of a bugle or trumpet tone.

1. Motion: Buzz the lips alone; then buzz them with the mouthpiece.

2. Vibration: Insert the mouthpiece into the hose and play as many tones as you can. Play different pitches by tightening and loosening the tension of your lips. For extra theatrical effect, swing the end of the hose around or wrap it around your body like a Sousaphone.

3. Amplification: Insert the funnel in the end of the hose and play again, noting the change of tone.

- Discuss the definition of *tremolo,* and identify the notation (𝄒) as a music symbol referring to articulations. Perform the *tremolo* by rapidly playing F over and over with hands alternating.

- Identify and listen to the chord changes in the bass part, using Skills Reinforcement on p. 380.

2a
- Learn and then perform the mallet accompaniment on p. 380 as the class sings "Ezekiel Saw the Wheel" **CD 19–16.**

Invite students to play in a Boomwhacker® ensemble. Have students

- Select the Boomwhackers® needed for *The Whacky Wheel Ensemble* (Low F, C, F, G, A, C).

- Gradually build the ostinato pattern at a medium tempo starting with 1st Boomer and Bass Boomer. Then, add 4th Boomer followed by 3rd Boomer. Finally, have your best rhythmic students add the 2nd Boomer part.

2c
- Perform *The Wacky Wheel Ensemble* as an accompaniment to "Ezekiel Saw the Wheel."

Invite students to play an accompaniment to "Ezekiel Saw the Wheel" on keyboard. See Skills Reinforcement on p. 380 and Resource Book p. H-28.

3 CLOSE

Element: TIMBRE ASSESSMENT

6b **Music Journal Writing** Select two or more instruments from each of the instrument sound families. Have students are to analyze and describe what happens to each instrument during the motion, vibration, and amplification steps in "The Life of a Sound."

SKILLS REINFORCEMENT

2c ▶ **Playing** Invite students to learn more about Boomwhackers®. Have them

- Determine the pitch of each Boomwhacker® by checking with a standard pitch source (piano). Ask them to describe how Boomwhackers® relate to one of the principles of the Three "Ls" of Pitch on p. 354.

- Experiment with different techniques for sounding the Boomwhackers®:
  - Hitting the tube (diagonally) on the floor.
  - Bouncing the tube on the floor vertically (as in the stamping tube tradition of Trinidad known as *bamboo tambo*).

- Use Boomwhackers® to build layered ostinatos such as those found in Unit 8: *Say It With Drums.*

TECHNOLOGY/MEDIA LINK

4c **Sequencing Software** Invite students to use the digital audio features of a sequencing program to record sounds.

- The syllable *ah,* sung for two seconds
- A wind instrument playing a long note
- A string instrument playing a short, accented note

After the sounds have been recorded into the sequencing program, have students use the digital audio editor to

- View the waveform of the sound.
- Analyze the attack of each sound and discuss the sound being set in motion. (The drum was hit, producing a loud attack.)
- Play back and manipulate each sound. (loop a part of it)

LESSON AT A GLANCE

Element Focus | **TIMBRE** Instruments made from locally available materials

Skill Objective | **CREATING** Make a homemade rattle and create a rattle composition

Connection Activity | **CULTURE** Discuss how instruments are made from locally available materials in different cultures

MATERIALS

- *Llactamanta*   **CD 19–18**
- rattles from various cultures
- student-made rattles

VOCABULARY

found sound

◆ ◆ ◆ ◆ National Standards ◆ ◆ ◆ ◆

4c Compose and arrange, using non-traditional sound sources and electronic media

6b Listen and analyze uses of timbre in music from diverse cultures

7a Students evaluate the music they perform

8b Identify ways music relates to science and math

MORE MUSIC CHOICES

For more experience with the sounds of natural instruments:

"El condor pasa," p. 46

Gamelan angklung, p. 384

Drums of the Iroquois and Sioux, p. 285

1 INTRODUCE

Discuss with students how local natural materials influence people's lifestyles, including their houses and musical instruments. (In locales where trees are dominant, both houses and drums may be made of wood.)

Nature's INSTRUMENTS

No matter where people live in the world, they make musical instruments out of whatever local materials are available.

Rattles from around the world show how people use different materials. Here are some examples.

Listen to *Llactamanta,* an Ecuadorian folk tune from the Andes mountains. It uses locally made instruments—the *ch'ajch'as* (llama toenail rattles) and the bamboo panpipes (see pages 46–47). Make your own rattle from available materials gathered from your house. Then, **create** a rhythm accompaniment to *Llactamanta.*

CD 19–18
Llactamanta

Ecuadorian Folk Tune

Other Andean instruments include winds: *quena, flauta, zampoñas;* strings: guitar, *mandolina,* and *charango;* percussion: *ch'ajch'as, guiro,* and bongos.

▲ Gourd rattle from Latin America

Basket rattles from Africa ▶

Bean maracas from the Caribbean ▶

382

Footnotes

CULTURAL CONNECTION

▶ **Bamboo Instruments** For interested students, suggest *The Bamboo Flute* by Garry Disher (Ticknor & Fields, 1993), a short novel about a boy who learns to play a bamboo flute.

Invite students to learn more about the growing of bamboo with *The Book of Bamboo* by David Farrelly (Sierra Club Books, 1984). Bamboo is featured in Japanese and Chinese artwork.

BUILDING SKILLS THROUGH MUSIC

▶ **Writing** Have students create a fictional location and an instrument that would be made with materials native to their location. They should then write a description of the location and the instrument.

SKILLS REINFORCEMENT

 ▶ **Listening** Write a list of some of the Andean instruments used in the recording of *Llactamanta* (*quena, flauta, zampoñas, guitarra, mandolina, chajchas, guiro,* bongos). Discuss the instruments with students. Then, have students

- Listen to *Llactamanta* **CD 19–18.**

- List the Andean instruments they hear, and what each instrument is playing (*chajchas*—steady rhythm; *zampoñas* [bamboo panpipes]—melody).

- Select one or two rattle and percussion rhythms from the music and notate it as an ostinato.

- Play the ostinato rhythms on homemade rattles with the recording.

Bamboo Instruments

Bamboo grows easily in warm and wet parts of the world, such as South America, much of Asia, and the South Pacific. Many musical instruments are made of bamboo. **Listen** again to the bamboo panpipes in *Llactamanta*.

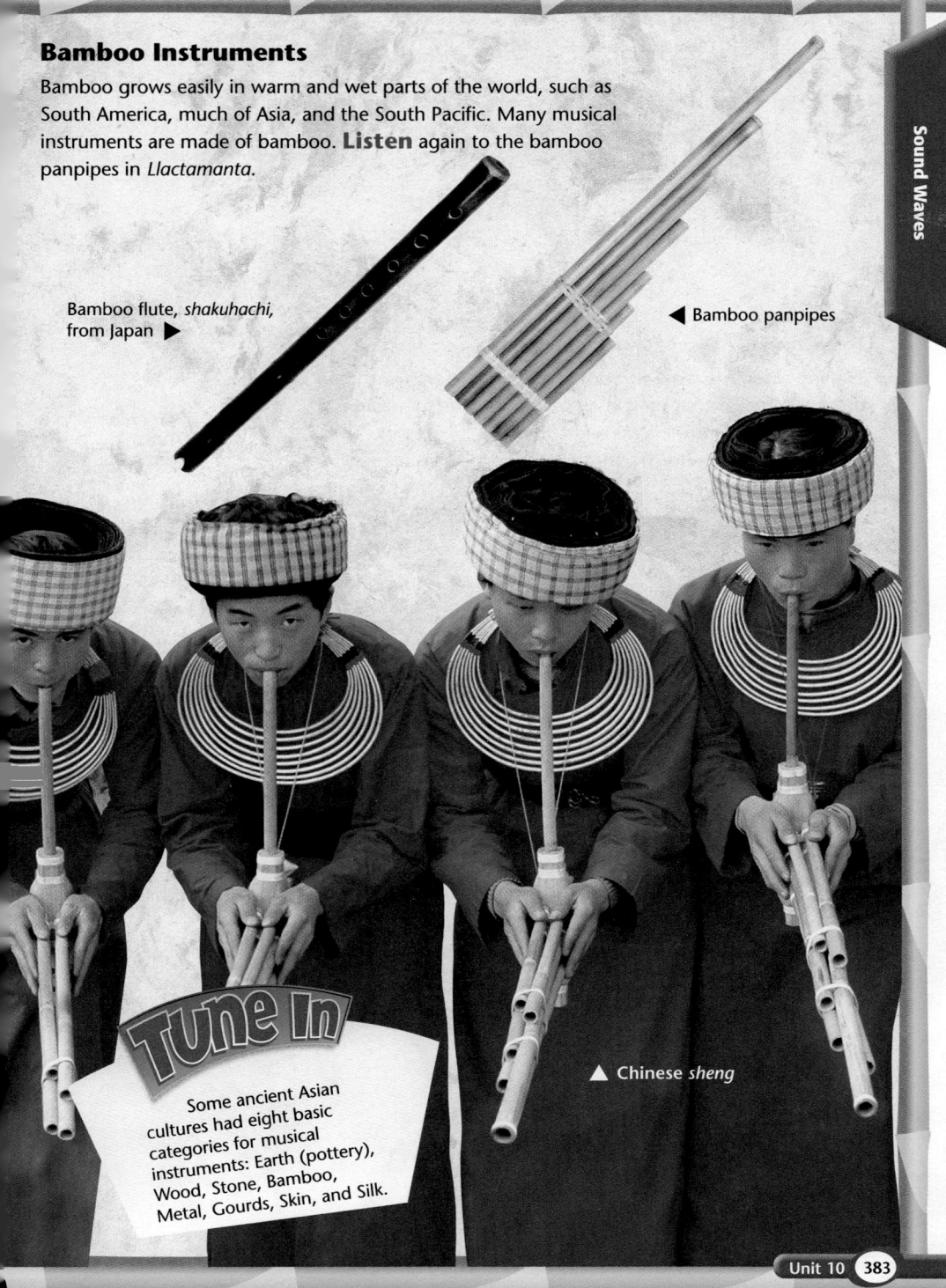

Bamboo flute, *shakuhachi*, from Japan ▶

◀ Bamboo panpipes

▲ Chinese *sheng*

Tune In

Some ancient Asian cultures had eight basic categories for musical instruments: Earth (pottery), Wood, Stone, Bamboo, Metal, Gourds, Skin, and Silk.

Sound Waves

Unit 10 **383**

2 DEVELOP

Have students read the information about instruments and rattles made by people throughout the world, pp. 382–383.

8b **ASK How would the stages of sound apply to the timbre of the rattles pictured on p. 382?** (See Lesson 7, p. 378. *Motion*: shake; *vibration*: beans, beads, rattle contents; *amplification*: rattle shell.)

Listening

6b Invite students to

- Listen to the recording of *Llactamanta* **CD 19-18,** which is music from the Andes mountains of South America.
- Identify when they hear these Andean instruments: *chajchas* (llama–toe rattles); *zampoñas* (bamboo panpipes).

Creating

4c Have students make their own rattles from locally available materials. Then, organize students into small groups and have them create rhythm compositions, using their rattles.

3 CLOSE

Element: TIMBRE ASSESSMENT

7a **Performance/Peer Critique** Have each group perform its rattle rhythm composition. Have students assess each composition, using the following criteria.

- Did the timbres of the rattles blend well together?
- Were the rhythms interesting and varied?
- Was the texture of the composition varied? (sometimes full, sometimes sparse)

ACROSS THE CURRICULUM

▶ **Social Studies** Invite students to create a bulletin board to display instruments made of local materials from different cultures and geographic regions around the world. Have students place pictures of instruments (bamboo flutes, African and Native American drums) on a world or climate map. Create a legend, organized by continent, that lists each instrument, country, and of what materials the instrument is made.

Students will learn of the close relationship between nature, climate, forests, and available materials to construct instruments (or homes). Share this project with the social studies and science classes.

TECHNOLOGY/MEDIA LINK

4c **CD-ROM** Encourage students to use the *Making More Music* software to create and notate the selected percussion or rattle rhythms from the recording *Llactamanta* **CD 19–18.** Have students

- Layer the percussion rhythms to create a fuller rhythmic texture.
- Create new rhythm tracks and add them to the layered mix.

LESSON AT A GLANCE

Element Focus   **TIMBRE** Gamelan timbres

Skill Objective   **LISTENING** Listen to gamelan timbres

Connection Activity   **RELATED ARTS** Discuss Balinese dance

MATERIALS
- *Gamelan angklung* (excerpt)   **CD 19–19**
- *Kebjar teruna* (excerpt)   **CD 19–20**
- tuned percussion instruments

VOCABULARY
gamelan   *angklung*

◆ ◆ ◆ ◆ **National Standards** ◆ ◆ ◆ ◆

4c Compose and arrange, using non-traditional sound sources and electronic media

6b Listen and analyze uses of timbre in music from diverse cultures

9a Describe characteristics of music genres from a variety of cultures

MORE MUSIC CHOICES
For more experience with the sounds of cultural instruments:

Hindewhu (whistle) solo, p. 269

"*Yo-shi nai*," p. 286

"*Banuwa*," p. 294

1 INTRODUCE

Invite students to read the information about the *gamelan angklung* and the Balinese gamelan, pp. 384–385. Discuss how the instruments in the gamelan work together for unity and variety.

Gamelan Orchestras

The people of Bali and Java play in gamelan orchestras.

The Indonesian **gamelan** consists of percussion, winds, and bell instruments that play as an orchestra. The gamelan is unique in its sound. The *gamelan angklung* is a smaller and lighter gamelan orchestra that plays in processions.

Listen to this example of *gamelan angklung*.

> A **gamelan** is an Indonesian orchestra consisting primarily of gongs, gong-chimes, metallophones, and drums.

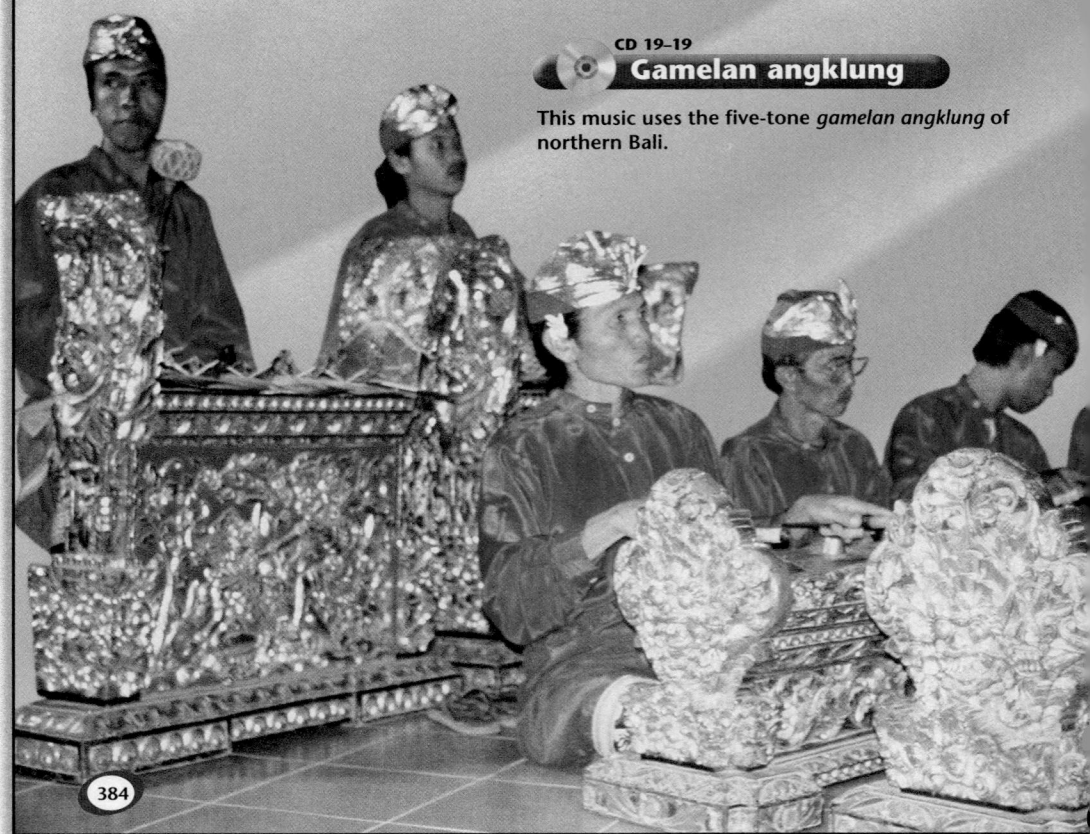

 CD 19–19
Gamelan angklung

This music uses the five-tone *gamelan angklung* of northern Bali.

384

Footnotes

ACROSS THE CURRICULUM

▶ **Social Studies** Provide a world globe for the class. Then invite students to circumnavigate the globe to find Bali. Go west from California. Keep going west, west, west across the Pacific. Stop at Asia; don't climb the Great Wall. Turn south and stop between the Pacific and Indian Oceans. Destination—Indonesia with 16,000 islands! Which one is Bali? Go south of Borneo and west of Java. You have arrived in beautiful Bali!

BUILDING SKILLS THROUGH MUSIC

▶ **Language** Divide the class into small groups. Have them create an "orchestra." They need to select instruments from world music, western orchestras, gamelan orchestras, and so on, to create their orchestra. Have them name their orchestra and write a description of their orchestra and reasons for selecting the instruments.

SPOTLIGHT ON

▶ **Balinese Dance** Invite students to explore Balinese dance and its relationship to the gamelan.

Balinese dance is known for its unique and stylized movements, and colorful and ornate costumes. In Bali, every village has a gamelan and a dance group. The gamelan frequently provides musical accompaniment for Balinese classical dance. Help students discover that every movement in Balinese dance is important and is designed to assist in telling the story. Dance movements are stylized and have meaning. For example, *ngaweh* means to "wave the hands."

One of the most famous of classic Balinese dances is the *Legong* dance. This dance, which portrays grace and femininity, is performed by two or three girls and is accompanied by a gamelan.

A Gamelan from Bali

Gamelans from the small island of Bali are generally more energetic than the gamelans of the island of Java. **Listen** for the variety of percussion instruments in *Kebjar teruna,* a piece for Balinese gamelan.

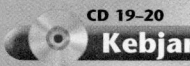
CD 19–20
Kebjar teruna

The *kebjar* is a dramatic Balinese dance in which a dancer interprets the different moods played by the gamelan.

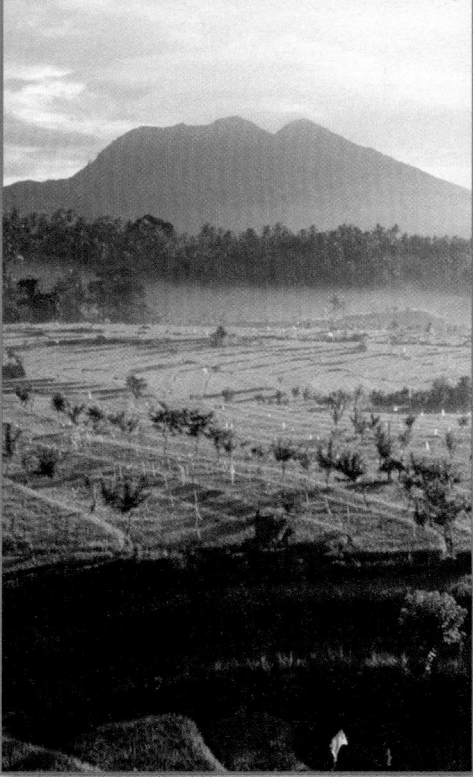
▲ **Terraced rice fields in Bali, Indonesia**

Tuned Percussion

Select a variety of percussion instruments that play pitches. Xylophone, glockenspiel, bells, and all pitched Orff instruments would be good choices.

When you have assembled a tuned percussion ensemble, you can **play** your instrument in a creative way.

- Explore your instrument. How do you create a sound? **Create** interesting rhythms with your instrument.

- Experiment with combining different timbres. When everyone is ready to start, one person may begin playing. Others should gradually join in and play together with what is already going on.

- After some time, stop the ensemble and **discuss** how to make it sound better; then **play** again.

2 DEVELOP

Listening

6b Have students listen to *Gamelan angklung* **CD 19–19** and then describe the timbres in the gamelan.

9a Play the recording of *Kebjar teruna* **CD 19–20** and then have students compare and contrast the two Balinese gamelan pieces. (*Gamelan angklung:* melodious quality, percussion and wind instruments; *Kebjar teruna:* rapid and energetic percussive sounds, audible steady beat)

Creating

4c Have students read the last two sections of p. 385. When the instruments have been assembled and the timbres have been explored, have students work together in small groups to create a tuned percussion piece that illustrates timbres similar to those of a gamelan. Ask each group to draw a graphic road map, or score, that outlines when each instrument will play and to name their composition. Challenge them to use variety in musical texture, dynamics, tempo, and rhythmic activity.

Playing

Help students recall the styles of the two gamelan pieces to which they have listened. Guide the class in deciding which instruments they will use to play each composition. Invite them to perform their gamelan compositions, using the scores they had created.

3 CLOSE

Element: TIMBRE **ASSESSMENT**

6b **Music Journal Writing** Have students listen to the gamelan listening excerpts in this lesson. Then, ask students to write a description of the timbres they heard in the gamelan in their journals.

CULTURAL CONNECTION

▶ **Musical Onomatopoeia** *Angklung* is the sound that an Indonesian bamboo shaker makes when shaken. Some other instruments named after their sound are Javanese *gong ageng, kempul, kenong, ketuk;* and the Ghanaian double bell, the *gankogui.* Challenge students to find other instruments that are named after their sound.

CHARACTER EDUCATION

▶ **Creativity** Discuss creativity. Creativity requires us to share part of ourselves with others. Successful group creating experiences require an environment in which people feel safe sharing their ideas; thus, cooperating, listening, respecting, contributing, and accepting are crucial elements if we are to be creative.

TECHNOLOGY/MEDIA LINK

4c **Sequencing Software** Help students use a digital audio sequencing program to create a collage of tuned percussion sounds. Have students, working in pairs,

- Perform and record a short sequence of sounds from one tuned percussion instrument. Save each recording as a sound file. Repeat this for each percussion instrument.

- Arrange the sound files in a collage at the computer workstation.

- Repeat sounds, arrange them in different orders, add digital effects, and save the new collage as a file.

- Play their work for the class, explaining how they organized and edited their composition.

Lesson	Elements	Skills	

LESSON 1

A Gospel Gift

pp. 392–395

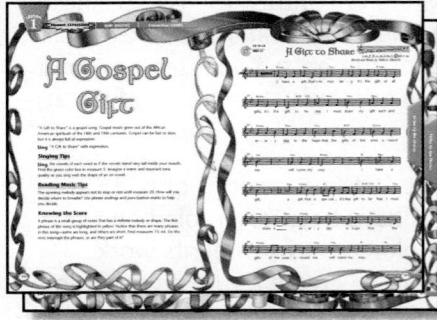

Element: Expression
Concept: Articulation
Focus: Expressive singing

Secondary Element
Rhythm: meter in 3

National Standards
1b 1c 1d 5a 7b 9a 9c

Skill: Singing
Objective: Sing text expressively through effective text delivery and appropriate tone quality

Secondary Skills
• **Listening** Listen to a gospel recording and discuss the style
• **Reading** Read melodic passages
• **Singing** Sing a gospel song expressively; organize a formal performance of the gospel song
• **Analyzing** Have students research and write reports on the history of gospel

SKILLS REINFORCEMENT
• **Listening** Listen to and recognize form (phrases, repetition, call and response)
• **Vocal Development** Develop inner hearing skills

LESSON 2

Rhythm Train

pp. 396–401

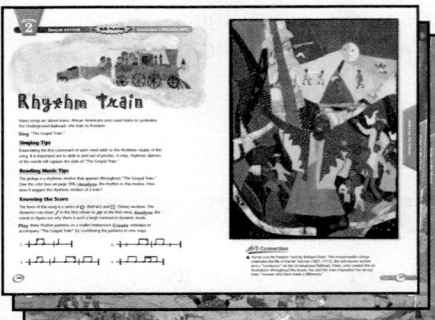

Element: Rhythm
Concept: Pattern
Focus: Dotted rhythms in $\frac{2}{4}$ meter

Secondary Element
Form: ABAB

National Standards
1a 1b 1d 2a 4c 5a 5c
6a 7a 7b

Skill: Playing
Objective: Read and play dotted rhythms and syncopation in $\frac{2}{4}$ meter

Secondary Skills
• **Listening** Listen for themes and dotted rhythms in a gospel song
• **Reading** Read repeating melodic and rhythmic patterns
• **Singing** Sing a song in gospel choir style
• **Moving** Learn nonlocomotor movements
• **Playing** Play and echo clap prominent train rhythms
• **Analyzing** Play each vocal part of a gospel song with a different sound to illustrate rhythmic complexity

• **Performing** Perform a gospel song and share proper etiquette in doing so

SKILLS REINFORCEMENT
• **Listening** Listen to and understand compositional elements (AB themes, ostinatos, embellishments, call and response)
• **Playing** Play rhythmic motives indicative of train sounds

LESSON 3

A Cajun Lullaby

pp. 402–407

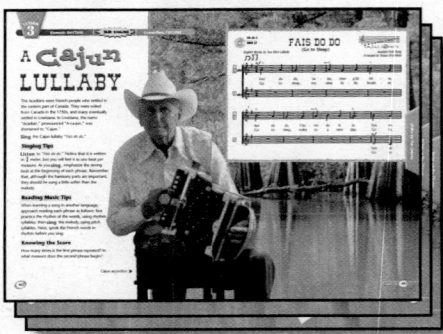

Element: Rhythm
Concept: Pattern
Focus: Dotted and tied rhythms in meter in 3

Secondary Element
Texture/Harmony: three-part harmony

National Standards
1b 5c 6a 7a 8b

Skill: Singing
Objective: Read and sing tied rhythms, with one beat to a measure in $\frac{3}{4}$ meter

Secondary Skills
• **Listening** Listen to a Cajun lullaby
• **Reading** Read and identify a rhythmic motive and how it functions in a Cajun song
• **Singing** Sing a lullaby in Cajun French
• **Analyzing** Discuss and read about Cajun culture
• **Performing** Invite Cajun musicians to perform in class
• **Moving** Discuss and possibly perform the Cajun two-step and waltz

SKILLS REINFORCEMENT
• **Creating** Create a hand-clapping routine to accompany a Cajun song
• **Guitar** Play an accompaniment with the Cajun "waltz strum" pattern

Connections

Music and Other Literature

Connection: Genre

Activity: Read about and discuss the history of gospel music

ACROSS THE CURRICULUM **Language Arts** Read story about sharing gifts

SPOTLIGHT ON
Gospel Facts on gospel music
The Performer Facts on gospel singer Mahalia Jackson

TEACHER TO TEACHER **Inner Hearing** Developing inner hearing skills

MOVEMENT **Nonlocomotor Movement** Perform synchronized choir movements to a gospel song

BUILDING SKILLS THROUGH MUSIC **Writing** Discuss the meaning behind lyrics

Song "A Gift to Share"

More Music Choices
"Ain't Gonna Let Nobody Turn Me 'Round," p. 85
"Sometimes I Feel Like a Motherless Child," p. 241
"This Little Light of Mine," p. 232

ASSESSMENT

Performance/Self Assessment Perform a gospel song with musical expression and videotape it

TECHNOLOGY/MEDIA LINK

Video Library Video on gospel singing
MIDI/Sequencing Software Experiment with tempo, isolate voice parts, teach harmony parts, and transpose the key of a gospel song

---

Connection: Language Arts

Activity: Read about and discuss metaphors in gospel music lyrics

SPOTLIGHT ON
Gospel Music Information about gospel style
Early Gospel Singers Facts on early gospel singers
Train Sounds Discover sounds that trains make
The Conductor Facts about Moses Hogan
The Performers Facts on the Moses Hogan Chorale

ACROSS THE CURRICULUM **Language Arts** Discuss lyrics in gospel music
Social Studies Discuss the Underground Railroad

CULTURAL CONNECTION **Spirituals** Discuss African American spirituals

AUDIENCE ETIQUETTE **Get There Early** Understand the importance of arriving early to a performance

MOVEMENT **Nonlocomoter Movement** Perform synchronized movements for a gospel performance

TEACHER TO TEACHER **MIDI Song File** Help students learn the song

BUILDING SKILLS THROUGH MUSIC **Writing** Discuss and use metaphors

Song "The Gospel Train"

More Music Choices
"Ezekiel Saw the Wheel," p. 379
"Glory, Glory, Hallelujah," p. 52

ASSESSMENT

Performance/Self Assessment Read, play, sing, and record a gospel song with dotted, syncopated rhythms

TECHNOLOGY/MEDIA LINK

MIDI/Sequencing Software Create ostinatos

Connection: Culture

Activity: Discuss Cajun culture, music, and language

ACROSS THE CURRICULUM **Science** Share a book on sleep

CULTURAL CONNECTION
Zydeco Discuss Zydeco and Cajun music
Cajun Food Discover spicy Cajun food

SPOTLIGHT ON
The Performer Facts on Cajun accordionist Clifton Chenier
Community Dances Background on the community dance "Fais do do"

MOVEMENT
Popular Dance Discuss the Cajun two-step and have students learn it
Nonlocomoter Movement Perform a synchronized swaying movement

TEACHER TO TEACHER **MIDI Song File** Help students learn the song

CHARACTER EDUCATION **Collaboration** Discuss how Zydeco music involves a combination of different cultures

MEETING INDIVIDUAL NEEDS **Using Technology** Learn vocal parts

BUILDING SKILLS THROUGH MUSIC **Health** Describe nightly rituals

Song *Fais do do* ("Go to Sleep")

More Music Choices
"Farewell to Tarwathie," p. 43
"Scarborough Fair," p. 95

ASSESSMENT

Performance/Self Assessment Read, sing, and videotape, or tape-record, a Cajun song in meter in 3

TECHNOLOGY/MEDIA LINK

MIDI/Sequencing Software Create a performance track of a Cajun song

Lesson	Elements	Skills

LESSON 4

A Song of Peace

pp. 408–411

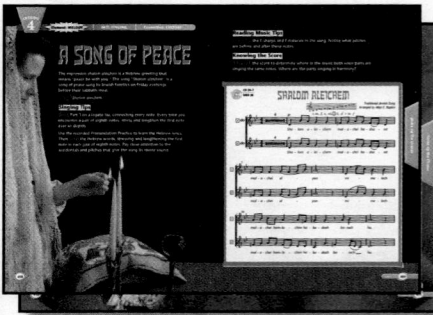

Element: Melody
Concept: Tonality
Focus: Harmonic minor melody

Secondary Element
Expression: dynamic markings

National Standards
1c 1d 6b 7a

Skill: Singing
Objective: Read and sing half steps between *ti-do, mi-fa,* and *si-la*

Secondary Skills
- **Listening** Listen to a Hebrew song and identify two themes
- **Reading** Read and sing a harmonic minor scale and melody with pitch syllables
- **Singing** Sing a Hebrew song in a *legato* style
- **Analyzing** Experiment with tempo changes
- **Performing** Perform a Hebrew song in concert

SKILLS REINFORCEMENT
- **Singing** Tips on singing the harmonic minor scale

LESSON 5

A Gift of Song

pp. 412–415

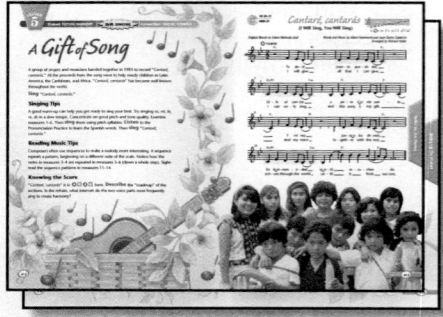

Element: Texture/Harmony
Concept: Harmony
Focus: Harmony in thirds and sixths

Secondary Element
Form: ABAB

National Standards
1c 1d 5a 6a

Skill: Singing
Objective: Read and sing harmony in thirds and sixths

Secondary Skills
- **Analyzing** Learn and discuss the Spanish lyrics of the song
- **Listening** Listen to a Spanish song with melodic sequences and harmony in thirds
- **Reading** Speak the pitch and rhythm syllables of a Spanish song
- **Singing** Sing the song in Spanish and then in English

SKILLS REINFORCEMENT
- **Singing** Tips on singing vowels and consonants

LESSON 6

A Sailing Song

pp. 416–421

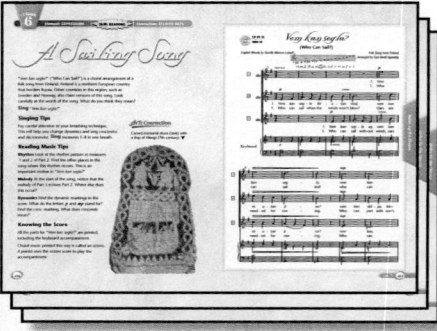

Element: Expression
Concept: Dynamics
Focus: Dynamics, *crescendo, descrescendo,* and other expressive markings in octavos

Secondary Element
Melody: harmonic and melodic minor scales

National Standards
1b 1c 1d 1e 5a 6a

Skill: Reading
Objective: Read an octavo score, and analyze choral text and melodic phrases with regard to musical expression

Secondary Skills
- **Analyzing** Study the relationship of text and melody of a song; make a list of onomatopoetic words
- **Listening** Listen to a Finnish song in three-part harmony
- **Reading** Read rhythm and pitch syllables for each vocal part; sing legato, following dynamic markings
- **Performing** Perform a song in various settings
- **Playing** Play two recorder accompaniments to a Finnish song

SKILLS REINFORCEMENT
- **Reading** Read a full octavo choral score
- **Singing** Learn to develop deep breathing for long phrasing
- **Recorder** Play a countermelody to a Finnish song

Connections

Music and Other Literature

Connection: Culture

Activity: Read about the cultural influences on Jewish music

TEACHER TO TEACHER
Singing Hebrew Singing tips
MIDI Song File Use the MIDI song file to help students learn the song

SPOTLIGHT ON **Hebrew Tradition** Background on the Jewish Sabbath

CULTURAL CONNECTION **Jewish Culture** Read about Jewish culture

ACROSS THE CURRICULUM **Language Arts** Share a book on being peaceful

BUILDING SKILLS THROUGH MUSIC **Social Studies** Discuss the influences of Jewish music

Song *"Shalom aleichem"*

More Music Choices
"Hava nagila," p. 153
"Hey, Ho! Nobody Home," p. 29

ASSESSMENT

Performance/Observation
Sing a Hebrew song in harmonic minor

TECHNOLOGY/MEDIA LINK
MIDI/Sequencing Software Compose enhancements for vocal performance in harmonic minor
Web Site Learn more about the music of Israel

Connection: Social Studies

Activity: Discuss ways to help people in need

ACROSS THE CURRICULUM **Social Studies** Discuss problems of local and world hunger; learn how the international community works together to fight hunger

SPOTLIGHT ON
"Cantaré, cantarás" **("I Will Sing, You Will Sing")** Information about a song recorded to raise money for charity
The Artist Facts on the Mexican painter Diego Rivera

CULTURAL CONNECTION **Visiting Spain** Discuss Spanish culture and art

TEACHER TO TEACHER **MIDI Song File** Use the MIDI song file to help students learn the song

BUILDING SKILLS THROUGH MUSIC **Visual Arts** Describe art through words

Song *"Cantaré, cantarás"* ("I Will Sing, You Will Sing")

More Music Choices
"El cóndor pasa," p. 46
"El payo," p. 145

ASSESSMENT

Performance/Self-Assessment Sing a song in Spanish with harmony

TECHNOLOGY/MEDIA LINK
MIDI/Sequencing Software Use the MIDI song file to explore form

---

Connection: Related Arts

Activity: Discuss the influences on Scandinavian art and folk objects

ACROSS THE CURRICULUM **Language Arts** Read and discuss a poem; help understand the meaning of text in music

SPOTLIGHT ON
The Long Ship Facts on the Scandinavian long ship
The Sea The importance of the sea in Scandinavian history

CULTURAL CONNECTION **Music and Singing in Scandinavia** Discuss singing in Scandinavia

TEACHER TO TEACHER
Singing Musically How text relates to the expression of a song
MIDI Song File Use the MIDI song file to help students learn the song

MEETING INDIVIDUAL NEEDS **Score Reading** Use notation or sequencing software to help students to learn how to read a score

BUILDING SKILLS THROUGH MUSIC **Social Studies** Discuss Scandinavian sea transportation

Song *"Vem kan segla?"* ("Who Can Sail?")

Poem "A Carelessly Crafted Raft"

More Music Choices
"You Are My Sunshine," p. 246
"Siyahamba," p. 212

ASSESSMENT

Music Journal Writing Read musical elements and notation in a Finnish folk song and write about the elements that contribute to musical expression

TECHNOLOGY/MEDIA LINK
Notation Software Create a notation score

Lesson	Elements	Skills	
LESSON 7 **Midnight Melodies** pp. 422–425 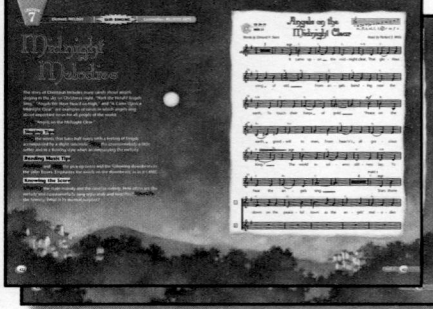	**Element: Melody** **Concept:** Countermelody **Focus:** Countermelody **Secondary Element** Articulation **National Standards** 1c 6a 6b 7b	**Skill: Singing** **Objective:** Sing a Christmas carol with a countermelody **Secondary Skills** • **Listening** Differentiate between a melody and a countermelody • **Analyzing** Analyze the melody and countermelody of a carol • **Reading** Read and discuss phrases, rhythms, accidentals, and the range of a carol • **Singing** Sing a carol paying attention to consonants and *legato* phrases • **Moving** Perform movements while singing a carol • **Performing** Formally perform a carol while remember proper	etiquette and technique **SKILLS REINFORCEMENT** • **Singing** Learn to sing consonants more effectively; gain proficiency in singing a *legato* melody • **MIDI Song File** Use a MIDI file to help students learn a carol
LESSON 8 **Sing a Joyous Carol** pp. 426–431 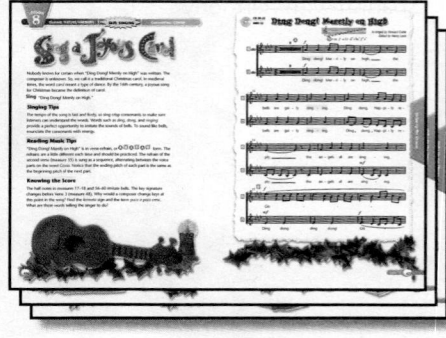	**Element:** **Texture/Harmony** **Concept:** Harmony **Focus:** Two-part harmony (soprano and alto), passing tones **Secondary Element** Expression: dynamics and articulation **National Standards** 1a 1c 1d 5a 6a	**Skill: Singing** **Objective:** Sing a two-part song that contains melismas **Secondary Skills** • **Listening** Listen to a recording to learn the parts of a carol • **Reading** Read and practice singing melismas • **Singing** Sing the song and practice singing the melismas and bell sounds • **Performing** Perform a carol with proper performance etiquette, technique, expression, and attention to detail	**SKILLS REINFORCEMENT** • **Vocal Development** Tips on singing long phrases with breath support • **Singing** Sing and enunciate bell sounds; tips on a choral warm-up exercise
LESSON 9 **Take a Little Trip** pp. 432–437 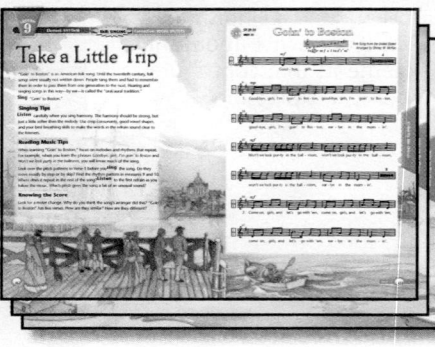	**Element: Rhythm** **Concept:** Pattern **Focus:** Rhythm patterns **Secondary Element** Melody: melodic sequence **National Standards** 1c 5b 6a 6b 6c 7b	**Skill: Singing** **Objective:** Sing rhythm patterns accurately and with clarity of diction **Secondary Skills** • **Listening** Listen to a recording of a folk song and discuss its form; develop critical listening skills • **Reading** Read the verse and refrain paying attention to the meter • **Singing** Sing a folk song while paying attention to consonant enunciation and phrasing • **Analyzing** Research other folk songs and ballads that tell a story • **Moving** Perform synchronized movements in concert	**SKILLS REINFORCEMENT** • **Enunciation and Pronunciation** Tips on these important vocal techniques

Connections	Music and Other Literature	

Connection: Related Arts
Activity: Art based on holiday themes

SPOTLIGHT ON
The Early Carol Discuss the history of the carol
Angels Discuss various meanings of the word *angel*

CULTURAL CONNECTION Holiday Celebrations Learn how other cultures celebrate holidays

ACROSS THE CURRICULUM Social Studies Discuss the history of the carol

TEACHER TO TEACHER *Legato* Phrases Learn to sing in a legato style

BUILDING SKILLS THROUGH MUSIC Writing Have students write their thoughts about an assessment

Song "Angels on the Midnight Clear"

More Music Choices
"Going upon the Mountain," p. 105
"Eres tú," p. 473
"Sing a Song of Peace," p. 66

ASSESSMENT

Performance/Peer Critique Perform a carol with movements paying attention to melody, countermelody, expression, and phrasing

TECHNOLOGY/MEDIA LINK
Multimedia Videotape and assess the performance of a carol

Connection: Genre
Activity: Read about and discuss the cultural background of caroling

ACROSS THE CURRICULUM Social Studies Read a book about an Alaskan Christmas; discuss history of specific carols

CULTURAL CONNECTION Caroling Discuss historical origins of caroling

TEACHER TO TEACHER
Melismas Tips on singing melismas
Raising the Level of Your Choir Challenge your choir to a higher level
MIDI Song File "Ding Dong! Merrily on High"

SPOTLIGHT ON Bells in Music Facts on the use of bells in music

CHARACTER EDUCATION Service Discuss the importance of charitable service

BUILDING SKILLS THROUGH MUSIC Social Studies Choose and write about a favorite carol

Song "Ding Dong! Merrily on High"

More Music Choices
"Caroling, Caroling," p. 458
"Gloria, Gloria," p. 459
"Good King Wenceslas," p. 460

ASSESSMENT

Performance/Observation Sing and tape-record a Christmas song with melismas and two-part harmony

TECHNOLOGY/MEDIA LINK
Notation Software Compose bell parts for a carol

Connection: Social Studies
Activity: Discuss the traditions and history of folk songs and ballads

ACROSS THE CURRICULUM Social Studies Share a book about Boston

SPOTLIGHT ON
Ballad Facts on the origins of ballads
The Conductor Background information on Henry Leck

CULTURAL CONNECTION
Folk Songs Discuss the heritage of folk songs
Social Dancing Facts on social dancing, frontier style (play parties)

MOVEMENT
Popular Dance Learn and perform dance movements to a folk song
Nonlocomotor Movement Learn other movements to a folk song

TEACHER TO TEACHER
Indianapolis Children's Choir Introduce this world-renowned choir
MIDI Song File "Goin' to Boston"

AUDIENCE ETIQUETTE Critical Listening Promote critical listening

BUILDING SKILLS THROUGH MUSIC Reading Paraphrase the verses of a song

Song "Goin' to Boston"

More Music Choices
"Red River Valley," p. 11
"Down in the Valley," p. 375
"Tom Dooley," p. 374

ASSESSMENT

Performance/Self-Assessment Sing a folk song in groups; evaluate the performance for rhythm, diction, and tempo

TECHNOLOGY/MEDIA LINK
Multimedia Videotape rehearsals of the class, or choir, to assess performance

INTRODUCING THE UNIT

When you *Strike Up the Chorus,* you are doing great things for students. Students have their instrument right there with them all the time. And they don't have to be the greatest singers in the world to use the power of singing to lift spirits. This unit gives you all the tools you need to put together great-sounding choral pieces. As students progress through this unit, they will be achieving higher skill levels in all aspects of performance. So strike up the chorus!

UNIT PROJECT

Read about scat singing on p. 386. "Just a Snap-Happy Blues" is based on scat singing, which is characterized by nonsense syllables.

Help your students create a list of nonsense syllables that could be used in music (for example, *doo-bee-doo-bee; sha-na-na; bop-shoo-op-shoo-op*). Encourage them to use syllables that will be easy to say and that will preserve the phrasing and accents in the music.

Listen to *It Don't Mean a Thing If It Ain't Got that Swing* **CD 19–21.** Invite students to list the nonsense syllables they heard in the piece.

Scat singing is often used to imitate instruments. Encourage your students to come up with their own vocalizations to sound like the following jazz instruments:

- Trumpet.
- Saxophone.
- Trombone.
- Drum set (also called a trap set).

Focus student attention on the choirs pictured on p. 387. Discuss the differences and similarities in the groups.

Invite students to name and discuss choirs that are familiar to them. This may include local and international groups.

Point out: choirs are usually made up of people who enjoy sharing their love of music with their audiences.

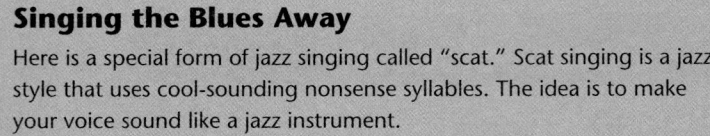

Singing the Blues Away

Here is a special form of jazz singing called "scat." Scat singing is a jazz style that uses cool-sounding nonsense syllables. The idea is to make your voice sound like a jazz instrument.

One of the most important jazz singers to adopt and use scat singing as part of his style was Mel Tormé [tohr-MAY].

Listen to Tormé's classic scat singing in *It Don't Mean a Thing If It Ain't Got that Swing.*

> **CD 19–21**
> ### It Don't Mean a Thing (If It Ain't Got That Swing)

by Duke Ellington
as performed by Mel Tormé

This performance also features jazz solo improvisations by the members of Mel Tormé's band.

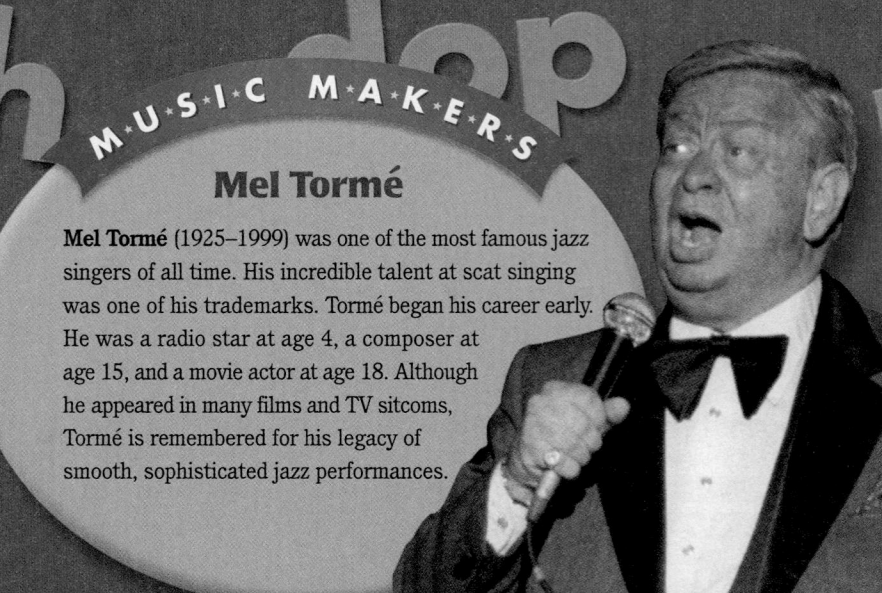

MUSIC MAKERS

Mel Tormé

Mel Tormé (1925–1999) was one of the most famous jazz singers of all time. His incredible talent at scat singing was one of his trademarks. Tormé began his career early. He was a radio star at age 4, a composer at age 15, and a movie actor at age 18. Although he appeared in many films and TV sitcoms, Tormé is remembered for his legacy of smooth, sophisticated jazz performances.

386

ACROSS THE CURRICULUM

Unit Highlights

▶ **LANGUAGE ARTS**

- Read about a young girl who learns to play the accordion from a street musician (p. 392)
- Become aware of metaphoric and descriptive language in gospel songs (p. 397)
- Read about ways to become a more peaceful person (p. 410)
- Investigate different aspects of shipbuilding (p. 416)
- Discuss descriptive language as found in choral texts (p. 419)

▶ **SOCIAL STUDIES**

- Learn about the Underground Railroad and some of the songs associated with it (p. 400)
- Discuss ways to help children or families in need (p. 412)

- Learn more about the agencies involved in the fight against world hunger (p. 414)
- Learn more about carols and carol singing (p. 424)
- Share information and write journal entries about holiday traditions (p. 426)
- Read the history of two Christmas carols (p. 429)
- Learn more about the impact that Boston has had on U.S. history (p. 432)

▶ **SCIENCE**

- Read about the body's need for sleep (p. 402)

UNIT 11

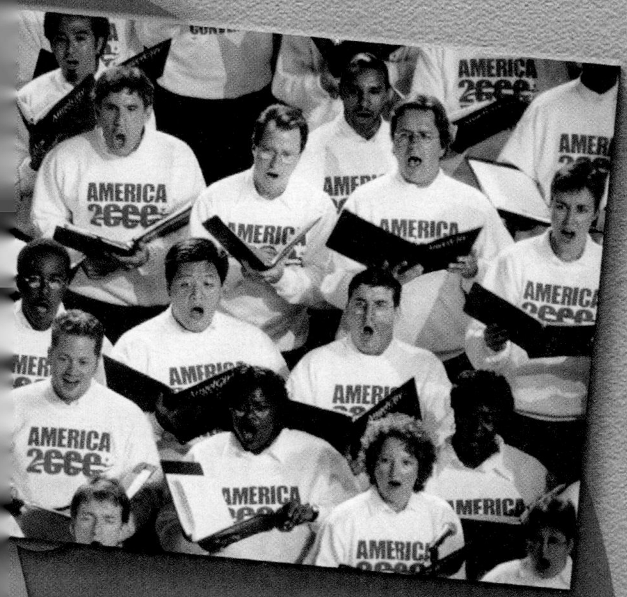

STRIKE UP THE CHORUS

Millions of people enjoy singing in choirs. Choirs perform in all styles—from folk to rock and from classical to jazz.

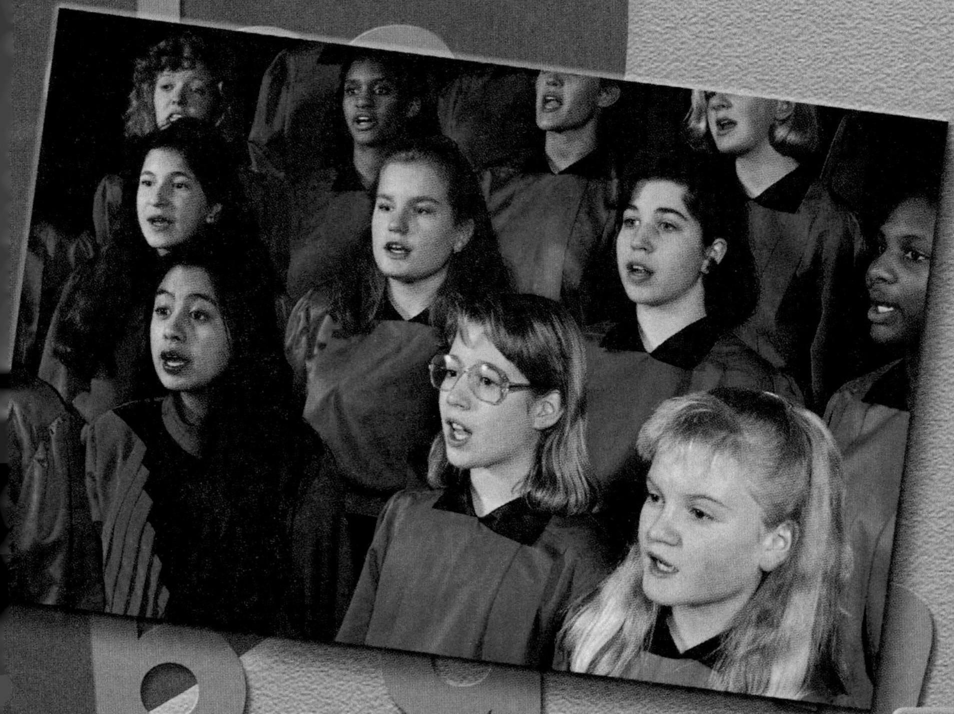

MUSIC SKILLS
ASSESSED IN THIS UNIT

Reading Music: Rhythm

Perform rhythms accurately while singing an arrangement of a folk song (p. 437)

Reading Music: Pitch

Sing an arrangement from an octavo (p. 421)

Performing Music: Singing

Evaluate a videotaped performance of an Acadian folk song (p. 407)

Observe and evaluate the performance of a specific scale and a traditional Jewish song (p. 411)

Sing a Hispanic song and evaluate the performance (p. 415)

Evaluate and discuss the performance of an arrangement of a song (p. 425)

Tape-record and discuss the performance of a song with two-part harmony (p. 431)

Performing Music: Playing

Evaluate performance factors after singing a three-part arrangement of a spiritual and accompanying it with an ostinato (p. 401)

Performance/Self-Assessment

Evaluate and discuss a videotaped performance (p. 395)

CULTURAL CONNECTION

Unit Highlights

▶ AFRICAN/AFRICAN AMERICAN

- The origins of African American spirituals (p. 397)
- "The Gospel Train" (p. 398)

▶ AMERICAN REGIONAL

- *Zydeco* music as one aspect of Cajun music (p. 403)
- *"Fais do do"* p. 403
- Cajun cooking as a separate genre (p. 404)
- The history of caroling (p. 426)
- "Goin' to Boston" (p. 433)
- Social dancing as an aspect of American frontier life (p. 434)

▶ EUROPEAN

- *"Shalom aleichem"* (p. 409)
- Jewish culture and music (p. 409)
- A few interesting facts about Spain (p. 413)
- *"Vem kan segla?"* (p. 417)
- Singing as an activity in Scandinavian countries (p. 417)

▶ HOLIDAYS

- An invitation to research Kwanzaa, Chanukah, and Ramadan (p. 423)

▶ FOLK SONGS

- The creation and transmission of folk songs by many different cultures (p. 433)

OPENING ACTIVITIES

MATERIALS

- "Just a Snap-Happy Blues"   **CD 19–22**

  Recording Routine:
  Intro (6 m.); vocal; coda

- Dance Directions for "Just a Snap-Happy Blues" p. 566

- *It Don't Mean a Thing (If It Ain't Got That Swing)* (excerpt)   **CD 19–21**

Listening

Have students listen to "Just a Snap-Happy Blues" **CD 19–22** while following the notation on pp. 388–389.

ASK What "special effects" do you notice in the song? (scat singing, accents, "scoops" up to pitches, finger snaps)

Invite students to discuss their observations with the class.

ASK What is the form of the song? (ABA)

Singing

Invite students to follow this routine to learn to sing "Just a Snap-Happy Blues."

- Have them first learn the unison part (mm. 1–24).
- Teach each voice part in mm. 25–48 to the entire class. Help students understand that each part is created from a short, repeated phrase.

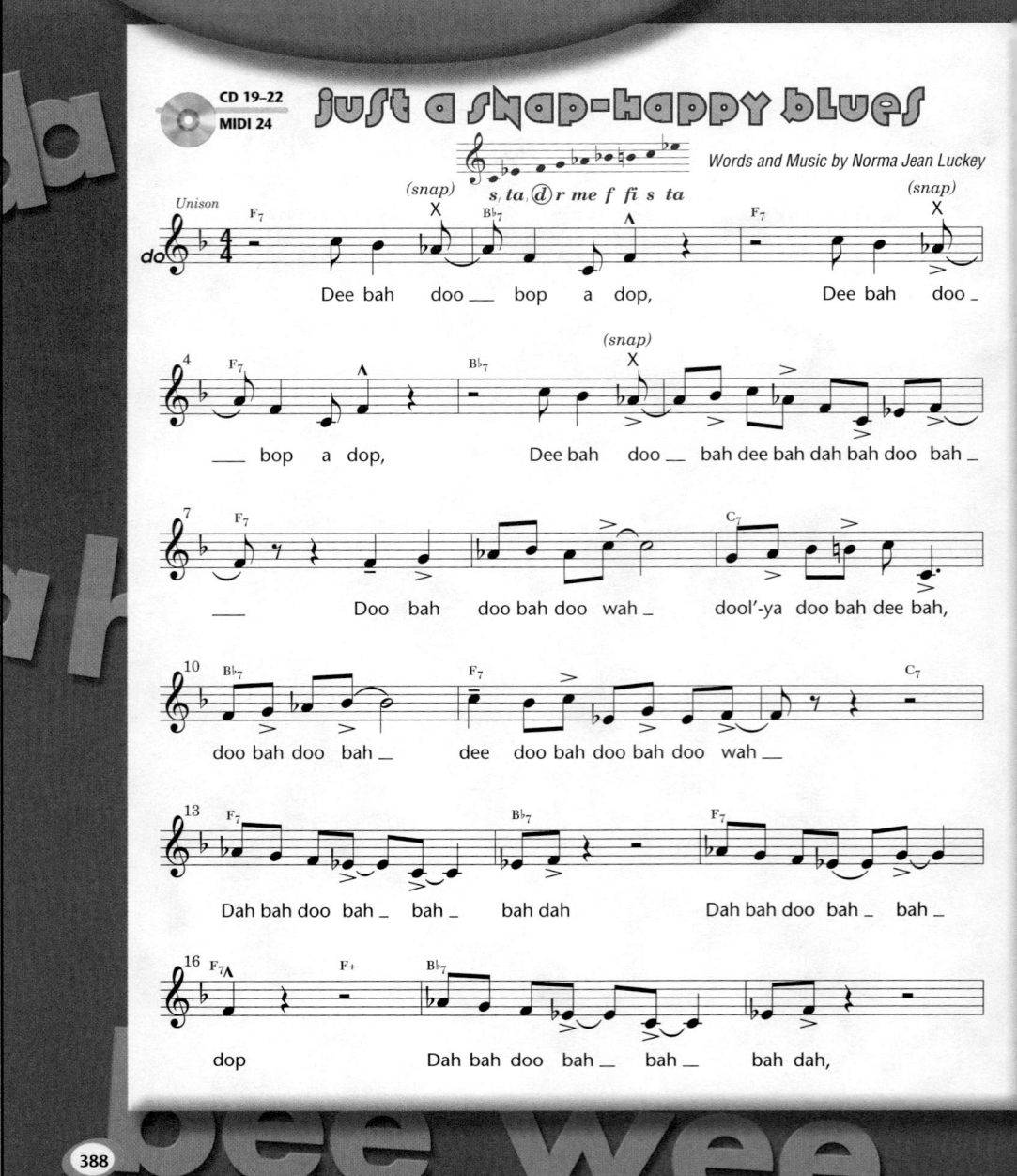

Sing 'n' Snap

Singing the blues doesn't mean you have to be sad.

Sing "Just a Snap-Happy Blues," a song that is sung entirely with scat syllables.

388

ASSESSMENT

Unit Highlights The lessons in this unit were chosen and developed to support the theme "Strike Up the Chorus." Each lesson, as always, presents a clear element focus, a skill objective, and an end-of-lesson assessment. The overall sequence of lessons, however, is organized according to this theme, rather than concept of skill development. In this context, formal assessment strategies, such as those presented in Units 1–6, are no longer applicable.

▶ **INFORMAL ASSESSMENTS**

At the close of each Teacher's Edition lesson in this unit, one of the following types of assessments is used to evaluate the learning of the key element focus or skill objective.

- Music Journal Writing (p. 421)
- Performance/Observation (pp. 411, 431)
- Performance/Peer Critique (p. 425)
- Performance/Self-Assessment (pp. 395, 401, 407, 415, 437)

▶ **RUBRICS**

Visit *www.sfsuccessnet.com* for rubrics to assess students' achievement in music skills.

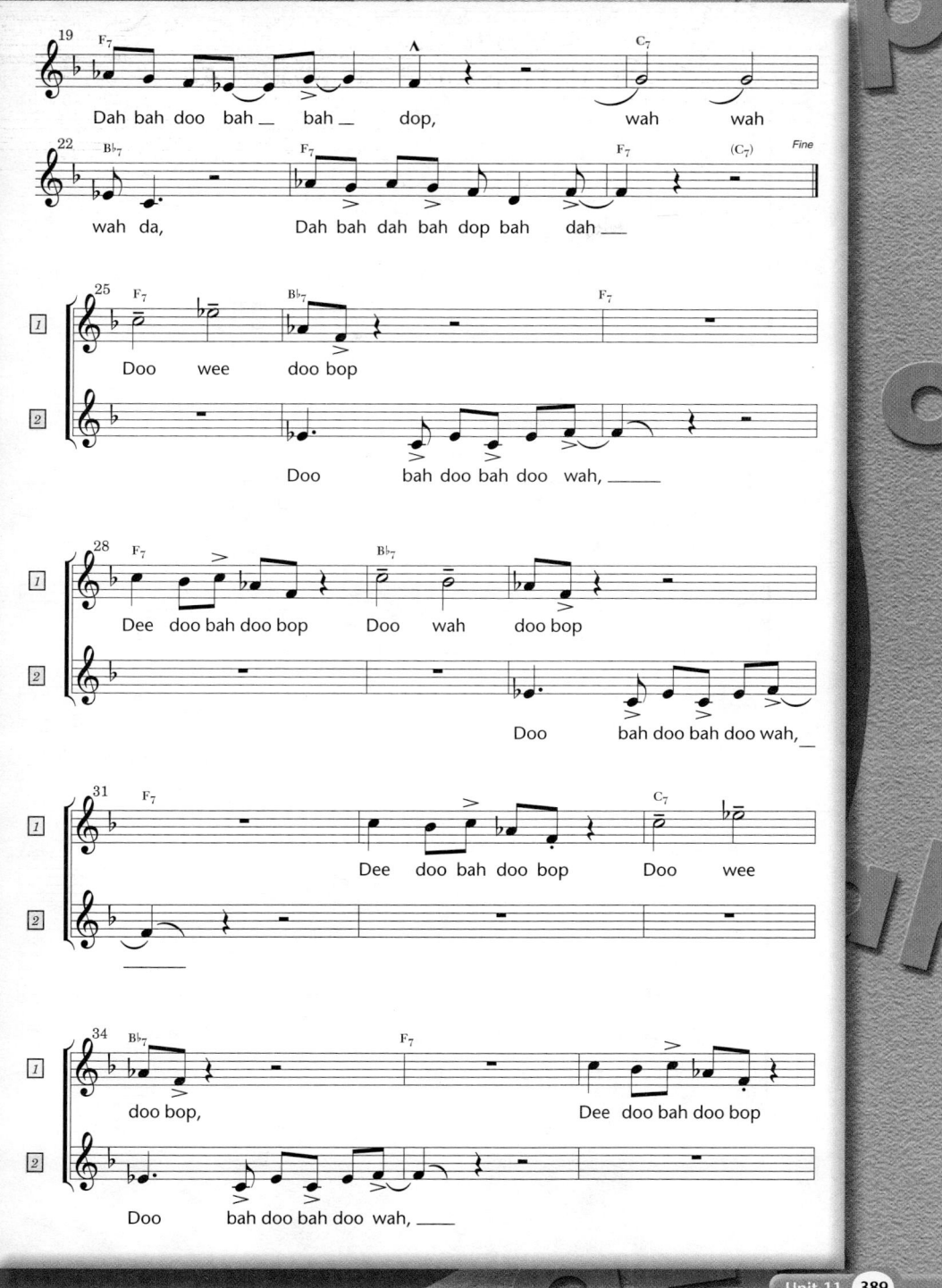

Reading

Have students read the words in rhythm on the unison section of "Just a Snap-Happy Blues."

- Encourage the students to add the accents and finger snaps as indicated.
- Remind students to "swing" the eighth note rhythms. (Written eighth notes appear to be evenly spaced, but when "swung," they are performed as though they were the first and last notes of a triplet.)
- Use as slow a tempo as needed to give your students time to read successfully.

Moving

Divide the class into three groups, one for each voice in "Just a Snap-Happy Blues." Have each group create a unique movement that will match either voice Part 1, 2, or 3.

After students have performed their movement for the class, invite all groups to perform with the recording. Help students recognize that some groups rest while others are moving.

See Dance Directions on p. 566 for other ideas.

TECHNOLOGY/MEDIA LINK

Unit Highlights

▶ **MIDI/SEQUENCING SOFTWARE**

- Learn a song by using the MIDI song file to manipulate various aspects of the song (p. 395)
- Create ostinatos and arrangements of a song using the MIDI file (p. 401)
- Create a performance track for a song using MIDI sequencing software (p. 407)
- Improvise and compose enhancements for the vocal performance of a song (p. 411)
- Use the MIDI file of a song to explore its form (p. 415)

▶ **MULTIMEDIA**

- Evaluate a videotaped class performance of a song (p. 425)
- Videotape rehearsals for the performance of a song and offer suggestions for improvement (p. 437)

▶ **NOTATION SOFTWARE**

- Score a computer version of a song using notation software (p. 421)
- Compose new bell parts for a song using notation software (p. 431)

Improvising

Help your students create their own scat singing to "Just a Snap-Happy Blues." For example, as the class sings Part 1, invite soloists to fill in rests (mm. 26–27, 30–31, etc.) with their own syllables.

Repeat the process for Parts 2 and 3.

Students can also fill in the rests with rhythms played on classroom or other percussion instruments.

Record and evaluate the most successful patterns. Use a tape or video recorder. Notate the patterns if possible.

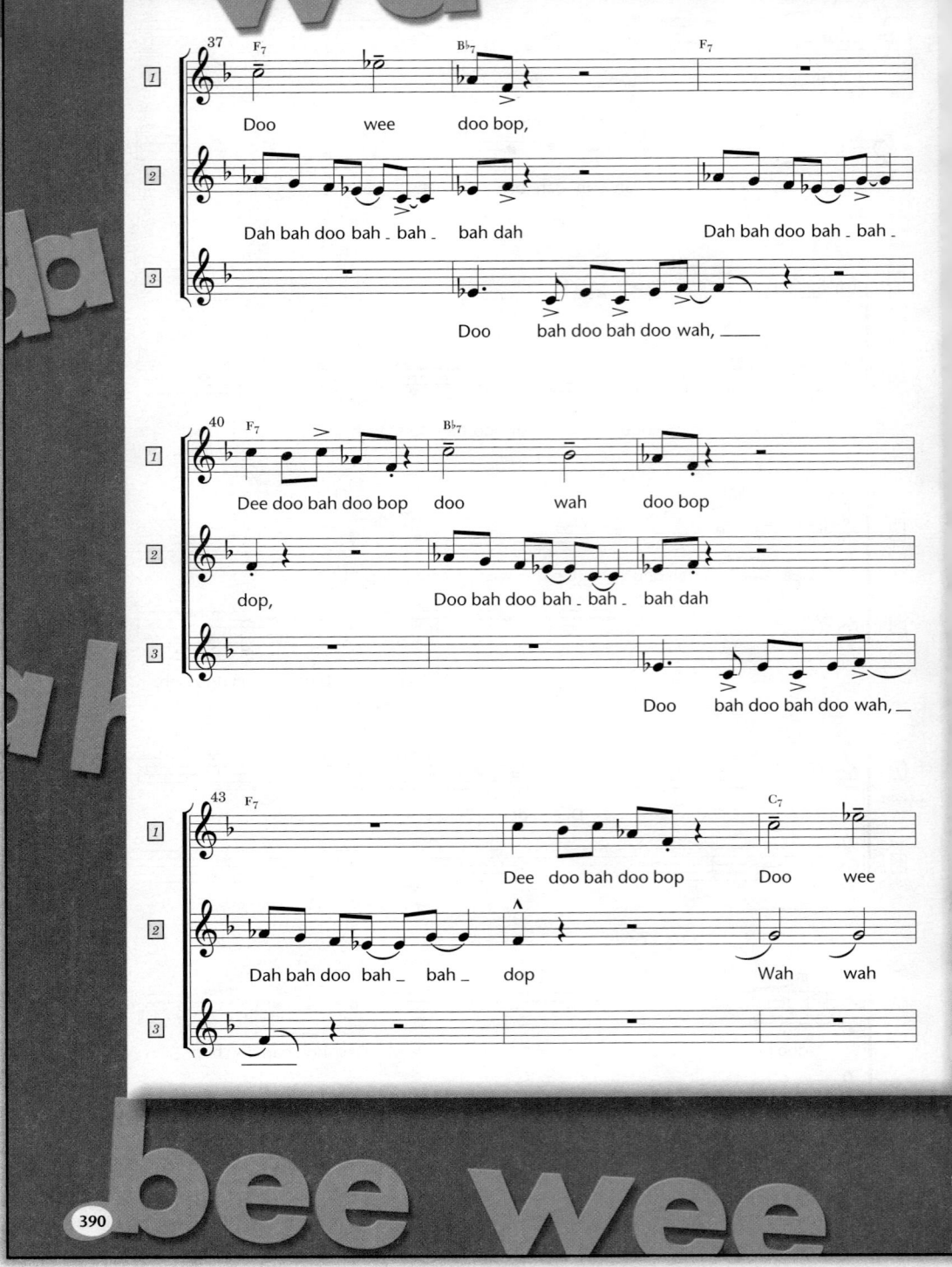

TECHNOLOGY/MEDIA LINK

▶ **VIDEO LIBRARY/DVD**

- See a video performance of a gospel choir (p. 395)

▶ **WEB SITE**

- Visit *www.sfsuccessnet.com* to learn more about the music of Israel (p. 411)

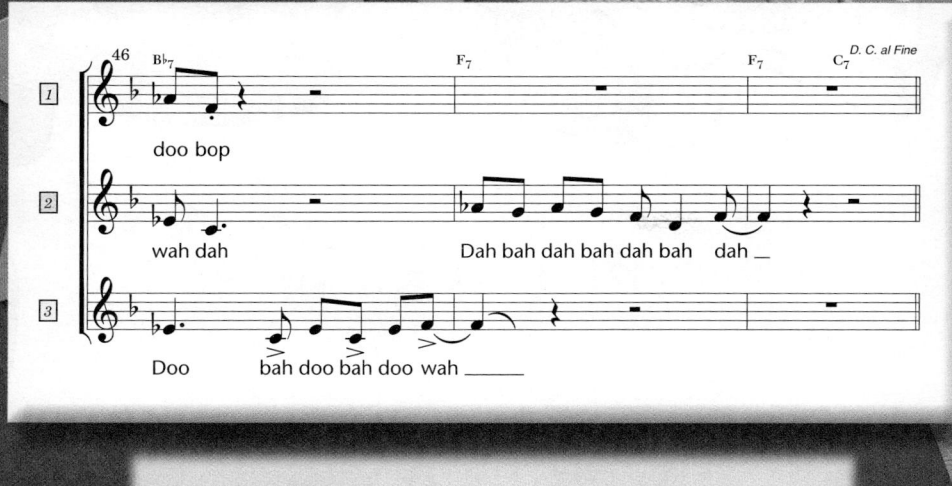

doo bop

wah dah   Dah bah dah bah dah bah   dah

Doo   bah doo bah doo wah

Snappy Moves

Create some jazzy moves for the blues tune "Just a Snap-Happy Blues." **Move** when you are singing. Freeze when the music rests.

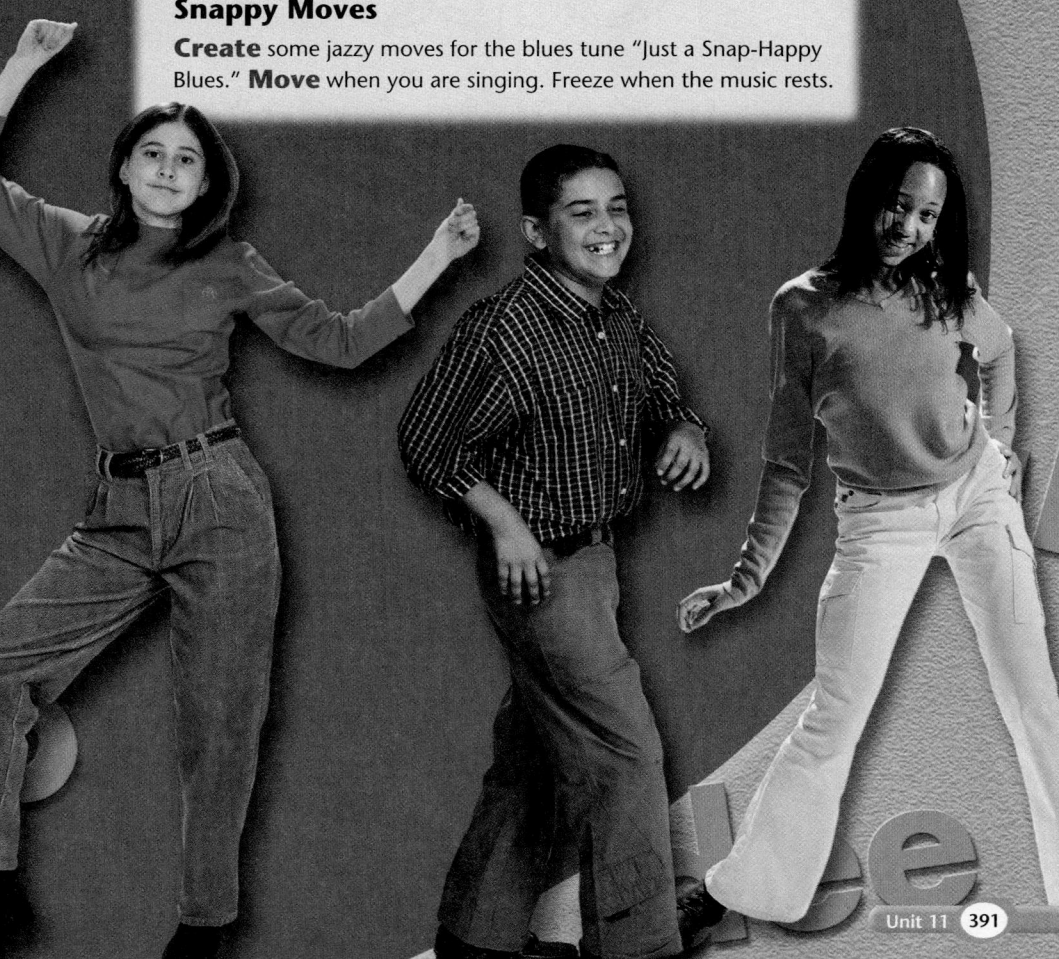

Unit 11 **391**

INNOVATIVE TEACHER SUPPORT FOR THIS UNIT

- **MAKING MUSIC DVD, Grade 6** contains video segments that support lessons, including signing and movement.
- **MAKING MUSIC with Movement and Dance** provides more opportunities for large group activities in music or physical education classes.
- **MAKING MUSIC with Technology** provides lesson plans for many technology applications; includes MIDI files.
- *¡A cantar!* features recorded songs and lessons from around the Spanish-speaking world; includes strategies for bilingual classes and for English-speaking teachers working with Spanish-speaking students.
- **Bridges to Asia** features recorded songs and lessons from Asian and Pacific region cultures.
- *www.sfsuccessnet.com* provides an online lesson planner to conveniently create lesson plans at school or at home. Includes rubrics for assessment, lesson modifications to meet the needs of all students, performance musicals based on program content, and more.

LESSON AT A GLANCE

Element Focus	**EXPRESSION** Expressive singing
Skill Objective	**SINGING** Sing text expressively through effective text delivery and appropriate tone quality
Connection Activity	**GENRE** Read about and discuss the history of gospel music

MATERIALS

- "A Gift to Share"   **CD 19-24**

  Recording Routine: Intro (4 m.); vocal

- *Glory, Glory, Hallelujah* (gospel)   **CD 3-29**

VOCABULARY

call and response   first and second endings
repeat sign   ornamentation

◆ ◆ ◆ National Standards ◆ ◆ ◆ ◆

1b Sing easy pieces with technical accuracy
1c Sing music from diverse genres
1d Sing music written in two parts
5a Read dotted notes in triple meter
7b Students use specific criteria for evaluating their own performances
9a Describe characteristics of music from a variety of genres
9c Compare, in several cultures, functions music serves

MORE MUSIC CHOICES

For more practice singing gospels or spirituals:
"Ain't Gonna Let Nobody Turn Me 'Round," p. 85
"Sometimes I Feel Like a Motherless Child," p. 241
"This Little Light of Mine," p. 232

A Gospel Gift

"A Gift to Share" is a gospel song. Gospel music grew out of the African American spirituals of the 18th and 19th centuries. Gospel can be fast or slow, but it is always full of expression.

Sing "A Gift to Share" with expression.

Singing Tips

Sing the vowels of each word as if the vowels stand very tall inside your mouth. Find the green color box in measure 5. Imagine a warm and resonant tone quality as you sing with the shape of an *ah* vowel.

Reading Music Tips

The opening melody appears not to stop or rest until measure 20. How will you decide where to breathe? Use phrase endings and punctuation marks to help you decide.

Knowing the Score

A phrase is a small group of notes that has a definite melody or shape. The first phrase of this song is highlighted in yellow. Notice that there are many phrases in this song—some are long, and others are short. Find measures 33–44. Do the rests interrupt the phrases, or are they part of it?

392

Footnotes

ACROSS THE CURRICULUM

▶ **Language Arts** Share the book *Gift* by Aliana Brodmann (Simon & Schuster, 1993) about a young girl who wants to spend her Chanukah money and finds a street musician who teaches her how to play the accordion (his gift to her). Invite students to write in their journals about the sharing of special talents and skills as gifts. Point out to students that this is different from giving a present. Ask students to think about what they could give someone as a special "gift."

BUILDING SKILLS THROUGH MUSIC

▶ **Writing** Have students read the lyrics of "A Gift to Share" and discuss the meaning of the words. Ask students to write 1–2 paragraphs reflecting on what it means to share the gift of being yourself.

SPOTLIGHT ON

▶ **Gospel** Black gospel music is African American Protestant sacred singing. It is associated with the twentieth-century sacred genre, which also includes white gospel music. In this style, vocalists embellish simple melodies with both full and falsetto voice. It is not uncommon for singers to hum, shout, growl, moan, whisper, scream, and cry. Singers add ornamentation, complex syncopations, blue notes or vocal slides, and freely repeated fragments of text. Some well-known gospel singers include Mahalia Jackson (see Spotlight On, p. 394), Marion Williams, Ray Charles, and Aretha Franklin. Accompaniments for gospel music include piano, Hammond organ, or guitar either alone or with bass, drums, and tambourine.

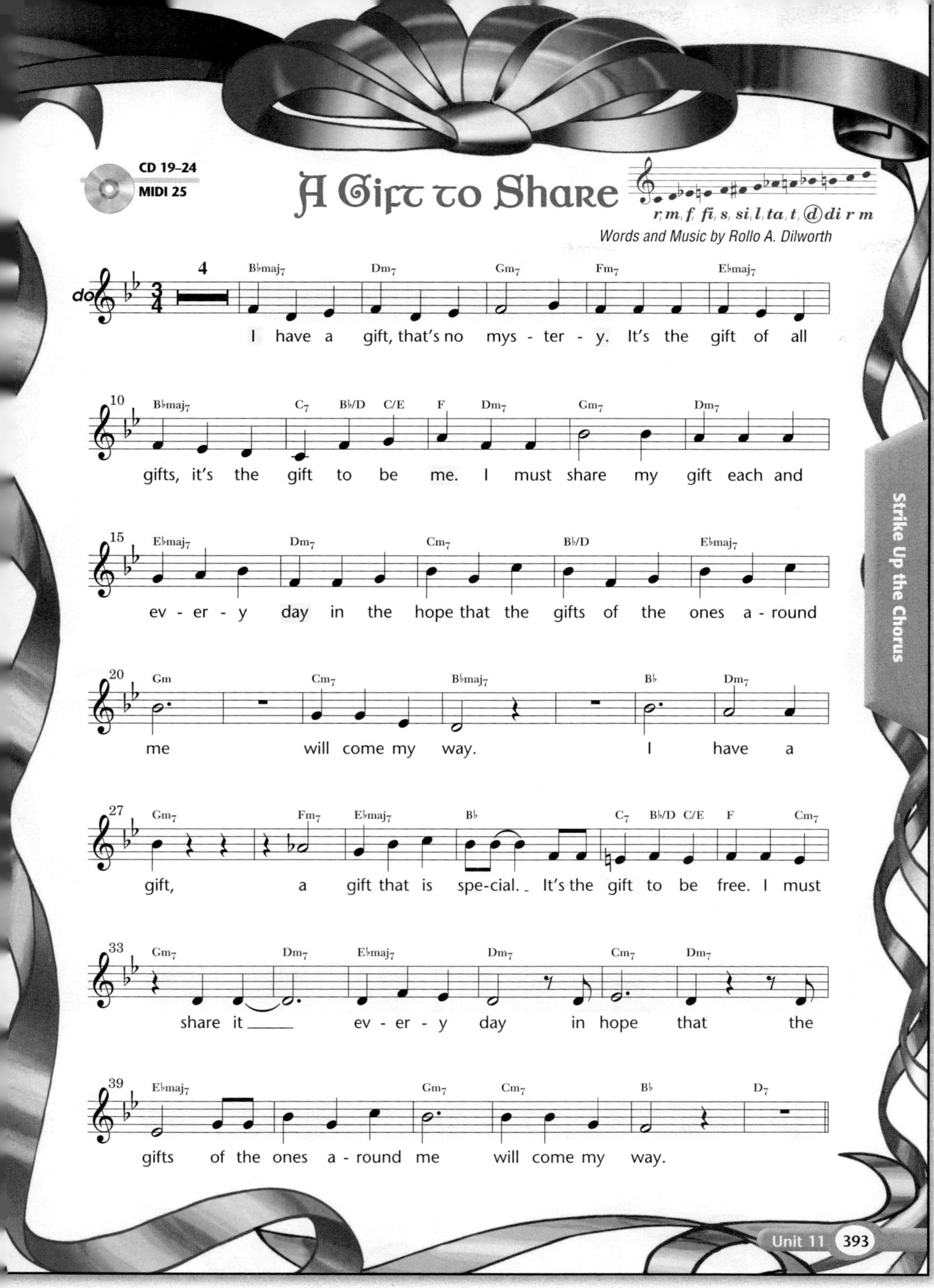

A Gift to Share

Words and Music by Rollo A. Dilworth

CD 19–24
MIDI 25

r m f fi s si l ta t @ di r m

I have a gift, that's no mys-ter-y. It's the gift of all

gifts, it's the gift to be me. I must share my gift each and

ev-er-y day in the hope that the gifts of the ones a-round

me will come my way. I have a

gift, a gift that is spe-cial. It's the gift to be free. I must

share it ___ ev-er-y day in hope that the

gifts of the ones a-round me will come my way.

Strike Up the Chorus

Unit 11 **393**

---

1 INTRODUCE

Read and discuss with students the history and purpose of African American gospel music as described on p. 392 and in Spotlight On, p. 392. Determine if gospel is sung by only a soloist, a choir, or both (both).

Have students read and discuss the lyrics of "A Gift to Share" and tell what the gifts are in the song (freedom, me). Lead students in a discussion of gifts by sharing the information in Across the Curriculum, p. 392.

2 DEVELOP

Listening

Play the gospel recording of *Glory, Glory, Hallelujah* **CD 3-29**, which features a gospel choir performing the song. Have students

- Describe the vocal style of the choir. (energetic, robust, big sound)
- Describe the vocal style of the soloist. (free style with improvisation on melody and rhythm, melodic ornamentation)

9a Share with students that gospel singers sing with freedom and expression (lots of ornamentation—adding extra notes to a particular word and note).

- Identify how the choir and soloist energize consonants.
- Identify why the soloist sometimes repeats text.
- Identify how and why rests interrupt the flow of the text and melody.

continued on page 394

SKILLS REINFORCEMENT

▶ **Listening** Students should be able to recognize phrases, phrase repetition, call and response, and first and second endings as ways of organizing a song. Help students notice that a phrase has a set number of measures. Awareness that phrases have an antecedent (musical question) and consequent (musical answer) arrangement helps singers understand the structural flow of a composition. Knowing the parts of a phrase helps singers recognize when a composer uses fragments of it to create new compositional material.

TEACHER TO TEACHER

▶ **Inner Hearing** Inner hearing is the ability to silently hear music in your head (melody, rhythm, harmony, and tonality) as you read music. It is one of the most important skills used by conductors, composers, and performing musicians and singers. The skill of sight-reading is based on inner hearing. Inner hearing is a skill that is necessary for developing accurate intonation, music reading, part-singing, and memorization.

Have students warm up using a variety of pitch syllable, scale, and chord interval exercises as a first step to developing an inner tonality. Help students focus on inner hearing before singing aloud; for example, before singing a musical passage. This technique can also be used throughout the choral rehearsal to focus attention on part-singing.

Lesson 1 Continued

Reading

Invite students to listen to "A Gift to Share" **CD 19-24.**

Have students

- Identify the melody in mm. 45–53 (Part 1).
- Identify the melody in mm. 54–73 (Part 2).
- Identify the first repeat sign (m. 74).
- Identify the call-and-response passage (mm. 74–77).
- Explain how the notes in the second ending differ from those in the first ending.

See Skills Reinforcement, p. 393, for practice listening for phrases and form.

Singing

Warm up the choir on *mi, do, re, mi* in several different keys. Then, have students say the rhythm syllables of "A Gift to Share, " mm. 5–20, feeling one beat to the bar.

Express beat 1 of each measure as if the duration of that beat was just a little bit longer: ONE, two, three. Have students

- Speak the text expressively (mm. 5–20), emphasizing the first beat of each measure.
- Sing the text expressively, emphasizing verbs, adjectives, and nouns.
- Sing a little softer on half and dotted half notes in the harmony parts, allowing the quarter notes in the harmony part to be heard.
- Sing the text, imagining the vowels of each word to be large inside the mouth, producing a warm vocal quality.

Have students sing "A Gift to Share" with the recording.

See Teacher to Teacher, p. 393, for information on how inner hearing helps students to sight-read better and Skills Reinforcement below, for more ideas about vocal development.

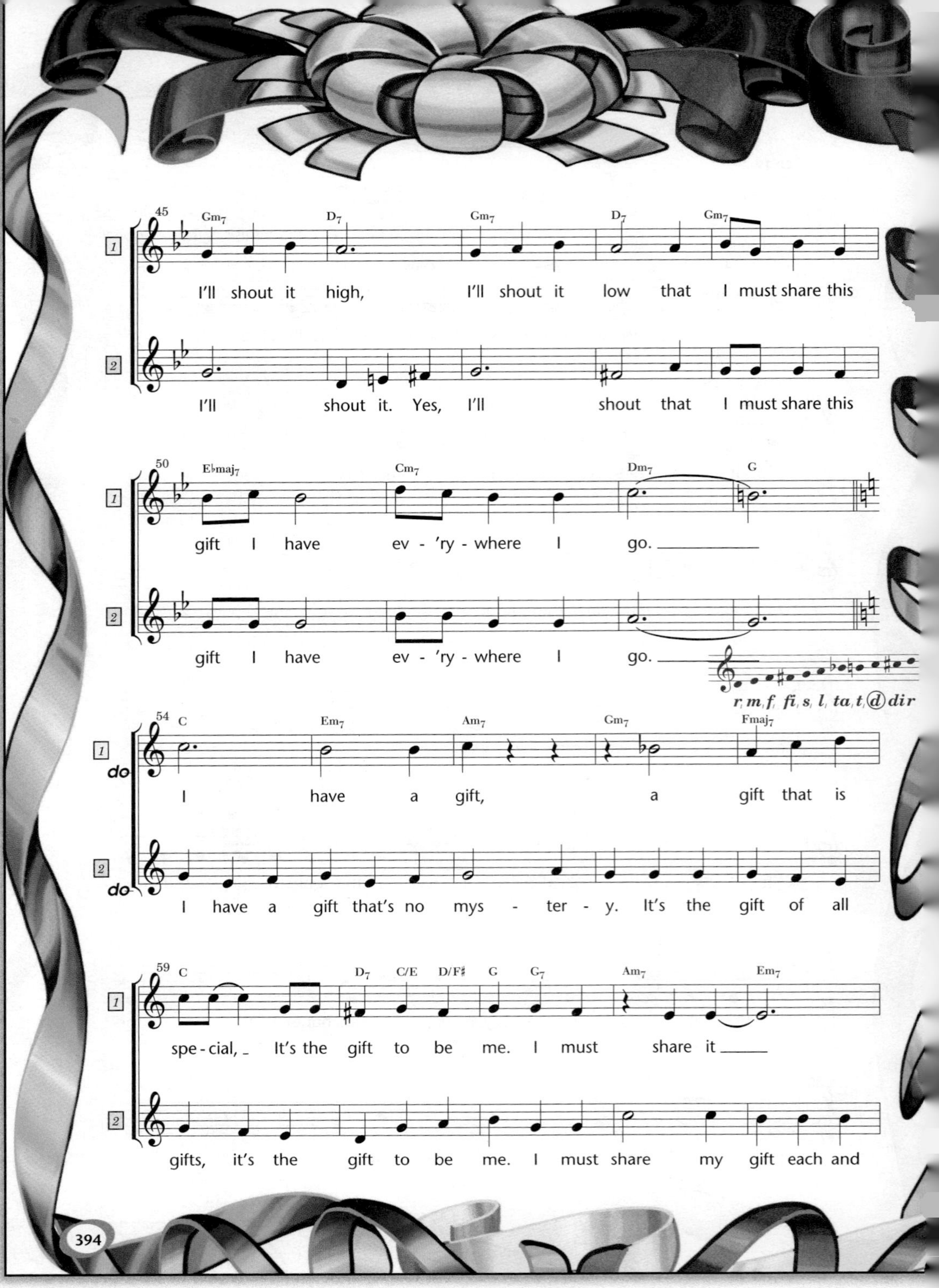

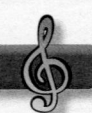

Footnotes

SPOTLIGHT ON

▶ **The Performer** Mahalia Jackson (1911–1972) was born in New Orleans, the third of four children. Her mother died when she was five. Her father sent her and one of her brothers to live with an aunt. By 1927, she had moved to Chicago and started to sing for her supper. She married, then opened a beauty shop, where she also sold flowers to churches and funeral homes. Many of her customers would try to blackmail her into singing at a funeral by refusing to buy her flowers unless she would sing. Jackson's recording of "Move On Up a Little Higher," in 1947, established her as the "Gospel Queen."

SKILLS REINFORCEMENT

▶ **Vocal Development** To assist students in developing better intonation (or key), play or sing a sustained tone while students internalize and then sing musical patterns against that tone. For example, playing a B♭ tonic while students internalize and then sing the opening phrase of "A Gift to Share" will focus students' attention on singing the melody in the key of B♭. It does not matter that the chords are changing, the B♭ tonic is still predominant.

To assist in memorizing a song, have students sing an entire choral score internally with the teacher conducting. Tell students that to internalize, think of humming, without actually humming. If they do this, they will hear the music in their heads.

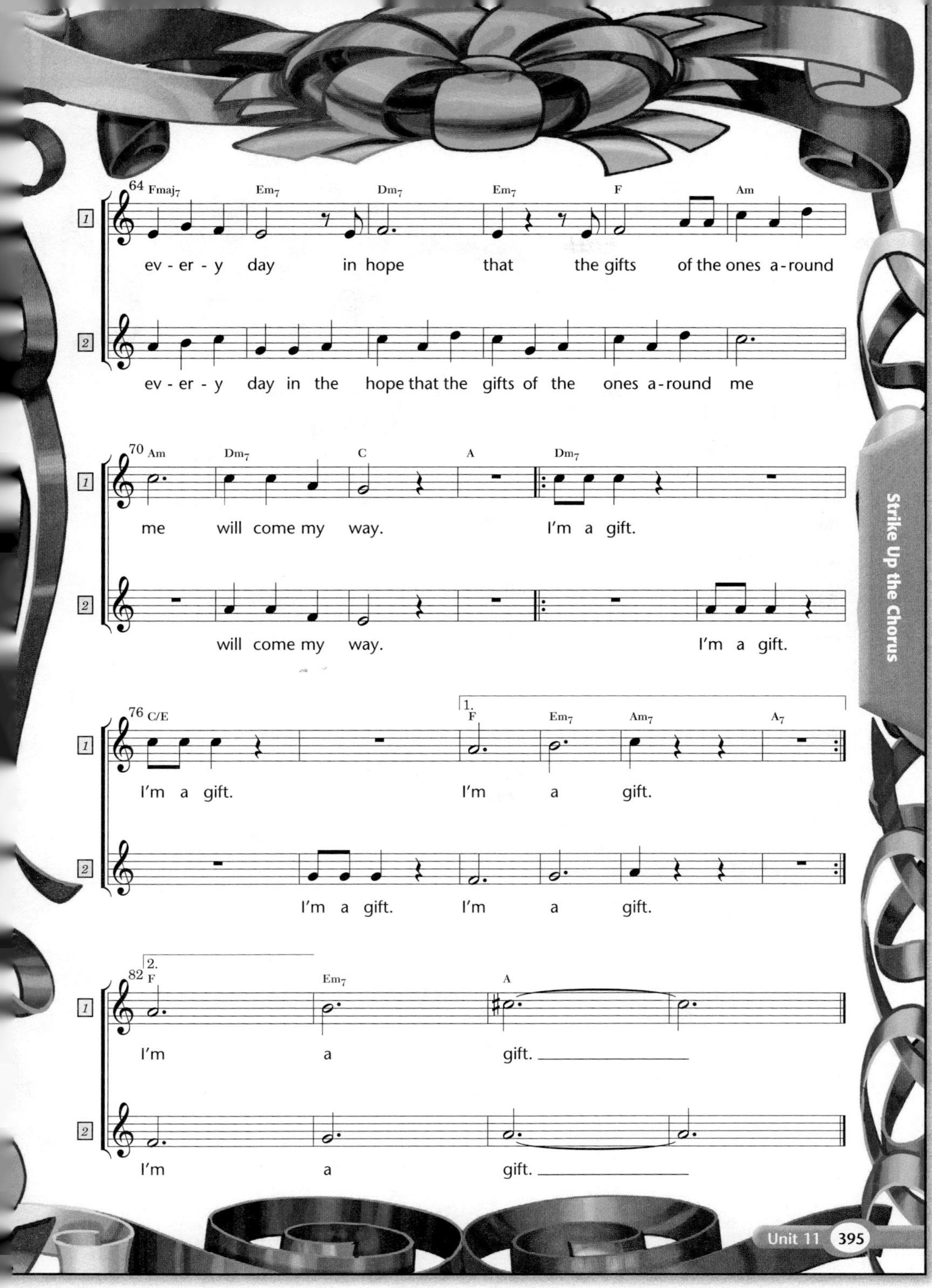

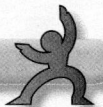

Musical notation (mm. 64–89, two parts)

| m. 64 | Fmaj7 | Em7 | Dm7 | Em7 | F | Am |

Part 1: ev-er-y day   in hope   that   the gifts   of the ones a-round

Part 2: ev-er-y day in the   hope that the   gifts of the   ones a-round me

| m. 70 | Am | Dm7 | C | A | Dm7 |

Part 1: me   will come my   way.   I'm a gift.

Part 2: will come my   way.   I'm a gift.

| m. 76 C/E | 1. F | Em7 | Am7 | A7 |

Part 1: I'm a gift.   I'm   a   gift.

Part 2: I'm a gift.   I'm   a   gift.

| m. 82 2. F | Em7 | A |

Part 1: I'm   a   gift. ____

Part 2: I'm   a   gift. ____

Analyzing

9a Have students read about the history of gospel music and its purpose. Revisit Spotlight On, p. 392. Students should listen to recordings of different gospel artists. The information that is gathered from these two activities can be made into written reports to be shared with the class.

Singing

9c For a final project, invite a gospel artist from the community to sing for the class and to talk about gospel music. Incorporate the nonlocomotor movements presented in Movement, below, into a performance of "A Gift to Share." Have students share some of their research on gospel music as part of the concert. Invite the gospel artist to be a part of a gospel concert. Guide students to learn and demonstrate appropriate large-ensemble performance techniques and concert etiquette during formal concerts. Videotape the concert for viewing and evaluating purposes.

3 CLOSE

Element: EXPRESSION — **ASSESSMENT**

7b Performance/Self-Assessment Play the concert videotape (see Singing, above) for the class, or have students sing "A Gift to Share" **CD 19-24** with attention to expression of the lyrics. Record the performance. Invite students to evaluate the effectiveness of their musical performance. Have them discuss their performance and musical expression, using the following criteria.

- Analyze the vocal quality for gospel style.
- Evaluate the clarity of diction.
- Evaluate the degree of expressive delivery of the words.
- Determine if the harmony parts are balanced.
- Determine if the tempo is appropriate for the text and style.

MOVEMENT

▶ **Nonlocomotor Movement** Synchronized choir movements are a part of the gospel choir experience. In "A Gift to Share," a swaying movement can be used beginning in m. 25. Have students initiate the swaying motion by shifting their weight to each heel in turn, on the first beat of each measure, and continuing the motion in that direction.

R–2–3   L–2–3

Keep the motion relaxed and subtle. Ask students to synchronize with each other (using tempo and meter as their guide). As students learn the song, develop new synchronized movements that the choir can use at a performance of "A Gift to Share."

TECHNOLOGY/MEDIA LINK

Video Library Invite students to see a gospel choir perform in the video, the *Total Experience Gospel Choir*.

MIDI/Sequencing Software The choral music in Unit 11 is accompanied by a MIDI song file for each song. Use these MIDI files to play the tempo slower, isolate vocal parts, teach the harmony parts, highlight difficult measures to repeat and practice, and transpose the key, if desired. These files will assist students in learning the music and in rehearsing for performance.

Use the MIDI song file for "A Gift to Share" to help students learn the song.

LESSON AT A GLANCE

Element Focus   **RHYTHM** Dotted rhythms in $\frac{2}{4}$ meter

Skill Objective   **PLAYING** Read and play dotted rhythms and syncopation in $\frac{2}{4}$ meter

Connection Activity   **LANGUAGE ARTS** Read about and discuss the use of metaphors in the lyrics of gospel music

MATERIALS

• "The Gospel Train"   CD 19-26
  Recording Routine: Intro (4 m.); refrain; v. 1; refrain; v. 2; refrain; v. 3; refrain
• nonpitched rhythm instruments

VOCABULARY

dotted rhythm   syncopation   pickup note   ostinato

◆ ◆ ◆ ◆ **National Standards** ◆ ◆ ◆ ◆

1a Sing accurately in small ensembles
1b Sing easy pieces with technical accuracy
1d Sing music written in three parts
2a Play instruments accurately in small ensembles
4c Compose, using traditional sound sources
5a Read dotted notes in duple meter
5c Identify standard notation symbols for expression
6a Listen and describe events in music using appropriate terms
7a Students evaluate the music they perform
7b Students use specific criteria for evaluating their own performances

MORE MUSIC CHOICES

For more practice singing gospel music or spirituals:
"Ezekiel Saw the Wheel," p. 379
"Glory, Glory, Hallelujah," p. 52

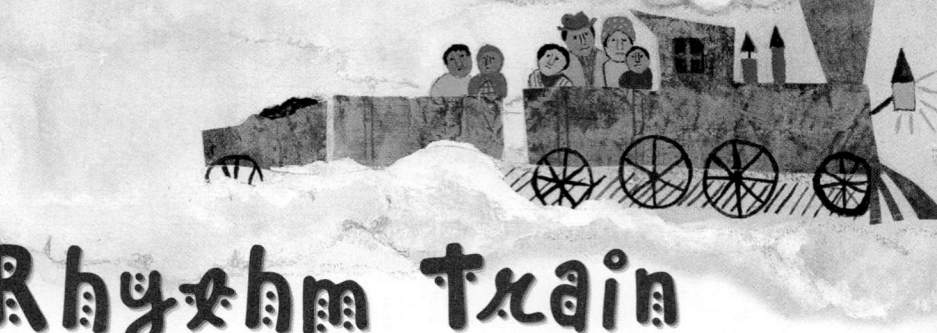

Rhythm Train

Many songs are about trains. African Americans once used trains to symbolize the Underground Railroad—the train to freedom.

Sing "The Gospel Train."

Singing Tips

Enunciating the first consonant of each word adds to the rhythmic vitality of this song. It is important not to slide in and out of pitches. A crisp, rhythmic delivery of the words will capture the style of "The Gospel Train."

Reading Music Tips

The pickup is a rhythmic motive that appears throughout "The Gospel Train." (See the color box on page 398.) **Analyze** the rhythm in this motive. How does it suggest the rhythmic motion of a train?

Knowing the Score

The form of this song is a series of **A** (Refrain) and **B** (Verse) sections. The dynamics vary from f in the first refrain to pp in the first verse. **Analyze** the words to figure out why there is such a large contrast in dynamic levels.

Play these rhythm patterns on a mallet instrument. **Create** ostinatos to accompany "The Gospel Train" by combining the patterns in new ways.

1. 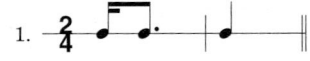   2.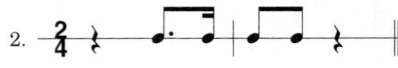

3. 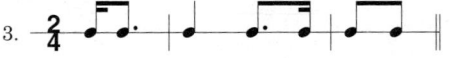   4.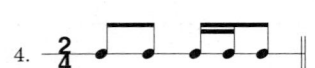

396

Footnotes

SKILLS REINFORCEMENT

▶ **Listening** Knowing how songs are constructed helps students sing with more musical awareness. Many gospel songs incorporate A and B themes, an ostinato, call and response, and embellished rhythms. Students should be encouraged to visually and aurally recognize these characteristics.

BUILDING SKILLS THROUGH MUSIC

▶ **Writing** Share the information from Introduce, p. 397. After a discussion about the use of metaphors in the song, have students write a sentence using one of the metaphors in the song effectively. Have them discuss other metaphors.

SPOTLIGHT ON

▶ **Gospel Music** Gospel, an informal, often spontaneous music style, began in the United States. It has call and response, shouts, and hand clapping. The Fisk University Choir popularized this music in its performances, but there was no publication of gospel music until 1875. This publication was *Gospel Songs*, collected by Philip Bliss.

▶ **Early Gospel Singers** Thomas Dorsey spent most of his life promoting gospel music. He worked with singers Ma Rainey, Sallie Martin, and Mother Willie Mae Ford Smith to popularize the art. Mahalia Jackson, one of the most famous gospel singers, is known for "What Could I Do?" and "City Called Heaven." Another gospel song, "Oh, Happy Day," became world famous. Today, gospel music is an important genre in the music market.

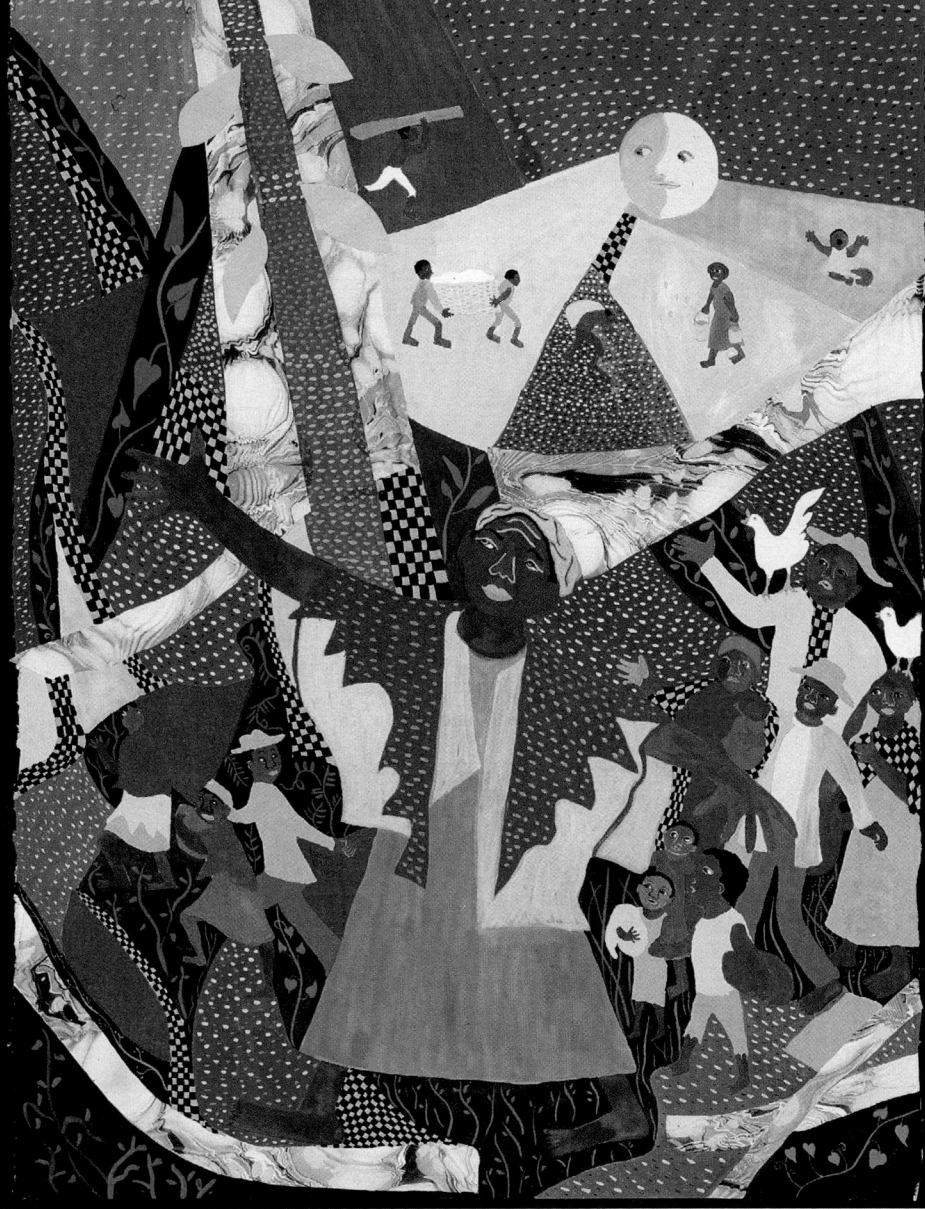

Arts Connection

▲ *Harriet and the Freedom Train* by Barbara Olsen. This mixed-media collage celebrates the life of Harriet Tubman (1821–1913), the anti-slavery activist and a "conductor" on the Underground Railroad. Olsen, who created the art illustrations throughout this lesson, has said her main inspiration has always been "women who have made a difference."

Unit 11 **397**

1 INTRODUCE

See Across the Curriculum below, and lead a discussion to explore the definition of a metaphor. Review the text in "The Gospel Train" and explain the following metaphors.

- *Get on board* (become a believer)
- *Gospel train* (the word of God)
- *I hear the wheels a-movin' through the land.* (The gospel message is being heard everywhere.)
- *Get your ticket* (make a commitment; join)
- *The fare is cheap and all can go.* (There is nothing to lose, and everybody is welcome.)

Share with students that trains offered symbolic metaphors to the Underground Railroad movement. Invite students to discuss these symbols and metaphors. Engage students in a discussion of the artwork *Harriet and the Freedom Train* on p. 397. Share information on the Underground Railroad and Harriet Tubman in Across the Curriculum, p. 400, and Skills Reinforcement, p. 398. Also see Unit 9 Lesson 8, beginning on p. 338.

2 DEVELOP

Listening

Play the Stereo Vocal recording of "The Gospel Train" **CD 19-26** and invite students to

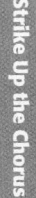

- Listen for the dotted rhythm on the words *get on* (Part 2) and *little.*
- Listen to Part 3 in mm. 9–12 and 13–16 for the imitation of an engine moving.
- Identify the number of themes in the song. (2; theme A is in mm. 1–8, and theme B is in mm. 9–16)

continued on page 398

ACROSS THE CURRICULUM

▶ **Language Arts** Storytelling is one of the oldest forms of communication. The words in many stories are often to be taken figuratively but not literally. Originally, gospel music was sung in the church, inspired by the gospel.

The metaphoric language of gospel music provides an opportunity to include the English department in the learning of these songs. The music department can perform gospel songs for the English department when descriptive language is studied.

Train Share the book *Locomotive: Building an Eight-Wheeler* by David Weitzman (Houghton Mifflin, 1999), and invite students to learn historical information about trains. Students will enjoy seeing the black-and-white renderings of trains across time.

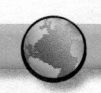

CULTURAL CONNECTION

▶ **Spirituals** Spirituals are American religious folk songs. African American spirituals were passed from generation to generation orally. Like gospel music, spirituals use call-and-response patterns and repeated refrains. These songs were sung in the nineteenth and twentieth centuries predominantly by African Americans but also by Americans of other races. They were the types of tunes heard at revivals and camp meetings. Many white spirituals were written down in shape-note publications such as the *Sacred Harp.*

Unit 11 *Strike Up the Chorus* **397**

Lesson 2 Continued

- Listen for which theme is harmonized at the end of the song. (theme A in mm. 45–53)
- Enjoy the performance by the Moses Hogan Chorale. See Spotlight On, p. 400, for information about this choir and Moses Hogan.

Reading

"The Gospel Train" has a great deal of melodic and rhythmic repetition. Students can learn the song efficiently by taking advantage of this characteristic. Have students

- Learn theme A (with pickup, mm. 1–8); sing theme A wherever it appears.
- Learn theme B (with pickup, mm. 9–16); sing theme B wherever it appears.
- Learn the ostinato part (Part 3, mm. 9–12); sing this part wherever it appears.

5c
- Learn Part 1 (mm. 1–2) and sing it wherever it appears; follow the same procedure for Part 3 (mm. 1–2).
- Learn the "conductor's" part (mm. 15–16) and sing it wherever it appears.

5a Invite students to look at the rhythm patterns on p. 396. Have them

- Echo clap the rhythm patterns as you model them.
- Sing the rhythm patterns, using rhythm syllables.
- Find these rhythms in the music and then sing selected phrases with these patterns.

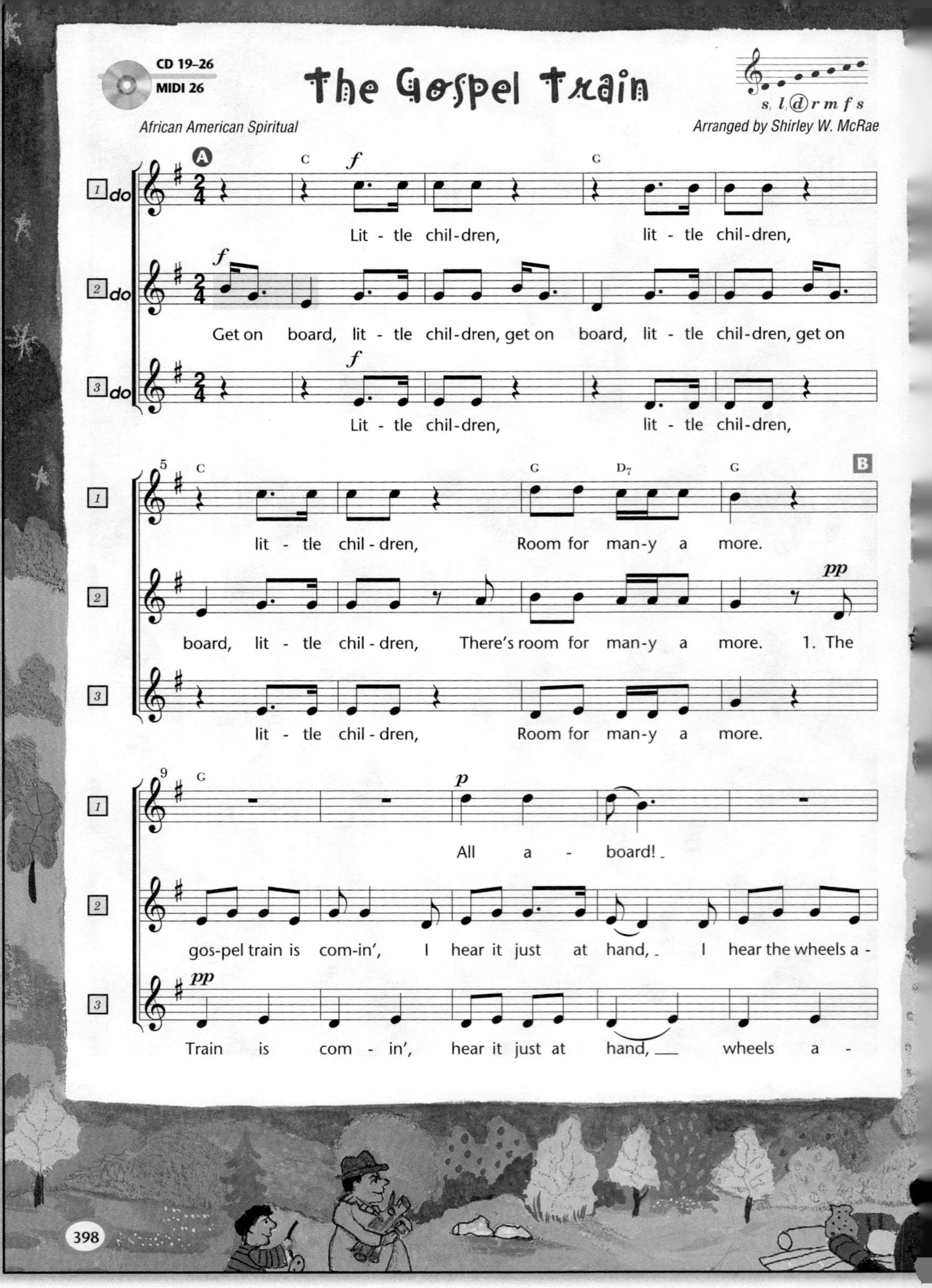

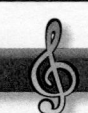

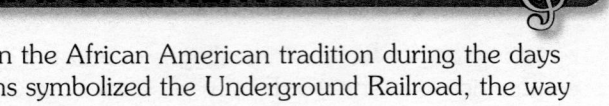

Footnotes

AUDIENCE ETIQUETTE

▶ **Get There Early** Students interested in attending a choral concert will understand the importance of an early arrival. Arriving early for a performance shows courtesy to the performers and other audience members. Help students list the advantages of arriving early. Audience members who arrive early have time to

- Find their seats and get comfortable.
- Read the program notes (if available) to learn more about the music or performers.
- Look at and examine the surroundings—the architecture of the building, the design of the stage and scenery, the lighting. How might these features affect the acoustics?
- Watch musicians on stage preparing for the performance or observe the set-up of instruments and equipment.

SKILLS REINFORCEMENT

▶ **Playing** In the African American tradition during the days of slavery, trains symbolized the Underground Railroad, the way to freedom.

Trains make strong rhythmic sounds as they roll along the train tracks, providing rhythmic ideas for songs. In "The Gospel Train," there are rhythmic motives that suggest rhythmic sounds a moving train would make. Have students perform these rhythmic motives on rhythm sticks to add excitement to the performance of the song. The rhythm patterns on p. 396 can be played as ostinatos or can be played in different combinations. Experiment with different sound sources for variety.

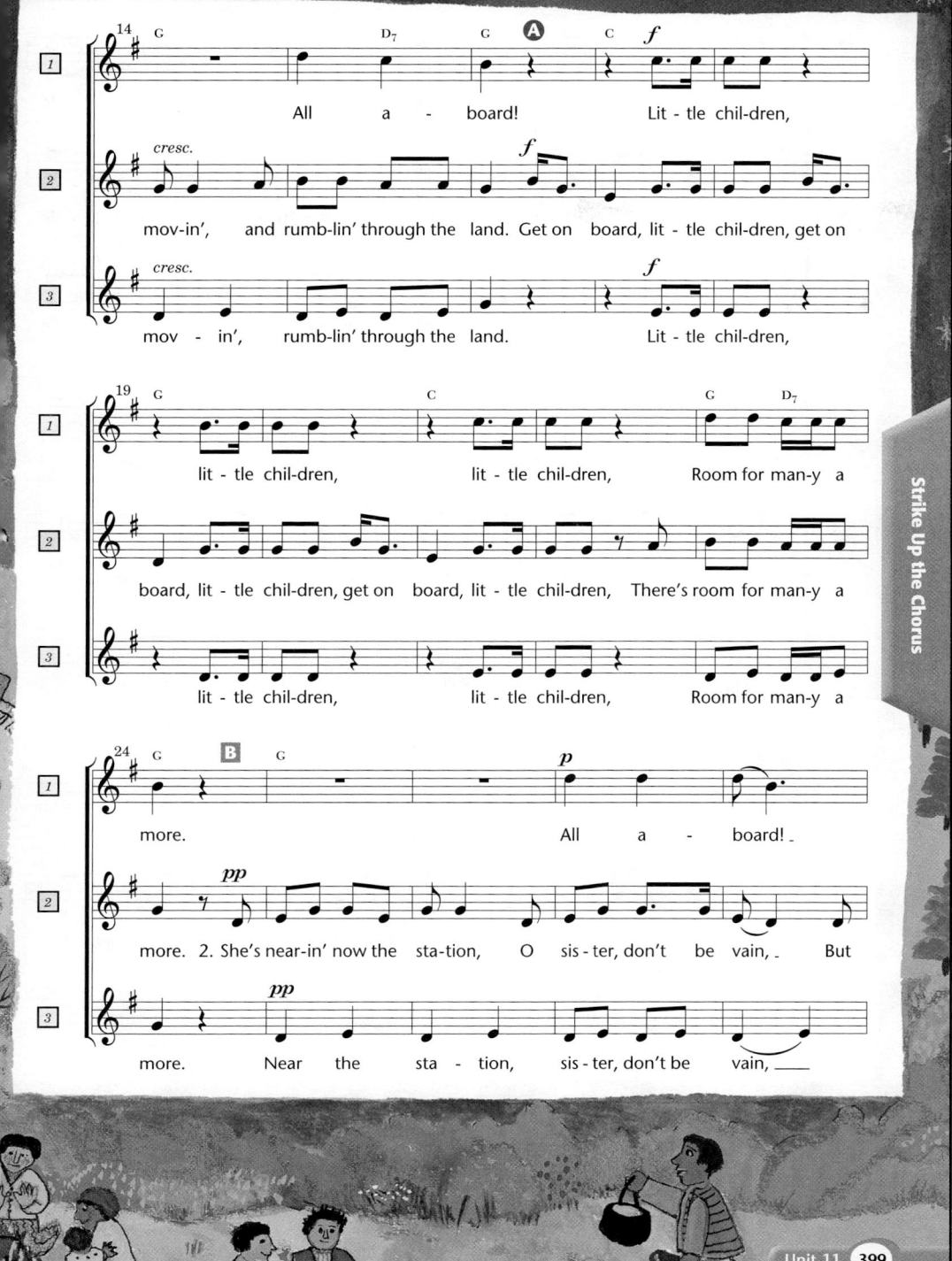

All a-board! Lit-tle chil-dren,

mov-in', and rumb-lin' through the land. Get on board, lit-tle chil-dren, get on

mov-in', rumb-lin' through the land. Lit-tle chil-dren,

lit-tle chil-dren, lit-tle chil-dren, Room for man-y a

board, lit-tle chil-dren, get on board, lit-tle chil-dren, There's room for man-y a

lit-tle chil-dren, lit-tle chil-dren, Room for man-y a

more. All a-board!

more. 2. She's near-in' now the sta-tion, O sis-ter, don't be vain, But

more. Near the sta-tion, sis-ter, don't be vain, _____

Strike Up the Chorus

Singing

Invite students to listen to "The Gospel Train" **CD 19-26** as they follow the music.

 Assist students in learning each part by having them sing each part with the recording.

Organize the class into groups and assign each group a part. Assist students in practicing and rehearsing parts, gradually introducing each part to the song.

Ask students to identify the music symbols referring to dynamics in the A theme (*f*) and the B theme (*pp*), and tell them they will need interpret them appropriately when performing. Tell students that performing the contrasting dynamics of both themes will add to the musical expression of the piece.

In addition, students should be certain that the A and B themes are dynamically a little louder than the harmony parts. The words *get on* and *little* should be sung with "elided" consonants (a consonant connected to a vowel); not "get on" or "Litt-le," but "ge-Ton" and "Li-Tle."

This technique will help emphasize the syncopated rhythm of the two words. Sing the ostinato in a plodding manner to imitate the train and the conductor's theme in legato style.

Moving

Students may wish to add the nonlocomotor movement suggestions in Movement below, to a performance of "The Gospel Train."

continued on page 400

SPOTLIGHT ON

▶ **Train Sounds** Discuss and list the types of sounds and rhythms that older trains make as they are moving. New electric trains don't make much sound, so think of old steam engines. Include the following *effects.*

- Straight eighth notes; start slow and *accelerando.* This may be vocalized as *chug-a, chug-a.*
- *Choo-choo* steam whistle.
- Locomotive whistle or horn: "*watch___ out___.*"
- Doppler effect: As a train approaches, its sound is normal. The moment the train passes, the sound drops in pitch. The sound waves are actually longer (lower in pitch) after the train passes by. A *crescendo* and *decrescendo* are part of this sound.

MOVEMENT

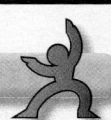

▶ **Nonlocomotor Movement** Gospel choirs perform synchronized movements as they sing in performance. "The Gospel Train" has an energy that lends itself to synchronized movements. A suggestion for synchronized motion during choral performance is this.

On the Chorus (B section): Students add hand claps on offbeats to the last two choruses.

On verse 1 (A section): Students slowly "pan" with their faces left to right for eight measures, as if they are watching the train pass by. Consider putting their hands to their brow, as well.

Create new movements for subsequent verses.

Playing

 Invite students to again look at the rhythms on p. 396. After distributing rhythm instruments to groups of students, have them

- Echo clap the rhythms as you model it.
- Play the rhythms, using body percussion.
- Play these rhythms on mallet instruments.
- Play these rhythms, when ready, as accompaniment to the recording of "The Gospel Train" **CD 19-26.**

Guide students to discover additional rhythms that trains create. Have students locate the train rhythms in the song (mm. 9–12). See Skills Reinforcement, p. 398, and Spotlight On, p. 399. Ask students to perform the rhythms as possible accompaniments to "The Gospel Train." Remind them that the rhythms on p. 396 will sound like train rhythms when played as ostinatos.

Invite students to explore the sounds that come from trains in Spotlight On, p. 399. Perform the sounds as rhythm patterns and ostinatos.

Analyzing

To help students understand the song's harmonic texture, assign groups a part and invite Part 1 to clap their line, Part 2 to tap rhythm sticks for their line, and Part 3 to speak *do* for every note of their line.

 ASK What other ways (other than singing) can you think of to perform the individual lines so the rhythmic differences can be heard? (use a drum, tap feet)

The activity above can be done in a circle, with three groups, or in a 1–2–3 sequence in a circle, so that students can hear and see the rhythmic complexity. Sing and record the song in one or more of the formations above.

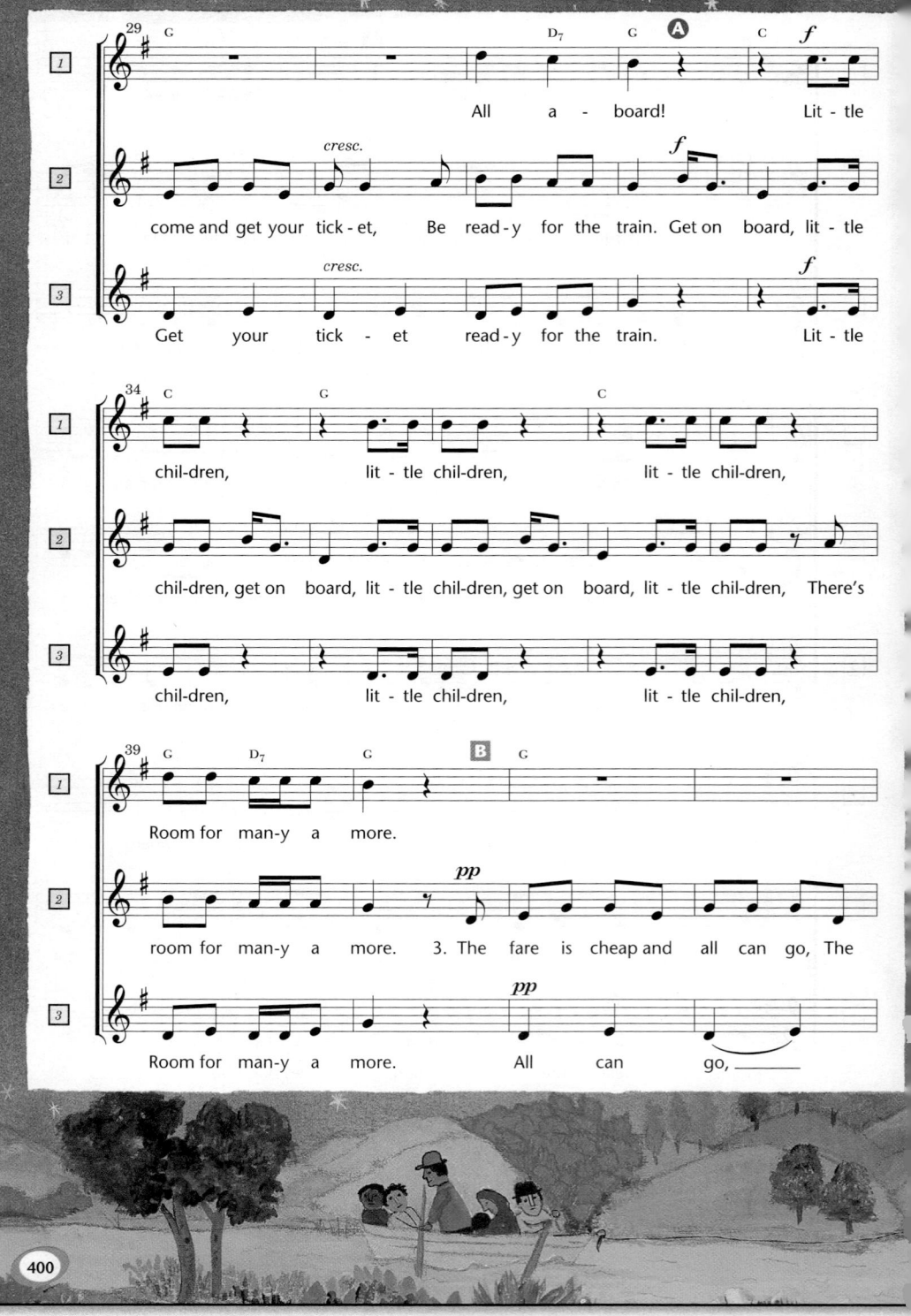

Footnotes

SPOTLIGHT ON

▶ **The Conductor** Moses Hogan (1957–2003) was born in New Orleans, Louisiana. Hogan graduated from the Oberlin Conservatory of Music in Ohio and studied at the Juilliard School in New York. As a concert pianist, he won the prestigious 28th Kosciuszko Foundation Chopin Competition. Hogan has over 70 choral works published for high school, college, church, and professional choirs, and is known for his many arrangements of spirituals.

▶ **The Performers** The Moses Hogan Chorale hails from New Orleans. It was started by Moses Hogan in 1980 and has become world renowned. The chorale has sung at the John F. Kennedy Center for the Performing Arts and the Sydney Opera House, as well as in churches, synagogues, and civic institutions. The chorale's members range in age from 19 to 69.

ACROSS THE CURRICULUM

▶ **Social Studies** The Underground Railroad was not underground, nor a railroad, but a network of aid to fugitives from slavery. As many as 100,000 slaves may have escaped in the years between the American Revolution and the Civil War. Harriet Tubman was a central figure in helping slaves escape to Canada. They were instructed to follow the stars that make up the constellation called the Big Dipper. A song based on this advice is "Follow the Drinkin' Gourd." (*Drinkin' Gourd* is a metaphor for Big Dipper.) Another song is "Steal Away." Part of the lyrics are *Steal away, steal away home, I ain't got long to stay here.* Slaves would travel at night to avoid being caught. They would look for houses with a single lantern at the front door as a signal that the house was a "safe house" where they could expect shelter and food before continuing north to freedom.

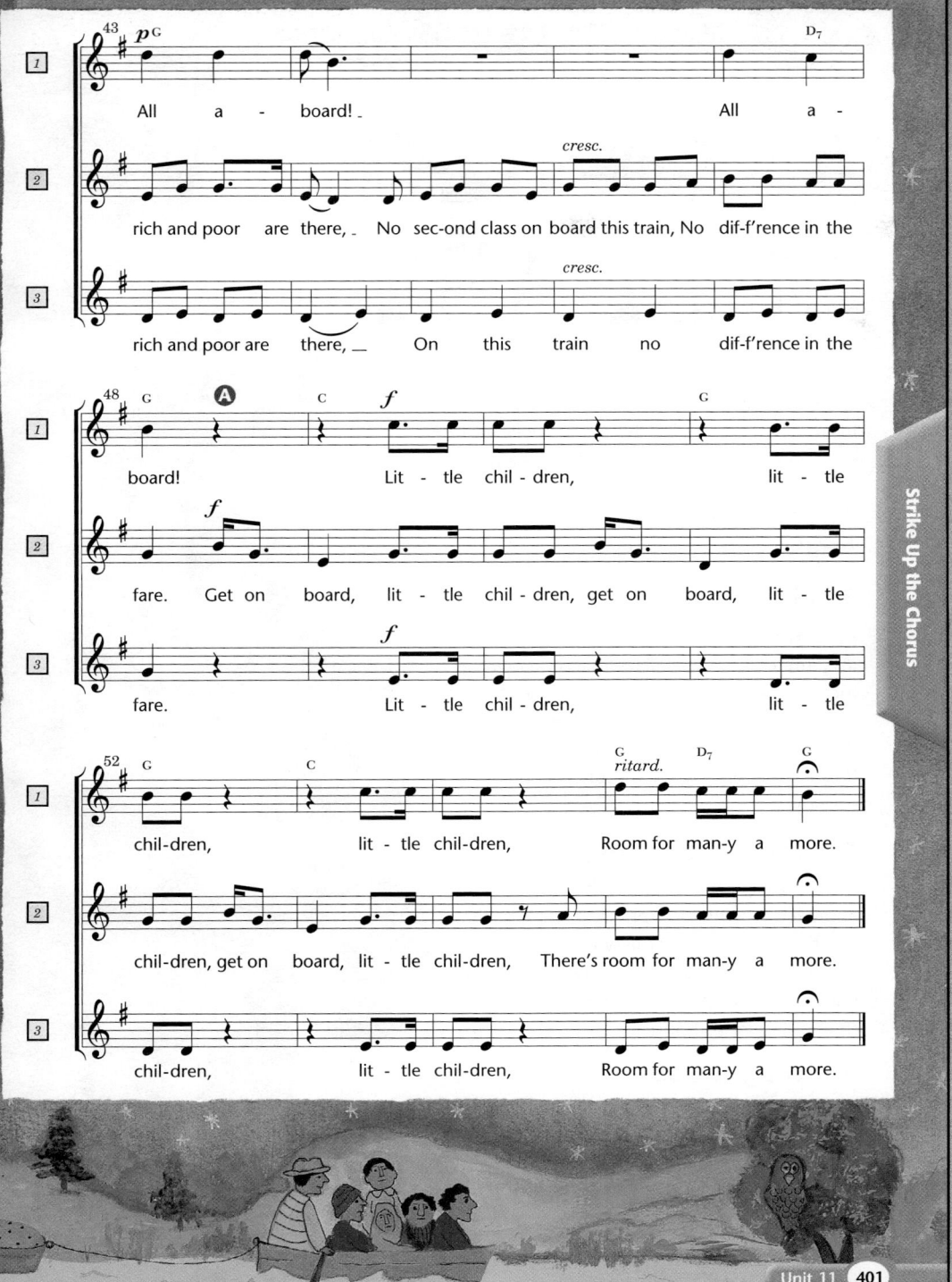

Unit 11 **401**

Performing

In addition to singing in the classroom, students may be interested in performing "The Gospel Train" at an informal or formal concert. Encourage students to set a high standard of performance suitable for a concert setting, and evaluate the quality of the music they sing. Share with students the proper performer etiquette for both rehearsals and concert performances.

Students may also be interested in attending choral concerts. Encourage students to attend live music concerts whenever possible. Guide them to exhibit audience concert etiquette as an actively involved listener during varied live performances. (See Audience Etiquette on p. 398.)

3 CLOSE

Skill: PLAYING   **ASSESSMENT**

Performance/Self-Assessment Have students sing "The Gospel Train," playing the dotted, syncopated rhythms on p. 396 as an ostinato on nonpitched instruments.

7a Have students

7b
- Evaluate the rhythmic accuracy of themes A and B.
- Evaluate the clarity and accuracy of the syncopated rhythms.
- Determine if Part 1 and Part 3 are rhythmically together in mm. 1–8.
- Determine if the style of singing for each part is rhythmically convincing.
- Evaluate their performance of contrasting dynamics in the themes and how these dynamics contributed to the effectiveness of the musical performance.
- Compare the Stereo Vocal recording to the student recording with regard to the four categories of assessment listed above.

TEACHER TO TEACHER

▶ **MIDI Song File** Use the MIDI song file of "The Gospel Train" to assist students in learning the song. Use the file to play the tempo more slowly, transpose the key, if desired, and play selected vocal parts and selected measures to help them learn the harmony and vocal parts more easily.

TECHNOLOGY/MEDIA LINK

MIDI/Sequencing Software Have students use the MIDI song file for "The Gospel Train" to experiment with creating ostinatos and arrangements of the song. Have them

- Create a new MIDI file and use cut and paste to copy selected rhythmic motives from the song into the new tracks.
- Cut and paste rhythms successively to create ostinatos. Do they sound like train rhythms?
- Layer tracks to build textures, then experiment with textures by deleting selected portions of tracks.

Afterwards, have students evaluate the results. Play selected arrangements for the class.

LESSON AT A GLANCE

Element Focus **RHYTHM** Dotted and tied rhythms in meter in 3

Skill Objective **SINGING** Read and sing tied rhythms, with one beat to a measure in $\frac{3}{4}$ meter

Connection Activity **CULTURE** Discuss Cajun culture, music, and language

MATERIALS

- "Fais do do" **CD 20-1**
- "Go to Sleep" **CD 20-2**
- **Pronunciation Practice/Translation** p. 540
  Recording Routine: Intro (6 m.); vocal; coda
- **Resource Book** p. A-31
- guitars

VOCABULARY

stretto *zydeco* *fais do do* Acadians *anacrusis*

◆ ◆ ◆ ◆ National Standards ◆ ◆ ◆ ◆

1b Sing easy pieces with technical accuracy
5c Identify standard notation symbols for pitch
6a Listen and describe events in music using appropriate terms
7a Students evaluate the music they perform
8b Identify ways music relates to social studies

MORE MUSIC CHOICES

For more practice singing in $\frac{3}{4}$:
"Farewell to Tarwathie," p. 43
"Scarborough Fair," p. 95

A Cajun LULLABY

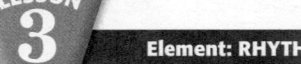

The Acadians were French people who settled in the eastern part of Canada. They were exiled from Canada in the 1750s, and many eventually settled in Louisiana. In Louisiana, the name "Acadian," pronounced "A-ca-jun," was shortened to "Cajun."

Sing the Cajun lullaby "Fais do do."

Singing Tips

Listen to "Fais do do." Notice that it is written in $\frac{3}{4}$ meter, but you will feel it as one beat per measure. As you **sing**, emphasize the strong beat at the beginning of each phrase. Remember that, although the harmony parts are important, they should be sung a little softer than the melody.

Reading Music Tips

When learning a song in another language, approach reading each phrase as follows: first practice the rhythm of the words, using rhythm syllables, then **sing** the melody, using pitch syllables. Next, speak the French words in rhythm before you sing.

Knowing the Score

How many times is the first phrase repeated? In what measure does the second phrase begin?

Cajun accordion ▶

Footnotes

ACROSS THE CURRICULUM

▶ **Science** Share the book *Sleep* by Alvin Silverstein, Virginia Silverstein, and Laura Silverstein Nunn (Franklin Watts, 1999), and invite students to study their bodies' need for sleep. Ask students to keep a sleep journal for a week. Do they get enough sleep? Too much? When are they more active?

BUILDING SKILLS THROUGH MUSIC

▶ **Health** Have students read the text to "Fais do do." Have them discuss the nightly routine prior to going to sleep (Mama brings sweet cake, daddy brings hot chocolate.) Building on the information from Across the Curriculum, have students write a description of their nightly ritual.

SKILLS REINFORCEMENT

▶ **Creating** Many videos depicting Cajun music traditions show listeners hand clapping along with the performers. Students can create a hand-clapping routine to accompany the song "Fais do do." Try out several routines created by students and discuss whether these might assist or inhibit their singing. Choose a hand-clapping pattern that complements simultaneous singing, and perform the song as a class.

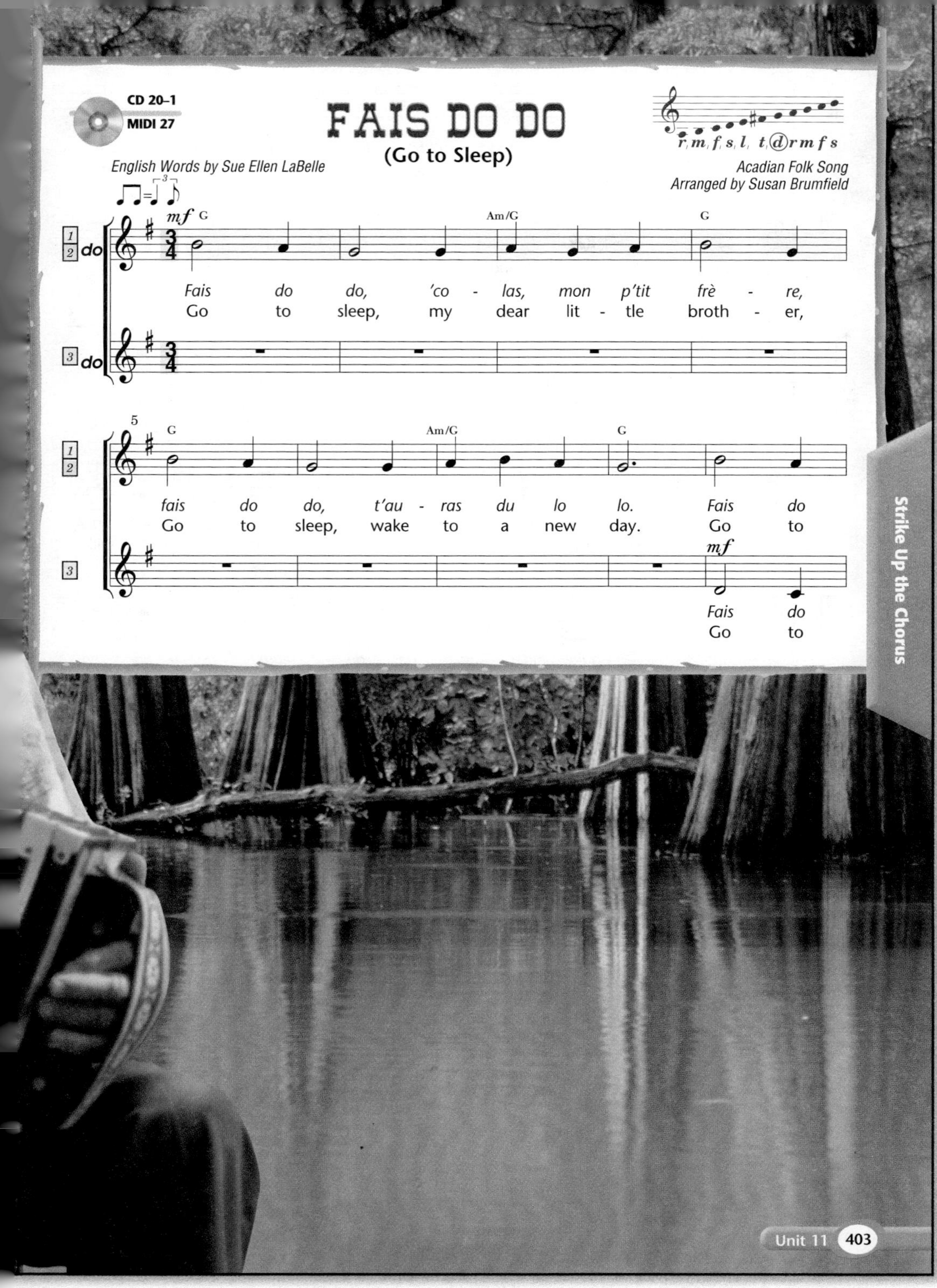

FAIS DO DO
(Go to Sleep)

English Words by Sue Ellen LaBelle

Acadian Folk Song
Arranged by Susan Brumfield

CD 20–1
MIDI 27

Fais do do, 'co - las, mon p'tit frè - re,
Go to sleep, my dear lit - tle broth - er,

fais do do, t'au - ras du lo lo.
Go to sleep, wake to a new day.

Fais do
Go to

Fais do
Go to

Strike Up the Chorus

1 INTRODUCE

Share with students the information on Cajun culture found in the Footnotes throughout this lesson. Discuss the French influence on the music, food, and language of the Cajuns.

Then, invite a French teacher to read the French text of *"Fais do do"* to the class; videotape his or her face. Play the vocal recording of *"Fais do do"* **CD 20-1** and ask the teacher to reread the text and explain what happens to initial and final vowels and consonants when they are sung.

2 DEVELOP

Listening

Play *"Fais do do"* **CD 20-1** and have students listen to

- How the music moves and feels as though it were one beat to the measure.

- The rhythm of the middle section (mm. 16–24). Then, identify and echo clap the rhythmic motive of this section. (See Reading on p. 394 for more activities using this motive.)

- How Parts 1 and 2 sing the same rhythm patterns in the harmony parts (mm. 9–32).

6a
- The *stretto* effect at mm. 33–36. (A *stretto* effect, pronounced STREH-toh, is an overlapping of exact rhythmic and melodic imitation; in this case, it occurs one measure later.)

- How the opening phrase revolves around *mi, re,* and *do.*

continued on page 404

CULTURAL CONNECTION

▶ *Zydeco* Zydeco music is one aspect of Cajun music. It is a form of music that began with African Americans in Cajun Louisiana. It is a combination of French and Cajun traditions, which includes blues, rhythm and blues, Caribbean music, and country and western. The instruments found in this music are the accordion, washboard, electric guitar, bass, and drums. Clifton Chenier (see Spotlight On, at right) is a well-known performer of *zydeco* music. "Don't Need a Ticket to Ride" is one of his songs.

SPOTLIGHT ON

▶ **The Performer** Accordion player Clifton Chenier mixed rhythm and blues, blues, and rock 'n' roll in his music. He helped introduce *zydeco* music to the pop music world. His gold tooth, cape, and crown contributed to his showmanship on stage. He was born to sharecropper parents in Louisiana. Chenier cited Fats Domino, Professor Longhair, and Joe and Jimmie Liggins as his influences. One of his first records was "Louisiana Stomp" in 1954. He mostly played rhythm and blues early in his career. By 1964, he recorded and toured playing *zydeco* music. Chenier suffered from ill health and died in 1987.

Reading

The middle section of *"Fais do do"* contains a prominent rhythmic motive with several interesting rhythm elements.

Invite students to find

- The tied rhythms for the voice parts. (mm. 16–17, 20–21, 40–45)
- The *stretto* section. (mm. 33–37)
- The repeat signs. (mm. 49 and 64)
- The section where all three voices are singing different pitches. (mm. 43–63)

Have a student write the rhythm pattern in mm. 16–17 (below) on the board and ask the class to clap and speak the pattern.

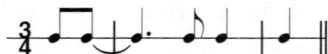

ASK What are the two eighth notes in m. 16 called? (pickup, or anacrusis)

How many times does the rhythm in mm. 17–18 occur in the middle section? (three)

SAY This dotted rhythm is the main element of the rhythmic motive in this section.

ASK What two or three musical elements add interest to the rhythmic motive? (The anacrusis tied to the dotted rhythm adds syncopation; a *crescendo–decrescendo* accompanies each motive.)

The melodic material for *"Fais do do"* **CD 20-1** centers on *mi, re, do* (mm. 1–2, 5–6, 9–10, 13–14 in the first refrain) and *mi, fa, so* (mm. 16–17, 18–19, 20–21, 23–24, 40–41, 42–43, and 44–45 in Part 3). Have students find these patterns and sight-sing them.

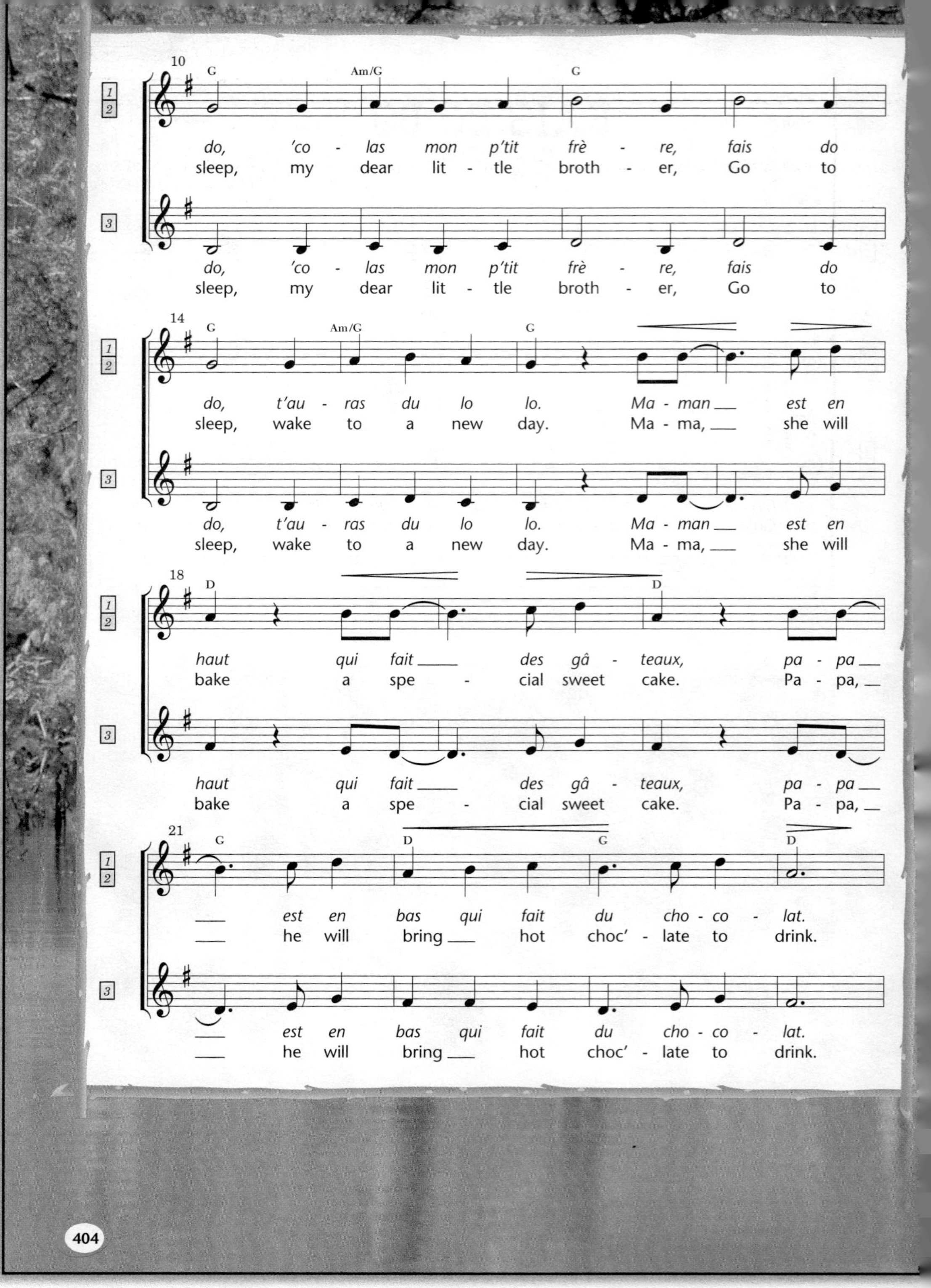

do, 'co - las mon p'tit frè - re, fais do
sleep, my dear lit - tle broth - er, Go to

do, 'co - las mon p'tit frè - re, fais do
sleep, my dear lit - tle broth - er, Go to

do, t'au - ras du lo lo. Ma - man ___ est en
sleep, wake to a new day. Ma - ma, ___ she will

do, t'au - ras du lo lo. Ma - man ___ est en
sleep, wake to a new day. Ma - ma, ___ she will

haut qui fait ___ des gâ - teaux, pa - pa ___
bake a spe - cial sweet cake. Pa - pa, ___

haut qui fait ___ des gâ - teaux, pa - pa ___
bake a spe - cial sweet cake. Pa - pa, ___

___ est en bas qui fait du cho - co - lat.
he will bring ___ hot choc' - late to drink.

___ est en bas qui fait du cho - co - lat.
he will bring ___ hot choc' - late to drink.

Footnotes

SKILLS REINFORCEMENT

▶ **Guitar** The song *"Fais do do"* is very well suited for guitar accompaniment. Use this Cajun "waltz strum" in the right hand. Practice the song using the strum alone with no chords (a silent "air strum"). When this step is fluent, practice the song with chord changes and no strum. When that step is fluent, play with the strum and the chords.

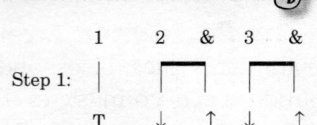

Step 1:

CULTURAL CONNECTION

▶ **Cajun Food** Cajuns, the descendants of the French Acadians, have always had interesting recipes, but most people never thought of Cajun food as a separate genre until about 1980, when chef Paul Prudhomme popularized blackened redfish. Since then, people have been interested in trying Cajun specialties. Most of the food is spicy. It is, however, spiced only with black pepper, cayenne pepper, and salt (not hot chiles and jalapeños).

Cajun food is known for its fresh local ingredients. Dishes usually contain seafood, vegetables, and rice. The seafood and vegetables are cooked in one pot and the rice in another.

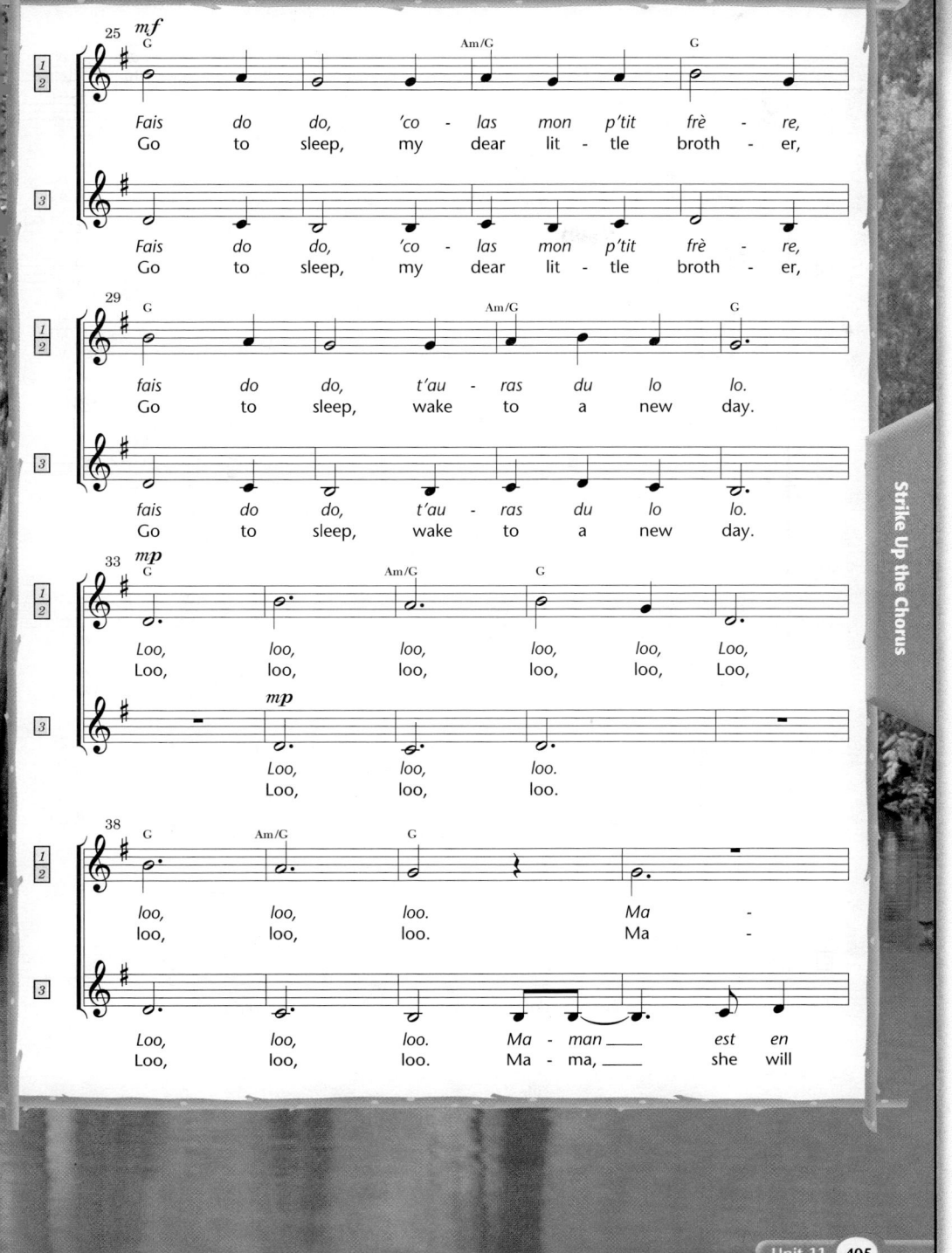

Fais do do, 'co - las mon p'tit frè - re,
Go to sleep, my dear lit - tle broth - er,

Fais do do, 'co - las mon p'tit frè - re,
Go to sleep, my dear lit - tle broth - er,

fais do do, t'au - ras du lo lo.
Go to sleep, wake to a new day.

fais do do, t'au - ras du lo lo.
Go to sleep, wake to a new day.

Loo, loo, loo, loo, loo, Loo,
Loo, loo, loo, loo, loo, Loo,

Loo, loo, loo.
Loo, loo, loo.

loo, loo, loo. Ma -
loo, loo, loo. Ma -

Loo, loo, loo. Ma - man ____ est en
Loo, loo, loo. Ma - ma, ____ she will

Strike Up the Chorus

Singing

1b Have students use the Pronunciation Practice Guide on Resource Book p. A-31. Then, have them listen to the Pronunciation Practice for part 1 **CD 20-4**, Part 2 **CD 20-5**, Part 3 **CD 20-6**, and learn to sing the song in French.

Play the video of the French teacher (see Introduce, p. 403) so that students can observe how the teacher's lips form the vowels and consonants. If there is no French teacher available, show part of a video in French to familiarize students visually with the formation of vowels in French.

Remind students of the singing tips on p. 402.

Analyzing

Understanding some aspects of the Cajun culture will help students sing *"Fais do do"* **CD 20-1** with more cultural awareness. Perhaps they can do a research report.

Have students

- Read about Cajun culture. See Cultural Connection, p. 404, and Spotlight On below.
- Read about how the French language influenced the Cajun language.
- **8b** Collect pictures of instruments used in Cajun music: fiddle, accordion, guitar, triangle, mandolin, and banjo.
- Read about Cajun music. See Cultural Connection and Spotlight On, p. 403.
- Find recordings of Cajun music and listen to them.

continued on page 406

 ## SPOTLIGHT ON

▶ **Community Dances** *"Fais do do,"* a lullaby in Cajun music, was also a community dance attended by the Acadian community. Parents brought their children to the dance, where the music helped children fall asleep. Favorite dances at these affairs were the two-step and waltz.

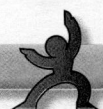 ## MOVEMENT

▶ **Popular Dance** Remind students of the Cajun two-step, p. 249, which is danced to the song "Jambalaya." The waltz is another favorite dance of the Acadians. Invite students to learn and then perform a traditional waltz step to *"Fais do do."*

▶ **Nonlocomotor Movement** Students can perform a synchronized swaying movement when performing *"Fais do do."* Have them sway back and forth in meter in 3. The right arm may also sway back and forth across the body.

Performing

If there are Cajun musicians in your community, invite them to accompany this song. They could also perform *zydeco* music as part of a concert on Cajun music. See Cultural Connection and Spotlight On, p. 403.

Cajun humor is funny and unusual and could be included in a program that lends itself to a multicultural concert format.

Moving

Discuss with students the love of dancing by the Acadian people. Share with them the anecdotal information about the *fais do do* community dance. See Spotlight On, p. 405.

If your school policy allows partner dancing, consider inviting a select group of students to demonstrate the waltz step to the class as they sing the song "*Fais do do*" **CD 20-1.** See Movement, p. 405.

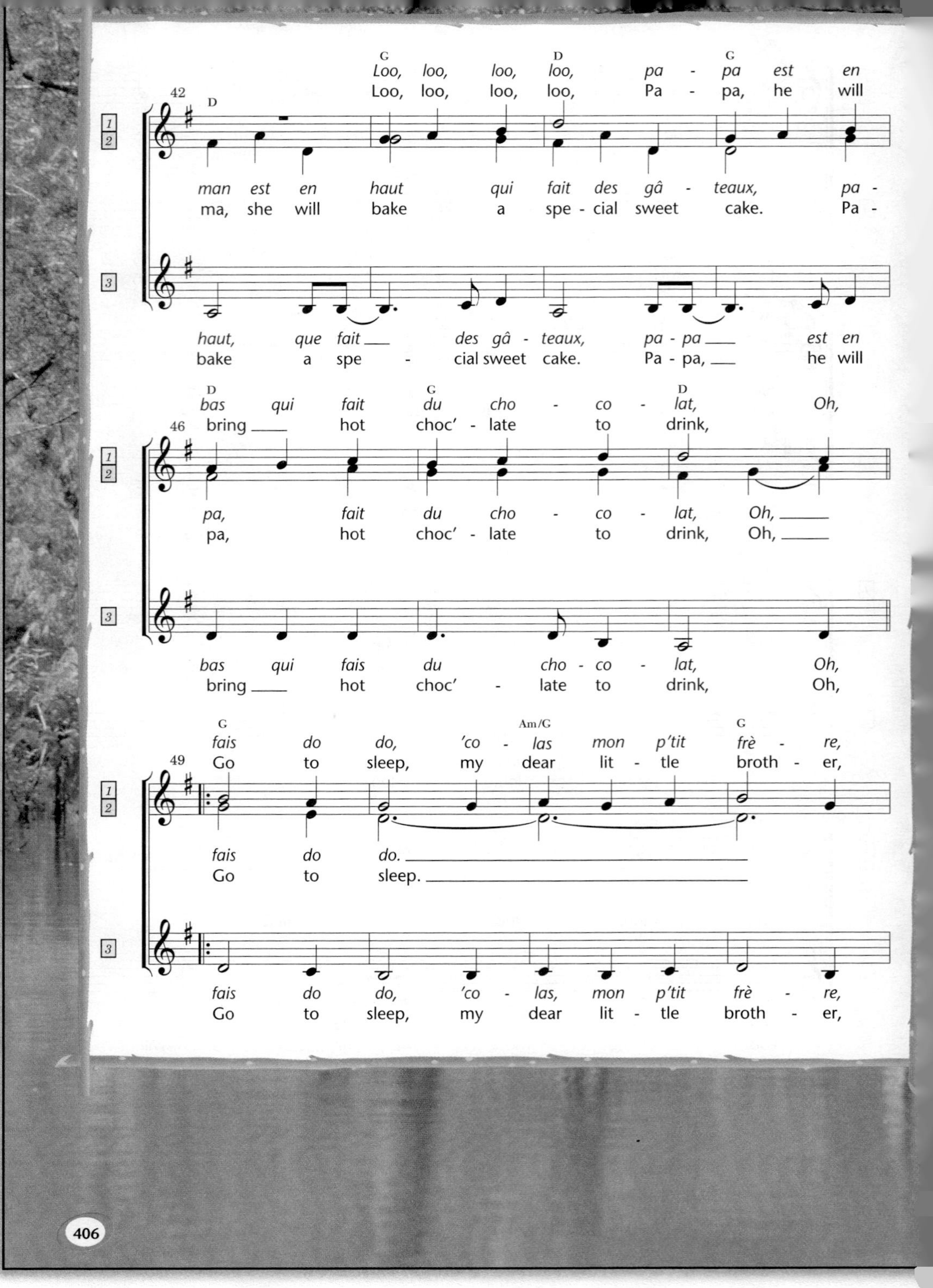

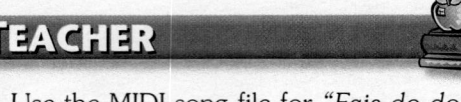

(Sheet music for "Fais do do," measures 42–51)

406

Footnotes

TEACHER TO TEACHER

▶ **MIDI Song File** Use the MIDI song file for "Fais do do" to assist students in learning this choral arrangement. Play the song at a slower tempo, isolate vocal parts, transpose the key, if desired, and select measures to assist students as they learn to sing the song.

CHARACTER EDUCATION

▶ **Collaboration** Discuss with students how *zydeco* music involves a combination of several musical cultures. Ask them

- What does it mean to collaborate? What is necessary for successful collaboration? (give and take, not always having things your way, relinquishing control, being able to see the good in others, being willing to share what you have or believe).
- To list situations in which people collaborate effectively. (members of a surgical team, melody and lyric writers)
- To describe situations in which they have collaborated with others to produce something.
- Why collaboration is valued as a character trait in our society? What are some ways they can collaborate with others to produce something different and good?

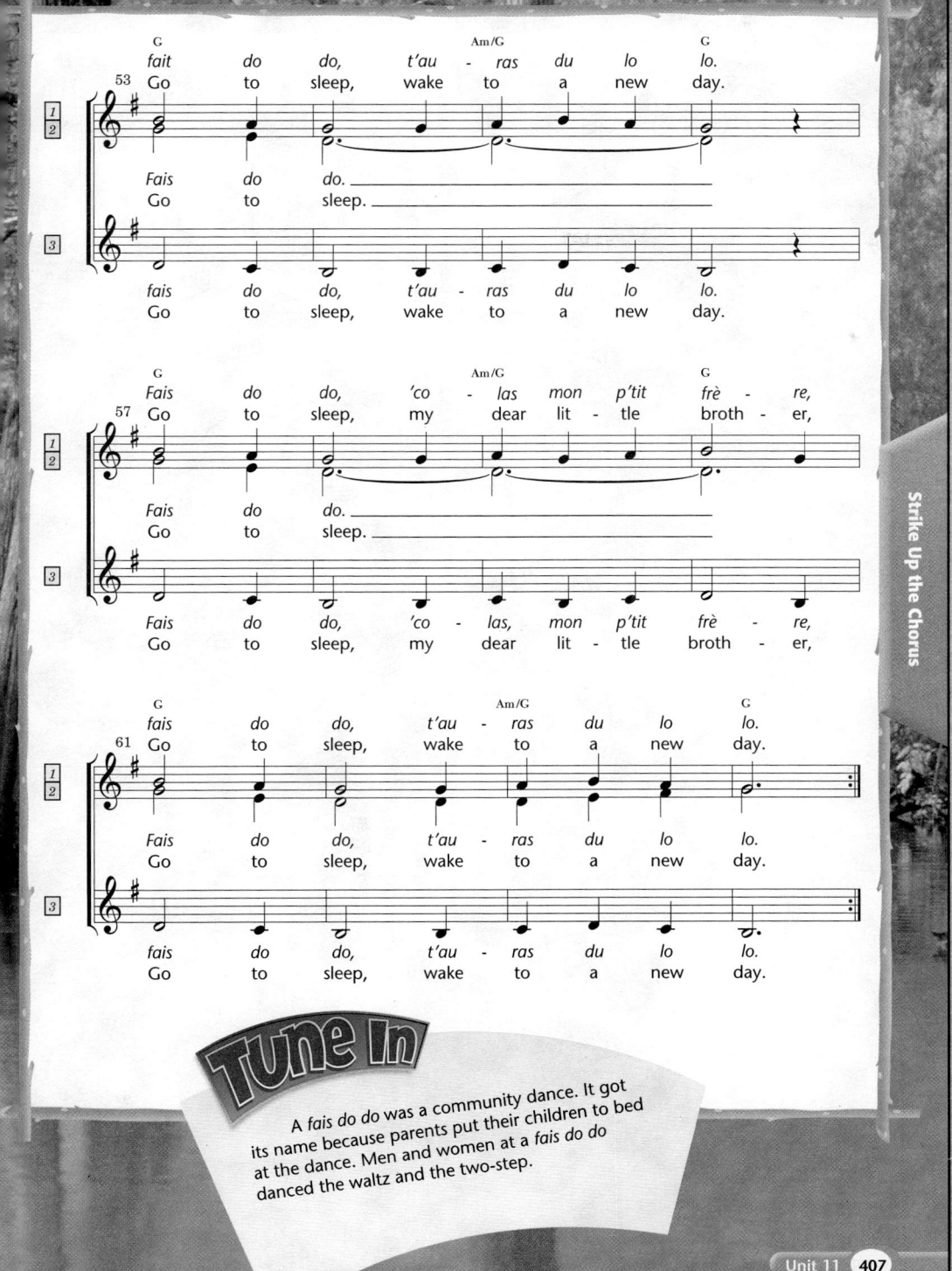

3 CLOSE

Skill: SINGING   **ASSESSMENT**

Performance/Self-Assessment Have students videotape or tape-record themselves singing *"Fais do do,"* with attention to clean dotted rhythms and a stress on the first beat.

7a Play the videotape/tape-recording back so that students can evaluate their performance for

- Singing dotted and tied rhythms in meter in 3.
- Performance of dynamic and expression markings.
- Clarity of French diction.
- Phrases for dynamic shape.
- Harmony parts for vocal balance.
- Correct posture for singing.

A *fais do do* was a community dance. It got its name because parents put their children to bed at the dance. Men and women at a *fais do do* danced the waltz and the two-step.

MEETING INDIVIDUAL NEEDS

▶ **Using Technology** Encourage students to use technology to learn vocal parts. The use of MIDI sequencing software and MIDI song files is one method of using technology.

Reinforcement Students having difficulty singing parts can use the MIDI song file to isolate a vocal part and slow down the tempo for easier singing. Repeat passages as needed.

On Target Students who know their vocal part can sing along with selected MIDI tracks that include the other vocal parts and instrumental accompaniment. As more tracks are added, challenge students to sing accurately, in time, and on pitch.

Challenge Students may wish to use the "score" mode of a sequencer to look at notation and practice ear training. Have students view a vocal part in score mode and sight-sing the part.

TECHNOLOGY/MEDIA LINK

MIDI/Sequencing Software Use MIDI sequencing software to create a performance track for the song *"Fais do do."* Duplicate the MIDI song file *"Fais do do"* and save it with a new name. Label the tracks for keyboard accompaniment and each of the voice parts. Remind students how to turn off and on individual tracks for MIDI playback. Divide the class into small groups and have students

- Listen to all of the MIDI tracks together while following their part in the book.
- Listen to their assigned part alone.
- Sing their part with the MIDI track for their part alone.
- Sing their part with all of the MIDI tracks together.

LESSON AT A GLANCE

Element Focus **MELODY** Harmonic-minor melody

Skill Objective **SINGING** Read and sing half steps between *ti-do, mi-fa,* and *si-la*

Connection **CULTURE** Read about the cultural influences
Activity on Jewish music

MATERIALS

- *"Shalom aleichem"* **CD 20-7**
  Recording Routine: Intro (4 m.); vocal; coda
- **Pronunciation Practice/Translation** p. 541
- **Resource Book** p. A-34
- keyboard

VOCABULARY

disjunct motion   conjunct motion

harmonic minor   embellishment

◆ ◆ ◆ ◆ National Standards ◆ ◆ ◆ ◆

1c Sing music from diverse cultures with appropriate expression
1d Sing music written in two parts
6b Listen and analyze uses of form in music from diverse cultures
7a Students evaluate the music they hear

MORE MUSIC CHOICES

For more practice singing in minor keys:

"Hava nagila," p. 153

"Hey, Ho! Nobody Home," p. 29

A SONG OF PEACE

The expression *shalom aleichem* is a Hebrew greeting that means "peace be with you." The song "Shalom aleichem" is a song of praise sung by Jewish families on Friday evenings before their Sabbath meal.

Sing *"Shalom aleichem."*

Singing Tips

Sing Part 1 on a legato *loo,* connecting every note. Every time you encounter a pair of eighth notes, stress and lengthen the first note ever so slightly.

Use the recorded Pronunciation Practice to learn the Hebrew lyrics. Then sing the Hebrew words, stressing and lengthening the first note in each pair of eighth notes. Pay close attention to the accidentals and pitches that give the song its minor sound.

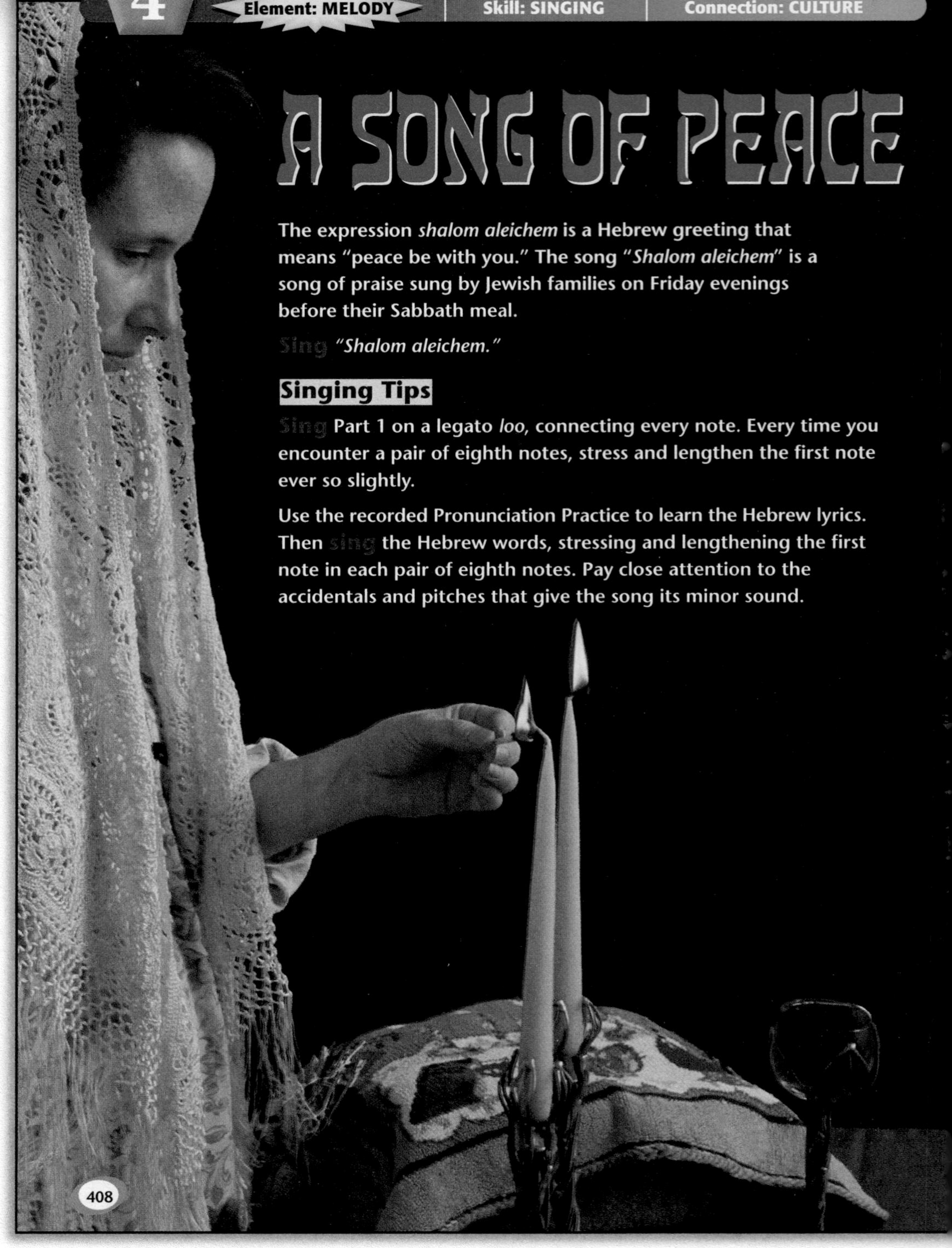

408

Footnotes

SKILLS REINFORCEMENT

▶ **Singing** To assist students in singing G-harmonic minor, have them sing these pitch sets as warm-ups as you play them on keyboard: G-harmonic-minor scale (G–A–B♭–C–D–E♭–F♯–G), G-minor chord (G–B♭–D), and the pitch sets (G-F♯-G) and (G-F♯-E♭-F♯-G). The use of the F-natural in *"Shalom aleichem"* introduces a modal tonality to the music. Add these sets to your warm-up: G-natural-minor scale (G–A–B♭–C–D–E♭–F–G), (G–F–G), and (G–F–E♭–F–G).

BUILDING SKILLS THROUGH MUSIC

▶ **Social Studies** Have students read the reference article about the music of Israel at *www.sfsuccessnet.com,* and answer this question: Based on your reading of the article, what are some of the factors that have influenced the many styles of Jewish music over time?

TEACHER TO TEACHER

▶ **Singing Hebrew** Singing in Hebrew is not difficult. Have students listen to the Pronunciation Practice tracks for *"Shalom aleichem"* **CD 20-9** and **CD 20-10** to assist them in learning the Hebrew words. However, if you are able to invite a Jewish student or a rabbi in the community who could teach the Hebrew, students could observe the lip formations and body language of the speaker. More importantly, singing many of the Hebraic melodies is not like singing melodies of other cultures. There is a tendency to sing from pitch to pitch with an ever so slightly slurred sound. It may seem mournful, yet is quite beautiful.

Reading Music Tips

Identify the F-sharps and F-naturals in the song. Notice what pitches are before and after these notes.

Knowing the Score

Analyze the score to determine where in the music both voice parts are singing the same notes. Where are the parts singing in harmony?

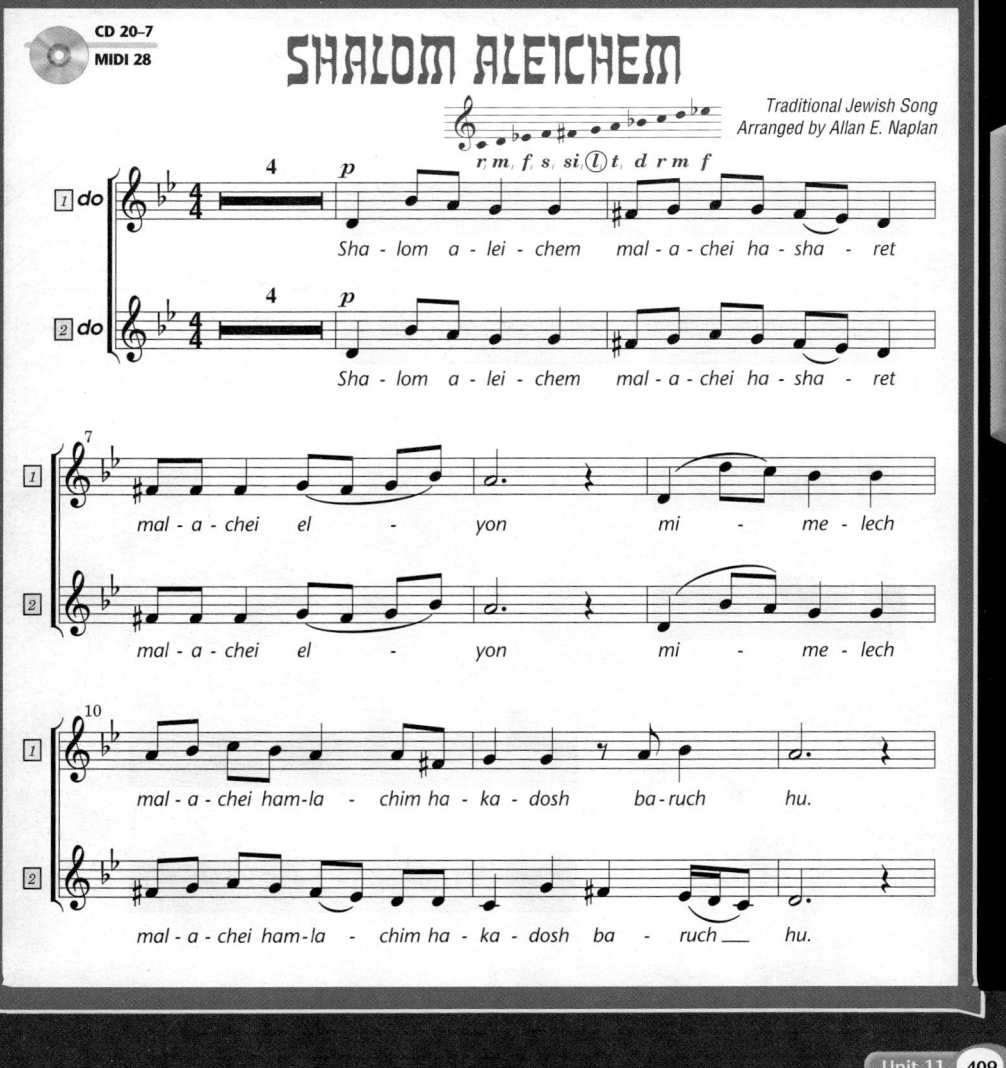

SHALOM ALEICHEM

Traditional Jewish Song
Arranged by Allan E. Naplan

Sha - lom a - lei - chem mal - a - chei ha - sha - ret

Sha - lom a - lei - chem mal - a - chei ha - sha - ret

mal - a - chei el - yon mi - me - lech

mal - a - chei el - yon mi - me - lech

mal - a - chei ham - la - chim ha - ka - dosh ba - ruch hu.

mal - a - chei ham - la - chim ha - ka - dosh ba - ruch hu.

1 INTRODUCE

Invite students to explore some of the traditions and culture of the Jewish people. Share information from the Footnotes throughout this lesson with students.

Tell students that there is no English translation for "Shalom aleichem" because it is not appropriate to the culture. See Resource Book p. A-34, for a literal translation.

Shalom means "peace." See Across the Curriculum, on p. 410, for activities that will encourage students to reflect on how to be peaceful people.

2 DEVELOP

Listening

6b Play the recording of "Shalom aleichem" **CD 20-7.**

Have students listen for

- Theme A. (mm. 5–12)
- Theme B. (mm. 13–20)
- Theme B harmonized. (mm. 22–29)

Play the recording again, inviting students to listen for embellished notes. (mm. 11, 18, 22–23, and 27)

Reading

"Shalom aleichem," written in G-harmonic minor, has a melody line with some large interval leaps (disjunct motion). The song also has passages with stepwise movement (conjunct motion).

Begin by having students sing a G-harmonic-minor scale (play the notes G, A, B♭, C, D, E♭, F♯, G).

Write mm. 5–9 on a staff on the board. Invite students to sing the pitch syllables, using hand signs.

See Skills Reinforcement, pp. 408 and 410, for reading and singing exercises.

continued on page 410

SPOTLIGHT ON

► **Hebrew Tradition** *Shabbat,* as it is called in Hebrew, is a day when weekday matters are set aside and higher pursuits are followed. It is the only ritual instituted in the *Torah*. The Sabbath is considered a "bride" or a "queen." The holiday begins with the lighting of the *Shabbat* candles by the woman of the house, no later than 18 minutes before sunset on Friday. The best dishes are set, nice clothes are worn, and a festive atmosphere is established. People eat and pray in a more leisurely manner than during the week. No work is allowed, including writing, erasing, weaving, and baking. People do, however, talk, walk, nap, and play games. Sabbath ends about 40 minutes after sunset (when three stars appear in the sky) on Saturday.

CULTURAL CONNECTION

► **Jewish Culture** Jewish people and their music find their roots in the Middle East, specifically in the land around present-day Israel (created in 1948). For centuries, Jews have lived among Eastern and Western cultures: the Western Mediterranean and North Africa, Europe, and the Americas. Moshe Denburg suggests that Jewish music defies a geographical location but has a unique property: intercultural synthesis. Because Jews have wandered the globe for thousands of years, they have assimilated foreign cultures into their art and daily lives. In short, Jewish music is cross-cultural—it has many faces.

Singing

1d Have students learn to sing *"Shalom aleichem"* in Hebrew using the Pronunciation Practice **CD 20-9** and **CD 20-10**, along with the Pronunciation Practice Guide on Resource Book p. A-34.

Invite students to sing *"Shalom aleichem"* **CD 20-7** in a *legato* style, with a slight bit of sliding from note to note to maintain the vocal style.

1c The long notes (dotted half and whole notes), should have a *crescendo* feeling, giving the melody line a sense of forward motion.

The sixteenth-note embellishments should be sung with rhythmic clarity. Vocally emphasizing the first eighth note of every two eight-note patterns supports the natural syllabic and word stress of the text. Each phrase should *crescendo* during the first measure and *decrescendo* during the second measure.

Analyzing

Since there is no tempo marking for this song, encourage students to experiment by singing it at different tempos. Try to "find" the tempo that seems to sound right for the text and the melodic character of the song.

Imagine the eighth notes having a little more forward motion than the longer notes, which should be slightly delayed.

Play the Stereo Vocal recording **CD 20-7** again and compare the students' performance with the recording.

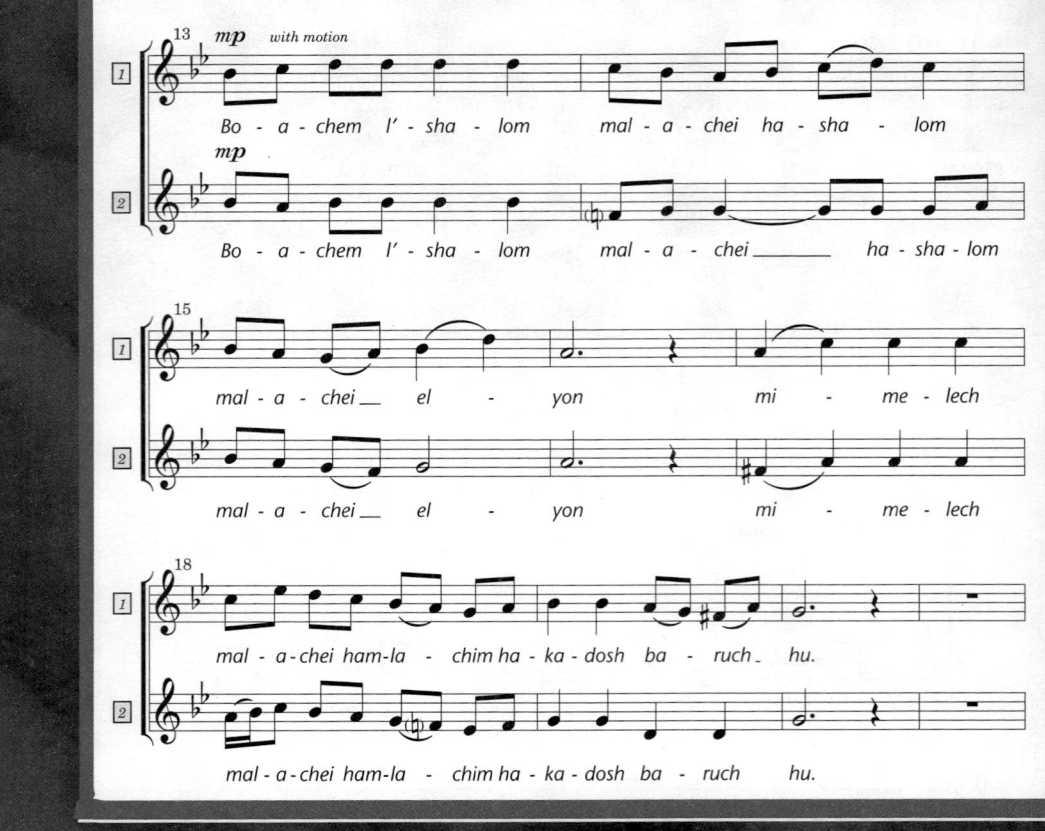

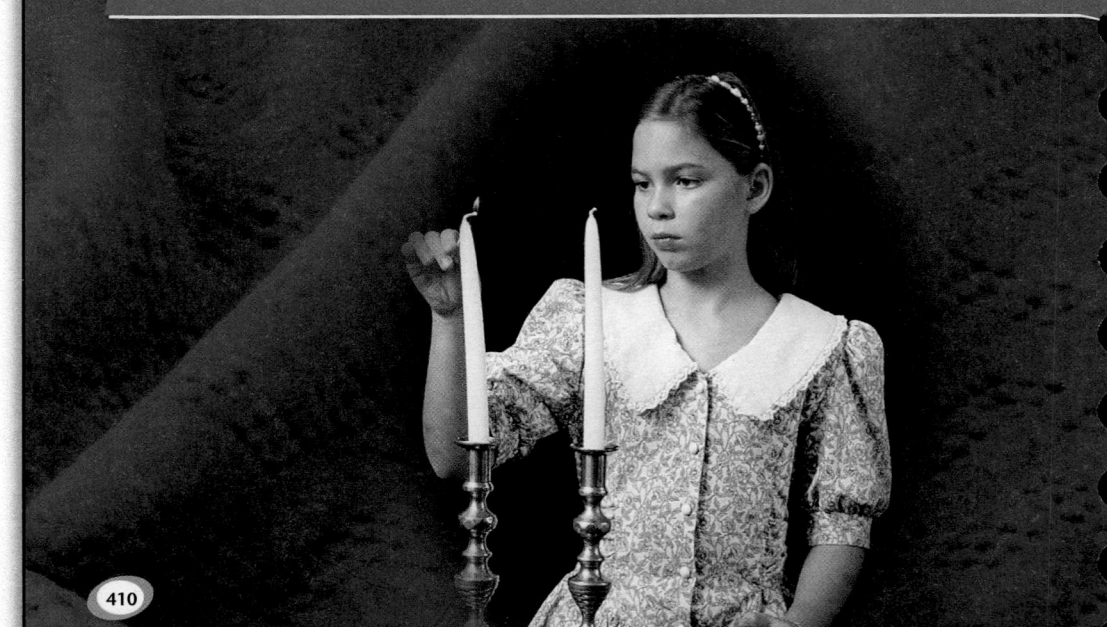

410

Footnotes

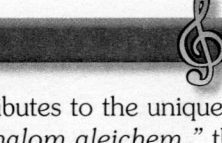

SKILLS REINFORCEMENT

▶ **Singing** The use of minor scales contributes to the unique sound of music from the Middle East. In *"Shalom aleichem,"* the G-harmonic-minor scale is prominent. Sing this scale, paying attention to the F♯-E♭ augmented second. Locate the passages in the song that use this interval and play them on the piano. Sing each phrase on a neutral syllable (*a, o,* or *ah*), flowing from note to note. There should be a slight sliding from pitch to pitch in order to capture the chantlike character of the song. Every time an F♯ occurs, sing it with more vocal weight because it is a "color note" and requires a vocal and textual emphasis. Help students to feel the pull from F♯-G (*si-la*) as well, as they sing this scale.

ACROSS THE CURRICULUM

▶ **Language Arts** Share the book *Make Someone Smile: And 40 More Ways to Be a Peaceful Person* by Judy Lalli (Free Spirit, 1996). Invite students to identify which of the 40 ideas they have done. Have them write an affirmation in their journals about some of the 40 ways they will attempt to integrate these ideas into their behavior.

Invite students to each identify one additional way that they can become more peaceful people. Bind these into a class book titled "More Ways to Be a Peaceful Person."

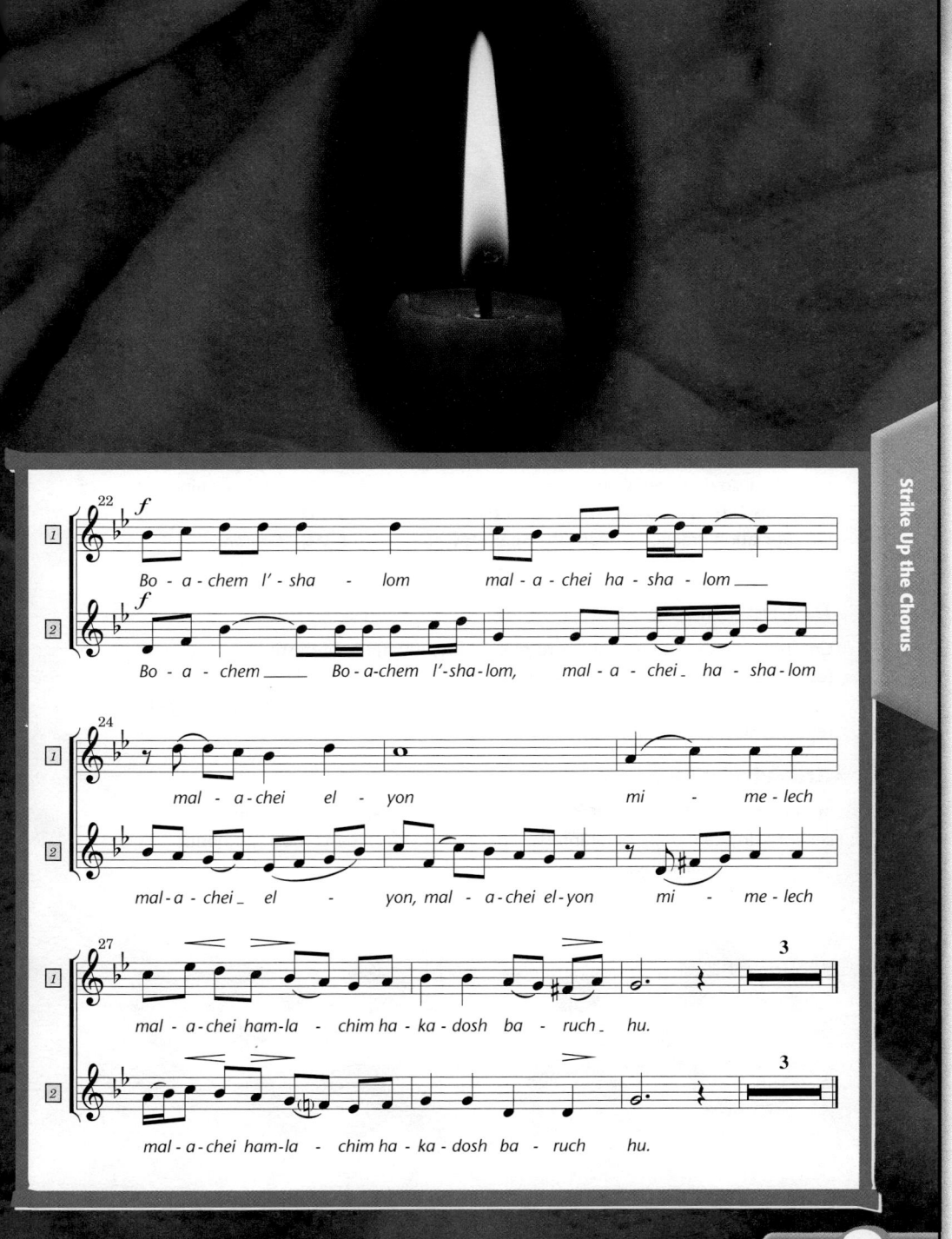

Bo - a - chem l' - sha - lom   mal - a - chei ha - sha - lom ___

Bo - a - chem ___ Bo - a - chem l' - sha - lom,   mal - a - chei _ ha - sha - lom

mal - a - chei el - yon   mi - me - lech

mal - a - chei _ el - yon, mal - a - chei el - yon   mi - me - lech

mal - a - chei ham - la - chim ha - ka - dosh ba - ruch _ hu.

mal - a - chei ham - la - chim ha - ka - dosh ba - ruch   hu.

Performing

When this song is sung for an audience, it would be useful to read the Hebrew text.

Introduce themes A and B separately and invite the audience to listen for the themes when they are harmonized in the song.

Programming this song could include several other Hebrew songs that depict activities in Jewish family life. Similarly, a group of other songs that highlight the daily life of another culture could also be part of the program.

3 CLOSE

Analyzing

Lead a discussion to review the G-harmonic-minor scale and melodic intervals in *"Shalom aleichem."*

7a Have students refer to their music notation and determine

- If the melody is in major or minor. (minor)
- If theme A has primarily disjunct or conjunct motion. (conjunct motion)
- What accidental appears that is not in the key signature. (F♯)
- The pitch syllable of that accidental. (*si*)

Element: MELODY — **ASSESSMENT**

Performance/Observation Ask students to sing the G-harmonic-minor scale (as you play along on the keyboard). Then, ask them to sing *"Shalom aleichem"* **CD 20-7.**

Observe and evaluate their performance. Observe their ability to sing the correct intervals with good intonation.

TEACHER TO TEACHER

▶ **MIDI Song File** Use the MIDI song file for *"Shalom aleichem"* to help students learn and practice the song. Play the tempo at a slower speed; isolate vocal parts; transpose the key; if desired, and use select measures to repeat and practice difficult parts.

TECHNOLOGY/MEDIA LINK

MIDI/Sequencing Software Open the MIDI song file for *"Shalom aleichem"* and challenge students to improvise/compose enhancements for the vocal performance. Begin with rhythmic ideas and extend to melodic ideas based on the harmonic-minor scale. Ask them to find MIDI voices that sound like instruments used in Jewish/Yiddish music (tambourine, clarinet, accordion, *shofar*). Ask them to find places in the song to add ostinatos or short music segments in the background.

Web Site Have students visit *www.sfsuccessnet.com* to learn more about the music of Israel.

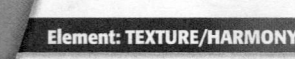

LESSON 5

LESSON AT A GLANCE

Element Focus **TEXTURE/HARMONY** Harmony in thirds and sixths

Skill Objective **SINGING** Read and sing harmony in thirds and sixths

Connection Activity **SOCIAL STUDIES** Discuss ways to help people in need

MATERIALS

- "Cantaré, cantarás" **CD 20-11**
- "I Will Sing, You Will Sing" (English) **CD 20-12**
- **Pronunciation Practice/Translation** p. 542
  Recording Routine: Intro (16 m.); verse; refrain; interlude (10 m.); refrain (two times)
- **Resource Book** p. A-35

VOCABULARY

verse	refrain	first and second ending
repeat sign	sequence	

◆ ◆ ◆ ◆ **National Standards** ◆ ◆ ◆ ◆
1c Sing music with appropriate expression
1d Sing music written in two parts
5a Read quarter and eighth notes in duple meter
6a Listen and describe events in music using appropriate terms

MORE MUSIC CHOICES

For more practice singing songs in Spanish:
"El cóndor pasa," p. 46
"El payo," p. 145

A Gift of Song

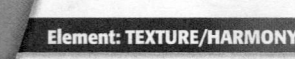

A group of singers and musicians banded together in 1985 to record "Cantaré, cantarás." All the proceeds from the song went to help needy children in Latin America, the Caribbean, and Africa. "Cantaré, cantarás" has become well known throughout the world.

Sing "Cantaré, cantarás."

Singing Tips

A good warm-up can help you get ready to sing your best. Try singing *so, mi, fa, re, do* in a slow tempo. Concentrate on good pitch and tone quality. Examine measures 1–6. Then **sing** them using pitch syllables. **Listen** to the Pronunciation Practice to learn the Spanish words. Then **sing** "Cantaré, cantarás."

Reading Music Tips

Composers often use sequences to make a melody more interesting. A sequence repeats a pattern, beginning on a different note of the scale. Notice how the notes in measures 3–4 are repeated in measures 5–6 (down a whole step). Sight-read the sequence patterns in measures 11–14.

Knowing the Score

"Cantaré, cantarás" is in Ⓐ Ⓑ Ⓐ Ⓑ form. **Describe** the "roadmap" of the sections. In the refrain, what intervals do the two voice parts most frequently sing to create harmony?

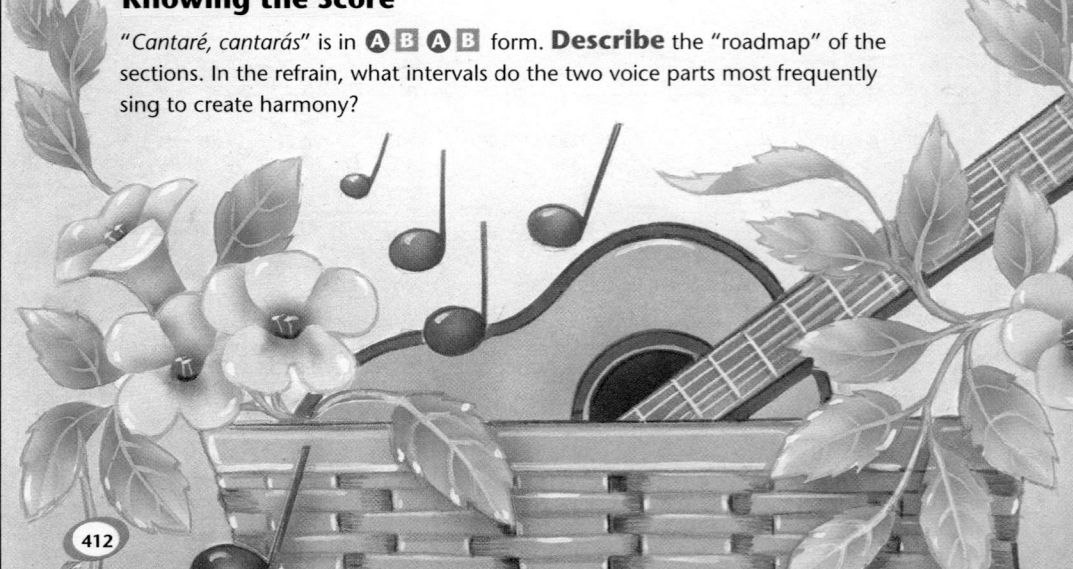

412

Footnotes

ACROSS THE CURRICULUM

▶ **Social Studies** Encourage students to discuss ways in which they can help a child or a family in need in their own community or elsewhere in the world. As they suggest ideas, list them on the board. Then, have students choose one idea and make it a class project for those who wish to participate.

BUILDING SKILLS THROUGH MUSIC

▶ **Visual Arts** Share the information on Diego Rivera from Spotlight On, p. 414. Ask students to look at *Calla Lily Vendor* on p. 415. Have them describe specific details in the painting using the elements of art.

SPOTLIGHT ON

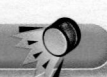

▶ **"Cantaré, cantarás" ("I Will Sing, You Will Sing")** In 1985, a group of artists, including Sergio Mendes, Vikki Carr, Plácido Domingo, Julio Iglesias, Miami Sound Machine, and José Feliciano, banded together to pledge their help to children of Latin America, the Caribbean, and Africa. Their foundation, Hermanos ("Brothers and Sisters"), has pledged that all proceeds from the sale of recordings of *"Cantaré, cantarás"* be used for supplies of food and medicine to those most in need. The deeply moving lyrics express the love and hope of people helping people. It is similar in feeling to "We Are the World," the children's song that seeks to promote unity and understanding between all peoples of the earth.

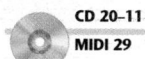

CD 20–11
MIDI 29

Cantaré, cantarás
(I Will Sing, You Will Sing)

English Words by Eileen Mahood-José

Words and Music by Albert Hammond and Juan Carlos Calderón
Arranged by Richard Kaller

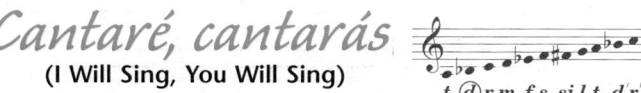

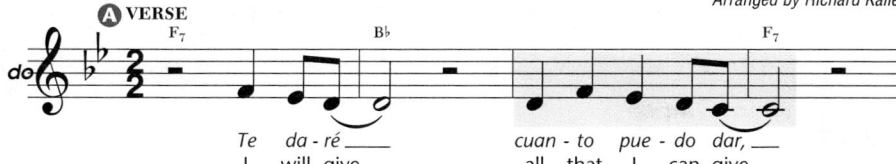

Te da-ré ___ cuan-to pue-do dar, ___
I will give ___ all that I can give, ___

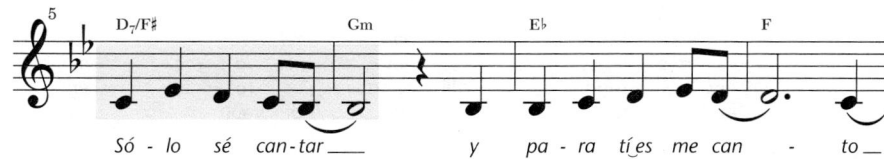

Só-lo sé can-tar ___ y pa-ra tí es me can - to ___
I can on-ly sing, ___ and this song is my gift. ___

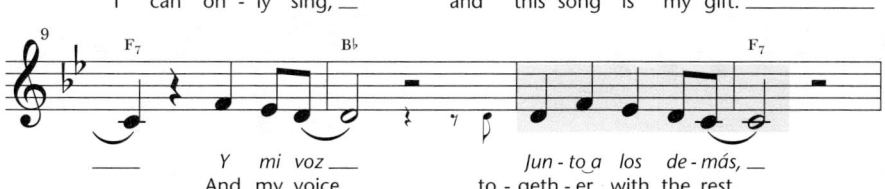

___ Y mi voz ___ Jun-to a los de-más, ___
___ And my voice ___ to-geth-er with the rest, ___

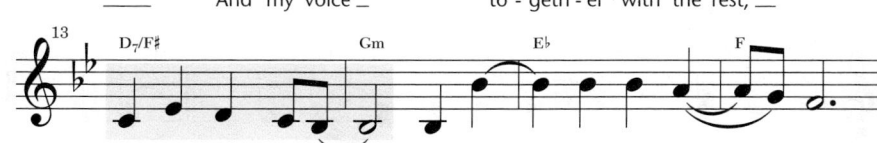

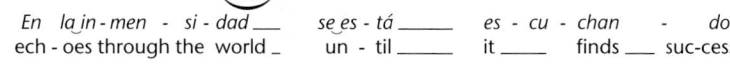

En la in-men - si-dad ___ se es-tá ___ es-cu-chan - do.
ech-oes through the world _ un-til ___ it ___ finds ___ suc-cess.

Strike Up the Chorus

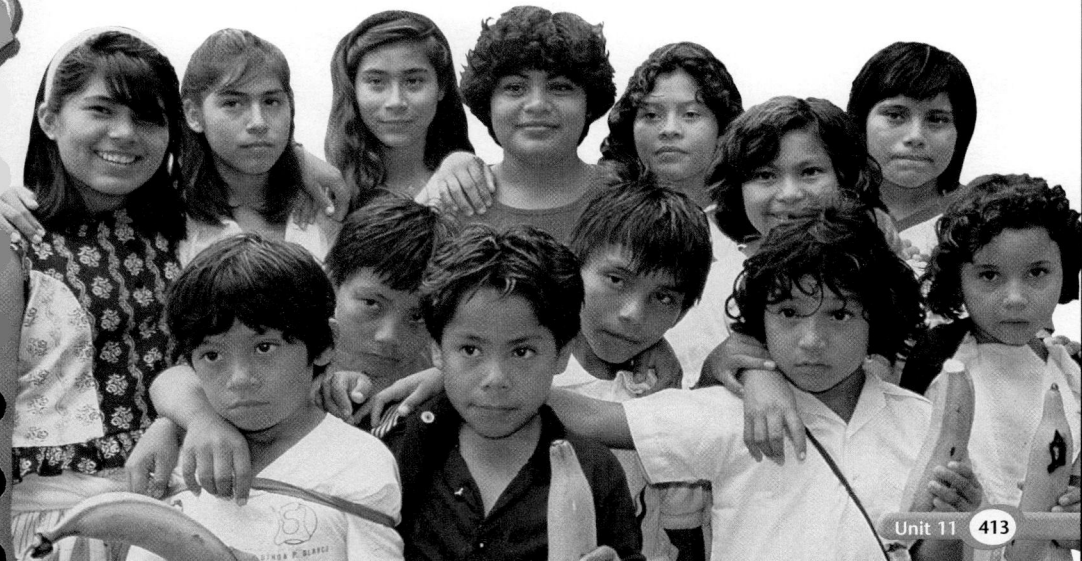

Unit 11 413

1 INTRODUCE

Invite students to listen to the recording of *"Cantaré, cantarás."* Share with students the information in Spotlight On, p. 412, and the reason why the song was recorded. Segue to a discussion on the problem of world hunger caused by poverty, and the role the United Nations takes in fighting world hunger. See Across the Curriculum, p. 414. Conclude by discussing ways to help people in need. Allow students to discover that the recording of *"Cantaré, cantarás"* was one solution to addressing the problem of world hunger.

Then invite students to look at the artwork, *Calla Lily Vendor*, on p. 415. Lead a discussion on artist Diego Rivera. See Spotlight On, p. 414. Discuss the cultural heritage of Spain. See Cultural Connection below. Ask students how culture and art can flourish in countries that face problems of poverty.

2 DEVELOP

Analyzing

Play the recording of *"Cantaré, cantarás"* **CD 20-11**. Note the modulation after the interlude.

Help students learn to sing the song in Spanish using the Pronunciation Practice **CD 20-14** (melody) and **CD 20-15** (harmony) along with the Pronunciation Practice Guide on Resource Book p. A-35.

Invite the Spanish teacher to read the Spanish text and provide a literal translation. Videotape the Spanish teacher's reading of the text.

Lead a discussion about the difference between a literal and a "free" translation of the text. (A free translation lends itself to singing English that makes poetic or artistic sense.)

continued on page 414

SKILLS REINFORCEMENT

▶ **Singing** In singing, the sound is carried by the vowels in words. Consonants define words and they can appear at the beginning, in the middle, and at the end of words. Depending upon the style of a song, both the vowels and the consonants are of equal importance, or one becomes more prominent. In *"Cantaré, cantarás,"* although the consonants are important, they should not obscure the importance of the vowels. In singing the Spanish in this song, the first consonant of each word should be enunciated quickly so that the vowel that follows is not obscured. The consonants should be sung gently, to accommodate the *legato* style of this song.

CULTURAL CONNECTION

▶ **Visiting Spain** Visiting Spain can be a spellbinding visual journey. It is a land of rich history and the home of such artists as Picasso, Miro, Dalí, and Goya. The countryside is dotted with great edifices, monasteries, and palaces. Spain has given the world both wonderful music and culinary delights. Spain's music includes *villancicos, flamenco* guitar music, and a rich history of folk music. On a visit to Spain, it would be important to sample two famous food dishes, *paella* (a stew) and *gazpacho* (a soup).

Lesson 5 Continued

Listening

Play the recording of *"Cantaré, cantarás"* **CD 20-11** and have students

- Listen for the melodic and rhythmic sequence in mm. 1–6 and mm. 9–14.
- Listen for the harmony in the refrain section.

- Raise their hands when the harmony part repeats.
- Identify the one harmonic interval in the refrain that is not a third or sixth. (Do not include unisons.) (a fourth, m. 23)
- Raise their hands when they hear rests in the music.

Reading

Most of the notes in this song move in a stepwise progression. Learning the individual melody and rhythm patterns will make learning the song easier. Invite students to

- Speak the rhythm syllables in mm. 1–8 and 9–16.
- Sing the pitch syllables in mm. 1–8 and 9–16.
- Speak the rhythm syllables in the refrain.
- Sing the pitch syllables in the refrain and discuss which pitch and rhythm patterns are similar and which are different.
- Discuss the purpose of the repeat signs and the first and second endings.

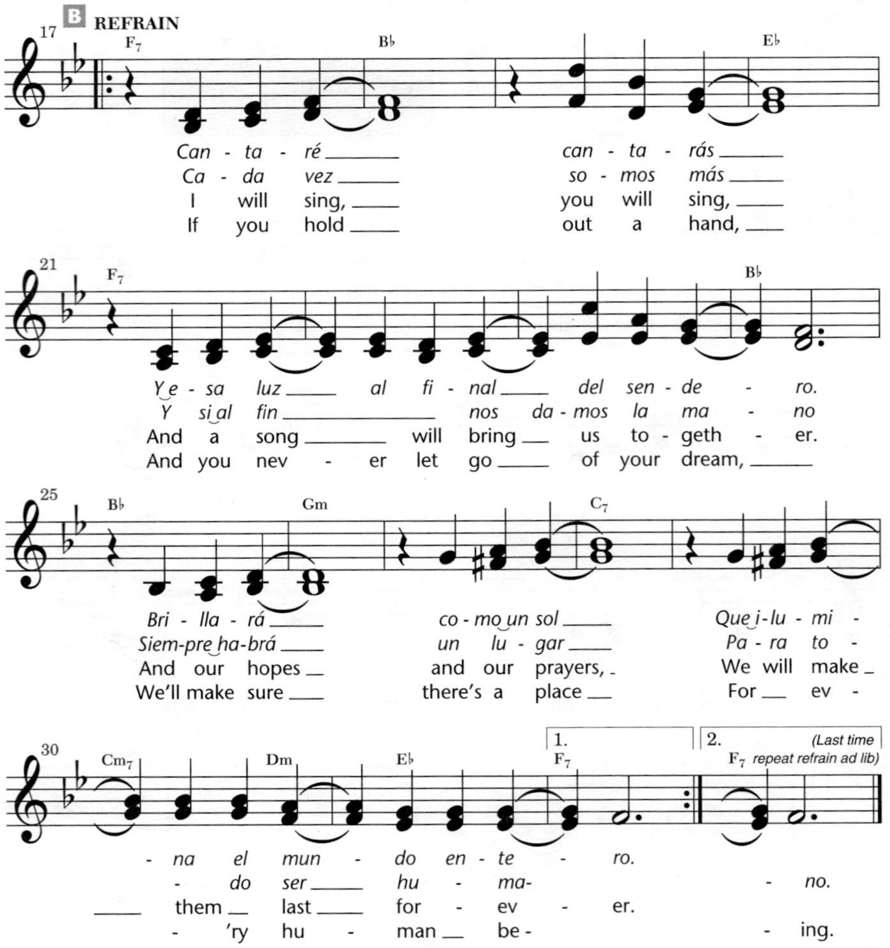

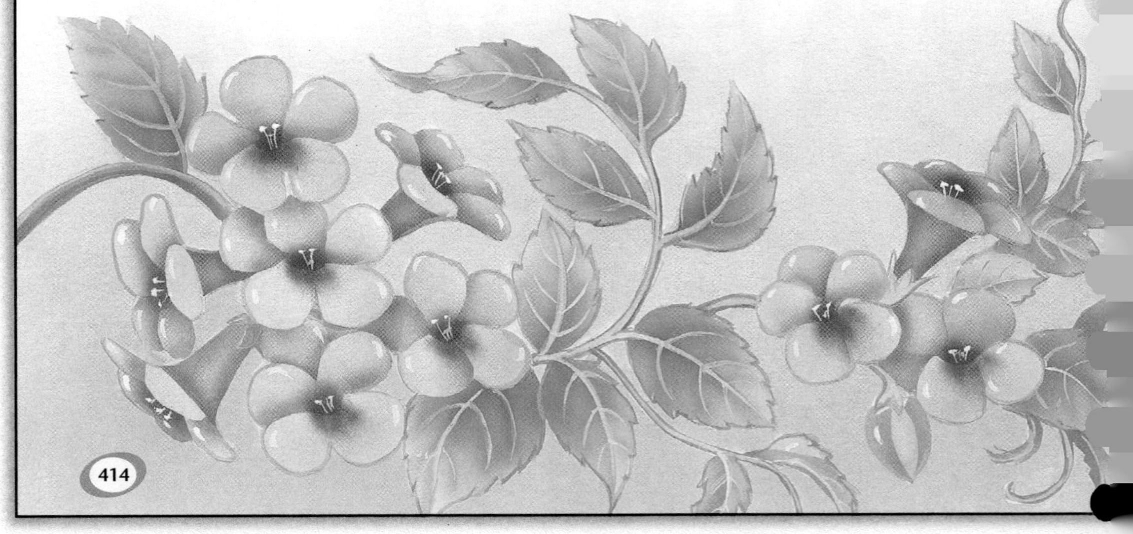

Footnotes

ACROSS THE CURRICULUM

▶ **Social Studies** Food is necessary for survival. Without proper nutrition, health, productivity, and physical and mental growth are at risk. Through the United Nations, countries around the world have addressed the world hunger problem. Today, its organizations work to assure that all people obtain proper nutrition. The Food and Agriculture Organization coordinates food policies. UNICEF, the World Health Organization, and the World Bank invest billions of dollars each year in agriculture, nutrition, and health matters. The World Food Program manages emergency food aid, and GATT (General Agreement Trade and Tariffs) assures free trade in food. These organizations have made inroads in world hunger, but more work is vital.

SPOTLIGHT ON

▶ **The Artist** Mexican mural painter Diego Rivera (1886–1957) enjoyed drawing from the time he was very young and took evening classes at the San Carlos Academy, enrolling full time at age 12. At age 20, he exhibited 26 works, which established him as an artist. In 1907, he went to Europe, where he was influenced by postmodernism and cubism, which he incorporated with his classic, precise, simplified, and colorful style of painting. Primarily a painter of Mexican history, he depicted subjects such as the earth, the farmer, the laborer, and some popular characters.

He returned to Mexico in 1921, becoming a revolutionary and joined the Mexican Communist Party in 1922. He married artist Frida Kahlo.

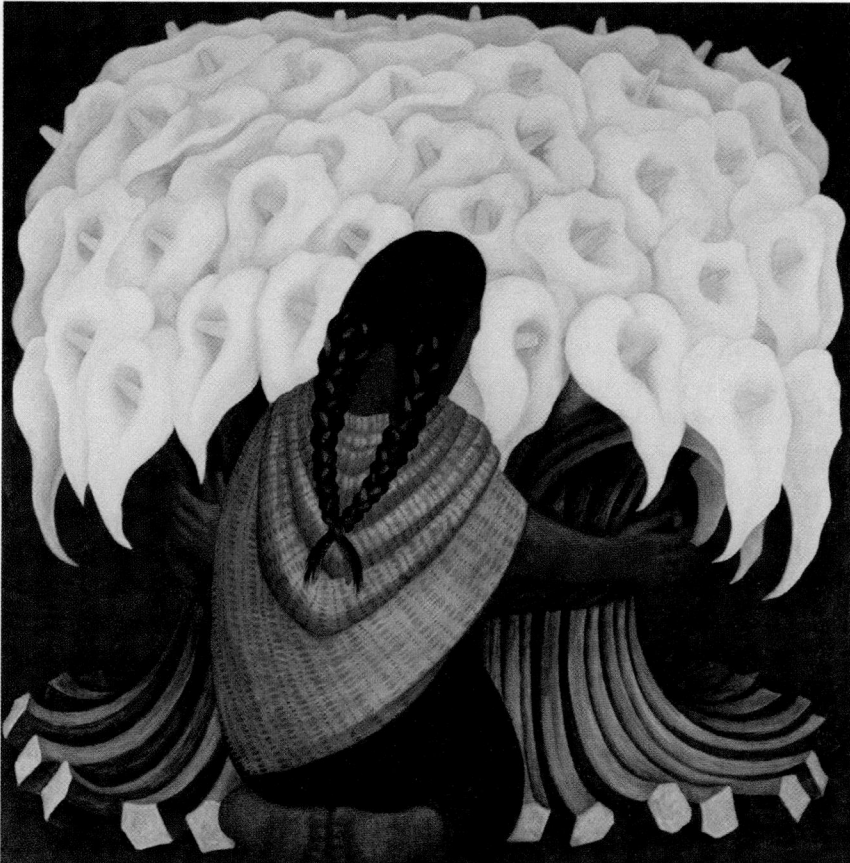

Singing

1c To capture the style of this song, emphasize the first quarter of each sequence pattern, *crescendo* slightly through the quarter notes, and *decrescendo* on the long notes, while keeping the phrase ending vocally energized.

1d While singing the harmony part, be certain Part 1 and Part 2 are dynamically balanced. Sing the refrain with an increased dynamic level and fuller-sounding voice.

3 CLOSE

Skill: SINGING   **ASSESSMENT**

Performance/Self-Assessment Have students sing *"Cantaré, cantarás"* **CD 20-11** as a class. Ask them to listen to their singing. Lead a discussion of their observations, asking the following questions.

- Were they able to sing the harmony in thirds and sixths in the refrain correctly?
- In what section of the song is the harmony sung in thirds and sixths? (refrain)
- In what measure do you find harmony that is not a third or sixth? (m. 23; a fourth)
- Were they able to sing the tied rhythms correctly?

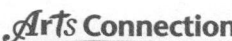

Arts **Connection**

▲ *Calla Lily Vendor* by Mexican artist Diego Rivera (1886–1957)

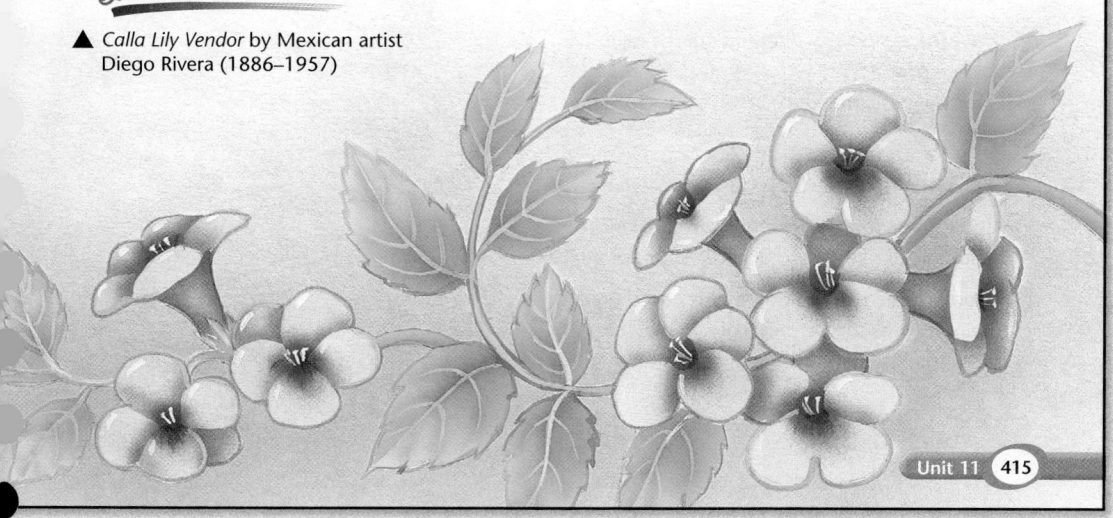

Unit 11 **415**

TEACHER TO TEACHER

▶ **MIDI Song File** Use the MIDI song file for *"Cantaré, cantarás"* to learn and practice the song. Use a slow tempo, isolate difficult measures, and use the file to teach the harmony parts.

TECHNOLOGY/MEDIA LINK

MIDI/Sequencing Software Have students use the MIDI song file for *"Cantaré, cantarás"* to explore the form of the song. Does the orchestration change from section to section? Change the instrumentation to get more variety in the form. Discuss other musical elements that can be changed to differentiate the form.

LESSON AT A GLANCE

Element Focus   **EXPRESSION** Dynamics, *crescendo*, *decrescendo*, and other expressive markings in octavos

Skill Objective   **READING** Read an octavo score, and analyze choral text and melodic phrases with regard to musical expression

Connection Activity   **RELATED ARTS** Discuss how the sea and sailing influenced Scandinavian art and folk objects

MATERIALS

- "*Vem kan segla?*"   **CD 20-16**
- "Who Can Sail?"   **CD 20-17**
  Recording Routine: Intro (8 m.); v. 1; v. 2; coda
- **Pronunciation Practice/Translation** p. 543
- "A Carelessly Crafted Raft" (poem)
- **Resource Book** p. A-36, J-15
- soprano and alto recorders, keyboard

VOCABULARY

onomatopoeia	metronome marking	*fermata*
texture	harmony	octavo

◆ ◆ ◆ ◆ National Standards ◆ ◆ ◆ ◆

1b Sing easy pieces with technical accuracy
1c Sing music with appropriate expression
1d Sing music written in three parts
1e In groups, sing moderately easy pieces with expression
5a Read dotted notes in triple meter
6a Listen and describe events in music using appropriate terms

MORE MUSIC CHOICES

For more practice singing harmony:
"You Are My Sunshine," p. 246
"*Siyahamba,*" p. 212

A Sailing Song

"*Vem kan segla?*" ("Who Can Sail?") is a choral arrangement of a folk song from Finland. Finland is a northern European country that borders Russia. Other countries in this region, such as Sweden and Norway, also claim versions of this song. Look carefully at the words of the song. What do you think they mean?

Sing "*Vem kan segla?*"

Singing Tips

Pay careful attention to your breathing technique. This will help you change dynamics and sing *crescendos* and *decrescendos*. **Sing** measures 1–8 in one breath.

Reading Music Tips

Rhythm Look at the rhythm pattern in measures 1 and 2 of Part 2. Find the other places in the song where this rhythm occurs. This is an important motive in "*Vem kan segla?*"

Melody At the start of the song, notice that the melody of Part 3 echoes Part 2. Where else does this occur?

Dynamics Find the dynamic markings in the score. What do the letters *p* and *mp* stand for? Find the *cresc.* marking. What does *crescendo* mean?

Knowing the Score

All the parts for "*Vem kan segla?*" are printed, including the keyboard accompaniment.

Choral music printed this way is called an *octavo*. A pianist uses the *octavo* score to play the accompaniment.

Arts Connection

Carved memorial stone (*stele*) with a ship of Vikings (7th century) ▼

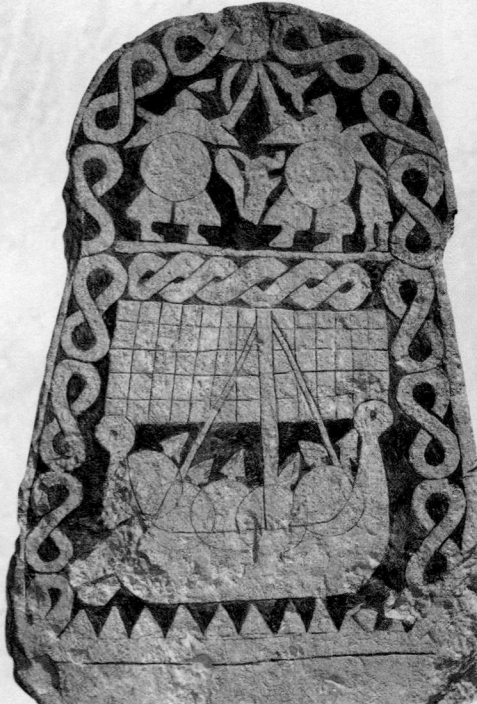

Footnotes

SKILLS REINFORCEMENT

▶ **Reading** Learning how to read a full score, such as an octavo, is a challenge for students. Use listening selections to focus on what students hear as they look at scores. Play "*Vem kan segla?*" **CD 20-16.** Each time students listen, they should focus on an instrument or vocal part.

BUILDING SKILLS THROUGH MUSIC

▶ **Social Studies** Share the information from Across the Curriculum, p. 416, and Spotlight On: The Long Ship, p. 417, about Scandinavia and sailing. Have students locate Scandinavian countries on a world map. Have them look at the bodies of water the ships had to traverse. Lead them in a discussion about the construction of ships and the reasons why engineers constructed the ships as they did.

ACROSS THE CURRICULUM

▶ **Language Arts** The sea and sailing are important to Scandinavian history, and shipbuilding was a serious craft. In contrast, have a student read to the class this fun poem on what might happen if we built a raft with less care than the Scandinavians. "A Carelessly Crafted Raft" by Lucinda Cave (*More Phonics Through Poetry*, GoodYear, 1997).

A Carelessly Crafted Raft

A carelessly crafted raft
Was caught in a hefty draft.
The wind swiftly shifted.
The raft luffed and drifted.
And afterward crashed on its aft.

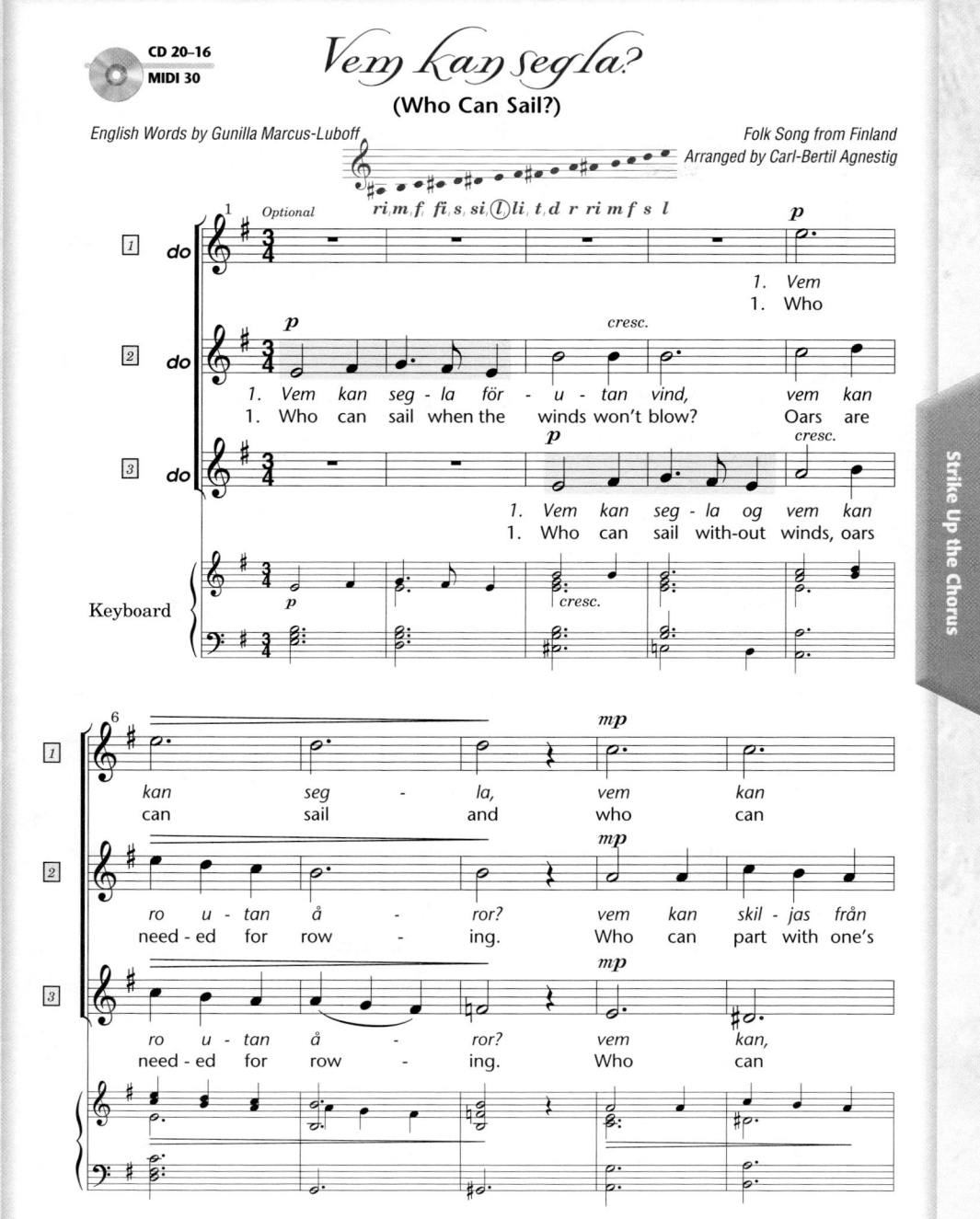

Vem kan segla?
(Who Can Sail?)

CD 20–16
MIDI 30

English Words by Gunilla Marcus-Luboff

Folk Song from Finland
Arranged by Carl-Bertil Agnestig

Strike Up the Chorus

1 INTRODUCE

Invite students to read about and view the Scandinavian art on pp. 416, 419, and 421. Guide students to discover the connection between Scandinavian art and the importance of sailing and the sea to the Scandinavian countries. Share Spotlight On below, and on p. 419, with students.

2 DEVELOP

Analyzing

Have students silently read the English text of *"Vem kan segla?"*

Lead a discussion about what the song means.

ASK Is the song about sailing? (no)

What is the relationship between the words about sailing and parting when tears are flowing? (The text is an example of an analogy, or a comparison.)

Introduce the melody (Part 1, mm. 1–16) by any of the following ways.

- Have a soloist sing it.
- Have a flute player from band play it.
- Play it on the piano.

Listening

Since this song is in three-part harmony, it is good aural discipline to be able to hear the three parts separately. Play the recording of *"Vem kan segla?"* **CD 20-16** three times.

On the first hearing, invite students to listen to the melody line (Parts 2 and 3).

 On the second hearing, invite students to focus on listening to the descant (Part 1).

On the third hearing, have students focus on listening to Part 2.

continued on page 418

▶ **The Long Ship** The long ship was a remarkable example of engineering skill. Developed by the Scandinavians around the eighth century, the boats were seaworthy and able to carry a large cargo. They could penetrate far into shallow inlets. These ships were very fast, able to move at speeds of eight knots per hour (about nine miles per hour). Long ships were both resilient and light, which was achieved by trimming the planking to two centimeters and by trimming all excess wood from the rib frames. Both ends of the long ship were drawn upward into symmetric, curved points, which enabled it to reverse directions without turning around. Rulers prized these ships, sometimes nicknamed "dragons." One such ship was excavated from a chieftan's burial mound.

CULTURAL CONNECTION

▶ **Music and Singing in Scandinavia** Singing is a popular activity in Scandinavian countries. In Sweden, a country with a small population of only 600,000, people enjoy singing in groups and church choirs. In addition to singing, adults who wish to learn to play an instrument in Sweden can join a study circle, subsidized by the Swedish government.

In contrast to this traditional singing, Finland and Sweden do not yet have a large number of rock, jazz, or folk music groups. This is changing. One of the recently popular Swedish groups receiving international attention is Roxette. Similarly, ABBA has also enjoyed international renown since their breakthrough in 1974 with the song "Waterloo."

Reading

Students can locate six different rhythmic motives in the score of *"Vem kan segla"* by using the worksheet on Resource Book p. J-15.

Divide the class into a three-part choir.

Separate the groups so that they can simultaneously

5a
- Speak the rhythm syllables for their part.
- Sight-sing the pitch syllables for their part.

Bring the three sections back together. Have the choir sing only the pitch syllables for their parts, as you slowly proceed, section by section.

ASK Where is the *fermata?* (in mm. 16 and 32)

What does the *fermata* mean? (hold the note longer than its written value)

Have students read Knowing the Score on p. 416. Then, guide students to explore reading a complete musical score, using the printed music for *"Vem kan segla?"* (pp. 417–420).

Introduce students to the vocabulary word *octavo* (a musical score for choral music in a special small-format layout). Have students examine the components of the score (the choral vocal parts [Parts 1, 2, and 3] joined as a *system,* and the keyboard accompaniment part).

Guide students to learn to read a score (following a score is called *score reading*) using Skills Reinforcement on p. 416.

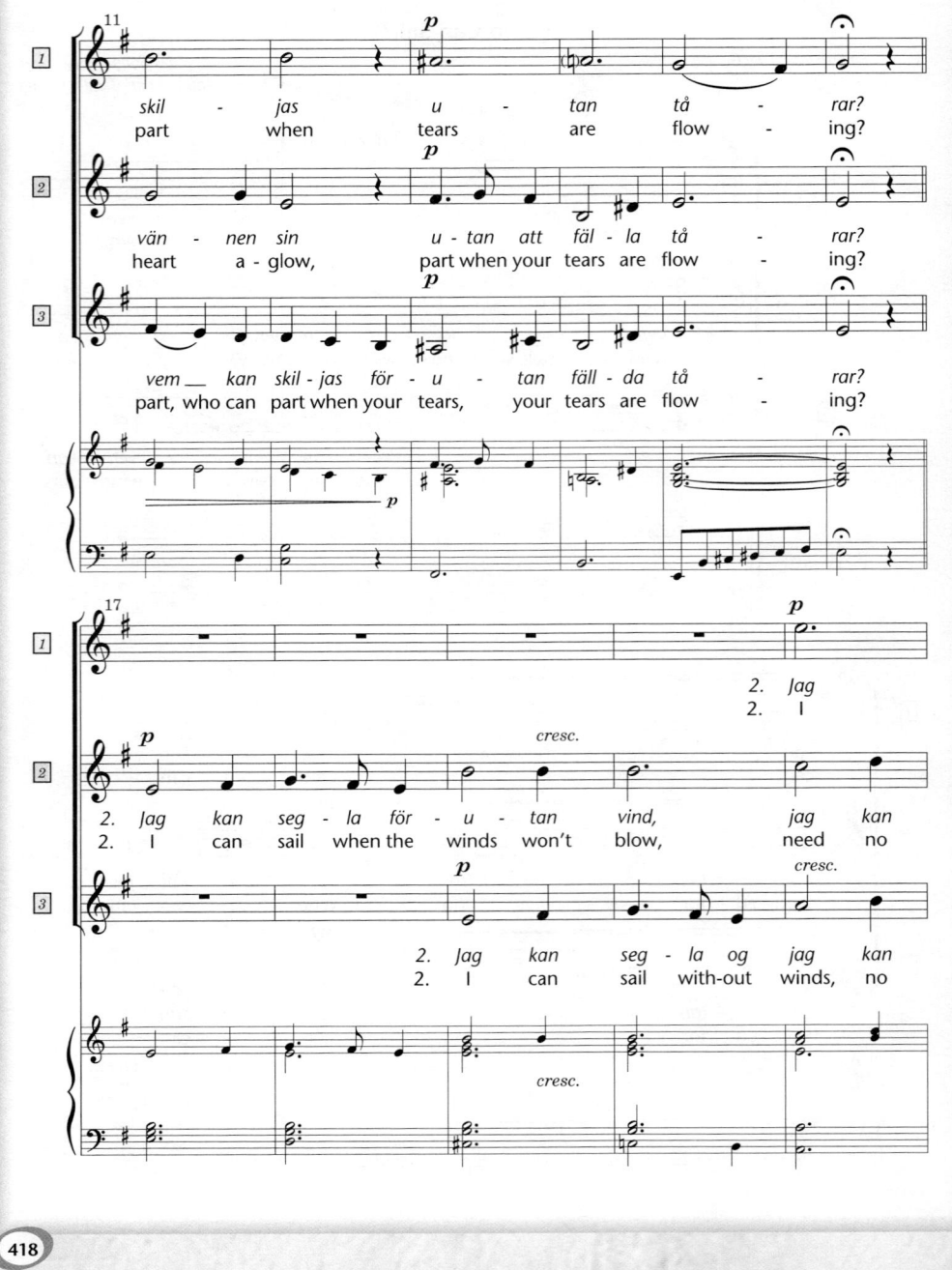

418

Footnotes

TEACHER TO TEACHER

▶ **Singing Musically** Being able to sing all the correct pitches and rhythms of a song does not make the performance musical. Even with dynamic contrast, the song may sound unconvincing. Knowing what the words of a text mean, however, will more likely produce musical results. To help students sing musically, it is useful to do the following preparation with texts.

- Study the words for meaning and emotional overtones.
- Practice reading the text expressively.
- Create strategies for teaching the syllabic and sense stress of each word.
- Say the words out loud and observe how you wish the vowels and consonants to sound.
- Record and evaluate your own performance.

SKILLS REINFORCEMENT

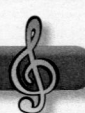

▶ **Singing** Correct deep breathing is important for good vocal support. While sitting, place your elbows on your knees and your chin in the palms of your hands, fingers along the side of your cheeks. Take a deep breath through your nose, as if you are smelling a hot apple pie. Notice the expansion of the entire area of your body where you wear a belt. You have just completed a deep-breathing exercise. Say each phrase in the song, using the above breathing technique, but sitting upright. Repeat the exercise, this time singing each phrase. Sing the song standing, incorporating deep breathing. Sing the song at slower tempos in order to develop good breath support. Try hissing each phrase at different tempos and still have some air remaining at the end of each phrase.

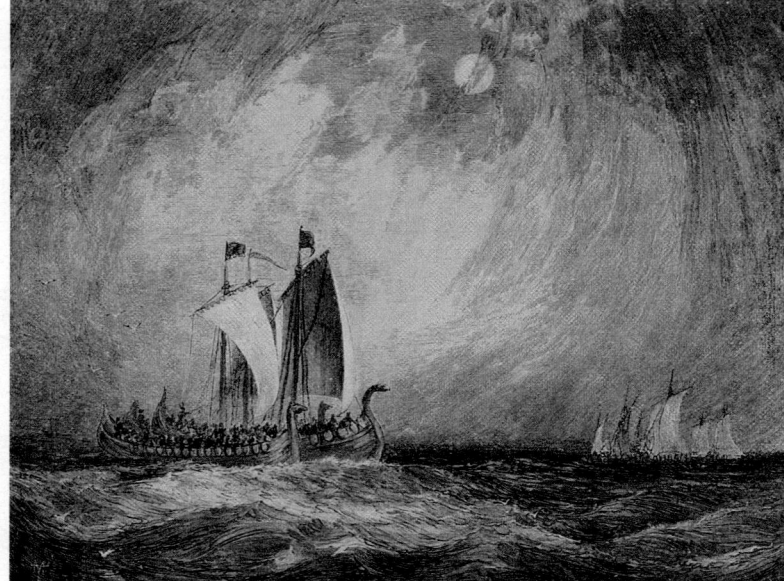

Arts Connection

▲ Two Norse ships at sea (Hand-colored woodcut)

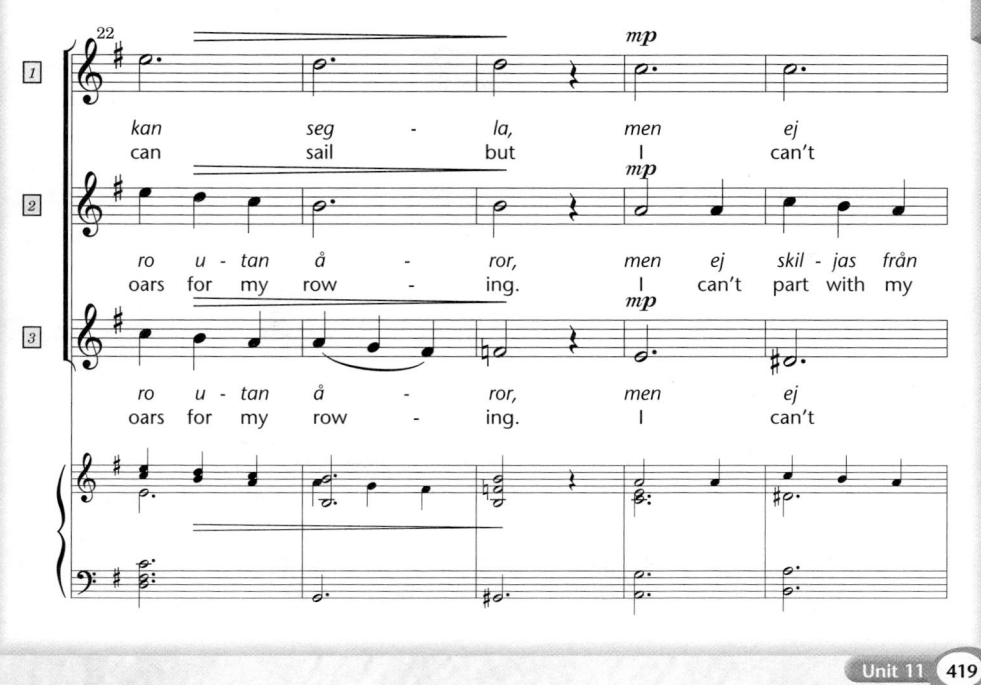

Unit 11 **419**

Reading

Tell students they are going to learn to sing *"Vem kan segla?"* **CD 20-16** expressively. There are several ways students can achieve expressive singing: through the text, dynamic shading, and harmonic interest.

Review the definition of the term *legato* with students and have them discuss why this song is best performed with *legato* articulation.

For the song *"Vem kan segla?,"* have students identify the music term referring to the articulation best suited to the song *(legato)* and understand how to interpret it when performing. (Smoothly connecting the notes when singing; taking deep breaths and singing phrases in one breath.)

For text, have students

- Sing *legato*.
- For onomatopoetic words such as *winds, blow,* and *flowing,* pronounce and enunciate them so that they sound like what they mean.

For dynamic shading:

- Follow the dynamic markings in the score.
- Each phrase must have dynamic direction; it must grow and fade, but with vocal energy.

For harmonic interest:

- When a voice has a moving part, it should be dynamically a bit louder (see mm. 6–7, 10–12).
- When notes are raised or lowered a half step in pitch, they should have a little more dynamic prominence (see mm. 10, 13–14, 24, 26, and 29–30).

Invite students to advance their choral singing by studying the text of the music, and then learn to sing words and phrases musically and with expression. See Teacher to Teacher on p. 418 for ideas on beginning this process.

continued on page 420

ACROSS THE CURRICULUM

▶ **Language Arts** Descriptive language is commonplace in many choral texts. Composers are drawn to texts that present their messages through the use of analogy, metaphor, simile, onomatopoeia, and colorful adjectives and adverbs. It is important that students understand the linguistic function and meaning of these poetic devices.

Discussions on text between the students and a visiting English or drama teacher can lead to informed performances that have the power to touch the listener musically.

SPOTLIGHT ON

▶ **Scandinavia and the Sea** The sea has played an important role in the culture and history of Scandinavia. The importance of the sea can be drawn from the earliest settlers of Scandinavia, through cave drawings showing Norse ships. The sea-worthiness of early Scandinavian sailors is also documented by the explorations of such characters as Leif Ericson, who reached the North American mainland around A.D. 1000.

Lesson 6 Continued

Students can also expand their vocal development by learning the technique of deep breathing. See Skills Reinforcement, p. 418, for more information.

Help students learn to sing *"Vem kan segla?"* in Finnish using the Pronunciation Practice **CD 20-19** and the Pronunciation Practice Guide on Resource Book p. A-36.

Analyzing

Discuss with students that descriptive language is common in choral texts. See Across the Curriculum, p. 419. One literary technique used in the lyrics of *"Vem kan segla?"* is *analogy*—comparing sailing *(when the winds won't blow)* with parting *(when the tears are flowing.)* The use of descriptive language gives the choral text a more poetic style.

Onomatopoeia (when the sound of a word suggests its meaning) is used in the words *winds (whin___sssss___)* and *blow (b-looooo___)*. Allow students to experiment in pronouncing these words, stressing syllables that associate its sound to the meaning.

Invite students to create a list of onomatopoetic words found in other songs. Encourage discussions about how the vowels and consonants of these words can be pronounced and enunciated to achieve meaningful expression. Propose a contest for the most expressive speaker.

Performing

It is important for students to hear *"Vem kan segla?"* **CD 20-16** performed in a variety of settings to aurally appreciate the melodic flow and the texture and harmony.

Before the final performance, have students

- Sing the song in block formation: descant, Part 1, and Part 2.

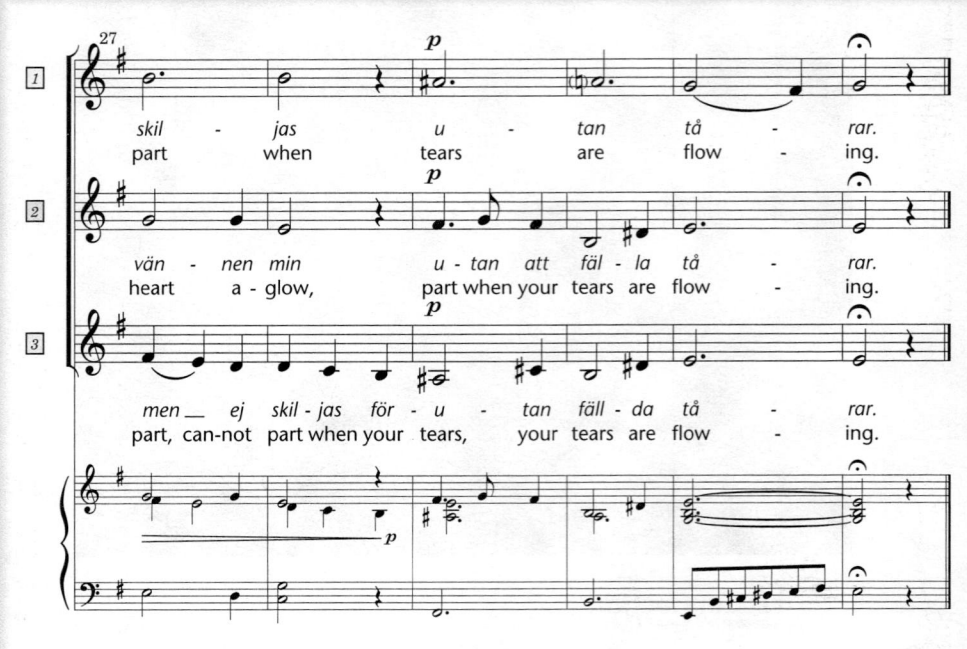

Playing the Recorder

Adding a recorder accompaniment to a choral piece adds variety to the vocal parts. Practice and then **play** this recorder part for *"Vem kan segla?"*

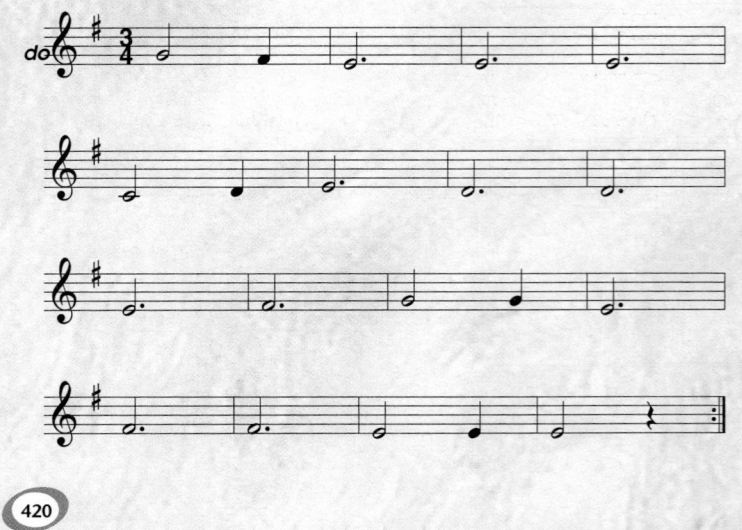

Footnotes

SKILLS REINFORCEMENT

► **Recorder** Have students play this countermelody to *"Vem kan segla?"* on alto recorder.

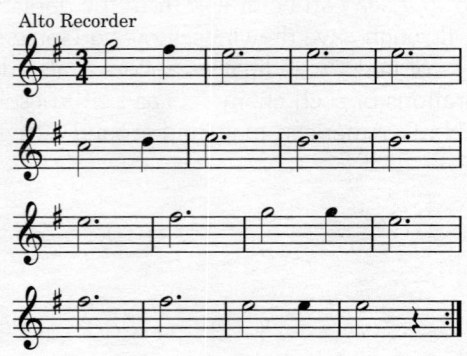

Alto Recorder

MEETING INDIVIDUAL NEEDS

► **Score Reading** Learning to read a score is a challenge for students. Invite students to use notation software, or sequencer (score editor), to assist them in learning to follow a score.

Reinforcement Open the MIDI song file for *"Vem kan segla?"* and view the notation on screen as it scrolls and as the MIDI file plays. Have them slow the tempo.

On Target Isolate and play back selected tracks (parts) of *"Vem kan segla?"* as they follow the notation on (computer) screen. Combining multiple tracks increases their challenge.

Challenge Discover that MIDI notation often looks more complex than printed notation, if the computer did not *quantize* the notation correctly.

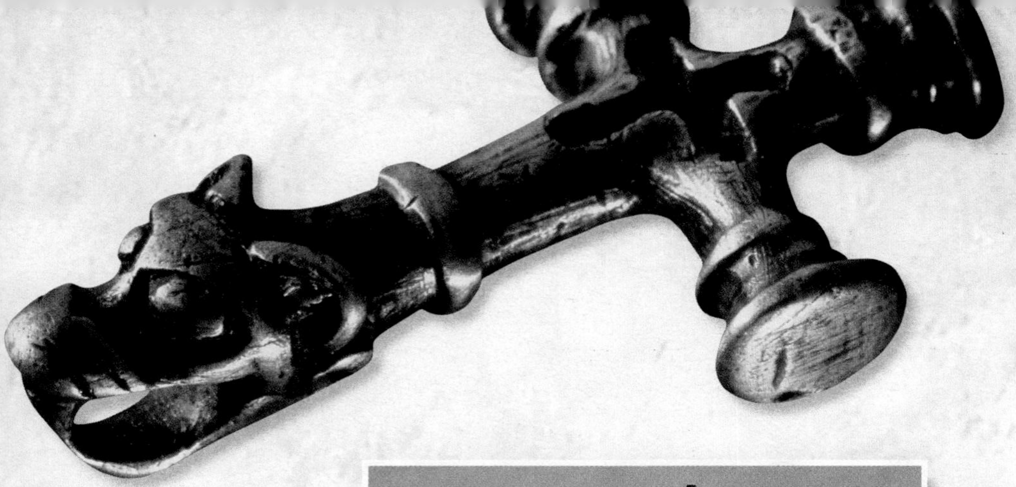

▲ *Thor's Hammer.* A Viking amulet from Iceland (10th century)

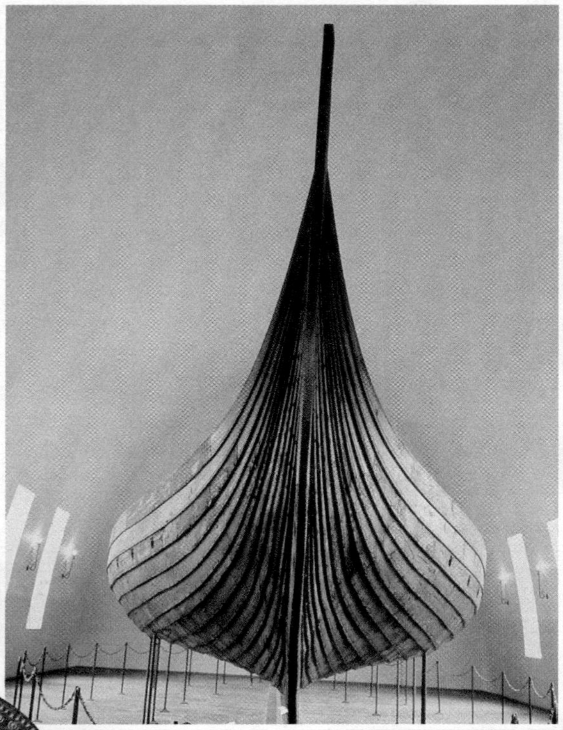

The Gokstad Ship. A Viking ship (9th century) ▶

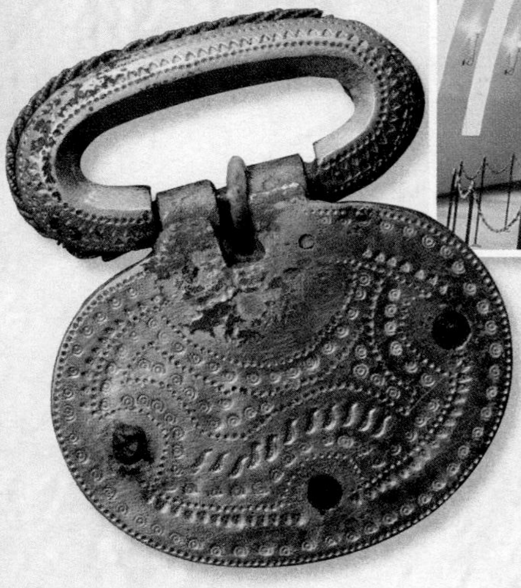

◀ A Scandinavian gilded bronze padlock (7th century)

- In the descant section, sing Parts 1 and 2 facing each other.

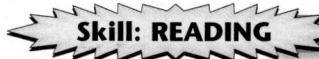

- Form three separate groups in different parts of the classroom and sing.
- Form three concentric circles and sing while walking in opposite directions.

Record each performance.

Playing

Invite students to learn two recorder accompaniments for *"Vem kan segla?"* The recorder accompaniments, in descant style, will enhance a live performance of this piece.

The soprano recorder accompaniment is found in the student text on p. 420. An accompaniment for alto recorder is found in Skills Reinforcement on p. 420.

3 CLOSE

Skill: READING   **ASSESSMENT**

Music Journal Writing Review with students the music reading concepts learned in studying *"Vem kan segla?"* Remind them of

- The function of an octavo. (a small-format choral score with all parts present)
- Components found in an octavo. (all vocal parts and accompaniment joined in a system)
- The poetic effect of descriptive language in choral text in the song. (analogy, onomatopoeia)
- Analyzing choral text and learning to sing words and musical phrases expressively based on the choral text.
- The expressive quality that dynamic and expressive markings add to musical performance. (dynamic marks, *crescendos, decrescendos,* and accidentals)

Have students listen to *"Vem kan segla?"* **CD 20-16.** Ask them to list in their music journals the markings in the octavo that indicate musical expression. Have students indicate exact measure numbers of the markings.

TEACHER TO TEACHER

▶ **MIDI Song File** Use the MIDI song file for *"Vem kan segla?"* to help students learn the song. Use this MIDI file to play the tempo slower, isolate vocal parts, teach the harmony parts, highlight difficult measures to repeat and practice, and transpose the key, if desired. This file will assist students in learning the music and in rehearsing for performance.

TECHNOLOGY/MEDIA LINK

Notation Software Challenge students to use notation software to score a computer version of *"Vem kan segla?"* Have students

- Set up the program for three staves, two treble and one bass.
- Choose the key of G (one sharp).
- Notate Part 1 and Part 2 of *"Vem kan segla?"* on the treble staves by selecting the desired rhythmic value and then clicking on the musical staff to choose the pitch.
- Notate a bass part by entering the lowest note of the keyboard part for each measure.
- Select a General MIDI voice for each of the three staves for computer playback.

LESSON AT A GLANCE

Element Focus   **MELODY** Countermelody

Skill Objective   **SINGING** Sing a Christmas carol with a countermelody

Connection Activity   **RELATED ARTS** Art based on holiday themes

MATERIALS
- "Angels on the Midnight Clear"   **CD 20-20**
  Recording Routine: Intro (6 m.); vocal; coda (after fermata)
- video camera (optional)

VOCABULARY

countermelody   anacrusis   fermata

> ◆ ◆ ◆ ◆ **National Standards** ◆ ◆ ◆ ◆
> **1c** Sing music with appropriate expression
> **6a** Listen and describe events in music using appropriate terms
> **6b** Listen and analyze uses of pitch and harmony in music from diverse genres
> **7b** Students use specific criteria for evaluating their own performances

MORE MUSIC CHOICES

For more practice with countermelodies:
"Going upon the Mountain," p. 105
"Eres tú," p. 473
"Sing a Song of Peace," p. 66

Midnight Melodies

The story of Christmas includes many carols about angels singing in the sky on Christmas night. "Hark the Herald Angels Sing," "Angels We Have Heard on High," and "It Came Upon a Midnight Clear" are examples of carols in which angels sing about important news for all people of the world.

Sing "Angels on the Midnight Clear."

Singing Tips

Sing the words that have half notes with a feeling of length accompanied by a slight *crescendo*. **Sing** the countermelody a little softer and in a flowing style when accompanying the melody.

Reading Music Tips

Analyze and **sing** the pick-up notes and the following downbeats in the color boxes. Emphasize the words on the downbeats, as in *it CAME*.

Knowing the Score

Identify the main melody and the countermelody. How often are the melody and countermelody sung separately and together? **Identify** the *fermata*. What is its musical purpose?

Footnotes

SPOTLIGHT ON

▶ **The Early Carol** Invite students to learn about the history of the carol. In the Middle Ages, the carol was a song of English origin, with text in English or Latin, and was usually about the Virgin Mary and Christmas. The medieval carol began with a *burden* (a refrain) followed by verses (stanzas). The burden was repeated after each verse. Today this form of composition is referred to as a strophic song—a song that has many verses and refrains all done to the same music.

BUILDING SKILLS THROUGH MUSIC

▶ **Writing** Have students write their thoughts from the assessment portion of the lesson. Ask them to write about the various methods used to help them learn the legato phrasing and which helped them the most.

SKILLS REINFORCEMENT

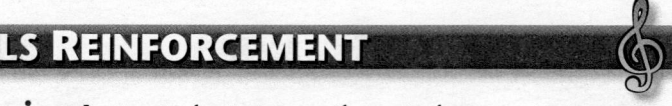

1c ▶ **Singing** Invite students to use these techniques to improve their singing of consonants. Singing consonants of words often suffers from either too much or too little enunciation. The result is either an unmusical performance, or a performance in which the audience cannot understand the words. In "Angels on a Midnight Clear," help students understand the difference between singing hard and gently sung consonants. For example, *It came* can be sung with force (hard) and the *t* and the *c* will be quite pronounced. However, since the meaning of the song's words and flow of the phrases do not call for hard consonants, ask students to sing the consonants clearly and gently—with little force. Additionally, ask students to let the consonants at the ends of words followed by words beginning with vowels elide or flow together to achieve smooth diction.

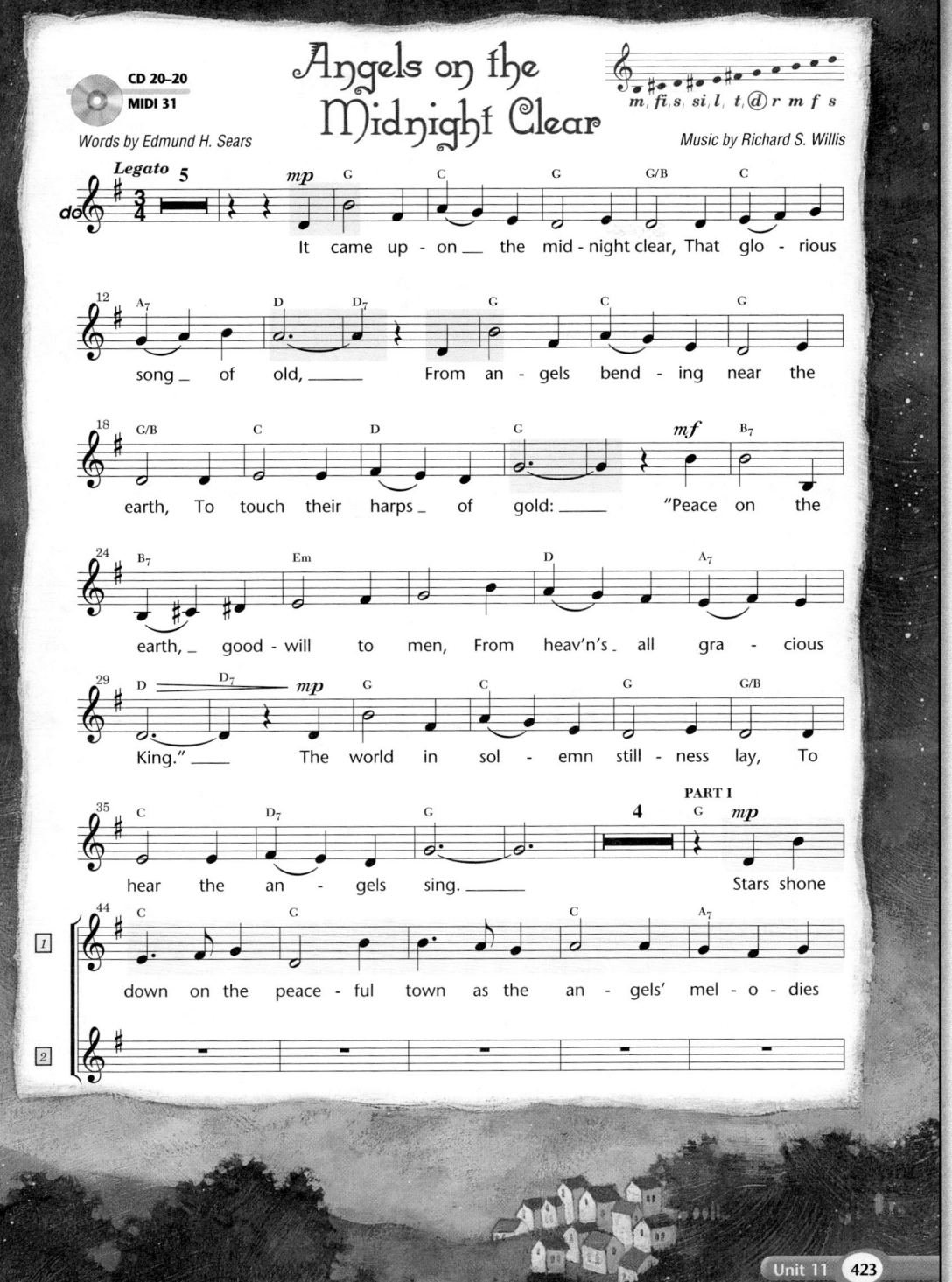

Angels on the Midnight Clear

Words by Edmund H. Sears

Music by Richard S. Willis

CD 20–20
MIDI 31

m fi si l, t @ r m f s

Legato

It came up-on __ the mid-night clear, That glo-rious song __ of old, _____ From an-gels bend-ing near the earth, To touch their harps __ of gold: _____ "Peace on the earth, __ good-will to men, From heav'n's __ all gra-cious King." _____ The world in sol-emn still-ness lay, To hear the an-gels sing. _____ Stars shone down on the peace-ful town as the an-gels' mel-o-dies

PART I

1 INTRODUCE

Invite students to look at the background art on pp. 422–425. Ask them how this scene might relate to Christmas. (A bright star at night signified the birth of Christ; accept other answers.) Tell students that many works of art have been inspired by Christmas.

Lead students in a discussion of how different cultures celebrate their holidays at year's end. (See Cultural Connection below.) Ask students to describe the works of art that depict their holidays.

Tell students that in this lesson they will sing a familiar Christmas carol along with a countermelody.

2 DEVELOP

Listening

ASK What is the definition of a countermelody? (a melody that runs counter to, or against, the melody) Refer students to the definition in the Glossary, p. 520. Guide them to discover that a countermelody adds harmonic interest to the melody.

Discuss with students how they might differentiate between a melody and countermelody as they listen to a song. (The melody is thematic and occurs first; the countermelody is a second melody that occurs at the same time, and counter to, the melody.)

6a Ask students to identify the melody and the countermelody as they listen to the recording of "Angels on the Midnight Clear" **CD 20-20.**

Analyzing

Invite students to analyze the melody and countermelody by looking at the notation of "Angels on the Midnight Clear" on pp. 423–425.

ASK What is the name of this famous Christmas carol? ("It Came upon a Midnight Clear")

continued on page 424

CULTURAL CONNECTION

▶ **Holiday Celebrations** Invite students to learn more about how different cultures celebrate holidays. Students may read about these holidays, bring information from home, or ask members of the community to visit the class and share stories and music of their holiday. Have students

- Discover the history of Kwanzaa, its traditions, songs and dances, food, and dress, and how it is celebrated.

- Learn about the history and purpose of Chanukah, and about its traditions, songs and dances, food, and dress. Find Chanukah greeting cards and discuss them.

- Learn about the traditions and fasting of the Muslim holiday of Ramadan. Discover that the end of Ramadan is celebrated by the Id-al-Fitr (Festival of Breaking).

TEACHER TO TEACHER

1c ▶ *Legato* **Phrases** Singing *legato* phrases can be a difficult concept to teach to students. Try using descriptive language such as similes or metaphors to capture the feeling and understanding of *legato* singing. Liken the flow of a musical phrase to "pearls strung on a golden chain" or "a sheet of water cascading over a dam." Say, "Imagine the words of each phrase are riding out of your mouth on a continuous column of air."

You can also liken *legato* singing to the analogy of a clothesline. The clothesline is the phrase. The hanging items are words. The clothespins are consonants. Don't break the line. If the line breaks, the clothes get muddy. (What the audience hears will be muddy.)

Lesson 7 Continued

6b Where, and in which parts, does the melody occur? (part 1, m. 6; part 2, m. 58)

Where, and in which parts, does the countermelody occur? (part 1, m. 43; part 1, m. 59)

Reading

SAY "Angels on the Midnight Clear" is in $\frac{3}{4}$ time, and many of the phrases begin on beat three. Then, have half the class find the beginning of each phrase and sing the first and second note. Have them identify the intervals (sixths, seconds, unisons) to determine how many are the same and different. Follow the same procedures for the countermelody with the second half of the class. Discuss what phrase-beginning intervals (sixths, seconds) are the same and different.

Have students identify which melody has

- Notes preceded with sharps. (melody, countermelody)
- Dotted-quarter notes. (countermelody)
- Eighth notes. (countermelody)
- Dotted-half notes tied to quarter notes. (melody)
- The widest vocal range. (the same, one octave: melody is b to b; countermelody is d to d)

Singing

1c Invite students to sing "Angels on the Midnight Clear." Using the techniques in Skills Reinforcement on p. 422 and p. 424, guide students to improve their singing of consonants and *legato* phrases.

Moving

Invite students to perform a movement as they sing "Angels on the Midnight Clear," reinforcing their singing and demonstrating appropriate large-ensemble performance techniques during an informal concert. Have them sing the song while standing in a circle so they can observe each other sing to maintain togetherness. As they sing, each student draws a rainbow arch with their right hand (left to right) to show (and influence) phrase shape.

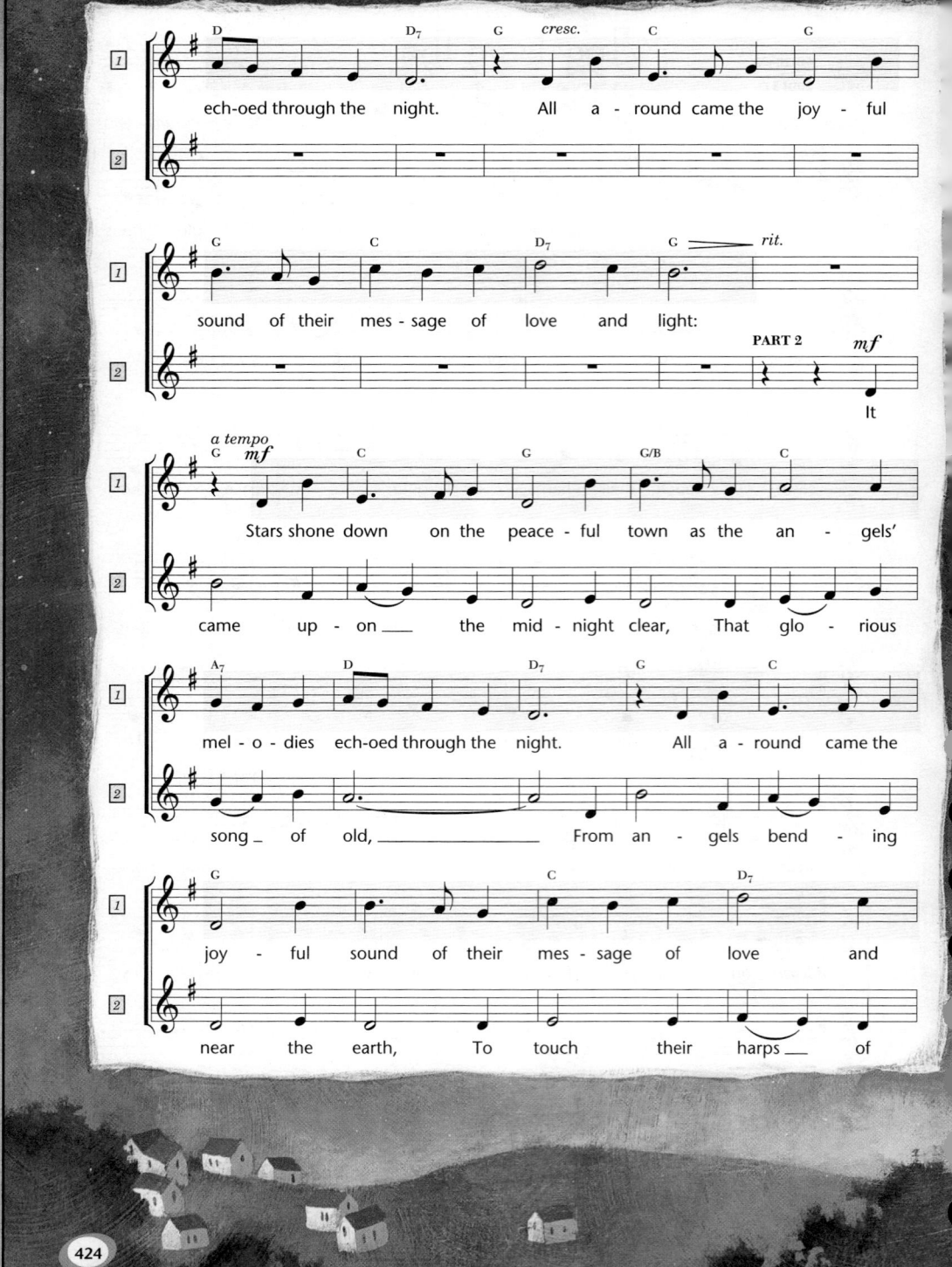

Footnotes

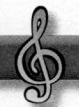

SKILLS REINFORCEMENT

1c ▶ **Singing** Help students gain proficiency in singing a *legato* melody when performing "Angels on the Midnight Clear" in a formal concert setting. Have them sing each phrase on *loo* or *loh*, encouraging them to vocally "paste the notes together." Connecting the notes in this way should be done in a flowing manner as the students move their right hand from left to right as if creating a rainbow. Have students identify the music symbols referring to tempo and interpret them appropriately when performing.

▶ **MIDI Song File** Use the MIDI song file for "Angels on the Midnight Clear" to help students learn and practice the song. You may isolate the vocal parts to learn the harmony and practice the song at a slow tempo.

ACROSS THE CURRICULUM

▶ **Social Studies** The carol is a song of English origin dating back to the Middle Ages. The texts could be sung in English or Latin or a mixture of the two. The texts were often about the Virgin Mary or Christmas. Today, the carol consists of stanzas (verses) sung to the same music, similar to a church hymn. See Spotlight On, p. 422, for information about early carols. Many early carols were danced as well as sung, and many of the tunes have a dance lilt.

Carols were often sung outside and may explain why today, carolers go caroling from house to house at Christmas time. Many countries in the world sing carols, and it is reported that the practice began with St. Francis of Assisi (approximately 1182–1226). He would set up a crib in church at Christmas time and the people would sing and dance around the crib.

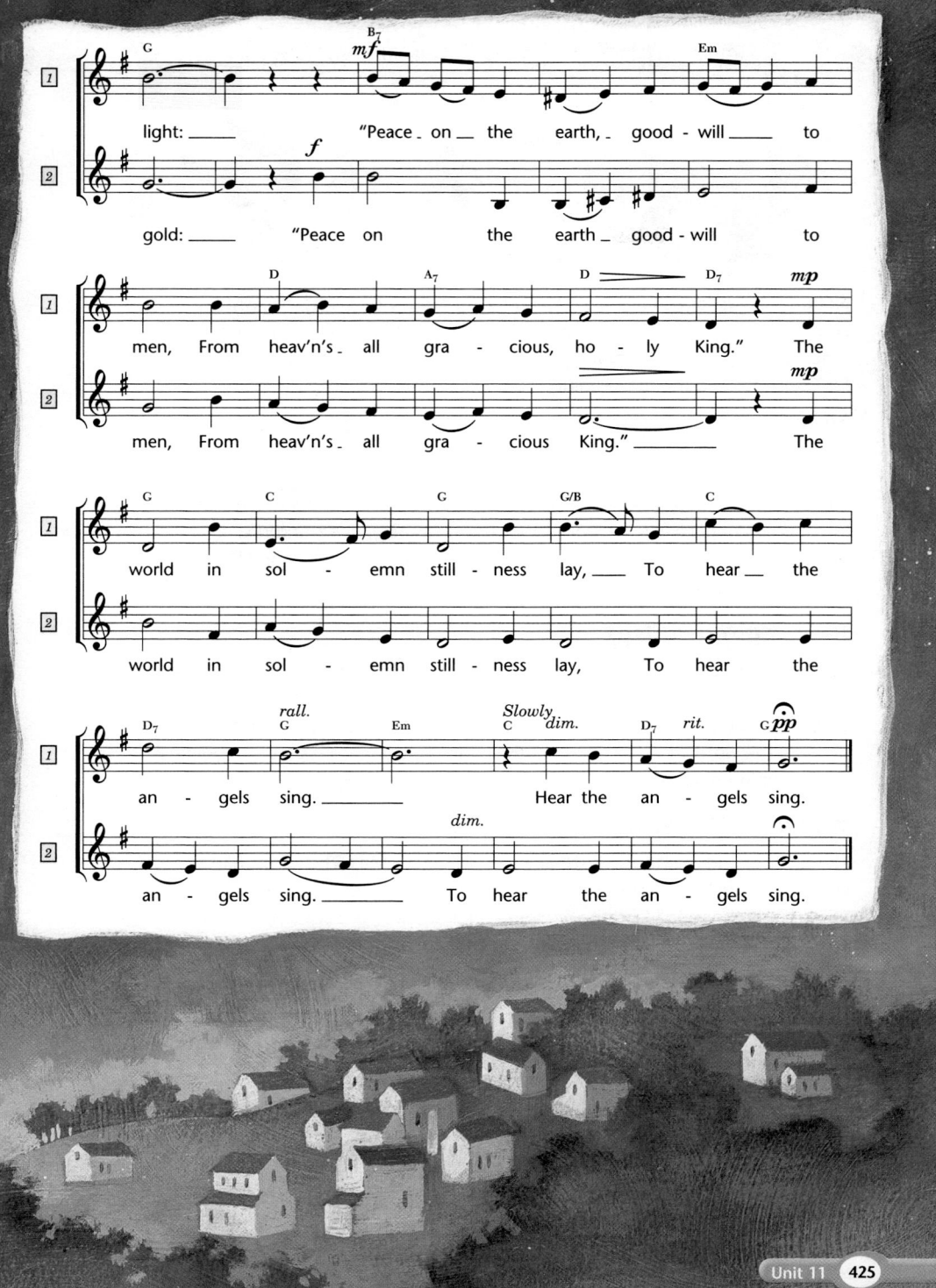

Then have half the class form a circle inside the larger circle, facing the larger circle; the inside circle sings the countermelody simultaneously with the melody, while both groups create phrase shapes with their hands.

When completed, have each circle form a straight line so that the inner-circle line can weave in and out of line two, while both lines sing their assigned melody. See Technology/Media Link below for videotaping the performance.

Performing

When performing "Angels on the Midnight Clear" for a formal concert, ask students to remember to demonstrate appropriate large–ensemble performance techniques (*legato* singing and phrasing) they learned earlier. For variety in performance options, the first part of the song could include the audience, while encircled by the choir. The choir then proceeds to the center aisle, singing the countermelody, creating two lines that face each side of the audience. Every other student in each line sings the melody while the remaining students sing the countermelody. A second verse could be added to the song for choir and audience, serving as a processional to get the singers on stage.

3 CLOSE

Skill: SINGING 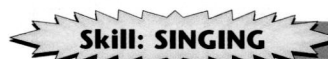 **ASSESSMENT**

1c **Performance/Peer Critique** As a class, have students sing "Angels on the Midnight Clear" and perform the movements in the Moving activity, p. 424.

7b As a class, have students evaluate and discuss their performance using the following criteria.

- The singing of both melodies were rhythmically correct.
- The countermelody was not as loud as the melody.
- All phrases were *legato*.
- All phrases had good rainbow-type shapes.
- All important words had appropriate vocal stress.

SPOTLIGHT ON

▶ **Angels** The word *angels* appears regularly in everyday conversation, but can mean different things. *Charlie's Angels* was a popular television show in the 1970s and movie in 2000. *You are an angel,* means you are a nice person or have done something nice for someone. When individuals look *angelic,* it means they look like angels. A *guardian angel* is an angel who watches over you—keeps you from harm. On Broadway, an *angel* is a person who invests enough money to underwrite the show's expenses. *Angels* that are sung about in Christmas carols refer to heavenly spirits. The angels in these songs are always in the sky, between heaven and earth. There is always more than one angel and they sing about the birth of Christ.

TECHNOLOGY/MEDIA LINK

7b **Multimedia** Invite students to videotape the class performance of "Angels on the Midnight Clear." After the performance has been taped, have the students view their movement and performance and evaluate themselves using the following criteria.

- The phrase singing matches the phrase shapes described by their hands.
- The melody and countermelody hand-shaped phrases are a clear representation of how the phrases vary in their shape and movement.
- The weaving activity is helpful in understanding how the two melodies harmonically relate to each other.

LESSON AT A GLANCE

Element Focus   **TEXTURE/HARMONY** Two-part harmony (soprano and alto), passing tones

Skill Objective   **SINGING** Sing a two-part song that contains melismas

Connection Activity   **GENRE** Read about and discuss the cultural and historical background of caroling

MATERIALS
- "Ding Dong! Merrily on High"   **CD 20-22**
  Recording Routine: Intro (8 m.); v. 1; v. 2; interlude (4 m.); v. 3

VOCABULARY

melisma	sequence	word painting
marcato	passing tones	

◆ ◆ ◆ ◆ **National Standards** ◆ ◆ ◆ ◆

1a Sing accurately with good breath control
1c Sing music with appropriate expression
1d Sing music written in two parts
5a Read eighth notes and dotted notes in duple meter
6a Listen and describe events in music using appropriate terms

MORE MUSIC CHOICES

For more practice singing Christmas songs:
"Caroling, Caroling," p. 458
"Gloria, Gloria," p. 459
"Good King Wenceslas," p. 460

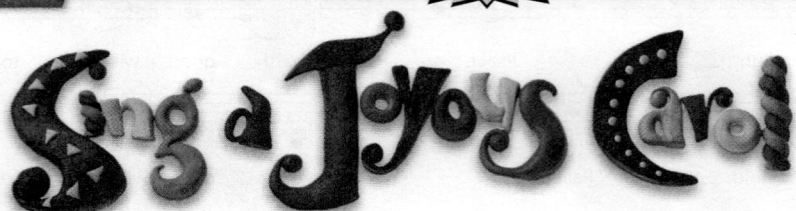

Sing a Joyous Carol

Nobody knows for certain when "Ding Dong! Merrily on High" was written. The composer is unknown. So, we call it a traditional Christmas carol. In medieval times, the word *carol* meant a type of dance. By the 16th century, a joyous song for Christmas became the definition of carol.

Sing "Ding Dong! Merrily on High."

Singing Tips

The tempo of the song is fast and lively, so sing crisp consonants to make sure listeners can understand the words. Words such as *ding, dong,* and *ringing* provide a perfect opportunity to imitate the sounds of bells. To sound like bells, enunciate the consonants with energy.

Reading Music Tips

"Ding Dong! Merrily on High" is in verse-refrain, or Ⓐ Ⓑ Ⓐ Ⓑ Ⓐ Ⓑ form. The refrains are a little different each time and should be practiced. The refrain of the second verse (measure 35) is sung as a sequence, alternating between the voice parts on the word *Gloria*. Notice that the ending pitch of each part is the same as the beginning pitch of the next part.

Knowing the Score

The half notes in measures 17–18 and 56–60 imitate bells. The key signature changes before Verse 3 (measure 48). Why would a composer change keys at this point in the song? Find the *fermata* sign and the term *poco a poco cresc.* What are these words telling the singer to do?

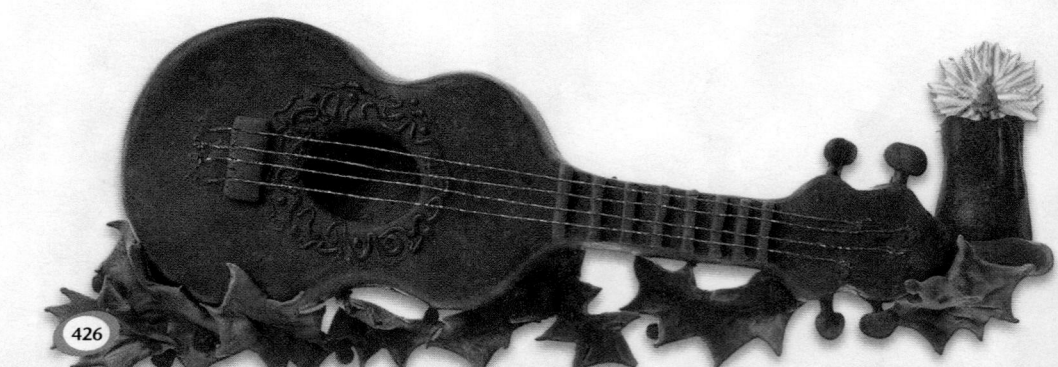

Footnotes

ACROSS THE CURRICULUM

▶ **Social Studies** Read aloud the book *Chinook Christmas* by Rudy Wiebe (Red Deer College, 1993) and invite students to consider Christmas in Alaska with the northern lights.

Invite students to share holiday traditions from their family. What happens when lots of family members get together to share a meal? Do they sing songs together? Ask students to write about their family traditions in their journals.

BUILDING SKILLS THROUGH MUSIC

▶ **Social Studies** Ask students to think about the carols that they know. List them on the board. Then, have them decide which carol is their favorite. Have students write a brief paragraph about why they chose that particular carol. Ask for volunteers to share their paragraphs.

CULTURAL CONNECTION

▶ **Caroling** Caroling is a singing activity that takes place in many countries at Christmas time. In the early days of American history, many churches did not allow carols in the worship service. Fortunately, caroling flourished outside the church. In the nineteenth and early twentieth centuries, members of British and American high society were carried about the town before sunrise in four-horse wagons to sing in front of the homes of their friends. Today, caroling includes singing outside peoples' homes, in hospitals, for senior citizens in assisted living facilities, and around the piano in homes throughout the United States.

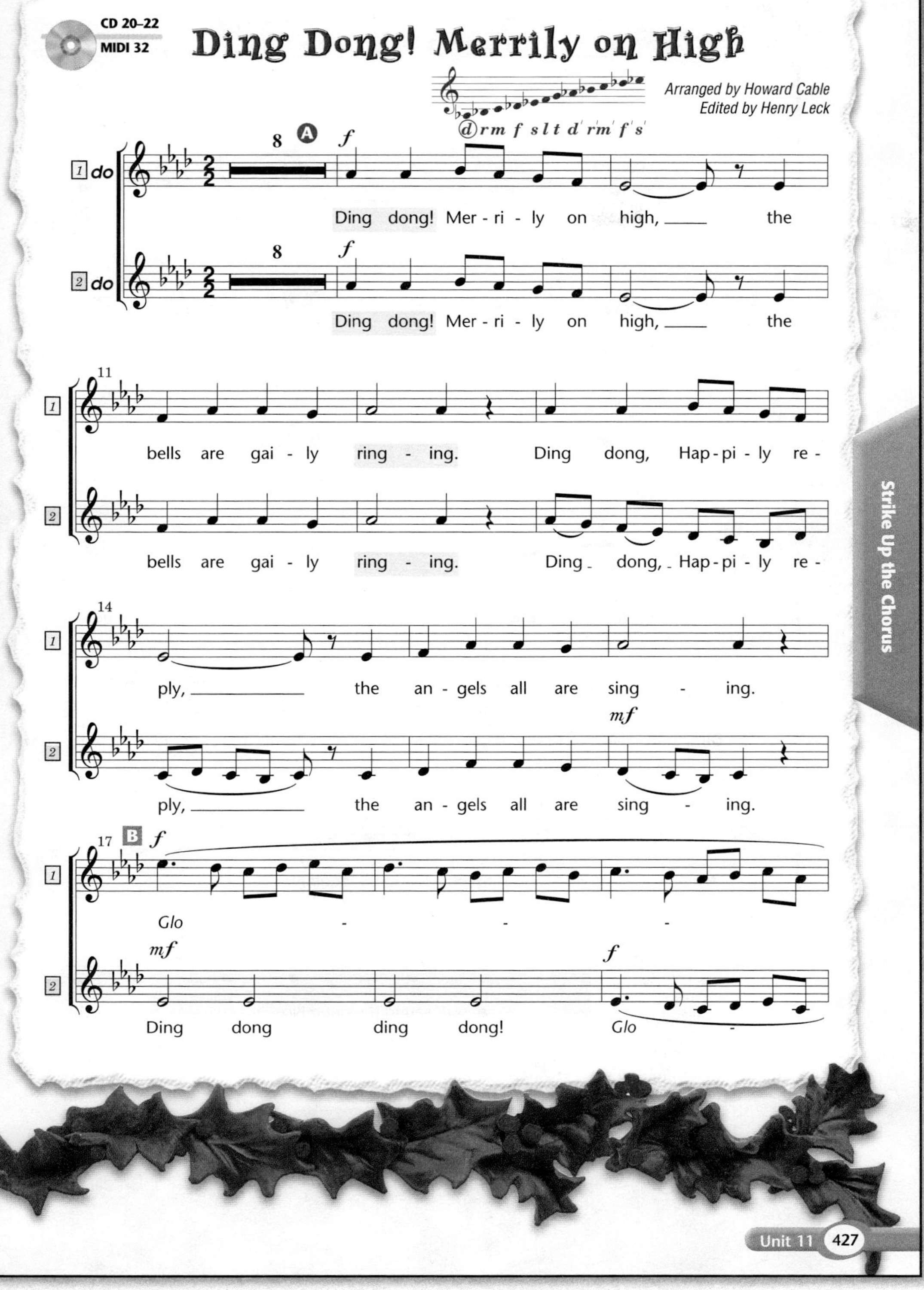

Ding Dong! Merrily on High

CD 20–22
MIDI 32

Arranged by Howard Cable
Edited by Henry Leck

(Music notation for Part 1 and Part 2)

A f

d' r m f s l t d' r m' f' s'

1 do — Ding dong! Mer-ri-ly on high, _____ the

2 do — Ding dong! Mer-ri-ly on high, _____ the

11
1 — bells are gai-ly ring-ing. Ding dong, Hap-pi-ly re-

2 — bells are gai-ly ring-ing. Ding dong, Hap-pi-ly re-

14
1 — ply, _____ the an-gels all are sing - ing.

2 — mf ply, _____ the an-gels all are sing - ing.

17 **B** f
1 — Glo - - -

2 — mf Ding dong ding dong! f Glo -

Strike Up the Chorus

1 INTRODUCE

Listen to the recording of "Ding Dong! Merrily on High" **CD 20-22**.

ASK What is it about this song that makes it sound joyous and merry? (The song is rhythmical and has repeated melodic runs called melismas. The musical style has a dancelike feel.)

Then, invite students to read about and discuss the historical and cultural background of caroling. See Across the Curriculum, p. 429, and Cultural Connection, p. 426. Additional information may be found in Unit 12 (pp. 458–461).

2 DEVELOP

Listening

Play the recording of "Ding Dong! Merrily on High" **CD 20-22** twice. During the first playing, have students look at the music in their book and

- Listen and follow the notes for Part 1. (soprano)
- Listen for repeated rhythm and melody patterns.
- Listen for when Part 1 sings the harmony part. (mm. 48–55)
- Listen for when Part 1 divides into two parts. (mm. 64–65)

During the second hearing, have students look at and follow the notes for Part 2 and listen for when

- Part 2 sings the same notes as Part 1. (mm. 9–12)
- Part 2 sings passing notes (example mm. 13–14). Passing notes are part of a melody progression but not part of the harmony.
- Part 2 has a duet with Part 1. (mm. 19–22, 40–42)

continued on page 428

SKILLS REINFORCEMENT

▶ **Vocal Development** Singing long phrases requires developing good breath support. Have students take a breath and hiss staccato-like *ss* for eight counts. After several repetitions, move to 10 counts, 12 counts, and then 14 counts. With practice, they will progress to 20 counts. Practice singing long phrases and ask students to hold the last note of the phrase for an additional four counts. This technique will make students conserve their air to hold the final note. During the singing of melismas (vocal runs), the breath can be used to help articulate the rhythmic shape of the phrase. For example, if the melisma is four sets of sixteenth-note patterns, the singers can start softly and *crescendo* while accenting the first note of each pattern.

TEACHER TO TEACHER

▶ **Raising the Level of Your Choir** There are several ways to introduce students to more challenging choral literature. Play recordings of pieces that you would like them to learn. Invite choirs from other schools to present programs at your school. Bring in guest conductors to work with your choir. Ask students to research the history of the composers and musical styles and report to the class. Have someone from the theater department read the text of the songs to the class and talk about their meanings. As students are learning a challenging song, record the rehearsal and ask them to critique their own progress.

Lesson 8 Continued

Reading

The arrangement of "Ding Dong! Merrily on High" is three verses with refrain.

The setting of the word *Gloria* is a good example of a melisma, sung on the *o* vowel. This melisma is a 5-measure sequence (mm. 17–22).

The rhythm and melody pattern in measure 17 is repeated four more times, only down a scale step each time.

For m. 17, on the word *Gloria,* have students

- Sight-read the rhythm syllables.
- Sight-sing the pitch syllables.
- Sing the word *Gloria.*

In effect, students have learned mm. 18–22.

Have the class sing Part 2, mm. 19–21. Here the word *Gloria* is set in a three-sequence pattern. (The third sequence is changed slightly.)

In mm. 35–40, the sequence pattern is handed back and forth between Part 1 and Part 2.

See Teacher to Teacher below for additional information on melismas.

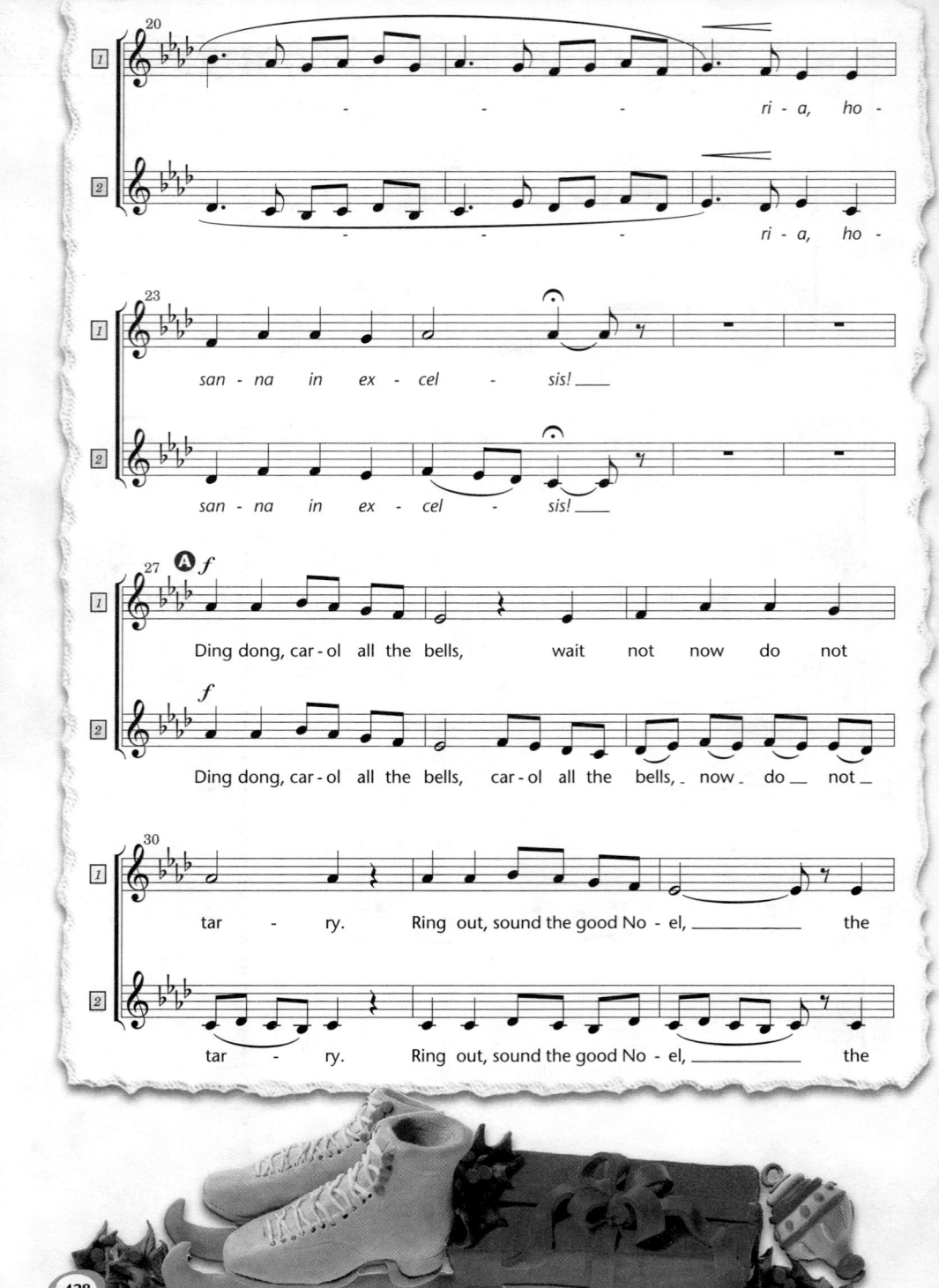

Footnotes

SKILLS REINFORCEMENT

▶ **Singing** Practice saying *ting,* creating a vocal accent on the *t*. After saying the *t,* say the *ing* as if humming it (creating a bell-like effect); put the two sounds together. Change the word to *ding* and follow the same procedure. Notice that the *t* and *d* are produced by the tip of the tongue pressing against the hard surface behind the upper teeth. Follow the same method, but sing *ting* and *ding* on pitch. Sing the passages in the song where *ding* and *dong* occur. Ask half the class to sing using a *d* for *ding* and *dong* and the other half a *t* for *ding* and *dong*. Notice that the two pronunciations combined give a clear and crisp production of the *d* consonant to the listener. When singing the *Gloria,* maintain the *o* position of the mouth.

TEACHER TO TEACHER

▶ **Melismas** Because "Ding Dong! Merrily on High" has numerous melismas (sometimes called "runs"), the song is vocally challenging. Students are likely to slide from pitch to pitch and may go flat. A good practice technique is to place an *h* in front of each repeated *o*. For example, *Glo—ho, ho, ho ho, ria.* When the singers are able to sing the entire pattern accurately and in tune, remove the *h* and have them sing *Glo—o–o-o-o-ria,* re-enunciating the *o* every time. If the pattern is sung lightly, with a *crescendo* through the eighth notes, and with good breath support, it will sound musically convincing.

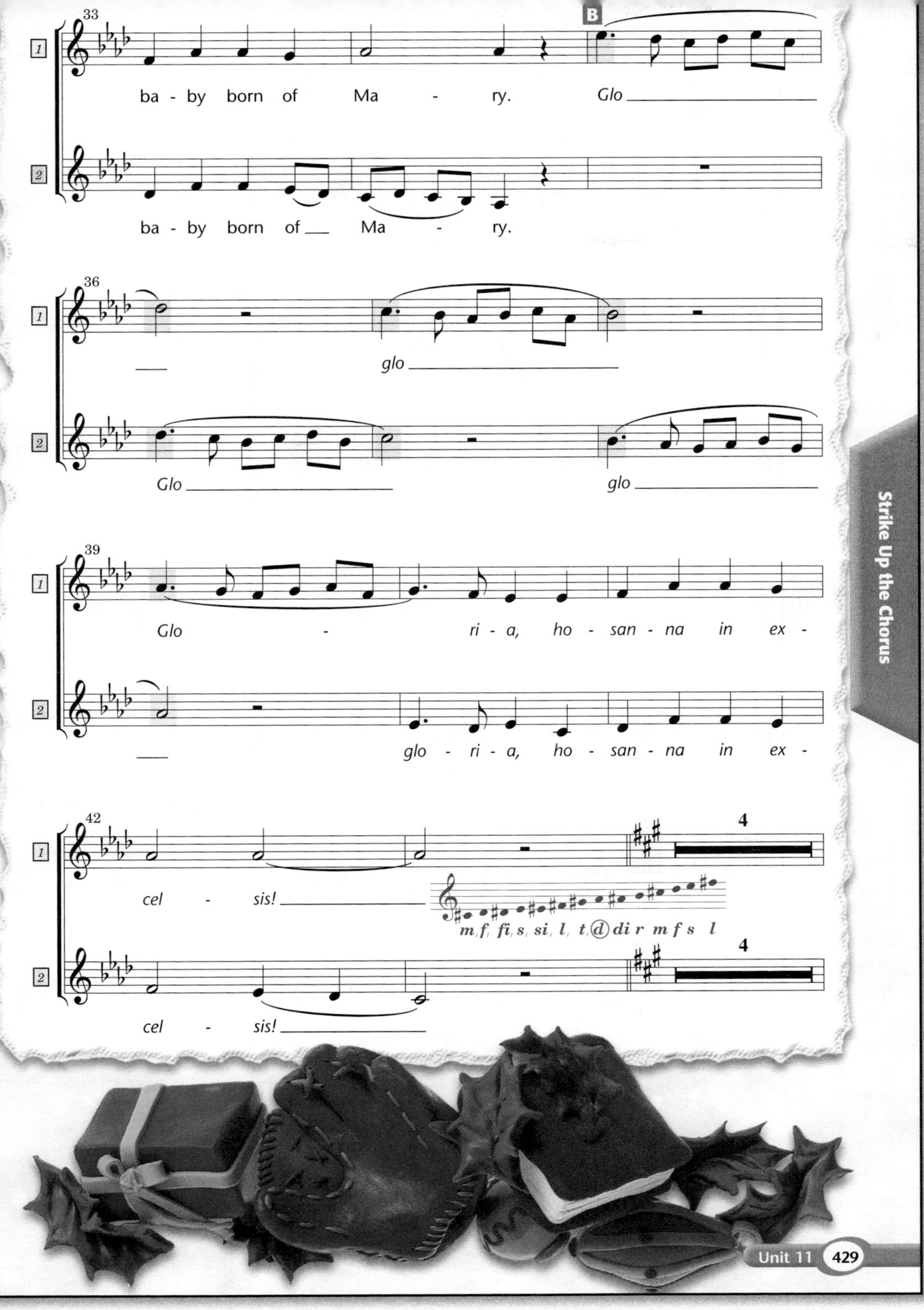

(Sheet music: measures 33–45 of "Ding Dong! Merrily on High," two vocal parts)

33 — **B**

Part 1: ba - by born of Ma - ry. Glo _____

Part 2: ba - by born of ___ Ma - ry.

36

Part 1: ___ glo _____

Part 2: Glo _____ glo _____

39

Part 1: Glo - ri - a, ho - san - na in ex -

Part 2: ___ glo - ri - a, ho - san - na in ex -

42

Part 1: cel - sis! _____

m f, fi, si, l, t (d) d i r m f s l

Part 2: cel - sis! _____

Singing

"Ding Dong! Merrily on High" **CD 20-22** is a joyous song. The melisma on *Gloria* is an example of word painting: the notes are supposed to look and sound like "a glorious or joyous feeling." Teacher to Teacher on p. 428 has more information on singing melismas on the word *Gloria*.

When singing this song, invite students to

- Sing each note with a light *marcato* style (a light accent on each note or word).

1c

- Sing *ding dong* with the tongue making firm contact on the hard surface behind the front teeth. (Techniques on how to vocalize bell effects on the words *ding dong* can be found in Skills Reinforcement on p. 428.)

- Sing *Gloria* with a very short break in sound between the dotted quarter and the following eighth note.

- Sing the song with a dancelike feeling and a light vocal quality.

Remind students to demonstrate these basic performance techniques as they perform independently, with accurate intonation.

Good breath support is required to sing the long phrases of the melisma. Skills Reinforcement on p. 427 has exercises on developing breath control.

continued on page 430

SPOTLIGHT ON

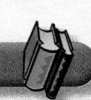

▶ **Bells in Music** What are some ways in which bells are used in music? In "Ding Dong! Merrily on High," the voices imitate the sound of bells. Bells are found throughout music in other ways. Handbells are used in classrooms. Bell choir ensembles play compositions specifically written for their ensemble. The idiophones in the orchestra include bells. Marching bands have bells. One of the most famous uses of bells in music is the ending of Tchaikovsky's *1812 Overture*. On special occasions real church bells have been used in the performance of this celebrated work.

ACROSS THE CURRICULUM

▶ **Social Studies** The history surrounding some of our best-known and often-sung Christmas carols is quite interesting. After learning that his son had been seriously wounded in the Civil War in 1863, Henry Wadsworth Longfellow wrote the poem "I Heard the Bells on Christmas Day"; the tune was added later. After visiting the Holy Land, Phillips Brooks wrote "O Little Town of Bethlehem." Three years later, Lewis Redner wrote the music.

Performing

"Ding Dong! Merrily on High" is ideally suited to be performed in a variety of venues, such as at a school assembly, evening concert performance, or during a visit to a nursing home or hospital. It can also be performed in a variety of ensembles, from a small *a cappella* chamber choir, to that of a large chorus performing with a concert band or orchestra. Remind students that in any formal or informal performance they still need to demonstrate appropriate small-ensemble or large ensemble performance techniques during these concerts.

A review of ensemble performance techniques would include singing with enthusiasm, with accurate intonation, diction, phrasing, and attention to style, articulations and dynamics. Tell students that a "musical" performance is an end result of much hard work by students and all involved. Remind students that their "performer etiquette" (similar to audience etiquette) is an important factor to a successful concert. As performers, students need to act professionally and appropriately. (Being attentive to the conductor, not talking or fooling around, standing erect, and performing to the best of their ability)

ASK How are some of the ways you could perform "Ding Dong! Merrily on High!" at a concert? (Accept a variety of answers and write them on the board.)

Tell students they can increase the effectiveness of their concert performance with the following performance scenarios.

- Sing in a circle around the audience.
- Intermix the soprano and alto singers throughout the circle.
- Ask students from the band to accompany the choir on trumpet, horn, trombone, or tuba.

Ask students if these concepts are an effective way to perform "Ding Dong! Merrily on High!"

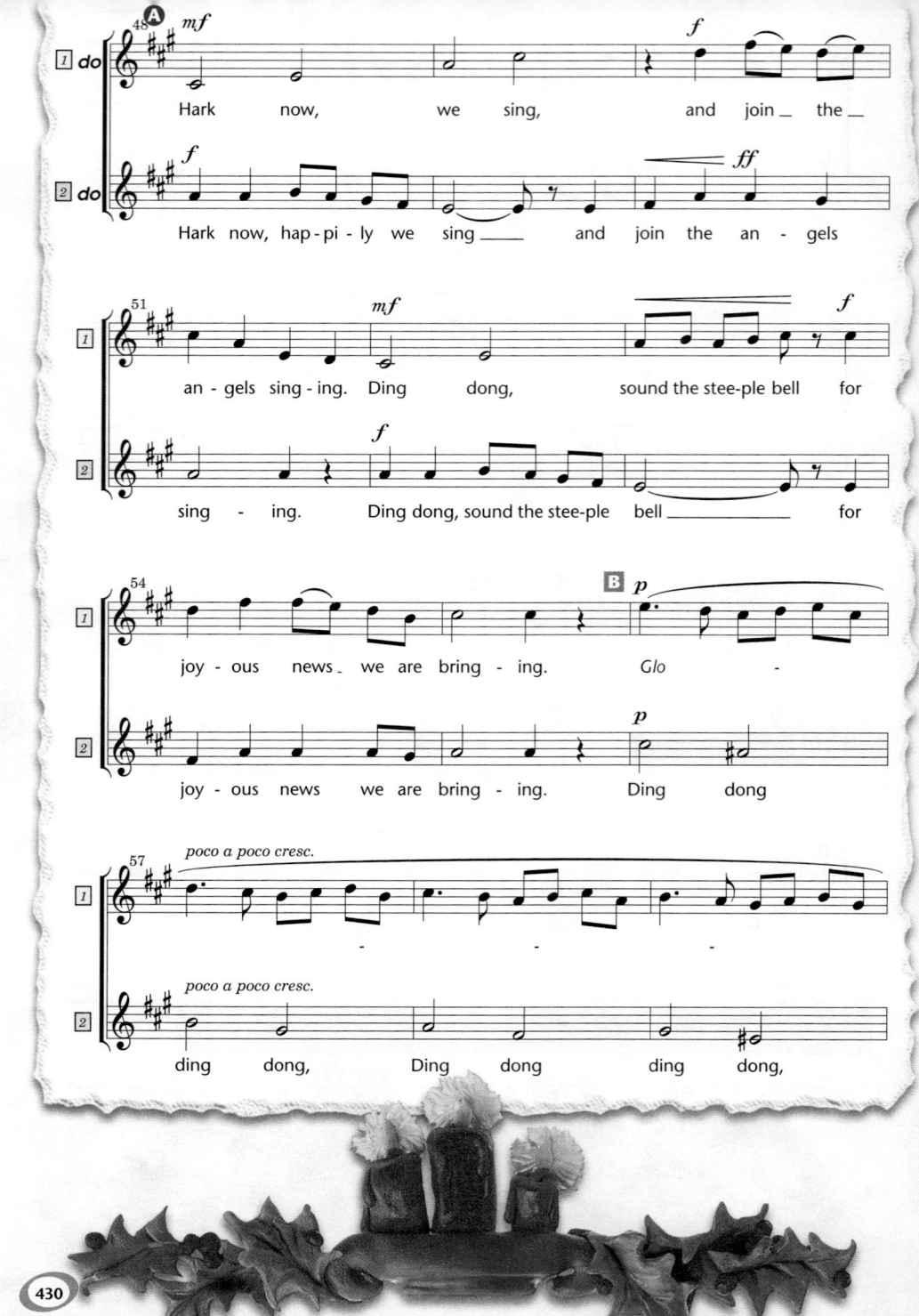

Footnotes

SKILLS REINFORCEMENT

▶ **Singing** Have students sing a rehearsal choral warm-up for this song. Sing descending thirds (a sequence) in the key of A♭ major and end with a cadence. (This is a simplified sequence from mm. 17–22.)

so–mi, fa–re, mi–do, re–ti, do–la, ti–so,
cadence: *so-so-do*

Add variety to the warm-up by having two groups alternate the singing of each sequence (group 1, group 2). Add movement to the warm-up by having the hand move away from the lips in a circular motion counting the number of sequences. (six) Alternate hands for each repetition (right hand, left hand). Add a second warm-up by starting on *mi*.

CHARACTER EDUCATION

▶ **Service** Discuss how caroling today typically involves groups of people singing for the enjoyment of others. Discuss the benefits of such an activity with students.

- Should service activities be instituted at certain times of the year (around holidays) or throughout the year?
- Encourage students to consider specific ways they can be of service to others as individuals and as a group (picking up trash, volunteering at the animal shelter, befriending a senior citizen, participating in fundraisers for charities).
- Challenge students to involve themselves in one service activity in the coming weeks. Following completion of their activities, discuss what they did and how they felt about it.
- What are the benefits of service for the one providing the service? For the recipients? Why should we serve others?

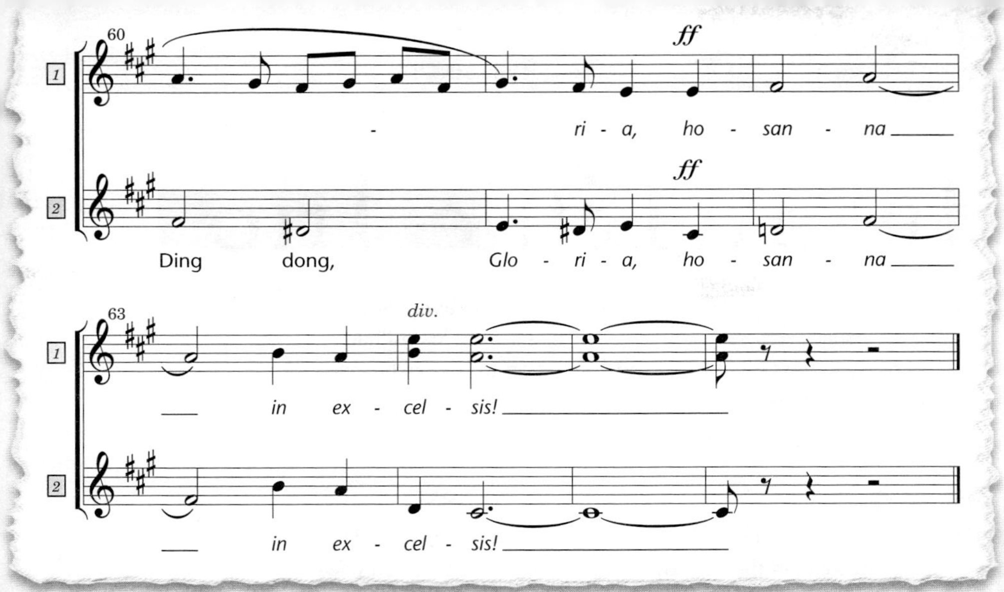

The music notation at top:

(Part 1) ...ri - a, ho - san - na____

(Part 2) Ding dong, Glo - ri - a, ho - san - na____

(measure 63, div.)

(Part 1) ____ in ex - cel - sis!____

(Part 2) ____ in ex - cel - sis!____

Unit 11 **431**

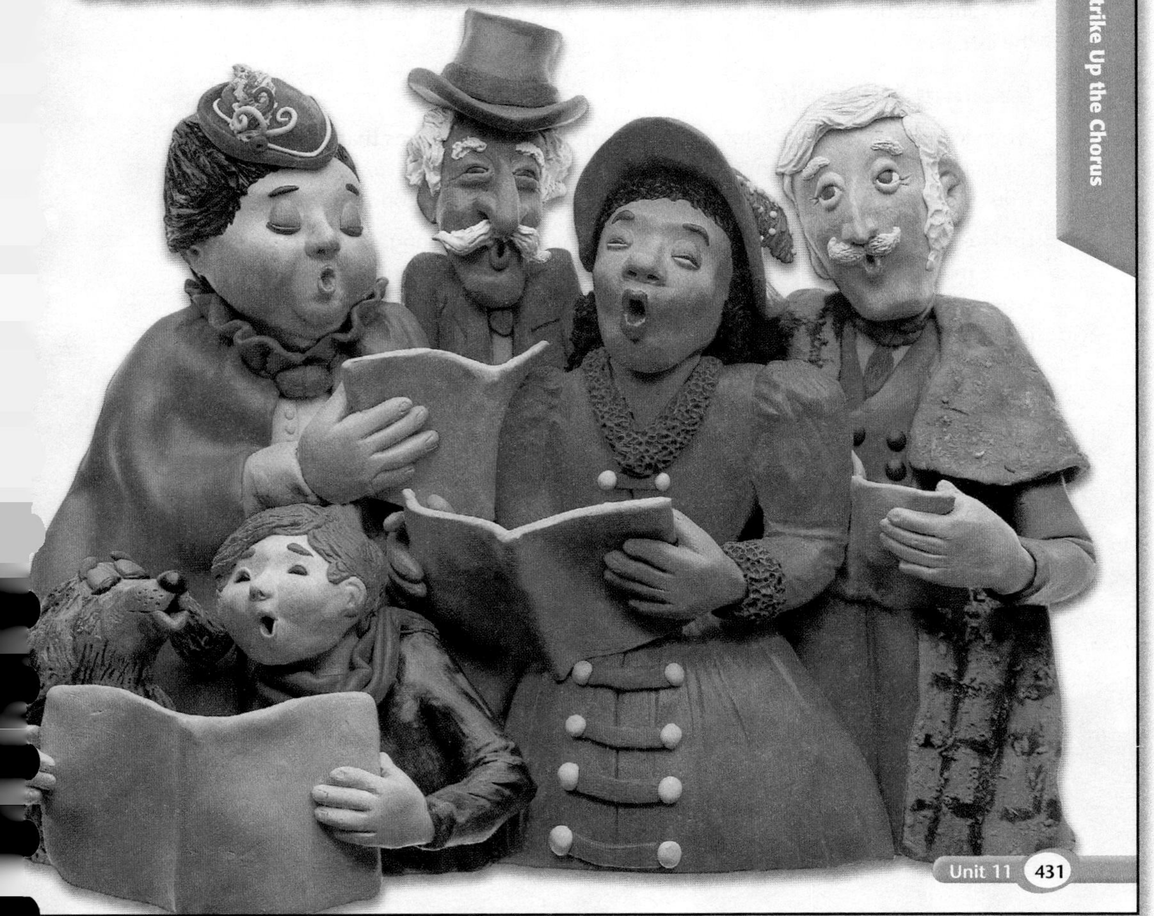

3 CLOSE

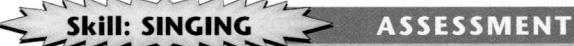

Skill: SINGING   **ASSESSMENT**

Performance/Observation As a class, have students sing and tape-record their performance of "Ding Dong! Merrily on High" **CD 20-22.** Observe students' ability to sing two-part harmony accurately. Listen to the performance and discuss it, based on the following criteria.

- Was each vocal part sung with energy?
- Were the rhythms and tempo accurate?
- Did the class maintain two-part harmony?
- Were the melismas sung cleanly?
- Were the sequences emphasized?
- Was the class able to make bell sounds on the words *ding* and *dong?*
- Did the class stop together on the *fermata?*

Congratulate the class on their singing "Ding Dong! Merrily on High." It is a challenging piece of music that raises the skill level of groups who meet the challenge.

TEACHER TO TEACHER

▶ **MIDI Song File** Use the MIDI song file for "Ding Dong! Merrily on High" to help students learn and practice the song. Use a slow tempo, isolate vocal parts, learn the harmony parts, select difficult sections for repetition and practice, and transpose the key, if desired.

TECHNOLOGY/MEDIA LINK

Notation Software Invite students to compose new bell parts for "Ding Dong! Merrily on High," using notation software. Divide the class into groups and assign the sections of the song to each group. (introduction, first interlude, final verse) Have students

- Use a music notation program to write bell parts in half notes.
- Use the key signature of the section.
- Use notes found in the vocal and accompaniment parts.
- Play their parts as the class sings that section.

LESSON AT A GLANCE

Element Focus   **RHYTHM** Rhythm patterns

Skill Objective   **SINGING** Sing rhythm patterns accurately and with clarity of diction

Connection Activity   **SOCIAL STUDIES** Discuss the traditions and history of folk songs and ballads

MATERIALS

- "Goin' to Boston"   CD 20-24

   Recording Routine: Intro (8 m.); v. 1; interlude (8 m.); v. 2; interlude (4 m.); v. 3; v. 4; interlude (4 m.); v. 5

- video camera (optional)

VOCABULARY

verse	refrain	major seventh
major second	play parties	

◆ ◆ ◆ ◆ National Standards ◆ ◆ ◆ ◆

1c Sing music with appropriate expression

5b Sightread melodies in treble clef

6a Listen and describe events in music using appropriate terms

6b Listen and analyze uses of pitch and form in music from diverse genre

6c Understand and use basic principles of rhythm and tonality in music analysis

7b Students use specific criteria for evaluating their own performances

MORE MUSIC CHOICES

For more practice singing American folk songs:

"Red River Valley," p. 11

"Down in the Valley," p. 375

"Tom Dooley," p. 374

Take a Little Trip

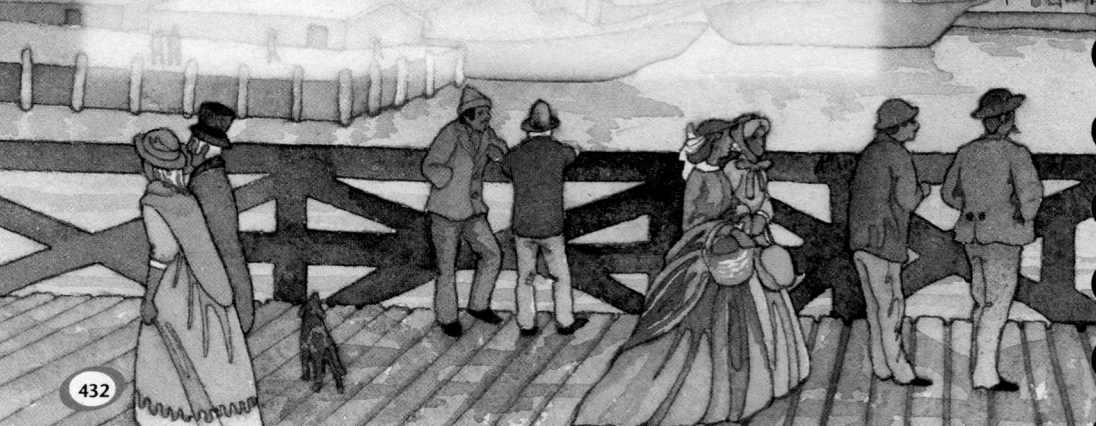

"Goin' to Boston" is an American folk song. Until the twentieth century, folk songs were usually not written down. People sang them and had to remember them in order to pass them from one generation to the next. Hearing and singing songs in this way—by ear—is called the "oral/aural tradition."

Sing "Goin' to Boston."

Singing Tips

Listen carefully when you sing harmony. The harmony should be strong, but just a little softer than the melody. Use crisp consonants, good vowel shapes, and your best breathing skills to make the words in the refrain sound clear to the listeners.

Reading Music Tips

When learning "Goin' to Boston," focus on melodies and rhythms that repeat. For example, when you learn the phrases *Goodbye, girls, I'm goin' to Boston* and *Won't we look purty in the ballroom,* you will know much of the song.

Look over the pitch patterns in Verse 1 before you **sing** the song. Do they move mostly by step or by skip? Find the rhythm pattern in measures 9 and 10. Where does it repeat in the rest of the song? **Listen** to the first refrain as you follow the music. Which pitch gives the song a bit of an unusual sound?

Knowing the Score

Look for a meter change. Why do you think the song's arranger did this? "Goin' to Boston" has five verses. How are they similar? How are they different?

432

Footnotes

ACROSS THE CURRICULUM

▶ **Social Studies** Share the book *Boston* by Deborah Kent (Children's Press, 1998) and invite students to learn about the city from this story.

Invite students to consider the impact that Boston has had on U.S. history. Useful books include *The American Revolution* by Joann Grote (Chelsea House, 1999) and *The Boston Tea Party* by Steven Kroll (Holiday House, 1998).

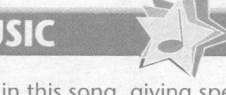

BUILDING SKILLS THROUGH MUSIC

▶ **Reading** Have students paraphrase the verses in this song, giving special attention to the sequence of events. Have them rewrite the ballad in their own words into a story.

SPOTLIGHT ON

▶ **Ballad** The ballad is a song composed in stanzas sung to a repeating tune that recounts a short, usually single-episode tale. Because a ballad tells a story, it is not unlike an epic song or fairy tale. The medieval ballad is the oldest, found in the late Middle Ages. Ballads can be found in England in the fourteenth century and in Scotland in the eighteenth century. They can be divided into four categories.

- Magical and marvelous
- Romantic and tragic
- Historical and legendary
- Humorous

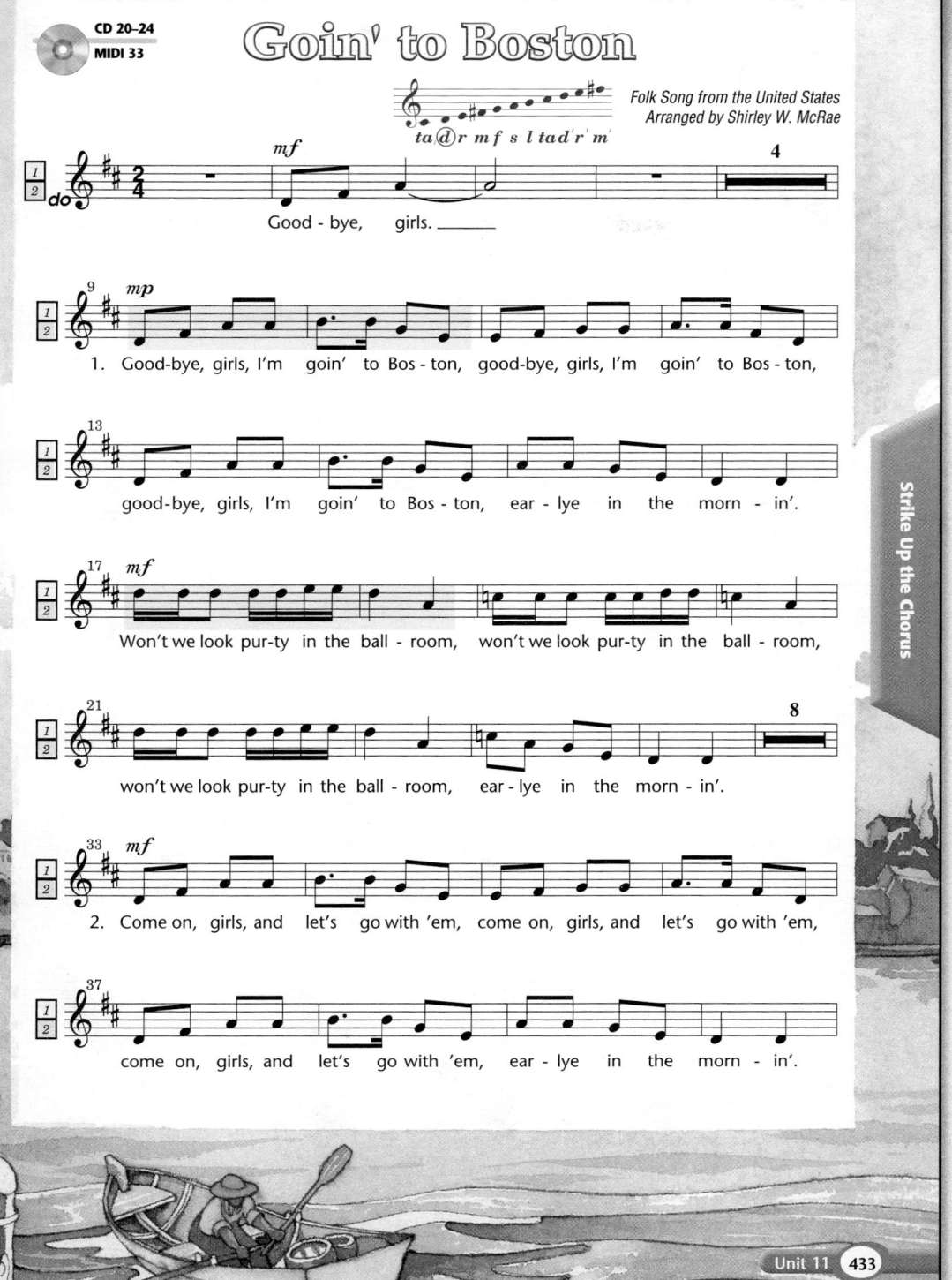

Goin' to Boston

CD 20–24
MIDI 33

Folk Song from the United States
Arranged by Shirley W. McRae

ta (d) r m f s l ta d r m

Good - bye, girls. _____

1. Good-bye, girls, I'm goin' to Bos - ton, good-bye, girls, I'm goin' to Bos - ton,

good-bye, girls, I'm goin' to Bos - ton, ear - lye in the morn - in'.

Won't we look pur-ty in the ball - room, won't we look pur-ty in the ball - room,

won't we look pur-ty in the ball - room, ear - lye in the morn - in'.

2. Come on, girls, and let's go with 'em, come on, girls, and let's go with 'em,

come on, girls, and let's go with 'em, ear - lye in the morn - in'.

Unit 11 **433**

1 INTRODUCE

Invite students to discuss the rich, historical tradition of folk songs and ballads. See Cultural Connection below, and Spotlight On, p. 432. Point out that our country is rich in this tradition (especially from Anglo-American roots), with songs such as "Goin' to Boston" and those listed under More Music Choices on p. 432.

Many folk songs and ballads tell a story. Invite a student to read the text of "Goin' to Boston" to the class.

Discuss the meaning of the verses in the song.

2 DEVELOP

Listening

Play the recording of "Goin' to Boston" **CD 20-24**. Have students follow the music in their books.

ASK How many times is the melodic idea in mm. 9–10 used in the verse (mm.9–16)? (two exactly; one additional time in sequence)

6a How many times is the melodic idea in mm. 17–18 used in the refrain (mm. 17–24)? (two exactly; one additional time in sequence)

How many verses are there? (five)

6c Does the verse or the refrain sound as if it is changing key? (refrain)

Which verse has a two-part section? (verse 3)

What changes in verse 4, the melody or the rhythm? (rhythm)

What happens to the meter in verse 4? (The meter alternates between meter in 5 and meter in 2.)

Guide students to identify the verses and refrain in the notation.

continued on page 434

▶ **Folk Songs** Folk songs are created by the peoples of many cultures. The subjects of folk songs are enormously varied. Folk songs are of interest to historians because they provide insights into what people thought and felt. They are often sung unaccompanied but sometimes use a single instrument played by the singer. Folk songs were generally not written down but were passed from one generation to the next orally. This transmission explains why there are so many versions of the same song. Each folk singer's changes would result in new interpretations of the song.

▶ **Singing** Enunciation is saying words so that all consonants and vowels can be understood and requires using lips, teeth, and tongue (articulators) correctly. Correct pronunciation is saying a word using the correct syllabic stress, for example, Boston (BOS-ton versus bos-TON). In singing, an additional problem occurs: the connection of a final consonant of a word to the initial vowel of the following word. For example, *Goodbye, Girls, I'm* could be sung with the following elision: *Goodbye, Girl, sI'm*, creating a mispronunciation of *I'm*. Guide students to find examples in the song where a word that ends in a consonant is followed by a word that begins with a vowel. What happens to the pronunciation?

Reading

5b Sing verse 4, paying attention to the $\frac{5}{8}$ time signature and measures.

Now, imagine that the extra beat simply allows more time for the action of "swinging your partner." Give the word a little more length for the swinging action, and it suddenly becomes much easier to understand the meter change and to read and perform the rhythms accurately.

On p. 436 (mm. 77–84), the song can also be performed as follows:

- Voice 1 continues with the melody (Part 2).

- Voice 2 continues singing harmony by singing the notes on the upper line one octave lower. Students singing this part can practice singing the notes one octave lower. This will be especially helpful for changing voices, since they will be in exactly the proper range.

- The voices can sing the music as written, and a lower voice added as suggested in the item above.

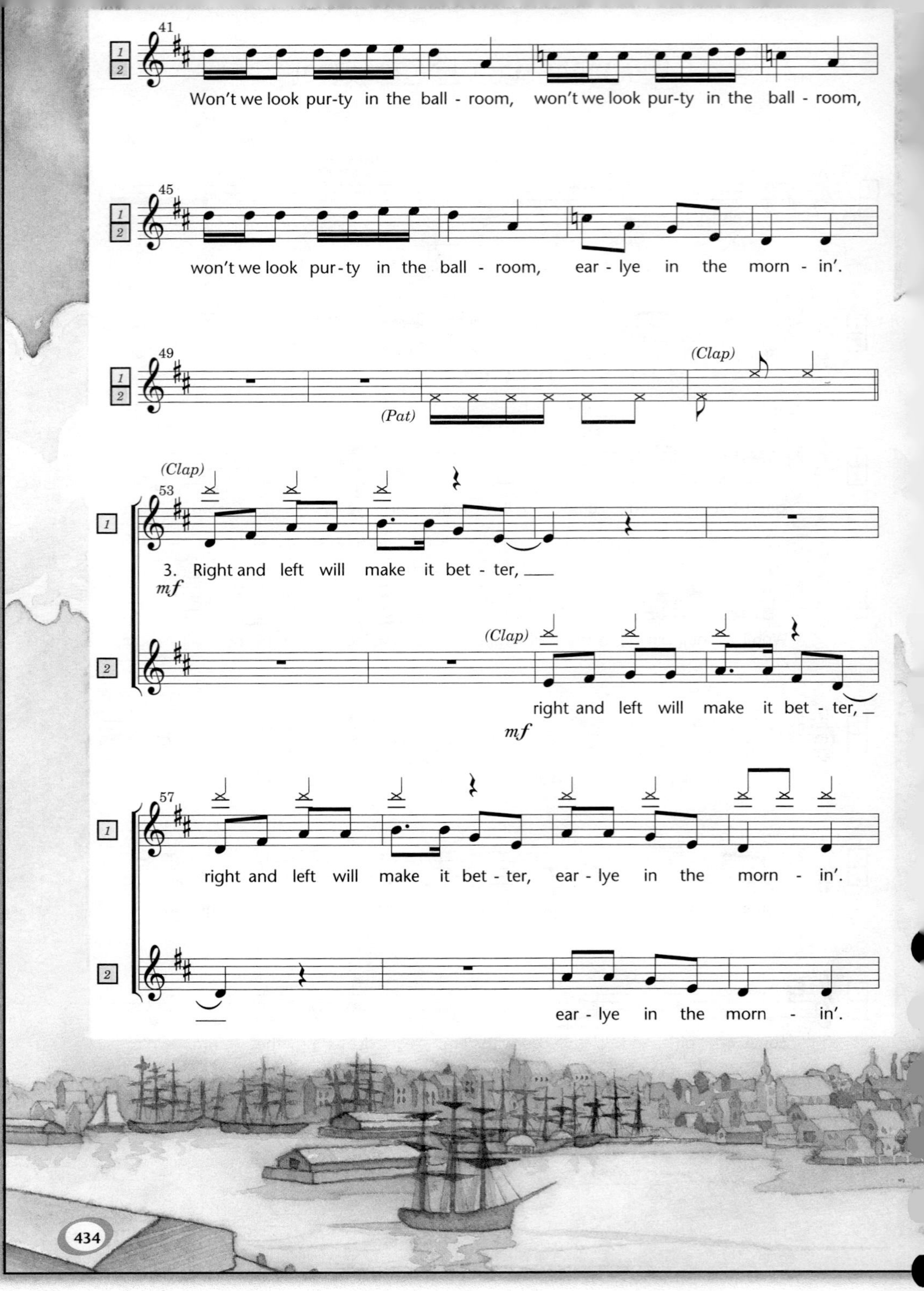

(Musical notation with lyrics:)

Won't we look pur-ty in the ball - room, won't we look pur-ty in the ball - room,

won't we look pur-ty in the ball - room, ear - lye in the morn - in'.

(Pat) (Clap)

(Clap)

3. Right and left will make it bet - ter, ___ *mf*

(Clap)

right and left will make it bet - ter, ___ *mf*

right and left will make it bet - ter, ear - lye in the morn - in'.

___ ear - lye in the morn - in'.

434

Footnotes

CULTURAL CONNECTION

▶ **Social Dancing** Social dances performed without instrumental accompaniment were a part of the American frontier. The texts to the songs in these frontier dances are generally based on poems and ballads. The dance was a matter of keeping step to the singing and going through various movements. Today, these social dances are danced by people of all ages. "Goin' to Boston" has the spirit of these social dances.

Teacher note: These social dances are described as play-parties in the lower grades. Older students may consider this as being juvenile, which is why they are referred to here as social dances.

MOVEMENT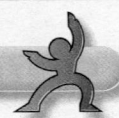

▶ **Popular Dance** Invite students to learn and then perform some of these dance movements to the song "Goin' to Boston" **CD 20-24.**

- Swinging partners by one hand or both.

- Advancing, retreating, and bowing to each other.

- Dancing in circles of four or eight.

- Promenading singly or in pairs, sometimes hand in hand or with crossed hands.

- Weaving back and forth between two rows of people going in opposite directions, clasping right and left hands alternately with those they meet.

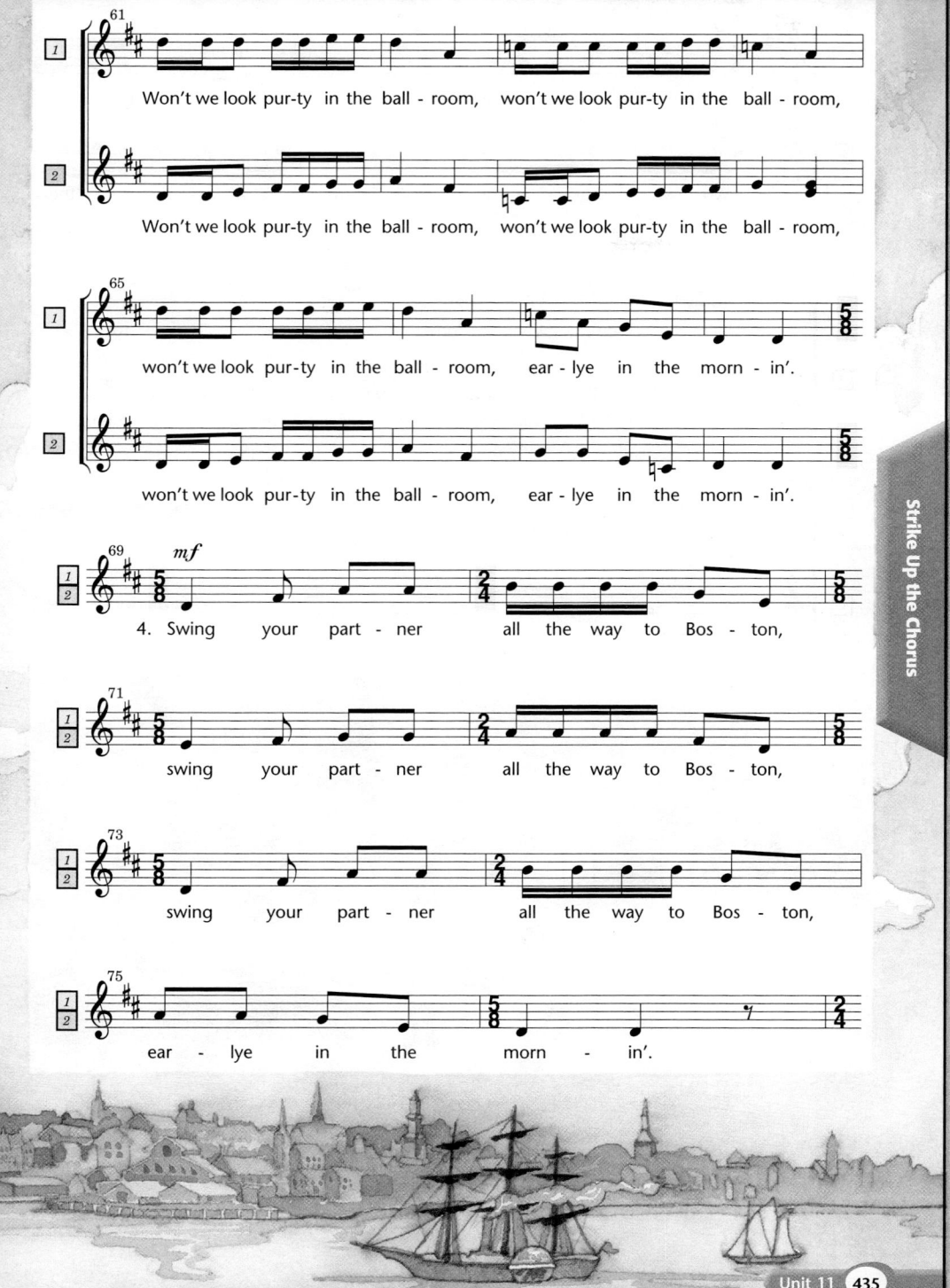

Won't we look pur-ty in the ball - room, won't we look pur-ty in the ball - room,

Won't we look pur-ty in the ball - room, won't we look pur-ty in the ball - room,

won't we look pur-ty in the ball - room, ear-lye in the morn - in'.

won't we look pur-ty in the ball - room, ear-lye in the morn - in'.

mf
4. Swing your part - ner all the way to Bos - ton,

swing your part - ner all the way to Bos - ton,

swing your part - ner all the way to Bos - ton,

ear - lye in the morn - in'.

Singing

Because there are five verses in "Goin' to Boston" **CD 20-24**, it is possible to alternate male and female voices (except verse 3) between girls and boys.

 All the consonant g's should be sung with energy. *Won't we look purty in the ballroom* must be clearly enunciated so all the consonants are heard. *Earlye in the mornin',* by contrast, should be sung *legato.* When singing the first four bars of verse 3, voice 1 must be certain to hold *better* for one and one-half beats.

Good facial expressions and sparkling eyes will enhance the telling of the story.

Analyzing

 Have students research other folk songs and ballads that tell a story. Have them determine if the songs are in verse and refrain style. Invite them to figure out if the verses are rhythmically and melodically the same or if they have variations.

See Skills Reinforcement, p. 433, for techniques on assisting students with enunciation and pronunciation of words in "Goin' to Boston."

continued on page 436

SPOTLIGHT ON

▶ **The Conductor** Henry Leck is the founder and conductor of the Indianapolis Children's Choir. As conductor of the choir, Leck has established the Indianapolis Children's Choir as one of the foremost children's choirs in the world. Some of the choral performances you have heard in *Silver Burdett MAKING MUSIC* are performed by the choir, including "Goin' to Boston."

TEACHER TO TEACHER

▶ **Indianapolis Children's Choir** Invite students to discover that some of the recordings they have listened to were performed by the Indianapolis Children's Choir. Use this choir and their recordings to illustrate the high level of performance of which students are capable. Here are some facts to share with students.

There are more than 1,000 children in the Indianapolis Children's Choir, comprising students of all ages, races, and creeds. The vocal quality and ability of the choir set the highest standards for choral performances by child choirs. The choir has traveled all over the world. Henry Leck is the founder and conductor.

Performing

Since "Goin' to Boston" (in its original form) is a play-party, students could sing it for a lower grade class that learned a play-party that goes with the song.

The two classes could perform together for a school function for parents and community. It could also be sung on a program of storytelling and folk songs.

Moving

"Goin' to Boston" **CD 20-24** is a song in the spirit of play-parties. It is suitable for a number of movement activities. The song is a rousing folk tune that has the spirit of a dance. The term *social dance* may be preferable, in the spirit of the American pioneer folk dance, to that of play-party, for older students.

See Movement, p. 434, for basic folk dance movement ideas that can be performed with "Goin' to Boston." These movements can be used as a starting point for students to create their own pioneer dance.

For synchronized movements that can be used with a chorus in performance, see Movement below.

Listening

As students learn to sing and perform "Goin' to Boston," they are developing critical listening skills required for performing and for listening in an audience. Students who practice active listening skills, including analysis and critique of music they hear in the classroom, will be more attentive at live performances. Guide students to develop and use critical listening skills before attending a concert performance. Use the tips in Audience Etiquette below, along with a preview of the music they will hear at the concert, to prepare students for a good listening experience. These will help students develop and exhibit concert etiquette as an actively involved listener during varied live performances.

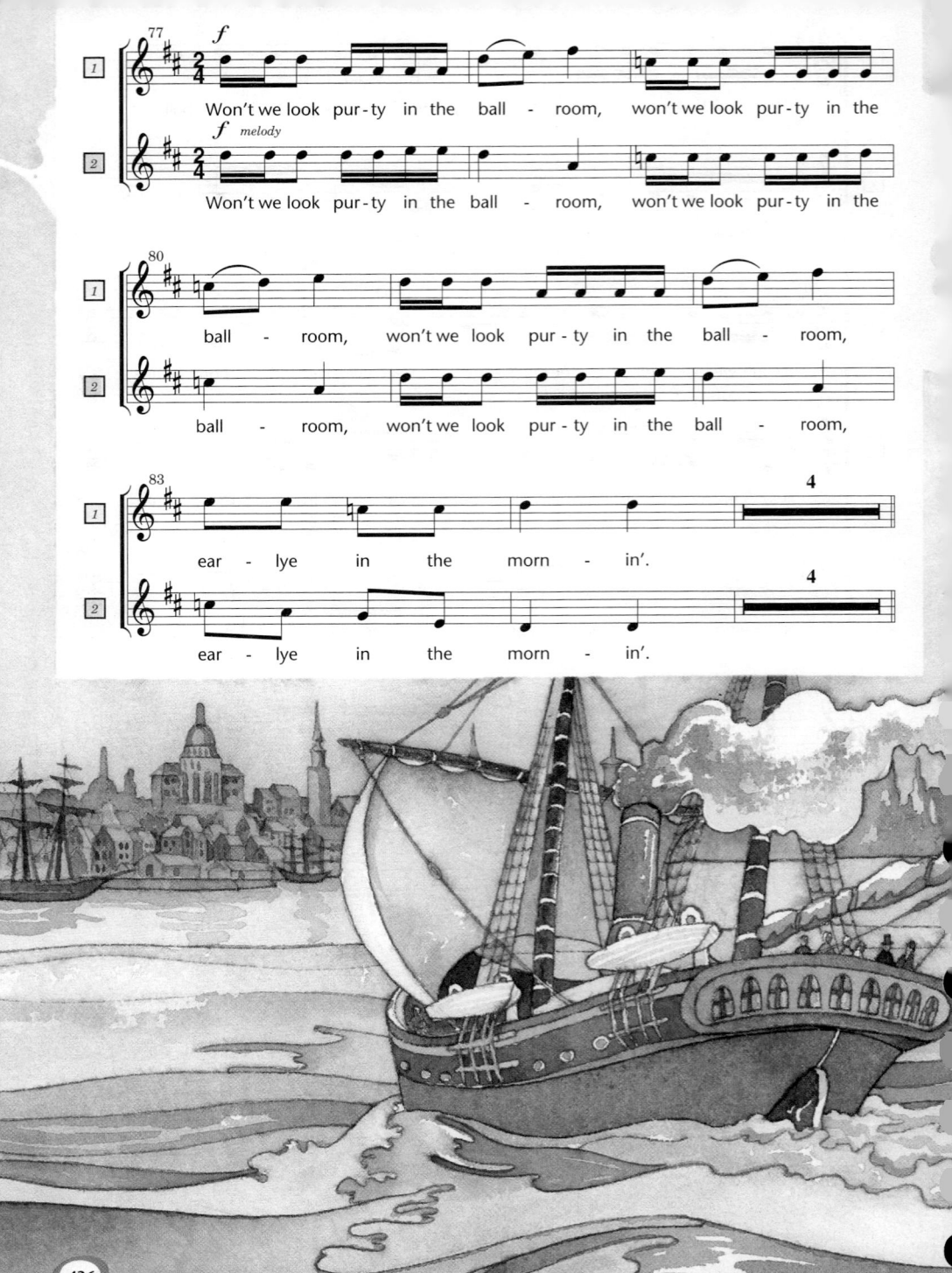

436

Footnotes

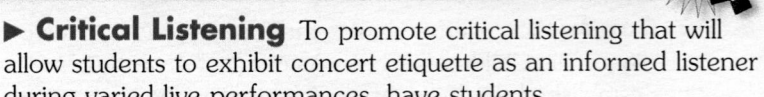

MOVEMENT

▶ **Nonlocomotor Movement** These synchronized movements may be used while singing "Goin' to Boston."

Dance Interludes: During the four-bar and eight-bar interludes, have the floor-level singers step forward and dance in the space downstage. Forward and back, and *do-si-do* are two good movements.

Claps: Perform claps as written. To get a good clapping sound, have students hold one hand slightly higher, and cupped. As the hands strike, move the hands upward. Elbows are away from the body. (top tier only, if space is cramped)

Pats and Claps: At mm. 51–52, there is notation for seven pats. Have the upper tiers pat the shoulders of the neighbor below them. Have the lowest tier perform the two claps.

AUDIENCE ETIQUETTE

▶ **Critical Listening** To promote critical listening that will allow students to exhibit concert etiquette as an informed listener during varied live performances, have students

- Use listening maps that illustrate form, dynamics, instrumentation, or other musical elements as they listen.

- Respond to music through movement to show the style, tempo, instrumentation, or other musical elements. Include patterned movements as well as creative movements.

- Respond to music in class by writing about what they hear in a listening log. Use effective questioning techniques to encourage students to respond to the music verbally. Students should include details in their responses, explain their thinking, and provide support for their answers.

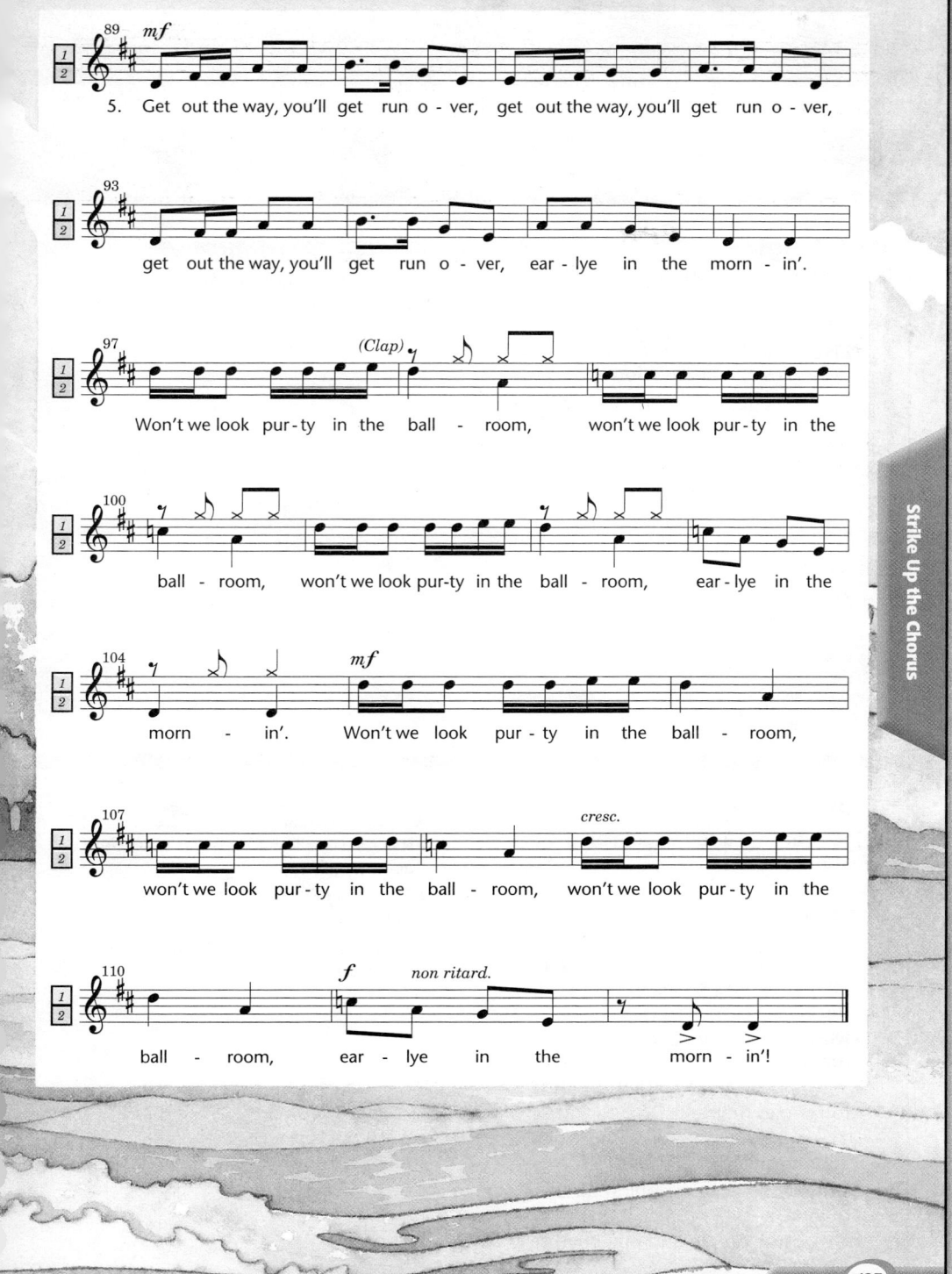

5. Get out the way, you'll get run o - ver, get out the way, you'll get run o - ver,

get out the way, you'll get run o - ver, ear - lye in the morn - in'.

(Clap)

Won't we look pur-ty in the ball - room, won't we look pur-ty in the

ball - room, won't we look pur-ty in the ball - room, ear - lye in the

morn - in'. Won't we look pur - ty in the ball - room,

won't we look pur - ty in the ball - room, won't we look pur - ty in the

ball - room, ear - lye in the morn - in'!

Unit 11 **437**

3 CLOSE

Skill: SINGING   **ASSESSMENT**

Performance/Self-Assessment Have students sing "Goin' to Boston" **CD 20-24** in parts. Divide the class into two groups. Have group 1 sing verse 1, and group 2 sing the refrain.

Invite each group to

- Listen for evenness of rhythm in the singing of the text.
- Listen for clarity of diction, particularly in the dotted rhythms.
- Listen for singing the full value of quarter notes.
- Listen for clarity of diction when singing sixteenth notes.
- Listen for steadiness of tempo when singing sixteenth notes.

TEACHER TO TEACHER

▶ **MIDI Song File** Use the MIDI song file for "Goin' to Boston" to help students learn and practice the song. Use a slow tempo, isolate vocal parts, teach harmony parts, select difficult sections to play and repeat, and transpose the key, if desired.

TECHNOLOGY/MEDIA LINK

Multimedia Have student volunteers videotape rehearsals of the class, or choir, performing "Goin' to Boston." Allow students to view the video and assess their performance. Using the video, demonstrate to students how to improve singing posture (and behavior) at a choral performance.

Unit 11   *Strike Up the Chorus*   **437**

Lesson	Elements	Skills

LESSON 1
A World United

pp. 442–443

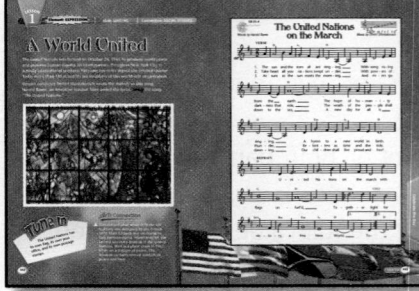

Element: Expression
Concept: Articulation
Focus: Dynamics, tempo, and articulation

Secondary Element
Form: verse-refrain form

National Standards
1a 1c 1e 6b 7a

Skill: Singing
Objective: Sing a song expressively

Secondary Skill
• **Listening** Listen for tempo, dynamics and articulation in a song

SKILLS REINFORCEMENT
• **Singing** Sing long phrases and sustained notes

LESSON 2
Celebrating People

pp. 444–447

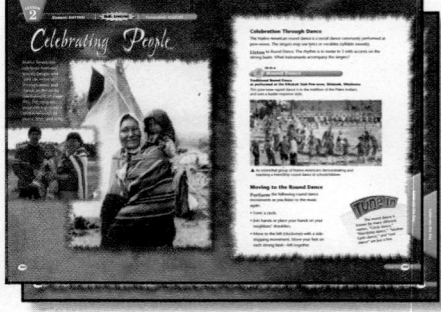

Element: Rhythm
Concept: Pattern
Focus: Sixteenth notes

Secondary Element
Melody: countermelody

National Standards
1a 1c 1d 5a 6b 7a

Skill: Singing
Objective: Sing a song containing sixteenth notes

Secondary Skills
• **Listening** Listen to the role percussion plays in a pow-wow; listen for contrasting sections in a piece of music
• **Movement** Dance to a Native American beat
• **Analyzing** Analyze rhythms and form road map
• **Singing** Sing a melody and countermelody
• **Movement** Learn signing for a song of peace
• **Creating** Create and play rhythm cards

SKILLS REINFORCEMENT
• **Recorder** Play a soprano recorder accompaniment
• **Reading** Read sixteenth-note patterns
• **Singing** Sing vocal chording as a warmup

LESSON 3
Halloween Treat

pp. 448–449

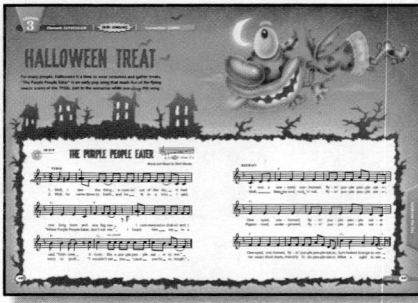

Element: Expression
Concept: Dynamics
Focus: Dynamics, articulation, and mood

Secondary Element
Rhythm: eighth notes and syncopation

National Standards
1a 2a 5a 6c

Skill: Singing
Objective: Sing a ballad with expression

Secondary Skills
• **Reading** Read quarter and eighth-note rhythms
• **Moving** Create and perform movements based on lyrics

SKILLS REINFORCEMENT
• **Recorder** Play an accompaniment on alto recorder

Connections	**Music and Other Literature**	
Connection: Science **Activity:** Read about and discuss the purpose of the United Nations **ACROSS THE CURRICULUM** **Social Studies** Read about and discuss the United Nations **SPOTLIGHT ON** **The Composer** Dmitri Shostakovich **The Artist** Marc Chagall **BUILDING SKILLS THROUGH MUSIC** **Social Studies** Identify influential events in history	**Song** "The United Nations on the March" **More Music Choices** "Bridges," p. 86 "At the Same Time," p. 115	**ASSESSMENT** **Performance/Peer Critique** Have students sing a song and assess their expression **TECHNOLOGY/MEDIA LINK** **Web Site** Access information on Dmitri Shostakovich
Connection: Culture **Activity:** Read about and discuss the themes of unity and peace in song lyrics **CULTURAL CONNECTION** **The Music of Pow-Wows** Background on Native American celebrations **MOVEMENT** **Signing** Background information on sign language **TEACHER TO TEACHER** **Changing Voice Techniques** Tips on boys' changing voices **SPOTLIGHT ON** **"I Am But a Small Voice"** Background information on the charitable purpose of this song **BUILDING SKILLS THROUGH MUSIC** **Reading** Interpret lyrics	**Song** "I Am But a Small Voice" **Listening Selection** *Round Dance* (excerpt) **More Music Choices** "A Brand New Day," p. 7 "*La mariposa,*" p. 58	**ASSESSMENT** **Performance/Peer Critique** Perform a song in groups **TECHNOLOGY/MEDIA LINK** **MIDI/Sequencing Software** Use digital audio to record a performance
Connection: Genre **Activity:** Create a dramatization for a ballad **CULTURAL CONNECTION** **Halloween** Origins of Halloween **ACROSS THE CURRICULUM** **Language Arts** Discuss H.G. Well's "War of the Worlds" **BUILDING SKILLS THROUGH MUSIC** **Visual Arts** Create an imaginary character based upon descriptive lyrics	**Song** "The Purple People Eater" **More Music Choices** "*Bắt kim thang,*" p. 13 *New Horizons in Music Appreciation,* p. 98	**ASSESSMENT** **Performance/Observation** Sing a ballad and observe expressive dynamics and articulation **TECHNOLOGY/MEDIA LINK** **CD-ROM** Use *Band-in-a-Box* to create accompaniments

Lesson	Elements	Skills

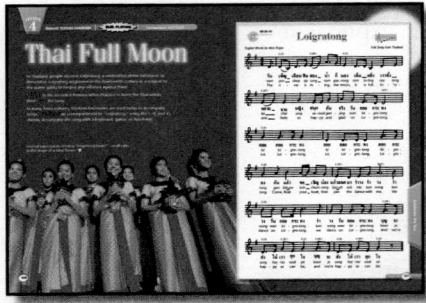

LESSON 4

Thai Full Moon

pp. 450–451

Element: Texture/Harmony
Concept: Harmony
Focus: Western harmony

Secondary Element
Rhythm: dotted-eighth rhythm patterns

National Standards
1c 2b 5a 7a

Skill: Playing
Objective: Accompany a non-Western melody with Western style accompaniment

Secondary Skills
• **Reading** Read repeating rhythm patterns
• **Singing** Sing a song in Thai

SKILLS REINFORCEMENT
• **Creating** Create an accompaniment for a song

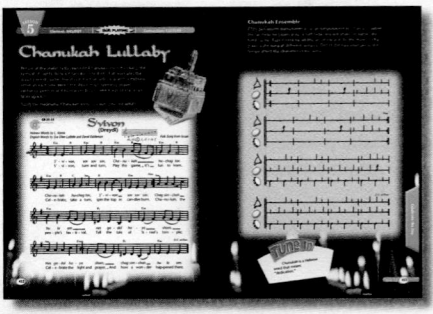

LESSON 5

Chanukah Lullaby

pp. 452–453

Element: Melody
Concept: Tonality
Focus: Harmonic minor

Secondary Element
Form: ABA

National Standards:
1c 2a 2b 6b

Skill: Playing
Objective: Play a song in harmonic minor

Secondary Skills
• **Singing** Sing a song with Hebrew lyrics in harmonic minor
• **Reading** Read and identify melodic elements in harmonic minor
• **Playing** Play a percussion ensemble accompaniment

SKILLS REINFORCEMENT
• **Playing** Play a melody in harmonic minor on bells or mallet instruments

---

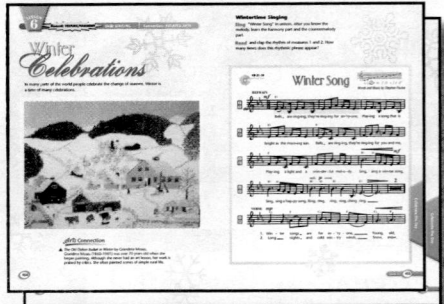

LESSON 6

Winter Celebrations

pp. 454–457

Element: Texture/Harmony
Concept: Texture
Focus: Polyphonic and homophonic textures

Secondary Element
Rhythm: $\frac{6}{8}$ meter

National Standards
1b 1d 2a 4c 5c 6b 6c 8a

Skill: Singing
Objective: Sing a song in two parts with different textures

Secondary Skills
• **Reading** Read rhythms in $\frac{6}{8}$ time
• **Singing** Sing a countermelody and harmonies and differentiate different textures
• **Listening** Listen to a contemporary work that pictures a horse-drawn sleigh

SKILLS REINFORCEMENT
• **Playing** Play a rhythm accompaniment that emulates a horse-drawn sleigh

---

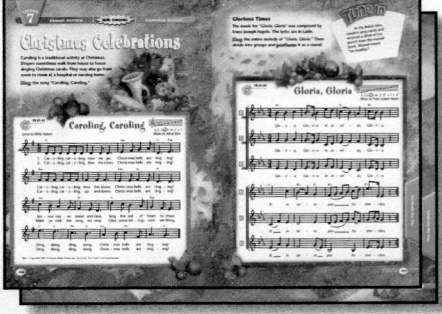

LESSON 7

Christmas Celebrations

pp. 458–461

Element: Rhythm
Concept: Meter
Focus: Meter $\frac{6}{8}$, $\frac{3}{4}$, $\frac{2}{2}$

Secondary Element
Timbre: instrumental (hand bells) and electronic

National Standards
1b 1d 2a 5a 5e 6a

Skill: Singing
Objective: Sing three Christmas songs in different meters

Secondary Skills
• **Singing** Sing a carol and identify any sequences and meter
• **Playing** Sing a song in three parts with bell accompaniment
• **Listening** Listen to a contemporary version of a classic carol

SKILLS REINFORCEMENT
• **Reading** Recognize and understand different meters
• **Percussion** Play rhythmic ostinatos to a carol
• **Bells** Play a bell accompaniment to a carol

Connections

Music and Other Literature

Connection: Culture
Activity: Explore Thai festival of *Loi Krathong*

CULTURAL CONNECTION — **Thai Language** Facts on the Thai language

SPOTLIGHT ON — **The Festival** Facts on the Thai festival *Loi Krathong*

SCHOOL TO HOME CONNECTION **CD-ROM** Research and write about Thai culture

BUILDING SKILLS THROUGH MUSIC **Science** Problem solving

Song *"Loigratong"*

More Music Choices
"Red River Valley," p. 11
"Everybody Loves Saturday Night," p. 296

ASSESSMENT

Performance/Self-Assessment Play a chord accompaniment on keyboard, guitar, Autoharp

TECHNOLOGY/MEDIA LINK
Web Site Explore the music of Thailand

Connection: Culture
Activity: Discuss the holiday Chanukah and the purpose of the *dreydl*

ACROSS THE CURRICULUM **Social Studies** Share background on Chanukah

SPOTLIGHT ON — *Dreydl* **Game** Instructions on how to play the *dreydl* game

BUILDING SKILLS THROUGH MUSIC **Math** Create a graph

Song "S'vivon" ("Dreydl")

More Music Choices
"Hey, Ho! Nobody Home," p. 28
"Sometimes I Feel Like a Motherless Child," p. 241

ASSESSMENT

Performance/Observation Play a melody on keyboard and identify it as harmonic minor

TECHNOLOGY/MEDIA LINK
CD-ROM *Use Band-in-a-Box* to experiment with tempo

Connection: Related Arts
Activity: Discuss the art of Grandma Moses

CULTURAL CONNECTION — **World Peace Bell**

SPOTLIGHT ON
The Artist Information on Grandma Moses and her paintings
Lieutenant Kijé Suite Facts on Prokofiev's music
The Composer Sergei Prokofiev

TEACHER TO TEACHER **Performing Suggestions** Tips on adding instruments to "Winter Song"

ACROSS THE CURRICULUM **Fine Art** Grandma Moses

BUILDING SKILLS THROUGH MUSIC **Visual Arts** Describe a piece of art

Song "Winter Song"

Listening Selection "Troika" from *Lieutenant Kije,* Op. 60

M·U·S·I·C M·A·K·E·R·S
Sergei Prokofiev

More Music Choices
"Lean on Me," p. 14
"Four Strong Winds," p. 170

ASSESSMENT

Performance/Self-Assessment Sing a song and identify its texture

TECHNOLOGY/MEDIA LINK
Web Site Explore information Prokofiev and other Russian composers

---

Connection: Culture
Activity: Read about and discuss the caroling traditions of Christmas

CULTURAL CONNECTION **Christmas Caroling** Historical background of caroling

TEACHER TO TEACHER **Assigning Harmony Parts** Assign vocal parts to match students' ability

SPOTLIGHT ON
King Wenceslas I Facts on this Czech king of Bohemia
Mannhiem Steamroller Background information on this prolific Christmas record label

SCHOOL TO HOME CONNECTION **Caroling** Caroling with family or friends

BUILDING SKILLS THROUGH MUSIC **Reading** Use a Story Map

Songs
"Caroling, Caroling"
"Gloria, Gloria"
"Good King Wenceslas"

Listening Selection *Good King Wenceslas*

More Music Choices
"Swanee," p. 118
"Greensleeves," p. 49

ASSESSMENT

Performance/Observation Sing holiday carols while walking

TECHNOLOGY/MEDIA LINK
MIDI/Sequencing Software Explore orchestration, rhythm, and ostinatos with a MIDI song file

---

Lesson	Elements	Skills	

LESSON 8 — Kwanzaa Joy
pp. 462–465

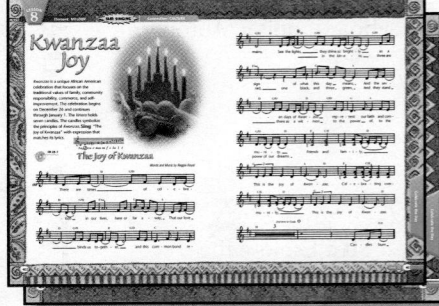

Element: Melody
Concept: Tonality
Focus: Key change or modulation

Secondary Element
Rhythm: eighth- and sixteenth-note rhythm patterns

National Standards
1a 2a 4a 6a 6c 7a 8b 9c

Skill: Singing
Objective: Sing a song with modulation

Secondary Skills
- **Listening** Listen to themes in a Kwanzaa song
- **Singing** Sing a song with a key change
- **Creating** Create call-and-response chants on Kwanzaa themes
- **Playing** Play a percussion accompaniment with *ritardandos* and *accelerandos*
- **Analyzing** Analyze a class performance of a Kwanzaa song

SKILLS REINFORCEMENT
- **Singing Triplets** Sing triplets accurately

LESSON 9 — Martin Luther King Day
pp. 466–471

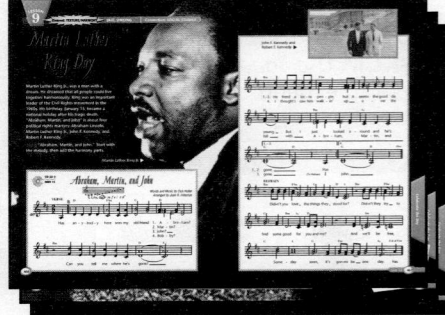

Element: Texture/Harmony
Concept: Harmony
Focus: Two- and three-part harmony

Secondary Element
Form: verse-refrain form

National Standards
1a 1d 5b 6c 8b

Skill: Singing
Objective: Sing songs in two- and three-part harmony

Secondary Skills
- **Listening** Listen to form, lyrics, harmony, homophonic texture in songs about civil rights
- **Singing** Sing a song about freedom in two parts; sing a song with a call and response
- **Playing** Play a recorder accompaniment
- **Analyzing** Analyze the form of a song
- **Moving** Create movements for a class performance
- **Creating** Create a new verse for a song
- **Reading** Read and analyze notation of a "system" and ledger lines

SKILLS REINFORCEMENT
- **Singing** Sing consonants and vowels with articulation
- **Reading** Read and analyze the relation between rhythm and lyrics
- **Recorder** Play a countermelody on recorder in the Resource Book

LESSON 10 — Valentines for Friends
pp. 472–479

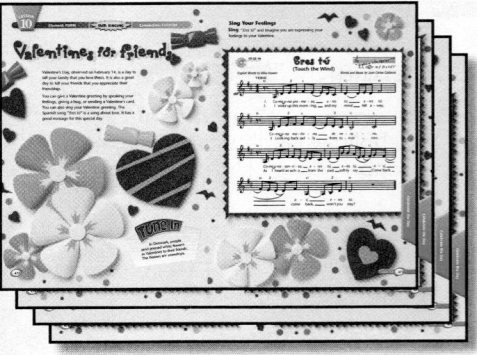

Element: Form
Concept: Form
Focus: Verse-refrain form

Secondary Element
Melody: countermelody

National Standards
1a 1c 1d 1e 2a 5e 6e

Skill: Singing
Objective: Sing two songs in verse-refrain form that have foreign language texts

Secondary Skills
- **Listening** Listen to a song and pay attention to its form
- **Singing** Sing a song in Spanish; sing a song with a recording in groups with harmonies and coutermelodies
- **Movement** Learn signing for words expressing love
- **Performing** Perform a song while exhibiting proper performance etiquette

SKILLS REINFORCEMENT
- **Reading** Read rhythm and melodies using respective syllable types
- **Recorder** Play an alto recorder accompaniment
- **Singing** Sing songs from various cultures; improve breath support over long phrases

Connections

Music and Other Literature

Connection: Culture

Activity: Discuss the meaning and customs of Kwanzaa

- **CULTURAL CONNECTION** — The Seven Principles of Kwanzaa The principles of Kwanzaa
- **TEACHER TO TEACHER** — Kwanzaa FAQ Questions and answers on Kwanzaa
- **ACROSS THE CURRICULUM** — Social Studies Share background on the Kwanzaa ceremony; symbolic items in the Kwanzaa celebration
- **SPOTLIGHT ON**
  Music in the Kwanzaa Ceremony Facts on Kwanzaa music
  The Composer Reggie Royal, composer of "The Joy of Kwanzaa"
- **SCHOOL TO HOME CONNECTION** — Kwanzaa Foods Ask students who celebrate Kwanzaa about the foods served
- **BUILDING SKILLS THROUGH MUSIC** — Reading Identify how music is used in holiday celebrations

Song "The Joy of Kwanzaa"

More Music Choices
"Go, My Son," p. 188
"One Moment in Time," p. 352
"Love in Any Language," p. 476

ASSESSMENT

Performance/Observation Sing a Kwanzaa song with eighth and sixteenth notes, and modulation

TECHNOLOGY/MEDIA LINK

Web Site Discover information on holiday music

Connection: Social Studies

Activity: Discuss Martin Luther King, Jr. John and Robert Kennedy, and Abraham Lincoln, and their fight for civil rights

- **MEETING INDIVIDUAL NEEDS** — English Language Learners Assist students in learning about Martin Luther King Jr.
- **ACROSS THE CURRICULUM** — Social Studies Discuss Abraham Lincoln and the Emancipation Proclamation; movements of the 1960s
- **SPOTLIGHT ON** — John F. Kennedy Facts about the president
  Martin Luther King, Jr. Information on Martin Luther King, Jr.
  Robert Kennedy Information on Robert F. Kennedy
- **CULTURAL CONNECTION** — Folk Music History Discuss folk music's role in the Civil Rights movement
  The Martin Luther King, Jr. Center Discuss this memorial
- **TEACHER TO TEACHER** — Teaching Three Parts Tips on teaching three-part harmony
- **BUILDING SKILLS THROUGH MUSIC** — Reading Identify literary devices in lyrics

Songs
"Abraham, Martin, and John"
"Free at Last"
"I Wish I Knew How It Would Feel to Be Free"

Listening Selections *I Wish I Knew How It Would Feel to Be Free* (excerpt)

M·U·S·I·C M·A·K·E·R·S
Billy Taylor

More Music Choices
"By the Waters of Babylon," p. 311
"Vem kan segla?" p. 417

ASSESSMENT

Performance/Self-Assessment Sing freedom songs in two- and three-part harmony

TECHNOLOGY/MEDIA LINK

MIDI/Sequencing Software Explore melodic contour and transposition using the MIDI song file

CD-ROM Use *Band-in-a-Box* to create an accompaniment

Connection: Culture

Activity: Explore the origins and traditions of Valentine's Day

- **CULTURAL CONNECTION** — E-mail Cards A new way to send Valentines
- **SPOTLIGHT ON**
  Valentine's Day; Valentine Traditions; Name-drawing The origins of sending Valentine cards
- **TEACHER TO TEACHER** — Long Phrases Tips on singing long phrases
  Singing and Posture Correct posture tips
- **ACROSS THE CURRICULUM** — Language Arts Different languages
- **MOVEMENT** — Signing Learn signing for a song
- **MEETING INDIVIDUAL NEEDS** — English Language Learner Say "I love you" in various languages
- **AUDIENCE ETIQUETTE** — Applause When to clap
- **CHARACTER EDUCATION** — Expressing Friendship Help students understand that making friends is a social skill
- **BUILDING SKILLS THROUGH MUSIC** — Reading Learn a phrase in foreign languages

Songs
"Eres tú" ("Touch the Wind")
"Love in Any Language"

More Music Choices
"Alexander's Ragtime Band," p. 136
"Jambalaya," p. 244
"Green, Green Grass of Home," p. 248

ASSESSMENT

Performance/Self-Assessment Sing a Valentine's song in verse-refrain form

TECHNOLOGY/MEDIA LINK

CD-ROM Use a CD-ROM encyclopedia to research Valentine's Day

Multimedia Produce a slide show based on a Valentine's theme

Lesson	Elements	Skills

LESSON 11
Birthdays and Anniversaries
pp. 480–481

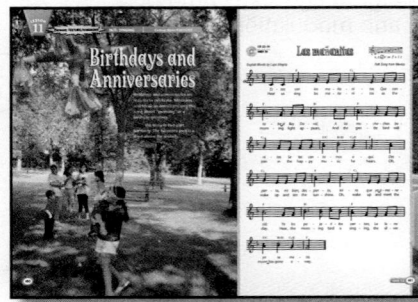

Element: Texture/Harmony
Concept: Harmony
Focus: Harmony in parallel thirds

Secondary Element
Rhythm: meter in 3

National Standards
1c 1d 2b

Skill: Singing
Objective: Sing a two-part song in parallel thirds

Secondary Skill
• **Playing** Create and play a chord accompaniment on guitar or keyboards

SKILLS REINFORCEMENT
• **Guitar** Play a strumming accompaniment
• **Keyboard** Play an accompaniment using the I, IV, and V7 chords
• **Improvisation** Use vocal chording to learn improvisation

---

LESSON 12
Carnaval Celebration
pp. 482–483

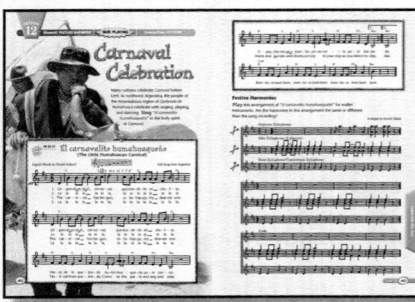

Element: Texture/Harmony
Concept: Harmony
Focus: Harmony in mallet accompaniment

Secondary Element
Rhythm: cut time

National Standards
1c 2a 2c 4a 7b

Skill: Playing
Objective: Play a mallet accompaniment

Secondary Skills
• **Analyzing** Identify first and second endings and the coda of a song
• **Singing** Sing a song in Spanish and identify syncopations in the rhythm
• **Playing** Perform a song on mallet instruments with non-pitched percussion accompaniment

SKILLS REINFORCEMENT
• **Playing** Help students with the harmony accompaniment of an Argentinian song

---

LESSON 13
Patriotism Sings
pp. 484–487

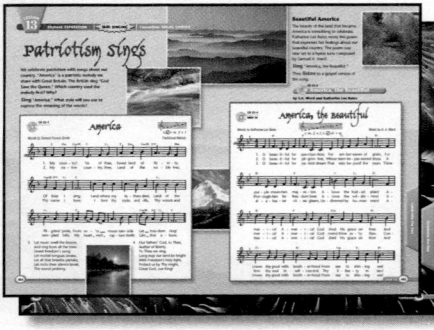

Element: Expression
Concept: Articulation
Focus: Slurs, *fermata*, dynamics, and mood

Secondary Element
Rhythm: dotted-quarter and dotted eighth rhythm patterns

National Standards
1d 1e 5a 5c 6b 7a

Skill: Singing
Objective: Sing three patriotic songs with expression

Secondary Skills
• **Singing** Sing and identify rhythmic patterns, sections, and expression in patriotic songs
• **Listening** Listen to a gospel version of a traditional American song
• **Analyzing** Analyze notation including fermata and anacrusis

SKILLS REINFORCEMENT
• **Playing** Play a rhythm accompaniment with a recording
• **Singing** Substitute notes when the vocal range is extreme
• **Keyboard** Play a keyboard accompaniment to a patriotic anthem

Connections

Music and Other Literature

Connection: Culture
Activity: Create a Mexican birthday piñata

- SPOTLIGHT ON   **Piñatas** Facts on this birthday tradition
- SCHOOL TO HOME CONNECTION   **Mini-piñata** Make a piñata at home
- BUILDING SKILLS THROUGH MUSIC   **Writing** Describe a birthday

Song "Las mañanitas" ("The Morning")

More Music Choices
"Así es mi tierra," p. 172

ASSESSMENT

Performance/Self-Assessment Sing a birthday song in harmony in thirds

TECHNOLOGY/MEDIA LINK
CD-ROM Use *Band-in-a-Box* to create Latin arrangements

Connection: Culture
Activity: Discover the celebration of Carnaval

- CULTURAL CONNECTION   **Immigration's Influence on Culture** Discuss the immigrant population's influence in Argentina
- ACROSS THE CURRICULUM   **Social Studies** Information on Argentinian culture
- BUILDING SKILLS THROUGH MUSIC   **Reading** Learn about Argentina

Song "El carnavalito humahuaqueño" ("The Little Humahuacan Carnival")

More Music Choices
"O lê lê O Bahía" p. 165
"Cuando pa' Chile me voy" p. 376
"La mariposa" p. 58

ASSESSMENT

Performance/Peer Critique Perform a mallet accompaniment with a recording

TECHNOLOGY/MEDIA LINK
Electronic Keyboard Use the auto accompaniment feature on a keyboard to create a appropriate accompaniment for the song

---

Connection: Social Studies
Activity: Discuss the history behind patriotic songs

- TEACHER TO TEACHER   **Keyboard Accompaniments** Chords
- CULTURAL CONNECTION   **"America"** Facts on "God Save the Queen"
- ACROSS THE CURRICULUM   **Social Studies** Discuss the War of 1812
- SPOTLIGHT ON   **The Author** Francis Scott Key
- CHARACTER EDUCATION   **Patriotism**
- SCHOOL TO HOME CONNECTION   **Pictures of America** Have students ask friends and family for photos of American culture
- BUILDING SKILLS THROUGH MUSIC   **Reading** Define unknown words

Songs
"America"
"America, the Beautiful"
"The Star-Spangled Banner"

Listening Selections
America, the Beautiful (Gospel)
L'union (excerpt)

More Music Choices
"Sing a Song of Peace," p. 66
"Strike Up the Band," p. 135

ASSESSMENT

Performance/Peer Critique Sing patriotic songs with musical expression

TECHNOLOGY/MEDIA LINK
Multimedia Create a slide show of pictures on a patriotic theme

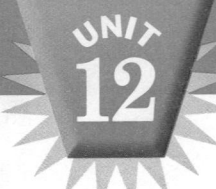

Introducing the Unit

Every culture in the world experiences the joy of celebrations. Music is a natural part of these events. This unit will guide students through the music of some familiar and not-so-familiar celebrations.

Unit Project

Help your students create a dance to *The "Body" Song.*

- Invite them to suggest hand motions and dance steps that could be performed while traveling around the room.
- Write suggestions on the board, then choose a performance order.
- Decide how long to perform each movement, keeping in mind that the song is in common time.
- Have students make a straight line and perform the dance as they walk around the room.

Focus student attention on the pictures on pp. 438-439.

ASK How is each dancer using his or her body? What do their movements tell you about the music to which they are dancing? What do you think each dancer is expressing? (Accept a variety of answers.)

Point out that dancers use their whole bodies to interpret music.

Invite students to discuss their experiences with dance or movement activities. Did they attend a memorable performance? Do they study dance at a local studio? Do their families have musical traditions that include dancing?

Your students may mention weddings, school dances, visiting performers and family reunions.

Discuss the nature of your students' experiences. Help them recognize that dance is used all over the world to express emotion and to celebrate cultural heritage.

Everybody's a Body

Our differences are what make us all wonderful and unique. Music helps us realize that all people are equal and deserving of respect.

The "Body" Song is in calypso style and reminds us that we are all somebody important.

Listen to *The "Body" Song* and its important message.

CD 21-1

The "Body" Song

by Brenda Russell
as performed by Al Jarreau
and Brenda Russell

The calypso style and steel drums create an exciting rhythmic beat in *The "Body" Song.*

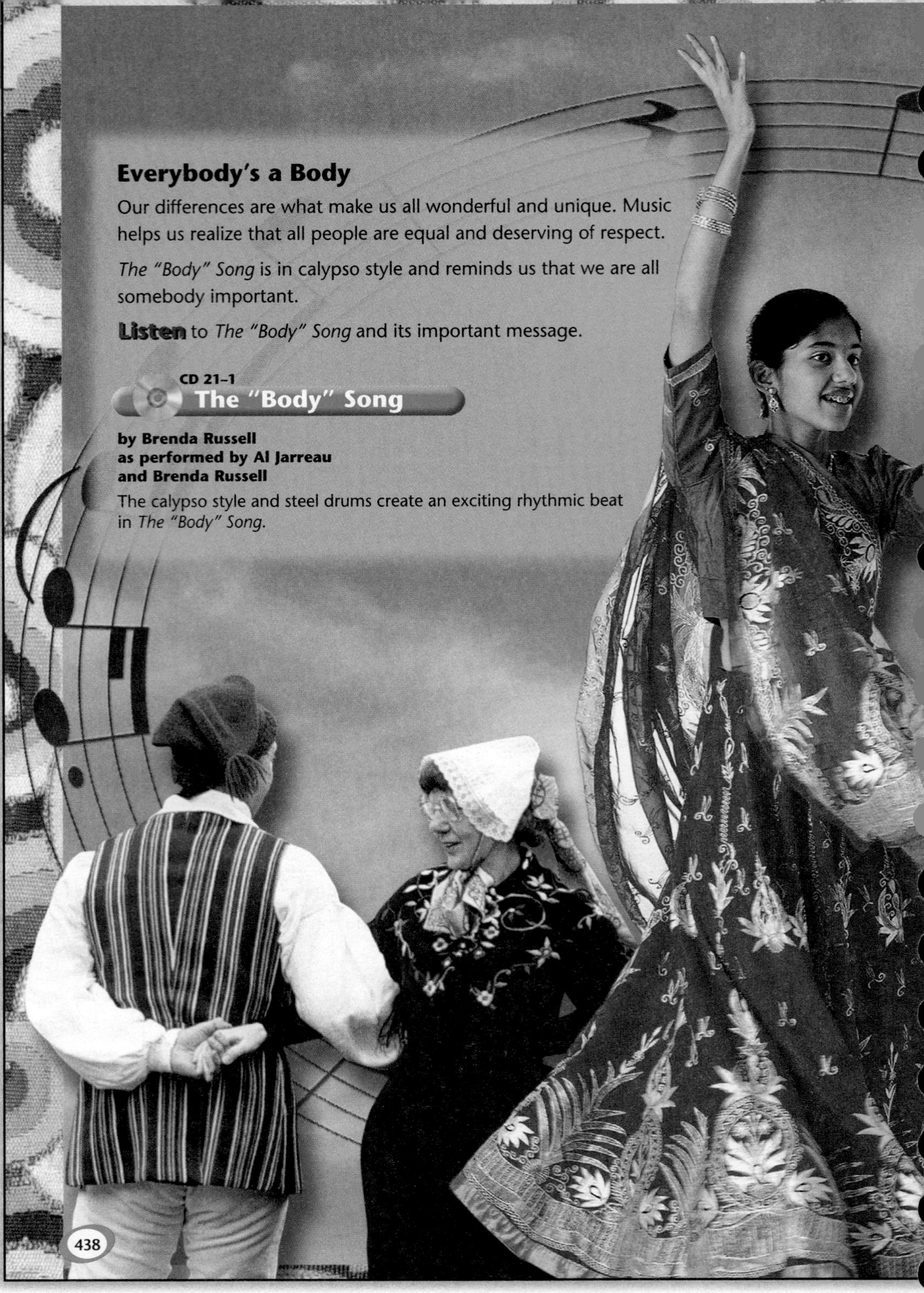

438

Across the Curriculum

Unit Highlights

▶ ART

- Becoming familiar with American and African American folk art (p. 455)

▶ LANGUAGE ARTS

- Learning about the broadcast in 1938 of War of the Worlds (p. 448)
- Examining how the phrase "I love you" is expressed in other languages (p. 474)
- Learning phrases of friendship in several different languages (p. 477)

▶ SOCIAL STUDIES

- Learning more about the role of the United Nations as an international peacekeeping organization (p. 442)
- Becoming aware of the Jewish holiday of Chanukah (p. 452)
- Learning more about the Kwanzaa ceremony (pp. 463, 464)
- Learning facts about the life of Abraham Lincoln (p. 466)
- Finding out about antiwar protests and the peace movement in the 1960s (p. 468)
- Using a song to begin learning some facts about Argentina (p. 483)
- Examining the War of 1812 and our national anthem (p. 485)

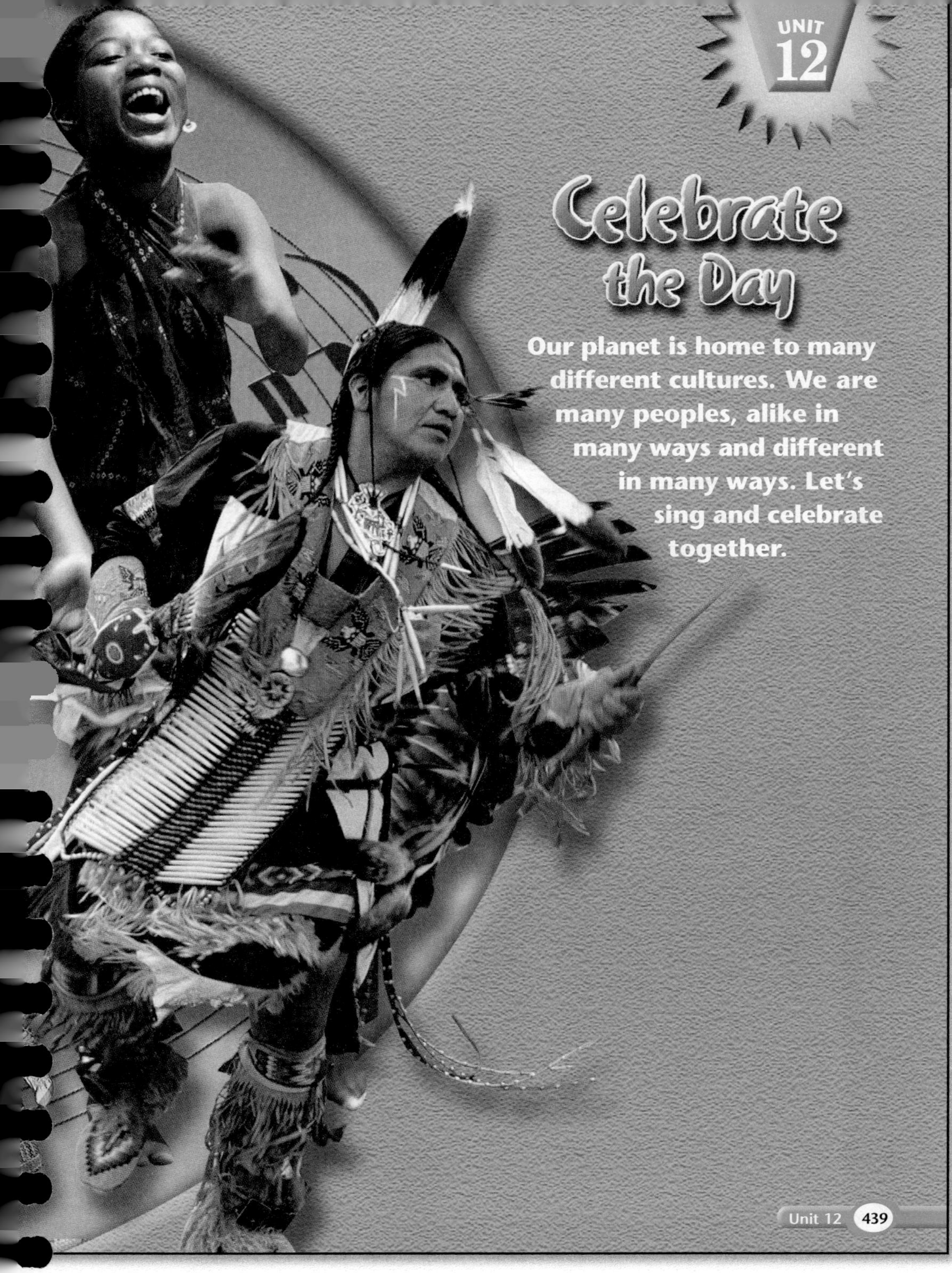

UNIT 12

Celebrate the Day

Our planet is home to many different cultures. We are many peoples, alike in many ways and different in many ways. Let's sing and celebrate together.

MUSIC SKILLS
ASSESSED IN THIS UNIT

Performing Music: Singing

- Assess the performance of a small group singing a song (p. 443)
- Evaluate group performances of a song (p. 447)
- Observe the proper interpretation of a ballad (p. 449)
- Determine the texture of a song (p. 457)
- Observe and evaluate a strolling performance of Christmas carols (p. 461)
- Observe and evaluate the performance of a song with a modulation (p. 465)
- Assess the performance of the class singing a song in two-part harmony (p. 471)
- Perform a song and record it on audiotape; determine the form of the song (p. 476)
- Perform a song expressively, under the direction of a student; critique the performance (p. 487)

Performing Music: Playing

- Provide accompaniment to a song and discuss its accuracy (p. 451)
- Play a melody accurately on a keyboard instrument; determine the key (p. 453)
- Perform the mallet accompaniment of a song (p. 483)

CULTURAL CONNECTION

Unit Highlights

▶ AFRICAN/AFRICAN AMERICAN

- Discuss the seven principles of Kwanzaa (p. 462)
- Learn about the King Center, founded by Coretta Scott King in memory of her husband, Martin Luther King Jr. (p. 469)

▶ AMERICAN REGIONAL

- Investigate the music of Native American pow-wows and the round dance (p. 444)
- Learn about the World Peace Bell, located in Newport, Kentucky (p. 454)
- Examine the style and lyrics of a protest song about four slain heroes (p. 467)
- Become aware that Valentine's Day cards can now be sent by e-mail (p. 472)

- Discuss the origins of the song "America" and its similarity to the British national anthem (p. 484)

▶ ASIAN; AUSTRALIAN

- Learn about Thai, the official language of Thailand (p. 450)

▶ SOUTH AMERICAN

- Become aware of the effects of immigration on Argentina (p. 482)

▶ EUROPEAN

- Explore the connection between All Hallow's Eve in Celtic Ireland and the origins of Halloween (p. 448)
- Learn some facts about the history of caroling and how it spread from England to the United States (p. 458)

OPENING ACTIVITIES

MATERIALS

- "Under the Same Sun"   **CD 21-2**

  Recording Routine: Intro (4 m.); refrain; v.1; refrain; v.2; refrain; bridge; refrain (refrain repeat ad lib)

- *The "Body" Song*   **CD 21-1**

Listening

Invite students to listen to "Under the Same Sun" **CD 21-2.**

ASK **What was repeated several times?** (The words *Though we dance to the beat…*)

Sing just the refrain for your students. Identify this as section A of the piece.

Listen to the song again, writing the sections of the song as they occur (ABABACAA).

Singing

Invite students to sing "Under the Same Sun" **CD 21–2** with the recording. Encourage them to

- Assign groups, soloists, and unison singing to different portions of the song.
- Decide on the order of performers. For example, a soloist might sing the first refrain, a small group sing the verse, and the entire class join in on the next refrain.

Reading

Help your students identify the direction of each phrase on pp. 440–441.

ASK **If you drew a line through the note heads of the first seven notes** *(Though we dance to the beat),* **what would it look like?** (An arch.)

Point out: the phrase begins and ends on the same pitch.

Have students take turns drawing the phrase shapes of the verse. Help them understand that ascending and descending phrases are paired. The descending phrases are like musical answers to the ascending phrases.

A Single Sun

We live under a single sun on a single planet.

Sing "Under the Same Sun," a song with another powerful message.

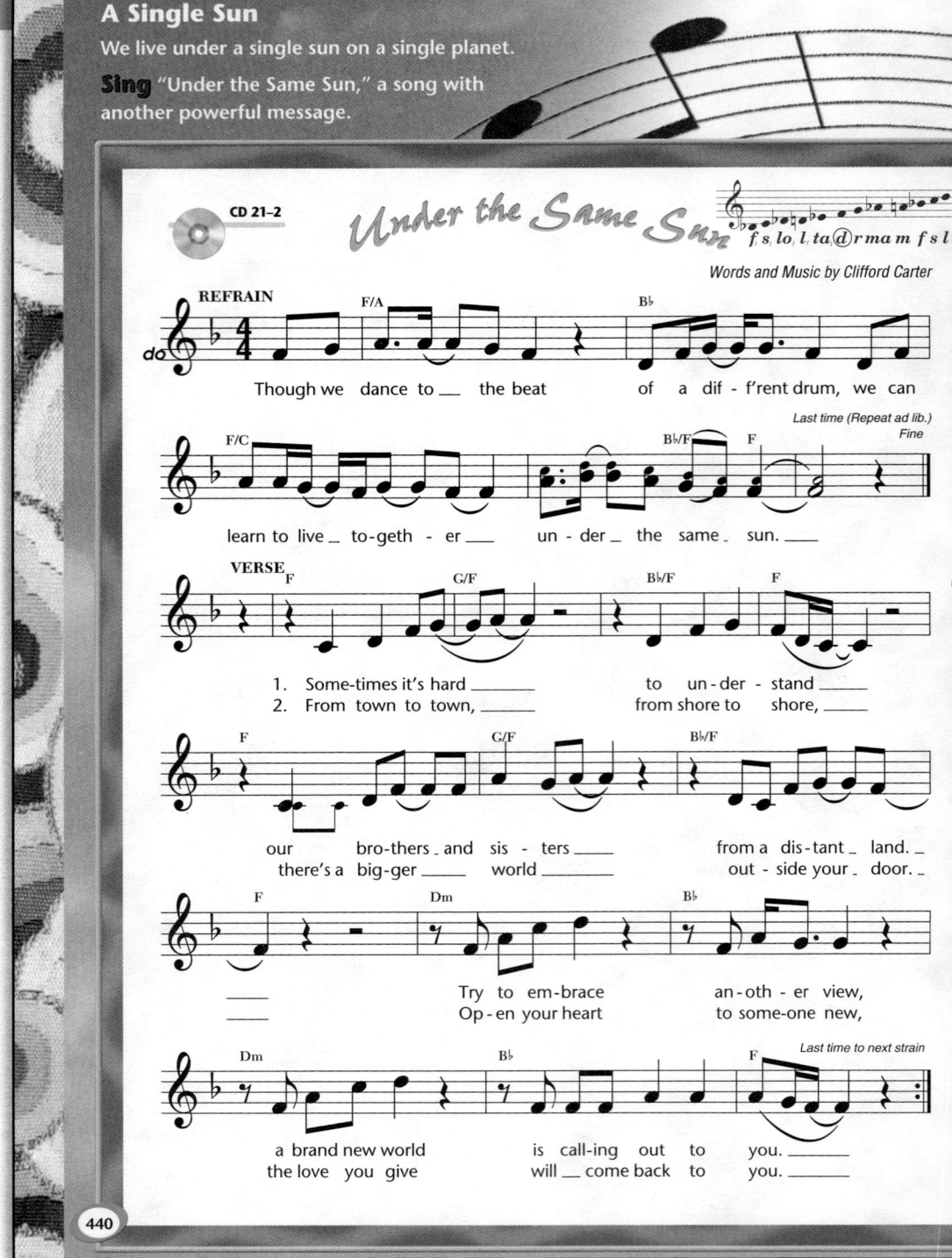

ASSESSMENT

Unit Highlights The lessons in this unit were chosen and developed to support the theme "Celebrate the Day." Each lesson, as always, presents a clear element focus, a skill objective, and an end-of-lesson assessment. The overall sequence of lessons, however, is organized according to this theme, rather than concept or skill development. In this context, formal assessment strategies, such as those presented in Units 1–6, are no longer applicable.

▶ **INFORMAL ASSESSMENTS**

At the close of each Teacher's Edition lesson in this unit, one of the following types of assessments is used to evaluate the learning of the key element focus or skill objective.

- Performance/Observation (pp. 449, 453, 461, 465)
- Performance/Peer Critique (pp. 443, 447, 483, 487)
- Performance/Self-Assessment (pp. 451, 457, 471, 476, 481)

▶ **RUBRICS**

Visit *www.sfsuccessnet.com* for rubrics to assess students' achievement in music skills.

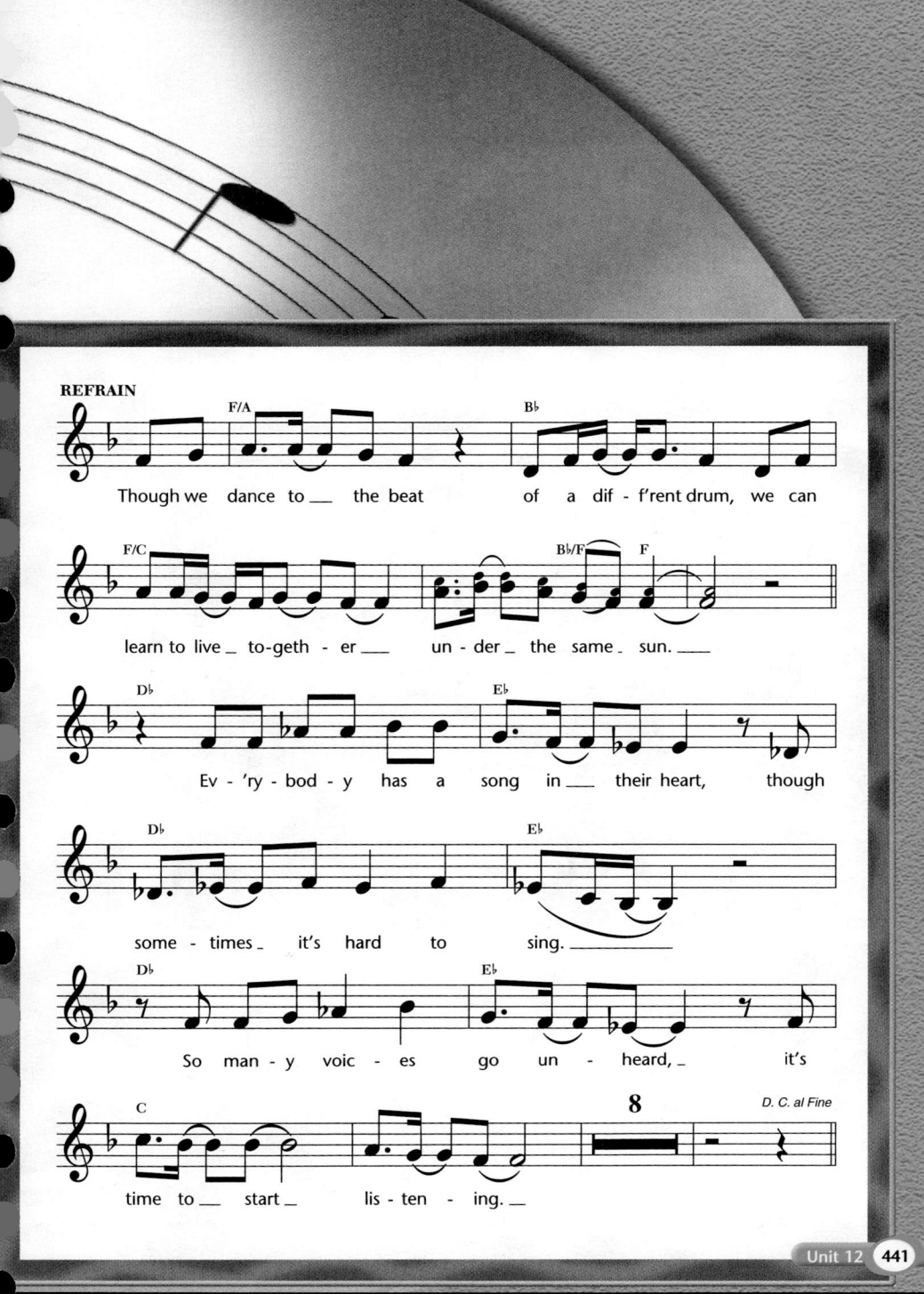

REFRAIN

Though we dance to __ the beat of a dif-f'rent drum, we can

learn to live _ to-geth - er __ un-der _ the same _ sun. __

Ev-'ry-bod-y has a song in __ their heart, though

some-times _ it's hard to sing. __

So man-y voic-es go un-heard, _ it's

time to __ start _ lis-ten - ing. __

D. C. al Fine

Moving

Have students create signing movements that express the meaning of the words of "Under the Same Sun." Have a few or all of the students perform these movements as they sing with the recording.

Improvising

Invite students to finish these sentences:

"It's easy to be friends with someone who…"

"It's hard to be friends with someone who… "

"We can learn to live together by… "

Let many students suggest different endings, then discuss the answers.

Have students choose a few favorite sentences. Let different students read them aloud before a performance of "Under the Same Sun."

INNOVATIVE TEACHER SUPPORT FOR THIS UNIT

- **MAKING MUSIC DVD, Grade 6** contains video segments that support lessons, including signing and movement.
- **MAKING MUSIC with Movement and Dance** provides more opportunities for large group activities in music or physical education classes.
- **MAKING MUSIC with Technology** provides lesson plans for many technology applications; includes MIDI files.
- **¡A cantar!** features recorded songs and lessons from around the Spanish-speaking world; includes strategies for bilingual classes and for English-speaking teachers working with Spanish-speaking students.
- **Bridges to Asia** features recorded songs and lessons from Asian and Pacific region cultures.
- *www.sfsuccessnet.com* provides an online lesson planner to conveniently create lesson plans at school or at home. Includes rubrics for assessment, lesson modifications to meet the needs of all students, performance musicals based on program content, and more.

TECHNOLOGY/MEDIA LINK

Unit Highlights

▶ **CD-ROM**

- Create different background accompaniments (p. 449)
- Experiment with the tempo of a song (p. 453)
- Create an arrangement to accompany a song (p. 471)
- Use a CD-ROM encyclopedia from the local library to learn more about Valentine's Day (p. 479)
- Create Latin arrangements to a song (p. 481)

▶ **ELECTRONIC KEYBOARD**

- Use a MIDI keyboard to create accompaniments (p. 483)

▶ **MIDI/SEQUENCING SOFTWARE**

- Record the performance of a song (p. 447)
- Explore orchestration and ostinatos in a song (p. 461)

- Use the MIDI file of a song to explore transposition, contour, and rhythm changes (p. 471)

▶ **MULTIMEDIA**

- Illustrate the lyrics of a song (p. 479)
- Organize a slide show of pictures (p. 487)

▶ **WEB SITE**

- Visit *www.sfsuccessnet.com* to learn more about the life and music of Dmitri Shostakovich and other Russian composers (p. 443)
- Explore the music of Thailand at (p. 451)
- Go to *www.sfsuccessnet.com* to learn more about Sergei Prokofiev and other Russian composers (p. 457)
- Learn more about holiday music at *www.sfsuccessnet.com* (p. 465)

LESSON AT A GLANCE

Element Focus — **EXPRESSION** Dynamics, tempo, and articulation

Skill Objective **SINGING** Sing a song expressively

Connection Activity **SOCIAL STUDIES** Read about and discuss the purpose of the United Nations

MATERIALS

- "The United Nations on the March"   **CD 21-4**
  Recording Routine: Intro (8 m.); v. 1; refrain; v. 2; refrain; interlude (8 m.); v. 3; coda

VOCABULARY

legato   *mezzo forte*   *ritardando*   modulation

◆ ◆ ◆ ◆ National Standards ◆ ◆ ◆ ◆

1a Sing accurately with good breath control
1c Sing music with appropriate expression
1e In groups, sing moderately easy pieces with expression
6b Listen and analyze uses of dynamics in music from diverse genres
7a Create standards for evaluating performances

MORE MUSIC CHOICES

For more practice in singing songs about unity:
"Bridges," p. 86
"At the Same Time," p. 115

1 INTRODUCE

Invite students to read about the United Nations on p. 442 and discuss the purpose of the United Nations in Across the Curriculum below.

Have students look at the photograph of Marc Chagall's stained glass window in the United Nations building. Ask them to locate a symbol of peace in the window (angel). See Spotlight On below, for information on Marc Chagall.

A World United

The United Nations was formed on October 24, 1945, to promote world peace and preserve human dignity. Its headquarters, though in New York City, is actually international territory. Fifty-one countries signed the original charter. Today more than 185 countries are members of this worldwide organization.

Russian composer Dmitri Shostakovich wrote the melody to this song. Harold Rome, an American teacher, later added the lyrics. **Sing** the song "The United Nations."

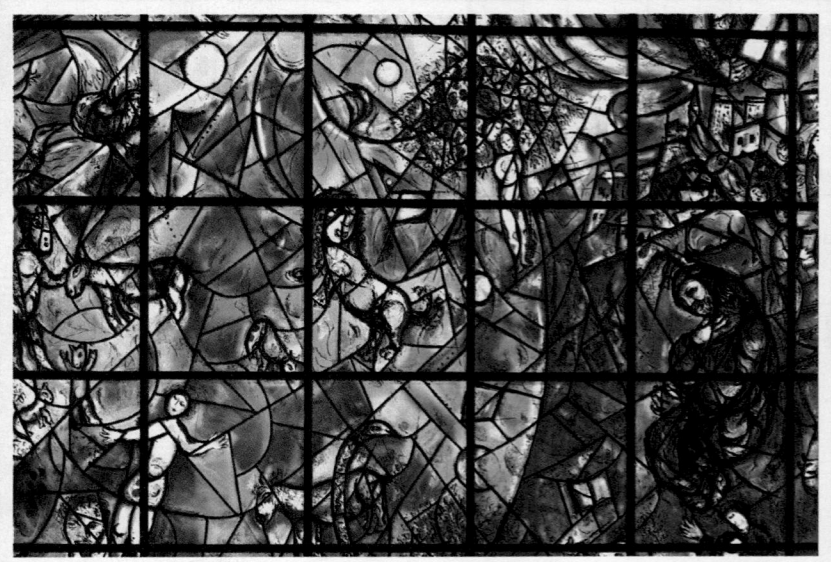

Tune In

The United Nations has its own flag, its own post office, and its own postage stamps.

Arts Connection

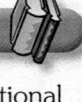

▲ This stained glass window in the UN building was designed by the French artist Marc Chagall as a memorial to Dag Hammarskjöld. Hammarskjöld, the second secretary-general of the United Nations, died in a plane crash in 1961 while on a mission of peace. The window contains several symbols of peace and love.

442

Footnotes

ACROSS THE CURRICULUM

▶ **Social Studies** The United Nations (UN) is an international peacekeeping organization with more than 185 member countries. It was founded in 1945 as a result of talks between the "Big Three"—the United States, Great Britain, and the U.S.S.R. United States president Franklin D. Roosevelt, British prime minister Winston Churchill, and Soviet leader Joseph Stalin envisioned the UN as a forum for discussing and resolving disputes before they grew out of control.

BUILDING SKILLS THROUGH MUSIC

▶ **Social Studies** Given the information that the United Nations was formed in 1945 as the result of talks between the U.S.A., U.S.S.R. and Great Britain, have students identify the events in world history at that time that would have influenced those talks.

SPOTLIGHT ON

▶ **The Composer** Composer Dmitri Shostakovich (1906–1975) lived in the U.S.S.R. and composed within the constraints imposed by Communist policies towards the arts. Shostakovich was named a Hero of the Soviet Union, and he received international praise for his later symphonic works.

▶ **The Artist** Marc Chagall (1887–1985) grew up in poverty in a small Russian town. He studied art in St. Petersburg and then in Paris. Chagall's early art depicted traditional Jewish life, folklore, and religious figures. In 1922, Chagall moved to Paris. He was one of the few artists to see his own work displayed at the Louvre during his lifetime. Chagall's work is also on display at the Paris Opera House, the National Museum in Paris, the Vatican, the Metropolitan Opera House, and the United Nations.

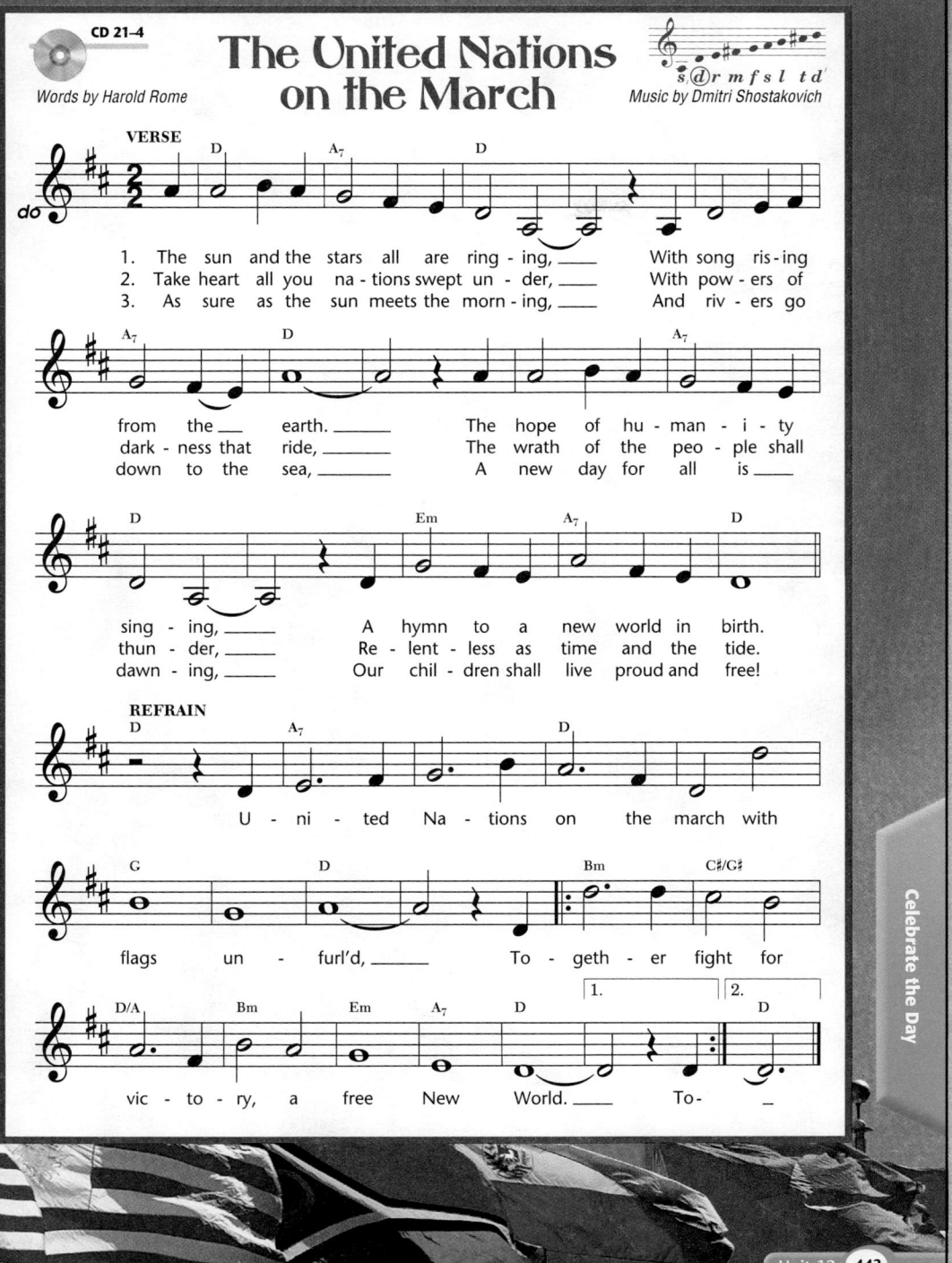

The United Nations on the March

Words by Harold Rome
Music by Dmitri Shostakovich

VERSE

1. The sun and the stars all are ring-ing, _____ With song ris-ing
2. Take heart all you na-tions swept un-der, _____ With pow-ers of
3. As sure as the sun meets the morn-ing, _____ And riv-ers go

from the __ earth. _____ The hope of hu-man-i-ty
dark-ness that ride, _____ The wrath of the peo-ple shall
down to the sea, _____ A new day for all is _____

sing-ing, _____ A hymn to a new world in birth.
thun-der, _____ Re-lent-less as time and the tide.
dawn-ing, _____ Our chil-dren shall live proud and free!

REFRAIN

U-ni-ted Na-tions on the march with

flags un-furl'd, _____ To-geth-er fight for

vic-to-ry, a free New World. _____ To-

Celebrate the Day

Unit 12 **443**

Listening

Have students listen to "The United Nations on the March" **CD 21-4.**

ASK Is the song performed *legato* or *staccato*? (*legato*)

Did the tempo remain the same throughout the song? (No; there were *ritardandos* in the interlude between verses 2 and 3 and in the coda.)

6b **Did the dynamic level remain the same throughout the song?** (Yes, it was *mezzo forte.*)

Explain that dynamics, tempo, and articulation add to the expressive qualities of the song.

Help students

- Locate the *ritardandos* in the interlude between the last two verses.
- Identify that the last verse is in a different key (modulation).

Singing

1c Invite students to sing "The United Nations on the March" **CD 21-4** with the recording.

Remind students to sing *legato* and to maintain a *mezzo forte* dynamic level throughout the song.

3 **CLOSE**

Element: EXPRESSION | **ASSESSMENT**

1e **Performance/Peer Critique** Organize the class into three groups. Have each group sing a different verse of "The United Nations on the March," with the entire class singing the refrain.

7a Have students assess each group's performance to determine if dynamics, tempo, and articulation were used to sing expressively.

SKILLS REINFORCEMENT

1a ▶ **Singing** Help students notice the long phrases (sustained notes followed by rests) in "The United Nations on the March." Have students

- Hold notes at each phrase ending for their full duration.
- Take a breath in the rests at the phrase endings.
- Use good diction. Practice sounding vowels and consonants in unison.
- Watch the sound of *ng.* Avoid the tendency to slide over the vowel and move to the *ng* too quickly. Practice holding the vowel and placing the final *ng* consonant on the release of the phrase.

TECHNOLOGY/MEDIA LINK

Web Site Go to *www.sfsuccessnet.com* to learn more about the life and music of Dmitri Shostakovich and other Russian composers.

Discuss how composers under the Soviet regime might have been influenced by the policies of the government. Ask students

- What did a composer do to earn a living? (composed music, taught in universities, conducted orchestras, performed)
- How did a composer earn money writing music? (Composers received commissions.)
- Who offered commissions to composers? (often, government art and music organizations)

LESSON AT A GLANCE

Element Focus   **RHYTHM** Sixteenth notes

Skill Objective   **SINGING** Sing a song containing sixteenth notes

Connection Activity   **CULTURE** Read about and discuss the themes of unity and peace in song lyrics

MATERIALS

- *Round Dance* (excerpt)   **CD 21-6**
- "I Am But a Small Voice"   **CD 21-7**

  Recording Routine: Intro (4 m.); vocal
- **Resource Book** pp. G-24, I-29
- rhythm cards and a selection of rhythm instruments, bass drum (optional)

VOCABULARY

slurs   ties   bar

◆ ◆ ◆ National Standards ◆ ◆ ◆

1a Sing accurately in small ensembles
1c Sing music from diverse cultures
1d Sing music written in two parts
5a Read sixteenth notes in duple meter
6b Listen and analyze uses of rhythm in music from diverse cultures
7a Students evaluate the music they hear

MORE MUSIC CHOICES

For more practice singing sixteenth notes:

"A Brand New Day," p. 7

"*La mariposa,*" p. 58

Celebrating People

Native Americans celebrate harmony among people and with the universe through music and dance, as shown by the example on page 445. The song on page 446 expresses a similar message of peace, love, and unity.

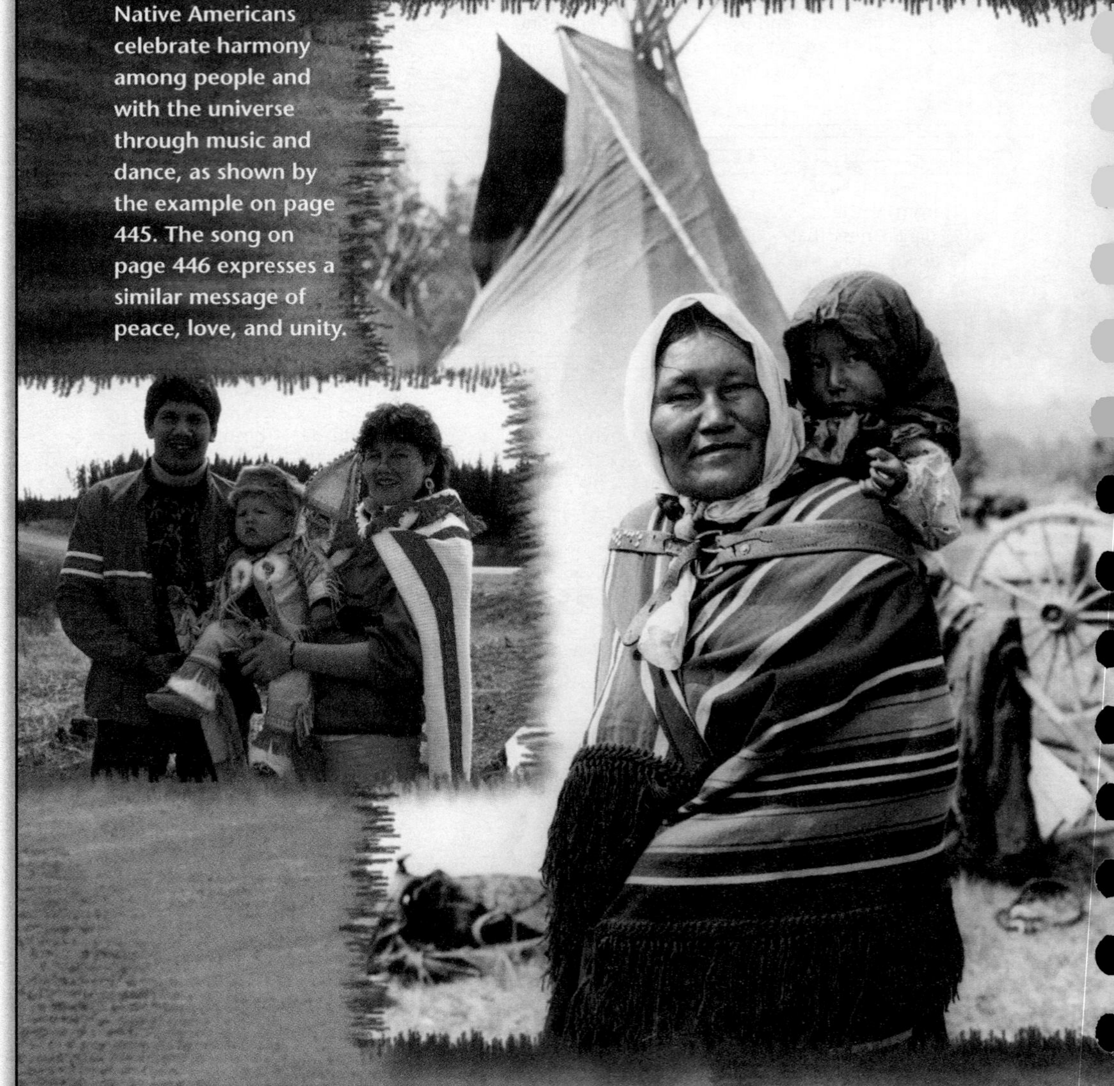

444

Footnotes

SKILLS REINFORCEMENT

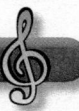

▶ **Recorder** Have students play a soprano recorder accompaniment for "I Am But a Small Voice" on Resource Book p. I-29.

BUILDING SKILLS THROUGH MUSIC

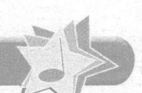

▶ **Reading** Have students write two or three sentences on what they believe is meant by the phrase *I am but a small voice,* as it is used in this song.

CULTURAL CONNECTION

▶ **The Music of Pow-Wows** Pow-wows are large gatherings where Native Americans celebrate their arts, crafts, food, music, dance, and culture. One theme of pow-wows is that of friendship and unity among people. Dance and singing are an important part of the pow-wow celebration.

The rhythm of the round dance is often based on eighth-note patterns or variation (triplet). The rhythm patterns are played on special large drums, called pow-wow drums, that are played by a group of people. (A pow-wow drum is shown on p. 187.)

For a fascinating look at the contemporary music and dance of Native Americans, see *Moving Within the Circle* by Bryan Burton (World Music Press, 2002).

Celebration Through Dance

The Native American round dance is a social dance commonly performed at pow-wows. The singers may use lyrics or vocables (syllable sounds).

Listen to *Round Dance*. The rhythm is in meter in 3 with accents on the strong beats. What instruments accompany the singers?

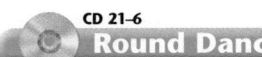
CD 21–6
Round Dance

**Traditional Round Dance
as performed at the Kihekah Steh Pow-wow, Skiatook, Oklahoma**
This pow-wow round dance is in the tradition of the Plains Indians and uses a leader-response style.

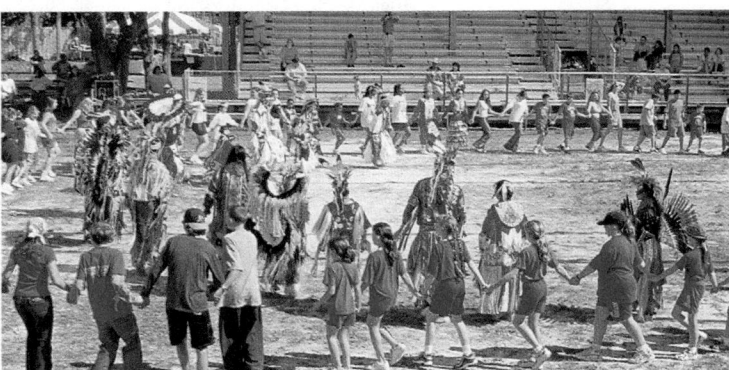

▲ An intertribal group of Native Americans demonstrating and teaching a friendship round dance to schoolchildren

Moving to the Round Dance

Perform the following round dance movements as you listen to the music again.

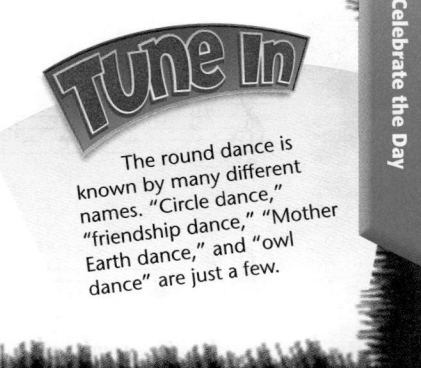
Tune In

The round dance is known by many different names. "Circle dance," "friendship dance," "Mother Earth dance," and "owl dance" are just a few.

• Form a circle.

• Join hands or place your hands on your neighbors' shoulders.

• Move to the left (clockwise) with a side-stepping movement. Move your feet on each strong beat—left-together.

Celebrate the Day

Unit 12 **445**

---

1 INTRODUCE

Ask students to read the text on p. 444 and then engage the class in a discussion about peace and unity. Invite students to read and discuss the lyrics of "I Am But a Small Voice," on p. 446, and identify the lyrics that relate to the themes of unity and peace.

2 DEVELOP

Listening

Invite students to read about the round dance on p. 445. Share with students the information in Cultural Connection on p. 444. Then, discuss the role of the pow-wow drum in the performance of the dance.

Play *Round Dance* **CD 21-6**. Help students discover that

6b
• The drums are playing accents on the strong beats in meter in 3.

• The singing is based on a leader-and-response form, with the leader starting and the others joining in.

Discuss with students how the pow-wow drum keeps the steady beat of the round dance. Point out that a large pow-wow drum is sometimes called the "sun drum" and the smaller hand drum is called the "moon drum."

Moving

Ask students to perform the movements described on p. 445 with *Round Dance* **CD 21-6**. If a large bass drum or other frame drums are available, select several students to perform eighth notes to accompany the round dance in pow-wow style.

continued on page 446

SKILLS REINFORCEMENT

5a ▶ **Reading** Guide students to correctly read sixteenth-note patterns grouped by beat. Copy the following rhythms from "I Am But a Small Voice" onto sheets of $8\frac{1}{2} \times 11$ inch paper. Invite students to use these "cards" to create 4-, 8-, or 16-beat rhythm patterns.

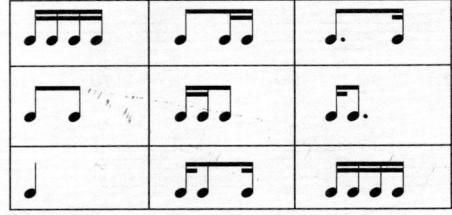

MOVEMENT

 ▶ **Signing** Sign language has been in use for almost 400 years. The manual alphabet was created in 1620, and the first school for the deaf was established in Paris in 1755. The first U.S. school for the deaf was established in 1817 by Laurent Clerc, whom some have called the most important deaf educator in history. American Sign Language uses signs made with the hands, facial expressions, body movement, and posture. It ranks fourth among the most commonly used languages in North America. Explore additional signing for "I Am But a Small Voice" on Resource Book p. G-24.

Unit 12 *Celebrate the Day* **445**

Analyzing

5a Have students examine "I Am But a Small Voice" to find groupings of sixteenth notes. Encourage students to draw imaginary circles around the sixteenth-note groupings in the song to identify each beat. See Skills Reinforcement on p. 445.

Help students follow the repeats, first and second endings, and *D.S. al Fine* in the song.

Listening

6b Invite students to listen to "I Am But a Small Voice" **CD 21-7** while following the music.

Help students discover that the song has four contrasting sections. Help them recognize that

- Section 1 is in unison; section 2 is in harmony.
- Section 3 is in unison; section 4 has a countermelody.
- Section 5 is an expanded section 1.
- Section 1 repeats.

Singing

Use the vocal chording warm-up in Skills Reinforcement below to prepare students' voices.

1c Invite students to sing the melody of "I Am But a Small Voice" **CD 21-7.**

Select a small group of students to sing the countermelody, which begins at the top of p. 447, with the recording.

Select a second small group of students to sing the harmony part, which begins on the fourth staff of the song, with the recording.

1d Encourage students to sing the song in harmony with the recording.

See Teacher to Teacher below for tips on changing voices.

No Voice Is Small

"I Am But a Small Voice" is a song with a message of peace and love.
Sing the song and reflect on the hope for peace in the world.

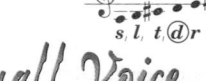

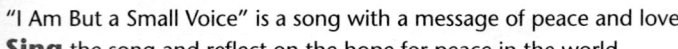

s, l, t, @r m f s lta t d'

CD 21-7

I Am But a Small Voice

Original Words by Odina E. Batnag   *English Words and Music by Roger Whittaker*

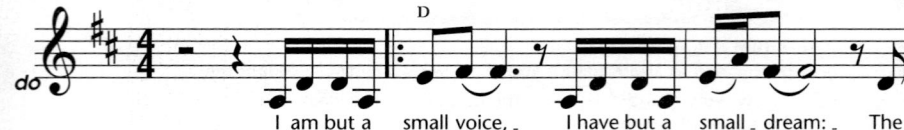

I am but a   small voice, _   I have but a   small _ dream: _   The
small voice, _   I have but a   small _ dream: _   To

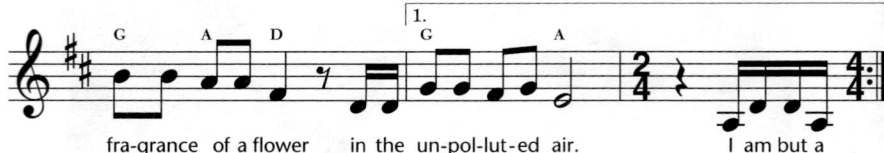

fra-grance of a flower   in the un-pol-lut-ed air.   I am but a
smile up - on the sun,   be __

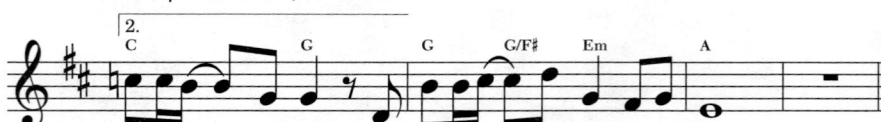

free to dance _ and sing,   Be   free to sing _ my song ev-'ry-where.

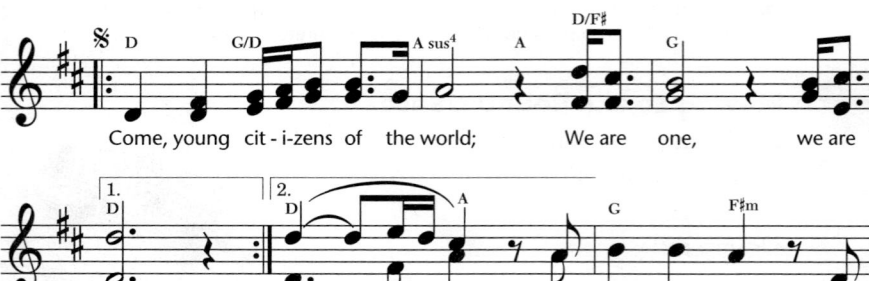

Come, young cit - i-zens of the world;   We are   one,   we are

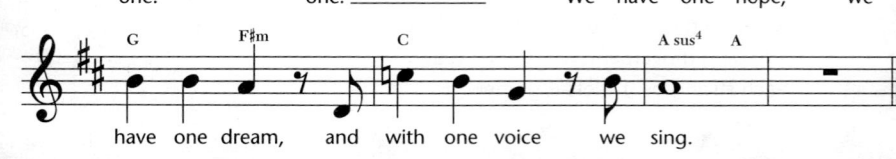

one.   one. __   We have one hope,   we

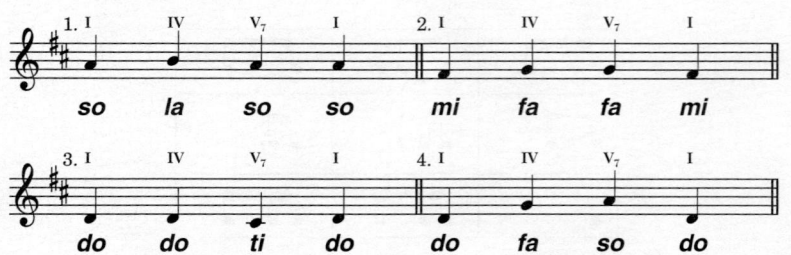

have one dream,   and   with one voice   we sing.

446

Footnotes

TEACHER TO TEACHER

▶ **Changing Voice Techniques** Boys with changing voices may want to sing "I Am But a Small Voice" in their new low register. Instead, encourage them to use their unchanged voice, giving the effect of a low treble register. Boys should also sing the opening in their unchanged voices because they will have the needed flexibility to navigate the large intervals in the first few measures. They can do this more easily if they are not flipping from changed to unchanged voice and vice versa. As the piece continues to the two-part section, give everyone an equal opportunity to sing the high part. Reinforce the value of continuing to sing in an unchanged voice for as long as possible. Doing so will help maintain vocal flexibility as they work through the coming changes.

SKILLS REINFORCEMENT

▶ **Singing** Encourage your students to do vocal chording as an opportunity to sing notes (as a warm-up) that will also train the ear to hear chords. Have students sing the notes below to a I-IV-V_7-I chord progression in D major. Use this as a warm-up to "I Am But a Small Voice."

1. I	IV	V_7	I	2. I	IV	V_7	I
so	la	so	so	mi	fa	fa	mi
3. I	IV	V_7	I	4. I	IV	V_7	I
do	do	ti	do	do	fa	so	do

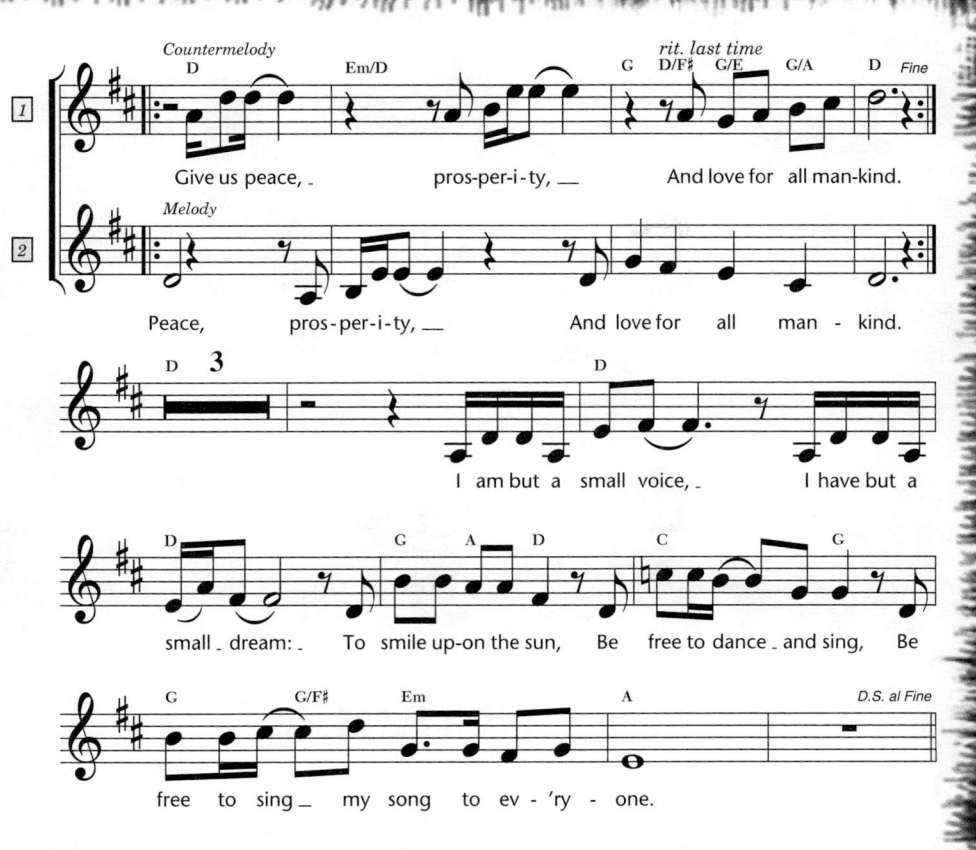

Give us peace, _ pros-per-i-ty, _ And love for all man-kind.

Peace, pros-per-i-ty, _ And love for all man - kind.

I am but a small voice, _ I have but a

small _ dream: _ To smile up-on the sun, Be free to dance _ and sing, Be

free to sing _ my song to ev - 'ry - one.

Signing a Message

Learn the three signs for the phrase, *I am but a small voice.* **Perform** the signs as you sing the song.

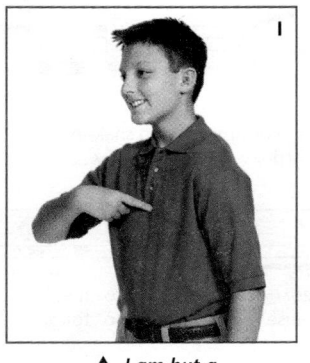

▲ *I am but a*

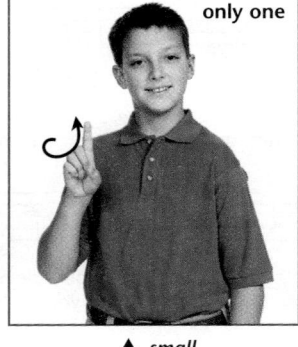

▲ *small*

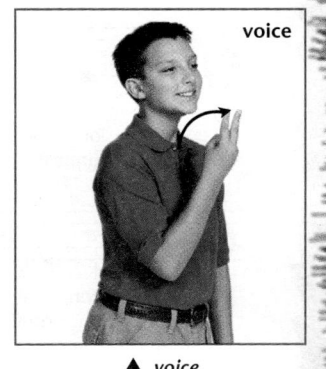

▲ *voice.*

Unit 12 447

Moving

Encourage students to learn the signs for "I Am But a Small Voice," p. 447. Find the places in the song where students can sign the words. Encourage students to perform the signs as they sing the song **CD 21-7.** For additional signing activities, see Resource Book p. G-24 and Movement on p. 445.

Playing

Have students learn a soprano recorder accompaniment for "I Am But a Small Voice" on Resource Book p. I-29.

Creating

Invite students to create rhythms using the cards described in Skills Reinforcement, p. 445. Inform students that each card represents one beat and that their rhythm should be four or eight beats long.

5a Divide the class into small groups and have each group

- Create a rhythm by placing the cards in order on the tray of the chalkboard or several music stands.
- Clap or play the rhythm on rhythm instruments.

Invite other members of the class to evaluate the performance.

3 CLOSE

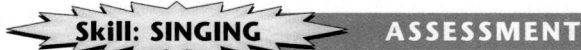

| Skill: SINGING | ASSESSMENT |

1a **Performance/Peer Critique** Divide the class into two groups and have each group perform "I Am But a Small Voice."

7a Invite each group to evaluate the other, using these criteria.

- Sixteenth-note rhythm patterns were sung correctly and clearly.
- Tied rhythms were performed accurately.
- Melody phrases were sung musically.
- The message was conveyed convincingly.

SPOTLIGHT ON

▶ **"I Am But a Small Voice"** In 1980, performer Roger Whittaker founded Children Helping Children, a songwriting contest sponsored by UNESCO (United Nations Educational, Scientific, and Cultural Organization). Children were asked to submit lyrics promoting peace and understanding. Whittaker agreed to set the words to music and to record the song. Over one million children from 57 nations entered the contest. The resulting song, "I Am But a Small Voice," was premiered at Radio City Music Hall in New York City in 1980. The lyrics were by Odina Batnag, a 13-year-old student from the Phillipines. The proceeds from record sales were given to UNESCO's program for handicapped children.

TECHNOLOGY/MEDIA LINK

MIDI/Sequencing Software Have students record their performance of "I Am But a Small Voice," using a digital audio recording program. Invite students to create a percussion accompaniment for the song. Students may perform a live percussion accompaniment and record it, using digital audio recording, or they may add a percussion track with MIDI sequencing. Students may play back their performances for self-assessment.

LESSON AT A GLANCE

Element Focus **EXPRESSION** Dynamics, articulation, and mood

Skill Objective **SINGING** Sing a ballad with expression

Connection Activity **GENRE** Create a dramatization for a ballad

MATERIALS

• "The Purple People Eater" **CD 21-9**
  Recording Routine: Intro (4 m.); v. 1; interlude (4 m.); v. 2; coda

• alto recorders

VOCABULARY

sequence   dynamics   articulation   timbre   ballad

◆ ◆ ◆ ◆ National Standards ◆ ◆ ◆ ◆

1a Sing accurately in large ensembles
2a Play instruments accurately alone
5a Read eighth and quarter notes in duple meter
6c Understand and use basic principles of chords in music analysis

MORE MUSIC CHOICES

For more songs and listenings based on humor:
"Bắt kim thang," p. 13
New Horizons in Music Appreciation, p. 98

1 INTRODUCE

Refer to Cultural Connection below, and engage students in a brief discussion of Halloween and the custom of dressing in costumes.

Tell students that the song "The Purple People Eater" is about fantasy dragons and flying saucers. The "purple people eater" would be an ideal subject for a Halloween costume.

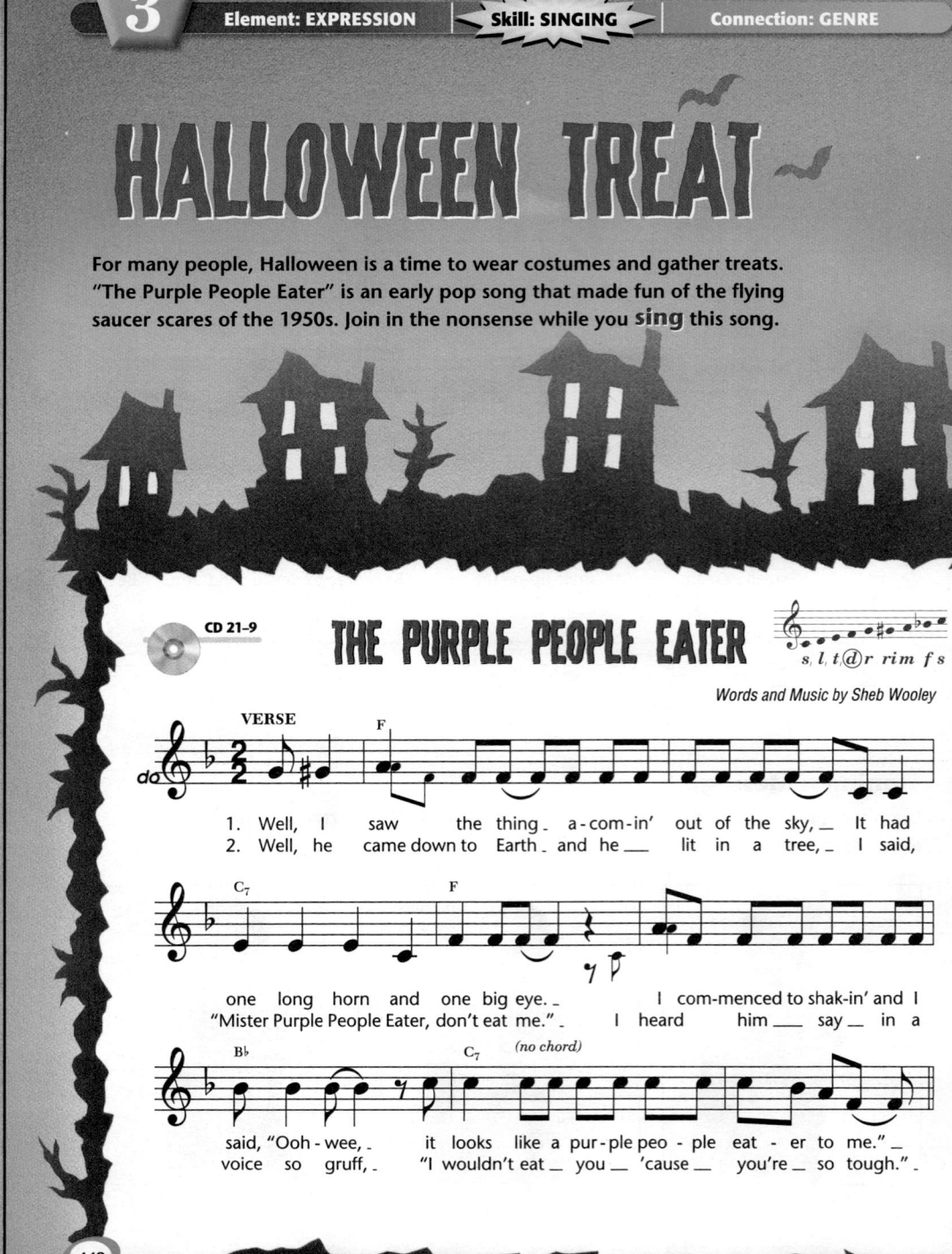

HALLOWEEN TREAT

For many people, Halloween is a time to wear costumes and gather treats. "The Purple People Eater" is an early pop song that made fun of the flying saucer scares of the 1950s. Join in the nonsense while you **sing** this song.

CD 21-9 THE PURPLE PEOPLE EATER

Words and Music by Sheb Wooley

VERSE

1. Well, I saw the thing a-com-in' out of the sky, It had
2. Well, he came down to Earth and he lit in a tree, I said,

one long horn and one big eye. I com-menced to shak-in' and I
"Mister Purple People Eater, don't eat me." I heard him say in a

said, "Ooh-wee, it looks like a pur-ple peo-ple eat-er to me."
voice so gruff, "I wouldn't eat you 'cause you're so tough."

448

Footnotes

CULTURAL CONNECTION

▶ **Halloween** The celebration of All Hallow's Eve began as early as 600 B.C. in Celtic Ireland. On October 31, the end of the Celtic summer and the beginning of the Celtic New Year, the Celts believed that spirits would visit their villages. To keep the spirits out of their villages, they darkened their houses, dressed in scary costumes, and paraded through the streets noisily. Trick or treating originated with the ancient Celts.

BUILDING SKILLS THROUGH MUSIC

▶ **Visual Arts** Have students identify the words in the song that describe the Purple People Eater. Have them create their own purple people eater that represents the description in the song.

ACROSS THE CURRICULUM

▶ **Language Arts** H. G. Wells wrote the story of an alien invasion, *War of the Worlds,* in 1898, long before space travel was even possible. Orson Welles turned the story into a radio drama broadcast on Halloween night 1938. Modeled after a news broadcast, Welles and others broadcast accounts of the alien invasion. Welles opened the program by announcing the show's contents were fictional. Nonetheless, thousands of people tuning in late panicked over the apparent invasion, jamming the streets, calling police, and protecting themselves from reported gas attacks. Welles's intention was to present an entertaining Halloween tale; however, the result was a landmark event in mass-media history.

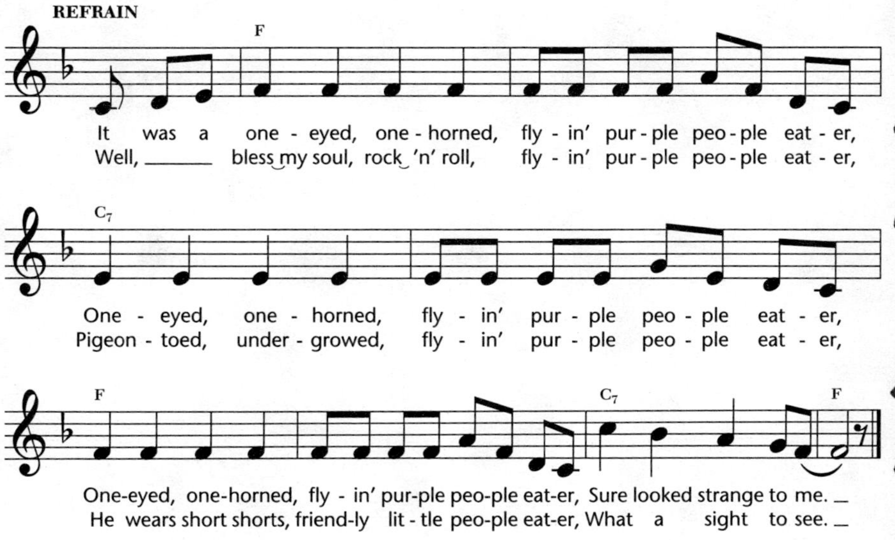

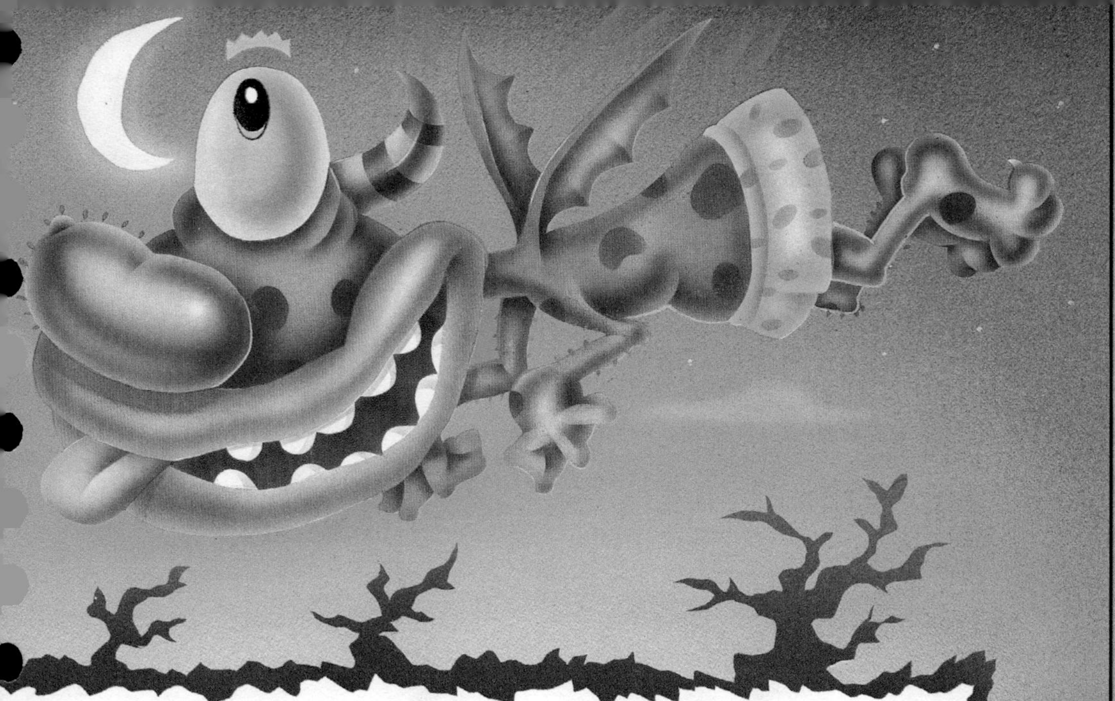

2 DEVELOP

Reading

5a Focus students' attention on the rhythm of the refrain on p. 449 and have them notice it uses all quarter and eighth notes except for the half note at the end.

Invite students to sight-read the rhythm of the refrain and the verse, first using rhythm syllables, then words.

Singing

1a Have students sing the song with the recording **CD 21-9.** Encourage students to experiment with dynamics, articulation, and mood as they sing the song again.

6c Encourage students to find a sequence in the refrain. (The second phrase of the refrain is a sequence of the first phrase, p. 449.)

Playing

Students can perform a countermelody on alto recorder to the song, as provided in Skills Reinforcement below.

Performing

Invite students to create a dramatization of the song, using the lyrics as inspiration.

Help students decide the number of characters needed, which part of the song will be sung by soloists and which part by the entire class, the type of movement needed by each character, and props and costumes.

3 CLOSE

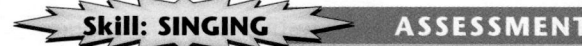

Skill: SINGING   **ASSESSMENT**

Performance/Observation Divide students into groups to perform their interpretation of the ballad. Observe whether they use expression—including dynamics, articulation, and mood—that is appropriate to the ballad.

REFRAIN

It was a one-eyed, one-horned, fly-in' pur-ple peo-ple eat-er,
Well, ___ bless my soul, rock 'n' roll, fly-in' pur-ple peo-ple eat-er,

One-eyed, one-horned, fly-in' pur-ple peo-ple eat-er,
Pigeon-toed, under-growed, fly-in' pur-ple peo-ple eat-er,

One-eyed, one-horned, fly-in' pur-ple peo-ple eat-er, Sure looked strange to me. _
He wears short shorts, friend-ly lit-tle peo-ple eat-er, What a sight to see. _

Celebrate the Day

Unit 12 **449**

SKILLS REINFORCEMENT

2a ► **Recorder** Students can play this accompaniment on the alto recorder to the verse of "The Purple People Eater." Have students practice mm. 2, 4, and 8 before trying to play with the recording **CD 21-9.**

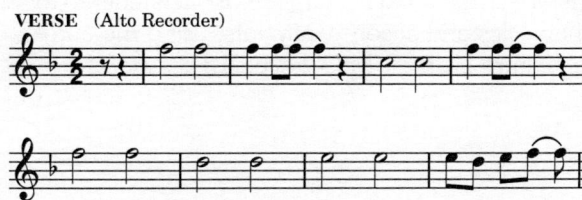

VERSE (Alto Recorder)

For a challenge, this accompaniment part can also be played with the refrain. Although the rhythms differ, the harmonies are the same.

TECHNOLOGY/MEDIA LINK

CD-ROM Ask students to create several different background accompaniments for "The Purple People Eater." Have them use *Band-in-a-Box* software to

- Take turns entering the song's chord progression into the computer.
- Experiment with singing the song with several different accompaniment styles. (Ask which style best fits the song.)
- Challenge students to use *Band-in-a-Box* to record and notate the song's melody. Suggest to students that it may be easier to enter the melody if they slow the tempo.

LESSON AT A GLANCE

Element Focus **TEXTURE/HARMONY** Western harmony

Skill Objective **PLAYING** Accompany a non-Western melody with Western-style accompaniment

Connection Activity **CULTURE** Explore the Thai festival of *Loi Krathong*

MATERIALS

- "*Loigratong*" (Thai)   **CD 21-11**
- "*Loigratong*" (English)   **CD 21-12**
  Recording Routine: Intro (4 m.); vocal; coda
- **Pronunciation Practice/Translation** p. 544
- **Resource Book** p. A-39
- guitar, keyboard, or Autoharp

VOCABULARY

lyrics   accompany   chords

> ◆ ◆ ◆ ◆ **National Standards** ◆ ◆ ◆ ◆
> **1c** Sing music from diverse cultures
> **2b** Perform easy instrumental pieces expressively
> **5a** Read dotted eighth notes in duple meter
> **7a** Students evaluate the music they perform

MORE MUSIC CHOICES

For more practice singing songs using I, IV, and V chords:
"Red River Valley," p. 11
"Everybody Loves Saturday Night," p. 296

1 INTRODUCE

Have students read about the festival of *Loi Krathong* (pronounced *Loigratong*, as in this song) on p. 450. *Loi Krathong* is a celebration of the full moon that is celebrated by the Thai people in November.

Share with students the information in Spotlight On, p. 451, and Cultural Connection below.

Thai Full Moon

In Thailand, people observe *Loigratong*, a celebration of the full moon, in November. *Loigratong* originated in the fourteenth century as a request to the water spirits to forgive any offenses against them.

Listen to the recorded Pronunciation Practice to learn the Thai words, then **sing** the song.

In many Asian cultures, Western harmonies are used today to accompany songs. **Perform** an accompaniment to "*Loigratong*," using the I, IV, and V$_7$ chords. Accompany the song with a keyboard, guitar, or Autoharp.

Festival participants holding "*Loigratong* boats"—small rafts in the shape of a lotus flower ▼

Footnotes

CULTURAL CONNECTION

▶ **Thai Language** Thai, the official language of Thailand, is a tonal language that uses words and vocal inflection. Thai has five inflections (tones) that alter the meaning of words—low, high, rising, falling, and monotone. The written language has 42 consonant characters (like letters) that represent 21 consonant sounds and 3 inflections. It also recognizes 28 combinations of 17 vowel characters. Tone markers are added to vowel and consonant characters to indicate vocal inflection.

BUILDING SKILLS THROUGH MUSIC

▶ **Science** Pose this problem to students: In order to plan a *Loi Krathong* celebration for next year, you must determine the date for the November full moon. Have students identify ways they can solve that problem.

SKILLS REINFORCEMENT

▶ **Creating** Ask students to create an accompaniment to "*Loigratong*," using the chords G, C, and D$_7$. Students may play these accompaniments on their choice of guitar, Autoharp, or keyboard. Discuss how rhythm and style changes in chord accompaniments affect the song's character. Invite students to explore additional styles and accompaniments, using the auto-accompaniment feature on their MIDI keyboards or *Band-in-a-Box* software.

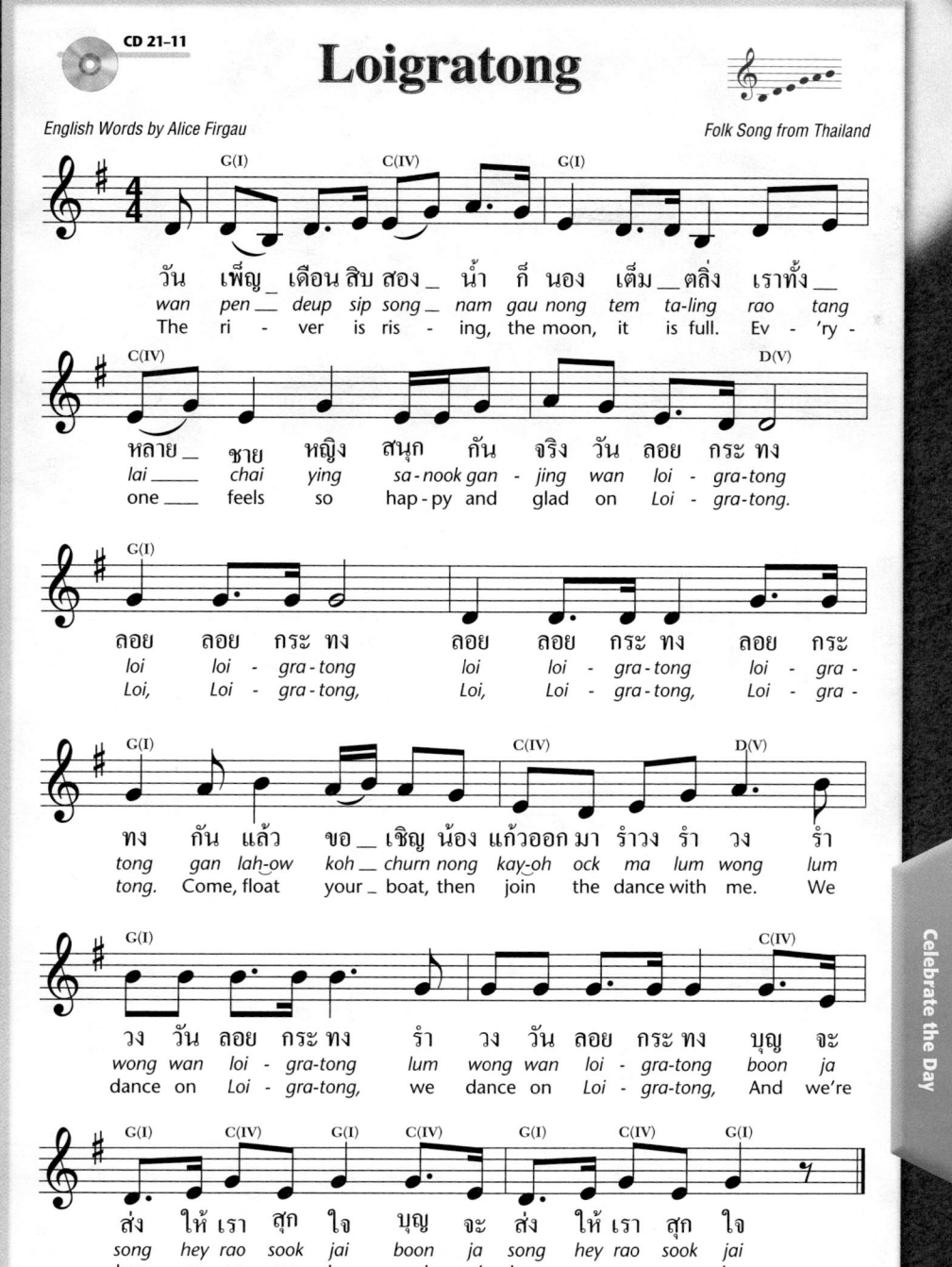

Loigratong

English Words by Alice Firgau

Folk Song from Thailand

วัน เพ็ญ เดือน สิบ สอง น้ำ ก็ นอง เต็ม ตลิ่ง เราทั้ง
wan pen deup sip song nam gau nong tem ta-ling rao tang
The ri - ver is ris - ing, the moon, it is full. Ev - 'ry -

หลาย ชาย หญิง สนุก กัน จริง วัน ลอย กระ ทง
lai chai ying sa-nook gan jing wan loi - gra-tong
one feels so hap-py and glad on Loi - gra-tong.

ลอย ลอย กระ ทง ลอย ลอย กระ ทง ลอย กระ
loi loi - gra-tong loi loi - gra-tong loi - gra -
Loi, Loi - gra-tong, Loi, Loi - gra-tong, Loi - gra -

ทง กัน แล้ว ขอ เชิญ น้อง แก้วออก มา รำวง รำ วง รำ
tong gan lah-ow koh churn nong kay-oh ock ma lum wong lum
tong. Come, float your boat, then join the dance with me. We

วง วัน ลอย กระ ทง รำ วง วัน ลอย กระ ทง บุญ จะ
wong wan loi - gra-tong lum wong wan loi - gra-tong boon ja
dance on Loi - gra-tong, we dance on Loi - gra-tong, And we're

ส่ง ให้ เรา สุก ใจ บุญ จะ ส่ง ให้ เรา สุก ใจ
song hey rao sook jai boon ja song hey rao sook jai
hap - py as can be, and we're hap - py as can be.

Unit 12 451

Celebrate the Day

2 DEVELOP

Reading

5a Direct students' attention to the rhythm patterns in *"Loigratong."* Have students

- Identify and clap repeating rhythm patterns.
- Find the location of a rhythm pattern as you clap it.
- Echo clap the song in phrases as you model it.

Singing

Use the Pronunciation Practice Guide on p. 544 and Resource Book p. A-39 to teach students the Thai text. Have students sing the Thai lyrics with the Pronunciation Practice **CD 21-14.**

1c Invite students to sing *"Loigratong"* with the Thai lyrics **CD 21-11** and then, in English **CD 21-12.**

Guide students to discern that the song is pentatonic.

Playing

Explain that popular music in Thailand and other Asian countries often has Western harmonies in the accompaniment.

2b Encourage students to practice the G (I), C (IV), and D (V) chords on guitar, keyboard, or Autoharp. Then, have them sing *"Loigratong"* while accompanying the song.

3 CLOSE

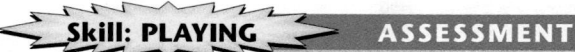 **Skill: PLAYING** — **ASSESSMENT**

7a **Performance/Self-Assessment** Invite students to accompany *"Loigratong"* with their choice of keyboard, guitar, or Autoharp while the class sings. Ask students to discuss the accuracy of their performance. Were chord changes made at the appropriate times?

SPOTLIGHT ON

▶ **The Festival** The Thai people celebrate *Loi Krathong* ("The Festival of Lights") on the days before and after the full moon (based on the lunar calendar). According to a thirteenth-century story, the celebration of *Loi Krathong* started when a young princess decorated a boat with candles and incense. She set it adrift, and it passed by a pavilion where her husband was hosting a party. All *Loi Krathong* celebrations involved setting beautifully decorated boats afloat at night. In the city of Chiang Mai, locals launch hot-air balloons to rid the town of its troubles. In the city of Tak, the people join their boats, or *krathongs*, together to create the illusion of necklaces floating on water.

SCHOOL TO HOME CONNECTION

▶ **Electronic Encyclopedia** Ask students to use an electronic encyclopedia in the local library to write a short report on Thai culture, music, or the *Loi Krathong* festival.

TECHNOLOGY/MEDIA LINK

Web Site Have students go to *www.sfsuccessnet.com* and explore the music of Thailand.

LESSON AT A GLANCE

Element Focus	**MELODY** Harmonic minor
Skill Objective	**PLAYING** Play a song in harmonic minor
Connection Activity	**CULTURE** Discuss the holiday Chanukah and the purpose of the *dreydl*

MATERIALS
- "S'vivon"   CD 21-15
- "Dreydl"   CD 21-16
  Recording Routine: Intro (4 m.); vocal; coda
- **Pronunciation Practice/Translation** p. 544
- **Resource Book** p. A-40
- triangle, tambourine, low drum, xylophones (2), glockenspiels (2), or melody bells

VOCABULARY

score   meter   harmonic minor   form

◆ ◆ ◆ ◆ **National Standards** ◆ ◆ ◆ ◆

1c Sing music from diverse cultures
2a Perform instrumental music from diverse cultures
2b Perform easy instrumental pieces with technical accuracy
6b Listen and analyze uses of pitch in music from diverse cultures

MORE MUSIC CHOICES

For more practice in singing songs in minor:
"Hey, Ho! Nobody Home," p. 28
"Sometimes I Feel Like a Motherless Child," p. 241

1 INTRODUCE

Invite students to discuss what they know about the traditions of Chanukah. Include information from Across the Curriculum below.

Inform students that *"S'vivon"* is Hebrew for *dreydl* and explain that a *dreydl* is a spinning top that Jewish children use to play a game.

Chanukah Lullaby

People of the Jewish faith celebrate Chanukah [HAHN-noo-kah], the Festival of Lights. During Chanukah, children of all ages play the *dreydl* [DREY-dl] game. The *dreydl* is a four-sided top with a Hebrew letter on each side. When the *dreydl* stops spinning, players exchange pennies and food according to which side of the *dreydl* faces upward.

Sing the traditional Chanukah song "S'vivon" [SEH-vee-vohn].

CD 21-15

S'vivon (Dreydl)

Hebrew Words by L. Kipnis
English Words by Sue Ellen LaBelle and David Eddleman

Folk Song from Israel

S' - vi - von,   sov sov sov,   Cha - nu - kah _____ hu - chag tov.
S' - vi - von,   turn and turn,   Play the game, it's _ fun to learn.

Cha - nu - kah   hu-chag tov,   S' - vi - von _____ sov sov sov.   Chag sim - chah _____
Cel - e - brate,   take a turn,   spin the top as   can - dles burn.   Cha - nu - kah, the

hu   la   am _____ nes   ga - dol ha - ya _____ sham. _____
peo - ple's   fes - ti - val,   Tell   the   tale   of   Is - rael's   tem - ple;

Nes ga - dol ha - ya   sham, _____ chag sim - chah _____ hu   la   am.
Cel - e - brate the   light and   prayer, _ And   how a   won - der   hap - pened there.

452

Footnotes

ACROSS THE CURRICULUM

▶ **Social Studies** Chanukah is a Jewish holiday that lasts for eight days and nights. Families celebrate the holiday in their homes by lighting one candle of the *menorah* each night until all candles are lit. Jewish families recite special prayers, sing songs, play Chanukah games, and exchange a gift each night. They may also eat traditional foods such as apple fritters and cookies, crispy potato latkes, and cheese-filled donuts.

BUILDING SKILLS THROUGH MUSIC

▶ **Math** Have students create a graph that is representative of the harmonic-minor scale. Using that model, they should be able to quickly identify the number of half steps between any two notes in the scale.

SPOTLIGHT ON

▶ **Dreydl Game** The *dreydl* is a four-sided spinning top with Hebrew letters carved on each side. The *dreydl* can be used to play a game for two or more players. Each player starts with several tokens. Each player puts a set amount of tokens into a *kupah*, or a collection pool. One player spins the *dreydl*, which falls on one of the letters. The player follows the directions below. The game continues until players lose all their tokens.

Nun	Tokens stay in the pool.
Gimel	Player wins the pool.
Hay	Player wins half the tokens in the pool.
Shin	Player loses tokens to the pool and must replace them before the next turn.

Chanukah Ensemble

Play percussion instruments as an accompaniment to *"S'vivon."* When the tambourine player plays a half note, you will shake, or rattle, the tambourine. Experiment by adding an *accelerando* to the music, or by playing the song at different tempos. **Describe** how changes to the tempo affect the character of the song.

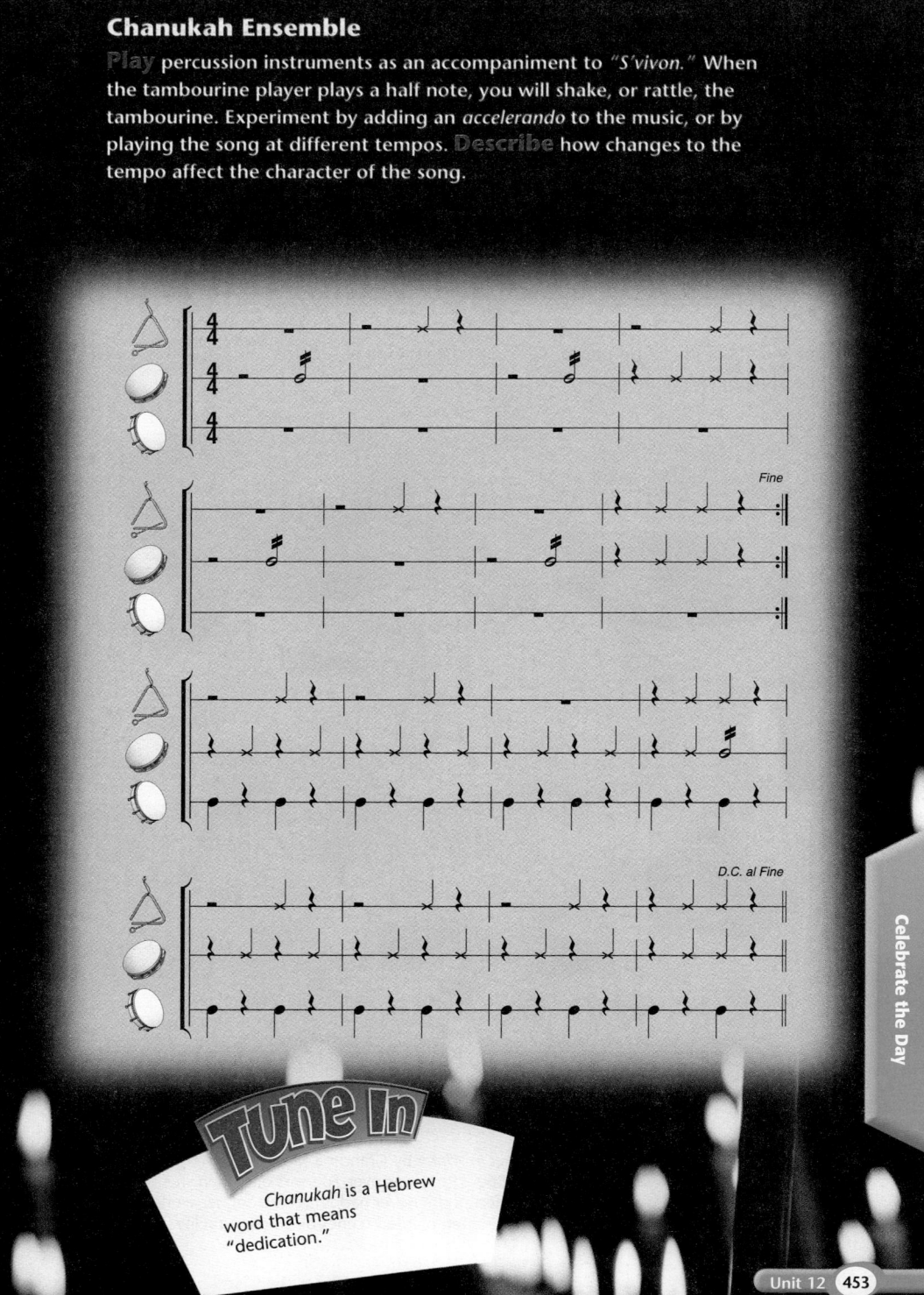

Chanukah is a Hebrew word that means "dedication."

2 DEVELOP

Singing

Invite students to sing the E-harmonic-minor scale as a warmup, using pitch syllables.

1c Using the Pronunciation Practice Guide on p. 544 and on Resource Book p. A-40, and the Pronunciation Practice **CD 21-18**, have students learn the Hebrew lyrics to the song. Then, sing the song with the recording **CD 21-15**.

1c Have students sing *"Dreydl,"* the English version of the song, with accompaniment **CD 21-16**.

Reading

6b Help students to discern that *"S'vivon"* is in the key of E minor. Have students identify and locate the elements that define the melody as E-harmonic minor. (The key signature of one sharp, the accidental D♯, and the first and last notes being E.)

Playing

2b Invite students to play the rhythm ensemble on p. 453 on percussion instruments. Explain that the slanted lines across the stem of the notes in the tambourine part indicate that the tambourine should sustain for two beats. (shake wrist for two beats)

2a Invite students to play the activities in Skills Reinforcement below. Then, ask students to perform the percussion accompaniment as they sing the song with the recording **CD 21-15**.

3 CLOSE

Skill: PLAYING — ASSESSMENT

Performance/Observation Invite students to play the melody of *"S'vivon"* on keyboard. Have them point out one musical element that defines the melody as E-harmonic minor. Observe students for pitch accuracy in their playing.

SKILLS REINFORCEMENT

2b ▶ **Playing** *"S'vivon"* is written in E minor. Students can play the song on melody bells, resonator bells, or keyboards.

Reinforcement Use a marked MIDI keyboard to assist students that may have difficulty remembering the notes of a piano keyboard. Have them locate and play the E-harmonic-minor scale before learning the melody. Pair experienced keyboard players with those needing assistance.

On Target Invite students to play the song in pairs—one to play the A sections (mm. 1–8) of the song, and another to play the B section (mm. 9–16) of the song. Have students play their accompaniments as the class sings the song.

Challenge Invite students to improvise a bell accompaniment (*obbligato*) to *"S'vivon."*

TECHNOLOGY/MEDIA LINK

CD-ROM Use *Band-in-a-Box* to experiment with tempo for *"S'vivon."* Have students

- Take turns entering the song's chord progression into the computer software, using *Band-in-a-Box*.
- Experiment with the tempo settings, gradually increasing the tempo.
- Perform the song with different tempo settings, singing faster and faster as the song progresses.

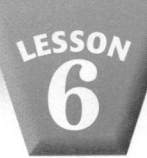

LESSON AT A GLANCE

Element Focus — **TEXTURE/HARMONY** Traditional and contemporary harmony; polyphonic and homophonic textures

Skill Objective — **SINGING** Sing a song in two parts with different textures

Connection Activity — **RELATED ARTS** Discuss the art of Grandma Moses

MATERIALS

- "Winter Song" — **CD 21-19**

  Recording Routine: Intro (4 m.); refrain; v. 1; refrain; v. 2; melody/countermelody

- "Troika" from *Lieutenant Kijé,* Op. 60 — **CD 21-21**

- hand chimes, resonator bells, jingle bells, tambourine, wrist bell, wood blocks (two sizes), shakers

VOCABULARY

texture	homophonic	polyphonic
countermelody	unison	

◆ ◆ ◆ ◆ National Standards ◆ ◆ ◆ ◆

1b Sing easy pieces with technical accuracy
1d Sing music written in two and three parts
2a Play instruments accurately alone and in small ensembles
4c Compose, using traditional sound sources
5c Identify standard notation symbols for rhythm
6b Listen and analyze uses of texture and rhythm timbre, and harmony in music from diverse genres
6c Understand and use basic principles of rhythm in music analysis
8a Show how different arts portray the same idea in unique ways

MORE MUSIC CHOICES

More songs in two-part harmony:

"Lean on Me," p. 14
"Four Strong Winds," p. 170

Winter Celebrations

In many parts of the world people celebrate the change of seasons. Winter is a time of many celebrations.

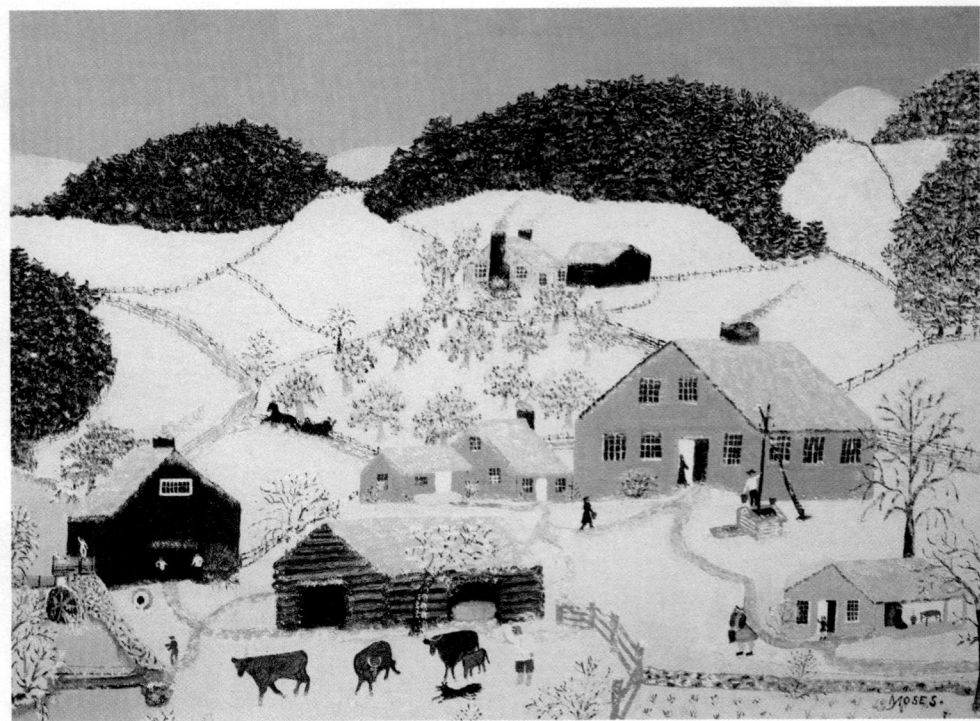

Arts Connection

▲ *The Old Oaken Bucket in Winter* by Grandma Moses. Grandma Moses (1860–1961) was over 70 years old when she began painting. Although she never had an art lesson, her work is praised by critics. She often painted scenes of simple rural life.

Footnotes

CULTURAL CONNECTION

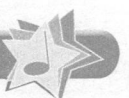

▶ **World Peace Bell** The world's largest swinging bell is the World Peace Bell located in Newport, Kentucky. It is decorated with images of the last millennium's accomplishments. The central image is of three children from different cultures holding hands. The bell measures 12 feet tall by 12 feet in diameter and weighs 66,000 pounds.

BUILDING SKILLS THROUGH MUSIC

▶ **Visual Arts** Have students read about Sergei Prokofiev on p. 457. Focus their attention on the portrait of Prokofiev by Pyotr Konchalosky and have them describe the color, form, and proportion of the painting, using art vocabulary.

SPOTLIGHT ON

▶ **The Artist** Anna Mary Robertson Moses (1860–1961) was fondly called "Grandma" because she was 78 years old when she started to paint. Grandma Moses, born in 1860, lived and worked on a New York farm most of her life. She started painting when she was forced to give up embroidery due to arthritis. Inspired by Currier and Ives prints and by her memories of her childhood, her artwork created nostalgia for simpler bygone days. Art collectors loved her depictions of rural life of the 1800s and early 1900s. Grandma Moses's paintings, such as *A Parade* (1949) and *Horse Shoeing* (1960), became known as American primitive art. Grandma Moses was 101 when she died in 1961.

Wintertime Singing

Sing "Winter Song" in unison. After you know the melody, learn the harmony part and the countermelody part.

Read and clap the rhythm of measures 1 and 2. How many times does this rhythmic phrase appear?

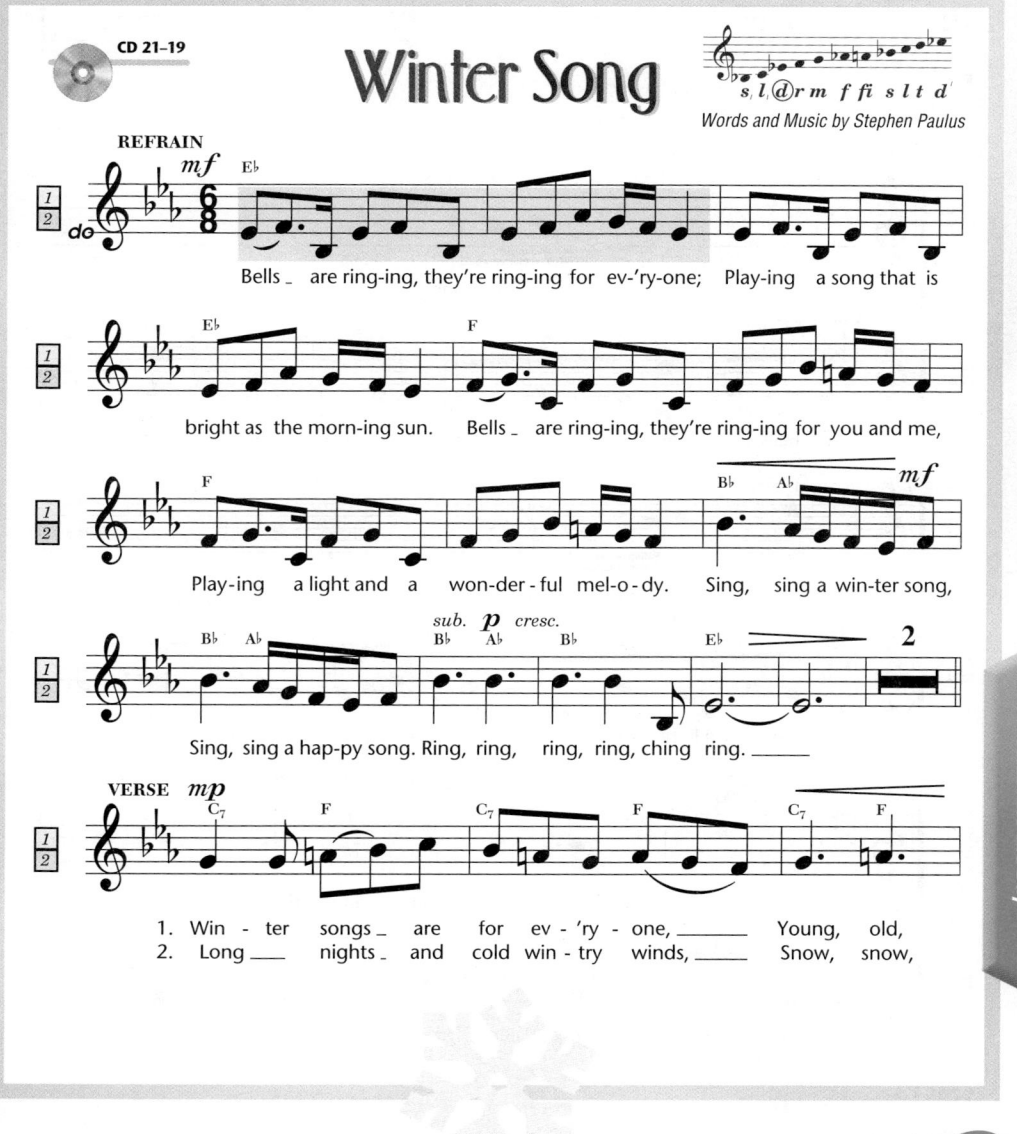

Celebrate the Day

1 INTRODUCE

Engage students in a short discussion about seasons and have them tell what their favorite season is and explain why it's their favorite.

8a Then, discuss the season of winter. Ask students to look at *The Old Oaken Bucket* by Grandma Moses on p. 454 and describe the winter scene. Share with students the information about the work and the artist, Grandma Moses, from Spotlight On, p. 454, and Across the Curriculum below.

Help students recognize why Grandma Moses's artwork was labeled primitive art.

2 DEVELOP

Reading

5c **ASK** What meter is "Winter Song"? ($\frac{6}{8}$)

Ask students to read and clap the rhythm for mm. 1 and 2. (Highlighted by the blue box.)

ASK **How many times does this rhythm phrase appear?** (6 times)

Invite students to play Stump the Class, by clapping a two-measure rhythm pattern found anywhere in "Winter Song." Ask the class to find the rhythm in the song.

When students are comfortable reading the rhythm patterns of all parts:

ASK **On the last measure of the fourth score/line, p. 455, there is a thick bar with the number 2 on it. What does it mean?** (two measures of rests)

Can you identify the music symbols referring to dynamics? (m. 1: *f*; m. 9: ——; m. 11: sub. *p*; m. 12 ——).

Can you identify the music terms referring to dynamics? (m. 11: sub. = subito; m. 11: cresc. = crescendo)

continued on page 456

TEACHER TO TEACHER

▶ **Performing Suggestions** Help students arrange a performance of "Winter Song" in a formal concert. They may want to add classroom instruments or change the voicing of the piece. Some ideas you might suggest:

2a • Play hand chimes/resonator bells whenever the words *ring, ring* occur. Play chords behind the singing, or play the melody on bells in place of the singing.

• Assign small groups to perform the verses. Part 1 may sing verse 1 alone, followed by Part 2 on verse 2.

4c • Compose a jingle bell ostinato to perform with the song. Help students decide when it occurs, when it stops, and if it alternates with other instrumental ostinatos. For example, a wrist bell might play mm. 1–8 and a tambourine mm. 9–14.

ACROSS THE CURRICULUM

▶ **Fine Art** Grandma Moses is a famous name in the field of folk art, also called primitive or native art. Primitive art includes paintings, sculptures, textiles, and other work created by an artist with little or no formal art training. Folk art is an important source of information about the past. The Museum of American Folk Art, in New York City, exhibits early 1800s portraiture (the painting of people in formal poses) and quilts as forms of folk art. Quilts were made by African American slaves to convey stories and secret messages. Made as wedding presents and signs of friendship, quilters sewed special messages or symbols into the quilt blocks.

Lesson 6 Continued

Can you identify the music terms referring to tempo? (three measures from the end: *rit.* = *ritardando*)

Invite students to identify the music symbol referring to tempo. (the *fermata* in the last line of the music) Have students interpret the tempo and dynamic symbols and terms when performing.

Singing

1b Invite students to sing the melody of "Winter Song" **CD 21-19** with the recording.

Direct students' attention to the harmony sections of the song and help them discover that

- Some sections of the song are in unison and others are in harmony.
- One of the harmony sections has a countermelody.

Invite a group of students to

- Sing the countermelody with the recording.
- Sing the harmony part beginning on the second staff of p. 456 with the recording.

1d Encourage students to sing the song in harmony with the recording.

6b **ASK** How many different textures did the composer use in this song? (two: homophonic and polyphonic)

Which section is polyphonic? (the section that added the countermelody)

Which sections are homophonic? (The second staff on the top of p. 456 and the last seven measures of the song with the lyrics *ring*.)

6c Help students discover that the "ring" section is a homophonic texture.

ASK Why is this a homophonic texture? (Because both parts are singing the same rhythm, the same words, and pitches within the same chord.)

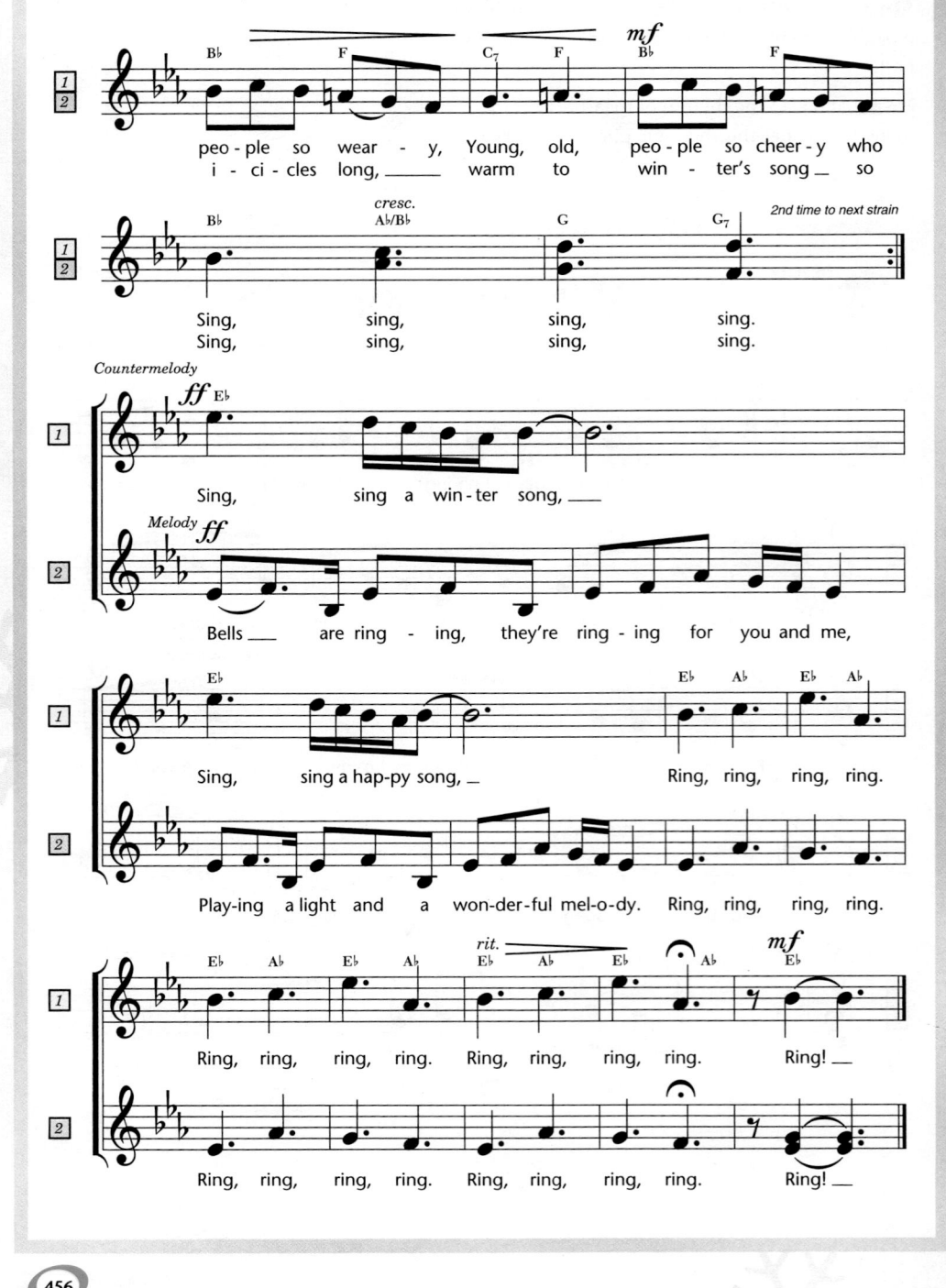

456

Footnotes

SKILLS REINFORCEMENT

2a ▶ **Playing** Have students play the rhythms below to the *allegro* section of *Troika* **CD 21-21** with the recording. Use two different size woodblocks. Hold the shakers (or maracas) in two hands. The shakers should be played "forward" on each beat; the offbeat eighth notes will occur naturally as the shakers are brought back.

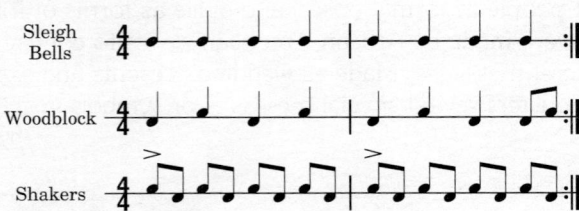

SPOTLIGHT ON

▶ *Lieutenant Kijé Suite* One of Prokofiev's most popular works was an orchestral suite adapted from the film score of the 1933 pro-Soviet film *Lieutenant Kijé*. Prokofiev had just moved to the U.S.S.R. from Paris and needed to produce a successful work of artistic propaganda to earn Soviet citizenship. He also needed to earn the favor of the Stalinist regime, which was beginning a campaign of terror that cost the lives of many of Prokofiev's friends and supporters. Although the movie flopped, he arranged the music into an orchestral suite, which became his first major U.S.S.R. success.

Troika Tune

Listen to this musical depiction of a *troika,* a Russian sleigh drawn by a team of three horses. How does the music convey the motion of the sleigh gliding across the snow-covered countryside?

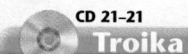
CD 21-21
Troika

from *Lieutenant Kijé*
by Sergei Prokofiev

Prokofiev composed this music in 1933 for a film about the daring adventures of a lieutenant in the Czar's army.

MUSIC MAKERS

Sergei Prokofiev

Composer **Sergei Prokofiev** (1891–1953) grew up in Ukraine on his family's farm. His mother, a talented piano player, sparked her son's interest in music with visits to the opera in Moscow. At the age of 11, Prokofiev received private lessons in music theory and composition. At the age of 13, he began his formal training in music at the St. Petersburg Conservatory, the leading music school in Russia.

Prokofiev composed for ballet (*Romeo and Juliet*), opera (*The Love of Three Oranges*), and the orchestra (*Lieutenant Kijé*).

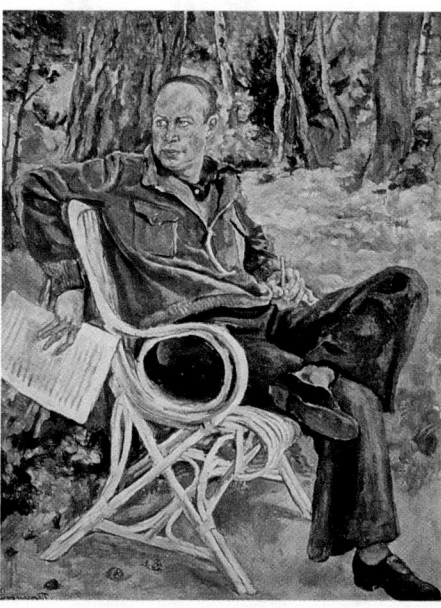

Arts Connection

▲ *Sergei Prokofiev* by Pyotr Konchalosky, 1934

Celebrate the Day

Unit 12 **457**

Listening

Remind students that riding in a horse-drawn sleigh is an old tradition, and an activity for people who live where it snows in the winter.

Have students read the text at the top of p. 457.

6b ASK As you listen to the introduction, does anything about the harmony strike you as being unusual? (The harmony and melody don't always sound traditional.)

Invite students to listen to *Troika* **CD 21-21.**

Share with students that Prokofiev was a twentieth-century composer who sometimes used contemporary harmonies.

ASK What instrument gives you the feeling that you are on a horse-drawn sleigh? (sleigh bells)

6c Invite students to listen to the rhythm patterns in *Troika* and help students identify the rhythms that suggest the motion of the sleigh. (The continuous eighth notes played by the strings, sometimes in *pizzicato,* suggest motion; the steady quarter-note beat of the sleigh bells suggests the steps of the horses.)

Encourage students to read about the composer, Sergei Prokofiev, on p. 457. Share additional background from Spotlight On, pp. 456 and 457.

3 CLOSE

Skill: SINGING **ASSESSMENT**

1d Performance/Self-Assessment Write the words *unison, polyphonic,* and *homophonic* on the board. Invite a volunteer to point to the appropriate texture as the class sings "Winter Song."

Divide the class into two groups, each singing one part. Have the class sing "Winter Song" and the volunteer points to the correct texture. Have the class swap parts and sing the song again.

Ask students to discuss their performance, and which textures required greater effort to sing accurately.

SPOTLIGHT ON

▶ **The Composer** Sergei Prokofiev (1891–1953) was one of the leaders of the Soviet proletarian school of composers. He began as a child prodigy and studied music under Rimsky-Korsakov in St. Petersburg. He wrote many pieces based on World War II themes; some evoked the heroic spirit of Soviet troops, others the tragic loss associated with warfare. *Peter and the Wolf,* his most famous work, was an immediate success at home and overseas. Famous personalities, including Eleanor Roosevelt, provided narration for several recordings. Although Prokofiev fell in and out of favor with the Communist Party, his artistic talent was recognized by the entire musical world. Prokofiev's work displayed a genius for melody and use of dissonance.

TECHNOLOGY/MEDIA LINK

Web Site Invite students to go to *www.sfsuccessnet.com* for more information on the life and music of Sergei Prokofiev and other Russian composers.

As with Dmitri Shostakovich, p. 443, remind students of the issues of composers creating music under the Soviet regime.

LESSON AT A GLANCE

Element Focus **RHYTHM** Meter: $\frac{6}{8}$, $\frac{3}{4}$, $\frac{2}{2}$

Skill Objective **SINGING** Sing three Christmas songs in different meters

Connection Activity **CULTURE** Read about and discuss caroling traditions of the Christmas holiday

MATERIALS

- "Caroling, Caroling" **CD 21-22**
  Recording Routine: Intro (4 m.); v. 1; interlude (4 m.); v. 2; interlude (4 m.); v. 1; coda
- "Gloria, Gloria" **CD 21-24**
  Recording Routine: Intro (8 m.); vocal (unison), interlude (4 m.); vocal 3-part round; coda
- **Pronunciation Practice/Translation** p. 545
- "Good King Wenceslas" **CD 21-27**
  Recording Routine: Intro (5 m.); five verses
- Good King Wenceslas **CD 21-29**
- **Resource Book** pp. A-41, C-7
- hand chimes or resonator bells/keyboard, finger cymbals or triangle

VOCABULARY

carol	sequence	octavo	staves
ostinato	countermelody	ballad	

◆◆◆ National Standards ◆◆◆

1b Sing easy pieces with technical accuracy
1d Sing music written in three parts
2a Play instruments accurately in small ensembles
5a Read quarter and eighth notes in alla breve time
5e In performance classes, sightread easy music
6a Listen and describe events in music using appropriate terms

MORE MUSIC CHOICES

For more practice with $\frac{2}{2}$ meter:
"Swanee," p. 118

For more practice with $\frac{6}{8}$ meter:
"Greensleeves," p. 49

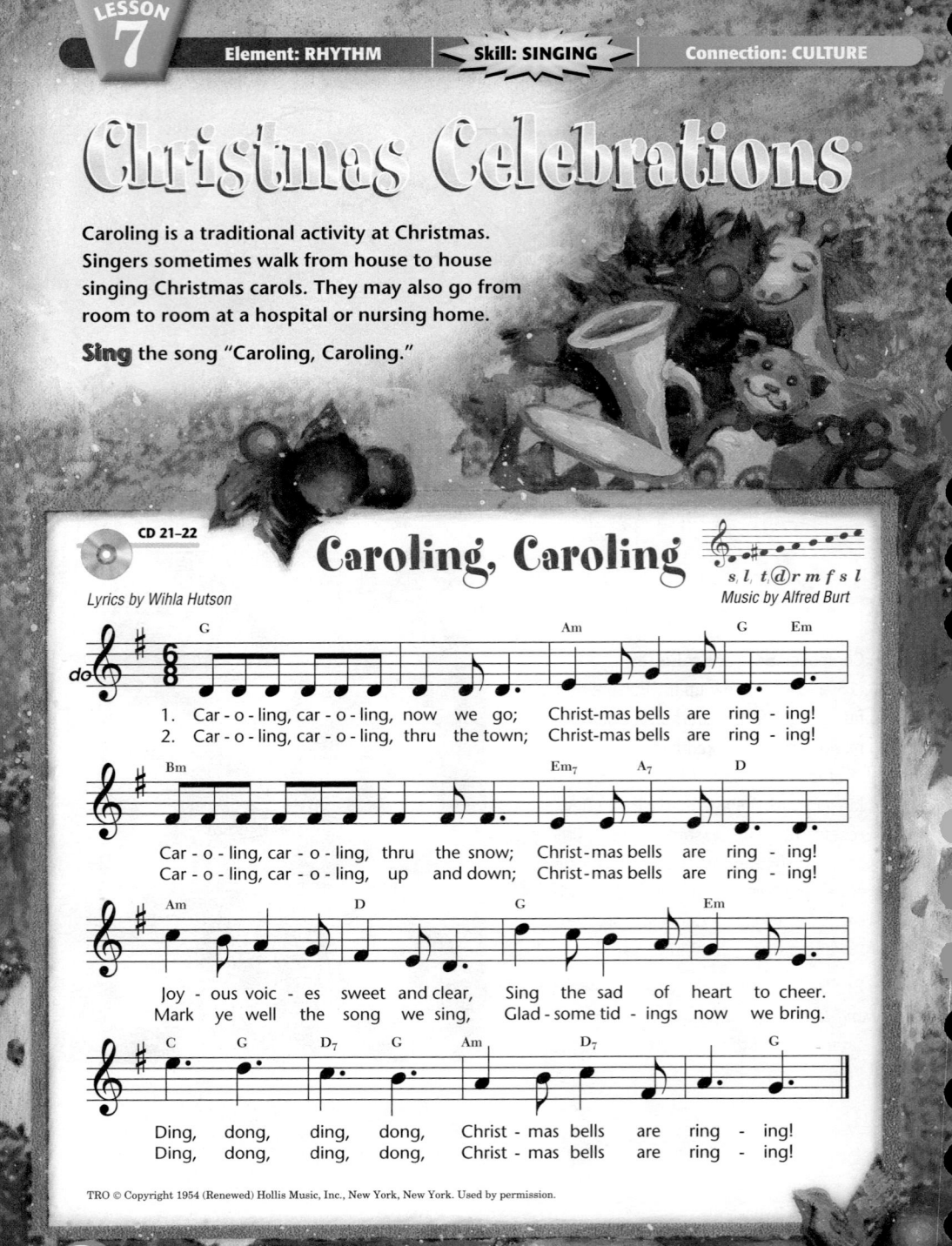

Christmas Celebrations

Caroling is a traditional activity at Christmas. Singers sometimes walk from house to house singing Christmas carols. They may also go from room to room at a hospital or nursing home.

Sing the song "Caroling, Caroling."

CD 21-22

Caroling, Caroling

Lyrics by Wihla Hutson
Music by Alfred Burt

s, l, t, @ r m f s l

1. Car-o-ling, car-o-ling, now we go; Christ-mas bells are ring-ing!
2. Car-o-ling, car-o-ling, thru the town; Christ-mas bells are ring-ing!

Car-o-ling, car-o-ling, thru the snow; Christ-mas bells are ring-ing!
Car-o-ling, car-o-ling, up and down; Christ-mas bells are ring-ing!

Joy-ous voic-es sweet and clear, Sing the sad of heart to cheer.
Mark ye well the song we sing, Glad-some tid-ings now we bring.

Ding, dong, ding, dong, Christ-mas bells are ring-ing!
Ding, dong, ding, dong, Christ-mas bells are ring-ing!

TRO © Copyright 1954 (Renewed) Hollis Music, Inc., New York, New York. Used by permission.

458

Footnotes

SKILLS REINFORCEMENT

▶ **Reading** Each of the three carols has a different meter, and each uses a different meter beat unit. For "Caroling, Caroling" the meter is $\frac{6}{8}$, "Gloria, Gloria" is $\frac{3}{4}$, and "Good King Wenceslas" uses $\frac{2}{2}$. Encourage students to say and then notate the following phrase in each of the three meters: *Tell me who's coming for dinner.* Have them decide which meter best fits the phrase.

BUILDING SKILLS THROUGH MUSIC

▶ **Reading** The lyrics of "Good King Wenceslas" can be difficult for students to understand. Using a Story Map (Resource Book, p. C-7), have students identify the characters, the setting, and the story line that is told in this song.

CULTURAL CONNECTION

▶ **Christmas Caroling** The first carols were written in England (1400s) and were associated with dancing. Dampened during the Protestant Reformation, carol singing re-emerged in England during the Victorian era. Many composers published new collections of carols to meet the growing demand for Christmastime carols. Victorian interest spread to the United States in the mid-1800s, where caroling was done from house to house. The British American Society had horse-drawn wagons take carolers to members' houses in predawn Christmas morning. The number of towns sponsoring caroling grew from 30 in 1918 to over 2,000 in 1928.

Glorious Times

The music for "Gloria, Gloria" was composed by Franz Joseph Haydn. The lyrics are in Latin.

Sing the entire melody of "Gloria, Gloria." Then divide into groups and **perform** it as a round.

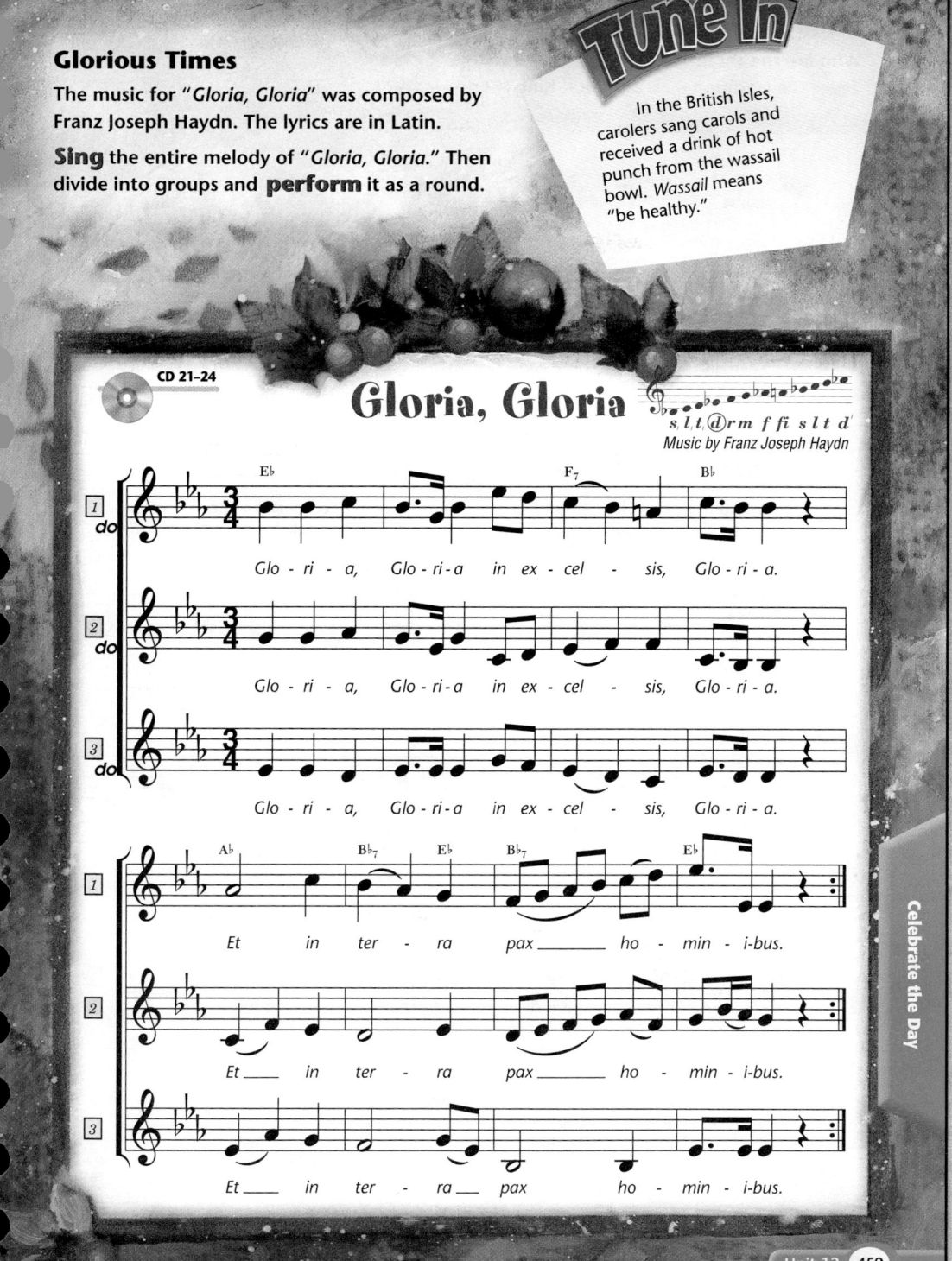

In the British Isles, carolers sang carols and received a drink of hot punch from the wassail bowl. *Wassail* means "be healthy."

CD 21-24

Gloria, Gloria

s, l, t, @ r m f fi s l t d'
Music by Franz Joseph Haydn

Glo - ri - a, Glo - ri - a in ex - cel - sis, Glo - ri - a.

Et in ter - ra pax _____ ho - min - i - bus.

Unit 12 459

1 INTRODUCE

Engage students in a discussion of caroling traditions and share with them information about caroling from Cultural Connection on p. 458. Explain that all three songs in this lesson are appropriate for caroling.

2 DEVELOP

Singing

5e Invite students to sight-read "Caroling, Caroling" **CD 21-22** with the recording.

6a **ASK Can you find any sequences in this song?** (Yes; mm. 9 and 10, and 11 and 12 form a sequence.)

What is the meter for this song? (⁶⁄₈)

Help students discover how the song fits the meter by having them read the lyrics to the song. Ask students to do the activity on meters in Skills Reinforcement on p. 458.

ASK Can the lyrics be sung in ⁴⁄₄ meter? (no)

Invite students to sing "Caroling, Caroling" **CD 21-22** with the recording.

As students look at the song *"Gloria, Gloria"* on p. 459, help them discover that it contains Latin lyrics and has three parts.

SAY The song is a round but is written in *octavo* style. Each part has a staff, and the staves are joined into systems.

ASK How many systems are on the page? (two)

How many staves are there per system? (three)

Use the Pronunciation Practice Guide on p. 545 and on Resource Book p. A-41, and the Pronunciation Practice **CD 21-26** to teach the song in Latin.

Invite students to sing Part 1, then Part 2, and finally Part 3 *"Gloria, Gloria"* **CD 21-22** with the recording. Assign a group to each part.

continued on page 460

TEACHER TO TEACHER

▶ **Assigning Harmony Parts** Since each of the three parts in *"Gloria, Gloria"* has a different range, singers should be assigned to a part that best fits their ranges.

- Part 1 has a range of an octave. Assign this part to singers who can easily sing from E♭ above middle C to E♭ top space.
- Part 2 has a range of an octave from B♭ below middle C to the B♭ above. Students who can sing these pitches comfortably should be assigned Part 2.
- Part 3 has the most limited range. It extends a seventh from the B♭ below middle C to the A♭ above with most of the pitches hovering between middle C and the G above. Assign boys with changing voices to this part.

SPOTLIGHT ON

▶ **King Wenceslas I** Wenceslas was the ruler of Bohemia (now the Czech Republic) from 907 to 929. He was known as a pious nobleman who worked for his people's religious and educational improvement. Wenceslas was murdered on his way to mass by his younger brother, Boleslav, who committed the act from anger about the takeover of Bohemia by the Germans. Peasants praying at Wenceslas's tomb reported many miracles. Boleslav moved the remains to the Church of St. Vitus in Prague in 932. King Wenceslas later became the patron saint of Bohemia and Czechoslovakia. His generosity and kindness are memorialized in J. M. Neale's Victorian carol "Good King Wenceslas."

1d Using the recording **CD 21-24,** have group 1 sing its part to the repeat sign, then add group 2, and finally add group 3. See Teacher to Teacher, p. 459, on assigning parts.

Playing

Help students organize resonator bells into the four chords required to accompany the song—E♭, A♭, B♭₇, F₇—and have students practice playing the chords. Or use an electronic keyboard with color-coded chords set on chimes or bell setting.

2a Invite students to sing the song in three parts with the resonator bell or keyboard accompaniment:

- Have the bells or keyboard play the song once through as an introduction.
- Add the voices in three parts.
- Conclude with the bells or keyboard playing the song as a coda.

Have students read the lyrics of "Good King Wenceslas" on p. 460.

ASK What do you call a song that tells a story? (a ballad)

1b Invite students to sing "Good King Wenceslas" **CD 21-27** with the recording. See Spotlight On, p. 459, for information on this king.

Help students discover that

- The song has four phrases, with the last phrase being one measure longer than the others.
- Each phrase has two sections, with each first section two measures long.
- The second two measures of the phrase answers the first two measures of the phrase.

5a Invite students to perform as a bell choir ensemble at an evening concert or school assembly using the accompaniment to "Good King Wenceslas" in Skills Reinforcement (Bells) below.

A Kingly Carol

Who are the three characters in this Christmas ballad?
Sing the traditional carol "Good King Wenceslas."

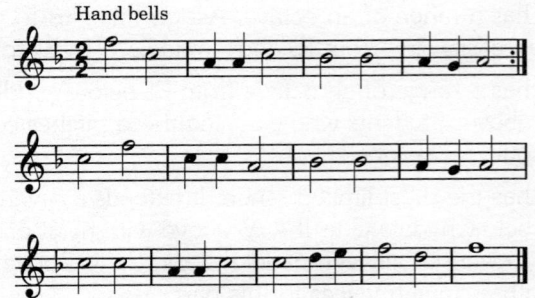

CD 21-27
MIDI 34

Good King Wenceslas
s, l, t, @ r m f s
Traditional

1. Good King Wen-ces-las looked out On the Feast of Ste-phen,
2. "Hith-er, page, and stand by me, If thou know'st it, tell-ing,

When the snow lay round a-bout, Deep and crisp and e-ven;
Yon-der pea-sant, who is he? Where and what his dwell-ing?"

Bright-ly shone the moon that night, Though the frost was cru-el,
"Sire, he lives a good league hence, Un-der-neath the moun-tain;

When a poor man came in sight, Gath-'ring win-ter fu-el.
Right a-gainst the for-est fence, By Saint Ag-nes' foun-tain."

3. "Bring me flesh and bring me wine, Bring me pinelogs hither,
   Thou and I will see him dine, When we bear them thither."
   Page and monarch forth they went, Forth they went together;
   Through the rude wind's wild lament, And the bitter weather.

4. "Sire, the night is darker now, And the wind blows stronger;
   Fails my heart, I know not how, I can go no longer."
   "Mark my footsteps, good my page! Tread thou in them boldly;
   Thou shalt find the winter's rage Freeze thy blood less coldly."

5. In his master's steps he trod, Where the snow lay dinted;
   Heat was in the very sod Which the saint had printed.
   Therefore, Christian folk, be sure, Wealth or rank possessing;
   Ye who now will bless the poor, Shall yourselves find blessing.

460

Footnotes

SKILLS REINFORCEMENT

▶ **Percussion** Invite students to play the rhythm ostinatos below on verses 1 and 5 of "Good King Wenceslas." They can be played on finger cymbals or triangle.

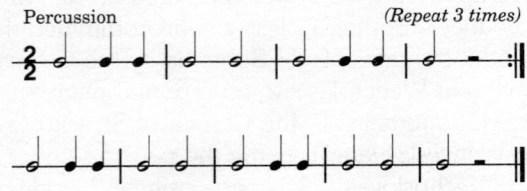

Percussion   *(Repeat 3 times)*

SKILLS REINFORCEMENT

▶ **Bells** Invite students to play this bell accompaniment on verses 1 and 5 of "Good King Wenceslas," using hand chimes or resonator bells.

Hand bells

The Good King Continues

Listen to this contemporary version of the same carol.

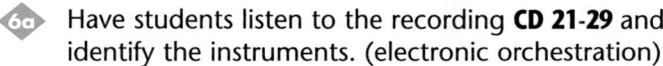

CD 21–29
Good King Wenceslas

Traditional Carol
as performed by Mannheim Steamroller
This arrangement features electronic timbres and
contemporary rhythms.

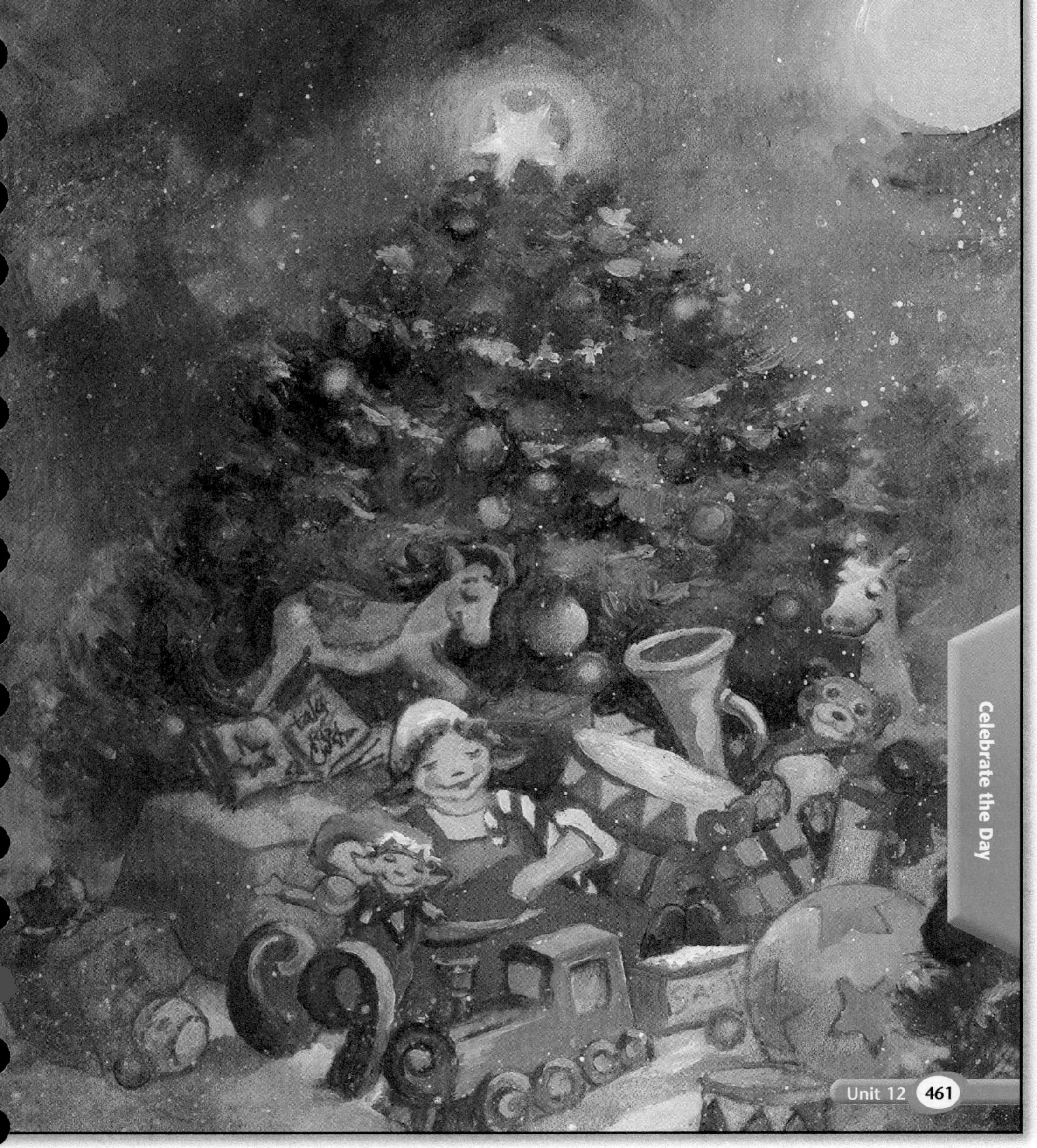

Add the percussion ensemble in Skills Reinforcement
(Percussion) on p. 460 to create additional variety and
interest in this concert performance of "Good King
Wenceslas."

Select two soloists or two small groups to sing the parts
of the king and the page, while the rest of the class
sings the story with the recording **CD 21-27.**

Listening

Inform students that "Good King Wenceslas" is a very
old carol, and Mannheim Steamroller has given it an
updated twist. See Spotlight On below.

6a Have students listen to the recording **CD 21-29** and
identify the instruments. (electronic orchestration)

**ASK How many times do you hear the ballad, and
what is different about the last time?** (four times;
voices were added)

**What rhythm ostinato do you hear repeated
throughout the music?**

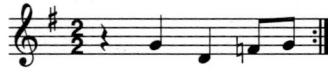

ASK Is the melody of the ostinato always the same?
(yes)

Playing

5a Invite students to sing or play the ostinato on melody
bells or keyboard as they listen to the recording
CD 21-29.

3 CLOSE

Skill: SINGING **ASSESSMENT**

Performance/Observation Have students sing
the carols as they walk through the halls. Remind them
of the importance of good tone quality and accurate
pitch, and to demonstrate appropriate small-ensemble
performance techniques during informal concerts.
Observe whether the meters and rhythms were performed accurately.

Celebrate the Day

Unit 12 **461**

SPOTLIGHT ON

▶ **Mannheim Steamroller** Chip Davis is the force behind
Mannheim Steamroller, a record label that has sold more
Christmas records than any other artist. Davis's creation introduced New Age music to the world. It is a combination of rock
and classical, electronic and acoustic. Davis records the material
in various locations, then mixes it with computerized sounds in a
recording studio. The name Mannheim pays homage to an eighteenth century orchestra known for introducing the Mannheim
crescendo to the classical music world. Davis's compositional and
recording techniques include the use of the *crescendo* to build
dynamic tension and excitement in his music.

SCHOOL TO HOME CONNECTION

▶ **Caroling** Ask students to discuss ideas with their family
about going caroling or about the class's visiting a children's hospital or nursing home to sing carols. Make proper arrangements.

TECHNOLOGY/MEDIA LINK

MIDI/Sequencing Software Use the MIDI song file of
"Good King Wenceslas" to explore orchestration and ostinatos in
the song. Ask students to

• Select new electronic instruments on tracks.

• Play the new orchestrations and discuss the differences.

• Add new rhythm or ostinato tracks to the arrangement.

Unit 12 *Celebrate the Day* **461**

LESSON AT A GLANCE

Element Focus   **MELODY** Key change or modulation

Skill Objective   **SINGING** Sing a song with a modulation

Connection Activity   **CULTURE** Read about and discuss the history, meaning, and customs of Kwanzaa

MATERIALS
- "The Joy of Kwanzaa"   **CD 22-1**
  Recording Routine: Intro (4 m.); vocal; coda
- percussion instruments

VOCABULARY

key	modulation	*rallentando*	*fermata*
ritardando	*accelerando*	triplet	

◆ ◆ ◆ ◆ National Standards ◆ ◆ ◆ ◆

1a Sing accurately in small and large ensembles
2a Play instruments accurately in small ensembles
4a Compose short pieces, demonstrating balance through music
6a Listen and describe events in music using appropriate terms
6c Understand and use basic principles of tonality in music analysis
7a Students evaluate the music they hear
8b Identify ways music relates to social studies
9c Compare, in several cultures, functions music serves

MORE MUSIC CHOICES

More songs that modulate:
"Go, My Son," p. 188
"One Moment in Time," p. 352
"Love in Any Language," p. 476

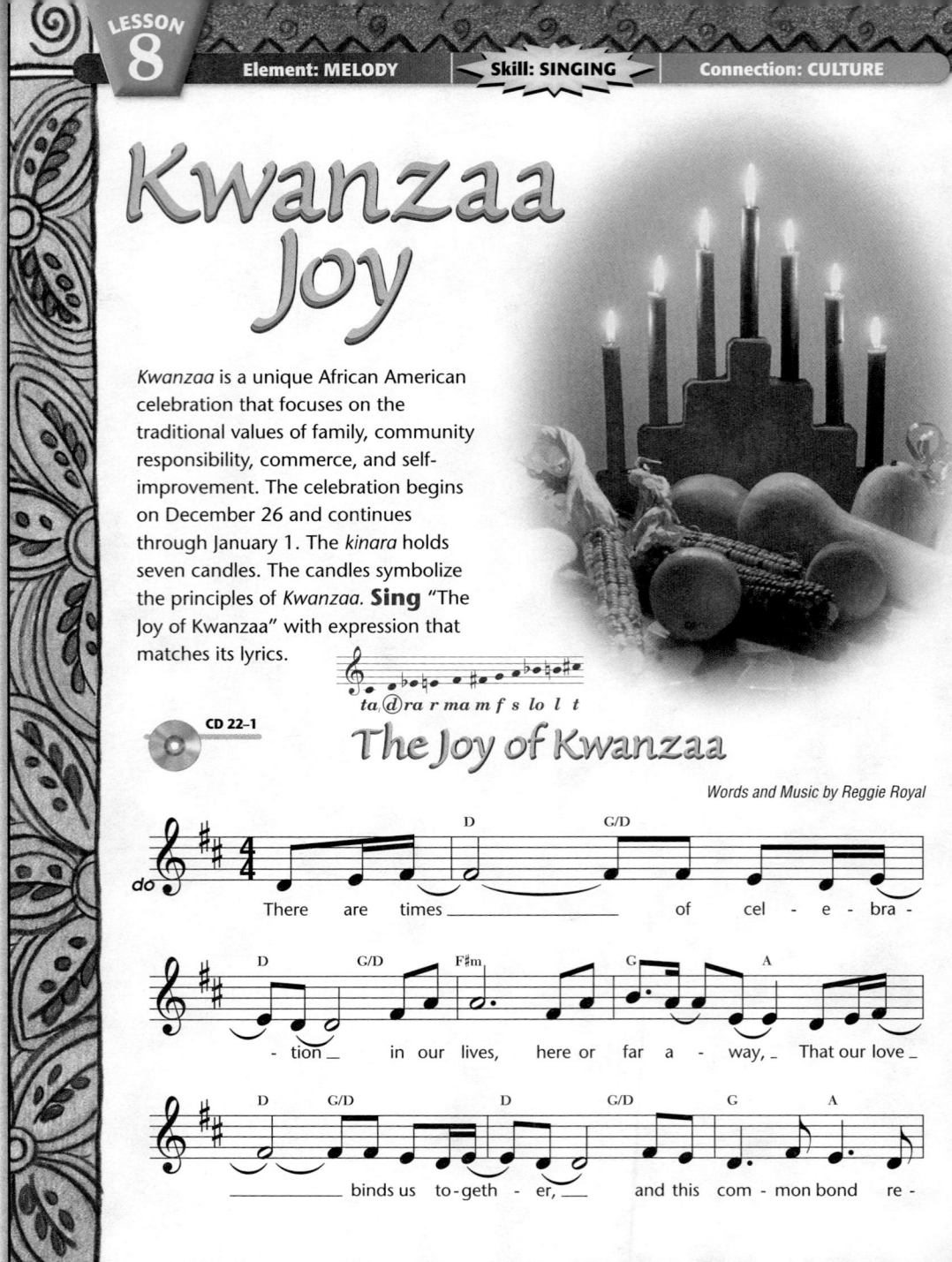

Kwanzaa Joy

Kwanzaa is a unique African American celebration that focuses on the traditional values of family, community responsibility, commerce, and self-improvement. The celebration begins on December 26 and continues through January 1. The *kinara* holds seven candles. The candles symbolize the principles of *Kwanzaa*. **Sing** "The Joy of Kwanzaa" with expression that matches its lyrics.

ta d r a r ma m f s lo l t

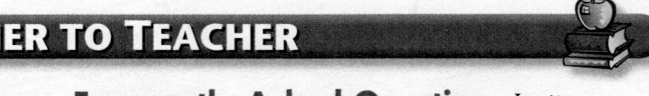
CD 22-1

The Joy of Kwanzaa

Words and Music by Reggie Royal

do

There are times _____ of cel - e - bra -

- tion _____ in our lives, here or far a - way, _____ That our love _____

_____ binds us to-geth - er, _____ and this com - mon bond re -

462

Footnotes

CULTURAL CONNECTION

▶ **The Seven Principles of Kwanzaa (*Nguzo Saba*)**
Dr. Karenga, the father of Kwanzaa, believed that African Americans of the past drew upon seven principles to survive. The seven principles are unity, self-determination, collective work and responsibility, cooperative economics, purpose, creativity, and faith. Adults are encouraged to discuss these principles with children during Kwanzaa celebrations. Discuss these principles with your students.

BUILDING SKILLS THROUGH MUSIC

▶ **Reading** Have students read the reference article on Holiday Music at **Take It to the Net** at *www.sfsuccessnet.com,* and then answer this question: What does this article identify as the three ways that music is used in the celebration of holidays?

TEACHER TO TEACHER

▶ **Kwanzaa Frequently Asked Questions** Invite students to learn about Kwanzaa. Ask students to make a list of words (under the headings *who, what, when, where*) and then create questions using the words. Following are some answers:

Dr. Maulana Ron Karenga started Kwanzaa on December 26, 1966, to dedicate a holiday to the African American experience and to celebrate African American heritage. Families and friends gather each night for a service honoring one Kwanzaa principle. They greet each other, exchange presents, and light candles in the *kinara,* or candleholder. The celebration lasts for seven days, in honor of the seven Kwanzaa principles.

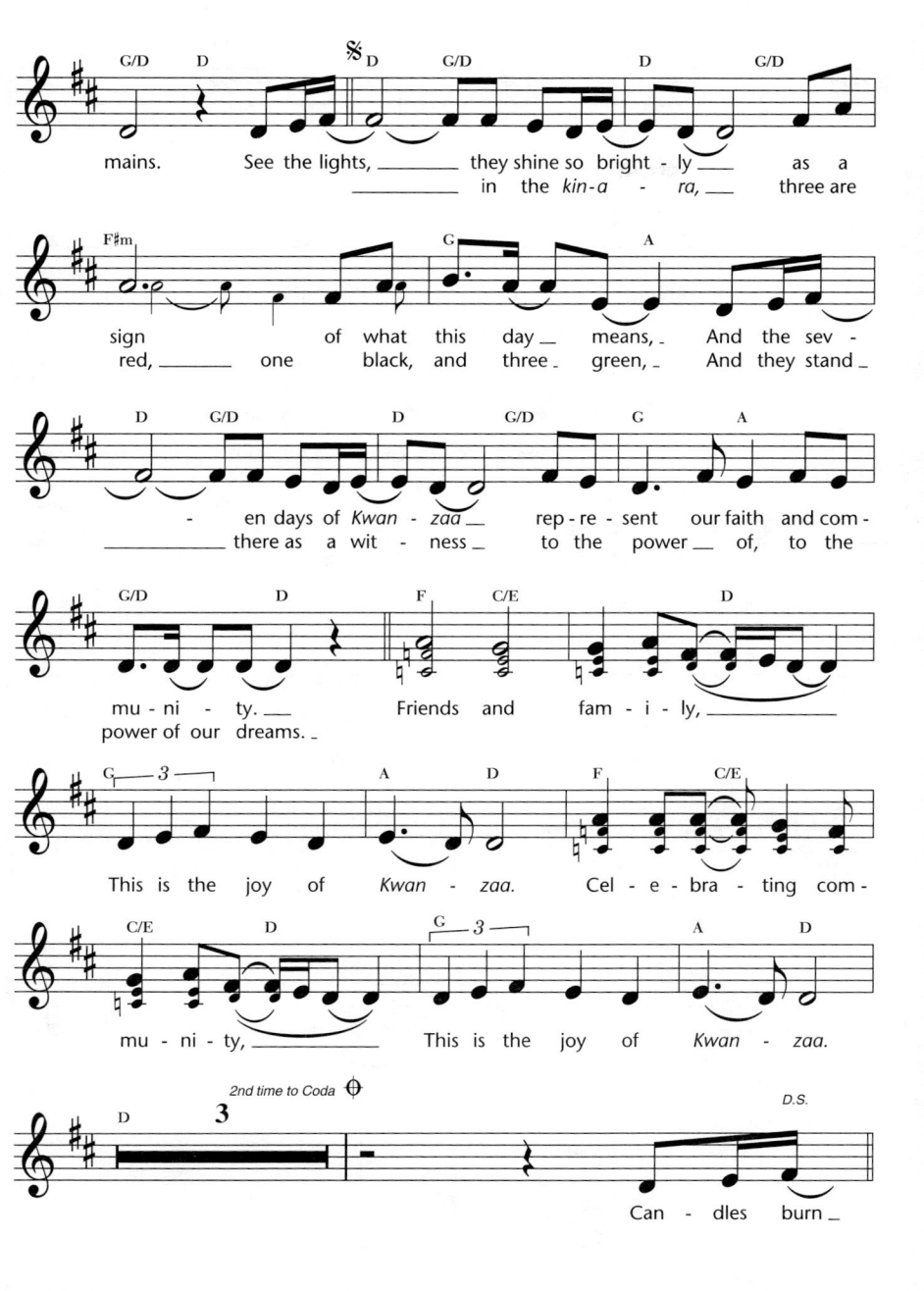

mains. See the lights, _____ they shine so bright - ly ____ as a
_____ in the *kin-a - ra*, ____ three are

sign _____ of what this day __ means, _ And the sev -
red, _____ one black, and three _ green, _ And they stand _

- en days of *Kwan - zaa* __ rep-re-sent our faith and com -
_____ there as a wit - ness _ to the power __ of, to the

mu - ni - ty. __ Friends and fam - i - ly, _____
power of our dreams. _

This is the joy of *Kwan - zaa.* Cel - e - bra - ting com -

mu - ni - ty, _____ This is the joy of *Kwan - zaa.*

2nd time to Coda

D.S.

Can - dles burn _

1 INTRODUCE

Have students read about Kwanzaa on p. 462. Discuss with students the history of Kwanzaa presented in Teacher to Teacher on p. 462 and its meaning in Across the Curriculum on p. 464. Tell students that music plays an important part in Kwanzaa (Spotlight On, p. 463) and its ceremonies (Across the Curriculum on p. 463). Then, discuss the seven principles of Kwanzaa in Cultural Connection on p. 462.

2 DEVELOP

Listening

Encourage students to listen to "The Joy of Kwanzaa" **CD 22-1** and follow the repeats and signs in the music.

6a Help students discover that the music has three different sections.

As they listen to the recording, have students raise their hands each time they hear the first theme (mm. 1–8) repeat.

Singing

1a Invite students to first sing the theme (mm. 1–8) and then, the entire song with the recording.

Have students locate the key change on p. 464.

ASK Is the new key higher or lower than the original key? (higher)

6c Help students discover that the song began in the key of D and moved to the key of E♭, which is a half-step higher.

Focus students' attention on the two measures before the key change. Explain that the key change actually begins in these measures and is called a *modulation*.

continued on page 464

ACROSS THE CURRICULUM

▶ **Social Studies** In the Kwanzaa ceremony, the family respects the Kwanzaa principles and honors its African heritage and ancestors. The family shares the Unity Cup, symbolizing the first principle of Kwanzaa and listens to a sacred text. The family then recites the African pledge and the American Pledge of Allegiance. The leader shares the symbolism of the African flag colors and candles to be lit. An inspirational speech using a Kwanzaa principle or example from African history follows. Then, the family lights the appropriate number of candles held by the *kinara*. The family honors its ancestors and rededicates their lives to the Kwanzaa principles. After the African pledge and a feast, they recite *"Harambee"* seven times to end the ceremony.

SPOTLIGHT ON

8b ▶ **Music in the Kwanzaa Ceremony** Music plays an important role in the Kwanzaa ceremony. Music is used to respect and honor the African heritage of Kwanzaa.

Family members begin the ceremony with African drumming or a song. The family sings a song before the inspirational speech. Finally, another song precedes the lighting of the candles on the *kinara*.

In addition to music for the ceremony, many popular songs have been written for the Kwanzaa holiday. These are similar in purpose to the carols written for Christmas. Songs are meant to be sung and enjoyed. Reggie Royal's "The Joy of Kwanzaa" is a song of celebration for the Kwanzaa holiday that students will enjoy singing.

ASK What happens to the text during the modulation? (It repeats the words *we can learn*.)

Explain to students that a modulation is a place where tempo changes may occur. A modulation can use a combination of tempo changes, such as

- *rallentando* (gradually slower)
- *fermata* (to hold a note)
- *accelerando* (gradually faster)

Although this performance does not use a tempo change at the modulation, invite students to explore how the tempo may be changed at this modulation. (a *rallentando* beginning at the words *we can learn*; to a *fermata* on B♭ and the word *learn*; followed by an *accelerando* on the word *unity*; back to the original tempo)

Creating

 Divide students into a few groups to create a simple call-and-response song or speech piece, using Kwanzaa questions or statements. (Subjects could include unity, self-determination, collective work and responsibility, cooperative economics, purpose, creativity, faith, *kinara*, libation, *umojo*, *mkeka*, *harambee*.)

Have each group

- Decide which subjects to include.
- Decide on the words and phrases.

Playing

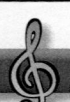 Invite students to add a percussion accompaniment to their song. Provide several instruments to choose from; if possible, include instruments indicative of Africa.

Encourage the groups to experiment with *rallentandos* (*ritardandos*) in their song.

Tell students they may also choose another option: *accelerando*.

ASK What do you think *accelerando* means? (to speed up)

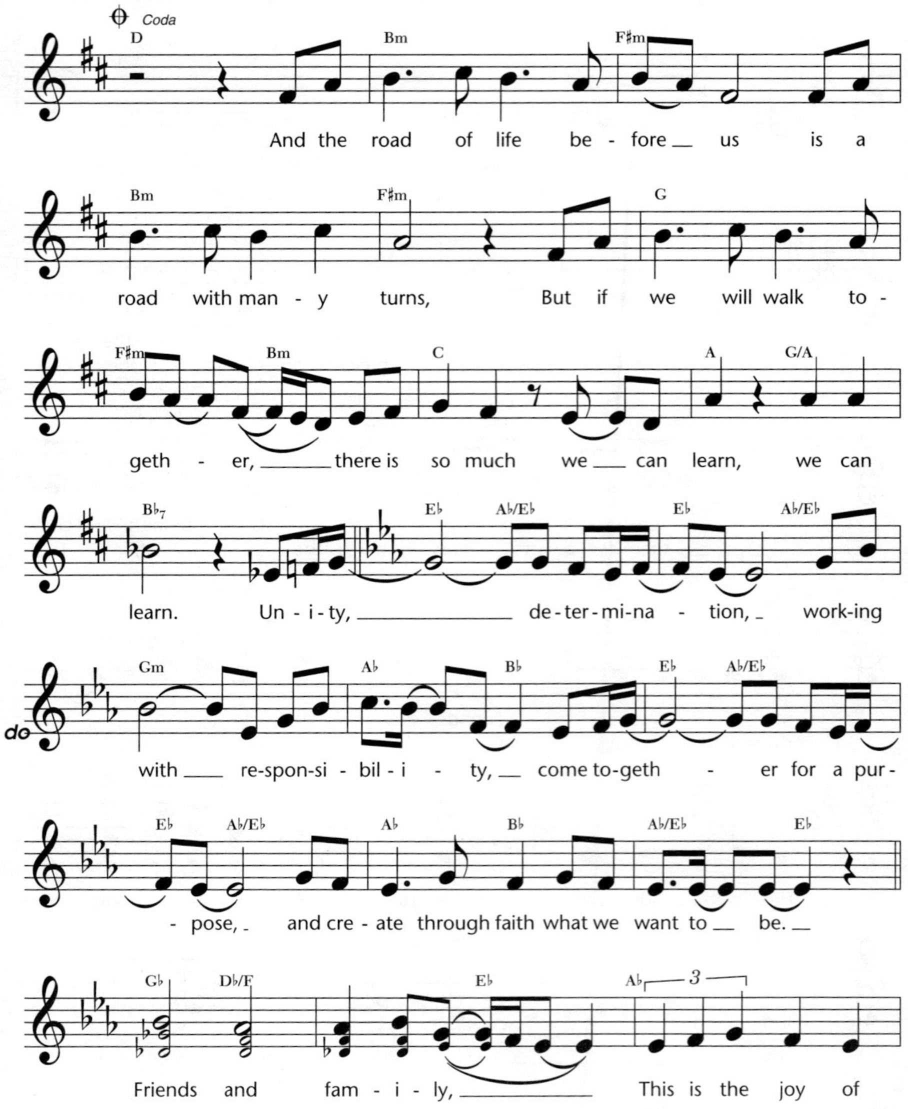

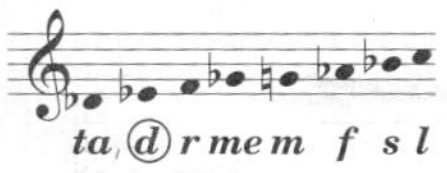

(Musical notation of "The Joy of Kwanzaa" with lyrics:)

And the road of life be - fore __ us is a
road with man - y turns, But if we will walk to -
geth - er, ___ there is so much we __ can learn, we can
learn. Un - i - ty, ___ de - ter - mi - na - tion, __ work-ing
with ___ re - spon - si - bil - i - ty, __ come to-geth - er for a pur-
- pose, __ and cre - ate through faith what we want to __ be. __
Friends and fam - i - ly, ___ This is the joy of

ta ⓓ r mem f s l

Take It to the Net Visit *www.sfsuccessnet.com* to learn more about holiday music.

464

Footnotes

ACROSS THE CURRICULUM

▶ **Social Studies** The Kwanzaa table utilizes a variety of ordinary items that represent greater things. Carefully prepared, the table is covered in the red, black, and green African American National flag. A straw mat, or *mkeka,* is laid on top of the table. The *kinara,* a candleholder that represents Africa, the root of all African American culture, sits on the *mkeka.* Seven candles in the *kinara*—1 black, 3 red, 3 green—symbolize the seven principles of Kwanzaa. Other symbolic items decorate the table: ears of corn symbolize children, and green plants symbolize unity with nature. Gifts of historical and cultural significance are laid on the table and exchanged at the end of the evening.

SKILLS REINFORCEMENT

▶ **Singing Triplets** The ending of "The Joy of Kwanzaa" introduces a new rhythm to the piece, a triplet. Your students may think there are five beats in the measure, as there appear to be five quarter notes in one measure. Note that the bracket and the number *3* appear only over three of the notes, not the last two. Listen to the rhythms in isolation. Have your students tap a steady beat as they listen. They will notice that the first three sounds do not line up with the beats. Define *triplet* as three notes that fit into a smaller number of beats. In this case, the triplet occupies two beats. Try saying, then singing, a three-syllable word *(syl-la-ble)* to pace the cadence, using appropriate rhythm syllables to complete the pattern.

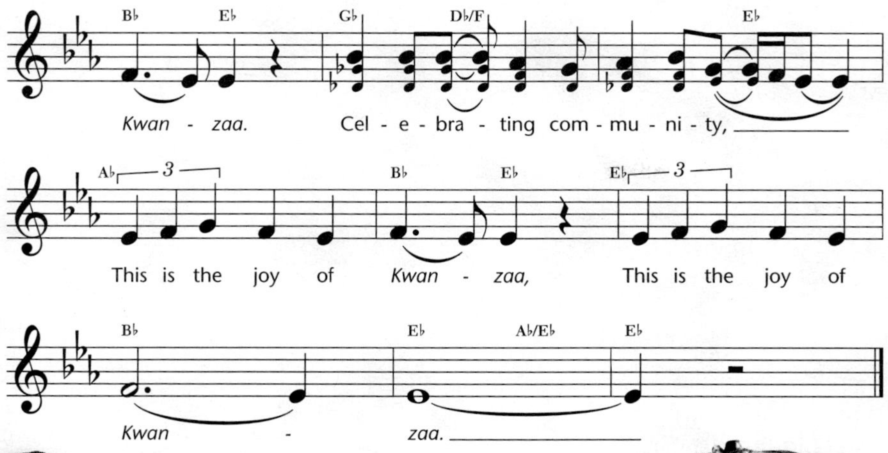

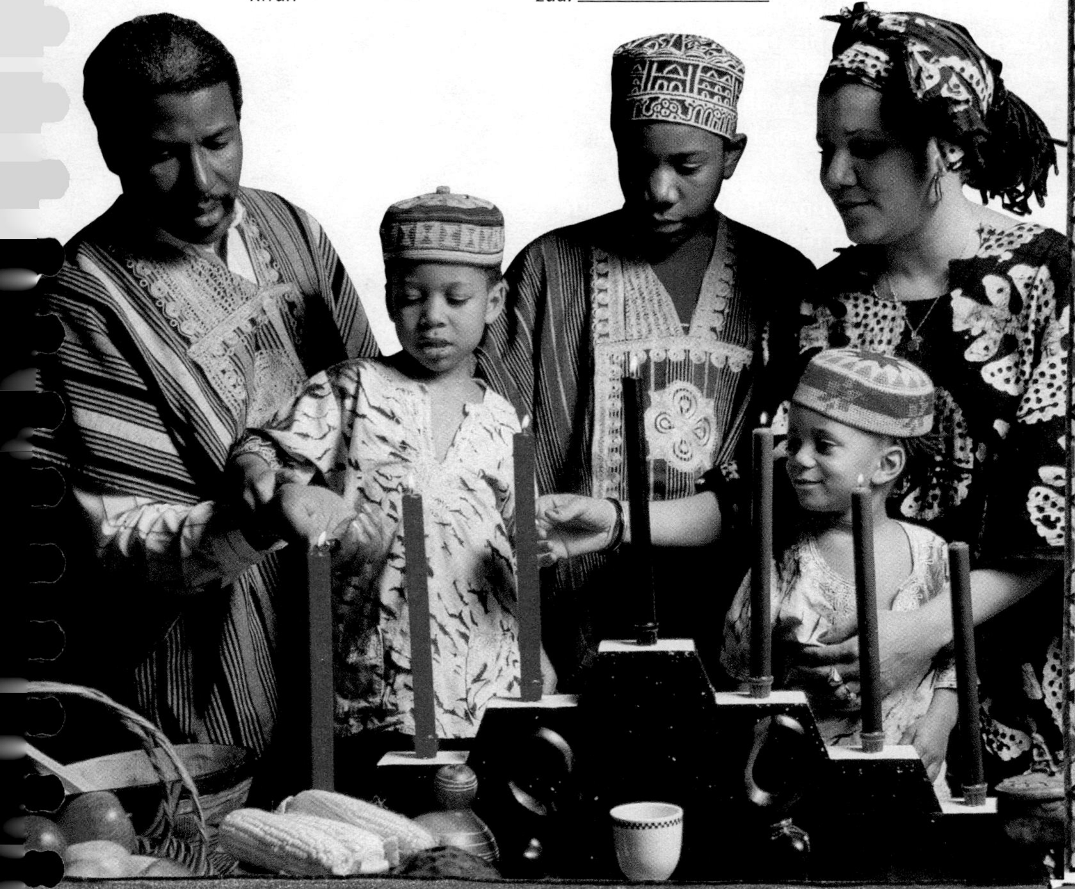

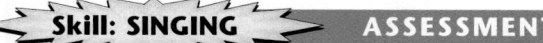

Kwan - zaa. Cel-e-bra-ting com-mu-ni-ty,

This is the joy of Kwan - zaa, This is the joy of

Kwan - zaa.

Groups may also want to use a *fermata*.

ASK What instruction does a *fermata* give? (to hold a note)

Give the groups time to work on their presentations, assisting them as needed to keep them on track. If time permits, encourage them to make visuals to enhance their performance. (a Kwanzaa table, Kwanzaa pictures, objects, costumes, posters)

Performing

Have each group make its presentation for the class.

Analyzing

7a At the conclusion of the performance, ask for positive comments from the class.

9c **ASK What principles of Kwanzaa did you demonstrate in your group presentation and in your group preparation?** (written on the board)

Give each group an opportunity to answer this question at the conclusion of their presentation.

After all groups have shared, discuss how the seven principles of Kwanzaa were or were not used for a successful group experience. Ask for additional insights students may want to share.

3 CLOSE

Skill: SINGING **ASSESSMENT**

1a **Performance/Observation** Have students present, as a class, "The Joy of Kwanzaa" with the recording **CD 22-1.** Observe and evaluate the group's success in performing the modulation. Did the class maintain proper intonation during the modulation?

Discuss with students additional tips on how to hear and sing a modulation. (One tip is to focus on the harmony, or chord, that an accompanying keyboard may emphasize.)

SPOTLIGHT ON

▶ **The Composer** Reggie Royal, composer of "The Joy of Kwanzaa," is a multitalented African American composer, performer, arranger, and musical director. His family encouraged his musical interests at a young age, and he began studying the piano at age four. At age eight, he was performing with the Florentine Opera Company and his church choir.

Royal has won the NAACP Image Award for Excellence in Theatre for his musical direction of *Five Guys Named Moe.* He has worked on Broadway shows and tours, including *Colors of Christmas, Smokey Joe's Cafe, Jelly's Last Jam,* and other musicals. Royal has also worked with Phil Collins, Natalie Cole, Brenda Russell, the Pointer Sisters, and other artists.

SCHOOL TO HOME CONNECTION

▶ **Kwanzaa Foods** Ask students who celebrate Kwanzaa at home to talk to the class about the foods that are served at Kwanzaa meals. Some of these traditional foods are sweet potatoes, okra, squash, yams, vegetable stew, and African foods such as benne cakes and sesame seed cookies. Southern dishes include sweet potato pie, fried okra, and black-eyed peas with ham.

TECHNOLOGY/MEDIA LINK

Web Site Have students go to *www.sfsuccessnet.com* to discover more about holiday music.

LESSON AT A GLANCE

Element Focus **TEXTURE/HARMONY** Two-part and three-part harmony

Skill Objective **SINGING** Sing songs in two- and three-part harmony

Connection Activity **SOCIAL STUDIES** Discuss Martin Luther King, Jr., John and Robert Kennedy, and Abraham Lincoln and their fight for civil rights

MATERIALS

• "Abraham, Martin, and John" **CD 22-3**
  Recording Routine: Intro (4 m.); v. 1; v. 2; v. 3; refrain; v. 4; coda

• "Free at Last" **CD 22-5**
  Recording Routine: Intro (4 m.); refrain; v. 1; refrain; v. 2; refrain; v. 3; refrain; coda

• "I Wish I Knew How It Would Feel to Be Free" **CD 22-8**
  Recording Routine: Intro (4 m.); v. 1; interlude (4 m.); v. 2; interlude (4 m.); v. 3; interlude (4 m.); v. 4; coda

• *I Wish I Knew How It Would Feel to Be Free* (excerpt) **CD 22-7**

• **Resource Book** p. I-31

• recorders

VOCABULARY

verse	refrain	call and response	ledger lines
texture	homophonic	system	octavo

◆ ◆ ◆ ◆ **National Standards** ◆ ◆ ◆ ◆

1a Sing accurately in small and large ensembles
1d Sing music written in two and three parts
5b Sightread melodies in treble and bass clefs
6c Understand and use basic principles of form, rhythm, and harmony
8b Identify ways music relates to social studies

MORE MUSIC CHOICES

For more practice with songs in two- and three-part harmony:
"By the Waters of Babylon," p. 311
"Vem kan segla?" p. 417

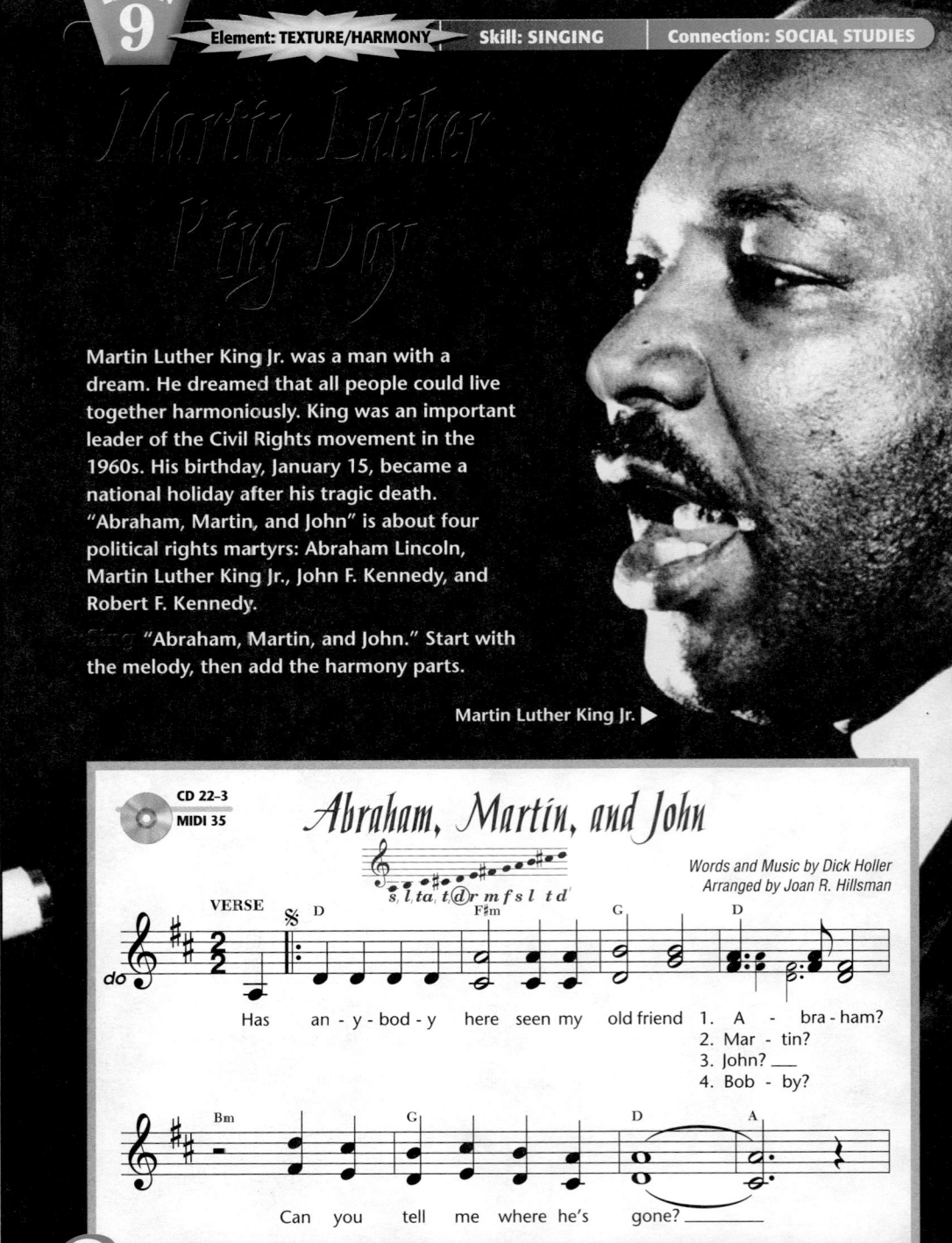

Element: TEXTURE/HARMONY   Skill: SINGING   Connection: SOCIAL STUDIES

Martin Luther King Day

Martin Luther King Jr. was a man with a dream. He dreamed that all people could live together harmoniously. King was an important leader of the Civil Rights movement in the 1960s. His birthday, January 15, became a national holiday after his tragic death. "Abraham, Martin, and John" is about four political rights martyrs: Abraham Lincoln, Martin Luther King Jr., John F. Kennedy, and Robert F. Kennedy.

Sing "Abraham, Martin, and John." Start with the melody, then add the harmony parts.

Martin Luther King Jr. ▶

CD 22-3
MIDI 35

Abraham, Martin, and John

Words and Music by Dick Holler
Arranged by Joan R. Hillsman

VERSE

Has an-y-bod-y here seen my old friend 1. A - bra - ham?
                                          2. Mar - tin?
                                          3. John? ___
                                          4. Bob - by?

Can you tell me where he's gone? ___

466

Footnotes

MEETING INDIVIDUAL NEEDS

▶ **English Language Learners** Invite students to have a conversation about the people featured in this song. Some students, especially those newer to the United States, may not know about the contributions of these individuals. You may also want to show pictures of the people profiled, as well as talk with students about the times in which they lived.

BUILDING SKILLS THROUGH MUSIC

▶ **Reading** The song "I Wish I Knew How It Would Feel to Be Free" has examples of both simile (verse 4) and metaphor (verses 1 and 2). Have students identify each and determine its meaning.

ACROSS THE CURRICULUM

▶ **Social Studies** Abraham Lincoln (1809–1865) grew up in both slave and free states; this shaped his views against slavery. He was against the Missouri Compromise of 1854, which allowed more slave states to enter the Union. He ran for president in 1860, having gained national attention in lively debates against Stephen Douglas. He followed the suggestion of an 11-year-old girl that he grow a beard to help him win the election. Lincoln's first trial as president was the secession of the Southern states from the Union, leading to the Civil War. Lincoln issued the Emancipation Proclamation in 1863, freeing slaves and effectively ending the practice of slavery. Lincoln was assassinated in 1865 as he watched a play at Ford's Theater in Washington, D.C.

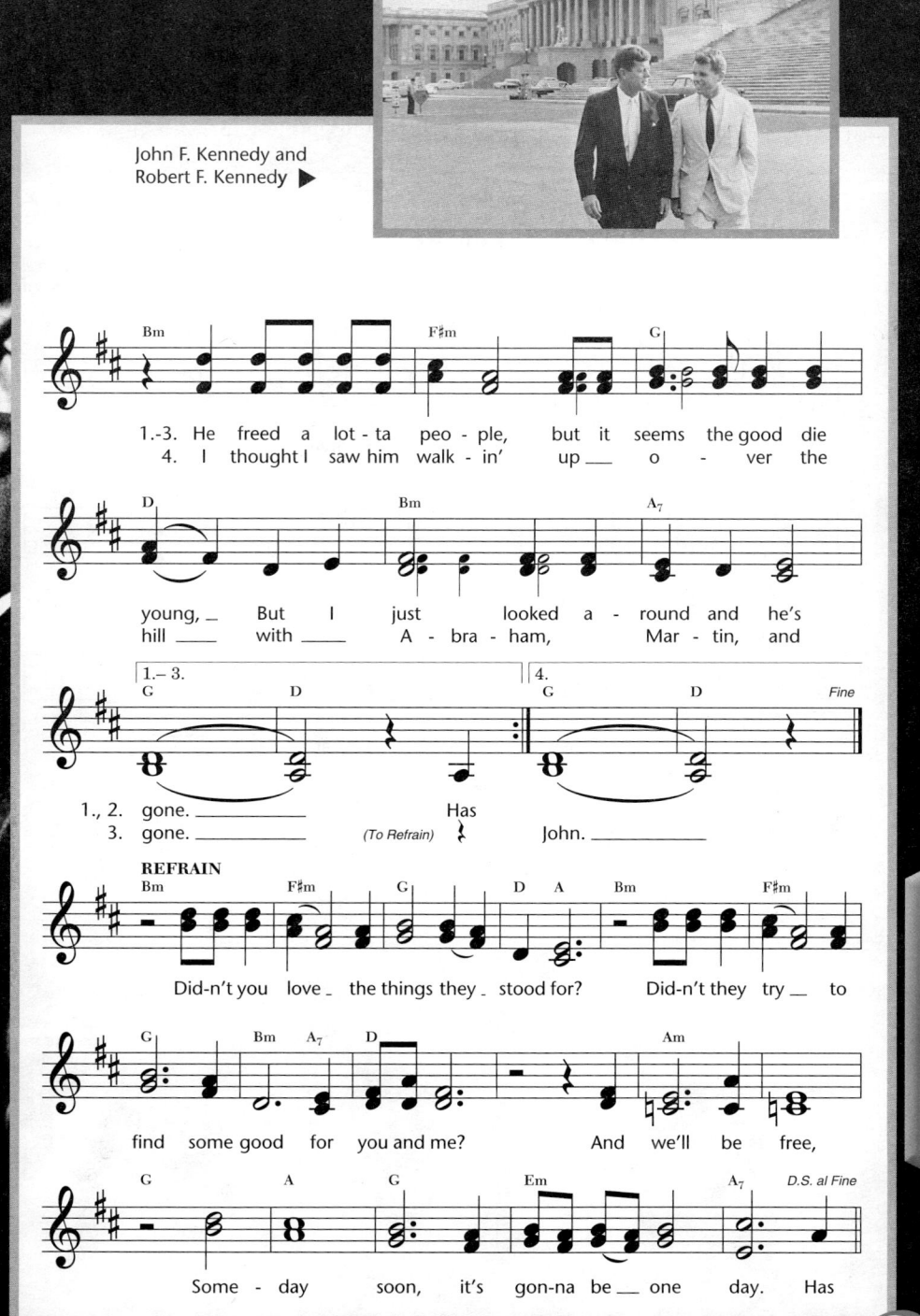

John F. Kennedy and
Robert F. Kennedy ▶

1.-3. He freed a lot-ta peo-ple, but it seems the good die
4. I thought I saw him walk-in' up __ o - ver the

young, __ But I just looked a - round and he's
hill __ with __ A - bra - ham, Mar - tin, and

1.- 3. **4.**
1., 2. gone. _____
3. gone. _____ *(To Refrain)* Has
John. _____

REFRAIN

Did-n't you love _ the things they _ stood for? Did-n't they try __ to

find some good for you and me? And we'll be free,

Some - day soon, it's gon-na be __ one day. Has

Unit 12 **467**

1 INTRODUCE

Ask students to read the text on p. 466. Lead a discussion on Abraham Lincoln, Martin Luther King Jr., John F. Kennedy, and Robert Kennedy. Share with students the information from Across the Curriculum on pp. 466 and 468; Spotlight On, pp. 467, 468, and 470; and Cultural Connection below, and on p. 469.

Explain that "Abraham, Martin, and John" is a song about four men who believed in and fought for civil rights. All four men were assassinated.

2 DEVELOP

Listening

6c With books closed, invite students to listen to "Abraham, Martin, and John" **CD 22-3.** Help students discover that

- Each verse is devoted to one of the heroes.
- The song uses only the individuals' first names.
- The song is in two-part song form (AB, verse/refrain).

Singing

1a Have students sing the melody of "Abraham, Martin, and John" with the recording. See Skills Reinforcement, on p. 469, for singing tips.

1d Divide the class into two groups. Invite one group to sing the harmony of the verse and the other to sing the harmony of the refrain with the recording.

Have students sing the song in two parts with the recording.

Playing

See Resource Book p. I-31 and invite students to play a countermelody on recorder to accompany "Abraham, Martin, and John" **CD 22-3.**

continued on page 468

Celebrate the Day

SPOTLIGHT ON

▶ **John F. Kennedy** John Fitzgerald Kennedy (1917–1963) was already a graduate of Harvard University, a World War II hero, and a Pulitzer Prize winner when he became the youngest president of the United States in 1960. During his presidency, he championed the cause of civil rights. He founded the Peace Corps and the Alliance for Progress to promote human rights and aid developing nations. After the Cuban missile crisis, he worked to end nuclear arms buildup. In 1963, he signed a nuclear test ban treaty and encouraged slowing the arms race. Kennedy was assassinated later that year. Millions of people across the world mourned his untimely death, but Kennedy's legacy as a peacemaker and humanitarian continue to inspire others to action.

CULTURAL CONNECTION

8b ▶ **Folk Music History** "Abraham, Martin, and John" was one of the most popular protest songs of the 1960s. The piece was written in folk style with chord progressions that revolve around the I, IV, and V chords. The words fall into a predictable pattern easily taught by rote. The song was often performed at large rallies, where everyone was encouraged to sing along. The contemporary message about four slain heroes allows us to reflect on the impact of Abraham, Martin, John, and Bobby Kennedy.

Analyzing

Direct students' attention to "Free at Last" on p. 468.

8b **ASK How are "Free at Last" and "Abraham, Martin, and John" related?** (Both songs are concerned with freedom.)

6c Help students observe that

- The song is also in verse/refrain form.
- The song begins and ends with the refrain.
- The verse uses call and response.
- **The verse is in two-part harmony, and the refrain is in three-part harmony.**

ASK How is the three-part harmony created? (The soloist sings the last phrase with the two-part choir.)

Singing

1a Invite students to sing the melody of "Free at Last" **CD 22-5** with the recording.

Help students discover that in the verse, the first measures of each response are the same, while the second measure is different.

1d Divide the class into two groups and invite one group to sing the harmony part of the responses with the recording. See Teacher to Teacher on p. 470.

Have students sing the response in harmony with the recording.

Select a soloist or small group of students to sing the solo, and have the rest of the class sing the responses of the verse with the recording. Help students recognize the similarities between the last phrase of the verse and the last phrase of the refrain.

Have the harmony group sing the harmony part of the refrain with the recording.

1d Encourage students to sing the entire song in harmony with the recording **CD 22-5.** See Skills Reinforcement on p. 471 for additional singing activities.

Precious Freedom

African American slaves frequently sang spirituals such as "Free at Last." Like Martin Luther King Jr., they looked forward to a day when they would have true feedom.

Sing "Free at Last." Take turns singing the solo sections of the song.

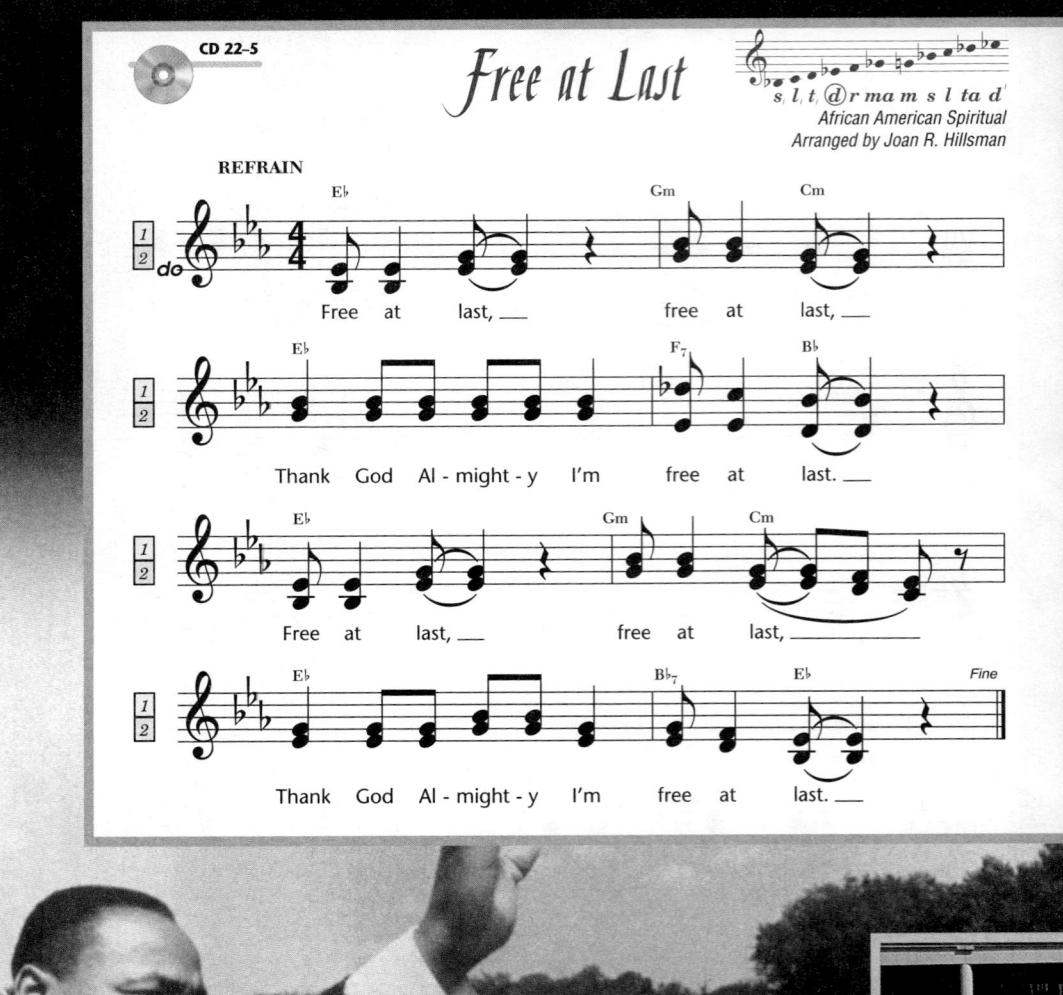

CD 22-5

Free at Last

African American Spiritual
Arranged by Joan R. Hillsman

468

Footnotes

SPOTLIGHT ON

▶ **Martin Luther King Jr.** The son of a Baptist preacher, Martin Luther King Jr. (1929–1968) rose to the heights of fame as a civil rights leader. He grew up in Atlanta, Georgia, in a culture dominated by segregation and racial inequality. As an adult, King formed the Southern Christian Leadership Conference, which advocated nonviolent protest of racial issues. When Rosa Parks was arrested for not giving up her bus seat to a white person, King responded by organizing a boycott of Montgomery buses. When civil rights legislation was making the rounds of Congress, King led the March on Washington to make his voice heard. King was assassinated for his beliefs in 1968, and his birthday was declared a national holiday in 1983.

ACROSS THE CURRICULUM

▶ **Social Studies** The 1960s peace movement prompted some of the decade's most memorable protests. The United States sent troops to oppose the spread of Communism in Vietnam. Young people turned their attention to U.S. involvement in the Vietnam conflict. Following Martin Luther King Jr.'s example, teenagers and college students organized nonviolent marches and concerts to voice their opinions. Over 250,000 people participated in the antiwar protest begun on November 15, 1969, in Washington, D.C. The protests continued until 1973, when President Richard Nixon finally withdrew American troops from the region after nearly two decades of involvement.

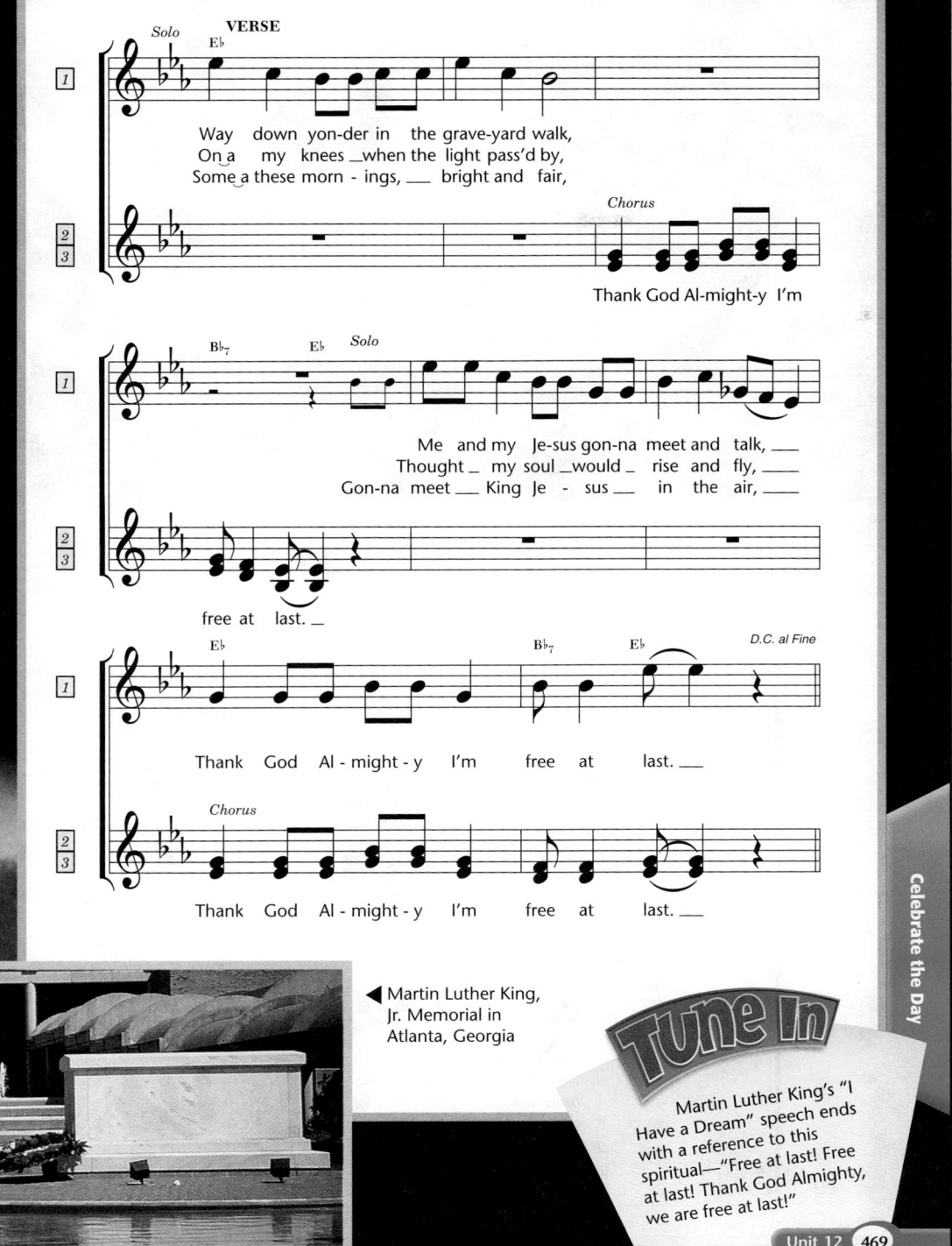

VERSE

Solo
Eb

Way down yon-der in the grave-yard walk,
On a my knees __ when the light pass'd by,
Some a these morn - ings, __ bright and fair,

Chorus

Thank God Al-might-y I'm

Bb7   Eb   Solo

Me and my Je-sus gon-na meet and talk, __
Thought _ my soul _ would _ rise and fly, __
Gon-na meet __ King Je - sus __ in the air, __

free at last. __

Eb   Bb7   Eb   D.C. al Fine

Thank God Al - might - y I'm free at last. __

Chorus

Thank God Al - might - y I'm free at last. __

◀ Martin Luther King, Jr. Memorial in Atlanta, Georgia

Tune In

Martin Luther King's "I Have a Dream" speech ends with a reference to this spiritual—"Free at last! Free at last! Thank God Almighty, we are free at last!"

Celebrate the Day

Moving

Invite students to suggest movement ideas for "Free at Last." (swaying side to side, clapping on certain beats)

ASK Should the soloist's movement be the same as that of the chorus? (No, it is more effective to have contrasting motion for the soloist.)

Divide the class into groups to work on movements for "Free at Last." Have students share their created movement with the class.

Encourage each group to teach their movement to the rest of the class, allowing the class to experiment with new moves.

 Have students perform "Free at Last" with the movements the class has created.

Creating

Encourage students to create new text for the verse of "Free at Last." Remind students that each new phrase must be eight counts long.

Suggest that students use the following ideas:

- Where is the singer, and what is the singer going to do?
- What time of day is it, and where is the singer going?
- When does an event take place, and whom will the singer meet at the event?

Encourage students to share their newly created verses. Have them choose a few to sing and then perform the new verses as a class.

Using information from Technology/Media Link on p. 471, encourage students to create an arrangement for "Free at Last." Have them experiment with different styles and then choose one to perform with movement and new verses.

continued on page 470

CULTURAL CONNECTION

▶ **The Martin Luther King Jr. Center** Coretta Scott King founded the King Center in 1968, in memory of her husband, Martin Luther King Jr. The Atlanta, Georgia, museum hosts more than one million visitors each year. Its goal is to preserve and protect the integrity of King's legacy. The King Center is part of the Martin Luther King Jr. National Historic Site, which includes King's birth home, the church where King and his father served, and the beautifully landscaped Peace Plaza. Visitors can also access a library and archives dedicated to King's work. The King Center is the headquarters of The National Holiday Advisory Committee, a group made of representatives from several states that discusses meaningful ways to celebrate King's birthday.

SKILLS REINFORCEMENT

▶ **Singing** Young singers often forget to hold the final vowel for the full count and pronounce the final consonant at the end of the final beat.

"Abraham, Martin, and John" Singing Tips
Every phrase of the verse ends in a consonant. Avoid closing on the *m* or *n* too early. Add the ending consonant almost as an afterthought.

Most phrases of the refrain end on a vowel. Hold the vowel sound without changing the shape of the mouth. Students who close their mouths before the end of the phrase will sound as if they are losing volume.

"Free at Last" Singing Tips
Perform a crisp *st* and take a breath before the next phrase. Listen closely for the solo part.

Listening

Invite students to listen to "I Wish I Knew How It Would Feel to Be Free" **CD 22-8** with books closed.

ASK What was the song about? (wanting to be free)

Was it sung in unison or harmony? (harmony)

Was it homophonic or polyphonic texture? (homophonic)

How many parts did you hear? (three)

Was the song in verse and refrain form? (no, verse or ballad form)

Reading

5b Have students focus on the music of "I Wish I Knew How It Would Feel to Be Free" and help them notice that

- One harmony part is written in the bass clef.
- The two staves are connected to form a *system*.

Explain that, in choral music, baritone and bass parts are written in the bass staff. Demonstrate the following:

- Draw two staves on the board, one above the other with space between them.
- Place a treble clef on the top staff and a bass clef on the bottom staff.
- Invite students to write the names of the lines and spaces on the treble staff.
- Draw a short line between the two staves and inform students that the line represents middle C.
- Have students discover that the name of the space above the bass clef is B and its top line is A.
- Encourage students to fill in the names of the rest of the lines and spaces of the bass staff.
- Challenge students to sight-read simple music in other clefs (bass clef) in various meters and keys (A♭). Using the first line of the bass clef, have students sight-read the rhythm. Then, give students the pitches (A♭, C, D♭) and ask them to sight-read the notated pitches.

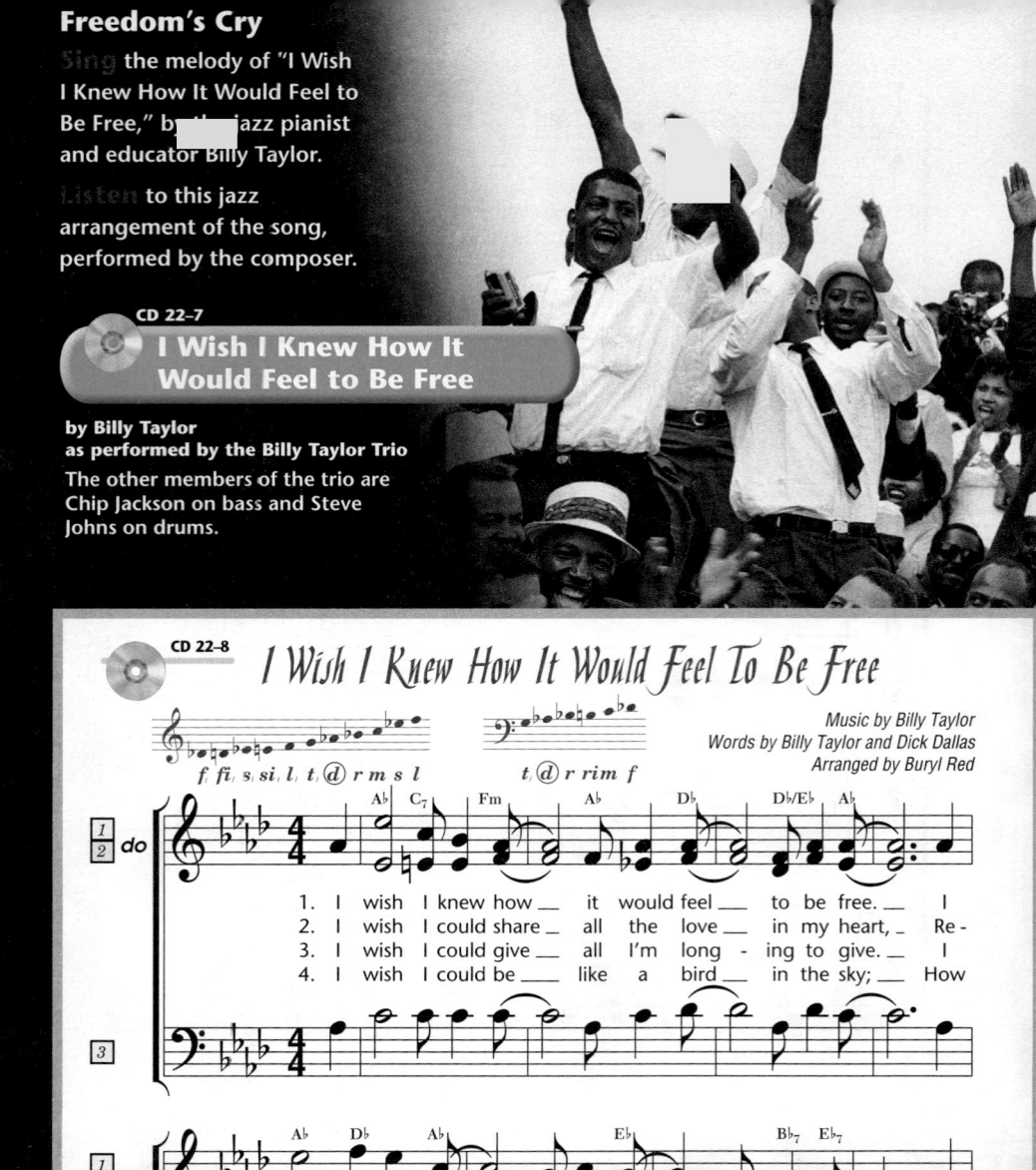

Freedom's Cry

Sing the melody of "I Wish I Knew How It Would Feel to Be Free," by the jazz pianist and educator Billy Taylor.

Listen to this jazz arrangement of the song, performed by the composer.

CD 22–7
I Wish I Knew How It Would Feel to Be Free

by Billy Taylor
as performed by the Billy Taylor Trio
The other members of the trio are Chip Jackson on bass and Steve Johns on drums.

CD 22–8
I Wish I Knew How It Would Feel To Be Free

Music by Billy Taylor
Words by Billy Taylor and Dick Dallas
Arranged by Buryl Red

1. I wish I knew how it would feel to be free. I
2. I wish I could share all the love in my heart, Re-
3. I wish I could give all I'm long - ing to give. I
4. I wish I could be like a bird in the sky; How

wish I could break all these chains hold - ing me. I
move all the bars that still keep us a - part. I
wish I could live like I'm long - ing to live. I
sweet it would be if I found I could fly. I'd

470

Footnotes

SPOTLIGHT ON

▶ **Robert Kennedy** John F. Kennedy's younger brother, Robert Kennedy (1925–1968), graduated from Harvard and joined him in the Navy during World War II. He gained national recognition during the Senate's 1955–57 investigation of Teamsters Union executives Jimmy Hoffa and David Beck. Appointed Attorney General of the United States when John Kennedy became president in 1960, Robert Kennedy fought racial discrimination and promoted civil rights legislation. He sent U.S. marshals and troops to enforce desegregation laws at the University of Mississippi in 1962. As a U.S. senator, he initiated programs to help underprivileged children, the disabled, and Brooklyn residents facing an economic depression. In 1968, Robert Kennedy ran for president but was assassinated on June 5 of that year.

TEACHER TO TEACHER

▶ **Teaching Three Parts** When teaching songs in more than two parts, it is a good idea to give singers opportunities to practice their part with each of the other parts. Here is a routine you might like to use with your students after they know their parts.

- Parts 1 and 2 sing a verse while Part 3 listens or sings its part quietly.
- Parts 1 and 3 sing a verse while Part 2 listens or sings its part quietly.
- Parts 2 and 3 sing a verse while Part 1 listens or sings its part quietly.

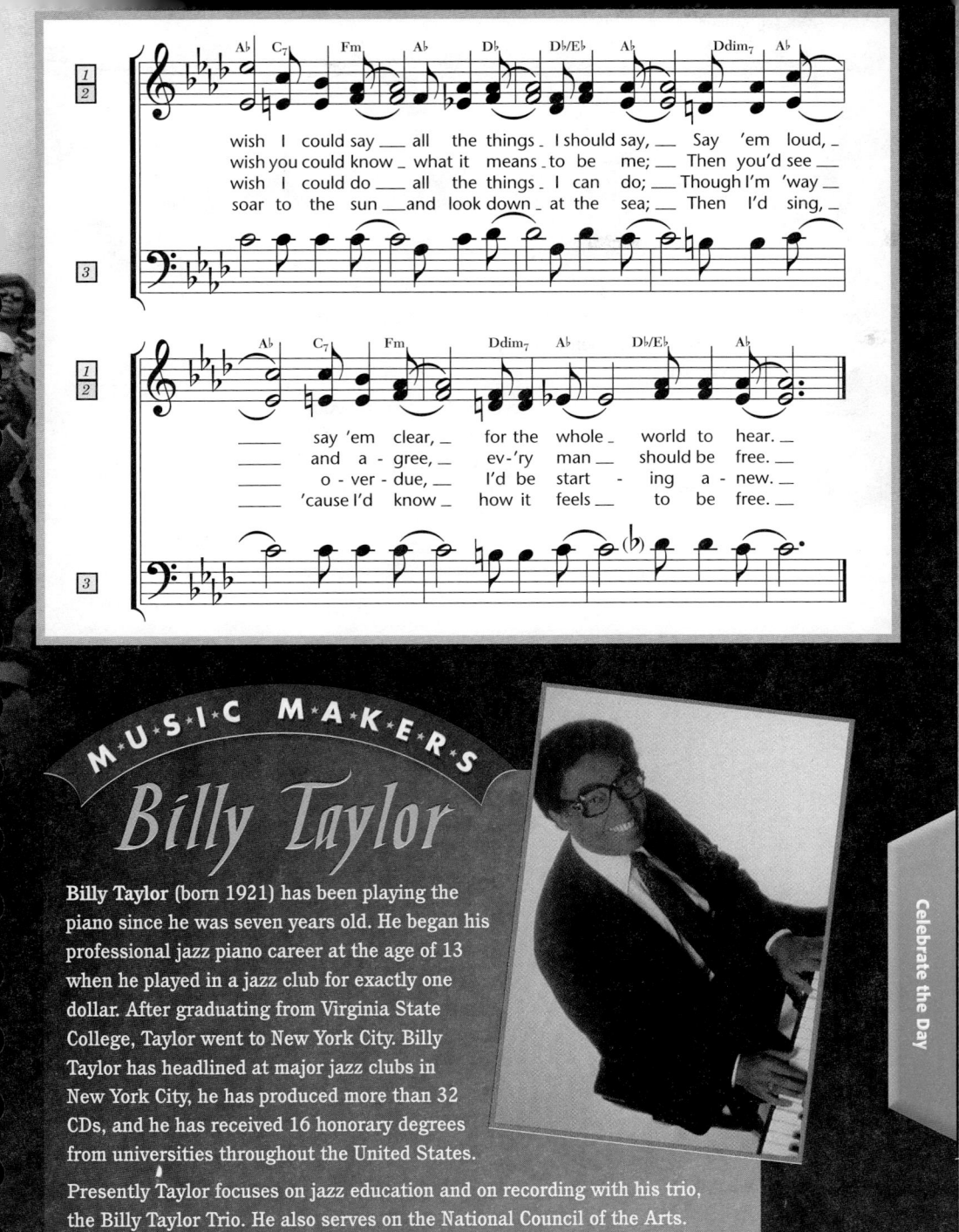

wish I could say ___ all the things. I should say, ___ Say 'em loud, ___
wish you could know ___ what it means to be me; ___ Then you'd see ___
wish I could do ___ all the things. I can do; ___ Though I'm 'way ___
soar to the sun ___ and look down at the sea; ___ Then I'd sing, ___

say 'em clear, ___ for the whole ___ world to hear. ___
and a-gree, ___ ev-'ry man ___ should be free. ___
o-ver-due, ___ I'd be start - ing a-new. ___
'cause I'd know ___ how it feels to be free. ___

M·U·S·I·C M·A·K·E·R·S

Billy Taylor

Billy Taylor (born 1921) has been playing the piano since he was seven years old. He began his professional jazz piano career at the age of 13 when he played in a jazz club for exactly one dollar. After graduating from Virginia State College, Taylor went to New York City. Billy Taylor has headlined at major jazz clubs in New York City, he has produced more than 32 CDs, and he has received 16 honorary degrees from universities throughout the United States.

Presently Taylor focuses on jazz education and on recording with his trio, the Billy Taylor Trio. He also serves on the National Council of the Arts.

Celebrate the Day

Unit 12 **471**

Explain to students that the short lines parallel to and above or below the staff are called *ledger lines*. These lines make it possible to indicate pitches that are not on the staff.

1a With the recording of "I Wish I Knew How It Would Feel to Be Free" **CD 22-8.**

1d

- Have students sing the melody of "I Wish I Knew How It Would Feel to Be Free."
- Invite boys to sing the baritone line. (Note: Some boys may have to sing the part an octave higher.)
- Invite boys to sing the harmony while girls sing the melody.
- Divide the girls into two groups and invite one group to sing the harmony part of the treble staff.
- Have students sing the song in three parts.

Invite students to read about Billy Taylor, on p. 471, and then listen to his recording of *I Wish I Knew How It Would Feel to Be Free* **CD 22-7.**

3 CLOSE

Element: TEXTURE/HARMONY **ASSESSMENT**

6c **Performance/Self-Assessment** Divide the class into two groups and assign each group a part in "Free at Last." Have the class sing "Free at Last" in harmony. Have each group switch parts and sing the song again in two parts. Ask students to assess each of their performances using the following criteria.

- Did you sing the harmony parts correctly and in tune?
- Did you pay attention to the melody and sing the harmony part softer than the melody part?
- Did you perform the rhythms accurately?

SKILLS REINFORCEMENT

▶ **Reading** Guide students to understand that the rhythm of a song is influenced by its lyrics. Have students perform the solo part to "Free at Last." Encourage them to speak the words before singing them. Invite students to experiment with the rhythm—should they "swing" the eighth notes or add syncopation? Singers take liberties with both the rhythm and the melody when singing solo sections of spirituals and gospel-like songs.

 ▶ **Recorder** Students can play a countermelody on recorder to accompany "Abraham, Martin, and John." See Resource Book p. I-31 for this arrangement, which features notes in the lower register.

TECHNOLOGY/MEDIA LINK

MIDI/Sequencing Software Use the MIDI song file of "Abraham, Martin, and John" to have students

- Explore transposing the song's key.
- Select the software program's graphic editor and examine the contour of the melody and other tracks.
- Explore graphic editing features. Have students experiment with making rhythmic changes by changing the length of notes or making melodic contour changes by changing the pitch.

CD-ROM Use *Band-in-a-Box* to create an arrangement to accompany "Free at Last." Have a student type in the chord symbols. Then, select a style and press play. Sing along.

LESSON AT A GLANCE

Element Focus   **FORM**   Verse-refrain form

Skill Objective   **SINGING**   Sing two songs in verse-refrain form that have foreign language texts

Connection Activity   **CULTURE**   Explore the origins and traditions of Valentine's Day

MATERIALS

- "Eres tú"   CD 22-10
- "Touch the Wind"   CD 22-11
  Recording Routine: Intro (5 m.); vocals; coda
- **Pronunciation Practice/Translation** p. 546
- "Love in Any Language"   CD 22-14
  Recording Routine: Intro (1 m.); vocal
- **Resource Book** pp. A-42, G-27
- alto recorders, tape recorder (optional)

VOCABULARY

verse-refrain form   countermelody   modulation

◆ ◆ ◆ ◆ National Standards ◆ ◆ ◆ ◆

1a Sing accurately in large ensembles
1c Sing music from diverse cultures
1d Sing music written in two parts
1e In groups, sing moderately easy pieces from memory
2a Play instruments accurately alone
5e In performance class, sightread easy music
6a Listen and describe events in music using appropriate terms

MORE MUSIC CHOICES

For more practice with countermelodies:
"Alexander's Ragtime Band," p. 136
For more songs with verse and refrain:
"Jambalaya," p. 244
"Green, Green Grass of Home," p. 248

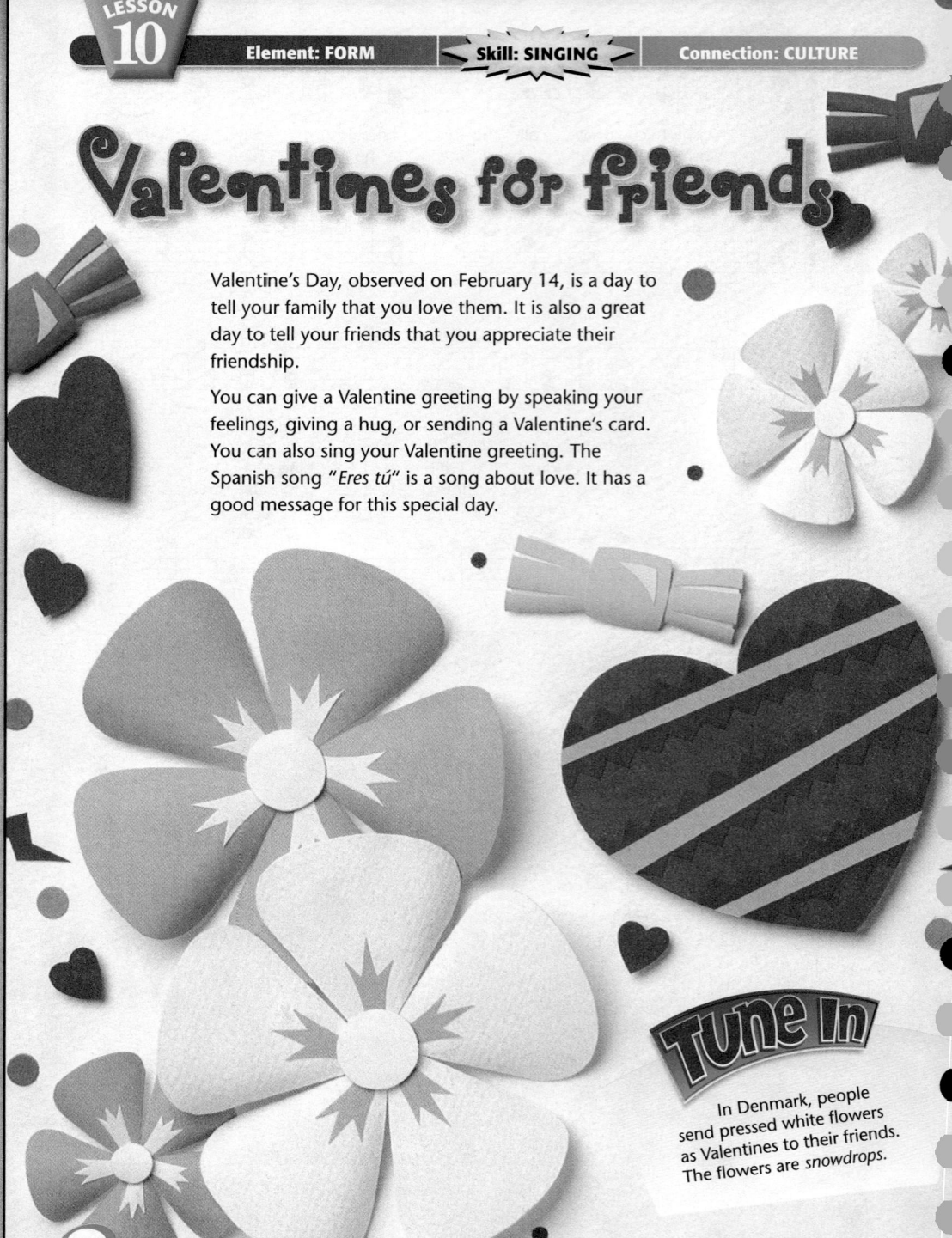

Valentines for friends

Valentine's Day, observed on February 14, is a day to tell your family that you love them. It is also a great day to tell your friends that you appreciate their friendship.

You can give a Valentine greeting by speaking your feelings, giving a hug, or sending a Valentine's card. You can also sing your Valentine greeting. The Spanish song "Eres tú" is a song about love. It has a good message for this special day.

Tune In

In Denmark, people send pressed white flowers as Valentines to their friends. The flowers are *snowdrops*.

472

Footnotes

CULTURAL CONNECTION

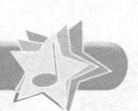

▶ **E-mail Cards** Share with students that Valentine's Day cards can now be sent by e-mail and the Internet. The wide availability of home computers has created a new option for sending mail. Many of your students can now send free animated greeting cards to anyone with an e-mail address. Some cards have animated characters, musical scores, and funny sight gags.

BUILDING SKILLS THROUGH MUSIC

▶ **Reading** Guide students in learning "Love In Any Language" and share Across the Curriculum on p. 477 with them. After students have learned the words "I love you" in French, Spanish, Russian, and Hebrew, have them research and share how to say the phrase in other languages. Have students sing the song again, substituting different languages.

SPOTLIGHT ON

▶ **Valentine's Day** Valentine was a Catholic priest who lived in Rome over 1700 years ago (A.D. 262). The Roman Emperor Claudius II forbade any soldier to marry or become engaged while serving in the army. Valentine refused to recognize this order, and he secretly married many couples affected by the decree. Unfortunately, he was discovered, arrested, and found guilty of treason. He was beheaded on the eve of February 14, the day before the Roman holiday *Lupercalia*. The Roman Catholic Church made Valentine a saint after his death. As Christianity spread throughout Europe, people celebrated St. Valentine's Day instead of *Lupercalia*.

Sing Your Feelings

Sing "Eres tú" and imagine you are expressing your feelings to your Valentine.

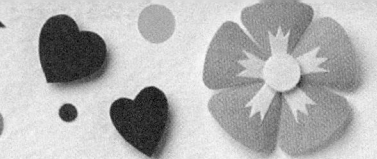

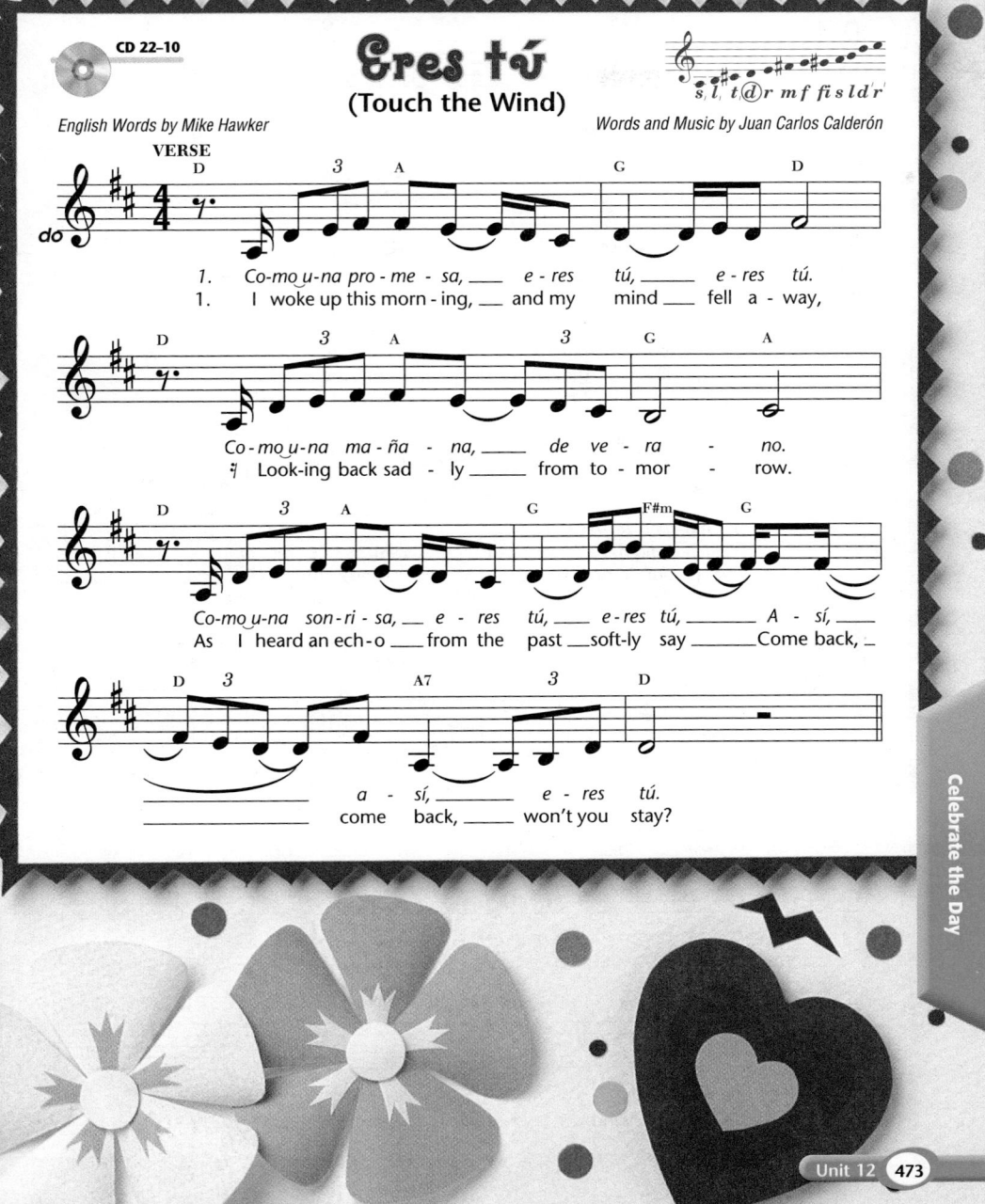

CD 22-10

Eres tú
(Touch the Wind)

English Words by Mike Hawker

Words and Music by Juan Carlos Calderón

VERSE

1. Co-mo u-na pro-me-sa, ___ e - res tú, ___ e - res tú.
1. I woke up this morn-ing, ___ and my mind ___ fell a - way,

Co-mo u-na ma-ña - na, ___ de ve-ra - no.
Look-ing back sad-ly ___ from to-mor - row.

Co-mo u-na son-ri-sa, ___ e - res tú, ___ e-res tú, ___ A - sí, ___
As I heard an ech-o ___ from the past ___ soft-ly say ___ Come back, ___

a - sí, ___ e - res tú.
come back, ___ won't you stay?

Celebrate the Day

Unit 12 **473**

1 INTRODUCE

Ask students if they know the origin of Valentine's Day. Have them read the information on p. 472. Share the information in Spotlight On, p. 472, about the background of the holiday.

Discuss the tradition of sending Valentine cards. For interesting facts on the sending of Valentines, see Spotlight On, pp. 475 and 478, and Cultural Connection on p. 472.

Tell students that although not all countries have a Valentine's Day, love and friendship are expressed in all cultures.

2 DEVELOP

Listening

Invite students to listen to "Eres tú" **CD 22-10** and have students notice that

- The song uses the verse-refrain form.
- The verse has two two-measure phrases followed by a four-measure phrase.
- Verses 1, 2, and 3 are all the same, although verse 1 is printed on a different page.
- The refrain is sung only after verses 2 and 3 and not after verse 1.
- The refrain repeats with a countermelody added.

Singing

Invite students to practice their sight-reading skills, using the procedure in Skills Reinforcement below. Use "Eres tú" and other songs to develop correct techniques important to vocal development. See Teacher to Teacher below, and on p. 475, and Skills Reinforcement on p. 476.

continued on page 474

SKILLS REINFORCEMENT

▶ Reading The first phrase of the refrain in "Eres tú" on p. 474 offers students an easy opportunity to try their music sight-reading skills. Have students

- Read the rhythm, using rhythm syllables.
- Read the melody, using pitch syllables.

Teach students the second phrase of the refrain by rote if they are unable to read it. Use rote to teach the verse.

TEACHER TO TEACHER

▶ Long Phrases Try these helpful tips for reminding students to sing long phrases.

- Trace the length of each phrase in the air as students sing. Invite them to join you.
- You may also show the phrase with both hands by pulling outwards on invisible taffy.

Whichever you choose, the physical movement will remind students to sing to the end of the phrase.

1c Invite students to learn to sing the Spanish text, using the Pronunciation Practice Guide on p. 546 and on Resource Book p. A-42 and the Pronunciation Practice **CD 22-13.**

Have students sing the melody of the refrain after verses 2 and 3 with the recording.

Encourage students to sing the verses of the song in Spanish with the recording **CD 22-10.**

Select a few students to sing the countermelody with the recording while the rest of the class sings the melody.

1d Invite students to sing the song with the countermelody in English with the recording **CD 22-11.**

Write the French, Spanish, Russian, and Hebrew translations of "I love you" on the board.

ASK Does anyone know how to say "I love you" in another language?

Invite those who can to write the phrase in that language on the board.

Refer to Across the Curriculum below to teach students how to pronounce the phrase "I love you" in other languages. See Across the Curriculum, p. 477, for additional phrases of friendship.

Demonstrate the American Sign Language (ASL) sign for "I love you," shown on p. 477, and encourage students to imitate it.

In a concert setting, *"Eres tú"* offers students the opportunity to perform expressively, from memory, a varied repertoire of music representing styles from diverse cultures. Students may also be interested in music from other cultures with vocal harmonies, in Skills Reinforcement below.

Playing

Invite students to accompany *"Eres tú"* on alto recorder. See Skills Reinforcement below.

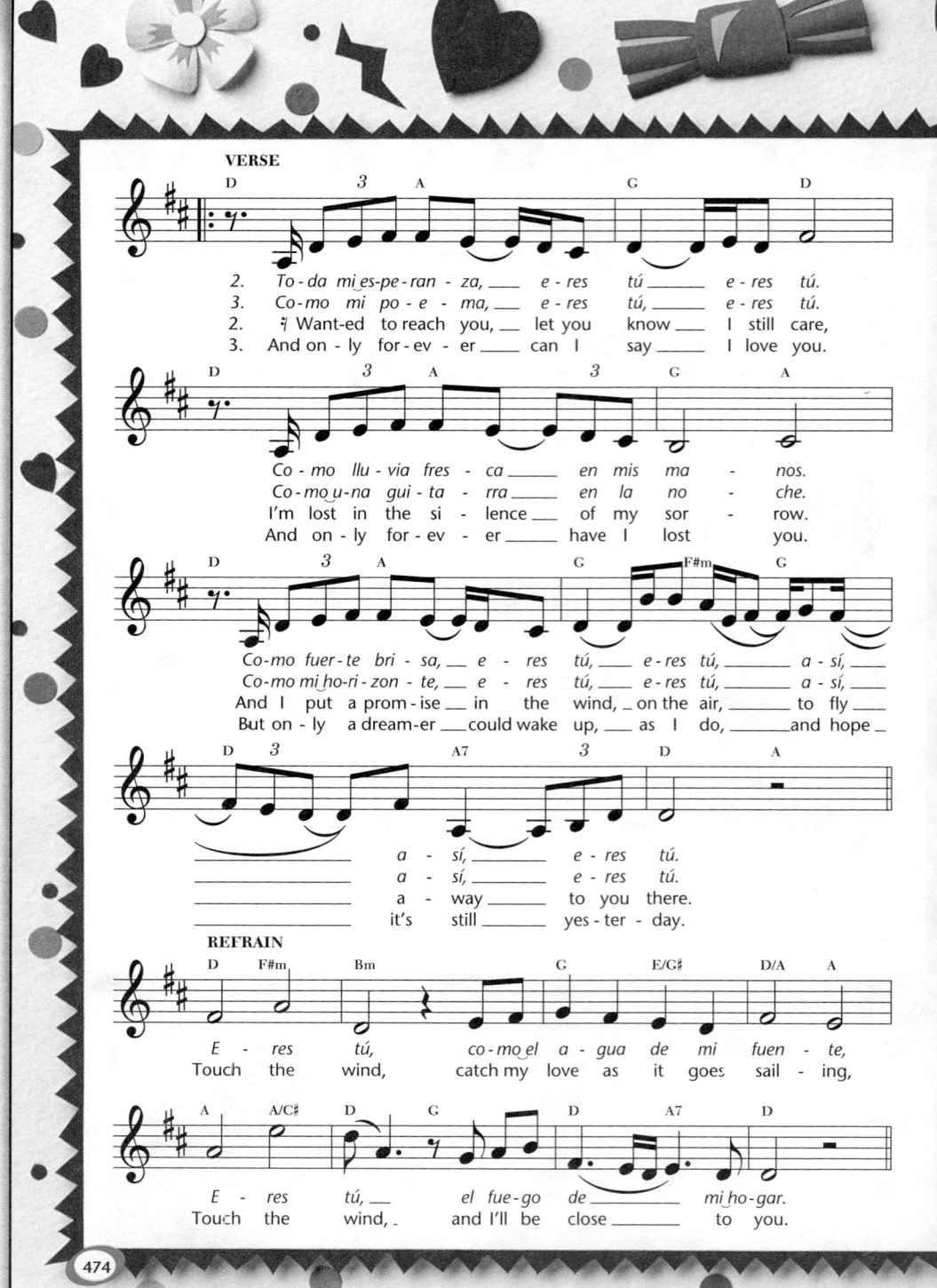

Footnotes

SKILLS REINFORCEMENT

► Recorder Invite students to get additional practice reading music for the alto recorder. Have students play this harmonic accompaniment during the verse of *"Eres tú."*

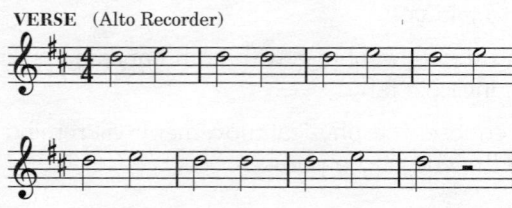

► Singing Students may wish to sing these songs from other cultures: *"Shalom aleichem"* on p. 409 (Israel); *"Habemos llegado"* on p. 174 (Puerto Rico); and *"Vem kan segla?"* on p. 417 (Finland).

ACROSS THE CURRICULUM

► Language Arts Valentine's Day is a good time to remind students that diverse cultures and countries often share common phrases. We express love with the words "I love you." Here is how that phrase is expressed in other languages.

Te amo	Spanish
Je t'aime	French
Ich liebe dich	German
Ti amo	Italian
Té amo	Portuguese

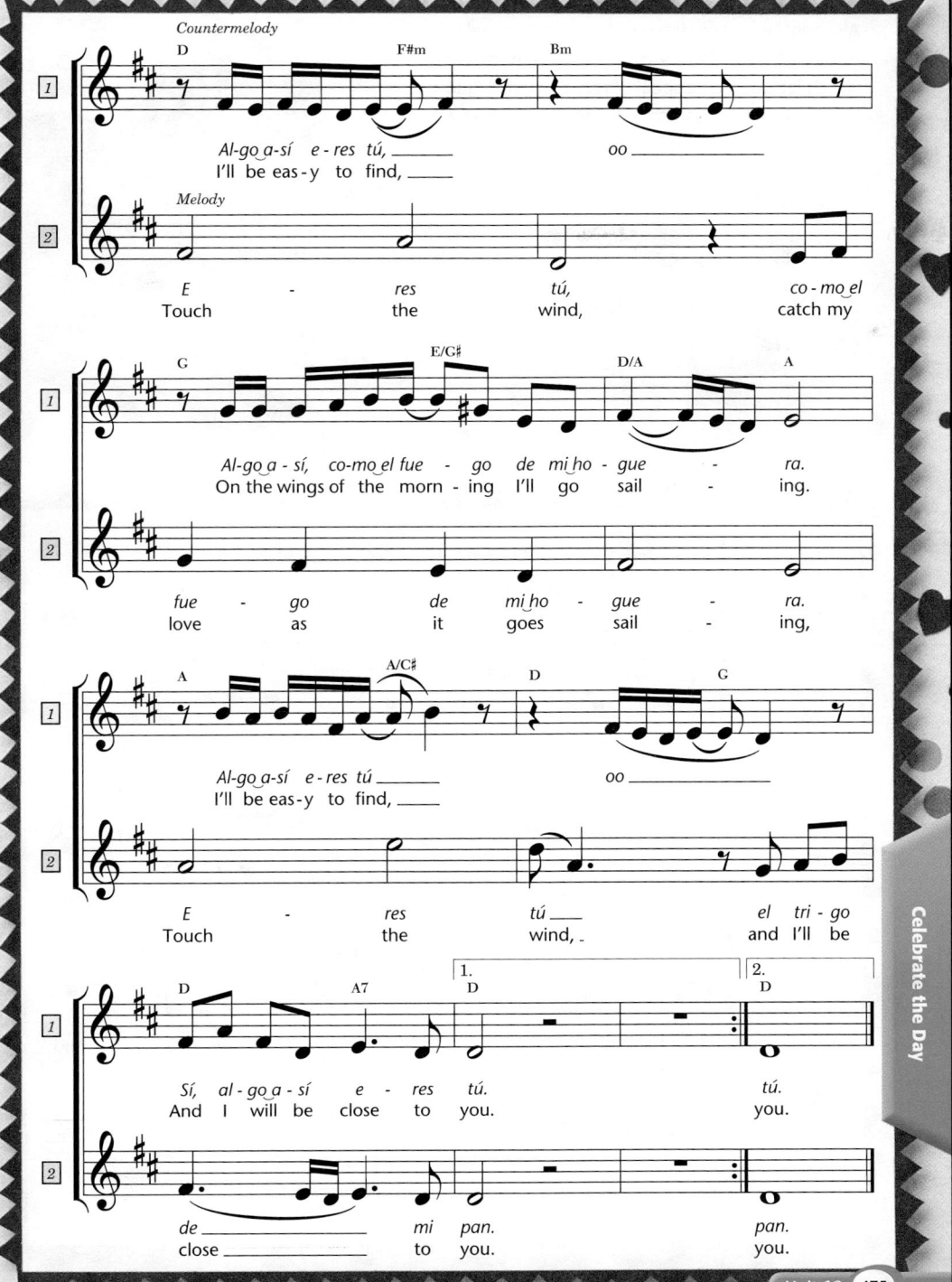

Celebrate the Day

Moving

 6a Invite students to listen to "Love in Any Language" **CD 22-14** with books closed and

- Discover what the song is about.
- Sign the ASL phrases when they hear the words in the song, p. 477.

With books open, help students follow the directions for signing the song.

Invite students to learn and perform the complete signing for "Love In Any Language." See Movement on p. 476 and on Resource Book p. G-27.

Singing

Encourage students to sing the refrain with the recording.

 6a Help students discover that

- The melody of the verse is the same each time it repeats, but the rhythm varies to fit the lyrics.
- The first part of the song is similar to an introduction.
- The verse starts after the refrain *We teach the young* p. 477.
- The key changes at the top of p. 479.

SAY The song modulates to a new key, beginning at the bottom of p. 478.

 1a Have students sing the entire song with the recording.

 1d Divide the class into two groups and have

- Group 1 sing the harmony part on the refrain on pp. 477 and 478.
- Group 2 sing the countermelody on p. 479 with the recording.

Invite students to sing "Love in Any Language" **CD 22-14** in two parts with the recording.

continued on page 476

SPOTLIGHT ON

▶ **Name-drawing** The Valentine tradition of sending cards to a sweetheart is based on an ancient tradition of *name-drawing,* in which young men drew girls' names from a hat to choose a "sweetheart" for the year. St. Valentine's Day was especially popular in the Middle Ages, when English knights sent Valentine messages, drawings, and poems to their ladies fair. Mass-produced Valentines were created in the 1800s and became popular in England and the United States. It became customary to send cards with short messages to friends and relatives, a tradition that is still alive today.

TEACHER TO TEACHER

1a ▶ **Singing and Posture** Help students prepare for a performance every time they sing. Have students monitor their body position and breathing techniques during every music class. Establish a "singing position" on the first day: torso straight but relaxed, hands at side if the individual is standing, face involved in activity. The students will look and sound better immediately, and they will gradually develop the habit of sitting or standing with good posture. Sixth-grade students want to look good when they sing, but they need an outside eye to guide them. Keep a video diary of their progress in maintaining good singing posture so that they can see the improvement.

These techniques will help students accomplish and demonstrate appropriate small- and large-ensemble performance techniques during formal and informal choral concerts

Performing

1a "Eres tú" and "Love in Any Language" are two songs that are concert favorites with audiences. Students will enjoy performing these songs for their peers at a small informal concert, such as a school assembly. Students may also wish to be a part of a larger formal evening concert for their parents and relatives, with combined music classes or school choir. In any case, students will benefit from the experience of learning to exhibit proper concert etiquette as an actively involved performer, and listener, during these varied live performances.

Have students keep a list of performance techniques that are appropriate for all concerts. The list can be divided into categories for small- and large-ensemble techniques and for formal and informal concerts. Lead a discussion of proper performer (and audience) etiquette, and have them add to the list.

1e
- Sing accurately, from memory, with good intonation, rhythm, and blend.
- Sing with proper posture and good breath support, singing long phrases where appropriate.
- Be attentive to the conductor, and your singing.
- Dress properly, as instructed by your conductor.
- Act professionally. Do not fool around during the concert.

3 CLOSE

Skill: SINGING   **ASSESSMENT**

1d **Performance/Self-Assessment** Invite students to choose which of the two songs they would like to perform and record. Have students

- Sing the song and record it on audiotape, if possible.
- Listen to the tape and write the form of the song (on paper), using the words *verse* and *refrain*.

A World of Love

Although we have different backgrounds and traditions, we all know what love is—no matter which language we speak. Practice saying "I love you" in French, Spanish, Russian, and Hebrew. Then **sing** the song "Love in Any Language."

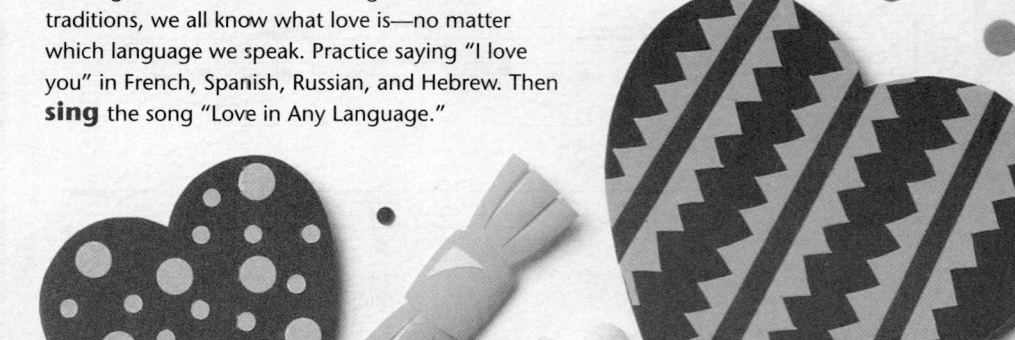

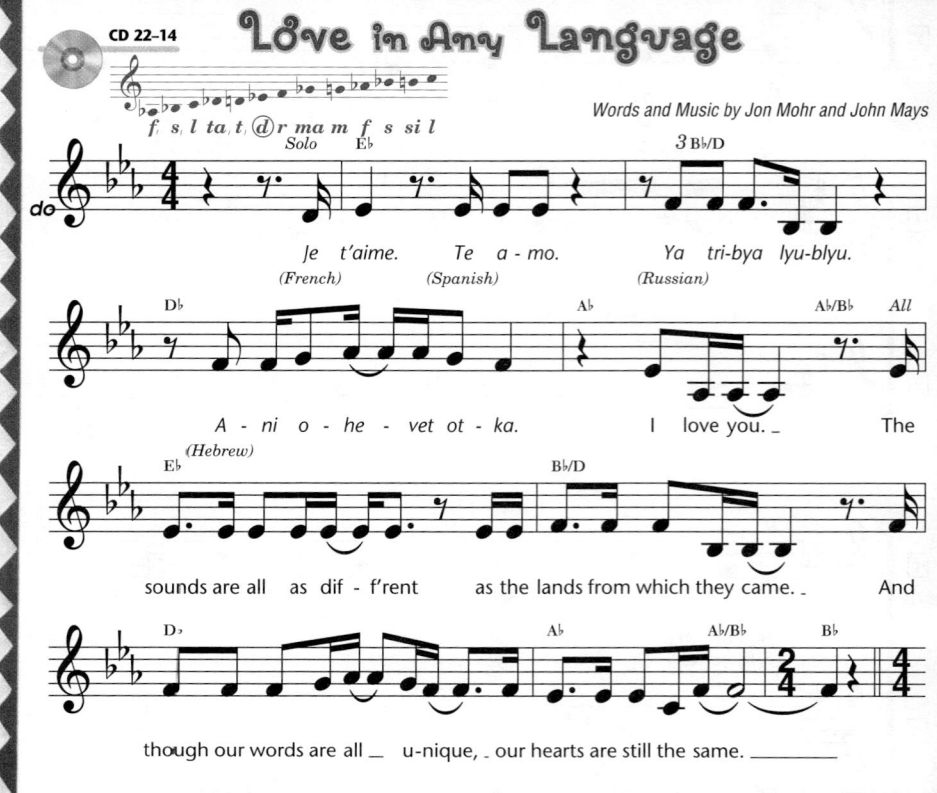

CD 22–14

Love in Any Language

Words and Music by Jon Mohr and John Mays

f, s, l, ta, t, @, r, ma, m, f, s, si, l
Solo   E♭   *3* B♭/D

do

Je t'aime.   Te a - mo.   Ya tri-bya lyu-blyu.
(French)   (Spanish)   (Russian)

D♭   A♭   A♭/B♭   *All*

A - ni o - he - vet ot - ka.   I love you. _   The
(Hebrew)

E♭   B♭/D

sounds are all as dif - f'rent   as the lands from which they came. _   And

D♭   A♭   A♭/B♭   B♭

though our words are all _ u-nique, _ our hearts are still the same. _____

476

Footnotes

SKILLS REINFORCEMENT

1a ▶ **Singing** You may find the following helpful in improving students' breath support when they are singing long phrases.

- Before singing, identify where each phrase starts and stops. This will help students predict the amount of breath they will need to sustain each line.
- Invite students to blow on invisible candles as long as each phrase lasts. Have them pretend that the candle is lit and that they can never blow out the light. As you play the recording, watch students' use of breath and their breathing techniques. Controlling air flow is an important element of singing.

MOVEMENT

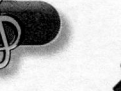

▶ **Signing** Students may be interested in expanding their knowledge of signing and in learning new signs. One opportunity to do this is in learning the signs for a song. The signing for "Love in Any Language" can be found on Resource Book p. G-27.

Inclusion of signing movements at an evening concert, or school performance, adds an important and dramatic dimension to the performance. Knowledge of signing also builds greater social awareness in students.

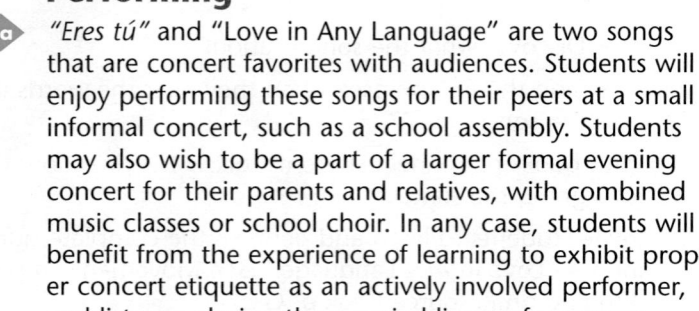

Signing with Love

Learn to sign these words as you sing "Love in Any Language."

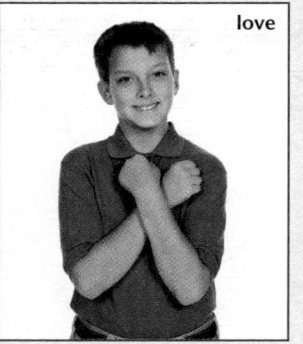
▲ Je t'aime

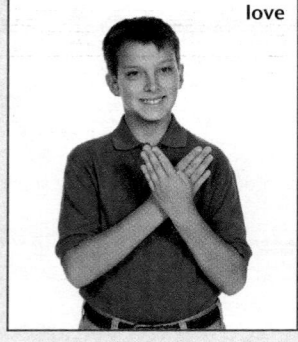
▲ Te amo

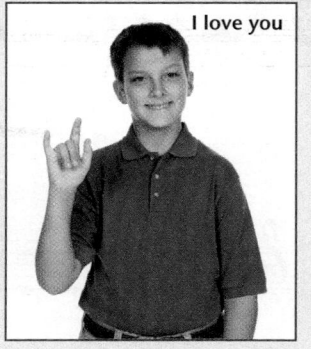
▲ I love you

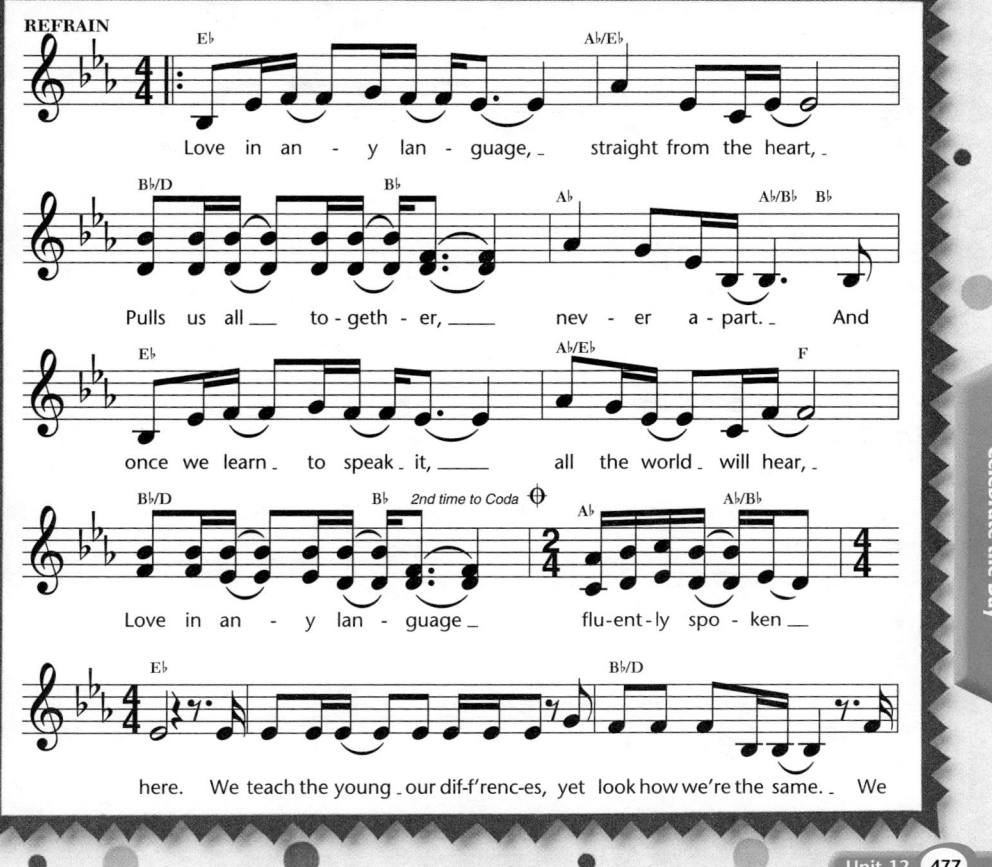

REFRAIN

Love in an - y lan - guage, _ straight from the heart, _

Pulls us all ___ to - geth - er, _____ nev - er a - part. _ And

once we learn _ to speak _ it, _____ all the world _ will hear, _

Love in an - y lan - guage _ flu - ent - ly spo - ken _____

here. We teach the young _ our dif-f'renc-es, yet look how we're the same. _ We

Celebrate the Day

- Self-assess their answers. (Do they have the right sequence and number of verses and refrains?)

If a tape recorder is not available, have students assess their peers' live performances.

A Look At
PRONUNCIATION PRACTICE TRACKS

The Pronunciation Practice tracks are recorded for your use in presenting high-quality non-English-language song demonstrations for your classroom.

In the interest of authenticity and accuracy, each model singer of the original text is a native of the country and language represented by the song.

Other helpful information about the Pronunciation Practice tracks:

- The length of phrases modeled is selected for optimum learning for each grade.
- In most cases, the Pronunciation Practice track is slower than the Stereo Vocal track, to facilitate easier learning of the non-English language.
- Not only will students learn the correct pronunciations, they will also be learning the way other languages are sung, including differences in timbre.
- It is possible for students to learn most of the non-English-language songs using only the Pronunciation Practice tracks.
- Use of the Pronunciation Practice track is a viable activity for a nonmusical substitute teacher to use in order for music learning to continue in your absence.

"Eres tú" Pronunciation Practice

Listen to the Pronunciation Practice track of *"Eres tú"* **CD 22-13.**

continued on page 478

MEETING INDIVIDUAL NEEDS

▶ **English Language Learners** Guide students to discover that a good way to express friendship to students from other countries is to learn a few words or phrases of the student's native language. Invite students in the class from other countries to write and speak these phrases in their native language. Invite teachers or persons in the community from other countries to visit the class and speak their native languages.

See Across the Curriculum in the next column for a list of foreign language phrases expressing greeting, friendship, and love.

ACROSS THE CURRICULUM

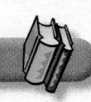

▶ **Language Arts** Have students learn these phrases of friendship. Ask native students or other teachers to help you pronounce these phrases.

English	Hello	How are you?	I like you I love you
French	Bonjour	Comment allez-vous?	Je vous aime Je t'aime
German	Hallo	Wie geht es Ihnen?	Ich mag Sie Ich liebe dich
Italian	Ciao	Como siete?	Li gradisco Ti amo
Portuguese	Ola	Como são você?	Eu gosto de te Té amo
Spanish	Hola	Cómo está usted?	Me gustas Te amo

A Look At
PHONETICS

The phonetics in this text offer a student-friendly and vocal-friendly rendition of the phonetic pronunciation. This simplified version is based on the type of written description a vocal instructor uses most often with this student age-group, desiring the most effectively sung vowel sounds.

When the foreign language sound has no English equivalent the closest English approximation will be used for the phonetics.

"Eres tú" Phonetics

Here is the refrain from *"Eres tú,"* as found in the Pronunciation Practice Guide, p. 546.

Eres tú

Pronunciation Practice

Refrain

Phrase 1. *E-res tú,*

eh-rehs too,

2. *co-mo el a-gua de mi fuen-te.*

koh-moh ehl ah-gwah deh mee fwehn-teh.

3. *E-res tú,*

eh-rehs too,

4. *el fue-go de mi ho-gar.*

ehl fweh-goh deh mee oh-gahr.

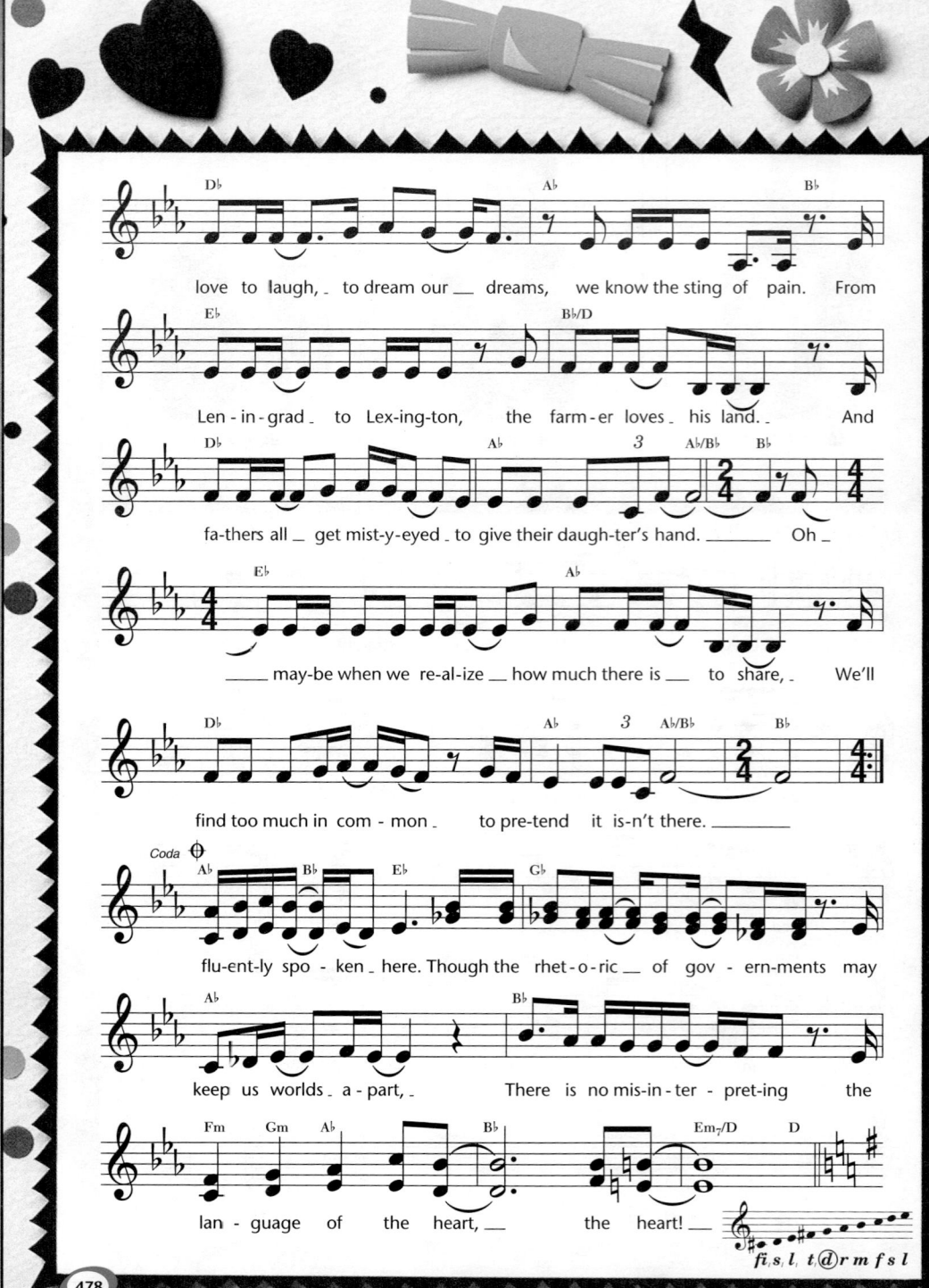

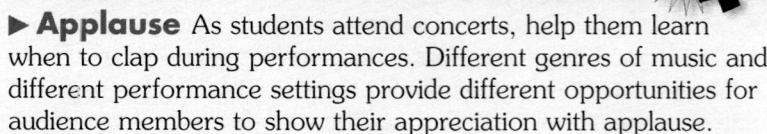

Footnotes

478

SPOTLIGHT ON

▶ **Valentine Traditions** Many interesting customs have developed around St. Valentine's Day.

- If a young lady receives clothing from a gentleman and keeps it, she will wed that young man.
- Wales: If you receive a wooden spoon with a heart, a key, or a keyhole, you have been told, "You unlock my heart."
- Whom will you marry? Say the names of potential suitors (or fair damsels) as you twist the stem off an apple. When the stem comes off, the name of the person you are saying at that moment is the one!
- Middle Ages: A man drew a name from a bowl and wore that name on his sleeve for a week. (That is where the expression "wearing your heart on your sleeve" came from.)

AUDIENCE ETIQUETTE

▶ **Applause** As students attend concerts, help them learn when to clap during performances. Different genres of music and different performance settings provide different opportunities for audience members to show their appreciation with applause.

- Orchestra/Concert Band/Instrumental Ensemble/Choir or Soloist—Do not clap between movements in a symphony or other multi-section piece of music. Wait until the conductor lowers his or her hands and steps off the podium before clapping.
- Jazz—During most jazz selections, players take turns improvising. It is appropriate to clap after each soloist is finished.
- Opera—During an opera, it is appropriate to clap after the overture, after an aria, and at the end of a scene or act.

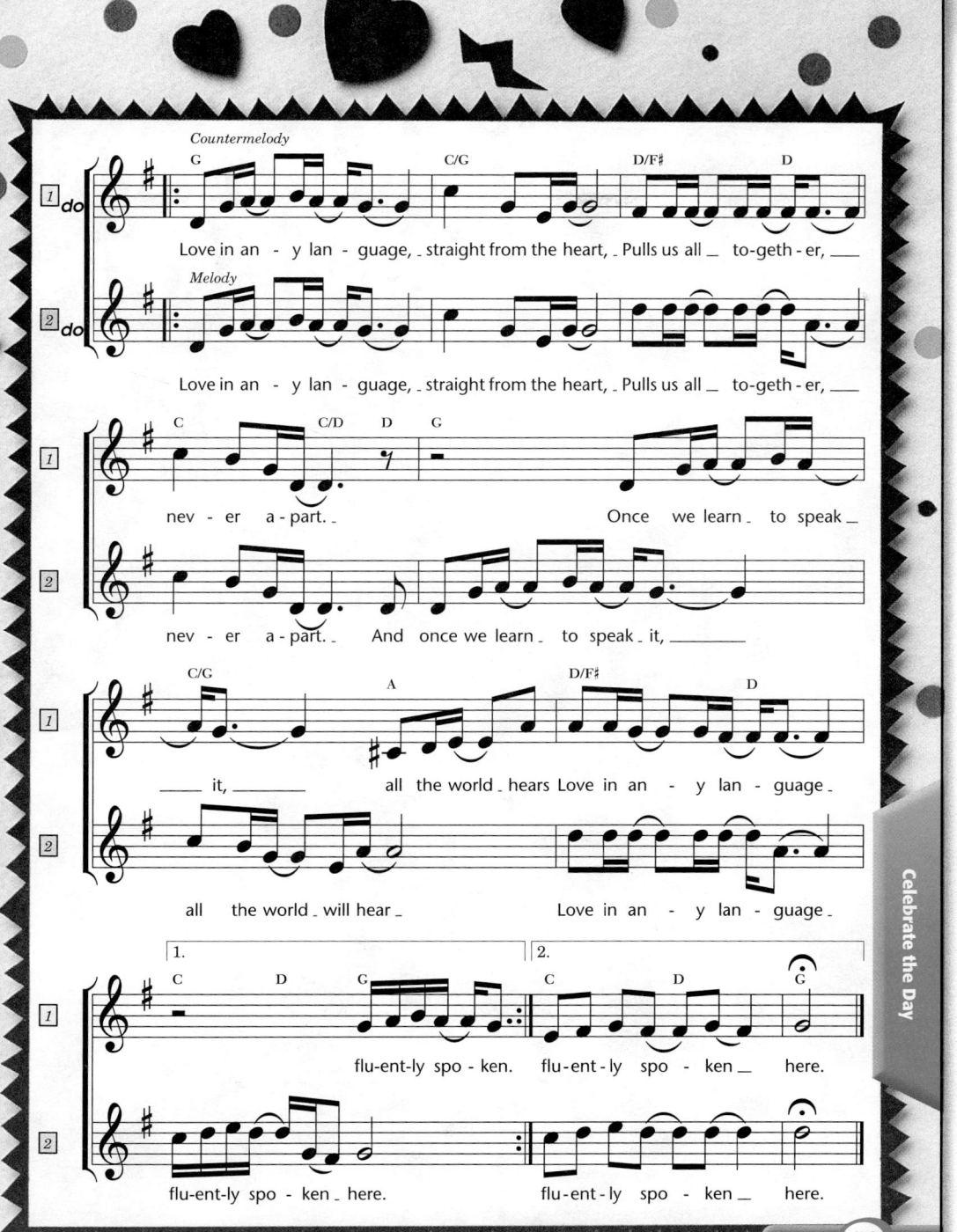

Love in an-y lan-guage, straight from the heart, Pulls us all __ to-geth-er, ___

nev-er a-part. __ Once we learn __ to speak __

nev-er a-part. And once we learn __ to speak __ it, ___

it, ___ all the world __ hears Love in an- y lan-guage.

all the world __ will hear __ Love in an- y lan-guage.

flu-ent-ly spo-ken. flu-ent-ly spo-ken __ here.

flu-ent-ly spo-ken __ here. flu-ent-ly spo-ken __ here.

A Look At TRANSLATIONS

Literal Translations A literal translation is a simple English translation of the foreign text. It is only meant to convey the meaning of the foreign text and is not meant for singing. You may want students to know that the literal translation does not express the cadence or beauty of the original language.

Literal translations are provided by professional language institutes or translators, language scholars, and professional nationals of the respective country. All attempts are made to respect native cultures.

"Eres tú" Literal Translation

Here is the refrain from *"Eres tú,"* in a literal translation.

Refrain
You are like the water in my fountain,
You are the fire in my hearth.
You are like the fire of my bonfire,
You are like the wheat of my bread.

English Lyrics The English lyrics of a song hope to transfer the original intent of the foreign language in a poetic and understandable English version. Lyrics hope to capture the mood of the song as well as the meaning. English verses are appropriate for singing.

"Eres tú" Lyrics

Here is the refrain from *"Eres tú,"* as English lyrics that can be sung.

Refrain

Touch the wind,

Catch my love as it goes sailing,

Touch the wind,

And I'll be close to you.

CHARACTER EDUCATION

▶ **Expressing Friendship** Guide students to understand that making friends is a social skill. Encourage students to discuss how they view friendship and how they wish to be treated.

Reinforcement Many students are shy and may appear to not be as popular or have as many friends as others. Invite them to exchange thoughts on what friendship means to each of them.

On Target Many students will feel that they are "cool" and have all the friends they need. Invite these students to examine how they act with their friends. Is there "give and take" in a friendship, or does someone mostly take? Ask them how they might change their actions so that their friendships grow and get better.

Challenge Invite students to challenge their current notions of friendship. Ask them if they can be friends with a shy person, or how a shy person might become more outgoing.

TECHNOLOGY/MEDIA LINK

CD-ROM Invite students to use a CD-ROM encyclopedia from their local library to learn more about Valentine's Day.

Multimedia Have students illustrate the lyrics of "Love in Any Language" using a slide show software program. Display the slides during a performance of the song.

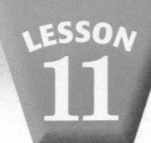

Birthdays and Anniversaries

Birthdays and anniversaries are reasons to celebrate. Mexicans and Mexican Americans sing this song about "morning" as a birthday greeting.

Sing the song in two-part harmony. The harmony part is a third above the melody.

480

LESSON AT A GLANCE

Element Focus **TEXTURE/HARMONY** Harmony in parallel thirds

Skill Objective **SINGING** Sing a two-part song in parallel thirds

Connection Activity **CULTURE** Create a Mexican birthday piñata

MATERIALS
- "Las mañanitas" (Spanish)   **CD 22-16**
- "Las mañanitas" (English)   **CD 22-17**
  Recording Routine: Intro (10 m.); vocal; interlude (10 m.); vocal; coda
- **Pronunciation Practice/Translation** p. 547
- **Resource Book** pp. A-45, H-30
- melody bells, guitars, keyboards

VOCABULARY
interval   thirds   parallel motion

◆ ◆ ◆ ◆ **National Standards** ◆ ◆ ◆ ◆

1c Sing music from diverse cultures
1d Sing music written in two parts
2b Perform easy instrumental pieces with technical accuracy

MORE MUSIC CHOICES
For more practice with harmony in thirds:
"Así es mi tierra," p. 172

1 INTRODUCE

Invite students to discuss family traditions for birthday celebrations. Explain that people in different countries celebrate birthdays differently. Most Mexican and other Hispanic people sing "Las mañanitas" as a birthday greeting. Tell students they will create a piñata, using the suggestions in School to Home Connection on p. 481. Share the information in Spotlight On below.

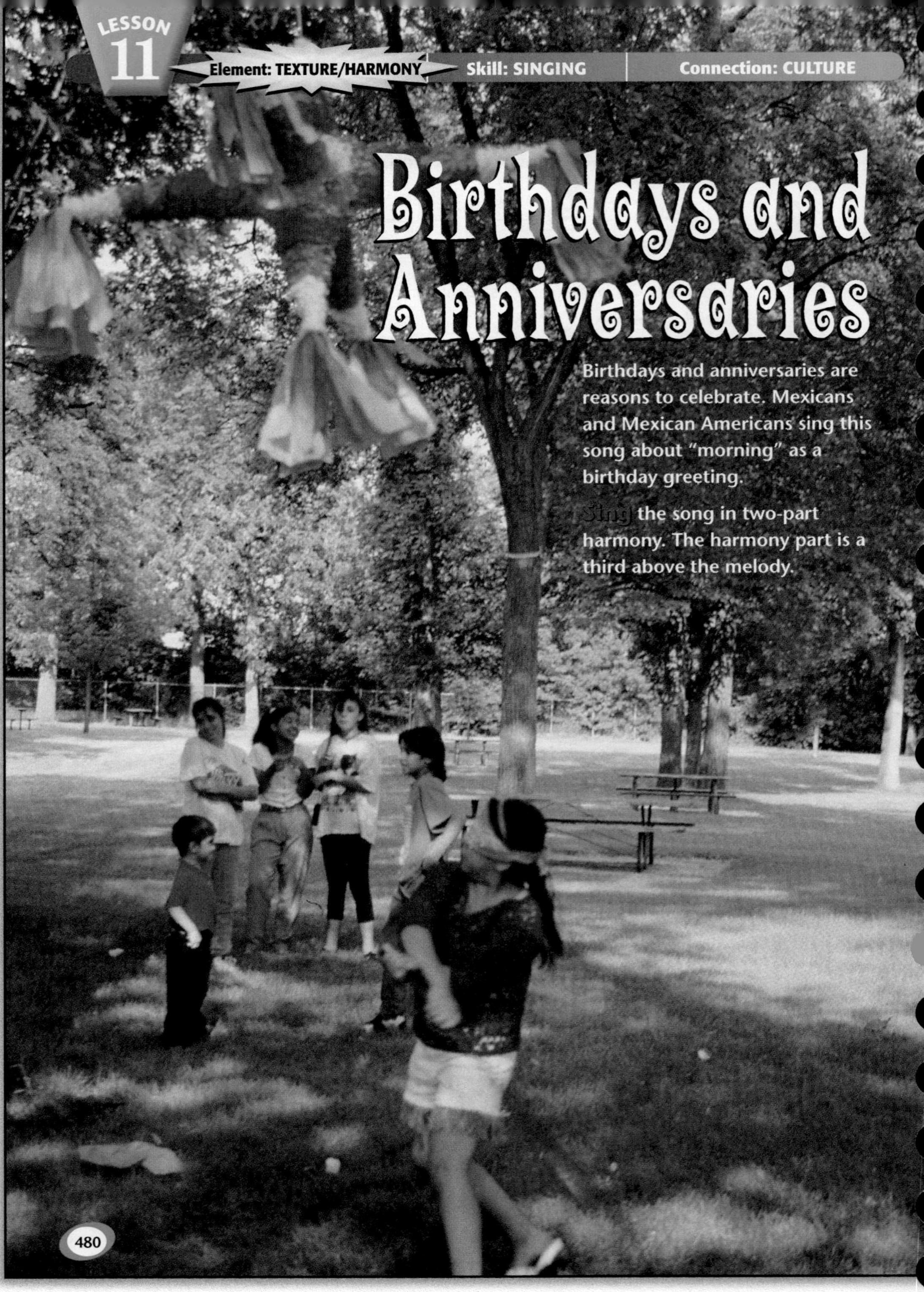

Footnotes

SPOTLIGHT ON

▶ **Piñatas** A popular centerpiece of many Spanish and Mexican birthdays is the piñata, a hollow papier-mâché animal stuffed with candy, toys, and trinkets. The piñata is hung above the heads of the party goers. Each person takes a turn hitting the piñata with a long stick while blindfolded. When it breaks, everyone rushes in to gather up its contents of coins, small toys, or pieces of candy.

BUILDING SKILLS THROUGH MUSIC

▶ **Writing** Have students develop a written description of how a birthday is celebrated in their household, demonstrating their ability to write a cohesive description of the day.

SKILLS REINFORCEMENT

▶ **Guitar** "Las mañanitas" is an ideal song for guitar accompaniment. It may be easier for students to play the song with a capo on the first fret and chording the song in E. Use a simple "thumb-strum-strum" in the right hand, one pattern per measure. Make use of this song by "serenading" class members on their birthdays, with the guitarist(s) standing near to the recipient.

▶ **Keyboard** Invite students to learn a keyboard accompaniment to "Las mañanitas" that uses the I, IV, and V_7 chords in F major. See Resource Book p. H-30 for this arrangement.

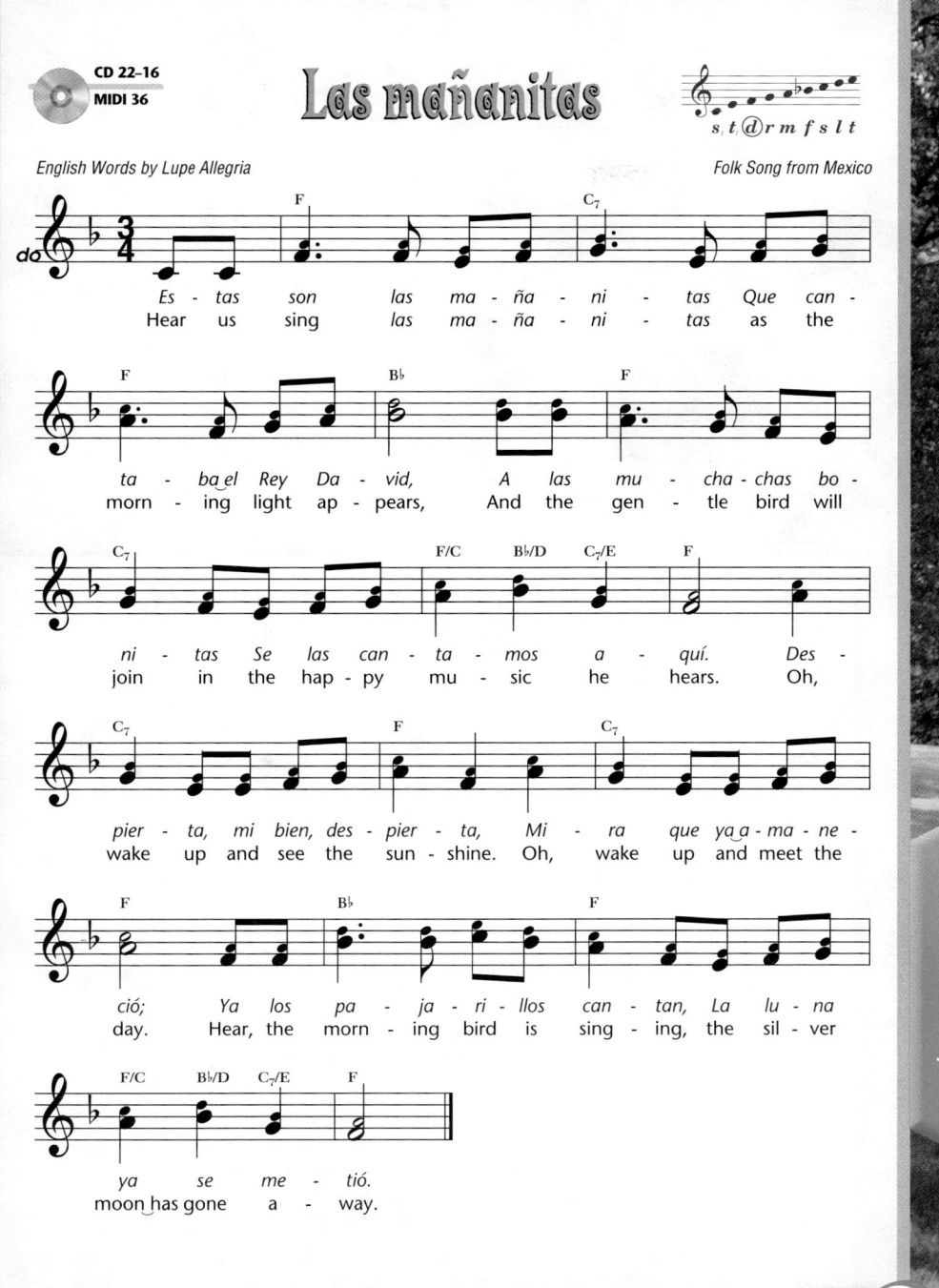

CD 22–16
MIDI 36

Las mañanitas

English Words by Lupe Allegria

Folk Song from Mexico

Es - tas son las ma - ña - ni - tas Que can -
Hear us sing las ma - ña - ni - tas as the

ta - ba el Rey Da - vid, A las mu - cha - chas bo -
morn - ing light ap - pears, And the gen - tle bird will

ni - tas Se las can - ta - mos a - quí. Des -
join in the hap - py mu - sic he hears. Oh,

pier - ta, mi bien, des - pier - ta, Mi - ra que ya a - ma - ne -
wake up and see the sun - shine. Oh, wake up and meet the

ció; Ya los pa - ja - ri - llos can - tan, La lu - na
day. Hear, the morn - ing bird is sing - ing, the sil - ver

ya se me - tió.
moon has gone a - way.

Celebrate the Day

Unit 12 **481**

2 DEVELOP

Singing

Have students learn the Spanish pronunciation by using the Pronunciation Practice Guide on p. 547 and on Resource Book p. A-45. Have them sing in Spanish with the Pronunciation Practice **CD 22-19** and **CD 20**.

1c Have students sing the melody in English with the recording **CD 22-17**.

1d Have students sing the harmony part with the recording **CD 22-16**.

ASK What do we call the distance between two notes? (an interval)

SAY On the staff, the interval from a space to the next space is a third and the interval from a line to the next line is also a third.

Guide students to discover that every interval in the harmony is a third, and that the thirds move parallel to each other. Tell students that this movement is called parallel motion. In this case, the harmony is in parallel thirds.

Playing

Have students find thirds on melody bells or keyboards.

ASK What chords are used to harmonize "Las mañanitas"? (F, B♭, and C₇)

2b Invite students to learn the guitar and keyboard accompaniment in Skills Reinforcement on p. 480, and on Resource Book p. H-30.

3 CLOSE

Element: TEXTURE/HARMONY — ASSESSMENT

Performance/Self-Assessment Invite students to sing "Las mañanitas" in harmony as a class. Allow students to break into groups to improve their singing of harmony. (Moving to a harmony note from the melody note and using a piano may help students.) Have students evaluate how they sang the harmony parts.

SKILLS REINFORCEMENT

▶ **Improvisation** Using vocal chording (see Skills Reinforcement, p. 446), students can begin vocal improvisation. Write the chord progression to the first eight measures of "Las mañanitas" on the board. (I, V₇, I, IV, I, V₇, I, IV, V₇, and I)

- Divide the class into three groups for vocal chording while the fourth group sings the melody to "Las mañanitas."
- Tell students to sing any note in the chord tone.
- Sing the melody while students sing their own harmonic accompaniments.
- Have students improvise different harmonic accompaniments.

SCHOOL TO HOME CONNECTION

▶ **Mini-piñata** Students can make a piñata at home or as a classroom project. Use cups with lids. Have students

- Push a pipe cleaner through the center of the bottom; bend the end so it will not pull out. Bend the other end to use as a hanger. (As a piñata, the cup will hang upside down.)
- Fill the cup with popcorn or candy.
- Replace the lid; decorate the piñata; hang it by the hanger.

TECHNOLOGY/MEDIA LINK

CD-ROM Have students create Latin arrangements to "Las mañanitas" using *Band-in-a-Box.*

LESSON AT A GLANCE

Element Focus **TEXTURE/HARMONY** Harmony in a mallet accompaniment

Skill Objective **PLAYING** Play a mallet accompaniment

Connection Activity **CULTURE** Discover the celebration of *Carnaval*

MATERIALS

- "*El carnavalito humahuaqueño*" **CD 22-21**
- "The Little Humahuacan Carnival" **CD 22-22**

  Recording Routine: Intro (8 m.); v. 1; interlude (4 m.); v. 2; coda

- **Pronunciation Practice/Translation** p. 547
- **Resource Book** pp. A-46, F-36
- mallet instruments, nonpitched percussion instruments

VOCABULARY

first and second endings   coda

ostinato   dissonance

◆ ◆ ◆ National Standards ◆ ◆ ◆

1c Sing music from diverse cultures

2a Play instruments accurately with good stick technique

2c Perform instrumental music from diverse cultures

4a Compose short pieces, demonstrating unity and variety through music

7b Students use specific criteria for evaluating their own performances

MORE MUSIC CHOICES

For other songs from South America sung in Spanish:

"*O lê lê O Bahía*" (Brazil), p. 165

"*Cuando pa' Chile me voy*" (Chile), p. 376

"*La mariposa*" (Bolivia), p. 58

1 INTRODUCE

Share with students the information in Cultural Connection below and Across the Curriculum, p. 483, on Argentinian culture.

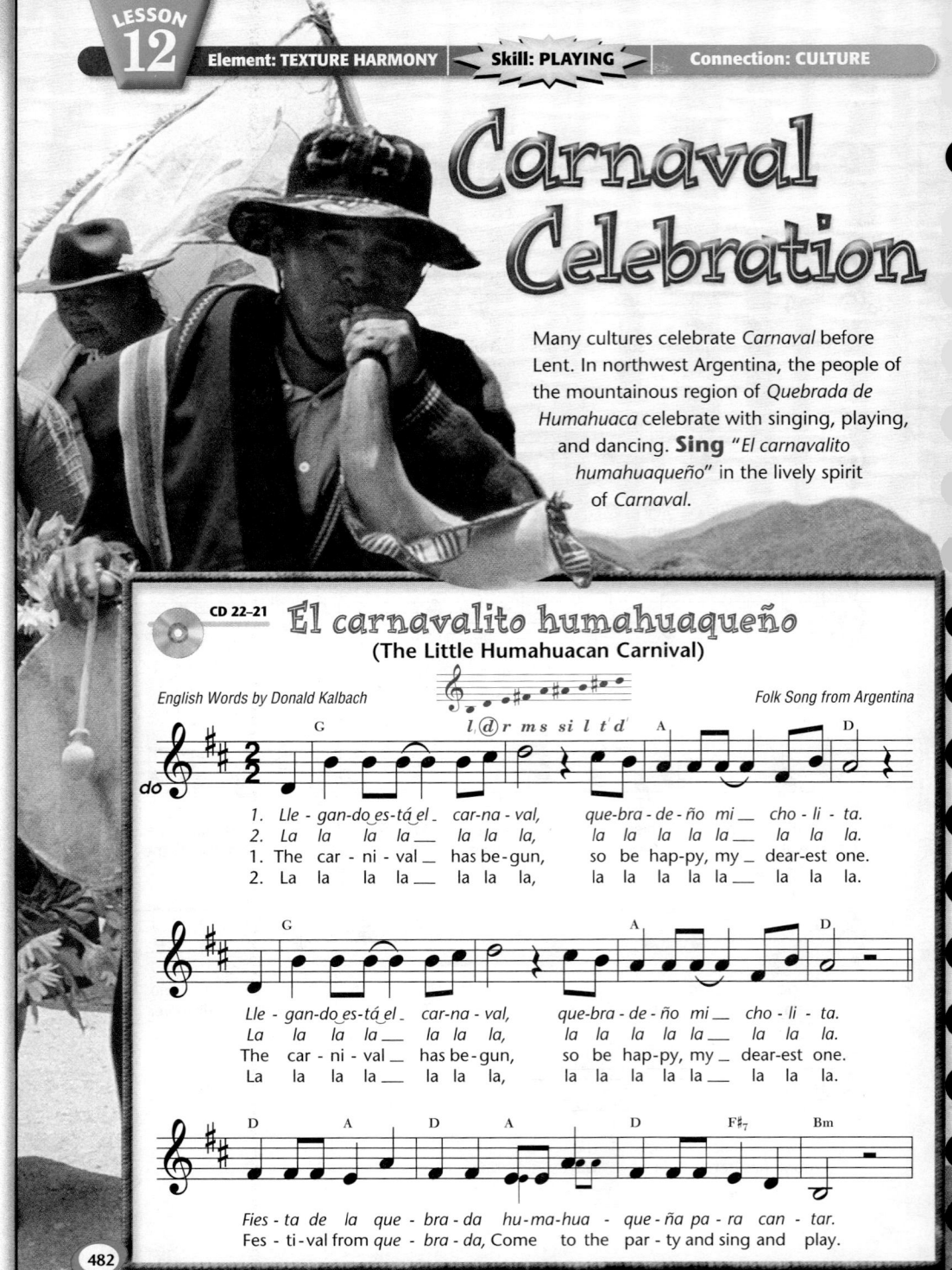

Carnaval Celebration

Many cultures celebrate *Carnaval* before Lent. In northwest Argentina, the people of the mountainous region of *Quebrada de Humahuaca* celebrate with singing, playing, and dancing. **Sing** "*El carnavalito humahuaqueño*" in the lively spirit of *Carnaval*.

CD 22-21 El carnavalito humahuaqueño
(The Little Humahuacan Carnival)

English Words by Donald Kalbach   *Folk Song from Argentina*

1. Lle - gan-do es-tá el _ car-na - val, que-bra - de - ño mi _ cho - li - ta.
2. La la la la, la la la, la la la la la la la la.
1. The car - ni - val _ has be-gun, so be hap-py, my _ dear-est one.
2. La la la la, la la la, la la la la la la la la.

Lle - gan-do es-tá el _ car-na - val, que-bra - de - ño mi _ cho - li - ta.
La la la la _ la la la, la la la la la _ la la la.
The car - ni - val _ has be-gun, so be hap-py, my _ dear-est one.
La la la la _ la la la, la la la la la _ la la la.

Fies - ta de la que - bra - da hu-ma-hua - que - ña pa - ra can - tar.
Fes - ti-val from *que - bra - da*, Come to the par - ty and sing and play.

482

Footnotes

CULTURAL CONNECTION

▶ **Immigration's Influence on Culture** Argentina's culture has its foundation in its immigrant population. This European influence contributed to the disappearance of pre-Columbian cultures. The European immigrant groups each adopted different roles. The Basque and Irish controlled sheep ranching, the Germans and Italians established farms, and the British invested in developing the country's economy.

BUILDING SKILLS THROUGH MUSIC

▶ **Reading** Working from the text information provided in the footnotes and in the student text, have students assemble all the information they can that helps them learn about Argentina, and organize that information using a graphic organizer of their choice from the Resource Book.

SKILLS REINFORCEMENT

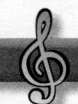

1a ▶ **Playing** To help students with the harmony played by the basses, echo-sing the bass and contrabass xylophone chord tones

2a for "*El carnavalito humahuaqueño*" on p. 483, using pitch syllables or note letter names before transferring to instruments. Although the rhythms for the alto xylophones are not difficult, invite students to first clap the rhythms, then clap and sing the top part of the chord, the middle note, and the lowest note before playing these notes on instruments. Two players can share the alto xylophone part, one playing the upper and middle notes, the other the lowest note. On knees, have students pat the rhythm of the soprano xylophone part before playing, noting that the ostinato occurs in mm. 3–4 and mm. 7–8.

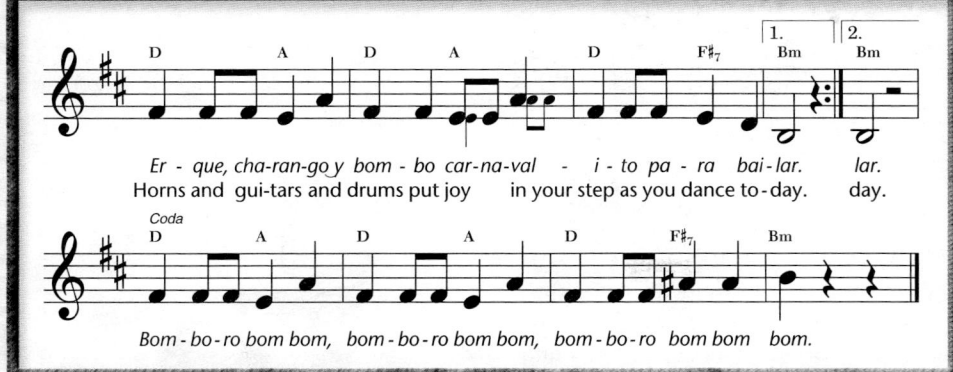

Er - que, cha-ran-go y bom - bo car-na-val - i - to pa - ra bai-lar. lar.
Horns and gui-tars and drums put joy in your step as you dance to-day. day.

Bom - bo - ro bom bom, bom - bo - ro bom bom, bom - bo - ro bom bom bom.

Festive Harmonies

Play this arrangement of "El carnavalito humahuaqueño" for mallet instruments. Are the harmonies in this arrangement the same or different than the song recording?

Arranged by Konnie Saliba

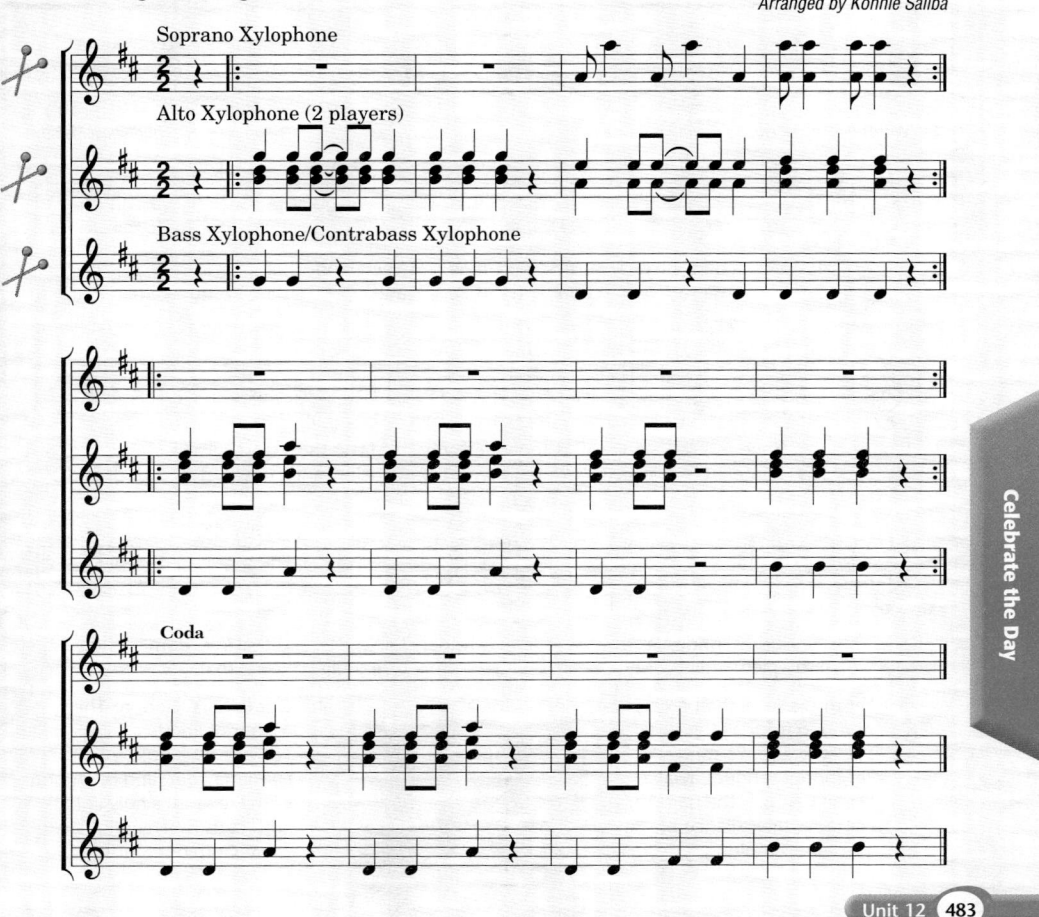

Unit 12 **483**

Celebrate the Day

2 DEVELOP

Analyzing

Ask students to look at the music and identify the first and second ending and the coda.

ASK What parts of the song are repeated? (mm. 1–4 repeated once; mm. 9–12 repeated once)

Singing

1c Invite students to listen to and sing "El carnavalito humahuaqueño" **CD 22-21.** Have them

- Use the Pronunciation Practice **CD 22-24** and Resource Book, p. A-46, to learn the Spanish.
- Sing with the recording and identify the syncopations.
- Sing the song again, clapping each measure that contains syncopated rhythms.

Playing

2a Guide students to discover the harmony in the alto xylophone part on p. 483. (G, D, and Bm chords.) Have students

4a - Perform a percussion ostinato in Resource Book, p. F-36, and then create ostinatos for nonpitched percussion instruments.

2c - Perform the song on mallet and percussion instruments.

3 CLOSE

Skill: PLAYING **ASSESSMENT**

2c **Performance/Peer Critique** Divide the class into groups. Ask each group to perform the mallet accom-
7b paniment with the recording. Afterwards, ask each group to critique its own performance, using the criteria below, and to offer suggestions for improvement.

- Were the chords (harmony) performed accurately?
- Were the rhythms accurate for each part?

ACROSS THE CURRICULUM

▶ **Social Studies** The Quebrada de Humahuaca is a very mountainous section of Argentina located in the northwest region. Humahuaca is the name of a town. The literal meaning of the word is *ravine*. The *erque (erke)* is a long horn used in the mountains, similar to a Swiss alpenhorn. The *charango* is a small guitar with five sets of double strings.

Meat dominates Argentina's menus, and meat means beef. Mixed grills *(parrillada)* serve up a cut of just about every part of the animal: tripe, intestines, and udders. It is a vegetarian's nightmare. Italian favorites, such as *gnocchi (ñoquis)* reflect the effects of immigration. Exquisite Argentine ice cream *(helado)* reflects the Italian influences. The sharing of *mate* is a symbol more than a beverage. The leaves of this plant are dried and used to make tea. To be offered this drink, is a sign of friendship.

TECHNOLOGY/MEDIA LINK

Electronic Keyboard Invite students to use the auto-accompaniment feature of their MIDI keyboard to create new accompaniments to "El carnavalito humahuaqueño." Have students identify auto-accompaniment styles that may be appropriate for the song. Ask them to perform the accompaniment, using one- and two-finger chords (typical of auto-accompaniment keyboards).

Have students vary the accompaniment style and tempo to discover how the character of the song may change. Students may wish to record their findings in their music journal. Invite students to perform their auto-accompaniment as the class sings the song.

LESSON AT A GLANCE

Element Focus   **EXPRESSION** Slurs, fermata, dynamics, and mood

Skill Objective   **SINGING** Sing a patriotic song with expression

Connection Activity   **SOCIAL STUDIES** Discuss the history behind patriotic songs

MATERIALS

- "America"   **CD 23-1**
  Recording Routine: Intro (4 m.); four verses with interludes (2 m.)
- "America, the Beautiful"   **CD 23-4**
  Recording Routine: Intro (4 m.); three verses
- "The Star-Spangled Banner"   **CD 23-6**
  Recording Routine: Intro (4 m.); three verses
- *America, the Beautiful* (gospel)   **CD 23-3**
- *L'union* (excerpt)   **CD 23-8**
- **Resource Book** p. H-31
- hand chimes or resonator bells (resonator bells must have one mallet per bell), keyboard

VOCABULARY

phrase   fermata

◆ ◆ ◆ National Standards ◆ ◆ ◆

1d Sing music written in two parts
1e In groups, sing moderately easy pieces with expression
5a Read dotted notes in triple meter
5c Identify standard notation symbols for expression
6b Listen and analyze uses of dynamics in music from diverse genres
7a Students evaluate the music they hear

MORE MUSIC CHOICES

For more practice singing about patriotism:
"Sing a Song of Peace," p. 66
"Strike Up the Band," p. 135

---

patriotism sings

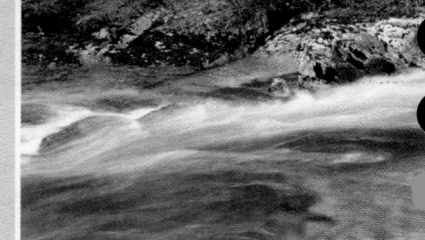

We celebrate patriotism with songs about our country. "America" is a patriotic melody we share with Great Britain. The British sing "God Save the Queen." Which country used the melody first? Why?

Sing "America." What style will you use to express the meaning of the words?

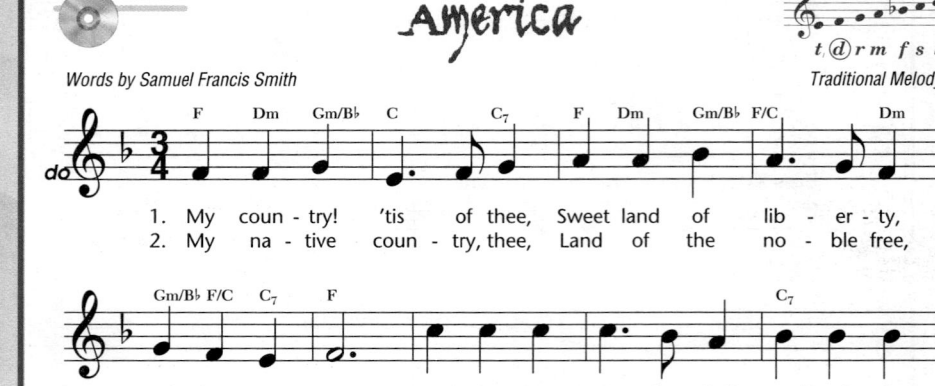

CD 23–1

America

Words by Samuel Francis Smith

Traditional Melody

t d r m f s l

1. My coun - try! 'tis of thee, Sweet land of lib - er - ty,
2. My na - tive coun - try, thee, Land of the no - ble free,

Of thee I sing; Land where my fa - thers died, Land of the
Thy name I love; I love thy rocks and rills, Thy woods and

Pil - grims' pride, From ev - 'ry __ moun - tain - side Let __ free - dom ring!
tem - pled hills; My heart __ with __ rap - ture thrills Like __ that a - bove.

3. Let music swell the breeze,
And ring from all the trees
Sweet freedom's song;
Let mortal tongues awake,
Let all that breathe partake,
Let rocks their silence break,
The sound prolong.

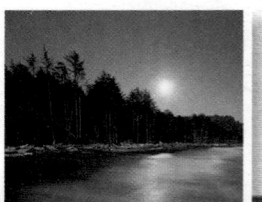

4. Our fathers' God, to Thee,
Author of liberty,
To Thee we sing;
Long may our land be bright
With Freedom's holy light,
Protect us by Thy might,
Great God, our King!

484

Footnotes

TEACHER TO TEACHER

▶ **Keyboard Accompaniments** If a teacher is not a trained pianist, playing the accompaniments to patriotic songs is a challenge. By playing chords with "added" bass notes (Gm/B♭), chord accompaniments to the songs will sound closer to their standard accompaniments. Popular music uses this method of notation (Gm/B♭) in comparison to music theory notation (ii6) and "inversion" nomenclature.

BUILDING SKILLS THROUGH MUSIC

▶ **Reading** Divide the class into groups. Assign each group one of the songs in the lesson. Have the groups write a list of all the words they do not recognize and determine definitions for them. Have the groups share the words and definitions from their song.

CULTURAL CONNECTION

▶ **"America"** The music to "America" is the same as the British national anthem, "God Save the Queen." When the British sing their anthem, it is traditional to change the words to reflect the current monarch. Here is the first verse of "God Save the Queen," first heard in 1744.

> God save our gracious Queen,
> Long live our noble Queen,
> God save the Queen!
> Send her victorious,
> Happy and glorious,
> Long to reign over us,
> God save the Queen!

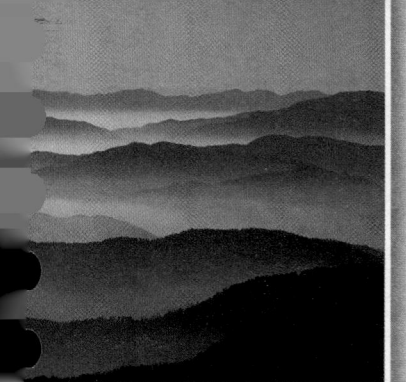

Beautiful America

The beauty of the land that became America is something to celebrate. Katharine Lee Bates wrote this poem that expresses her feelings about our beautiful country. The poem was later set to a hymn tune composed by Samuel A. Ward.

Sing "America, the Beautiful."

Then **listen** to a gospel version of the song.

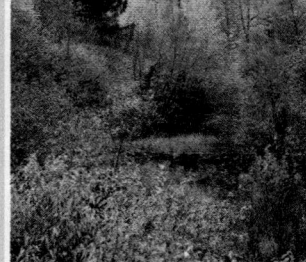

CD 23-3
America, the Beautiful

by S.A. Ward and Katharine Lee Bates

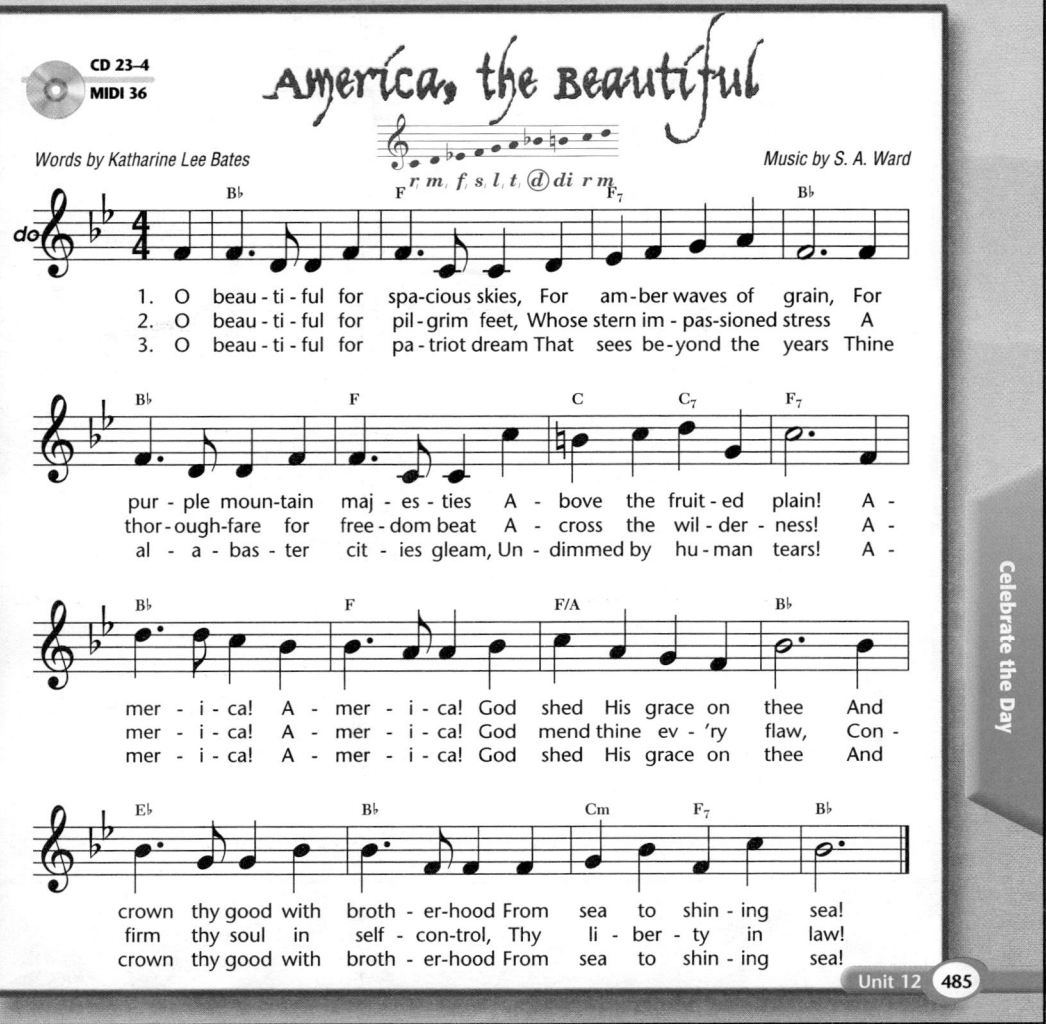

CD 23-4
MIDI 36

America, the Beautiful

Words by Katharine Lee Bates

Music by S. A. Ward

1. O beau-ti-ful for spa-cious skies, For am-ber waves of grain, For
2. O beau-ti-ful for pil-grim feet, Whose stern im-pas-sioned stress A
3. O beau-ti-ful for pa-triot dream That sees be-yond the years Thine

pur-ple moun-tain maj-es-ties A-bove the fruit-ed plain! A-
thor-ough-fare for free-dom beat A-cross the wil-der-ness! A-
al-a-bas-ter cit-ies gleam, Un-dimmed by hu-man tears! A-

mer-i-ca! A-mer-i-ca! God shed His grace on thee And
mer-i-ca! A-mer-i-ca! God mend thine ev-'ry flaw, Con-
mer-i-ca! A-mer-i-ca! God shed His grace on thee And

crown thy good with broth-er-hood From sea to shin-ing sea!
firm thy soul in self-con-trol, Thy li-ber-ty in law!
crown thy good with broth-er-hood From sea to shin-ing sea!

Unit 12 485

Celebrate the Day

continued on page 486

1 INTRODUCE

Encourage students to create a list of patriotic holidays on the board and discuss the history associated with each one. (Independence Day, Veterans Day, Presidents Day, Memorial Day, Flag Day)

Encourage students to read and discuss the information on p. 484.

2 DEVELOP

Singing

1e Invite students to sing "America" **CD 23-1** with the recording.

5a Write the rhythm for the second measure of "America" on the board and have students identify the measures that have the same rhythm pattern. (mm. 2, 4, 8, 10, and 12)

Have students quietly clap the rhythm each time it occurs as they sing the song with the recording.

Invite students to sing "America, the Beautiful" **CD 23-4** with the recording. Have students read p. 485.

ASK How many sections are in the song? (two)

Help students discover that "America" has one phrase of six measures and one phrase of eight measures.

Help students discover that the first section uses more dotted rhythms than the second.

ASK How would using various dynamics make the song more expressive? (make the listener feel proud, thoughtful, jubilant)

Encourage students to sing the song again, following the director's dynamic cues.

ACROSS THE CURRICULUM

▶ **Social Studies** The War of 1812, the "second war for independence," involved Native American, British, and American troops. Unresolved issues from the Revolutionary War, laws preventing free access to British ports, and the capture of almost 400 American ships and crews in two years, led to the United States's declaring war on Britain on June 18, 1812. Battles occurred in Canada, the United States, and on the Great Lakes. Following the 1814 American victory at Fort McHenry, the British retreated. Diplomats in Europe signed a peace treaty ending the war. However, news did not reach the United States until mid-1815, too late to prevent the Battle of New Orleans.

Students can learn more about our national anthem in *The Star-Spangled Banner (Cornerstones of Freedom)* by Deborah Kent (Children's Press, 1995).

SKILLS REINFORCEMENT

▶ **Playing** Invite students to play this rhythm accompaniment on drums to *L'union* **CD 23-8**, p. 487. It will be a challenge to start at the correct place and to play along with the recording. Students will have fun trying.

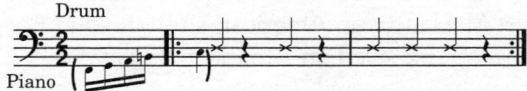

Drum

Piano

Playing

Invite students to learn a keyboard accompaniment to "America, the Beautiful." See Skills Reinforcement on p. 487 and Resource Book p. H-31.

Listening

6b Listen to *America, the Beautiful* **CD 23-3** sung by a gospel choir. Describe this version. (It has a pop beat and orchestration; the choir is very expressive; the vocalist freely uses melodic ornamentation; it's a different musical style.)

5a Write the rhythm for the anacrusis (and following downbeat) of "The Star-Spangled Banner" on the board. Have students identify the measures that have the same rhythm pattern. Remind students that the first measure occurs on the word *say!* (mm. 2, 8, and 10)

Singing

Invite students to sing the melody of "The Star-Spangled Banner" **CD 23-6** on pp. 486–487 with the recording. Lightly clap the rhythm pattern (shown on the board) when it occurs.

Have students observe the slurs on certain pairs of notes. Inform students that, in this case, these are performed by slightly accenting the beginning note of the slur and singing the last note (or notes) a bit softer.

Invite students to sing the last two lines of the song, beginning with the anacrusis on the word *Oh,* without the slurs. Then, sing these lines with slurs.

ASK How does singing the slurred notes without slurs affect its character? (It sounds choppy; it doesn't sound natural. The slur makes it sound correct.)

5c Draw attention to the *fermata* on p. 487 and have students interpret it. (Hold the note until the conductor releases it.)

Have students look at p. 486 and find where the harmony part of "The Star-Spangled Banner" begins. (on the last beat of p. 486)

Our National Anthem

"The Star-Spangled Banner" was written when our young country was struggling to retain its freedom. We should all reflect on the freedom and opportunities we now enjoy in the United States.

Sing our National Anthem.

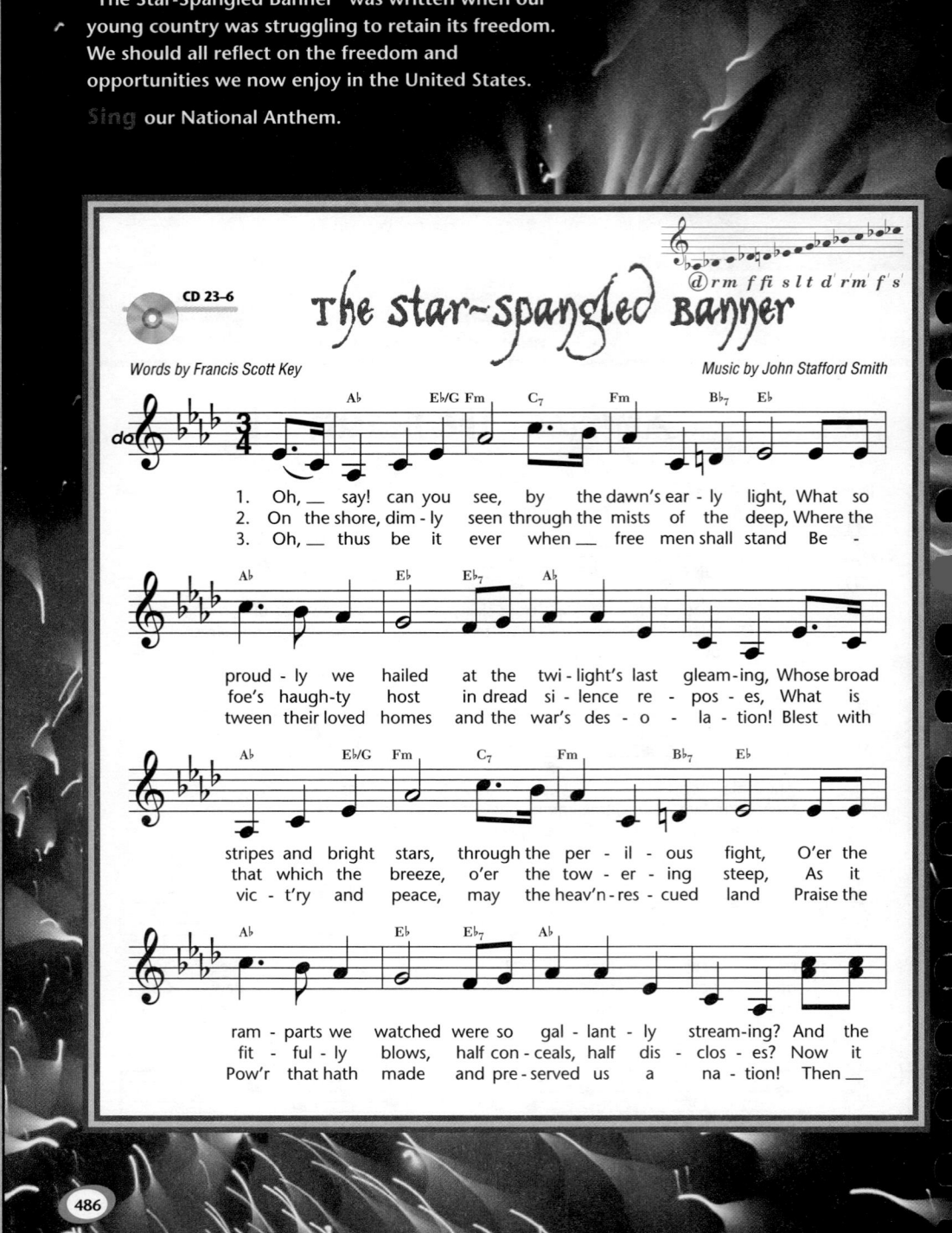

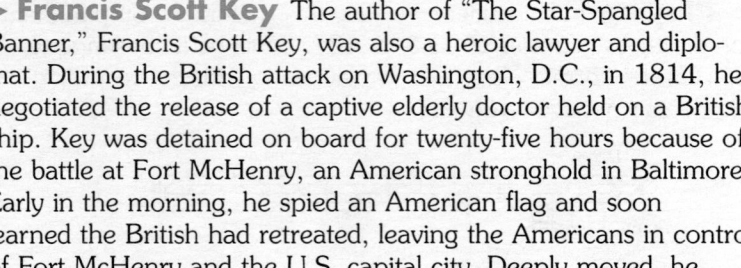

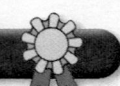

SPOTLIGHT ON

▶ **Francis Scott Key** The author of "The Star-Spangled Banner," Francis Scott Key, was also a heroic lawyer and diplomat. During the British attack on Washington, D.C., in 1814, he negotiated the release of a captive elderly doctor held on a British ship. Key was detained on board for twenty-five hours because of the battle at Fort McHenry, an American stronghold in Baltimore. Early in the morning, he spied an American flag and soon learned the British had retreated, leaving the Americans in control of Fort McHenry and the U.S. capital city. Deeply moved, he scribbled a poem about the event on the back of an envelope in his pocket. The poem was published in 1814 to be sung to the tune "Anacreon in Heaven" and became the U.S. national anthem on March 3, 1931.

CHARACTER EDUCATION

▶ **Patriotism** Discuss with students what it means to be patriotic. Encourage students to describe specific behaviors that lead them to believe someone is patriotic. For Americans, part of being patriotic involves participating in various activities associated with living in a democracy. (voting, jury duty, contributing to charity, expressing public opinion, writing to politicians, running for public office) Why are these activities important? Why do people choose not to participate in these activities? What are ways you can show your patriotism? Encourage students to talk with people of varying ages (senior citizen, middle-aged, young adult) about patriotism. Do people demonstrate patriotism differently now than when these adults were your age? How was patriotism encouraged? If differences exist between current and past practices, what has shaped these differences? (Wars often affect patriotism in people.)

A Patriotic Celebration

The selection below, by the American composer and pianist Louis Moreau Gottschalk, is a musical celebration of America.

Listen for three familiar melodies. Can you name them?

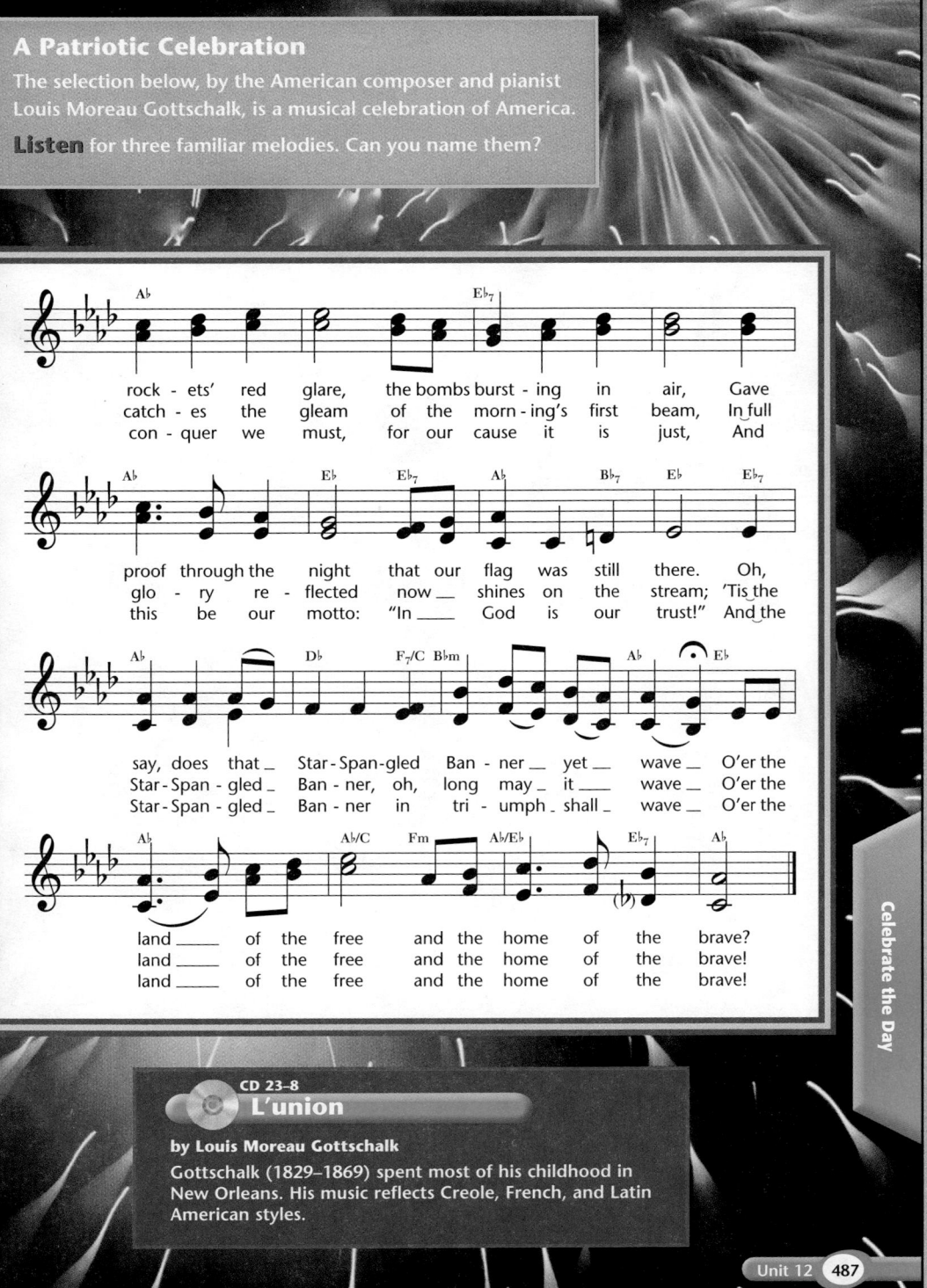

rock - ets' red glare, the bombs burst - ing in air, Gave In full
catch - es the gleam of the morn - ing's first beam, Gave In full
con - quer we must, for our cause it is just, And

proof through the night that our flag was still there. Oh,
glo - ry re - flected now __ shines on the stream; 'Tis the
this be our motto: "In _____ God is our trust!" And the

say, does that _ Star - Span - gled Ban - ner __ yet __ wave __ O'er the
Star - Span - gled _ Ban - ner, oh, long may _ it ___ wave __ O'er the
Star - Span - gled _ Ban - ner in tri - umph · shall _ wave __ O'er the

land _____ of the free and the home of the brave?
land _____ of the free and the home of the brave!
land _____ of the free and the home of the brave!

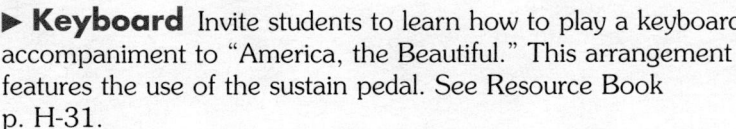

CD 23–8

L'union

by Louis Moreau Gottschalk

Gottschalk (1829–1869) spent most of his childhood in New Orleans. His music reflects Creole, French, and Latin American styles.

Celebrate the Day

Unit 12 **487**

Singing

 Invite students to sing the harmony part of the second section with the recording **CD 23-6.**

Select a group of students to sing the harmony part while the class sings the melody with the recording.

See Skills Reinforcement below, for tips on assisting students having difficulty singing the range.

Listening

Have students listen to *L'union* **CD 23-8** by Louis Moreau Gottschalk.

Guide students to hear the three melodies: (1) "The Star-Spangled Banner" (1:40); (2) "Columbia" (3:33); and (3) "Yankee Doodle" (5:25).

Invite students to play a rhythm accompaniment to *L'union,* in Skills Reinforcement on p. 485.

3 CLOSE

Skill: SINGING **ASSESSMENT**

Performance/Peer Critique Divide students into two groups, letting them choose volunteers to be their director. Allow them time to discuss how they will use dynamics to enhance their performance. Have each group perform "The Star-Spangled Banner." Encourage all students to perform with expression, using dynamics, phrasing, and good singing technique. Remind them to observe the *fermata* on the word *wave.*

Ask the listening group to critique the performance, using these criteria: Did the group demonstrate

- Noticeable dynamics appropriate to mood of the song?
- Good phrasing and performance of slurs?
- Proper interpretation of the fermata?

SKILLS REINFORCEMENT

▶ **Singing** The melody of "The Star-Spangled Banner" requires a range of an octave and a fifth. Many young singers are incapable of singing both extremes of this range; therefore, our national anthem is difficult for them to perform. Students for whom the A♭ below middle C is low may substitute the middle C for the A♭, making the song easier to sing. Note: The range of "The Star-Spangled Banner" is only one step wider than "Silent Night."

▶ **Keyboard** Invite students to learn how to play a keyboard accompaniment to "America, the Beautiful." This arrangement features the use of the sustain pedal. *See* Resource Book p. H-31.

SCHOOL TO HOME CONNECTION

▶ **Pictures of America** Ask parents or other family members of students to lend pictures of various places, landscapes, landmarks, and people in America. Have students bring in pictures (put their name on back) for a multimedia presentation.

TECHNOLOGY/MEDIA LINK

Multimedia Organize a slide show of pictures to accompany the singing of "The Star-Spangled Banner," "America," and "America, the Beautiful" at concerts and performances. Use overheads or slide projectors to project images. If you have access to computers with presentation software, scan pictures into a scanner and have students create a multimedia presentation, using the computer software.

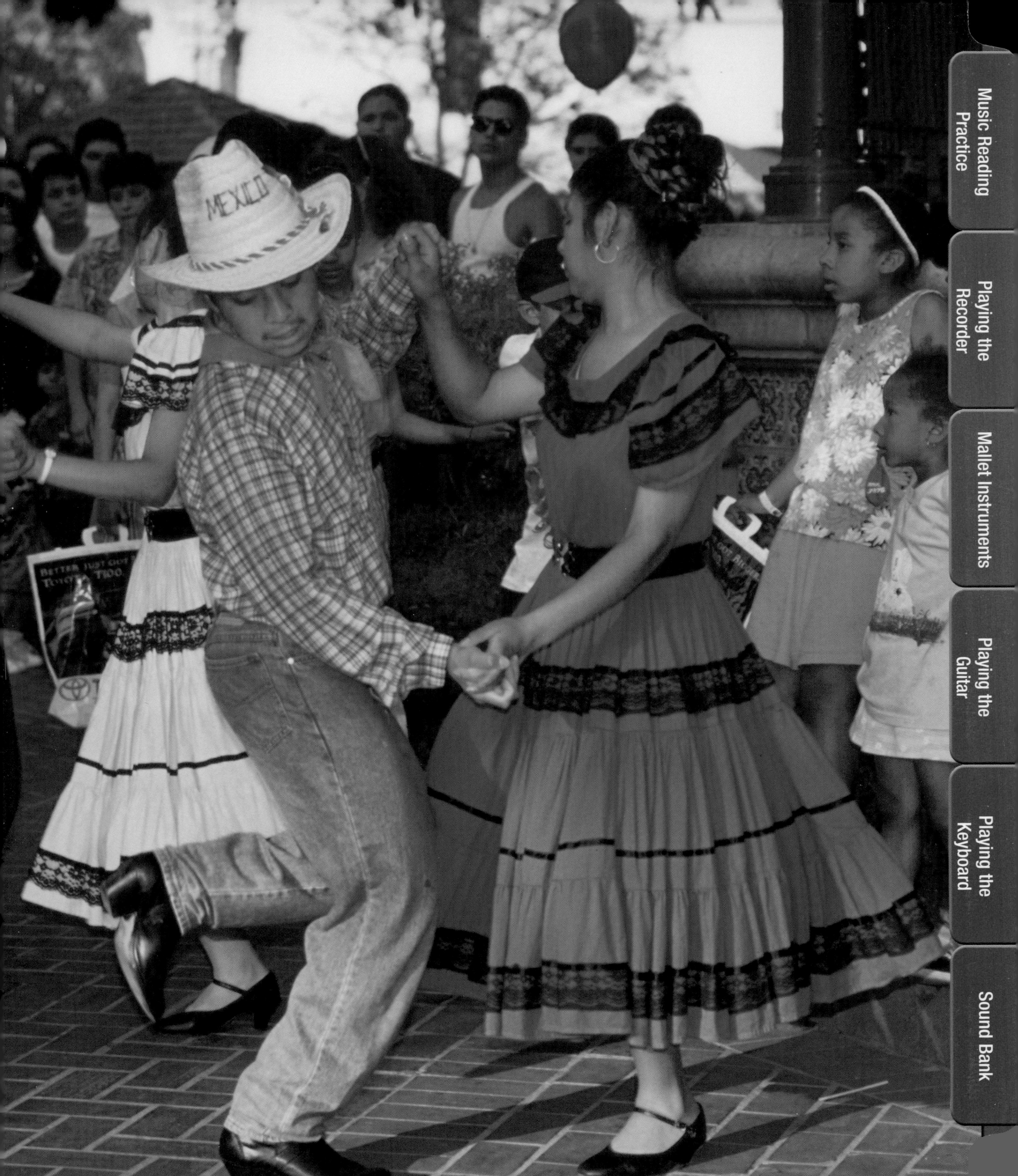

Music Reading Practice

Playing the Recorder

Mallet Instruments

Playing the Guitar

Playing the Keyboard

Sound Bank

SILVER·BURDETT

Making Music

CONTENTS

Student Resources

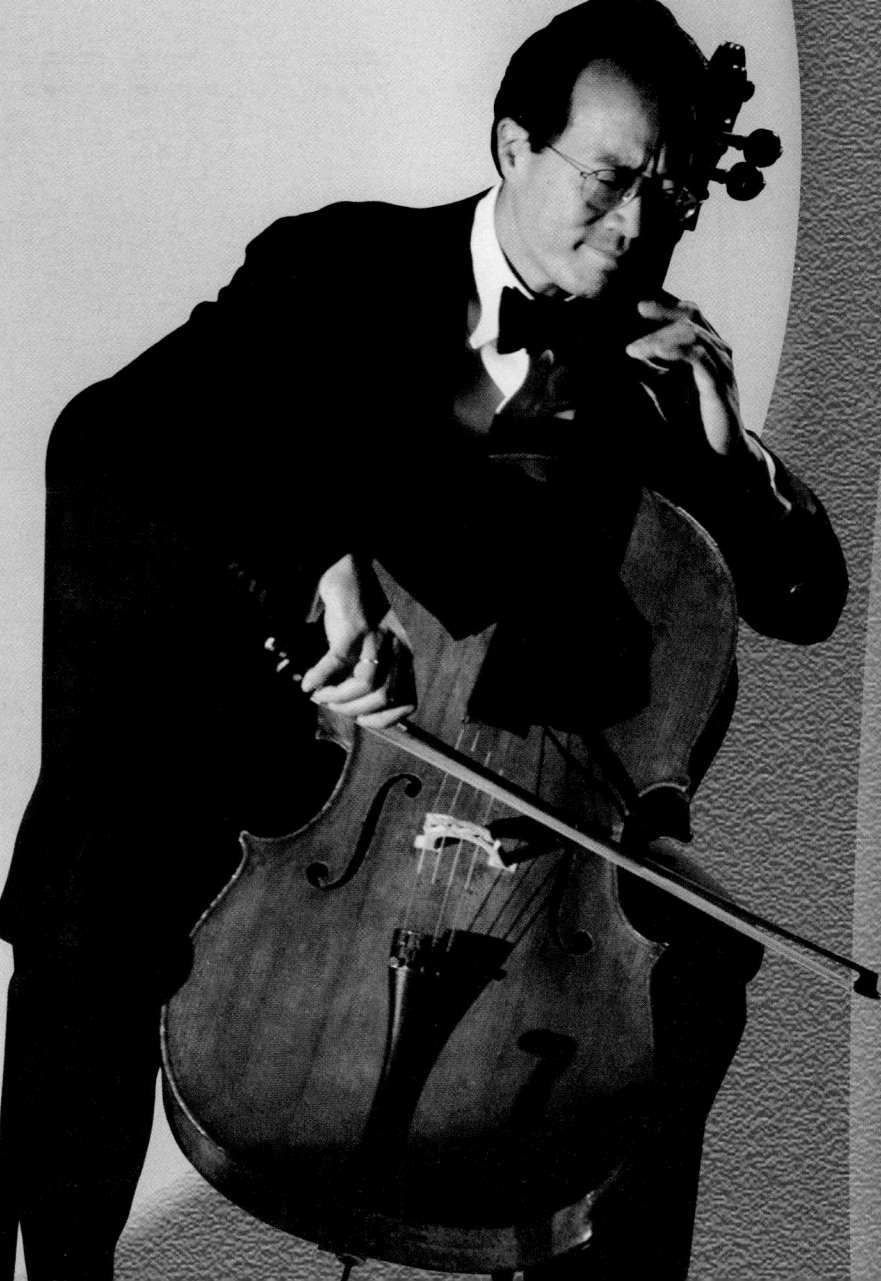

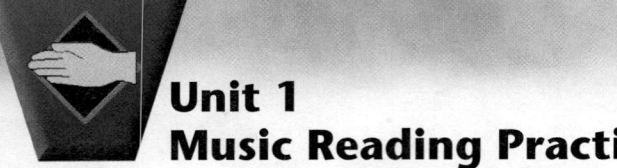

Unit 1
Music Reading Practice

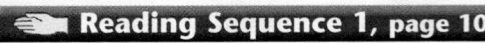
Reading Sequence 1, page 10

Note: For an overview and description of the Music Reading Practice section, see "Reading Sequence Formats" below.

MATERIALS

- "Red River Valley," p. 11   **CD 1-6**
- Reading Sequence 1
  Rhythm part (woodblock)   **CD 1-8**
  Rhythm part with accompaniment   **CD 1-9**
  Accompaniment only   **CD 1-10**
- **Resource Book** pp. D-2, E-2
- nonpitched percussion instruments

Rhythm: Review ♩, ♫, ♪, and Ties

Play the recording of "Red River Valley" **CD 1-6**. Guide students to realize that the opening refrain is at a slower tempo than the rest of the song. Then direct students to Reading Sequence 1 and have them

- Listen to the recording while tapping the beat. Ask students to identify the measures where the tempo changes (m. 7) and ties (mm. 2, 6, 10, 14) occur.
- Compare the pickups (anacruses) in Reading Sequence 1 with the song notation.
- Conduct in meter in 4 and say the rhythm syllables of Reading Sequence 1. Then have students tap the rhythm while providing a contrasting audible beat.

Reading Sequence 2, page 12

MATERIALS

- "Bắt kim thang," p. 13   **CD 1-13**
- Reading Sequence 2
  Rhythm part (woodblock)   **CD 1-17**
  Rhythm part with accompaniment   **CD 1-18**
  Accompaniment only   **CD 1-19**
- **Resource Book** pp. D-3, E-3
- nonpitched percussion instruments

Rhythm: Review ♬, ♪♪, ♪♪, and Upbeats

Invite students to conduct in meter in 2 as they listen to "Bắt kim thang" **CD 1-13.** Have them

- Tap the beat and say the rhythm syllables.
- Clap the rhythm pattern and say the rhythm syllables.
- Tap the beat and say the rhythm syllables for the counter-rhythm on p. 13.

Direct students to Reading Sequence 2 and have them tap the beat and perform Reading Sequence 2 using rhythm syllables.

Divide the class into three groups. Have

- Group 1 tap the beat.
- Group 2 clap Reading Sequence 2.
- Group 3 sing the song.

Ask students to switch parts until everyone has performed each activity.

Reading Sequence 1, page 10

CD 1–8
MIDI 38

Rhythm: Review ♩, ♫, ♪, and Ties

As you conduct in meter in 4, use rhythm syllables to **read** and **perform** this counter-rhythm for "Red River Valley." Note how the ties change the rhythm.

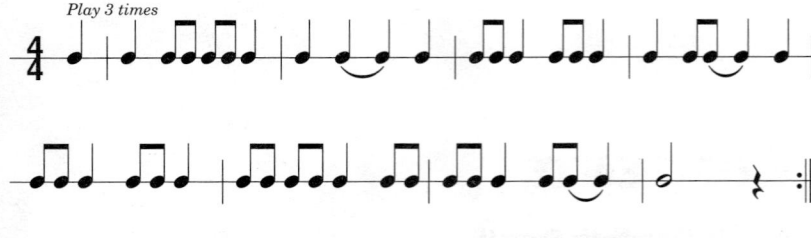

Play 3 times

Reading Sequence 2, page 12

CD 1–17
MIDI 39

Rhythm: Review ♬, ♪♪, ♪♪, and Upbeats

Read and **perform** this counter-rhythm for "Bắt kim thang," using rhythm syllables.

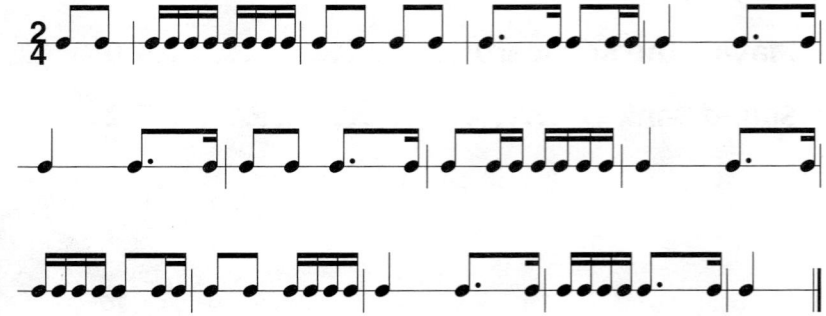

488

Footnotes

▶ **Reading Sequence Formats** The music reading program in Units 1–6 develops fundamental musical concepts and reading skills. You may reinforce and extend your students' music reading experiences using the 24 Reading Sequences of the Music Reading Practice section in the student text. These exercises are also available as blackline masters in the Resource Book for creating overhead transparencies, student worksheets, and assessment activities.

▶ **From Duo to Trio (Reading Sequence 1)** Divide the class into 3 groups. Play the recording of "Red River Valley" **CD 1-6** and have group one sing the song, group two conduct in meter in 4, and group three tap the Reading Sequence 1 rhythm.

▶ **Preparation (Reading Sequence 2)** Ask students to tap the beat, say the rhythm syllables, and clap the rhythms for "Bắt kim thang" and the Show What You Know counter-rhythm on p. 13. The rhythms appear in different combinations to provide thorough practice.

Reading Sequence 3, page 18
CD 2–3
MIDI 40

Melody: Reading Melodic Patterns

Using pitch syllables, **read** and **sing** this countermelody for "Bury Me Not on the Lone Prairie."

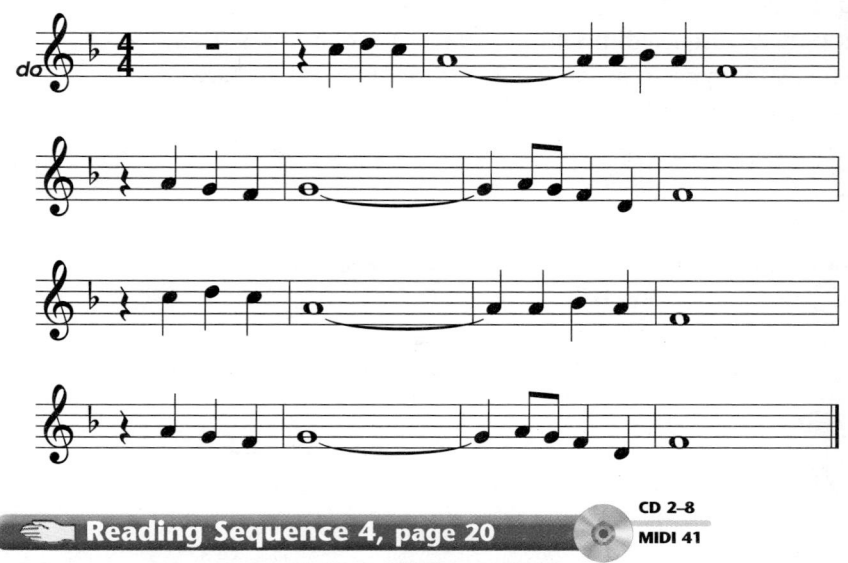

Reading Sequence 4, page 20
CD 2–8
MIDI 41

Melody: Reading Melodic Contour

Read and **sing** this countermelody for "Gonna Build a Mountain," using pitch syllables.

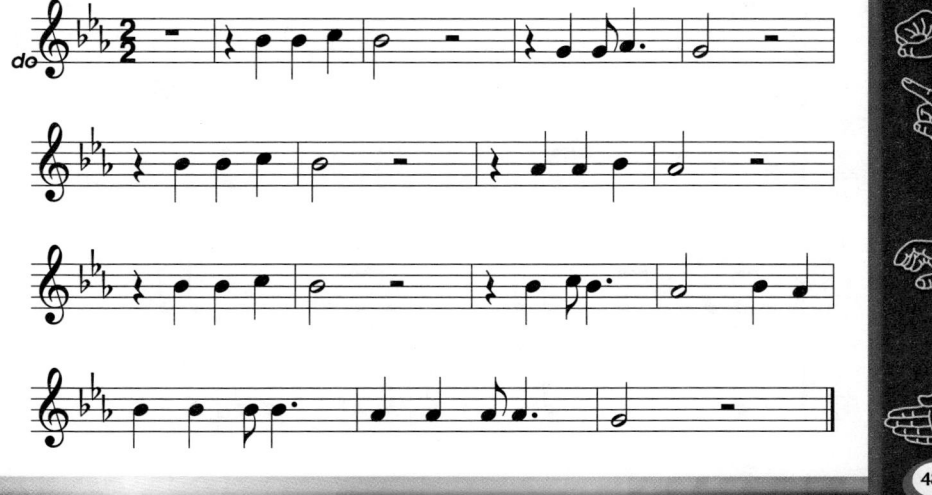

489

Reading Sequence 3, page 18

Note: See "Using the MIDI Files" in the Footnotes for suggestions on implementing this feature.

MATERIALS
- "Bury Me Not on the Lone Prairie," p. 19   **CD 2-1**
- Reading Sequence 3
  Melody part   **CD 2-3**
  Melody part with accompaniment   **CD 2-4**
  Accompaniment only   **CD 2-5**
- **Resource Book** pp. D-4, E-4

Melody: Reading Melodic Patterns

Invite students to locate all of the ties in "Bury Me Not on the Lone Prairie" (mm. 2, 6, 10, 11, 14). Have students

- Conduct in meter in 4 as they listen to the recording **CD 2-1.**
- Conduct and sing the pitch syllables.

Direct students to Reading Sequence 3. Have students

- Conduct and say the rhythm syllables.
- Conduct and sing the pitch syllables.

Play the recording **CD 2-3** as students conduct and sing pitch syllables for Reading Sequence 3. Divide the class into two groups. Have group one sing the melody of the song and group two sing the countermelody. Then have students switch parts.

Reading Sequence 4, page 20

MATERIALS
- "Gonna Build a Mountain," p. 21   **CD 2-6**
- Reading Sequence 4
  Melody part   **CD 2-8**
  Melody part with accompaniment   **CD 2-9**
  Accompaniment only   **CD 2-10**
- **Resource Book** pp. D-5, E-5

Melody: Reading Melodic Contour

Play the recording of "Gonna Build a Mountain" **CD 2-6**. Have students review conducting in both meter in 4 and meter in 2 as they listen. Direct students to Reading Sequence 4. Have students

- Conduct in meter in 2 and perform Rhythm Sequence 4 using rhythm syllables.
- Identify identical and similar melodic patterns.
- Identify that the melodic contour of phrase 4 (mostly descending) differs from all other patterns.
- Trace the melodic contour of each pattern as they sing pitch syllables.

▶ **Using the MIDI Files** MIDI files are provided for all Reading Sequence exercises. Each file contains individual tracks for specific melody or rhythm parts, as noted in the corresponding exercise on the pupil page, and a full accompaniment for the song on which the exercise is based. As an instructional tool, the files can be used to isolate individual parts, accompany any combination of parts, and transpose the pitches or change the tempo of the exercise and accompaniment.

▶ **Echo Song (Reading Sequence 3)** "Bury Me Not on the Lone Prairie" may be sung as an echo song. Divide the class into two groups. Group one begins. Group two starts on beat two of measure two. Discuss the similarities and differences between an echo song and a countermelody.

▶ **New Words (Reading Sequence 4)** Ask students, in small groups, to create new lyrics for Reading Sequence 4. For example, *I'm gon-na build* for the first pattern, or *a lit-tle hill* for the second. Have each group sing their lyrics with the recording.

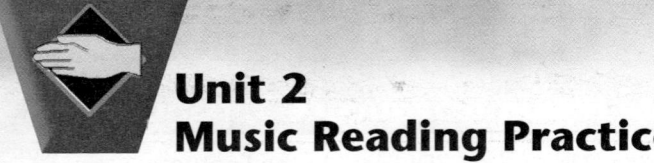

Unit 2
Music Reading Practice

👆 Reading Sequence 5, page 42

MATERIALS

- "Farewell to Tarwathie," p. 43 — **CD 3-1**
- Reading Sequence 5
  Rhythm part (claves) — **CD 3-3**
  Rhythm part with accompaniment — **CD 3-4**
  Accompaniment only — **CD 3-5**
- **Resource Book** pp. D-6, E-6
- nonpitched percussion instruments, metronome

Rhythm: Reading Rhythms in 3/4

Invite students to identify the number of phrases in verse 1 of "Farewell to Tarwathie." Have students locate the three phrases that begin with the same anacrusis.

Play the recording of "Farewell to Tarwathie" **CD 3-1.** Have a student find the ♩ beat tempo (approximately 132 bpm) using a metronome. Have students conduct in meter in 3 and say the rhythm syllables for the song at that tempo. Direct students to Reading Sequence 5. Have them

- Locate all dotted rhythm patterns.
- Conduct and say the rhythm patterns using rhythm syllables.

Divide the class into two groups. Let group one clap all even-numbered measures; let group two tap all odd-numbered measures. Then have students switch parts.

👆 Reading Sequence 6, page 44

MATERIALS

- "Barb'ry Allen," p. 44 — **CD 3-8**
- Reading Sequence 6
  Rhythm Part 1 (cowbell) — **CD 3-9**
  Rhythm Part 2 (woodblock) — **CD 3-10**
  Rhythm Parts 1 and 2 — **CD 3-11**
  Rhythm Parts 1 and 2 with accompaniment — **CD 3-12**
  Accompaniment only — **CD 3-13**
- **Resource Book** pp. D-7, E-7
- nonpitched percussion instruments

Rhythm: Reading Rhythms in 3/4

Using a metronome and the recording of "Barb'ry Allen" **CD 3-8,** help students determine that this ballad is not sung at a strict tempo. Review the number of phrases in "Barb'ry Allen" and point out that each phrase begins with a single *ti* anacrusis. Have students

- Locate all dotted rhythms in the song.
- Conduct and say the rhythm syllables in the song.

Direct students to Reading Sequence 6. Have them

- Compare the phrases in the song to the phrases in Reading Sequence 6.
- Locate all dotted rhythms.
- Perform Reading Sequence 6 using rhythm syllables as they conduct in meter in 3.

👆 Reading Sequence 5, page 42 — **CD 3–3 / MIDI 42**

Rhythm: Reading Rhythms in 3/4

Find the dotted-rhythm patterns below. As you conduct a three-beat pattern, use rhythm syllables to **read** the rhythms. Then **perform** them as an accompaniment for "Farewell to Tarwathie."

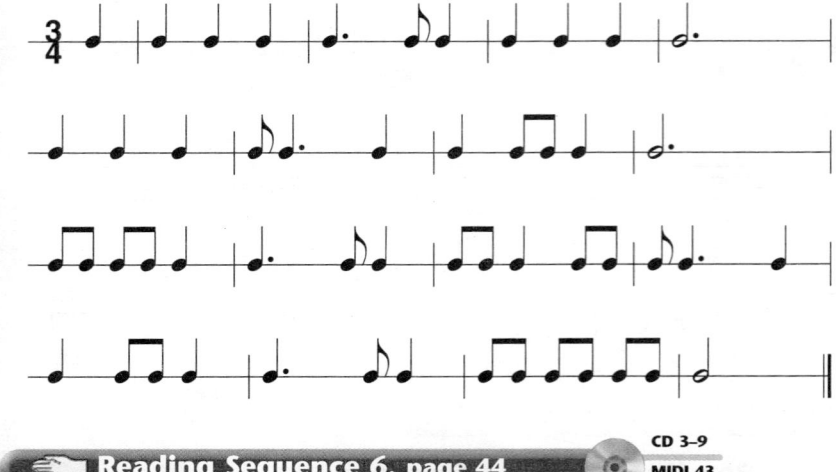

👆 Reading Sequence 6, page 44 — **CD 3–9 / MIDI 43**

Rhythm: Reading Rhythms in 3/4

Using rhythm syllables, **read** and **perform** these rhythms for "Barb'ry Allen."

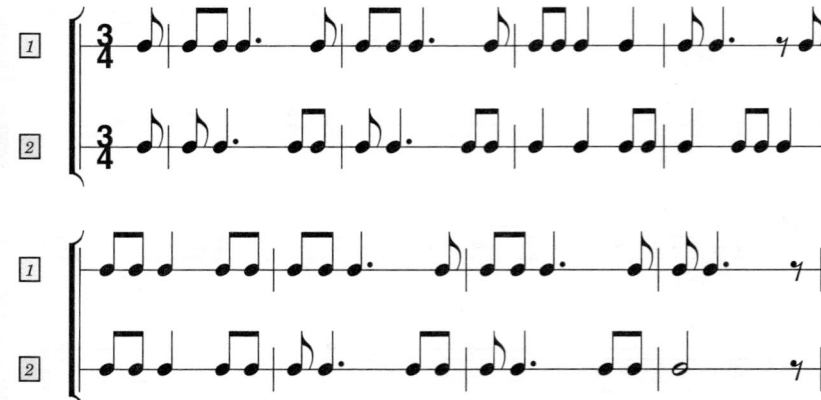

Footnotes

▶ **Changing Tempos (Reading Sequences 5 & 6)** "Farewell to Tarwathie" and "Barb'ry Allen" are both in triple meter, but are performed at different tempos. Have students experiment with different tempos as they conduct in meter in 3. Using rhythm syllables, perform the exercises in Music Reading Worksheet 5, exercises 2 and 3, found in Resource Book p. D-6.

▶ **Comparing Rhythms (Reading Sequences 5 & 6)** "Farewell to Tarwathie" and "Barb'ry Allen" contain the ♩.♪ and ♪♩. rhythms and three different rhythmic pickups (upbeats). Compare the dotted rhythms and pickups in Reading Sequences 5 and 6. Extend the practice of these rhythms by dividing the class into two groups and having one group clap Reading Sequence 5 while the other group taps Reading Sequence 6 two times.

Reading Sequence 7, page 56

CD 4–5
MIDI 44

Melody: Reading a Major Scale

Using pitch syllables and hand signs, **read** and **sing** this countermelody for "*Adiós, amigos.*"

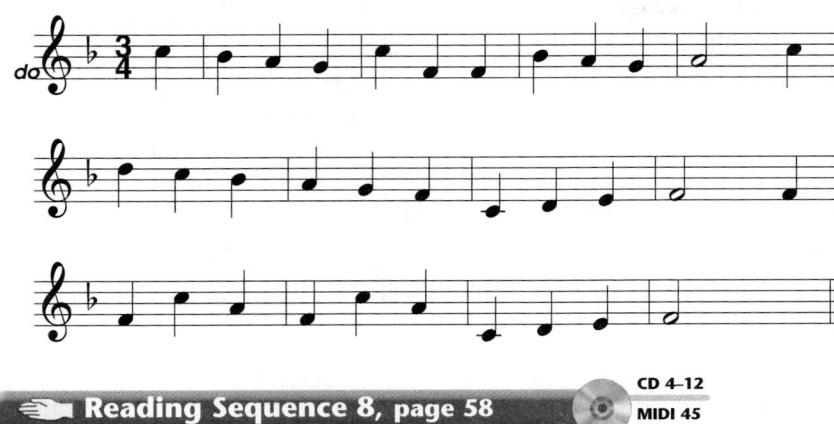

Reading Sequence 8, page 58

CD 4–12
MIDI 45

Melody: Reading a Minor Scale

As you tap a steady beat, use pitch syllables to silently **read** and **sing** this countermelody for "*La mariposa.*" This will help develop your inner hearing.

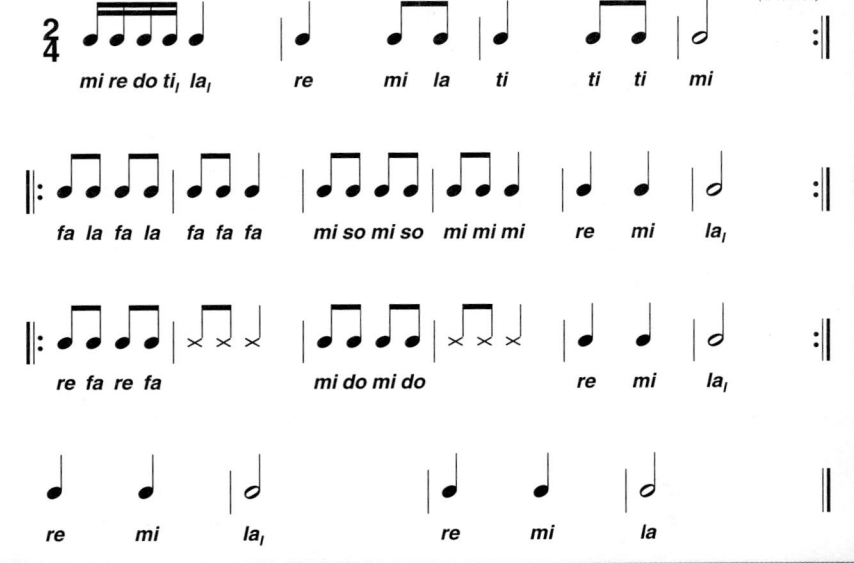

491

▶ **Changing Keys (Reading Sequence 7)** The countermelody for "*Adiós, amigos*" is written in the same key as the song notation and recording. Let higher-voiced singers sing the countermelody with the recording. Change the key to D-*do* or C-*do* to accommodate lower singers' voices.

▶ **Repeating Melodies (Reading Sequence 8)** Remind students that the first phrase of Reading Sequence 8 must be sung four times. Phrases two and three are sung twice. The last measure in phrase three is performed a total of three times.

Reading Sequence 7, page 56

MATERIALS
- "*Adiós, amigos,*" p. 57   **CD 4-3**
- Reading Sequence 7
  Melody part   **CD 4-5**
  Melody part with accompaniment   **CD 4-6**
  Accompaniment only   **CD 4-7**
- **Resource Book** pp. D-8, E-8

Melody: Reading a Major Scale

Invite students to conduct in meter in 3 as they sing "*Adiós, amigos.*" Review the *do* diatonic scale at the bottom of p. 56 in the student text. Ask students to sing the scale ascending and descending. Direct students to Reading Sequence 7 and have them

- Read the rhythm patterns using rhythm syllables as they conduct in meter in 3.
- Sing the countermelody using pitch syllables and hand-signs.
- Sing Reading Sequence 7 while listening to "*Adiós amigos*" **CD 4-3.**

Ask one group of students to sing the countermelody using pitch syllables while another group sings the song.

Reading Sequence 8, page 58

MATERIALS
- "*La mariposa,*" p. 58   **CD 4-8**
- Reading Sequence 8
  Melody part   **CD 4-12**
  Melody part with accompaniment   **CD 4-13**
  Accompaniment only   **CD 4-14**
- **Resource Book** pp. D-9, E-9

Melody: Reading a Minor Scale

Review the minor scale (shaded) on p. 58 in the student text. Have students sing the scale first using pitch syllables, then (absolute) pitch names.

Invite students to review the section form of "*La mariposa.*" Ask students to sing the song, first with lyrics, then using pitch syllables. Direct students to Reading Sequence 8. Have them

- Read the rhythm patterns and identify the number of times each section will be performed.
- Sing the countermelody at reading tempo, using pitch syllables and handsigns.
- Sing the countermelody while listening to "*La mariposa*" **CD 4-8.**

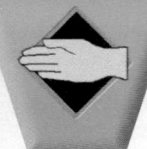

Unit 3
Music Reading Practice

Reading Sequence 9, page 80

MATERIALS

- *"Do, Re, Mi, Fa,"* p. 80 — **CD 5-8**
- Reading Sequence 9
  Rhythm Part 1 (woodblock) — **CD 5-10**
  Rhythm Part 2 (cowbell) — **CD 5-11**
  Rhythm Part 3 (triangle) — **CD 5-12**
  Rhythm Parts 1, 2, and 3 — **CD 5-13**
  Rhythm Parts 1, 2 and 3 with accompaniment — **CD 5-14**
  Accompaniment only — **CD 5-15**
- **Resource Book** pp. D-10, E-10
- nonpitched percussion instruments

Rhythm: Reading Augmentation and Diminution

Review augmentation and diminution. Have students

- Sing *"Do, Re, Mi, Fa"* as they conduct in meter in 4.
- Sing and conduct an augmented version and a diminished version of the melody.

Direct students to Reading Sequence 9. Invite students to

- Conduct in meter in 4 and read the counter-rhythm.
- Read and perform the augmented and diminished parts.

Divide the class into three groups to read and perform the three versions simultaneously. (See "Figure It Out" in the Footnotes.) Perform again while listening to the recording of *"Do, Re, Mi, Fa"* (use the canon performance) **CD 5-8.**

Reading Sequence 10, page 82

MATERIALS

- *"Hava nashira,"* p. 82 — **CD 5-16**
- Reading Sequence 10
  Rhythm Part 1 (triangle) — **CD 5-19**
  Rhythm Part 2 (woodblock) — **CD 5-20**
  Rhythm Parts 1 and 2 — **CD 5-21**
  Rhythm Parts 1 and 2 with accompaniment — **CD 5-22**
  Accompaniment only — **CD 5-23**
- **Resource Book** pp. D-11, E-11
- nonpitched percussion instruments

Rhythm: Reading Augmentation and Diminution

Review the rhythmic augmentation and diminution of *"Hava nashira."* Have students write an augmentation and diminution of the first two measures and the last two measures of the song.

Have students use rhythm syllables and tap the beat as they

- Read Part 1 in Reading Sequence 9.
- Read Part 2 in the reading sequence.

Divide the class into two groups. Have students read the exercises simultaneously. Next, play the recording of *"Hava nashira"* **CD 5-16** while students perform the parts. Have students identify which part is an augmentation and which is a diminution of *"Hava nashira."*

Reading Sequence 9, page 80 — CD 5-10 / MIDI 46

Rhythm: Reading Augmentation and Diminution

Using rhythm syllables, **read** and **perform** this three-part rhythm accompaniment for *"Do, Re, Mi, Fa."*

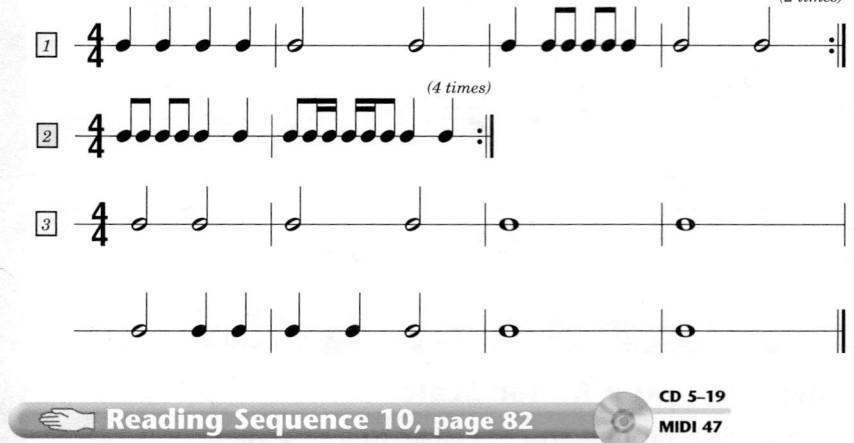

Reading Sequence 10, page 82 — CD 5-19 / MIDI 47

Rhythm: Reading Augmentation and Diminution

As you lightly tap the beat, use rhythm syllables to **read** and **perform** this two-part rhythm accompaniment for *"Hava nashira."*

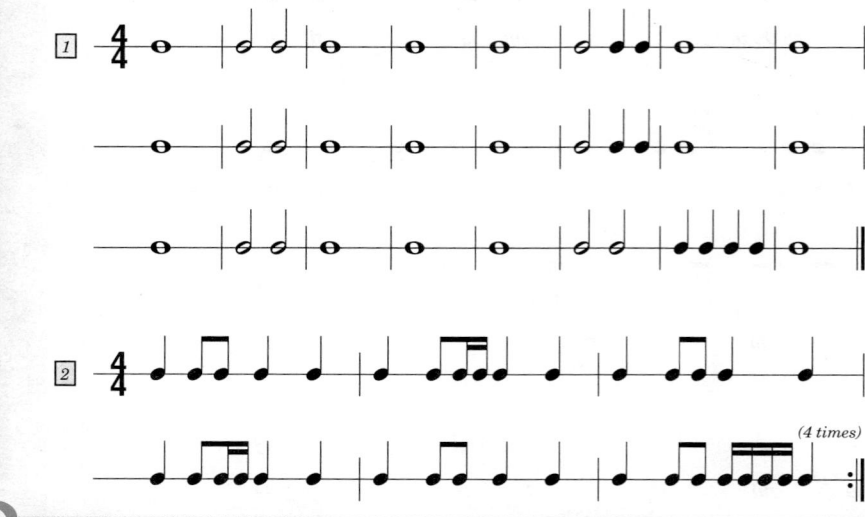

Footnotes

▶ **Figure It Out (Reading Sequence 9)** Help students to figure out how many times they need to perform the diminished part in order to match one performance of the counter-rhythm. Then have them figure out how many times they need to perform the counter-rhythm in order to match one performance of the augmented part.

▶ **A Performance Trio (Reading Sequence 10)** Divide the class into three groups. Assign the original rhythm, and the augmented and diminished parts to the groups. Perform all notations simultaneously, rotating each group through each notation. You may also begin with the original rhythm and then add the other notations in canon.

Reading Sequence 11, page 94   CD 6–6 · MIDI 48

Melody: Reading in Modes

Using pitch syllables and hand signs, **read** and **sing** this minor countermelody for "Scarborough Fair," which is in dorian mode.

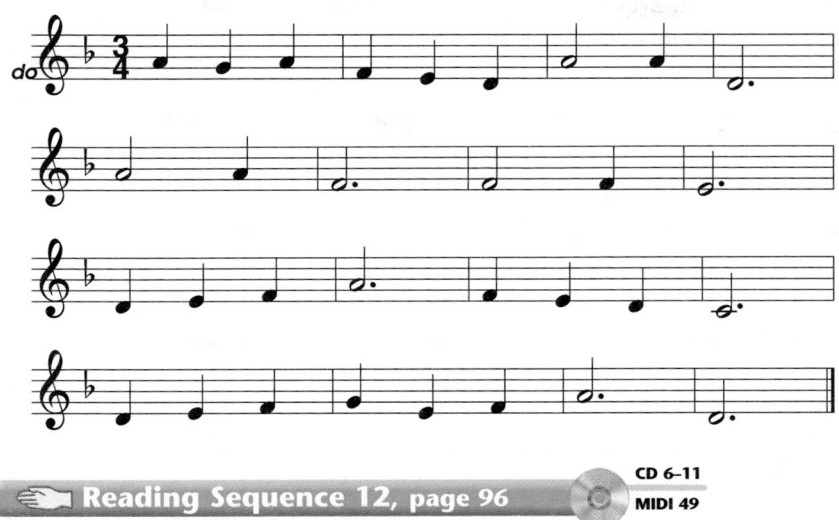

 Reading Sequence 12, page 96   CD 6–11 · MIDI 49

Melody: Reading in Mixolydian Mode

Locate the measures that are identical in each phrase. How are the last two measures of each phrase alike, or different? Then, use pitch syllables to **read** and **sing** this countermelody for "Harrison Town."

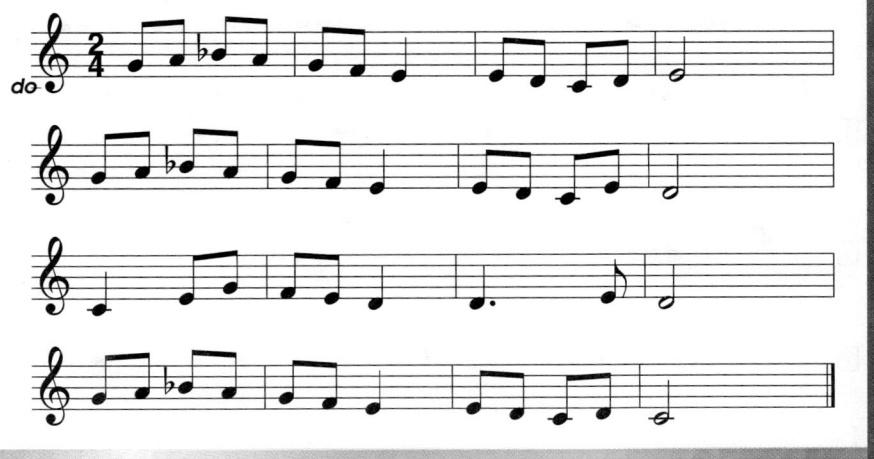

493

▶ **Practice Reading *fi* (Reading Sequence 11)** Use handsigns to read this *fi* exercise.

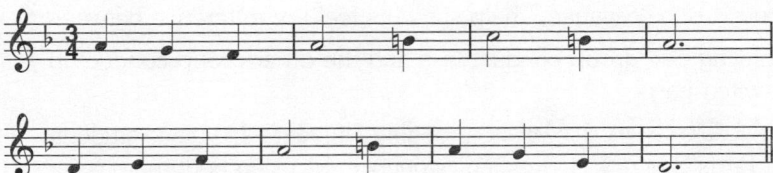

▶ **Practice Reading *ta* (Reading Sequence 12)** "Harrison Town" contains some difficult intervals using the new pitch *ta* (*so-ta* and *ta-fa*). Students should first sing the stepwise intervals in this exercise. Then, to make the *so-ta* interval in "Harrison Town" easier for students to read and sing, guide students to sing all *la* pitches silently "inside" their head. This skill is referred to as "inner hearing." In this exercise, students should sing the syllables of the song normally ("outside"). Each time they come to a *la* syllable, they sing the *la* syllable silently "inside."

 Reading Sequence 11, page 94

MATERIALS

- "Scarborough Fair," p. 95   **CD 6-4**
- Reading Sequence 11
  Melody part   **CD 6-6**
  Melody part with accompaniment   **CD 6-7**
  Accompaniment only   **CD 6-8**
- **Resource Book** pp. D-12, E-12

Melody: Reading in Dorian Mode

Review the song "Scarborough Fair." Then review the pitch syllable *fi*. On the board, have students create a pitch set of all the pitches in the song, lowest to highest, on a musical staff. Invite them to sing the pitch set using pitch syllables and handsigns, ascending and descending. Using Reading Music Worksheet 11 in Resource Book pp. D-12 and D-13, have students play the dorian mode on a barred instrument or piano, using D as *la*₁. Then have them write the dorian mode on their worksheet.

Invite students to read Reading Sequence 11 using pitch syllables and handsigns. Ask them to repeat the exercise with the syllable *loo*. Use this as a countermelody for "Scarborough Fair." Use the exercise in the Footnote, "Practice Reading *fi*" for more practice.

 Reading Sequence 12, page 96

MATERIALS

- "Harrison Town," p. 97   **CD 6-9**
- Reading Sequence 12
  Melody part   **CD 6-11**
  Melody part with accompaniment   **CD 6-12**
  Accompaniment only   **CD 6-13**
- **Resource Book** pp. D-14, E-13

Melody: Reading in Mixolydian Mode

Review the mixolydian mode. Have students sing pitch syllables for the scale on p. 96 in the student text using handsigns. Perform the scale ascending and descending. Have students

- Identify the rhythmic similarities, melodic similarites, and differences in Reading Sequence 12.
- Sing the exercise using pitch syllables and handsigns; provide an audible beat at the reading tempo.
- Sing the exercise as a countermelody to "Harrison Town" **CD 6-9.**

Divide the class into two groups. Ask the first group to sing the song while the other group sings the exercise as a countermelody. Then ask them to switch parts.

Unit 4
Music Reading Practice

Reading Sequence 13, page 118

MATERIALS

- "Swanee," p. 118 — **CD 7-3**
- Reading Sequence 13
  Rhythm part (woodblock) — **CD 7-5**
  Rhythm part with accompaniment — **CD 7-6**
  Accompaniment only — **CD 7-7**
- **Resource Book** pp. D-16, E-14
- nonpitched percussion instruments, woodblock, drum, claves, metronome

Rhythm: Reading Rhythms in ²∕₂

Review ²∕₂ meter and cut time by inviting students to conduct in meter in 2 as they listen to "Swanee" **CD 7-3.** Lead students through the activity presented in "²∕₂ Meter and Cut Time Review" in the Footnotes. Direct students to Reading Sequence 13 and have them

- Conduct in meter in 2 and read the rhythm syllables.
- Play Reading Sequence 13 on a woodblock while one student plays the half-note beat on a drum.
- Play the rhythm for "Swanee" on claves while someone plays the counter-rhythm on the woodblock.
- Sing "Swanee" while clapping Reading Sequence 13.

Review with students the relationship between ²∕₂ meter and cut-time ¢ on p. 119 of the student text.

Reading Sequence 14, page 120

MATERIALS

- "One Morning in May," p. 121 — **CD 7-8**
- Reading Sequence 14
  Rhythm Part 1 (woodblock) — **CD 7-10**
  Rhythm Part 2 (triangle) — **CD 7-11**
  Rhythm Parts 1 and 2 — **CD 7-12**
  Rhythm Parts 1 and 2 with accompaniment — **CD 7-13**
  Accompaniment only — **CD 7-14**
- **Resource Book** pp. D-17, E-15
- nonpitched percussion instruments

Rhythm: Reading Rhythms in ³∕₈

Review ³∕₈ meter by having students tap an ♪ beat while performing "One Morning in May" using rhythm syllables. Direct students to Reading Sequence 14. Have them conduct the ♪ beat and say rhythm syllables while they

- Read Rhythm Part 2.
- Read Rhythm Part 1.

Divide the class into two groups. Have Group 1 read and perform Rhythm Part 1 using body percussion; have Group 2 read and perform Rhythm Part 2 using an alternate body percussion. Ask students to switch parts. Repeat the exercise, but have students read and perform the rhythms simultaneously as they silently say the rhythm syllables. This exercise develops students' inner-hearing skills.

Reading Sequence 13, page 118
CD 7–5
MIDI 50

Rhythm: Reading Rhythms in ²∕₂

As you conduct in meter in 2, use rhythm syllables to **read** and **perform** this counter-rhythm for "Swanee."

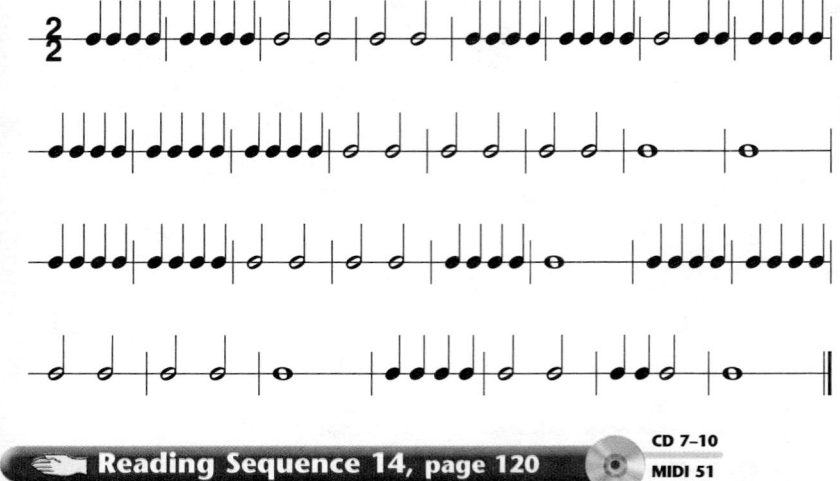

Reading Sequence 14, page 120
CD 7–10
MIDI 51

Rhythm: Reading Rhythms in ³∕₈

Using rhythm syllables, **read** and **perform** this two-part rhythm accompaniment for "One Morning in May."

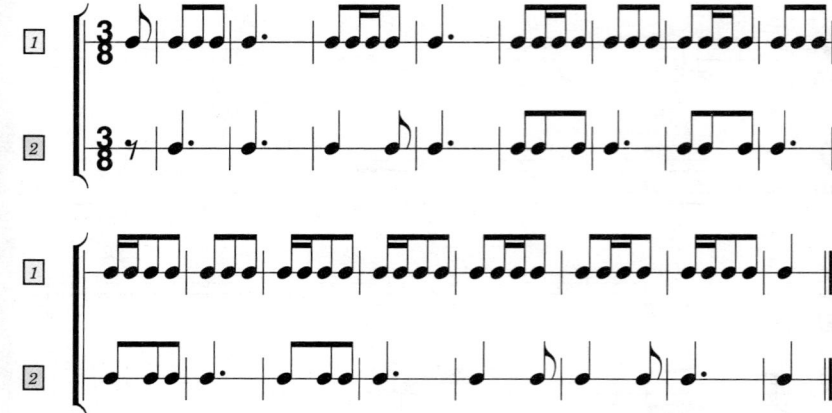

Footnotes

▶ **²∕₂ Meter and Cut Time Review (Reading Sequence 13)** Following the opening activity, divide the class into two groups. Set a metronome at ♩ = 72 bpm. As both groups sing "Swanee," help students feel the difference between ²∕₂ and ⁴∕₄ meter by having one group conduct in ²∕₂ and the other group conduct in ⁴∕₄. Ask students to switch parts.

▶ **Two Parts At Once in ³∕₈ Meter (Reading Sequence 14)** Have students perform Rhythm Parts 2 and 1 in Reading Sequence 14 using body percussion. Ask them to switch rhythm parts using an alternate body percussion for each part. Challenge students to perform the rhythms simultaneously by themselves. Ask them to use their left hand for Rhythm Part 2 and their right hand for Rhythm Part 1.

Reading Sequence 15, page 130 CD 7–27 MIDI 52

Melody: Reading in Harmonic Minor

Read and **sing** this countermelody for *"Lo yisa,"* using hand signs and pitch syllables.

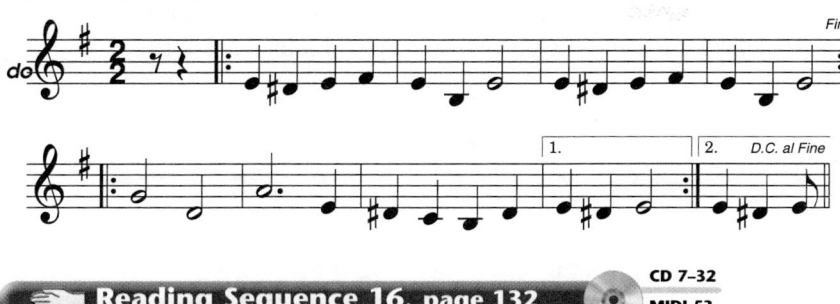

Reading Sequence 16, page 132 CD 7–32 MIDI 53

Melody: Reading Melodic Sequences

Identify the melodic sequence in this countermelody for *"Alleluia."* Then, **read** and **sing** it using pitch syllables.

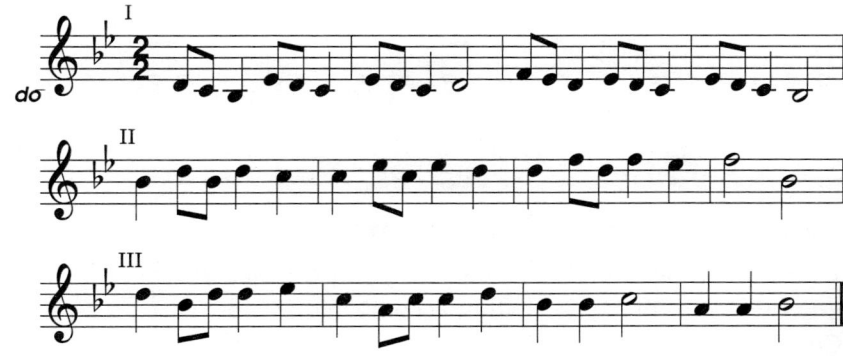

495

Reading Sequence 15, page 130

MATERIALS

- *"Lo yisa,"* p. 130   **CD 7-23**
- Reading Sequence 15
  Melody part   **CD 7-27**
  Melody part with accompaniment   **CD 7-28**
  Accompaniment only   **CD 7-29**
- **Resource Book** pp. D-18, E-16

Melody: Reading in Harmonic Minor

Review the harmonic minor scale and *si* by having the students sing *"Lo yisa"* first with lyrics, then with handsigns and pitch syllables. Write the harmonic minor scale on the board using E-*la,* extending from *mi*₁ to *mi*. See "Harmonic Minor Scale from *mi*₁ to *mi*" in the Footnotes.

Prepare students to read Reading Sequence 15 by pointing out patterns using *si,* found in the countermelody for *"Lo yisa."* Direct students to Reading Sequence 15. Have them

- Locate and sing all patterns using *si.*
- Sing the countermelody using pitch syllables and handsigns.

Divide the class into two groups. Using pitch syllables, ask students to sing *"Lo yisa"* and Reading Sequence 15.

Reading Sequence 16, page 132

MATERIALS

- *"Alleluia,"* p. 133   **CD 7-30**
- Reading Sequence 16
  Melody part   **CD 7-32**
  Melody part with accompaniment   **CD 7-33**
  Accompaniment only   **CD 7-34**
- **Resource Book** pp. D-19, E-17

Melody: Reading Melodic Sequences

Have the students sing the three-part canon, "Alleluia." Review melodic sequence in mm. 5-7 and mm. 9-10. Direct students to Reading Sequence 16. (See "Determining the Length of Melodic Sequences" in the Footnotes.) Have students identify melodic sequences as ascending and descending: Part I, mm. 1-2 (ascending); mm. 3-4 (descending). Part II: mm. 1-3 (ascending). Part III: mm. 1-2 (descending).

Have students sing the first pitch of each pattern forming a melodic sequence. Ask students to sing each part using handsigns and pitch syllables, then as a three-voice canon. Play the recording of "Alleluia" **CD 7-30** as an accompaniment to Reading Sequence 16.

▶ **The Harmonic Minor Scale from *mi*₁ to *mi*** (Reading Sequence 15)
Have students sing the scale starting on *la*₁. Go up to *mi,* then down to *mi*₁ and back to *la.* Prepare the patterns *la*₁-*si*₁-*la*₁; *la*₁-*si*₁-*fa*₁-*mi*₁-*si*₁-*la*₁. Review intervals *do-la*₁-*re-la*₁ as preparation for reading the final phrase.

▶ **Determining the Length of the Melodic Sequences** (Reading Sequence 16) There are two sizes of melodic sequence patterns. Have students analyze Part II and identify the number of beats used in each sequence pattern (1 m.) and Part I sequence length as 1 beat (in $\frac{2}{2}$) or 2 beats (in $\frac{4}{4}$). Let them determine which length is used for Part III (1 m.) After the students have sung this countermelody as a three-part canon with the recording **CD 7-30,** divide the class into 6 groups and challenge students to perform the exercise as a 6-part *a cappella* canon.

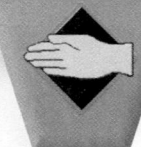

Unit 5
Music Reading Practice

Reading Sequence 17, page 156

MATERIALS

- "Let Us Sing Together," p. 156   **CD 8-28**
- Reading Sequence 17
  Rhythm part (woodblock)   **CD 8-30**
  Rhythm part with accompaniment   **CD 8-31**
  Accompaniment only   **CD 8-32**
- **Resource Book** pp. D-20, E-18
- nonpitched percussion instruments

Rhythm: Reading ♪ ♩ ♪ Syncopation

Review the ♪ ♩ ♪ syncopation by having students clap and say the rhythm of "Let Us Sing Together" while they tap the beat with their feet. On p. 157 in the student text, have the students find the rhythm that they were tapping. Use percussion instruments to play the four-part rhythm exercise.

Direct students to Reading Sequence 17. Have them

- Tap the beat with their feet as they read, clap, and say rhythm syllables for the counter-rhythm for "Let Us Sing Together."
- Read and perform Reading Sequence 17 in four-part canon using four different timbres.

Reading Sequence 18, page 158

MATERIALS

- "Lost My Gold Ring," p. 158   **CD 9-1**
- Reading Sequence 18
  Rhythm Part 1 (tambourine)   **CD 9-3**
  Rhythm Part 2 (woodblock)   **CD 9-4**
  Rhythm Part 3 (cowbell)   **CD 9-5**
  Rhythm Parts 1, 2, and 3   **CD 9-6**
  Rhythm Parts 1, 2, and 3 with accompaniment   **CD 9-7**
  Accompaniment only   **CD 9-8**
- **Resource Book** pp. D-21, E-19
- nonpitched percussion instruments

Rhythm: Reading ♫ ♩ Syncopation

Review ♫ ♩ syncopation by having students listen to, sing, and then clap the rhythm of "Lost My Gold Ring." Direct students to Reading Sequence 18. Have students

- Identify the measures in which all ♫ ♩ syncopations occur. (Part 1: mm. 1, 3; Part 2: m. 4; Part 3: m. 2)
- Identify the measures in which all ♪ ♩ ♪ syncopations occur. (Part 1: m. 2; Part 2: m. 3; Part 3: m. 1)
- Use ♩ = 72 bpm to tap the beat with their foot and clap each of the four-measure rhythms.

After students can perform the rhythm parts, have them listen to "Lost My Gold Ring" **CD 9-1** and clap each of the rhythm parts, in turn.

Reading Sequence 17, page 156   **CD 8–30**   **MIDI 54**

Rhythm: Reading ♪ ♩ ♪ Syncopation

Using rhythm syllables, **read** and **perform** this counter-rhythm for "Let Us Sing Together." As you do so, tap a steady beat with your foot.

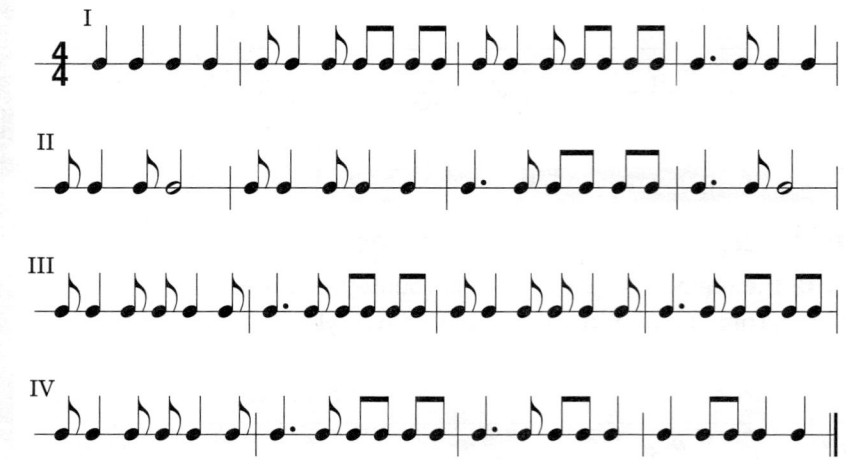

Reading Sequence 18, page 158   **CD 9–3**   **MIDI 55**

Rhythm: Reading ♫ ♩ Syncopation

Tap a steady beat with your foot. Using rhythm syllables, **read** and **perform** this three-part rhythm accompaniment for "Lost My Gold Ring."

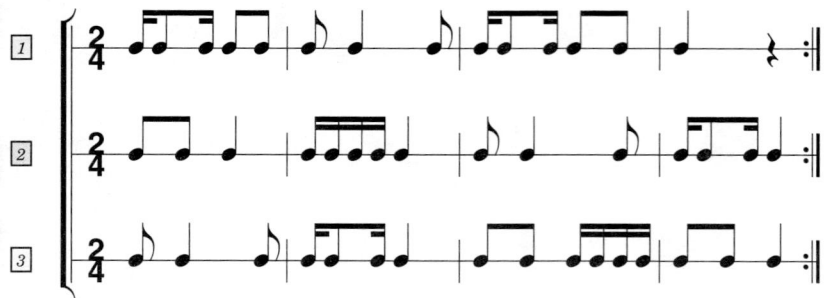

Footnotes

▶ **Practicing ♪ ♩ ♪ Syncopation: A Double Canon** (**Reading Sequence 17**) Divide the class into two large groups, A and B. Subdivide each group into four more groups I, II, III, and IV. Large group A performs the song "Let Us Sing Together" in four-part canon. Large group B performs the "Let Us Sing Together" counter-rhythm in four-part canon. Then have students switch parts.

▶ **Performing Routine** (**Reading Sequence 18**) When performing Reading Sequence 18 with the recording of "Lost My Gold Ring" **CD 9-1**, have students tap the beat during the introduction, then clap the three parts (1, then 2, then 3) a total of two times. Alternatively, divide the class into three groups; let each group play one of the parts. Students may also use three different non-pitched percussion instruments to perform the parts.

Reading Sequence 19, page 164

CD 9–18
MIDI 56

Melody: Reading Intervals (Seconds and Thirds)

Using hand signs and pitch syllables, **read** and **sing** this countermelody for "O lê lê O Bahía."

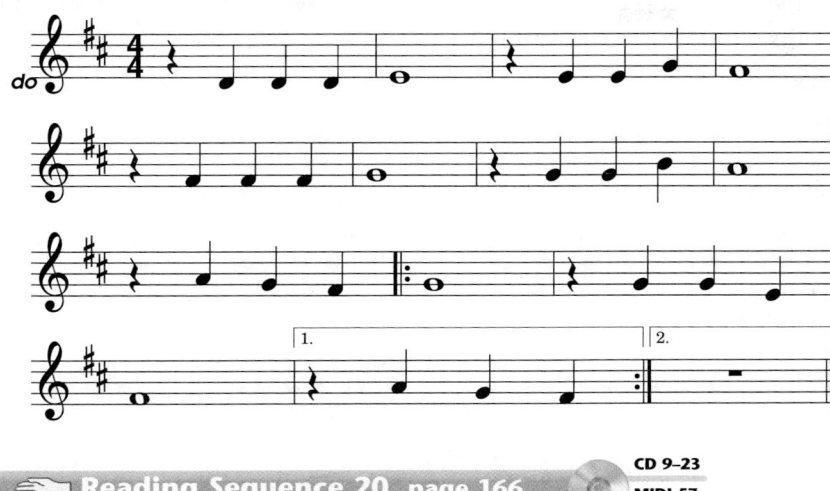

Reading Sequence 20, page 166

CD 9–23
MIDI 57

Melody: Reading Intervals (Major)

Locate and sing the intervals of a third, a fourth, a fifth, and an octave in this exercise. Then, using pitch syllables, **read** and **sing** it as a countermelody for "Like a Bird."

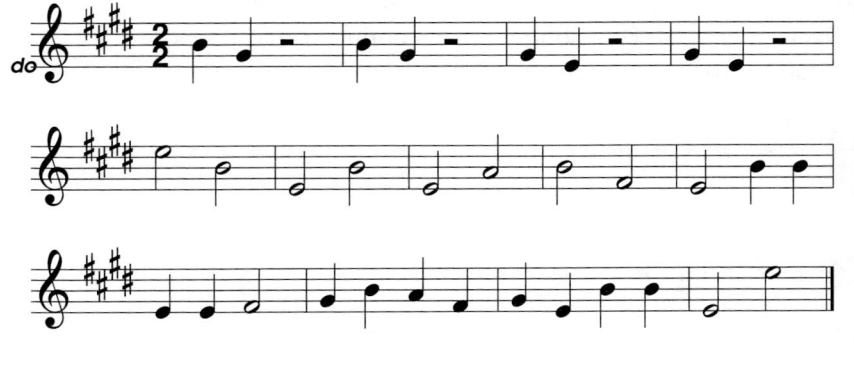

497

▶ **Practicing Major and Minor Thirds (Reading Sequence 19)** Help students hear the difference between major and minor thirds. Have them first sing all 3rds in the major scale ascending, then descending. Divide the class into 2 groups. Group 1 sings *mi-do*; Group 2 sings *fa-re* at the same starting pitch as the *mi-do* group. Continue singing the remaining 3rds until they find the matching major 3rds (*la-fa*; *ti-so*). Repeat to find the matching minor 3rds (*fa-re*; *so-mi*; *re⎮-ti*).

▶ **Preparing Interval Reading in Major (Reading Sequence 20)** Provide aural and visual preparation for students by writing the E-major scale on the board and conducting an interval warm-up from the staff. Be sure to focus on the major and minor 3rds, perfect 4ths and 5ths and octaves in Reading Sequence 20.

Reading Sequence 19, page 164

MATERIALS

- "O lê lê O Bahía," p. 165 — **CD 9-14**
- Reading Sequence 19
  Melody part — **CD 9-18**
  Melody part with accompaniment — **CD 9-19**
  Accompaniment only — **CD 9-20**
- **Resource Book** pp. D-22, E-20

Melody: Reading Intervals (Seconds and Thirds)

Have students sing "O lê lê O Bahía" while conducting in meter in 4. Review major and minor seconds in the major scale, on p. 166 in the student text. Using the chart, have students identify major and minor seconds in the major scale. Direct their attention to Reading Sequence 19. Have students

- Identify major and minor seconds.

Help students discover the major and minor thirds in the major scale. (major 3rds: *do-mi* and *fa-la*; minor 3rds: *re-fa*; *mi-so*.) Use "Practicing Major and Minor Thirds" in the Footnotes to assist the students. Then have students

- Locate all major and minor 3rds in Reading Sequence 19.
- Tap the beat as students show handsigns and sing pitch syllables for the countermelody for "O lê lê O Bahía."

Divide the class into two groups. Ask Group 1 to sing "O lê lê O Bahía" while Group 2 sings the countermelody. Have students switch parts.

Reading Sequence 20, page 166

MATERIALS

- "Like a Bird," p. 167 — **CD 9-21**
- Reading Sequence 20
  Melody part — **CD 9-23**
  Melody part with accompaniment — **CD 9-24**
  Accompaniment only — **CD 9-25**
- **Resource Book** pp. D-23, E-21

Melody: Reading Intervals (Major)

Invite students to conduct in $\frac{2}{2}$ as they sing "Like a Bird" in unison, and then as a three-part canon. Have students

- Locate and sing an octave, perfect 4th, perfect 5th, and minor third (*so-mi*) in the song notation.
- Identify a major 3rd above *do* (*mi*).

Direct students to Reading Sequence 20. Have them

- Locate and sing all major and minor 3rds, perfect 4ths and 5ths, and octaves.
- Conduct in $\frac{2}{2}$ as they use pitch syllables to read and sing the countermelody.
- Sing Reading Sequence 20 with the recording of "Like a Bird" **CD 9-21.**

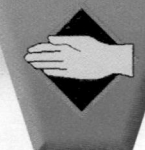

Unit 6
Music Reading Practice

Reading Sequence 21, page 194

MATERIALS

• "Paths of Victory," p. 195	**CD 10-30**
• Reading Sequence 21	
Rhythm part (woodblock)	**CD 10-33**
Rhythm part with accompaniment	**CD 10-34**
Accompaniment only	**CD 10-35**
• **Resource Book** pp. D-24, E-22	
• nonpitched percussion instruments	

Rhythm: Reading Syncopation

Review the 3+3+2 syncopated pattern on p. 194 of the student text by having students listen to "Paths of Victory" **CD 10-30**, as they tap the beat, and softly say the *ta-ti-ta-ti-ta* pattern throughout. Direct students to Reading Sequence 21. Have them

- Analyze the counter-rhythm for identical measures (mm. 1, 3, 5, 7, 10, 11 12).
- Lightly tap an ♪ beat as they read and say the rhythm syllables.
- Conduct in meter in 4 and say the rhythm syllables.

Invite students to play the beat using claves as the class claps the counter-rhythm.

Reading Sequence 22, page 196

MATERIALS

• "New Hungarian Folk Song," p. 196	**CD 10-35**
• Reading Sequence 22	
Rhythm part (woodblock)	**CD 10-37**
Rhythm part with accompaniment	**CD 10-38**
Accompaniment only	**CD 10-39**
• **Resource Book** pp. D-25, E-23	
• nonpitched percussion instruments, tambourine, hand drum	

Rhythm: Reading Mixed Meter

Have students sing and conduct "New Hungarian Folk Song" to review ⁴⁄₄ and ²⁄₄ metric changes. Direct students to Reading Sequence 22. Have them

- Locate and analyze identical rhythms in the four phrases (mm. 2, 4; mm. 4, 7; mm. 6, 8)
- Conduct, read, and perform Reading Sequence 22 using rhythm syllables.
- Lightly clap the counter-rhythm as you tap the beat for the students.
- Lightly clap the rhythm while listening to "New Hungarian Folk Song" **CD 10-35**.

Draw attention to the dynamic markings. Have students perform on the tambourine and hand drum, and determine which instrument best suits the performance of dynamics.

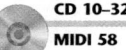

Reading Sequence 21, page 194
CD 10-32
MIDI 58

Rhythm: Reading Syncopation

Using rhythm syllables, **read** and **perform** this syncopated counter-rhythm for "Paths of Victory." Conduct in meter in 4 as you say the syllables.

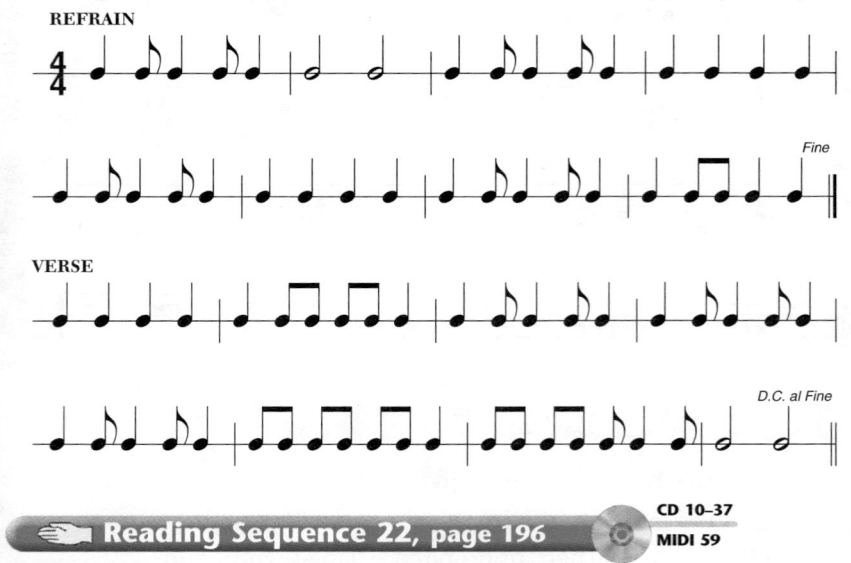

Reading Sequence 22, page 196
CD 10-37
MIDI 59

Rhythm: Reading Mixed Meter

Using rhythm syllables, **read** and **perform** this counter-rhythm for "New Hungarian Folk Song." Then, conduct it, paying close attention to the meter changes.

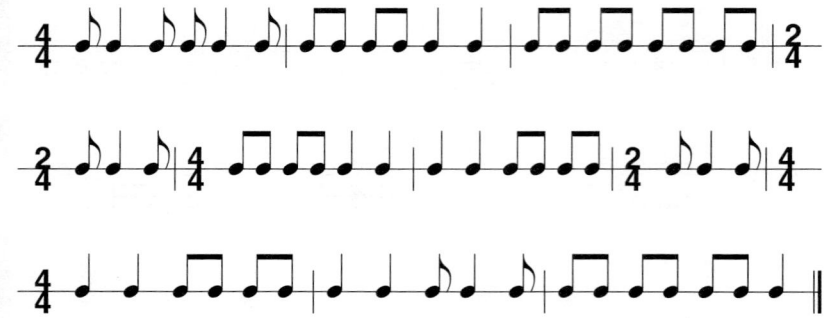

498

Footnotes

▶ **A Different Syncopation (Reading Sequence 21)** Up to now, syncopations with ♪ and ♩ notes have been ♪ ♩ ♪ combinations. In this lesson, the rhythmic values are reversed: ♩ ♪ ♩ ♪, typically found in guitar accompaniments. Help students understand this difference by having them perform both rhythm patterns to the song: (1) ♪ ♩ ♪ ♩ ♩ and (2) ♩ ♪ ♩ ♪ ♩.

▶ **More Mixed Meter Practice (Reading Sequence 22)** Provide additional mixed meter practice for students by having them conduct and read, and then clap the Reading Sequence 22 as you tap the beat for the students.

Reading Sequence 23, page 204

CD 11–6
MIDI 60

Melody: Reading Intervals (Fourths and Fifths)

Using hand signs and pitch syllables, **read** and **sing** this melody for "Blue Mountain Lake." **Identify** and **sing** the intervals of fourths and fifths.

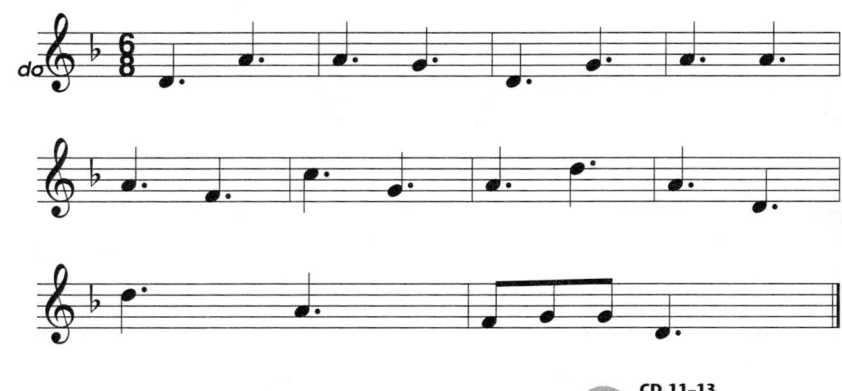

Reading Sequence 24, page 206

CD 11–13
MIDI 61

Melody: Reading Intervals (Harmonic Minor)

Using pitch syllables and hand signs, **read** and **sing** this countermelody for "*Kyrie*."

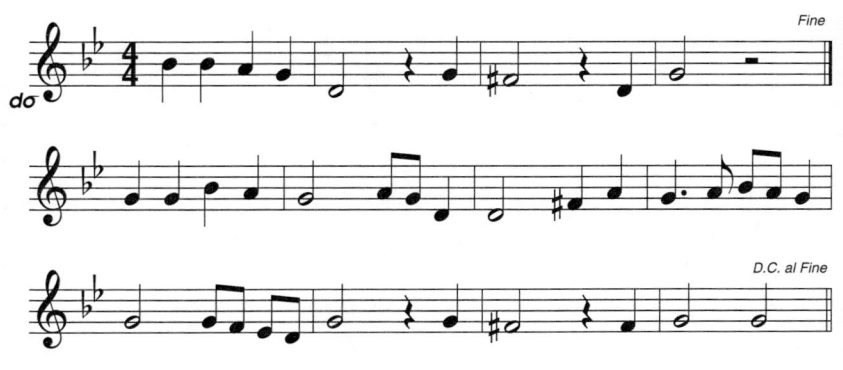

499

▶ **Preparing Harmonic Minor and Interval Reading (Reading Sequence 24)** Prepare students to successfully read this exercise by writing a G-har-monic minor tone set on the staff. Then conduct a melodic warmup focusing on the intervals *re-la; la-re; si-mi; mi-si;* and *si-ti* in the following patterns.

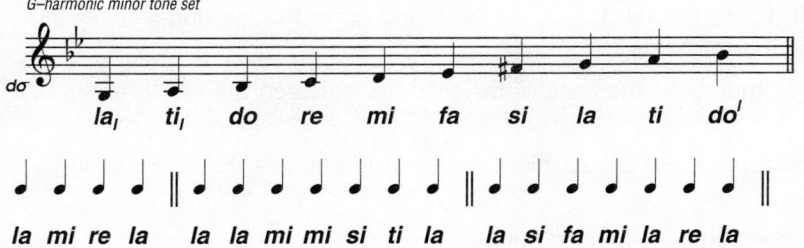

Reading Sequence 23, page 204

MATERIALS

• "Blue Mountain Lake," p. 205	**CD 11-4**
• Reading Sequence 23	
Melody part	**CD 11-6**
Melody part with accompaniment	**CD 11-7**
Accompaniment only	**CD 11-8**
• **Resource Book** pp. D-26, E-24	

Melody: Reading Intervals (Fourths and Fifths)

Conduct a review of major and minor 2nds and 3rds. Draw a vertical tone ladder (*la,* to *la*) on the board. Help students identify a 4th above *la,* (*re*) and the 4th above *mi* (*la*). Bracket the 4ths to the left of the ladder. Repeat, having students identify a 5th below *la* (*re*) and the 5th below *mi* (*la,*). Have students sing "Blue Mountain Lake" and identify all of the 4ths and 5ths. Direct students to Reading Sequence 23. Have them

- Identify all intervals of 4ths and 5ths.
- Use handsigns and pitch syllables to read Reading Sequence 23.
- Sing Reading Sequence 23 as they listen to the recording of "Blue Mountain Lake" **CD 11-4.**

Reading Sequence 24, page 206

MATERIALS

• "Kyrie," p. 206	**CD 11-11**
• Reading Sequence 24	
Melody part	**CD 11-13**
Melody part with accompaniment	**CD 11-14**
Accompaniment only	**CD 11-15**
• **Resource Book** pp. D-27, E-25	

Melody: Reading Intervals (Harmonic Minor)

Review the harmonic minor (scale) by having students sing "*Kyrie*" using pitch syllables. Write the tone set on the staff. Extend the tone set and conduct a reading warmup (See "Preparing Harmonic Minor and Interval Reading" in the Footnotes.) Direct students to Reading Sequence 23. Have them

- Identify and sing perfect 4ths (m. 3: *la-mi/mi-la*) and perfect 5ths (m. 3: *re-la/la-re*).
- Isolate and sing the melodic patterns using *si.*
- Use pitch syllables and handsigns to sing the countermelody. Lower voices should use the descending melody to low G. Higher voices sing the melody ending on second-line G.
- Sing the countermelody with the recording of "*Kyrie*" **CD 11-11.**

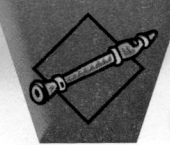

Playing the Recorder

MATERIALS
- *Nele's Dances, No. 17*   **CD 23-9**
- *Nele's Dances, No. 18*   **CD 23-10**
- **Resource Book** pp. I-1 through I-32
- soprano and alto recorders

VOCABULARY
countermelody

ACTIVITIES

Getting Ready

Have students look at the picture of the soprano and alto recorders. If an alto recorder is available, students can experiment with playing it using the soprano fingerings. For example, have some students play G on the soprano recorder while others play the alto using the same G fingering.

ASK How is the sound of the note played on the alto recorder different from the sound of the note played on the soprano recorder? (The sound of the note played on the alto recorder is lower.)

Now have some students play low C on their soprano recorder while others play the soprano G fingering on the alto recorder. They should hear that they are now playing the same note. Explain to students that the soprano recorder always sounds one octave higher than written while the alto recorder sounds as written.

Have students use the illustrations on p. 500 to review the fingerings for G, A, B, high C, and high D. Remind students to

- Cover holes securely.
- Whisper *daah* on each note.
- Blow gently.

Beginning with "B-A-G" Plus Two

Prepare students to play the soprano recorder countermelody for "Bridges" on p. 501. Have them

- Sing the letter names of the notes in rhythm.
- Sing the letter names of the notes while fingering their recorders.

Then have students play the recorder countermelody.

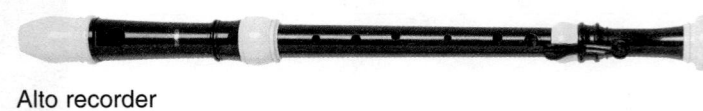

Recorders come in different sizes. As seen in this picture, the soprano recorder is smaller than the alto recorder. Both instruments use the same set of fingerings but produce different pitches. The fingerings below are for soprano recorder.

Alto recorder

Soprano recorder

Getting Ready

Look at the diagram for the note G. Using your left hand, cover the holes that are darkened. Press hard enough so that the holes make a light mark on each finger and thumb. Cover the tip of the mouthpiece with your lips. Blow gently as you whisper *daah*. **Play** a steady beat on the note G. After you can play G, try practicing A, B, high C, and high D. The diagrams will help with finger placement.

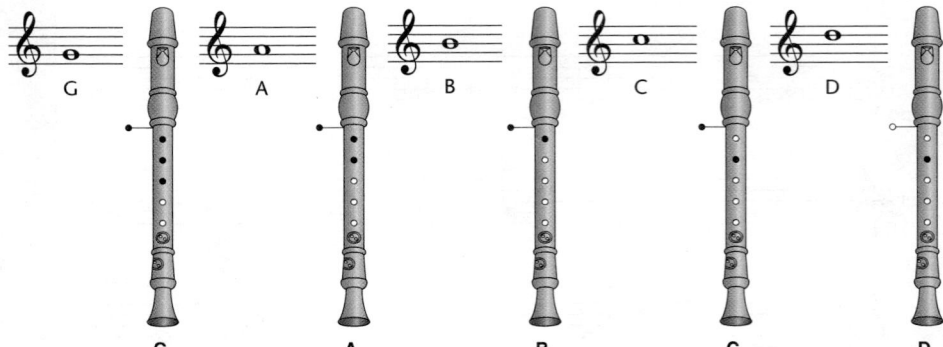

Beginning with "B-A-G" Plus Two

Now that you can play B, A, G, high C, and high D, **play** this simplified melody of "Bridges," page 86. Does the recorder part move mostly by steps, leaps, or repeats?

Footnotes

▶ **Recorder Playing Position** Here are some general guidelines for proper recorder technique.

- Hold the recorder at about a 45 degree angle with the holes facing out and the single thumb hole closer to the body.
- Place the left thumb on the hole in the back and curve the left fingers over the first, second, and third holes.
- Place the right thumb on the back of the recorder between the fourth and fifth holes.
- When covering holes, use the cushions (pads) of the fingers. Fingers should be slightly curved.
- Each hole is covered by a specific finger.
- Rest the mouthpiece lightly on the lower lip.
- Press the upper lip against the mouthpiece with a slight amount of pressure.

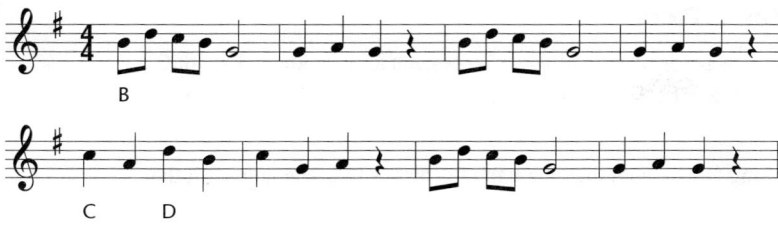

B

C   D

Building Right-Hand Strength

Here are two pairs of new notes: D and E; F and C. As you practice these note pairs, cover the holes securely with your fingers flat, not arched, and whisper *daah*. When playing notes in the low register of the recorder, remember to use very little air.

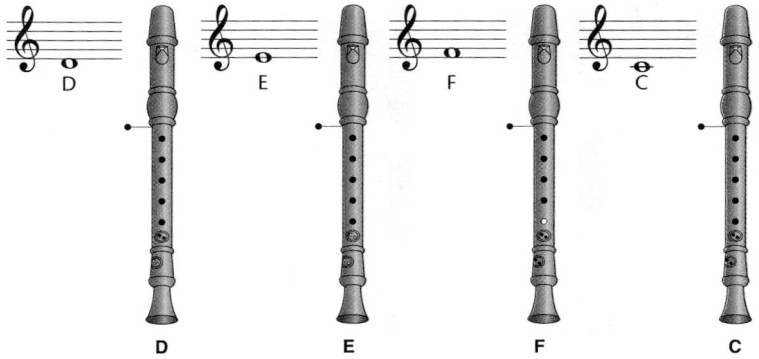

D   E   F   C

D   E   F   C

After learning D and E, **play** the melody of "Peace Like a River," page 190. Be sure to whisper *daah* gently in the style of the music. The two phrases of this song are written below so you can begin to practice.

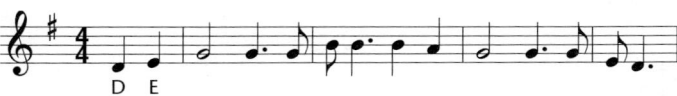

D E

Play this part for the recorder throughout the song "*Adiós, amigos*," page 57. It uses F and C. How is it the same as the melody on the recording?

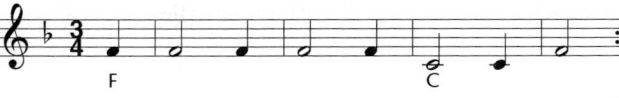

F   C

501

Encourage students to practice their recorders at home. See Resource Book pp. I-10 and I-11 for student copies of this countermelody.

As students are reviewing how to play the soprano recorder, some students may wish to learn to play the alto. Relate the alto recorder to the soprano recorder. Alto recorder countermelodies can be found throughout the Resource Book and Teacher Edition. For students who would like to learn the alto recorder, a countermelody for "Bridges" that uses C, D, and E can be found on Resource Book p. I-10.

Building Right-Hand Strength

Have students practice playing E, D and F, C note pairs. Make sure they understand that they have to add only one finger when leaping from F down to C.

In order to help students with building right hand strength, point out the following:

- Very little air is needed when playing notes in the low register.

- When first playing notes that use the right hand, students may forget to completely cover the left hand holes.

- Students should check that all their fingers are firmly covering the necessary holes.

After students have practiced E, D and F, C note pairs, have them play the two pieces found on p. 501.

For additional practice, students can play ostinatos and countermelodies found in the Teacher's Edition and Resource Book for the following songs.

- "Do, Re, Mi, Fa," p. 80
- "Let Us Sing Together," p. 156
- "*Corta la caña,*" Resource Book pp. I-26, I-27

▶ **Care of Plastic Recorders** After playing, dry the interior with a swab such as a large feather or small cloth attached to a cleaning rod. If the mouthpiece becomes clogged, blow into the recorder while covering the top hole or window of the mouthpiece. Plastic recorders can be washed in the top shelf of most dishwashers or by hand with warm soapy water. Be sure to rinse and dry the recorder after washing.

▶ **Care of Wood Recorders** Warm up the instrument before playing. Each time you play, take the recorder apart and dry the inside with a swab. Do not expose the wood recorder to extreme temperature changes or water. Use cork grease sparingly for easier assembly of the instrument and to prevent the cork from drying. Wood recorders will require a "break in" period.

▶ **Inclusion** A soprano recorder is available for students with finger disabilities. Sections are put together and the holes are rotated and plugged according to the needs of the player.

continued on page 502

Learning Notes in Pairs

Direct students' attention to the fingerings for F#, G#, and B♭ on p. 502.

Relate these new fingerings to those learned previously: F# to G; G# to A; and B to B♭.

Have students learn the half step rule for notes with accidentals. They should read the directions for the half-step rule and experiment with the fingerings for F#, G#, and B♭.

New Recorder Challenges

In addition to the recorder challenges found on p. 502, students can practice these notes by playing the following countermelodies found in the Resource Book.

- "Give My Regards to Broadway," p. I-5
- *"El payo,"* p. I-14
- "Strike Up the Band," p. I-13

Learning Notes in Pairs

Try learning these new notes paired with some notes you already know: F# with G, G# with A, and B♭ with B. This half-step rule will help you remember how to finger F# and G#.

Think of the fingering for the note that is a half step higher than the note with the accidental.

Skip a hole on your recorder and then cover the next two holes.

If you are attempting to play G#, think of the fingering for A. Leave the next hole uncovered and then cover the following two holes. Check the diagram below to see if you have fingered G# correctly. Use the same rule to learn to play F# and B♭. What notes will you think about first?

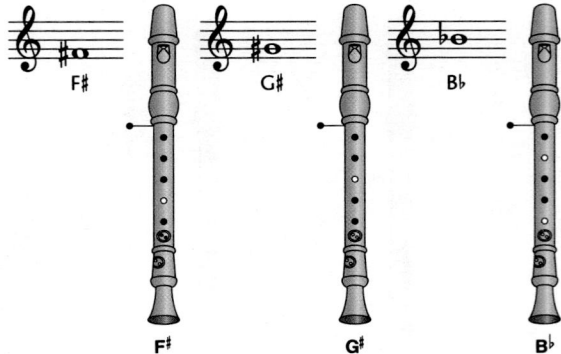

New Recorder Challenges

After learning F#, **play** this ostinato from "Hey, Ho! Nobody Home," page 28. Is it easier to play from E up to F# or from G down to F#?

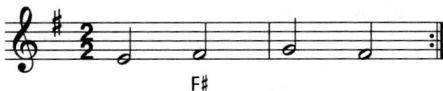

When you can play G# and B♭, **play** the verse of "You Are My Sunshine," page 246. Before playing with the recording, practice each phrase slowly. Remember to **sing** the refrain.

502

Footnotes

▶ **Recorder Identification** If possible, each student should have his or her own recorder. To help identify the instruments, use an electric engraving tool to carve the initials or name of each student on the recorder below the thumb hole. As an alternative, have students place a unique sticker on the front of their recorders below the window.

▶ **Fingering Systems** Soprano recorders are made with either Baroque (English) or German fingering systems. The Baroque recorder can be identified as having a smaller fourth hole and a larger fifth hole while the German recorder has a larger fourth hole and a smaller fifth hole. Although the Baroque recorder requires students to learn cross or forked fingering, this recorder has better octave and chromatic intonation. Baroque (English) fingering is used throughout the recorder program in MAKING MUSIC.

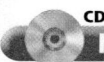

The Virtuoso Recorder

Michala Petri is one of the world's best recorder performers. She is called a virtuoso because her technical and artistic playing are at a very high level. **Listen** to her skillful playing on these contemporary pieces.

CD 23–9, 10

Nele's Dances, No. 17 and No. 18

by Thomas Koppel
as performed by Michala Petri

Koppel, a Danish composer, wrote *Nele's Dances* specifically for Michala Petri and her virtuoso recorder playing.

Recorder Fingerings

This fingering chart will help you learn alto recorder fingerings by relating them to the soprano recorder.

Soprano Recorder

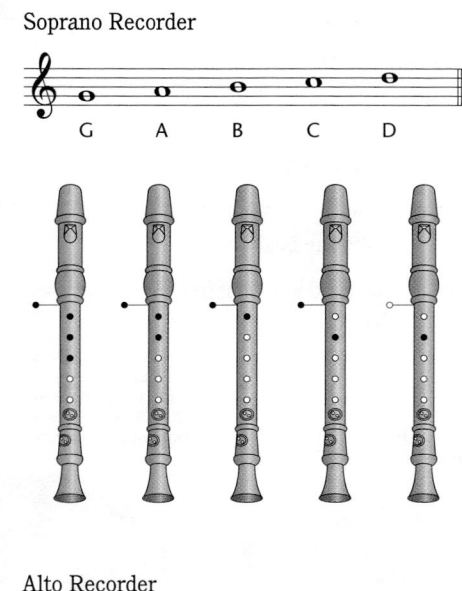

G   A   B   C   D

Alto Recorder

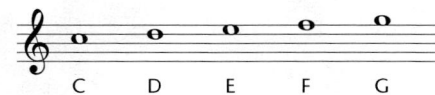

C   D   E   F   G

(503)

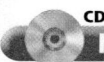

The Virtuoso Recorder

Invite students to listen to Michala Petri's performance of *Nele's Dances, No. 17 and No. 18* **CD 23-9** and **23-10**. Have students discuss aspects of her performance such as the quality of her tone and the dexterity of her fingers.

Recorder Fingerings

Have students compare the fingerings of the alto and soprano recorders. Use the illustrations on p. 503 to reinforce understanding.

▶ **Listening** Provide students with opportunities to listen to music that includes a recorder or similar aerophone. Some examples to choose from are

• "Scarborough Fair," **CD 3-13**, recorder
• *Paddy Whack*, **CD 13-14**, penny whistle
• *Brolga*, **CD 11-12**, didgeridoo
• "La mariposa," **CD 2-7**, panpipes

▶ **Band-in-A-Box** Set up the computer, keyboard, and *Band-in-a-Box* software. Using the style button, have students select a style from the blues category. Enter chords in the key of G following a 12-bar blues progression.

For each chord in the progression, students should identify the notes that comprise the chord. For example: G = G, B, D. Have students improvise a melody on their recorders for each measure using the chord tones.

Playing the Recorder (503)

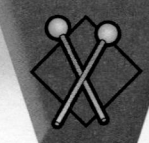

Mallet Instruments

MATERIALS

- "Hey, Ho! Nobody Home," p. 28
- "Evening Chaconne," p. 202 **CD 11-3**
- "Autumn" (poem), p. 193
- **Resource Book** pp. F-1 through F-38
- soprano and alto glockenspiels; soprano, alto, and bass xylophones; soprano, alto, and bass metallophones; a variety of mallets

VOCABULARY

bordun

ACTIVITIES

Moving and Playing

Upper grade students may have varying levels of ability and experience. Prepare them for coordinated playing of Orff mallet instruments with movement, body percussion, and small percussion practice. Have students pat a steady beat with both hands on their legs, then have them pat with alternating hands. When students show proficiency, have them pat with a crossover movement left, right, then left-over-right. These movement activities help prepare students to play simple, alternating, and crossover borduns on xylophones, metallophones, and glockenspiels. It is also beneficial to pat tricky rhythm patterns before playing them on instruments.

Listening

Choosing Mallets Have students read about mallets on p. 504 of the student text. Then demonstrate the various timbres that can be produced when different mallets are used on the instruments. For example, play a metallophone with a soft yarn-headed mallet. Then play with a hard rubber-headed mallet. Have students compare the timbres.

Improvising

Mallet instruments can be used creatively and to reinforce music reading skills. Instruments can be set up in the following scales.

- C *do* pentatonic: C-D-E-G-A
- F *do* pentatonic: F-G-A-C-D
- G *do* pentatonic: G-A-B-D-E
- e *la* pentatonic: e-g-a-b-d
- d *la* pentatonic: d-f-g-a-c
- D dorian mode: D-e-f-g-a-b-c-D
- G mixolydian mode: G-a-b-c-d-e-f-G

Have students improvise with specific rhythms on unspecified pitches. The rhythms used can be derived from words in poetry, song lyrics, or other sources.

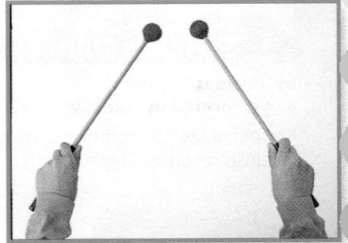

Mallet Instruments

Playing Mallets

When using mallets to play barred instruments, follow these simple suggestions.

Holding the Mallets

Fold your fingers and thumbs around the mallet handle—the thumb should lie alongside the handle, but the pointer finger should not sit on top of the mallet. The backs of your hands should face the ceiling. Grip the handles on the hand grips, but not at the very end. (Smaller hands may need to grip further up toward the mallet head.) Elbows should hang easily at your sides. Avoid elbows that stick out to the side or hug the body.

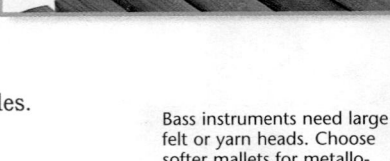

Striking the Bars

Strike each bar at its center, not at either end. Let your mallet strike quickly and then bounce away. If you let the mallet stay on the bar, the sound is stopped.

Matching Mallets to Instruments

It is important to choose the appropriate mallet for each instrument to make the best sound.

For special effects, use hard wood mallets or mallet handles.

Glockenspiels need small wood, hard rubber, or composition heads. ▼

Alto/soprano xylophones need medium-sized felt or yarn heads with a hard core. Alto/soprano metallophones need the same, but with a softer core. ▼

Bass instruments need large felt or yarn heads. Choose softer mallets for metallophones, and harder mallets for xylophones.

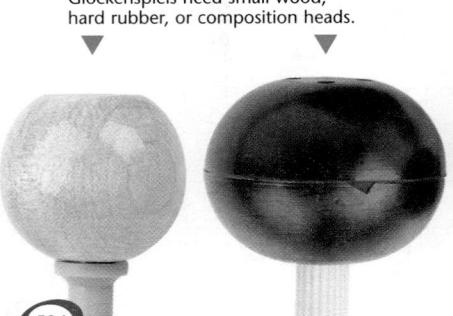
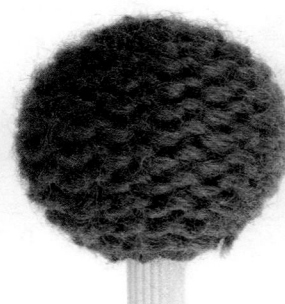
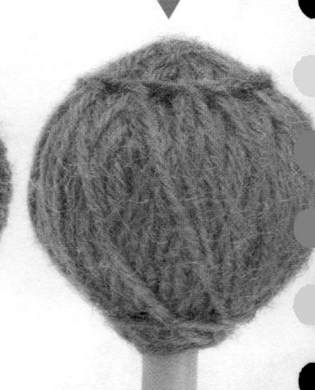

Footnotes

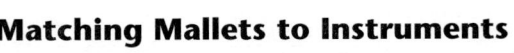

▶ **Care of Mallet Instruments** Show students how to set up the instruments in specific scales. Have them lift the bars up carefully with two hands, one hand at each end of the bar. Caution them to make sure the nails that hold the bars in place do not get bent. Explain to students that the bars are being removed so that they can make "good" sounding music together. Have students practice walking to the instruments by "moon-walking" slowly around them. They should not step over the instruments because their toes can easily get hooked on them and cause injury to the student and damage to the instrument.

▶ **Position and Technique** Students should kneel, stand, or sit in front of an instrument. Have them hold the mallets by wrapping their fingers in a relaxed way over and around the grip of the mallet, arms slightly away from their sides. Have students strike the bars at the center and "pull" the sound from the instrument with a light, upward, and buoyant stroke. If students push downward into the bars, the vibration of the bars will be muted, making a dull sound.

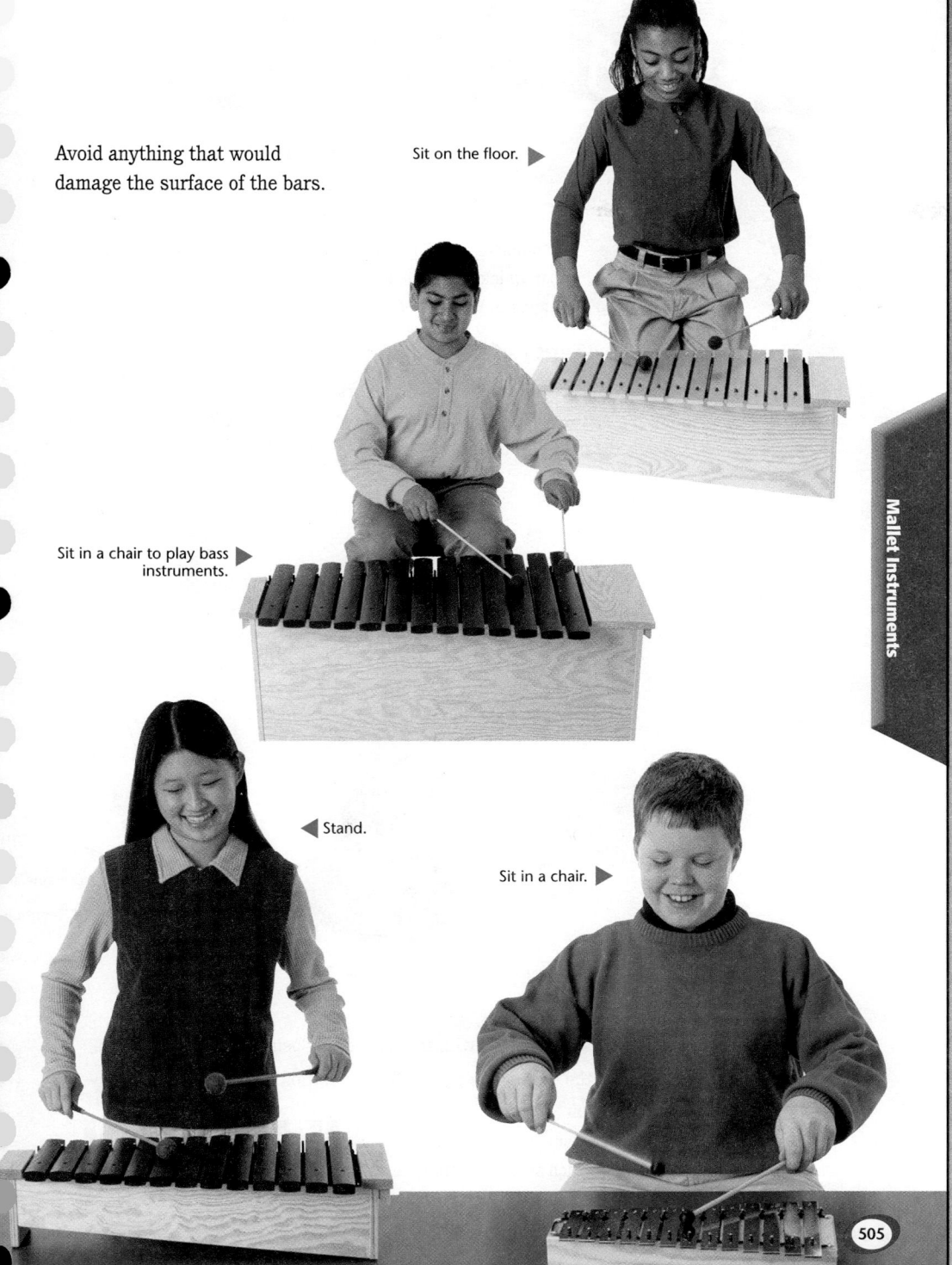

Avoid anything that would damage the surface of the bars.

Sit on the floor. ▶

◀ Sit in a chair to play bass instruments.

◀ Stand.

Sit in a chair. ▶

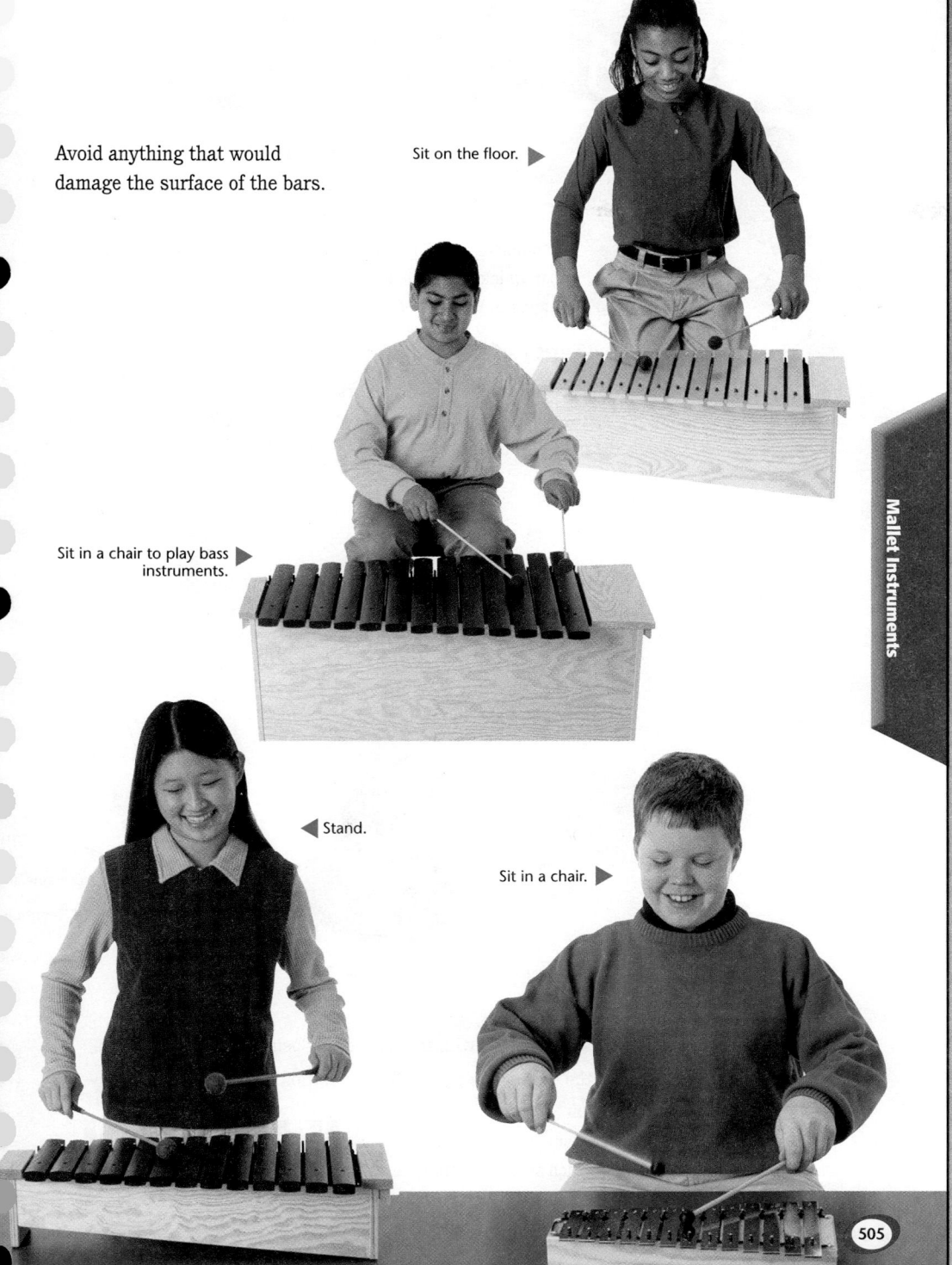

(505)

The instruments can also be used to play sound effects to enhance meaning in poetry. Have students read the poem "Autumn" on p. 193. Invite them to explore non-tonal setups on glockenspiels, metallophones, and xylophones. Encourage students to use various mallet types and techniques, such as *glissandos*, to illustrate words of the poem such as *cascade down*, *autumn breeze*, and *delicate ballet*.

Playing Borduns

A simple bordun is the first and fifth pitches of a scale played together or alternated. In *do* pentatonic on C, the bordun would be C and G. In d *la* pentatonic, the bordun would be d and a. Students should always use two hands when playing.

Have students play the alto metallophone and bass metallophone simple borduns on p. 29 as the class sings "Hey, Ho! Nobody Home" on p. 28. Invite them to experiment with playing with various types of mallets.

Playing Harmony

Play the recording of "Evening Chaconne" **CD 11-3** on p. 202. Assign instrument parts to the students. As students listen, have them follow the score and pat the rhythm of their assigned parts, emulating the gestures necessary for playing the instruments.

Encourage students who are assigned to the glockenspiel parts to determine what right-left malleting pattern they will use to make their part easier to play.

Students who are assigned to play the bass line will experience performing a descending parallel harmony.

Creating

Students can create tonal or atonal compositions using works of fine art as inspiration. The painting on p. 415 in the student text, *Calla Lily Vendor*, has discernable patterns, rhythm, shape, texture, and direction. Have students, individually or in a group, experiment with a variety of timbres on the mallet instruments. Then have them create graphic scores that map the form, texture, rhythm, and melody of their works. Invite them to perform for the class.

▶ **Orff Instrumentarium** See Resource Book p. F-37 for a key to instrument abbreviations on a score. Set up the instruments in the classroom as an ensemble, grouping the families together in the following manner. Place a bass xylophone for you to play in the center, facing the group. On the left, set up the soprano and alto glockenspiels in two rows. Similarly, to the right, set up the soprano and alto metallophones, with a bass metallophone in a third row. Set up the xylophones in similar formation to the metallophones. Then set up other percussion and drums to the right and behind the xylophones.

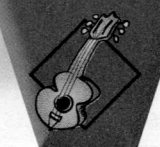

Playing the Guitar

MATERIALS

Guitars

Sound Bank, pp. 512-519   **CD 23-28**

"Mama Don't 'Low," p. 358   **CD 18-6**

"Sometimes I Feel Like a Motherless Child,"
p. 241   **CD 12-17**

This section introduces three types of guitars and their parts, some characteristic applications, and proper playing position.

Why Play the Guitar?

Ask students if they know anyone, a family member or friend, who plays the guitar. Briefly discuss when the instrument is played by this person.

ASK When have you seen a guitar played other than in this class? (Accept all answers.)

Types of Guitars

Ask students to remove guitars from their cases. Point out the major parts of the instrument as captioned in the student text. Ask students to locate these parts on their guitars. Ask how their guitars compare to the types shown on p. 506.

Write out a list of acoustic guitar parts on the board or distribute to help students remember the parts of the guitar and their purpose.

- **Soundhole:** Allows the string vibrations amplified in the resonator to project outward.
- **Bridge:** Allows vibrations to enter the resonator.
- **Tuning pegs:** Tighten and loosen the strings to change pitch.
- **Nut:** Keeps strings spaced properly on the fingerboard above the frets, and takes some of the string tension off the tuning pegs.

Add the following list for electric guitar.

- **Pick-ups:** Pick up, or amplify, the string vibrations, since there is no resonance on a solid body guitar.
- **Tone/volume controls:** Change the sensitivity of the pickups.
- **Tremelo arm:** Allows string tension to be controlled by the right hand.

Discuss with students some of the many uses of the guitar in music. Suggestions include as accompaniment for voices, as a rhythm instrument, or a melodic or "lead" instrument. Also briefly discuss in which music styles the guitar is used. Suggestions include classical, folk, blues, rock, and alternative.

Use the listening selections listed in the Materials section to explore the sound of the different instruments.

Tuning the Guitar

Explain string numbers with students. Refer to strings by size or thickness until the students learn their numbers. Allow students a few moments to strum the strings with the right thumb. Have the class play and count each string one at a time.

Playing the Guitar

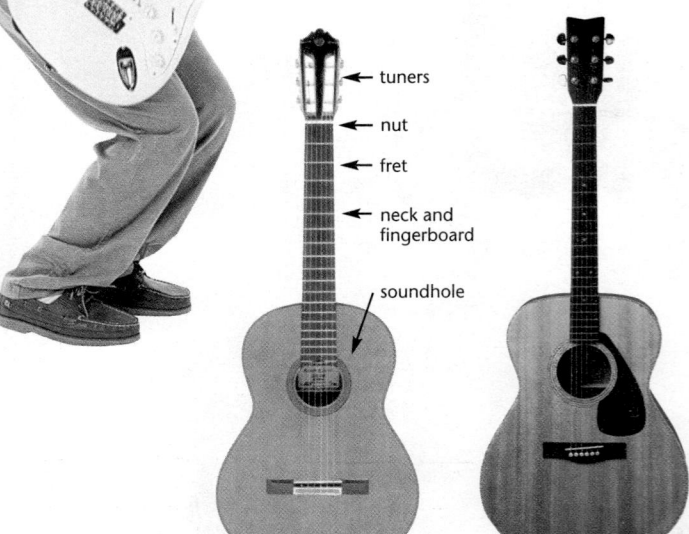

Why Play the Guitar?

The guitar is a very popular and versatile instrument. Once you learn some basics, you can create your own "musical voice" in the special way you play the guitar. You can quickly learn some of these basics by following the suggestions included in these pages.

Types of Guitars

There are three types of guitars—nylon-string classical, steel-string acoustic, and electric. Look at these photographs and learn the names of their parts:

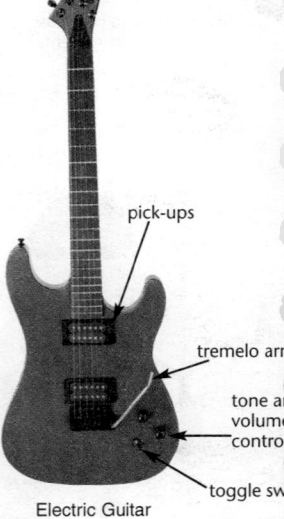

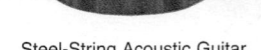

← tuners

← nut

← fret

← neck and fingerboard

soundhole

pick-ups

tremelo arm

tone and volume controls

toggle switch

Nylon-String Classical Guitar   Steel-String Acoustic Guitar   Electric Guitar

Tuning the Guitar

- Guitar strings are numbered 1, 2, 3, 4, 5, 6, with the sixth string being the lowest in pitch.
- You can tune the guitar using the keys of the piano. The illustration below shows what keys to use for tuning each guitar string.
- You can also tune your guitar by using an electronic tuner, which allows you to "see" when each string is in tune.

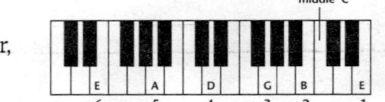

middle C

E   A   D   G   B   E
6   5   4   3   2   1

Footnotes

▶ **A Short History of the Guitar** The guitar has been traced back to ancient Egypt. It became very popular in Europe during the Renaissance, and its features slowly changed, as it grew larger and acquired more strings. The guitar was widely used in the United States by the mid-nineteenth century, and by the mid-twentieth century it had become, and still remains, the most popular musical instrument.

Some important developments in the guitar during the twentieth century include 1) the invention of the dreadnaught-style steel string guitar; 2) the use of nylon strings on the classical guitar beginning after World War II; and 3) the invention of the electric guitar.

There are virtuoso performers associated with every type of guitar. Classical guitarists include Andrés Segovia and Christopher Parkening. Steel string acoustic guitarists include Doc Watson and John Renbourn. Electric guitarists include Jimi Hendrix and Eric Clapton.

- You can also tune the guitar by using a method called relative tuning. Follow these steps:

1. Tune the sixth, or lowest-pitched, string to E on the piano or pitch pipe.

2. Press the sixth string on fret 5 and pluck it with your right thumb, producing the note A, which you use to tune the next, or fifth, string.

3. Reach your right hand over to the tuning keys, and turn the fifth-string key until the two sounds match. Now the fifth string is in tune.

4. Press the fifth string on fret 5, and use the pitch to tune the fourth string, repeating the tuning process as before.

5. Press the fourth string on fret 5, and use the pitch to tune the third string.

6. Press the third string on fret 4, and use the pitch to tune the second string.

7. Press the second string on fret 5, and use the pitch to tune the first string. Now you are in tune!

The Best Playing Positions

There are three ways to hold your guitar comfortably and correctly. Notice the different ways that are pictured here:

- Always raise the guitar neck slightly, because this allows the left hand to play chords without extra tension and effort.

- Always keep the front of the guitar completely vertical, because this also helps the left hand to play chords easily.

- You can also play standing up with the help of a guitar strap, but make sure to keep the neck slanted slightly upwards, and hold the guitar high enough so that it is not difficult to see what you are doing.

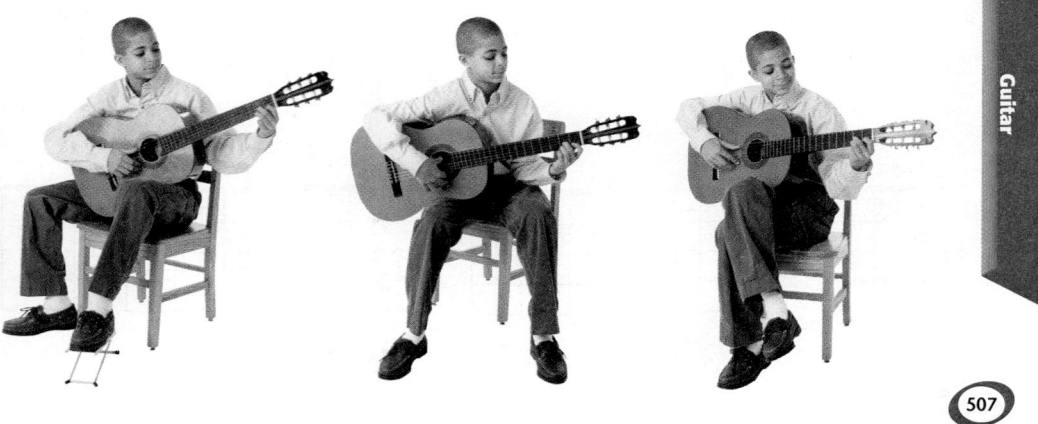

507

Guitar

ASK Do all the guitars sound the same? (They won't if the guitars aren't tuned.)

Explain the general rules for using tuning pegs: Tightening the string *raises* the pitch. The player turns the tuning peg away from himself or herself. Loosening the string *lowers* the pitch. The player turns the tuning peg toward him or her.

Then have students practice tuning with a keyboard. Make sure the process is *aural*. In other words, ask students whether strings need to be higher or lower to match the target pitch, and therefore if the strings should be tightened or loosened.

Consider using an electronic tuner for those students who are visual learners.

Demonstrate relative tuning following the steps on p. 507. This is the method that students will most likely use the most as they continue learning, so practice the steps carefully. Since this process introduces left-hand technique, draw the students' attention to the specific area that the fingers press in each fret (i.e., in the space above an indicated fret, rather than directly on it).

The Best Playing Positions

It is best for the students to use a proper playing position from the very beginning. Have the class read the instructions on p. 507. Then, referring to the photographs on p. 507, ask students to experiment until they find the position that is most comfortable for them.

Point out the optimal position of the neck, which properly aligns the left-hand for chording.

The inside of the right elbow should straddle the widest part of the guitar body, and the right hand should be placed directly over the sound hole.

Playing the Guitar

▶ **Reading Guitar Chord Diagrams** Observe the detailed chord diagram on p. 508. Help students identify the various features of these diagrams. The best way to help students orient the diagrams to what they see on their own guitars is to have them hold the guitar vertically at an arm's distance, then turn it so that they are looking squarely at its front.

continued on page 508

Playing Basics

Have students wrap the thumb of the left hand around the neck of the guitar as they practice the right thumb strum described above. Then teach a strum which uses the thumb and index finger. Explain that the thumb will play the bass note on string 6, and the rest of the strings are scraped with the nail of the index finger, using a smooth downward motion. Try these basic patterns with your students.

Thumb-Strum-Thumb-Strum ($\frac{2}{4}$, $\frac{4}{4}$, and $\frac{6}{8}$ meter)

Thumb-Strum-Strum ($\frac{3}{4}$ meter)

As before, practice playing as a group first. Then ask each student to play the strum individually. It is important that each student hears himself or herself individually. This builds confidence and a discriminating ear. Students should aim for increased accuracy and speed with practice.

For more advanced strumming patterns, try the cajun waltz, calypso, rhythm and blues, and compound brush strums. Diagrams are provided below and on the next page.

Ask students to select one song from the textbook that could be played with one of these strums.

Playing Guitar Chords

To begin developing left hand technique, have the students observe and then repeat the numbering of the left-hand fingers, as illustrated on p. 508.

Remind students to press the strings down only before actually playing the strings to reduce finger fatigue. When not playing, the fingertips can be simply rested on the appropriate strings.

Guitar Chords Used in This Book

Ask students to look at the chords fingered on p. 508. Have them locate the fingers on the neck, keeping the fingers of the left hand relaxed and "round," with space between the guitar neck and the hand. For each chord, give students a moment to find the position, then have them strum the chord as a group and then individually.

Strum Diagrams

Rhythm-and-Blues Strum

Use the thumb to brush the down strings while you count. Add a fuller strum on "f" by scraping all the nails of the fingers across the strings in a downward motion. Finally, play on the bass notes on "T."

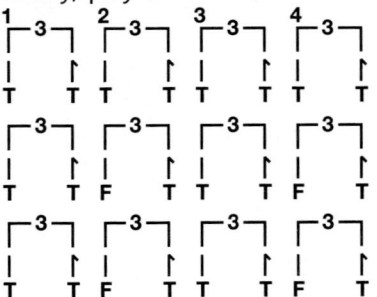

Playing Basics

Here is some basic information on how to play the guitar:

- The left-hand fingers press the strings on the frets to produce chords, which are used to accompany songs.
- The right-hand thumb brushes the strings to make the sounds.
- You may also use a "pick," a small triangular-shaped piece of soft plastic, to play the strings with your right hand.
- Notice how the left-hand fingers are numbered; you will use these numbers when you begin reading the guitar chords.

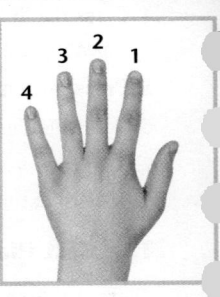

Playing Guitar Chords

- All chords have note names—these are indicated in many song scores in this book. The position of the chord names tells you what chords you will use, and when you will be changing chords in the song. They look like this:

Guitar Chords Used in This Book

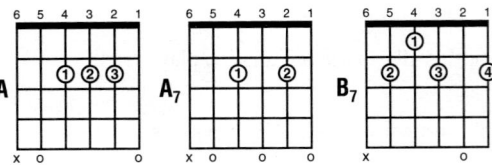

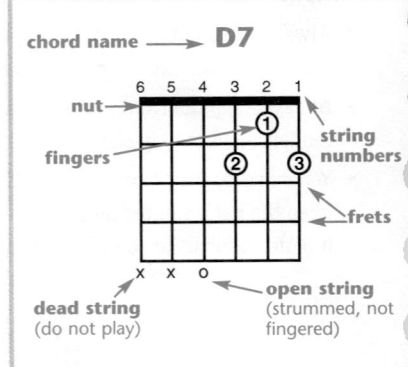

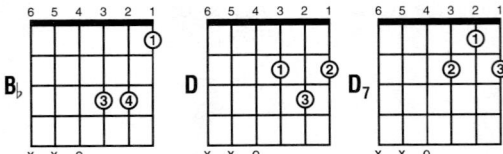

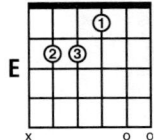 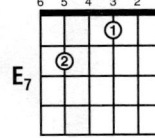 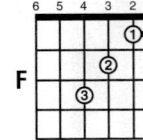 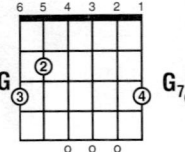 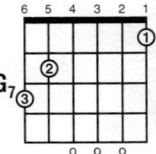 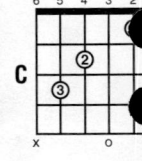

Footnotes

▶ **Developing a Repertoire** Below is a list of songs in the student text that can be played well on the guitar. Create special sections in these songs such as interludes that will showcase your guitar players.

Songs in the Key of C
Cuando pa' Chile me voy, p. 376   *Má teodora*, p. 301
Water Come A Me Eye, p. 300   Lost My Gold Ring, p. 158

Songs in the Key of G or D
By the Waters of Babylon, p. 311   Give a Little Love, p. 140
Down in the Valley, p. 375   *Ise oluwa*, p. 230
Everybody Loves Saturday Night, p. 296

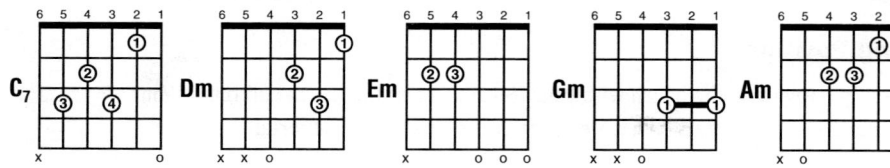

Using a Capo

- A capo is a clamp-like device that allows guitarists to use easy, first-position guitar chords to play songs in virtually any key (changing the key of a song is called transposing).

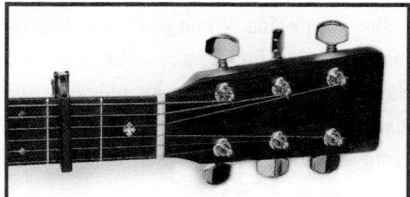

How You Can Tell You're Improving

You are improving if you answer "yes" to more and more of these questions:

- Can you make chord changes without looking?
- Can you play at an even tempo?
- Can you sing along while you play?
- Do your fingertips hurt less when you play?
- Can you play for longer periods of time?
- Can you play some songs from memory?

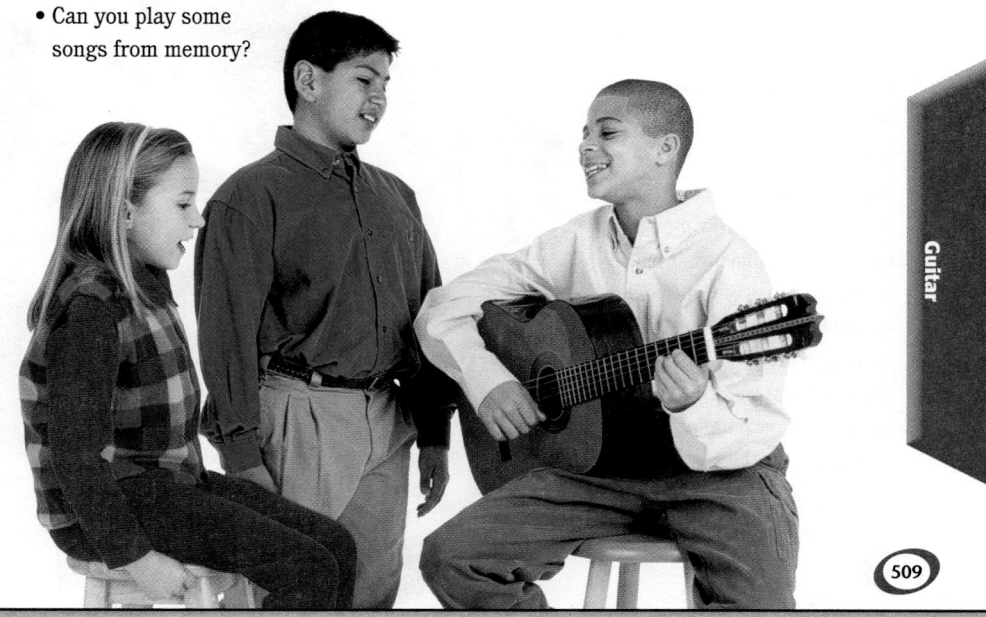

(509)

Using a Capo

Have students take out their capos or distribute them. Explain that using a capo on a fret transposes a song up by half steps. Demonstrate how to attach one to the neck of the guitar. Point out that the capo should be parallel to the fret on the guitar neck, so that the transposing is even for each string. Have students look at the photograph on p. 509. Point out that the capo is behind the second fret. Therefore, the key of the song moves up two half steps, or one whole step.

Explain that the fingerings for the chords remain the same when using a capo; students should simply move their hand positions up the number of frets taken by the capo and play the same chords.

Have students tune their instruments without the capo. Then select a song that the students have mastered, and have them transpose the song a whole step using the capo. Observe correct placement of the capo.

How You Can Tell You're Improving

Review the questions in this section at the end of each lesson. Also review posture and technique at each lesson. Individual weekly assessments are useful in determining which students may need extra help.

Strum Diagrams

Cajun Waltz Strum

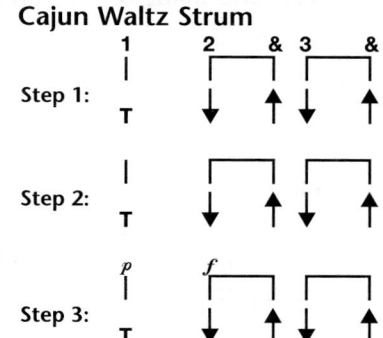

Compound Brush Strum

First, play this rhythm on the middle strings of the guitar with short, quick downstrokes of your index finger:

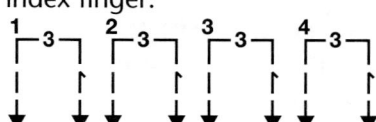

Now, add an upstroke with your index finger in between each downstroke.

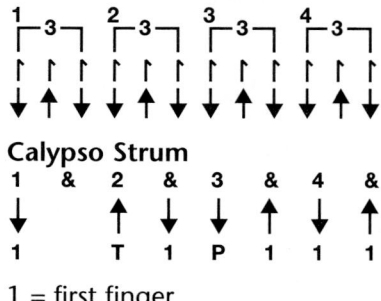

Calypso Strum

1	&	2	&	3	&	4	&
↓		↑	↓	↓	↑	↓	↑
1		T	1	P	1	1	1

1 = first finger
T = thumb
P = palm, slapping down on strings

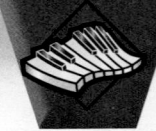

Playing the Keyboard

MATERIALS
- Textbook
- Keyboards

This section is designed to assist you in class piano instruction, in addition to or in place of private instruction.

Sitting Position

Have each student (or as many as you have keyboards) sit facing the keyboard, as far forward on the bench as is necessary for the student's feet to reach the floor. The edge of the bench should touch just below the top of the leg. If a student's feet do not comfortably reach the floor when he or she is properly seated, provide a large telephone book or other support for under the feet. It is important that the upper body be high enough for the forearms to be on the same level as the keyboard, with wrists parallel to the keyboard.

Hand Position

Have students stand with arms down at the side. Have them look down and observe the shape of the hand in a relaxed position. Then, ask students to sit at the keyboard and put their hands above the keys, holding their hands loosely in that same position. You can ask them to lightly swing their elbows to check flexibility. Point out that the curved fingers need to rest far enough in on the keys so that the thumb touches a white key.

If necessary, have students switch places so that all have a chance to find their playing position.

Finger Numbers

Ask students to hold up their hands and count off 1, 2, 3, 4 and 5, while wiggling that finger. You may wish to have students count off each hand separately first, and then together.

Fingering for Steps and Skips

Ask students to look at the diagrams at the top of p. 511. Then, after checking students for proper playing position, ask them to play the patterns first individually, then as a group. Have students switch places if necessary so that all have a turn.

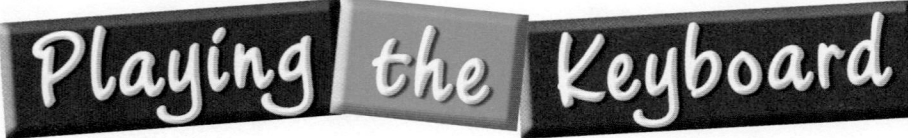

Sitting Position

Sit slightly forward on the bench with your feet resting on the floor at all times. Your knees should be just under the front edge of the keyboard. Sit comfortably.

Hand Position

Your hand position is the shape of your hand as it hangs naturally at your side. When you bring your hand up to the keyboard, your fingers should be slightly curved at the middle joint and the wrist should be parallel to the keyboard. Your elbows should be flexible as they hang near your side. Do not "hug" your elbows too close to your sides.

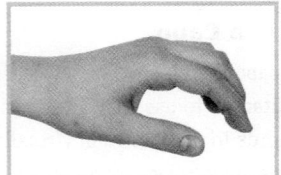

Finger Numbers

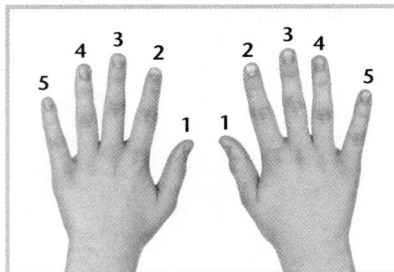

Fingering for Steps and Skips

You have learned that melodies move by steps, by leaps (skips), and by repeats. How a melody moves determines the fingering to be used to play that melody on the keyboard. The examples, on page 511, show the relationship between right/left movement on the keyboard and up/down movement on the staff.

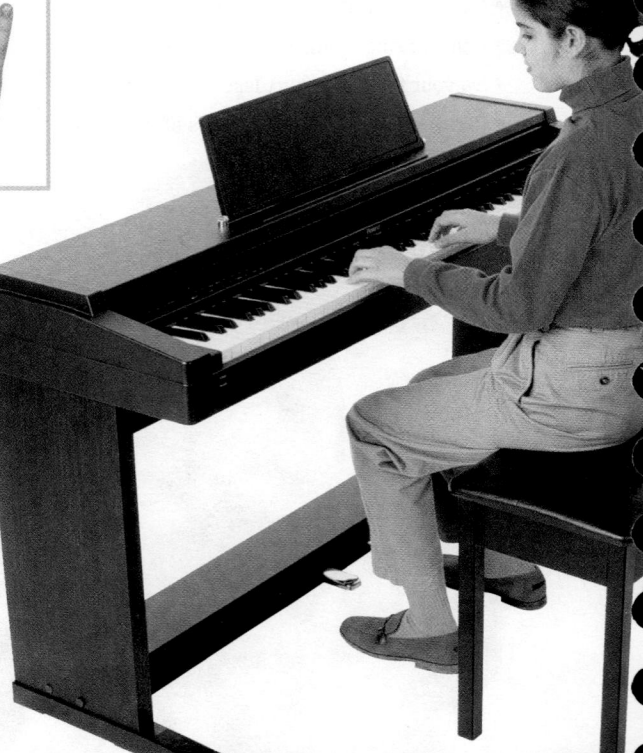

 Footnotes

▶ **Chording** Many songs can be accompanied with just three or four chords. Consider teaching the class root position chords for C, G, D, and Am. Have students experiment with I-IV-V-I chord progressions (G-C-D-G), and expand to include the minor ii chord progression (G-C-Am-D-G). When students master this exercise, consider teaching this chord pattern in a I IV_4^6 ii V^6 I inversion pattern.

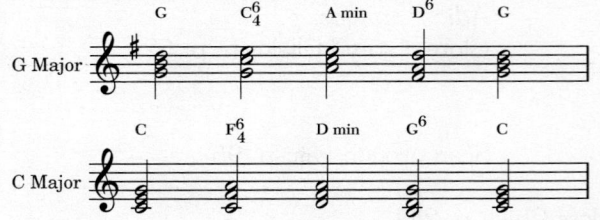

Teach other white-key chord progressions (C-F-G-C, and C-F-Dm-G-C) as the class gains skill.

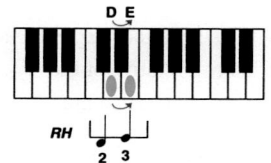 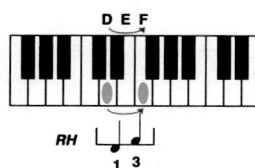 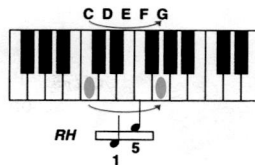

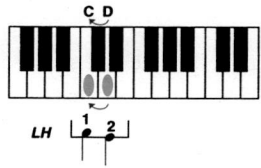 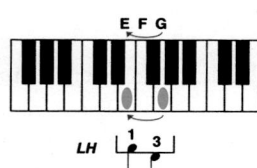 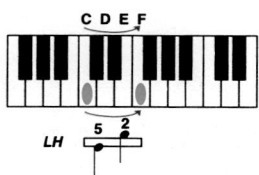

Three-Line Reading

Play the following examples. Determine a logical fingering before you begin each one.

RH　　Begin on E:

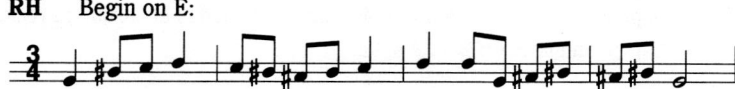

LH　　Begin on F:

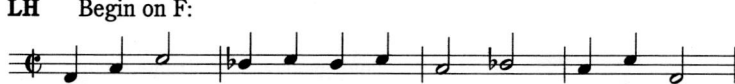

Playing from Treble and Bass Clefs

When singing music, you have learned to follow the upward/downward direction of a melody and to determine if it moves by step, by leap, or if it stays on a repeated tone. When playing music, you must read music in the same way as well as determine where to play the notes on the keyboard. Each note in printed music indicates one place, and only one place, where it can be played. **Play** the following examples in the treble and bass clefs.

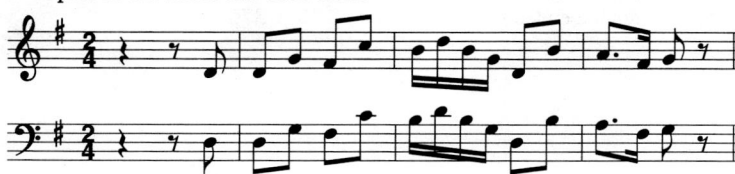

(511)

Three-Line Reading

Ask students to look at the three-line examples on p. 511. Point out the last measure in each example. Note that the last pitch and the first pitch of the patterns are the same.

ASK What is the distance between the highest and lowest note? (a fifth)

Have students place their hands in position, noting the accidentals in the pattern.

Check each student for proper playing position, then ask them to play each pattern as a group.

ASK In what meter is the first example? ($\frac{3}{4}$) The second? (cut time)

　　Is this duple or triple meter? (triple/duple)

Playing from Treble and Bass Clefs

Ask students to look at the examples at the bottom of p. 511, and find the lowest and highest notes in each example. Point out that those pitches will use the outer fingers of the hand. Check each student for proper playing position, then ask them to play each line separately, then together. Again, have students switch places if necessary so that all have a turn.

ASK What do you notice about the melody patterns? (They are the same for each hand.)

As a review, consider duplicating the pattern at the bottom of the page and asking the students to mark the fingering numbers above each pitch. Remind them to pay attention to which clef and hand they are working with in making their determination.

▶ **Integrating the Curriculum** Students may be interested in maintaining a bulletin board filled with images of famous keyboard players past and present. Performers may be grouped according to time period, style, or specific instrument. The bulletin board may be updated as the year progresses. Encourage students to bring in photographs or articles of the performers to include in the class bulletin board.

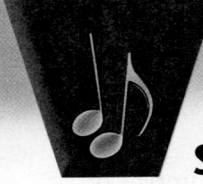

Sound Bank

MATERIALS
- Sound Bank   **CD 23**, tracks 11-49

VOCABULARY

percussion	vibration	pitch	resonance
timbre	tension	bow	reed
valve			

USING THE SOUND BANK

Sound Bank is a glossary of the principal instruments discussed in this book. Text, pictures, and recordings are designed to be used together to help students integrate the definitions, illustrations, and sounds.

Ready Reference When an instrument is studied in the book, reinforce the learning by having students

- Look at the illustration.
- Listen to the sound.
- Read the definition.

Evaluation Test students' comprehension by playing the recorded examples in random order and having students respond orally or on paper.

Instrument Families The instruments shown in the student text are listed alphabetically but are divided into families—strings (orange), percussion (blue), woodwinds (purple), and brass (green). The color codes will help students immediately identify the family to which an instrument belongs.

ACTIVITIES

Vibrations and Sound

SAY All sound sources make vibrations. Vibrations are back-and-forth movements that come to our ears through the air. Our ears "hear" the vibrations as sound.

To demonstrate vibration, hit a cymbal or pluck the free end of a ruler that is braced on a desk.

Use the following instruments for additional demonstrations of vibration and sound. Allow students to touch the instruments lightly, in order to feel as well as see the vibrations.

- drumhead
- Autoharp strings
- guitar strings
- piano strings

Guide students in experimenting with other classroom percussion instruments to feel vibrations. Point out that

- On some instruments, the vibrations may be obvious.
- On others, such as the maracas, the vibrations may be very delicate and difficult to feel. (On the sand blocks, they cannot be felt at all.)

See p. 514 for another experiment with vibrations.

Sound Bank

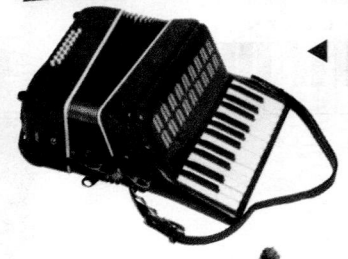

◄ **Accordion** A keyboard instrument with bellows that expand and compress to produce sound. The concertina is a relative of the accordion and has buttons. The accordion and concertina are popular in European and Cajun music. CD 23-11 p. 245

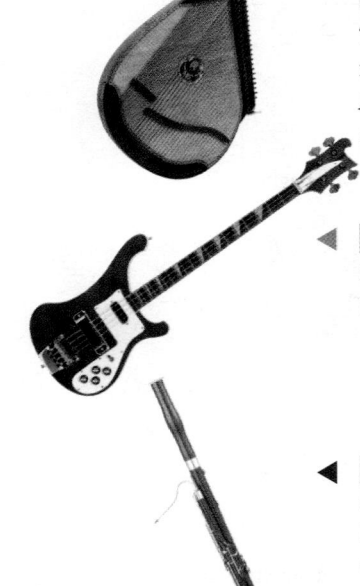

◄ **Bandura** A traditional string instrument of Ukraine that sounds similar to a harpsichord. Each string produces only one pitch. There are no frets as with a guitar. A bandurist usually plucks notes with the fingers or a pick. The left hand plays bass notes. *Banduras* range in size from treble to bass and have 30 to 60 strings. CD 23-12 p. 103

◄ **Bass Guitar** An electric guitar with four bass strings played by plucking. The bass guitar plays bass lines and is important in rock, pop, and jazz. CD 23-13 p. 92

◄ **Bassoon** A large, tube-shaped woodwind instrument with a double reed. Lower notes on the bassoon can be gruff or comical. Higher notes are softer, sweeter, and more gentle-sounding. CD 23-14 p. 354

◄ **Bodhrán** [boh-RAHN] An Irish wood-frame drum played with a double-ended small stick. CD 23-15 p. 276

   Instrument Key: strings   percussion   woodwind   brass   keyboard

---

Footnotes

▶ **Playing Percussion Instruments** Almost anything that makes noise can be used as a percussion instrument. Percussion instruments can be struck, shaken, or scraped.

- Struck: most percussion instruments; struck with hands, mallets, sticks
- Shaken: maracas (seeds or pebbles strike the inside)
- Scraped: sand blocks, guiro

The percussion section of a concert band or a symphony orchestra is usually placed toward the rear, since it can be heard easily. In addition to adding specific effects and colors to the ensemble, percussion instruments help provide a rhythmic foundation.

Percussion instruments can also be grouped according to those that make a definite pitch (timpani, mallet percussion) and those that produce a sound of indefinite pitch (drums, maracas, triangle).

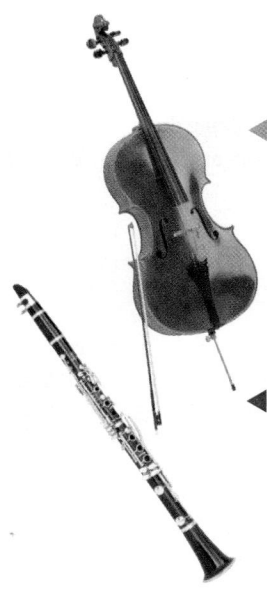

Cello [CHEH-loh] A large, wooden string instrument played with a bow or by plucking the strings. The player sits with the cello between the knees. The cello has a low, rich-sounding, warm tone. CD 23–16 p. 355

Clarinet A wind instrument shaped like a long cylinder with a flare at the end. It is usually made of wood and has a reed in the mouthpiece. Low notes on the clarinet are soft and mellow. The highest notes are clear and resonant. CD 23–17 p. 355

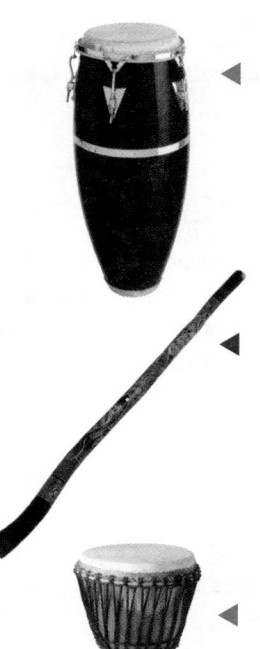

Conga [KOHN-gah] An Afro-Cuban drum with a long, barrel-shaped body. Conga drums come in several sizes: the smaller *quinto*, the standard *conga*, and the larger *tumba*. A *tumbador* is a conga player. The conga is struck with the fingers and the palms of the hands. CD 23–18 p. 264

Didgeridoo [dih-jehr-ee-DOO] A long, hollow tube made from a Eucalyptus tree, played with the breath and vibrating lips like the tuba. The *didgeridoo* is a traditional instrument of the Aborigines in Australia. Players use circular breathing to create drone tones. CD 23–19 p. 271

Djembe [JEHM-beh] An African, medium-sized drum made from an animal hide stretched across a wooden frame. CD 23–20 p. 231

Most instruments appear on the page indicated. In a few instances, the reference is to a family of instruments.

Timbre

SAY Every instrument—and every voice—has its own timbre. Usually, we can tell who is speaking or what is being played just by the sound—we don't even have to look. Let's listen to the timbres of our voices.

Divide the class into two parts. Face the "listeners" away from the "speakers." Have the

- Speakers take turns saying the same sentence or phrase at about the same dynamic level.
- Listeners try to identify the speaker from the timbre.
- Groups switch roles.

Turn this activity into a game by keeping score.

Repeat this activity, using instruments featured in the Sound Bank. Use the recordings to review, if necessary.

Resonance

SAY Resonance can make sounds louder and fuller. Let's try this experiment to hear resonance.

Have students

- Say something—"hello," or their names—into the air.
- Say the same thing into a resonating chamber—an empty cardboard box or an empty wastebasket.

ASK **What happened to the sound?** (It got louder and fuller.)

Making a Pitch

ASK **Some of the percussion instruments pictured in your book have a definite pitch. Can you tell which they are?** (mbira, steel drums, tabla, timpani, xylophone)

SAY Other percussion instruments have an indefinite pitch, although some can make high or low sounds. The conga, for instance, is larger than the doumbek and makes a lower sound.

SAY The pitch of an instrument results from the number of vibrations: the more vibrations, the higher the pitch. The pitch can be made higher or lower in three ways: size, tension, and thickness. If the sound sources are equal in two of the ways, the third will determine the pitch.

continued on page 514

▶ **Playing String Instruments** String instruments make sounds when the strings vibrate. The strings are stretched over sound boxes of various shapes. Most string instruments are held between chin and shoulder or rested on the floor. Some, such as the guitar and harp, are plucked or strummed with the fingers or a pick. The orchestral strings (violin, viola, cello, and string bass) may also be plucked or even strummed, but they are usually bowed.

String players press the strings with their left hand to make different pitches. The right hand draws the bow across the strings or plucks the strings, creating sound. String players (including guitarists) must do two very different things—one with each hand—to make music.

During the eighteenth century, the string family became the foundation of the orchestra. A symphony orchestra today might have 20 to 30 violins (divided between "first" and "second"), 8 to 12 violas, 8 to 12 cellos, and 6 to 10 string basses.

Size

SAY A large drum makes a lower sound than a small drum. A large dog barks at a lower pitch than a small dog. You might also be able to see how size determines pitch in your own family: A man's voice will sound lower than your own voice or a woman's voice.

Tension

SAY Tension means tightness; the tighter you make the string or the drumhead, for instance, the higher the pitch.

ASK On some instruments, like the triangle, the player can't change the tension. How can the player get different pitches? (by using larger or smaller triangles)

Guide students in experimenting with tension using rubber bands.

ASK What happens to the sound of a rubber band when you pull it to make it longer—increase the tension? (The pitch gets higher.)

Is the sound loud? (no) **Is it attractive?** (no) **How can it be made louder and more attractive?** (Add resonance.)

Have students work in pairs to demonstrate tension, pitch, and resonance. One student stretches a rubber band across the open end of a glass, cup, or box. Another student plucks the rubber band.

SAY When resonance is added, it is easier to hear the sound of the rubber band.

ASK How can you raise the pitch? (Stretch the rubber band more.)

What happens to the sound when the rubber band is stretched? (It gets higher.) **When it is relaxed?** (It gets lower.)

Thickness

Experiment by playing individual strings of an Autoharp or a guitar.

ASK What happens when you pluck a string that is thicker? (It makes a lower sound.) **Thinner?** (It makes a higher sound.)

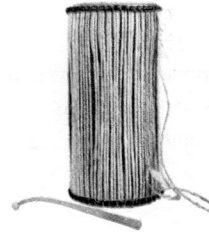

Donno [doh-noh] An hourglass-shaped talking drum played with an L-shaped stick. The *donno* is also known as a *dundun*. CD 23–21 p. 231

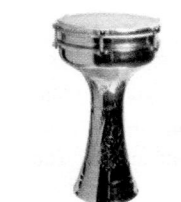

Dombak [DOM-bak] A Middle Eastern, goblet-shaped drum that produces a deep bass ("dom") and a high, sharp tone ("bak"). The *dombak* is also known as a *dombek*, *tombak*, and *darabukka*. It is sometimes spelled *doumbek*. CD 23–22 p. 308

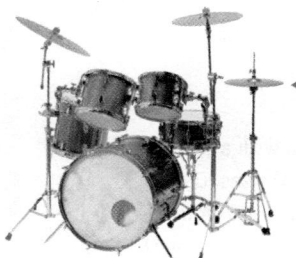

Drums (Trap Set) A drum set (or "kit") consisting of bass and snare drums, tom toms, hi-hat, and cymbals. The drum set is important in all forms of rock, pop, and jazz. CD 23–23 p. 256

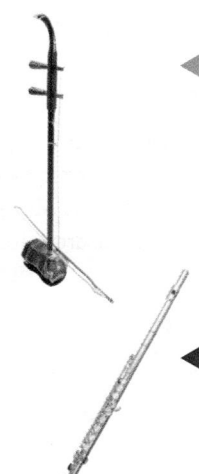

Erhu [EHR-hoo] A two-string Chinese instrument. It is played by a bow with the hand inserted between the two strings. The *erhu* sounds something like a violin and is an important instrument in modern Chinese orchestras. CD 23–24 p. 103

Flute A small metal instrument shaped like a pipe. The player holds the flute sideways and blows across an open mouthpiece. The flute's sound is pure and clear. CD 23–25 p. 355

514 Instrument Key: strings   percussion   woodwind   brass   keyboard

Footnotes

▶ **Playing Woodwind Instruments** All wind instruments make sound when the air inside them vibrates. The tubes and bells of wind instruments contain the vibrating air and give the sound resonance. Woodwind players make sounds by blowing across a hole (flute), by vibrating a reed (clarinet, saxophone), or by vibrating two reeds against each other (oboe, bassoon). The player changes the size of the instrument, making it longer or shorter by opening or closing holes along the instrument's length.

Flutes, oboes, and bassoons can be traced back to the 1400s. Composers since the 1700s have incorporated them in the orchestra because each woodwind is easily capable of playing melodies and because each brings a unique timbre to the orchestra. Clarinets are relatively new and were not added to the orchestra until the late eighteenth century (the time of Mozart and Haydn). Although the recorder is a woodwind instrument, it was replaced by the more popular and more powerful flute in the 1700s. The saxophone is used mostly in stage bands, jazz ensembles, and concert bands.

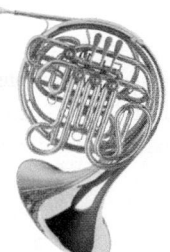

◀ **French Horn** A medium-sized instrument made of coiled brass tubing with a large bell at one end. The player holds the horn on his or her lap and keeps one hand inside the bell. The horn has a mellow, warm tone. CD 23–26 p. 356

◀ *Gankogui* [gahn-KO-gwee] A handmade, iron, double bell found in Ghana and other African countries. The bell is held in the "weak" hand and struck on the edge of the opening with the side of a stick. CD 23–27 p. 231

◀ **Guitar (Electric)** An electronic six-string instrument that is strummed or plucked with a pick. It requires an amplifier to be heard. The electric guitar plays chords and melodies, and is important in rock and pop music. CD 23–28 p. 374

◀ **Kendang** [KEN-dang] An Indonesian, barrel-shaped, double-headed drum. The *kendang*, sometimes spelled *kendhang*, is similar to the *mridangam* of southern India and plays a leading role in the gamelan orchestra. CD 23–29 p. 276

◀ **Koto** [KOH-toh] A Japanese instrument of 13 to 17, and sometimes up to 25 strings. It is known as the national instrument of Japan. The player kneels on the floor. Sound is produced by plucking the silk strings with a bamboo, bone, or ivory pick. CD 23–30 p. 302

Most instruments appear on the page indicated. In a few instances, the reference is to a family of instruments. **515**

▶ **Playing Brass Instruments** Brass players make the air inside the instrument vibrate by buzzing their lips against the mouthpiece. The lips must be tight and the air forced through them.

Brass players change pitches by tightening their lips even more or by pressing one valve or a combination of valves (except the trombone, although valve trombones can sometimes be found). Each time a valve is pressed, another length of tubing is added, changing the instrument's size by making it longer.

Although brass instruments existed from the 1400s, they are the last instrumental family to become full-fledged members of the orchestra. Prior to the early 1800s, brass instruments were used only for special effects or on special occasions. As the orchestra became larger, however, more brass instruments were included. Now, it is common to see two to four of each member of the family. Due to its mellow sound and ease of blending, the French horn, derived from the hunting horn, won acceptance before the others.

Playing Keyboard Instruments

The piano, organ, and synthesizer are keyboard instruments. All keyboard instruments are played the same way, but the sound is made in different ways.

SAY When the piano keys are pushed down, padded hammers strike the strings inside the instrument, in much the same way that the bars are struck on the glockenspiel and marimba.

Demonstrate, if possible, by exposing the inside mechanism of a piano, allowing students to see the hammers strike the strings.

SAY When electronic keyboard or electronic organ keys are pushed down, circuits in the machine are turned on in a way that makes sound. Both instruments are really synthesizers, since these circuits can be made to produce many different sounds, even some not available in nature.

Playing Longer and Shorter Sounds

ASK Which percussion instruments make sounds that last for a short time? (conga, *djembe, donno, doumbek, gankogui, kendhang, kpanlogo, mridangam,* snare drum, *tabla*)

How can you make the sound of a drum longer? (by hitting it repeatedly, as in a roll on the snare drum)

Experimenting with Sound

Some instruments can be played in more than one way. For instance, an Autoharp can be played by

- Strumming in the usual way, using a pick or, for comfort, a door stop.
- Striking the strings with a mallet.
- Scraping with a guitar pick or other object.
- Plucking individual strings.

ASK Can you use an instrument to make a sound like corn popping, or trees rustling, or a sound of your choice? (Allow students to experiment with different ways to play the instruments as well as different volumes.)

When students have discovered how to create sounds in new ways or to imitate another sound, encourage them to create sound effects to accompany a poem in the book.

For another sound experiment, have students try to make a bottle "play." They should use a bottle with a small neck and blow across the top toward the other side, trying to aim the air so that it is split in half.

ASK Are there any instruments in the Sound Bank that make sound the same way? (Yes; the modern flute is played that way.)

continued on page 516

ORCHESTRA INSTRUMENTS FEATURED IN THE SOUND BANK

Flute The modern flute had its origins in the pipe, used in ancient Greece and Rome. The tones produced by the flute are sweet and mellow and are often used by composers to carry the melody. Its range is from middle C to three octaves above. Agile and responsive, the flute can play difficult passages. It is especially effective as a solo instrument. Most symphony orchestras today have three flutes and sometimes as many as five.

Clarinet The clarinet, invented at the beginning of the eighteenth century, is related to the ancient single-reed *chalumeau*. The clarinet is one of the most important instruments of the orchestra. Today's symphony orchestra has two or three clarinets. The instrument's four distinct registers give it a great range of expression, making it particularly well suited to solo work.

Bassoon This versatile instrument was invented in the sixteenth century and used in the orchestra as early as 1674. It was not until the eighteenth century, however, that it became a regular member of the symphony orchestra. There are usually two bassoons in the modern-day symphony orchestra. Because of its great range, the bassoonist can play both bass and tenor parts. Its lower register is dark and rich, while the upper register has a penetrating and plaintive tone quality.

French Horn The French horn is descended from the hunting horn, which is coiled but, unlike the French horn, has no valves. It is believed that the French horn was introduced into the orchestra around 1664. The French horn blends well with other instruments. It is especially well suited to slow, sustained melodies, although it is capable of a variety of expressions. Today's symphony orchestra usually has four French horns.

Trumpet The modern-day trumpet dates back 5,000 years to China and India. The ancient Aztecs and Egyptians also used it, but it was not until 1815 that the piston valve system was added, making it possible for the player to play all notes in any key with ease. The trumpet has a clear, brilliant tone and is often used in loud fanfares or to add a martial flavor to the music. While it can also be played softly, most composers prefer its full, brilliant tones.

Trombone One of the oldest of musical instruments, the trombone is a direct descendant of the Moorish *sackbut*. It became a part of the symphony orchestra in the nineteenth century. The trombone has an extremely powerful tone, giving it a stately, often majestic quality. Today the instrument is popular in marching and military bands and in popular music and jazz. Today's symphony orchestra usually has three trombones.

Tuba The tuba first appeared in German military bands in the 1820s. Although it has the reputation of being rather weighty, it can be agile and graceful. It has occasionally been featured as a virtuoso soloist.

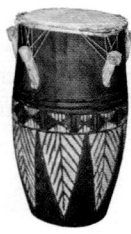

Kpanlogo [pahn-LOH-go] A barrel-shaped drum, carved from a single tree, found among the Ga people of Ghana, West Africa. The antelope-hide drum head is held tight by wooden stakes driven into the sides of the drum. CD 23–31 p. 277

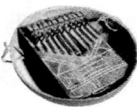

Mbira [mm-BEE-rah] An African finger xylophone of 5 to 30 or more thin metal, wood, or cane tongues attached to a sounding board. The tongues are plucked with the thumbs and fingers to produce a sound similar to that of a xylophone. CD 23–32 p. 27

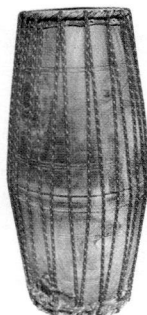

Mridangam [MREE-dan-gam] A double-headed, barrel-shaped drum that is made of wood with animal hide drawn across the top. The *mridangam* is the classic drum of southern India and is primarily used for accompanying the *vena*, flute, violin, or voice. CD 23–33 p. 305

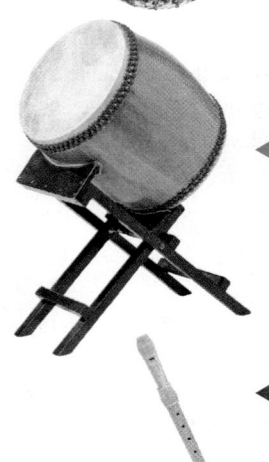

Odaiko [oh-DIE-ko] A large drum from Japan that is struck with large cylindrical sticks. One of several Japanese drums played in the tradition of *taiko*. CD 23–34 p. 277

Recorder A simple wind instrument made of wood or plastic with a "whistle" mouthpiece. Recorders come in many sizes and have a gentle, hollow sound. CD 23–35 p. 370

(516) Instrument Key: strings | percussion | woodwind | brass | keyboard

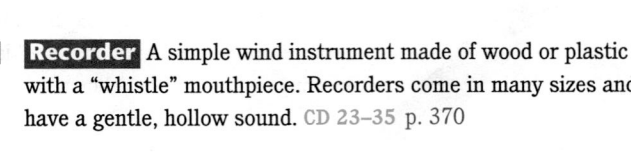

Footnotes

Band Instruments Featured in the Sound Bank

▶ **Saxophone** Saxophones were invented by Adolphe Sax, a Belgian, around 1840. Sax may have been experimenting with reed mouthpieces on brass instruments that are now obsolete. Saxophones were intended for military bands and became extremely popular in France. The instrument is popular now in concert bands, dance bands, and jazz ensembles. It has still to find a permanent place in the symphony orchestra, however, probably because it sometimes overpowers other instruments.

▶ **Drums (trap set)** This is an arrangement of drums played by one sitting player. The bass drum is played by one foot through a pedal arrangement, the hi-hat (a pair of cymbals) played by the other. There are also two to four drums—a snare drum and tom-tom(s). There might also be several suspended cymbals of different sizes. Trap sets are very popular in dance bands, jazz ensembles, and rock ensembles.

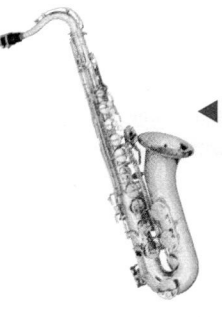 ◄ **Saxophone** The saxophone is a member of the woodwind family and is made of metal. Sound is made by blowing air into a mouthpiece with a reed and pressing keys to play different pitches. CD 23–36 p. 355

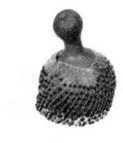 ◄ **Shekere** [SHEH-keh-reh] A large, calabash-gourd rattle with outside netting and shells. This West African rattle is either hit against the thigh or the hand. CD 23–37 p. 231

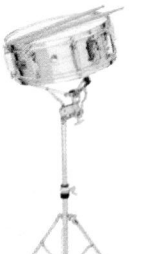 ◄ **Snare Drum** A small, cylinder-shaped drum with two heads. Snares are stretched across the bottom head to create a vibrating sound. A snare drum is played with drumsticks and plays non-pitched rhythm patterns. CD 23–38 p. 362

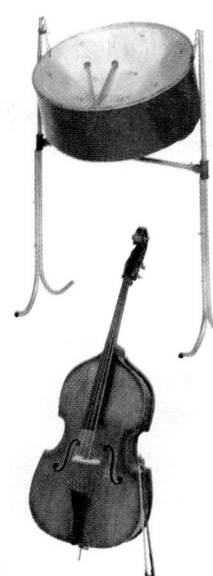 ◄ **Steel Drums** Steel drums are fashioned from oil drums and the top surfaces are shaped into facets that sound musical pitches when struck by mallets. Steel drums have a unique sound and are popular in the islands of the Caribbean. CD 23–39 p. 299

◄ **String Bass** This is the largest of the string instruments. It is often played standing. The bass strings produce low bass tones and are either bowed or plucked. It is played in orchestral, jazz, and pop music. CD 23–40 p. 355

Most instruments appear on the page indicated. In a few instances, the reference is to a family of instruments. **517**

Sound Bank

Band Instruments Featured in the Sound Bank

▶ **Guitar** Forerunners of the guitar are traceable to early Babylonian and Egyptian instruments. Early guitars had strings made of gut or silk. Today, the classical, or Spanish, guitar has nylon strings (the lower three wrapped with fine wire). The strings can also be metal. The six-string guitar probably originated in Italy before 1780 and spread through Europe by the early 1800s. When played softly, the guitar is gentle and sweet. When played more loudly, it sounds lush and full. The electric guitar is much louder than the acoustic guitar and can also make many special sounds. In the United States and in much of Europe, the electric guitar serves as the basic instrument in rock ensembles.

▶ **Bass Guitar** An electronic bass instrument that is capable of much more power than the string bass, the bass guitar is used to provide a bass line in jazz and rock music.

Timpani Introduced into Europe by the Turks in the fifteenth century, timpani were used at first with trumpets in cavalry bands. They began to be included in the orchestra during the latter part of the seventeenth century. Today's symphony orchestra usually has four timpani. The player must have an unusually good sense of pitch, since he or she is required to make changes in tuning during the course of a concert—frequently when the orchestra is playing in a different key!

Snare Drum The snare drum has had a long military history. It is now an indispensable member of the percussion section of the band and orchestra. The player can produce an explosive sound by striking the center of the head; a light, clicking sound by striking the rim; or an air of mystery and suspense by using the most difficult stroke—the roll. The instrument is ideal for bringing clarity to rhythm patterns, no matter how fast or intricate they may be.

Xylophone The xylophone can be traced back to primitive peoples in Asia, Africa, and America. Its oldest forms were a few slabs of wood or fragments of stone of different sizes, laid on ropes of straw and tuned to make a scale. In Europe, the xylophone was in use in the sixteenth century, mainly for special effects or novelty. It was not until the second half of the nineteenth century that improvements in the tone of the instrument led to its place as a bonafide member of the percussion section of most symphony orchestras.

Violin The violin as we know it today was perfected more than 300 years ago. The finest instruments were made in the sixteenth, seventeenth, and early eighteenth centuries in Italy by the Amati, Stradivari, and Guarneri families. The violin has the beauty and warmth of the human voice, but at the same time it is capable of expressing a great range of moods and effects, which makes it an ideal solo instrument.

Cello The cello is correctly named *violoncello*, an Italian word meaning "little big-viol." It is a little more than twice as long and twice as wide as the violin and has a range of almost four octaves. In the orchestra, the cello usually plays the bass line of music. However, it is often called upon to play in the upper registers. The cello's rich, melancholy voice is an indispensable part of any symphony orchestra.

String Bass The bass is known by several different names—string bass, bass viol, double bass (because it "doubles" the bass line played by the cello). The bass is the lowest-pitched instrument of the orchestral string section. It forms a foundation for the music of the orchestra and is used only occasionally for solo work. It can be useful for suggesting a mood or for introducing an effect. It is an important member of jazz ensembles as well as orchestra ensembles.

continued on page 518

Sound Bank

INSTRUMENTS FEATURED IN THE RECORDINGS

Many of the listening selections, songs, and illustrations in this book may be used to supplement the lessons on timbre. See the specific references below for selected instruments in the Sound Bank.

- ACCORDION: *Sellenger's Round* **CD 3-14**
  Illustration: p. 402

- BANDURA: *Shchedryk* **CD 6-20**
  Illustration: p. 103

- BASS GUITAR: "Birthday" **CD 6-1**
  Illustration: p. 92

- BASSOON: *Wedding Day at Troldhaugen* **CD 1-5**
  Illustration: p. 354

- BODHRAN: *Paddy Whack* **CD 16-16**
  Illustration: p. 276

- CELLO: "*Shalom aleichiem*" **CD 20-7**
  Illustration: p. 355

- CLARINET: "Tom Dooley" **CD 19-7**
  Illustration: p. 355

- CONGA: *Ti mon bo* **CD 17-3**
  Illustration: p. 356

- DIDGERIDOO: *Brolga* **CD 2-17**
  Illustration: p. 271

- DJEMBE: "*Ise oluwa*" **CD 12-3**
  Illustration: p. 231

- DONNO: "*Kelo aba w'ye*" **CD 14-20**
  Illustration: p. 231

- DOMBAK: *Yemeni Baglamis Telli Basina* **CD 15-36**
  Illustration: p. 308

- DRUMS: *Lost River* **CD 14-15**
  Illustration: p. 283

- ERHU: *The Moon Mirrored in the Pool* **CD 6-19**
  Illustration: p. 103

- FLUTE: "Peace Like a River" **CD 10-26**
  Illustration: p. 355

- FRENCH HORN: *The Blue Danube* **CD 10-29**
  Illustration: p. 356

- GANKOGUI: "Take Time in Life" **CD 14-22**
  Illustration: p. 231

- GUITAR: "Birthday" **CD 6-1**
  Illustration: p. 151

- KENDANG: *Kebjar teruna* **CD 19-20** (The kendang is an Indonesian drum found in gamelan orchestras. It is not prominent in the recording.)
  Illustration: p. 276

- KOTO: "*Asadoya*" **CD 15-17**
  Illustration: p. 515

- KPANLOGO: *Kpanlogo for 2* **CD 16-7**
  Illustration: p. 277

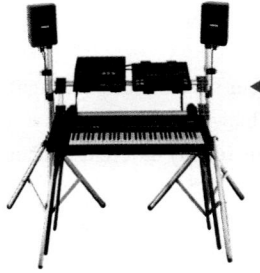

Synthesizer An electronic keyboard instrument found in many styles of rock and pop music. Synthesizers create sounds through electronic synthesis and can produce many instrument sounds. CD 23–41 p. 356

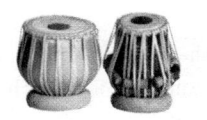

Tabla [TAH-blah] Drums used in the classical music of northern India, similar to the timpani. *Tablas* produce pitched and nonpitched sounds by being played on different parts of the drumhead. CD 23–42 p. 277

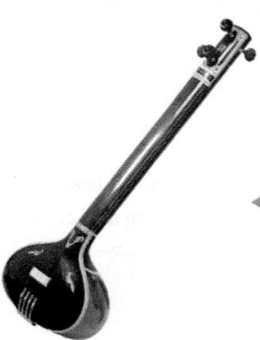

Tamboura [TAM-boo-rah] A four-string drone instrument popular in India. The *tamboura* strings are tuned to the intervals of an octave and a fifth, and are played in a continuous drone style. CD 23–43 p. 304

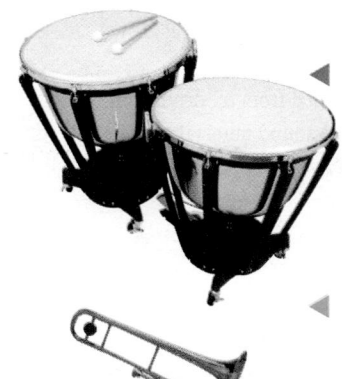

Timpani Large, pot-shaped drums, also called kettledrums. The timpani can be tuned to specific pitches. Several timpani are used to play melody patterns. CD 23–44 p. 356

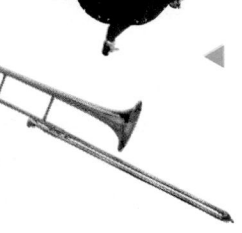

Trombone A large brass instrument with a bell at one end of the tubing. Pitch is changed by moving a long slide on the side of the instrument. The trombone is found in bands, orchestras, and jazz ensembles. CD 23–45 p. 356

(518) **Instrument Key:** strings percussion woodwind brass keyboard

Footnotes

 Active Listening At the same time that they are listening to the recorded Sound Bank or supplementary examples, students should also look at the illustration of the instrument either in the Sound Bank or on the cited page. This will help them to remember the sound of the instrument when they see it, and vice versa. Reinforcing this association will help students' future listening.

Begin with two examples. Test students' ability to differentiate the instruments. Use dissimilar sounds at first, then gradually make them more similar.

When several instruments are learned in this way, divide the class into teams and have students challenge each other. Keep score of correct answers.

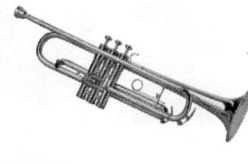

Trumpet A small brass instrument with a bell (a flared opening) at one end of its coiled tubing. The player presses valves to change pitch. The sound of the trumpet is bold and bright. CD 23–46 p. 356

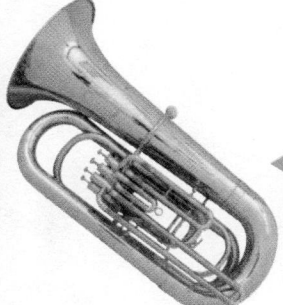

Tuba The largest brass instrument, with a large bell that points upward. The player changes the pitch by pressing valves. The tuba's sound is very low, deep, and sturdy. CD 23–47 p. 362

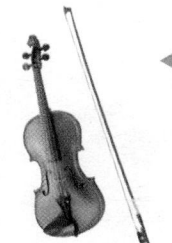

Violin The smallest string instrument in a Western orchestra. It is held under the player's chin and is bowed or plucked. The violin's tone can be brilliant, warm, harsh, or mellow. CD 23–48 p. 355

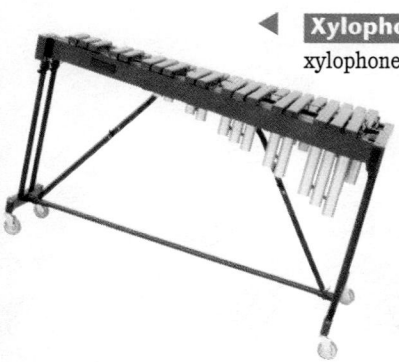

Xylophone A keyboard of wooden bars played with mallets. The xylophone has a bright, brittle sound. CD 23–49 p. 356

Most instruments appear on the page indicated. In a few instances, the reference is to a family of instruments.

- MBIRA: *Chigamba* **CD 2-21**
  Illustration: p. 27
- MRIDANGAM: *Kriti: gan ganapate*
  Illustration: p. 516
- ODAIKO DRUM: *Lion* **CD 15-21**
  Illustration: p. 277
- RECORDER: "Scarborough Fair" **CD 6-4**
  Illustration: p. 370
- SAXOPHONE: "Hey, Ho! Nobody Home" **CD 2-22**
  Illustration: p. 355
- SHEKERE: "By The Waters of Babylon" **CD 16-1**
  Illustration: p. 231
- SNARE DRUM: *Fanfare for Freedom* **CD 8-4**
  Illustration: p. 362
- STEEL DRUMS: *Gidden riddum* **CD 15-9**
  Illustration: p. 310
- STRING BASS: *Orchestral Suite No. 2* **CD 10-28**
  Illustration: p. 355
- SYNTHESIZER: *This Is Your Night* (Dance Mix) **CD 18-21**
  Illustration: p. 356
- TABLA: *Máru-bihág* **CD 15-22**
  Illustration: p. 277
- TAMBOURA: *Máru-bihág* **CD 15-22**
  Illustration: p. 518
- TIMPANI: *Pictures at an Exhibition,* "The Great Gate of Kiev" **CD 8-27**
  Illustration: p. 356
- TROMBONE: *Finlandia* **CD 5-3**
  Illustration: p. 356
- TRUMPET: *Prince of Denmark's March* **CD 3-30**
  Illustration: p. 356
- TUBA: *Galliard battaglia* **CD 18-11**
  Illustration: p. 362
- VIOLIN: *The Four Seasons, Concerto No. 2,* "Summer," Movement 3 **CD 6-18**
  Illustration: p. 355
- XYLOPHONE: *Evening Chaconne* **CD 13-10**
  Illustration: p. 356

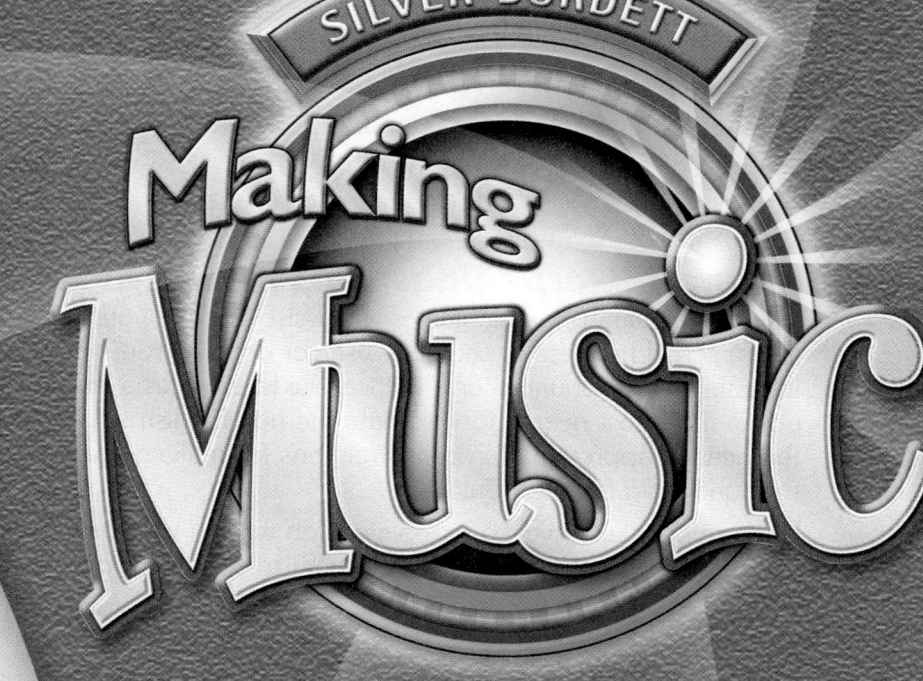

CONTENTS

Teacher Resources

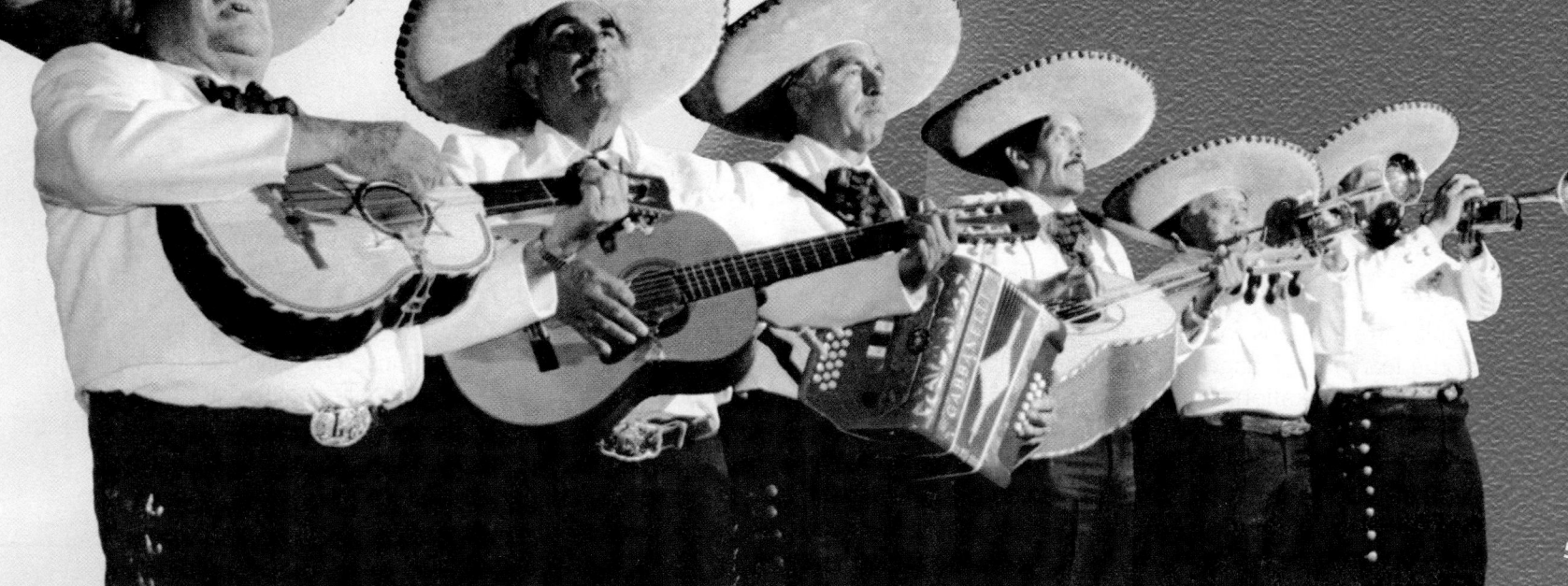

Pronunciation Practice

Phonetic Respellings for Pronunciation of Non-English Songs

These simplified phonetic guides will assist you and your students in pronouncing non-English words. All pronunciation phonetics are matched to those of the native singer on the Pronunciation Practice Track and have been verified by the CP Language Institute. The Pronunciation Practice Guide provides a phonetic respelling in syllabic form, based on sounds in the English language that most nearly approximate the non-English sounds. When words do not have an English equivalent, we have provided the nearest approximation or instructions for making the sound. The Key to Pronunciation below refers to the system used in the Pronunciation Practice Guides.

Where possible, vowel sounds have been written with beautiful vocal tones in mind. For example, it is difficult to sing a sustained long *i* sound. Instead students are taught to sustain an *ah* sound, adding a small touch of *ee* to the release of the vowel.

Key to Pronunciation

ah	as in f<u>a</u>ther		(m)	French nasal <u>m</u>, not articulated as a distinct letter but as an open nasal sound
ah_ee	as in l<u>i</u>ght (diphthong; a long *ah* sound with a hint of *ee* at close)		n	as in <u>n</u>ote
aw	as in <u>aw</u>e		(n)	French nasal <u>n</u>, not articulated as a distinct letter, but as an open nasal sound.
eh_ee	as in d<u>ay</u> (diphthong; a long *eh* sound with a hint of *ee* at close)		(ng)	as in sa<u>ng</u> (sometimes sounded as a prolonged nasal tone)
b	as in <u>b</u>utton		oh	as in t<u>o</u>ne
ch	as in <u>ch</u>urch		oo	as in sp<u>oo</u>n
d	as in <u>d</u>ad		ow	as in p<u>ow</u>der
dj	as in ju<u>dg</u>e		p	as in <u>p</u>at
ee	as in s<u>ee</u>d		r	as in <u>r</u>an
eh	as in l<u>e</u>t		(r)	as in tu<u>r</u>n (combined with another vowel sound in German)
ew	used for French <u>u</u> (pronounce a bright *ee* and round the lips as if to whistle)		rr	rolled <u>r</u>
f	as in <u>f</u>ace		rrrr	extended trilled <u>r</u>
g	as in <u>g</u>oat		s	as in <u>s</u>ong
h	as in <u>h</u>at		t	as in <u>t</u>ell
hkh	guttural, aspirant <u>h</u> of German, Hebrew <u>ch</u>, and Spanish <u>j</u>		th	as in <u>th</u>at
ih	as in f<u>i</u>t		thh	as in fea<u>th</u>er
I	as in l<u>i</u>ght (a harsh *i* sound, where possible an *ah_ee* has been suggested for singing the I sound)		uh	as in <u>u</u>p
			v	as in <u>v</u>an
k	as in <u>k</u>ite		w	as in <u>w</u>ay
l	as in <u>l</u>et		wh	as in <u>wh</u>at
ll	prolonged <u>l</u> sound		y	as in <u>y</u>es (not a vowel sound)
m	as in <u>m</u>an		z	as in <u>z</u>one
			zh	as in a<u>z</u>ure

English Translations by CP Language Institute

The English translations for these songs were provided by CP Language Institute. For over two decades, the Institute has been one of the leading language consultants for clients in the New York City area and in other locations. The Institute specializes in translation, interpretation, typesetting, graphic design, language instruction, and voice overs. Its highly qualified staff of native translators guided and monitored the pronunciation and recording of each Pronunciation Track for Silver Burdett MAKING MUSIC.

and Translations

Bắt kim thang (Setting Up the Golden Ladder), p. 13 CD 1-16

Traditional Song from Vietnam

Pronunciation Practice

Verse 1

Phrase 1. *Bắt kim thang cà lang bí rợ.*
buhk'n kihm tayng kah layng bee ruhr.

2. *Cột qua kèo kèo qua cột.*
koht'n kwah kay‿oh kay‿oh kwah koht'n.

3. *Chú bán dầu qua cầu mà té.*
choo bayn yee‿oh kwah kah‿oh mah teh‿ehr.

4. *Chú bán ếch ở lại làm chi.*
choo bayn eht'n ehr II‿ee lehm chee.

5. *Con le le đánh trống thổi kèn.*
kohn leh‿eer leh‿eer duhn trawng thoh-ee kehn.

6. *Con bìm bịp thổi*
kohn bihm bihp'm thoh‿ee

7. *tò tí te tò te.*
taw tee teh‿ehr taw teh‿ehr.

Translation

Verse 1

Set up a ladder—a golden ladder.
Jump to the right, jump to the left.
Hey, look at the oil vendor!
He just fell from the bridge!
Oh, the frog vendor is afraid to cross it.
The *le le* bird is playing his drum and trumpet.
The *bim bip* bird is singing the notes "to ti te."

Magnolia, p. 16 CD 1-25

Words and Music by Tish Hinojosa

Pronunciation Practice

Verse 1

Phrase 1. *Tem-pra-no‿en la ma-ña-na‿un pa-ja-ri-to can-ta,*
tehm-prah-noh‿ehn lah mah-nyah-nah‿oon pah-hah-ree-toh kahn-tah,

2. *des-pier-ta la mag-no-li-a.*
dehs-pee‿ehrr-tah lah mahg-noh-lee-ah.

3. *Su can-ción me ha-bla,*
soo kahn-see‿ohn meh ah-blah,

4. *dul-ce y tan cla-ra,*
dool-seh ee tahn klah-rrah,

5. *ba-jo la mag-no-li-a.*
bah-hoh lah mahg-noh-lee-ah.

6. *Flor blan-ca‿y bo-ni-ta*
flohr blahn-kah‿ee boh-nee-tah

7. *ho-jas bien bri-lla-das,*
oh-hahs bee‿ehn bree-yah-dahs,

8. *cre-cen en mag-no-li-a.*
kreh-sehn ehn mahg-noh-lee-ah.

9. *En pri-ma-ve-ra so-la,*
ehn prree-mah-veh-rrah soh-lah,

10. *yo sue-ño por ho-ras,*
yoh soo‿weh-nyoh pohr oh-rrahs,

11. *ba-jo la mag-no-li-a.*
bah-hoh lah mahg-noh-lee-ah.

12. *Hmm y mi-ro‿el cie-la‿a-llá.*
hmm ee mee-roh‿ehl see‿eh-lah‿ah-yah.

13. *Hmm y pien-so to-do‿a-mar.*
hmm ee pee‿ehn-soh toh-doh‿ah-mahr.

14. *El vien-to bai-la mag-no-li-a por mí.*
ehl vee‿ehn-toh bah‿ee-lah mahg-noh-lee-ah pohrr mee.

Translation

Verse 1   Early in the morning there is a bird singing,
a bird singing. The magnolia tree wakes up.
Its song speaks to me so clearly and sweetly
Under the magnolia tree. White beautiful flowers
and shiny leaves grow on the magnolia tree.
Only in spring, I dream for hours
under the magnolia tree.
Hmm, and I look at the sky above.
Hmm, and I think I love everything,
the wind makes the magnolia dance for me.

Magnolia, p. 16 CD 1-25 *(continued)*
Words and Music by Tish Hinojosa

Pronunciation Practice

Verse 2

Phrase

1. *Ve-ra-no se a-ca-ba*
   veh-rah-noh seh ah-kah-bah

2. *tam-bién el jue-go pa-ra,*
   tahm-bee͜ehn ehl wheh-goh pah-rrah,

3. *ba-jo la mag-no-li-a.*
   bah-hoh lah mahg-noh-lee-ah.

4. *Ho-jas caen de͜e-to-ño,*
   oh-hahs kahn deh͜eh-toh-nyoh,

5. *a-nun-cian-do͜in-vier-no,*
   ah-noon-see͜ahn-doh͜een-vee͜ehrr-noh,

6. *ba-jo la mag-no-li-a.*
   bah-hoh lah mahg-noh-lee-ah.

7. *Mi͜her-ma-ni-ta͜y yo con*
   mee͜ehrr-mah-nee-tah͜ee yoh kohn

8. *té y de-sa-yu-no,*
   teh ee deh-sah-yoo-noh,

9. *ba-jo la mag-no-li-a.*
   bah-hoh lah mahg-noh-lee-ah.

10. *Pre-ten-dien-do ho-jas,*
    preh-tehn-dee͜ehn-doh oh-yahs,

11. *ta-cos bien sa-bro-sos,*
    tah-kohs bee͜ehn sah-brroh-sohs,

12. *ba-jo la mag-no-li-a.*
    bah-hoh lah mahg-noh-lee-ah.

13. *Hmm vie-nen a vi-si-tar.*
    hmm vee͜eh-nehn ah vee-see-tahr.

14. *Hmm John, Rin-go, George, y Paul.*
    hmm Jahn, Reen-goh, Jorj, ee Pahl.

15. *Ri-en-do ve-mos mag-no-li-a bai-lar.*
    ree-ehn-doh veh-mohs mahg-noh-lee-ah
    bah͜ee-lahr.

Translation

Verse 2 The summer comes to an end,
and the games stop too, under the magnolia.
Autumn leaves start falling,
announcing the coming winter under the magnolia
   tree.
my sister and I have tea and breakfast
under the magnolia tree.
Full of leaves, very tasty tacos*
under the magnolia.
Hmm, here they come to visit
John, Ringo, George, and Paul,
Laughing we see the magnolia dance.

Tacos—fried tortilla stuffed with cheese, pork,
chicken, etc.

El condor pasa, p. 46 CD 3-19
Music by Daniel Almonica Robles

Pronunciation Practice

Verse 1

Phrase 1. *El a-mor co-mo_un con-dor ba-ja-rá,*
ehl ah-mohr koh-moh_oon kohn-dohr
bah-hah-rah,

2. *mi co-ra-zón,*
mee koh-rah-sohn,

3. *gol-pea-rá,*
gohl-pee_yah-rah,

4. *des-pués se_i-rá.*
dehs-pwehs seh_ee-rah.

5. *La lu-na_en el de-sier-to bri-lla-rá.*
lah loo-nah_ehn ehl deh-syehr-toh
bree-yah-rah.

6. *Tú ven-drás.*
too vehn-drahs.

7. *So-la-men-te_un be-so,*
soh-lah-mehn-teh_oon beh-soh,

8. *me de-ja-rás.*
meh deh-hah-rahs.

9. *¿Quién sa-be si ma-ña-na vol-ve-rás,*
kee_ihn sah-beh see mah-nyah-nah
vohl-veh-rahs,

10. *qué ha-rás,*
keh hah-rahs,

11. *no pen-sa-rás?*
noh pehn-sah-rahs?

12. *Yo sé que nun-ca vol-ve-rás,*
yoh seh keh noon-kah vohl-veh-rahs,

13. *más pien-so que*
mahs pee_yehn-soh keh

14. *no vi-vi-ré*
noh bee-bee-ray

15. *co-mo po-dré.*
koh-moh poh-dreh.

Translation

Love like a condor will come down;
My heart will hit, then it will leave, m m m m.
The moon in the desert will shine;
You will come, only a kiss you will leave me, m m m m.

La paloma se fué (The Dove That Flew Away), p. 51 CD 3-25, 26

Folk Song from Puerto Rico

Pronunciation Practice

Phrase 1. *¿Se-ño-res no han vis-to*
seh-nyoh-rehs noh_ahn vee-stoh

2. *la pa-lo-ma que vo-ló del pa-lo-mar?*
lah pah-loh-mah keh voh-loh dehl
pah-loh-mahrr?

3. *¿Se-ño-res no han vis-to*
seh-nyoh-rehs noh_ahn vee-stoh

4. *la pa-lo-ma que vo-ló del pa-lo-mar?*
lah pah-loh-mah keh voh-loh dehl
pah-loh-mahrr?

5. *Se fué la pa-lo-ma, se fué la pa-lo-ma,*
seh fweh lah pah-loh-mah, seh fweh lah
pah-loh-mah,

6. *se fué pa-ra no vol-ver.*
seh fweh pah-rah noh vohl-vehrr.

7. *Se fué la pa-lo-ma, se fué la pa-lo-ma,*
seh fweh lah pah-loh-mah, seh fweh lah
pah-loh-mah,

8. *se fué pa-ra no vol-ver.*
seh fweh pah-rah noh vohl-vehrr.

Translation

Gentlemen, have you not seen the dove that flew from the birdhouse?
Gentlemen, have you not seen the dove that flew from the birdhouse?
The dove left, the dove left, it left never to return,
The dove left, the dove left, it left never to return.

Adiós, amigos (Goodbye, My Friends), p. 57 CD 4-4

Folk Song from New Mexico

Pronunciation Practice

Verse 1

Phrase 1. *A-diós a-mi-gos,*
ah-dee_ohs ah-mee-gohs,

2. *que duer-man muy bien,*
keh dwehrr-mahn moo_ee bee_ehn,

3. *Que vie-nen los án-ge-les*
keh vee_eh-nehn lohs ahn-heh-lehs

4. *pa-ra guar-dar.*
pah-rrah gwahrr-dahrr.

5. *A-diós, a-diós,*
ah-dee_ohs, ah-dee_ohs,

6. *a-diós, a-diós.*
ah-dee_ohs, ah-dee_ohs.

Translation

Verse 1 Goodbye, friends, sleep very well.
The angels are coming to keep guard.
Goodbye, Goodbye, Goodbye.

La mariposa (The Butterfly), p. 58 CD 4-11
Folk Song from Bolivia

Pronunciation Practice

Chorus

Phrase 1. *La la la la lai la lai la lai la lai lai lai lai lai,*
lah lah lah lah lah_ee lah lah_ee lah lah_ee lah
lah_ee lah_ee lah_ee lah_ee lah_ee,

2. *La la la la lai la lai la lai la lai la la la la la
lai lai lai.*
lah lah lah lah lah_ee lah lah_ee lah lah_ee lah
lah_ee lah lah lah lah lah lah_ee lah_ee
lah_ee.

Verse 1

Phrase 1. *Al son de las ma-tra-cas*
ahl sohn deh lahs mah-trah-kahs

2. *to-dos can-tan y bai-lan*
toh-thos kahn-tahn ee bah_ee-lahn

3. *La mo-re-na-da.*
lah moh-reh-nah-dah.

4. *Con las pal-mas,*
kohn lahs pahl-mahs,

5. *Con los ta-cos.*
kohn lohs tah-kohs.

6. *¡Vi-va la fies-ta!*
vee-vah lah fyehs-tah!

Translation

Everybody sings and dances the morenada to the beat of
the rattles.

With your hands, with your heels. Hurray for the party!

Hurray for the party! Hurray for the party!

Yü guang guang (Moonlight Lullaby), p. 60 CD 4-18
Folk Song from Hong Kong

Pronunciation Practice

Phrase 1. *Yü gwahng gwahng*
yew gwahng gwahng

2. *tsee-oo day-ee tong*
tsee-oo day-ee tahng

3. *Hah tzai nay gwai gwai*
hah tzah_ee neh gwah_ee gwah_ee

4. *fuhn lah-oo tchong*
fuhn lah-oo tchahng

5. *teeng dsee-yoo ah mah*
tehng tsee-yoo ah mah

6. *yee_oo gong tsah(p) yong law*
yee_oo gahng tsah pyoong law

7. *ah yeh tai ngow*
ah yeh tah_een (n)yow

8. *koy tsü(ng) sahn gong.*
kuh_ee tsuh(ng) sahn gahng.

Translation

The moonlight is shining on the earth;

You are a nice baby—go to sleep.

Tomorrow your mom will plant young rice seedlings;

Your grandfather will watch the cattle going up the hill.

Hava nashira (Sing and Be Joyful), p. 82 CD 5-18

Folk Song from Israel

Pronunciation Practice

Phrase 1. *Ha-va na-shir-a, shir hal-le-lu-jah.*
         hah-vah nah-shee-rah, sheer hah-leh-loo-yah.

       2. *Ha-va na-shir-a, shir hal-le-lu-jah.*
         hah-vah nah-shee-rah, sheer hah-leh-loo-yah.

       3. *Ha-va na-shir-a, shir hal-le-lu-jah.*
         hah-vah nah-shee-rah, sheer hah-leh-loo-yah.

Translation

Now come with singing, sing "Hallelujah!"

Dona nobis pacem, p. 125 CD 7-19

Traditional Canon

Pronunciation Practice

Phrase 1. *Do-na no-bis pa-cem, pa-cem,*
         doh-nah noh-bees pah-chehm, pah-chehm,

       2. *Do-na no-bis pa-cem.*
         doh-nah noh-bees pah-chehm.

       3. *Do-na no-bis pa-cem,*
         doh-nah noh-bees pah-chehm,

       4. *Do-na no-bis pa-cem.*
         doh-nah noh-bees pah-chehm.

       5. *Do-na no-bis pa-cem,*
         doh-nah noh-bees pah-chehm,

       6. *Do-na no-bis pa-cem.*
         doh-nah noh-bees pah-chehm.

Translation

Give us peace, peace
Give us peace.
Give us peace,
Give us peace.
Give us peace,
Give us peace.

Lo yisa (Vine and Fig Tree), p. 130 CD 7-26

Hebrew Words from the Book of Isaiah
Music by Shalom Altman

Pronunciation Practice

Verse 1

Phrase 1. *Lo yi-sa goy el goy che-rev,*
         loh yee-sah goy ehl goy hkheh-rehv,

       2. *Lo yil-m'-du od mil-cha-ma.*
         loh yihl-muh-doo ohd mihl-hkhah-mah.

       3. *Lo yi-sa goy el goy che-rev,*
         loh yee-sah goy ehl goy hkheh-rehv,

       4. *Lo yil-m'-du od mil-cha-ma.*
         loh yihl-muh-doo ohd mihl-hkhah-mah.

       5. *Lo yi-sa goy el goy che-rev,*
         loh yee-sah goy ehl goy hkheh-rehv,

       6. *Lo yil-m'-du od mil-cha-ma.*
         loh yihl-muh-doo ohd mihl-hkhah-mah.

Translation

Verse 1 Nation shall not lift up sword against nation,
         neither shall they learn war any more.

El payo (The Cowpoke), p. 145 CD 8-11

Folk Song from Mexico

Pronunciation Practice

Verse 1

Phrase 1. *Es-ta-bá＿un pa-yo sen-ta-do.*
ehs-tah-bah＿oon pah-yoh sehn-tah-thoh.

2. *En tran-cas de＿un co-rral;*
ehn trahn-kahs deh＿oon koh-rahl;

3. *Y＿el ma-yor-do-mo le di-jo,*
ee＿yehl mah-yohr-doh-moh leh dee-hoh,

4. *"No es-tés tris-te, Ni-co-lás."*
"noh ehs-tehs trees-teh, nee-koh-lahs."

5. *"Si quie-res que no＿es-té tris-te*
"see kee＿eh-rehs keh noh＿ehs-teh trees-teh

6. *Lo que pi-da me＿has de dar."*
loh keh pee-tha meh＿ahs deh dahr."

7. *Y＿el ma-yor-do-mo le di-jo,*
ee＿yehl mah-yohr-doh-moh leh dee-hoh,

8. *"Ve pi-dien-do, Ni-co-lás."*
"veh pee-dee＿ehn-do, nee-koh-lahs."

Verse 2

Phrase 1. *"Necesito treinta pesos,*
"neh-seh-see-toh treh＿een-tah peh-sohs,

2. *Una cuera y un gabán."*
oon-ah koo＿eh-rah ee＿oon gah-bahn."

3. *Y＿el mayordomo le dijo,*
ee＿yehl mah-yohr-doh-moh leh dee-hoh,

4. *"No＿hay dinero, Ni-co-lás."*
"noh＿ah＿ee dee-neh-roh, nee-koh-lahs."

5. *"Ne-ce-si-to trein-ta pesos*
"neh-seh-see-toh treh＿een-tah peh-sohs

6. *Pa-ra po-der-me ca-sar."*
pah-rah poh-dehrr-meh kah-sahr."

7. *Y＿el ma-yor-do-mo le di-jo,*
ee＿yehl mah-yohr-doh-moh leh dee-hoh,

8. *"Ni＿un real ten-go, Ni-co-lás."*
"nee＿oon reh＿ahl tehn-goh, nee-koh-las."

Translation

Verse 1 A churlish fellow was sitting
on the gate posts of a corral,
and the foreman told him,
"Don't be sad, Nicholas."
"If you wish that I not be sad
whatever I may ask for, you must give me."
And the foreman told him,
"Start asking, Nicholas."

Verse 2 "I need thirty pesos,
A leather jacket, and an overcoat."
And the foreman told him,
"There is no money, Nicholas."
"I need thirty pesos
So that I can marry."
And the foreman told him,
"I don't have even a dime, Nicholas."

Hava nagila, p. 153 CD 8-25

Jewish Folk Song

Pronunciation Practice

Phrase
1. *Ha-va na-gi-la, ha-va na-gi-la,*
   hah-vah nah-gee-lah, hah-vah nah-gee-lah,

2. *ha-va na-gi-la, v'-nis-m'-cha.*
   hah-vah nah-gee-lah, veh-nees-meh-hkhah.

3. *Ha-va n'-ra-n'-na, ha-va n'-ra-n'-na,*
   hah-vah neh-rrah-neh-nah, hah-vah neh-rrah-neh-nah,

4. *ha-va n'-ra-n'-na, v'-nis-m'-cha.*
   hah-vah neh-rrah-neh-nah, veh-nees-meh-hkhah.

5. *U-ru, u-ru a-chim,*
   oo-roo, oo-roo ah-hkheem,

6. *u-ru a-chim b'-lev sa-me-ach, u-ru a-chim b'lev sa-me-ach,*
   oo-roo ah-hkheem beh-lehv sah-meh-ahkh,
   oo-roo ah-hkheem beh-lehv sah-meh-ahkh,

7. *u-ru a-chim b'-lev sa-me-ach, u-ru a-chim b'lev sa-me-ach,*
   oo-roo ah-hkheem beh-lehv sah-meh-ahkh,
   oo-roo ah-hkheem beh-lehv sah-meh-ahkh,

8. *u-ru a-chim, u-ru a-chim b'lev sa-me-ach.*
   oo-roo ah-hkheem, oo-roo ah-hkheem beh-lehv sah-meh-ahkh.

Translation

Come, let us sing and be happy. Wake up, brothers, with a happy heart.

O lê lê O Bahía (O Le O La), p. 165 CD 9-17

Folk Song from Brazil

Pronunciation Practice

Phrase
1. *Da Ba-hí-a me man-da-ram*
   dah bah-ee-ah mee mahn-dah-rahm

2. *O lê lê O Ba-hí-a*
   oh leh leh oh bah-ee-ah

3. *Um ces-ti-nho de ca-já,*
   oom sehs-tchee-nyoh djeh kah-zhah,

4. *O lê lê O Ba-hí-a*
   oh leh leh oh bah-ee-ah

5. *E man-da-ram per-gun-tar*
   ee mahn-dah-rahm pehr-goon-tahr

6. *O lê lê O Ba-hí-a,*
   oh leh leh oh bah-ee-ah,

7. *Se eu que-ri-a me ca-sar.*
   see oh kee_eh-ree-ah mee kah-sahr.

8. *O lê lê O Ba-hí-a,*
   oh leh leh oh bah-ee-ah,

9. *O le o la, O lê lê O Ba-hí-a,*
   oh leh oh lah, oh leh leh oh bah-ee-ah,

10. *O le o la, O lê lê O Ba-hí-a.*
    oh leh oh lah, oh leh leh oh bah-ee-ah.

Translation

It was sent to me from Bahia,
A basket full of cajás,*
And they asked me
If I wanted to get married.

*Cajá—The golden-yellow, plumlike fruit of the *cajàzeiro*. It has a sourish aromatic flavor, and a faint smell of turpentine.

Así es mi tierra (This Is My Land), p. 172 CD 9-33

Words and Music Ignacio Fernandez Esperón

Pronunciation Practice

Phrase
1. *A-sí es mi tie-rra,*
   ah-see ehs mee tyeh-rrah,

2. *mo-re-ni-ta y lu-mi-no-sa;*
   moh-reh-nee-tah ee loo-mee-noh-sah;

3. *A-sí es mi tie-rra,*
   ah-see ehs mee tyeh-rrah,

4. *tie-ne el al-ma he-cha de a-mor.*
   tyeh-nehl ahl-mah eh-chah deh ah-mohr.

5. *A-sí es mi tie-rra,*
   ah-see ehs mee tyeh-rrah,

6. *a-bun-dan-te y ge-ne-ro-sa;*
   ah-boon-dahn-teh heh-neh-roh-sah;

7. *¡Ay, tie-rra mí-a*
   ah ee, tyeh-rrah mee-ah

8. *co-mo es gra-to tu ca-lor!*
   koh-moh ehs grah-toh too kah-lohr!

9. *Sus al-bo-ra-das*
   suhs ahl-bor-rah-thahs

10. *tan lle-ni-tas, de a-le-grí-a.*
    thahn yeh-nee-tahs, deh ah-leh-gree-ah.

11. *Sus se-re-na-tas*
    suhs seh-reh-nah-tahs

12. *tan pro-pi-ci as al a-mor.*
    thahn proh-pee-cee ahs ahl ah-mohr.

13. *A-sí es mi tie-rra,*
    ah-see ehs mee tyeh-rrah,

14. *flor de la me-lan-co-lí-a.*
    flohr deh lah meh-lahn-koh-lee-ah.

15. *¡Ay, tie-rra mí-a*
    ah ee, tyeh-rrah mee-ah

16. *co-mo es gra-to tu ca-lor!*
    koh-moh ehs grah-toh too kah-lohr!

Translation

This is my land, both sun-bronzed and bright,
This is my land, with a soul made for love.
This is my land, abundant and generous,
Oh, my land, how pleasant is your warmth!
Your dawnings are so full of joy,
And your serenades are well suited for love.
This is my land, flower of sadness,
Oh, my land, how pleasant is your warmth!

Habemos llegado (We Have Arrived), p. 174 CD 10-4

Folk Song from Puerto Rico

Pronunciation Practice

Verse 1

Phrase 1. *Ha-be-mos lle-ga-do_a su_a-ma-do ho-gar.*
ah-beh-mohs djeh-gah-doh_ah soo_ah-mah-doh
oh-gahrr.

2. *Ha-be-mos lle-ga-do_a su_a-ma-do ho-gar.*
ah-beh-mohs djeh-gah-doh_ah soo_ah-mah-doh
oh-gahrr.

3. *Con con-chas, con per-las, con bri-sas del
mar;*
kohn kohn-chahs, kohn pehrr-lahs, kohn
brree-sahs dehl mahrr;

4. *Con con-chas, con per-las, con bri-sas del
mar.*
kohn kohn-chahs, kohn pehrr-lahs, kohn
brree-sahs dehl mahrr.

Verse 2

Phrase 1. *Oí-ga-me, se-ño-ra, le ven-go_a can-tar.*
oh_ee-gah-meh, seh-nyoh-rah, leh vehn-
goh_ah kahn-tahrr.

2. *Oí-ga-me, se-ño-ra, le ven-go_a can-tar.*
oh_ee-gah-meh, seh-nyoh-rah, leh vehn-
goh_ah kahn-tahrr.

3. *Que_es u-na pro-me-sa que quie-ro pa-gar;*
keh_ehs oo-nah proh-meh-sah keh kyeh-roh
pah-gahrr;

4. *Que_es u-na pro-me-sa que quie-ro pa-gar.*
keh_ehs oo-nah proh-meh-sah keh kyeh-roh
pah-gahrr.

Translation

We have arrived at your beloved home.
We have arrived at your beloved home.
With shells, with pearls, with breezes from the sea;
With shells, with pearls, with breezes from the sea.

Listen to me, lady, I come to sing to you.
Listen to me, lady, I come to sing to you.
This is a promise that I want to keep,
This is a promise that I want to keep.

Siyahamba, p. 212 CD 11-23

Traditional Freedom Song from South Africa

Pronunciation Practice

Verse 1

Phrase

1. *Si-ya-hamb'-e-ku-kha-nye-ni kwen-khos'.*
   see-yah-hahm-beh-koo-khah-nyeh-nee
   kgwehn-kohs.

2. *Si-ya-hamb'-e-ku-kha-nye-ni kwen-khos'.*
   see-yah-hahm-beh-koo-khah-nyeh-nee
   kgwehn-kohs.

3. *Si-ya-hamb'-e-ku-kha-nye-ni kwen-khos'.*
   see-yah-hahm-beh-koo-khah-nyeh-nee
   kgwehn-kohs.

4. *Si-ya-hamb'-e-ku-kha-nye-ni kwen-khos'.*
   see-yah-hahm-beh-koo-khah-nyeh-nee
   kgwehn-kohs.

5. *Si-ya-ham-ba Si-ya-ham-ba*
   see-yah-hahm-bah see-yah-hahm-bah

6. *Si-ya-hamb'-e-ku-kha-nye-ni kwen-khos'.*
   see-yah-hahm-beh-koo-khah-nyeh-nee
   kgwehn-kohs.

7. *Si-ya-ham-ba Si-ya-ham-ba*
   see-yah-hahm-bah see-yah-hahm-bah

8. *Si-ya-hamb'-e-ku-kha-nye-ni kwen-khos'.*
   see-yah-hahm-beh-koo-khah-nyeh-nee
   kgwehn-kohs.

Translation

Phrase 1-4 Light—of God. We are walking in the light of God.

Phrase 5 We are walking, we are walking,

Phrase 6 Light—of God. We are walking in the light of God.

Phrase 7 We are walking, we are walking,

Phrase 8 Light—of God. We are walking in the light of God.

Ise oluwa, p. 230 CD 12-5

Yoruba Folk Song from Nigeria

Pronunciation Practice

Verse 1

Phrase

1. *I-se o-lu-wa*
   ee-sheh oh-loo-wah

2. *ko le ba-je-oh;*
   koh leh bah-jeh-oh;

3. *I-se o-lu-wa*
   ee-sheh oh-loo-wah

4. *ko le ba-je-oh.*
   koh leh bah-jeh-oh.

5. *Ko le ba-je-oh,*
   koh leh bah-jeh-oh,

6. *ko le ba-je-oh.*
   koh leh bah-jeh-oh.

7. *I-se o-lu-wa*
   ee-sheh oh-loo-wah

8. *ko le ba-je-oh.*
   koh leh bah-jeh-oh.

9. *I-se o-lu-wa*
   ee-sheh oh-loo-wah

10. *ko le ba-je-oh.*
    koh leh bah-jeh-oh.

Translation

Ise oluwa—The work of God

Verse 1 The work of God will never be destroyed.
It can never be destroyed.
The work of God will never be destroyed.

Riendo el río corre (Run, Run, River), p. 263 CD 13-27

Words and Music by Tish Hinojosa

Pronunciation Practice

Refrain

Phrase 1. *Co-rre, co-rre,*
     koh-rreh, koh-rreh,

    2. *co-rre⌣el río,*
     koh-rreh⌣ehl ree⌣oh,

    3. *Ri-en-do⌣el rí-o co-rre.*
     ree-ehn-doh⌣ehl rree-oh koh-rreh.

    4. *Co-rre, co-rre,*
     koh-rreh, koh-rreh,

    5. *co-rre⌣el río,*
     koh-rreh⌣ehl ree⌣oh,

    6. *Ri-en-do⌣el rí-o co-rre.*
     rree-ehn-doh⌣ehl rree-oh koh-rreh.

Verse 1

Phrase 1. *Cuén-ta-me de las mon-ta-ñas*
     kwehn-tah-meh deh lahs mohn-tah-nyahs

    2. *de tu em-pe-sar,*
     deh too ehm-peh-sahrr,

    3. *Cuén-ta-me de pie-dra⌣y pe-na*
     kwehn-tah-meh deh pyeh-drah⌣ee peh-nah

    4. *que lle-vas al mar.*
     keh djeh-vahs ahl mahrr.

Verse 2

Phrase 1. *Sa-bes tú de la dis-tan-cia*
     sah-behs too-deh lah dees-tahn-see⌣yah

    2. *que pien-sas al-can-zar,*
     keh pyehn-sahs ahl-kahn-sahrr,

    3. *Co-mo sue-ño de la lu-na*
     koh-moh-sweh-nyoh deh lah loo-nah

    4. *que me das pa-ra so-ñar.*
     keh meh dahs pah-rah soh-nyahrr.

Refrain

Phrase 1. *Co-rre, co-rre,*
     koh-rreh, koh-rreh,

    2. *corre⌣el río,*
     koh-rreh⌣ehl ree⌣oh,

    3. *Ri-en-do⌣el rí-o co-rre.*
     rree-ehn-doh⌣ehl ree-oh koh-rreh.

    4. *Co-rre, co-rre,*
     koh-rreh, koh-rreh,

    5. *corre⌣el río,*
     koh-rreh⌣ehl ree⌣oh,

    6. *Ri-en-do⌣el rí-o co-rre.*
     rree-ehn-doh⌣ehl ree-oh koh-rreh.

Translation

Refrain [It] runs, [it] runs, [it] runs the river. Laughing, the river runs.

Verse 1 Tell me about the mountains of your origins;
    Tell me about the rocks and sorrows you carry to the sea.

Verse 2 You know about the distance you will reach
    Like a moon's dream you give something to dream about.

Banuwa, p. 294 CD 15-3
Folk Song from Liberia

Pronunciation Practice

Phrase 1. *Ba-nu-wa, ba-nu-wa, ba-nu-wa yo.*
bah-noo-wah, bah-noo-wah, bah-noo-wah yoh.

2. *Ba-nu-wa, ba-nu-wa, ba-nu-wa yo.*
bah-noo-wah, bah-noo-wah, bah-noo-wah yoh.

3. *Ba-nu-wa, ba-nu-wa, ba-nu-wa yo.*
bah-noo-wah, bah-noo-wah, bah-noo-wah yoh.

4. *A-la-no, neh-ni a-la-no.*
ah-lah-noh, neh-nee ah-lah-noh.

5. *A-la-no, neh-ni a-la-no.*
ah-lah-noh, neh-nee ah-lah-noh.

Translation

Do not cry, do not cry, don't cry, little girl.

Má Teodora, p. 301 CD 15-15
Folk Song from Cuba

Pronunciation Practice

Unison and Melody

Phrase 1. *¿Dón-de_es-tá la Má Teo-do-ra?*
dohn-deh_ehs-tah lah mah teh_oh-doh-rah?

2. *Rajando la le-ña_es-tá.*
rah-hahn-doh lah leh-nyehs-tah.

3. *¿Con su pa-lo_y su ban-do la?*
kohn soo pah-loh_ee soo bahn-doh lah?

4. *Ra-jan-do la le-ña_es-tá.*
rah-hahn-doh lah leh-nyehs-tah.

5. *¿Dón-de_es-tá que no la ve-o?*
dohn-deh_ehs-tah keh noh lah veh-oh?

6. *Ra-jan-do la le-ña_es-tá.*
rah-hahn-doh lah leh-nyehs-tah.

7. *Ra-jan-do la le-ña_es-tá.*
rah-hahn-doh lah leh-nyehs-tah.

8. *Ra-jan-do la le-ña_es-tá.*
rah-hahn-doh lah leh-nyehs-tah.

Translation

Where is Má Teodora?
She is chopping up the firewood.
With her shovel and bandore?
She is chopping up the firewood.
Where is she that I can't see her?
She is chopping up the firewood.

Má Teodora, p. 301 CD 15-15 *(continued)*

Pronunciation Practice

Unison and Harmony

Phrase 1. *¿Don-de es-tá la Má Teo-do-ra?*
dohn-deh ehs-tah lah mah teh oh-doh-rah?

2. *Rajando la le-ña es-tá.*
rah-hahn-doh lah leh-nyehs-tah.

3. *¿Con su pa-lo y su ban-do-la?*
kohn soo pah-loh ee soo bahn-doh-lah?

4. *Ra-jan-do la le-ña es-tá.*
rah-hahn-doh lah leh-nyehs-tah.

5. *¿Don-de es-tá que no la ve-o?*
dohn-deh ehs-tah keh noh lah veh-oh?

6. *Ra-jan-do la le-ña es-tá.*
rah-hahn-doh lah leh-nyehs-tah.

7. *Ra-jan-do la le-ña es-tá.*
rah-hahn-doh lah leh-nyehs-tah.

8. *Ra-jan-do la le-ña es-tá.*
rah-hahn-doh lah leh-nyehs-tah.

Asadoya, p. 303 CD 15-20
Folk Song from Okinawa

Pronunciation Practice

Phrase 1. *A A-sa-do-ya nu*
ah ah-sah-doo-yah noo

2. *Ku-ya-ma ni yo*
koo-yah-mah nee yoh

3. *sa yu-i yu-i,*
sah yoo-ee yoo-ee,

4. *A-n chu-ra sa na*
ah-(n) choo-rah sah nah

5. *u-ma-ri ba-shi-o.*
oo-mah-ree bah-shee-oh.

6. *Ma-ta ha-ri-nu*
mah-tah hah-ree-noo

7. *chin-da-ra, ka-nu-sya-ma yo.*
cheen-dah-rah, kah-noo-shyah-mah yoh.

Translation

Okinawan lyrics:
Ah, Kuyama of the house of Asadoya,
So beautiful you were born,
My dear, my darling (?).

Japanese lyrics:
Ah, you are a pretty wild rose,
Blooming lonely in the prairie,
When it gets dark
I really hate to go,
Leaving you here alone.

Alumot (Sheaves of Grain), p. 306 CD 15-29

Harvest Song from Israel

Pronunciation Practice

Phrase 1. *Ye-la-dim na-gi-la*
yeh-lah-deem nah-gee-lah

      2. *ve-na-sov bim-cho-lot!*
veh-nah-sohv beem-hoh-loht!

      3. *Shi-bo-lim hiv-shi-lu.*
shee-boh-leem heev-shee-loo.

      4. *Ne´ e-sof a-lu-mot!*
neh heh-sohv ah-loo-moht!

      5. *A-lu-mot shel za-hav,*
ah-loo-moht shehl zah-hahv,

      6. *ha-sa-deh ra-chav, ra-chav.*
hah-sah-deh rah-hahv, rah-hahv.

      7. *Ba-sa-deh u-va-nir,*
bah-sah-deh oo-vah-nihrr,

      8. *shi-ru ze-mer la-ka-tsir!*
shee-rroo zeh-mehrr lah-kah-tsihrr!

Translation

Children, rejoice and circle in a dance
Sheaves have ripened!
Let us gather them.
Sheaves of gold, the field—wide, wide
In the field—and on the tilled grounds,
Sing a song to the reapers!

Oye, p. 336 CD 17–7

By Jim Papoulis

Pronunciation Practice

Verse 1
Phrase 1. *Es-tán só-los, llo-ran-do*
eh-stahn soh-lohs, djoh-rahn-doh

      2. *en si-len-cio, en la_os-cu-ri-dad.*
ehn see-lehn-see-oh, ehn lah_oh-skoo-ree-dahd.

      3. *Es-tán so-ñan-do, de-se-an-do*
eh-stahn soh-nyahn-doh, deh-seh-ahn-doh

      4. *con es-per-an-za, por la_op-or-tun-i-dad.*
kohn eh-speh-rahn-sah, pohrr lah_oh-pohrr-
too-nee-dahd.

      5. *Es-cú-cha-los, es-cú-cha-los, ell-os te lla-man.*
ehs-koo-chah-lohs, ehs-koo-chah-lohs, eh-djohs
teh djah-mahn.

Refrain
Phrase 1. *Oye.*
oh-yeh.

Verse 2
Phrase 1. *Es-cú-cha-los, mí-ra-los*
ehs-koo-chah-lohs, mee-rah-lohs

      2. *es-cu-cha lo que tra-tan de de-cir.*
ehs-koo-chah loh keh trah-tahn deh deh-seer.

      3. *Es-tán en bús-que-da, del ca-mi-no*
eh-stahn ehn boo-skeh-dah, dehl kah-mee-noh

      4. *pe-que-ñas vo-ces, lla-man-do-te.*
peh-keh-nyahs voh-sehs, djah-mahn-doh-teh.

Translation

Verse 1   He is alone, crying
in silence, in the dark.
He is dreaming, wishing
with hope for the opportunity.
Listen to them, listen to them, they call you.

Refrain   Listen.

Verse 2   Listen to them, look at them.
Listen to what they try to tell you.
They are in search of the way,
little voices, calling you.

Corta la caña (Head for the Canefields), p. 364 CD 18-17

Folk Song from Puerto Rico

Pronunciation Practice

Phrase 1. *Yo ven-go de mon-te_a-den-tro*
yoh vehn-goh deh mohn-teh_ah-dehn-troh

2. *de cor-tar ca-ña, ca-ñe-ro,*
deh kohrr-tahrr kah-nyah, kah-nyeh-rroh,

3. *por más ca-ña que se cor-te*
pohrr mahs kah-nyah keh seh kohrr-teh

4. *nun-ca se ga-na_el di-ne-ro.*
noon-kah seh gah-nah_ehl dee-neh-rroh.

5. *To-do_el mun-do la pro-cla-ma*
toh-doh_ehl moon-doh lah proh-klah-mah

6. *que_es muy fá-cil de cor-tar,*
keh_ehs moo-ee fah-seel deh kohrr-tahr,

7. *cuan-do se ja-la la mo-cha*
kwahn-doh seh hah-lah lah moh-chah

8. *na-die quie-re tra-ba-jar.*
nah-dee_eh kee_eh-rreh trah-vah-hahrr.

9. *Cor-ta la ca-ña, ca-ñe-ro,*
kohrr-tah lah kah-nyah, ka-nyeh-rroh,

10. *cór-ta-la.*
kohrr-tah-lah.

11. *Cor-ta la ca-ña, ca-ñe-ro,*
kohrr-tah lah kah-nyah, ka-nyeh-rroh,

12. *cór-ta-la.*
kohrr-tah-lah.

Translation

I come from inside the sugar cane fields.
After cutting sugar cane, cane cutter,
No matter how much sugar cane one cuts
One never earns enough money.
Everyone says that it is very easy to cut;
When it comes time to swing the machete nobody
   wants to work.
Cut the sugar cane, cane cutter, cut it.

Cuando pa' Chile me voy (Leavin' for Chile), p. 376 CD 19-14

Cueca from Chile

Pronunciation Practice

Verse 1

Phrase 1. *Cuan-do pa' Chi-le me voy,*
kwahn-doh pah chee-leh meh voi,

2. *Cru-zan-do la cor-di-lle-ra,*
kroo-sahn-doh lah kohr-dee-yeh-rah,

3. *Cuan-do pa' Chi-le me voy,*
kwahn-doh pah chee-leh meh voi,

4. *Cru-zan-do la cor-di-lle-ra,*
kroo-sahn-doh lah kohr-dee-yeh-rah,

5. *La-te_el co-ra-zón con-ten-to,*
lah-teh_ehl koh-rah-sohn kohn-tehn-toh,

6. *Pues u-na chi-le-na me_es-pe-ra.*
pwehs oo-nah chee-leh-nah meh_ehs-peh-rah.

7. *La-te_el co-ra-zón con-ten-to,*
lah-teh_ehl koh-rah-sohn kohn-tehn-toh,

8. *Pues u-na chi-le-na me_es-pe-ra.*
pwehs oo-nah chee-leh-nah meh_ehs-peh-rah.

9. *Y cuan-do vuel-vo de Chi-le,*
ee kwahn-doh vwehl-voh deh chee-leh,

10. *En-tre ce-rros y que-bra-das,*
ehn-treh seh-rohs ee keh-brah-thahs,

11. *Y cuan-do vuel-vo de Chi-le,*
ee kwahn-doh vwehl-voh deh chee-leh,

12. *En-tre ce-rros y que-bra-das,*
ehn-treh seh-rohs ee keh-brah-thahs,

13. *La-te_el co-ra-zón con-ten-to,*
lah-teh_ehl koh-rah-sohn kohn-tehn-toh,

14. *Pues me_es-pe-ra u-na cu-ya-na.*
pwehs meh_es-peh-rah oo-nah koo-yah-nah.

15. *La-te_el co-ra-zón con-ten-to,*
lah-teh_ehl koh-rah-sohn kohn-tehn-toh,

16. *Pues me_es-pe-ra u-na cu-ya-na.*
pwehs meh_es-peh-rah oo-nah koo-yah-nah.

Refrain

Phrase 1. *Vi-van el bai-le y la dan-za,*
vee-vahn ehl bI-leh ee lah dahn-sah,

2. *vi-van la cue-ca_y la zam-ba,*
vee-vahn lah kweh-kah_ee lah sahm-bah,

3. *Dos pun-tas tie-ne_el ca-mi-no*
dohs poon-tahs tyeh-neh_ehl kah-mee-noh

4. *y_en las dos al-guien me_a-guar-da.*
ee_ehn lahs dohs ahl-ghee_yehn me_ah-gwahr-thah.

Translation

Verse 1

When I go to Chile crossing the mountain range
and when I come back from Chile among hills and brooks,
My heart beats happy, for a Chilean awaits me
My heart beats happy, for a Cuyean awaits me
Long live dance and dance. Long live the Cueca and
    the Zamba.
Two ends has the road and in both someone awaits me.

Verse 2

I dance the Cueca in Chile,
I dance the Zamba in Cuyo,
In Chile with the Chilean girls,
with the others in Calingasta.
Sad life, happy life is the muleteer's life.
There are small sorrows in the road, and there is laughter
    at the end of the path.

*The words "baile" and "danza" are synonyms; both
stand for the English word "dance."*

Cuando pa' Chile me voy (Leavin' for Chile), p. 376 CD 19-14 *(continued)*

Pronunciation Practice

    5. *Dos pun-tas tie-ne_el ca-mi-no*
       dohs poon-tahs tyeh-neh_ehl kah-mee-noh

    6. *y_en las dos al-guien me_a-guar-da.*
       ee_ehn lahs dohs ahl-ghee_yehn me_ah-gwahr-
       thah.

Verse 2

Phrase 1. *En Chi-le bai-lo la cue-ca,*
         ehn chee-leh bI-loh lah kweh-kah,

    2. *En Cu-yo bai-lo la zam-ba,*
       ehn koo-joh bI-loh lah sahm-bah,

    3. *En Chi-le bai-lo la cue-ca,*
       ehn chee-leh bI-loh lah kweh-kah,

    4. *En Cu-yo bai-lo la zam-ba,*
       ehn koo-joh bI-loh lah sahm-bah,

    5. *En Chi-le con las chi-le-nas,*
       ehn chee-leh kohn lahs chee-leh-nahs,

    6. *Con las o-tras en Ca-lin-ga-sta.*
       kohn lahs oh-trahs ehn kah-leen-gah-stah.

    7. *En Chi-le con las chi-le-nas,*
       ehn chee-leh kohn lahs chee-leh-nahs,

    8. *Con las o-tras en Ca-lin-ga-sta.*
       kohn lahs oh-trahs ehn kah-leen-gah-stah.

    9. *Vi-da triste, vi-da a-le-gre,*
       vee-thah trees-teh, vee-thah ah-leh-greh,

  10. *Es la vi-da del a-rri-er-o,*
       ehs lah vee-thah dehl ah-rree-eh-roh,

  11. *Vi-da triste, vi-da a-le-gre,*
       vee-thah trees-teh, vee-thah ah-leh-greh,

  12. *Es la vi-da del a-rri-e-ro,*
       ehs lah vee-thah dehl ah-rree-eh-roh,

  13. *Pe-ni-tas en el ca-mi-no,*
       peh-nee-tahs ehn ehl kah-mee-noh,

  14. *Y ri-sas al fin del sen-de-ro.*
       ee ree-sahs ahl feen dehl sehn-deh-roh.

  15. *Pe-ni-tas en el ca-mi-no,*
       peh-nee-tahs ehn ehl kah-mee-noh,

  16. *Y ri-sas al fin del sen-de-ro.*
       ee ree-sahs ahl feen dehl sehn-deh-roh.

Refrain (Repeat)

Fais do do (Go to Sleep), p. 403 CD 20-4, 5
Acadian Folk Song

Pronunciation Practice

Vocal Part 1

Phrase 1. *Fais do do, 'co-las mon p'tit frè-re,*
feh doh doh, koh-lah, mo(n) p'tee freh-ruh,

2. *fais do do, t'au-ras du lo lo.*
feh doh doh, toh-rah doo loh loh.

3. *Ma-man est en haut*
mah-maw eh taw(n) oh

4. *qui fait des gâ-teaux,*
kee feh doo gah-toh,

5. *pa-pa est en bas qui fait du cho-co-lat.*
pah-paw eh taw(n) bah kee feh doo shah-koh-lah.

6. *Fais do do, 'co-las mon p'tit frè-re,*
feh doh doh, koh-lah mo(n) p'tee freh-ruh,

7. *fais do do, t'au ras du lo lo.*
feh doh doh, toh rah doo loh loh.

8. *pa-pa est en bas, qui fait du cho-co-lat.*
pah-paw eh taw(n) bah, kee feh doo shah-koh-lah.

9. *Oh, fais do do, 'co-las mon p'tit frè-re,*
oh feh doh doh, koh-lah mo(n) p'tee freh-ruh,

10. *Fais do do, t'au-ras du lo lo.*
feh doh doh, toh-rah doo loh loh.

Vocal Part 2

Phrase 1. *Fais do do, 'co-las, mon p'tit frè-re,*
feh doh doh, koh-lah, mo(n) p'tee freh-ruh,

2. *fais do do, t'au ras du lo lo.*
feh doh doh, toh rah doo loh loh.

3. *Ma-man est en haut*
mah-maw eh taw(n) oh

4. *qui fait des gâ-teaux,*
kee feh doo gah-toh,

5. *pa-pa est en bas qui fait du cho-co-lat.*
pah-paw eh taw(n) bah kee feh doo shah-koh-lah.

6. *Fais do do, 'co-las mon p'tit frè-re,*
feh doh doh, koh-lah mo(n) p'tee freh-ruh,

7. *fais do do, t'au-ras du lo lo.*
feh doh doh, toh-rah doo loh loh.

8. *Ma-man est en haut*
mah-maw eh taw(n) oh

Translation

Go to sleep, my baby brother
Go to sleep, and wake up to treats.

Mommy is upstairs, baking some cookies.
Daddy is downstairs, making some goodies.

Go to sleep, my baby brother.
Go to sleep, and wake up to treats.

Oh, go to sleep, my baby brother,
Go to sleep, and wake up to treats.

Fais do do (Go to Sleep), p. 403 CD 20-4, 5 *(continued)*

Pronunciation Practice

9. *qui fait des gâ-teaux,*
   kee feh doo gah-toh,

10. *pa-pa, fait du cho-co-lat.*
    pah-paw, feh doo shah-koh-lah,

11. *Oh, fais do do, t'au-ras du lo lo.*
    oh, feh doh doh, toh-rah doo loh loh.

Vocal Part 3

Phrase 1. *Fais do do, 'Co-las, mon p'tit frè-re,*
   feh doh doh, koh-lah, mo(n) p'tee freh-ruh,

2. *fais do do, t'au-ras du lo lo.*
   feh doh doh, toh-rah doo loh loh.

3. *Ma-man est en haut*
   mah-maw eh taw(n) oh

4. *qui fait des gâ-teaux,*
   kee feh doo gah-toh,

5. *pa-pa est en bas qui fait du cho-co-lat.*
   pah-paw eh taw(n) bah kee feh doo shah-koh-lah.

6. *Fais do do, 'co-las mon p'tit frè-re,*
   feh doh doh, koh-lah mo(n) p'tee freh-ruh,

7. *fais do do, t'au-ras du lo lo.*
   feh doh doh, toh-rah doo loh loh.

8. *Ma-man est en haut,*
   mah-maw eh taw(n) oh,

9. *qui fait des gâ-teaux,*
   kee feh doo gah-toh,

10. *pa-pa est en bas qui fait du cho-co-lat.*
    pah-paw eh taw(n) bah kee feh doo shah-koh-lah.

11. *Oh, fais do do, 'co-las mon p'tit frè-re,*
    oh, feh doh doh, koh-lah mo(n) p'tee freh-ruh,

12. *fais do do, t'au-ras du lo lo.*
    feh doh doh, toh-rah doo loh loh.

Shalom aleichem, p. 409 CD 20-9

Traditional Jewish Song

Pronunciation Practice

Phrase 1. *Sha-lom a-lei-chem mal-a-chei ha-sha-ret*
   shah-lohm ah-leh-hkhehm mahl-ah-hkheh ah-shah reht

2. *mal-a-chei el-yon*
   mahl-ah-hkheh ehl-yohn

3. *mi me-lech mal-a-chei ham-la-chim*
   mee meh-lehkh mahl-ah-hkheh hahm-lah-hkheem

4. *ha-ka-dosh ba-ruch hu*
   hah-kah-dohsh bah-roohkh hoo

5. *Bo-a-chem l´-sha-lom*
   boh-ah-hkhehm luh-shah-lohm

6. *mal-a-chei ha-sha-lom*
   mahl-ah-hkheh hah-shah-lohm

7. *mal-a-chei el-yon*
   mahl-ah-hkheh ehl-yohn

8. *mi-me-lech mal-a-chei ham-la-chim*
   mee-meh-lehkh mahl-ah-hkheh hahm-lah-hkheem

9. *ha-ka-dosh ba-ruch hu*
   hah-kah-dohsh bah-roohkh hoo

10. *Bo-a-chem bo-a-chem l´-sha-lom*
    boh-ah-hkhehm boh-ah-hkhehm luh-shah-lohm

11. *mal-a-chei ha-sha-lom*
    mahl-ah-hkheh hah-shah-lohm

12. *mal-a-chei el-yon*
    mahl-ah-hkheh ehl-yohn

13. *mal-a-chei el-yon*
    mahl-ah-hkheh ehl-yohn

14. *mi-me-lech mal-a-chei ham-la-chim*
    mee meh-lehkh mahl-ah-hkheh hahm-lah-hkheem

15. *ha-ka-dosh ba-ruch hu*
    hah-kah-dohsh bah-roohkh hoo

Translation

Peace be with you, ministering angels, angels of the most high, the Supreme King of Kings, the Holy One blessed be He.

May your coming be in peace, angels of the Most High, the Supreme King of Kings, the Holy one, blessed be He.

Cantaré, cantarás (I Will Sing, You Will Sing), p. 413 CD 20-14

Words and Music by Albert Hammond and Juan Carlos Calderón

Pronunciation Practice

Verse 1

Phrase   1. *Te da-ré*
             teh dah-reh

        2. *cuan-to pue-do dar,*
             kwahn-toh pweh-thoh dahr,

        3. *Só-lo sé can-tar*
             soh-loh seh kahn-tahr

        4. *y pa-ra tí_es mi can-to*
             ee pah-rah tee_ehs mee kahn-toh

        5. *Y mi voz,*
             ee mee vohs,

        6. *Jun-to_a los de-más,*
             hoon-toh_ah lohs deh-mahs,

        7. *En la_in-men-si-dad*
             ehn lah_een-mehn-see-thath

        8. *se_es-tá es-cu-chan-do.*
             seh_ehs-tah ehs-koo-chahn-doh.

Refrain

Phrase   1. *Can-ta-ré*
             kahn-tah-reh

        2. *can-ta-rás*
             kahn-tah-rahs

        3. *Y_e-sa luz al fi-nal*
             ee_eh-sah loos ahl fee-nahl

        4. *del sen-de-ro.*
             dehl sehn-deh-roh.

        5. *Bri-lla-rá*
             bree-yah-rah

        6. *co-mo_un sol*
             koh-moh_oon sohl

        7. *Que_i-lu-mi-na el mun-do en-te-ro.*
             keh_ee-loo-mee-nah ehl moon-doh ehn-teh-roh.

        8. *Ca-da vez*
             kah-thah vehs

        9. *so-mos más*
             soh-mohs mahs

   10. *Y si_al fin nos da-mos la ma-no*
             ee see_ahl feen nohs dah-mohs lah mah-noh

   11. *Siem-pre_ha-brá*
             see_ehm-preh ah-brah

   12. *un lu-gar*
             oon loo-gahr

   13. *Pa-ra to-do ser hu-ma-no.*
             pah-rah toh-doh sehr oo-mah-noh.

Translation

Verse 1   I will give you all I can give.
I only know how to sing, and my song is for you.
And my voice, together with others
in the immensity, is being heard.

Refrain   I will sing, you will sing,
and that light at the end of the path
will shine like the sun illuminating
the whole world.
We are more and more.
And if we, at last, hold our hands,
there will always be a place for
each and every human being.

Vem kan segla? (Who Can Sail?), p. 407 CD 20-19

Folk Song from Sweden

Pronunciation Practice

PART 1
Verse 1
Phrase 1. *Vem kan seg-la,*
vehm kahn see-gklah,

2. *vem kan skil-jas*
vehm kahn sheel-ee_yahs

3. *u-tan tå-rar?*
yew-tahn toh-rahrr?

Verse 2
Phrase 1. *Jag kan seg-la,*
yahg kahn see-gklah,

2. *men ej skil-jas*
mehn eh sheel-ee_yahs

3. *u-tan tå-rar.*
yew-tahn toh-rahrr.

PART 2
Verse 1
Phrase 1. *Vem kan seg-la för-u-tan vind,*
vehm kahn see-gklah fehr-yew-tahn veend,

2. *vem kan ro u-tan å-ror?*
vehm kahn roo yew-tahn oh-roorr?

3. *vem kan skil-jas från vän-nen sin*
vehm kahn sheel-ee_yahs frahn vehn-nehn seen

4. *u-tan att fäl-la tå-rar?*
yew-tahn aht fehl-lah toh-rahrr?

Verse 2
Phrase 1. *Jag kan seg-la för-u-tan vind,*
yahgk kahn see-gklah fohr-yew-tahn veend,

2. *jag kan ro u-tan å-ror,*
yahgk kahn roh yew-tahn oh-roorr,

3. *men ej skil-jas från vän-nen min*
mehn eh sheel-ee_yahs frohn vehn-nehn meen

4. *u-tan att fäl-la tå-rar.*
yew-tahn aht fehl-lah toh-rahrr.

PART 3
Verse 1
Phrase 1. *Vem kan seg-la og*
vehm kahn see-gklah oh

2. *vem kan ro u-tan å-ror?*
vehm kahn roo yew-tahn oh-roorr?

3. *vem kan, vem kan skil-jas*
vehm kahn, vehm kahn sheel-ee_yahs

4. *för-u-tan fäll-da tå-rar?*
fehr-yew-tahn fehl-dah toh-rahrr?

Verse 2
Phrase 1. *Jag kan seg-la og*
yahgk kahn see-gklah oh

2. *jag kan ro u-tan å-ror,*
yahgk kahn roh yew-tahn oh-roorr,

3. *men ej, men ej skil-jas*
mehn eh, mehn eh sheel-ee_yahs

4. *för-u-tan fäll-da tå-rar.*
fohr-yew-tahn fehl-dah toh-rahrr

Translation

Part 1 Verse 1
Who can sail, who can part without tears?

Part 1 Verse 2 I can sail, but not part without tears.

Part 2 Verse 1 Who can sail without wind, who can row without oars? Who can part from his friend without shedding tears?

Part 2 Verse 2 I can sail without wind, I can row without oars, but not part from friend of mine without shedding tears.

Part 3 Verse 1 Who can sail and who can row without oars? Who can, who can part without fallen tears?

Part 3 Verse 2 I can sail and I can row without oars but not part without shedding tears.

Loigratong, p. 451 CD 21-14
Folk Song from Thailand

Pronunciation Practice

Phrase 1. *Wan pen deup sip song*
          wahn peh(n) duhp sihp sahng

2. *nam gau nong tem ta-ling*
   nahm goh nahng tehm tah-leeng

3. *rao tang lai chai ying*
   rah_ow tahng lah_ee shah_ee yeeng

4. *sa-nook gan-jing wan loi-gra-tong*
   sah-nook gahn-jeeng wahn loy-krah-tuhng

5. *loi loi-gra-tong loi loi-gra-tong*
   loy loy-krah-tuhng loy loy-krah-tuhng

6. *loi-gra-tong gan lah-ow*
   loy-krah-tuhng gahn lah-ow

7. *koh churn nong kay_oh ock ma lum wong*
   koh chuhrn nahng key_oh ohk mah luhm
   wahng

8. *lum wong wan loi-gra-tong lum wong wan loi-gra-tong*
   luhm wahng wahn loy-krah-tuhng luhm wahng
   wahn loy-krah-tuhng

9. *boon ja song hey rao sook jai*
   boon jah sahng heh_ee rah_ow sook jah_ee

10. *boon ja song hey rao sook jai*
    boon jah sahng heh_ee rah_ow sook jah_ee

oy = as in b<u>oy</u>

Translation

When the moon is full on the twelfth month
the river water rises up to the banks.
All men and women enjoy the day,
floating the gratong.
The ladies come out and dance
and float the gratong.
Good things will make us happy.

S´vivon (Dreydl), p. 452 CD 21-18
Folk Song from Israel. Hebrew Words by L. Kipnis
English words by Sue Ellen LaBelle and David Eddleman

Pronunciation Practice

Phrase 1. *S´-vi-von, sov, sov, sov,*
          seh-vee-vahn, sahv, sahv, sahv,

2. *Cha-nu-kah hu-chag tov.*
   hah-noo-kah hoo-hkhahg tahv.

3. *Cha-nu-kah hu chag tov,*
   hkhah-noo-kah hoo-hkhahg tahv,

4. *S´-vi-von sov, sov, sov.*
   seh-vee-vahn sahv, sahv, sahv.

5. *Chag sim-chah hu la am*
   hahg seem-hkhah hoo lah ahm

6. *nes ga-dol ha-ya sham.*
   nehs gah-dohl hah-yah shahm.

7. *nes ga-dol ha-ya sham,*
   nehs gah-dohl hah-yah shahm,

8. *chag sim-chah hu la am.*
   hkhahg seem-hkhah hoo lah ahm.

Translation

Little dreydl, spin, spin, spin,
Chanukah is a day of great joy;
Great was the miracle that happened there.
Spin, little dreydl, spin, spin, spin.

Gloria, Gloria, p. 459 CD 21-26
Music from Franz Joseph Haydn

Pronunciation Practice

Part 1

Phrase 1. *Glo-ri-a, Glo-ri-a*
gloh-ree-ah, gloh-ree-ah

2. *in ex-cel-sis Glo-ri-a*
een ex-shehl-sees gloh-ree-ah

3. *Et in ter-ra*
eht een tehr-rah

4. *pax ho-mi-ni-bus.*
pahx oh-mee-nee-boos.

Part 2

Phrase 1. *Glo-ri-a, Glo-ri-a*
gloh-ree-ah, gloh-ree-ah

2. *in ex-cel-sis Glo-ri-a*
een ex-shehl-sees gloh-ree-ah

3. *Et in ter-ra*
eht een tehr-rah

4. *pax ho-mi-ni-bus.*
pahx oh-mee-nee-boos.

Part 3

Phrase 1. *Glo-ri-a, Glo-ri-a*
gloh-ree-ah, gloh-ree-ah

2. *in ex-cel-sis Glo-ri-a*
een ex-shehl-sees gloh-ree-ah

3. *Et in ter-ra*
eht een tehr-rah

4. *pax ho-mi-ni-bus.*
pahx oh-mee-nee-boos.

Translation

Glory in the highest, and peace to men on earth.

Eres tú (Touch the Wind), p. 473 CD 22-13
Music by Juan Carlos Calderón

Pronunciation Practice

Verse 1

Phrase 1. *Co-mo͜u-na pro-me-sa, e-res tú, e-res tú.*
koh-moh͜oo-nah proh-meh-sah, eh-rehs too,
eh-rehs too.

2. *Co-mo͜u-na ma-ña-na, de ve-ra-no.*
koh-moh͜oo-nah mah-nyah-nah, deh
veh-rah-noh.

3. *Co-mo͜u-na son-ri-sa, e-res tú, e-res tú,*
koh-moh͜oo-nah sohn-rhee-sa, eh-rehs too,
eh-rehs too,

4. *A-sí, a-sí, e-res tú.*
ah-see, ah-see, eh-rehs too.

Translation

Verse 1 You are like a promise, you are
Like a summer morning.
Like a smile you are,
That's the way you are,
That's the way you are.

Eres tú (Touch the Wind), p. 473 CD 22-13 *(continued)*

Pronunciation Practice

Verse 2

Phrase 1. *To-da mi_es-pe-ran-za, e-res tú, e-res tú.*
toh-thah mee_ehs-peh-rahn-sah, eh-rehs too, eh-rehs too.

2. *Co-mo llu-via fres-ca en mis ma-nos.*
koh-moh yoo-vee_ah frehs-kah ehn mees mah-nohs.

3. *Co-mo fuer-te bri-sa, e-res tú, e-res tú,*
koh-moh fwehr-teh bree-sah, eh-rehs too, eh-rehs too,

4. *a-sí, a-sí, e-res tú.*
ah-see, ah-see, eh-rehs too.

Refrain

Phrase 1. *E-res tú,*
eh-rehs too,

2. *co-mo_el a-gua de mi fuen-te.*
koh-moh_ehl ah-gwah deh mee fwehn-teh.

3. *E-res tú,*
eh-rehs too,

4. *el fue-go de mi_ho-gar.*
ehl fweh-goh deh mee_oh-gahr.

Verse 3

Phrase 1. *Co-mo mi po-e-ma, e-res tú, e-res tú.*
koh-moh mee poh-eh-mah, eh-rehs too, eh-rehs too.

2. *Co-mo_u-na gui-ta-rra en la no-che.*
koh-moh_oo-nah ghee-tah-rrah ehn lah noh-cheh.

3. *Co-mo mi ho-ri-zon-te, e-res tú, e-res tú,*
koh-moh mee oh-ree-zohn-teh, eh-rehs too, eh-rehs too,

4. *a-sí, a-sí, e-res tú.*
ah-see, ah-see, eh-rehs too.

Refrain

Phrase 1. *Al-go_a-sí e-res tú,*
ahl-goh_ah-see eh-rehs too,

2. *oo*
oo

3. *Al-go_a-sí, co-mo_el fue-go*
ahl-goh_ah-see, koh-moh_ehl fweh-goh

4. *de mi_ho-gue-ra.*
deh mee_oh-geh-rrah.

5. *Al-go_a-sí e-res tú,*
ahl-goh_ah-see eh-rehs too,

6. *oo*
oo

7. *Sí, al-go_a-sí e-res tú,*
see, ahl-goh_ah-see eh-rehs too,

Translation

Verse 2 You are all my hope, you are
Like fresh rain in my hands.
Like a strong breeze you are,
That's the way you are,
That's the way you are.

Verse 3 You are like a poem, you are
Like a guitar in the night.
Like my horizon you are,
That's the way you are.
That's the way you are.

Refrain
You are like the water in my fountain,
You are the fire of my hearth.
You are like the fire of my bonfire,
You are like the wheat of my bread.

Countermelody
You are something like that, oo,
Something like that, the fire of my hearth,
You are something like that, oo,
Yes, you are something like that.

Las mañanitas, p. 481 CD 22-19, 20
Folk Song from Mexico

Pronunciation Practice

Phrase
1. *Es-tas son las ma-ña-ni-tas*
   ehs-tahs sohn lahs mah-nyah-nee-tahs

2. *Que can-ta-ba ̮el Rey Da-vid,*
   keh kahn-tah-bah ̮ehl reh dah-veed,

3. *A las mu-cha-chas bo-ni-tas*
   ah lahs moo-chah-chahs boh-nee-tahs

4. *Se las can-ta-mos a-quí.*
   seh lahs kahn-tah-mohs ah-kee.

5. *Des-pier-ta, mi bien, des-pier-ta,*
   dehs pyehr-tah, mee byehn, dehs-pyehr-tah,

6. *Mi-ra que ya ̮a-ma-ne-ció;*
   mee-rah keh yah ̮ah-mah-neh-see ̮oh;

7. *Ya los pa-ja-ri-llos can-tan,*
   yah lohs pah-hah-ree-yohs kahn-tahn,

8. *La lu-na ya se me-tió.*
   lah loo-nah yah seh meh tee ̮oh.

Translation

These are the mañanitas* that
King David sang, to the beautiful girls.
We sing them here.
Wake up, my love, wake up. Look the day has
   already broken,
and the birds are already singing.
The moon has already hidden.

Mañanitas—morning songs

El carnavalito humahuaqueño
(The Little Humahuacan Carnival), p. 482 CD 22-23
Folk Song from Argentina

Pronunciation Practice

Phrase
1. *Lle-gan-do ̮es-tá ̮el car-na-val,*
   djeh-gahn-doh ̮ehs-tah ̮ehl kahr-nah-vahl,

2. *que-bra-de-ño mi cho-li-ta.*
   keh-brah-deh-nyoh mee choh-lee-tah.

3. *Lle-gan-do ̮es-tá ̮el car-na-val,*
   djeh-gahn-doh ̮ehs-tah ̮ehl kahr-nah-vahl,

4. *que-bra-de-ño mi cho-li-ta.*
   keh-brah-deh-nyoh mee choh-lee-tah.

5. *Fies-ta de la que-bra-da*
   fyeh-stah deh lah keh-brah-thah

6. *hu-ma-hua-que-ña pa-ra can-tar.*
   oo-mah-wah-keh-nyah pah-rah kahn-tahr.

7. *Er-que, cha-ran-go ̮y bom-bo*
   ehr-keh, chah-rahn-goh ̮ee bohm-boh

8. *car-na-val-i-to pa-ra bai-lar.*
   kahr-nah-vah-lee-toh pah-rah bah ̮ee-lahr.

9. *Bom-bo-ro bom-bom, bom-bo-ro bom-bom,*
   bom-bo-ro bom bom bom.
   bohm-boh-roh bohm-bohm, bohm-boh-roh
   bohm-bohm, bohm-boh-roh bohm bohm bohm.

Translation

The carnival is coming,
quebradeño, my honey.
The carnival is coming,
quebradeño, my honey.

The party of the broken
humahuaqueña is for singing.
The horn, guitar and drum;
the carnival is for dancing.

La, la, la, la, la, la, la, la,
la, la, la, la, la, la, la,
La, la, la, la, la, la, la, la,
la, la, la, la, la, la, la.

The party of the broken
humahuaqueña is for singing.
The horn, guitar and drum;
the carnival is for dancing.

Movement Glossary

A

action words Words (verbs) that readily evoke movement. Examples include freeze, flutter, melt, pop, crumple, swivel, creep, ripple, dart, explode.

allemande left In square or contra dances, corners grasp left forearms, wrists, hands or elbows and walk around clockwise back to place. They bend left elbows and pull away a bit.

allemande right is the same movement using right forearms, etc.

arch Two people raise one or two joined hands for others to duck under.

B

ballroom A partner hold in which the man's right arm is around the woman with his right hand with his right hand firmly in the middle of her back.

basket or basket hold Dancers join hands with second person on either side, not those beside them. Baskets can be formed in front of the body or in back. Longer arms may be on top, or arms may weave with left arm under and right over, or vice versa.

bend A basic stationary movement, bend brings two body parts closer together. The opposite of stretch, bend is done in the joints of the body.

body percussion Sounds produced by the contact of two or more body parts.

pat body percussion in which both hands tap the thighs simultaneously or alternately.

> **clap** body percussion in which hands strike
>
> **snap** body percussion in which the sound is produced by friction between the thumb and third finger
>
> **stamp** body percussion in which the foot strikes the floor

bow In classroom dances, an acknowledgment of the partner with a dip of the head or a quick bend at the waist. Although in traditional dances, the man may bow more dramatically while the woman acknowledges with a bend of knees or curtsey, the simple bow described here is appropriate for both genders.

buzz step (or **buzz turn**) A movement with a down-up motion in an uneven rhythm (slow-quick). When turning clockwise, dancers step on right foot with slightly bent knee, then push with ball of left foot as though on a scooter. Use opposite footwork for counterclockwise. Movement is smooth with feet close to the floor and no leaps. Dancers keep the outsides of their right feet close.

C

CW, CCW Movement directions clockwise and counterclockwise (see listings).

cast off Dancers at head of longways set, turn away from each other and lead their lines around the outside to the foot of the set.

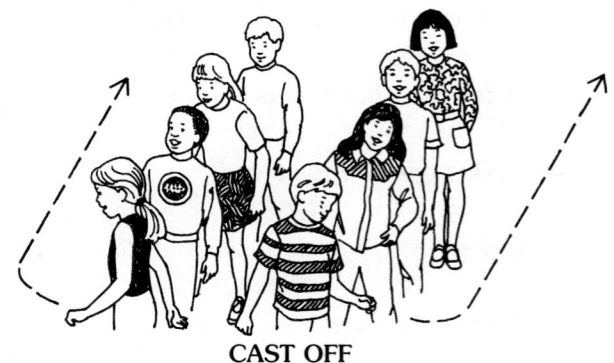

CAST OFF

circle formation A dance in a ring with hands joined or not. Examples of circles include single, double, concentric, and closed, and open (see individual listings.)

classroom choreography A dance pattern arranged for successful teaching in school settings. It may be based on traditional movements, but made more appropriate for schoolchildren. (See traditional dance)

clockwise A movement direction that progresses as do the hands of the clock, or around the circle to the left. Referred to in most dance notes as CW.

close A movement when the free foot comes up next to the supporting foot and takes weight. Also referred to as "together," as in step-together.

closed circle A circular formation that has no beginning or end. Hands may be joined or not.

collapse A basic stationary movement, collapse is the complete release of the body or body part into gravity.

concentric-circle formation Closed circles within circles, sometimes each moving to a different pattern or in opposite directions. Hands may be joined or not.

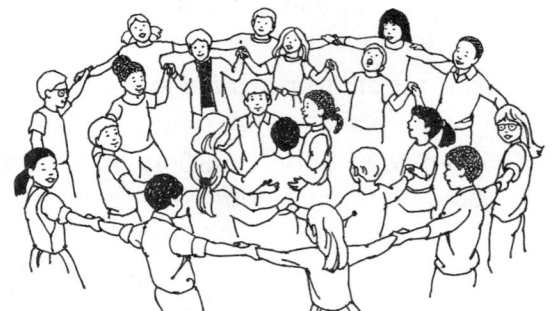

CONCENTRIC-CIRCLE FORMATION

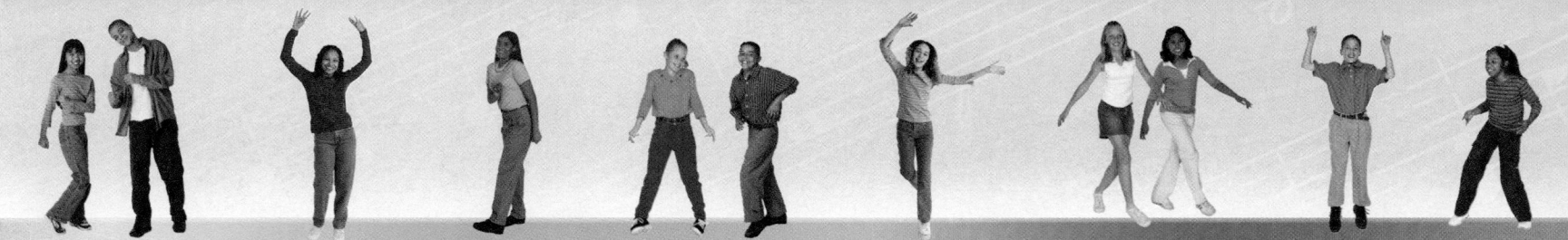

contra dance A traditional dance form, originally from the U.S. New England region. It is called "contra" because it is usually performed in longways sets with partners opposite (from the French contre).

contrast The diversity or variety between adjacent movements or patterns.

corner In contra dance or square dance, the person next to you who is not your partner.

counterclockwise A movement direction that progresses opposite to the hands of the clock, or around the circle to the right. Referred to in most dance notes as CCW.

crawl A basic locomotor movement, crawl is a weight transfer on a low level in space, using hands and knees or hands and feet.

creative dance Within the context of music education, a form of dance which develops skills related to the elements and concepts of movement while exploring possibilities for kinesthetic self-expression.

D

direction The spatial orientation of the line of motion. Directions include forward, backward, sideways, up and down.

do-si-do Dancers face and pass right or left shoulders, then go around each other back-to-back and return backwards, with no turns, to place. Originally and sometimes still called in square dancing do-sa-do (named for the French dos-á-dos or back-to-back).

double circle A couple formation in which partners stand side-by-side facing the same direction, or front-to-front with one person's back to the center and the other facing into the center.

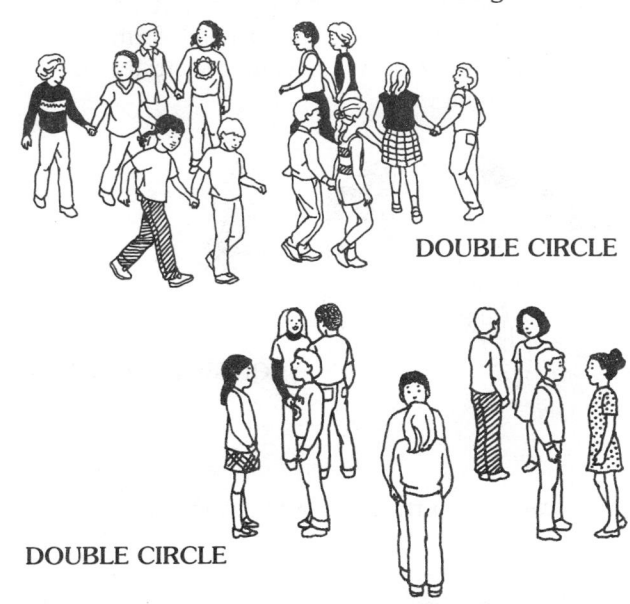

DOUBLE CIRCLE

DOUBLE CIRCLE

E

effort actions The Twentieth Century movement theorist Rudolf van Laban's terms referring to basic qualities of movement. The eight effort actions are: slash, press, thrust (punch), glide, wring, flick, float and tap (dab). (See individual listings.)

elbow swing (or **elbow turn**) Two dancers link right or left elbows and move in a circle.

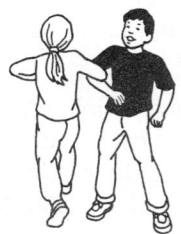

ELBOW SWING

energy One of the basic elements of dance, energy provides the "texture" or "color" of movement. Although variously described through the terms force, dynamics, weight, and movement qualities, energy refers to the way muscular power is used to produce qualities of motion.

entrance/exit The range of possibilities for entering and leaving the performing space.

F

flick A light, quick movement which is scattered or curved; one of the Laban effort actions. An example is the quick movement of butterfly wings.

float A light, slow, drifting movement; one of the Laban effort actions. An example is the movement of astronauts in outer space.

focus The direction of attention in movement. Focus most commonly refers to the gaze of the eyes.

formation Arrangement of dancers in the space. Examples include scattered, line, circle, Sicilian circle, concentric circle, double circle, longways set, square set.

G

gallop A basic locomotor movement with a forward step and a closing step in an uneven rhythm (slow-quick or quick-slow). Either of the steps can be leaps. The leading foot does not alternate. It is also possible to gallop backward.

general space (also **shared space**) The larger space in which movement can occur.

gesture A movement of a single part of the body usually on the periphery. Examples include a nod of the head, a tap of the foot, a wave. Gestures can have predetermined meanings, many of these translate worldwide.

glide A smooth, sustained, linear movement; one of the Laban effort actions. An example is the movement of skating or sledding.

grand right and left (also **right and left grand** or **grand chain**) A movement sequence in which partners progress around the circle in opposite directions by joining right hands and pulling past each other's right shoulder, then giving left hands to next person and passing left shoulders. They continue to alternate rights and lefts until they meet their partner, or the seventh or eighth person, as designated in the dance pattern.

grapevine pattern or step An intertwining 4-step movement pattern that can have several combinations and move clockwise or counterclockwise: step to side/cross in front/step to side/cross in back, or cross in front/step to side/cross in back/step to side, or other weaving patterns. In country-western "line" dances, grapevine means a 3-step pattern: side/back/side/touch.

group shape (group design) The sculptural grouping of more than one body in space, also known as "tableau," "portrait," or "stage picture."

H

hand holds Different ways to connect hands for dancing. Examples include ballroom, basket, pinkie, skater's, T, V, and W. (See individual listings.)

HAND HOLDS

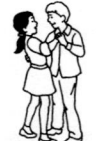 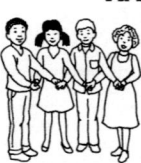 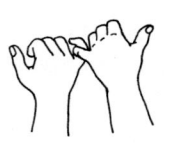 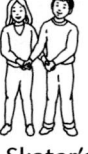

Ballroom   Basket   Pinkie   Skater's

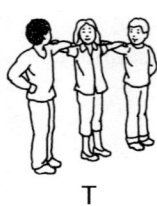 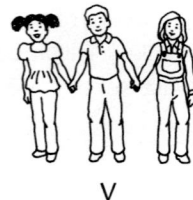 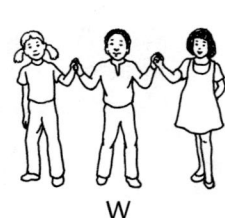

T   V   W

hand jive A nonlocomotor movement activity in which hand motions are performed to the musical beats.

head couple (or **top couple**) In a longways set, the couple closest to the band and caller or CD player and teacher.

hop A basic locomotor movement in even beat that has a takeoff and landing from one foot to the same foot.

I

improvise Movement that is created spontaneously, ranging from free-form to highly structured form. Improvisation always has an element of chance.

in place Movements performed without traveling.

J

jig A musical meter in $\frac{6}{8}$ as well as a set dance or solo exhibition dance, traditionally from the British Isles, in $\frac{6}{8}$ meter.

jump A basic locomotor movement in even beat that has a take-off and landing from one or both feet to both feet.

L

leader/follower In this versatile relationship, the follower imitates or copies the movement of a leader. The imitation can be sequential or simultaneous. Simultaneous leader/follower exercises can be done as mirrors where the leaders and followers are face-to-face, or as shadows where the followers are behind the leader. (See individual listings.)

leap A basic locomotor movement in even beat that has a take-off from one foot with a landing on the other, usually higher than that of a walk or run.

levels High, medium, and low areas of space.

line A formation in which dancers are side by side, facing the same direction. Hands are joined, using a variety of hand-holds. Lines can be short and straight or long and curved (sometimes called **open circles**).

locomotor movement (or **traveling movement**) Movement that carries the body from place to place using a transfer of weight. Examples include run, walk, skip, hop, jump, gallop, turn, crawl, and leap. (See individual listings.)

longways/contra set A dance formation that consists of partners facing in two parallel lines. The part closest to the caller and the music is the top or head, farthest away is the bottom or foot. Dancers travel up toward the top, or down toward the bottom.

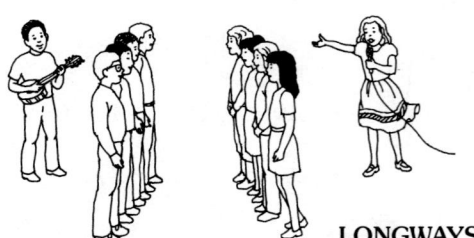

LONGWAYS / CONTRA SET

M

march To walk with a rhythmic stride to the steady beat.

mirror To follow in unison the movements of a partner or leader as if looking in a mirror.

mixer A group dance or singing game in which participants change partners each time the pattern repeats.

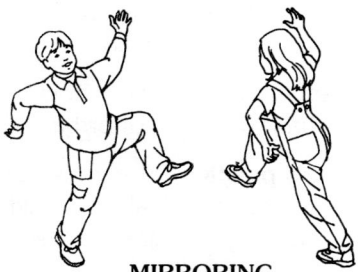

MIRRORING

movement echo Echoing repeats or copies a movement after the movement is done by a leader.

movement exploration To experiment with movements using variations on time, space, and energy.

movement phrase Similar to a grammatical phrase, a movement phrase is a natural grouping of movements with a sense of completion.

movement qualities Styles of movement created by the way force is used to begin and continue the actions.

> **percussive** characterized by sharp, forceful, explosive attack.
>
> **suspended** movement characterized by a momentary hanging of the body or a body part in space, followed by a collapse to gravity.
>
> **sustained** movement begun and continued with smooth, even force.
>
> **vibratory** movement in which the body or body part(s) shivers and or shakes as a result of rapid contractions and releases of muscles.

movement rondo Like the musical form, a movement rondo alternates contrasting movements or patterns with a recurring movement or pattern. For example, ABACAD.

N

nonlocomotor movement (or **stationary movement**) Movements that do not involve traveling from place to place. Some examples are bend, drop, swing, and twist.

O

open circle A nonclosed circular formation that has a leader at one or both ends.

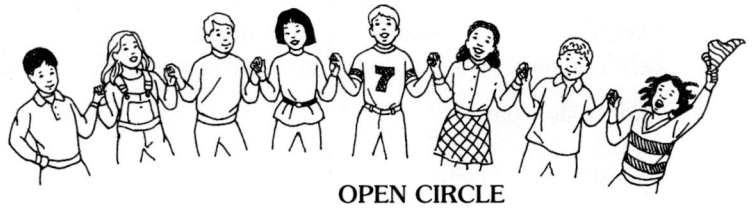

OPEN CIRCLE

P

pathway The line or trajectory created by movement in the air or on the floor. Spatial (air) pathways or floor pathways may be straight or curved.

pattern The smallest unit of form. Pattern usually involves several movements and makes use of repetition.

patterned dances Dances with a prescribed sequence of steps and/or movements.

peel off The movement enacted when individuals in a single file or column reach a designated spot and turn back down the line alternately to the right or left.

personal space (or **self space**) The sphere or "bubble" of space that immediately surrounds the body in stillness or motion.

pinkie hold A hand hold, usually in the W position, in which little fingers are joined. Generally it is right under and left over ("right under the leftovers"). (See **hand holds**.)

pivot A turn clockwise or counterclockwise on the ball of one or both feet.

play-party A music game, originating in nineteenth-century U.S. in response to religious prohibitions against dancing. Traditionally, the accompaniment was only singing and foot stomping, as the fiddle was "the devil's instrument."

press A strong, slow, sustained linear movement where the force is focused in direction; one of the Laban effort actions. An example is the movement of rowing a boat.

progression Mostly in contra dances and those of the British Isles, the movement of each couple is to the next position in the set.

promenade A figure in which partners join hands and walk together around the circle.

promenade position (or **skater's position**) A partner position in which individuals stand side by side, facing the same direction, with right hands joined over left hands in front of the body. There are also other promenade positions; this is best for school-age students.

pull A basic stationary movement that moves toward the center of the body. Beginning with a stretch, pull moves into a bend with the use of force.

push A basic stationary movement that moves away from the center of the body. Beginning with a bend, push extends into a stretch with the use of force.

R

reel A musical meter in $\frac{4}{4}$ as well as a set dance from the British Isles and the U.S. in $\frac{4}{4}$ meter. A reel is also a way to join arms in traditional longways dances, sometimes called "strip the willow."

right-hand star A figure in which four or more dancers join right hands and circle clockwise. A left-hand star goes counterclockwise. Also called a wheel, a mill, or right-hands-across, hands may be joined by piling them in the middle, grasping the one opposite, or holding the wrist ahead.

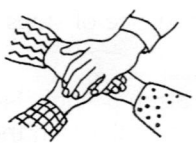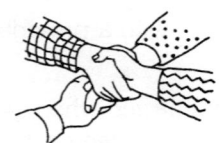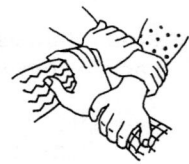

RIGHT-HAND STAR

ring Another way to refer to circle formations, especially in historic dances.

run A basic locomotor movement in even rhythm that transfers weight from one foot to the other with a moment when both feet are off the ground.

 S

sashay (or **chassé, side gallop, slide, slip**) A sideways locomotor movement in uneven rhythm (slow-quick, slow-quick) in a side-close, side-close pattern.

scattered formation A random arrangement of dancers within the assigned space.

set An arrangement of dancers in square, longways, or groups-of-three formations. Also refers to the setting step, or balance step, in English country dances.

shadow To imitate the movements of a person from behind him or her.

shape The sculptural line or design of one or more bodies in space. (See **group shape**.)

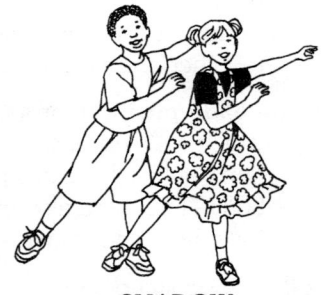

SHADOW

Sicilian circle A dance formation in which couples face other couples around the circle, with one pair facing and progressing counterclockwise, the other facing and progressing clockwise.

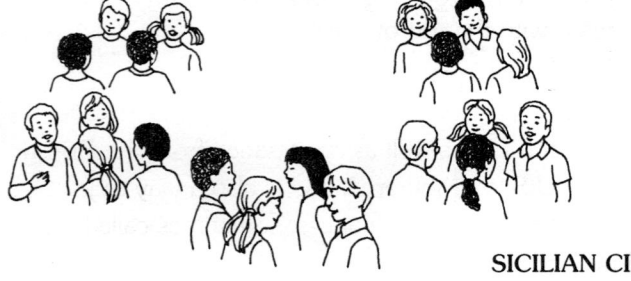

SICILIAN CIRCLE

single circle A ring formation with dancers usually facing the center of the circle; hands may be joined or not.

skater's hold A partner hold in which right hands join over left hands in front of or behind the body. (See **hand holds**.)

skater's position (or **promenade position**) A partner position where individuals stand side by side, facing same direction, with right hands joined over left hands in front of or behind the body.

skip A basic locomotor movement that combines a step and a hop with alternating feet in an uneven rhythm (slow-quick, slow-quick).

slash A sharp, strong, curved movement; one of the Laban effort actions. An example is the movement of whirling helicopter blades.

slide See sashay.

space A basic dance element, referring to the area through which one moves.

square dance A traditional U.S. form performed by four couples in a four-sided or box formation.

square set An arrangement of four couples in an imaginary box formation, each couple standing on a different side of the box, all facing center. In U.S. and British Isles squares, couple 1 has its back to the music, then count counterclockwise for couples 2, 3, and 4. Couples 1 and 3 are head couples, 2 and 4 are side couples.

stage directions:

    down stage portion of the performance area closest to the audience.

    stage left portion of stage area to left of performer.

    stage right portion of the performance area to right of performer.

    up stage portion of the performance area most distant from the audience.

stamp As used in patterned dances, placing the foot firmly on the floor and lifting it slightly so as not to take weight (see also stomp); the next movement is done on the same foot. As body percussion, a stamp takes weight.

stationary movement (or **nonlocomotor movement**) Movement done in place. Stationary movement does not travel. Examples include bend, stretch, twist, swing, sway, push/pull, and collapse. (See individual entries.)

step-close A step pattern in which the dancer steps on one foot and brings the other foot beside the first foot (step-together), taking the weight also on the second foot.

step-hop A basic step pattern that includes a step and a hop in an even rhythm.

step in place Walking without traveling through space.

step-together See step-close.

step-touch A step pattern where the dancer steps on one foot and brings the other foot beside the first foot, touching it to the floor but not putting weight on it.

stomp As used in patterned dances, placing the foot firmly on the floor and taking weight on it. (See also **stamp**.) The next movement will be on the other foot.

stretch A basic stationary movement in which there is full extension of a body part or the whole body.

sway A stationary movement that moves side to side, or front and back. Sway is a gentle, rocking movement of one body part or the whole body shifting weight in place.

swing A basic stationary movement that occurs when the body or a body part moves in an arc or circle. Swinging includes several phases: the release of the body/body part into gravity, and the lift and suspension of the body/body part on the other side of the arc.

swing As used in patterned dances, turning with various hand or arm holds such as a two-hand swing or elbow swing. Also, swing is a nonlocomotor movement in which one knee lifts as its foot lightly swings across the other leg. Also, swing is, of course, the popular couple dance that used to be called the jitterbug.

T

T hold The shoulder hold in which dancers, usually in a circle formation, place their hands on their neighbors' nearest shoulders. Arms are somewhat extended to form a "T." (See **hand holds**.)

tap A quick, light, staccato movement which moves to one point; one of the Laban effort actions. An example is the movement of knocking on the door.

thrust A fast, strong, linear movement that moves to one point; one of the Laban effort actions. An example is the movement of a karate blow.

top of the set The end of the set closest to the band and caller or the music source.

traditional dances Dances that have roots in a culture, or have been passed down through generations mostly unchanged, or have some claim to historical accuracy.

turn A locomotor movement that indicates the body revolving around its vertical axis while traveling through space. Turning can be done while walking, skipping, hopping, galloping, or leaping.

twist A nonlocomotor movement in which the body or body part rotates on its axis.

two-step A movement pattern in which the dancer steps forward on the first foot, closes with the second foot, steps forward again on the first foot, and holds for a beat. It may also be done in other directions.

U

unison movement Two or more dancers performing the same movement at the same time.

V

V hold A partner or group position in which individuals stand side by side with hands joined and held down, making "Vs" between them. (See **hand holds**.)

W

W hold A partner or group position in which individuals stand side by side with hands joined at shoulder level and elbows down, making "Ws" between them. (See **hand holds**.)

walk A basic locomotor movement in even rhythm in which weight is transferred from one foot to the other, keeping continual contact with the floor. There is a wide range of possibilities for varying the walk. Examples include character walks, inventive walks, walks of varying tempos and directions, and walks expressing various emotions.

weaving (or **winding**) A movement pattern in which some dancers go around other dancers who are standing still, often with arms raised in arches or windows.

weight The concept of weight includes several different meanings. In the context of transferring weight, it refers to the downward force of the vertical axis of the body as it moves in space. Laban's use of the term refers to weight as the intensity of force used in the muscles as in light or heavy. Weight can also refer to the quality of the body giving in to gravity or allowing gravity to work on it.

wring A strong, sustained, twisting movement; one of the Laban effort actions. An example is the movement of squeezing water from a towel.

wring the dishrag Partners face, joining two hands and swinging them overhead in the same direction to complete a circle while turning the bodies back-to-back and ending up face-to-face.

Dance Directions

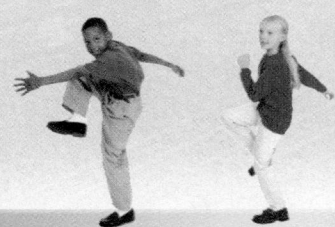

Red River Valley, p. 11 CD 1-11

Choreography by Sanna Longden, based on notes from the Kentucky Dance Institute

Routine: Intro (2 m.); v. 1; refrain; interlude (8 m.); v. 2; refrain; interlude (8 m.); refrain; coda

Formation: Divide the class into groups of three. Each trio gets together with another trio and, with one trio facing the other, makes a circle, holding hands. The circles of six people should be arranged in a "circle," as well. For example, if there are four circles of six, place them at 12, 3, 6, and 9 o'clock positions.

Part 1	Verse 1
Measures 1–2	• Each trio greets the trio they are facing.
Measures 3–4	• All six join hands in a circle and move to the left (4 beats) and right (4 beats).
Measures 5–6	• Center person turns with the person on their right, using elbows, 2 hands, ballroom hold, etc.
Measures 7–8	• Center person turns with the person on their left.
Part 2	Refrain
Measures 9–10	• Each trio moves to its right to pass by the other threesome and progresses to the next trio coming toward them along the circle.
Measures 11–12	• New groups of six join hands and repeat the circling as in Part 1.
Measures 13–14	• The four outside students make a right-hand-star (see Movement Glossary, p. 552).
Measures 15–16	• The center students pass right shoulders in a do-si-do (see Movement Glossary, p. 549).
Part 3	Instrumental
Measures 13–14	• The right-hand person in each trio changes places by passing right shoulders and joining the other trio.
Measures 15–16	• The left-hand person in each trio changes places by passing right shoulders and joining the other trio.

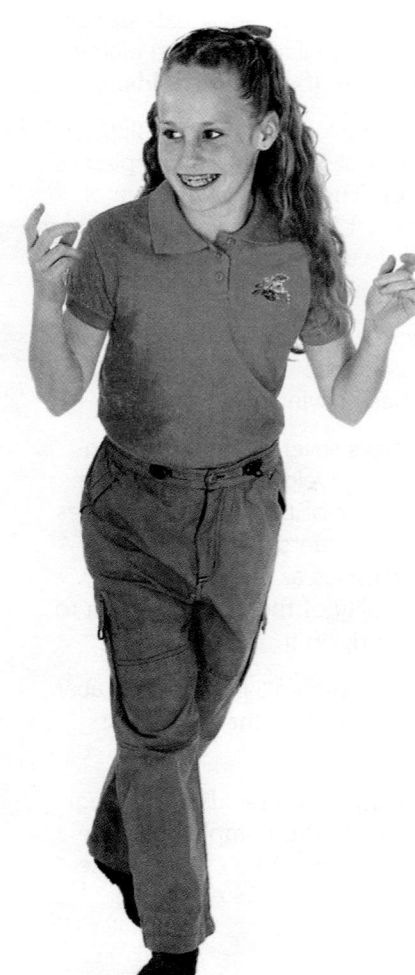

Dance repeats with Verse 2, Refrain, and Instrumental sections as above. On the last Refrain, do Part 1 again. *Coda:* Same six people make a right-hand star. Finish with a "Yee-hah!"

Sellenger's Round, p. 44 CD 3-14

English Dance from "The English Dancing Master," by John Playford
Contributed by Sanna Longden, based on multiple sources

Routine: (Instrumental) Intro (4); part 1 (ABB); part 2 (ABB); part 3 (ABB); part 4 (ABB). (Practice track repeats entire routine.)

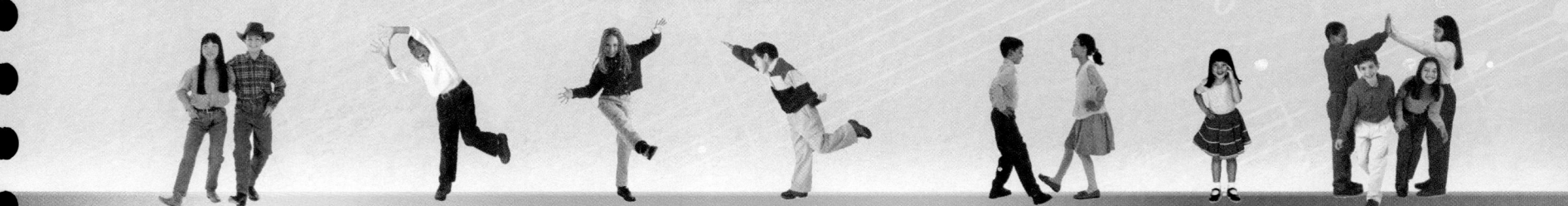

Sellenger's Round first appeared in John Playford's 1670 edition of *The English Dancing Master.* Like many dances by Playford, it is in rondo form.

Formation: Divide the class into pairs. Boy or girl pairs are traditional, but not necessary. Have students form a single circle of partners, with the "girl" on the right of the "boy." All face center, with hands joined down at sides in V-hold position (see Movement Glossary, p. 553).

Part 1: Circling (A)

Measures 1–8
- Students circle to the left with 8 sashay or side-gallop steps, then repeat to the right.

Chorus (B)

Measures 9–10
- Students dance into center with 2 two-steps: right-left-right-and, left-right-left-and. (See Movement Glossary.)

Measures 11–12
- Students move backwards to place right foot, left foot, right foot, left foot.

Measures 13–14
- Partners face each other, and dance 2 two-steps in place: right-left-right-and, left-right-left-and.

Measures 15–16
- Each person turns to his or her right in 4 counts.

- Students repeat chorus.

Part 2: Up a Double and Back (A)

Measures 1–2
- All join hands and move toward center: right foot, left foot, right foot, touch.

Measures 3–4
- All move in a double back to place: left foot, right foot, left foot, touch.

Measures 5–8
- Students repeat mm. 1–4.

Chorus (B)
- Students repeat chorus movements above.

Part 3: Siding (A)

Measures 1–8
- Partners walk toward each other, right shoulder to right shoulder: right foot, left foot, right foot, touch; then back away, left foot, right foot, left foot, touch. Repeat for mm. 5–8.

Chorus (B)
- Students repeat movements for first chorus.

Part 4: Arming (A)

Measures 1–8
- Partners do a right elbow turn for 8 counts, then a left elbow turn for 8 counts.

Chorus (B)
- Students repeat movements for first chorus.

It is customary in *Sellenger's Round* to end the dance with a repeat of Part 1. However, this recording offers enough music for a repeat of Parts 2 and 3, ending with a final chorus and an elegant bow.

Kerenski, p. 78 CD 5-4

Collected and notated by Sanna Longden

Routine: Intro, v. 1 (ABC); v. 2 (ABC); v. 3 (ABC); v. 4 (ABC)

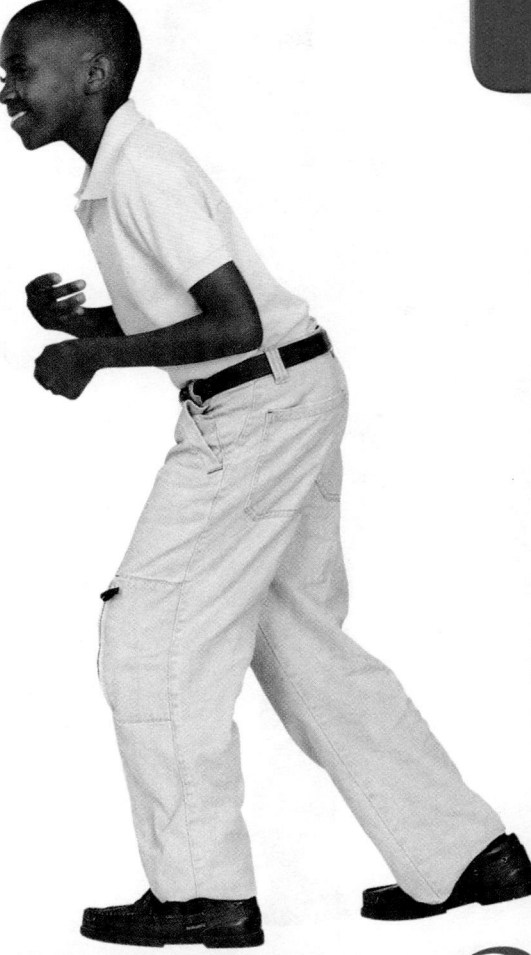

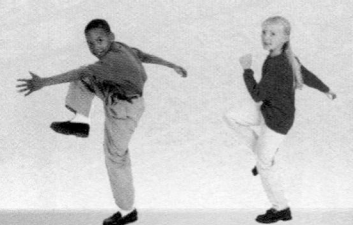

Kerenski was popular in Finland during the 1920s and is still performed today. It is similar to a well-known Russian dance and there is a good reason for this similarity—Finland was part of Russia from 1809 to 1917. Some of the Russian aristocracy had summer homes in Finland, so the local folk had opportunities to learn Russian social dances. This Finnish version of the dance was named for Alexander Feodorovich Kerenski, a premier of Soviet Russia.

Formation: Divide the class into pairs. Students will stand as couples, in ballroom dance position or with both hands joined, scattered around the dance space, ready to move counterclockwise around the floor.

A Section

Measures 1–2	• Pairs step side, together, side, together. Boys begin on left foot, girls on right foot.
Measures 3–4	• Students walk four steps forward.
Measures 5–8	• Students repeat mm. 1–4 but end with a touch (no weight on the foot).
Measures 9–16	• Pairs repeat mm. 1–8 in the opposite direction, with opposite footwork. Students keep the same position, just turning their faces in the direction they are moving.

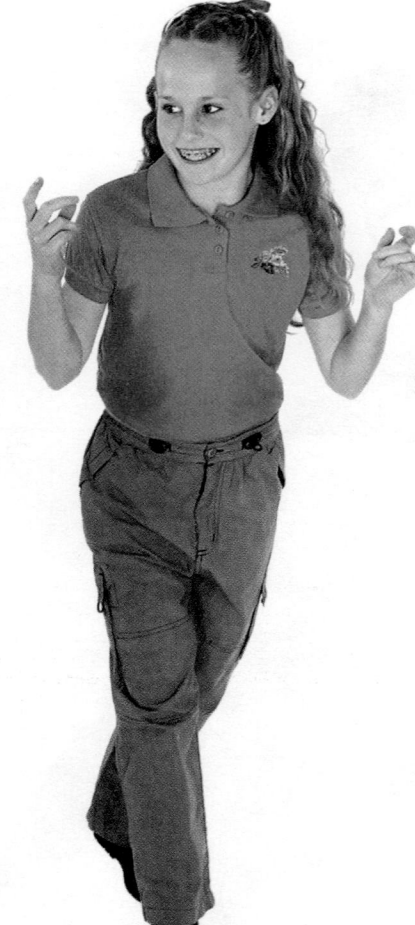

B Section

Pairs join inside hands at shoulder height and face counterclockwise.

Measures 17–18	• Starting with the outside foot, students move as follows: step, lift, step, lift.
Measures 19–20	• Partners turn away from each other and take 2 walking steps or 1 two-step, then turn back with 2 walking steps or 1 two-step.
Measures 21–24	• Students repeat mm. 17–20.

C Section

Boys face out, girls face center. Both have hands on hips, or boys can beckon to partners as girls indicate "no" by shaking index fingers in Measures 25–28. Reverse roles in mm. 29–32.

Measures 25–28	• Boys move backward into center. Girls follow, moving forward. Both take 3 step-hops or 6 walking steps, then 3 stomps.
Measures 29–32	• Repeat mm. 25–28. This time, girls move backward and boys move forward.
Measures 33–40	• Partners go to ballroom position and perform 8 smooth turning two-steps or polka steps moving in the line of dance. A simpler alternative is to have partners go to skater's position or crossed-hands hold (see Movement Glossary, p. 552), then move counterclockwise with 8 two-steps or 16 walking steps.

Hit Me with a Hot Note and Watch Me Bounce, p. 112 CD 6-31

Choreography by Wendy Taucher

Routine: Intro (4 m.); v. 1; v. 2; bridge; v. 3.; coda

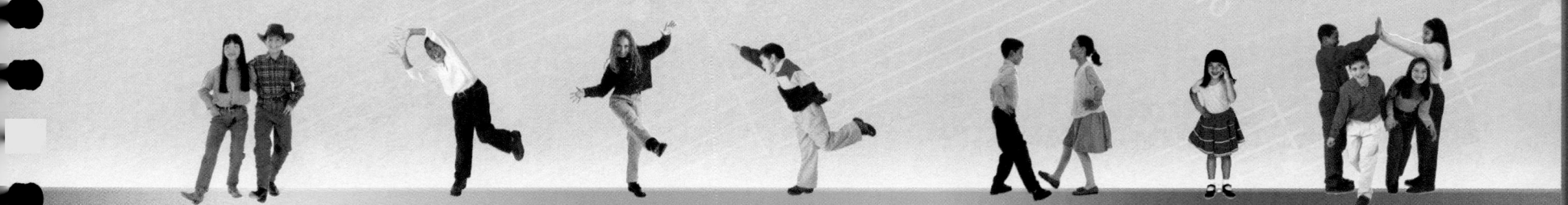

Directions

Write on index cards these body movements students can perform: bounce head, shake hands, move arms, bounce elbows, move torso, bounce on toes. Put the cards in a container. Invite students to think of ways to keep the beat in groups of 8 counts.

Divide the class into two groups. One group will be the "beat keepers;" the other group will be the "movers." Draw one "mover" card at a time, and have the "movers" perform the movement named on the card, while the "beat keepers" keep the beat with the movements decided on by the class. Repeat the activity, having students switch roles.

Encourage students to perform only the movement named on the card, keeping the rest of the body still.

Hava nagila, p. 153 CD 8-23

Contributed and notated by Sanna Longden

Routine: Intro (4 m.); vocal; interlude (4 m.); vocal

People dance the *hora* as they sing "Hava nagila." The dance came to Israel in the early twentieth century when the land was called Palestine. (Israel became a nation in 1948.) It was brought by settlers from Romania, where horas are popular circle dances. In fact, the word hora means "circle dance." The Israeli hora was originally done in closed circles with hands joined and held down at the sides in a V hold position or with hands on neighbors' shoulders in a T hold position (see Movement Glossary, p. 553). In Israel, the traditional hora moves clockwise, although today horas can move in any direction. The hora has a six-beat pattern, while "Hava nagila" has four beats per measure, so two times through the dance pattern will take three measures of music. People also dance the hora with other songs. See "Alumot" on p. 306.

Formation: Students stand in a closed circle, facing center, hands joined down at sides in a V hold position or on neighbors' shoulders in a T hold position. In a large group, there may be two or more concentric circles (see Movement Glossary, p. 548), each going in the opposite direction from the circle in front of it.

Directions • Students step onto left foot, then step onto right foot, crossing over in front or in back, step onto left foot again, lift right foot while bouncing or hopping on left foot, step onto right foot, then lift left foot while bouncing or hopping on right foot.

Version Two • Students leap onto left foot, then leap onto right foot, crossing over in front or in back, jump on both feet, kick right foot while hopping on left foot, jump on both feet, then kick left foot while hopping on right foot.

Así es mi tierra, p. 172 CD 9-35

Arranged and notated by Sanna Longden, based on traditional dances

Routine: Intro (4 m.); vocal (AABA); vocal (AABA); coda

The movements for this dance come from the people who live on both sides of the Mexico-United States border. Just like examples of "world music," which may combine elements from several cultures, *norteño* (nor-TEH-nyoh) dances combine the vigorous northern Mexican style with U.S. and European steps. This *"Así es mi tierra"* dance is typical of Tex-Mex polkas.

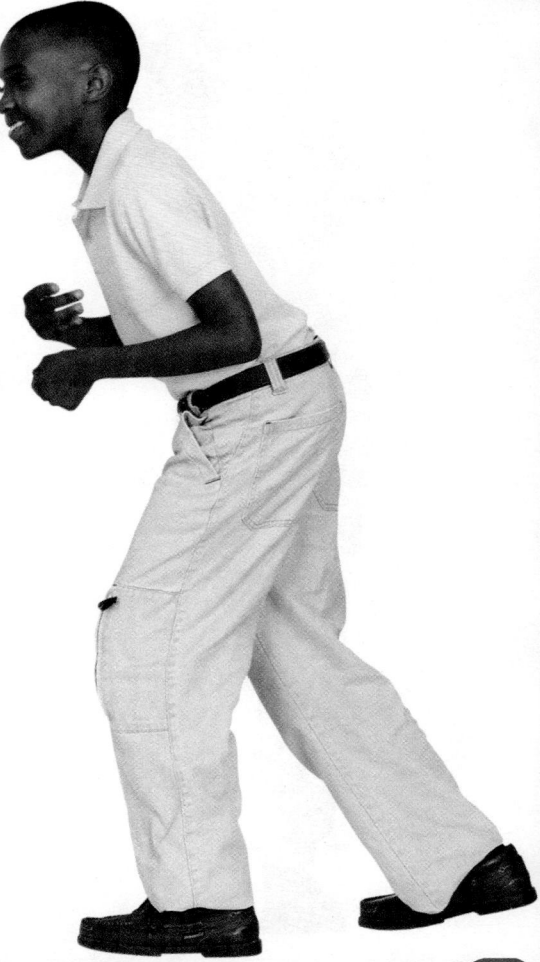

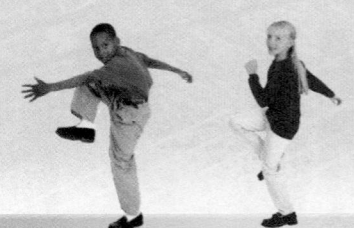

Formation: Divide the class into pairs and have students stand in a longways set (see Movement Glossary, p. 550) for four couples. Assign each couple a number, 1 to 4, starting with the pair at the top of the set. Boys have left shoulders toward the music source. Girls face them with right shoulders toward the music source.

Styling: This pleasant song allows for a somewhat slower pace and pauses between polkas. Girls hold "skirts" out at sides and do fancy flourishes ("skirt work"); boys hook thumbs in handsome "belt buckles." Have students use polka steps, two-steps, or just walking steps.

Introduction   Girls do "skirt work," while swaying in place. Boys also stand in place, swaying slightly.

A Section Part 1—Forward and Backward

Measures 1–3   *Así_es mi tierra, morenita_y luminosa;*
  * The downbeat of m. 1 is on the word *tierra*. Partners take 3 polka steps toward each other. Boys begin on left foot, girls on right.

Measure 4–7   *Así_es mi tierra, tiene_el alma hecha de_amor.*
  * Boys stamp right foot, girls stamp left foot (no weight on stamped foot), then move backward, 3 polka steps away from partner, starting on the stamped foot.

Measure 8   *Así_es mi*
  * Boys stamp left foot, girls stamp right foot.

Measures 9–16   *tierra, abundante_y . . . calor!*
  * Students repeat mm. 1–8.

A Section Part 2—Exchanging Partners

Measures 1–4   *Así_es mi tierra, morenita_y luminosa; Así_es mi*
  * Boy 1 in each set takes girl 1 to the foot of set and leaves her there in 8 sashay steps (see Movement Glossary, p. 552).

Measures 5–8   *tierra, tiene_el alma_hecha de_amor. Asi_es mi*
  * Same boy takes girl 4 from the foot of the set to the top of the set (girl 1's former spot) with 8 sashay steps.

Measures 9–12   *tierra, abundante_y generosa; ¡Ay, tierra*
  * Boy 4 takes girl 1 back to the top of the set (above girl 4), in 8 sashay steps.

Measures 13–15   *mía como_es grato tu calor!*
  * Boy 4 takes girl 4 back to her original place at bottom of set. (Students shift in a natural way to fill empty positions.)

B Section Part 3—Elbow Turns

Measures 16–23   *Sus alboradas . . . al amor.*
  * All partners do right-elbow turns for 4 polka steps, then left-elbow turns for 4 polka steps.

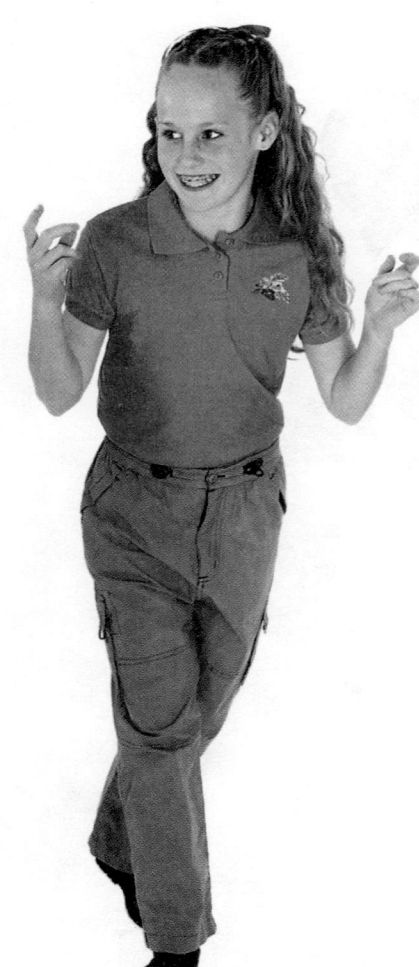

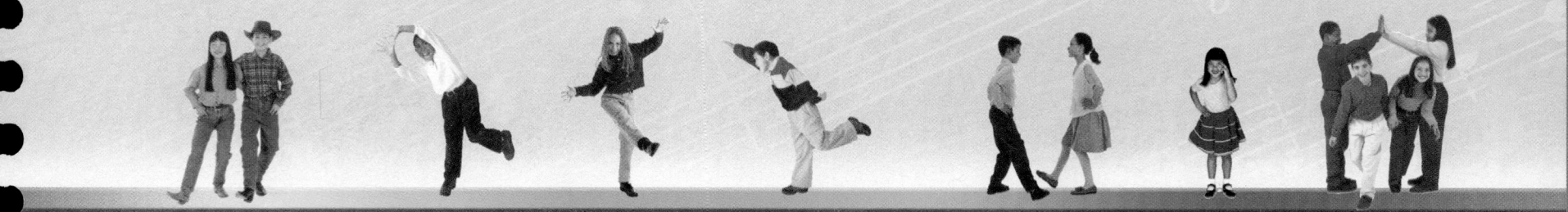

A Section Part 4—Cast off and do-si-do

Measures 24–32 *Así_es mi tierra, . . . como es grato tu calor!*

- Pair 1 in each set casts off (see Movement Glossary, p. 548), and travels down the outside of the set to the bottom with 8 polka steps, while pairs 2, 3, and 4 do a right-shoulder do-si-do (see Movement Glossary, p. 548) for 4 polka steps, then repeat with left shoulders. As they dance, they shift positions, so couple 2 becomes the top couple to begin the dance again.

Mary Ann, p. 180 CD 10–10

Arranged and notated by Sanna Longden

Routine: Intro (4 m.); v. 1; interlude (4 m.); interlude (4 m.); v. 3; coda

When people dance in the West Indies, they usually do not follow special patterns—they just move to the music! Students can start with this basic calypso step, then improvise some steps of their own.

Formation: Divide the class into pairs, and have students scatter around the dance space, partners facing or not.

Styling: Encourage students to keep steps small and underneath the body. Advise them to relax shoulders and soften knees, but maintain an upright torso. Their arms do not hang straight down, but dangle at sides with elbows slightly bent, moving gently along with rest of body.

Basic Step
- Students step with right foot in front of left and a small hip twist (count 1), step left foot in place (count 2), step right foot next to left foot (count 3), and step left foot in place (count 4). This pattern can also start on left foot. Students may repeat the basic step as many times as desired. To start on the opposite foot, students should touch with no weight instead of stepping on count 4. Here are some variations students can try.

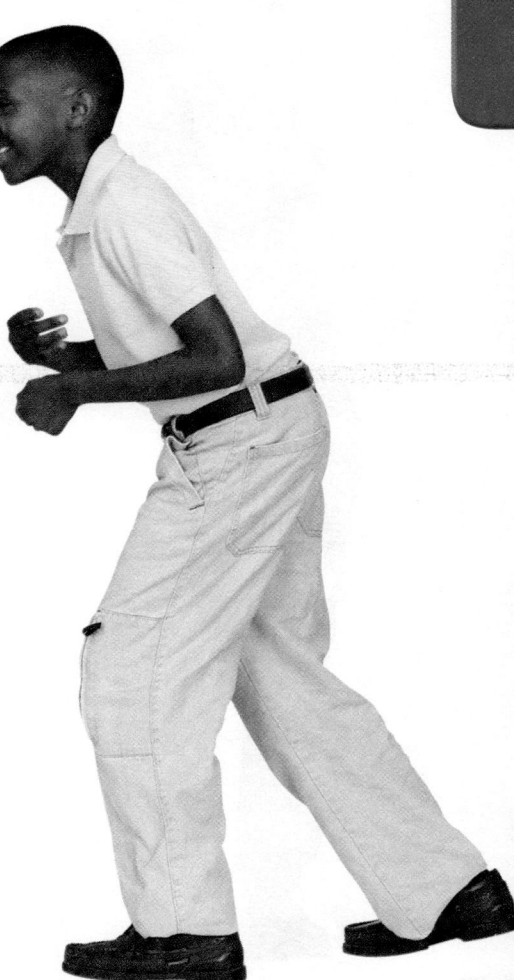

Measures 1–8 *Side-by-Side*
- Partners stand side by side and perform 4 basic steps on the same or opposite feet, then switch the starting feet for 4 more basic steps.

Face-to-Face
- Partners face each other and perform 4 basic steps, with one partner moving forward, the other moving backward. Then partners switch starting feet and direction for 4 more basic steps.

Switch Positions
- Partners do 4 basic steps side by side, then 4 basic steps face-to-face.

Do-Si-Do
- One partner does a do-si-do around the other with 4 basic steps, while the other dances in place. Then partners switch roles.

Double Do-Si-Do
- Partners do-si-do around each other in 4 basic steps, passing right shoulders, then do-si-do around each other passing left shoulders for 4 more basic steps.

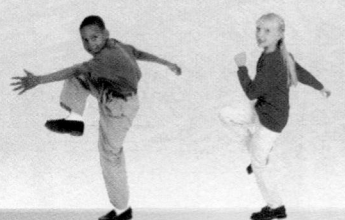

Face-and-Turn

- Partners face each other and perform 4 basic steps, then both turn alone in a full circle for 4 more basic steps.

Measures 9–16
- Partners separate and move around the dance space among the other dancers. They progress forward with 8 basic steps, starting with either the right or left foot, then switching to opposite footwork after measure 4. To cover more ground, they can take a bigger step on each count 1. On measure 8, everyone should stop near a new partner. Each new partner will inspire new ways of using the basic step.

Interlude
- New partners greet each other by circling face to face with basic steps.

Coda
- All dance toward the center of the dance space with basic steps, ending in a happy group.

Four Potatoes Medley, p. 205 CD 11-9, 11-10

Contra dance arranged and notated by Sanna Longden

Recording Routine: *Four Potatoes only:* (Instrumental) A B A B A B A B; then as performed for the remainder of the medley.

This contra dance is based on the *Pam and Pat Reel*. Contra dancing (which gets its name from the position of the two opposing lines or, in French, *contre*) is a popular form of social dance in the United States, a modified form of English country dances brought by the first New England settlers. There are myriad patterns, both traditional and contemporary.

Formation: Divide the class into pairs, and have students stand in a longways set (see Movement Glossary, p. 550) of 6–10 couples. Callers should call the movements 4–8 beats ahead of time.

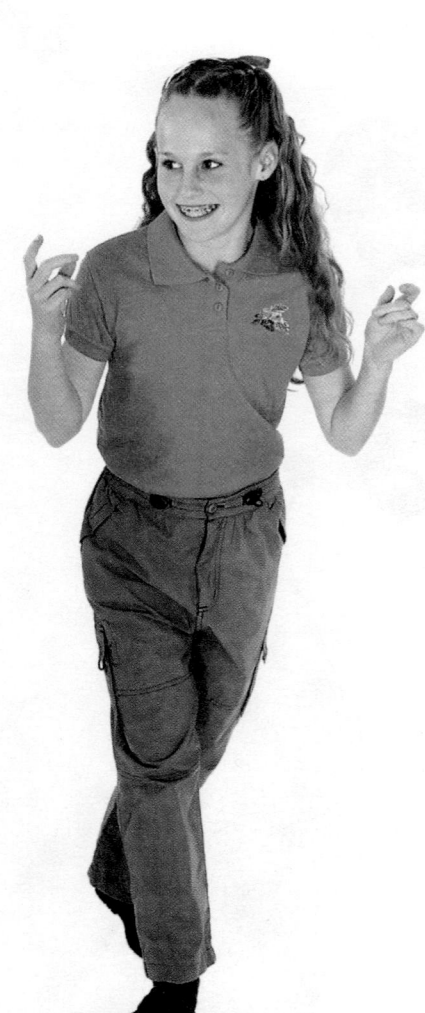

A Section

Counts 1–8
- Partners walk toward each other for 4 counts, bow quickly, and walk backward 4 counts.

Counts 9–16
- Partners hook right elbows and walk 8 steps clockwise back to place.

Counts 17–24
- Students repeat counts 1–8.

Counts 25–32
- Partners hook left elbows and walk 8 steps counterclockwise back to place.

B Section

Counts 1–8
- First two couples make a right-hand-star (see Movement Glossary, p. 552), then the next two couples, then the next two, and so forth. All walk 8 steps clockwise back to place.

Counts 9–16
- Same couples make left-hand-stars, then walk 8 steps counterclockwise back to place.

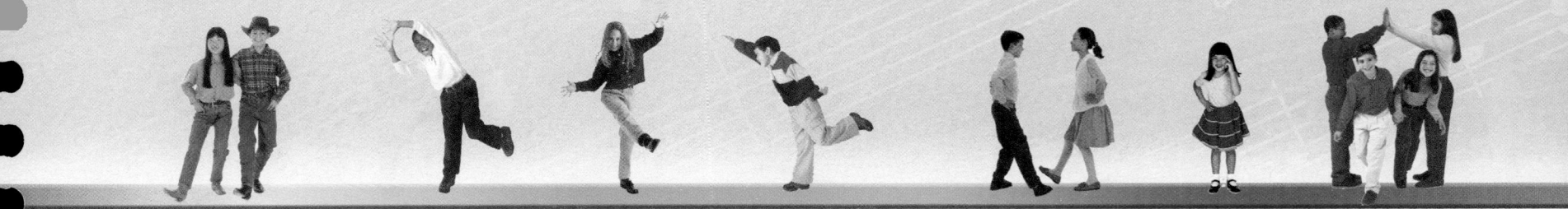

Kpanlogo for 2, p. 296 CD 15-6

Notated by Sanna Longden, based on notes of Dick Oakes and Tony Shay

Routine: As performed

"Highlife" is the generic name for a type of West African dance that is a combination of European social dance and indigenous folk movements. This highlife is arranged from dances of the Ewe, Ga, Ashanti, and Yoruba tribes of Ghana. The movements provided here are only suggestions—figures may vary from student to student.

Formation: Students scatter individually around the room, facing center. Have them bend elbows at sides, forearms parallel to floor and held loosely, forefingers pointing down, knees soft. Movements are loose and relaxed.

Basic Step	• With weight on left leg, students touch right heel toward center with toe pointing up and point at right toe with right index finger (Count 1). Then they step on right foot with bent knees (Count 2). Students repeat with opposite foot and finger work, which completes one basic step. Students may wish to start the dance with 8 basic steps.
Variations	Students may add these ideas to the basic footwork.
Sawing	• Students hold palms down, left above right, knees bent, and saw out and down, then in and back for 4 measures.
Egg Beating	• Students keep knees bent, and make a mixing motion with one hand under the opposite elbow for 2 measures, then switch mixing hand and "mixing bowl" arm for 2 measures.
Small Drum	• Students do 3 basic steps, then lift in place, and pantomime beating a drum, hands moving up and down in front of them.
Large Drum	• Students do 3 basic steps, then lift in place, and pantomime beating a big bass drum, hands moving side to side in front of them.
Big Chicken	• Students spread knees, put hands on waist, and "flap" their elbows in and out.
Flying Chicken	• Elbows to side and palms to floor, students do 2 basic steps in and 2 out.
Swimming in Place	• Students do exaggerated "crawl stroke," feet together, knees bent.
Swimming to Center	• Same as "swimming in place," but move forward.
Swimming Back Out	• Same as "swimming in place," but move backward.

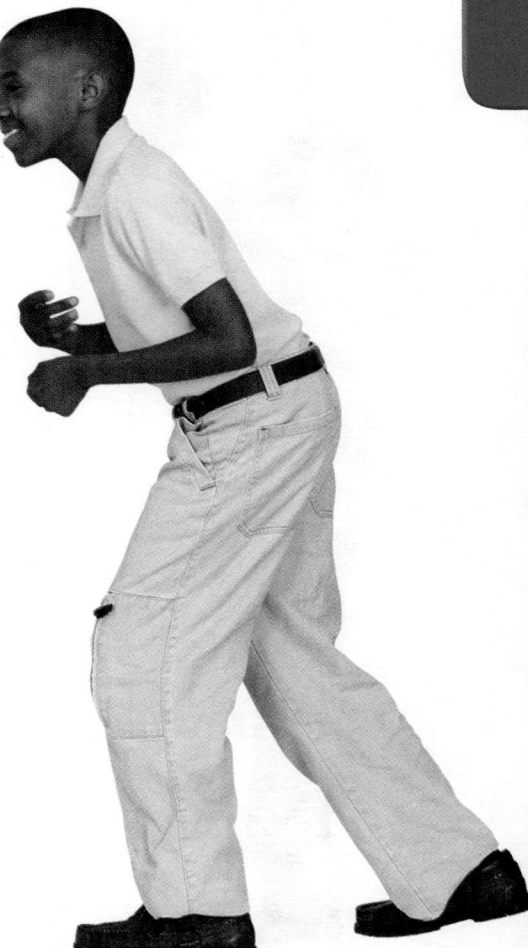

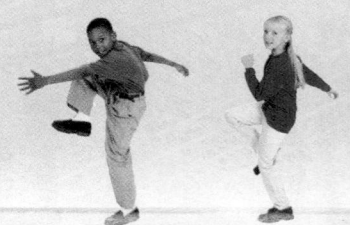

Dham dhamak dham samelu, p. 305 CD 15-24

Notated by Sanna Longden, based on traditional dance figures

Routine: As performed

This dance, called *Raas,* is a stick dance from the Gujerati region of India. It is often performed at festivals such as Indian New Year, which comes in late October or early November. The sticks are often decorated with painted bands of red, orange, yellow, and other colors. The dancers wear colorful clothing, with red as the dominant color. The dance is often done to *garba* music. The songs are usually about the harvest and festive occasions. It has a strong, hypnotic beat like rock music and may go on for 15–30 minutes. The dance can also be performed to rock or disco music.

Formation: Divide the class into pairs. Students may stand in a circle of partners or in a longways set (See Movement Glossary, p. 550). If students are in a circle, one partner has his or her back to center of circle, while the other is facing center. Ideally, each person has two sturdy sticks (about 18–24 inches long). Classroom rhythm sticks work well.

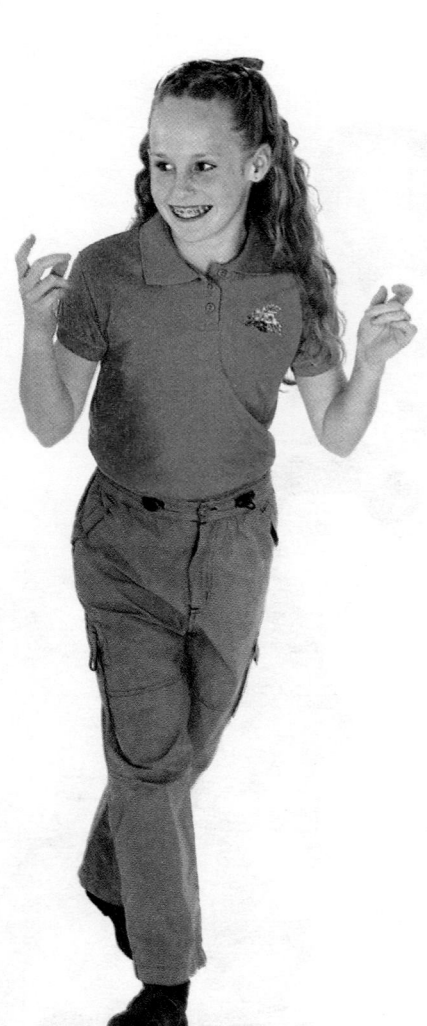

Footwork	• Students step on right foot, touch left toe next to right foot, step on left foot, touch right toe next to left foot. Students may also begin on left foot. There are five step-touches in each pattern. On each touch, students hit sticks together.
Stick-Work	Begin on vocal.
Step-Touch 1	• Students hit own sticks at their right side.
Step-Touch 2	• Students keep sticks parallel and close together and lean them diagonally to the right to hit partner's sticks.
Step-Touch 3	• Students repeat step-touch 2, leaning sticks to the left.
Step-Touch 4	• Students hit own sticks at their left side.
Step-Touch 5	• Students hit their right stick against their partner's right stick. They may wish to spin around individually after they tap sticks.

This dance may also be done as a mixer. If this is the case, each student will move to the left during each new step-touch 1. They will become partners with the next person on their left, and be ready to tap sticks with their new partner on step-touch 2.

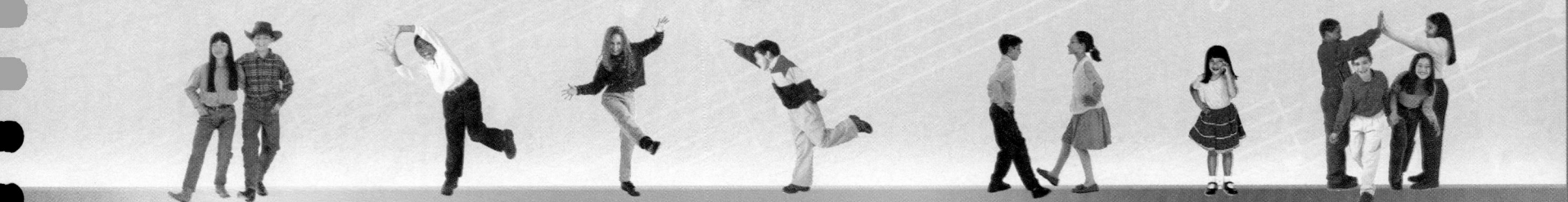

Alumot, p. 306 CD 15-30

Hora notated by Sanna Longden

Routine: Intro (4 m.); vocal 1; interlude (4 m.); vocal 2; coda

Al yadee, p. 308 CD 15-34

Debke notated by Sanna Longden

Routine: Intro (4 m.); verse; interlude (12 m.); interlude (12 m.); verse

Both the *hora* and the *debke* come from the Middle East. The steps are quite similar, but there are some interesting differences in style. The *hora* came to Israel in the early twentieth century when the land was called Palestine. The dance was originally from Romania, where horas are popular circle dances. In fact, the word *hora* means "circle dance." The Israeli *hora* was originally done in closed circles with hands joined and held down at the sides in a V hold position, or with hands on neighbors' shoulders in a T hold position. In Israel, the traditional *hora* moves to the left (clockwise), although now *horas* move in any direction. The steps are high and joyous, with leaps and kicks.

The *debke* (sometimes called *debky*) is one of the most common types of Arab dance. The word means "line dance," and traditional *debkes* are often done in short lines. Dancers generally join hands down at sides in a V hold position, and they move shoulder to shoulder in a tight counterclockwise formation. Although the step pattern is almost the same as the Israeli *hora,* steps for the *debke* are more vertical, sharp and powerful, with stamps and knee movements. Both the *hora* and *debke* have a 6-beat pattern danced to songs with 4 beats per measure.

Basic *Hora*	Students move clockwise as follows: step on left foot, step on right foot, step on left foot, lift or kick right foot, step on right foot, and lift or kick left foot. (See also dance directions for *Hava nagila*, p. 557)
Basic *Debke*	Students move counterclockwise as follows: step on right foot, step on left foot, step on right foot, stamp left foot, step on left foot, stamp right foot.

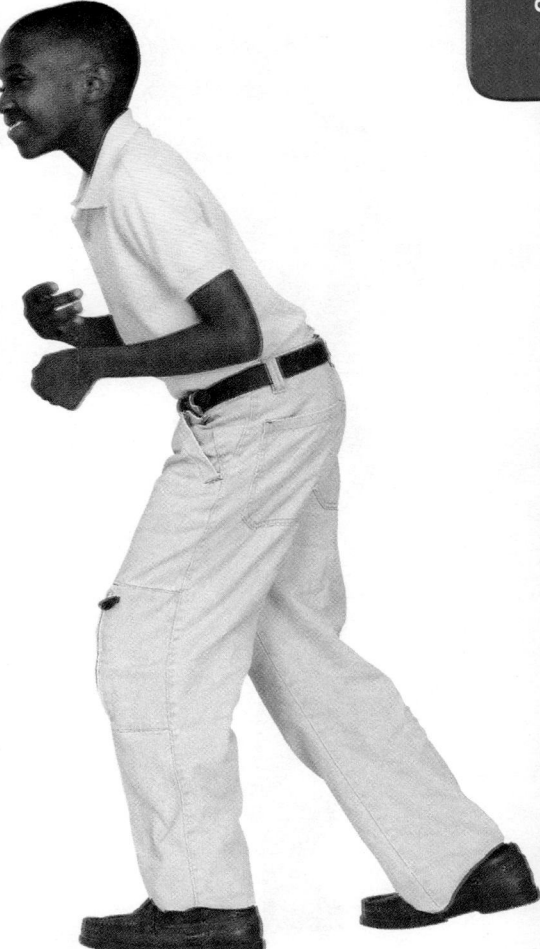

On My Way, p. 313 CD 16-4

Choreography by Susan Thomasson

Routine: Intro (4 m.); vocal AABA; coda

A Section

Measures 1–16	• Students step to right side with right foot, with knees bent and body leaning slightly to the right, tap left foot behind right foot and snap fingers, step to left side with left foot, with knees bent and body leaning slightly to the left, tap right foot behind left foot and snap fingers (mm. 1–8). Repeat movements to the end of the section (mm. 9–18).

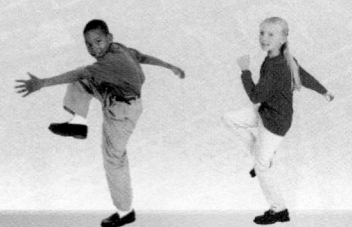

B Section

Measures 17–18   *And as I'm goin' along,*
- Students lunge (right knee bent, left knee straight) to right diagonal corner, bringing the right arm straight up with palm down as they lunge. They watch their arm as it goes up.

Measures 19–20   *I carry with me*
- Students repeat mm. 17–18 but to the left.

Measures 21–22   *promises that can't go wrong,*
- Starting with closed fists, students flick hands open to a high diagonal, right hand on count 1, left hand on count 3. They repeat this move in m. 6.

Measures 23–24   *As I travel on*
- Students repeat mm. 17–18.

Measures 25–26   *As I travel on my*
- Students repeat mm. 19–20.

Measures 27–28   *way. (rest)*
- Students step together and center body.

A Section

Measures 29–36   • Students repeat first A section, mm. 1–8.

B Section

Measures 37–48   • Students repeat first B section, mm. 17–24.

Paddy Whack, p. 327 CD 16-16

Arranged by Sanna Longden, based on traditional solo jig movements

Routine: (Instrumental) Intro; A (16 m.); A (16 m.); B (16 m.); B (16 m.); coda (8 m.)

Students can dance an Irish jig to *Paddy Whack*. Irish dancers often compete in dance contests. In order to win a competition, dancers must move in certain ways. Dance champions keep their torsos very upright, hold their arms and hands straight down at their sides, curl their hands into fists and anchor them against their thighs, point their toes, and take small, sharp steps and kicks.

Formation: All dancers face the same direction, standing still, waiting for the music to begin.

A Section

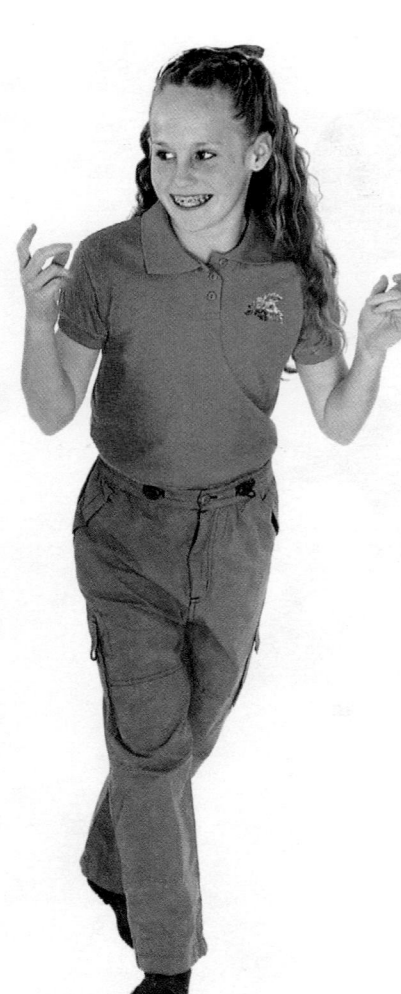

Measure 1   • Students stand on left foot, touch right toe in front, and hop on left foot as right foot kicks out and up.

Measure 2   • Students take 4 quick steps in place (right-left-right-left) and hold for 2 counts.

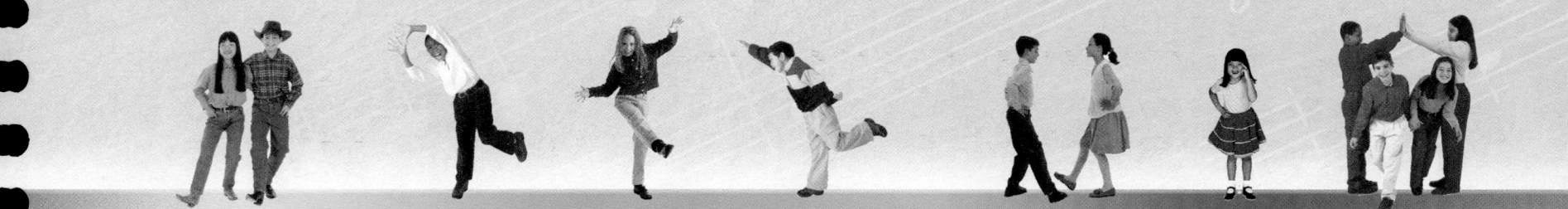

Measures 3–6	• Students repeat mm. 1–2 twice.
Measure 7	• Students stand on left foot, touch right toe in front and hop on left foot as right foot kicks out and up.
Measure 8	• Students stomp with weight on right foot, and hold on both feet.
A Section	• Students repeat A section movements, starting with touch on left toe.

B Section

Measures 1–4	• Students slide to right as follows: side-close, side-close, side-close, side-touch. They repeat, then slide to left in the same pattern and repeat.
Measures 5–8	• Students repeat mm. 1–4.

B Section

Measures 1–8	• Students take 4 skips forward, then 4 skips backward, then repeat skips in and out.
Coda	• Students bend in a bow for 4 beats, then come up in 4 beats. Hands are straight down at sides; feet are spread with R heel touching L instep.

Mama Don't 'Low, p. 358 CD 18-6

Arranged and notated by Sanna Longden, based on traditional dance figures

Routine: Intro (8 m.); v. 1; v. 2; coda

Some early settlers from England, Ireland, and Scotland emigrated to the Appalachian Mountains, bringing their music and dances with them. One of the friendliest types of dance is the *Sicilian Circle*, which people still enjoy today. This is a Sicilian Circle dance, composed of traditional figures. The pattern of a Sicilian Circle dance varies with the experience of the dancers, the plans and pleasure of the caller, and the point of the activity. Here are some easy and fun figures for "Mama Don't 'Low."

Formation: Divide the class into pairs. Couples face couples in a circle around the dance space. One pair faces and moves clockwise, the other counterclockwise. In mixed-gender pairs, (not necessary for this dance), girls are on the right of boys. The person directly across the circle is the "opposite."

Styling: Remind students to move lightly to the music, rather than marching. So that the dance will be successful, encourage students to listen to the musical phrases, anticipate the next figure, and be supportive of all partners.

Calling: The caller "calls" the next figure that the dancers are supposed to do. Callers should cue 4 to 8 beats ahead to give dancers time to position themselves. It is helpful to have the pattern written on cards and to have the cards safely in hand for reminders. Callers may vary the pattern to keep dancers alert and listening. To offer choices, variations for each figure are included—dance figures can be mixed and matched to the musical phrases.

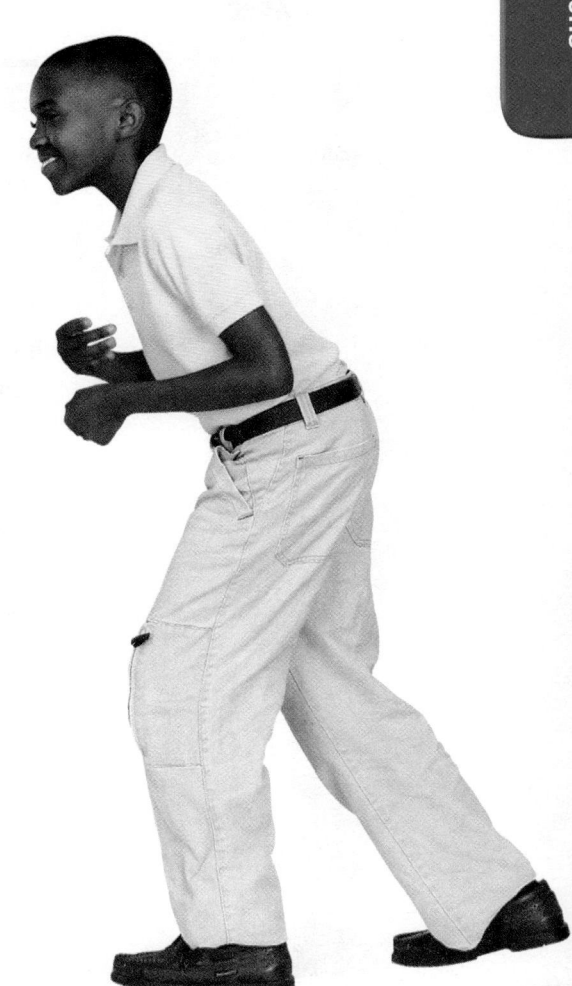

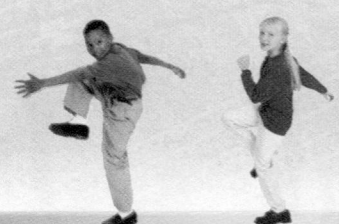

Measures 1–4	***Mama don't 'low no guitar playin' 'round here,***
	• Each set of 4 walks clockwise in a right-hand-star (See Movement Glossary, p. 533) for 8 counts. Variation: Each set of 4 joins hands and circles clockwise for 8 counts.
Measures 5–8	***Mama don't 'low no guitar playin' 'round here,***
	• Each set walks counterclockwise in a left-hand-star for 8 counts. Variation: Each set circles counterclockwise for 8 counts.
Measures 9–10	***I don't care what Mama don't 'low, Gonna***
	• Each student does a right-elbow swing with their opposite for 4 counts.
Measures 11–12	***play my guitar anyhow,***
	• Each student does a left-elbow swing with their partner for 4 counts.
	• Variation for mm. 9–12: Each student does a right-shoulder do-si-do with their opposite for 8 counts.
Measures 13–16	***Mama don't 'low no guitar playin' 'round here.***
	• Each set of partners moves forward, passing right shoulders with the opposite partners, and goes toward an oncoming pair for 8 counts.
	• Variation: Partners moving clockwise raise their inside hands in an arch over the partners who duck under while moving counterclockwise toward the next pair.

Just a Snap-Happy Blues, p. 388 CD 19-22

Choreography by Judith Thompson-Barthwell

Routine: Intro (4 m.); vocal A (24 m.); vocal B (12 m.); vocal C (12 m.); vocal A (24 m.); coda

Encourage students to create movements for "Just a Snap-Happy Blues." Here are some suggestions to get them started.

Formation: Have students stand in one group as a chorus. Divide the chorus into 3 sections, vocal part 1, vocal part 2, and vocal part 3. As students sing, have them perform the following movements. Make sure there is enough space between students to allow for arm and foot movements.

Section A Unison

Measures 1–2	• Students stamp right foot, then left foot on first two rest beats, then snap as indicated in the song and hold.
Measures 3–6	• Students repeat mm. 1–2 twice.
Measures 7–8	• Students step side-to-side: right foot, left foot, right foot, snap fingers, left foot, snap fingers, right foot, snap fingers.
Measures 9–12	• Students step side-to-side: left foot, snap fingers, right foot, snap fingers.
Measures 13–14	• Students cross right foot over left (count 1) and turn all the way around (counts 2-3-4). They face front (count 1), freeze, and hold (counts 2-3-4).

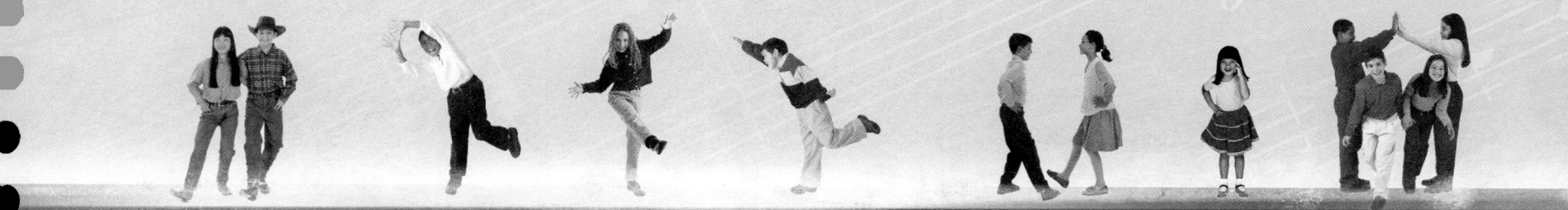

Measures 15–16 • Students step sideways, starting with either foot: step, touch, step, touch, step, touch, step, touch.

Measures 17–20 • Students repeat mm. 13–16.

Measures 21–22 • Students lift right arm out to the side, then left arm out to the side, then put arms down and freeze.

Measures 23–24 • Students repeat mm. 15–16.

Section B Vocal part 1

Measures 25–26 • Students bring right arm up in a "jazz hand" (arm stretched out front with fingers spread open and palm facing front), raise left arm up in a "jazz hand," then bring both arms down, and freeze.

Measures 27–28 • Students freeze (counts 1-2-3-4), then point index fingers up, wagging them side-to-side with the beat (counts 1-2-3-4).

Measures 29–36 • Repeat mm. 25–28.

Section B Vocal Part 2

Measures 25–26 • Students freeze (counts 1-2-3-4), then walk forward 3 steps (counts 1-2-3) and touch (count 4).

Measures 27–28 • Students walk backward (counts 1-2-3-4), then freeze (counts 1-2-3-4).

Measures 29–36 • Repeat mm. 25–28.

Section C Vocal Part 1

Measures 37–48 • Repeat section A.

Section C Vocal Part 2

Measures 37–38 • Students cross right foot over left (count 1) and turn all the way around (counts 2-3-4). They face front (count 1), freeze, and hold (counts 2-3-4).

Measures 39–40 • Students step sideways, starting with either foot: step, touch, step, touch, step, touch, step, touch.

Measures 41–44 • Students repeat mm. 37–40.

Measures 45–46 • Students lift right arm out to the side, then left arm out to the side, then put arms down and freeze.

Measures 47–48 • Students repeat mm. 15–16.

Section C Vocal Part 3

Measures 37–48 • Perform section B vocal part 2, mm. 25–28.

Section A Unison

Measures 1–24 • All students perform section A.

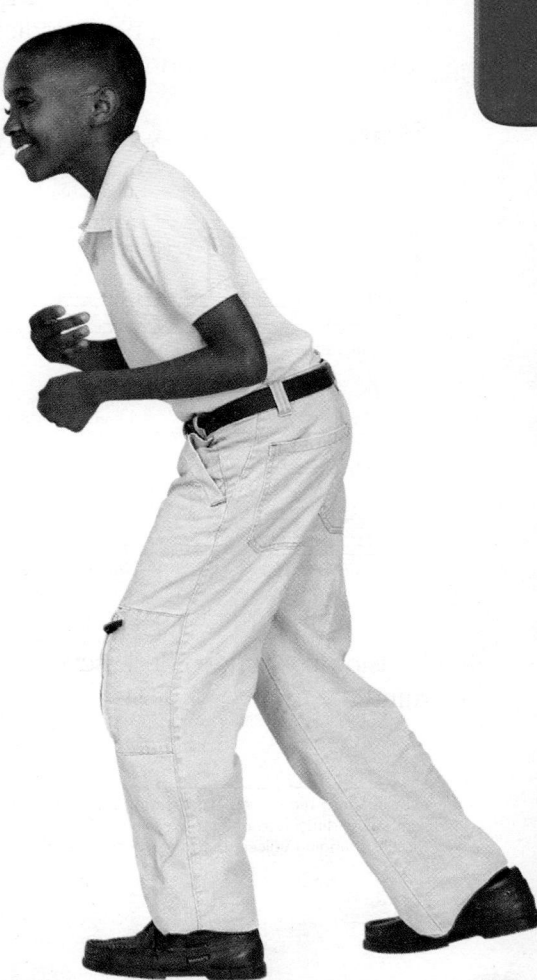

Adolescent Voice

Introduction

The care and training of the adolescent voice is of primary importance. If proper vocal habits can be achieved in the adolescent years, a lifetime of healthy singing will result. These pages present practical information about the changing voice and how the young voice can be developed during maturation.

Male Voice Classification and Part Assignments

Certain developmental stages of adolescent male voices can be identified during puberty, but several criteria must be taken into account. **Range** (not including *falsetto*) is the single most potent indicator of voice development. Other important criteria are *tessitura* (most comfortable singing area of the range), **voice quality** (amount of natural breathiness and constriction; resonance characteristics), **register development** (modal, *falsetto*, whistle registers; also lift point: where the *falsetto* register begins*), and **average speaking voice pitch.**

Voice classification involves applying these criteria in assigning voice parts to different developmental stages. This range/*tessitura* chart identifies the developmental stages for males. (The bracketed notes indicate *tessituras*; the term *baritone* does not connote adult sound.)

Stages of the Changing Voice

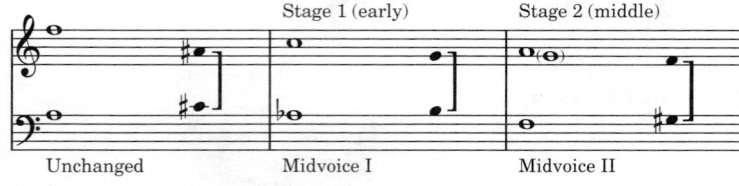

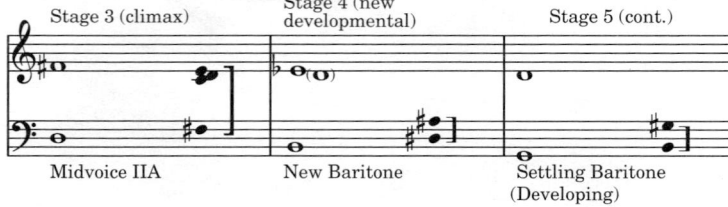

In using the range chart, several points should be kept in mind.

---

*The *falsetto* register emerges during Midvoice II. The lift point or beginning of the *falsetto* is sometimes difficult to detect, especially in trained voices or those just beginning the stage. For rapidly changing voices, the *falsetto* may be difficult to produce, particularly in the range C^4–G^4.

- Lower limits of ranges move down generally by plateaus of thirds.

- There tends to be more stability and less individual variation in the lower range limits throughout the different stages.

- In the upper pitch limits, there are great variations (even in individuals) throughout Midvoice I, II, and IIA; but stabilization takes place in the New Baritone stage.

- The stages represent transitions that may last a few weeks, a few months, or in some cases—a year or longer.

The sequence of changes may also be thought of in the following way.

Early	Middle	Climax	New Development
Midvoice I	Midvoice II	Midvoice IIA	New Baritone Settling (Developing) Baritone

Group voice-testing procedures have been developed to help the teacher identify the various stages of change. (See Group Testing Procedures, p. 570.)

In the sixth, seventh, and eighth grades, one finds many voices in the Midvoice II, Midvoice IIA, and the New Developing Baritone stages. There may be exceptions to this, but there are no true basses or tenors at this point. (Some voices may begin to approximate these classifications, but most voices must still mature a great deal.) In a choral setting, consider the stages in terms of high, middle, and low.

High	Middle	Low
Unchanged	Midvoice II	New Baritone
Midvoice I	Midvoice IIA	Settling (Developing) Baritone

Have the boys sing "America," p. 484, in the key of C or B. The low voices (those singing in the lower octave) can be grouped together. Now transpose the song to the key of F or G. The high voices will be easy to separate because they will sing very easily in this range:

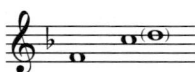

Their voices will be lighter and less mature.

The remaining voices will sound very strong in the key of B♭ or A singing in the following range:

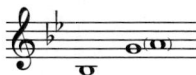

These are Midvoice II's and IIA's. The keys that work best for these stages are C, B, and B♭. Low voices will double the pitches one octave below.

Group lighter voices together (Unchanged and Midvoice I) and place in a section where they can sing an upper part easily. The following diagram shows one way to seat students in a mixed choir arrangement.

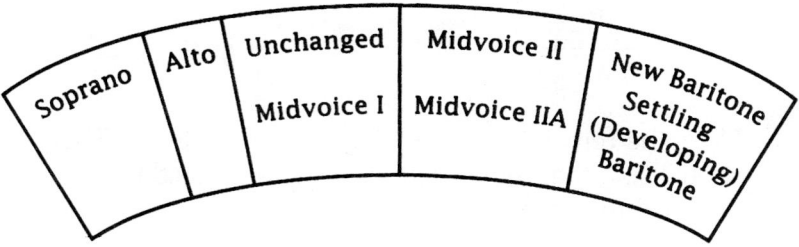

If the changing voices are grouped properly, students can be assigned to parts that fit their singing ranges and *tessituras*. Not all parts of each song will necessarily fit these stages, but certain sections or parts will. Sometimes notes must be changed or omitted for certain voices, but if the teacher understands the range capabilities of each student, songs that match the criteria mentioned earlier can be selected.

Unison and two- and three-part songs often do not offer part-assignment flexibility; however, the principles of finding "singable" areas within all songs still apply. Unison songs are especially troublesome. Try to find tunes with a composite range of a sixth or minor seventh.

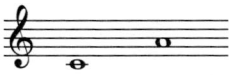

Baritones can double these pitches one octave lower. Although Midvoice II's may have some trouble in this key, they will be able to sing most of the notes.

Composite Vocal Ranges

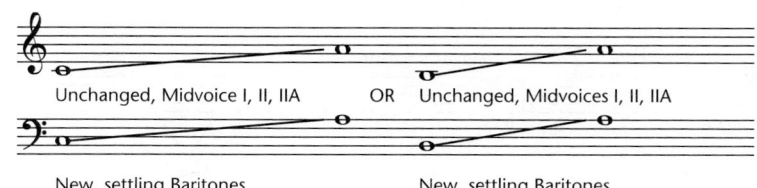

For boys' choruses, apply the same principles of the group audition process from which four-part divisions can easily be derived.

Tenor 1 = Unchanged, Midvoice I's

Tenor 2 = Midvoice I's, Midvoice II's, and some Midvoice IIA's

Baritone 1 = Midvoice IIA's, New Baritones

Baritone 2 = Settling (Developing) Baritones (Basses)

In the first few meetings of the class, however, the teacher may wish to divide the group into three parts—high, medium, and low.

High—Unchanged, Midvoice I's

Medium—Midvoice II's, some IIA's (if the upper register is still stronger than the lower register)

Low—New Baritones, Settling (Developing) Baritones

Female Voice Classification and Part Assignments

Girls' voices do not undergo the dramatic changes that boys' voices do during puberty; however, care must be taken to help them develop good vocal habits during this period. The female vocal folds do lengthen and grow, and the thyroid cartilage shows more vertical growth than it does in males. While the Adam's apple is not as prominent in girls as it is in boys, this does not mean that maturation is not occurring. In the seventh and eighth grades, girls' voices begin to show distinct personal qualities, and the chest, middle, and head registers become more obvious. There is less variability in the range of girls' voices. Therefore, there is more flexibility in assigning choral parts. Guard against assigning them exclusively to one part, such as alto. It is essential that their entire vocal range be developed and exercised. Girls' voices do not approximate or equal the adult alto or soprano classification during junior high years.

The chart shows the typical female range during seventh and eighth grades as well as register lift points.

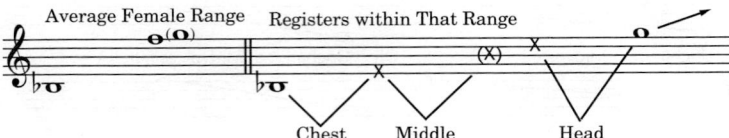

Average Female Range   Registers within That Range

Chest   Middle   Head

It is important that the chest register not be carried too high; that is, to the breaking point, typically.

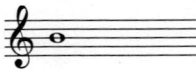

This often occurs when girls sing too heavily in the alto range.

Have girls alternate singing soprano and alto parts so that they exercise their voices through the normal pitch range. Exclusive assignment to alto may harm the growth of the range and cause voice-pushing, forcing, and neglecting the upper part of the range. (See Group Testing Procedures below.)

After the girls have been assigned to two groups, they can sing either the high or the low treble part.

Group Testing Procedures

Individual and group voice testing are crucial processes that need to take place in every choral class. The following practical approach will permit the teacher to classify students (both girls and boys) by voice parts.

1. Divide the class into two groups—boys and girls.

2. Have both groups sing "America," p. 484, in the key of C (B♭ will also work if there are boys who are physically more mature in the class). The primary range of a sixth fits the vocal ranges reasonably well for all parts (with changed voices singing an octave below the rest).

3. Have the boys sing alone in the key of C or B♭. Listen for voices singing in the octave below middle C. These are your New and Settling Baritones. (Some Midvoice IIAs will sing some notes in the lower octave, and some will not match pitch. Assign them to the upper tenor or baritone line.) Check for boys singing in *falsetto* register; some Midvoice II's and Midvoice IIA's and even baritones do this.

4. Have the baritones sing as a group. Listen for notes sounding below the correct pitch. If you have chosen voices that have not yet reached the baritone stage, you

will hear their sound above the pitch level being sung by the others.

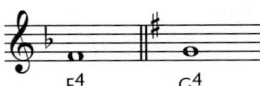

F4   G4

5. Have the other boys sing "America" in F or G. Note those who sing in the upper octave with ease and light vocal quality. These are Midvoice I's and Unchanged Voices. They should be assigned to alto in an SATB mixed chorus situation or possibly tenor if the range is high and does not go below G³ or A³. Watch for boys singing in *falsetto*; some may be Midvoice IIs or baritones. Expect to hear some voices doubling the pitch an octave below. (Midvoice II's will do this.)

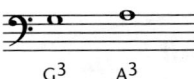

G3   A3

6. Have the remaining voices sing "America" in B♭. They should sing their notes with ease. They should be assigned the tenor part.

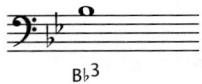

B♭3

7. Have the girls sing "America" in C or B♭. Note those who have the strongest voices and sing the notes with ease. Then have them sing "America" again in F or G, noting those girls who have the strongest, most mature voices and are not forcing the sound. Voices identified in both segments may be divided evenly between the soprano and alto parts. Listen for balance, uniformity, and clarity of sound between the groups. Voices identified in the low key but not in the upper key should be assigned to alto and vice versa for those identified in the upper key but not in the lower key. Assign the rest evenly to the alto part and soprano parts.

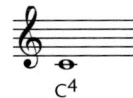

C4

8. Have the girls sing in several keys (low to high). There should not be much difference in balance or quality of sound between the two groups, although the soprano may be lighter in quality.

9. Finally, have all sing "America" in B♭, B, or C.

This procedure will enable you to establish a positive rapport with the students immediately. Voices can be assigned parts, and a lesson in "voice maturation" can be given in a practical, applied setting. Students are interested in understanding the growth process in their singing voices and will listen attentively if they are involved throughout the audition process. Most will achieve some degree of success and will look forward to the next class with enthusiasm.

Principles for Voice Development

- Establish proper body alignment and breathing for singing.

- Help students achieve the proper coordination between subglottic air pressure, extrinsic and intrinsic muscular control of the vocal folds, and articulation within the resonance areas. This will happen if students do not allow excessive tension to develop in the jaw and throat areas.

- Begin exercises in the area of the students' range that is most comfortable, regardless of the variety of stages of vocal development in the class.

- Give enough vocal practice in the proper modal registers (normal voice ranges) as the voices develop.

- Teach the students to understand the process of voice maturation and to consider the changing voice a healthy, natural phenomenon.

- Teach the students to listen for resonant tones and good pitch, and to feel relaxation in the breathing process.

- Help students (particularly Midvoice II's, IIA's, New Baritones, and Settling Baritones) develop the transition area between modal (chest) register and *falsetto* (C^4–G^4 in particular).

- Develop exercises to improve pitch agility. (See Vocalises, p. 572.)

- Have students work for precise vowel and consonant articulation.

- Help students watch for visible and audible signs of vocal stress. Avoid practicing for too long a period of time.

- Be aware of the need for motivation and other psychological aspects of singing.

- Always give positive reinforcement to student efforts. Be supportive and honest throughout all aspects of singing.

Teaching Good Body Alignment

Proper body alignment ensures increased efficiency of the vocal and breathing mechanism. Below are two basic techniques for teaching good posture.

- Rest the body weight easily on the balls of the feet. Stand with the feet a little apart, one foot slightly in front of the other.

- Raise the arms above the head, then lower them slowly (still extended) on either side of the body, with chest up and shoulders back. As the students raise their arms, have them rise to tiptoes, then return to normal as the arms descend. Rest on heels with weight evenly distributed and be sure the students are relaxed. This will ensure proper body balance and good body position for singing.

Teaching Correct Breathing

Have the students

- Place hand on abdomen and expel air, utilizing hissing sound. Feel relaxation response, or release, upon inhalation.

- Slowly inhale by audibly sucking air in through slightly puckered lips. Count to four or indicate the length of the inhalation by conducting beats. At the end of inhalation, expel the air by making a hissing sound, *ssss*. Inhalation and expiration should be considered a continuous action.

- Repeat and check for relaxation in the upper body and throat.

- Suck air for a count of two. Exhale and connect with a voiced (sung) sound, *sah*—at a comfortable pitch for all voices.

- Inhale and then expel the air on a whispered *hah*. This eliminates the lip area as the focal point and permits feeling the upward flow of air in the back of the throat. Next, inhale on a whispered *ah* and exhale, connecting immediately with *hah* on a comfortable tone.

- Gradually eliminate the whispered *ah* inhalation. Along with the elimination of inspiratory air noise, there should develop a well-coordinated intercostal, diaphragmatic-abdominal action that serves to direct the air pressure at the proper rate and intensity through the glottis. The resulting tone should be rich and unforced.

Vocalises for the Changing Voice

These exercises begin in the composite range for changing male voices. They will work well with girls' developing voices, but should be transposed higher (girls only) to account for the female pitch range. While it is good for an SATB choir to begin with these pitches, at some point brief vocalises should be done with girls separate from the boys. For adolescent girls it is very important to devise vocalises, such as *arpeggios,* to exercise register transitions and to develop vocal efficiency throughout the singing range. Over time, this can easily be done in the mixed chorus situation.

Repeat each exercise several times in a moderate tempo at the given pitch. Then continue, raising the starting pitch by half steps until the upper limit of the vocal range is reached. For flexibility, increase the tempo of each exercise.

Exercise 1   To energize sound:

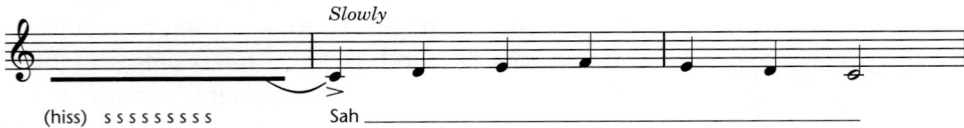

Exercise 2   To develop energy:

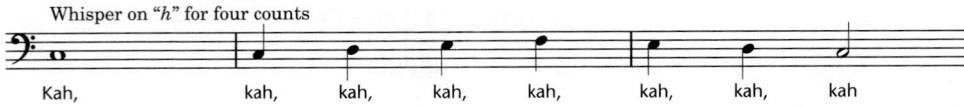

Exercise 3   To build resonance and projection:

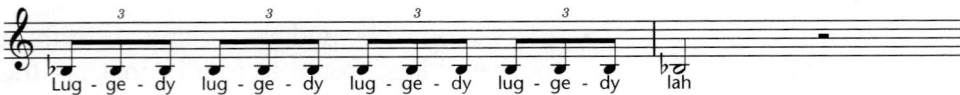

Exercise 4   For flexible jaw, vital sound projection, and proper energy level:

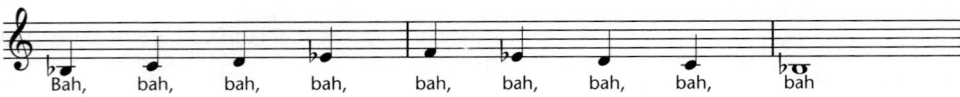

Exercise 5   To develop glottic pressure and breath support:

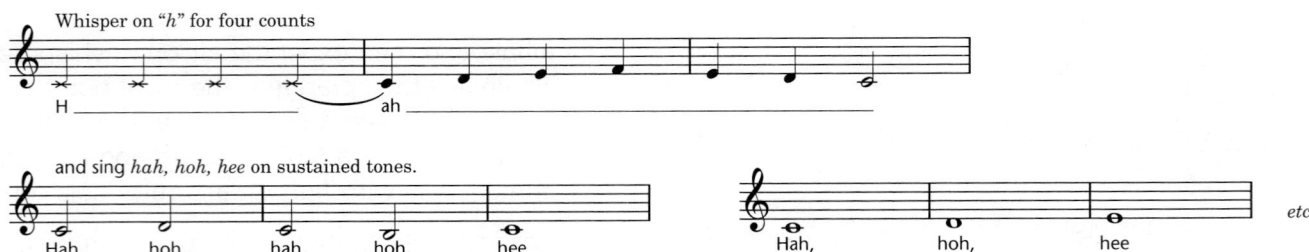

Exercise 6   For lightness, good vocal cord approximation for expanding the range, and rhythmic-pitch agility:

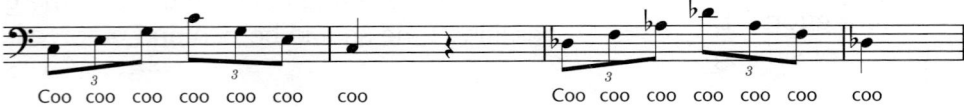

Exercise 7 For precise articulation, pitch agility, and energy:

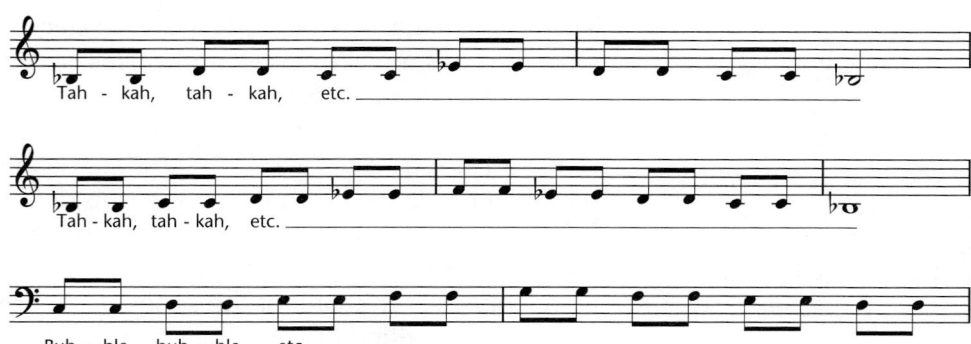

Tah - kah, tah - kah, etc. _____

Tah - kah, tah - kah, etc. _____

Bub - ble, bub - ble, etc. _____

Exercise 8 For sustained notes with gradual *crescendos, decrescendos,* and dynamic control:

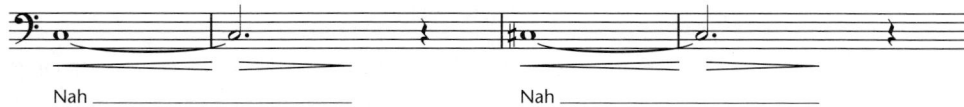

Nah _____   Nah _____

Exercise 9 For lip articulation, lightness, and building consistency throughout range without strain:

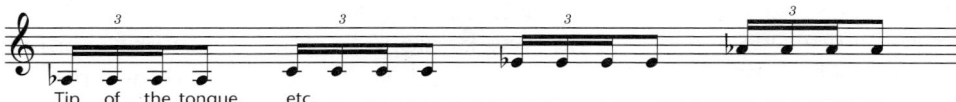

Tip of the tongue, etc. _____

Exercise 10 For resonance and pitch agility:

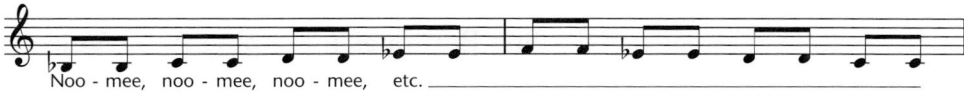

Noo - mee, noo - mee, noo - mee, etc. _____

Exercise 11 For consistent tone throughout the range, dynamic flexibility, and developing richness and depth in tone:

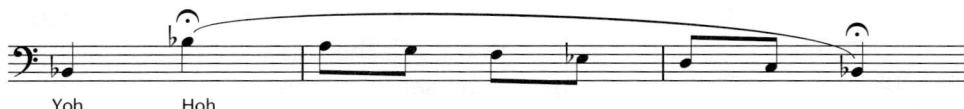

Yoh   Hoh _____

Exercise 12 For rhythmic flexibility:

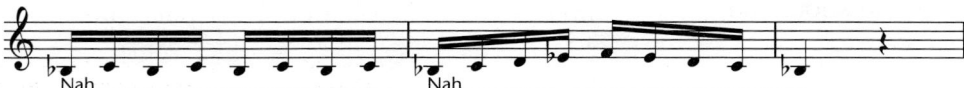

Nah _____   Nah _____

Song Analyses for Changing Male Voices

All of the songs presented in this text have been analyzed for meeting the unique needs of changing male voices. It is important to note that some accommodation has to be made for the various voice change stages so that adolescent singers will experience success in classroom singing activities. Due to the developmental process, primarily of the larynx and vocal tract, the capabilities of individual voices can vary quite widely, thus the reason for suggesting specific options for these voices with *every* song.

The following observations for each voice change stage can assist in modifying ranges, changing octaves or part assignments, and so on, to ensure the successful performance of each song:

Midvoice I

These voices are in the first stage of change, and thus are losing higher pitches in the range, notably C^5–F^5. Avoid singing pitches in this part of the range. Often singers can produce the notes, but must strain to do so. This causes many vocal problems, especially later in the maturation process. Stay in the comfortable *tessitura* as much as possible. In some case, when the top part is very high, the Midvoice I can double the pitches one octave below. See the charts for suggestions.

Midvoice II

The second stage of change presents many challenges. These voices should be singing primarily in the G^3–F^4 range, although some can handle higher *tessituras* in the early part of this stage. Some voices may have an easy transition to *falsetto* (lift point typically G^4–B^4). Other voices may have trouble even producing the *falsetto* register. Check the charts for performance suggestions. Some transposition may be possible, or doubling higher parts an octave below. Sometimes some sections or individual notes may have to be eliminated. There are a variety of performance options, however, and voices in this stage should be encouraged to creatively explore possibilities.

Midvoice IIA

This is the climax of voice change. The stage does not last long (perhaps a few months in most cases). Voices are extremely vulnerable during this time and care must be taken to ensure good breath support and efficiency. A good range for these voices is E^3–C^4 (D^4), although some individuals might be able to produce notes outside this parameter. Explore performance options. Some alto parts might fit the range, and many lower parts of three-voice arrangements work very well. In many of the songs of this text, chorus versus verse writing can be taken into account. Midvoice IIAs may sing both or either section and still receive much satisfaction. The song charts offer a variety of performance options.

New Baritone

The New Baritone range offers a number of possibilities for performance. Top parts and in some cases alto can be sung an octave lower. Melodic writing often suits this voice. One must avoid singing A^3–D^4 (E^4), as a *tessitura*. Some three-part songs (part III) in this text contain this high range. It is better to assign Midvoice IIs and IIAs to this part and allow the New Baritone to sing the top or in some cases the middle part an octave below. This avoids strain, poor intonation, and inaccurate pitch acuity. If the performance options are followed, most of the songs in this text can be sung quite easily.

Settling Baritones (Emerging Adult Voice)

Basically these voices are gaining flexibility and range during this stage. Some may have tendencies toward tenor or baritone, but still do not have adult capabilities. Individuals may be able to sing lower or higher parts with ease, while some will have difficulties producing *falsetto* in the C^4–G^4 range. In regard, the same is true for New Baritones; thus, some of the same suggestions for New Baritone, particularly about avoiding high *tessituras,* apply to this voice change stage. The significant differences between the two stages are that Settling Baritones often have much lower ranges and are more flexible in upper pitch areas.

Composite Vocal Ranges

Song Title	Midvoice I	Midvoice II	Midvoice IIA	New Baritone	Settling Baritone
Abraham, Martin, and John, p. 466	alto	alto •refrain top pt	alto •refrain top pt	•alto	•alto
Adiós, amigos, p. 57	omit high Ds	•last line	•same as II as written	•	•
Ain't Gonna Let Nobody Turn Me 'Round, p. 85		•	•	•	•
Al yadee, p. 308				•	•
Alexander's Ragtime Band, p. 136	+pt1	+pt1	+pt1	•either pt	•either pt
Alleluia, p. 133	•line 2	•line 2, 1st 2m of line 3	•line 2, 1st 2m of line 3	••line 2, m1–2	••line 2, m1–2
Alumot, p. 306				•	•
America, p. 484	transpose to B♭ or B, basses sing octave lower				
America, the Beautiful, p. 485	•line 2, last 3m	•line 2, last 3m •lines 3, 4	same as II	•, last 3m••	•, last 3m••
Angels on the Midnight Clear, p. 423	p1 melody then pt2	p1 melody then pt2, omit high Bs, •"Peace on"	p1 •melody then pt1, omit low B & C♯ in m24	p1 •melody then •pt2	same as N.B.
Asadoya, p. 303	omit high Ds	•lines 1–3	•lines 1–3	•	•
Así es mi tierra, p. 172	pt2, alto	•pt1 except last 2m	•pt2 except last 2m	•pt2 alto	•pt2 alto
At the Same Time, p. 115		•p. 1 lines 5–6 •p.2 lines 6–8 •p.3 lines 1-3,6	same as II	•lines 1-4 ••lines 5, 6 ••lines 1–5 p2	same as N.B.
Banuwa, p. 294	any part	p2 alto, pt2 p2, 3 alto/pt3	•last line	•	•
Barb'ry Allen, p. 44			•	•	•
Bắt kim thang, p. 13			•	•	•
Birthday, p. 90	section B, pts2 or 3	•section A, B, C, as written pt2	+section A, C, section B pt3	•+B section	•+B section
Blue Mountain Lake, p. 205		•lines 3, 4	•	•	•
Blue Skies, p. 88		•pt2 B lines 1–2	•	•	•
Boil Them Cabbage Down, p. 370	•	•	•	•	•
Brand New Day, A, p. 7	+verse	•+refrain	•	•refrain	•refrain
Bridges, p. 86	omit high Ds	•omit low Ds	•	•	•
Bury Me Not on the Lone Prairie, p. 19		•sing middle C as written	•	•	•
By the Waters of Babylon, p. 311	any part	lower notes	sing lower notes	•	•
Cantaré, cantarás, p. 413	melody +alto	•last 2 verses	+last 2 verses	•	•
Caroling, Caroling, p. 458	omit m3, line 2, m1,3 line 3, m1,2 line 4	•lines 3, 4	•	•	•
Corta la caña, p. 364	•refrain	•	•	•	•
Cowboys' Christmas Ball, p. 239	omit high Ds	•	•	•	•
Cuando pa' Chile me voy, p. 376	+refrain alto	•	•	•alto	•alto
Dance for the Nations, p. 122		•line 2	•line 2	•	•
Ding Dong! Merrily on High, p. 427	pt2	+pt2	•pt2	•pt3	•pt3
Do, Re, Mi, Fa, p. 80		•	•	•	•
Dona Nobis Pacem, p. 125	omit lines 3–4	•omit low Ds	•	•	•
Don't Be Cruel, p. 255		•	•	•	•
Don't Cry for Me, Argentina, p. 74	alto	•when upper notes not comfortable	•	•	•
Down in the Valley, p. 375				•	•
Downtown, p. 258		•p2	•after 1st 2 lines	•	•

Key:
- • = melody or part to be sung one octave lower
- •• = melody or part to be sung two octaves lower
- + = sing only this section
- m = measure number
- p = page
- pt = part

Song Title	Midvoice I	Midvoice II	Midvoice IIA	New Baritone	Settling Baritone
El carnavalito humahuaqueño, p. 482		•lines 1–2 except Ds	same as II	•	•
El condor pasa, p. 46			•B sect last line as written	•	•
El payo, p. 145	+lines 1,2	•last 2 lines	•last 2 lines	•	•
Eres tú, p. 473	pt2 refrain	refrain omit lines 1, 2, pt1	same as II	•	•
Everybody Loves Saturday Night, p. 296				•	•
Ezekiel Saw the Wheel, p. 379	alto	•top part	•top part	•melody or alto	•melody or alto
Fais do do, p. 403	pt2	pt3	pt3	•	•
Farewell to Tarwathie, p. 43	omit high Ds, Es	•	•	•	•
Four Strong Winds, p. 170	+pt2	•top part	•top part	•melody	•melody
Free at Last, p. 468	alto	•refrain top pt, alto as written	same as II	•refrain alto •verse pts 2 or 3	•refrain alto +verse pts2 or 3
Gift to Share, A, p. 393	pt2	+•pt section 2	+•pt section upper pt	•	•
Give a Little Love, p. 140		+2nd ending	+2nd ending	•	•
Give My Regards to Broadway, p. 39			•	•	•
Gloria, Gloria, p. 459	pts 2&3	•lines 3,4	•	•	•
Glory, Glory, Hallelujah, p. 52			•	•	•
Go, My Son, p. 188	•pt2, bottom line m1–2	•p2	•p2	•	•
Goin' to Boston, p. 433	omit m17-22 pt2	•p1, lines 4,5 •p2, lines 1,2 •p3 lines 1,2 •p4 top part •p5	same as II	•pt2	•pt2
Going upon the Mountain, p. 105		•verse except m7–8, •counter melody 1 & 2	same as II	•	•
Gonna Build a Mountain, p. 21		•m9–11	•m9–11	•	•
Good King Wenceslas, p. 460	melody	•m1–2, line 3 •last 3m, line 4	same as II	•	•
Gospel Train, The, p. 398	pts 2 or 3	•pt3	•pt3	•pts 2 or 3	•pts 2 or 3
Green, Green Grass of Home, p. 248	omit high Ds	•except for line 1	•except for line 1	•	•
Greensleeves, p. 49	omit high Ds	•refrain	•refrain	•	•
Habemos llegado, p. 174		alto, omit m1–8	•unison, alto on chorus	•	•
Harrison Town, p. 97		•line 4, m1 •line 5	same as II	•	•
Hava nagila, p. 153	omit high Ds	•beginning m2, line 4	same as II	•	•
Hava nashira, p. 82	omit high Ds	•lines 2,3	•lines 2,3	•	•
Hey, Ho! Nobody Home, p. 28				•	•
Hit Me with A Hot Note and Watch Me Bounce, p. 112			B♭, C too high	•	•
I Am But a Small Voice, p. 446	alto	•top part, other notes as written	same as II	•alto	•alto
I Got Rhythm, p. 101		omit low Ds	•	•	•
I Walk the Unfrequented Road, p. 79		omit high Bs & Cs	same as II	•	•
I Wish I Knew How It Would Feel to Be Free, p. 470	alto	pt3	pt2 or 3	•pts 2 or 3	•pts 2 or 3
I've Been Everywhere, p. 226		bottom line refrain alto	•except for bottom line, refrain	•	•
Ise Oluwa, p. 230	alto	bottom pt	bottom pt	•	•
It's Time, p. 274		•pt1 except line 2, alto	•pt1 except line 2, alto	•alto p2, pt2	•alto p2, pt2
Jambalaya, p. 244		•refrain except last 3 notes	same as II	•	•
Joy of Kwanzaa, The, p. 462	any part	lower pts	•upper pts	•any pt	•any pt
Just a Snap-Happy Blues, p. 388	ptI or II	ptII or III •pt1	ptII or III •pt1	•pt2	•pt2
Kelo aba w'ye, p. 290	either pt	either pt	•	•	•

Key:
- • = melody or part to be sung one octave lower
- •• = melody or part to be sung two octaves lower
- + = sing only this section
- m = measure number
- p = page
- pt = part

Song Title	Midvoice I	Midvoice II	Midvoice IIA	New Baritone	Settling Baritone
Key to the Highway, p. 243		•line 2, last 2m	•	•	•
Kyrie, p. 206	Ds too high	•		•	•
La mariposa, p. 58		omit line 3	omit line 3	•	•
Las mañanitas, p. 481	lower notes	•upper notes	•lower notes	•lower notes	•lower notes
La paloma se fué, p. 51	either pt on refrain	+alto, pt2 on refrain	•verse; alto, pt2 on refrain	•verse; •alto on refrain option: •melody	same as N.B.
Lean on Me, p. 14	refrain; alto	•melody on refrain	same as II	•melody then alto on refrain	same as N.B.
Let Us Sing Together, p. 156		•line 3	•line 3	•	•
Like a Bird, p. 167	omit high C♯ through E	•except m2,3, line 4	•	•	•
Lo yisa, p. 130		•lines 2,3	•lines 2,3	•	•
Loigratong, p. 451		•line 5	•line 5	•	•
Lost My Gold Ring, p. 158				•	•
Love in Any Language, p. 476	refrain: alto	refrain: alto •p4	same as II	•alto	•alto
Má Teodora, p. 301	alto	response: alto	response: alto	•	•
Magnolia, p. 16			•omit low Cs	•	•
Mama Don't 'Low, p. 358	omit high Ds	•	•	•	•
Mary Ann, p. 180	+pt2	•pt1	•pt1 or 2	•	•
Mr. Tambourine Man, p. 150		+line 4 of refrain & verse	•+refrain	•	•
My Dear Companion, p. 23			•	•	•
Nana Kru, p. 282		•line 2	•line 2	•	•
New Hungarian Folk Song, p. 196		some *falsetto* notes	some *falsetto* notes	•	•
O lê lê O Bahía, p. 165		•line 2, m1,2	•line 2	•	•
Old Chisholm Trail, The, p. 237		•lines 1–2, •refrain except m5, line 3	•lines 1–2 & refrain	•	•
On My Way, p. 313	alto	alto p2,3	alto p2,3	•	•
One Moment in Time, p. 352	omit lines 3,7 •last 3 notes	•	•	•	•
One Morning in May, p. 121		•lines 2,3	•lines 2,3	•	•
Oye, p. 336		alto on last line & refrain	same as II	•pt1 or 2	•pt1 or 2
Paths of Victory, p. 195		+verse •line 6	•except last line	+	•
Peace Like a River, p. 190	+alto	+alto	alto or •upper pt	•either pt	•either pt
Purple People Eater, The, p. 448		•line 3 •p1 last 3m •p2 last 2m	•	•	•
Red River Valley, p. 11			•	•	•
Rhythm Is Gonna Get You, The, p. 348		•verse	•	•	•
Riendo el río corre, p. 263	•verse except coda	same as II	•	•	
Rock and Roll Is Here to Stay, p. 36		•Cs & Ds too low	•	•	•
Run! Run! Hide!, p. 340	pt2	pt2	pt2	•	•
S'vivon, p. 452		omit high Cs, Bs	omit high Bs, Cs	•	•
Scarborough Fair, p. 95	omit high Ds	•lines 2,3	•	•	•
Scattin' A-Round, p. 160		•line 2, 1st 2 notes	same as II	•	•
Shalom aleichem, p. 409	pt2	•pt1	•pt1	•	•
Sing a Song of Peace, p. 66	sing pt1	pt1	pt1	+pts1 or 2	•pts1 or 2
Siyahamba, p. 212	alto or pt3	alto	alto	•	•
Skye Boat Song, p. 372	omit high Ds	•	•	•	•
Sometimes I Feel Like a Motherless Child, p. 241	alto	alto	alto or •top pt	•	•

Key:

- • = melody or part to be sung one octave lower
- •• = melody or part to be sung two octaves lower
- + = sing only this section
- m = measure number
- p = page
- pt = part

Song Title	Midvoice I	Midvoice II	Midvoice IIA	New Baritone	Settling Baritone
Star-Spangled Banner, The, p. 486	alto	•top part beg. last beat p1	same as II	•	•
Strike Up the Band, p. 135		•lines 4–6,8	same as II	•	•
Summertime, p. 250		•except m4, line 1; m12, line 3; m13–14, line 4; last 2 lines	same as II	•	•
Sun Gonna Shine, p. 242				•	•
Surfin' U.S.A., p. 260	+line 4, p1, 2	•except line 4, p1, 2	same as II	•	•
Swanee, p. 118		•m12–18, last line except last 2m	•except for line 5	•	•
Take Time in Life, p. 292		•lower pt	•lower pt	•bottom 2 pts	•bottom 2 pts
There Is Love Somewhere, p. 318		omit high As & Bs if uncomfortable	•	•	•
This Is My Song, p. 77	omit high Ds	•	•	•	•
This Little Light of Mine, p. 232	alto	•both pts	•both pts	•	•
Tom Dooley, p. 374			•	•	•
Under the Same Sun, p. 440	lower notes	•+refrain upper notes	same as II	•	•
United Nations on the March, The, p. 443	omit high Ds	+refrain; omit high Cs & Ds	same as II	•	•
Vem kan segla?, p. 417	pt3	•pt1	•pt1	•pt3	•pt3
Vive l'amour, p. 176	+alto pt	+alto pt	+alto pt	•	•
Wai bamba, p. 26		•pt2	•pt2	••pt2	••pt2
Water Come a Me Eye, p. 300	either pt	•m1–2 each line response: alto	same as II	•either pt	•either pt
Water Is Wide, The, p. 228	alto	alto	alto	•melody	•melody
What a Wonderful World, p. 62	alto or sop pt p2	alto, p2	alto p2	•	•
Winter Song, p. 455	pt2	+•pt1, p2	•p1 lines 4, 5 •pt1, p2	•	•
Worried Man Blues, p. 371		•except lines 2–3	•	•	•
Yo-shi nai, p. 286			•	•	•
You Are My Sunshine, p. 246	omit m1–2, line 4	•verse except for 1st note	same as II	•	•
Your Friends Shall Be the Tall Wind, p. 201		•line 3 & last line	•		
Your Life Is Now, p. 4		•	•	•	•
Yü guang guang, p. 60		B♭ high	B♭ high	•	•

Key:

•	= melody or part to be sung one octave lower	+	= sing only this section	p	= page
••	= melody or part to be sung two octaves lower	m	= measure number	pt	= part

Teacher Notes

RESEARCH
Validates the Program

MAKING MUSIC Research Base

Silver Burdett MAKING MUSIC incorporates the rich tradition and history of a company that has served the music education profession for almost 120 years. Because this experience has been merged with applications of the most recent research on learning in music, teachers may safely rely on the curriculum, instructional models, and methods that comprise the program. The strong, empirical base of the program is strengthened by the considerable number of authors who are themselves researchers in music teaching and learning and have published works in their specific fields. Many of the authors have specialized in and researched areas such as curriculum design, perception, acquisition of music skills, and repertoire for music learning. Authors for Orff Process, Listening Maps, Signing, Child Voice, Adolescent Voice, and other specific areas, a Multicultural Advisory Panel, and a Teacher Advisory Panel also helped to shape MAKING MUSIC.

Research documents the ways in which children perceive and respond to music, how individuals approach the task of learning, and how they gain insights through involvement with music materials. MAKING MUSIC takes into account that every child is inherently musical and has the potential for musical growth. It also reflects the research in how that growth occurs. For example, MAKING MUSIC recognizes that children go through several stages in their ability to sing accurately and expressively. Therefore the program provides effective strategies and materials for nurturing vocal growth at every stage of development.

Research in music learning shows that students often understand a concept before they can accurately perform the related skill. For example, the concept of beat is often attained at a fairly young age, but the ability to maintain a steady beat at a variety of speeds or tempos does not occur until around the age of nine. MAKING MUSIC was created to distinguish between skills development and conceptual understandings. Skills strands are introduced, developed slowly, and practiced over time. Analogous concepts are introduced and interwoven as appropriate so that meaning is not separated from practice.

According to Howard Gardner, children come to school already knowing a great deal about music. Children are usually able to apply to music the concepts of loud/soft, high/low, fast/slow, and long/short. They respond readily to style and can often name different styles. They know the names and sounds of many instruments and are eager to manipulate sounds to create interesting effects and patterns. Students are open to a wide range of music. They have a strong sense of the syntax of music from their own cultures. Most importantly, they do not question whether they are musical but naturally employ the human language of music.

> **MAKING MUSIC**
> **takes into account that**
> **every student is inherently**
> **musical and has the potential**
> **for musical growth.**

When children begin formal schooling, the challenge for the music educator is to ensure that children grow musically from their intuitive knowledge to discipline-specific knowledge. The National Standards for Arts Education provide guidelines for this process. These standards, issued by MENC: National Association for Music Education, identify the music elements and skills that should be covered at each grade level, and these same elements and skills form the foundation of MAKING MUSIC.

Activities for skills development, written by many excellent teachers who understand the development of music skills, are woven through the series. Complementing the skills strand is an in-depth focus on concept development. MAKING MUSIC has dedicated an entire section of each grade to the development of music elements and skills, using an appropriate and pedagogically sound sequence. Elements are introduced through discovery, expanded, assessed, reviewed, and applied, using new materials that demand increasingly sophisticated listening and perception.

Skills Acquisition

- Many research studies related to music skills acquisition have agreed that students learn more about music when they use keyboards. This has proven to be true for both elementary and middle school students. Therefore, a keyboard skills strand has been incorporated into grades K-8 of MAKING MUSIC.
- In another skills area, the Listening Map Transparencies included in this program are visuals designed to represent musical sounds. By using simplified scores students are provided a greater awareness of specific elements of music. Listening map transparencies in MAKING MUSIC are of this type, and while they illustrate the sound, they are careful not to apply any subjective meanings to the listening selections.
- Common sense tells us that reading notation, or in the case of songs, reading notation with lyrics simultaneously, can be a difficult skill to acquire. MAKING MUSIC always prints songs (with lyrics and notation) against a white background. Also, color-coded identification of vocal parts is placed before the music staff begins instead of surprinting the actual vocal part.

Assessment Practices

- Recent research also suggests that assessment practices reflect and document the range of behaviors specific to the discipline being studied. Studies on the value of written assessment as a self-teaching tool have encouraged the addition of writing projects to lessons. Ideas for reflective thinking and self-assessment through maintenance are particularly appropriate to music instruction. Ideas for use of video, audio, and written entries that may comprise portfolios are given throughout the series.

Contemporary/Popular Music

- One aspect of student motivation and involvement in music learning is subjective task value, which includes attraction as a source of enjoyment for its own sake. Music preference and attitude studies show that students prefer music styles that are popular and regarded as their own. The shift to preference for popular music may begin as early as age five or six. MAKING MUSIC offers students contemporary and popular music that speaks to students' interests outside the classroom, while it also offers more traditional, multicultural, and "classical" selections than any other program. Interviews

with popular musicians of proven ability and appeal further relate students' daily music with music learning and help them recognize the commitment necessary to become a "pro."

Culturally Diverse Music

- MAKING MUSIC also recognizes that music literature representing a diversity of cultures and countries is an important contributor to multicultural education, now mandated in many schools.

> **The inclusion of music literature from a student's own culture increases his or her sense of self-esteem.**

With the advancement of cultural pluralism, there is increased necessity for students to understand and appreciate music of cultures different from their own. Also, the inclusion of music literature from a student's own culture increases his or her sense of self-esteem. Research shows that students learn more and have a greater appreciation for diversity in music when they are actively involved. MAKING MUSIC actively involves students in music literature from many different cultures and countries.

Teaching Style Concepts

- Studies have confirmed the effectiveness of teaching style concepts by comparing pieces and excerpts of the style being studied as well as pieces of a contrasting style. This practice is incorporated into all levels of MAKING MUSIC.

Music Literacy

- MAKING MUSIC is a program that sustains students' interest as it brings them to music literacy and proficiency. Research on these different factors has been integrated into MAKING MUSIC by authors who were selected for their strong credentials in the various fields of music learning. This outstanding group of music professionals has created a program with which teachers can accomplish the goal of all music instruction—enthusiastic, musically literate students capable of a lifetime of active involvement in music.

QUALITY RECORDINGS in the Classroom

Today's Children and the Contemporary Sound

Since first becoming aware of its power, people throughout the ages have listened to music through "mental earphones." These earphones have always delivered music to us with sound that originates from the technological, environmental, and social conditions of the era. Whether a log drum in the jungles of Africa or a harpsichord in an eighteenth-century French drawing room, the sound of an instrument is fashioned by the available material from which it was made, the shape to which that material was transformed, the way in which the performer plays, and the site of the performance. The social context in which the music takes place also influences our way of listening. In church, at a high tea, in a salon, at a sporting event—each of these situations influences how we hear and respond to music.

Though we may not like to think of music as a product of technology, it nevertheless is colored by technology in critical and profound ways. The electronic organ, for example, has changed the sound of African American music so much that its special "electric" tone color has become a natural part of our perception of the gospel sound.

Electronics has had a deep and lasting impact on the ways we listen to music. Whether we listen through sound speakers or a headset, in an arena or in a Broadway theater, music is often heard through electronic reproduction. Even symphony concerts and opera performances, once the haven for unamplified performances, are sometimes assisted

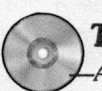 **True To The Music**
—A Commentary by Buryl Red

Few musicians are as well known in nearly every niche of the music industry as Buryl Red. He has an international reputation as a composer, arranger, conductor, and producer. Not surprisingly, he is also a staunch advocate of music education, serving most recently as Executive Producer of recordings for Silver Burdett MAKING MUSIC. The following article contains his beliefs regarding the role and purpose of recordings in music education, both past and present.

through subtle electronic enhancement. This "electronicization" of contemporary music has produced a generation of children steeped in the electronically amplified sound. Such children have difficulty as they first encounter the traditional venues of the concert hall and opera house when amplification is not being employed. The sound, to these children, sounds somehow distant and without presence. The common complaint is, "It isn't loud enough!" Some of these children grow up to become recording engineers who have never heard the sound of a real acoustic violin or flute or piano. Having never been to a concert, they are unacquainted with the pure sound of those instruments unembellished by electronic wizardry. Even some adult concertgoers are beginning to complain that the Mahler symphony they hear in the concert hall is not as compelling sonically as what they hear on their CD players at home.

These, then, are our children—reared in a new tradition and accustomed to a

sound that their elders did not experience as they grew up. So in presenting recordings to today's children, especially in a classroom series, it is of greatest importance that those recordings have the intensity and energy that young contemporary ears want to experience and have come to expect. In MAKING MUSIC, the full weight of modern recording technology has been brought to bear on the wonderful songs that are the backbone and strength of this program. Instrumental tracks have been created that favorably compare to the sound of recordings children hear at home and on the street.

Recording for Authenticity in All Cultures and Styles

In MAKING MUSIC, concern and sensitivity have gone into the recordings to ensure that they provide authenticity in the program's multicultural songs and listening selections. Care has been taken to create recorded performances that reflect the style and conditions of each culture. Recording an ethnic selection involves making subtle choices. In recording a blues song, for example, I must ask myself a number of questions: Is the song a blues from the old folk tradition? Is it a modern blues composed for a Broadway show? Is it a hybrid of the two, or perhaps something in-between? Once that has been decided, an arrangement must be written to create that exact sound and flavor, and the performance and recording must represent the subtleties of the particular tradition. The days are now past when that traditional blues song can be recorded with flute, harp, and vibraphone and sung by young children who do not represent and cannot produce the sound of the singers who would sing that blues song. We might record it, but our children wouldn't "buy" it.

I believe, too, that as we recognize and respect the styles of various non-Western cultures and ethnic groups, we must be equally zealous in maintaining the stylistic integrity of the varied musical expressions of Western cultures. Presenting a song from a Broadway musical would mean that we have recorded the tune as it sounds on Broadway rather than as it would sound were it recorded in some concocted manner that suits "children's music." We have made a very special effort to represent the traditions of all types of music in their proper context.

The Myth of Children's Music

The recordings of contemporary popular music in MAKING MUSIC sound like contemporary popular music rather than watered-down imitations. In the not-so-distant past, such imitations served to make this style of music more suitable as "children's music" or, worse, "textbook music." We have too long subscribed to the idea that music for children must be "dumbed down" to ensure that they grasp it easily. That idea may be one of the most damaging of myths about children and their ability to hear and perceive music aesthetically. Children are eager to demonstrate that they can handle almost any music that excites them; textbook recordings have, in the past, often failed to do this.

I don't believe there is such a thing as "children's music." There is only music that reaches out and touches people, both young and old. A friend once pointed out to me that children's music is any music that children enjoy singing or hearing. Children need not be talked down to musically. They are capable of listening to and enjoying pieces that may strike adults as technically complex, because they listen with open ears and no preconceived notions. These pieces need to be recorded for them with full attention to their expressive content, authenticity, and validity. Even if the purpose of the arrangement is to place emphasis on a particular musical concept, we do not want to say that the performance of the music itself doesn't really matter, or that it doesn't need to be artistically or emotionally convincing. Even with those pieces that have been composed with a pedagogical point in mind, we want to communicate to our young audience the emotional impact of the music. After all, isn't that what it's all about?

> **...children's music is any music that children enjoy singing or hearing.**

Most children already have some skill in perceiving stylistic differences in music by the time they arrive at school. They know the difference between a pop song and a rap, for example. It is equally important to present music that is not so familiar to them, such as concert (or "serious") music, folk music from diverse cultures, and music from distant historical periods. To do that properly, these styles must be presented with equal intensity, as well as emotional and artistic integrity. If this is not done, children will gain the impression that music recorded offhandedly or with obvious lack of care has no feeling and is not worthy of attention. That would

do a great deal of harm. For this reason, all genres of music must be presented within their broadest definitions. For example, African American music is so rich in its varied styles that even a spiritual can be presented in many different ways, all of which are valid from historical viewpoints. That spiritual might have been performed as a church or field song, or an Underground Railroad song in the nineteenth century. Today it might be performed as a gospel song.

Recording Performances

Recordings in MAKING MUSIC contain performances that capture this integrity and intensity. We asked our instrumentalists and singers to perform with the same attention to artistic detail that they would bring to any concert, recording date, or theatrical performance. The music dominated and the musicians played more than dots on paper. They paid attention to the stylistic and dynamic nuances of any professional performance. There were *rubatos* and *ritardandos*, shades of loud and soft, and the artists lent their own deeply felt interpretations. In short, the performers came to the studio to make *real* music. Best of all, thanks to the superb quality of the arrangements and original compositions, we were freed from the "jingle" sound that has for too many years dominated the educational music recording field.

Communication is what good musical performance is, and we tried never to forget it. Often this effort to communicate the style and feeling of the music determined the choice of vocalists. In the majority of cases we featured children's choruses on the song selections, but at times we realized that children's voices could not always communicate the energy and the intensity of the music—in a gospel song, for instance. In such situations it was clear that adult voices could more adequately acquaint children with the goal we were aiming for—to demonstrate what the music is really supposed to sound like. Appropriately, both children and adults have often been used together, a very felicitous combination.

In using adult voices, only the very best from their stylistic fields were chosen to perform for these recordings. A song from India called for singers who were associated with a Hindu temple, who knew the song from personal experience, and who knew how it was supposed to be sung. An African song brought in singers from the African continent— singers such as South African stars Thuli Dumakude and Blondie Chaplin, who brought true authenticity and feeling to the music.

Folk songs from South America were beautifully recreated by the group Andes Mata, who arrived at the studio with panpipes and *charangos*. When we wanted a more contemporary South American sound, we found the best in Gustavo Moretto, whose studies in this country have led to his recognition as a serious concert composer in the United States but who is considered a pop and jazz performer in South America.

For an African American gospel song, we chose performers who could represent that style impeccably— Carol Woods, for example, one of our finest African American singing stars of Broadway and film.

Other world-class musicians whom we involved in these recordings were Yomo Toro, the great guitarist well known in the Latino community; Joseph Joubert, who has been musical director for Judy Collins and accompanist for Wynton Marsalis, Kathleen Battle, and Ben Vereen; and Linda Twine, who has conducted such hit musicals as *Jelly's Last Jam*, *Big River*, and *The Wiz*.

Notation—A Matter of Interpretation

In many ways we are just beginning to be comfortable with other ways of producing sound. This is an issue, especially in vocal music, for those of us who have been schooled in the purest Western choral tradition, which includes jazz and pop styles as well as the Western "classical" tradition. The multicultural movement has shown us that there are other equally valid ways of producing vocal sound, although some of these styles may make us uncomfortable because of our lack of experience with them. Our first impulse is to try to notate the songs and melodies of these non-Western cultures. Notation was conceived and developed specifically to record on paper the music of Western Europe. Unfortunately, most non-Western music cannot be contained, rhythmically or tonally, within the Western notational system.

It's a dilemma. But I feel we have been too much a slave to notation in past music series. After all, even within the context of Western music of all eras and styles—especially in jazz and popular music—music is rarely performed exactly as it is printed on the page. Music is dependent on an interpretation by a performer, unless the composer has written for a computer and has been in control of every nuance. This is why we have chosen the very best performers to make these recordings. We know that their interpretations will be valid ones, even though there might be elements that another musician might have done a little differently. I think we have addressed very well that dilemma between notation and interpretation and provided an example for every student of the ways in which notation becomes a "blueprint" for performance without being a dictator.

Pick-A-Track™ vs. Stereo Performance Track

The Pick-A-Track technique, introduced over two decades ago by Silver Burdett, was handy for teaching songs using the recorded voices and then "dialing them out" so that children in the classroom could sing the song with the instrumental track only. Teachers loved this recording feature. The problem with Pick-A-Track is that it is unnatural. Music is not naturally heard the way it is presented in Pick-A-Track. When you attend a live performance, the sound from the singers and the instrumentalists is heard from roughly the same source. No one hears the singers' sound coming from one sole spot and the instrumentalists from another.

A better way of dealing with the "voices versus instrumentalists" question is provided by the stereo vocal and the stereo performance tracks. In the stereo vocal, the sound is recorded and mixed just as it is in commercial recordings, providing a rich, full stereo sound that has depth, balance, and clarity. Songs in MAKING MUSIC are recorded as full stereo vocals with techniques used in the best commercial recordings.

A Philosophy of Recording

We have approached the recording process of MAKING MUSIC with a definite philosophy in mind: to create recordings that are true to the music—recordings that will stimulate a child's interest and create an exciting response in a way that the old textbook recording philosophy, with its super-simple accompaniments, basic harmonic structure, unmusical interpretations, and babyish singers, did not. We know now that children need to be able to hear "classroom" music in the same aurally exciting way they hear their favorite recording artists.

Classroom Management

As we know, unresolved classroom discipline and management issues can often be at the heart of teacher stress and dissatisfaction. How can we begin to improve our own music classroom discipline and management strategies in order to increase student learning and also increase our own happiness and satisfaction in our classrooms?

Creating Positive Environments for Musical Learning

The rewards of teaching music to young students are obvious, but may deserve focus here as we balance a discussion of the ever-present discipline and management concerns in many of our music classrooms. We music teachers enjoy frequent reminders of the success of our hard work in the classroom. Among these joys are the treasured moments when we actually see and hear evidence of our students' musical development—the satisfying sounds of their active music making; their faces reflecting their hard work and accompanying sense of personal and group accomplishment; the pride of increasing music skills and knowledge; and, of course, our group performance goals well met and received. However, we also know that these and other rewarding moments don't come easily. They are often accompanied by recurring challenges involving music classroom discipline and management.

As music teachers, we are aware of the need for constructive suggestions and direct action toward improving our music classroom environments. Evidence of successful hard work in this area often includes the following teacher-centered events:

- careful pre-thought and classroom organizational planning

- the establishment and practice of positive and effective discipline and management techniques

- consistent expectations and appropriate reinforcement of students' efforts

- reflection with other teachers resulting in classroom experimentation, growth, and development of discipline and management skills throughout one's career.

Simply put, many music teachers seek some guidance about their discipline and management practices including the enhancement of communication skills and relationships with students. Furthermore, they need to talk and listen to one another, especially those closest to the problems at hand.

The following sections of this article will offer a variety of practical suggestions and strategies for planning/organizing, implementing, evaluating, and reflecting upon discipline and management techniques in the classroom.

Organizing for a Successful Year (Pre-planning)

Try some of the following ideas for increased organization and communication at your school site.

- **Plan ahead for less performance stress.**
  Meet with your appropriate school-site administrator before the school year begins. Outline your needs for rehearsal space, dates, and times, as well as tentative dates and times for actual performances and assemblies. Once you have these agreed dates, be sure they actually appear on the school's master calendar. Create a brief flyer with this information to share with classroom teachers, administrators, and parents. Make it known that all is scheduled.

- **Toot your own horn.**
  Share a one-page description that highlights selected activities and learning which will take place in your classroom. Be sure to list performance dates. Share this information at faculty meetings. The more opportunities you have in which you can share your teaching with others, the better. Invite peers and administrators to your classroom to witness what the students can do in music class.

- **Open the door to communication about music's solid role within the entire school curriculum.**
  Invite administrators, school board members, parents, and classroom teachers to join in your performance efforts. Administrators might be willing to greet parents. Other teachers might be willing to narrate or join your efforts by displaying at actual performances student artwork, poetry, and other projects related to your performance themes and song texts.

Music Classroom Tips: Selected Strategies for Positive Environments

One overriding goal within a well-managed, positive learning environment is the development of individual student self-discipline and self-control. The following suggestions are also meant to increase your positive interactions with the students, and students with each other.

- **Avoid chaos upon entry to the music classroom.**

  Many teachers experience problems with misbehavior right at the start of the music lesson. What may be needed is a non-verbal focus activity. Try posting a chart with interesting, different ways for students to enter your classroom each day. For example, "Walk in very slow motion, no talking… and be seated by the end of the metallophone music." Greet your class outside the door, point to the sign, and start the entry. Be sure to reward students who follow the suggestion. You might ask students to think of interesting ways to enter. For example, "Tip-toe to the table, get your music books, open to page 53, and wave." Write these suggestions on cards and start a collection of ideas!

- **Every good meal has a tempting menu!**

  Create a very brief outline "menu" of your lesson. Write key words (make them interesting) on the board and go over the plan with the students. Let them know where the lesson is going. For example, "New partner dance from a surprise desert country" or "New note on the recorder=?" Menus provide a way to keep the class moving forward time-wise and, at the same time, involve students in looking forward to what will happen next.

- **Use your classroom space to increase student focus.**

  Consider using different areas of your classroom for different general music activities. These areas can be very close together. For example, students may learn that musical listening is near the AV equipment, recorder practice and reading/notation drill is near a chart area, movement is in an open space, related children's literature and dramatization is in a reading/visuals corner, and Orff instruments are in another corner. If you do not have your own music room, consider how this idea can be adapted to other classroom spaces, usually within more confined spaces. Simply changing direction and focus may be a way of increasing interest in your lesson activities.

Specific Activity Tips

- **Singing**

  Behavior problems often occur when students do not know what to do next, particularly when beginning new song material using printed music. Try asking students to work with a partner to survey a new song by saying to them, "Point to the first ending and show your partner where we are" or "Point to the words of the song text as we listen to the CD recording" or "Point to the words as we say them together in rhythm," and so on. You might also say, "I may stop the recording. If I do, please silently show your partner where we are in the music. Then we will go on." Also, ask students to take turns with a partner and read song texts aloud, or sing phrases back and forth for extra practice. Reward pairs who can do this well.

- **Movement**

  Many teachers desire to teach movement on a frequent basis but may dread the possible chaos. You may wish to try the following.

  Bus Stop Designate a known area in the front of your room (for example, in front of the piano or table) as the "bus stop." During movement activities where students must find a partner, there are two simple rules— no one can say no if asked, and if you cannot find a partner, simply go to the "bus stop" and wait. The first person you meet there is your partner, as the person can't say no.

  Specific Commands Students can misuse a lot of valuable class time to form one or more dance circles. Try saying to them, "We need a standing-up single circle in the middle of our space by the time I finish counting to 10. Please go there without talking. Let's see if you can do it. Let me know when you are ready." Then count to "10" slowly. Look away and let the students tell you the circle is ready. Lavish them with praise. If unsuccessful, have the class do it again. They will want to please you.

- **Listening**

  Try structuring your music listening episode into three parts by using simple non-verbal cues and known responses (depending on the type of listening you are doing). For example, if students are listening to a recorded instrument featured within pictures in the student books, tell them, "We will have a signal for three things. When you see one finger up, listen quietly. Two fingers up means you are to point to the picture of the

Aim for increasingly positive feedback!

instrument you hear. Three fingers up means you are to write the name of the instrument and some words describing its sound." Observe how closely students pay attention to your non-verbal signals!

- **Instrument Buddies**
Most of us must have our students share Orff and other classroom percussion instruments. Pair up students (including those with special needs) with another before instruments are assigned. One student plays while the other watches and sings. When it is time to change instrument players, take a moment of class time for the first buddy to "teach" their part to the next. Buddies can also help the new players by conducting the actual playing motion, steady beat, and so on. Students can then repeat the same routine by going to different instruments, always with the former "player" teaching the new player.

When things go wrong, consider. . .

- **Are you as positive as you think you are?**
Research points to the fact that effective teachers make positive comments approximately three out of four times to their students. Video tape yourself on a typical day and tally your comments to your students (negative, positive, neutral). You may be surprised!

- **Aim for increasingly positive feedback.**
Provide positive comments for student behavior that are actually appropriate for the task at hand. These positive re-enforcements do not need to be artificial or forced in nature and can include a nod of the head, a "thumbs-up," and a smile. Verbal comments can include "That recorder descant is really coming along," or "Way to go! I didn't have to ask you to put away the instruments." Aim to increase your positive comments in class, and your students will in turn desire to behave in order to hear your praise. Remember to reserve praise for true growth and effort.

Try the following.

- **Younger children**
Choose an indestructible item such as a beanbag, stuffed animal, plastic cup, and so on. Keep this colorful item in the same place, visible to all students to the front and side of the classroom. Teach your students that the object will be handed to anyone who is talking, off-task,

and so on. If given the item, they must hold it silently until they stop what they are doing and are willing to join the group again. They simply must put the object back in its regular place. Then, when and if a student misbehaves, simply hand the student the object (saying nothing) and let them determine when to physically put it back. Follow up with a discussion with that student (after class) about what behavior they changed.

- **Older children**
Sometimes a student must be isolated from the group. Make this isolation time productive by putting that student to work. Provide a piece of paper with two columns. One is "What went wrong today," the other is "What I will do next time instead." After class, discuss the student's responses, tear up the "wrong" side, and have the student keep (or send to the parent with return signature and/or phone call home) the "What I will do next time instead" side.

> **Remember you are not alone!**

Invite discussion and reflection about discipline and management.

Remember, you are not alone. Many teachers report that some of their best solutions to discipline and management problems come from other teachers—music teachers, classroom teachers, and specialists. Try the following suggestions.

- Don't depend on others to start a dialogue on this subject! Invite a peer to listen to your situation and give you feedback and suggestions. Let them know how it went when you implemented suggestions. Keep track of things that work well. Offer the same help to them and others in person, over the phone, via e-mail, and so on. We often can help others more than we can help ourselves, and, in doing so, end up solving some of our own challenges along the way.

- Ask your school-site administrator and music/arts coordinators for professional time to observe others teach and exchange discipline strategies.

- Request that decision-makers create opportunities at professional growth days and meetings for teachers to talk to other teachers about discipline and management ideas. Encourage teachers to share their strengths in this area.

- Reach out to student teachers and new teachers who many times are in great need of your experience with discipline and management. Offer to mentor others.

MEETING INDIVIDUAL NEEDS

INCLUSION

Legislative mandates have resulted in hundreds of thousands of children with disabilities receiving a free, appropriate education—a free, appropriate music education—that had previously been denied to them. Children with disabilities are now singing, playing instruments, listening to music, dancing, and making friends in inclusive music classrooms.

Since the passage of *The Individuals with Disabilities Education Act* (formerly *The Education for All Handicapped Children Act of 1975*), concerned parents, guardians, teachers, administrators, and other professionals have continuously worked to provide in inclusive settings the highest quality education for children with and without disabilities. These efforts are documented by a wealth of printed literature, clinics, and in-service programs that focus on educational opportunities that will result in children with disabilities living maximally independent, happy, and productive lives in their homes, schools, and communities.

> **A challenge of inclusive classrooms is to maintain the highest expectations for each student.**

Music can enrich the quality of life of all children, and children with disabilities can participate, or partially participate, in the same meaningful music activities as their peers. The inclusive music classroom may be the only opportunity for children with disabilities to learn music skills and apply knowledge that will enhance the quality of their musical lives. In some cases, children with disabilities may be gifted or musically talented. Because of the high emphasis on verbal and motor skills in school, these children are not easily identified.

A challenge of inclusive classrooms is to maintain the highest expectations for each student and to carefully observe, assess, and nurture a wide range of music responses, from the simple to the more complex. Children may be different in many ways, but what remains constant are the long-term values that we hold for their well-being, happiness, and musical development.

Collaboration, Communication, and Support

The long-term effectiveness of any music program for a child with disabilities requires communication and collaboration with others who are knowledgeable about the individual. Time spent at the beginning of the school year, and ongoing contact, can build an important support group for the student as well as the music teacher. The particular type of disability category is relatively unimportant compared to knowing pertinent information about the student's safety. Information that will specifically affect instructional decisions includes the nature of any physical disabilities or health impairments, medications, or medical procedures.

Children with disabilities are important resources because they can communicate ways in which the teacher can structure activities for inclusion. In conversations with others, no matter how brief, teachers should inform parents (and others, including the child) about the child's successes in the music classroom—no matter how small they may seem at the time.

Teachers should communicate music and social goals to classroom aides and define the ways in which they can help the child progress socially and musically. Likewise, it is important that tolerance and social problem solving are taught to classrooms of students throughout the year. Students without disabilities should be taught when and how to help their disabled peers, although each student with a disability should be given every opportunity to participate successfully and as independently as possible.

Planning and Implementing Lessons

Children with and without disabilities are exposed to essentially the same music curriculum for each grade level, and expectations should be high for each child. A flexible curriculum that provides multiple ways of expressing competency and achievement will not lower standards. Specific adaptations for any child should be minimal and in keeping with the intent of the lesson and the lesson's activities. In some cases, adaptations that are necessary to meet the individual needs of a child may be appropriate for all students and can be incorporated easily into the lesson.

Well-established teaching principles apply to teaching all children in every situation, and yet the success of each child's learning is dependent upon individualizing those principles. Some examples of these principles are:

- knowing what is important to teach and when

- knowing what will motivate a child

- knowing when and what kind of questions or tasks to ask of a child

- knowing when and how to give a child feedback

- knowing how to teach skills, knowledge, and confidence.

Individualizing instruction remains at the core of excellence in teaching and learning. Planning individually focused accommodations facilitates instruction that is aligned with the music curriculum and relevant to individual needs.

Strategies

Here are several principles and specific strategies to consider in planning and implementing lessons.

- Encourage children to perform music, even simple choral accompaniments or improvisation, at home when they are alone or for family and friends.

- Provide opportunities to make choices and decisions about music and music making that are similar to those that are given to non-disabled peers.

- Provide frequent opportunities for social interactions with peers in small groups and with a kind partner.

- Communicate and greet the child in the same manner as you would other children of the same age from the same class. Monitor your proximity and interactions with the child and make adjustments when needed.

- Use small groups and partners early in the school year. Place no more than one child with a disability in any group, along with kind, sensitive children who are good musical models.

- Analyze sequences and implement relevant steps that move from simple tasks to more complex ones. Even the simplest task should be experienced in an age-appropriate context.

- Provide an adequate range of examples to exemplify a concept.

- Provide adequate practice across activities that are interesting and engaging. When children perform a rhythm or sing a phrase correctly, have them repeat that experience as a class, in small groups, individually, and in a variety of related activities.

- Although some children may have specific behavioral programs that require individual procedures, develop a set of classroom rules, routines, and management techniques that are consistently applied with all children.

- Teach children what to do when they lose their place or make a mistake. Good musicians develop skills for recovering from errors.

- Give individual specific praise and corrective feedback as a matter of routine.

- If a child cannot participate fully, develop minimal adaptations to allow him or her to participate as completely and independently as possible.

- Some children may have difficulty with tasks involving printed materials (such as tracing musical phrases or locating music symbols). Single word cues at the beginning of lines may help organize the search. Have children work in pairs on some occasions, tracing and locating symbols and words together.

- Have children with physical disabilities play a variety of instruments and instrumental parts for accompaniments and in ensembles. First, observe physical movements as children perform simple and more complex patterns on different "silent instruments." Then provide choices of instruments that you know the children will be able to play, and give them choices of rhythms they have performed successfully during "silent practice."

- In many cases, assessment can be the same as for non-disabled students. In other cases, children simply may need more time or a change in the assessment context or modality. Alternative forms of assessment might include providing a cassette tape recorder, an enlarged version of printed material, an extended time, a separate room, a scribe, a reader, a computer, or a sign-language interpreter. In all cases, assessment should be consistent with the individual goals that are set for the child and should include both effort and individual achievement.

- If peer tutors are used, help them understand the importance of showing sensitivity about how and when to help their peers with disabilities.

- In some cases, teacher aides may provide support for students with more severe disabilities. Instruct aides as to how and when to help. The aide should allow the child to participate as independently as possible. Children who come with aides from special education classrooms should arrive for class and leave class at the same time as their non-disabled peers.

> **Individualizing instruction remains at the core of excellence in teaching and learning.**

Teaching for Thinking

Graphic organizers are overt strategies that can help make students' thinking visible and concrete by organizing information visually. They employ various levels of thinking skills and effectively advance vocabulary and concept development.

The main objective of teaching for thinking is to help children understand how they know what they know. Critical thinking can be taught, practiced, learned, and assessed. There is much to think about in music, and teaching for thinking should be an integral part of the music program.

Teaching for thinking can happen simply and in a few minutes through modeling the thinking process. Think aloud about the content of a lesson or problem and how you would solve it. For example, "I'm not sure which of these instruments I want to use for the accompaniment. Let me think about their sounds as I try them out to see how each would fit the style of the song." Structure brief, but frequent opportunities for students to practice thinking and to talk about their decisions with partners or in small groups.

Before students can think creatively and critically, however, they must have a solid knowledge base of meaningful concepts and ideas and a basic understanding of their connections and relationships. As you work with the strategies listed below, carefully choose activity material, concepts, and ideas that students have thoroughly learned. Remember that thinking critically can involve active music making as well as verbal activities.

GRAPHIC ORGANIZERS

Graphic organizers are overt strategies that can help make students' thinking visible and concrete by organizing information visually. They employ various levels of thinking skills and effectively advance vocabulary and concept development. They can be used by individuals, pairs, and small groups or with the whole class as an instructional tool, extension activity, or evaluation.

It is important to model the process for using the graphic organizers before asking the children to use them on their own. Adapt materials to meet your specific purpose. It is not necessary to fill in all the spaces each time. If necessary, add lines or boxes to accommodate the needed information.

The graphic organizers found in the Resource Book can be made into transparencies for use on the overhead projector or reproduced. They may include any of the following: Story Map, Semantic Map, Comparison Chart, Venn Diagram, KWHL Chart, and Semantic Feature Analysis Chart.

STORY MAP

Story maps are simple vertical flow charts that identify the main story elements. They are usually a post-reading or post-listening activity, but can also be used as a formula for creating a story. They can also be used with ballads, such as "Don Gato," and program music, such as Peter and the Wolf.

Key Elements of Story Maps

WHEN (time)

WHERE (place)

WHO (characters)

WHAT (the dilemma that the main characters try to solve)

HOW (the series of steps taken to solve the problem)

ENDING (the resolution of the story's problem and new understandings created by it)

Teaching Sequence

1. Using a transparency of the story map, explain to the students that using a story map will help them see how the parts of a story or ballad fit together and help them remember the story line. Discuss the map headings to make sure the students understand them.

2. Listen to a ballad, stopping at the end of each verse to discuss the story map headings and fill in any information. Ask students, "Were the WHO, WHAT, WHERE, and WHEN introduced? Was the problem introduced? Could you infer any information?" Sometimes the information isn't available in the lyrics.

3. It is important to have the students predict and summarize each time. Have students give reasons for their predictions. Ask questions sequentially and logically so that the students can identify the most important information in the story.

4. Now listen to the selection all the way through and discuss their responses.

5. After they have worked through several story maps with your help, have students work in pairs or small groups to map another ballad or to create one of their own. Always discuss the completed map with them, leading them to think about how all the parts of the story are related.

SEMANTIC MAP

A semantic map graphically illustrates the relationships among a group of words or concepts. Surrounding the central concept are categories related to it.

Teaching Sequence

1. Select a central word or concept related to the lesson and write it in the center circle; for example, classroom instruments.

2. Ask the children to think of words related to the central word and write them down on a sheet of paper.

3. Select children to share orally some of the words they have written. List these on the chalkboard. Assist the children in categorizing the words and naming the categories. To reinforce or assess concepts previously taught, provide the category headings and ask the children to list related words under the appropriate headings.

4. Discuss the map and, most importantly, help children understand how they arrived at their choices. Help them think about their thinking (meta-cognition).

COMPARISON CHART

A comparison chart simply lists how two things are alike and how they are different by writing similarities in the left-hand column and differences in the right-hand column.

VENN DIAGRAM

With two overlapping circles, Venn diagrams illustrate the relationships among categories of items as students examine unique characteristics and common characteristics.

Teaching Sequence

1. Select two categories that share common characteristics familiar to your children, such as two songs.

2. Label each circle with its category or composition title.

3. Ask the children to suggest items or words that belong in at least one of the categories. If the word belongs in only one category, place it in the outer area of that circle. If it is common to more than one category, write it in the overlapping area of the circles.

KWHL CHART

A KWHL chart is used for gathering and organizing information. It is helpful as a pre- and post-reading or pre- and post-listening activity for the recorded interviews.

Teaching Sequence

1. K stands for **what I already know**. In the first box list what is already known about the subject being studied or the person to be interviewed.

2. W stands for **what I want to know**. Help the students generate questions about the subject matter or develop interview questions for the individual to be interviewed and list them in the second box.

3. H stands for **how am I going to learn this**. Help students brainstorm and list ways to learn; for example, read books or magazines, watch videos, interview someone, and listen to recorded interviews. In the third box, write the method(s) they are going to use.

4. L stands for **what I learned**. In the last column list the information gathered from reading, listening, and so on. Review the questions listed in the second box to see if they were answered sufficiently.

SEMANTIC FEATURE ANALYSIS CHART

Semantic maps show how items or words are alike. Semantic feature analysis shows how they are alike and different by using a grid design to graphically display the common features. In this way, items can be compared and contrasted by specific features or characteristics.

Teaching Sequence

1. Begin with a list of known words that share several common features. Write these in the left-hand column; for example, musical instruments.

2. Ask students to suggest features common to several of the words. Write the features in a row across the top of the grid; for example, metal, wood, strings.

3. Complete the grid by putting plus (+) or yes, or minus (–) or no, beside each word beneath each feature to indicate if a word does or does not incorporate a listed feature. Students may find a feature that may not apply precisely to one or more words in the category. Use this discovery as a spark for lively discussion.

4. Encourage students to discuss the unique meaning of each word. Point out that no two words share exactly the same pattern of features.

Character Education in Our Music Classroom

"What does it mean to teach children lifelong skills to develop positive character traits? Are we now responsible to teach this, too?"

Toward Lifelong Skill Development

Among the many terms currently used around the nation to describe lifelong skill goals toward positive character development are the following: trustworthiness, truthfulness, listening to others, achieving your personal best, responsibility, effort, perseverance, friendship, controlling anger, fairness, cooperation, conflict management and resolution, and citizenship.

Most of us are in agreement that our students need repeated opportunities in continuing to develop these and other positive character traits. We recognize that our students may naturally exercise these lifelong skills as members of their families, as participants in their class and school communities, and as future adult members and citizens of their surrounding community, state, and nation. But what responsibility do we have as teachers to make sure these concepts and skills are taught? Why does this responsibility have to be added to our list of things to accomplish in the music classroom?

As music teachers, we may naturally feel overwhelmed in tackling such skill development because of the multiple requirements and accountability systems we already must meet and document. Furthermore, we may be frustrated by what we believe to be powerfully negative influences of the media, popular culture, and trends in youth social behavior on any efforts toward the development of a child's good character— character that was once primarily developed and shaped at home and within many forms of religious education and community life.

At the same time, we also know that we already provide many opportunities toward character skill development through activities in our daily music classroom. We may simply need to highlight ways to communicate what is innate in our music classroom learning environments in order to point out the natural connections to the character development of our students.

> **When you build character, you must address. . . the head, the heart, and the hand.**

Toward this goal, it may be helpful to understand what it means to educate character in others. It has been said that teaching good character involves teaching toward knowing the good, loving the good, and doing the good. These are powerfully motivating concepts which move many educators, administrators, parents, community and religious leaders, and other child advocates toward educative action designed to benefit the common good of not only the child, but of our entire society.

Of course, there are many approaches to action in meeting these goals. One truth may be that there is more involved than just saying and reminding children of good character words and traits. When you build character, you must address the cognitive, the emotional, and the behavioral—the head, the heart, and the hand. Music learning activity, as we know, involves all three realms. In so doing, it provides daily opportunities for our students to develop good character traits and skills.

The remainder of this article will offer you specific connections between selected character or lifelong skills concepts and concrete examples found in music classroom activities. What is important here are not the specific terms themselves, but rather the overall concepts and connections. We hope these connections may serve to help you in your communications with others about how music education is vitally linked to and an active reinforcement of character education for children.

Connections Involving Self

Responsibility We require students to arrive on time, put away their supplies, follow directions, be well-behaved, and and prepared musically. Successful musical rehearsal and performance requires and rewards personal responsibility toward a group effort.

Curiosity Students are exercising this trait when they are asked to find the new note and its fingering on the recorder, figure out what beats are missing in a particular measure, guess the cultural origin of a recorded listening segment, and so on. When we ask older students to explore and find out information about instruments, composers, styles of music, or have them ask new probing questions about what they play, sing, or hear, students are exercising their curiosity in an active, productive manner.

Effort and Perseverance The act of practicing music alone or in a group requires continual effort and the exercise of perseverance. Students cannot give up on practicing and must "try again and again" if they are to improve the musical sound. Music teachers motivate by modeling these traits for their students, as music making itself is a natural composite of both perseverance and effort.

Courage When we praise and reward students for their ability to overcome being self-conscious and nervous in performance, we are helping them develop this trait of courage. The need for courage never ends. In reviewing how far a student or group has come, we are pointing out that courage is what this effort demanded in order to succeed. Also, many music teachers teach about famous composers and performing artists who overcame impossible odds to develop their skills and performance talents. Determination and resolve are companion traits with courage.

Connections Involving Others

Listening to Others The ability to listen is at the heart of all musicianship. Cooperative group projects and partner work in music class involve shared decision-making and compromise. Students must listen to the teacher for direction and criticism, as well as to one another in order to complete a specific group project or task. Also, we listen to others making music to learn how to make music for others and with others.

Friendship One of the best motivators for student participation in music and music performance groups is reported simply as, "We get to make friends." Research indicates that many at-risk students value school because of their participation in music. Friendships in the music classroom often naturally evolve from working together toward a rewarding common goal. A community of friends is established because our stu-

dents enjoy working with others who enjoy the same things they do.

Caring Students help other students to learn music, critique and support others' efforts, and take care of one another within the larger group. Students are actively caring for one another when they offer to help, lend a hand to and include students with special needs, and understand when others need their assistance.

> *The ability to listen is at the heart of all musicianship.*

Cooperation All music making requires active cooperation with the leader and other performers. Students are exercising this skill continually in the music classroom by making sound together, moving, trading instruments, picking partners, setting up and cleaning up, and countless other activities.

We ask our students to share and work together in the music classroom. We model and expect students to be fair to others as we give everyone a turn. We ask students to work out their different points of view in making decisions for a group project. We say to younger children, "Show me that you and your partner know how to share and put away the instruments." Many music teachers ask older students to work out a class problem and lead others to do the same.

Truthfulness We encourage our students to critique one another with the goal of helping others improve their music making. We ask students to tell us the truth about what they think of a

performance. "Which part needs to be louder?" "What needs to be done for this to sound better?" "Where's the hard part and what do we need to do to be able to play or sing it?"

Flexibility and Sense of Humor We can teach our students to be flexible by modeling this trait ourselves, especially in our ability to laugh at our mistakes and the world around us. We model flexibility by accepting human error, being accommodating, and adapting to the needs of individuals and the group. Many teachers and students learn to exercise this important skill when working with students with special needs. We learn to adapt and not be inflexible in demanding that all students do musical tasks in the same way. We are open to students who often think of alternative ways to make music as they compose and experiment with musical sounds.

Controlling Anger Students are asked to exercise individual control over their physical and emotional reactions to others and less-than-perfect events in the music classroom. We ask and reward students for controlling themselves and being patient with others during music making.

Building Community and Citizenship A well-managed music classroom is a model for future adult citizenship in the larger community. In this classroom, individuals have a role to add to the composite community effort by learning their part through hard work and self-discipline, directly participating in constructive and creative action with others, electing and supporting leaders, respecting the rights of the majority, and caring about the overall goal and effort of the many. Simply put, students work toward projects and performance in community, every member offering an important and valued addition to the whole.

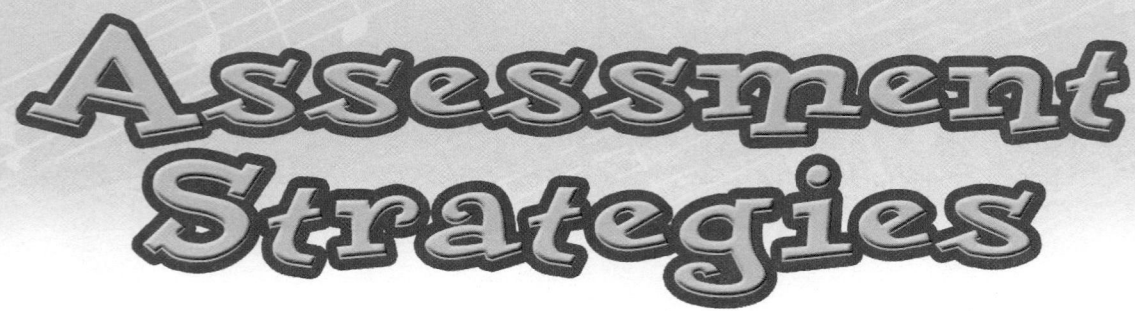

Evaluation Criteria and Procedures Built Into MAKING MUSIC

At every grade level of MAKING MUSIC, evaluation criteria (referred to as assessments throughout the program) are provided within lessons and at the ends of units. Assessments incorporated into each lesson affect perceptions of students, teachers, administrators, and all who care about what is accomplished by studying music, and they serve to provide essential information about what students achieve from taking a music course based on MAKING MUSIC.

Because individual teachers seldom have the time or resources to develop truly comprehensive assessments, and because effective assessments must include a rich diversity of methods and strategies that encourage all students to be successful, the authors and editors of MAKING MUSIC have incorporated the following types of assessment into the program.

• Observations

Teachers observe individuals, small groups, or the entire class during an activity to assess some aspect of student learning. Students may also observe one another for peer assessment. Possibilities for observations include checklists of elements or skills, anecdotal comments, and student performances.

• Performances

Teachers assess progress on or attainment of skills and behaviors through individual or group performances, including composition, movement activities, sound pieces, projects, demonstrations, cooperative learning, and, of course, all performing skills.

• Self-Assessments

Students are asked to think about themselves as musicians. These self-assessments may include descriptions of things they have learned to do well, are continuing to work on, are planning to do, or would like to learn. Self-assessments may be reflections, checklists, journal writing, interest inventories, attitudinal surveys, or descriptions of students' feelings and values.

• Interviews

Teachers formally or informally talk with students individually or in groups in order to better understand students' thinking processes and attitudes. Interviews may be conferences or discussions that demonstrate processing, problem solving, critical thinking, and so on.

• Music Journals/Journal Writing

Opportunities are provided for students to write as they formulate, organize, internalize, and evaluate concepts. Writing provides a good record of the student's thinking, an indicator of what the student is learning and how the student feels. Writing may be a separate activity or may be part of a larger project. Journals may include students' written evaluations of music, specific assignments, or actual compositions. Musical compositions may be in the form of notated compositions, compositional sketches, or graphic notations.

• Audio Journals and Video Journals

Opportunities are provided for students to make recordings of their performances, interviews, and so on. A student's audio or video journal may be a record of his or her "critical incidents" in music making or listening.

• Portfolios

A music portfolio will include examples of a student's musical work. Examples may include representative work, "best" work, mandatory assignments, and so on. Examples often reflect the variety of contexts in which the learning occurs. Portfolios in music might include audio recordings, video recordings, photos, graphic notation leading to actual notation, examples of tests or "What Do You Hear?" exercises, graphic organizers, and so on. Teachers may have students develop individual portfolios or may create group portfolios for the whole class.

Assessments demonstrate what is accomplished by studying music and show what students learn from a course using MAKING MUSIC.

• What Do You Hear?

Cognitive assessments provide an objective way to measure students' understanding of music concepts. "What Do You Hear?" exercises are provided at *every* grade level. They include blackline masters for student answer sheets and recorded excerpts that the student must listen to and analyze.

• Reaction Letters or Reaction Memos

Students might be asked to write letters to "Old Dan Tucker" or to the Boys Choir of Harlem or to Mozart. In setting up the activity, the Teacher's Edition provides the "stem" to get the student started, such as "I wish I could be part of your group because...." Also, students might write reaction letters or memos to each other regarding their work in class.

• Peer Critiques

Students might provide, either by discussion or in writing, critiques of interviews, in-process work, final work, or performances.

• Written Assessments

Written assessments include quizzes and tests, activity sheets, and graphic organizers. Opportunities for assessment using written language are found at the ends of units and within each lesson of MAKING MUSIC, where they help to focus the entire lesson and help teachers and students to conceptualize the learning that is taking place.

• Attitude Inventory

Students respond to a checklist or provide written responses to music. Attitude inventories may be used as pretests and posttests to learning. In this way, teachers learn the attitudes students had before studying a particular selection and compare it to how students' attitudes might have changed.

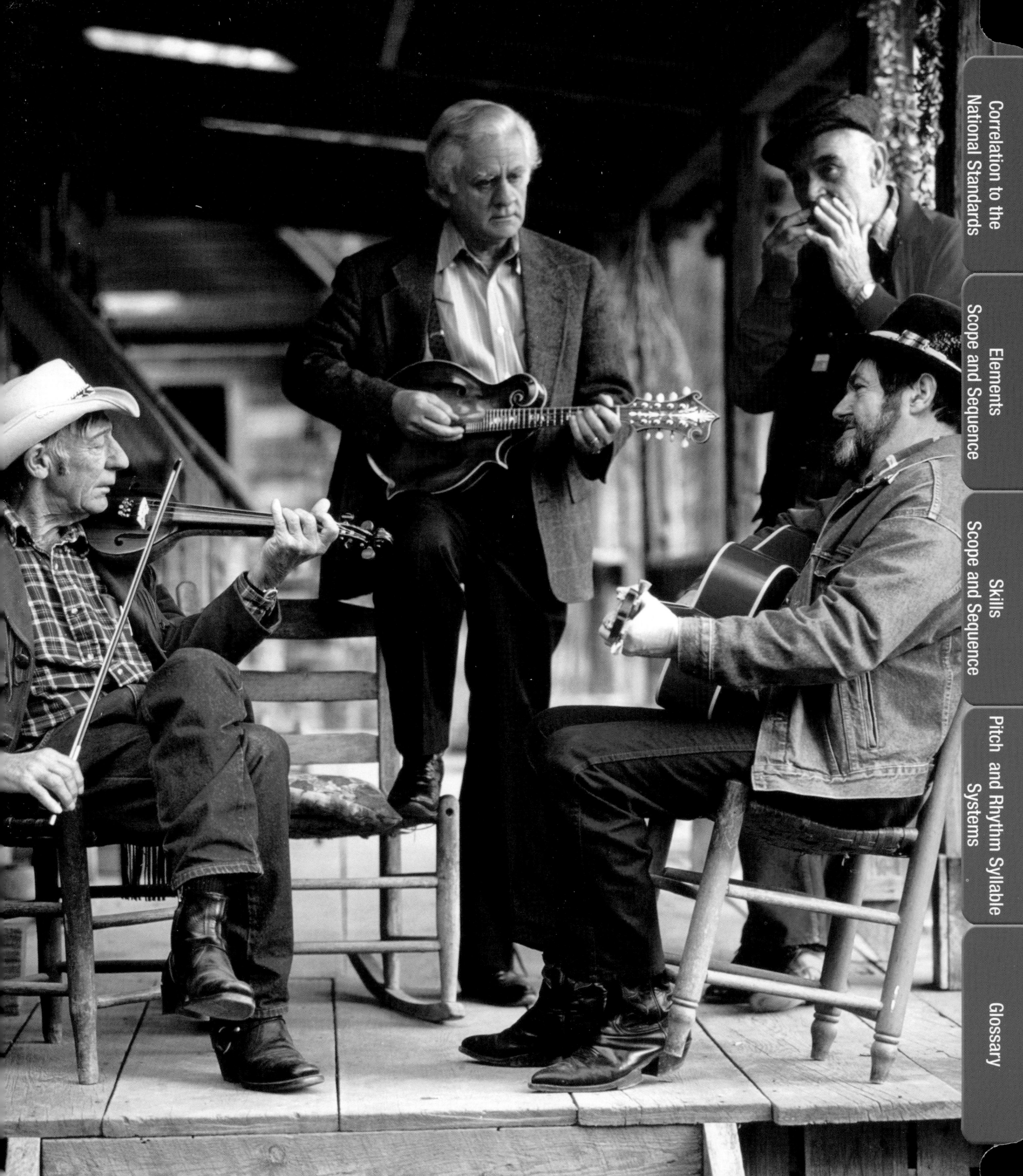

Correlation to the
National Standards

Elements
Scope and Sequence

Skills
Scope and Sequence

Pitch and Rhythm Syllable
Systems

Glossary

Correlation to the
National Standards

Elements
Scope and Sequence

Skills
Scope and Sequence

Pitch and Rhythm Syllable
Systems

Glossary

SILVER·BURDETT
Making Music

Planning and Reference Tools

CONTENTS

"Because music is a basic expression of human culture, every student should have access to a balanced, comprehensive, and sequential program of study in music." This goal, as expressed by the authors of the National Standards for Arts Education, is the driving force behind MAKING MUSIC and the correlation chart below. The chart, and the corresponding on-page National Standards references in this Teacher's Edition (shown with the icon ◆1a◆), will provide valuable assistance in tracking your students' progress and making this goal a reality.

Organization

The National Standards have been developed and organized according to two specific grade-level clusters: Grades K–4 and Grades 5–8. Within each cluster, students may work towards a degree of competency in the skills described in any of the Standards. Full competency, however, is not expected until students have exited the last grade of each cluster. The process of meeting each Standard, then, is a cumulative one in which some Standards may not be fully applicable until the last grade of the cluster.

The page references in the chart below reflect this understanding. The musical activities presented in the earlier grades of MAKING MUSIC engage students in developmentally appropriate learning experiences, which are designed to prepare students to achieve specific Standards by the end of Grades 4 and 8.

Content Standard	Achievement Standard	Teacher's Edition Page
1 Singing, alone and with others, a varied repertoire of music	**1a** Students sing accurately and with good breath control throughout their singing ranges, alone and in small and large ensembles	7–10, 19, 20, 23, 27, 29, 51, 53, 89, 97, 100, 123, 126–129, 135, 160, 163, 173, 174, 203, 234, 318, 337, 359, 371, 373, 375, 376, 399, 443, 447, 449, 463, 465, 467–469, 471, 475, 476
	1b Students sing with expression and technical accuracy a repertoire of vocal literature with a level of difficulty of 2, on a scale of 1 to 6, including some songs performed from memory	8, 23, 68, 69, 78, 79, 165, 241, 394, 399, 405, 419, 456, 460
	1c Students sing music representing diverse genres and cultures, with expression appropriate for the work being performed	13, 15, 17, 27, 48, 49, 51, 54, 56, 59, 61, 83, 85, 115, 116, 126, 129, 141, 145, 153, 159, 173, 191, 193, 197, 207, 213, 215, 217, 218, 233, 234, 238, 239, 245, 247, 251, 261, 264, 291, 295, 296, 301, 303, 307, 308, 309, 311, 321, 341, 349, 394, 410, 415, 419, 422, 424, 425, 429, 435, 443, 446, 451, 453, 481
	1d Students sing music written in two and three parts	15, 68, 80, 83, 84, 107, 133, 137, 161, 171, 173, 174, 177, 181, 207, 214, 230, 241, 295, 299, 301, 341, 380, 394, 399, 410, 415, 421, 446, 456, 457, 460, 467, 468, 471, 473, 475, 481, 487

Used by permission of MENC: The National Association for Music Education

Content Standard	Achievement Standard	Teacher's Edition Page
	1e Students who participate in a choral ensemble sing with expression and technical accuracy a varied repertoire of vocal literature with a level of difficulty of 3, on a scale of 1 to 6, including some songs performed from memory	342, 419, 443, 476, 485
2 **Performing on instruments, alone and with others, a varied repertoire of music**	**2a** Students perform on at least one instrument[1] accurately and independently, alone and in small and large ensembles, with good posture, good playing position, and good breath, bow, or stick control	18, 26, 28, 29, 42, 53, 58, 59, 77, 94, 107, 132, 135, 140, 144, 145, 174, 194–196, 198, 199, 204, 238, 241, 243, 256–258, 276, 278, 281, 282, 318, 337, 359, 361, 366, 369–372, 374, 375, 379, 380, 381, 400, 449, 453, 455, 456, 460, 464, 473
	2b Students perform with expression and technical accuracy on at least one string, wind, percussion, or classroom instrument a repertoire of instrumental literature with a level of difficulty of 2, on a scale of 1 to 6	50, 51, 100, 127, 176, 183, 207, 289, 291, 292, 293, 299, 300, 376, 451, 453, 481
	2c Students perform music representing diverse genres and cultures, with expression appropriate for the work being performed	69, 142, 152, 182, 199, 230, 236, 252, 263, 265, 277, 278, 282, 285, 290, 296, 297, 300, 301, 304, 309, 310, 311, 329, 333–335, 348, 349, 361, 363, 366, 381
	2d Students play by ear simple melodies on a melodic instrument and simple accompaniments on a harmonic instrument	67, 87, 89, 92, 93, 233, 238, 239, 243, 260, 300, 317
	2e Students who participate in an instrumental ensemble or class perform with expression and technical accuracy a varied repertoire of instrumental literature with a level of difficulty of 3, on a scale of 1 to 6, including some solos performed from memory	51, 165, 201
3 **Improvising melodies, variations, and accompaniments**	**3a** Students improvise simple harmonic accompaniments	94, 141, 175
	3b Students improvise melodic embellishments and simple rhythmic and melodic variations on given pentatonic melodies and melodies in major keys	54, 64, 100, 234, 252, 278, 303, 359, 360
	3c Students improvise short melodies, unaccompanied and over given rhythmic accompaniments, each in a consistent style, meter, and tonality	93, 252, 253, 259

Content Standard	Achievement Standard	Teacher's Edition Page
4 Composing and arranging music within specified guidelines	**4a** Students compose short pieces within specified guidelines,[2] demonstrating how the elements of music are used to achieve unity and variety, tension and release, and balance	16, 17, 79, 123, 243, 283, 290, 293, 464
	4b Students arrange simple pieces for voices or instruments other than those for which the pieces were written	29, 171, 209, 229
	4c Students use a variety of traditional and nontraditional sound sources and electronic media when composing and arranging	27, 29, 40, 43, 51, 53, 65, 97, 103, 119, 123, 135, 161, 162, 167, 169, 183, 193, 197, 199, 201, 203, 208, 209, 215, 229, 259, 261, 265, 297, 301, 329, 335, 373, 381, 383, 385, 400, 455
5 Reading and notating music	**5a** Students read whole, half, quarter, eighth, sixteenth, and dotted notes and rests in 2/4, 3/4, 4/4, 6/8, 3/8, and *alla breve* meter signatures	11, 13, 19, 43, 45, 67, 96, 97, 119, 121, 123, 125, 129, 133, 137, 157, 159, 167, 195–197, 201, 211, 245, 282, 290, 308, 309, 318, 321, 329, 333, 340, 345, 394, 398, 414, 418, 429, 445–447, 449, 451, 460, 461, 485, 486
	5b Students read at sight simple melodies in both the treble and bass clefs	21, 57, 59, 83, 125, 126, 167, 205, 470
	5c Students identify and define standard notation symbols for pitch, rhythm, dynamics, tempo, articulation, and expression	19, 57, 77–79, 91, 92, 97, 119, 153, 159, 167, 214, 295, 342, 398, 404, 455, 486
	5d Students use standard notation to record their musical ideas and the musical ideas of others	11, 42, 131, 155, 167
	5e Students who participate in a choral or instrumental ensemble or class sightread, accurately and expressively, music with a level of difficulty of 2, on a scale of 1 to 6	131, 165, 342, 459, 473
6 Listening to, analyzing, and describing music	**6a** Students describe specific music events[3] in a given aural example, using appropriate terminology	7, 11, 15, 17, 27, 54, 67, 69, 89, 97, 121, 129, 131, 153, 155, 161, 164, 165, 169, 209, 217, 233, 234, 256, 258, 261, 269–271, 305, 327, 333, 337, 340, 345, 355, 357, 397, 403, 414, 417, 423, 427, 433, 459, 461, 463, 473, 475
	6b Students analyze the uses of elements of music in aural examples representing diverse genres and cultures	8, 13, 19, 21, 25, 27, 30, 39, 41–45, 47–49, 51, 57, 59, 61, 63, 65, 77, 90, 91, 93, 99, 101, 103, 119, 126, 131, 136, 139, 143, 159, 163, 169, 171, 173, 174, 177, 190, 192, 195, 199, 200, 205, 207, 209–211, 218, 219, 231, 233, 235, 237, 238, 242, 243, 256, 261, 269–271, 277, 281, 283, 285, 289, 291, 292, 297, 305, 317, 319, 321, 324, 325, 337, 349, 357, 361, 363, 365, 369, 377, 380–383, 385, 409, 424, 443, 445, 446, 453, 456, 457, 486

Content Standard	Achievement Standard	Teacher's Edition Page
	6c Students demonstrate knowledge of the basic principles of meter, rhythm, tonality, intervals, chords, and harmonic progressions in their analyses of music	19, 21, 81, 83, 87, 99, 114–116, 118, 119, 121, 129, 131, 133, 135, 157, 161, 163, 177, 199, 201, 204, 205, 345, 433, 449, 456, 457, 463, 467, 468, 471
Evaluating music and music performances	**7a** Students develop criteria for evaluating the quality and effectiveness of music performances and compositions and apply the criteria in their personal listening and performing	25, 85, 93, 117, 171, 279, 325, 383, 401, 407, 411, 443, 447, 451, 465, 487
	7b Students evaluate the quality and effectiveness of their own and others' performances, compositions, arrangements, and improvisations by applying specific criteria appropriate for the style of the music and offer constructive suggestions for improvement	23, 116, 117, 143, 197, 203, 215, 311, 327, 335, 337, 347, 373, 395, 401, 425, 437
Understanding relationships between music, the other arts, and disciplines outside the arts	**8a** Students compare in two or more arts how the characteristic materials of each art[4] can be used to transform similar events, scenes, emotions, or ideas into works of art	40, 49, 52–54, 134, 209, 218, 219, 237, 239, 250, 302, 455
	8b Students describe ways in which the principles and subject matter of other disciplines taught in the school are interrelated with those of music[5]	7, 11, 22, 23, 40, 41, 44, 45, 47, 48, 62, 80, 81, 84, 86–88, 94, 98, 99, 105, 115–118, 120, 129, 132, 133, 162, 169, 191, 194, 195, 197, 200, 201, 213, 217, 218, 311, 323, 324, 330–335, 339, 340, 354–356, 359, 362–364, 366, 375, 376, 378, 379, 382, 405, 463, 467, 468
Understanding music in relation to history and culture	**9a** Students describe distinguishing characteristics of representative music genres and styles from a variety of cultures[6]	44, 58, 61, 85, 103, 120, 130, 137, 156, 191, 240, 241, 247, 248, 255, 258, 263, 265, 270, 271, 281, 283, 303, 304, 308, 334, 346, 385, 393, 395
	9b Students classify by genre and style (and, if applicable, by historical period, composer, and title) a varied body of exemplary (that is, high–quality and characteristic) musical works and explain the characteristics that cause each work to be considered exemplary	25, 30, 87, 92, 174, 211, 231, 252, 331
	9c Students compare, in several cultures of the world, functions music serves, roles of musicians,[7] and conditions under which music is typically performed	233, 234, 270, 277, 285, 290, 291, 294, 297, 302, 319, 323, 324, 338, 339, 346, 347, 395, 465

1. E.g., band or orchestra instrument, keyboard instrument, fretted instrument, electronic instrument
2. E.g., a particular style, form, instrumentation, compositional technique
3. E.g., entry of oboe, change of meter, return of refrain
4. I.e., sound in music, visual stimuli in visual arts, movement in dance, human interrelationships in theatre
5. E.g., language arts: issues to be considered in setting texts to music; mathematics: frequency ratios of intervals; sciences: the human hearing process and hazards to hearing; social studies: historical and social events and movements chronicled in or influenced by musical works
6. E.g., jazz, mariachi, gamelan
7. E.g., lead guitarist in a rock band, composer of jingles for commercials, singer in Peking opera

ELEMENTS Scope and Sequence

	K	1	2	
Expression				
Dynamics	Loud/soft Getting louder/getting softer Soft dynamics	Loud/soft Getting louder/getting softer	Loud/soft Dynamics and dynamic markings including *p*, *f*, *crescendo/ decrescendo* Getting louder/getting softer Sudden changes	
Tempo	Fast/slow Getting faster/getting slower Changes in tempo	Fast/slow Getting faster/getting slower Changes in tempo	Getting faster/getting slower Tempo markings: *fermata* ⌢ Changes in tempo	
Articulation	Smooth and connected Short and detached *Legato/staccato*	Smooth and connected Short and detached *Legato/staccato*	Smooth and connected Short and detached *Legato/staccato* Accents	
Mood	Variety of moods	Variety of moods	Variety of moods	
Rhythm				
Beat	Steady beat Steady beat/no beat Beat/rhythm Beat/silent beat (rest)	Steady beat Steady beat/no beat Beat/rhythm Sound/silence Beat/silent beat (rest)	Steady beat Steady beat/no beat Beat/rhythm Beat/offbeat	
Duration	Long and short sounds Longer/shorter One sound per beat = ♩ Two sounds per beat = ♫	Longer/shorter One sound per beat = ♩ Two sounds per beat = ♫ No sound on a beat = 𝄽	Longer/shorter Tie One sound per beat = ♩ Two sounds per beat = ♫ No sound on a beat = 𝄽 Four sounds on a beat = ♬♬ ♩	
Meter	Strong beat/weak beat	Strong beat/weak beat Meter in 2 Meter in 3	Strong beat/weak beat Meter in 2 $\frac{2}{4}$ meter Meter in 3 $\frac{3}{4}$ meter	

3	4	5	6
Dynamics and dynamic markings including *p*, *f*, *crescendo/ decrescendo*, sudden changes (*subito*, *p*, *f*), *mezzo* (*mp*, *mf*), *pp*, *ff* Dynamic contrasts Dynamics as an expressive choice	Dynamics and dynamic markings including *crescendo/decrescendo*, *subito*, *p*, *f*, *mezzo* (*mp*, *mf*), *pp*, *ff* Changes in dynamics Appropriateness of dynamic choices Dynamics as an expressive choice	Dynamics and dynamic markings including *crescendo/decrescendo*, *subito*, *p*, *f*, *mezzo* (*mp*, *mf*), *pp*, *ff* Changes in dynamics Appropriateness of dynamic choices Dynamics as an expressive choice	Dynamics and dynamic markings including *crescendo/decrescendo*, *subito*, *p*, *f*, *mezzo* (*mp*, *mf*), *pp*, *ff* Balancing dynamics Changes in dynamics Appropriateness of dynamic choices Dynamics as an expressive choice
Tempos and tempo markings including *accelerando*, *ritardando*, *allegro*, *moderato*, *adagio* Changes in tempo Tempo as an expressive choice	Tempos and tempo markings including *accelerando*, *presto*, *andante*, *subito* Changes in tempo Sudden changes in tempo Appropriateness of tempo choices Tempo as an expressive choice	Tempos and tempo markings including *allegretto*, *lento* Changes in tempo Appropriateness of tempo choices Tempo as an expressive choice	Tempos and tempo markings including *rubato*, *fermata* ⌒ Changes in tempo Appropriateness of tempo choices Tempo as an expressive choice
Articulations and articulation markings including *legato/ staccato*, accents, *pizzicato/arco* Articulation as an expressive choice	Articulations and articulation markings including *legato/ staccato*, accents, *pizzicato/arco*, various slurs, *marcato* Phrasing Articulation as an expressive choice	Articulations and articulation markings including *legato/ staccato*, accents, *pizzicato/arco*, various slurs, *marcato* Articulation as an expressive choice	Articulations and articulation markings including *legato/ staccato*, accents, *pizzicato/arco*, various slurs, *marcato* Vocal/instrumental methods Articulation as an expressive choice
Variety of moods	Variety of moods	Variety of moods	Variety of moods
Beat/rhythm Beat/offbeat Upbeat	Beat/offbeat Upbeat	Beat/offbeat Upbeat Backbeat	Backbeat Anacrusis
Tie	Tie	Tie Augmentation Diminution	Tie Augmentation Diminution Relative duration
2/4, 3/4, 4/4 meters	2/4, 3/4, 4/4, 6/8 meters Changes in meter	2/4, 3/4, 4/4, 6/8 meters Meter in 5 Meter in 7 Mixed meter	2/4, 3/4, 4/4, 6/8, 3/8, 2/2 meters Mixed meter Compound meters Changing meters

	K	1	2
Pattern	Sound/silence Same/different Combinations including: ♩ , ♫ , 𝄽 Repeated patterns	Sound/silence Same/different Ostinato Combinations including: ♩ , ♫ , 𝄽 Repeated patterns	Ostinato Combinations including: ♩ , ♫ , 𝄽 , ♩. , 𝅘𝅥𝅯𝅘𝅥𝅯𝅘𝅥𝅯𝅘𝅥𝅯	

Form

Phrase Form	Same/different phrases Echo (imitation) Call and response Introduction	Same/different phrases Question/answer phrase Long and short phrases Echo (imitation) Call and response Repetition/contrast Phrase forms including: ab, aba Introduction and coda Cumulative song	Same/different phrases Question/answer phrase Long and short phrases Repetition/contrast Phrase forms including: ab, aba, aaba, aabb Solo/chorus Call and response Introduction and coda Cumulative song	

Section Form	Same/different sections	Same/different sections
		Introduction and coda
		Verse/refrain (AB)
		Section forms including: AB
		  (binary), ABA
			Same/different sections
			Introduction and coda
			Verse/refrain (AB)
			D.C. al fine (ABA)
			Section forms including: AB, ABA,
			  AABA, ABACA (rondo)	

Composite Form				

Melody

| **Pitch & Direction** | High/low
Higher/lower
Upward/downward
Low to high
High to low | High/low
Higher/lower
Upward/downward
Low to high
High to low
Steps, skips, and repeated pitches | Melodic direction
Higher/lower
Upward/downward
Steps, leaps, and repeated pitches | |

3	4	5	6
Ostinato Even and uneven rhythm patterns (dotted rhythms) Syncopation/no syncopation Combinations including [rhythm notation]	Even and uneven rhythm patterns (dotted rhythms) Syncopation/no syncopation Combinations including [rhythm notation] Swing eighths	Even and uneven rhythm patterns (dotted rhythms) Syncopation/no syncopation Motive Combinations in simple meter: [rhythm notation] Combinations in compound meter: [rhythm notation] Combinations of 2 and 3 in mixed meter: [rhythm notation] and [rhythm notation]	Syncopation Motive Combinations in duple meter: [rhythm notation] Combinations in compound meter: [rhythm notation] Combinations of 2 and 3 in mixed meter: [rhythm notation] and [rhythm notation] Layered patterns Rock 'n' roll shuffle Even rock rhythms
Question/answer phrase Long and short phrases Repetition/contrast Phrase forms including ab, aba, aaba, aabb Solo/chorus Call and response Introduction, interlude, and coda Cumulative song	Question/answer phrase Long and short phrases Repetition/contrast Motive Phrase forms including ab, aba, aaba, aabb Solo/chorus Call and response Introduction, interlude, and coda Cumulative song Ballad	Question/answer phrase Long and short phrases Repetition/contrast Motive Phrase forms including ab, aba, aaba, aabb, abac Solo/chorus Call and response Introduction, interlude, and coda Ballad 12-bar blues	Motive Phrase forms including ab, aba, aaba, abbb, aabb, abac Solo/chorus Call and response Introduction, interlude, and coda Ballad 12-bar blues Canons and rounds Fugue
Same/different sections Introduction and coda Interlude Verse/refrain (AB) *D.C. al fine* (ABA) First and second endings *D.S. al fine* Section forms including AB, ABA, AABA, ABACA (rondo)	Introduction and coda Interlude Verse/refrain (AB) *D.C. al fine* (ABA) First and second endings *D.S. al fine* Section forms including AB, ABA, AABA, ABACA (rondo) Theme/variations	Section forms including AB, ABA, AABA, ABACA Theme/variations March Overture Finale Movement	Section forms including AB, ABA, AABA, ABACA, ABCA, AABAA Theme/variations Overture Finale Movement Through-composed Fugue Minuet and Trio Bridge
	Opera, operetta, musical theater, piano prelude, symphony	Opera, operetta, musical theater, piano prelude, symphony, sonata-allegro, concerto	Opera, operetta, musical theater, piano prelude, symphony, sonata-allegro, concerto
Melodic sequence Melodic direction Steps, skips, and repeated pitches Intervals: unison, octave Pitch letter names	Melodic imitation Melodic sequence Melodic contour Steps, skips, and repeated pitches Intervals: unison, octave, third Pitch letter names Range and register Definite and indefinite pitch	Melodic imitation Melodic sequence Melodic contour Intervals: unison, second, third, fourth, fifth, sixth, seventh, octave Pitch letter names Range and register Definite and indefinite pitch Ornamentation Whole and half steps	Intervals: unison, second, third, fourth, fifth, sixth, seventh, octave Pitch letter names Range and register Definite and indefinite pitch Ornamentation Whole and half steps Accidentals Blues notes Manipulation of pitches as compositional devices: sequence, repetition, contrast; melodic ideas and development; theme, motive, melodic ostinato

Melody (continued)	K	1	2	
Tonality		Tonal center *do*-pentatonic	Tonal center *do*-pentatonic *la*-pentatonic	
Pattern	Same/different	Same/different Combinations including *so-mi, la,* *so-mi-la, do, so-mi-la-do*	Same/different Motive Pentatonic pitch patterns, including *so-mi, so-mi-la, do, so-mi-la-do,* *mi-re-do, re, la-so-mi-re-do*	
Timbre **Environmental**	Nature sounds Found sounds Machine sounds	Nature sounds Found sounds Machine sounds	Nature sounds Found sounds Machine sounds	
Vocal	Various tone qualities produced by individuals and groups Individual: sing, speak, shout, whisper	Various tone qualities produced by individuals and groups Individual: sing, speak, shout, whisper; adult, child	Various tone qualities produced by individuals and groups Individual: male, female, child Group: duet, trio, quartet, chorus	

3	**4**	**5**	**6**
Tonal center *do*-pentatonic *la*-pentatonic *so*-pentatonic Major/minor	Tonal center Key signature *do*-pentatonic *la*-pentatonic *so*-pentatonic Major/minor Whole and half steps Scales: pentatonic, major, minor Changes of key (modulation)	Tonal center Key signature *do*-pentatonic *la*-pentatonic *so*-pentatonic Major/minor Whole and half steps Scales: pentatonic, major, natural minor, harmonic minor Modes: aeolian, dorian, mixolydian Changes of key (modulation) Cadence	Major/minor Whole and half steps Scales: pentatonic, chromatic, major, natural minor, harmonic minor, whole-tone, blues Modes: aeolian, dorian, mixolydian Atonality (chance music) Changes of key (modulation)
Motive Melodic ostinato Pentatonic pitch patterns, including *mi-re-do, so-mi-re-do, la-so-mi-re-do, so₁-la₁-do-re-mi-so-la-do¹*	Motive Melodic ostinato Melodic sequence Diatonic pitch patterns including *la-so-mi-re-do, la₁, so₁, do¹, so-do¹, fa¹, so₁-la₁-do-re-mi-fa-so-la-do¹, ti*	Motive Melodic ostinato Melodic sequence Diatonic pitch patterns including *la-so-mi-re-do, la₁, so₁, do¹, so-do¹, fa¹, so₁-la₁-do-re-mi-fa-so-la-do¹, ti* *la* diatonic (natural minor) *si* in melodic minor *ti* in dorian mode *te* in mixolydian mode	Motive Melodic ostinato Melodic sequence Melodic repetition Motive manipulation Diatonic pitch patterns including *so₁-la₁-do-re-mi-fa-so-la-ti-do¹* *la* diatonic (natural minor) *si* in melodic minor *ti* in dorian mode *te* in mixolydian mode Pitches in compositional devices: sequence, retrograde, imitation, inversion, repetition, transposition, modulation
Nature sounds Found sounds Machine sounds	Nature sounds Found sounds Machine sounds	Nature sounds Found sounds Machine sounds	Nature sounds Found sounds Machine sounds Elemental acoustics Sound quality determined by the sound source Sound quality affected by the material, shape, and size of the source Sound quality affected by the way the sound is produced
Various tone qualities produced by individuals and groups Individual: male, female, child Group: duet, trio, quartet, chorus	Various tone qualities produced by individuals and groups Individual: soprano, alto, tenor, bass Group: large and small ensembles Vocal blending *A capella* singing Variety of vocal styles including: opera, operetta, musical theater, and popular singers	Various tone qualities produced by individuals and groups Individual: soprano, alto, tenor, bass Group: large and small ensembles Vocal blending *A capella* singing Variety of vocal styles including: opera, operetta, musical theater, and popular singers Vocal production	Various tone qualities produced by individuals and groups Individual: soprano, alto, tenor, bass Group: large and small ensembles Vocal blending *A capella* singing Variety of vocal styles including: opera, operetta, musical theater, and popular singers Vocal production Vocal production and style of diverse cultures

Elements Scope and Sequence

Timbre (continued)	K	1	2
Instrumental	Body percussion Classroom percussion Various tone qualities produced by individual instruments and groups of instruments Individual instruments including flute, trumpet, snare drum, piano, guitar Group: large and small ensembles	Body percussion Classroom percussion Various tone qualities produced by individual instruments and groups of instruments Tuned percussion Individual instruments including trombone, violin, timpani, trumpet, clarinet, flute Group: large and small ensembles	Various tone qualities produced by individual instruments and groups of instruments Individual instruments including timpani, clarinet, African percussion, trumpet Group: large and small ensembles Families: strings, percussion, winds Instrumentation from diverse cultures
Electronic			Synthesized sounds

Texture & Harmony

	K	1	2
Texture	One sound/more than one sound Accompaniment/no accompaniment Layers of sound Thick/thin	One sound/more than one sound Accompaniment/no accompaniment Layers of sound Thick/thin Ostinato Bordun	Accompaniment/no accompaniment Layers of sound Thick/thin Ostinato Bordun
Harmony			

3	4	5	6
Various tone qualities produced by individual instruments and groups of instruments Individual instruments Group: large and small ensembles Families: strings, percussion, winds, keyboards Instrumentation from diverse cultures including: Cambodian pinpeat orchestra, Irish instruments, Japanese instruments	Various tone qualities produced by individual instruments and groups of instruments Individual instruments Group: large and small ensembles including orchestra, concert band, *jarocho, gamelan,* symphony orchestra Families: strings, percussion, winds, keyboards Instruments from diverse cultures including: Irish instruments, Indian instruments, Chinese instruments	Various tone qualities produced by individual instruments and groups of instruments Individual instruments Group: large and small ensembles including orchestra, symphony orchestra, *jarocho, gamelan,* bands (marching, symphonic, dance, military, rock) Families: strings (chordophones), percussion (idiophones and membranophones), winds (aerophones)	Various tone qualities produced by individual instruments and groups of instruments Individual instruments Group: large and small ensembles including orchestra, symphony orchestra, concert band, *jarocho, gamelan,* bands (marching, symphonic, dance, military, rock), jug band Families: strings (chordophones), percussion (idiophones and membranophones), winds (aerophones) Folk instruments Instrument making: student-made instruments Instruments from diverse cultures including: West African percussion, Middle Eastern percussion, Caribbean percussion, drums from around the world
Synthesized sounds	Synthesized sounds Electric guitar	Synthesized sounds Electric guitar	Synthesized sounds Electric guitar Sampling
Layers of sound Thick/thin Ostinato Partner songs Echo songs Countermelodies and descants	Layers of sound Thick/thin Ostinato Partner songs Echo songs Countermelodies and descants Rounds and canons Monophonic, homophonic, polyphonic textures	Ostinato Partner songs Countermelodies and descants Rounds and canons Monophonic, homophonic, polyphonic textures	Ostinato Partner songs Countermelodies and descants Rounds and canons Change in texture density Combining independent melodies Monophonic, homophonic, polyphonic textures

Harmony/no harmony
Unison/chordal harmony
Major/minor
Chord changes including:
    I–V_7
2-part singing
	Harmony/no harmony
	Unison/chordal harmony
	Major/minor
	Chord changes including:
	    I–V_7
	    I–IV
	    I–IV–V_7
	Chord roots
	2-part singing
	Harmony in thirds and sixths
	Harmonic styles including: parallel and contrary motion
		Major/minor
		Chord changes including:
		    I–V_7
		    I–IV
		    I–IV–I–V_7
		    I–IV–V_7
		Construction of triads and other chords
		Chord intervals: root, third, fifth, seventh
		Chord progressions
		Cadence
		2-part singing
		Harmony in thirds and sixths
		3-part singing
		Harmonic styles including: organum, parallel motion, contrary motion, countermelodies
			Major/minor triads and inversions
			Chord changes including:
			    I–V_7
			    I–IV
			    I–IV–I–V_7
			    I–IV–V_7
			Construction of triads and other chords
			Chord intervals: root, third, fifth, seventh
			Chord progressions
			Cadence
			2-part harmony
			Harmony in thirds and sixths
			3-part harmony
			SATB
			Harmonic styles including: organum, parallel motion, contrary motion, countermelodies

Skills Scope and Sequence

	K	**1**	**2**	
Singing **Vocal Development**	Vocal range C4–A4; *tessitura* D4–A4 Engage in vocal exploration using speaking, singing, calling, and whispering Engage in vocal exploration using high, middle, and low registers Explore producing head voice sounds and sustaining tones Engage in vocal exploration using descending and ascending *glissandi* on vowel *oo* Expand vocal range upward Sing a variety of simple songs in various keys and meters, alone and with a group Practice good vocal health	Vocal range D4–D5; *tessitura* D4–B4 Engage in vocal exploration using speaking, singing, calling, and whispering and descending and ascending *glissandi* Engage in vocal exploration using high, middle, and low registers Develop head voice sounds in the upper register and sustain tones Expand vocal range upward Develop good singing posture Sing a variety of simple songs in various keys and meters, alone and with a group Practice good vocal health	Vocal range C4–D5; *tessitura* D4–B4 Engage in vocal exploration, blending chest and head voice throughout the vocal range to produce uniform tonal quality in each register Practice producing head voice sounds in the upper register and sustaining tones Expand vocal range upward Practice good singing posture Sing a variety of simple songs in various keys and meters, alone and with a group, responding to cues from a conductor Practice good vocal health	
Intonation	Develop aural perception of different tones, patterns, and/or sounds Develop inner hearing of rhythms, tones, patterns, and melodies Develop pitch matching skills	Develop aural perception and inner hearing of different tones, patterns, rhythms, melodies, and/or sounds Develop pitch matching skills for *so-mi*, *so-la-so-mi*, and *do* Develop aural perception of melodic steps and skips	Develop aural perception and inner hearing skills Develop resonance singing on a neutral syllable (*oo*) Practice pitch matching for *mi-so-la* and expand to include *do-re-mi* Develop aural perception of home tone or tonal center Develop correct intonation singing *do*-pentatonic songs	
Expression	Sing songs using dynamics of *mp*	Sing songs using dynamics of *mp*	Expand dynamics range *mp–mf*, maintaining appropriate vocal quality Develop articulation skills of singing with connected and separated notes (legato and staccato) Develop singing in complete phrases with energy and direction Practice singing ritardando following a conductor	
Part Singing	Sing melodic echoes and dialogue songs	Sing melodic patterns in echo and call-and-response forms	Sing melodic patterns in echo and call-and-response forms Perform speech pieces in canon Sing simple drones and melodic ostinatos	
Diction	Develop good diction through modeling	Develop good diction through modeling Sing on a neutral syllable (*oo*) to develop resonant singing	Improve good diction through modeling Sing on a neutral syllable (*oo*) to develop resonant singing	
Song Repertoire	Sing songs representing genres and styles from diverse cultures Memorize a repertoire of songs	Sing songs representing genres and styles from diverse cultures Memorize a repertoire of songs	Sing songs representing genres and styles from diverse cultures Memorize a repertoire of songs	

3	4	5	6
Vocal range B3–E5; *tessitura* D4–D5 Engage in vocal exploration, blending chest and head voice throughout the vocal range to produce uniform tonal quality in each register Expand vocal range upward Develop correct breathing techniques Practice good singing posture Sing a variety of songs in various keys and meters, alone and with a group, responding to cues from a conductor Practice good vocal health	Vocal range A3–G5; *tessitura* C4–D5 Expand core vocal range Practice blending chest and head voice throughout the vocal range to produce uniform tonal quality in each register Develop deep breathing skills and breath control Practice good sitting and standing postures for singing Build confidence in solo singing Sing with sensitivity to blend in a group or choral ensemble, responding to cues from a conductor Practice good vocal health	Vocal range A3–G5; *tessitura* C4–D5 Sing vocalises using basic arpeggios to expand core vocal range Perform warm-up exercises and sing vocalises to prepare for singing Practice blending chest and head voice throughout the vocal range to produce uniform tonal quality in each register Improve deep breathing skills and breath control Build confidence in solo singing Refine good sitting and standing postures for singing Sing with sensitivity to blend in a group or choral ensemble, responding to cues from a conductor Practice good vocal health	Average vocal range G3–G5; *tessitura* D4–D5 Understand and adapt vocal range to accommodate changing voices Perform warm-up exercises and sing *mi-re-do* and *do-re-mi-fa-so* vocalises in varied keys Practice blending chest and head voice throughout the vocal range Refine deep breathing skills, breath control, and staggered breathing techniques for long notes or phrases Refine good sitting and standing postures for singing Build confidence in solo singing Sing with sensitivity to blend in a choral ensemble, responding to cues from a conductor Practice good vocal health
Develop aural perception and inner hearing skills Develop resonance singing on a neutral syllable (*oo*) Develop pitch matching skills Develop correct intonation singing *do-*, *la-*, and *so-* pentatonic songs Develop octave singing	Develop aural perception and inner hearing skills Develop correct intonation, singing extended pentatonic patterns and scales Develop singing half steps in tune using *do*-pentatonic scale Identify and sing *do*-pentatonic intervals	Develop aural perception and inner hearing skills Perform vocalises to improve resonance and placement Sing with correct intonation Identify and sing intervals in *do*-pentatonic and major scales	Develop aural perception and inner hearing skills Perform vocalises to improve resonance and placement Sing with correct intonation Recognize change of mode Sing dorian and mixolydian modes and harmonic minor scales Identify natural and harmonic minor scales
Expand dynamics range *p–mp–mf–f*, maintaining appropriate vocal quality Practice singing complete phrases on neutral syllables	Expand dynamics range, maintaining appropriate vocal quality Develop *legato* singing	Develop techniques for incorporating *crescendo* and *diminuendo* into singing expressively while maintaining the appropriate tempo Practice *legato* singing Develop *staccato* singing using proper breath support Sing songs using appropriate phrasing	Expand dynamics range, incorporating *crescendo* and *diminuendo* into singing expressively while maintaining the appropriate tempo Practice *legato* and *staccato* singing Sing with *rubato* while maintaining the appropriate dynamic level Sing using appropriate phrasing Sing major scales, arpeggios, and chords
Sing echo songs, melodic ostinatos, partner songs, rounds, countermelodies, descants, and easy 2-part canons Add harmony to songs by singing chord roots	Sing melodic ostinatos, partner songs, rounds, canons, descants, countermelodies, and 2-part songs Add harmony to songs by singing chord roots Add harmonic endings to songs in preparation for singing parallel harmonies Experience 3-part singing	Sing melodic ostinatos, partner songs, rounds, canons, countermelodies, descants, and 2- and 3-part songs Add harmony to songs by singing chord roots and 2- and 3-part chordal accompaniments using the following chords: I, IV, V$_7$, I Sing in parallel thirds	Sing melodic ostinatos, partner songs, rounds, canons, countermelodies, descants, and 2- and 3-part songs Add harmony to songs by singing chord roots and 2- and 3-part chordal accompaniments in major and minor modes using the following chords: I, IV, V$_7$, I; i, V$_7$ Sing in parallel thirds and sixths
Develop correct production of uniform vowel sounds and well-articulated consonants Sing on a neutral syllable (*oo*) to develop resonant singing	Sing vocalises of pure vowels: *a(ah)*, *e(eh)*, *i(ee)*, *o(oh)*, and *u(oo)* to develop resonant singing Practice correct production of uniform vowel sounds Develop correct articulation of consonant *r* Develop correct articulation of voiced and unvoiced consonants	Refine correct production of uniform vowel sounds Practice correct articulation of consonant *r* and voiced and unvoiced consonants Develop correct articulation of diphthongs Learn and apply basic rules for correct English diction	Refine correct production of uniform vowel sounds Refine correct articulation of consonant *r* and voiced and unvoiced consonants Practice correct articulation of diphthongs Develop techniques for singing sustained words correctly
Sing songs representing genres and styles from diverse cultures Memorize a repertoire of songs	Sing songs representing genres and styles from diverse cultures Memorize a repertoire of songs	Sing music from diverse genres and cultures, with appropriate expression and tone quality Memorize a repertoire of songs	Sing music from diverse genres and cultures, with appropriate expression and tone quality Memorize a repertoire of songs

	K	**1**	**2**	
Playing **Percussion** **(Mallets, unpitched, drumming)**	Explore timbre possibilities using body percussion and nonpitched instruments Learn correct playing techniques for pitched and nonpitched percussion Use instruments as "sound effects" for stories, poems, and dramatizations Play a steady beat using bilateral motions Play rhythm patterns on nonpitched percussion instruments, individually and in unison with others Play melodic patterns on mallet instruments Play and invent simple rhythm patterns Use patterns as introductions, interludes, and codas for songs and speech pieces	Expand instrumental sound resources, playing each with appropriate technique Explore techniques for playing mallet instruments and nonpitched percussion Use body percussion in different levels Play a steady beat using bilateral and alternating motions Imitate and invent rhythmic and melodic patterns, individually and in unison with others Play melodic patterns (ostinatos, melodic fragments) Play elemental harmonies (simple bordun) Repeat simple rhythmic and melodic patterns to accompany songs Play instruments in combination with each other (ensemble) Incorporate expressive elements into playing Develop awareness of timbre categories: woods, metals, shakers, scrapers, and so on	Play a steady beat and strong beat using bilateral and alternating lateral motions Play rhythmic patterns and ostinatos from notation Imitate and invent rhythmic and melodic patterns both in isolation and to accompany songs, speech pieces, and movement Develop basic mallet techniques Play melodic patterns to accompany songs (ostinatos, melodic fragments) Play simple melodies by rote on mallet instruments Play elemental harmonies (simple bordun, moving bordun, crossover bordun) Play instruments in groups (ensemble)	
String Instruments **(Autoharp, Guitar)**			Play one-chord and two-chord strums on the Autoharp	

Develop "crossover" mallet technique for playing borduns and ostinatos Play accompaniments for songs and speech pieces using body percussion, nonpitched percussion, and/or mallet instruments. Play combined patterns in ensemble to accompany songs, speech pieces, and movement, including borduns, melodic ostinatos, rhythmic ostinatos, and melodic/rhythmic fragments Develop a knowledge base for selecting accompaniment instruments appropriate to the style and culture of a song Develop original accompaniments as a group	Refine mallet techniques Include syncopation in rhythmic and melodic patterns Use body percussion and/or non-pitched percussion instruments to perform rhythm rounds, and create question/answer rhythmic phrases Use mallet instruments, keyboard, and/or recorder to create question/answer rhythmic phrases Play accompaniments on mallet instruments involving two chords—I–V, I–VI, I–VII Develop familiarity with chromatic structure of the keyboard Play melodies on mallet instruments by rote and by reading Develop simple instrumental pieces	Include offbeat rhythms in rhythmic and melodic patterns Play accompaniments on mallet instruments involving the I–IV–V$_7$ harmonic progression Develop more extended instrumental pieces. Include opportunities for rhythmic and/or melodic solos (composed or improvised) Provide opportunities for individuals to play small pieces alone, demonstrating good technique and style Develop ability to play culture-specific instruments and styles; e.g., various African drumming genres	Incorporate harmonization into the development of accompaniments using mallet instruments Play accompaniments on mallet instruments involving the I–IV–V$_7$ harmonic progression Expand familiarity and capability with culture-specific styles and instruments Provide opportunities for individuals to play small pieces alone, demonstrating good technique and style Develop ability to play culture-specific instruments and styles; e.g., various African drumming genres Play basic rock rhythm patterns with popular songs
Play two-chord Autoharp accompaniments for songs using simple strums	Play Autoharp accompaniments, both major and minor, using three chords and simple strums Identify types of guitars (nylon-string classical, steel-string acoustic, electric) Identify parts of the guitar Tune the guitar from a piano Develop proper guitar playing posture Use finger numbers for the left-hand Learn how to form chords Learn fundamental right-hand techniques (basic strumming patterns, picking) Learn fundamental left-hand techniques (chords A, D, E$_7$, G, C, D$_7$) Learn half chords Learn techniques for smooth transitions between chords Learn open tuning Begin use of the capo Create simple accompaniments to songs including short introductions, refrains, and ostinatos Play songs in the keys of C, D, and G	Play Autoharp accompaniments, both major and minor, using three or more chords Review types of guitars (nylon-string classical, steel-string acoustic, electric) Review parts of the guitar Tune the guitar using relative tuning Reinforce proper guitar playing posture (three different approaches) Learn to read chord diagrams Review and reinforce techniques for smooth transitions between chords Continue using the capo Play common chord progressions Learn alternative playing techniques Continue to learn and use open tuning Learn classic songs from guitar repertoire Continue left-hand techniques (review chords and learn A$_7$, E$_7$, G$_7$, Em, Am, Dm) Create accompaniments to songs including introductions, verses, refrains, and ostinatos Play songs in the keys C, D, G, F, Em, and Dm Discuss guidelines for improving practice time Discuss guidelines of self-assessment of skill progress	Use Autoharp accompaniments in conjunction with other string band instruments such as guitar Review parts of the guitar Tune the guitar from a piano Tune the guitar using relative tuning Reinforce proper guitar playing posture (three different approaches) Review and learn to read chord diagrams Review and reinforce techniques for smooth transitions between chords Continue using the capo Learn right-hand techniques (strumming patterns, picking) Continue to learn and use open tuning Learn alternating bass string technique Play music from the classical, pop, and folk genres Begin playing the electric guitar Learn to use mallet chords Continue left-hand techniques (review chords and learn Bm, B$_7$, B♭, Gm) Create accompaniments to songs including introductions, verses, refrains, and ostinatos Play songs in the keys C, D, G, F, and several minor keys

Skills Scope and Sequence

	K	1	2	
Keyboard and MIDI	Identify black and white keys Maintain a steady beat Locate high and low sounds Play with supported index fingers Identify and play basic pulse Use timbre to identify range Play a two-handed accompaniment Discover and play pitches that move up and pitches that repeat Play strong beats Play an ostinato Play repeated phrases	Play with supported fingers Discover and play rhythm patterns Identify and play high and low sounds Accompany reinforcing a steady beat Play an ostinato Play call-and-response melodies Play a melodic phrase with ascending and descending skips Play a two-handed accompaniment Play a refrain	Play a two-handed accompaniment using supported index fingers Identify and play specific pitches Play duet accompaniments Read prestaff notation Discover and play *mi-re-do* patterns Determine melodic direction and play steps, skips, and repeats Determine appropriate finger numbers Play phrases using *do-re-mi-so* Play an ostinato Play melodies Accompany in various styles Read note values	
Recorder				

| --- | --- | --- | --- |
| Read prestaff notation
Read finger numbers and note values
Play rhythm patterns to show high and low sounds on specific pitches
Read a five-line staff
Show timbre by playing a duet accompaniment
Play sixteenth notes
Play accompaniments using harmonic intervals
Play extended range with melodies divided between hands
Identify and accompany songs in different meters
Play broken chord accompaniments
Play melodies with an octave range
Play I and V$_7$ chords | Review prestaff notation
Review five-line reading and fingering
Identify and play same and different phrases
Play triads
Expand five-finger position to achieve "closest position"
Play ensembles
Play walking bass lines
Play broken chord accompaniments
Improvise using pentatonic scales
Play fingering shifts
Play melodies with a large stretch
Play ♩. ♪ rhythm patterns
Play using thumb crossing
Improvise on a given pentascale and rhythmic pattern
Play I, IV, and V$_7$ chords | Review five-line reading and fingering
Play syncopated rhythm patterns
Play two-handed broken chords
Play a strumming accompaniment
Play a descant
Play a tritone accompaniment for blues
Play a two-handed accompaniment with crush notes
Play a three-part round
"Comp" a blues accompaniment
Improvise on a blues pentascale and scat syllables
Play an accompaniment using triplets
Play an introduction and an interlude | Review five-line reading and fingering
Play a rhythmic ostinato
Play a harmonic ostinato
Play a broken-chord accompaniment
Play a tritone blues accompaniment
Determine and play different dynamic levels
Play a strumming accompaniment
Determine and play multiple fingering positions
Play a countermelody using finger crossing
Play closest position chords
Play a trio
Play I, IV, and V$_7$ chords
Play a piano piece |
| Read notes B, A, G, E, D
Play with holes properly covered
Use proper hand position with left hand on top
Play with the pads of slightly curved fingers
Move fingers together
Play one-, two-, and three-note tonal patterns, ostinatos, and countermelodies
Show phrases by breathing
Blend sound with other recorder players
Blend sound with singers and/or other instruments | Read new notes C', D', and F♯
Play with holes properly covered
Use proper hand position with left hand on top
Play with the pads of slightly curved fingers
Move fingers together
Build right-hand strength
Play two-, three-, four-, and five-note tonal patterns, ostinatos, melodies, and countermelodies
Play syncopated rhythm patterns
Play melodic phrases using steps, skips, and repeats
Accompany 2-chord songs in keys G, D
Create ostinatos
Create introductions and interludes
Improvise using notes E, G, A, B
Show phrases by breathing
Blend sound with other recorder players
Blend sound with singers and/or other instruments
Blend harmony with melody | Read new notes G♯, C, F, and B♭
Improve playing and breathing techniques and hand dexterity
Develop right-hand strength
Play melodic phrases using steps, skips, and repeats
Play ostinatos, abbreviated melodies, melodies, and countermelodies
Play syncopated rhythm patterns
Play contrasting sections
Play a phrase of a round as an ostinato
Play partner songs
Create introductions, interludes, and codas
Improvise in major and *la*-pentatonic (G and *e*)
Create ostinatos
Create melodies based upon a rhythm
Practice proper articulation
Blend sound with other performers
Practice proper breathing and phrasing
Blend harmony with melody
Learn to read ahead
Listen to recorder music played in different styles | Read the new note E'
Introduce alto recorder
Read C, D, E, F, and G for alto recorder
Improve playing and breathing techniques and hand dexterity
Play ostinatos, abbreviated melodies, melodies, and countermelodies
Blend sound with other performers
Blend harmony with melody
Play enharmonic tones
Play a phrase of a round as an ostinato
Play ensemble recorder music
Play vocal scores for recorder consort
Play partner songs
Create ostinatos
Improvise in phrases as contrasting sections to melodies
Improvise 12-bar blues in A using pentatonic scale tones A, C, D, E, and G
Improvise recorder parts following chord progressions
Create melodies based upon a rhythm
Practice proper articulation
Refine playing in the low register
Add breath marks at phrase endings and practice proper breathing and phrasing
Learn to read ahead
Listen to recorder music played in different styles |

	K	**1**	**2**
Creating **Improvising**	Improvise patterns, using sound and movement Improvise rhythmic ostinato accompaniments Improvise introductions to songs, stories, poems, and dramatizations, using patterns of sound and movement Explore a range of sound possibilities with voices, body percussion, instruments, and environmental and electronic sound sources Improvise sound pieces to describe moods or images Improvise sound pieces and/or sound effects to accompany stories, poems, and songs	Improvise simple rhythms, using sound and movement, in call-and-response form Improvise a contrasting or B section in an AB or ABA form, using sound and/or movement Improvise rhythmic, melodic, and movement patterns and use as accompaniments to songs and speech pieces Improvise, using sound and movement, backgrounds or settings for poems, stories, songs, and speech pieces Use tempo and dynamic changes and contrasts in improvisations Improvise simple sound pieces for voices, body percussion, instruments, and environmental and electronic sounds	Improvise the b phrase in an aaba form Improvise body percussion patterns to accompany songs or speech pieces Invent strumming patterns for one-chord Autoharp accompaniments Improvise melodic phrases using the pentatonic scale Improvise sound pieces and music to accompany movement, poetry, and storytelling, using a variety of media, including technology sources
Composing	Create movements and dramatizations for songs and poems Create new words and movements for familiar songs Compose soundscapes for voices, body percussion, instruments, and environmental sounds	Compose, using sound and movement, backgrounds or settings for poems, stories, songs, and speech pieces Create introductions for songs and speech pieces, using sound and movement Invent systems for notating musical ideas Compose original verses to familiar songs Use tempo and dynamic changes and contrasts in compositions Compose simple sound pieces for voices, body percussion, instruments, and environmental and electronic sounds	Create settings, sound effects, or accompaniments for songs, poems, dances, and speech and creative movement pieces, using a variety of sound sources and movement ideas Compose simple AB and ABA pieces, using sound and movement Compose introductions and codas for songs and speech pieces, using sound and movement Compose B and C sections to create an ABACA piece Compose and notate rhythmic and melodic ostinato accompaniments to pentatonic melodies, using classroom percussion or technology sources

Reading/Notating

| **Rhythm** | Beat icons
Long/short icons | Interpret icons representing beat/strong beat, long/short, and tempo and dynamic changes

Durations including:
♩, 𝄾, ♫
Follow and create listening charts | Iconic notation

Durations including:
♩, 𝄾, ♫, ♬, 𝅗𝅥
Meters including: $\frac{2}{4}$, $\frac{3}{4}$
Tie |

3	4	5	6
Improvise contrasting B and C sections in a rondo (ABACA) form, using sound and movement Improvise rhythmic, melodic, and movement ostinatos in accompaniments for songs or speech pieces Improvise simple pieces that show thick and thin texture contrasts; use movement to show texture Improvise simple melodies based on the pentatonic scale Use variation in dynamics, tempo, and articulation in improvisations Experiment with various electronic and environmental sound sources and alternative ways to play instruments	Use melodic sequences in improvisations Improvise music to accompany movement or dance Improvise introductions, codas, and interludes Improvise melodies in major and minor Improvise simple sound and movement variations on a theme Improvise pieces in rondo (ABACA) form, using a variety of sound sources, including technology and movement Invent playing techniques (strumming, mallet) for I-V and I-IV accompaniments	Improvise extended phrases in question/answer form, using movement, rhythms, and melody Improvise melodies over accompaniments, using the I, IV, and V chords Improvise melodies, using various scales Experiment with strumming or other playing techniques to create rhythmic variety in chordal accompaniments	Use melodic sequences in improvisations Improvise answer phrases when given question phrases Improvise music to accompany movement and movement to accompany music Improvise chordal accompaniments for familiar songs Use given and original motives and themes as the basis for improvising with sound and movement Use acoustic and electronic instruments to improvise melodies over given chord patterns including rock and blues
Compose accompaniments and dramatizations for songs and readings, using a variety of sound sources and movements Compose rhythmic, melodic, and movement ostinatos in accompaniments for songs or speech pieces Compose simple melodies based on the pentatonic scale Create AB, ABA, and ABACA pieces, using speech, instruments, voices, and movement Compose and notate two short rhythm pieces that can be performed together as partners Compose simple pieces that show thick and thin texture contrasts; use movement to show texture Use variation in dynamics, tempo, and articulation in compositions Compose simple percussion and wind instrument pieces to explore sound sources and timbres	Compose music to accompany movement or dance Compose accompaniments of or backgrounds and dramatizations for songs, poems, and stories, using music and movement Create, notate, and perform a pentatonic melody Create and perform speech, rhythm, and movement canons Compose introductions, codas, and interludes Use melodic sequences in compositions Create, notate, and perform rhythmic, speech, or movement variations on a theme Compose pieces in rondo (ABACA) form, using a variety of movement and sound sources, including technology options	Compose and arrange accompaniments for songs, poems, stories, and dramas, using music and movement Compose, notate, and perform compositions in AB, ABA, and ABACA forms Compose a music or movement theme and variations on the theme Compose, notate, and perform melodies in major and minor mode, using various media, including technology Invent a scale, using classroom instruments and technology options, and compose a melody using that scale	Compose, notate, and perform original songs, instrumental works, speech pieces, and dramatizations Compose music to accompany dance or dramatic presentations Use given and original motives and themes as the basis for composing with sound and movement Compose chordal accompaniments for familiar songs Create new verses for a song Invent new arrangements of simple pieces, using voices, acoustic instruments, or electronic instruments other than those for which the music was originally written Compose and notate short arrangements, using computer software Experiment with found sounds and new sound sources to create music Compose accompaniments in different musical styles using auto-accompaniment on MIDI keyboards
Durations including: (rhythmic notation) Meters including: 2/4, 3/4, 4/4	Upbeat Durations including: (rhythmic notation) Meters including: 2/4, 3/4, 4/4	Upbeat Durations including: (rhythmic notation) Meters including: 2/4, 3/4, 4/4, 6/8	Steady beat/back beat Durations including: (rhythmic notation) (tied notes) Meters including: 2/4, 3/4, 4/4, 2/2, 6/8 Compound, changing, and asymmetrical meters Syncopation

	K	1	2
Melody	Upward/downward melodic motion icons Preparation for *so-mi* patterns	Interpret icons representing melodic motion Patterns including: *so-mi, so-mi-la, so-mi-la-do* *do*-pentatonic in C, F, G for playing on mallet instruments	Patterns including: *so-mi, so-mi-la, so-mi-la-do, mi-re-do, so-mi-re-do, la-so-mi-re-do* *do*-pentatonic in C, F, and G *la*-pentatonic in e

Listening/Analyzing/Describing

	K	1	2
	Respond to characteristics of phrase form: same and different Respond to characteristics of rhythm: steady beats, strong beats, silent beats, long/short sounds, repeated rhythm patterns Respond to characteristics of melodies: high/low pitches; upward/downward melodic direction; repeated melodic patterns Identify accompaniment/no accompaniment Identify environmental sounds: animals, machines, and weather Identify instrumental sounds of classroom percussion instruments, keyboards, flute, and trumpet Identify differences between vocal sounds: speaking, singing, shouting, whispering, humming Respond to expressive qualities in music: fast/slow and loud/soft Listen to music of diverse cultures and styles Demonstrate appropriate audience behavior while observing classroom performances Discuss appropriate audience behaviors	Respond to characteristics of phrase form: same/different, call and response, and solo/chorus Respond to characteristics of sectional form: verse and refrain Respond to characteristics of rhythm: steady beats, strong beats, silent beats, absence of beats, long and short sounds, rhythm patterns Respond to characteristics of melody: high/low pitches, upward/downward direction, melodic patterns Identify and describe various accompaniments Identify various found sounds Identify sounds of nonpitched and pitched percussion instruments; trombone, violin, flute, clarinet, and trumpet Identify vocal timbres: male, female, child Identify qualities of speech, singing, shouting, whispering Respond to expressive qualities in music: fast, slow, and changing tempos; loud, soft, and changing dynamics Describe mood and style in a variety of music Identify music of diverse cultures and styles Listen to music that suggests a story or subject Demonstrate appropriate audience behavior while observing classroom performances Discuss appropriate audience behaviors	Identify characteristics of phrase form: same and different, call and response, aab, and aaba Identify characteristics of sectional form: verse and refrain, AB, ABA, and ABACA Identify rhythmic elements: steady beat, long and short sounds, repeated rhythm patterns, $\frac{2}{4}$, $\frac{3}{4}$ meters Identify high/low pitches, steps/skips, melodic direction, and melodic patterns Contrast styles of two pieces Identify melodic and rhythmic ostinatos Identify vocal timbres of individuals and groups: male, female, child Identify various instrumental timbres, including nonpitched and pitched percussion, strings, woodwinds, brass, and electronic instruments Respond to expressive qualities in music: fast, slow, and changing tempos; loud, soft, and changing dynamics Perceive and respond to articulation changes (*legato* and *staccato*) Identify and respond to section changes Describe mood and style in a variety of music Identify music of diverse cultures and styles Listen to music that suggests a story or subject Demonstrate appropriate audience behavior while observing classroom performances Discuss appropriate audience behaviors

3	4	5	6
Patterns including: *mi-re-do*, *so-mi-re-do*, *la-so-mi-re-do*, *la₁*, *so₁*, *do¹*, *so₁-la₁-do-re-mi-so-la-do¹* *do*-pentatonic scale *la*-pentatonic scale *so*-pentatonic scale Letter names for pitches	*do*-pentachordal Patterns including: *la-so-mi-re-do*, *la₁*, *so₁*, *so-do¹*, *fa, ti, so₁-la₁-do-re-mi-fa-so-la-ti-do¹* *do*-pentatonic scale *la*-pentatonic scale *so*-pentatonic scale Letter names for pitches	Major/minor diatonic Dorian Mixolydian *do*-pentachordal Patterns including: *la-so-mi-re-do*, *fa, so₁-la₁-do-re-mi-fa-so-la-ti-do¹* *do*-pentatonic scale *la*-pentatonic scale *so*-pentatonic scale Letter names for pitches	Half/whole steps Accidentals; intervals Ornamentation Major/minor scales Pitch sets (12-tone, whole-tone) Motive Repetition and contrast *do*-pentatonic scale *la*-pentatonic scale *so*-pentatonic scale Letter names for pitches
Identify AB, ABA, AABB, and ABACA forms Identify rhythmic elements: steady beat, $\frac{2}{4}$ and $\frac{3}{4}$ meters, patterns Identify same/different, longer/shorter, higher/lower, upward/downward, louder/softer, faster/slower Identify patterns and themes Identify chord changes in two-chord songs Distinguish between major and minor tonality Analyze and describe how tempo, dynamics, and timbre affect the mood of a piece Identify various vocal timbres of individual performers and groups Identify instrument families in the orchestra: strings, woodwinds, brass, percussion Respond to expressive qualities in music: fast, slow, and changing tempos; loud, soft, and changing dynamics Identify music of diverse cultures and styles Listen to program and nonprogram music Listen to standard orchestral and chamber music Demonstrate appropriate audience behavior while observing classroom performances Discuss appropriate audience behaviors	Identify form in instrumental pieces Identify rhythmic elements in $\frac{2}{4}$, $\frac{3}{4}$, and $\frac{4}{4}$ meters Identify same/different, longer/shorter, higher/lower, upward/downward, louder/softer Distinguish between major and minor tonality Analyze and describe how tempo, dynamics, and timbre affect the mood of a piece Identify vocal timbres of groups Identify individual instruments Identify families of instruments from diverse cultures: strings, woodwinds, brass, percussion Analyze and describe differences between orchestra and band sound Respond to expressive qualities in music: fast, slow, and changing tempos; loud, soft, and changing dynamics Compare and describe the elements of style in two contrasting pieces Analyze music of diverse cultures and styles Analyze standard orchestral and chamber music Listen to choral works Demonstrate appropriate audience behavior while observing classroom performances Discuss appropriate audience behaviors	Identify and analyze sectional, theme and variations, and ABACA/rondo form Identify rhythmic elements of meter in $\frac{2}{4}$, $\frac{3}{4}$, $\frac{4}{4}$, and $\frac{6}{8}$ Identify chords Distinguish between major, minor, and other modes Analyze and compare rhythmic elements in terms of steady beat, meter, rhythm patterns, and relative duration Analyze and compare melodic structure in terms of movement, contour, sequence, phrase, cadence, and mode Analyze and compare pieces in terms of texture and chordal and linear harmony Identify timbres of individual singing voices and vocal ensembles Identify timbres of individual instruments and ensembles Respond to expressive qualities in music: fast, slow, and changing tempos; loud, soft, and changing dynamics Respond to show form in music Respond to show interpretation of lyrics in music Analyze and compare elements of style in several contrasting pieces Analyze music of diverse cultures and styles Identify complete sections from longer musical forms Compare program and absolute music Listen to chamber groups Demonstrate appropriate audience behavior while observing classroom performances Discuss appropriate audience behaviors	Identify repetition and contrast Identify sectional forms: AB, ABA, ABACA/rondo, and theme and variations Identify chords Distinguish between major, minor, and other modes Identify intervals: thirds and sixths Identify cadence Identify and describe how the words of a song affect the form and expressive qualities Identify *rubato* Recognize appropriateness of tempo choices Identify tempo category for selection: *largo, adagio, andante, moderato, allegro, vivace, presto, prestissimo* Discern individual and group timbres Discern vocal timbres from a variety of cultures Identify similarities and differences among string instruments from different cultures Move to show form, melodic contour, tempo changes, and changes in dynamics Respond to expressive qualities in music: fast, slow, and changing tempos; loud, soft, and changing dynamics Identify and describe style differences determined by rhythm, melody, and timbre Analyze music of diverse cultures and styles Recognize composite forms: opera, cantata, mass, and others Identify dance styles Recognize and describe a variety of vocal styles Identify various styles of drumming Demonstrate appropriate audience behavior while observing classroom performances Discuss appropriate audience behavior while listening to peers and guest musicians perform for the class

	K	1	2
Moving			
Nonlocomotor	Acquire a repertoire of nonlocomotor movements: pat, clap, stamp, bend, stretch, twist, shake Perform nonlocomotor motions in finger plays and action songs	Practice basic repertoire of nonlocomotor movements in finger plays and action songs Develop these alternating patterns: pat-clap, pat-tap, pat-stamp	Practice nonlocomotor movements Practice alternating patterns Develop repertoire of bilateral movements: snap and hand jive motions
Locomotor	Develop a repertoire of locomotor movements: walk, run, hop, jump, twirl Coordinate locomotor movements during singing games and circle dances	Practice basic locomotor movements: walk, run, hop, jump, twirl Practice coordinating locomotor movements during singing games and circle dances Develop these locomotor movements: skip, slide, leap, gallop	Practice basic locomotor movements during singing games and circle dances Develop facility with basic patterned locomotor movements: line and folk dances
Time	Perform creative movements while exploring concepts of time: rhythm (pulse, beat, speed-time or tempo); accent (light or strong); and duration (length)	Perform creative movements while exploring concepts of time: rhythm, accent, tempo, and duration	Perform creative movements while exploring concepts of time: rhythm, accent, tempo, and duration
Space	Perform creative movements while exploring concepts of space: level (low, middle, high); direction (forward, backward, sideways, up, down); size (large or small); place-pathways (on the floor, in the air); focus	Perform creative movements while exploring concepts of space: level, direction, size, place-pathways, focus	Perform creative movements while exploring concepts of space: level, direction; size, place-pathways, focus
Energy	Perform creative movements while exploring concepts of energy: attack (smooth, sharp); weight (heavy, light); strength/tension (tight, loose); flow (sudden or sustained, bound or free) Experiment with qualities of movement including effort actions such as flick, tap, thrust, slash, float, glide	Perform creative movements while exploring concepts of energy: attack, weight, strength/tension, and flow Experiment with qualities of movement including effort actions such as flick, tap, thrust, slash, float, glide	Perform creative movements while exploring concepts of energy: attack, weight, strength/tension, and flow Experiment with qualities of movement including effort actions such as thrust, slash, float, glide, wring, press

3	4	5	6
Refine nonlocomotor movements Practice alternating patterns Develop these alternating patterns: clap-snap, stamp-snap, pat-clap-snap Practice bilateral movements	Refine nonlocomotor movements Refine alternating patterns Develop these alternating patterns: alternating snap, stamp-pat-clap, stamp-pat-clap Refine bilateral movements	Refine nonlocomotor movements Refine alternating patterns Develop these alternating patterns: alternating pat-snap, clap-snap, stamp-snap, pat-clap-snap, stamp-pat-clap-snap Refine bilateral movements	Refine nonlocomotor movements Refine alternating patterns Refine bilateral movements
Practice basic locomotor movements Practice patterned locomotor movements in singing games; circle, line, and folk dances Develop this pattern of locomotor movement: square dance	Refine basic locomotor movements Practice patterned locomotor movements Develop these patterns of locomotor movements: social and popular (or contemporary) dances	Refine basic locomotor movements Refine patterned locomotor movements Develop these patterns of locomotor movements: social and popular (or contemporary) dances	Refine locomotor movements Refine patterned locomotor movements Develop these patterns of locomotor movements: social and popular (or contemporary) dances
Perform creative movements while exploring concepts of time: rhythm, accent, tempo, and duration	Perform creative movements while exploring concepts of time: rhythm, accent, tempo, and duration	Perform creative movements while exploring concepts of time: rhythm, accent, tempo, and duration	Perform creative movements while exploring concepts of time: rhythm, accent, tempo, and duration
Perform creative movements while exploring concepts of space: level, direction; size, place-pathways, focus	Perform creative movements while exploring concepts of space: level, direction; size, place-pathways, focus	Perform creative movements while exploring concepts of space: level, direction; size, place-pathways, focus	Perform creative movements while exploring concepts of space: level, direction; size, place-pathways, focus
Perform creative movements while exploring concepts of energy: attack, weight, strength/tension, and flow Experiment with qualities of movement including effort actions such as thrust, slash, float, glide, wring, press	Perform creative movements while exploring concepts of energy: attack, weight, strength/tension, and flow Experiment with qualities of movement including effort actions such as thrust, slash, float, glide, wring, press	Perform creative movements while exploring concepts of energy: attack, weight, strength/tension, and flow Experiment with qualities of movement including effort actions such as thrust, slash, float, glide, wring, press	Perform creative movements while exploring concepts of energy: attack, weight, strength/tension, and flow Experiment with qualities of movement including effort actions such as thrust, slash, float, glide, wring, press

Skills
Scope and Sequence

Pitch Syllable Systems

Several systems of both pitch and rhythm syllables are available for use in the music classroom. The purpose of using syllables is to ensure that students develop the ability to associate musical notation with a corresponding sound. When choosing a system, consider the developmental level of the students and the ease with which they can achieve success. Also, take into account consistency between grade levels and performance-based music programs.

Solfeggio or solfa

There are two types of solfége systems. Both systems use the following syllables and their chromatic alterations.

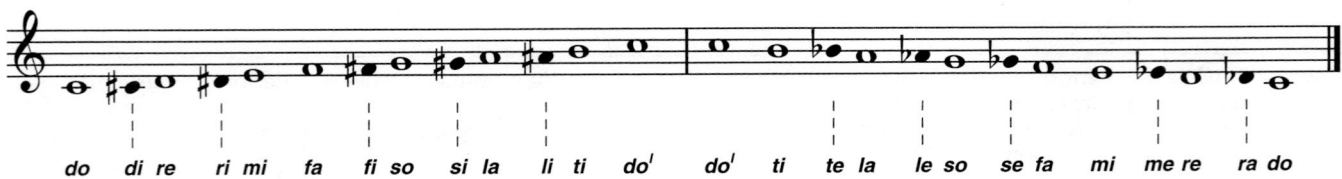

| do | di | re | ri | mi | fa | fi | so | si | la | li | ti | do' | do' | ti | te | la | le | so | se | fa | mi | me | re | ra | do |

Moveable do

The syllable *do* is the tonic pitch in any major key. Minor keys are based on *la*. The advantage to this system is that it establishes patterns that can easily be adapted to any key (for example, a minor third always exists between *so* and *mi,* and there is always a half-step between *mi* and *fa*). This method tends to favor early success particularly for younger students, since the introduction of letter names and key signatures can be postponed until a more age-appropriate time.

Moveable Major Scale

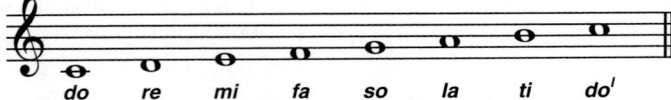

| do | re | mi | fa | so | la | ti | do' |

Relative Harmonic Minor Scale

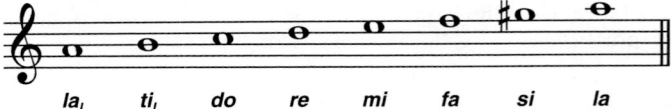

| la₁ | ti₁ | do | re | mi | fa | si | la |

Fixed do

The pitch C is always *do*, regardless of key. Proponents of this system argue that it more accurately represents true music reading, since the lines and spaces of the staff are always associated with the same sound. Knowledge of key signatures is required for success with this system.

Fixed Major Scale

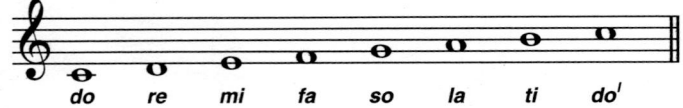

| do | re | mi | fa | so | la | ti | do' |

Fixed Harmonic Minor Scale

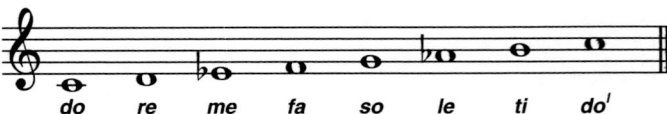

| do | re | me | fa | so | le | ti | do' |

Moveable Numbers

Similar to moveable *do,* this system uses numbers (usually 1–7) with 1 functioning as the tonic. Students can often achieve success early on because of their familiarity with numbers, although the numbers themselves can be less musical to sing than *solfa* syllables. This system does not allow for half step alteration, and rhythmic accuracy can be a factor when using 7.

Moveable Major Scale – Numbers

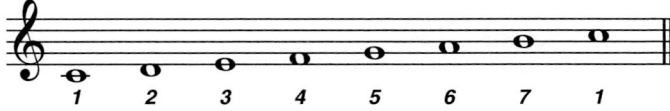

Moveable Harmonic Minor Scale – Numbers

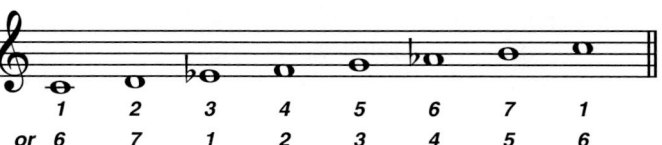

Fixed Numbers

Similar to fixed *do,* the numbers correspond to a specific pitch class. C is usually 0 and this advanced system is often reserved for twelve-tone music.

Fixed Major Scale – Numbers

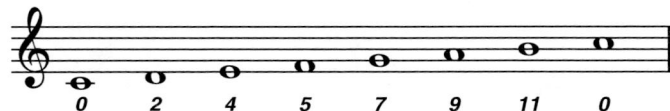

Neutral Syllable

This system uses a neutral syllable such as *la, lu, du,* etc. It is most beneficial for students who are already proficient readers and possess a strong aural sense of intervallic relationships. These students appreciate the lack of need to transfer pitches to any type of syllable.

Rhythm Syllable Systems

	Traditional	Kodály-based	Gordon
	This numbers-based method reinforces meter by starting each measure with *1*. Each beat is numbered and subdivisions of the beat are represented by the use of syllables *&* and *e*. A variation of this system uses *ta, te, la,* and *lee*. The most widely used system in instrumental music programs, this method is less singable because it incorporates multi-syllable numbers.	Although Zoltán Kodály used these syllables, they were developed by Emil Chevé in nineteenth century France. Rather than using numbers, each beat is represented by *ta*. Subdivision of the beat is based on *ti* and each rhythmic pattern is assigned a distinct syllable. This method lends itself to singing and/or playing patterns without having to distort melodies by using numbers.	Gordon's syllables are designed to promote audiation, or the ability to hear a musical sound when looking at notation. Like the Kodály-based syllables, the use of *du, da,* and *de* are easily singable.
Simple Meter			
♩	1	ta	du
♫	1-& OR 1-*te*	ti-ti	du-da
♬♬	1-e-&-a OR 1-ta-te-ta	ti-ri-ti-ri OR ti-ka-ti-ka	du-ta-de-ta
♪♫	1-&-a OR 1-te-ta	ti-ti-ri OR ti-ti-ka	du-de-ta
♫♪	1-e-& OR 1-ta-te	ti-ri-ti OR ti-ka-ti	du-da-de
♫♪	1-e-a OR 1-ta-ta	ti-ri-ti OR ti-ka-ti	du-ta-ta
♪. ♪	1-a OR 1-ta	teem-ri OR teem-ka	du-ta
♫♪.	1-e OR 1-ta	ti-reem OR tik-um	du-ta
♩	1-2	ta-am OR to-o	du-
♩.♪	1-2 & OR 1-2 te	tam ti	du de
♪ ♩.	1 &-2 OR 1 te-2	ti tam	du de
♪♩♪	1 &-2 & OR 1 te-2 te	syn-co-pa OR ti ta ti	du-du de
♩.	1-2-3	ta-a-am OR to-o-om	du-u-u
o	1-2-3-4	ta-a-a-am OR toe	du-u-u-u

Compound Meter

	1	ta	du
♩.	1	ta	du
♫♪	1-&-a OR 1-la-lee	ti-ti-ti	du-da-di
♬♬	1-e-&-a-&-a OR 1-ta-la-ta-lee-ta	ti-ri-ti-ri-ti-ri OR ti-ka-ti-ka-ti-ka	du-ta-da-ta-di-ta
♬♪	1-e-&-& OR 1-ta-la-lee	ti-ri-ti-ti OR ti-ka-ti-ti	du-ta-da-di
♪♬	1-&-a-& OR 1-la-ta-lee	ti-ti-ri-ti OR ti-ti-ka-ti	du-da-ta-di
♪.♬	1-e-& OR 1 -ta-lee	teem-ri-ti OR teem-ka-ti	du-ta-di

Breath Impulse

A variation of the traditional method, the breath impulse system uses numbers to represent each beat in a measure. When performing longer durations or sustained notes, the numbers are extended *(Wu-un, Two-oo,* and so on) with pulses of air that correspond to the underlying rhythmic pulse. The pulses vary to achieve the correct subdivision *(Wu-uh-uh-un* for sixteenth notes; *Wu-uh-un* for compound meter). Supporters of this method maintain that it emphasizes rhythmic subdivision, promotes good breath control, and contributes to success in vibrato development. This method is more widely used by instrumental teachers, since it does not lend itself to singing melodies expressively.

Rhythm Syllable Systems

Glossary

A

a cappella Vocal music performed without instrumental accompaniment.

AB form A musical plan that has two different parts, or sections.

ABA form A musical plan that has three sections. The first and last sections are the same. The middle section is different.

accelerando A gradual increase in tempo.

accent (>) A single tone or chord that is performed louder than those around it.

accompaniment The musical background, such as chords and rhythms, that supports the melody.

acoustics The science of the production, control, and transmission of sound.

aerophone Instrument that produces sound by a vibrating air column. The aerophone family includes woodwinds, brass, organs, and the human voice.

alto A female voice, the range of which lies below that of the soprano.

antiphonal "Sound against sound," or one group echoing or answering another.

augmentation Rhythm that is notated to be twice as slow.

B

backbeat The strong offbeat in a measure, such as the snare drum playing on beats 2 and 4 in rock rhythms.

ballad A folk song that tells a story, often with many verses. In pop music, a slow, lyric song that is often about love.

band A balanced group of instruments, consisting of woodwinds, brass, and percussion.

bar lines The vertical lines on the staff, used to mark off groupings of beats.

baritone A male voice, the range of which lies between that of the tenor and the bass.

beat A repeating pulse that can be felt in most music.

blues A style of music that has emotional lyrics; slow, offbeat rhythms; and improvised singing and playing.

boogie-woogie A special blues progression that uses blues chords and swing rhythm. Boogie-woogie is sometimes called "eight-to-the-bar."

brass A group of wind instruments now or originally made of brass— including trumpets, French horns, trombones, and tubas—used in bands and orchestras.

C

cadence A group of chords or notes at the end of a phrase or piece that give a feeling of pausing or finishing.

call and response A style of performance in which a leader plays or sings a call, and a group responds.

canon A form in which each part performs the melody entering at different times on the same or different pitches.

cantata A large dramatic work, sometimes of a religious nature, for choir and instruments. Many cantatas contain solo and chorus sections with continuous narration (recitative).

choir Commonly used to mean a group of singers performing together. Also a group of instruments, as in a brass *choir*.

chord Three or more different tones played or sung simultaneously.

chord progression The order of chords in a segment of a piece of music.

chordophone An instrument that produces sound by vibrating strings. The chordophone family includes the orchestral strings, guitar, and piano.

chorus A large group of singers.

chromatic scale A scale consisting of 12 consecutive half steps.

composer A person who creates pieces of music by putting sounds together in his or her own way.

compound meter A meter in which the beat is subdivided into three equal parts. Usually, the dotted quarter note gets the beat.

concerto A piece for a solo instrument with orchestra, usually in three movements.

contour The "shape" of a melody, made by the way it moves upward and downward in steps and leaps and by repeated tones.

contrast Two or more things that are different. In music, for example, slow is a *contrast* to fast; section A is a *contrast* to section B.

countermelody A melody that runs counter to, or against, the main melody.

crescendo (———) Gradually getting louder.

cut time ($\frac{2}{2}$ or ¢) A meter of two beats per measure. The half note gets the beat. This is also called $\frac{2}{2}$ meter

D

decrescendo (———) Gradually getting softer.

diction The pronunciation and enunciation of words in singing or speaking.

diminution Rhythm that is notated to be twice as fast.

disco Dance music of the 1970s that marked the beginnings of today's dance genre. Named after "discothèques" (dance clubs), disco was dominated by its straight steady beat played by the bass drum.

DJ A "disc jockey," who plays (spins) records for dance parties. Today's DJs produce, write, and "mix" music in the styles of dance, techno, and hip-hop music.

downbeat The strong beat in music. The first, accented beat of the measure.

duet A piece written to be played or sung by two performers.

duple meter A meter of two beats per measure.

duration The length of a sound, from very short to very long.

dynamics The degrees of loudness and softness of sound.

E

electrophone An instrument that produces sound either electronically or digitally with no acoustic generation. The electrophone family includes electronic keyboards, synthesizers, and samplers.

elements The parts out of which whole works of art are made. For example, music uses the *elements* of melody, rhythm, texture, tone color, form; painting uses line, color, space; and so on.

ensemble A group of musicians (players or singers) performing together. Also the instruments or voices of such a group.

F

fanfare A tune for one or more brass instruments; it is usually short and made of strong, accented passages. A *fanfare* is often used to announce someone or something.

form The structure of a composition; the way its musical materials are organized.

forte A dynamic marking (*f*) indicating loud.

fugue A musical form in which the main melody is stated in one voice and then is imitated by two or more voices, each entering successively.

G

gamelan An Indonesian ensembles consisting primarily of gongs, gong-chimes, metallophones, and drums.

gospel An African American style of music that combines jazz rhythms and blues singing with religious music. It may be accompanied by hand clapping, swaying, foot stomping, and other movements.

ground bass A bass line that continually repeats throughout a composition.

H

harmony Two or more different tones sounding at the same time. Harmony is most often structured around stylistic and historical rules and principles.

hexachordal An arrangement of six tones in a row with no skip, corresponding to tones 1, 2, 3, 4, 5, and 6 of the major scale.

highlife A musical style that combines elements of traditional African styles and jazz. Some common instruments are saxophones, brass, electric guitars, and percussion.

homophonic A musical texture consisting of a melody supported by harmony.

G

idiophone An instrument that produces sound by vibration of the body of the instrument. The idiophone family includes cymbals, bells, and wood blocks.

imitation Successive restatements of a musical idea in different voices.

improvise To make up music as it is performed.

instrumentation The number and kinds of instruments used in a composition.

interlude Music played between verses of a song or sections of a composition.

interval The distance between two notes.

introduction The opening section of a piece of music. In a song, music played before the singing begins.

J

jazz A style that grew out of the music of African Americans, then took many different substyles, such as big band, boogie, cool jazz, swing, bebop, Chicago, and New Orleans. It features solo improvisations over a set harmonic progression.

K

key The scale on which a piece of music is based, named for its tonic, or "home" tone.

key signature The musical symbol set, comprised of sharps or flats placed on the staff, that defines the key of a piece of music.

L

leap To move from one tone to another, skipping over the tone(s) in-between.

legato Notes that are connected to each other and played or sung smoothly.

lyrics The words of a song.

M

major scale An arrangement of eight tones in a scale according to the following steps: whole, whole, half, whole, whole, whole, half.

marcato A musical direction to perform in a marked or emphasized manner; often in reference to a melody.

measure In notation, one or more grouping of beats set off by bar lines.

medium Any material used in creating a work of art, such as the instrument(s) used in writing a piece of music.

melodic contour The shape of a musical phrase.

melodic sequence The repetition of a melodic pattern, usually at different stepwise pitch levels.

melody A line of single tones that move upward, downward, and repeat; a tune.

membranophone An instrument that produces sound by vibration of a stretched membrane or skin. The membranophone family includes most drums.

meter The organization of beats into groups, most often in sets of two or three.

meter signature The symbol, such as $\frac{2}{4}$ or $\frac{6}{8}$, that tells how many of what type of notes are in each measure. For instance, $\frac{2}{4}$ means there are two quarter notes (or their equivalent) in each measure.

minor scale Any of several arrangements of eight tones in a scale in which the scale begins and ends on *la* (the tonic), one and one-half steps down from the home tone *(do).* For example, in natural minor: whole, half, whole, whole, half, whole, whole.

mixed meter The use of more than one time signature in a piece of music.

mode A musical scale with a specific set of half-steps and whole steps that give it a unique sound.

modulate To change keys within a piece of music.

monophonic A musical texture consisting of a single melodic part.

mood The feeling that a piece of music gives. The *mood* of a lullaby is quiet and gentle.

motive A short musical idea that repeats throughout a composition.

musical expression The qualities of music that determine emotional content. Some of these qualities are loud, soft, slow, and fast.

N

new wave A popular style of rock in the 1980s that was heavily influenced by electronic music, drum machines, and synthesizers.

O

octave The distance from one note to the next note that has the same letter name. On the staff, there are eight lines and spaces between the notes in an octave.

offbeat A beat other than the strong beat.

opera A musical play in which most of the speaking lines are sung.

operetta A musical play, often similar to an opera but usually less serious. In an *operetta* most of the dialogue is spoken.

orchestra A performing group of various instruments. The term can be applied to many different ensembles, such as the Western symphony orchestra or the Chinese string orchestra.

orchestration *See instrumentation.*

ostinato A musical idea that is continually repeated. Ostinatos can be melodic, rhythmic, or harmonic.

overture A piece of music originally designed to be played before the beginning of an opera or musical play, often containing melodies that will be heard later in the work.

P

parody A humorous imitation.

partner songs Two or more different songs that can be sung at the same time, creating harmony.

pentachordal scale An arrangement of five tones in a row with no skip, corresponding to tones 1, 2, 3, 4, and 5 of the major scale.

pentatonic A scale consisting of five tones. A common pentatonic scale corresponds to tones 1, 2, 3, 5, and 6 of the major scale.

percussion A group of pitched or nonpitched instruments that are played by striking with mallets, beaters, and so on, or by shaking.

phrase A musical unit comparable to a sentence. Each phrase expresses a thought ending with a sense of pause or closure.

pitch The identification of a tone with respect to highness or lowness.

plainsong Monophonic chant sung usually with even rhythm using Latin texts. *Plainsong* is one of the earliest examples of notated music.

polyphonic A musical texture in which two or more melodic parts occur at the same time. This creates layers of harmony.

power chords Chords containing only a root and fifth (no third), often used by rock guitarists.

Q

question-and-answer drumming An African style of playing rhythms. A leader plays a phrase (the question), which is answered by other phrases from the group (the answer).

quodlibet A piece in which each voice sings its own line over and over, the lines harmonizing as in a round.

R

range In a melody, the span from the lowest tone to the highest tone.

recitative A sung narration with *rubato* tempo and minimal accompaniment, used to carry the story forward.

refrain The part of a song that repeats, using the same melody and words.

reggae A Caribbean style of rock music popularized by Bob Marley. Offbeat rhythms are prominent in this style.

register The pitch location of a group of tones. For example, if the tones in a group are all high sounds, they are all high sounds, they are in a high *register*.

repetition Music that is the same, or nearly the same, as music heard previously.

rhythm The way movement is organized in a piece of music, using beat, no beat, long and short sounds, meter, accents, no accents, tempo, syncopation, and so on.

ritardando (*rit.*) A gradual decrease in tempo.

ritornello The instrumental section of an opera, cantata, or other vocal piece.

rondo A musical form in which the main musical idea, A, is repeated, with contrasting sections in between (ABACA).

root position A chord in which the pitch called the root is the lowest note of the chord. For example, C is the root of a C chord.

round A composition in which two or more parts enter in succession with the same melody.

rubato A change of tempo in which the music pushes ahead and/or pulls back slightly to allow greater expression.

S

salsa A Latin style of music with syncopated bass lines, energetic percussion rhythms, and vibrant horn parts and vocal harmonies. Popularized by Tito Puente in the 1940s, *salsa* is still popular today.

scale (mode) An arrangement of pitches from lower to higher, according to a specific pattern of intervals.

scat singing A special style of jazz singing that uses nonsense syllables to sing instrument-like melodic lines.

score Written music or notation of a composition, with each of the vocal or instrumental parts appearing in vertical alignment.

sequence See *melodic sequence*.

sforzando (*sfz*) A sudden accent on a note or chord.

shanty A sailor's song.

sight-reading The ability to read music accurately the first time.

simple meter A meter in which the beat is subdivided into two equal parts. Usually, the quarter note gets the beat.

slur Notation placed above or below a group of notes to indicate that they should be played legato.

solo Music for a single singer or player, often with an accompaniment.

soprano The highest range of the female voice.

staccato (♩) Notes that are short and separated from each other.

steady beat A regular pulse.

step A movement from one tone to another, upward or downward, without skipping scale tones in between.

strings A term used to refer to stringed instruments that are played by plucking, bowing, or strumming.

strong beat The first beat in a measure, sometimes called the downbeat.

style A description given to music that has a special character or sound derived from the way it uses its musical elements—melody, rhythm, timbre, harmony, texture, and form.

subject The main theme, or melody, in a fugue. The subject is contrasted by the episode.

suite A musical form consisting of a collection of short pieces for a solo instrument.

symphony A large, usually lengthy, piece of art music for a full Western orchestra. The term is also sometimes used to mean "symphony orchestra."

syncopation A term used to describe accented rhythms that are off the beat.

T

techno and dance music A contemporary style of music created with electronic keyboards, synthesizers, and samplers. The music has a strong dance beat, bass line, and melodic patterns.

tempo The speed of the beat.

tenor The highest-pitched adult male voice.

texture The layering of sounds to create a thick or thin quality in music.

theme An important melody that occurs several times in a piece of music.

theme and variations A composition, each section of which is an alteration of the initial theme.

tie (♩‿♩) A symbol that joins two notes of the same pitch together to make the sound longer.

timbre The tone color, or unique sound, of an instrument or voice.

time line An African rhythm in which a pattern repeats and becomes the main beat that holds the music together.

time signature ($\frac{4}{4}$) The musical symbol that indicates how many beats are in a measure (top number) and which note gets the beat (bottom number).

tonal center The key in which a piece of music is written. Often the tonal center will be the first or last note of a piece.

tone row An early twentieth-century composition technique in which the pitches of the chromatic scale are ordered in a non-tonal way.

tonic The home tone of a scale. In a major scale, the tonic is *do*.

triad A three-note chord.

triple meter A meter of three beats per measure.

tutti An Italian word meaning "all," used in orchestral works to indicate that a section is to be played by the whole orchestra.

U

unison The same pitch sounded by more than one source.

V

variant In form, a section that repeats but is varied slightly. For example, a *variant* of an A section would be indicated by A^1.

variation A significant change in a musical theme.

verse The part of a song that repeats, using the same melody but different words.

W

whole-tone scale A consecutive succession of six tones, each a whole step apart.

627a

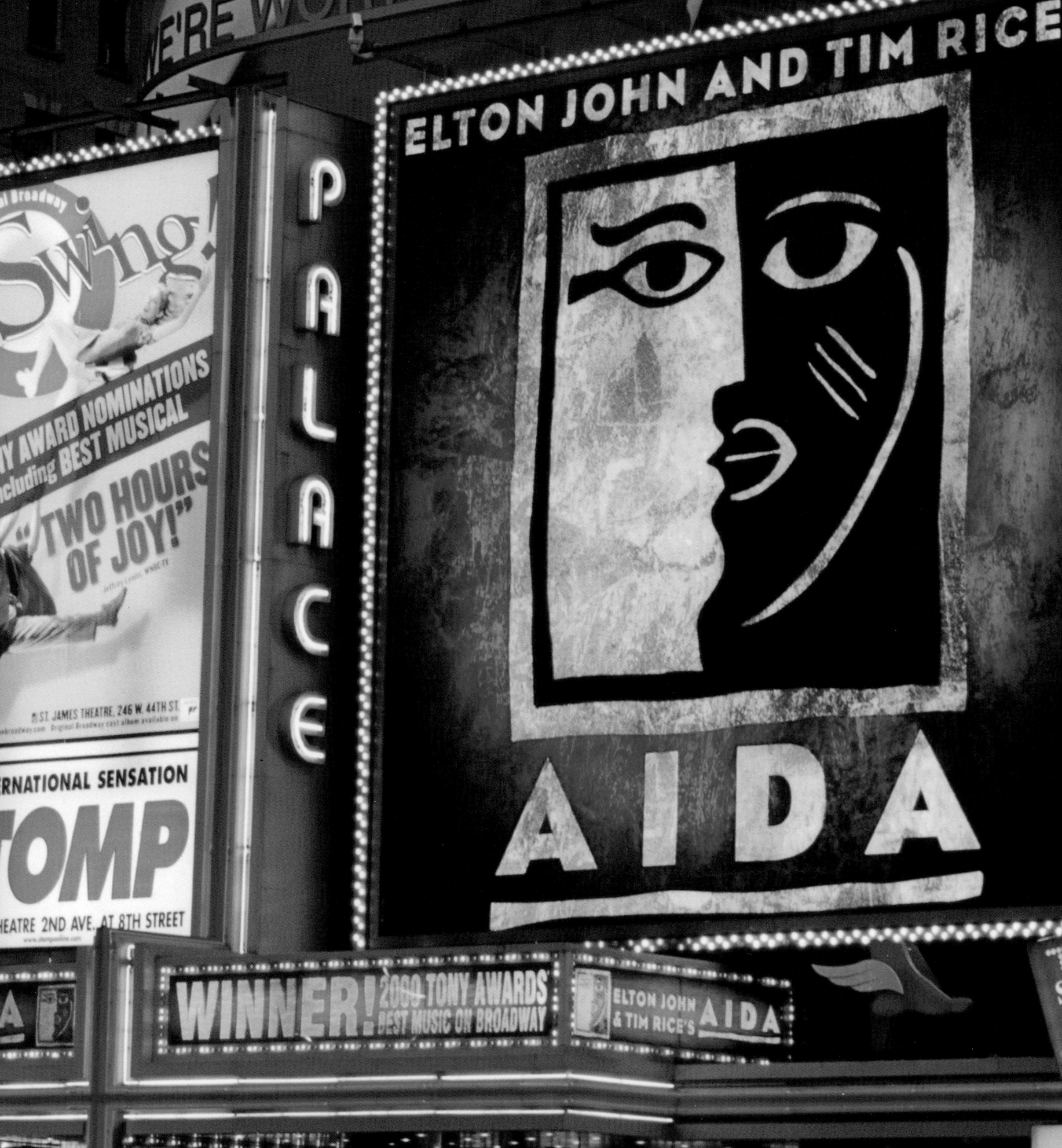

Themes Index

Pitch and Rhythm Index

Recorder Index

Classified Index

Listening Index

Song and Speech Piece Index

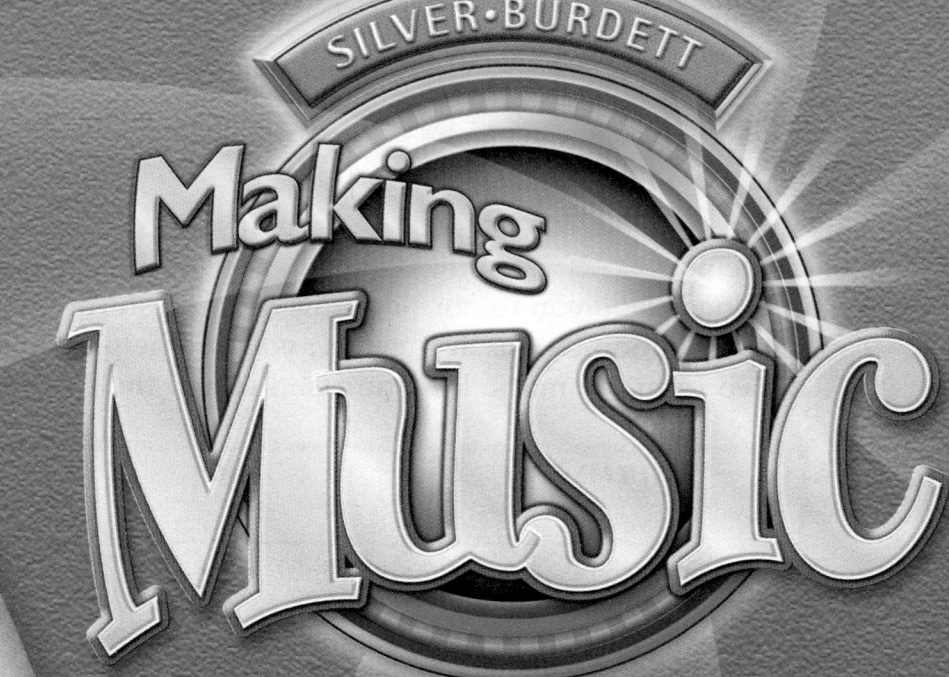

CONTENTS

Indexes

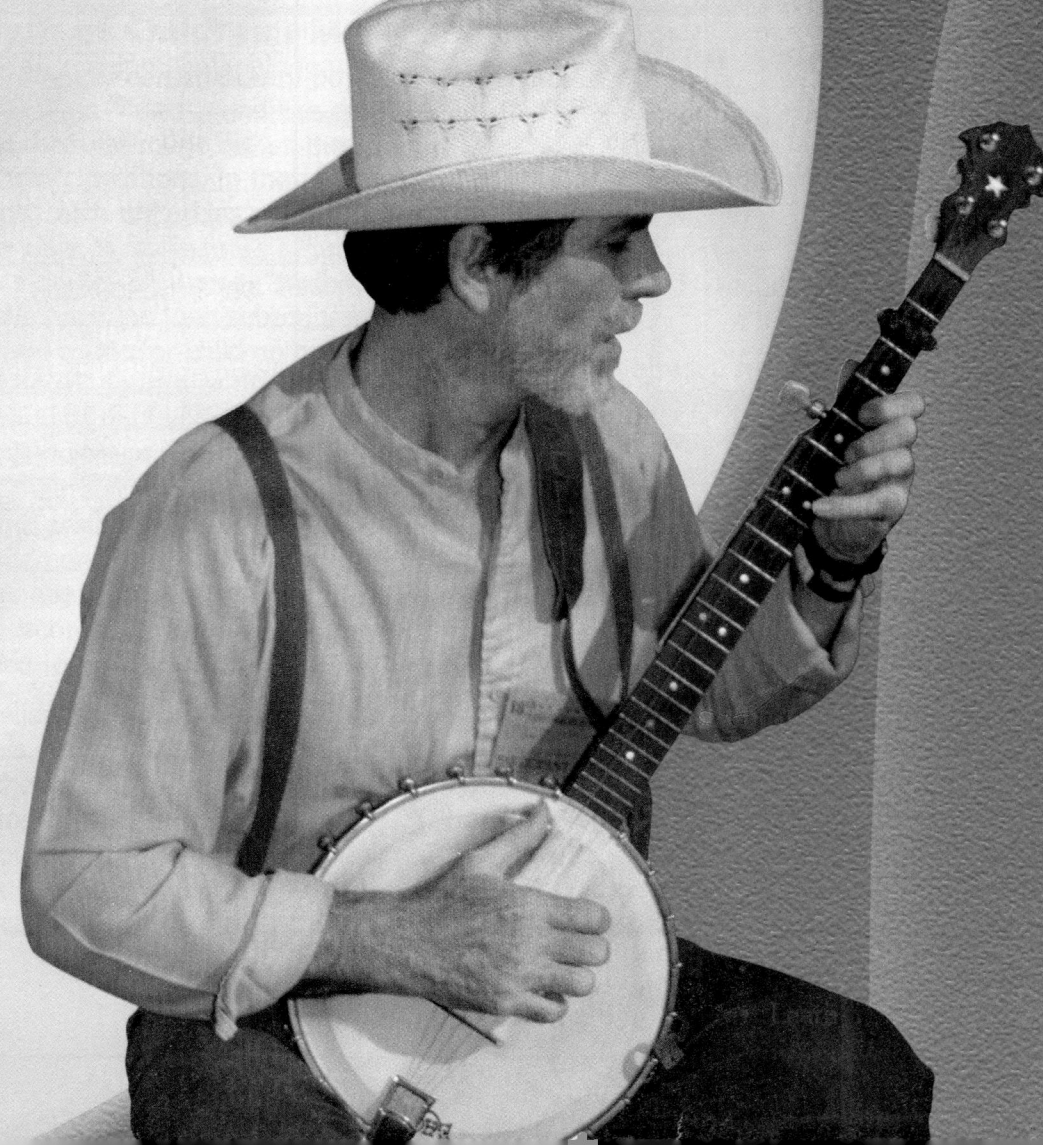

627b

THEMES INDEX

The content of MAKING MUSIC can be used to support teaching thematically in an integrated curriculum. This list shows many of the topical ideas teachers might use from this program. We encourage you to consider this list as a starting point only, a framework that can be enlarged upon easily. In this way, you can help deepen the meaning that your students derive from the music literature and enrich their work in other disciplines.

THEME	PAGE
Adventure	43
American History	11, 19, 57, 76, 83, 97, 156, 232, 234, 241, 370, 371, 398, 484, 485, 486
Animals, Birds, Insects	13, 23, 46, 57, 88, 167, 196, 316, 318
Birthdays and Anniversaries	90, 92, 481
Black History Month	85, 190, 232, 234, 235, 468, 470
Celebrations	9, 26, 274, 450, 451, 481
Cowboys	11, 19, 145, 246, 247
Dancing	58, 90, 122, 153, 154, 157, 182, 192, 265, 301, 305, 307, 308, 309, 320, 321, 322, 323, 324, 325, 326, 327, 333, 334, 368, 369, 440
December Holidays	103, 426, 452, 458, 459, 460, 461, 462
Dreams and Ideals	21, 86, 101, 115, 140, 188, 195, 201, 274, 352, 413, 440, 446
Drumming	186, 272, 273, 276, 277, 278, 279, 280, 281, 282, 283, 284, 285, 286, 287, 288, 289, 290, 291, 292, 293, 295, 297, 298, 299, 303, 304, 309, 310
Enslaved Peoples	338, 339, 340, 396, 397, 398
Fall and Winter	16, 40, 41, 60, 76, 193, 447, 454, 455
Families/Home	4, 16, 28, 248, 274, 292

THEME	PAGE
Famous People	6, 34, 40, 72, 73, 93, 114, 188, 224, 225, 246, 247, 256, 257, 261, 262, 332, 338, 339, 348, 365
Feelings	7, 28, 49, 52, 82, 95, 103, 115, 140, 145, 190, 240, 241, 242, 243, 246, 255, 258, 274, 371, 376, 470, 473, 476
Freedom	7, 85, 139, 166, 212, 311, 338, 339, 340, 396, 397, 466, 468, 470
Friendship	14, 23, 57, 63, 115, 170, 176, 201, 246, 255, 308
Halloween	448
Harvest	60, 76, 306
Humor	80, 145, 165, 244, 448
Instruments in Songs	135, 136, 139, 150, 156, 358, 370
Lost Love	95, 170, 300, 303
Lullabies Around the World	60, 403, 452
Mountains, Rivers, and Valleys	11, 21, 118, 191, 192, 263, 283, 374, 375, 451
Native Americans	61, 186, 188, 270, 284, 285, 286, 287, 444, 445
One Wonderful World	62, 115, 413, 440, 442, 443, 445, 446, 476
Patriotism	66, 135, 163, 172, 484, 485, 486
Peace	66, 115, 131, 190, 409, 446

THEME	PAGE
People at Work	22, 150, 204, 320, 364, 367, 376
Poems	6, 7, 40, 41, 122, 170, 185, 193
Power of Music	101, 104, 112, 258, 344, 345, 348, 350
Saying Goodbye	11, 43, 57, 205, 272
Science, Math, and Music	330, 331, 354, 355, 356, 362, 363, 366, 367, 378
Seas, Oceans, Beaches	43, 180, 260, 345
Spring and Summer	16, 60, 121, 250, 252
Stars, Sun, Moon	208, 450, 451
Traveling	43, 76, 97, 195, 212, 226, 228, 234, 243, 313, 372, 376, 398, 433
Trees	16, 131, 157
United Nations	442, 443
Valentine's Day	472, 473, 476
Weather	40, 41, 88, 102, 170, 332, 372

THEME	PAGE

Pitch and Rhythm Index

The Pitch and Rhythm Index provides a listing of songs for teaching specific pitches and rhythms. Specific measure numbers are indicated in parentheses when the rhythms or pitches apply to only a portion of a song. The letter *a* indicates that the anacrusis to the measure is included.

The Pitch Index is organized by the teaching sequence used in MAKING MUSIC. Pitch categories are listed in the order in which they are presented in the series.

The Rhythm Index is also organized by the teaching sequence used in MAKING MUSIC. The songs or portions of songs that are listed contain only rhythms that have been taught up to that point in the sequence.

An asterisk (*) next to a song title indicates that the song is used to present the pitch or rhythm in this grade level.

Pitch

so-mi

mi so
Downtown (m. 18, 20, 22), p. 258

la

mi so la
El cóndor pasa (m. a3–4, a7–8), p. 46
Hey, Ho! Nobody Home (m. 1–2, 7–8), p. 28
La paloma se fué (m. 1–2, a5–6), p. 51

do

do mi so la
Old Chisholm Trail, The (m. 1–4), p. 237

do mi so
Cowboys' Christmas Ball (m. 1–2), p. 239
Free at Last (m. 1–2), p. 468
Harrison Town (m. a1–2, a5–6, a13–14), p. 97
Lost My Gold Ring (m. 1–2), p. 158
Mama Don't 'Low (m. 5–8), p. 358

re

do re mi
At the Same Time (m. 1–2), p. 115
Fais do do (m. 1–16, 25–32, part 1–2), p. 403
Give My Regards to Broadway (m. 19–32), p. 39
Going Upon the Mountain (Melody only), p. 105
Scattin' A-Round (Variations on Row 3) (m. 1–2, 9–10, 17–18), p. 160
There Is Love Somewhere (m. 1–4, 13–16), p. 318

do re mi so
Don't Be Cruel (m. a1–8, coda), p. 255
Free at Last (m. 5–8), p. 468
Going Upon the Mountain (Melody only), p. 105
Going Upon the Mountain (m. a9–16), p. 105
My Dear Companion (m. 13–16, 29–33), p. 23
Paths of Victory (m. 5–8), p. 195

do re mi so la
Asadoya (m. 1–3), p. 303
Barb'ry Allen (m. a7–8), p. 44
Ezekiel Saw the Wheel (m. verse, melody, m. 17–24), p. 379
Joy of Kwanzaa, The (m. 1–16), p. 462
My Dear Companion (m. 5–8, 21–24), p. 23
Old Chisholm Trail, The (, m. a7–8), p. 237
Under the Same Sun (m. 14–18 of verse), p. 440
Your Life Is Now (m. 14–18), p. 4

re mi so la
Jambalaya (On The Bayou) (m. a1–3), p. 244
New Hungarian Folk Song (m. 3–8), p. 196
There Is Love Somewhere (m. 5–8), p. 318

la₁

la₁ do re mi
Ain't Gonna Let Nobody Turn Me 'Round, p. 85
I've Been Everywhere (m. 1–4), p. 226
Skye Boat Song (m. 9–16), p. 372
Sometimes I Feel Like a Motherless Child (m. 1–6), p. 241
Your Life Is Now (m. 13–20), p. 4

la₁ do re mi so
El carnavalito humahuaqueño (Melody only), p. 482
El carnavalito humahuaqueño (m. 9–16), p. 482
Go, My Son (final: *mi*), p. 188
On My Way (m. 1–8, 9–16 uppervoice), p. 313

la₁ do re mi so la
New Hungarian Folk Song, p. 196

la₁ do mi so
My Dear Companion (m. 1–4, 9–12, 25–28), p. 23

la₁ do mi
Your Life Is Now (m. 1–2 of refrain), p. 4

so₁

so₁ la₁ do
Mama Don't 'Low (m. 13–16), p. 358

so₁ la₁ do re
I Got Rhythm (m. 1–4, 17–20), p. 101
Water Is Wide, The (m. 13–16), p. 228

so₁ la₁ do re mi
Asadoya (m. 7–9), p. 303
At the Same Time (m. 1–8), p. 115
Bắt kim thang (final: *do*), p. 13
Blue Skies (m. 1–15, 25–32), p. 88
Bury Me Not on the Lone Prairie (m. 5–8, 13–16), p. 19
Farewell to Tarwathie (m. a1–8, a13–16), p. 43
Glory, Glory, Hallelujah (m. 1–8), p. 52
Gonna Build a Mountain (m. 1–8), p. 21
Gospel Train, The (Part II), p. 398
Gospel Train, The (Part III), p. 398
Key to the Highway (m. 1–2), p. 243
Loigratong (m. 5–12), p. 451
Paths of Victory (m. 1–4, 9–12), p. 195
Peace Like a River (Melody) (final: *do*), p. 190
Swanee (m. 1–7, 17–24), p. 118
This Little Light of Mine (m. 21–36), p. 232
Tom Dooley (final: *do*), p. 374
Under the Same Sun (m. 6 –13 of verse), p. 440
Water Is Wide, The (m. 1–4), p. 228
Worried Man Blues (final: *do*), p. 371
Your Life Is Now (m. 1–8), p. 4

so₁ la₁ do re mi so
Glory, Glory, Hallelujah (m. 9–12), p. 52

Paths of Victory (final: *do*), p. 195
Skye Boat Song, p. 372

so₁ la₁ do re mi so la
Bury Me Not on the Lone Prairie (Melody only) (final: *do*), p. 19
Farewell to Tarwathie (final: *do*), p. 43
Glory, Glory, Hallelujah (m. 13–16), p. 52
Your Life Is Now (m. 1–11), p. 4

so₁ la₁ do mi
Mama Don't 'Low (m. 1–4), p. 358

so₁ do
Adiós, amigos (m. a9–12), p. 57

so₁ do re mi
Ezekiel Saw the Wheel (m. refrain, melody, m. 1–16), p. 379
You Are My Sunshine (m. 1–2), p. 246

so₁ do re mi so la
Ezekiel Saw the Wheel (final: *do*), p. 379

so₁ mi
Bắt kim thang (m. 11), p. 13

mi₁ so₁ la₁ do re
Loigratong (m. 1–4), p. 451

mi₁ so₁ la₁ do mi
Run! Run! Hide! (m. part 2, 1–8, 18–37), p. 340

do¹

do re mi so la do¹
Asadoya (m. 4–5), p. 303
Don't Be Cruel (m. 5–12), p. 255
Going Upon the Mountain (final: *do*), p. 105

do mi so do¹
Star-Spangled Banner, The (m. 1–2, 7–11, 6–17), p. 486

mi so la do¹
El cóndor pasa (m. a11–12, a15–16), p. 46
Going Upon the Mountain (m. 1–4), p. 105
Kelo aba w'ye (final: *mi*), p. 290

mi so do¹
Water Come a Me Eye (m. calls: m. 9–10, 13–14), p. 300

so la do¹
Banuwa (m. 13–16 of melody), p. 294
Don't Be Cruel (m. 1–4), p. 255
Free at Last (m. 9–10), p. 468
Going Upon the Mountain (m. 1–2, 5–6), p. 105
Ise oluwa (m. 9–12), p. 230
It's Time (m. 5, 7, 9), p. 274

la₁ do re mi so la do¹
By the Waters of Babylon (m. 9–13), p. 311

Recorder Index

Classified Index

V

VOCAL DEVELOPMENT. *See also Skills Reinforcement: Singing; Texture/Harmony: Part Songs.*

Classified Index

Acknowledgments and Credits

Design and Electronic Production: Kirchoff/Wohlberg, Inc.
Listening Maps and Music Reading Practice: MediaLynx Design Group
Photo Research: Feldman & Associates, Inc. and Kirchoff/Wohlberg, Inc.
Every effort has been made to obtain permission for all photographs found in this book and to make full acknowledgment for their use. Omissions brought to our attention will be corrected in subsequent editions.

Illustration Credits

xii Chi Chung; 1 David Diaz; 7 John Hovell; 8 John Hovell; 9 John Hovell; 10 Ron Himler; 12 Chi Chung; 19 Christin Ranger; 31 Tony Nuccio; 33 Christin Ranger; 38 Steve Barbaria; 42 Andrew Wheatcroft; 46 Donna Perrone; 48 Vilma Ortiz-Dillon; 56 Andrea Z. Tachiera; 60 Jean & Mou-Sien Tseng; 70 Steve Barbaria; 71 Andrew Wheatcroft; 78 Tom Leonard; 79 Chi Chung; 80 Joe Boddy; 82 Joe Boddy; 88 Jeffrey Lindberg; 90 Tom Leonard; 95 Tom Leonard; 108 Jeffrey Lindberg; 109 Joe Boddy; 110 Adair Payne; 112 Adair Payne; 114 John Hovell; 120 Ron Himler; 123 Barbara Cousins; 130 Craig Spearing; 144 Fian Arroyo; 146 Wendy Rasmussen; 148 Carol Wyatt; 150 Carol Wyatt; 153 Bradley Clark; 163 Michael Di Giorgio; 164 Craig Spearing; 165 Craig Spearing; 170 Marion Eldridge; 173 Carmen L. Garza; 179 Michael Di Giorgio; 180 Nora Koerber; 182 Nora Koerber; 184 Craig Spearing; 191 Phoebe Beasley; 192 Phoebe Beasley; 200 Bobbi Pratte (Tull); 204 Guy Porfirio; 206 David Diaz; 212 Roseanne Kaloustian; 213 Michael Di Giorgio; 220 David Diaz; 222 Obadinah Heavner; 236 Arvis Stewart; 250 Larry Johnson; 252 Larry Johnson; 272 Shane Reiswig; 274 Shane Reiswig; 290 Patti Green; 292 Patti Green; 297 Tony Nuccio; 306 Fiona King; 312 Sarah Larson; 314 Sarah Larson; 323 John Hovell; 324 John Hovell; 332 Cathy Diefendorf; 334 Vilma Ortiz-Dillon; 344 John Hovell; 346 John Hovell; 350 Dorothea Taylor Palmer; 352 Dorothea Taylor Palmer; 357 Tony Nuccio; 378 Paul Gourhan; 392 George Hamblin; 394 George Hamblin; 396 Barbara Olson; 397 Barbara Olson; 398 Barbara Olson; 400 Barbara Olson; 412 Rosiland Solomon; 414 Rosiland Solomon; 422 Linda Wingerter; 424 Linda Wingerter; 426 Obadinah Heavner; 427 Obadinah Heavner; 428 Obadinah Heavner; 429 Obadinah Heavner; 430 Obadinah Heavner; 431 Obadinah Heavner; 432 Arvis Stewart; 434 Arvis Stewart; 436 Arvis Stewart; 447 Michael Di Giorgio; 448 Cameron Eagle; 458 Marni Backer; 460 Marni Backer; 462 Gail Piazza; 464 Gail Piazza; 472 Sally Jo Vitsky; 474 Sally Jo Vitsky; 476 Sally Jo Vitsky; 477 Michael Di Giorgio; 478 Sally Jo Vitsky

Photograph Credits

Every effort has been made to secure permission and provide appropriate credit for photographic material. The publisher deeply regrets any omission and pledges to correct errors called to its attention in subsequent editions. Unless otherwise acknowledged, all photographs are the property of Scott Foresman, a division of Pearson Education. Photo locators denoted as follows: Top (T), Center (C), Bottom (B), Left (L), Right (R), Background (Bkgd)

xii Ebet Roberts Photography; 2 (CL) Paul Natkin/Photo Reserve; 2 Paul Natkin/Photo Reserve; 2 © Peter Cade/Getty Images/Stone; 2 © Brooke Slezak/Getty Images/Stone; 2 Jane Faircloth/TRANSPARENCIES, Inc.; 2 Claudia Dhimitri/Viesti Collection, Inc.; 4 Tony Freeman/PhotoEdit; 4 Viesti Collection, Inc.; 6 Fotos International/Getty Images; 9 Paul Natkin/Photo Reserve; 14 John T. Wong/Index Stock Imagery/PictureQuest; 16 Peter Smithers/Corbis; 20 © Randy Wells/Getty Images/Stone; 20 Dean Conger/Corbis; 20 SuperStock; 22 (BL) Tim Barnwell Photography; 22 James L. Amos/Corbis; 23 Christe's Images/SuperStock; 24 (CL) G Salter/Lebrecht Collection; 24 EPA/David de la Paz/AP/Wide World Photos; 25 (BR) © Jon B. Petersen/Jon B. Petersen Photography, Inc.; 25 (BR) © Sheldan Collins/Corbis; 25 (CR) © 2002 Jack Vartoogian ALL RIGHTS RESERVED/Jack Vartoogian/Photographer; 25 (TR) "Sacred Harp Singin" 1974, Embroidery, Ethel Wright Mohamed Stitchery Museum/Mama's Dream World, Belzoni, Mississippi; 26 L. Reemer; 30 Purchased with funds from Lily Auchincloss in honor of John I.H. Baur/Whitney Museum of American Art; 32 Paul Natkin/Photo Reserve; 33 John T. Wong/Index Stock Imagery/PictureQuest; 34 Lambert/Getty Images; 34 Mark Hadley/London Features; 34 The Granger Collection, New York; 34 Photofest; 34 SuperStock; 34 The Granger Collection, New York; 35 H. Armstrong Roberts; 36 Jane Faircloth/TRANSPARENCIES, Inc.; 40 Bettmann/Corbis; 41 David David Gallery/SuperStock; 44 Liam Blake/Panoramic Images; 46 Robert Frerck/Odyssey Productions; 46 The Granger Collection, New York; 50 (TCR) Trío Musical by Obed Gómez; 54 Milton Montenegro/PhotoDisc; 54 Rita Maas/Getty Images; 54 © Larry Stein/Black Star Publishing/PictureQuest; 56 (Bkgd) Chris Cheadle/The Image Bank/Getty Images; 62 SuperStock; 65 Bettmann/Corbis; 66 Gavin Graham Gallery, London/Bridgeman Art Library, London/SuperStock; 66 SuperStock; 68 SuperStock; 71 Robert Frerck/Odyssey Productions; 72 Cincergi Pictures/Kobal Collection; 72 Photofest; 72 Martha Swope/Getty Images; 72 Kobal Collection; 76 (BL) Natalia Linsén/Otava Publishing Company Ltd., Helsinki, Finland; 76 © Nick Gunderson/Getty Images/Stone; 78 (Bkgd) © Toshihiko Chinami/The Image Bank/Getty Images; 78 Hulton Getty Picture Library/Stone; 79 Tony Freeman/PhotoEdit; 79 Joe Viesti/Viesti Collection, Inc.; 83 Lebrecht Collection; 92 ©Ben Margot/AP/Wide World Photos; 93 Photofest; 94 Zdenek Chrapek/Lebrecht Collection; 96 © Pat O'Hara/Getty Images/Stone; 98 The Granger Collection, New York; 99 Getty Images; 102 Lebrecht Collection; 103 David Allen Brandt/Getty Images/Stone; 104 (R) MaryAnn & Bryan Hemphill/Index Stock Imagery; 104 (BC) Jane Wooster Scott/SuperStock; 105 (BR) © Michael Ochs Archives.com/Michael Ochs Archives; 106 (TR) Getty Images; 106 (BL) MaryAnn & Bryan Hemphill/Index Stock Imagery; 109 Getty Images; 112 Courtesy of Ann Hampton Callaway; 112 Courtesy of Michael Rafter; 114 AL TIELEMANS/SPORTS ILLUSTRATED; 118 Mark Barrett/Silver Image; 122 SuperStock; 124 (Bkgd) © Todd Gipstein/National Geographic Image Collection/Getty Images; 127 (CR) © 2005 Copyright: © Succession Picasso/ARS/© Christie's Images,New York; 130 (T) UN/DPI; 130 (Bkgd) Getty Images; 132 (BR) © Archivo Iconografico, S.A./Corbis; 132 László Zombory; 134 Museum of Art, Carnegie Institute, Pittsburgh, Pennsylvania/SuperStock. © 2002 Artists Rights Society (ARS), New York/ADAGP, Paris; 139 Everett Johnson/Getty Images; 139 Lebrecht Collection; 140 S. Pierce/Getty Images; 143 Ebet Roberts Photography; 144 (Bkgd) © B.S.P.I./Corbis; 144 (TR) © Kelly-Mooney Photography/Corbis; 147 Ebet Roberts Photography; 148 Hulton-Deutsch Collection/Corbis; 148 Terry Oblander; 149 London Features; 149 Photofest; 149 Bettmann/Corbis; 152 Paul A Souders/Corbis; 155 Ali Schafler/AP/Wide World; 156 © Bettmann/Corbis; 158 Frank Driggs/Getty Images; 158 Walter Sanders/Getty Images; 159 The Granger Collection, New York; 160 Lebrecht Collection; 161 Chris Stock/Lebrecht Collection; 162 J Sohm/Image Works; 162 Lebrecht Collection; 166 © Craig Aurness/Corbis; 166 Alan Williams/Photo Researchers, Inc.; 168 Music Division, The New York Public Library for the Performing Arts, Astor, Lenox and Tilden Foundations/New York Public Library Picture Collection; 169 The Granger Collection, New York; 169 Lebrecht Collection; 170 Roger Ressmeyer/Corbis; 176 Corbis; 178 Suzanne Plunkett/AP/Wide World; 186 Salvino Campos Photography; 186 © Kent & Donna Dannen; 187 © Michael Crummet; 188 Photofest; 188 Peter Turnley/Corbis; 189 J. Pat Carter/Getty Images; 189 Bettmann/Corbis; 192 Corbis; 194 Charles Gatewood/Image Works; 197 Courtesy of the Nemeth family; 198 Bill Aron/PhotoEdit; 199 Bill Aron/PhotoEdit; 202 PhotoLink/PhotoDisc; 208 Stedelijk Museum, Amsterdam, Holland/© 2002 The Pollock-Krasner Foundation/Artists Rights Society (ARS), New York/SuperStock; 208 Estate of Hans Namuth. Pollock-Krasner House and Study Center; 209 Getty Images; 209 © 1960 Henmar Press, Inc., used by permission/C. F. Peters Corp./Lebrecht Collection; 210 © M. Angelo/Corbis; 211 Arne Hodalic/Corbis; 216 Photofest; 217 Getty Images; 218 CBS Photo Archive/Getty Images; 220 The Granger Collection, New York; 221 Graham Salter/Lebrecht Collection; 222 Getty Images; 222 Kevin Schafer/Corbis; 222 Keren Su/China Span; 223 Alan L. Mayor; 223 Reuters Newmedia Inc/Corbis; 223 Tettoni, Cassio & Assoc. Pte Ltd Photobank/Viesti Collection, Inc.; 224 Photofest; 224 Bruce Fier/© Panoramic Images, Chicago; 224 Frank Driggs/Getty Images; 224 Getty Images; 226 Getty Images; 227 MGM Records/Getty Images; 227 Culver Pictures Inc.; 227 AP/Wide World; 227 Photofest; 228 The Granger Collection, New York; 231 ASZA.com; 231 MaryAnn & Bryan Hemphill/Index Stock Photos; 234 The Granger Collection, New York; 235 Frank Driggs/Getty Images; 237 (T) Buffalo Bill Historical Center, Cody, WY; 7.69/Buffalo Bill Historical Center; 238 (CC) Jenne Magafan, Cowboy Dance or Fiesta de Vaqueros, © Smithsonian American Art Museum, Washington, DC/Art Resource, NY; 240 Lebrecht Collection; 242 © Messerschmidt/Getty Images; 244 Chris Stock/Lebrecht Collection; 244 Larry Miller; 246 Bettmann/Corbis; 247 AP/Wide World; 249 Alan L. Mayor; 249 A. Ramey/PhotoEdit; 249 Reuters Newmedia Inc/Corbis; 251 AP/Wide World; 254 Bettmann/Corbis; 256 (BR) Getty Images;

256 Romilly Lockyer/Getty Images; 257 Bettmann/Corbis; 259 (TL) M Peters; 260 Rick Doyle/Corbis; 261 Hulton-Deutsch Collection/Corbis; 262 Ebet Roberts Photography; 262 AP/Wide World; 262 Albans/AP/Wide World; 262 Ebet Roberts Photography; 262 AP/Wide World; 262 Reuters Newmedia Inc./Corbis; 264 Jack Vartoogian; 267 OnTour Enterprises; 268 Ebet Roberts Photography; 268 Vanina Lucchesi/© AFP; 269 The Granger Collection, New York; 270 Shamshahrin Shamsudin/© AFP; 270 Ebet Roberts Photography; 270 © John Running; 271 Paul A. Souders/Corbis; 272 G. Salter/Lebrecht Collection; 272 Getty Images; 272 SuperStock; 272 H. Luther; 272 Erich Lessing/Museum of Mankind, London, Great Britain/Art Resource, NY; 272 Chris Stock/Lebrecht Collection; 272 Ghana Goods; 276 Chris Stock/Lebrecht Collection; 276 T. Bognar; 276 A. Tovy; 277 SuperStock; 277 Abigail Hadeed/Visuals Concepts; 277 Jack Vartoogian; 278 The Stock Market; 278 Aldo Tutino/Art Resource, NY; 280 Corbis; 280 The Newark Museum/Art Resource, NY; 282 © Bruno De Hogues/Getty Images/Stone; 282 Aldo Tutino/Art Resource, NY; 284 The Bowers Museum of Cultural Art/Corbis; 284 Nathan Benn/Corbis; 284 Dan Polin/Lights, Words, and Music; 285 David Young Wolff/PhotoEdit; 286 Porterfield/Chickering/Photo Researchers, Inc.; 286 © 2000 John Running; 288 Robert Freck/Odyssey Productions; 291 Courtesy of Will Schmid; 293 Corbis; 294 © Victor Englebert; 295 © Victor Englebert; 296 © Victor Englebert; 299 Doug Armand/Stone; 300 © Victor Englebert; 302 Janette Ostier Gallery, Paris, France/Giraudon, Paris/SuperStock; 304 Corbis; 305 B. Gibbs; 307 © Richard T. Nowitz; 310 H. Rogers; 310 Library of Congress; 312 © 2000 Carol Rosegg; 312 Courtesy of Brian Crawley; 316 Joe McDonald/Corbis; 317 Corbis; 318 © AFP; 319 AP/Wide World; 319 Courtesy of David "Dakota" Sanchez; 320 Glover with yellow shirt/Getty Images; 322 Steven Senne/AP/Wide World; 323 Rowntree/Hulton Getty Picture Library/Stone; 323 Musee d'Orsay, Paris/Giraudon, Paris/SuperStock; 324 © Gerrit Greve/Corbis; 326 Alastair Muir/Lebrecht Collection; 328 Lois Greenfield; 328 Ousama Ayoub/© AFP; 330 Paul Warchol Photography; 330 © Richard Payne; 331 Courtesy of Walter Vangreen; 334 AFP/Corbis; 336 (TR) Jamey Smith, North Shore Country Day School, Winnetka, IL/The Foundation for Small Voices; 337 (BR) The Foundation for Small Voices; 338 Hulton Getty Picture Library/Stone; 339 Hulton Getty Picture Library/Getty Images; 344 Photofest; 347 Photofest; 350 © Paul Mozell/Stock, Boston, Inc./PictureQuest; 350 Jim Britt/Archive Photos; 350 Daemmrich Photography; 356 Yamaha Corporation of America; 359 Corbis; 359 C Squared Studios/PhotoDisc; 361 Courtesy of Vanguard Records; 365 Mitchell Gerber/Corbis; 366 Betty Freeman/Lebrecht Collection; 367 Mark Burnett/Stock Boston; 368 Ebet Roberts Photography; 370 Spencer Grant/PhotoEdit; 371 The Granger Collection, New York; 372 Getty Images; 373 Kevin Schafer/Corbis; 382 Chris Stock/Lebrecht Collection; 382 H. Rogers; 383 Keren Su/China Span; 384 J. Highet/Lebrecht Collection; 385 © Gian Berto Vanni/Corbis; 386 AP/Wide World; 386 David Young Wolff/PhotoEdit; 386 Corbis; 402 Owen Franklin/Corbis; 402 Eastcott/Momatiuk/Photo Researchers, Inc.; 408 Bill Aron/Photo Researchers, Inc.; 410 Bill Aron/Photo Researchers, Inc.; 410 H. Rogers; 411 S. Solum/PhotoLink/PhotoDisc; 413 Jeff Greenberg/Unicorn Stock Photos; 415 Archivo Iconografico, S.A./Corbis; 416 Archivo Iconografico, S.A./Corbis; 419 North Wind Picture Archives; 421 Werner Forman/Art Resource, NY; 421 Werner Forman/Art Resource, NY; 421 © Archivo Iconografico SA/Corbis; 438 Tom Bean; 438 Mark D. Phillips/Photo Researchers, Inc.; 438 Chip and Rosa Maria de la Cueva Peterson; 438 The Granger Collection, New York; 442 Viesti Collection, Inc.; 442 UN/DPI Photo by T. Chen; 444 © Lionel Delevingne/Stock Boston/PictureQuest; 444 © Underwood & Underwood/Corbis; 445 © Marilyn "Angel" Wynn/Nativestock; 450 Tettoni, Cassio & Assoc. Pte Ltd Photobank/Viesti Collection, Inc.; 452 Doug Martin/Photo Researchers, Inc.; 452 H. Wiesenhofer/PhotoLink/PhotoDisc; 454 Grandma Moses: The Old Oaken Bucket in Winter Copyright © 1953 (renewed 1981), Grandma Moses Properties Co., NY, Geoffrey Clements/Corbis; 457 Lebrecht Collection; 462 Lawrence Midgale/Photo Researchers, Inc.; 465 Chester Higgins Jr./Photo Researchers, Inc.; 466 SuperStock; 467 Corbis; 468 Jean Higgins/Unicorn Stock Photos; 468 TimePix; 470 © Flip Schulke/Corbis; 471 Carol Weinberg; 480 Chip and Rosa Maria de la Cueva Peterson; 482 (L) Jorge Luis Campos Fotografias; 484 Shogoro/Photonica; 484 Bruce Heinemann/PhotoDisc; 484 Russell Illig/PhotoDisc; 484 Alex L. Fradkin/PhotoDisc; 485 Bruce Heinemann/PhotoDisc; 486 Akira Inoue/Photonica; 512 Felicia Martinez/PhotoEdit; 515 Erich Lessing/Museum of Mankind, London, Great Britain/Art Resource, NY; TAB 1 ©Gary Conner/PhotoEdit; TAB 2 ©Lindsay Hebberd/Corbis; TAB 3 ©Tom Raymond/Getty Images; TAB 4 ©Bob Krist/Corbis

Acknowledgments

Credits and appreciation are due publishers and copyright owners for use of the following: 4: "Your Life Is Now" Words and Music by John Mellencamp and George Green. Copyright © 1998 Belmont Mall Publishing, EMI April Music Inc. and Katsback Music. This arrangement Copyright © 2001 Belmont Mall Publishing, EMI April Music Inc. and Katsback Music. All Rights on behalf of Belmont Mall Publishing administered by Sony/ATV Music Publishing, 8 Music Square West, Nashville, TN 37203. All Rights on behalf of Katsback Music Administered by EMI April Music Inc. International Copyright Secured. All Rights Reserved. Used by Permission. 6: "Youth" from *Collected Poems* by Langston Hughes. Copyright © 1994 by the Estate of Langston Hughes. Reprinted by permission of Alfred A. Knopf, a division of Random House Inc. 7: "A Brand New Day" Words and Music by Luther Vandross. © 1975 WB Music Corp. (ASCAP). All Rights Reserved. Used by Permission. WARNER BROS. PUBLICATIONS U.S. INC., Miami, FL 33014. 13: "Bắt kim thang" (Setting Up the Golden Ladder) English Words © 1998 Silver Burdett Ginn. 14: "Lean On Me" Words and Music by Bill Withers. © 1972 (Renewed) Interior Music (BMI). All Rights Reserved. Used by Permission. WARNER BROS. PUBLICATIONS U.S. INC., Miami, FL 33014. 16: "Magnolia" Words and Music by Tish Hinojosa. © 1996 WB Music Corp. (ASCAP) & Manazo Music (ASCAP). All Rights administered by WB Music Corp. All Rights Reserved. Used by Permission. WARNER BROS. PUBLICATIONS U.S. INC., Miami, FL 33014. 21: "Gonna Build a Mountain" From the Musical Production *Stop the World-I Want to Get Off*. Words and Music by Leslie Bricusse and Anthony Newley. © Copyright 1961 (Renewed) TRO Essex Music Ltd., London, England. TRO-Ludlow Music, Inc., New York, New York, controls all publication rights for the U.S.A. and Canada. Used by Permission. 23: "My Dear Companion" Words and Music by Jean Ritchie. © 1976 Jean Ritchie, Geordie Music Publishing Co. Reprinted with permission. 26: "Wai bamba" a Shona Wedding Song from *Let Your Voice Be Heard!: Songs from Ghana and Zimbabwe* by Abraham Kobina Adzenya, Dumisani Maraire and Judith Cook Tucker. Courtesy of World Music Press. 36: "Rock and Roll Is Here To Stay" Words and Music by David White. © 1957 by Singular Publishing Co. Copyright Renewed by Arc Music Corporation. All Rights Reserved. Used by Permission. International Copyright Secured. 41: "Stopping by Woods on a Snowy Evening" from *The Poetry of Robert Frost*, Edward Connery Lathem, editor. Copyright 1923, © 1969 by Henry Holt and Co. © 1951 by Robert Frost. Reprinted by permission of Henry Holt and Co., LLC. 43: "Farewell to Tarwathie" (Adieu to My Comrades) from *The Singing Islands* by Peggy Seeger and Ewan McColl. © 1960 (Renewed) EMI Mills Music, Ltd. All Rights Reserved. Used by Permission. WARNER BROS. PUBLICATIONS U.S. INC., Miami, FL 33014. 46: "El condor pasa" Music by Daniel Almonica Robles. English Words © 1995 Silver Burdett Ginn. 51: "La paloma se fué" (The Dove that Flew Away) © 1988 Alejandro Jimenez/World Music Press. Publisher World Music Press/Judith Cook Tucker. 57: "Adiós, amigos" (Goodbye, My Friends) English Words © 2002 Pearson Education, Inc. 58: "La mariposa" (The Butterfly) English Words © 1991 Silver Burdett Ginn. 60: "Yü guang guang" (Moonlight Lullaby) English Words © 1991 Silver Burdett Ginn. 62: "What A Wonderful World" featured in the Motion Picture *Good Morning Vietnam*. Words and Music by George David Weiss and Bob Thiele. Copyright © 1967 Range Road Music Inc., Quartet Music Inc., and Abilene Music, Inc. Copyright Renewed. This arrangement Copyright © 2001 by Range Road Music Inc., Quartet Music Inc., and Abilene Music, Inc. Rights for George David Weiss assigned to Abilene Music, Inc. All Rights Reserved. Used by Permission. WARNER BROS. PUBLICATIONS U.S. INC., Miami, FL 33014 and Hal Leonard Corporation. 66: "Sing a Song of Peace" Music by Al Jacobs, Arranged by Jill Gallina, Words by Jill Gallina, Words "This Is My Country" by Don Raye. Copyright © 1991 by Shawnee Press, Inc. (ASCAP) International Copyright Secured. All Rights Reserved. Reprinted by Permission. 74: "Don't Cry for Me, Argentina" Music by Andrew Lloyd Webber. Words by Tim Rice. © 1976, 1977 Evita Music Ltd. All Rights for U.S. and Canada controlled and administered by Universal-MCA Music Publishing, a division of Universal Studios, Inc. All Rights Reserved. Used by Permission. WARNER BROS. PUBLICATIONS U.S. INC., Miami FL 33014. 79: "I Walk the Unfrequented Road" Words by Frederick L. Hosmer from *We Sing of Life* by Vincent Silliman. Copyright © 1955 The American Ethical Union. Reprinted by permission. 80: "Do, Re, Mi, Fa" from *150 Rounds and Canons*. Reprinted by permission of Boosey & Hawkes, Inc. 85: "Ain't Gonna Let Nobody Turn Me 'Round" © 2002 Pearson Education, Inc. 86: "Bridges" Words and Music by Bill Staines. © 1983 Mineral River Music (BMI)/Administered by Bug Music. All Rights Reserved. Used by Permission. 88: "Blue Skies" from Betsy featured in *Blue Skies*. Words and Music by Irving Berlin. Copyright © 1927 by Irving Berlin. Copyright Renewed. This arrangement © Copyright 2001 by the Estate of Irving Berlin. International Copyright Secured. All Rights Reserved. Used by Permission. 90: "Birthday" Words and Music by John Lennon and Paul McCartney. Copyright © 1968 Sony/ATV Songs LLC. Copyright Renewed. This arrangement Copyright © 2001 Sony/ATV Songs LLC. All Rights Administered by Sony/ATV Music Publishing, 8 Music Square West, Nashville, TN 37203. International Copyright Secured. All Rights Reserved. Used by Permission. 92: From "Birthday" Words and Music by John Lennon and Paul McCartney. Copyright © 1968 Sony/ATV Songs LLC. Copyright Renewed. This arrangement Copyright © 2001 Sony/ATV Songs LLC. All Rights Administered by Sony/ATV Music Publishing, 8 Music Square West, Nashville, TN 37203. International Copyright Secured. All Rights Reserved. Used by Permission. 97: "Harrison Town" © 2002 Pearson Education, Inc. 101: "I Got Rhythm" Words by Ira Gershwin, Music by George Gershwin. 1930 (Renewed) WB Music Corp. All Rights Reserved. Used by Permission. WARNER BROS. PUBLICATIONS U.S. INC., Miami, FL 33014. 105: "Going upon the Mountain" from *Folk Songs and Singing Games of the Illionis Ozarks* compiled by David McIntosh, edited by Dale Whiteside. © 1974 by Southern Illinois University Press. Reprinted by permission. 112: "Hit Me with a Hot Note and Watch Me Bounce" Words by Don George, Music by Duke Ellington. © 1945 (Renewed). EMI Robbins Catalog Inc. All Rights Reserved. Used by Permission. WARNER BROS. PUBLICATIONS U.S. INC., Miami, FL 33014. 115: "At The Same Time" Words and Music by Ann Hampton Callaway. © 1997 WB Music Corp. (ASCAP), Halaron Music (ASCAP), Emmanuel Music Corp. (ASCAP) & Works Of Heart Publishing (ASCAP). All Rights administered by WB Music Corp. All Rights Reserved. Used by Permission. WARNER BROS. PUBLICATIONS U.S. INC., Miami, FL 33014. 118: "Swanee" Words by Irving Caesar, Music by George Gershwin. © 1919 (Renewed) WB Music Corp. & Irving Caesar Music Corp. All Rights administered by WB Music Corp. All Rights Reserved. Used by Permission. WARNER BROS. PUBLICATIONS U.S. INC., Miami, FL 33014. 122: "Dance for the Nations" Words and Music by John (J) Krumm. Used with permission of the author. 122: "Celebration" by Alonzo Lopez from *Whispering Wind* edited by Terry Allen. Copyright © 1972 by the Institute of American Indian Arts. Reprinted by permission of Doubleday, a division of Random House, Inc. 133: "Alleluia" responsory from Bernstein's Mass. Music by Leonard Berstein. 135: "Strike Up the Band" Words by Ira Gershwin. Music by George Gershwin. © 1927 (Renewed) WB Music Corp. All Rights Reserved. Used by Permission. WARNER BROS. PUBLICATIONS U.S. INC., Miami, FL 33014. 136: "Alexander's Ragtime Band" Words and Music by Irving Berlin. Copyright 1911 by Irving Berlin. Arrangement Copyright 1938 by Irving Berlin. Copyright renewed. International Copyright Secured. All Rights Reserved. Used by Permission. 140: "Give a Little Love" Words and Music by Al Hammond & Diane Warren. © 1986 Albert Hammond Music and Realsongs. All Rights o/b/o Albert Hammond Music administered by WB Music Corp. All Rights Reserved. Used by Permission. WARNER BROS. PUBLICATIONS INC., Miami, FL 33014. 145: "El payo" (The Cowpoke) English Words © 1995 Silver Burdett Ginn. 150: "Mr. Tambourine Man" Words and Music by Bob Dylan. Copyright © 1964, 1965 Warner Bros., Inc. Copyright © renewed 1992, 1993 by Special Rider Music. International Copyright Secured. All Rights Reserved. Reprinted by Permission of Music Sales Corporate (ASCAP). 160: "Scattin' A-Round" Arrangement © 2002 Pearson Education, Inc. 168: From *Lyric Suite* by Alban Berg. 1927 (Renewed) Universal Edition. All Rights Reserved. Used by Permission of EUROPEAN AMERICAN MUSIC DISTRIBUTORS LLC, Sole U.S. and Canadian Agent for Universal Edition. 170: "Four Strong Winds" from *Song to a Seagull*. Words and Music by Ian Tyson. © 1963 (Renewed) Four Strong Winds Music Ltd. (ASCAP). All Rights administered by WB Music Corp. All Rights Reserved. Used by Permission. WARNER BROS. PUBLICATIONS U.S. INC., Miami, FL 33014. 170: "The Wind" by James Reeves. © James Reeves from *Complete Poems for Children* (Classic Mammoth). Reprinted by permission of the James Reeves Estate. 172: "Así es mi tierra" (This Is My Land) Words and Music by Ignacío Fernandez Esperón. Copyright © 2003 by Promotora Hispano Americana De Musica, S.A. All Rights Administered by Peer International Corporation. International Copyright Secured. All Rights Reserved. Used by Permission. English version by Silver Burdett Ginn. 174: "Habemos llegado" English Words © 2005 Pearson Education, Inc. 176: "Vive l'amour" Arrangement © 1995 Silver Burdett Ginn. 180: "Mary Ann" © 2002 Pearson Education, Inc. 188: "Go, My Son" Words and music by Burson-Nofchissey. © 1969 by Kirt Olson dba Blue Eagle Music, assigned 1988 to Tantara Music. (ASCAP). 190: "Peace Like a River" Arrangement © 1995 Silver Burdett Ginn. 193: "Autumn" by John Hayden from *Rainbow Collection, Stories and Poetry* by Young People, edited by Joan Korenblit and Kathie Janger, 1989. Reprinted by permission. 195: "Paths of Victory" Words and Music by Bob Dylan. Copyright © 1954 Warner Bros. Copyright Renewed 1992 by Special Rider Music. International Copyright Secured. All Rights Reserved. Reprinted by permission of Music Sales Corporation (ASCAP). 196: "New Hungarian Folk Song" from *Mikrokosmos* (Bartok). © Copyright 1940 by Hawkes & Son (London) Ltd. Copyright Renewed. Definitive corrected edition © Copyright 1987 by Hawkes & Son (London) Ltd. Reprinted by permission of Boosey & Hawkes, Inc. 199: From "El Salón México" Music by Aaron Copland. Reprinted by permission of Boosey and Hawkes, Inc. 201: "Your Friends Shall Be the Tall Wind" Words by Fannie Stearns Davis, Music by Emma Lou Diemer. © 1970, 1973, 1979. Gemini Press. Inc. Reprinted by permission. 202: "Evening Chaconne" © 2002 Pearson Education, Inc. 205: "Blue Mountain Lake" © 2002 Pearson Education, Inc. 212: "Siyahamba" Arrangement © 2002 Pearson Education, Inc. 214: "Roads Go Ever Ever On" from The Hobbit by J.R.R. Tolkien. Copyright © 1966 by J.R.R. Tolkien. Copyright © renewed 1994 by Christopher R. Tolkien, John F.R. Tolkien and Priscilla M.A.R. Tolkien. Reprinted by permission of Houghton Mifflin Company and HarperCollins Publishers Ltd. All Rights Reserved. 216: "Alleluia" from Bernstein's *Mass* by Leonard Bernstein. All Rights Reserved. Reprinted by permission of Boosey & Hawkes, Inc. 218: From "Overture to Candide" Music by Leonard Bernstein. Reprinted by permission of Boosey and Hawkes, Inc. 225: "America's Music" © 2002 Pearson Education, Inc. 226: "I've Been Everywhere" Words and Music by Geoff Mack. Copyright © 1962 by Belinda Music (Australia) Pty. Ltd. Copyright Renewed. This arrangement Copyright © 2003 by Belinda Music (Australia) Pty Ltd. All Rights Administered by Unichappell Music Inc. International Copyright Secured. All Rights Reserved. Used by Permission. 228: "The Water Is Wide" Arrangement © 2002 Pearson Education, Inc. 230: "Ise oluwa" Yoruba *Folk Song From Nigeria*, arranged by Nitanju Bolade Casel. © 1989 Nitanju Bolade Casel, Clear Ice Music. Used by Permission. 232: "This Little Light of Mine" Arrangement © 2002 Pearson Education, Inc. 237: "The Old Chisholm Trail" © 1995 Silver Burdett Ginn. 242: "Sun Gonna Shine" Traditional, arranged and adapted by John Fahey. Copyright © Tortoise Music (ASCAP). Reprinted by permission. 243: "Key to the Highway" Words and Music by Charles Segar and Big Bill Broonzy. 1941, 1944, © 1971 (Copyrights Renewed). Universal-Duchess Music Corp. All Rights Reserved. Used by Permission. WARNER BROS. PUBLICATION U.S. INC., Miami, FL 33014. 244: "Jambalaya (On The Bayou)" Words and Music by Hank Williams. 1952 (Renewed). Acuff-Rose Music, Inc. and Hiriam Music for the USA. All Rights outside USA controlled by Acuff-Rose Music Inc. All Rights Reserved. Used by Permission. WARNER BROS. PUBLICATIONS U.S. INC., Miami, FL 33014. 246: "You Are My Sunshine" Words and Music by Jimmie Davis and Charles Mitchell. Copyright 1930 by Peer International Corporation. This arrangement Copyright © 2001 by Peer International Corporation. Copyright Renewed. International Copyright Secured. All Rights Reserved. Reprinted by permission. 248: "Green, Green Grass of Home" Words and Music by Curly Putnam. Copyright © 1965 Sony/ATV Songs LLC. Copyright Renewed. This arrangement Copyright © 2001 Sony/ATV Songs LLC. All Rights administered by Sony/ATV Music Publishing, 8 Music Square West, Nashville, TN 37203. International Copyright Secured. All Rights Reserved. Used by Permission. 250: "Summertime" Music by George Gershwin, Words by DuBose and Dorothy Heyward and Ira Gershwin. 1935 (Renewed © 1962) George Gershwin Music, Ira Gershwin Music and DuBose and Dorothy Heyward Memorial Fund. All rights administered by WB Music Corp. All Rights Reserved. Used by Permission. WARNER BROS. PUBLICATIONS U.S. INC., Miami, FL 33014. 255: "Don't Be Cruel (To A Heart That's True)" Words and Music by Otis Blackwell and Elvis

Presley. Copyright © 1956 by Unart Music Corporation and Elvis Presley Music, Inc. Copyright Renewed and Assigned to Elvis Presley Music. This arrangement Copyright © 2001 by Elvis Presley Music. All Rights Administered by Cherry River Music Co. and Chrysalis Songs. International Copyright Secured. All Rights Reserved. Used by Permission. 258: "Downtown" Words and Music by Anthony Hatch. © 1964 (Renewed) Welbeck Music Ltd., London. All Rights for U.S.A. and Canada controlled and administered by Universal-MCA Music Publishing, a Division of Universal Studios, Inc. All Rights Reserved. Used by Permission. WARNER BROS. PUBLICATIONS U.S. INC., Miami, FL 33014. 260: "Surfin' U.S.A." Words by Brian Wilson, Music by Chuck Berry. Copyright © 1958, 1963 (Renewed) by Arc Music Corporation (BMI) and Isalee Music Inc. (BMI). This arrangement Copyright © 2003 by Arc Music Corporation (BMI) and Isalee Music Inc. (BMI) International Copyright secured. All Rights Reserved. Used by Permission. 263: "Riendo el río corre" (Run, Run, River) WB MUSIC CORP. Warner Chappell Music Inc. English version by Pearson Education, Inc. 274: "It's Time" Words and Music by Lebo M., John Van Tongeren, and Jay Rifkin. © 1995 Walt Disney Music Company and Wonderland Music Company, Inc. All Rights Reserved. Reprinted by permission. 276: "World Music Drumming" Excerpts used in student book pp. 276–311, from *World Music Drumming* by Will Schmid. Published by Hal Leonard Corporation. Reprinted by permission. 286: "Yo-shi nai" a Navaho dance song, collected by David McAllister, published in Enemy Way Music: A Study of Social and Esthetic Values as Seen in Navaho Music, Cambridge, MA, 1954; published by the museum. Recorded by David P. McAllister. Used with permission. 290: "Kelo aba w'ye" Traditional Ga Song from Ghana, Arranged by W.K. Amoaku. © 1971 by Schott Musik International. © renewed. All Rights Reserved. Used by Permission of European American Music Distributors LLC, sole U.S. and Canadian agent for Schott Musik International. 292: "Take Time in Life" Copyright © 1962 CRS, Transferred to World Around Songs, 20 Colberts Creek Rd., Burnsville, NC 28714. Reprinted by permission. 301: "Ma Teodora" English Words © 2002 Pearson Education, Inc. 303: "Asadoya" English Words Used by Permission of Bruce Saylor. 306: "Alumot" (Sheaves of Grain) English Words © 2002 Pearson Education, Inc. 308: "Al yadee" Words adapted by Sally Monsour from New Dimensions in Music: Mastering Music, Teacher's Edition by Robert A. Choate et al., p. 160 Copyright © 1960 by Sally Monsour. Reprinted by Permission. 313: "On My Way" Words by Brian Crawley, Music by Jeanine Tesori, arranged by Michael Rafter, from the Musical, Violet. 1998. Used by Permission. 320: "Now That's Tap" Words and Music by Reg E. Gaines, Daryl Waters, Zane Mark. © 10-G Publishing (ASCAP), DMW Music (ASCAP) and Zenox Music Publishing (ASCAP). All Rights administered by WB Music Corp. (ASCAP). All Rights Reserved. Used by Permission. WARNER BROS. PUBLICATION S U.S. INC., Miami, FL 33014. 328: "Sha Sha Sha" © 2002 Pearson Education, Inc. 336: "Oye" by Jim Papoulis. "Oye" is from the project Sounds of a Better World, all proceeds go to Children's Charities. soundsofabetterworld.org. Reprinted by permission. 340: "Run! Run! Hide!" arranged by Linda Twine. This arrangement copyright © 2000 by Hinshaw Music, Inc., Chapel Hill, NC, 27514. International Copyright Secured. All Rights Reserved. Copying or reproducing this publication in whole or in part violates the Federal Copyright Law. This arrangement is printed with the permission of the publisher. 348: "Rhythm is Gonna Get You" Words and Music by Gloria M. Estefan and Enrique Garcia. © 1987 Foreign Imported Productions & Publishing, Inc. (BMI) International Rights Secured. All Rights Reserved. Reprinted by permission. 352: "One Moment in Time" Words and Music by Albert Hammond and John Bettis. © 1987 Albert Hammond Music & John Bettis Music. All Rights o/b/o John Bettis Music administered by WB Music Corp. All Rights Reserved. Used by Permission. WARNER BROS. PUBLICATIONS U.S. INC., Miami, FL 33014. 364: "Corta la caña"(Head for the Canefields) English Words © 1995 Silver Burdett Ginn. 371: "Worried Man Blues" from *Folk Blues* by Jerry Silverman. © Saw Mill Music Corp. Used by Permission. All Rights Reserved. 372: "Skye Boat Song" Words by Sir Harold Boulton, arranged by Annie MacLeod. © 1958 (Renewed) Summy-Birchard Music, a division of Summy-Birchard, Inc., All Rights Reserved. Used by Permission. WARNER BROS. PUBLICATIONS, U.S. Inc., Miami, FL 33014. 376: "Cuando pa' Chile me voy" (Leavin' for Chile) English Words © 1995 Silver Burdett Ginn. 388: "Just a Snap-Happy Blues" © 2002 Pearson Education, Inc. 393: "A Gift to Share" © 2002 Pearson Education, Inc.

398: "The Gospel Train" arranged by Shirley W. McRae, edited by Henry H. Leck, 1994. Copyright Transferred 2000, Colla Voce Music, Inc., 4600 Sunset Avenue, #83, Indianapolis, IN 46208. Reprinted by permission of Colla Voce Music, Inc. 403: "Fais do do" (Go to Sleep) Arrangement © 2002 Pearson Education, Inc. 409: "Shalom aleichem" Arrangement © 2002 Pearson Education, Inc. 413: "Cantaré, cantaras" (I Will Sing, You Will Sing) Words and Music by Albert Hammond, Anahi and Juan Carlos Calderón. Copyright © 1985 Irving Music, Inc., Calquin Music, EMI April Music, Inc., and Albert Hammond Enterprises Inc. All Rights o/b/o Albert Hammond Enterprises Inc., administered by Music of Windswept. All Rights Reserved. Used by Permission. WARNER BROS. PUBLICATIONS U.S. INC., Miami, FL. 33014 and Hal Leonard Corporation. 416: "A Carelessly Crafted Raft" by Lucinda Cave. Copyright © 1997 by Lucinda Cave. Reprinted by permission of the author. 417: "Vem kan segla?" (Who Can Sail?) Finnish Folk Song. Reprinted by permission. Copyright Walton Music Corp. 423: "Angels On the Midnight Clear" Music by Richard Willis, Words by Edmund H. Sears. Arranged by Catherine Bennett. Copyright © 1987 by Shawnee Press, Inc. International Copyright Secured. All Rights Reserved. Reprinted by Permission. 427: "Ding-Dong! Merrily on High" Words by G.R. Woodward. Arranged by Howard Cable, edited by Henry Leck. Copyright © 1993 by Brassworks Music, Inc. This arrangement Copyright © 1994 by Brassworks Music, Inc. International Copyright Secured. All Rights Reserved. Reprinted by permission of Canadian Brass. 433: "Goin' to Boston" Edited by Henry H. Leck. Copyright Transferred 2000, Colla Voce Music, Inc., 4600 Sunset Avenue, #83, Indianapolis, IN 46208. Reprinted by permission of Colla Voce Music, Inc. 440: "Under the Same Sun" Words and Music by Clifford Carter, 1995. Reprinted by permission. 443: "United Nations on the March, The" from *Songs That Changed the World*, Edited by Wanda Willson Whitman. Crown Publishers, Inc., New York. Copyright © 1969 by Wanda Willson Whitman. 446: "I Am But A Small Voice" original Words by Odina E. Batnag; English Words and Music by Roger Whittaker. Copyright © 1983 BMG Songs Inc. and BMG Music Publishing Ltd. (PRS). This arrangement Copyright © 2001 BMG Songs, Inc. and BMG Music Publishing Ltd. (PRS). All Rights administered by BMG Songs, Inc. International Copyright Secured. All Rights Reserved. Used by Permission. 448: "The Purple People Eater" Words and Music by Sheb Wooley. Reprinted by permission. 451: "Loigratong" English Words © 1998 Silver Burdett Ginn. 452: "S'vivon" (Dreydl) verse by L. Kipnis from The New Jewish Song Book, compiled and edited by Harry Coopersmith, 1965. © Behrman House, Inc., reprinted with permission. www.behrmanhouse.com. English version by Pearson Education, Inc. 455: "Winter Song" Words and Music by Stephen Paulus. Copyright © 1976 by Carl Fischer LLC. International Copyright Secured. All Rights Reserved. Reprinted by permission. 458: "Caroling, Caroling" Words by Wihla Hutson, Music by Alfred Burt. TRO-© Copyright 1954 (Renewed) 1957 (Renewed) Hollis Music, Inc., New York, NY. Used by Permission. 462: "Joy of Kwanzaa" Words and Music by Reggie Royal. Reijiro Music. Reprinted by permission. 466: "Abraham, Martin and John" Words and Music by Dick Holler; arranged by Joan R. Hills. © 1968, 1979 Regent Music Corporation. All Rights Reserved. International Copyright Secured. WARNER BROS. PUBLICATIONS, INC. 468: "Free at Last" Arrangement © 1995 Silver Burdett Ginn. 470: "I Wish I Knew How It Would Feel To Be Free" Music by Billy Taylor, Words and Music by Billy Taylor and Dick Dallas. Copyright © 1964 and 1968 by Duane Music Inc. Reprinted with permission. 473: "Eres tú" (Touch the Wind) Words and Music by Juan Calderón, English Words by Michael Hawker. © 1972 (Renewed) Ed. Musicales PolyGram-Discorama. All Rights for United States and Canada controlled and administered by Universal PolyGram International Publishing, Inc. All Rights Reserved. Used by Permission. WARNER BROS. PUBLICATIONS U.S. INC., Miami, FL 33014. 476: "Love in Any Language" Words and Music by John Mohr and John Mays. Copyright © 1986 by Jonathan Mark Music, Birdwing Music, Sutton Hill Music. All Rights Reserved. 481: "Las mañanitas" from *Children's Songs from Mexico*. © Alfred Publishing Co. Inc. Used with permission of the publisher. 482: "El carnavalito humahuaqueño" English Words © 2005 Pearson Education, Inc. The editors of Scott Foresman have made every attempt to verify the source of "Lo yisa" (p. 130), but were unable to do so. Every effort has been made to locate all copyright holders of material used in this book. If any errors or omissions have occurred, corrections will be made.

Teacher Notes

Teacher Notes

Teacher Notes

Teacher Notes

LISTENING INDEX

Listening Selections by Composer

Listening Selections by Title

Listening Index

Selected Listenings

Montages
Drums from Around the World, p. 277 CD 14-12
Drums of the Iroquois and Sioux, p. 285 CD 14-16
Sound Waves Montage, p. 354 CD 18-4
Vocal Styles Around the World, p. 61 CD 4-19
Vocal Timbres Around the World, p. 170 CD 9-27

Dances
Al yadee, p. 308 CD 15-34
Al yadee (practice tempo), p. 308 CD 15-35
Alumot, p. 306 CD 15-30
Alumot (practice tempo), p. 306 CD 15-31
Así es mi tierra, p. 172 CD 9-35
Así es mi tierra (practice tempo), p. 172 CD 9-36
Dham dhamak dham samelu, p. 305 CD 15-24
Dham dhamak dham samelu (practice tempo), p. 305 CD 15-25
Four Potatoes Medley, p. 205 CD 11-9
Four Potatoes Medley (practice tempo), p. 205 CD 11-10
Hava nagila, p. 153 CD 8-23
Hava nagila (practice tempo), p. 153 CD 8-26
Hit Me with a Hot Note and Watch Me Bounce, p. 112 CD 6-31
Hit Me with a Hot Note and Watch Me Bounce (practice tempo), p. 112 CD 6-32
Kerenski, p. 78 CD 5-4
Kerenski (practice tempo), p. 78 CD 5-5
Kpanlogo for 2 (practice tempo), p. 296 CD 15-7
Mama Don't 'Low, p. 358 CD 18-6
Mama Don't 'Low (practice tempo), p. 358 CD 18-8
Mary Ann, p. 180 CD 10-10
Mary Ann (practice tempo), p. 180 CD 10-12
Paddy Whack, p. 327 CD 16-16
Paddy Whack (practice tempo), p. 327 CD 16-17
Red River Valley, p. 11 CD 1-11
Red River Valley (practice tempo), p. 11 CD 1-12
Sellenger's Round, p. 44 CD 3-14
Sellenger's Round (practice tempo), p. 44 CD 3-15

Recorded Interviews
Interview with Ann Hampton Callaway and Michael Rafter, p. 113 CD 6-33
Interview with David "Dakota" Sanchez, p. 319 CD 16-10
Interview with Jeanine Tesori and Brian Crawley, p. 312 CD 16-3
Interview with Linda Twine, p. 339 CD 17-10
Interview with Petula Clark, p. 259 CD 13-20
Interview with Valerie Dee Naranjo, p. 186 CD 10-23
Interview with William Schuman, p. 83 CD 5-24

Recorded Poems and Stories
Stopping by Woods on a Snowy Evening (poem), p. 40 CD 2-36

SONG AND SPEECH

PIECE INDEX